DISORDERS OF HEMOGLOBIN

Genetics, Pathophysiology, and Clinical Management

SECOND EDITION

This book is a completely revised new edition of the definitive reference on disorders of hemoglobin. Authored by world-renowned experts, the book focuses on basic science aspects and clinical features of hemoglobinopathies, covering diagnosis, treatment, and future applications of current research. While the second edition continues to address the important molecular, cellular, and genetic components, coverage of clinical issues has been significantly expanded, and there is more practical emphasis on diagnosis and management throughout.

The book opens with a review of the scientific underpinnings. Pathophysiology of common hemoglobin disorders is discussed next in an entirely new section devoted to vascular biology, the erythrocyte membrane, nitric oxide biology, and hemolysis. Four sections deal with α and β thalassemia, sickle cell disease, and related conditions, followed by special topics. The second edition concludes with current and developing approaches to treatment, incorporating new agents for iron chelation, methods to induce fetal hemoglobin production, novel treatment approaches, stem cell transplantation, and progress in gene therapy.

Martin H. Steinberg is Professor of Medicine, Pediatrics, Pathology and Laboratory Medicine at Boston University School of Medicine and Director of the Center of Excellence in Sickle Cell Disease at Boston Medical Center. He received his BA from Cornell University and an MD from Tufts University School of Medicine. Dr. Steinberg is a diplomat of the American Board of Internal Medicine in the subspecialty of Hematology, a Fellow of the American Association for the Advancement of Science and a member of the American Society for Clinical Investigation and Association of American Physicians.

Dr. Steinberg's research and clinical interests are focused on disorders of the red blood cell with a special emphasis on sickle cell disease and inherited disorders of hemoglobin. His current work focuses on genotype-phenotype relationships in sickle cell disease and thalassemia, and how multiple genes influence the phenotype of disease. Dr. Steinberg has published nearly 300 articles in his areas of interest and has edited three textbooks that focus on the basic science and clinical aspects of sickle cell disease and other disorders of the hemoglobin molecule.

He has served as a scientific consultant for the American Heart Association, FDA, NIH, NSF, Doris Duke Charitable Foundation, US-Israel Binational Science Foundation, Wellcome Trust, Telethon2002, ISERM, Accreditation Council for Graduate Medical Education, and the Department of Veterans Affairs, and served on the editorial boards of the *American Journal of Hematology, American Journal of the Medical Sciences, BMC Medical Genetics, Haematologica, Journal of Laboratory and Clinical Medicine* and *Hemoglobin.*

Bernard G. Forget is a distinguished physician scientist in Hematology, nationally and internationally recognized for research accomplishments in the field of Molecular Hematology pertaining to the molecular biology of gene expression in blood cells and the molecular basis of hereditary disorders of the red blood cell, including hemoglobinopathies. He is the co-author with Dr. H. F. Bunn of a highly respected textbook entitled *Hemoglobin: Molecular, Genetic and Clinical Aspects*, (WB Saunders Co., Philadelphia, 1986). He is the senior author of a large number of scientific publications in the field of Molecular Hematology and red blood cell disorders, published in leading journals He has also co-authored a number of chapters on thalassemia and other red blood cell disorders in various leading hematology textbooks.

Douglas R. Higgs qualified in medicine at King's College Hospital Medical School in 1974 and trained as a haematologist. He joined the MRC Molecular Haematology Unit (Oxford) in 1977 and is currently Professor of Molecular Haematology at the University of Oxford and Director of the MRC Molecular Haematology Unit. The current interests of the Unit are (i) to understand the processes of lineage commitment in haemopoiesis with particular emphasis on erythropoiesis (ii) to understand how the globin genes are activated and regulated during normal erythropoiesis (iii) to study the human genetic diseases affecting these processes. The main interest of his own laboratory has been to understand how the human alpha globin genes are regulated from their natural chromosomal environment in the telomeric region of 16p13.3. Recently the group has characterised the terminal 2 Mb of chromosome 16 and concentrated on understanding how gene expression is influenced by epigenetic modifications of this region (e.g. chromatin structure, histone acetylation, methylation, timing of replication, nuclear positioning) and the proteins that mediate these processes.

David J. Weatherall is currently Regius Professor of Medicine Emeritus, University of Oxford and Chancellor, Keele University, Keele, UK. His major research contributions have been in the elucidation of the clinical, biochemical and molecular characteristics of the thalassaemias and their related disorders, the population genetics of these conditions, and the application of this information to the development of programmes for the prevention and management of these diseases in the developing countries.

DISORDERS OF HEMOGLOBIN

Genetics, Pathophysiology, and Clinical Management

SECOND EDITION

Edited by

Martin H. Steinberg
Boston University School of Medicine

Bernard G. Forget
Yale University School of Medicine

Douglas R. Higgs
University of Oxford

David J. Weatherall
University of Oxford

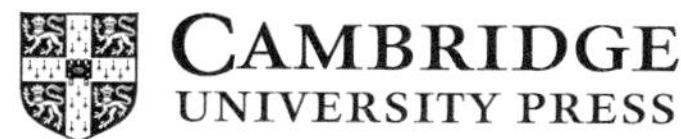

CAMBRIDGE UNIVERSITY PRESS
Cambridge, New York, Melbourne, Madrid, Cape Town, Singapore, São Paulo, Delhi

Cambridge University Press
32 Avenue of the Americas, New York, NY 10013-2473, USA

www.cambridge.org
Information on this title: www.cambridge.org/9780521875196

First published 2009

Printed in the United States of America

A catalog record for this publication is available from the British Library.

Library of Congress Cataloging in Publication data

Disorders of hemoglobin : genetics, pathophysiology, and clinical
management / [edited by] Martin H. Steinberg . . . [et al.]. – 2nd ed.
p. ; cm.
Includes bibliographical references and index.
ISBN 978-0-521-87519-6 (hardback)
1. Hemoglobinopathy. I. Steinberg, Martin H.
[DNLM: 1. Hemoglobinopathies – genetics. 2. Hemoglobinopathies – physiopathology.
3. Hemoglobinopathies – therapy. WH 190 D612 2009]
RC641.7.H35D575 2009
616.1′51 – dc22 2008032334

ISBN 978-0-521-87519-6 hardback

Contents

List of Contributors

Foreword

H. Franklin Bunn, MD
Professor of Medicine
Division of Hematology
Brigham and Women's Hospital
Harvard Medical School
Boston, MA

Preface

Martin H. Steinberg, MD

Bernard G. Forget, MD

Douglas R. Higgs, MD, FRS

Sir David J. Weatherall, MD, FRS

Introduction

Sir David J. Weatherall, MD, FRS
Emeritus Professor of Medicine (University of Oxford)
Weatherall Institute of Molecular Medicine
University of Oxford
John Radcliffe Hospital
Headington, Oxford, UK

SECTION ONE. The Molecular, Cellular, and Genetic Basis of Hemoglobin Disorders

Douglas R. Higgs, MD, FRS
Professor of Molecular Haematology and Director of the MRC Molecular Haematology Unit (University of Oxford)
MRC Molecular Haematology Unit
Weatherall Institute of Molecular Medicine
University of Oxford
John Radcliffe Hospital
Headington, Oxford, UK

Bernard G. Forget, MD
Professor of Medicine and Genetics
Director, Hematology Training Program
Section of Hematology
Department of Medicine
Yale University School of Medicine
New Haven, CT

Chapter 1: A Developmental Approach to Hematopoiesis

Elaine Dzierzak, PhD
Professor of Developmental Biology
Erasmus Stem Cell Institute
Erasmus Medical Center
Rotterdam, The Netherlands

Chapter 2: Erythropoiesis

Sjaak Philipsen, PhD
Professor of Genomics of Cell Differentiation
Department of Cell Biology
Erasmus University Medical Center
Rotterdam, The Netherlands

William G. Wood, PhD
Professor of Haematology
MRC Molecular Haematology Unit
Weatherall Institute of Molecular Medicine
University of Oxford
John Radcliffe Hospital
Headington, Oxford, UK

Chapter 3: The Normal Structure and Regulation of Human Globin Gene Clusters

Bernard G. Forget, MD.

Ross C. Hardison, PhD
T. Ming Chu Professor of Biochemistry and Molecular Biology
The Pennsylvania State University
University Park, PA

Chapter 4: Nuclear Factors That Regulate Erythropoiesis

Gerd A. Blobel, MD, PhD
Professor of Pediatrics
Division of Hematology
The Children's Hospital of Philadelphia
University of Pennsylvania School of Medicine
Philadelphia, PA

Mitchell J. Weiss, MD, PhD
Associate Professor of Pediatrics
Division of Hematology
The Children's Hospital of Philadelphia
University of Pennsylvania School of Medicine
Philadelphia, PA

Chapter 5: Molecular and Cellular Basis of Hemoglobin Switching

George Stamatoyannopoulos, MD, Dr Sci
Professor of Medicine and Genome Sciences
Director, Markey Molecular Medicine Center
University of Washington School of Medicine
Seattle, WA

Patrick A. Navas, PhD
Research Assistant Professor
Division of Medical Genetics
Department of Medicine
University of Washington School of Medicine
Seattle, WA

Qiliang Li, PhD
Research Professor of Medicine
Division of Medical Genetics
Department of Medicine
University of Washington School of Medicine
Seattle, WA

Chapter 6: Structure and Function of Hemoglobin and Its Dysfunction in Sickle Cell Disease

Daniel B. Kim-Shapiro, PhD
Professor of Physics
Department of Physics
Wake Forest University
Olin Physical Laboratory
Winston Salem, NC

Chapter 7: Hemoglobins of the Embryo, Fetus, and Adult

Martin H. Steinberg, MD
Professor of Medicine
Pediatrics, Pathology and Laboratory Medicine
Boston University School of Medicine
Boston, MA

Ronald L. Nagel, MD
New York, NY

SECTION TWO. Pathophysiology of Hemoglobin and Its Disorders

Martin H. Steinberg, MD

Chapter 8: Rheology and Vascular Pathobiology in Sickle Cell Disease and Thalassemia

Dhananjay K. Kaul, PhD
Professor of Medicine
Division of Hematology
Albert Einstein College of Medicine
Bronx, NY

Chapter 9: The Erythrocyte Membrane

Patrick G. Gallagher, MD
Professor of Pediatrics
Section of Perinatal Medicine
Yale University School of Medicine
New Haven, CT

Clinton H. Joiner, MD, PhD
Professor of Pediatrics
Children's Hospital Medical Center
Cincinnati, OH

Chapter 10: The Biology of Vascular Nitric Oxide

Jane A. Leopold, MD
Associate Professor of Medicine
Cardiovascular Medicine Division
Department of Medicine
Brigham and Women's Hospital
Boston, MA

Joseph Loscalzo, MD, PhD
Hersey Professor of the Theory and Practice of Medicine
Chairman, Department of Medicine
Brigham and Women's Hospital
Boston, MA

Chapter 11: Mechanisms and Clinical Complications of Hemolysis in Sickle Cell Disease and Thalassemia

Gregory J. Kato, MD
Director, Sickle Cell Vascular Disease Unit
Vascular Therapeutic Section
Vascular Medicine Branch
National Institutes of Health
Bethesda, MD

Mark T. Gladwin, MD
Professor of Medicine
Division Chief, Pulmonary, Allergy, and Critical Care Medicine
University of Pittsburgh Medical Center
Director, Hemostasis and Vascular Biology Research Institute
University of Pittsburgh
Pittsburgh, PA

Chapter 12: Animal Models of Hemoglobinopathies and Thalassemia

Mary Fabry, PhD
Professor of Medicine
Division of Hematology
Albert Einstein College of Medicine
Bronx, NY

SECTION THREE. α Thalassemia

Douglas R. Higgs, MD, FRS

Chapter 13: The Molecular Basis of α Thalassemia

Douglas R. Higgs, MD, FRS

Chapter 14: The Pathophysiology and Clinical Features of α Thalassemia

Douglas R. Higgs, MD, FRS

Chapter 15: Unusual Types of α Thalassemia

Douglas R. Higgs, MD, FRS.

Veronica J. Buckle, MD
MRC Senior Scientist
MRC Molecular Haematology Unit
Weatherall Institute of Molecular Medicine
University of Oxford
John Radcliffe Hospital
Headington, Oxford, UK

Richard Gibbons, MD
University Lecturer and Honorary
Consultant Clinical Geneticist
Weatherall Institute of Molecular Medicine
University of Oxford
John Radcliffe Hospital
Headington, Oxford, UK

David Steensma, MD
Associate Professor of Medicine and Oncology
Consultant, Division of Hematology
Mayo Clinic
Rochester, MN

SECTION FOUR. The β Thalassemias

Bernard G. Forget, MD

Chapter 16: The Molecular Basis of β Thalassemia, δβ Thalassemia, and Hereditary Persistence of Fetal Hemoglobin

Swee Lay Thein, MD
Professor of Molecular Haematology
Head, Division of Gene and Cell Based Therapy
King's College London School of Medicine and King's College Hospital
London, UK

William G. Wood, PhD

Chapter 17: Clinical Aspects of β Thalassemia and Related Disorders

Nancy F. Olivieri, MD
Senior Scientist
Division of Clinical Investigation and Human Physiology
University Health Network
Toronto General Hospital
Toronto, ON, Canada

Sir David J. Weatherall, MD, FRS

Chapter 18: Hemoglobin E Disorders

Suthat Fucharoen, MD
Director, Thalassemia Research Center
Institute of Science and Technology for Research and Development
Mahidol University
Salaya Campus
Puttamonthon, Nakornpathom, Thailand

Sir David J. Weatherall, MD, FRS

SECTION FIVE. Sickle Cell Disease

Martin H. Steinberg, MD

Chapter 19: Clinical and Pathophysiological Aspects of Sickle Cell Anemia

Martin H. Steinberg, MD.

Kwaku Ohene-Frempong, MD
Professor of Pediatrics
Hematology
The Children's Hospital of Philadelphia
Philadelphia, PA

Matthew M. Heeney, MD
Instructor in Pediatrics
Harvard Medical School
Boston, MA

Chapter 20: Sickle Cell Pain: Biology, Etiology, and Treatment

Samir K. Ballas, MD
Professor of Medicine and Pediatrics
Thomas Jefferson University
Philadelphia, PA

James R. Eckman, MD
Professor of Medicine
Comprehensive Sickle Cell Center
Emory University School of Medicine
Atlanta, GA

Chapter 21: Hemoglobin SC Disease and Hemoglobin C Disorders

Martin H. Steinberg, MD

Ronald L. Nagel, MD

Chapter 22: Sickle Cell Trait

Martin H. Steinberg, MD

Chapter 23: Other Sickle Hemoglobinopathies

Martin H. Steinberg, MD

SECTION SIX. Other Clinically Important Disorders of Hemoglobin

Martin H. Steinberg, MD

Chapter 24: Unstable Hemoglobins, Hemoglobins with Altered Oxygen Affinity, Hemoglobin M, and Other Variants of Clinical and Biological Interest

Martin H. Steinberg, MD

Ronald L. Nagel, MD

Chapter 25: Dyshemoglobinemias

Neeraj Agarwal, MD
Assistant Professor, Oncology Division
University of Utah, School of Medicine
Salt Lake City, UT

Ronald L. Nagel, MD

Josef T. Prchal, MD
Professor of Medicine
Internal Medicine
Hematology Division
University of Utah
Salt Lake City, UT

SECTION SEVEN. Special Topics in Hemoglobinopathies

Martin H. Steinberg, MD

Chapter 26: Population Genetics and Global Health Burden

Sir David J. Weatherall, MD, FRS

Thomas N. Williams, PhD
Wellcome Trust Senior Clinical Fellow
Kenya Medical Research Institute/Wellcome Trust Programme
Centre for Geographic Medical Research
Kilifi District Hospital
Kilifi, Kenya

Chapter 27: Genetic Modulation of Sickle Cell Disease and Thalassemia

Martin H. Steinberg, MD

Ronald L. Nagel, MD

Chapter 28: Laboratory Methods for Diagnosis and Evaluation of Hemoglobin Disorders

Mary Fabry, PhD

John M. Old, MD
Consultant Clinical Scientist
National Haemoglobinopathy Reference Laboratory
Oxford Haemophilia Centre
Churchill Hospital
Oxford, UK

SECTION EIGHT. New Approaches to the Treatment of Hemoglobinopathies and Thalassemia

Martin H. Steinberg, MD

Chapter 29: Transfusion and Iron Chelation Therapy in Thalassemia and Sickle Cell Disease

Janet L. Kwiatkowski, MD
Assistant Professor of Pediatrics
Division of Hematology
The Children's Hospital of Philadelphia
Philadelphia, PA

John B. Porter, MA, MD, FRCP, FRCPath
Professor of Haematology
Department of Haematology
University College London
London, UK

Chapter 30: Induction of Fetal Hemoglobin in the Treatment of Sickle Cell Disease and β Thalassemia

Yogen Saunthararajah, MD
Associate Professor
Cleveland Clinic/University of Illinois at Chicago
Twissing Cancer Institute
Cleveland, OH

George F. Atweh, MD
Koch Professor of Medicine
Director, Division of Hematology/Oncology
Director, Barrett Cancer Center
University of Cincinnati College of Medicine
Cincinnati, OH

Chapter 31: Novel Approaches to Treatment

Kirkwood A. Pritchard Jr., PhD
Professor of Pediatric Surgery
Medical College of Wisconsin
Milwaukee, WI

Alicia Rivera, PhD
Instructor of Pediatrics
Harvard Medical School
Boston, MA

Cheryl Hillery, MD
Blood Center of Wisconsin
Associate Professor
Pediatrics and Medicine
Medical College of Wisconsin
Milwaukee, WI

Carlo Brugnara, MD
Professor of Pathology
Harvard Medical School
Children's Hospital
Boston, MA

Chapter 32: Stem Cell Transplantation

Emanuele Angelucci, MD
Associate Professor
Head, Hematology Department and BMT Centre
Armando Businco Cancer Centre
Cagliari, Italy

Mark Walters, MD
Director, Blood and Marrow Transplantation Program
Children's Hospital Oakland Research Institute
Oakland, CA

Chapter 33: Prospects for Gene Therapy of Sickle Cell Disease and Thalassemia

Derek A. Persons, MD
Assistant Member
Department of Hematology
Division of Experimental Hematology
St. Jude Children's Research Hospital
Memphis, TN

Brian P. Sorrentino, MD
Member
Department of Hematology
Director, Division of Experimental Hematology
St. Jude Children's Research Hospital
Memphis, TN

Arthur W. Nienhuis, MD
Member
Department of Hematology
Division of Experimental Hematology
St. Jude Children's Research Hospital
Memphis, TN

Foreword

H. Franklin Bunn

The study of hemoglobin continues to be a rewarding endeavor. Cumulative progress since the turn of the last century has laid cornerstones in protein chemistry and molecular genetics and has provided a wealth of insight into the pathogenesis of some of the world's most prevalent and devastating disorders. The first edition of *Disorders of Hemoglobin,* published 8 years ago, was a comprehensive compilation and analysis of the basic science of hemoglobin and its application to the thalassemias, sickle cell disease, and other globin mutants that spawn a wide range of clinical phenotypes. This second edition now presents an updated overview of all aspects of the hemoglobin story as well as a detailed account of the impressive advances that have been made in biochemistry, genetics, and clinical investigation.

Hemoglobin boasts a proud history. By the end of the nineteenth century, it was well established that hemoglobin was a composite of protein and heme that could reversibly bind oxygen and that this substance was found in almost all living creatures. Entry into the twentieth century marked the dawn of quantitative physiology, biochemistry, and the application of the scientific method to medicine. All three of these developing disciplines owe their early impetus to hemoglobin and the lessons learned from this remarkable molecule. Physiologists from Scandinavia (Bohr and Krogh) and England (Barcroft, the Haldanes, and Roughton) made accurate equilibrium and kinetic measurements of oxygen–hemoglobin binding as a function of pH and thereby provided a mechanistic understanding of the reciprocal transport of oxygen from lung to tissues and of acid waste from tissues to lung. These early contributions set the stage for an appreciation of how the homeostasis of the organism depends on the orderly integration of its organ systems.

The fledgling science of biochemistry was given a jump start by the studies of Adair and Svedberg, which established that hemoglobin is a uniform protein with a large but narrowly defined molecular weight and was therefore, like sodium chloride and glucose, a bona fide molecule. Hemoglobin and its cousin myoglobin were the first proteins whose structures were solved at high resolution by X-ray crystallography by Perutz and Kendrew, respectively, thereby, providing an opportunity for detailed exploration of structure–function relationships. Hemoglobin was the first multisubunit protein to be understood at the molecular level and therefore was the model system used by Monod, Changeux, and Wyman for establishing the principles of allostery, which dictate the regulation of a broad range of enzymes, receptors, transcription factors, and so on.

The linkage of specific diseases to abnormalities of specific molecules began with Pauling's demonstration in 1949 that patients with sickle cells have hemoglobin with an altered surface charge. Within 8 years, Ingram demonstrated that sickle hemoglobin differs from normal hemoglobin only by a substitution of valine for glutamic acid in the sixth residue of the β-globin subunit. This was the first example of how an abnormal gene can change the structure of a protein and, therefore, verified in a most satisfying way the Beadle–Tatum one gene–one enzyme hypothesis.

During the last quarter of the twentieth century, with the development of recombinant DNA technology and genomics, hemoglobin again became *primus inter pares* among biological molecules. Indeed, the human globin genes were among the first to be molecularly cloned and sequenced. This soon led to the identification of a wide range of globin gene mutants responsible for the α and β thalassemias. Understanding the mechanisms by which these genotypes impair globin biosynthesis provided insight into the diverse clinical manifestations encountered in patients with different types of thalassemia. In addition, the evolving knowledge of human globin genes enabled the development of molecular techniques for antenatal diagnosis and polymorphism-based population studies, both of which were then applied to many other disorders.

To date, more than 1,000 hemoglobin variants have been discovered and characterized. Study of these variants, so amply documented in this book, established the principle of how a mutant genotype alters the function of the protein it encodes, which in turn can lead to a distinct clinical phenotype. This linkage is at the heart of how molecular genetics impacts our understanding of pathophysiological mechanisms.

Thus, hemoglobin held center stage in the biomedical discoveries of the twentieth century, and, in the new millenium, there is no indication that the pace has slackened. This book begins with authoritative and up-to-date coverage of all aspects of hemoglobin, beginning with overviews of erythropoiesis, globin gene regulation, and structure–function relationships. Subsequent sections of the book are devoted to in-depth coverage of the thalassemias, sickle cell disease, and other hemoglobinopathies. A recurrent theme is how understanding pathophysiology at the molecular level has informed the design and development of novel, rationally based therapy.

This second edition incorporates a number of advances that have been made in the past 8 years. Chapter 4 describes the important insights that have accrued from the discovery of α-hemoglobin stabilizing protein (AHSP), the chaparone that protects the α-hemoglobin subunit during assembly of the tetramer. Chapters 6, 10, and 11 include new information on nitric oxide and its controversial roles in allosteric modulation of hemoglobin function and in the pathophysiology of sickle cell disease and other types of hemolytic anemia. Chapter 27 presents recent information on the contribution of genetic polymorphisms to the clinical phenotypes of sickle cell disease and thalassemia. The last 4 chapters cover the development of oral iron chelators as well as bolder therapeutic strategies, including impressive progress in globin gene therapy.

The creative energy that continues to bear down on all aspects of hemoglobin research is well represented by the impressive list of basic and clinical investigators who have contributed to this book. As in any field at the cutting edge of science, controversies enrich the scientific dialogue among hemoglobinologists. In carefully reading chapters on closely related topics, the thoughtful reader will adopt a policy of caveat emptor, appreciating that strongly held opinions need to be vetted by both experimentation and alternative hypotheses. This proviso notwithstanding, *Disorders of Hemoglobin* offers authoritative and comprehensive coverage of one of the most exciting and fruitful areas at the interface of bioscience and clinical medicine.

Preface

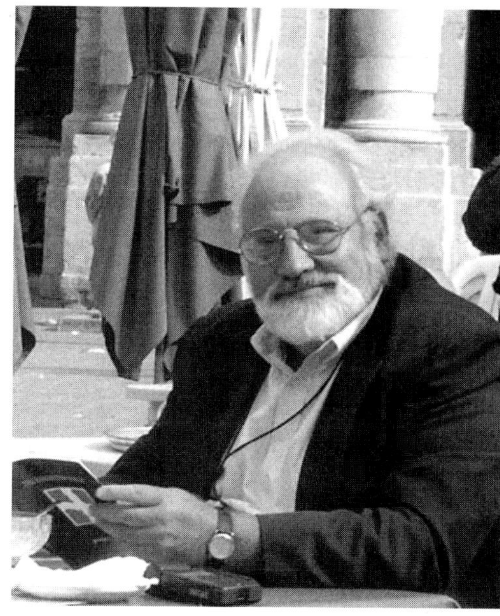

Eight years have passed since this monograph first appeared, and the advances in basic, translational, and clinical research during this interval justify a new edition. To conserve space and avoid duplicating our first edition, we review very briefly historical aspects, summarize established older information, and focus on the progress of the past 8 years. Although some older references are retained, we have tried to focus on the literature since 2001. In expanding our coverage of clinical issues, we also have decreased the length of the book by considering together pathophysiological features common to many hemoglobin disorders such as vasculopathy, erythrocyte membrane damage, and mechanisms of hemolysis. More than half of the contributors to this volume are either new authors or previous authors addressing different topics; David Weatherall has joined the editorial team.

Hemoglobin has been an interest of basic and translational scientists, clinicians, and clinical diagnostic laboratories. So, we continue to address the molecular, cellular, genetic, diagnostic, and clinical aspects of hemoglobin disorders. When applicable, we provide practical recommendations for diagnosis and treatment. The first section of the book again focuses on molecular, cellular, and genetic aspects of hemoglobin and includes discussions of developmental hematopoiesis, erythropoiesis, globin genes and their regulation, minor normal hemoglobins, and an update on new structural and functional features of normal and variant hemoglobins. Pathophysiology of hemoglobin disorders follows, with new chapters on vascular biology, the erythrocyte membrane, the biology of nitric oxide, mechanisms of hemolysis, and how animal models of disease provide new pathophysiological insights. Four sections deal with diagnosis, complications, and treatment of α thalassemia, β thalassemia, and related conditions, including hemoglobin E diseases, sickle cell disease, and less common genetic and acquired hemoglobin disorders. This is followed by special topics such as population genetics and the health burden of hemoglobin disorders, the genetic modulation of sickle cell disease and thalassemia, and developments in laboratory detection, including antenatal diagnosis. Finally, current and developing approaches to treatment, incorporating new agents for iron chelation, methods to induce fetal hemoglobin production, novel treatment approaches such as antioxidants, antiinflammatory agents, enhancement of nitric oxide effects, and agents that modulate membrane cation and water transport are discussed, concluding with the use of stem cell transplantation and progress in gene therapy.

Ronald L. Nagel (pictured), a coeditor of the first edition, has retired as Irving D. Karpas Professor of Medicine, Physiology and Biophysics and Head of the Division of Hematology at Albert Einstein College of Medicine. Although no longer a coeditor of this monograph, his influence in the field is felt in most chapters. His contributions to the structure, function, pathophysiology, and genetics of hemoglobin disorders are vast and time tested. The editors, and the field of hematology, will miss his scientific insight and originality.

The Editors

Introduction

David J. Weatherall

A few years ago, an eminent British professor of medicine, while reviewing a new edition of a well-known textbook of medicine, suggested that works of this type were becoming valueless because they were already out of date by the time they were published. His derogatory comments went further: Having taken the trouble to weigh the book, he suggested that volumes of this type would suffer the same fate as dinosaurs and become extinct by collapsing under their excessive weight. Even allowing for this bizarre and completely erroneous view of the biological fate of the dinosaurs, does this argument carry any weight beyond its metaphorical context?

Undoubtedly, there is feeling rife among medical publishers that the day of the major monograph in the biological sciences may be coming to an end. They argue that there is so much information online that the need for works of this type is becoming increasingly limited. Is this really the case? Although it is impossible to deny that the long gestation of monographs of this type may lead to the omission of the occasional "breakthrough" in a field, it seems very important that in any rapidly moving area of the biomedical sciences there is a regular and broad critical review of where it has got to and how it has been modified by recent advances. Not uncommonly in medical research and practice, today's breakthrough is tomorrow's breakdown.

Is the hemoglobin field moving rapidly? This was another question that had to be considered by the editors of this new edition. As judged by the amount of space given to disorders of the red cell in current journals, the volume of work in this field seems to have declined considerably over recent years. A visitor from outer space, browsing through the journals, might be excused for wondering how Homo sapiens transfers oxygen to their tissues. Hence, it might have been perceived that there is insufficient material to warrant this new edition.

A broader review of the field over recent years suggests, however, that this is not the case. There undoubtedly have been major advances in our understanding of the regulation of hematopoiesis, some of which have important implications for a better understanding of the pathophysiology of the hemoglobin disorders that may, in the longer term, lead to more definitive approaches to their management. Furthermore, there have also been dramatic developments in many areas of genome technology that have direct application to the many unanswered questions of the hemoglobin field, not in the least the reasons for the remarkable phenotypic variation of its diseases. Of even greater importance, there has been a genuine increase in the appreciation of the major public health burden that these diseases are likely to cause in the future. This is particularly relevant to the poorer countries of the world in which the epidemiological transition following improvements in nutrition and basic public health is resulting in a reduction in neonatal and childhood mortality; many babies with severe hemoglobin disorders who would previously have died in early life are now surviving to present for diagnosis and management.

It is only in the last few years that these public health issues have been recognized by the major international health agencies. In 2002, the World Health Organization (WHO) published a report, *Genomics and World Health*, in which the hemoglobin disorders were described as a prime example of how the new technology of molecular genetics can be applied for the benefit of poorer countries. At the 118th session of the WHO Executive Board, held in 2006, the sickle cell disorders and thalassemias were formally recognized as major health burdens that required immediate action. In 2007, it was decided to include the hemoglobin disorders in the Global Burden of Disease Program, an international study conducted under the auspices of several universities, the WHO, the Bill and Melinda Gates Foundation, the World Bank, and others that attempts to define the relative global burden posed by each of the major diseases. Previous versions of this work have undoubtedly had a major influence on developing healthcare policies by governments and international healthcare agencies.

Clearly, this new edition is appearing at the same time as a major drive to define the most appropriate ways of controlling and managing the hemoglobin disorders, particularly in the developing countries, and to determine the most cost-effective and efficient ways of approaching this problem. We hope, therefore, that this updated distillation of knowledge about the scientific, clinical, and epidemiological aspects of this field will be of value to scientists and clinicians, not only to those in wealthier countries but particularly to those who are attempting to cope with these diseases with limited resources in the developing countries of the world.

There is also an important message for our younger readers. There are still some extraordinarily exciting areas of this field to be pursued, not in the least a better understanding of the reasons for the remarkable clinical diversity of all the hemoglobin disorders; a better appreciation of their pathophysiology at the molecular level with respect to novel approaches for their more definitive management; and an understanding of the long-neglected role of the environment in their clinical diversity, the cellular mechanisms whereby protection against malaria has resulted in their extremely high frequency, how current knowledge of their diagnosis and control may be applied in the poorer countries of the world, and many other stimulating questions. Currently, the hemoglobin field offers challenges ranging from basic cell and molecular biology through clinical research at the bedside to epidemiology, public health, and the social sciences.

Finally, we thank Cambridge University Press and particularly Beth Barry and more recently Larry Fox for continued support of this project. We are also extremely grateful to the authors from many parts of the world who have willingly given their time to writing parts of this new edition, and for the personal help that we have received from Liz Rose, during its preparation. It is particularly gratifying to be able to report that the marriages of the four editors have survived another edition.

SECTION ONE

THE MOLECULAR, CELLULAR, AND GENETIC BASIS OF HEMOGLOBIN DISORDERS

Douglas R. Higgs and Bernard G. Forget

Over the past 30 years we have become familiar with the way in which different types of hemoglobin are expressed at different stages of development. In the human embryo the main hemoglobins include Hb Portland ($\zeta_2\gamma_2$), Hb Gower I ($\zeta_2\varepsilon_2$), and Gower II ($\alpha_2\varepsilon_2$). In the fetus, HbF ($\alpha_2\gamma_2$) predominates and in the adult, HbA ($\alpha_2\beta_2$) makes up the majority of hemoglobin in red cells. These simple facts belie the complexity of the cellular and molecular processes that bring about these beautifully coordinated changes in the patterns of globin gene expression throughout development.

To understand these phenomena we have to consider the individual components including 1) the origins of erythroid cells in development, 2) the processes by which erythroid cells differentiate to mature red cells at each developmental stage, and 3) the molecular events that produce the patterns of gene expression we observe.

Two different types of erythroid cells are observed during development. The first erythroid cells to be seen in the developing embryo are located in the blood islands of the yolk sac. These primitive erythroid cells are morphologically different from the definitive erythroid cells made in the fetal liver and bone marrow and contain predominantly embryonic hemoglobins. Somewhat later during embryonic development, definitive erythroid and other hematopoietic cells originate from multipotent cells identified in a part of the embryo that lies near the dorsal aorta, in the region close to where the kidneys first develop: the so-called aorta-gonads-mesonephros (AGM) region. It is thought that the cells that are destined to provide fetal- (liver) and adult- (bone marrow) derived red cells originate from AGM cells, although the ultimate origin of hematopoietic stem cells is still a matter of controversy. In the first trimester of pregnancy, fetal erythroid cells derived predominantly from hematopoiesis in the liver contain mainly HbF with small amounts of embryonic hemoglobin. There are no circumstances in which expression of embryonic globins persists at high levels or becomes substantially reactivated in fetal or adult life, although low levels of ζ-globin chains are present in the most severe form of α thalassemia. Until approximately the time of birth, fetal cells continue to make predominantly HbF but switch to making HbA between 30 and 40 weeks postconception. In contrast to the situation in embryonic cells, there are many conditions in which HbF synthesis persists or becomes reactivated in adult red cells. The simplest explanation for all of these observations is that the switch from embryonic to fetal–adult patterns of hemoglobin synthesis involves the replacement of embryonic cells (with one program of expression) by definitive cells (with a different program of expression). In contrast, the switch from fetal to adult hemoglobin expression takes place in definitive cells so this represents a true change in the molecular program within a single lineage of erythroid progenitor cells.

At present we do not know when during development the embryonic and fetal programs are established in the differentiating hematopoietic cells. Furthermore we do not fully understand by what mechanisms the programs of globin gene expression are initiated or maintained. Perhaps the greatest progress toward such an understanding has been to identify key regulatory molecules, including transcription factors, cofactors, and chromatin-associated proteins that play important roles in specifying the formation of erythroid cells from multipotent hematopoietic stem cells. Of greatest importance in this area has been the characterization of the tissue-restricted zinc finger proteins (GATA-1 and GATA-2), their cofactors (FOG-1 and FOG-2), the b-Zip family of proteins (NF-E2, Nrf1, Nrf2, Nrf3, Bach1 and Bach2), and the erythroid Krüppel-like factors (EKLF and FKLF). Experiments in which GATA-1, GATA-2, and FOG-1 have been inactivated in the mouse genome show that these proteins play a major role in establishing the erythroid lineage and allowing differentiation to mature red cells.

A major focus of interest over the past 20 years has been to understand how these developmental programs are played out on the α- and β-globin gene clusters. We now know that in most mammals in each cluster the globin genes are arranged along the chromosome in the order in which the genes are expressed in development: the α-like globin gene cluster on chromosome 16 (ζ-α_2-α_1-) and the β-like globin gene cluster on chromosome 11 (ε-$^G\gamma$-$^A\gamma$-δ-β-), suggesting that gene order may be important in unfolding this program. Expression of each cluster is dependent on remote regulatory elements, originally identified as DNase I hypersensitive sites in the chromatin of nucleated erythroid cells. In the α-globin gene cluster there is a single regulatory element (RE or HS -40) that lies 40 kb upstream of the gene complex, and in the β-globin gene cluster there are five major hypersensitive sites, collectively referred to as the β-globin locus control region (β-LCR) lying 5–20 kb upstream of the locus. Again, many details remain unknown but it appears that the ζ and ε genes are switched on in embryonic cells and are largely off in definitive cells in which they cannot be substantially reactivated. With regard to the switch from γ- to β-globin gene expression during fetal development and neonatal life, the situation is complex. There is strong evidence for autonomous silencing of the γ genes, in a manner analogous to that of the ε gene, but it also appears that there may exist some degree of competition between the γ- and β-globin genes that is modified by the transcriptional milieu, which can change dramatically during this time of development, with the balance tipped toward γ-globin gene expression in fetal life and β-globin gene expression in adult life. The balance between γ- and β-globin gene expression may be altered in vivo (in hereditary persistence of fetal hemoglobin and other hemoglobinopathies) as well as in various experimental systems. Changes in the repertoire or amounts of transcription factors may influence the switch from γ- to β-globin gene expression. For example, without EKLF the β-globin genes cannot be fully activated during development. Alternatively, alterations in the arrangement of the β-LCR and the γ- and β-like genes with respect to each other may alter the pattern of switching. The precise molecular mechanisms underlying these changes are still poorly understood but it seems unlikely that changes in the patterns of globin gene expression are only brought about through changes in the repertoire of *trans*-acting factors present in embryonic, fetal, and adult red cells, as originally proposed; however, they may be influenced by other epigenetic changes in the chromosome (e.g., chromatin structure and modification, replication timing, and methylation).

Despite our continuing interest and frustrated attempts to fathom how the entire globin clusters are regulated, we do know a lot about the structure and function of individual genes. The globin genes have provided the paradigm for understanding the general arrangement of mammalian genes including their promoters, exons, introns, and processing signals. Furthermore, the mechanisms by which these genes are transcribed into pre-RNA, processed into mature RNA, and translated into protein are now understood in detail. This brings us back in a full circle to where modern molecular biology started by establishing the structure and function of the proteins that are expressed by globin genes. Hemoglobin was one of the first proteins whose amino acid sequence and crystal structure were solved, which in turn led to a complete understanding of how it captures, transports, and releases oxygen. Given the very large number of natural mutants of hemoglobin that have now been identified it also provides an unsurpassed example of how mutations can give rise to "molecular diseases," the best example still being sickle cell disease.

Even with this apparent depth of knowledge, there are still surprises. We know from theory and experiment that erythrocytes containing embryonic hemoglobins and fetal hemoglobins have a higher affinity for oxygen than those containing adult hemoglobin. Traditionally we have surmised that this enables the developing fetus to acquire oxygen more efficiently from the maternal circulation, a seemingly important consideration. We have known for many years, however, that the babies of mothers whose blood contains mainly fetal (high-affinity) hemoglobin are entirely normal. Similarly, thanks to experimental work in model systems, we know that mice, which by design only make embryonic hemoglobin throughout fetal and adult life, survive normally and thrive as adults. Presumably the complex system of hemoglobin switching that keeps investigators so busy has been molded in very subtle ways by natural selection. So why do we pursue this subject with such enthusiasm? There are two main reasons. The first is that the globin system still provides the most thoroughly studied and comprehensively understood example of mammalian gene expression we have. If there are undiscovered general principles governing the regulation of mammalian genes, then analysis of globin gene expression is likely to elucidate them. The second is that understanding how these genes are controlled offers the best hope of developing strategies to ameliorate or cure the many thousands of severely affected patients who inherit defects in the structure or production of the α- and β-like globin chains that make up embryonic, fetal, and adult hemoglobins.

The following seven chapters trace the genesis of hemoglobin, from the earliest appearance of erythroid cells during development, through the nuclear factors that govern its synthesis, the evolution of globin genes, their organization and switching, to the production of hemoglobin and its functions in the erythrocyte.

1

A Developmental Approach to Hematopoiesis

Elaine Dzierzak

INTRODUCTION AND GENERAL CONSIDERATIONS

During mammalian development, the first morphologically recognizable blood cells in the conceptus are those of the erythroid lineage. The early production of erythroid lineage cells in the yolk sac is required for the development of the vertebrate embryo. These blood cells are short-lived, however. In contrast, long-term adult hematopoiesis results from a complex cell lineage differentiation hierarchy that produces at least eight functionally distinct lineages of differentiated blood cells. The founder cells for this hierarchy are the hematopoietic stem cells (HSCs), which undergo progressive differentiation, proliferation, and restriction in lineage potential. The adult blood system is constantly replenished throughout adult life from rare HSCs harbored in the bone marrow. The field of "developmental hematopoiesis" investigates how this complex adult system is generated in the conceptus. Current research interests in this field include 1) the embryonic origins, cell lineage relationships, and functions of the cells within the multiple embryonic hematopoietic compartments; 2) the changing developmental microenvironments that support hematopoietic (stem) cell growth; and 3) the molecular programming of the hematopoietic system during ontogeny. This chapter will focus on our current knowledge concerning the embryonic beginnings of the adult hematopoietic system. Insights emerging from such a developmental approach should lead to novel molecular and cellular manipulations that could aid in the ex vivo generation and/or expansion of HSCs and progenitors for clinical use in transplantations for leukemias or blood-related genetic disease.

ONTOGENY OF THE HEMATOPOIETIC SYSTEM

Developmental studies provide insight into the initiation, growth, and function of cells in the wide variety of adult tissues. The cellular interactions and molecular programs governing tissue development are conserved throughout evolution, as revealed in a variety of animal models ranging from invertebrates to mammalian vertebrates. Similarly, conserved developmental principles also govern the generation of the hematopoietic system. Our current knowledge of the embryonic origins of the adult hematopoietic system has been gained from the study of nonmammalian vertebrate embryos such as frogs and birds[1,2] and the widely used mammalian vertebrate model, the mouse.[3] These cumulative results have provided wide support for multiple de novo hematopoietic specification events, at least three independent embryonic origins of hematopoiesis, and for the colonization theory of hematopoiesis. The variety of in vivo and in vitro hematopoietic assays and the ease of genetic manipulation of mice have significantly expanded our molecular knowledge of mammalian blood development. Studies of human embryonic hematopoiesis are further facilitated through xenotransplantation studies of human cells into mice[4] and induced hematopoietic differentiation of embryonic stem cells (ESCs) (mouse and human).[5,6] Thus, a more dynamic view of human embryonic hematopoiesis has been realized.

Initiation and Appearance of Hematopoietic Cells

Mesoderm

The hematopoietic system is one of the earliest tissues to develop during ontogeny. It is derived from the mesodermal germ layer of the conceptus, and in the human this embryonic stage is referred to as the "mesoblastic" period.[7] The mesoderm forms through an inductive interaction between the ectodermal and endodermal germ layers during the midblastula stage (Fig. 1.1A). Much of our knowledge of mesoderm induction comes from studies of amphibian embryos in which the manipulation, grafting, and culture of embryos are facilitated by their large size and development outside the mother. Nieuwkoop[8] was the first to demonstrate that culture of the amphibian midblastula stage animal cap (ectoderm) alone leads to the production of epidermis, whereas coculture of the animal cap with the vegetal pole (endoderm) leads to the generation of mesodermal structures such as muscle, notochord, heart, pronephros, and blood (Fig. 1.1B). Cell lineage mapping studies show that mesodermal cells are formed from the presumptive ectoderm that receives signals from the underlying vegetal component and presumptive endoderm.[9,10] Recent studies suggest that the earliest hematopoietic mesoderm is derived from a specialized mesendodermal layer of cells.[11,12] Animal cap assays have identified mesoderm-inducing factors including transforming growth factor–β_1 (TGFβ_1) family members BMP-4, activin, and Vg1, and members of the fibroblast growth factor (FGF) family.[11–13] The production (by endodermal cells) of these factors and their graded distribution suggest that they act as morphogens. Together with the

A

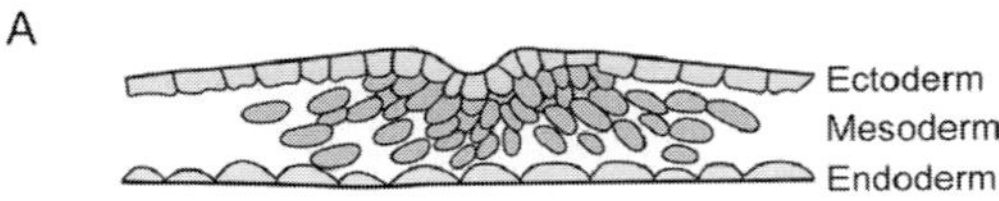

B

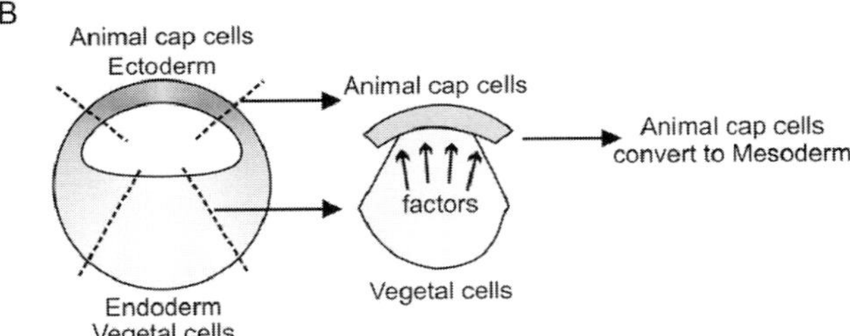

Figure 1.1. Schematic diagram of germ layer development in vertebrate embryos. **(A)** Mesoderm arises from an inductive interaction between ectoderm and endoderm. **(B)** Experimental scheme in Xenopus embryos that shows that mesodermal cells arise from the ectoderm (animal cap cells) under the inductive influence of the endodermal vegetal fragment.[10] (See color plate 1.1.)

extensive rearrangements of cell movement during gastrulation, different lineages of mesoderm are formed: dorsal, paraxial, lateral, and ventral. Numerous secreted factors (as well as transcription factors and adhesion molecules) play roles in this patterning of mesoderm.[12,14]

Similarly, mesoderm induction is the first step leading to the specification of hematopoietic cells in the mammalian conceptus. Mesoderm induction occurs in the primitive streak of the mouse conceptus beginning at embryonic day (E) 6.5/7.0. Single-cell marking of the presumptive mesoderm in the mouse epiblast showed that the first mesoderm emerging from the posterior primitive streak contributes to extraembryonic hematopoietic tissue, that is, yolk sac and allantois[15] (Fig. 1.2A). Mesodermal derivatives within the rostral embryo body arise from epiblast cells that ingress through the anterior primitive streak. Thereafter, cells that give rise to lateral blood-forming mesoderm of the anterior trunk (Fig. 1.2B) transit through the primitive streak. Mesoderm emigrating from more caudal regions of the streak forms the mesoderm of the remaining trunk regions.[16] Interestingly, the entire epiblast of the early- and midstreak stage mouse embryo contains hemogenic potential, but that potential is later restricted to the trunk and posterior region of the embryo.[17] Thus, induction of prospective hematopoietic mesoderm is conserved between vertebrate species.[16]

Extraembryonic Hematopoiesis: Yolk Sac

Yolk sac blood islands containing primitive erythrocytes are detectable in the mouse conceptus at E7.5[18] and in the human conceptus at approximately 16–20 days of gestation.[19] Mesodermal cells migrate to this extraembryonic site and come in close contact with the endoderm. As shown in avian embryos, interaction with the endoderm is required for the initiation of hematopoiesis.[20] Several endodermally produced developmental factors and morphogens in the chick[21] and the Indian hedgehog factor produced by the endoderm in mouse embryo cultures[22,23] play inductive roles in patterning hematopoietic mesoderm.

The close temporal and spatial appearance of hematopoietic and endothelial cells in the yolk sac has led to speculation of a common mesoderm precursor cell for these two lineages, the hemangioblast.[24,25] Indeed, the shared expression of markers such as Flk-1 (KDR), SCL, and CD34 by hematopoietic cells and endothelial cells and the complete lack of endothelial and hematopoietic cells in Flk-1-deficient embryos support the existence of hemangioblasts in the mammalian conceptus.[26–28]

ESC hematopoietic differentiation cultures have facilitated the isolation and characterization of hemangioblasts. Stepwise differentiation of ESCs toward the mesodermal lineage and thereafter to hematopoietic and endothelial lineages closely parallels such development in the yolk sac.[29] Under controlled culture conditions, ESCs differentiate to form cells expressing Brachyury, a well-known mesodermal marker. Brachyury expression in mouse ESCs is upregulated following exposure to mesodermal inducing factors such as FGF, TGF-β_1, and BMP-4. Shortly thereafter these cells express Flk-1 and have potential to differentiate to angioblasts and SCL$^+$CD34$^+$ blast colony–forming cells (BLCFC)[30] The ESC-derived BLCFCs are considered to be hemangioblasts. This cell type has also been identified in the early mouse embryo. At E7.5 Brachyury$^+$ cells become Flk1$^+$. When put in culture, these cells (and a small fraction of the Brachyury$^+$Flk1$^-$ cells) exhibit the functional properties of BLCFC.[31] Additional studies have

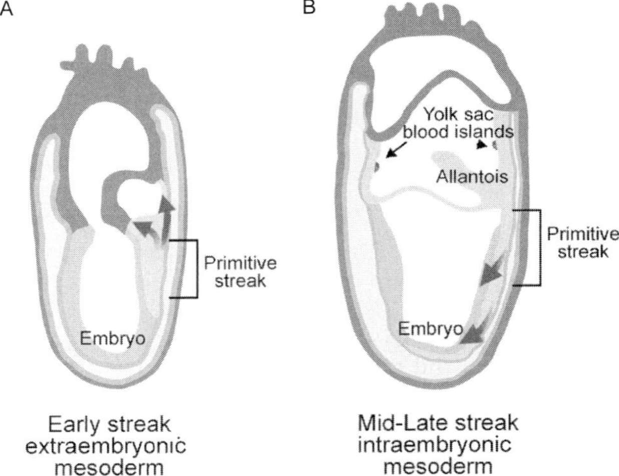

Figure 1.2. Mesodermal migration during mouse embryogenesis. **(A)** Schematic diagram of a mouse conceptus at the early primitive streak stage. Emerging from the posterior primitive streak are waves of yolk sac mesoderm migrating to form this extraembryonic tissues. Slightly later, this mesoderm also forms the allantois. Hemangioblasts are found in the posterior primitive streak. **(B)** Schematic diagram of a mouse conceptus at the mid–late primitive streak stage. Mesoderm emerging from the anterior primitive streak forms the paraxial and lateral mesoderm of the trunk region of the embryo (mesoderm for the prospective PAS/AGM region). At this stage the allantois is visible, as are the first primitive erythroid cells in the yolk sac blood islands. (Drawings adapted from ref. 3.) (See color plate 1.2.)

established that subsequent SCL expression can be used to isolate the hemangioblast from angioblasts.[26] Surprisingly, hemangioblasts in vivo are localized not in yolk sac but in the posterior primitive streak[31] (Fig. 1.2A). As they migrate to the yolk sac they become committed endothelial and hematopoietic progenitors and several of these cells contribute to the formation of each blood island.[32] Studies with human ESCs and other animal models further demonstrate the existence of hemangioblasts in the earliest stages of mesoderm and blood development, and there are some suggestions that hemangioblasts may persist in postnatal stages.[26]

Extraembryonic Hematopoiesis: Chorion, Allantois, and Placenta

The placenta has long been recognized as a site where hematopoietic cells are harbored and circulate; however, it is only recently that this tissue was shown to possess hemogenic properties.[33,34] Placenta organogenesis is initiated through the fusion of the chorionic membrane with the allantois, both derived from the extraembryonic mesoderm. The growth of this highly vascularized extraembryonic tissue is a cooperative effort between fetus and mother, allowing nutrients to be delivered to the fetus and wastes exported to the mother.

The hemogenic properties of the allantois were initially studied in avian embryos. The avian allantois, before it becomes vascularized, contains clusters of hematopoietic cells resembling blood islands[35] and, upon grafting, forms adult blood and endothelium.[36] In contrast, initial grafting studies of the mouse allantois did not reveal erythroid lineage contribution in vivo, although a small population of erythroid cells was found in cultured tissues.[37] Recently, both the mouse allantois and chorion have been shown to possess intrinsic hematopoietic potential that is not dependent on chorioallantoic fusion.[33,34] Mouse allantois and chorion tissues contain multilineage hematopoietic potential as shown by colony–forming unit-culture (CFU-C) assays. They express the Runx1 transcription factor, a molecule required for hematopoietic induction. The rudiments of the prospective placenta are hemogenic before the vascular continuity between the allantois and yolk sac is established, and thus are thought to generate de novo hematopoietic cells. In addition, soon after the formation of the placenta, potent hematopoietic progenitor and stem cell activity can be found at high frequency in this tissue.[38–40] It remains to be determined what percentages of these hematopoietic cells are de novo generated in the placenta and whether placental cells contribute long term to the adult hematopoietic system.

Intraembryonic Hematopoiesis: Paraaortic Splanchnopleura/Aorta-Gonad-Mesonephros

In the mid-1970s, amphibian and avian embryo culture and grafting approaches were used extensively to study

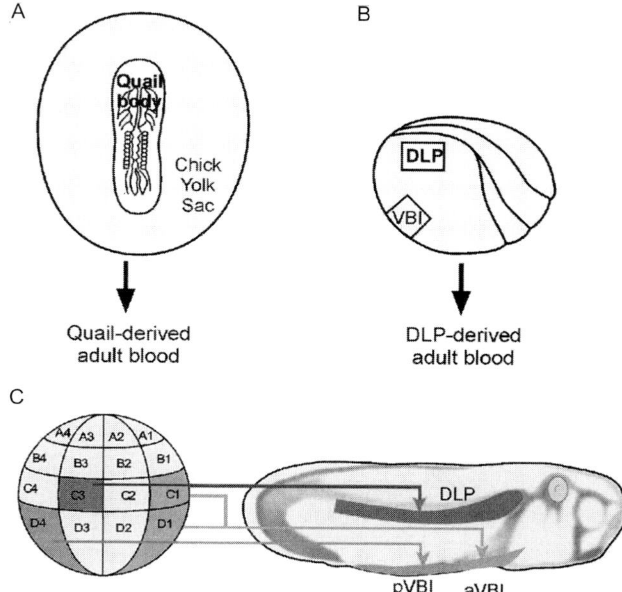

Figure 1.3. Nonmammalian vertebrate embryo–grafting experiments used for determining the origin of the adult hematopoietic system. **(A)** A schematic diagram of the avian embryo grafting strategy in which quail embryo bodies were grafted onto chick yolk sacs at the precirculation stage of development. **(B)** A schematic diagram of the amphibian embryo grafting strategy in which genetically marked dorsal lateral plate (DLP) or ventral blood island (VBI) regions were transplanted onto unmarked Xenopus or Rana embryos. **(C)** Genetic marking experiment in 32 blastomere Xenopus embryo (left). Marking of the C3 blastomere, D4 blastomere, and C1 and D1 blastomeres allowed the tracing of progeny cells to the DLP, pVBi, and aVBI, respectively, at the larval stage (right). (Drawings adapted from ref. 3.) (See color plate 1.3.)

cell fate, morphogenesis, and organogenesis. In the avian species, grafts between quail and chick embryos or between different strains of chicks were used to create chimeras in which the embryonic origins of adult blood cells were determined.[1,41] Donor-specific nucleolar or immunohistochemical markers determined whether the differentiated adult blood cells were derived from the graft or the recipient. For example, yolk sac chimeras were constructed by grafting a quail embryo body onto the extraembryonic area of a chick blastodisk (Fig. 1.3A). The combined results of many such experiments[41–44] led to the following conclusions: 1) the first emergence of hematopoietic cells is extraembryonic, in the yolk sac; 2) slightly later, hematopoietic cells emerge both extraembryonically and intraembryonically; and 3) intraembryonically derived hematopoietic cells are permanent contributors to the adult hematopoietic system. Most extraembryonically derived hematopoietic cells become extinct. Furthermore, multipotential hematopoietic progenitors as assayed in in vitro clonal cultures are associated with the dorsal aorta of avian embryos.[45] The close association of hematopoietic cell clusters and endothelial cells on the ventral aspect of the dorsal aorta[41] led to the hypothesis that hematopoietic cells are derived from endothelial cells. Indeed, when chick aortic endothelial cells are labeled in situ with lipophilic dye during prehematopoietic stages,[46,47] labeled intraaortic hematopoietic clusters are found 1 day later, thus demonstrating a precursor–progeny relationship between endothelial cells and hematopoietic clusters.[2]

Similarly, chimeric embryo studies in amphibians have demonstrated independent intraembryonic and extraembryonic mesodermally derived sites of hematopoiesis.[48–50] Using DNA content as a marker, chimeric frog embryos were generated by reciprocal grafting of the ventral blood island (VBI) region (a region analogous to avian and mammalian yolk sac) and the dorsal lateral plate (DLP) (a region analogous to the avian intraembryonic region containing the dorsal aorta) from diploid and triploid embryos (Fig. 1.3B). Again, the ventral mesodermal yolk sac analog produces the first hematopoietic cells, and slightly later, the dorsal mesodermal intrabody compartment generates adult hematopoietic cells. Unlike birds, some ventrally derived hematopoietic cells persist to adult stages and appear to contribute to red and white blood cell populations.[48,49] The specific localization of intrabody hematopoiesis has been found to be associated with the dorsal aorta and pronephros, with the most abundant hematopoiesis in the pronephros.[51] Indeed, lineage-tracing experiments in which individual blastomeres in the 32-cell stage embryo are marked show that the blastomeres contributing to the formation of the VBIs (anterior and posterior) are distinct from each other and from the blastomere that contributes to the formation of the DLP[52] (Fig. 1.3C). Moreover, in early embryos the prospective hematopoietic cells in the VBI (primitive) and DLP (adult) can be reprogrammed to an adult or primitive hematopoietic fate. The programs become fixed at a later time point and are thought to become restricted through regulatory interactions from the local environment.[53] Thus, there are three distinct origins of prospective hematopoietic cells in Xenopus that are influenced by the local microenvironment. Similarly, in the early-stage mammalian embryo, there are at least three distinct mesodermal tissue origins of hematopoietic cells, the yolk sac, intraembryonic aorta-gonad-mesonephros (AGM) region, and the chorioallantoic placenta (and possibly the vitelline and umbilical vessels) (Fig. 1.4A). The AGM region de novo produces the first adult type HSCs[54–55] (reviewed in Dzierzak[56]). This intraembryonic region contains a single central aorta surrounded by the differentiated urogenital tissue (Fig. 1.4B). At early developmental stages, the AGM is identified as the paraaortic splanchnopleura (PAS)[57]) and consists of the paired dorsal aortae and the surrounding mesenchyme adjacent to the gut endoderm.

The establishment of the vascular connection between the mouse embryo body and the extraembryonic sites at E8.25[37] precludes the identification of extra-versus intraembryonically derived hematopoietic cells. Potent hematopoietic progenitors CFU-spleen (S)[58] B lymphoid,[59] and multipotent (erythroid-myeloid-lymphoid) hematopoietic progenitors[60] have been found in the E9 PAS/AGM region. At slightly later stages of mouse embryogenesis (E10), adult-type HSCs are autonomously generated in the AGM region[54,55] and more specifically the dorsal aorta.[61]

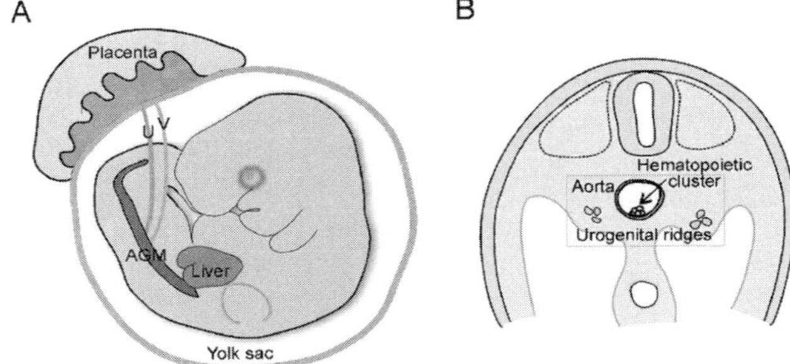

Figure 1.4. Sites of hematopoietic activity in the midgestation mouse conceptus. **(A)** A whole E10.5 mouse conceptus is shown. The placenta, AGM, yolk sac, and the vitelline (V) and umbilical (U) vessels harbor and/or generate hematopoietic cells at this time. **(B)** Transverse section through the AGM region of an E10.5 mouse embryo is shown. The dorsal aorta is located in the midline, with the neural tube on the dorsal and gut on the ventral side. The urogenital ridges laterally flank the aorta. Hematopoietic cell clusters are found in the lumen of the dorsal aorta as they emerge from the ventral hemogenic endothelium. (See color plate 1.4.)

As reported in a wide range of species,[41,52,62,63] hematopoietic foci appear as clusters adhering tightly along the ventral wall of the dorsal aorta (Fig. 1.4B). Cell surface markers, such as CD34 and CD31,[63,64] are shared between the hematopoietic cell clusters and endothelial cells. Both cell types also express the Runx1 (AML1, CBFα2) transcription factor,[65] which is required for definitive hematopoiesis[66,67] and the Sca-1 marker used for sorting adult HSCs.[68] Thus, the PAS/AGM region plays an important role as an early and potent intraembryonic site of hematopoiesis. Hemogenic potential is localized to a subset of endothelial cells lining the wall of the dorsal aorta. Interestingly, the other major vasculature (umbilical and vitelline vessels) of the mouse embryo also contain hematopoietic clusters and it is thought that potent hematopoietic cells emerge from hemogenic endothelium in the midgestation vasculature.

Secondary Hematopoietic Territories: Liver and Bone Marrow

In mammalian species, the liver serves as a temporary hematopoietic territory during fetal stages of development. The colonization theory of hematopoiesis first suggested that the hematopoietic cells generated within the extraembryonic yolk sac migrate and colonize the fetal liver and then later move to the bone marrow where they contribute to adult hematopoiesis.[69] Now included in the colonization theory of the fetal liver are the potent hematopoietic cells generated in the PAS/AGM and allantois/chorion/placenta (Fig. 1.5). Abundant evidence from coculture experiments and quantitative temporal and spatial analyses of hematopoietic progenitors/stem cells supports the currently accepted dogma that fetal liver does not de novo generate hematopoietic cells but instead is seeded with cells from these generating tissues.[3] Moreover, the demonstration that mouse embryos with a deficiency of β_1-integrin contain normal yolk sac hematopoiesis but lack fetal liver hematopoiesis provides the first genetic

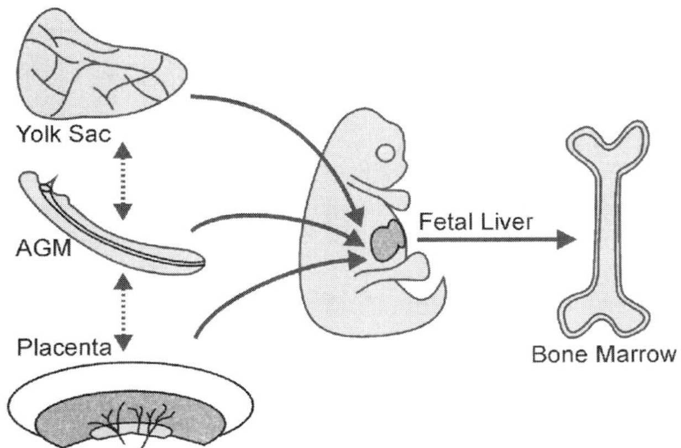

Figure 1.5. Sites of hematopoiesis and possible migration and colonization events during mouse embryonic development. It is generally accepted that migration to the fetal liver and adult bone marrow occurs, as indicated by the solid arrows. Cell migration between the embryonic tissues (yolk sac, AGM, and placenta) generating different types of hematopoietic cells is as yet undetermined (dotted arrows).

evidence that adhesion/homing molecules play a role in the colonization process.[70,71] In addition to providing a niche for harboring hematopoietic cells, the fetal liver expands and differentiates the newly emigrated cells, particularly directing differentiation toward the erythroid lineage.[72] Colonization with hematopoietic progenitors begins at late E9[73,74] and HSCs appear at E11 in the mouse fetal liver.[56,75] The liver remains a hematopoietic niche until birth when the hematopoietic cells again migrate and colonize the newly established trabecular spaces in the long bones, the so-called bone marrow. In the human fetal liver, CD34+ hematopoietic progenitors appear at 30 days of gestation and hematopoiesis continues in this tissue only until 20 weeks of gestation. At week 10, the bone trabeculae are being established and marrow hematopoiesis commences 1 week later.[19]

The Embryonic Hematopoietic Hierarchy

The complex lineage relationships of the cells within the adult mammalian hematopoietic hierarchy are well known and are based on results of in vivo and in vitro differentiation assays of bone marrow cells[76] (see Table 1.1 for assay descriptions). These assays measure the maturational progression of cells at the base and branch points of the hematopoietic system all the way through to the terminally differentiated cells of all the distinct blood lineages. The stem cells and progenitors measured by in vitro hematopoietic assays such as CFU-C, fetal thymic organ culture, stromal cocultures, CAFC and LT-CIC, and in vivo transplantation approaches for CFU-S and short-term and long-term repopulating HSCs have led to a placement of these cells within the "textbook" depiction of the hierarchy for adult hematopoiesis. Molecules expressed by distinct hematopoietic lineages and undifferentiated hematopoietic progenitor and stem cells have been instrumental

Table 1.1. Assays to detect hematopoietic cells in the mouse cconceptus

Cell type	Hematopoietic assay	Method	Lineage	Reference
Erythroid–myeloid progenitor	CFU-C	In vitro culture for 5–14 d in semisolid medium with growth factors	Erythrocytes, macrophages, granulocytes, mast	77
Erythroid–myeloid progenitor	CFU-S	In vivo transplantation into lethally irradiated adult recipients leading to macroscopic spleen colony formation at 8–16 d	Erythrocytes, macrophages, granulocytes	58
T-lymphoid progenitor	Fetal thymic organ culture/OP9-delta coculture	In vitro culture with T-depleted thymus for 9–21 d or coculture with delta producing stromal line	T lymphoid	60, 94
B-lymphoid progenitor	Stromal coculture	In vitro 14-d coculture with IL-7 and stromal cells	B lymphoid	60, 95
Multipotent progenitor	Single-cell multipotential assay	A two-step in vitro culture. Tissue explants/cells cultured on S17 or OP9 cells followed by CFU-C and B/T lymphoid assay or in vivo transplantation to immunodeficient adults	Erythroid, myeloid, B and T lymphoid	60
Neonatal repopulating HSC	Neonatal liver transplantation	In vivo transplantation directly in the liver of 1-day-old hematopoietic ablated recipients. Yields long-term, multilineage repopulation	All hematopoietic lineages	111
Adult repopulating HSC	Adult transplantation	In vivo transplantation into lethally irradiated adult recipients. Yields long-term, high-level, multilineage repopulation	All hematopoietic lineages	55, 75, 123

in assigning direct precursor–progeny relationships and prospectively isolating the cells within the adult hierarchy.

The adult hierarchy begins with the HSC and proceeds unidirectionally, with restrictive events occurring throughout hematopoietic differentiation to produce all the differentiated cells in the hematopoietic system. Although these events are represented by discrete cells in the hierarchy, it is most likely that there is a continuum of cells between these landmarks. Indeed, use of the Flt3 receptor tyrosine kinase surface marker along with many other well-studied markers has redefined the early branch points of the adult hierarchy and the subsets of cells committing to myeloid and lymphoid lineages.[77] With the description of further markers to identify additional intermediate cell subsets, it may be possible to determine all the molecular events needed for the differentiation of entire adult hematopoietic system and the transit time necessary for differentiation to the next subset.

Until recently, little was known about the embryonic hematopoietic hierarchy.[3] Although the adult hematopoietic system is usually in a state of equilibrium, the hematopoietic system of the embryo is vastly different: It must de novo generate the entire hematopoietic system, generate these cells within a short span of time in several mesodermally derived microenvironments (yolk sac, amnion/chorion/placenta, and PAS/AGM), and promote the sequential migration, colonization, and maintenance of hematopoietic cells in yet other microenvironments (liver, circulation, other) before they are finally localized in the bone marrow of the adult (Fig. 1.5). Additionally, different subsets of hematopoietic cells exist in the embryo, possess unique functions, and are not long-lived. Thus, to model the embryonic hematopoietic hierarchy cell origins, precursor–progeny relationships and lifespans of the hematopoietic cells throughout ontogeny must be established. A description of the types of terminally differentiated cells, committed progenitors, immature progenitors, and HSCs existing within the mouse conceptus, and in some cases the human conceptus, is provided here.

Erythropoiesis

Histological sectioning reveals that cells of the erythroid lineage are the earliest differentiated hematopoietic cells in the human and mouse conceptus. Primitive erythroblasts are observed in the yolk sac blood islands of the human at E16–20,[78] and mouse at E7.0/7.5.[18,79,80] In human embryos, up to 100% of all nucleated blood cells at 4–8 weeks of gestation are erythropoietic. These cells are found in the chorial and umbilical vessels, liver sinusoids, and other intraembryonic blood vessels. A switch to enucleated definitive erythropoietic cells occurs at 7–10 weeks of gestation in the blood, and slightly earlier in the fetal liver[78] (Fig. 1.6). Similarly, in the mouse, nucleated primitive erythropoietic cells predominate in the yolk sac and fetal liver until a switch

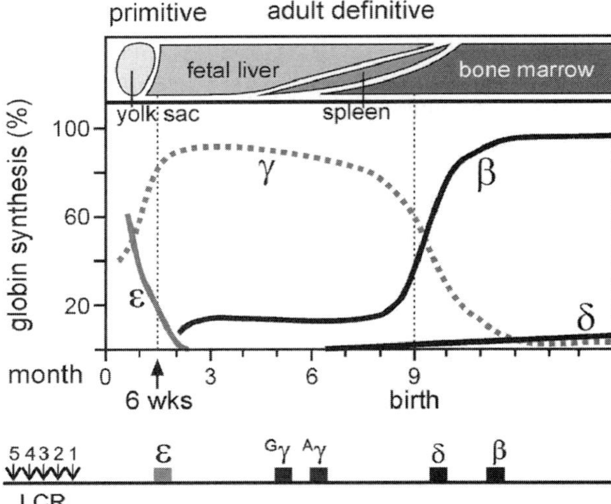

Figure 1.6. Developmental expression of the human globin genes. Sites of primitive and definitive hematopoiesis throughout development are shown. Sequential waves of ε (epsilon), γ (gamma), and β (beta) globin synthesis begin with ε-globin expression in the first month of human development, followed by γ-globin expression in the fetal stage, to just after birth when β-globin becomes the predominant hemoglobin type in definitive erythroid cells. The chromosomal organization of the genes of the human β-globin locus is in a linear arrangement that correlates with developmental expression. The arrows indicate the DNase1 hypersensitive sites of the LCR (locus control region), which is a region important for globin gene regulation.

from primitive to definitive cell types occurs between E10 and E12.[81,82]

In both species, the switch from primitive to definitive erythropoiesis is characterized by changes in the expression of the developmentally regulated fetal and adult globin genes (reviewed in refs. 83, 84 [Fig. 1.6]). Individual erythroid progenitors from ESC differentiation cultures can give rise to both fetal and adult erythroid cells[85] and single fetal liver cells can switch from a fetal to adult globin gene expression program.[86] The general populations of mature erythroid cells, however, are derived from developmentally separate stem cell populations in the embryo.[80,87] Moreover, the receptor tyrosine c-kit appears to be required for fetal liver hematopoiesis but not yolk sac erythropoiesis,[88] suggesting the origins of primitive and definitive erythroid cells from distinct and differentially regulated hematopoietic progenitor/stem cell populations. Additional molecular differences in primitive and definitive erythropoietic programs, particularly in the requirements for erythropoietic growth factors such as erythropoietin and transcription factors (GATA-1 and EKLF) are well documented.[89]

Myelopoiesis

The first cells of the monocyte–macrophage lineage appear in human conceptuses at 4–5 weeks in gestation.[78] Monocytes are routinely represented in human embryos at approximately a 1%–4% frequency in nucleated blood populations after 11 weeks of gestation. Interestingly, macrophages can be found in early human blood smears only until approximately 14 weeks of gestation. This is consistent with findings in the mouse that two separate lineages of macrophages are thought to develop in ontogeny: primitive macrophages and the monocytic lineage of macrophages.[90] In the mouse, primitive macrophages (which begin to appear at E9 in the yolk sac) are thought to arise from a local precursor and not a monocytic progenitor. These primitive macrophages proliferate and colonize other embryonic tissues. In contrast, adult macrophages do not circulate through the blood. These cells of the monocytic lineage begin to appear in the fetal liver and yolk sac at E10. Thus, the ontogeny of the monocyte–macrophage is different in the early embryo compared with its later developmental stages and it has been suggested that adult macrophages are the progeny of monocytic precursors from the AGM.[91]

Lymphopoiesis

The production of lymphoid cells begins in the human at 7–10 weeks of gestation.[78] Small lymphocytes are found in the blood: 0.2% of nucleated cells at weeks 9–10 and 14% after 14 weeks. Large lymphocytes represent 3%–5% of nucleated blood cells after 11 weeks of gestation. No lymphoid cells are found in the yolk sac, although the presence of lymphoid progenitors has not been examined. Lymphopoiesis begins in the human fetal liver, thymus, gut-associated lymphoid tissue, and lymph plexuses at approximately 7 weeks of gestation, whereas the bone lymphocytes are found only at week 12.

Extensive analyses on the development of lymphoid progenitors have been performed in the mouse. Although no functional lymphocytes are found in the mouse conceptus at early gestational stages, cells with lymphoid potential are present. E8.5 yolk sac contains T lymphoid potential when cultured in depleted fetal thymic explants.[92,93] B lymphoid potential is found in the embryo body (E9.5) and subsequently the yolk sac (E10) of the mouse conceptus by coculturing such cells in the presence of stromal cells.[94] Dissection of the PAS/AGM region has revealed the presence of an AA4.1-positive progenitor for the B1a lineage of B cells as early as E8.5.[59,60] A two-step culture system with E7.5 mouse embryo tissues has demonstrated multipotential lymphoid progenitors in the intraembryonic PAS but not in the yolk sac. Only beginning at E8.5 does the yolk sac acquire such multipotential lymphoid activity,[57] suggesting that PAS-generated multipotential lymphoid progenitors may migrate to the yolk sac after E8.5 when the intra- and extraembryonic circulation is connected. Alternatively, the yolk sac may be capable of producing such progenitors de novo but 1 day later than the PAS. At E10, multipotent B-lymphoid progenitors are found in the circulation, reach a maximum number at E12, and are undetectable in the blood at E14.[95] B-cell precursors are detected in the fetal liver at E14 and in the embryonic marrow at E15.

Interestingly, adult mouse bone marrow and fetal liver HSC–enriched populations exhibit different T- and B-lymphoid lineage potentials. In the T-lymphoid lineage, fetal liver but not bone marrow HSCs produce Vγ3 and Vγ4 T-cell receptor–positive subsets.[96] Such T cells can also be cultured from yolk sac after E8.5.[93,96] Similarly in the B-lymphoid lineage, the B1a subset of cells is produced by fetal liver,[97] yolk sac,[98] and PAS,[59] but not by adult bone marrow. It is interesting to propose that the distinct B1a–B cell subset, as well as Vγ3–4 T-cell subsets, may be the product of a special subset of developmentally regulated progenitors or HSCs in the PAS of the early embryo. It is not known whether such lymphoid subsets and progenitors exist in human embryos.

Erythroid–Myeloid Progenitors: CFU-C

The early presence of hematopoietic progenitors within the developing mouse yolk sac was established using in vitro culture approaches developed initially for measuring the hematopoietic potential of adult mammalian bone marrow. The culture of yolk sac cells in semisolid medium in the presence of colony-stimulating factors revealed the presence of erythroid and granulocyte–macrophage progenitors beginning at E7.[69,99] Burst-forming unit-E (BFU-E) and CFU-Mix are also found in the yolk sac at E8,[99] and mast cell precursors are found at E9.5.[100] At E8.25, following the first wave of primitive erythropoiesis and before the circulation is established, myeloid progenitors are detected in the yolk sac.[101] After the circulation is established myeloid progenitors are also found in the trunk region.[89] Tissue explant culture prior to CFU-C assay reveals that both the E8 yolk sac and E8 PAS contains cells with potential to become myeloid progenitors.[57] Similar cultures of precirculation allantoides[34] also revealed cells with myeloid potential. By E9 the placenta contains an abundance of myeloid progenitors.[38] Analyses of two mutant mice, *Cdh5*$^{-/-}$ and *Ncx1*$^{-/-}$, have provided strong in vivo evidence for the de novo production of definitive myeloid progenitors in the yolk sac. In *Cdh5*$^{-/-}$ conceptuses there is no vascular connection, whereas in *Ncx1*$^{-/-}$ conceptuses the vitelline vessels are intact but there is no heartbeat to promote the circulation between the yolk sac and embryo body. Similar numbers of myeloid progenitors were found in the E9.5 *Cdh5*$^{-/-}$ yolk sac compared with wild-type conceptuses, although macrophage and mixed colony–forming progenitors were decreased in number.[102,103] In *Ncx1*$^{-/-}$ conceptuses, the numbers of myeloid progenitors of all types in the yolk sac were found to be equivalent to the cumulative number of progenitors in the *Ncx1*$^{+/+}$ conceptuses in all anatomical sites.[103] No progenitors were found in the *Ncx1*$^{-/-}$ PAS, suggesting that the yolk sac normally generates all of these progenitors and distributes them to the PAS and liver. Alternatively, Ncx1-deficient conceptuses, which lack hemodynamic stress, do not produce the proper signals to induce myeloid progenitor formation in the PAS.[104] Thus, several types of definitive myeloid progenitors are generated de novo in the yolk sac and also in the chorioallantoic placenta and PAS/AGM.

In the human, yolk sac hematopoiesis covers the period from midweek 3 in gestation to week 8. BFU-Es have been found at early stages in the yolk sac but begin to decrease in frequency at week 5, when the fetal liver BFU-E frequency increases,[105] thus suggesting a colonization of the fetal liver by yolk sac progenitors. Along with erythroid progenitors, the yolk sac and embryo body have been found to contain clonogenic myeloid progenitors and erythroid–myeloid multipotent progenitors at 25–50 days into human gestation.[106,107] At the 4- to 5-week stage of gestation, a discrete population of several hundred cells bearing the cell surface phenotype of immature hematopoietic cells ($CD45^+$, $CD34^+$, $CD31^+$, and $CD38^-$) are found adhering to the ventral endothelium of the dorsal aorta.[63,107] These clusters are similar to those described in the chick and mouse. Interestingly, when these cell clusters are cocultured with bone marrow stromal cells and assayed in methylcellulose for CFU-Cs, they yield many progenitors and large multilineage hematopoietic colonies.[63]

Erythroid–Myeloid Progenitors: CFU-S

To determine whether the more immature hematopoietic progenitor compartment of the adult hierarchy is present early during embryonic development, in vivo transplantation analyses for CFU-S have been performed in irradiated mice. CFU-S are immature erythroid–myeloid progenitors that yield macroscopic colonies on the spleens of lethally irradiated mice 9–14 days following transplantation.[108,109] Beginning at E9, statistically significant numbers of CFU-S are found both in the yolk sac and PAS/AGM.[58,69] It is difficult to determine from which tissue these in vivo progenitors originate because the vascular connection between the yolk sac and embryo body is made at E8.5. The absolute numbers of CFU-S from the developing mouse embryo up to late E10 reveal that the AGM region contains more CFU-S than the yolk sac.[54,58] When an organ culture step is used before in vivo transplantation of yolk sac or AGM, the numbers of AGM CFU-S increase substantially, whereas only a slight increase in yolk sac CFU-S numbers is observed.[54] Thus, the AGM region is the more potent generator of CFU-S. CFU-S are localized to both the aorta subregion and urogenital subregion of the AGM and are also found in the vitelline and umbilical arteries.[109]

Erythroid-Myeloid-Lymphoid Multipotential Progenitors

Within the mouse embryo, these in vitro progenitors are found at E7.5 within the intrabody PAS/AGM region by a two-step culture system, 1 full day earlier than in the yolk sac.[57] Results of temporal studies suggest that preliver intrabody hematopoiesis is more complex and potent than extraembryonic yolk sac blood formation, and such PAS-generated multipotent progenitors may seed the yolk sac after the circulation is established at E8.5. The multipotential progenitors in the E8–9 PAS have also been tested in vivo for CFU-S and adult repopulating HSC activity. In vivo, these cells do not repopulate lethally irradiated adult recipient mice short term or long term after transplantation; however, they do contribute to long-term, low-level hematopoiesis following transplantation into immunocompromised adult recipients. These results suggest that they are not fully competent adult HSCs but could be candidates pre–stem cell population. Similarly, the human AGM but not the yolk sac contains multipotent progenitors beginning at day 24 in gestation. They express CD34, and $CD34^+$ hematopoietic cell clusters begin to appear on the ventral wall of the dorsal aorta at day 27. These multipotent cells could be HSCs or precursors of such cells.[19,28,110]

Neonatal Repopulating Hematopoietic Stem Cells

A more potent in vivo repopulating multilineage hematopoietic cell has been described through the use of another transplantation assay. Neonatal mice from pregnant dams treated with busulfan (for myeloablation to enhance engraftment) were injected (directly into the liver at the time of birth) with yolk sac or PAS/AGM cells. When E9 $CD34^+$c-kit^+ cells from E9 yolk sac and E9 PAS/AGM were transplanted in this manner, both were capable of multilineage engraftment and secondary engraftment into adult lethally irradiated recipient mice.[111] Neither of these sorted populations could repopulate primary adult lethally irradiated recipients nor engraft the hematopoietic system of the primary neonatal recipient to 100%. Because the yolk sac contains more neonatal repopulating cells than the PAS/AGM, these investigators suggest that the yolk sac may be the generating source. Previous studies have suggested that the early-stage yolk sac cells can indeed lead to long-term hematopoiesis when transferred into embryonic recipients, either transplacentally or into the yolk sac cavity.[112,113] These studies showed donor yolk sac–derived cells in the erythroid and lymphoid lineages, respectively, of fully developed adults. Thus, neonatal/fetal repopulating cells are long-lived multilineage progenitors that have the potential to become competent adult-type HSCs when exposed to the appropriate microenvironment.

Hematopoietic Stem Cells

At the base of the adult hematopoietic hierarchy are HSCs. They are defined by their ability to high-level, multilineage, long-term repopulate irradiated adult mouse recipients. The presence of differentiated hematopoietic cells and many restricted, multipotent and in vivo immature hematopoietic progenitors in the PAS/AGM region, yolk sac, and chorioallantoic placenta of the mouse conceptus leads to the prediction (within the context of the adult hematopoietic hierarchy) that HSCs should be present from the onset of embryonic hematopoiesis at E7.0/7.5. In mouse embryos, however, the first adult repopulating HSCs are found only beginning at E10 in the AGM region[55] and at E11 in the yolk sac[55,69,70] and placenta.[39,40] Organ explant culture before in vivo transplantation has revealed that the AGM region is the first tissue to generate autonomously HSCs.[54] The yolk sac and placenta may subsequently be seeded by AGM-generated HSCs, or alternatively, these tissues may be capable of de novo generating their own HSCs.

Direct Precursors to the Hematopoietic Lineages

Primitive erythroid cells arise from hemangioblasts, whereas the "definitive" classes of hematopoietic progenitor stem cells are thought to arise through different precursors, the so-called "hemogenic endothelium." Discrete subsets of vascular endothelial cells in the conceptus exhibit hemogenic potential.[25] Cross-species immunohistochemical studies have shown hematopoietic clusters tightly adherent to the ventral endothelium of the dorsal aorta and that of the umbilical and umbilical arteries[2] (Fig. 1.4B). The first appearance of hematopoietic clusters is in parallel to the appearance of the first definitive HSCs that can be detected. In the chick embryo, metabolic lineage tracing (AcLDL-DiI) or retroviral labeling of endothelial cells prior to hematopoietic cell appearance has confirmed the endothelial–hematopoietic lineage relationship of aortic hematopoietic clusters.[46,47] Similar marking attempts in ex utero cultured E10 mouse embryos show AcLDL-DiI$^+$ definitive erythroid cells in the circulation 12 hours after intracardiac injection and marking of aortic endothelium.[114] The phenotypic profile and spatial localization of HSCs in the AGM are also supportive of hemogenic endothelium as the direct precursor to definitive hematopoietic cells. All AGM HSCs are CD45$^+$, Ly-6A (Sca-1) GFP$^+$, c-kit$^+$CD34$^+$, Runx1$^+$, SCL$^+$, and Gata2$^+$.[68,115–119] These markers (with the exception of CD45) are also expressed by some or all endothelial cells in the ventral aspect of the dorsal aorta at E10/11. Most or all AGM HSCs express cell surface vascular endothelial cadherin,[117,120] which is typically thought of as an endothelial marker. Interestingly, not all the cells in the hematopoietic clusters express the same hematopoietic markers: Only some cells express CD41$^+$[121] or the *Ly-6A GFP* transgene,[122] indicating that some cells in the clusters take on the HSC fate whereas others are fated to be progenitors. Studies in the mouse conceptus have identified hematopoietic clusters on both the ventral and dorsal aspects of the dorsal aorta.[123] Functional studies indicate that definitive hematopoietic progenitors reside on both aspects of the aorta, but only the ventral aspect contains fully potent HSCs.[123] Thus, there appear to be subsets of hemogenic endothelium.

In contrast, some studies suggest that HSCs are derived from mesenchyme located directly underneath endothelial cells in the ventral aspect of the dorsal aorta, or in discrete patches ventral–lateral to the dorsal aorta (subaortic patches). In Runx1-haploinsufficient AGMs, HSCs are present within the Runx1-expressing mesenchymal cells underlying the ventral aspect of the dorsal aorta (as defined by the phenotype CD45$^-$, CD31$^-$, and vascular endothelial cadherin$^-$). AGM cells similarly sorted from wild-type embryos did not contain HSCs,[117] suggesting that HSCs are normally localized in the aortic endothelium. When cells from the subaortic patches (CD45$^-$ckit$^+$AA4.1$^+$) are transplanted into immunodeficient adult recipients, some long-term repopulating activity was found but the level of engraftment was low, ranging from 0.4% to 1.9%.[124] These cells are not as potent as the Runx1$^+$ or Ly-6A (Sca-1) GFP$^+$ aortic endothelial/cluster HSCs that provide up to 100% engraftment of irradiated adult recipients.[68,117] The hematopoietic cells localized in the subaortic patches may be precursors to the fully potent HSCs found in the aortic endothelial hematopoietic clusters or may represent differentiated progeny of hemogenic endothelium that have ingressed (as in the chick embryo) into this site. Together, these mouse data strongly indicate that the direct precursors of HSCs are predominantly hemogenic endothelial cells. In addition, the vascular endothelium of the human embryo has blood-forming potential.[125]

A Model of the Embryonic Hematopoietic Hierarchy

The appearance of terminally differentiated primitive erythrocytes in the mouse conceptus 3 days before the appearance of adult-type HSCs is the antithesis of the adult hematopoietic hierarchy. In the conceptus, the stepwise progressive appearance of distinct cells with increasingly complex hematopoietic potential supports a model in which the embryonic hematopoietic system is not a single-lineage differentiation hierarchy but is instead many hierarchies. It is a continuum of hematopoietic fate determining events occurring within distinct subsets of presumptive hemogenic mesoderm that specify a variety of temporally and spatially separate precursor cells – hemangioblasts and hemogenic endothelium (Fig. 1.7). Dependent on developmental time and position within the extra- and intraembryonic tissues (yolk sac, placenta, and AGM), cells emerge with different hematopoietic potentials. Thus, the embryonic hematopoietic hierarchy is modeled on the appearance of functionally different cells without indications for lineage relationships. Although it is clear that "hemangioblasts" and hemogenic endothelium play roles, further results are necessary to determine whether the wide range of hematopoietic activities in the conceptus are achieved directly through hematopoietic fate

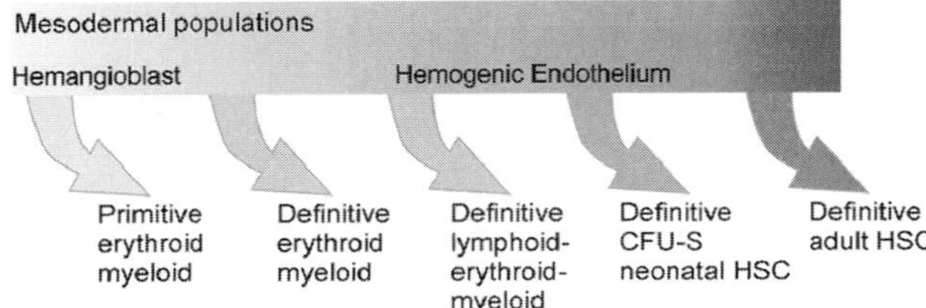

Figure 1.7. The early embryonic/developmental hematopoietic hierarchy is unlike that of the adult. The temporal appearance of hematopoietic cells in the mouse conceptus suggests that many of these cells do not arise from an HSC but instead they arise directly from mesodermal populations that go through a hemangioblast and/or hemogenic endothelial intermediate. Thereafter, hematopoietic fate is acquired and hematopoietic cells are generated. The sequential appearance of primitive erythroid–myeloid cells, followed by increasingly more complex definitive hematopoietic cells and finally the appearance of definitive HSCs is contrary to adult hematopoietic differentiation hierarchy with the expected precursor–progeny relationships. Instead, the hematopoietic system in the embryo is generated at least five independent times in different mesodermal populations.

determination events in a variety of nonhematopoietic precursors (hemangioblasts and different subsets of hemogenic endothelium) or through the acquisition of more complex hematopoietic activities imposed by the microenvironment after hematopoietic fate determination of a small cohort of similarly active cells. In the human conceptus, the sequential appearance of differentiated and more complex hematopoietic progenitors is consistent with what has been observed in the mouse conceptus.[106,107] Moreover, the distribution of these hematopoietic cells occurs similarly in the yolk sac, AGM, liver, spleen, and bone marrow (the hematopoietic activity of the placenta is predicted but is as yet uncertain (Fig. 1.8).

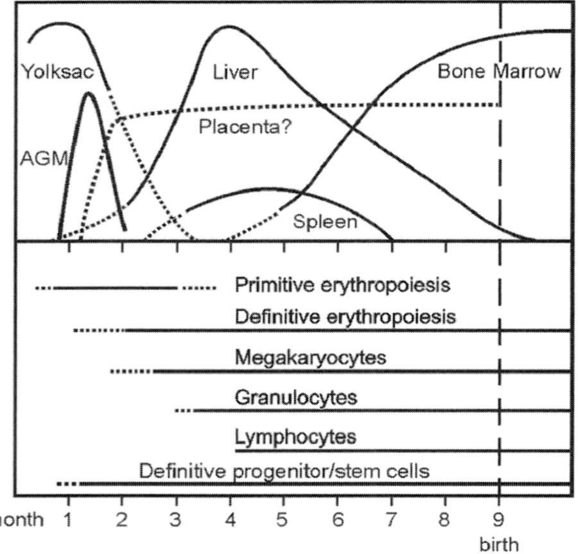

Figure 1.8. The sites of hematopoietic activity and the temporal appearance of the distinct hematopoietic lineages in the human embryo. There is a general correspondence of the hematopoietic sites and the temporal appearance of hematopoietic cells between the human and the mouse embryo. (Figure adapted from ref. 196.)

Hematopoietic Colonization and Migration During Development

Until 1965 it was thought that the hematopoietic populations found in adult vertebrates were intrinsically generated in tissues such as the liver, spleen, bone marrow, thymus, and bursa of Fabricius (only found in avian species). A paradigm shift occurred when it was shown that hematopoietic cells generated in earlier embryonic tissues colonized these secondary hematopoietic tissues. The generating sources of the hematopoietic cells are likely to be one or more of these tissues: the yolk sac, PAS/AGM, and chorioallantoic placenta. In this section a summary of the findings demonstrating the migration of hematopoietic cells during development is provided.

Avian

The results of experiments by Moore and Owen,[126] in which parabiosed chick embryos were examined, suggested that the thymus, spleen, bursa of Fabricius, and bone marrow were colonized by blood-borne cells. Definitive proof that the hematopoietic cells in adult tissues are extrinsically derived comes from the quail–chick and chick–chick embryo grafting experiments. Initial experiments focused on the colonization of the grafted thymus and spleen rudiments with embryonic hematopoietic precursors.[41,44] Each tissue rudiment provided the stroma or microenvironment for the seeding and differentiation of extrinsic precursors. Interestingly, it was found that several short periodic waves of lymphoid precursors enter the thymus, whereas a single long wave of precursors enter and colonize the bursa.[127] These studies showed that the tissue rudiments exhibited limited times of receptivity for emigrating hematopoietic cells and suggested the emergence of progenitors at several discrete developmental times.

Similarly, the ontogeny of the multilineage hematopoietic system was examined in embryo grafting experiments in which yolk sac chimeras were made (reviewed in ref. 1 and references therein) (Fig. 1.3A). The sites of de novo hematopoietic cell emergence were determined to be the yolk sac and the intraembryonic region containing the dorsal aorta. Only very briefly in early stages of embryogenesis do yolk sac–born erythrocytes predominate in the blood. Subsequently, intrabody-born erythrocytes rapidly predominate and red cells from the yolk sac disappear completely by the hatching stage. At least two generations of hemoglobin-producing cells were observed: the first from yolk sac–derived cells and the second from yolk sac– and intrabody-derived cells. During embryonic stages a small number of intrabody-derived cells can be found in the yolk sac and likewise, a small number of yolk sac–derived macrophage-like (microglial) cells can be found intraembryonically in the eye and in the brain. These cellular exchanges are thought to occur through the circulation of small populations or subsets of hematopoietic cells that may serve a specialized, short-lived function. In the adult, the originating source of adult blood was confirmed to be the intrabody region. When the prevascularized quail allantoic bud was grafted in the coelom of a chick host, cells of both the hematopoietic and endothelial lineages were found in the bone marrow of the host.[36] Thus, the bone marrow is seeded by hematopoietic and endothelial precursors that arise in situ in the allantois. Hence, the allantois- as well as the paraaortic-derived cells of the avian embryo migrate and seed the adult blood system.

Amphibians

Waves of colonization are also observed in the amphibian model system. Embryo grafting experiments show that the larval liver is colonized by intrabody-derived hematopoietic cells.[128] The liver is thought to be seeded by intrabody cells that migrate through the interstitium because intrabody cells are not found in the circulation. Interstitial migration of cells is an efficient means of cell distribution within the amphibian embryo body and has been found to occur even before the completion of the vascular network.[50] Support for interstitial migration has been provided recently in the zebrafish. $CD41^+$ hematopoietic cells in the interstitium enter the circulation by intravasation via the posterior cardinal veins.[129] In later stages of amphibian development, near the time of metamorphosis, intrabody-derived hematopoietic clones fluctuate in their contribution to the liver and some ventral blood island–derived clones are detected[128,130] but do not become the predominant cell type.

Mammals

In contrast to the ease of in vitro culture and manipulation of amphibian and avian embryos for the analysis of hematopoietic cell migration and colonization, the in utero inaccessibility of the mouse conceptus necessitates the use of other approaches for these studies. Some of the first experiments probing hematopoietic migration and colonization involved culturing whole E7 mouse embryo bodies in the presence or absence of the yolk sac.[69] After 2 days, tissues were dissected and analyzed for granulocyte–macrophage colony formation. Only embryo bodies that retained their yolk sac were able to give rise to hematopoietic cells, suggesting that the yolk sac is the only embryonic site producing hematopoietic cells that colonize the liver rudiment. This experiment, as well as those examining the kinetics of CFC production in the yolk sac and fetal liver, suggests a dependence of early fetal hepatic hematopoiesis on an influx of exogenous yolk sac–derived cells.[69,80,99] Other researchers have demonstrated that at late E9 fetal liver is populated by yolk sac–derived erythroid cells when these tissues are cultured adjacent to each other.[131] Recently, studies in mouse conceptuses deficient for *Cdh5* and *Ncx1* genes suggest migration of yolk sac–derived myeloid progenitors to the embryo body.[102,103] In the absence of a vascular connection or heartbeat to promote the circulation, myeloid progenitors of all types were found in the yolk sac but not the embryo body. This suggests that the yolk sac normally generates all of these myeloid progenitors and distributes them to the PAS/AGM and liver. It is possible, however, that the PAS/AGM requires the normal stimulus of hemodynamic stress present in the wild-type conditions to generate these progenitors. Moreover, these experiments are limited to analysis of only very early tissues, and thus cannot take into account the multiple waves of hematopoietic cell generation and migration seen in the nonvertebrate species, particularly those that give rise to the adult hematopoietic system.

Spatial and temporal quantitative analyses for CFU-C, CFU-S, and HSCs in the mouse conceptus provide strong support for migration of AGM, yolk sac, and placental-derived cells to the fetal liver.[39,54,58,75] Data on B lymphopoiesis in the mouse conceptus suggest migration of these cells to the fetal liver through the circulation.[95] The spleen and thymus are seeded either directly from the generating tissues or from the fetal liver.[132,133] As found in avian embryos, the early classes of mouse hematopoietic cells (those defined by hematopoietic activity less potent than an HSC's and with limited life span) may provide maturation signals to the rudiments of the secondary hematopoietic territories in the mouse to promote their growth and receptivity for the later generated HSCs.[134,135]

There is convincing evidence that integrins play an important role in the embryo in the colonization of secondary hematopoietic territories. Mouse embryos lacking β_1-integrin die during preimplantation stages of gestation.[70] Chimeric embryos with β_1-integrin$^{-/-}$ ESCs were generated to examine its role during later stages of hematopoietic ontogeny.[71] Although the yolk sac was found to contain normal numbers of hematopoietic cells derived from the β_1-integrin$^{-/-}$ ESCs, the fetal liver did not contain any β_1-integrin–deficient hematopoietic cells. The clonogenic potential of the yolk sac hematopoietic cells was normal, and such cells were found in the circulation of embryos until E15. These results strongly suggest that β_1-integrin is required for the successful migration of hematopoietic cells to the fetal liver. Additionally, and in accordance with a role for β_1-integrin in adult hematopoietic cell migration, no β_1-integrin–deficient hematopoietic cells were found in the thymus, bone marrow, or blood of adult chimeric mice.

To trace the lineage of cells in the mouse conceptus that give rise to the permanent hematopoietic system in the adult, molecular marking using the Cre-lox recombination system[136] has been attempted. This in vivo marking technology is based on the expression of a marker transgene (*Rosa 26* locus inserted fluorescent or enzymatic gene) that is activated through the excision of a stop sequence positioned between two lox recombination sites. Cre recombinase performs the recombination event in specific cells depending on transcriptional regulatory elements driving its expression and the activity of Cre recombinase (Cre-ERT), which can be controlled in a temporal manner by administration of tamoxifen. Thus, hematopoietic cells can be marked within a specific window of developmental time and the progeny of these marked cells can be followed through later fetal and adult stages. When the SCL (expressed in endothelial cells and definitive HSCs[118]) and Runx1 (expressed in all definitive hematopoietic cells, hemogenic endothelium, and some mesenchymal cells[117]) regulatory elements were used to direct Cre-ERT expression and early and midgestation mouse conceptuses were exposed to tamoxifen, approximately 10% of the bone marrow cells in the adult expressed the marker.[137,138] These results indicate that the progeny of SCL- and Runx1-expressing cells in the mouse conceptus migrate to the adult bone marrow and contribute to adult hematopoiesis. Thus, the progeny of hematopoietic cells generated in the embryo (tissue origin as yet unknown) migrate to the bone marrow where they reside and contribute to hematopoiesis through adult life.

Molecular Aspects of Embryonic (Primitive) and Adult (Definitive) Hematopoiesis

Molecular interactions regulate the generation of the hematopoietic system. Some of these interactions include developmental signaling pathways, transcription factors, and chromatin remodeling factors. Induction events are orchestrated by the signaling pathways that "turn on or off" transcription factors that regulate the expression of specific panels of genes (genetic programs) associated with hematopoietic fate and function. Moreover, the genetic programs are controlled by a limited number of epigenetic regulators (chromatin modifiers) that confer a "cell-specific molecular memory" and thus maintain the hematopoietic fate of the cell. The microenvironments in the mouse conceptus where hematopoietic cells are generated (yolk sac, PAS/AGM, and chorioallantoic placenta) differ from each other and from the secondary hematopoietic territories (fetal liver and adult bone marrow) that promote maintenance, self-renewal, and/or differentiation of hematopoietic progenitor and stem cells. Thus, beginning with the cell extrinsic influences of morphogens and factors emanating from the surrounding cellular environment, developmental signaling pathways are triggered and activate distinct but overlapping genetic (and epigenetic) programs to direct hematopoietic development in the mouse conceptus.

Our understanding of the molecular programming of the hematopoietic system throughout ontogeny has been profoundly influenced by the use of gene-targeting technologies in mouse ESCs.[139] The ability to generate mice with mutations in any chosen gene has resulted in the identification of numerous signaling pathways, transcription factors and epigenetic regulators that are critical for the development of the hematopoietic system. The most striking hematopoietic defects found are genetic mutations that affect both primitive and definitive hematopoiesis and mutations that profoundly affect definitive but not primitive hematopoiesis. Because the deletion of some hematopoietic genes results in anemia and early embryonic lethality, study of the affects of such genes at the later developmental stages is facilitated by chimeric mouse generation with homozygous mutant ESCs and also conditional gene targeting strategies.

Functional differences in the cells that make up the primitive (embryonic) and definitive (adult) hematopoietic systems predicted differences in molecular programming through development. Prime examples include the developmental regulation of the globin genes (α and β)[83] in primitive and definitive erythroid cells and the T- and B-cell receptor genes ($V\gamma3$-$V\gamma4$ and B1a, respectively) in fetal lymphoid cells.[96,97] These programs are regulated at the level of the HSC and thus suggest distinct developmental subsets of HSCs (dependent on the stem cell source and/or local microenvironment). Genes involved in hematopoietic specification also may be developmentally regulated in mesodermal cells as they emerge from the primitive streak and move to the extraembryonic yolk sac (ventral mesoderm) and intraembryonic PAS/AGM (lateral mesoderm). Thus, the genetic programs leading to hematopoietic specification overlap to a large degree but also possess unique features related to hematopoietic potential, function, site, and life span.

This section and Table 1.2 summarize some of the signaling pathways, transcription factors, and epigenetic factors that most affect the development of the embryonic and adult hematopoietic systems.

Signaling Pathways

Hematopoietic specification occurs shortly following the onset of mesoderm formation. The effects of various factors of the TGFβ_1 superfamily and FGF family of genes in mesoderm and blood formation[13,140] have been revealed in the Xenopus embryo model. The TGFβ_1 superfamily member, BMP-4, acts as a ventralizing molecule within the mesoderm (the region known to form hematopoietic cells). BMP-4 also induces the expression of *Mix.1*, a gene that has been shown to induce hematopoiesis in the Xenopus animal cap assay.[53,141] Interestingly, the three blood compartments (aVBI, pVBI, and DLP) are specified from mesoderm that encounters different concentrations of BMP-4[142] and the timing of expression of pivotal hematopoietic transcription factors (SCL, LMO2, and Runx1) is controlled by FGF.[143]

Similar to the interactions between endoderm and prospective hematopoietic mesoderm in Xenopus, such interactions are also necessary for hemogenic induction in the chick embryo. Blood island generation occurs only when the mesothelial and endoderm germ layers are cultured together – when cultured separately no primitive erythroblasts form.[20,21,144] Somitic mesoderm, which normally only contributes to endothelium in the dorsal aspect of

Table 1.2. Molecules involved in early mouse hematopoietic development

Class	Gene	Phenotype	Reference
Developmental growth factor/signaling pathway	TGFβ$_1$	Lethal at E9.5–11.5, defects in hematopoiesis and vascular network formation	149
	BMP-4	Lethal at gastrula stage, no mesodermal differentiation. Later embryonic lethal, decreased yolk sac (YS) mesoderm formation and decreased erythropoiesis. Expressed in cells underlying aortic hematopoietic clusters	122, 148, 152
	Flk-1/VEGF	Lethal at E8.5–9.5, defective in YS blood island and vessel formation, severe decrease in YS progenitor cell number and no definitive hematopoiesis	27, 154, 155
	Notch1	Conceptuses die at E10, almost normal numbers of YS primitive erythroid and erythroid–myeloid progenitors, but no AGM hematopoiesis or HSCs. Notch1 and Delta-like 4, and Jagged 1 and 2 expressed in aortic endothelium	157, 158
	c-kit/SF	Severe mutants lethal at E16, deficiencies in hematopoietic cells, CFU-S, primordial germ cells and melanocytes	88, 161, 162
Transcription factor	SCL	Lethal at E9.5, deficient in primitive and definitive hematopoiesis and defective in angiogenesis	165, 169
	GATA-2	Lethal at E10.5, severe FL anemia. Relatively normal YS hematopoiesis but decreased CFU-C. No AGM HSCs or aortic clusters	115, 116, 178
	Runx1	Lethal at E12, complete absence of definitive progenitors and HSCs and aortic clusters. Primitive hematopoiesis relatively normal	65, 66, 67, 117, 181
Epigenetic factor	Mel-18,	Enhanced HSC self-renewal	190
	Mph1/Rae28	Embryonic lethal due to insufficient hematopoiesis	191
	Bmi-1	Self-renewal defect in FL HSCs	192
	Mll	Complete lack of definitive hematopoiesis in the conceptus and early embryonic lethality	195

the dorsal aorta and not to the ventral endothelium or hematopoietic clusters, can be reprogrammed to assume the latter fates following transient exposure to endoderm prior to grafting.[21] Several signaling molecules, including vascular endothelial growth factor (VEGF), basic (b)FGF, and TGFβ$_1$ could substitute for this endodermal signal[21] and the overexpression of BMP-4 has been found to influence mesodermal subtype formation.[145] Thus, graded expression patterns of factors specify unique subsets of mesoderm including the presumptive hematopoietic mesoderm.[14]

Studies in the mouse conceptus also show that contact with visceral endoderm is necessary for primitive hematopoiesis in yolk sac explants. Exposure of prospective neurectoderm to endoderm or heparin–acrylic beads soaked in Indian Hedgehog (Ihh) could respecify this normally nonhematopoietic tissue to hematopoietic fate.[22,23] Ihh is normally produced by the visceral endoderm, and this expression pattern, together with the explant data, suggests that Ihh signaling is essential for primitive erythropoiesis. Ihh signaling is essential for hematopoiesis in the zebra fish equivalent of the AGM and is at the beginning of a signaling cascade for blood cell formation in the dorsal aorta that includes the downstream effectors VEGF, Notch, GATA-2, and Runx1.[146] Although deletion of Ihh or its receptor Smoothened (Smo) in mice does not eliminate primitive erythropoiesis in the yolk sac, it does profoundly affect yolk sac vascularization[147] and may also affect the AGM region.

In the mouse VEGF/Flk-1, FGF, and TGFβ$_1$ (and family members) are generally thought of as ventralizing factors. ESC differentiation cultures and gene-targeting studies reveal a role for the VEGF/Flk-1 and TGFβ$_1$ signaling axes in vasculogenesis and hematopoiesis.[27,148] In the TGFβ$_1$ homozygous null condition, perinatal lethality occurs in 50% of the embryos between E9.5 and E11.5.[149] The initial differentiation of endothelial cells from mesoderm occurs, but there is no organization of these cells into a vascular network. Defects in yolk sac vasculogenesis and hematopoiesis appear to be responsible for embryonic death, although the severity of the endothelial and hematopoietic cell defects do not always correlate. TGFβ$_1$ signaling in the hematopoietic system suggests complex effects (indirect and/or redundant), because it is a member of the large TGFβ_1 superfamily that interacts through an array of receptors and intracellular Smad proteins.[150]

Another TGFβ_1 family member, BMP-4, plays a role in early stages of mouse hematopoiesis. It induces the in vitro hematopoietic differentiation of ESCs.[151] Gene targeting supports a role for BMP-4 in specification of hematopoietic mesoderm. Mouse embryos deficient for BMP-4 usually die at the time of gastrulation with little or no mesodermal differentiation.[148] The few BMP-4–deficient embryos that do survive to slightly later ontogenic stages show profound decreases in mesoderm formation and erythropoiesis in the yolk sac, indicating a strict requirement for BMP-4 in the formation of the ventral-most mesoderm. BMP-4 can influence hematopoietic cell formation from the presumptive anterior head fold, normally a nonhematopoietic portion of the mouse epiblast.[17] When added to AGM explant cultures, BMP-4 increases the number of HSCs.[122] Interestingly, BMP-4 is localized in the mesenchyme underlying aortic clusters in the mouse[122] and human[152] embryo and thus appears to be an important effector in hematopoietic specification and growth. It controls the expression of some pivotal hematopoietic transcription factors such as SCL and GATA-1 (reviewed in ref. 153).

Mouse embryos deficient in the VEGF/Flk-1 signaling axis exhibit more severe and consistent defects than TGFβ_1-deficient embryos. All Flk-1–deficient embryos die between E8.5 and E9.5.[27] They are defective in the production of yolk sac blood islands and vessel formation, and the numbers of hematopoietic progenitors are dramatically reduced. A *LacZ* marker gene inserted in the *Flk-1* gene allowed tracking of endothelial and hematopoietic cell formation in embryos. Those embryos lacking functional Flk-1 expressed the *LacZ* marker appropriately in the developing mesoderm. However, these expressing cells accumulated in the amnion instead of the areas of blood island formation, suggesting the requirement for Flk-1 as early as the formation and/or migration of the yolk sac mesodermal cells. The gene for VEGF, the ligand of Flk-1, has also been mutated. The generation of chimeric embryos with VEGF $^{+/-}$ ESCs results in embryonic lethality at E11, defective vasculogenesis, and a substantially reduced number of yolk sac red blood cells.[154,155] VEGF can direct the in vitro differentiation of ESCs to both endothelial and hematopoietic lineages.[156] Flk-1 is expressed by presumptive hemangioblasts, as shown by ESC studies and analyses of early-stage mouse conceptuses in the posterior region of the primitive streak.[30,31,156]

Although gene targeting of all these signaling molecules results in defects in both primitive and definitive hematopoiesis, Notch1 signaling in the mouse conceptus has been found to be selectively important for AGM (adult definitive) but not yolk sac (primitive) hematopoiesis. Notch1-deficient mouse conceptuses die at E10 and contain almost normal numbers of yolk sac primitive erythroid and erythroid–myeloid progenitors, but have no AGM hematopoiesis or HSCs.[157] Notch1, Notch4, and their ligands Delta-like 4, Jagged 1, and Jagged 2 are expressed in endothelial cells lining the dorsal aorta.[158] Mutations that affect Notch signaling in zebra fish eliminate Runx1 expression and hematopoietic cluster formation in the AGM.[146,159] Overexpression of Runx1 in Notch signaling mutants in both zebrafish and mice restores AGM hematopoiesis.[159,160] Thus, Notch1 appears to be a unique and pivotal factor in the onset of AGM definitive hematopoiesis.

c-kit is a receptor tyrosine kinase closely related to Flk-1. Many natural mutations for c-kit, and its ligand, steel factor (SF), have been found in mice. W and Sl strains of mice, respectively, mutant for these genes,[161,162] exhibit deficiencies in hematopoiesis, primordial germ cells, and melanocytes. The most severe mutations result in embryonic lethality beginning at E16. Yolk sac primitive erythropoiesis is not affected, but definitive CFU-S progenitors and mast cells are absent. SF has been shown to act as a proliferative[88,163] or antiapoptotic[164] agent in hematopoietic progenitors and CFU-S. Thus, c-kit/SF signaling is required for normal definitive hematopoiesis and may play a role in clonogenicity of early hematopoietic progenitors or, as in primordial germ cells and melanocytes, play a role in definitive hematopoietic progenitor migration.

Transcription Factors

The SCL transcription factor (basic helix-loop-helix family) is known to play a pivotal role in the production of all hematopoietic cells in the embryo as shown by gene targeting in the mouse.[165–169] SCL$^{-/-}$ mouse conceptuses die at E9.0 of a complete absence of blood formation. Unlike TGFβ_1 and Flk-1, SCL is not required for all endothelial cell and vascular formation; yolk sac capillaries are initiated. Vitelline vessel formation, however, is blocked and subsequent angiogenesis in the yolk sac is defective. A transgenic rescue of the hematopoietic defects in SCL$^{-/-}$ embryos confirms that SCL is necessary for embryonic angiogenesis.[169] Interestingly, ectopic injection of RNA encoding the SCL hematopoietic transcription factor specifies normally nonhematopoietic pronephric mesoderm to become hematopoietic.[170] The graded expression of this hematopoietic transcription factor may initiate the normal spatial borders of hematopoiesis in the different mesodermally derived regions of the embryo. Differentiation studies using SCL$^{-/-}$ ESCs indicate that this factor is essential for hematopoietic differentiation and vascular remodeling, playing a role in the hematopoietic commitment of the hemangioblast.[171] Similarly gene-targeted deletion of the *LMO2* gene results in a phenotype identical to that of SCL$^{-/-}$ embryos.[172,173] It has been found that the LMO2 protein heterodimerizes with the SCL protein forming a transcriptional regulatory complex.[174,175]

GATA-2 is a member of GATA (DNA-binding motif) transcription factor family of genes. The GATA factors are highly conserved among all vertebrate species. Along with GATA-1 and GATA-3, studies in mammalian cell lines have shown that GATA-2 plays a role in transcriptional regulation within the hematopoietic system.[176,177] Specifically, GATA-2 is thought to act in HSCs and progenitors, due to its specific expression pattern. Mice lacking the transcription factor GATA-2 suffer from slightly reduced primitive erythropoiesis and a complete lack of other committed progenitors and HSCs and die at E10.5.[178] GATA-2 is expressed in the aortic endothelium[116] and is thought to affect the expansion of the hemogenic population emerging from these cells.[115] Interestingly, GATA-2 haploinsufficiency profoundly decreases the number of AGM HSCs, but yolk sac HSCs are only slightly affected. The tissue differences suggest a developmental timing component in the requirement of HSCs for GATA-2, different tissue-specific interacting partners for GATA-2, and/or different downstream targets. Nonetheless, GATA-2 is strictly required for adult (definitive) hematopoiesis and is expendable for embryonic (primitive) erythropoiesis. GATA-2 is thought to work together with SCL and the Ets transcription factor Fli-1 in recursive gene regulatory circuit in early mouse hematopoietic development.[179,180]

The *CBF* transcription factor genes are the most frequent targets of chromosomal rearrangements in human leukemias and were thus suggested to function in the hematopoietic system. Runx1 (also called CBFα2 and AML-1) and CBFβ_1 form a heterodimeric factor that interacts through Runx1 DNA-binding domain to bind the core enhancer motif present in a number of hematopoietic-specific genes. Targeted mutagenesis revealed that *Runx1* and *CBFβ_1* genes[66,67,181] are required for definitive but not primitive hematopoiesis – embryos present with a complete lack of definitive hematopoietic progenitors and HSCs, fetal liver anemia, and embryonic lethality occurring after E11.5.[66,67,182] Yolk sac vessels and primitive erythropoiesis appear normal in these embryos. *Runx1* appears to act at the level of proliferation, generation, or maintenance of definitive hematopoietic progenitor and/or stem cells. Insertion of a *LacZ* maker gene into the *Runx1* locus[65] shows Runx1 expression ventrally in the mesenchyme, endothelium, and hematopoietic clusters of the dorsal aorta,[65,117] confirming a role in the establishment of the first adult-type HSCs.

Haploinsufficiency of *Runx1* leads to an early increase in AGM HSCs when these are directly isolated from the embryo and transplanted into irradiated adult mice.[65,117,182,183] When hematopoietic tissues of *Runx1*$^{+/-}$ conceptuses are first cultured as explants and then transplanted, they display interesting differential responses to *Runx1* haploinsufficiency. HSCs were profoundly decreased in AGM explants but were increased in both yolk sac and placenta, suggesting that different regulatory networks, downstream targets, interacting molecules, or altered developmental timing are operative in these tissues.[183] The Ets family transcription factor, PU.1, which is required for definitive hematopoiesis, is a critical downstream target of Runx1.[184] Also, studies have shown that the hematopoietic cytokine gene *IL-3* is a target of Runx1 and that IL-3 affects AGM HSC numbers.[183] As a pivotal factor in HSC ontogeny, transcriptional regulation of Runx1 requires the recruitment of a SCL/LMO2/Ldb-1 complex to its intronic enhancer sequence. This enhancer targets all definitive HSCs in the mouse embryo, suggesting that it integrates the other major hematopoietic transcriptional networks to initiate HSC generation.[179]

Thus, an understanding of how the master regulators are controlled and fine-tuned with respect to their levels in different hematopoietic subpopulations and sites will provide insight into the genetic network that governs hematopoietic emergence in the conceptus. By analogy to the ESC program,[185] it may be possible to establish hematopoietic identity in nonhematopoietic cells with just a small set of factors (Runx1, GATA, Ets, and SCL).

Epigenetic Factors

Lineage-specific gene expression programs are not only controlled at the level of transcription factor recruitment, but are coordinated and maintained in an active or repressed state of expression through the involvement of chromatin modifiers.[186] Cellular memory enables cells to maintain a specific lineage fate over many cell divisions and involves epigenetic modifications that include DNA methylation and histone acetylation. Groups of proteins called the polycomb group (PcG) and trithorax group (trxG) proteins, recruit histone deacetylases and methyltransferases and are well conserved in evolution in many different species. PcG proteins are transcriptional repressors and trxG proteins are transcriptional activators during development. These proteins associate with chromatin at specific loci but their core proteins do not bind DNA. The importance of PcG protein in development was recognized through their role in maintaining a silent state of *Hox* gene expression.[187] *Hox* genes are known to be important in the hematopoietic system. When *Hox* genes are overexpressed in HSCs, they proliferate extensively, increasing their pool size.[188] Although PcG proteins are involved in many loci in a variety of stem cells, most studies investigating the role of PcG and trxG proteins in HSCs focus on fetal liver and adult bone marrow–derived HSCs.

The PcG protein Ezh2 is found in a complex with histone deacetylases. Ezh2, together with Eed protein, also binds DNA methyltransferases.[187] These complexes are thought to be involved in the initiation of gene repression and act functionally to preserve HSC quality and prevent HSC exhaustion after trauma.[189] Several other PcG proteins affecting HSC self-renewal are thought to maintain gene repression. These include Mel-18, Mph1/Rae28, and Bmi-1.[190–192] Homozygous deficiency of Mel-18 leads to enhanced HSC self-renewal; Mph1/Rae28 deficiency is embryonic lethal due to insufficient hematopoiesis during development; and Bmi1-deficient fetal liver HSCs are impaired in self-renewal.

An example of a trxG protein involved in hematopoiesis is the *Mll* gene. MLL1 is a histone methyltransferase.[193,194] It is misexpressed following chromosomal translocation in acute leukemias. Moreover, gene targeting of *Mll1* in the mouse results in a complete lack of definitive hematopoiesis in the conceptus and early embryonic lethality.[195] Thus, the control of HSC self-renewal by PcG and trxG proteins supports a role for epigenetic modifications in the homeostasis of the hematopoietic system as it is initiated in the mouse conceptus, and such mechanisms most likely play a role in the initiation and maintenance of some leukemias.

IMPLICATIONS OF EMBRYONIC HEMATOPOIESIS FOR POTENTIAL CLINICAL APPLICATION IN HUMAN BLOOD-RELATED THERAPIES

Significant progress continues to be made in the field of developmental hematopoiesis. The previous dogma concerning the origins of the adult mammalian hematopoietic system in the yolk sac has given way to a new understanding of multiple and independent sites of hematopoietic generation in the early- and midgestation conceptus. The initiation of the first multipotential hematopoietic progenitors and adult-type HSCs is now known to occur in the intraembryonic PAS/AGM. The placenta has been shown to be a potent generator of hematopoietic cells, and perhaps other yet untested embryonic tissues may also possess hematopoietic potential. The molecular programming within the variety of hematopoietic cells and embryonic compartments begins to reveal differences in developmental levels and timing of expression of pivotal hematopoietic transcription factors and the heritable genetic program that defines specific hematopoietic fate. The in vitro production of hematopoietic cells from factor-directed ESC differentiation cultures is improving due to knowledge obtained from results of molecular and cellular studies on the normal in vivo embryonic development of hematopoietic cells. Together with the long-anticipated direct precursor to hematopoietic cells, the hemangioblast, the rapid acceptance of hemogenic endothelium as the predominant precursor to definitive adult hematopoietic cells suggests a new strategy for hematopoietic cell production – one that would involve the isolation, expansion, and induction of hemogenic endothelium, perhaps from adult vasculature, to establish HSC fate. Through further knowledge of the cells and molecules that lead to the normal generation of the adult hematopoietic system, we can continue to improve medical strategies for the treatment of blood-related genetic diseases and leukemia.

ACKNOWLEDGMENTS

The author thanks laboratory members (past and present) and researchers in the field for insightful discussions leading to this chapter. The research in my laboratory is supported by the Netherlands Medical Sciences Research Organization (VICI 916-36-601), the Netherlands Innovative Research Program (BSIK SCDD 03038), and the National Institutes of Health (R37 DK54077).

REFERENCES

1. Dieterlen-Lievre F, Le Douarin NM. Developmental rules in the hematopoietic and immune systems of birds: how general are they? *Seminars in Developmental Biology* 1993;4(6): 325–32.
2. Jaffredo T, Nottingham W, Liddiard K, Bollerot K, Pouget C, de Bruijn M. From hemangioblast to hematopoietic stem cell: an endothelial connection? *Exp Hematol* 2005;33(9):1029–40.
3. Dzierzak E, Speck NA. Of lineage and legacy: the development of mammalian hematopoietic stem cells. *Nat Immunol* 2008;9(2):129–36.
4. McKenzie JL, Gan OI, Doedens M, Wang JC, Dick JE. Individual stem cells with highly variable proliferation and self-renewal properties comprise the human hematopoietic stem cell compartment. *Nat Immunol* 2006;7(11):1225–33.
5. Park C, Lugus JJ, Choi K. Stepwise commitment from embryonic stem to hematopoietic and endothelial cells. *Curr Top Dev Biol* 2005;66:1–36.
6. Zambidis ET, Peault B, Park TS, Bunz F, Civin CI. Hematopoietic differentiation of human embryonic stem cells progresses through sequential hematoendothelial, primitive, and definitive stages resembling human yolk sac development. *Blood* 2005;106(3):860–70.
7. Miale J. Laboratory medicine Hematology. Sixth edition ed. St. Louis: The C. V. Mosby Company; 1982.
8. Nieuwkoop P. The formation of mesoderm in Urodelean amphibians. I. Induction by the endoderm. *Roux Arch Entw Mech Org* 1969;162:341–73.
9. Dale L, Smith JC, Slack JM. Mesoderm induction in Xenopus laevis: a quantitative study using a cell lineage label and tissue-specific antibodies. *J Embryol Exp Morphol* 1985;89:289–312.
10. Nieuwkoop P, Ubbels G. The formation of mesoderm in Urodelean amphibians. IV. Quantitative evidence for the purely 'ectodermal' origin of the entire mesoderm and of the pharyngeal endoderm. *Roux Arch Entw Mech Org* 1972;169:185–99.
11. Rodaway A, Patient R. Mesendoderm. an ancient germ layer? *Cell* 2001;105(2):169–72.
12. Wardle FC, Smith JC. Transcriptional regulation of mesendoderm formation in Xenopus. *Semin Cell Dev Biol* 2006;17(1): 99–109.
13. Smith JC. Mesoderm-inducing factors in early vertebrate development. *Embo J* 1993;12(12):4463–70.
14. Stennard F, Ryan K, Gurdon JB. Markers of vertebrate mesoderm induction. *Curr Opin Genet Dev* 1997;7(5):620–7.
15. Lawson KA, Meneses JJ, Pedersen RA. Clonal analysis of epiblast fate during germ layer formation in the mouse embryo. *Development* 1991;113(3):891–911.
16. Kinder SJ, Tsang TE, Quinlan GA, Hadjantonakis AK, Nagy A, Tam PP. The orderly allocation of mesodermal cells to the extraembryonic structures and the anteroposterior axis during gastrulation of the mouse embryo. *Development* 1999;126(21):4691–701.

17. Kanatsu M, Nishikawa SI. In vitro analysis of epiblast tissue potency for hematopoietic cell differentiation. *Development* 1996;122(3):823–30.
18. Russell ES, Bernstein SE. Blood and blood formation. In: Green EL, ed. Biology of the laboratory mouse. 2nd ed. New York: McGraw-Hill; 1966:351–72.
19. Tavian M, Peault B. Embryonic development of the human hematopoietic system. *Int J Dev Biol* 2005;49(2–3):243–50.
20. Miura Y, Wilt FH. Tissue interaction and the formation of the first erythroblasts of the chick embryo. *Dev Biol* 1969; 19(2):201–11.
21. Pardanaud L, Dieterlen-Lievre F. Manipulation of the angiopoietic/hemangiopoietic commitment in the avian embryo. *Development* 1999;126(4):617–27.
22. Belaoussoff M, Farrington SM, Baron MH. Hematopoietic induction and respecification of A-P identity by visceral endoderm signaling in the mouse embryo. *Development* 1998;125(24):5009–18.
23. Dyer MA, Farrington SM, Mohn D, Munday JR, Baron MH. Indian hedgehog activates hematopoiesis and vasculogenesis and can respecify prospective neurectodermal cell fate in the mouse embryo. *Development* 2001;128(10):1717–30.
24. Murray P. The development in vitro of the blood of the early chick embryo. *Proc Roy Soc London* 1932;11:497–521.
25. Sabin F. Studies on the origin of blood vessels and of red blood corpuscles as seen in the living blastoderm of chicks during the second day of incubation. *Carnegie Inst Wash Pub # 272, Contrib Embryol* 1920;9:214.
26. Park C, Ma YD, Choi K. Evidence for the hemangioblast. *Exp Hematol* 2005;33(9):965–70.
27. Shalaby F, Rossant J, Yamaguchi TP, et al. Failure of blood-island formation and vasculogenesis in Flk-1-deficient mice. *Nature* 1995;376(6535):62–6.
28. Tavian M, Hallais MF, Peault B. Emergence of intraembryonic hematopoietic precursors in the pre-liver human embryo. *Development* 1999;126(4):793–803.
29. Palis J, Robertson S, Kennedy M, Wall C, Keller G. Development of erythroid and myeloid progenitors in the yolk sac and embryo proper of the mouse. *Development* 1999; 126(22):5073–84.
30. Fehling HJ, Lacaud G, Kubo A, et al. Tracking mesoderm induction and its specification to the hemangioblast during embryonic stem cell differentiation. *Development* 2003; 130(17):4217–27.
31. Huber TL, Kouskoff V, Fehling HJ, Palis J, Keller G. Haemangioblast commitment is initiated in the primitive streak of the mouse embryo. *Nature* 2004;432(7017):625–30.
32. Ueno H, Weissman IL. Clonal analysis of mouse development reveals a polyclonal origin for yolk sac blood islands. *Dev Cell* 2006;11(4):519–33.
33. Corbel C, Salaun J, Belo-Diabangouaya P, Dieterlen-Lievre F. Hematopoietic potential of the pre-fusion allantois. *Dev Biol* 2007;301(2):478–88.
34. Zeigler BM, Sugiyama D, Chen M, Guo Y, Downs KM, Speck NA. The allantois and chorion, when isolated before circulation or chorio-allantoic fusion, have hematopoietic potential. *Development* 2006;133(21):4183–92.
35. Caprioli A, Minko K, Drevon C, Eichmann A, Dieterlen-Lievre F, Jaffredo T. Hemangioblast commitment in the avian allantois: cellular and molecular aspects. *Dev Biol* 2001;238(1):64–78.
36. Caprioli A, Jaffredo T, Gautier R, Dubourg C, Dieterlen-Lievre F. Blood-borne seeding by hematopoietic and endothelial precursors from the allantois. *Proc Natl Acad Sci U S A* 1998;95(4):1641–6.
37. Downs KM. The murine allantois. *Curr Top Dev Biol* 1998;39:1–33.
38. Alvarez-Silva M, Belo-Diabangouaya P, Salaun J, Dieterlen-Lievre F. Mouse placenta is a major hematopoietic organ. *Development* 2003;130(22):5437–44.
39. Gekas C, Dieterlen-Lievre F, Orkin SH, Mikkola HK. The placenta is a niche for hematopoietic stem cells. *Dev Cell* 2005;8(3):365–75.
40. Ottersbach K, Dzierzak E. The murine placenta contains hematopoietic stem cells within the vascular labyrinth region. *Dev Cell* 2005;8(3):377–87.
41. Dieterlen-Lievre F. On the origin of haemopoietic stem cells in the avian embryo: an experimental approach. *J Embryol Exp Morphol* 1975;33(3):607–19.
42. Beaupain D, Martin C, Dieterlen-Lievre F. Are developmental hemoglobin changes related to the origin of stem cells and site of erythropoiesis? *Blood* 1979;53(2):212–25.
43. Dieterlen-Lievre F, Martin C. Diffuse intraembryonic hemopoiesis in normal and chimeric avian development. *Dev Biol* 1981;88(1):180–91.
44. Martin C, Beaupain D, Dieterlen-Lievre F. Developmental relationships between vitelline and intra-embryonic haemopoiesis studied in avian 'yolk sac chimaeras'. *Cell Differ* 1978;7(3):115–30.
45. Cormier F, Dieterlen-Lievre F. The wall of the chick embryo aorta harbours M-CFC, G-CFC, GM-CFC and BFU-E. *Development* 1988;102(2):279–85.
46. Jaffredo T, Gautier R, Brajeul V, Dieterlen-Lievre F. Tracing the progeny of the aortic hemangioblast in the avian embryo. *Dev Biol* 2000;224(2):204–14.
47. Jaffredo T, Gautier R, Eichmann A, Dieterlen-Lievre F. Intraaortic hemopoietic cells are derived from endothelial cells during ontogeny. *Development* 1998;125(22):4575–83.
48. Kau CL, Turpen JB. Dual contribution of embryonic ventral blood island and dorsal lateral plate mesoderm during ontogeny of hemopoietic cells in Xenopus laevis. *J Immunol* 1983;131(5):2262–6.
49. Maeno M, Tochinai S, Katagiri C. Differential participation of ventral and dorsolateral mesoderms in the hemopoiesis of Xenopus, as revealed in diploid-triploid or interspecific chimeras. *Dev Biol* 1985;110(2):503–8.
50. Turpen JB, Knudson CM, Hoefen PS. The early ontogeny of hematopoietic cells studied by grafting cytogenetically labeled tissue anlagen: localization of a prospective stem cell compartment. *Dev Biol* 1981;85(1):99–112.
51. Turpen JB, Knudson CM. Ontogeny of hematopoietic cells in Rana pipiens: precursor cell migration during embryogenesis. *Dev Biol* 1982;89(1):138–51.
52. Ciau-Uitz A, Walmsley M, Patient R. Distinct origins of adult and embryonic blood in Xenopus. *Cell* 2000;102(6):787–96.
53. Turpen JB, Kelley CM, Mead PE, Zon LI. Bipotential primitive-definitive hematopoietic progenitors in the vertebrate embryo. *Immunity* 1997;7(3):325–34.

54. Medvinsky A, Dzierzak E. Definitive hematopoiesis is autonomously initiated by the AGM region. *Cell* 1996;86(6): 897–906.
55. Muller AM, Medvinsky A, Strouboulis J, Grosveld F, Dzierzak E. Development of hematopoietic stem cell activity in the mouse embryo. *Immunity* 1994;1(4):291–301.
56. Dzierzak E. The emergence of definitive hematopoietic stem cells in the mammal. *Curr Opin Hematol* 2005;12(3):197–202.
57. Cumano A, Dieterlen-Lievre F, Godin I. Lymphoid potential, probed before circulation in mouse, is restricted to caudal intraembryonic splanchnopleura. *Cell* 1996;86(6):907–16.
58. Medvinsky AL, Samoylina NL, Müller AM, Dzierzak E. An early pre-liver intraembryonic source of CFU-S in the developing mouse. *Nature* 364; 64–67.
59. Godin IE, Garcia-Porrero JA, Coutinho A, Dieterlen-Lievre F, Marcos MA. Para-aortic splanchnopleura from early mouse embryos contains B1a cell progenitors. *Nature* 1993;364(6432):67–70.
60. Godin I, Dieterlen-Lievre F, Cumano A. Emergence of multipotent hemopoietic cells in the yolk sac and paraaortic splanchnopleura in mouse embryos, beginning at 8.5 days postcoitus. *Proc Natl Acad Sci U S A* 1995;92(3):773–7.
61. de Bruijn MF, Speck NA, Peeters MC, Dzierzak E. Definitive hematopoietic stem cells first develop within the major arterial regions of the mouse embryo. *Embo J* 2000;19(11):2465–74.
62. Garcia-Porrero JA, Godin IE, Dieterlen-Lievre F. Potential intraembryonic hemogenic sites at pre-liver stages in the mouse. *Anat Embryol (Berl)* 1995;192(5):425–35.
63. Tavian M, Coulombel L, Luton D, Clemente HS, Dieterlen-Lievre F, Peault B. Aorta-associated CD34+ hematopoietic cells in the early human embryo. *Blood* 1996;87(1):67–72.
64. Wood HB, May G, Healy L, Enver T, Morriss-Kay GM. CD34 expression patterns during early mouse development are related to modes of blood vessel formation and reveal additional sites of hematopoiesis. *Blood* 1997;90(6):2300–11.
65. North T, Gu TL, Stacy T, et al. Cbfa2 is required for the formation of intra-aortic hematopoietic clusters. *Development* 1999;126(11):2563–75.
66. Okuda T, van Deursen J, Hiebert SW, Grosveld G, Downing JR. AML1, the target of multiple chromosomal translocations in human leukemia, is essential for normal fetal liver hematopoiesis. *Cell* 1996;84(2):321–30.
67. Wang Q, Stacy T, Binder M, Marin-Padilla M, Sharpe AH, Speck NA. Disruption of the Cbfa2 gene causes necrosis and hemorrhaging in the central nervous system and blocks definitive hematopoiesis. *Proc Natl Acad Sci U S A* 1996;93(8):3444–9.
68. de Bruijn MF, Ma X, Robin C, Ottersbach K, Sanchez MJ, Dzierzak E. Hematopoietic stem cells localize to the endothelial cell layer in the midgestation mouse aorta. *Immunity* 2002;16(5):673–83.
69. Moore MA, Metcalf D. Ontogeny of the haemopoietic system: yolk sac origin of in vivo and in vitro colony forming cells in the developing mouse embryo. *Br J Haematol* 1970;18(3):279–96.
70. Fassler R, Meyer M. Consequences of lack of beta 1 integrin gene expression in mice. *Genes Dev* 1995;9(15):1896–908.
71. Hirsch E, Iglesias A, Potocnik AJ, Hartmann U, Fassler R. Impaired migration but not differentiation of haematopoietic stem cells in the absence of beta1 integrins. *Nature* 1996;380(6570):171–5.
72. Ema H, Nakauchi H. Expansion of hematopoietic stem cells in the developing liver of a mouse embryo. *Blood* 2000;95(7):2284–8.
73. Houssaint E. Differentiation of the mouse hepatic primordium. II. Extrinsic origin of the haemopoietic cell line. *Cell Differ* 1981;10(5):243–52.
74. Johnson GR, Moore MA. Role of stem cell migration in initiation of mouse foetal liver haemopoiesis. *Nature* 1975;258(5537):726–8.
75. Kumaravelu P, Hook L, Morrison AM, et al. Quantitative developmental anatomy of definitive haematopoietic stem cells/long-term repopulating units (HSC/RUs): role of the aorta-gonad- mesonephros (AGM) region and the yolk sac in colonisation of the mouse embryonic liver. *Development* 2002;129(21):4891–9.
76. Metcalf D. The hemopoietic colony stimulating factors. Amsterdam: Elsevier Science Publishers B. V.; 1984.
77. Adolfsson J, Borge OJ, Bryder D, et al. Upregulation of Flt3 expression within the bone marrow Lin(-)Sca1(+)c-kit(+) stem cell compartment is accompanied by loss of self-renewal capacity. *Immunity* 2001;15(4):659–69.
78. Kelemen E, Calvo W, Fliedner T. Atlas of Human Hemopoietic Development. Berlin: Springer-Verlag; 1979.
79. Ferkowicz MJ, Yoder MC. Blood island formation: longstanding observations and modern interpretations. *Exp Hematol* 2005;33(9):1041–7.
80. Wong PM, Chung SW, Reicheld SM, Chui DH. Hemoglobin switching during murine embryonic development: evidence for two populations of embryonic erythropoietic progenitor cells. *Blood* 1986;67(3):716–21.
81. Kovach JS, Marks PA, Russell ES, Epler H. Erythroid cell development in fetal mice: ultrastructural characteristics and hemoglobin synthesis. *J Mol Biol* 1967;25(1):131–42.
82. Rifkind RA, Chui D, Epler H. An ultrastructural study of early morphogenetic events during the establishment of fetal hepatic erythropoiesis. *J Cell Biol* 1969;40(2):343–65.
83. Grosveld F, Dillon N, Higgs D. The regulation of human globin gene expression. *Baillieres Clin Haematol* 1993;6(1): 31–55.
84. Russell ES. Hereditary anemias of the mouse: a review for geneticists. *Adv Genet* 1979;20:357–459.
85. Kennedy M, Firpo M, Choi K, et al. A common precursor for primitive erythropoiesis and definitive haematopoiesis. *Nature* 1997;386(6624):488–93.
86. Wijgerde M, Grosveld F, Fraser P. Transcription complex stability and chromatin dynamics in vivo. *Nature* 1995; 377(6546):209–13.
87. Nakano T, Kodama H, Honjo T. In vitro development of primitive and definitive erythrocytes from different precursors. *Science* 1996;272(5262):722–4.
88. Ogawa M, Matsuzaki Y, Nishikawa S, et al. Expression and function of c-kit in hemopoietic progenitor cells. *J Exp Med* 1991;174(1):63–71.
89. McGrath KE, Palis J. Hematopoiesis in the yolk sac: more than meets the eye. *Exp Hematol* 2005;33(9):1021–8.
90. Naito M, Umeda S, Yamamoto T, et al. Development, differentiation, and phenotypic heterogeneity of murine tissue macrophages. *J Leukoc Biol* 1996;59(2):133–8.
91. Bonifer C, Faust N, Geiger H, Muller AM. Developmental changes in the differentiation capacity of haematopoietic stem cells. *Immunol Today* 1998;19(5):236–41.

92. Eren R, Zharhary D, Abel L, Globerson A. Ontogeny of T cells: development of pre-T cells from fetal liver and yolk sac in the thymus microenvironment. *Cell Immunol* 1987;108(1):76–84.
93. Liu CP, Auerbach R. In vitro development of murine T cells from prethymic and preliver embryonic yolk sac hematopoietic stem cells. *Development* 1991;113(4):1315–23.
94. Ogawa M, Nishikawa S, Ikuta K, et al. B cell ontogeny in murine embryo studied by a culture system with the monolayer of a stromal cell clone, ST2: B cell progenitor develops first in the embryonal body rather than in the yolk sac. *Embo J* 1988;7(5):1337–43.
95. Delassus S, Cumano A. Circulation of hematopoietic progenitors in the mouse embryo. *Immunity* 1996;4(1):97–106.
96. Ikuta K, Kina T, MacNeil I, et al. A developmental switch in thymic lymphocyte maturation potential occurs at the level of hematopoietic stem cells. *Cell* 1990;62(5):863–74.
97. Herzenberg LA, Stall AM, Lalor PA, et al. The Ly-1 B cell lineage. *Immunol Rev* 1986;93:81–102.
98. Cumano A, Furlonger C, Paige CJ. Differentiation and characterization of B-cell precursors detected in the yolk sac and embryo body of embryos beginning at the 10- to 12-somite stage. *Proc Natl Acad Sci U S A* 1993;90(14):6429–33.
99. Johnson GR, Barker DC. Erythroid progenitor cells and stimulating factors during murine embryonic and fetal development. *Exp Hematol* 1985;13(3):200–8.
100. Sonoda T, Hayashi C, Kitamura Y. Presence of mast cell precursors in the yolk sac of mice. *Dev Biol* 1983;97(1):89–94.
101. Ferkowicz MJ, Starr M, Xie X, et al. CD41 expression defines the onset of primitive and definitive hematopoiesis in the murine embryo. *Development* 2003;130(18):4393–403.
102. Rampon C, Huber P. Multilineage hematopoietic progenitor activity generated autonomously in the mouse yolk sac: analysis using angiogenesis-defective embryos. *Int J Dev Biol* 2003;47(4):273–80.
103. Lux CT, Yoshimoto M, McGrath K, Conway SJ, Palis J, Yoder MC. All primitive and definitive hematopoietic progenitor cells emerging prior to E10 in the mouse embryo are products of the yolk sac. *Blood* 2007.
104. Yashiro K, Shiratori H, Hamada H. Haemodynamics determined by a genetic programme govern asymmetric development of the aortic arch. *Nature* 2007;450(7167):285–8.
105. Migliaccio G, Migliaccio AR, Petti S, et al. Human embryonic hemopoiesis. Kinetics of progenitors and precursors underlying the yolk sac–liver transition. *J Clin Invest* 1986;78(1):51–60.
106. Huyhn A, Dommergues M, Izac B, et al. Characterization of hematopoietic progenitors from human yolk sacs and embryos. *Blood* 1995;86(12):4474–85.
107. Peault B. Hematopoietic stem cell emergence in embryonic life: developmental hematology revisited. *J Hematother* 1996;5(4):369–78.
108. Till JE, Mc CE. A direct measurement of the radiation sensitivity of normal mouse bone marrow cells. *Radiat Res* 1961;14:213–22.
109. de Bruijn MF, Peeters MC, Luteijn T, Visser P, Speck NA, Dzierzak E. CFU-S(11) activity does not localize solely with the aorta in the aorta-gonad-mesonephros region. *Blood* 2000;96(8):2902–4.
110. Tavian M, Robin C, Coulombel L, Peault B. The human embryo, but not its yolk sac, generates lympho-myeloid stem cells: mapping multipotent hematopoietic cell fate in intraembryonic mesoderm. *Immunity* 2001;15(3):487–95.
111. Yoder MC, Hiatt K, Dutt P, Mukherjee P, Bodine DM, Orlic D. Characterization of definitive lymphohematopoietic stem cells in the day 9 murine yolk sac. *Immunity* 1997;7(3):335–44.
112. Toles JF, Chui DH, Belbeck LW, Starr E, Barker JE. Hemopoietic stem cells in murine embryonic yolk sac and peripheral blood. *Proc Natl Acad Sci U S A* 1989;86(19):7456–9.
113. Weissman I VP, R Gardner. Fetal hematopoietic origins of the adult hematolymphoid system. Cold Spring Harbor: Cold Spring Harbor Laboratory; 1978.
114. Sugiyama D, Ogawa M, Hirose I, Jaffredo T, Arai K, Tsuji K. Erythropoiesis from acetyl LDL incorporating endothelial cells at the preliver stage. *Blood* 2003;101(12):4733–8.
115. Ling KW, Ottersbach K, van Hamburg JP, et al. GATA-2 plays two functionally distinct roles during the ontogeny of hematopoietic stem cells. *J Exp Med* 2004;200(7):871–82.
116. Minegishi N, Ohta J, Yamagiwa H, et al. The mouse GATA-2 gene is expressed in the para-aortic splanchnopleura and aorta-gonads and mesonephros region. *Blood* 1999;93(12):4196–207.
117. North TE, de Bruijn MF, Stacy T, et al. Runx1 expression marks long-term repopulating hematopoietic stem cells in the midgestation mouse embryo. *Immunity* 2002;16(5):661–72.
118. Sanchez MJ, Bockamp EO, Miller J, Gambardella L, Green AR. Selective rescue of early haematopoietic progenitors in Scl(−/−) mice by expressing Scl under the control of a stem cell enhancer. *Development* 2001;128(23):4815–27.
119. Sanchez MJ, Holmes A, Miles C, Dzierzak E. Characterization of the first definitive hematopoietic stem cells in the AGM and liver of the mouse embryo. *Immunity* 1996;5(6):513–25.
120. Taoudi S, Morrison AM, Inoue H, Gribi R, Ure J, Medvinsky A. Progressive divergence of definitive haematopoietic stem cells from the endothelial compartment does not depend on contact with the foetal liver. *Development* 2005;132(18):4179–91.
121. Ody C, Vaigot P, Quere P, Imhof BA, Corbel C. Glycoprotein IIb-IIIa is expressed on avian multilineage hematopoietic progenitor cells. *Blood* 1999;93(9):2898–906.
122. Durand C, Robin C, Bollerot K, Baron MH, Ottersbach K, Dzierzak E. Embryonic stromal clones reveal developmental regulators of definitive hematopoietic stem cells. *Proc Natl Acad Sci U S A* 2007;104(52):20838–43.
123. Taoudi S, Medvinsky A. Functional identification of the hematopoietic stem cell niche in the ventral domain of the embryonic dorsal aorta. *Proc Natl Acad Sci U S A* 2007;104(22):9399–403.
124. Bertrand JY, Giroux S, Golub R, et al. Characterization of purified intraembryonic hematopoietic stem cells as a tool to define their site of origin. *Proc Natl Acad Sci U S A* 2005;102(1):134–9.
125. Oberlin E, Tavian M, Blazsek I, Peault B. Blood-forming potential of vascular endothelium in the human embryo. *Development* 2002;129(17):4147–57.
126. Moore MA, Owen JJ. Experimental studies on the development of the thymus. *J Exp Med* 1967;126(4):715–26.
127. Le Douarin NM, Dieterlen-Lievre F, Oliver PD. Ontogeny of primary lymphoid organs and lymphoid stem cells. *Am J Anat* 1984;170(3):261–99.

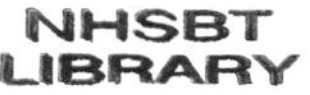

128. Chen XD, Turpen JB. Intraembryonic origin of hepatic hematopoiesis in Xenopus laevis. *J Immunol* 1995;154(6):2557–67.
129. Kissa K, Murayama E, Zapata A, et al. Live imaging of emerging hematopoietic stem cells and early thymus colonization. *Blood* 2008;111(3):1147–56.
130. Bechtold TE, Smith PB, Turpen JB. Differential stem cell contributions to thymocyte succession during development of Xenopus laevis. *J Immunol* 1992;148(10):2975–82.
131. Cudennec CA, Thiery JP, Le Douarin NM. In vitro induction of adult erythropoiesis in early mouse yolk sac. *Proc Natl Acad Sci U S A* 1981;78(4):2412–6.
132. Bertrand JY, Desanti GE, Lo-Man R, Leclerc C, Cumano A, Golub R. Fetal spleen stroma drives macrophage commitment. *Development* 2006;133(18):3619–28.
133. Yokota T, Huang J, Tavian M, et al. Tracing the first waves of lymphopoiesis in mice. *Development* 2006;133(10):2041–51.
134. Jotereau FV, Le Douarin NM. Demonstration of a cyclic renewal of the lymphocyte precursor cells in the quail thymus during embryonic and perinatal life. *J Immunol* 1982;129(5):1869–77.
135. van Ewijk W, Hollander G, Terhorst C, Wang B. Stepwise development of thymic microenvironments in vivo is regulated by thymocyte subsets. *Development* 2000;127(8):1583–91.
136. Xie H, Ye M, Feng R, Graf T. Stepwise reprogramming of B cells into macrophages. *Cell* 2004;117(5):663–76.
137. Gothert JR, Gustin SE, Hall MA, et al. In vivo fate-tracing studies using the Scl stem cell enhancer: embryonic hematopoietic stem cells significantly contribute to adult hematopoiesis. *Blood* 2005;105(7):2724–32.
138. Samokhvalov IM, Samokhvalova NI, Nishikawa S. Cell tracing shows the contribution of the yolk sac to adult haematopoiesis. *Nature* 2007;446(7139):1056–61.
139. Abbott A. Biologists claim Nobel prize with a knock-out. *Nature* 2007;449(7163):642.
140. Dale L, Howes G, Price BM, Smith JC. Bone morphogenetic protein 4: a ventralizing factor in early Xenopus development. *Development* 1992;115(2):573–85.
141. Mead PE, Brivanlou IH, Kelley CM, Zon LI. BMP-4-responsive regulation of dorsal-ventral patterning by the homeobox protein Mix.1. *Nature* 1996;382(6589):357–60.
142. Walmsley M, Ciau-Uitz A, Patient R. Adult and embryonic blood and endothelium derive from distinct precursor populations which are differentially programmed by BMP in Xenopus. *Development* 2002;129(24):5683–95.
143. Walmsley M, Cleaver D, Patient R. Fibroblast growth factor controls the timing of Scl, Lmo2, and Runx1 expression during embryonic blood development. *Blood* 2008;111(3):1157–66.
144. Wilt FH. Erythropoiesis in the Chick Embryo: The Role of Endoderm. *Science* 1965;147:1588–90.
145. Tonegawa A, Funayama N, Ueno N, Takahashi Y. Mesodermal subdivision along the mediolateral axis in chicken controlled by different concentrations of BMP-4. *Development* 1997;124(10):1975–84.
146. Gering M, Patient R. Hedgehog signaling is required for adult blood stem cell formation in zebrafish embryos. *Dev Cell* 2005;8(3):389–400.
147. Byrd N, Becker S, Maye P, et al. Hedgehog is required for murine yolk sac angiogenesis. *Development* 2002;129(2):361–72.
148. Winnier G, Blessing M, Labosky PA, Hogan BL. Bone morphogenetic protein-4 is required for mesoderm formation and patterning in the mouse. *Genes Dev* 1995;9(17):2105–16.
149. Dickson MC, Martin JS, Cousins FM, Kulkarni AB, Karlsson S, Akhurst RJ. Defective haematopoiesis and vasculogenesis in transforming growth factor-beta 1 knock out mice. *Development* 1995;121(6):1845–54.
150. Karlsson G, Blank U, Moody JL, et al. Smad4 is critical for self-renewal of hematopoietic stem cells. *J Exp Med* 2007;204(3):467–74.
151. Johansson BM, Wiles MV. Evidence for involvement of activin A and bone morphogenetic protein 4 in mammalian mesoderm and hematopoietic development. *Mol Cell Biol* 1995;15(1):141–51.
152. Marshall CJ, Kinnon C, Thrasher AJ. Polarized expression of bone morphogenetic protein-4 in the human aorta-gonad-mesonephros region. *Blood* 2000;96(4):1591–3.
153. Sadlon TJ, Lewis ID, D'Andrea RJ. BMP4: its role in development of the hematopoietic system and potential as a hematopoietic growth factor. *Stem Cells* 2004;22(4):457–74.
154. Carmeliet P, Ferreira V, Breier G, et al. Abnormal blood vessel development and lethality in embryos lacking a single VEGF allele. *Nature* 1996;380(6573):435–9.
155. Ferrara N, Carver-Moore K, Chen H, et al. Heterozygous embryonic lethality induced by targeted inactivation of the VEGF gene. *Nature* 1996;380(6573):439–42.
156. Choi K, Kennedy M, Kazarov A, Papadimitriou JC, Keller G. A common precursor for hematopoietic and endothelial cells. *Development* 1998;125(4):725–32.
157. Kumano K, Chiba S, Kunisato A, et al. Notch1 but not Notch2 is essential for generating hematopoietic stem cells from endothelial cells. *Immunity* 2003;18(5):699–711.
158. Robert-Moreno A, Espinosa L, de la Pompa JL, Bigas A. RBPjkappa-dependent Notch function regulates Gata2 and is essential for the formation of intra-embryonic hematopoietic cells. *Development* 2005;132(5):1117–26.
159. Burns CE, Traver D, Mayhall E, Shepard JL, Zon LI. Hematopoietic stem cell fate is established by the Notch-Runx pathway. *Genes Dev* 2005;19(19):2331–42.
160. Nakagawa M, Ichikawa M, Kumano K, et al. AML1/Runx1 rescues Notch1-null mutation-induced deficiency of para-aortic splanchnopleural hematopoiesis. *Blood* 2006;108(10):3329–34.
161. Bernstein A. Molecular genetic approaches to the elucidation of hematopoietic stem cell function. *Stem Cells* 1993;11 Suppl 2:31–5.
162. Witte ON. Steel locus defines new multipotent growth factor. *Cell* 1990;63(1):5–6.
163. Okada S, Nakauchi H, Nagayoshi K, et al. Enrichment and characterization of murine hematopoietic stem cells that express c-kit molecule. *Blood* 1991;78(7):1706–12.
164. Hassan HT, Zander A. Stem cell factor as a survival and growth factor in human normal and malignant hematopoiesis. *Acta Haematol* 1996;95(3–4):257–62.
165. Porcher C, Swat W, Rockwell K, Fujiwara Y, Alt FW, Orkin SH. The T cell leukemia oncoprotein SCL/tal-1 is essential for development of all hematopoietic lineages. *Cell* 1996;86(1):47–57.

166. Robb L, Elwood NJ, Elefanty AG, et al. The scl gene product is required for the generation of all hematopoietic lineages in the adult mouse. *Embo J* 1996;15(16):4123–9.
167. Robb L, Lyons I, Li R, et al. Absence of yolk sac hematopoiesis from mice with a targeted disruption of the scl gene. *Proc Natl Acad Sci U S A* 1995;92(15):7075–9.
168. Shivdasani RA, Mayer EL, Orkin SH. Absence of blood formation in mice lacking the T-cell leukaemia oncoprotein tal-1/SCL. *Nature* 1995;373(6513):432–4.
169. Visvader JE, Fujiwara Y, Orkin SH. Unsuspected role for the T-cell leukemia protein SCL/tal-1 in vascular development. *Genes Dev* 1998;12(4):473–9.
170. Gering M, Rodaway AR, Gottgens B, Patient RK, Green AR. The SCL gene specifies haemangioblast development from early mesoderm. *Embo J* 1998;17(14):4029–45.
171. D'Souza SL, Elefanty AG, Keller G. SCL/Tal-1 is essential for hematopoietic commitment of the hemangioblast but not for its development. *Blood* 2005;105(10):3862–70.
172. Warren AJ, Colledge WH, Carlton MB, Evans MJ, Smith AJ, Rabbitts TH. The oncogenic cysteine-rich LIM domain protein rbtn2 is essential for erythroid development. *Cell* 1994;78(1):45–57.
173. Yamada Y, Warren AJ, Dobson C, Forster A, Pannell R, Rabbitts TH. The T cell leukemia LIM protein Lmo2 is necessary for adult mouse hematopoiesis. *Proc Natl Acad Sci U S A* 1998;95(7):3890–5.
174. Landry JR, Kinston S, Knezevic K, Donaldson IJ, Green AR, Gottgens B. Fli1, Elf1, and Ets1 regulate the proximal promoter of the LMO2 gene in endothelial cells. *Blood* 2005; 106(8):2680–7.
175. Wadman IA, Osada H, Grutz GG, et al. The LIM-only protein Lmo2 is a bridging molecule assembling an erythroid, DNA-binding complex which includes the TAL1, E47, GATA-1 and Ldb1/NLI proteins. *Embo J* 1997;16(11):3145–57.
176. Jippo T, Mizuno H, Xu Z, Nomura S, Yamamoto M, Kitamura Y. Abundant expression of transcription factor GATA-2 in proliferating but not in differentiated mast cells in tissues of mice: demonstration by in situ hybridization. *Blood* 1996;87(3):993–8.
177. Labbaye C, Valtieri M, Barberi T, et al. Differential expression and functional role of GATA-2, NF-E2, and GATA-1 in normal adult hematopoiesis. *J Clin Invest* 1995;95(5):2346–58.
178. Tsai FY, Keller G, Kuo FC, et al. An early haematopoietic defect in mice lacking the transcription factor GATA-2. *Nature* 1994;371(6494):221–6.
179. Nottingham WT, Jarratt A, Burgess M, et al. Runx1-mediated hematopoietic stem-cell emergence is controlled by a Gata/Ets/SCL-regulated enhancer. *Blood* 2007;110(13):4188–97.
180. Pimanda JE, Ottersbach K, Knezevic K, et al. Gata2, Fli1, and Scl form a recursively wired gene-regulatory circuit during early hematopoietic development. *Proc Natl Acad Sci U S A* 2007;104(45):17692–7.
181. Wang Q, Stacy T, Miller JD, et al. The CBFbeta subunit is essential for CBFalpha2 (AML1) function in vivo. *Cell* 1996;87(4):697–708.
182. Cai Z, de Bruijn M, Ma X, et al. Haploinsufficiency of AML1 affects the temporal and spatial generation of hematopoietic stem cells in the mouse embryo. *Immunity* 2000;13(4):423–31.
183. Robin C, Ottersbach K, Durand C, et al. An unexpected role for IL-3 in the embryonic development of hematopoietic stem cells. *Dev Cell* 2006;11(2):171–80.
184. Huang G, Zhang P, Hirai H, et al. PU.1 is a major downstream target of AML1 (RUNX1) in adult mouse hematopoiesis. *Nat Genet* 2008;40(1):51–60.
185. Takahashi K, Yamanaka S. Induction of pluripotent stem cells from mouse embryonic and adult fibroblast cultures by defined factors. *Cell* 2006;126(4):663–76.
186. Fisher AG, Merkenschlager M. Gene silencing, cell fate and nuclear organisation. *Curr Opin Genet Dev* 2002;12(2): 193–7.
187. Cao R, Zhang Y. The functions of E(Z)/EZH2-mediated methylation of lysine 27 in histone H3. *Curr Opin Genet Dev* 2004;14(2):155–64.
188. Owens BM, Hawley RG. HOX and non-HOX homeobox genes in leukemic hematopoiesis. *Stem Cells* 2002;20(5):364–79.
189. Kamminga LM, Bystrykh LV, de Boer A, et al. The Polycomb group gene Ezh2 prevents hematopoietic stem cell exhaustion. *Blood* 2006;107(5):2170–9.
190. Kajiume T, Ninomiya Y, Ishihara H, Kanno R, Kanno M. Polycomb group gene mel-18 modulates the self-renewal activity and cell cycle status of hematopoietic stem cells. *Exp Hematol* 2004;32(6):571–8.
191. Ohta H, Sawada A, Kim JY, et al. Polycomb group gene rae28 is required for sustaining activity of hematopoietic stem cells. *J Exp Med* 2002;195(6):759–70.
192. Park IK, Qian D, Kiel M, et al. Bmi-1 is required for maintenance of adult self-renewing haematopoietic stem cells. *Nature* 2003;423(6937):302–5.
193. Milne TA, Briggs SD, Brock HW, et al. MLL targets SET domain methyltransferase activity to Hox gene promoters. *Mol Cell* 2002;10(5):1107–17.
194. Nakamura T, Mori T, Tada S, et al. ALL-1 is a histone methyltransferase that assembles a supercomplex of proteins involved in transcriptional regulation. *Mol Cell* 2002; 10(5):1119–28.
195. Ernst P, Fisher JK, Avery W, Wade S, Foy D, Korsmeyer SJ. Definitive hematopoiesis requires the mixed-lineage leukemia gene. *Dev Cell* 2004;6(3):437–43.
196. Rifkind R, Bank A, Marks P, al. e. *Fundamentals of Hematology*. 2nd ed. Chicago: Year Book Medical Publishers; 1980.

2

Erythropoiesis

Sjaak Philipsen and William G. Wood

INTRODUCTION

Erythropoiesis involves the production of mature enucleated erythrocytes from committed erythroid progenitor cells, which in turn are derived from multilineage progenitors and ultimately from the hematopoietic stem cell (HSC). In human the mature erythrocytes turn over at a rate of approximately 1% per day and it can be estimated that maintaining the red blood cell count in an adult requires approximately 2.4×10^6 new erythrocytes to be produced each second. It is not surprising, therefore, that the regulation of erythropoiesis is a complex, multifaceted process that has to cope with not only maintaining the steady state but also with providing reserves to cope rapidly with increased demand as a result of physiological or pathological demands. In this chapter we will consider the developmental origins of red cell production, their differentiation from HSCs as well as production of the hormone erythropoietin. We will examine how erythropoietin responds to tissue hypoxia and exerts its effect through cell surface receptors on erythroid cells to trigger a number of cell signaling cascades to maintain, through critical transcription factors, the survival, proliferation, and maturation of the erythron.

ERYTHROPOIESIS DURING DEVELOPMENT

The first erythrocytes appearing during vertebrate development are known as primitive erythrocytes. These cells are produced by a transient first wave of hematopoiesis, which is almost entirely dedicated to the production of primitive red cells. Primitive erythropoiesis has been studied in evolutionary distant vertebrates, in particular in fish, amphibians, birds, and mammals. Despite the considerable anatomical differences between the developing embryos of these phyla, primitive erythropoiesis appears to be a remarkably conserved process allowing observations made in lower vertebrates to be extrapolated – with care – to mammals. The establishment of blood circulation is important to provide oxygen and nutrients to the developing embryo. Primitive erythrocytes are relatively large cells characterized by the expression of embryonic globins. In mammals, these are the only erythroid cells that retain their nucleus when they enter the circulation. Definitive hematopoiesis gives rise to all hematopoietic lineages and replenishes the hematopoietic compartment throughout the lifespan of the organism. In fish, amphibians, and birds the definitive erythrocytes remain nucleated. Mammalian definitive erythrocytes expel their nucleus before they enter the circulation. Definitive erythrocytes are smaller than primitive erythrocytes and express fetal/adult globins. We will now describe the main features of erythropoiesis in fish (zebrafish, *Danio rerio*), amphibians (African clawed frog, *Xenopus laevis*), birds (chicken, *Gallus gallus*) and mammals (mouse, *Mus musculus*, and human, *Homo sapiens*).

ZEBRAFISH (*Danio rerio*)

The zebrafish has become a popular model organism to study early vertebrate development in particular. Large numbers of fertilized eggs can be obtained easily. The eggs are transparent and development of the embryos can therefore be monitored without any interference. Development proceeds rapidly: from the fertilized egg to hatched fry takes only 72 hours. Large collections of mutants are available that have been generated through forward genetic screens, using insertional, radiation-induced and *N*-ethyl-*N*-nitrosourea–mediated mutagenesis.[1] Effective "knock-down" of specific proteins can be achieved by injecting antisense-modified oligonucleotides, known as morpholinos, into fertilized eggs.[2] The morpholinos are designed to bind to the translation initiation site or a splice junction of a particular RNA molecule, thereby preventing the synthesis of protein. With the zebrafish genome sequence at hand, one can thus perform a very quick functional analysis of any protein of interest. To distinguish the morpholino-injected fish from genetic mutants, they are called "morphants".[3] Complementary proteins can be overexpressed through the injection of RNA synthesized in vitro. Finally, fish transmitting transgenes through the germline can be obtained by injection of linearized plasmids, albeit with low efficiency.[4] Nevertheless, useful reporter strains have been generated in this way, for instance lines expressing green fluorescent protein in the endothelial cells of the vasculature[5] and in erythroid cells.[6,7] Such transgenic reporter fish provide easy visualization of mutants and morphants in which erythroid development is disturbed. From the forward genetic screens, approximately 25 complementation groups affecting blood formation have been identified.[10] These groups fall into categories ranging from defective HSC generation (e.g., the *cloche* mutant affecting an as yet unidentified gene[11]), arrested erythroid development (e.g., the *vlas tepes* mutant affecting the *GATA-1* gene[12]) to structural defects in erythrocytes (e.g., the *sauternes* mutant affecting the *alas2* gene[13]) and the *retsina* mutant affecting the *band3* gene.[14] Often, mutations in the orthologous genes are associated with human hematological disorders, which has led to the notion that the zebrafish provides useful models for human diseases.[15]

SITES OF ERYTHROPOIESIS IN THE ZEBRAFISH

The first erythroid cells arise in an area known as the intermediate cell mass, first evident at 16 hours postfertilization. This structure is a derivative of the lateral plate mesoderm that first appears approximately 10 hours postfertilization, at the end of gastrulation and the start of somatogenesis. The first erythroid cells become visible at 22 hours postfertilization and enter the circulation at 24 hours postfertilization. The primitive erythroid cells express embryonic *α-like* and *β-like globin* genes.[16] Although the anatomical location of the intermediate cell mass is not obviously related to the extraembryonic location in the yolk sac of the primitive erythroid progenitors in mammals, the intermediate cell mass is derived from two paraxial stripes of mesoderm arising during gastrulation, a location analogous to the mammalian site. Similar to mammals, the first definitive hematopoietic cells appear in the ventral wall of the dorsal aorta, approximately 48 hours postfertilization.[17] These cells can be identified by the expression of transcription factors such as runx1 and myb.[18–20] setting them apart from the primitive erythroid cells, which can be identified by the expression of embryonic globins.[16] In the adult zebrafish, the kidney is the site of erythropoiesis. This is clearly different from the situation in mammals, in which the bone marrow is the main site of adult erythropoiesis. Possibly, the production of erythropoietin (Epo), the main hormone regulating erythropoiesis, in the mammalian kidney is a remnant of the erythropoietic function of this organ in their ancestors.[21]

ERYTHROPOIESIS IN *Xenopus*

There is a long tradition of using the African clawed frog *Xenopus laevis* as a model system to study vertebrate development.[22] *Xenopus* eggs are polarized, and unlike mammals, the cells in the early embryo are highly organized as a result of oriented cleavage planes.[23] Thus, lineage-tracing experiments can be performed in 32-cell stage embryos by injecting single blastomeres with a reporter, such as a fluorescent dye or in vitro synthesized RNA encoding β-galactosidase. This has been applied to demonstrate that primitive hematopoiesis and definitive hematopoiesis are derived from independent cell lineages.[24,25] *Xenopus laevis* has a tetraploid genome, which limits its use in genetic experiments due to the presence of a duplicate copy of each gene, which may or may not have identical functions. Its close relative *Xenopus tropicalis* has a diploid genome and is therefore increasingly used by developmental biologists.[26] The full scala of molecular tools can be applied to *Xenopus*, similar to zebrafish. An advantage of *Xenopus* is that morpholino-mediated knockdown and RNA-mediated protein overexpression can be targeted to single blastomeres at the 32-cell stage. In this way, gene function can be studied more specifically in the lineage giving rise to the tissue of interest, without interfering directly with the rest of the embryo. Primitive erythropoiesis in *Xenopus* occurs in structures known as ventral blood islands (VBIs), which can be further subdivided into anterior and posterior VBIs. VBIs are analogous to the mammalian yolk sac blood islands, although they are an integral part of the embryo. Anterior VBIs are derived from mesodermal cells originating from the C1 and D1 blastomeres, whereas posterior VBIs are derived from the D4 blastomere. Definitive hematopoietic cells are derived from a single blastomere, C3, which gives rise to a mesodermal structure known as the dorsal lateral plate.[24] The dorsal lateral plate serves as an intermediate structure; after extensive cell migration and tissue remodeling, the first definitive hematopoietic cells are observed as hematopoietic clusters closely associated with the ventral wall of the dorsal aorta.[25] Anatomically, the dorsal lateral plate is the equivalent of the paraaortic splanchnopleura in mammals.[27] Later in development and during adult life, the liver and spleen are the main sites of erythropoiesis; there is no evidence for hematopoietic activity in the bone marrow.[28] At all stages, erythroid cells of *Xenopus* remain nucleated.

ERYTHROID DEVELOPMENT IN THE CHICKEN (*Gallus gallus*)

Developing avian embryos are easily accessible and can be subjected to experimental manipulation in ovo. A particularly powerful procedure is the grafting of quail tissue in orthopic or ectopic locations in the chick embryo. Quail-derived cells can be traced later in the developing chimeric embryos with species-specific monoclonal antibodies.[29,30] The most extreme version of this grafting procedure is the replacement of the entire chick embryo by the quail embryo. Such experiments performed with embryos isolated before the onset of circulation revealed that definitive hematopoiesis arises intraembryonically, independent of the first wave of extraembryonic primitive hematopoiesis.[31] Thus, primitive erythrocytes are formed in the yolk sac blood islands from stem cells generated in situ. Definitive HSCs are born in the ventral side of the dorsal aorta. Furthermore, it has been demonstrated that the allantois, an endodermal and mesodermal embryonic appendage, is also a source of definitive HSCs.[32] The bone marrow is seeded with HSCs as soon as it is formed and is the location of erythropoiesis in the adult bird.[33,34] Like in the other model organisms, primitive chicken erythrocytes express embryonic globins, whereas definitive cells express adult-type globins.[35,36] Remarkably, definitive erythrocytes of birds remain nucleated, despite the high demand for oxygen during flight. Possibly, the highly efficient respiratory system of birds alleviates the need for enucleated erythrocytes to support their high metabolic rate.

Although the chicken is a great experimental system to investigate early developmental processes, genetic approaches can only be applied to a very limited extent in this organism. The chicken has therefore not become a widely used model system to study erythropoiesis in vivo. Nevertheless, lineage-tracing studies combined with detailed morphological analyses are still expected to contribute significantly to the understanding of the ontogeny of vertebrate hematopoiesis.[37]

MAMMALIAN ERYTHROPOIESIS

The first erythroid cells appearing during mammalian development emerge in the extraembryonic location of the yolk sac (Fig. 2.1a,b). These cells are formed in close association with the endothelial lining of the emerging blood vessels, before the vasculature is connected to the embryo and the onset of blood circulation.[38] Once released in the bloodstream, the macrocytic primitive erythrocytes retain proliferative capacity and mitotic figures are observed in the circulating blood of early mammalian embryos (Fig. 2.1c).[39] Intravascular erythropoiesis is not normally observed at any other developmental stage; both fetal and adult erythrocytes are enucleated before they enter the circulation. The view has long been held that primitive erythrocytes remain nucleated and that they disappear from the circulation very quickly during the embryonic to fetal transition period. Until recently, the fate of these cells was a mystery, but more recent work has shown that the primitive cells in fact enucleate very efficiently between days 12.5 and 14.5 of mouse development, resulting in macrocytic, enucleated, erythrocytes.[40] At this stage, the first fetal liver-derived definitive erythrocytes appear in the circulation and their numbers increase rapidly (Fig. 2.1e–h). This has made it particularly difficult to trace the remaining primitive erythrocytes. The use of transgenes that specifically label the primitive cells with a green fluorescent reporter protein has demonstrated that the primitive cells are a stable population that persist through the end of gestation.[40] The primitive cells are characterized by the expression of embryonic globins (εy, βh1, and ζ in the mouse, ε, γ, and ζ in human) resulting in a variety of hemoglobin tetramers in man ($\zeta_2\varepsilon_2$ (Gower1); $\alpha_2\varepsilon_2$ (Gower2), $\zeta_2\gamma_2$ (Portland1) $\zeta_2\beta_2$ (Portland2)). Mice immediately switch to adult globins when definitive erythropoiesis starts in the fetal liver. Expression of a specific fetal β-like-globin (γ-globin) is a feature of anthropoid primates. Hemoglobin tetramers consisting of α- and γ-globin chains ($\alpha_2\gamma_2$) are known as fetal hemoglobin (HbF) in humans. These specialized hemoglobins allow the developing fetus to extract oxygen more efficiently from the maternal blood. Near the time of birth, the site of erythropoiesis switches to the bone marrow and the spleen. Humans rely mainly on the bone marrow for steady-state adult erythropoiesis, but in mice the spleen remains an important erythropoietic organ during adult life (Fig. 2.1k,l). Under stress conditions, for instance caused by low oxygen pressure or anemia, the spleen is used to expand the erythropoietic capacity in both species.[41] Fetal globin expression is silenced in adult erythropoiesis. Hemoglobin tetramers composed of α- and β-globin ($\alpha_2\beta_2$, HbA) account for approximately 97% of all hemoglobin in adult erythrocytes. HbA_2 ($\alpha_2\delta_2$) and HbF account, respectively, for approximately 2% and <1% of total hemoglobin in most adults. HbF is restricted to a few cells, termed F cells, in normal adults.[42] Clonal analysis has shown that F cells are derived from the same progenitor cells as the cells containing adult globin, which rules out that fetal and adult stem cell lineages coexist.[43] Some individuals maintain higher levels of HbF throughout adult life. This condition is known as hereditary persistence of fetal hemoglobin (HPFH) and is caused in the majority of cases by deletions in the β-*globin* locus, but also by point mutations in the γ-*globin* gene promoters.[44] In rare cases, the HPFH phenotype does not segregate with the β-*globin* locus, suggesting a *trans*-regulatory mechanism (see also Chapter 14). The HPFH condition is not clinically manifest, but it is a factor ameliorating the effects of β thalassemia and sickle cell disease. Reactivation of γ-*globin* expression in adults with these disorders is therefore a very attractive therapeutic approach, because the majority of patients will have normal γ-globin genes that they have switched off after birth. Despite the fact that mice do not have a fetal *β-like* globin gene, the γ-globin genes in human β-*globin* locus transgenes are expressed in the early fetal liver, and silenced later in development.[45,46] Furthermore, γ-*globin* transgenes with HPFH mutations in the promoter recreate the HPFH condition in mice.[47,48] The use of transgenic mice for the study of human globin gene regulation is described in detail in Chapter 5.

ERYTHROID DIFFERENTIATION

Erythroid cells are derived from HSCs but the path they follow is still a matter of debate (Fig. 2.2).[49] There is no evidence for direct feedback of committed progenitors to the HSC compartment since the number of stem and early progenitor cells is little affected by extreme fluctuations in numbers of end-stage cells of any of the lineages. This protects the stem cell compartment from depletion by differentiation. Indeed, lineage fate decisions may be a more stochastic process in which there are probabilities of outcome dictating differentiation among the various lineages while the fate of an individual cell remains undirected and unpredictable.[50] The interplay of the internal transcription program and epigenetic alterations (such as DNA methylation and chromatin modifications) on the one hand with the external environment (such as localized growth factor concentrations and cell–cell interactions) on the other is complex as discussed extensively in Chapter 1.

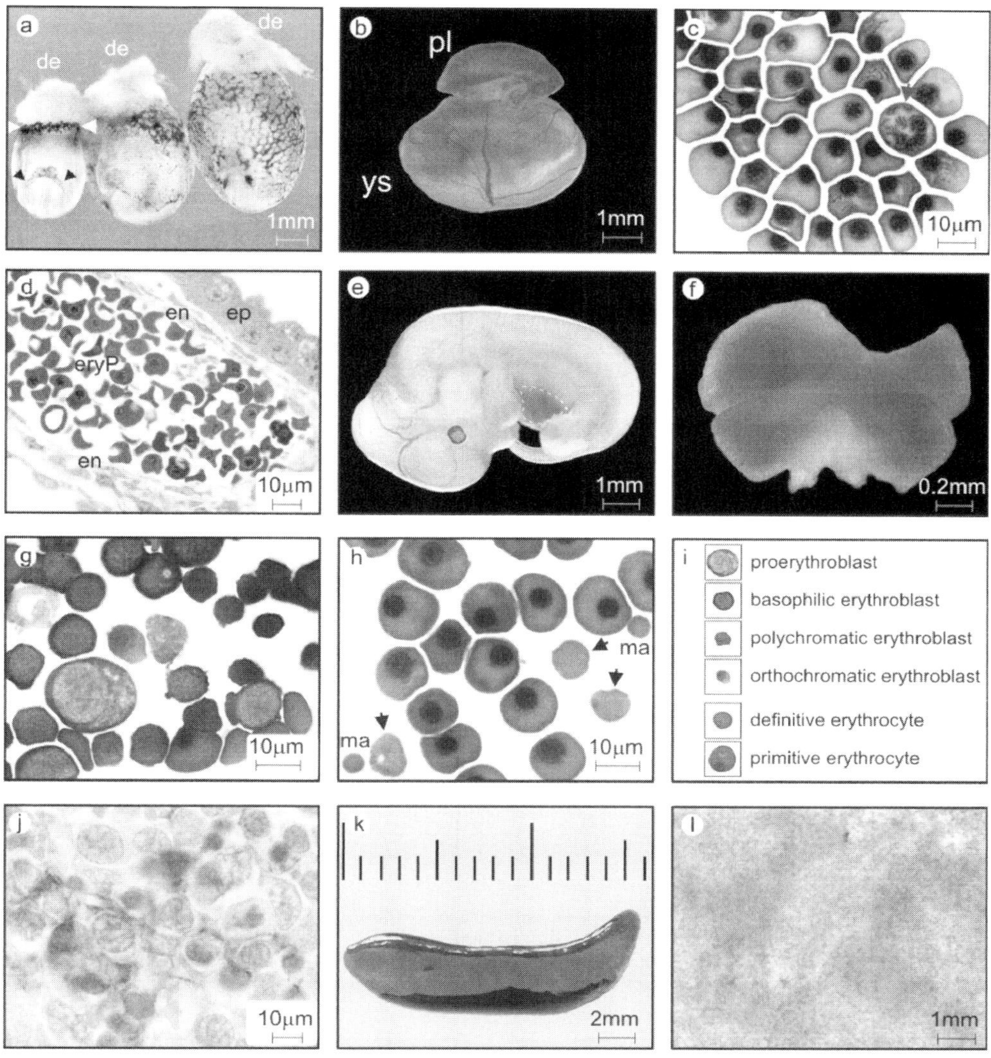

Figure 2.1. Erythropoiesis during mouse development. **(a)** E8.5 embryos, inside their yolk sacs, carrying a *LacZ* reporter gene driven by β*-globin* regulatory elements. Erythroid cells appear dark after staining for LacZ activity. White arrowheads point at the blood islands emerging as a ring at the top of the yolk sac. These are spreading through the developing vasculature, illustrated by the two embryos on the right that are progressively more advanced in development. The black arrowheads indicate the linear heart tube that already appears to contain erythroid cells before the yolk sac cells have reached the embryo. de = decidua, remaining maternal tissue. **(b)** E11.5 embryo inside its yolk sac. The blood-filled yolk sac vasculature is apparent. ys = yolk sac; pl = placenta. **(c)** Cytospin of E11.5 peripheral blood, stained with dianisidine and histological dyes.[207] Nuclei are dark, the hemoglobin-filled cytoplasm brown. Red arrow: cell in mitosis. **(d)** Section of a yolk sac vessel at E12.5, stained with toluidine/methylene blue. eryP = primitive erythrocytes; en = endothelial cells; ep = columnar epithelial cells. **(e)** E12.5 mouse embryo; the fetal liver area is indicated by a dotted line. **(f)** E12.5 fetal liver. **(g)** Cytospin of E12.5 fetal liver cells, stained as in (c). **(h)** Cytospin of E12.5 blood, stained as in (c). ma = contaminating maternal erythrocyte **(i)** key to (g) and (h). **(j)** Erythroblastic island in E13.5 fetal liver. The cytoplasmic extensions of the central macrophage (stained with the F4/80 antibody [brown]) are surrounding erythroid cells at various stages of differentiation. **(k)** Spleen of an adult mouse. **(l)** Section of adult mouse spleen stained as in (c). Red pulp, containing the erythroid cells, is stained brown; white pulp is stained blue. (See color plate 2.1.)

Early progenitors are capable of giving rise to multilineage colonies but whether there is a fixed order to cell fate decisions (i.e., at each stage a cell has limited choices) or whether there is greater plasticity to a cell's potential fates remains to be resolved. Among the models proposed, the one put forward by the Weissman group has been perhaps the most accepted (Fig. 2.2). It posits a decision between two fates at each step in differentiation, thereby gradually diminishing the lineage potential. The initial decision separates the lymphoid and myeloid lineages with commitment to either a common lymphoid progenitor (CLP) or a common myeloid progenitor (CMP). The CLP can give rise to either B or T lymphocytes whereas the fate of the CMP is to give rise to either of two bipotential cells,

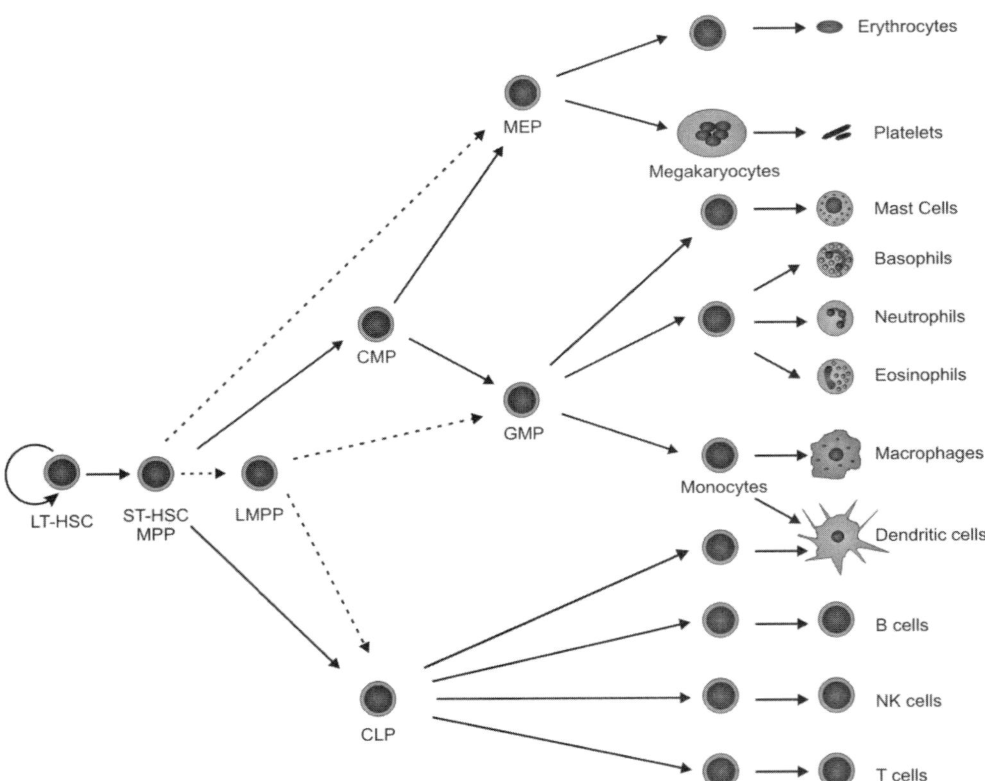

Figure 2.2. Possible pathways of hematopoietic differentiation from the HSC. In the scheme proposed by the Weissman group[51–53] (solid arrows), multipotential progenitors (MPP or short-term HSC [ST-HSC]) give rise to either a CLP or a CMP, which in turn gives rise to either a GMP (equivalent to CFU-GM) or an MEP. The scheme suggested by Adolfsson et al.[54] (dotted arrows) involves the generation of MEPs directly from the MPP/ST-HSC, whereas a LMPP has the potential to generate both CLPs and GMPs. These schemes are not necessarily exclusive and alternate schemes have been proposed (see text). LT-HSC = long-term HSC; NK cell = natural killer cell. Adapted from ref. 148.

the colony-forming unit (CFU)–granulocyte macrophage (GM) (ultimately producing macrophages or granulocytes) or the CFU-erythrocyte/megakaryocyte (E/Meg) leading to erythrocyte or megakaryocyte cells.[51–53] Alternate schemes have been proposed. Adolfsson et al.[54] first identified a highly proliferative lymphoid primed multipotent progenitor (LMPP) with GM potential but that was devoid of the ability to adopt erythroid or megakaryocytic lineage fates (Fig. 2.2). Transcription profiling confirmed a close relationship of early lymphoid and early GM precursors and Meg/E cells showed an early divergence and their own gene expression signature.[55,56] Cells expressing a *Gata-1* or *Pu.1* reporter gene have also been used to analyze early hemopoietic differentiation. *Gata-1* and *Pu.1* are mutually antagonistic, inhibiting each other's expression and transactivation domains and are believed to be critical in GM/lymphoid versus Meg/E lineage commitment. *Pu.1* is expressed in the HSC and upregulated expression of the *Pu.1* reporter was observed in progenitors that included granulocyte-macrophage–lymphoid progenitors (LMPP or GMLP) as well as CMPs. In contrast, cells marked by a *Gata-1* reporter gene gave rise to CMPs that could generate megakaryocyte–erythroid progenitors (MEPs) and granulocyte–macrophage progenitors (GMPs). These various schemes are discussed and compared by Ye and Graf[57] and Murre.[58]

Populations of cells corresponding to these progenitors can be purified by fluorescence-activated cell sorting (FACS) based on the expression of various cell surface markers, and the lineage output of these cells is determined by the phenotype of the colonies emerging from colony assays in the presence of growth factors. The results, therefore, are dependent on the cell surface markers chosen and on the assumption that the culture conditions are adequate to identify all lineage potentials of an individual cell. The differentiation schemes described previously demonstrate possible routes to terminal differentiation without precluding alternatives and need not represent the preferred route in vivo, as opposed to the in vitro route imposed by the experimental conditions. They are qualitative (or semiquantitative) assessments of the possible outputs, but to know what occurs in the in vivo processes would require a quantitative audit of stem and progenitor cell outputs that is beyond what is currently attainable.

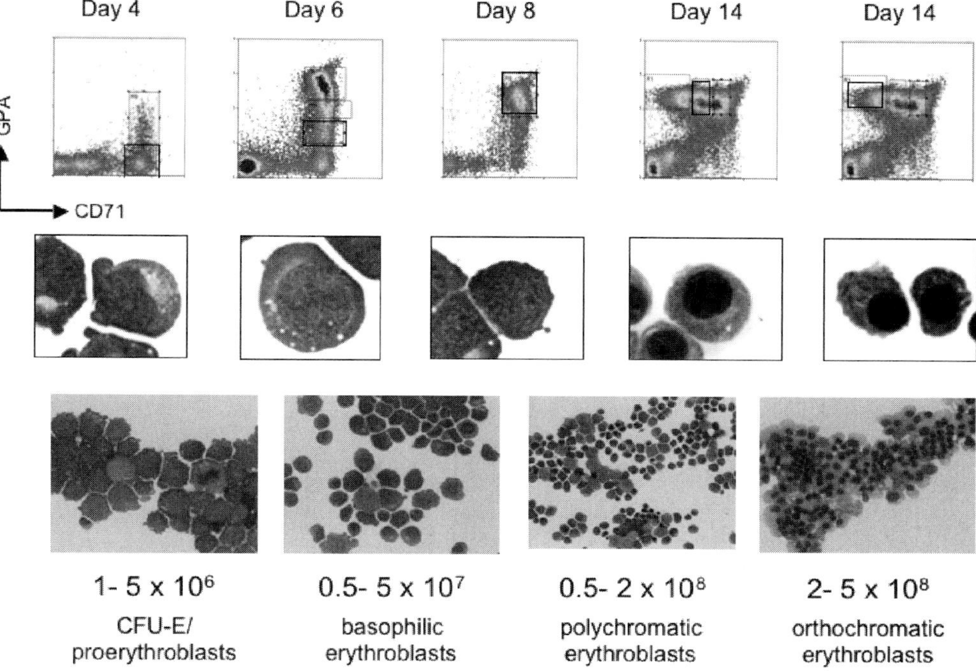

Figure 2.3. Purification of human erythroblasts. Top: FACS analysis of human erythroblasts grown in vitro by the method of Fibach et al;[61] days refers to the time in phase 2 of culture. Middle: High-power view of cells sorted from the gate shown as a bold rectangle in the plot above. Bottom: Low-power view of the same sorted cells, together with representative cell numbers obtainable from mononuclear cells from 1 U of blood. (See color plate 2.3.)

ERYTHROID PROGENITORS

The earliest erythroid progenitor identified is the burst-forming unit-erythroid (BFU-E), so called because of its appearance; the earliest progeny are motile, giving rise to a multisubunit colony (or burst). These appear as large colonies containing up to several thousand hemoglobinized cells after 5–8 (mouse) or 10–14 (human) days in methylcellulose cultures. Their growth is dependent on several growth factors of which stem cell factor ([SCF] also known as Steel factor or Kit ligand), thrombopoietin (Tpo), interleukin-3 (IL-3), IL-11, and Flt3 ligand are among the most important. They are not initially dependent on Epo, which may be withheld for a few days but then becomes essential to complete terminal differentiation to hemoglobinized cells. BFU-E occur at a frequency of 40–120/10^5 bone marrow cells and also circulate in the peripheral blood at a frequency of 10–40/10^5 light density mononuclear cells.[59]

The late erythroid progenitors, CFU-erythroid (CFU-E), consist of small colonies of 16– 125 cells that appear after 2–3 (mouse) or 5–8 (human) days in culture. They are approximately 5–8 times as abundant as BFU-E in bone marrow and, under normal circumstances, they do not appear in the circulation. The division of erythroid progenitors into BFU-Es and CFU-Es is useful, but somewhat arbitrary because it masks the fact that there is a continuum of progenitors from the earliest multisubunit BFU-Es to late BFU-Es (large single colonies) to the smallest colonies derived from late CFU-Es. As progenitors undergo this differentiation process their numbers increase, with their proliferative potential simultaneously decreasing.

LIQUID CULTURE OF ERYTHROID CELLS

After the development of semisolid cultures for the growth of BFU-E and CFU-E, a number of techniques have been described for the production of erythroblasts in liquid cultures.[60–62] The cells proliferate and differentiate in a one-phase or two-phase system and although culture conditions differ in each protocol, SCF, Epo, dexamethasone, and transferrin are commonly present, frequently supplemented by insulin or insulin-like growth factor–I (IGF-I). The starting material may be CD34 positive cells or mononuclear cells. Discarded buffy coat samples obtained from a blood bank may produce a total of up to 5×10^8 erythroblasts from 1 U with a purity of up to 90% (Fig. 2.3). The great advantage of these techniques is that they allow the production of large numbers of erythroblasts from peripheral blood samples, enabling functional analyses of normal or abnormal erythropoiesis without the need for bone marrow sampling. In addition, erythroid cultures can also be obtained using mouse or human embryonic stem cells as the starting material,[63–65] and there has been significant progress in development of culture techniques that enable large-scale production of fully matured human

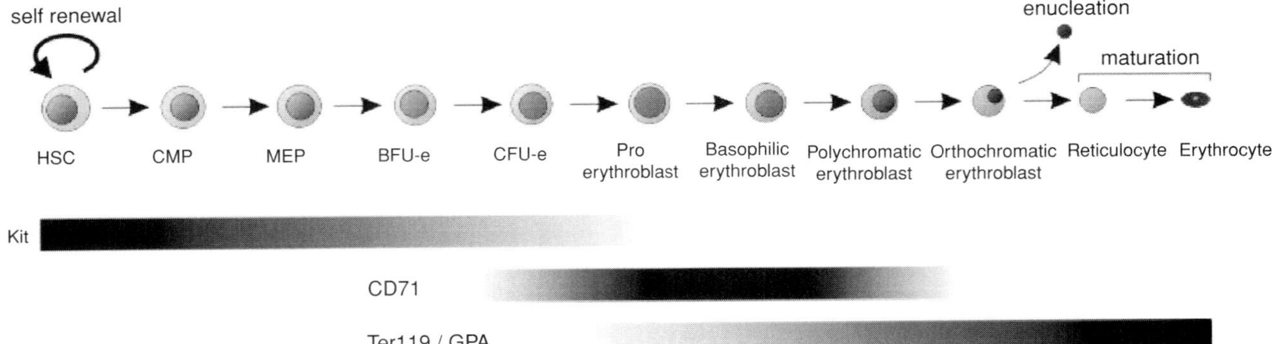

Figure 2.4. Schematic representation of the erythroid differentiation series in the mouse. The expression of the most commonly used cell surface markers to identify the various stages is indicated by the bars. Gray = low expression; black = high expression. Cells at the CFU-E and proerythroblast stages are the most sensitive to, and dependent on, the presence of Epo. We refer to Chapter 1 for a description of cell surface markers used to characterize the HSC compartment.

erythrocytes.[66,67] Although this raises the prospects of producing completely defined erythrocytes for transfusion purposes, it is prohibitively expensive and a daunting task to generate the vast numbers of cells required for clinical practice.[68]

ERYTHROID CELL PURIFICATION

Purification techniques for populations highly enriched for CFU-E/Megs have been described for both human[53] and murine[51] bone marrow, but purifying BFU-E alone has been less successful. CFU-E can be obtained as a pure population, either by physical techniques[69] or by FACS. CD36 positive cells with very high levels of CD71 (transferrin receptor) expression but negative for glycophorin A define the CFU-E population (Fig. 2.4). Low levels of glycophorin A appear at the proerythroblast stage and increase, reaching maximum fluorescence levels in basophilic erythroblasts. CD71 remains high throughout this phase but then declines as maturation proceeds, becoming undetectable in orthochromatic erythroblasts and reticulocytes, whereas glycophorin A levels are maintained. Thus, the stages of erythroid maturation from CFU-E onward can be analyzed, quantitated, and even sorted by this method. Because this results in a rather crude division of the differentiation stages, there remains the need for additional cell surface markers to define these in more detail.

REGULATION OF ERYTHROPOIESIS

It is clear that in hypoxia or anemia, increased output of red cells is strongly correlated with the levels of circulating Epo; however, the earliest erythroid progenitors are responsive to a number of hemopoietic cytokines including Tpo, GM-CSF, IL-3, and IL-11, and in particular to SCF. SCF binds to its receptor Kit, a tyrosine kinase that signals through several pathways including phosphoinositide-3 (PI-3) kinase, Src kinases, and phospholipase Cγ (see later), after dimerization and autophosphorylation. At later stages, SCF acts synergistically with Epo in the proliferation and expansion of the developing erythroid progenitors and may play a role in phosphorylating the EpoR itself.[70]

HYPOXIA SENSING

In response to reduced oxygen availability, the body responds in many ways, such as increasing Epo production, by altering the glycolytic pathway, and by inducing new blood vessel formation via the vascular endothelial growth factor and upregulating transferrin receptor levels. But how is hypoxia sensed and measured? Hypoxia response elements are found in many different genes, displaying a range of tissue-specific expression patterns. The elements are bound by a heterodimeric transcription factor 1 (HIF1), comprising HIF1-α (the regulatory partner) and HIF1-β (identical to the aryl hydrocarbon receptor translocator protein).[71] Under normoxic conditions, prolyl residues in HIF1-α become hydroxylated, targeting it for binding by the von Hippel–Lindau ubiquitin ligase complex.[72] This results in proteolytic destruction of HIF1-α by the proteasome. The hydroxylases responsible have an absolute requirement for dioxygen, thus linking their function to the availability of molecular oxygen.[73] Hypoxia, therefore, suppresses the hydroxylation allowing the assembly of a transcriptionally active HIF1 complex. In the kidney and liver, a cooperative interaction of HIF with hepatic nuclear factor-4, including recruitment of the coactivator CBP/p300, occurs in the 3′ end of the *Epo* gene, leading to a significant increase in transcription (Fig. 2.5).[74,75]

ERYTHROPOIETIN

A humoral factor controlling red cell production was first demonstrated in 1906, its source was shown to be the kidney, and the Epo protein was purified in 1977.[76] When the *Epo* gene was cloned, a hypoxia response element was identified in the DNA at its 3′ end and it soon became clear that this element was not restricted to this gene but that a specific, sensitive hypoxia response was a general feature of mammalian cells.[77] Epo acts on its receptor to trigger several different signal transduction systems, which allow the survival, proliferation, and maturation of the erythroid cells.[78] In the absence of Epo, the cells rapidly undergo apoptosis and the antiapoptotic function of Epo is clearly an important facet of its action.[39] The main initial site of Epo production is the fetal liver, with production largely switching to the kidney shortly after birth. Under normoxic conditions, little or no Epo mRNA is detectable in the kidneys but hypoxia results in its accumulation within 30 min in the peritubular interstitial cells and levels can increase 200-fold over baseline.[79] Epo is a 166–amino acid, 34.4-kD glycoprotein found in serum at baseline levels of 1–30 mU/mL that can be elevated 1000-fold by severe anemia. It contains approximately 40% carbohydrate, rich in sialic acid residues, and has a half-life of 7–8 hours in plasma, whereas nonglycosylated Epo is cleared rapidly from the circulation.

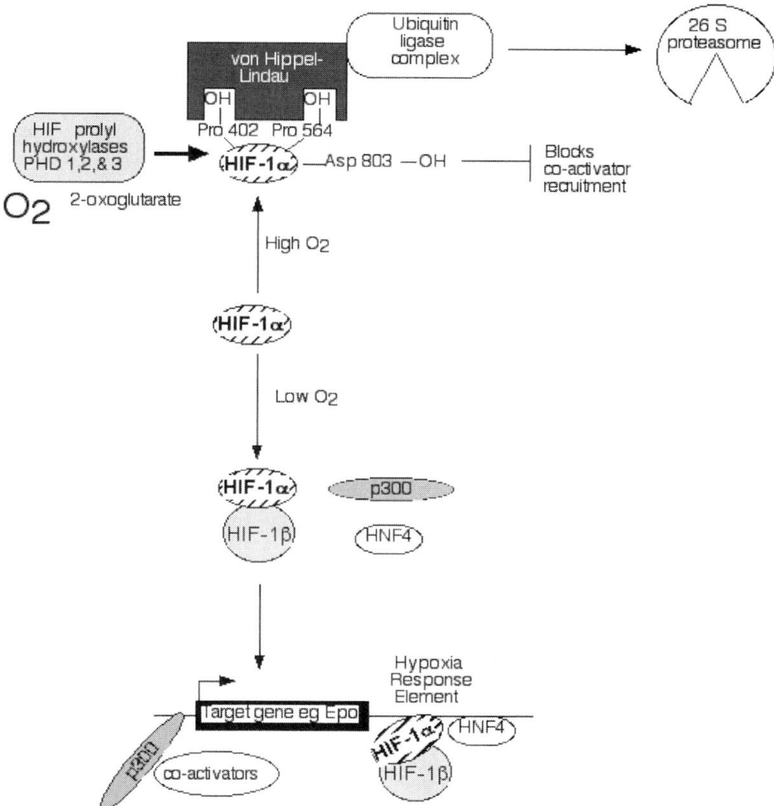

Figure 2.5. The regulation of *Epo* gene expression. The *Epo* gene is primarily regulated by HIF. The HIF1α subunit is highly unstable under normal or raised oxygen levels and is readily hydroxylated by the three HIF prolyl hydroxylases, PHD1-3, reactions which are directly dependent on oxygen. Hydroxylated HIF1α is rapidly destroyed by the proteasome after binding to the von Hippel–Lindau protein and ubiquitination. Under low oxygen conditions, HIF1α binds with the stable but limiting HIF1β subunit and translocates to hypoxia response elements in its target genes including, in the kidney, the *Epo* gene. In conjunction with other transcription factors and coactivators such as CBP/p300, gene expression is activated.

The cloning of the *Epo* gene allowed expression of a recombinant human Epo in mammalian cells that could be harvested for clinical use. It immediately found therapeutic application in end-stage renal disease. Its use has now expanded to many neoplastic (hematological and nonhematological) conditions associated with anemia as an underlying condition or as a result of cytotoxic treatment. Modified forms of Epo, with a higher carbohydrate content and longer half-lives in vivo have been developed and approved for clinical usage, and small-molecule Epo mimetics with higher affinity for the EpoR are under investigation.[80,81]

ERYTHROPOIETIN RECEPTOR AND CELL SIGNALING

Epo exerts its effects on erythroid cells via the EpoR. The low numbers (20–50) of EpoRs on BFU-E explain the relative Epo nonresponsiveness of these cells, and much higher levels (300–500) are found in CFU-E, proerythroblasts, and basophilic erythroblasts. The EpoR is a member of a cytokine receptor superfamily that includes growth hormone, prolactin, G-CSF, GM-CSF, and M-CSF receptors.[82] The 507–amino acid molecule contains an N-terminal extracellular domain consisting of a fibronectin type III repeat divided into two subdomains, each containing two cysteine residues that form an intradomain disulfide bond. A highly conserved WSXWS motif lies close to the transmembrane segment. The intracellular C-terminal end of the molecule contains eight tyrosine residues with potential for phosphorylation, associated with the binding of several proteins containing Src homology 2 (SH2) domains. Knock-in mice with a truncation of the final 108 amino acids of this domain, including seven of the Tyr residues (EpoR-H), as well as the same truncation plus a Y343F substitution (EpoR-HM), are viable and fertile with normal hematology.[83] Abnormalities in signaling under low Epo levels and under stress suggest that redundancy in signal transduction means that this part of the receptor is not essential for red cell production.[84,85] The EpoR exists in a nonliganded dimeric form which, on binding Epo, undergoes a conformational change bringing together the intracellular parts of the dimer (Fig. 2.6). Bound to the EpoR, close to the transmembrane region, is the tyrosine kinase Janus kinase 2 (JAK2). Increasing the proximity of the JAK2 molecules activates them to transphosphorylate each other and also to phosphorylate the tyrosine residues on the EpoR itself. This provides docking sites for signal transducers and activators of transcription proteins (STAT, principally STAT

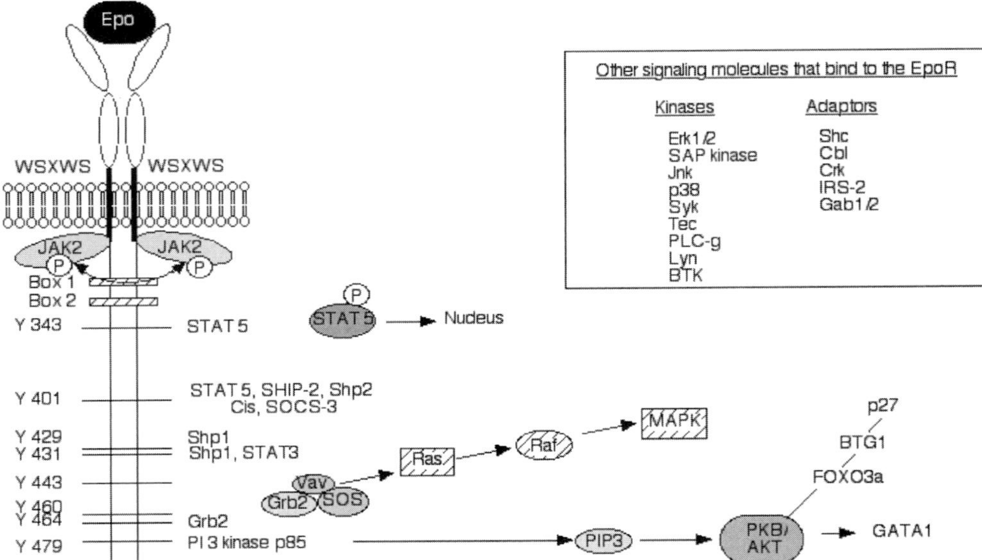

Figure 2.6. Schematic diagram of the Epo receptor showing some of the signal transduction pathways initiated when Epo binds. Multiple signals are transduced and many have been observed only in cell lines rather than in primary erythroblasts. The complexity and redundancy is demonstrated by the lack of an erythroid phenotype when many of the molecules are mutated or knocked out in mice. For a more detailed discussion see ref. 208.

5a and 5b in erythroid cells) to bind via their SH2 domains. They too become phosphorylated by JAK2 kinase, whereupon the STATs dimerize and move to the nucleus to stimulate gene transcription.

Phosphorylation of the EpoR allows the recruitment of other proteins containing SH2 domains to the receptor, including SHP1, SHP2, SHIP, PI-3 kinase, Lnk, PLC-γ, and suppressor of cytokine signaling, which contribute to alternative transduction pathways having effector or repressor effects on erythropoiesis. The Ras-mitogen-activated protein kinase and PI-3 kinase transduction pathways in particular appear to play important roles in erythroid cell production. Protein kinase B or AKT is a major downstream effector of PI-3 kinase–activated by Epo binding and is responsible for phosphorylation of a serine residue in GATA-1, a transcription factor necessary for maturation of the erythroid cells.[86,87] Germline mutations of some of these components suggest overlap or redundancy of function,[88] which makes the interpretation of results complex, and a phenotype may only be exposed under stress conditions or at early stages in development when erythropoiesis is maximal. Understanding the relative contributions of each pathway to red cell proliferation and maturation will be an important consideration of future research (Fig. 2.6). The effects of dysregulated signal transduction on red cell production are graphically illustrated by patients with mutations in the C-terminal inhibitory domain of the EpoR, causing erythrocytosis,[89,90] and patients with activating mutations in the JAK2 kinase, causing polycythemia vera.[91,92]

Epo signaling is negatively regulated by suppressor of cytokine signaling proteins and several phosphatases, including SHP1, SHP2, and protein tyrosine phosphatase 1B, which can modulate the activity of JAK2 kinase. Null mutants of some of these regulators may display increased numbers of erythroid progenitors or increased sensitivity to Epo levels, but a complete understanding of their regulatory roles awaits further analysis. Among the target genes of Epo stimulation, antiapoptotic genes have an important role. In particular, *Bcl-X$_L$* expression is markedly stimulated by Epo via STAT5, acting principally at the later stages of erythroid maturation.[93,94] Bcl-X$_L$ knockout mice die at approximately embryonic day 13 (E13), displaying apoptotic hematopoietic cells in the fetal liver.[95] Ablation of Bcl-X$_L$ in erythroid cells causes anemia in adult mice,[93,94] although it is still under debate whether Bcl-X$_L$ mediates the antiapoptotic effects of Epo.[93]

KNOCKOUT PHENOTYPES OF SIGNAL TRANSDUCTION MOLECULES INVOLVED IN ERYTHROPOIESIS

The central role of Epo and the EpoR in red cell production is emphasized by the similarity of the phenotypes of animals homozygous for their knockouts.[39,96] In both cases, there are reduced numbers of primitive erythrocytes but the embryos die at E12.5–13.5 due to a failure of definitive erythropoiesis. The fetal liver contains both BFU-E and CFU-E, in increased numbers in Epo$^{-/-}$ embryos, indicating that erythroid cells can develop to this stage without Epo signaling. The survival, proliferation, and terminal differentiation of these cells are dependent on Epo and the transduction of its signals. JAK2 knockout homozygotes die a day earlier than Epo and EpoR knockouts with fewer erythroid progenitors, suggesting that signaling via JAK2 operates earlier in erythropoiesis.[97,98] In contrast, mice deficient in STAT5a and 5b are viable, albeit with reduced numbers of early erythroblasts, particularly in fetal life in which erythropoiesis is maximal.[99] Bcl-x null mice die at day 13 with a neuronal and hemopoietic phenotype.[95] Mice with a conditional knockout of Bcl-x exhibited splenic erythroblastosis and severe anemia due to apoptosis of late-stage erythroblasts.[93,94] Day 14.5 mice deficient for the p85a subunit of PI-3 kinase are pale with a marked reduction of mature erythrocytes in their peripheral blood. Furthermore, the absolute number and frequency of both BFU-E and CFU-E are reduced in *p85*$^{-/-}$ fetal livers compared with wild-type controls, which is associated with reduced proliferation.[100] Complete deletion of the *SCF* gene or its receptor tyrosine kinase Kit results in death at E14–16 from severe anemia.[101]

OTHER HORMONAL INFLUENCES ON ERYTHROPOIESIS

A positive effect of androgenic steroids on erythropoiesis has long been recognized and used in the treatment of various disorders with red cell production failures, including renal disease before the introduction of recombinant Epo. Their activity includes increased Epo production in vivo[102,103] and increased numbers of BFU-E and CFU-E in vitro.[104,105] Glucocorticoids, such as dexamethasone, massively increase erythroid progenitor proliferation in cell culture systems from chick, mouse, and human hemopoietic cells.[60,106] Removal of dexamethasone is necessary to move from the proliferation stage to erythroblast maturation in some in vitro systems[107] but not others.[61] That thyroid disorders are frequently associated with anemia and modulation of erythropoiesis, particularly by triiodothyronine, is long established,[108,109] possibly acting through a receptor with β_2 adrenergic properties.[110] In proliferation/maturation systems, T_3 reduces proliferation, increases maturation, and may play a role in enucleation.[107] T_3 signaling through the nuclear receptor TRα is also essential for the transient spleen erythropoiesis in the mouse at birth.[111] Cortisol, estrogen, and progesterone do not promote erythropoiesis. The effects of insulin, IGF-I, and IGF-II, frequently included in in vitro systems, remain to be clarified.

STEADY-STATE ERYTHROPOIESIS

Erythrocytes represent the most common cell type in adult blood. Human blood contains approximately 5×10^6 erythrocytes/μL (normal range 4.7–6.1 $\times 10^6$ for males and 4.2–5.4 $\times 10^6$ for females); these cells have an average lifespan of 120 days. Erythroid cells at the terminal stages of differentiation have shed their nucleus, endoplasmic reticulum, and mitochondria, and consequently they are no longer able to proliferate. To maintain the red blood cell count in approximately 5 L of blood of an adult individual, approximately 2.4×10^6 new erythrocytes have to be produced each second. The new cells enter the circulation as reticulocytes that are still engaged in protein translation. In humans, it takes approximately 1 week for reticulocytes to complete the maturation process. In the bone marrow, a series of intermediate erythroid precursors can be recognized that progressively gain erythroid characteristics (Fig. 2.4). Development from the proerythroblast to the reticulocyte involves four–five rapid cell divisions, resulting in a progressive reduction in cell size. Mature erythrocytes have a diameter of only 6–8 μm. Their small size and biconcave shape create a large surface area for gas exchange and allow the cells to enter the microcapillaries in the tissues.

ERYTHROBLASTIC ISLANDS ARE THE STRUCTURAL UNITS OF DEFINITIVE ERYTHROPOIESIS

In the bone marrow, the structural unit where erythropoiesis takes place is termed the erythroblastic island.[112] It consists of a central macrophage (also known as the nurse cell) surrounded by differentiating erythroid progenitors. Erythroblastic islands are also found in the mouse fetal liver (Fig. 2.1j), but a role for an analogous structure has not been identified in yolk sac erythropoiesis. The fact that yolk sac cells enter the circulation while they are still nucleated, a process in which the macrophage plays an important role, supports the notion that primitive erythropoiesis does not take place in islands. Efficient enucleation of definitive cells can be observed in vitro in colony assays and bulk cultures of primary cells, in the absence of macrophages. Macrophages are formed during primitive hematopoiesis, and it will therefore require further investigation to determine the role of these cells in primitive erythropoiesis. A number of proteins on the surface of the macrophage and the erythroblasts mediate interactions between the macrophage and the erythroblasts, and between the erythroblasts themselves.

The erythroblast–macrophage protein ([EMP] or macrophage–erythroblast attacher [MAEA]) is expressed on both cell types and mediates adhesion between the cells. Maea knockout mice survive until birth, displaying defects in terminal erythroid maturation.[113] Formation of erythroblastic islands is impaired and Maea null macrophages appear to lack the extensive cytoplasmic extensions typical of mature macrophages. Maea null macrophages are unable to interact with wild-type erythroblasts. In contrast, Maea null erythroblasts can interact with wild-type macrophages, but this does not rescue the enucleation defect of these erythroblasts. In enucleating wild-type erythroblasts, Maea colocalizes with F-actin aggregates present at the constriction between the extruding nucleus and the reticulocyte. The actin cytoskeleton in Maea null erythroblasts is predominantly localized to the cell membrane, and very little cytoplasmic actin is observed. Maea-deficient macrophages display condensed, less organized actin filaments and are unable to efficiently develop long cytoplasmic extensions. Collectively, it can be concluded that Maea is required for the organization of the erythroblastic island and for efficient enucleation of erythroblasts.

Maea is likely involved in the organization of the actin cytoskeleton in both macrophages and erythroblasts. Of note, disruption of F-actin bundles with cytochalasin D treatment inhibits enucleation.[114] Furthermore, ablation of paladin (Plld), a protein involved in the organization of the actin cytoskeleton, causes a dramatic reduction in the number of definitive fetal liver erythrocytes. Plld-deficient macrophages are unable to interact with erythroblasts,[115] providing evidence for autonomous macrophage-specific functions in the islands. This is further emphasized by studies of Dnase2a knockout mice. This lysosomal enzyme digests the large amounts of DNA taken up by the macrophages when they engulf the nuclei expelled from the erythroblasts. Dnase2a-deficient macrophages accumulate nuclear DNA from phagocytosed nuclei and appear to lose progressively the ability to support erythropoiesis. At E17.5, Dnase2a knockout fetuses are severely anemic, owing to the failure of definitive erythropoiesis, and no surviving newborn animals are found. Transplantation experiments demonstrated that Dnase2a$^{-/-}$ erythroid cells can develop to mature erythrocytes, supporting the notion that the primary defect is in the macrophage lineage.[116] Induction of interferon (IFN)-α expression in the affected macrophages appears to be the primary cause of the lethal anemia as breeding of the Dnase2a-deficient mice to mice deficient in the type I IFN receptor resulted in compound mutants that were born healthy.[117]

The role of other cell adhesion molecules and interactions with extracellular matrix proteins such as laminin and fibronectin is less clearly defined. Erythroblasts express α_4 (*Itga4*)/CD29/β_1 integrin (*Itgb1*), and the CD242 ([*Icam4*] LW blood group) counterreceptor. Macrophages express CD51 (α_V integrin, *Itgav*) and the vascular cell adhesion molecule 1 (Vcam1) counter receptor. Perturbation of the integrin system can adversely affect erythroblastic island formation[118] and stress erythropoiesis,[119] but the generic role of cell adhesion in tissue integrity and the considerable potential for redundancy precludes the assignment of specific functions to individual factors.

A role for signaling between erythroid cells in the island has been most convincingly demonstrated for death ligand–death receptor interactions. Erythroid cells express the CD95 (*Fas*) death receptor throughout differentiation. Only mature cells express the ligand CD95L (*Fasl*), but these cells are insensitive to Fas signaling. In contrast, immature cells activate proapoptotic proteases in response to Fasl exposure. The levels of the essential transcription factors Tal1 and Gata1 are reduced through cleavage by activated caspases, most notably by caspase 3 (Casp3).[120–122] This cleavage will stop progression along the erythroid differentiation pathway and may induce cell death. A decreased survival rate of erythroid progenitor cells is a hallmark of many acquired and hereditary anemias. Patients with rheumatoid arthritis develop anemia in approximately 50% of cases, and treatment with a blocking antibody directed against the death receptor ligand TNFα improved the anemia and decreased the elevated numbers of apoptotic erythroid progenitors in the bone marrow.[123] An increased rate of apoptosis is also observed in β thalassemia patients. This results in a phenomenon known as ineffective erythropoiesis.[123–126] Up to 80% of erythroid progenitors may be lost due to apoptosis occurring at the polychromatic erythroblast stage.[125] Precipitating α-globin chains may accelerate the apoptotic response.[126] The apoptotic erythroblasts are cleared very rapidly by macrophages. These cells are activated by increased IFNγ levels in approximately one-third of the patients,[127] and this may contribute to the quantitative differences in ineffective erythropoiesis between different patients. In normal erythropoiesis, expelled nuclei are also phagocytosed very rapidly by the central macrophages. Once released, the nuclei contain very low levels of adenosine triphosphate and start to expose phosphatidylserine on their surface very quickly because it requires energy to maintain phosphatidylserine exclusively localized to the inner leaflet of the cell membrane. Surface exposure of phosphatidylserine is an early event in apoptosis and serves as an "eat me" signal for apoptotic cells. This signal is also used for the engulfment of expelled nuclei by the macrophages.[128]

Mice overexpressing the Gata1 transcription factor in late erythroblasts have provided genetic evidence for the occurrence of signaling in the erythroblastic island. Pancellular overexpression of Gata1 causes impaired terminal differentiation, resulting in an embryonic lethal anemia; however, Gata1-overexpressing erythroid cells differentiate normally in vivo when wild-type cells are present, indicating that these cells produce a red cell differentiation signal (REDS) that rescues the defect in Gata1-overexpressing cells.[129] Genetic experiments, combining a tissue-specific Cre/loxP system and X inactivation, were used to produce mice in which half the erythroid cells overexpress Gata1 and half are Gata1 null. These embryos are anemic and die by E14, supporting a homotypic signaling mechanism in which mature erythroid cells produce REDS.[130] The REDS mechanism is reminiscent of the death receptor–death ligand interactions occurring in the erythroblastic island, but whether these are the same or parallel pathways remains to be proven; the large number of possible death receptor–death ligand combinations has not yet been exhaustively tested.[130]

STRESS ERYTHROPOIESIS

Under steady-state conditions, approximately 1% of the erythrocytes are cleared every day and replaced by new cells. Remarkably, the rate of erythropoiesis can increase very significantly from this base line level in response to hypoxia. Hypoxic stress occurs when adequate oxygen supply to all tissues is compromised by insufficient numbers of functional erythrocytes. In a natural setting, this occurs when traveling from sea level to high altitudes. In the clinic, hypoxic stress is a major problem in the large variety of clinical conditions that have anemia as a hallmark. Increasing red cell production is the primary response to counteract hypoxic stress. Epo production in the kidneys is directly regulated by tissue oxygen tension through the activity of the hypoxia-inducible transcription factor complex, discussed earlier in this chapter. It is estimated that less then 10% of the EpoR molecules are liganded with Epo under normal conditions.[131] Because Epo levels may increase up to a 1,000-fold under conditions of severe tissue hypoxia,[77] increased occupancy of EpoR molecules appears to contribute directly to the higher erythropoietic rate. Although Epo is the main regulator of red cell production, other factors have an auxiliary role in the expansion of the erythroid progenitor compartment through their support of progenitor self-renewal. In particular, bone morphogenetic protein-4 ([Bmp4]/Smad5,[132] Stat5,[133] SCF (Kit ligand, Kitl)/Kit,[134] and the glucocorticoid receptor (GR)[135] are known to be involved. The analysis of mouse mutants has revealed distinct requirements for stress erythropoiesis, thus setting it apart from steady-state erythropoiesis. Mice with mutations in the intracellular domain of the EpoR, or expressing EpoR at a reduced level, display virtually normal steady-state erythropoiesis but have an impaired stress erythropoietic response.[83] EpoR signaling promotes erythropoiesis, but it also triggers events that counteract this activity. Mutations that affect this negative feedback loop may result in erythrocytosis. Hyperactive Jak2, the major cytoplasmic target of EpoR that activates multiple downstream pathways, causes polycythemia vera.[91,92] Mice lacking Lnk, a negative regulator of Jak2 activity, display increased numbers of erythroid progenitors and an enhanced response to erythropoietic stress.[136] Shifting the balance between the negative and positive effects of EpoR signaling may therefore be another factor contributing to the increased rate of erythropoiesis under hypoxic stress. The up to 100-fold increase in the numbers of BFU-Es and CFU-Es that occurs in the mouse spleen upon erythropoietic stress is due to the increase of a distinct type of BFU-Es that are unique to the spleen. Steady-state BFU-Es require, in addition to Epo, at least one other growth factor such as SCF. In contrast, high Epo levels alone suffice for stress BFU-E. Their formation is dependent on the Bmp4/Smad5 axis: *Flexed tail* mice, carrying a mutation in Smad5, have an inadequate stress response and are unable to form stress BFU-E.[132] The earlier observation that a GR-dependent progenitor is responsible for the stress response suggests that stress BFU-Es also require an intact GR.[135]

A decreased apoptotic rate of erythroid progenitors may also contribute to the increase in red cell production that occurs under erythropoietic stress. It is believed that under steady-state conditions up to 60% of proerythroblasts succumb to apoptosis in the mouse spleen.[137] Mice deficient for the Stat5 transcription factor, the major downstream signaling target of EpoR, have a blunted stress erythropoietic response. The erythroid progenitors have an increased rate of apoptosis attributed to their failure to upregulate expression of the antiapoptotic Bcl-X_L protein.[99,133] Furthermore, the Fas/Fasl death receptor–death ligand system has been proposed to regulate erythroid homeostasis.[120] Under stress conditions, expression of Fas and Fasl is reduced in erythroid cells and this may therefore contribute to the enhanced survival of these cells observed under these conditions. Interestingly, the expression of Fas and Fasl is repressed by Epo, further indicating that the survival function of the EpoR/Stat5 pathway is an important modulator of the erythropoietic rate.[137]

TRANSCRIPTIONAL REGULATION OF ERYTHROPOIESIS

TRANSCRIPTION FACTORS REQUIRED FOR THE STEM CELL/EARLY PROGENITOR COMPARTMENT AFFECT ERYTHROPOIESIS

A wide variety of transcription factors is known to be involved in the establishment of hematopoietic cell lineages. For example, Tal1, a basic helix-loop-helix transcription factor, and Lmo2, a LIM-domain transcription factor, are critical for the onset of hematopoiesis because null embryos show complete absence of primitive and definitive hematopoiesis.[138–141] The zinc-finger transcription factor Gata2 is also essential for the early stages of hematopoiesis. Both primitive and definitive hematopoiesis are abrogated when the *Gata2* gene is deleted, and it appears to play a role in the proliferation of the early precursors rather than in their differentiation.[142,143] Runx1 is crucial for the early stages of definitive hematopoiesis. In Runx1 null embryos yolk sac hematopoiesis is normal but fetal liver hematopoiesis is absent.[144] Once multipotent progenitors arise from the HSC and proliferate, the process of lineage restriction starts. The first step in this process involves restriction to either the myeloid or the lymphoid lineage. A number of transcription factors that are preferentially expressed in cells destined to one of those fates have been identified but few have been extensively studied. Pu.1, a member of the Ets family of transcription factors, is the best-studied transcription factor known to be involved in lineage restriction at this stage. Pu.1's effect on lineage commitment is dependent on its expression level: A high level of expression leads to commitment to the myeloid lineage whereas lower levels of expression lead to commitment to the lymphoid lineage.[145–147]

Thus, due to their role in the stem cell/progenitor compartment, inactivation of these factors also affects erythropoiesis. Because the number of transcription factors with identifiable functions during hematopoiesis is too vast to allow a thorough discussion of every one of them, we will focus on two examples of factors with an important role in terminal differentiation of erythroid cells. As erythroid cells proceed through differentiation, their nucleus becomes progressively condensed and they shut down expression of many genes that are no longer required. Upregulation of erythroid-specific genes therefore occurs in an increasingly repressive environment, providing a particular challenge to the transcriptional regulators. The role of several transcriptional regulators in erythropoiesis has been mentioned in previous sections of this chapter. Here, we will discuss the transcription factor Gata1, which is essential for expansion and survival of erythroid progenitors, and erythroid Krüppel-like factor (EKLF), a transcription factor required for terminal erythroid differentiation, in more detail because these proteins provide the best-studied examples of erythroid transcriptional regulators.

GATA1

Gata1 is expressed in primitive and definitive erythroid cells and in megakaryocytes, eosinophils, mast cells, dendritic cells, and in the Sertoli cells of the testis.[148] Gene targeting studies have shown that Gata1 is essential for normal erythropoiesis. Gata1 null mouse embryos die of severe anemia between E10.5 and E11.5.[149] Gata1 knockdown embryos (Gata1.05), which express only approximately 5% of the wild-type Gata1 levels, also show an arrest of primitive erythropoiesis and die between E11.5 and E12.5.[150] Other Gata1 knockdown mice (Gata1-low),[151] which express approximately 20% of the wild-type Gata1 levels, show a somewhat milder phenotype. Despite the fact that the majority of Gata1-low mice die between E13.5 and E14.5, due to ineffective primitive and definitive erythroid differentiation, some are born alive (2% of the expected 25%) and a small number survive to adulthood. These mice are anemic at birth but they recover from the anemia and have a normal lifespan. From the analysis of these different mouse models a direct relationship between the expression levels of Gata1 and the severity of the phenotype is evident. Based on the observation that Gata1 null erythroid cells undergo apoptosis, it has been suggested that Gata1 is directly involved in cell survival. One of the known target genes of Gata1 is *Bcl-X*$_L$, a gene encoding an antiapoptotic protein.[152] Another possible Gata1 function is the regulation of G_1/S cell cycle progression. Cell cycle control is very important for erythroid differentiation because progenitors must be able to proliferate to proceed through development, but for terminal differentiation to occur cells must exit the cell cycle.[153] This idea is reinforced by the identification of a variety of Gata1 target genes involved in cell cycle regulation.[154]

Gata1 has also been implicated in the reprogramming of hematopoietic precursors. Forced expression of Gata1 was shown to reprogram myeloblasts and CD34$^+$ bone marrow cells to develop into eosinophils.[155,156] Furthermore, forced expression of Gata1 was also shown to reprogram GMPs to give rise to erythroid, eosinophilic, and basophilic-like cells.[157] Another report[158] shows that ectopic Gata1 expression guides hematopoietic precursors to commitment to the erythrocyte megakaryocytic lineage. Gata1 is known to interact with a variety of cofactors and other transcription factors. Gata1 can homodimerize[159] and has been shown to interact with transcription factors such as EKLF/Sp1,[160] Fog1,[161] PU.1,[162] Rb,[153] and CBP/p300.[163,164] Interestingly, Gata1 can form different protein complexes with distinct transcriptional activity.[165] Gata1 can interact via FOG-1 with the repressive MeCP1 complex, which results in the formation of a complex with histone deacetylase activity that binds to repressed early hematopoietic genes and genes of the eosinophilic lineage. Gata1 can also interact with the essential hematopoietic transcription factor Gfi1b and bind to repressed proliferative genes, while an activating complex of Gata1 with Tal1, and Ldb1 was found at the enhancer of the active erythroid *EKLF* gene. Gata1 also interacts with the Mediator complex, which forms a bridge between transcriptional activators and RNA polymerase II. The mediator subunit Med1 is a coactivator of Gata1 during erythroid development.[166] Thus, Gata1 can acts as a repressor and an activator, regulating multiple target genes that are essential for normal erythropoiesis.[154,167]

GATA-1 MUTATIONS IN HUMAN DISEASE

Mutations in the N-terminal transactivation domain and the N-finger of GATA-1 have been linked to human disease (Fig. 2.7a,b). Missense mutations in the N-finger of GATA-1 have been found in patients with X-linked thrombocytopenia and anemia. The majority of these mutations affect the FOG-1 interaction surface of the N-finger (Fig. 2.7b), adversely affecting the binding of FOG-1.[168–173] This further emphasizes the importance of the FOG-1–GATA-1 interaction. One mutation, R216Q, displays normal FOG-1 interaction. Compared with wild-type GATA-1, this mutant binds with comparable affinity to single GATA sites but with decreased affinity to palindromic sites.[168,172] This indicates that the DNA binding properties of the N-finger contribute to the overall function of GATA-1. The severity of disease depends on the particular mutation: D218G results in macrothrombocytopenia and mild dyserythropoietic features but no marked anemia, whereas D218Y is a more severe mutation resulting in deep macrothrombocytopenia, marked anemia, and early mortality.[170] These phenotypic differences correlate well with the stronger loss of affinity of the D218Y mutant for FOG-1 binding, compared with the D218G mutant. Another class of mutations affects the N terminus of the protein, resulting in the synthesis of a shorter isoform of GATA-1 lacking the first 84 amino acids (GATA-1s; Fig. 2.7a). Acquired mutations leading to the formation of GATA-1s are associated with megakaryoblastic leukemia in the context of trisomy 21 (Down syndrome).[174] One family with a germline GATA-1s mutation has been described. Affected individuals displayed macrocytic anemia and were often neutropenic, but no signs of megakaryoblastic leukemia were observed.[175] In summary, only a few mutations in GATA-1 causing human disease have been reported thus far. This likely reflects the lethality of mutations affecting the function of GATA-1 more severely, as can be deduced from the studies in the mouse.

EKLF

Expression of the EKLF or Klf1 transcription factor is largely restricted to the erythroid cell lineage, where it is present in both primitive and definitive cells.[176] The promoter of the *EKLF* gene contains a functional binding site for the transcription factor Gata1, suggesting that the expression of EKLF is dependent on and downstream of Gata1.[177] EKLF binds DNA at CACC-boxes, which are found in many erythroid gene promoters.[178] EKLF specifically binds the sequence 5′-CCA CAC CCT-3′.[179] The strong affinity for this specific site is illustrated by β thalassemia patients who carry mutations in the EKLF binding site in the *β-globin* promoter. The loss in specificity for binding of EKLF strongly reduces the expression of *β-globin.*[180–182] Furthermore, EKLF has a higher affinity for the human *β-globin* promoter then the *γ-globin* promoter, which has a similar but not identical CACC-box.[183] To determine the role of EKLF in vivo, the gene has been knocked out in mice.[184,185] Mice heterozygous for the EKLF gene appear completely healthy. In the absence of EKLF, however, the developing fetuses die around E14 (Fig. 2.8a,b). The primitive erythroid cells function sufficiently for normal survival of the EKLF knockout mice during embryonic development up to approximately E12. The expression of embryonic globins is not influenced by the absence EKLF (Fig. 2.8c), even though EKLF binds these genes in vivo.[186] When the embryos switch to definitive erythropoiesis in the fetal liver, EKLF null mutants rapidly develop fatal anemia, because of a deficiency in β-globin expression. This is in contrast to α-globin expression that is not dependent on EKLF. Remarkably, the number of CFU-E in the EKLF null fetal livers is similar of those found in wild-type fetal livers, showing that EKLF deficiency causes a very late erythroid defect.[184,185] Furthermore, fetal liver–derived erythroid cells of $EKLF^{-/-}$ fetuses have an abnormal morphology, and most of the cells retain a nucleus. Interestingly, definitive erythroid cells of mice with deleted adult *β-globin* genes have morphological abnormalities that are more like those found in human β thalassemia than those found in $EKLF^{-/-}$ fetuses.[187] This was the first indication that the adult *β-globin* genes are not the only target genes of EKLF. Stronger evidence that nonglobin EKLF target genes contribute to the definitive red blood cell abnormalities and prenatal death in $EKLF^{-/-}$ fetuses came from a transgenic rescue study. $EKLF^{-/-}$ mice could not be rescued by expression of exogenous human γ-globin. Despite efficient production of hybrid hemoglobin, consisting of mouse α- and human γ-globin in the fetal livers, hemolysis was not corrected and survival was not prolonged.[188] This strongly suggested that EKLF regulates more essential genes in erythropoiesis. Indeed, genome-wide expression analyses of $EKLF^{-/-}$ erythroid cells have demonstrated that EKLF activates the expression of many other erythroid-specific genes. Although there are some indications that EKLF may repress transcription in some contexts,[189,190] the genome-wide expression analyses provided little evidence that EKLF acts as a repressor.[191–193] Examples of genes activated by EKLF are the gene encoding AHSP, a protein involved in stabilization of free α-globin chains, and genes encoding proteins associated with the erythroid cell membrane, such as band 4.9/dematin. These proteins are important for the function and stability of the erythrocytes, and consistent with this notion EKLF null primitive erythrocytes were found to display morphological abnormalities (Fig. 2.8d,e). In addition, EKLF appears to have a role in cell cycle regulation linked to the proliferation arrest required for terminal differentiation.[194]

Thus, EKLF is an activator of essential erythroid genes that are upregulated during terminal erythroid differentiation. This suggests that mutations affecting the function of the EKLF transcription factor would have a major impact on the severity of disease in thalassemia and sickle cell

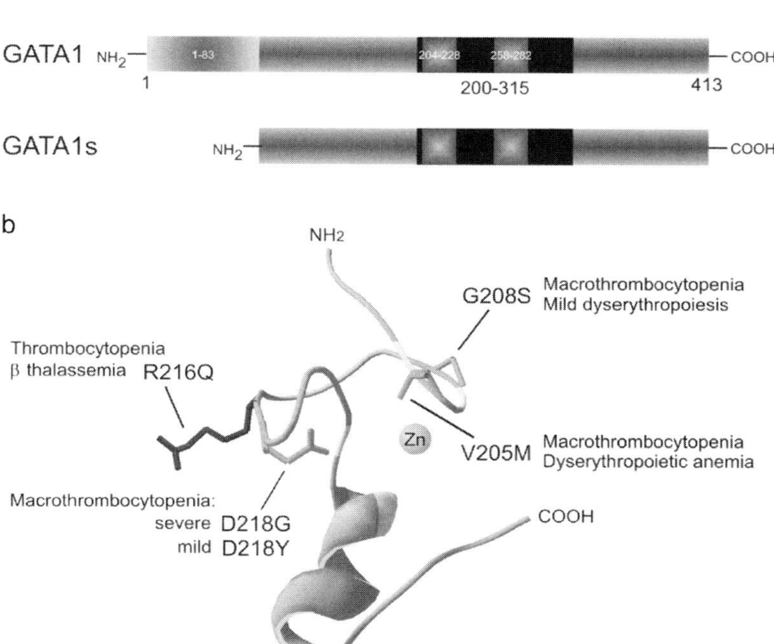

Figure 2.7. Mutations in the GATA-1 transcription factor associated with human disease. **(a)** Schematic drawing of the GATA-1 protein with the N-terminal transactivation domain, lacking in the GATA-1s isoform, and the N- and C-terminal zinc fingers indicated. **(b)** Three-dimensional structure of the N-terminal zinc finger, with the positions of disease-causing mutations shown. Mutation of arginine 216 to glutamine (R216Q) affects DNA binding; the other mutations affect interactions with the essential GATA-1 cofactor FOG-1. (Adapted from ref. 148.)

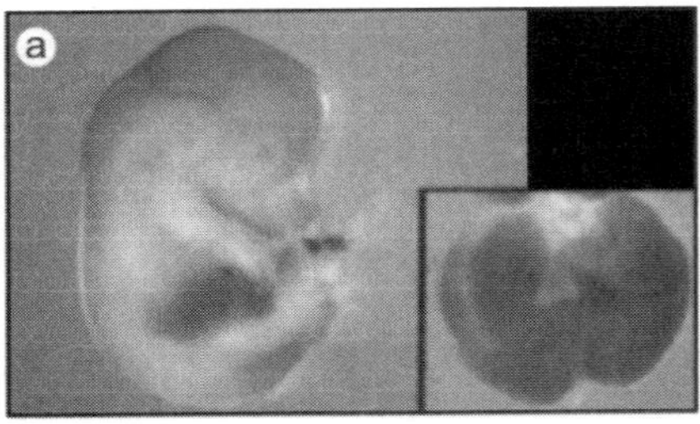

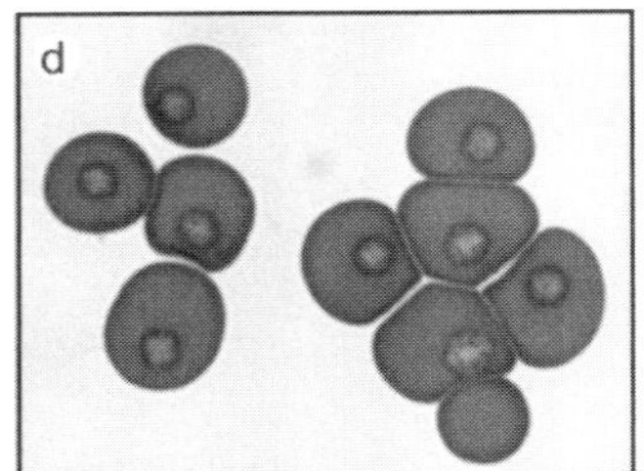

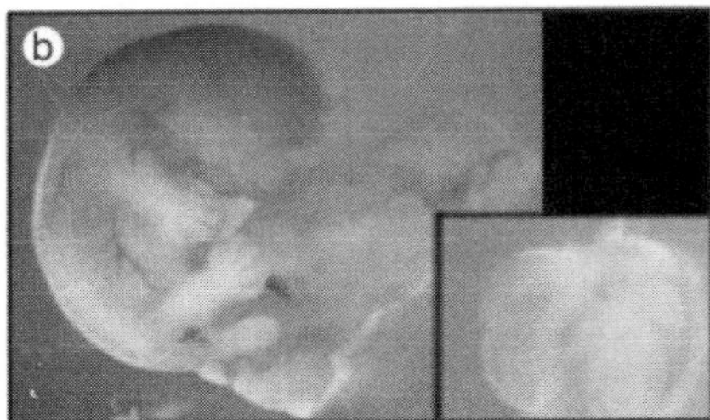

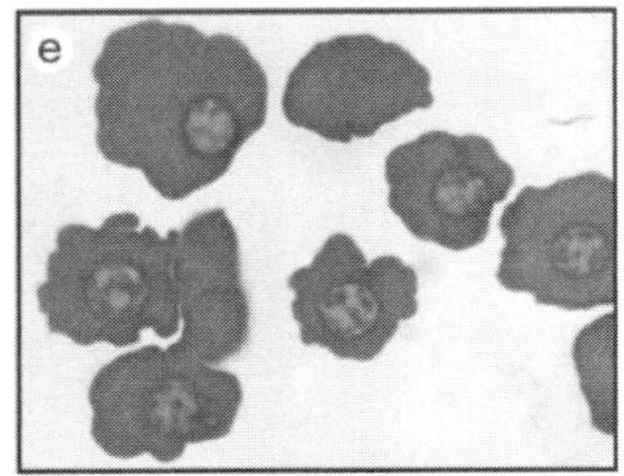

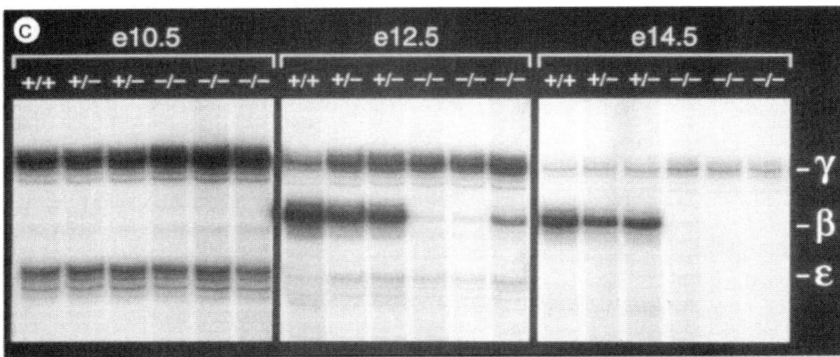

Figure 2.8. Phenotype of EKLF knockout fetuses. **(a)** E13.5 wild-type fetus. Inset: fetal liver. **(b)** E13.5 EKLF knockout fetus, displaying obvious pallor of the fetal liver (inset). **(c)** Mice carrying a human β-globin locus transgene were crossed with EKLF knockout mice. Expression analysis of the human *β-like globin* genes is shown at various gestational ages. Note that in the EKLF knockout background (–/–) the adult *β-globin* gene fails to be activated, whereas expression of the embryonic *ε-globin* and *fetal γ-globin* genes is not affected. **(d)** Cytospin of E12.5 blood from wild-type fetus, displaying primitive erythrocytes. **(e)** Cytospin of E12.5 blood from EKLF knockout fetus displaying primitive erythrocytes. Note the irregular shape of the cell membranes, compared with (d). ((d) and (e) Adapted from ref. 191.) (See color plate 2.8.)

anemia patients. Thus far, mutations in *EKLF* have not been found in the human population, but the experimental data suggest that it is worth investigating the occurrence of such mutations.

EKLF AFFECTS CHROMATIN CONFORMATION IN ERYTHROID CELLS

DNA is packaged in chromatin, which has a repressive effect on transcription. A number of complexes have been described that counteract this repressive effect. One of these complexes is the SWI/SNF complex; an adenosine triphosphate–dependent chromatin-remodeling complex that changes the chromatin structure by altering DNA–histone contacts within nucleosomes. EKLF requires a SWI/SNF-related chromatin-remodeling complex for transactivation of the *β-globin* gene when the DNA template is packaged in chromatin.[195] The EKLF-SWI/SNF complex generates a transcriptionally active β-globin promoter in vitro. The SWI/SNF complex contains homologs of the yeast BRG1, BAF170, BAF155, and BAF47 proteins, and a subunit that is unique to higher eukaryotes, BAF57. EKLF is necessary for recruitment of two of these subunits, BRG1 and BAF170, near the transcription initiation site of the β-globin promoter, suggesting that the complex uses EKLF for specific targeting.[196] We note that BRG1-mutant mice display an erythroid phenotype that bears similarity to that of EKLF null mutants.[197] In addition to interactions with SWI/SNF complex, EKLF works together with other nuclear factors, and interactions with Gata1, CBP/p300, Sin3A, and histone deacetylase 1 have been described.[160,189,198,199] Interestingly, both EKLF and Gata1 are involved in the spatial organization of the *β-globin* locus, bringing remote regulatory elements in the vicinity of the active promoters of the globin genes.[200,201] We refer to Chapter 4 for a detailed discussion of the regulation of *globin* gene expression.

GENE EXPRESSION DURING ERYTHROID MATURATION

As erythroid maturation proceeds, red cell protein synthesis becomes more concentrated on hemoglobin production. In general, mRNAs encoding red cell proteins are upregulated after erythroid commitment, including red cell membrane proteins, blood group antigens, glycolytic enzymes, carbonic anhydrase and enzymes of the heme synthesis pathway. Globin gene transcription occurs from the proerythroblast stage onward, reaching a maximum in polychromatic erythroblasts before declining in orthochromatic erythroblasts. The high stability of globin RNA results in the accumulation of approximately 20,000 copies per cell which, as a result of selective destruction of nonglobin RNAs, comprise more than 90% of the mRNA in reticulocytes. Globin chain synthesis parallels mRNA accumulation. The changes in gene expression may be found in Goh et al.[202] and Keller et al.[203] and effects on cell cycle regulatory genes in Fang et al.[84] A catalogue of erythroid gene expression may be found at http://hembase.niddk.nih.gov. Finally, mass spectrometry–based analysis of the erythrocyte proteome has identified 751 proteins.[204–206] This unexpected complexity forms the basis for future research aimed at understanding how red blood cells actually work.

REFERENCES

1. Driever W, Solnica-Krezel L, Schier AF, et al. A genetic screen for mutations affecting embryogenesis in zebrafish. *Development.* 1996;123:37–46.
2. Heasman J, Kofron M, Wylie C. Beta-catenin signaling activity dissected in the early Xenopus embryo: a novel antisense approach. *Dev Biol.* 2000;222(1):124–134.
3. Ekker SC. Morphants: a new systematic vertebrate functional genomics approach. *Yeast.* 2000;17(4):302–306.
4. Stuart GW, McMurray JV, Westerfield M. Replication, integration and stable germ-line transmission of foreign sequences injected into early zebrafish embryos. *Development.* 1988;103(2):403–412.
5. Motoike T, Loughna S, Perens E, et al. Universal GFP reporter for the study of vascular development. *Genesis.* 2000;28(2):75–81.
6. Long Q, Meng A, Wang H, Jessen JR, Farrell MJ, Lin S. GATA-1 expression pattern can be recapitulated in living transgenic zebrafish using GFP reporter gene. *Development.* 1997;124(20):4105–4111.
7. Kobayashi M, Nishikawa K, Yamamoto M. Hematopoietic regulatory domain of gata1 gene is positively regulated by GATA1 protein in zebrafish embryos. *Development.* 2001;128(12):2341–2350.
8. Bahary N, Zon LI. Use of the zebrafish (Danio rerio) to define hematopoiesis. *Stem Cells.* 1998;16(2):89–98.
9. Orkin SH, Zon LI. Genetics of erythropoiesis: induced mutations in mice and zebrafish. *Annu Rev Genet.* 1997;31:33–60.
10. Weinstein BM, Schier AF, Abdelilah S, et al. Hematopoietic mutations in the zebrafish. *Development.* 1996;123:303–309.
11. Stainier DY, Weinstein BM, Detrich HW 3rd, Zon LI, Fishman MC. Cloche, an early acting zebrafish gene, is required by both the endothelial and hematopoietic lineages. *Development.* 1995;121(10):3141–3150.
12. Lyons SE, Lawson ND, Lei L, Bennett PE, Weinstein BM, Liu PP. A nonsense mutation in zebrafish gata1 causes the bloodless phenotype in vlad tepes. *Proc Natl Acad Sci USA.* 2002;99(8):5454–5459.
13. Brownlie A, Donovan A, Pratt SJ, et al. Positional cloning of the zebrafish sauternes gene: a model for congenital sideroblastic anaemia. *Nat Genet.* 1998;20(3):244–250.
14. Paw BH, Davidson AJ, Zhou Y, et al. Cell-specific mitotic defect and dyserythropoiesis associated with erythroid band 3 deficiency. *Nat Genet.* 2003;34(1):59–64.
15. Barut BA, Zon LI. Realizing the potential of zebrafish as a model for human disease. *Physiol Genomics.* 2000;2(2):49–51.
16. Brownlie A, Hersey C, Oates AC, et al. Characterization of embryonic globin genes of the zebrafish. *Dev Biol.* 2003;255(1):48–61.
17. Murayama E, Kissa K, Zapata A, et al. Tracing hematopoietic precursor migration to successive hematopoietic organs during zebrafish development. *Immunity.* 2006;25(6):963–975.
18. Burns CE, DeBlasio T, Zhou Y, Zhang J, Zon L, Nimer SD. Isolation and characterization of runxa and runxb, zebrafish members of the runt family of transcriptional regulators. *Exp Hematol.* 2002;30(12):1381–1389.
19. Kalev–Zylinska ML, Horsfield JA, Flores MV, et al. Runx1 is required for zebrafish blood and vessel development and expression of a human RUNX1-CBF2T1 transgene advances a model for studies of leukemogenesis. *Development.* 2002;129(8):2015–2030.
20. Thompson MA, Ransom DG, Pratt SJ, et al. The cloche and spadetail genes differentially affect hematopoiesis and vasculogenesis. *Dev Biol.* 1998;197(2):248–269.
21. Paffett-Lugassy N, Hsia N, Fraenkel PG, et al. Functional conservation of erythropoietin signaling in zebrafish. *Blood.* 2007;110(7):2718–2726.
22. Tata JR. Early metamorphic competence of Xenopus larvae. *Dev Biol.* 1968;18(5):415–440.
23. Nieuwkoop PD. The organization center of the amphibian embryo: its origin, spatial organization, and morphogenetic action. *Adv Morphog.* 1973;10:1–39.
24. Ciau-Uitz A, Walmsley M, Patient R. Distinct origins of adult and embryonic blood in Xenopus. *Cell.* 2000;102(6):787–796.
25. Walmsley M, Ciau-Uitz A, Patient R. Adult and embryonic blood and endothelium derive from distinct precursor populations which are differentially programmed by BMP in Xenopus. *Development.* 2002;129(24):5683–5695.
26. Beck CW, Slack JM. An amphibian with ambition: a new role for Xenopus in the 21st century. *Genome Biol.* 2001;2(10):REVIEWS1029.
27. Godin IE, Garcia-Porrero JA, Coutinho A, Dieterlen-Lievre F, Marcos MA. Para-aortic splanchnopleura from early mouse embryos contains B1a cell progenitors. *Nature.* 1993;364(6432):67–70.
28. Chegini N, Aleporou V, Bell G, Hilder VA, Maclean N. Production and fate of erythroid cells in anaemic Xenopus laevis. *J Cell Sci.* 1979;35:403–415.
29. Guillemot FP, Oliver PD, Peault BM, Le Douarin NM. Cells expressing Ia antigens in the avian thymus. *J Exp Med.* 1984;160(6):1803–1819.
30. Peault BM, Thiery JP, Le Douarin NM. Surface marker for hemopoietic and endothelial cell lineages in quail that is defined by a monoclonal antibody. *Proc Natl Acad Sci USA.* 1983;80(10):2976–2980.
31. Dieterlen-Lievre F. On the origin of haemopoietic stem cells in the avian embryo: an experimental approach. *J Embryol Exp Morphol.* 1975;33(3):607–619.
32. Caprioli A, Jaffredo T, Gautier R, Dubourg C, Dieterlen-Lievre F. Blood-borne seeding by hematopoietic and endothelial precursors from the allantois. *Proc Natl Acad Sci USA.* 1998;95(4):1641–1646.

33. Samarut J, Bouabdelli M. In vitro development of CFU-E and BFU-E in cultures of embryonic and postembryonic chicken hematopoietic cells. *J Cell Physiol.* 1980;105(3):553–563.
34. Szenberg A. Ontogeny of myelopoietic precursor cells in the chicken embryo. *Adv Exp Med Biol.* 1977;88:3–11.
35. Dolan M, Sugarman BJ, Dodgson JB, Engel JD. Chromosomal arrangement of the chicken beta-type globin genes. *Cell.* 1981;24(3):669–677.
36. Hansen DA, Seftor EA, DeKloe J, McCabe JB, Tobin AJ. Developmental regulation of globin and nonglobin messenger RNAs in avian erythroid cells. *Dev Biol.* 1984;102(2):278–289.
37. Dieterlen-Lievre F, Pouget C, Bollerot K, Jaffredo T. Are intra-aortic hemopoietic cells derived from endothelial cells during ontogeny? *Trends Cardiovasc Med.* 2006;16(4):128–139.
38. Brotherton TW, Chui DH, Gauldie J, Patterson M. Hemoglobin ontogeny during normal mouse fetal development. *Proc Natl Acad Sci USA.* 1979;76(6):2853–2857.
39. Lin CS, Lim SK, D'Agati V, Costantini F. Differential effects of an erythropoietin receptor gene disruption on primitive and definitive erythropoiesis. *Genes Dev.* 1996;10(2):154–164.
40. Fraser ST, Isern J, Baron MH. Maturation and enucleation of primitive erythroblasts during mouse embryogenesis is accompanied by changes in cell-surface antigen expression. *Blood.* 2007;109(1):343–352.
41. Socolovsky M. Molecular insights into stress erythropoiesis. *Curr Opin Hematol.* 2007;14(3):215–224.
42. Boyer SH, Belding TK, Margolet L, Noyes AN. Fetal hemoglobin restriction to a few erythrocytes (F cells) in normal human adults. *Science.* 1975;188(4186):361–363.
43. Papayannopoulou T, Brice M, Stamatoyannopoulos G. Hemoglobin F synthesis in vitro: evidence for control at the level of primitive erythroid stem cells. *Proc Natl Acad Sci USA.* 1977;74(7):2923–2927.
44. Stamatoyannopoulos G. Control of globin gene expression during development and erythroid differentiation. *Exp Hematol.* 2005;33(3):259–271.
45. Dillon N, Grosveld F. Human gamma-globin genes silenced independently of other genes in the betaglobin locus. *Nature.* 1991;350(6315):252–254.
46. Strouboulis J, Dillon N, Grosveld F. Developmental regulation of a complete 70-kb human beta-globin locus in transgenic mice. *Genes Dev.* 1992;6(10):1857–1864.
47. Berry M, Grosveld F, Dillon N. A single point mutation is the cause of the Greek form of hereditary persistence of fetal haemoglobin. *Nature.* 1992;358(6386):499–502.
48. Peterson KR, Li QL, Clegg CH, et al. Use of yeast artificial chromosomes (YACs) in studies of mammalian development: production of beta-globin locus YAC mice carrying human globin developmental mutants. *Proc Natl Acad Sci USA.* 1995;92(12):5655–5659.
49. Buza-Vidas N, Luc S, Jacobsen SE. Delineation of the earliest lineage commitment steps of haematopoietic stem cells: new developments, controversies and major challenges. *Curr Opin Hematol.* 2007;14(4):315–321.
50. Hu M, Krause D, Greaves M, et al. Multilineage gene expression precedes commitment in the hemopoietic system. *Genes Dev.* 1997;11(6):774–785.
51. Akashi K, Traver D, Miyamoto T, Weissman IL. A clonogenic common myeloid progenitor that gives rise to all myeloid lineages. *Nature.* 2000;404(6774):193–197.
52. Kondo M, Weissman IL, Akashi K. Identification of clonogenic common lymphoid progenitors in mouse bone marrow. *Cell.* 1997;91(5):661–672.
53. Manz MG, Miyamoto T, Akashi K, Weissman IL. Prospective isolation of human clonogenic common myeloid progenitors. *Proc Natl Acad Sci USA.* 2002;99(18):11872–11877.
54. Adolfsson J, Mansson R, Buza-Vidas N, et al. Identification of Flt3+lympho-myeloid stem cells lacking erythro-megakaryocytic potential a revised road map for adult blood lineage commitment. *Cell.* 2005;121(2):295–306.
55. Mansson R, Hultquist A, Luc S, et al. Molecular evidence for hierarchical transcriptional lineage priming in fetal and adult stem cells and multipotent progenitors. *Immunity.* 2007;26(4):407–419.
56. Pronk CJH, Rossi DJ, Mansson R, et al. Elucidation of the phenotypic, functional and molecular topography of a myeloerythroid progenitor cell hierarchy. *Cell Stem Cell.* 2007;1:428–442.
57. Ye M, Graf T. Early decisions in lymphoid development. *Curr Opin Immunol.* 2007;19(2):123–128.
58. Murre C. Defining the pathways of early adult hematopoiesis. *Cell Stem Cell.* 2007;1:357–358.
59. Migliaccio A, Papayannopoulou T. Erythropoiesis. In: Steinberg MH, Forget BG, Higgs DR, Nagel RL, eds. *Disorders of Hemoglobin: Genetics, Pathophysiology and Clinical Management.* Cambridge, UK: Cambridge University Press; 2001:52–71.
60. Dolznig H, Boulme F, Stangl K, et al. Establishment of normal, terminally differentiating mouse erythroid progenitors: molecular characterization by cDNA arrays. *Faseb J.* 2001;15(8):1442–1444.
61. Fibach E, Manor D, Oppenheim A, Rachmilewitz EA. Proliferation and maturation of human erythroid progenitors in liquid culture. *Blood.* 1989;73(1):100–103.
62. Migliaccio G, Di Pietro R, di Giacomo V, et al. In vitro mass production of human erythroid cells from the blood of normal donors and of thalassemic patients. *Blood Cells Mol Dis.* 2002;28(2):169–180.
63. Pilat S, Carotta S, Schiedlmeier B, et al. HOXB4 enforces equivalent fates of ES-cell-derived and adult hematopoietic cells. *Proc Natl Acad Sci USA.* 2005;102(34):12101–12106.
64. Carotta S, Pilat S, Mairhofer A, et al. Directed differentiation and mass cultivation of pure erythroid progenitors from mouse embryonic stem cells. *Blood.* 2004;104(6):1873–1880.
65. Olivier EN, Qiu C, Velho M, Hirsch RE, Bouhassira EE. Large-scale production of embryonic red blood cells from human embryonic stem cells. *Exp Hematol.* 2006;34(12):1635–1642.
66. Neildez-Nguyen TM, Wajcman H, Marden MC, et al. Human erythroid cells produced ex vivo at large scale differentiate into red blood cells in vivo. *Nat Biotechnol.* 2002;20(5):467–472.
67. Giarratana MC, Kobari L, Lapillonne H, et al. Ex vivo generation of fully mature human red blood cells from hematopoietic stem cells. *Nat Biotechnol.* 2005;23(1):69–74.
68. Douay L, Andreu G. Ex vivo production of human red blood cells from hematopoietic stem cells: what is the future in transfusion? *Transfus Med Rev.* 2007;21(2):91–100.
69. Nijhof W, Wierenga PK. Isolation and characterization of the erythroid progenitor cell: CFU-E. *J Cell Biol.* 1983;96(2):386–392.

70. Wu H, Klingmuller U, Besmer P, Lodish HF. Interaction of the erythropoietin and stem-cell-factor receptors. *Nature.* 1995;377(6546):242–246.
71. Wang GL, Jiang BH, Rue EA, Semenza GL. Hypoxia-inducible factor 1 is a basic-helix-loop-helix-PAS heterodimer regulated by cellular O2 tension. *Proc Natl Acad Sci USA.* 1995;92(12):5510–5514.
72. Jaakkola P, Mole DR, Tian YM, et al. Targeting of HIF-alpha to the von Hippel-Lindau ubiquitylation complex by O2-regulated prolyl hydroxylation. *Science.* 2001;292(5516):468–472.
73. Schofield CJ, Ratcliffe PJ. Oxygen sensing by HIF hydroxylases. *Nat Rev Mol Cell Biol.* 2004;5(5):343–354.
74. Bunn HF, Gu J, Huang LE, Park JW, Zhu H. Erythropoietin: a model system for studying oxygendependent gene regulation. *J Exp Biol.* 1998;201(Pt 8):1197–1201.
75. Galson DL, Tsuchiya T, Tendler DS, et al. The orphan receptor hepatic nuclear factor 4 functions as a transcriptional activator for tissue-specific and hypoxia-specific erythropoietin gene expression and is antagonized by EAR3/COUP-TF1. *Mol Cell Biol.* 1995;15(4):2135–2144.
76. Fisher JW. Erythropoietin: physiology and pharmacology update. *Exp Biol Med (Maywood).* 2003;228(1):1–14.
77. Ebert BL, Bunn HF. Regulation of the erythropoietin gene. *Blood.* 1999;94(6):1864–1877.
78. Wojchowski DM, Gregory RC, Miller CP, Pandit AK, Pircher TJ. Signal transduction in the erythropoietin receptor system. *Exp Cell Res.* 1999;253(1):143–156.
79. Suzuki N, Obara N, Yamamoto M. Use of gene-manipulated mice in the study of erythropoietin gene expression. *Meth Enzymol.* 2007;435:157–177.
80. Bunn HF. New agents that stimulate erythropoiesis. *Blood.* 2007;109(3):868–873.
81. Jelkmann W. Erythropoietin after a century of research: younger than ever. *Eur J Haematol.* 2007;78(3):183–205.
82. Watowich SS, Wu H, Socolovsky M, Klingmuller U, Constantinescu SN, Lodish HF. Cytokine receptor signal transduction and the control of hematopoietic cell development. *Annu Rev Cell Dev Biol.* 1996;12:91–128.
83. Zang H, Sato K, Nakajima H, McKay C, Ney PA, Ihle JN. The distal region and receptor tyrosines of the Epo receptor are non-essential for in vivo erythropoiesis. *Embo J.* 2001;20(12):3156–3166.
84. Fang J, Menon M, Kapelle W, et al. EPO modulation of cell-cycle regulatory genes, and cell division, in primary bone marrow erythroblasts. *Blood.* 2007;110:2361–2370.
85. Li K, Menon MP, Karur VG, Hegde S, Wojchowski DM. Attenuated signaling by a phosphotyrosine-null Epo receptor form in primary erythroid progenitor cells. *Blood.* 2003;102(9):3147–3153.
86. Kadri Z, Maouche-Chretien L, Rooke HM, et al. Phosphatidylinositol 3-kinase/Akt induced by erythropoietin renders the erythroid differentiation factor GATA-1 competent for TIMP-1 gene transactivation. *Mol Cell Biol.* 2005;25(17):7412–7422.
87. Zhao W, Kitidis C, Fleming MD, Lodish HF, Ghaffari S. Erythropoietin stimulates phosphorylation and activation of GATA-1 via the PI3-kinase/AKT signaling pathway. *Blood.* 2006;107(3):907–915.
88. Rooke HM, Orkin SH. Phosphorylation of Gata1 at serine residues 72, 142, and 310 is not essential for hematopoiesis in vivo. *Blood.* 2006;107(9):3527–3530.
89. Kralovics R, Indrak K, Stopka T, Berman BW, Prchal JF, Prchal JT. Two new EPO receptor mutations: truncated EPO receptors are most frequently associated with primary familial and congenital polycythemias. *Blood.* 1997;90(5):2057–2061.
90. de la Chapelle A, Sistonen P, Lehvaslaiho H, Ikkala E, Juvonen E. Familial erythrocytosis genetically linked to erythropoietin receptor gene. *Lancet.* 1993;341(8837):82–84.
91. Baxter EJ, Scott LM, Campbell PJ, et al. Acquired mutation of the tyrosine kinase JAK2 in human myeloproliferative disorders. *Lancet.* 2005;365(9464):1054–1061.
92. James C, Ugo V, Le Couedic JP, et al. A unique clonal JAK2 mutation leading to constitutive signalling causes polycythaemia vera. *Nature.* 2005;434(7037):1144–1148.
93. Rhodes MM, Kopsombut P, Bondurant MC, Price JO, Koury MJ. Bcl-x(L) prevents apoptosis of late stage erythroblasts but does not mediate the antiapoptotic effect of erythropoietin. *Blood.* 2005;106(5):1857–1863.
94. Wagner KU, Claudio E, Rucker EB 3rd, et al. Conditional deletion of the Bcl-x gene from erythroid cells results in hemolytic anemia and profound splenomegaly. *Development.* 2000;127(22):4949–4958.
95. Motoyama N, Wang F, Roth KA, et al. Massive cell death of immature hematopoietic cells and neurons in Bcl-x-deficient mice. *Science.* 1995;267(5203):1506–1510.
96. Wu H, Liu X, Jaenisch R, Lodish HF. Generation of committed erythroid BFU-E and CFU-E progenitors does not require erythropoietin or the erythropoietin receptor. *Cell.* 1995;83(1):59–67.
97. Neubauer H, Cumano A, Muller M, Wu H, Huffstadt U, Pfeffer K. Jak2 deficiency defines an essential developmental checkpoint in definitive hematopoiesis. *Cell.* 1998;93(3):397–409.
98. Parganas E, Wang D, Stravopodis D, et al. Jak2 is essential for signaling through a variety of cytokine receptors. *Cell.* 1998;93(3):385–395.
99. Socolovsky M, Fallon AE, Wang S, Brugnara C, Lodish HF. Fetal anemia and apoptosis of red cell progenitors in Stat5a−/−5b−/− mice: a direct role for Stat5 in Bcl-X(L) induction. *Cell.* 1999;98(2):181–191.
100. Huddleston H, Tan B, Yang FC, et al. Functional p85alpha gene is required for normal murine fetal erythropoiesis. *Blood.* 2003;102(1):142–145.
101. Munugalavadla V, Kapur R. Role of c-Kit and erythropoietin receptor in erythropoiesis. *Crit Rev Oncol Hematol.* 2005;54(1):63–75.
102. Blanchard KL, Acquaviva AM, Galson DL, Bunn HF. Hypoxic induction of the human erythropoietin gene: cooperation between the promoter and enhancer, each of which contains steroid receptor response elements. *Mol Cell Biol.* 1992;12(12):5373–5385.
103. Gordon AS, Zanjani ED, Levere RD, Kappas A. Stimulation of mammalian erythropoiesis by 5beta-H steroid metabolites. *Proc Natl Acad Sci USA.* 1970;65(4):919–924.
104. Singer JW, Adamson JW. Steroids and hematopoiesis. II. The effect of steroids on in vitro erythroid colony growth:

evidence for different target cells for different classes of steroids. *J Cell Physiol.* 1976;88(2):135–143.

105. Singer JW, Samuels AI, Adamson JW. Steroids and hematopoiesis. I. The effect of steroids on in vitro erythroid colony growth: structure/activity relationships. *J Cell Physiol.* 1976;88(2):127–134.
106. von Lindern M, Zauner W, Mellitzer G, et al. The glucocorticoid receptor cooperates with the erythropoietin receptor and c-Kit to enhance and sustain proliferation of erythroid progenitors in vitro. *Blood.* 1999;94(2):550–559.
107. Leberbauer C, Boulme F, Unfried G, Huber J, Beug H, Mullner EW. Different steroids co-regulate longterm expansion versus terminal differentiation in primary human erythroid progenitors. *Blood.* 2005;105(1):85–94.
108. Dainiak N, Hoffman R, Maffei LA, Forget BG. Potentiation of human erythropoiesis in vitro by thyroid hormone. *Nature.* 1978;272(5650):260–262.
109. Golde DW, Bersch N, Chopra IJ, Cline MJ. Thyroid hormones stimulate erythropoiesis in vitro. *Br J Haematol.* 1977;37(2):173–177.
110. Popovic WJ, Brown JE, Adamson JW. The influence of thyroid hormones on in vitro erythropoiesis. Mediation by a receptor with beta adrenergic properties. *J Clin Invest.* 1977;60(4):907–913.
111. Angelin-Duclos C, Domenget C, Kolbus A, Beug H, Jurdic P, Samarut J. Thyroid hormone T3 acting through the thyroid hormone alpha receptor is necessary for implementation of erythropoiesis in the neonatal spleen environment in the mouse. *Development.* 2005;132(5):925–934.
112. Bessis M. L'ilot erythroblastique, unite fonctionnelle de la moelle osseuse. *Rev Hematol.* 1958;13(1):8–11.
113. Soni S, Bala S, Gwynn B, Sahr KE, Peters LL, Hanspal M. Absence of erythroblast macrophage protein (Emp) leads to failure of erythroblast nuclear extrusion. *J Biol Chem.* 2006;281(29):20181–20189.
114. Koury ST, Koury MJ, Bondurant MC. Cytoskeletal distribution and function during the maturation and enucleation of mammalian erythroblasts. *J Cell Biol.* 1989;109(6 Pt 1):3005–3013.
115. Liu XS, Li XH, Wang Y, et al. Disruption of palladin leads to defects in definitive erythropoiesis by interfering erythroblastic island formation in mouse fetal liver. *Blood.* 2007;110:870–876.
116. Kawane K, Fukuyama H, Kondoh G, et al. Requirement of DNase II for definitive erythropoiesis in the mouse fetal liver. *Science.* 2001;292(5521):1546–1549.
117. Yoshida H, Okabe Y, Kawane K, Fukuyama H, Nagata S. Lethal anemia caused by interferon-beta produced in mouse embryos carrying undigested DNA. *Nat Immunol.* 2005;6(1):49–56.
118. Lee G, Lo A, Short SA, et al. Targeted gene deletion demonstrates that the cell adhesion molecule ICAM-4 is critical for erythroblastic island formation. *Blood.* 2006;108(6):2064–2071.
119. Scott LM, Priestley GV, Papayannopoulou T. Deletion of alpha4 integrins from adult hematopoietic cells reveals roles in homeostasis, regeneration, and homing. *Mol Cell Biol.* 2003;23(24):9349–9360.
120. De Maria R, Zeuner A, Eramo A, et al. Negative regulation of erythropoiesis by caspase-mediated cleavage of GATA-1. *Nature.* 1999;401(6752):489–493.
121. Ribeil JA, Zermati Y, Vandekerckhove J, et al. Hsp70 regulates erythropoiesis by preventing caspase-3-mediated cleavage of GATA-1. *Nature.* 2007;445(7123):102–105.
122. Zeuner A, Eramo A, Testa U, et al. Control of erythroid cell production via caspase-mediated cleavage of transcription factor SCL/Tal-1. *Cell Death Differ.* 2003;10(8):905–913.
123. Papadaki HA, Kritikos HD, Valatas V, Boumpas DT, Eliopoulos GD. Anemia of chronic disease in rheumatoid arthritis is associated with increased apoptosis of bone marrow erythroid cells: improvement following anti-tumor necrosis factor-alpha antibody therapy. *Blood.* 2002;100(2):474–482.
124. Centis F, Tabellini L, Lucarelli G, et al. The importance of erythroid expansion in determining the extent of apoptosis in erythroid precursors in patients with beta-thalassemia major. *Blood.* 2000;96(10):3624–3629.
125. Mathias LA, Fisher TC, Zeng L, et al. Ineffective erythropoiesis in beta-thalassemia major is due to apoptosis at the polychromatophilic normoblast stage. *Exp Hematol.* 2000;28(12):1343–1353.
126. Pootrakul P, Sirankapracha P, Hemsorach S, et al. A correlation of erythrokinetics, ineffective erythropoiesis, and erythroid precursor apoptosis in thai patients with thalassemia. *Blood.* 2000;96(7):2606–2612.
127. Wanachiwanawin W, Wiener E, Siripanyaphinyo U, et al. Serum levels of tumor necrosis factor-alpha, interleukin-1, and interferon-gamma in beta(o)-thalassemia/HbE and their clinical significance. *J Interferon Cytokine Res.* 1999;19(2):105–111.
128. Yoshida H, Kawane K, Koike M, Mori Y, Uchiyama Y, Nagata S. Phosphatidylserine-dependent engulfment by macrophages of nuclei from erythroid precursor cells. *Nature.* 2005;437(7059):754–758.
129. Whyatt D, Lindeboom F, Karis A, et al. An intrinsic but cell-nonautonomous defect in GATA-1-overexpressing mouse erythroid cells. *Nature.* 2000;406(6795):519–524.
130. Gutierrez L, Lindeboom F, Langeveld A, Grosveld F, Philipsen S, Whyatt D. Homotypic signalling regulates Gata1 activity in the erythroblastic island. *Development.* 2004;131(13):3183–3193.
131. Syed RS, Reid SW, Li C, et al. Efficiency of signalling through cytokine receptors depends critically on receptor orientation. *Nature.* 1998;395(6701):511–516.
132. Lenox LE, Perry JM, Paulson RF. BMP4 and Madh5 regulate the erythroid response to acute anemia. *Blood.* 2005;105(7):2741–2748.
133. Socolovsky M, Nam H, Fleming MD, Haase VH, Brugnara C, Lodish HF. Ineffective erythropoiesis in Stat5a(−/−)5b(−/−) mice due to decreased survival of early erythroblasts. *Blood.* 2001;98(12):3261–3273.
134. Menon MP, Karur V, Bogacheva O, Bogachev O, Cuetara B, Wojchowski DM. Signals for stress erythropoiesis are integrated via an erythropoietin receptor–phosphotyrosine-343-Stat5 axis. *J Clin Invest.* 2006;116(3):683–694.
135. Bauer A, Tronche F, Wessely O, et al. The glucocorticoid receptor is required for stress erythropoiesis. *Genes Dev.* 1999;13(22):2996–3002.
136. Tong W, Zhang J, Lodish HF. Lnk inhibits erythropoiesis and Epo-dependent JAK2 activation and downstream signaling pathways. *Blood.* 2005;105(12):4604–4612.
137. Liu Y, Pop R, Sadegh C, Brugnara C, Haase VH, Socolovsky M. Suppression of Fas-FasL coexpression by erythropoietin

mediates erythroblast expansion during the erythropoietic stress response in vivo. *Blood.* 2006;108(1):123–133.
138. Shivdasani RA, Mayer EL, Orkin SH. Absence of blood formation in mice lacking the T-cell leukaemia oncoprotein tal-1/SCL. *Nature.* 1995;373(6513):432–434.
139. Porcher C, Swat W, Rockwell K, Fujiwara Y, Alt FW, Orkin SH. The T cell leukemia oncoprotein SCL/tal-1 is essential for development of all hematopoietic lineages. *Cell.* 1996;86(1):47–57.
140. Robb L, Lyons I, Li R, et al. Absence of yolk sac hematopoiesis from mice with a targeted disruption of the scl gene. *Proc Natl Acad Sci USA.* 1995;92(15):7075–7079.
141. Robb L, Elwood NJ, Elefanty AG, et al. The scl gene product is required for the generation of all hematopoietic lineages in the adult mouse. *EMBO J.* 1996;15(16):4123–4129.
142. Tsai FY, Keller G, Kuo FC, et al. An early haematopoietic defect in mice lacking the transcription factor GATA-2. *Nature.* 1994;371(6494):221–226.
143. Tsai FY, Orkin SH. Transcription factor GATA-2 is required for proliferation/survival of early hematopoietic cells and mast cell formation, but not for erythroid and myeloid terminal differentiation. *Blood.* 1997;89(10):3636–3643.
144. Okuda T, van Deursen J, Hiebert SW, Grosveld G, Downing JR. AML1, the target of multiple chromosomal translocations in human leukemia, is essential for normal fetal liver hematopoiesis. *Cell.* 1996;84(2):321–330.
145. Huang G, Zhang P, Hirai H, et al. PU.1 is a major downstream target of AML1 (RUNX1) in adult mouse hematopoiesis. *Nat Genet.* 2008;40:51–60.
146. Nerlov C, Graf T. PU.1 induces myeloid lineage commitment in multipotent hematopoietic progenitors. *Genes Dev.* 1998;12(15):2403–2412.
147. Scott EW, Simon MC, Anastasi J, Singh H. Requirement of transcription factor PU.1 in the development of multiple hematopoietic lineages. *Science.* 1994;265(5178):1573–1577.
148. Ferreira R, Ohneda K, Yamamoto M, Philipsen S. GATA1 function, a paradigm for transcription factors in hematopoiesis. *Mol Cell Biol.* 2005;25(4):1215–1227.
149. Fujiwara Y, Browne CP, Cunniff K, Goff SC, Orkin SH. Arrested development of embryonic red cell precursors in mouse embryos lacking transcription factor GATA-1. *Proc Natl Acad Sci USA.* 1996;93(22):12355–12358.
150. Takahashi S, Onodera K, Motohashi H, et al. Arrest in primitive erythroid cell development caused by promoter-specific disruption of the GATA-1 gene. *J Biol Chem.* 1997;272(19):12611–12615.
151. McDevitt MA, Shivdasani RA, Fujiwara Y, Yang H, Orkin SH. A "knockdown" mutation created by ciselement gene targeting reveals the dependence of erythroid cell maturation on the level of transcription factor GATA-1. *Proc Natl Acad Sci USA.* 1997;94(13):6781–6785.
152. Gregory T, Yu C, Ma A, Orkin SH, Blobel GA, Weiss MJ. GATA-1 and erythropoietin cooperate to promote erythroid cell survival by regulating bcl-xL expression. *Blood.* 1999;94(1):87–96.
153. Whyatt DJ, Karis A, Harkes IC, et al. The level of the tissue-specific factor GATA-1 affects the cell-cycle machinery. *Genes Funct.* 1997;1(1):11–24.
154. Rylski M, Welch JJ, Chen YY, et al. GATA-1-mediated proliferation arrest during erythroid maturation. *Mol Cell Biol.* 2003;23(14):5031–5042.
155. Kulessa H, Frampton J, Graf T. GATA-1 reprograms avian myelomonocytic cell lines into eosinophils, thromboblasts, and erythroblasts. *Genes Dev.* 1995;9(10):1250–1262.
156. Hirasawa R, Shimizu R, Takahashi S, et al. Essential and instructive roles of GATA factors in eosinophil development. *J Exp Med.* 2002;195(11):1379–1386.
157. Heyworth C, Gale K, Dexter M, May G, Enver T. A GATA-2/estrogen receptor chimera functions as a ligand-dependent negative regulator of self-renewal. *Genes Dev.* 1999;13(14):1847–1860.
158. Iwasaki H, Mizuno S, Wells RA, Cantor AB, Watanabe S, Akashi K. GATA-1 converts lymphoid and myelomonocytic progenitors into the megakaryocyte/erythrocyte lineages. *Immunity.* 2003;19(3):451–462.
159. Crossley M, Merika M, Orkin SH. Self-association of the erythroid transcription factor GATA-1 mediated by its zinc finger domains. *Mol Cell Biol.* 1995;15(5):2448–2456.
160. Merika M, Orkin SH. Functional synergy and physical interactions of the erythroid transcription factor GATA-1 with the Kruppel family proteins Sp1 and EKLF. *Mol Cell Biol.* 1995;15(5):2437–2447.
161. Tsang AP, Visvader JE, Turner CA, et al. FOG, a multitype zinc finger protein, acts as a cofactor for transcription factor GATA-1 in erythroid and megakaryocytic differentiation. *Cell.* 1997;90(1):109–19.
162. Rekhtman N, Radparvar F, Evans T, Skoultchi AI. Direct interaction of hematopoietic transcription factors PU.1 and GATA-1: functional antagonism in erythroid cells. *Genes Dev.* 1999;13(11):1398–1411.
163. Boyes J, Byfield P, Nakatani Y, Ogryzko V. Regulation of activity of the transcription factor GATA-1 by acetylation. *Nature.* 1998;396(6711):594–598.
164. Blobel GA, Nakajima T, Eckner R, Montminy M, Orkin SH. CREB-binding protein cooperates with transcription factor GATA-1 and is required for erythroid differentiation. *Proc Natl Acad Sci USA.* 1998;95(5):2061–2066.
165. Rodriguez P, Bonte E, Krijgsveld J, et al. GATA-1 forms distinct activating and repressive complexes in erythroid cells. *EMBO J.* 2005;24(13):2354–2366.
166. Stumpf M, Waskow C, Krotschel M, et al. The mediator complex functions as a coactivator for GATA-1 in erythropoiesis via subunit Med1/TRAP220. *Proc Natl Acad Sci USA.* 2006;103(49):18504–18509.
167. Welch JJ, Watts JA, Vakoc CR, et al. Global regulation of erythroid gene expression by transcription factor GATA-1. *Blood.* 2004;104(10):3136–3147.
168. Tubman VN, Levine JE, Campagna DR, et al. X-linked gray platelet syndrome due to a GATA1 Arg216Gln mutation. *Blood.* 2007;109(8):3297–3299.
169. Freson K, Devriendt K, Matthijs G, et al. Platelet characteristics in patients with X-linked macrothrombocytopenia because of a novel GATA1 mutation. *Blood.* 2001;98(1):85–92.
170. Freson K, Matthijs G, Thys C, et al. Different substitutions at residue D218 of the X-linked transcription factor GATA1 lead to altered clinical severity of macrothrombocytopenia and anemia and are associated with variable skewed X inactivation. *Hum Mol Genet.* 2002;11(2):147–152.
171. Nichols KE, Crispino JD, Poncz M, et al. Familial dyserythropoietic anaemia and thrombocytopenia due to an inherited mutation in GATA1. *Nat Genet.* 2000;24(3):266–270.

172. Yu C, Niakan KK, Matsushita M, Stamatoyannopoulos G, Orkin SH, Raskind WH. X-linked thrombocytopenia with thalassemia from a mutation in the amino finger of GATA-1 affecting DNA binding rather than FOG-1 interaction. *Blood.* 2002;100(6):2040–2045.
173. Balduini CL, Pecci A, Loffredo G, et al. Effects of the R216Q mutation of GATA-1 on erythropoiesis and megakaryocytopoiesis. *Thromb Haemost.* 2004;91(1):129–140.
174. Wechsler J, Greene M, McDevitt MA, et al. Acquired mutations in GATA1 in the megakaryoblastic leukemia of Down syndrome. *Nat Genet.* 2002;32(1):148–152.
175. Hollanda LM, Lima CS, Cunha AF, et al. An inherited mutation leading to production of only the short isoform of GATA-1 is associated with impaired erythropoiesis. *Nat Genet.* 2006;38(7):807–812.
176. Southwood CM, Downs KM, Bieker JJ. Erythroid Kruppel-like factor exhibits an early and sequentially localized pattern of expression during mammalian erythroid ontogeny. *Dev Dyn.* 1996;206(3):248–259.
177. Crossley M, Tsang AP, Bieker JJ, Orkin SH. Regulation of the erythroid Kruppel-like factor (EKLF) gene promoter by the erythroid transcription factor GATA-1. *J Biol Chem.* 1994;269(22):15440–15444.
178. Philipsen S, Talbot D, Fraser P, Grosveld F. The beta-globin dominant control region: hypersensitive site 2. *EMBO J.* 1990;9(7):2159–2167.
179. Miller IJ, Bieker JJ. A novel, erythroid cell-specific murine transcription factor that binds to the CACCC element and is related to the Kruppel family of nuclear proteins. *Mol Cell Biol.* 1993;13(5):2776–2786.
180. Faustino P, Lavinha J, Marini MG, Moi P. beta-Thalassemia mutation at –90C–>T impairs the interaction of the proximal CACCC box with both erythroid and nonerythroid factors. *Blood.* 1996;88(8):3248–3249.
181. Feng WC, Southwood CM, Bieker JJ. Analyses of beta-thalassemia mutant DNA interactions with erythroid Kruppel-like factor (EKLF), an erythroid cell-specific transcription factor. *J Biol Chem.* 1994;269(2):1493–1500.
182. Orkin SH, Antonarakis SE, Kazazian HH, Jr. Base substitution at position -88 in a beta-thalassemic globin gene. Further evidence for the role of distal promoter element ACACCC. *J Biol Chem.* 1984;259(14):8679–8681.
183. Donze D, Townes TM, Bieker JJ. Role of erythroid Kruppel-like factor in human gamma- to beta-globin gene switching. *J Biol Chem.* 1995;270(4):1955–1959.
184. Perkins AC, Sharpe AH, Orkin SH. Lethal beta-thalassaemia in mice lacking the erythroid CACCC transcription factor EKLF. *Nature.* 1995;375(6529):318–322.
185. Nuez B, Michalovich D, Bygrave A, Ploemacher R, Grosveld F. Defective haematopoiesis in fetal liver resulting from inactivation of the EKLF gene. *Nature.* 1995;375(6529):316–318.
186. Zhou D, Pawlik KM, Ren J, Sun CW, Townes TM. Differential binding of erythroid Krupple-like factor to embryonic/fetal globin gene promoters during development. *J Biol Chem.* 2006;281(23):16052–16057.
187. Yang B, Kirby S, Lewis J, Detloff PJ, Maeda N, Smithies O. A mouse model for beta-thalassemia. *Proc Natl Acad Sci USA.*1995;92(25):11608–11612.
188. Perkins AC, Peterson KR, Stamatoyannopoulos G, Witkowska HE, Orkin SH. Fetal expression of a human Agamma globin transgene rescues globin chain imbalance but not hemolysis in EKLF null mouse embryos. *Blood.* 2000;95(5):1827–1833.
189. Chen X, Bieker JJ. Stage-specific repression by the EKLF transcriptional activator. *Mol Cell Biol.* 2004;24(23):10416–10424.
190. Siatecka M, Xue L, Bieker JJ. Sumoylation of EKLF promotes transcriptional repression and is involved in inhibition of megakaryopoiesis. *Mol Cell Biol.* 2007;27(24):8547–8560.
191. Drissen R, von Lindern M, Kolbus A, et al. The erythroid phenotype of EKLF-null mice: defects in hemoglobin metabolism and membrane stability. *Mol Cell Biol.* 2005; 25(12):5205–5214.
192. Hodge D, Coghill E, Keys J, et al. A global role for EKLF in definitive and primitive erythropoiesis. *Blood.* 2006;107(8): 3359–3370.
193. Nilson DG, Sabatino DE, Bodine DM, Gallagher PG. Major erythrocyte membrane protein genes in EKLF-deficient mice. *Exp Hematol.* 2006;34(6):705–712.
194. Tallack MR, Keys JR, Perkins AC. Erythroid Kruppel-like factor regulates the G1 cyclin dependent kinase inhibitor p18INK4c. *J Mol Biol.* 2007;369(2):313–321.
195. Armstrong JA, Bieker JJ, Emerson BM. A SWI/SNF-related chromatin remodeling complex, E-RC1, is required for tissue-specific transcriptional regulation by EKLF in vitro. *Cell.* 1998;95(1):93–104.
196. Kadam S, McAlpine GS, Phelan ML, Kingston RE, Jones KA, Emerson BM. Functional selectivity of recombinant mammalian SWI/SNF subunits. *Genes Dev.* 2000;14(19):2441–2451.
197. Bultman SJ, Gebuhr TC, Magnuson T. A Brg1 mutation that uncouples ATPase activity from chromatin remodeling reveals an essential role for SWI/SNF-related complexes in beta-globin expression and erythroid development. *Genes Dev.* 2005;19(23):2849–2861.
198. Zhang W, Kadam S, Emerson BM, Bieker JJ. Site-specific acetylation by p300 or CREB binding protein regulates erythroid Kruppel-like factor transcriptional activity via its interaction with the SWI-SNF complex. *Mol Cell Biol.* 2001;21(7):2413–2422.
199. Gregory RC, Taxman DJ, Seshasayee D, Kensinger MH, Bieker JJ, Wojchowski DM. Functional interaction of GATA1 with erythroid Kruppel-like factor and Sp1 at defined erythroid promoters. *Blood.* 1996;87(5):1793–1801.
200. Drissen R, Palstra RJ, Gillemans N, et al. The active spatial organization of the beta-globin locus requires the transcription factor EKLF. *Genes Dev.* 2004;18(20):2485–2490.
201. Vakoc CR, Letting DL, Gheldof N, et al. Proximity among distant regulatory elements at the beta-globin locus requires GATA-1 and FOG-1. *Mol Cell.* 2005;17(3):453–462.
202. Goh SH, Josleyn M, Lee YT, et al. The human reticulocyte transcriptome. *Physiol Genomics.* 2007;30(2):172–178.
203. Keller MA, Addya S, Vadigepalli R, et al. Transcriptional regulatory network analysis of developing human erythroid progenitors reveals patterns of coregulation and potential transcriptional regulators. *Physiol Genomics.* 2006;28(1): 114–128.
204. Goodman SR, Kurdia A, Ammann L, Kakhniashvili D, Daescu O. The human red blood cell proteome and interactome. *Exp Biol Med (Maywood).* 2007;232(11):1391–1408.

205. Kakhniashvili DG, Bulla LA, Jr., Goodman SR. The human erythrocyte proteome: analysis by ion trap mass spectrometry. *Mol Cell Proteomics.* 2004;3(5):501–509.
206. Pasini EM, Kirkegaard M, Mortensen P, Lutz HU, Thomas AW, Mann M. In-depth analysis of the membrane and cytosolic proteome of red blood cells. *Blood.* 2006;108(3):791–801.
207. Beug H, Palmieri S, Freudenstein C, Zentgraf H, Graf T. Hormone-dependent terminal differentiation in vitro of chicken erythroleukemia cells transformed by ts mutants of avian erythroblastosis virus. *Cell.* 1982;28(4):907–919.
208. Richmond TD, Chohan M, Barber DL. Turning cells red: signal transduction mediated by erythropoietin. *Trends Cell Biol.* 2005;15(3):146–155.

3

The Normal Structure and Regulation of Human Globin Gene Clusters

Bernard G. Forget and Ross C. Hardison

The genes encoding the different globin chains of hemoglobin are members of an ancient gene family. In this chapter we will review the structural features of the globin genes, with particular attention to the sequences needed for proper regulation of gene expression. Some of these have been well conserved during mammalian evolution and therefore are likely to provide a common function in many mammals. Others are only found in higher primates and may play roles in lineage-specific regulation. We will first describe the structural characteristics of the human globin genes and then provide a comparative analysis of the genomic contexts, regulatory regions, and evolutionary conservation of features present in the globin gene clusters.

NUMBER AND CHROMOSOMAL LOCALIZATION OF HUMAN GLOBIN GENES

Hemoglobin is a heterotetramer that contains two polypeptide subunits related to the α-globin gene subfamily (referred to here as α-like globins) and two polypeptide subunits related to the β-globin gene subfamily (β-like globins). Globin polypeptides bind heme, which in turn allows the hemoglobin in erythrocytes to bind oxygen reversibly and transport it from the lungs to respiring tissues. In humans, as in all vertebrate species studied, different α-like and β-like globin chains are synthesized at progressive stages of development to produce hemoglobins characteristic of primitive (embryonic) and definitive (fetal and adult) erythroid cells (Fig. 3.1).

Before precise knowledge of globin gene organization was gained by gene mapping and molecular cloning, a general picture of the number and arrangement of the human globin genes emerged from the genetic analysis of normal and abnormal hemoglobins and their pattern of inheritance. The number and subunit composition of the different normal human hemoglobins (Fig. 3.1) suggested that there must exist at least one globin gene for each of the different globin chains: α, β, γ, δ, ε, and ζ. Evidence from the study of hemoglobin variants and the biochemical heterogeneity of the chains in fetal hemoglobin (HbF) showed that the α- and γ-globin genes were duplicated. Persons were identified whose red cells contained more than two structurally different α-globin chains that could be best explained by duplication of the α-globin gene locus, and the characterization of the structurally different $^{G}\gamma$- and $^{A}\gamma$-globin chains of HbF imposed a requirement for duplication of the γ-globin gene locus.

Studies of the pattern of inheritance of hemoglobin variants from persons carrying both an α chain and a β chain variant revealed that the α- and β-globin genes are on different chromosomes (or very widely separated if on the same chromosome). Variants of α-globin and β-globin chains were always observed to segregate independently in offspring of doubly affected parents (reviewed in ref. 1). Linkage of the various β-like globin genes to one another was established from the study of interesting hemoglobin variants that contained fused globin chains, presumably resulting from nonhomologous crossover between different β-like globin genes. Characterization of Hb Lepore,[2] with its δβ fusion chain, established that the δ-globin gene was linked to and located on the 5′ (or N-terminal) side of the β-globin gene. Analysis of Hb Kenya,[3] with its $^{A}\gamma\beta$ fusion chain, provided evidence for linkage of the $^{A}\gamma$ gene, and presumably the $^{G}\gamma$ gene as well, to the 5′ side of the δ- and β-globin genes.

Thus, the general arrangement of the globin genes that emerged from these various genetic analyses can be represented as illustrated in Figure 3.1. It was also assumed, but unsupported by genetic evidence, that the embryonic α-like (ζ) and β-like (ε) globin genes were likely to be linked to the loci encoding their adult counterparts.

By using rodent–human somatic hybrid cells containing only one or a few human chromosomes, Deisseroth and colleagues[4,5] clearly established that the human α- and β-globin genes resided on different chromosomes. The α-like globin genes are located on chromosome 16, whereas the β-like globin genes are on chromosome 11. The latter results were obtained by hybridizing a solution of total cellular DNA from the various somatic hybrid cells to radioactive cDNAs, synthesized from α- and β-globin mRNAs by reverse transcriptase. These results were later confirmed and extended by various groups using the gene mapping procedure of Southern blot analysis with DNA from various hybrid cell lines containing different translocations or deletions of the involved chromosomes.

These studies also localized the globin gene loci to specific regions on their respective chromosomes: the β-globin gene cluster to the short arm of chromosome 11, and the α-globin gene cluster to the short arm of chromosome 16 (Fig. 3.1). These chromosomal assignments were further confirmed and refined by in situ hybridization of radioactive cloned globin gene probes to metaphase chromosomes and by fluorescence-based in situ hybridization. Thus, the β-globin gene cluster was assigned to 11p15.5 and the

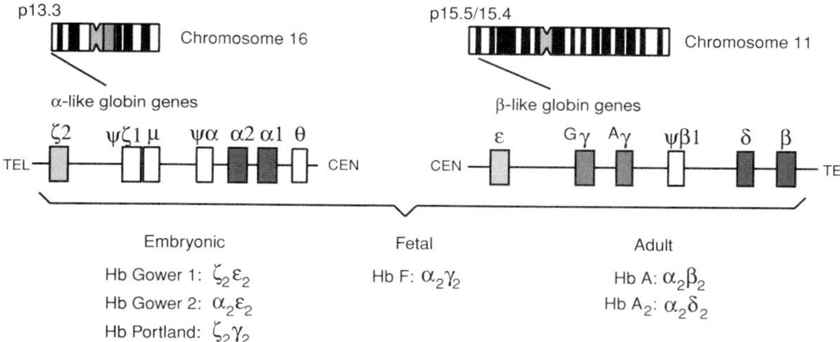

Figure 3.1. Basic organization of human globin gene complexes. The locations of the α-globin gene complex very close to the telomere of the short arm of chromosome 16 and the β-globin gene complex on the short arm of chromosome 11 are shown at the top. The genes are shown as boxes on the second line, named according to the globin polypeptide that is encoded. In both diagrams, the 5′–3′ transcriptional orientation is from left to right. Note that the orientations with respect to the centromere (CEN) and telomere (TEL) are opposite; the α-like globin genes are transcribed toward CEN, whereas the β-like globin genes are transcribed toward TEL. The composition of hemoglobins produced at progressive developmental stages is given at the bottom.

α-globin gene cluster to 16p13.3. Subsequent DNA sequencing of entire human chromosomes and alignment with maps of chromosome bands places the β-globin gene cluster in 11p15.4. The α-globin gene cluster is only approximately 150 kb from the telomere of the short arm of chromosome 16.

GLOBIN GENE STRUCTURE: INTRONS AND THEIR REMOVAL

The coding region of each globin gene in humans and other vertebrates is interrupted at two positions by stretches of noncoding DNA called intervening sequences (IVSs) or introns.[6] In the β-like globin genes, the introns interrupt the sequence between codons 30 and 31 and between codons 104 and 105; in the α-globin gene family, the intervening sequences interrupt the coding sequence between codons 31 and 32 and between codons 99 and 100 (Fig. 3.2.A). Although the precise codon position numbers at which the interruption occurs differ between the α- and β-like globin genes, the introns occur at precisely the same position in the aligned primary sequence of the α- and β-globin chains. Thus, given the likely possibility that the α- and β-globin gene families originally evolved from a single ancestral globin gene,[7] these gene sequences are homologous, and we infer that the presence of the introns at these positions predates the separation of α-globin and β-globin genes approximately 500 million years ago (in an ancestral jawed vertebrate). The first intervening sequence (IVS-1) is shorter than the second intervening sequence (IVS-2) in both α- and β-globin genes, but IVS-2 of the human β-globin gene is much larger than that of the α-globin gene (Fig. 3.2.A).

The pattern of intron sizes of the ζ-like globin genes differs from that of the other α-like globin genes. Whereas the introns in the α and ψα genes are small, that is, fewer than 150 bp, those of the ζ and ψζ genes are larger.[8] Furthermore, the first introns of the ζ and ψζ genes are much larger than their second introns; in fact they are 8–10 times larger than the first introns of any other globin gene.

The presence of intervening sequences that interrupt the coding sequences of structural genes imposes a requirement for some cellular process to remove these sequences in the mature mRNA. As illustrated in Figure 3.2.B, intervening sequences are transcribed into globin (and other) precursor mRNA molecules,[9] but they are subsequently excised and the proper ends of the coding sequences joined to yield the mature mRNA.[10] This posttranscriptional processing of mRNA precursors to remove introns has been termed splicing. A crucial prerequisite for the proper splicing of globin (and other) precursor mRNA molecules is the presence of specific nucleotide sequences at the junctions between coding sequences (exons) and intervening sequences (introns). Comparison of these sequences in many different genes has permitted the derivation of two different consensus sequences, which are almost universally found at the 5′ (donor) and 3′ (acceptor) splice sites of introns.[11,12] The consensus sequences thus derived are shown in Figure 3.2A, along with the consensus surrounding the branch point A involved in the initiation of splicing. The dinucleotides GT and AG shown in boldface, at the 5′ and 3′ ends, respectively, of the intron, are essentially invariant and are thought to be absolutely required for proper splicing. This is the so-called GT-AG rule. Rare examples have been described in which GC instead of GT is found at the donor splice site junction.

The importance of these consensus sequences is underscored by the fact that mutations that either alter them or create similar consensus sequences at new sites in a globin gene can lead to abnormal processing of globin mRNA precursors; these constitute the molecular basis for many types of thalassemia (Chapters 13 and 16). Throughout this chapter we will refer to human mutations that affect some aspect of the pathway for gene expression. Readers desiring more information may want to use databases such as HbVar (http://www.bx.psu.edu)[13] or the Phencode project (http://phencode.bx.psu.edu)[14] to find positions, genotypes, and phenotypes for the greater than 1,000 known globin gene variants.

DETAILED CHROMOSOMAL ORGANIZATION OF THE HUMAN GLOBIN GENES

A precise picture of the chromosomal organization of the α- and β-like human globin gene clusters, with respect to the number of structural loci and intergenic distances, was obtained by a number of different techniques: 1) restriction

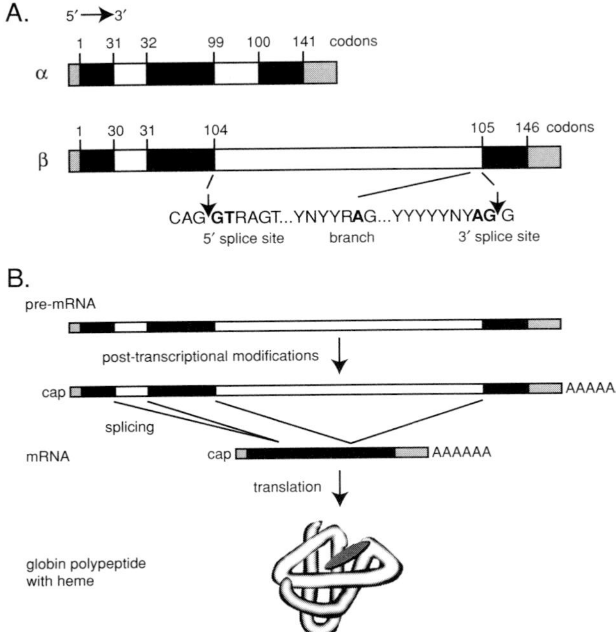

Figure 3.2. Structure and expression pathway of globin genes. (**A**) General structure of globin genes. The coding sequences of all globin genes in humans and other animals are separated by two introns (white boxes) into three exons. The first exon has a short 5′ untranslated region (gray box) followed by a coding region (black box). All of the central exon codes for protein, whereas the third exon begins with coding sequences and ends with a 3′ untranslated region. The relative sizes of the portions of the genes are indicated by the sizes of the boxes, and codon numbers are given above the boxes. The consensus sequence for critical sequences used in splicing are shown under the second intron of the β-globin gene, and similar sequences are present in all introns. The vertical arrows show the splice site junctions within the consensus sequences where cleavage occurs during the process of joining the exons. (**B**) The pathway for expression of globin genes. The RNA transcript is shown with short boxes corresponding to the untranslated regions (gray), coding regions (black), and introns (white) as in (A), with processing and splicing steps occurring in the nucleus to form the mature mRNA. The mRNA is translated in the cytoplasm to generate a globin polypeptide to which the heme (gray disk) will bind. The diagram of the folded globin structure was provided by Dr. John Blamire at the Brooklyn College of the City University of New York.

endonuclease mapping of genomic DNA (e.g., refs. 15, 16) using the gel blotting procedure of Southern,[17] and, 2) gene isolation and sequencing using recombinant DNA technology (e.g., ref. 18). Sets of overlapping genomic DNA fragments spanning the entire α- and β-globin gene clusters were obtained by gene cloning, initially in bacteriophage λ and larger fragments in cosmid vectors. Detailed analysis of these recombinant DNA clones and complete DNA sequencing led to the determination of the gene organization illustrated in Figure 3.3. Some results were expected, such as the finding of single δ- and β-globin gene loci and duplication of the α- and γ-globin gene loci. In addition, single loci for the embryonic ζ- and ε-globin chains were found linked to the α- and β-globin gene clusters, respectively. It is noteworthy that the genes in each cluster are in the same transcriptional orientation and are arranged, in a 5′ to 3′ direction, in the same order as their expression during development.

An unexpected finding was the presence in the globin gene clusters of additional gene-like structures with sequence homology and an exon–intron structure similar to the actively expressed globin genes. These DNA segments have been called pseudogenes.[19] One, called ψβ1, is in the β-like globin gene cluster between the γ- and δ-globin genes. At least two (and possibly four) are in the α-like globin gene cluster. The two clear examples are ψζ1 and ψα1, located between the active ζ-globin and α-globin genes (Fig. 3.3). All three (ψβ1, ψζ1, and ψα1) are characterized by the presence of one or more mutations that render them incapable of encoding a functional globin chain. This inability to encode a functional globin polypeptide does not necessarily render the pseudogenes inactive for transcription. The pseudogene ψβ1 is transcribed and spliced, as shown by several spliced expressed sequence tags, whereas no evidence has been provided that ψα1 is transcribed. These pseudogenes appear to have arisen by gene duplication events within the globin gene clusters followed by mutation and inactivation of the duplicated gene and subsequent accumulation of additional mutations through loss of selective pressure.

Two other α-like globin genes have been identified and characterized in the α-globin gene cluster, but their roles, if any, in encoding globin polypeptides are still uncertain. The θ-globin gene is located to the 3′ or C-terminal side of the duplicated α-globin genes.[20] It is more closely related to the α-globin genes than to the ζ-globin genes and is expressed at low levels in erythroid cells.[21,22] Clear homologs to the θ-globin gene are found in the homologous position in other mammalian α-like globin gene clusters. The μ-globin gene is located just 3′ of the ψζ1-globin pseudogene;[23,24] it was initially called ψα2[25] but with more accurate sequencing it is clear that this gene does not contain mutations that would render it inactive. It is a distant relative, being equally divergent from both α-globin and ζ-globin genes. Its closest relatives are the α^D-globin genes, which are actively expressed in red cells of reptiles and birds.[24,26] DNA sequences similar to that of the human μ-globin gene are found in other mammals, but in some species, such as mouse, the sequence has diverged so much that no obvious gene structure is found. Thus the presence of the θ-globin gene is conserved in all mammals examined but the μ-globin gene has been lost in some but not all lineages. Transcripts from both the θ-globin gene and the μ-globin gene are produced and spliced in erythroid cells, albeit at much lower levels than the α-globin gene. Curiously, no hemoglobin containing the θ-globin chain or the μ-globin chain has been identified, even by sensitive mass spectrometry.[23] Furthermore, the predicted structure (translated amino acid sequence) of the θ-globin chain suggests that it would be unlikely to function normally as a hemoglobin subunit.[27] Thus these genes remain a puzzle. They tend to be retained over mammalian

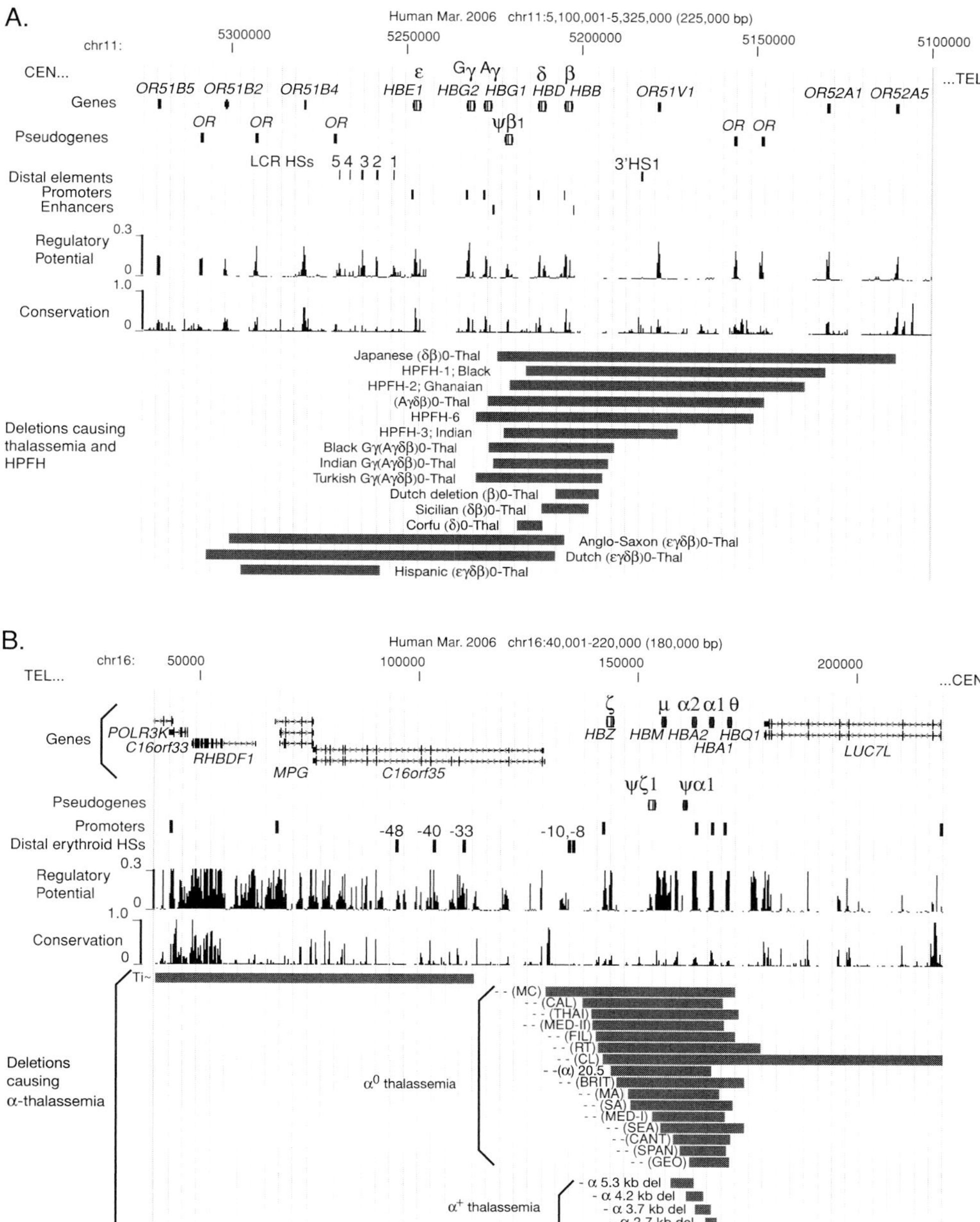

Figure 3.3. Detailed maps of the human globin gene complexes, including genomic features and representative deletions. (**A**) Detailed map of the β-like globin gene complex and surrounding olfactory receptor genes. The globin genes are named both by the encoded globin polypeptide and the official gene name. Pseudogenes are shown on a line below the genes. The known *cis*-regulatory modules are separated into distal elements such as the locus control region (shown as five DNase hypersensitive sites or HSs), promoters and enhancers close to the 3′ ends of *HBG1* and *HBB*. The next two tracks show two features derived from multiple alignments of the human genomic sequence with sequences from six other placental mammals (chimpanzee, rhesus macaque, mouse, rat, dog, and cow). The regulatory potential measures the similarity of patterns in the alignments to those that are distinctive for known regulatory regions versus neutral DNA.[57] The conservation score estimates the likelihood that an alignment is in the most constrained portion of the genome, likely reflecting purifying selection (phastCons).[56] Positions of deletions that cause δβ thalassemia or hereditary persistence of fetal hemoglobin (HPFH) are shown in the lower portion. (**B**) Detailed map of the α-like globin gene complex and surrounding genes. The conventions and tracks are similar to those in (A) Positions of the distal erythroid HSs are from Hughes et al.[26] The deletions are grouped by those with deletion of a single α-globin gene (α^+ thalassemia), deletion of both α-globin genes (α^0 thalassemia), and a representative deletion (Ti∼) that removes the distal enhancer (HS-40) but no structural genes. Coordinates of the deletions were provided by Dr. Jim Hughes. These figures were generated starting with output from the UCSC Genome Browser,[121] using the following tracks in addition to ones already mentioned: UCSC Known Genes,[122] ORegAnno for *cis*-regulatory modules,[123] and Locus Variants for the deletions.[14] For panel A, the Genome Browser output was rotated 180° so that the 5′–3′ transcriptional orientation is left to right (note that the genome coordinates are decreasing from left to right). Both figures were edited for clarity.

evolution, suggesting that their sequences are constrained to preserve some function. They are expressed at the RNA level but do not appear to be translated into a polypeptide. Perhaps they or their RNA transcripts play some role that has yet to be discovered.

GENOMIC CONTEXT OF THE α-GLOBIN AND β-GLOBIN GENE CLUSTERS

The separation of α- and β-globin gene clusters to different chromosomes has allowed them to diverge into strikingly different genomic contexts, with paradoxical consequences for our understanding of their regulation. Given that all contemporary vertebrates have developmentally regulated hemoglobin genes encoding proteins used for oxygen transport in erythrocytes, it would have been reasonable to expect that the molecular mechanisms of globin gene regulation would be conserved in vertebrates. Certainly, the coordinated and balanced expression of α- and β-globin genes to produce the heterotypic tetramer $\alpha_2\beta_2$ in erythrocytes should be a particularly easy aspect of regulation to explain. Because the two genes would have been identical after the initial duplication in the ancestral vertebrate, with identical regulatory elements, it is parsimonious to expect selection to keep the regulatory elements very similar.

Much has changed between the α- and β-like globin gene clusters since their duplication. Not only are they now on separate chromosomes in birds and mammals, but in mammals they are in radically different genomic contexts.[28] A major determinant of the genomic environment is the G+C content. A G+C-rich DNA segment has a high mole fraction of the nucleotides guanidylic acid (G) and cytidylic acid (C), whereas an A+T-rich DNA segment has a high mole fraction of the nucleotides adenylic acid (A) and thymidylic acid (T). The G+C content for the human genome on average is low (~41%) but some segments can be much lower or higher, ranging from 30% to 65% in 20-kb windows.[29] Regions that are G+C rich tend to be enriched in genes, and those genes tend to be expressed in a broad range of tissues. They also tend to have islands with an abundance of the dinucleotide CpG.[30] This is in stark contrast to the bulk of the genome, which has very few CpGs because these are the sites for DNA methylation, and substitution of CpG to TpG or CpA is very rapid on an evolutionary time scale (as much as 10 times faster than the rates of other substitutions). The CpG islands are thus short regions (a few hundred base pairs) in which the CpG dinucleotides are not methylated; these have been associated with important functions such as promoters for transcription.

The β-globin gene clusters in humans and other mammals are A+T rich, with no CpG islands,[31] whereas the α-like globin gene clusters are highly G+C rich, with multiple CpG islands.[32] This correlates with several important differences in the structure and regulation of the two gene clusters. Tissue-specific gene expression of the β-like globin genes is correlated with an increased accessibility of the chromatin only in expressing cells,[33] and hence "opening" of a chromatin domain is a key step in activation of these genes. In contrast, there are the α-like globin genes, which are in constitutively open chromatin.[28] The β-globin gene cluster is subject to tissue-specific DNA methylation,[34] but, in keeping with the presence of CpG islands, the α-globin gene cluster is not methylated in any cell type.[35] The β-globin gene clusters are replicated early in S phase only in cells expressing them, whereas the human α-globin genes are replicated early in all cells.[36–38] Thus, the mammalian α-globin genes have several characteristics associated with constitutively expressed "housekeeping" genes. The strikingly different genomic contexts of the two gene clusters affect several aspects of DNA and chromatin metabolism, including timing of replication, extent of methylation, and the type of chromatin into which the loci are packaged. Rather than selecting for similarities to ensure coordinate and balanced expression, the processes of evolution at these two loci have made them quite different. The full implications of these differences may not yet be known. For instance, the two "healthy" genes with no known function in the α-like globin gene cluster, θ and μ, are themselves CpG islands. Could this be a clue to a role for these genes outside the conventional one of coding for proteins?

The types of genes that surround the α-like and β-like globin gene clusters are quite different (Fig. 3.3). The β-like globin gene cluster is surrounded by olfactory receptor (*OR*) genes, which encode G protein–coupled receptors expressed in olfactory epithelium.[39] Several *OR* gene clusters containing approximately 1,000 genes and pseudogenes are found in the human genome. The *OR* gene cluster surrounding the β-like globin genes is a particularly large one, with approximately 100 genes extending almost 1 million bp (Mb) past *HBB* (the β-globin gene) and over 3 Mb toward the centromere from *HBE1* (the ε-globin gene). This arrangement is found in homologous regions in mammals and in chickens. Thus the erythroid-specific regulation of the β-like globin gene cluster is exerted in a chromosomal environment that is largely devoted to olfactory-specific expression. Perhaps this has had an impact on selection for a particularly powerful enhancer, to override the olfactory-specific regulation. As shown in Figure 3.3A, some deletions causing δβ thalassemia or hereditary persistence of fetal hemoglobin not only remove β-like globin genes, but they also fuse the remaining genes with sequences close to an *OR* gene. The phenotype of patients carrying such deletions may be explained in part by bringing positive or negative regulatory elements normally associated with *OR* genes into proximity of the β-like globin genes[40–41] (see Chapter 16).

In contrast, the α-like globin genes are surrounded by a variety of genes (Fig. 3.3.B), many of which are widely expressed and carry out fundamental roles in cellular metabolism and physiology, such as *MPG* (encoding the DNA repair enzyme methyl purine glycosylase) and *POLR3K* (encoding a subunit of RNA polymerase III).[42] Although the α-like globin gene cluster and surrounding DNA is in constitutively open chromatin, histones are hyperacetylated (another mark of active loci) in erythroid cells in a more restricted region encompassing the globin genes and their regulatory sequences.[43] The regions homologous to that surrounding the α-like globin gene cluster have undergone inter- and intrachromosomal rearrangements in various vertebrate lineages, but the genes from *POLR3K* through *HBQ1* have remained together in all species examined from fish to mammals.[44] This suggests that this region encompasses all the sequences needed in *cis* for appropriate regulation of the α-like globin genes.

Despite these many differences between α-like and β-like globin gene clusters in mammals, the appropriate genes are still expressed coordinately between the two loci, resulting in balanced production of α-like and β-like globins needed for the synthesis of normal hemoglobins. The mechanisms that accomplish this task still elude our understanding.

One important aspect that is common to the genomic contexts of both gene clusters is the presence of distal strong enhancers. The discovery of these enhancers was aided by mapping of deletions that result in β thalassemia or α thalassemia, which are inherited deficiencies in the amount of β-globin or α-globin, respectively (see Chapters 13 and 16). A number of these deletions removed distal sequences but retained all the globin genes, such as the deletions associated with Hispanic $(\varepsilon\gamma\delta\beta)^0$ thalassemia and the Ti~ α^0 thalassemia (Fig. 3.3), as well as other deletions (Figs. 13.7 and 16.5). Within the deleted intervals are critical long-range enhancers needed for high-level expression of any gene in the linked globin gene clusters. These are the locus control region (LCR) for the β-globin gene cluster and HS-40 or major regulatory element for the α-globin gene cluster. Thus regulation of expression of globin genes involves DNA sequences both close to the genes (proximal) and as much as 70 kb away from the genes (distal). These will be examined in more detail in the next section.

EVOLUTIONARY INSIGHTS INTO REGULATION OF GLOBIN GENE CLUSTERS

Motivation

One avenue for improving the conditions of patients with hemoglobinopathies could involve regulation of expression of the globin genes. This hope is based on the normal human variation in phenotypes presented for a given mutant genotype. For example, patients with naturally higher concentrations of HbF ($\alpha_2\gamma_2$) in their erythrocytes tend to have milder symptoms of either sickle cell disease or β thalassemia (Chapters 17 and 19). The α-globin gene status can affect the severity of β thalassemia, with more balanced production of α-globin and β-globin associated with milder disease. Thus considerable effort has gone into studying the stage-specific expression of the globin genes, with a long-term goal of enhancing or restoring production of embryonic or fetal hemoglobins in adult life or reducing expression of deleterious alleles. Although no current treatment by gene therapy is in practice as of this writing, much effort continues in this area. The use of hydroxyurea in the treatment of sickle cell disease is an outgrowth of studies on mechanisms of regulation of globin genes. Current studies aim to discover more sophisticated and directed pharmacological methods for enhancing production of embryonic and fetal hemoglobins.

Studies over the past three decades have revealed much about the regulation of the human globin genes. In this section, we will summarize some of the information about DNA sequences needed in *cis* (i.e., on the same chromosome) for regulation of the globin genes. Chapter 4 will cover the proteins interacting with these regulatory DNA sequences.

Common versus Lineage-specific Regulation

Comparison of noncoding genomic DNA sequences among related species is a powerful approach to identifying and better understanding *cis*-regulatory modules (CRMs). It is important to distinguish, however, what is similar and what is distinctive about the patterns of regulated expression of the genes in the species being compared. If one is searching for CRMs that perform a function common to most or all mammals, then conservation across all mammals and evidence of strong constraint in noncoding DNA will provide good candidates for further experimental tests (e.g., refs. 45–47). Such constrained noncoding sequences can have within them short, almost invariant regions that frequently correspond to transcription factor binding sites. These have been called phylogenetic footprints.[48] If one is studying a type of regulation that only occurs in higher primates, then searching for sequences conserved in other mammalian orders will be futile. Instead, the search should focus on sequences conserved in the species with a common mode of regulation but which differ from the homologous regions in species with a different regulation. These have been called differential phylogenetic footprints.[49]

Regulatory features of globin genes common to many vertebrate species include tissue specificity and some aspects of developmental specificity. Expression of the α-like and β-like globin genes in all vertebrate species examined is restricted to the erythroid lineage. Thus some determinants of tissue specificity should be common to all these genes. One example is binding by the transcription factor GATA-1. As will be detailed in the following sections, the promoter, enhancers, or both for all globin genes have binding sites for GATA-1. Another feature common to all mammals is the expression of the ε-globin and ζ-globin genes exclusively in primitive erythroid cells, which are produced during embryonic life. Thus one might expect determinants of embryonic expression to be conserved in many species. Indeed, conservation of the upstream promoter regions of these genes in eutherian mammals is more extensive than is seen for other promoters in their globin gene clusters.[50]

An example of lineage-specific regulation is the recruitment of the γ-globin genes for expression in fetal erythroid cells. In most eutherian mammals, the γ-globin genes are expressed in primitive erythroid cells, similar to the ε-globin gene, and the β-globin gene is expressed in definitive erythroid cells both during fetal and adult life. Simian primates, including humans, express the γ-globin genes during fetal erythropoiesis, and the expression of the β-globin gene is delayed. The extent of delay varies in different primate clades, but in humans it is largely delayed until just before birth. Thus when examining interspecies alignments of the regulatory regions of the β-globin gene (*HBB*) and the γ-globin genes (*HBG1* and *HBG2*), one will be seeing a combination of CRMs used in common (e.g., for adult erythroid expression of *HBB*) and in a lineage-specific manner (e.g., fetal expression of *HBG1*).

Quantitative Analysis of Sequence Alignments

Alignments of genomic DNA sequences reveal the segments that are similar between species, and often these reflect homology (descent from a common ancestor). These sequence matches tend to have the highest similarity in the protein-coding exons, but significant stretches of noncoding sequences also align between mammalian species (for globin gene complexes, see refs. 51–53). Further analysis is required to discern which sequence matches simply reflect common ancestry (aligned neutral DNA) versus those in sequences that are under constraint (sequences with a common function).[54,55]

Several bioinformatic tools have been developed to help interpret the alignments of multiple sequences. Results from two of these, each analyzing alignments of several mammals (human, chimpanzee, rhesus macaque, mouse, rat, dog, cow, and sometimes additional ones), are shown in Figure 3.3. The Conservation track plots the phastCons score at each position of the human sequence. This score is an estimate of the posterior probability that a given nucleotide is in the most strongly constrained (i.e., most slowly changing) portion of the genome.[56] Higher scores are associated with a greater likelihood that a position or region is under strong purifying selection. Sequences that are needed for a feature that is common to these several placental mammals would be expected to have a high Conservation score.

A discriminatory analysis of the multiple alignments was used to generate a Regulatory Potential score.[57] This machine-learning approach estimates the likelihood that a given aligning segment is a CRM, given the frequency of patterns in the alignments that are distinctive for CRMs as opposed to neutral DNA. The patterns are strings of alignment columns, and their discriminatory power is determined by the frequency of the patterns in training sets of alignments in CRMs compared with alignments in neutral DNA. Although the Regulatory Potential score is influenced by features in addition to constraint, it is designed for finding CRMs that are common among species.

Basal Promoters

Promoters are DNA sequences needed for accurate initiation of transcription. For some promoters including the globin gene promoters, one DNA segment interacts with RNA polymerase II and its accessory factors (such as TFIID and TFIIB) to determine the start site of transcription; this is the basal promoter.[58] Five motifs have been associated with basal promoters, and these are found in the promoters of human globin genes (Fig. 3.4.A). They include the familiar TATA box to which TBP binds, along with the BRE to which TFIIB binds and the Inr and DPE motifs to which components of TFIID bind.[58]

Early studies revealed the presence of the ATAAA motif approximately 25–30 bp 5′ to the start site of transcription of the globin genes,[59] and this is by far the most restricted in its consensus, that is, this motif appears to be under evolutionary constraint in globin genes. Recent studies on other promoters are revealing the roles of additional motifs close to the start site of transcription, but on both sides. Matches to these motifs can be found readily at the appropriate positions in the human globin genes (Fig. 3.4.A). The motifs other than TATA do not have well-defined consensus sequences, either for genes in general or for the human globin genes, and thus their presence alone may not signify function. Also, only the TATA box, Inr, and DPE show evidence of constraint in homologs in other mammalian species (Fig. 3.5.A, conservation track). Each of the motifs except BRE has been implicated in function by finding a mutation in at least one case of β thalassemia. Every base in the TATA box has been altered in one or another β thalassemia, and mutations in Inr, MTE, and DPE also are associated with β thalassemia (Fig. 3.5.A, Compilation of Human Disease Variants and Other Mutations). The BRE overlaps with the β-direct repeat element (βDRE), which is a *cis*-regulatory element bound by βDRF and demonstrated to function in regulation of the β-globin gene by mutagenesis and expression in transfected cells.[60] Thus, the mutagenesis data (natural and directed) indicate that all five motifs are important for appropriate expression of the β-globin gene. The presence of similar motifs in the basal promoters for other human globin genes suggests that they are active in these genes as well.

Although it is common to describe promoters recognized by RNA polymerase II by the motifs shown in Figure 3.4.A, it is important to realize that this is true for only a minority of human genes. Globin gene promoters

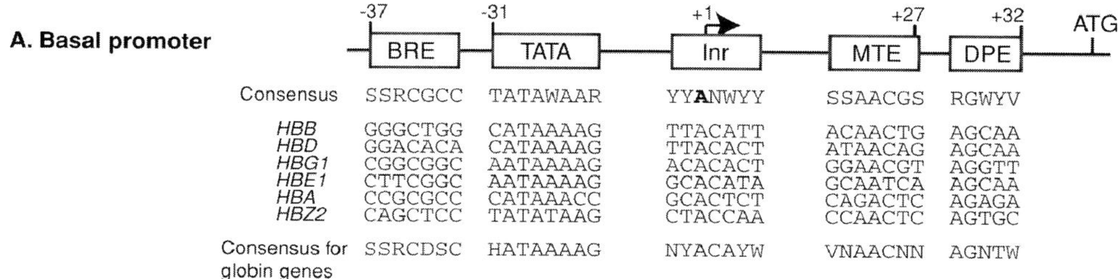

B. Upstream regulation

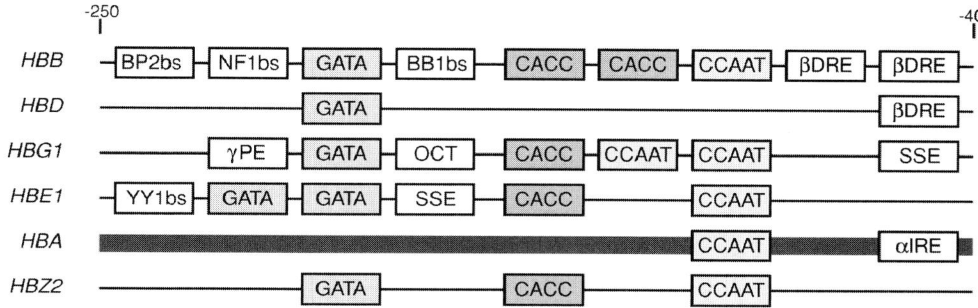

C. Proximal enhancers 3′ to genes

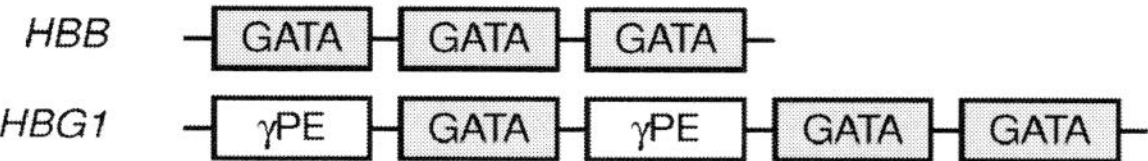

D. Distal positive regulators 5′ to genes

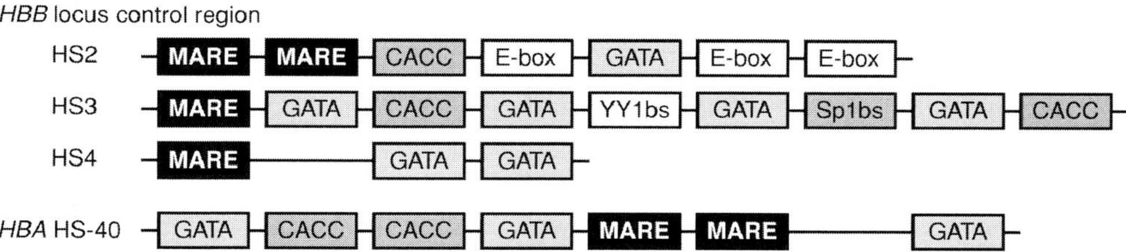

Figure 3.4. Motifs and binding sites in *cis*-regulatory modules of globin genes. (**A**) Motifs in the basal promoter, based on those defined in the review by Maston et al.[58] Numbers along the top are relative to the transcription start site as +1, and ATG denotes the translation start site. The top consensus sequence is from Maston et al. Corresponding positions in the globin genes are given for each motif, followed by the consensus derived for the globin genes. Symbols for ambiguous nucleotides are S = C or G, W = A or T, R = A or G, Y = C or T, D = A or G or T, H = A or C or T, V = A or C or G, and N = A or C or G or T. (**B**) Motifs in the regulatory regions immediately upstream of the basal promoters. Motifs are indicated by sequence (CCAAT, CACC, and GATA), the name of the element (βDRE, αIRE, γPE, and OCT) or the protein name followed by bs for "binding site" (BP2bs, NF1bs, and BB1bs). Boxes for motifs found in several upstream regions are shaded. The boxes were placed in the correct order but spacing is not indicated. The thick line for the *HBA* upstream regions (both *HBA1* and *HBA2*) denotes that it is a CpG island. (**C**) Motifs in the proximal enhancers. (**D**) Motifs in distal positive regulators, including three hypersensitive sites of the β-globin LCR and HS-40 for the α-globin gene cluster.

fall into the category of promoters with well-defined TATA boxes at a restricted location and one major start site for transcription. Recent studies show that these comprise a small minority of promoters, perhaps only 10%–20%. Most promoters are CpG islands with no obvious TATA box, and in some cases they have a broad distribution of start sites.[61]

Upstream Regulatory Sequences

Adjacent to the basal promoter is the upstream regulatory region,[58] which in globin genes runs from approximately positions -40 to -250 (Fig. 3.4.B). Only one motif in this region is found in all the highly expressed globin genes: the CCAAT box. Proteins such as NF-Y and CP1 bind to this

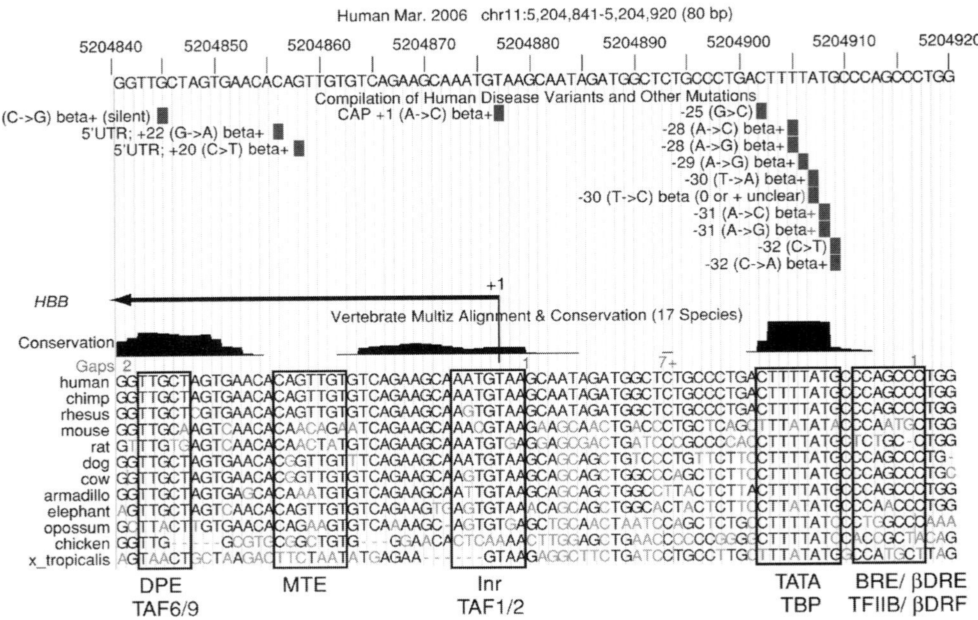

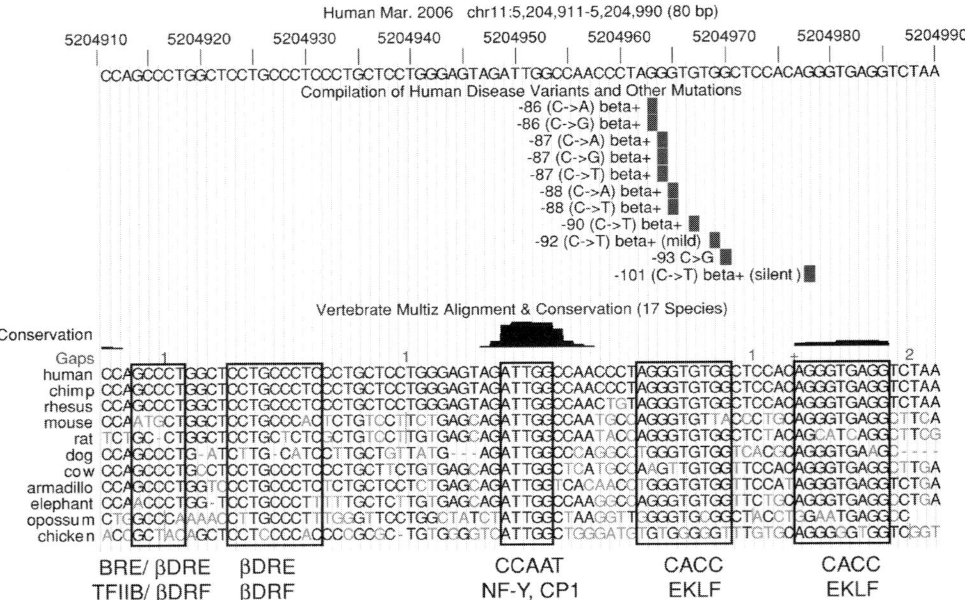

Figure 3.5. Conservation and mutations in globin gene promoters. (**A**) Basal promoter and (**B**) upstream promoter for *HBB*. In each panel, the sequence of an 80-bp segment is shown, along with positions of mutations associated with β thalassemia, conservation scores, and alignments with many mammals, chicken, and frog (*X. tropicalis*). The display is from the UCSC Genome Browser in genome coordinates (top line), and the direction of transcription is from right to left (opposite that used in previous figures). The start site of transcription is denoted by the vertical line leading to a leftward arrow. Boxes are drawn around motifs, which are labeled by name and proteins that bind to them (bottom line in each panel).

motif,[62,63] and it has been implicated in promoter function because of its presence in many promoters and the results of mutagenesis and binding studies.[59] It is missing from the δ-globin gene (*HBD*) promoter, but this gene is expressed at a low level (~1%–2% of *HBB*).

Two motifs are found in many but not all promoters. One is the CACC box, which is bound by transcription factors in the Krüppel-like zinc finger class (KLF). The first erythroid KLF discovered was erythroid Krüppel-like factor, which binds to the CACC box in the *HBB* promoter and is needed for erythropoiesis.[64,65] The CACC boxes in globin promoters tend to be highly conserved in other mammals, albeit not as constrained as the CCAAT box (Fig. 3.5.B). Mutations in almost every position in the proximal CACC box have been associated with β thalassemia (Fig. 3.5.B). Thus many lines of evidence point to the importance of this motif. Other KLFs may bind to the CACC boxes in other globin gene promoters, such as FKLF or KLF13[66] for the *HBG1* and *HBG2* promoters.

The other motif occurring frequently in upstream regulatory regions is WGATAR, the binding site for GATA-1 and related proteins (Fig. 3.4.B). GATA-1 plays a critical role in erythroid-specific gene activation and repression,[67–69] and the binding sites in these upstream regions have been implicated in positive regulation of the respective genes.[70,71] The GATA-1 binding sites upstream of *HBE1*, *HBG1*, *HBG2*, and *HBZ2* are conserved in most mammals, but the ones upstream of *HBB* are not. GATA-1 binds to the promoter regions of β-globin genes in both human[63] and mouse,[72] but the binding site motif occurs in different places in the two promoters.[73] This is an example of alterations in the binding site being associated with changes in the pattern of regulation, such as the delay in onset of expression in humans.

A different set of binding sites is distinctive to each type of gene. For instance, βDRF[60] and BB1-binding protein[72,74] have been implicated in the regulation of the β-globin gene but not other globin genes (Fig. 3.4.B). Both binding sites are conserved in many placental mammals (Fig. 3.5.B).[73] Likewise, binding of OCT1 and γPE has been shown for the upstream regions of γ-globin genes but not others.[75]

The *cis*-elements close to the γ-globin genes are key determinants of fetal compared with embryonic expression. One of the clearest demonstrations of this is from transgenic mouse experiments in which a construct containing an LCR is used to enhance expression of globin genes. The γ-globin gene of prosimians, that is, the bushbaby galago, is expressed embryonically, and when it is included in the test construct in transgenic mice, the transgene is also expressed embryonically. In contrast, a human γ-globin gene, normally expressed during fetal life in humans, is expressed fetally when transferred into transgenic mice in an otherwise identical construct.[76] Thus one would expect to find alterations in the regulatory regions of anthropoid (monkey, ape, and human) γ-globin genes that are associated with this change in stage specificity (i.e., sequences that are conserved in anthropoid primates but are different in prosimians and nonprimate mammals). Examination of aligned sequences for differential phylogenetic footprints[49] led to the identification of a stage selector element in the human γ-globin gene promoter (Fig. 3.4.B). The stage selector element is a binding site for a factor called the stage selector protein, which has been implicated in the differential expression of γ- and β-globin genes.[77] Additional DNA sequences that bind several proteins have been implicated in fetal silencing of the γ-globin gene.[49]

Parallel protein-binding and mutagenesis studies led to the discovery of a novel protein that binds to an element called the γPE, in the upstream regulatory region of the γ-globin genes, which has also been implicated in regulation of this gene.[75]

The most distinctive globin gene promoters are those of the α-globin genes (*HBA1* and *HBA2*). These promoters are CpG islands, and among the hemoglobin genes, only those encoding α-globin have this feature. (The θ-globin and μ-globin genes also have promoters in CpG islands, but as discussed previously, it is not clear that they encode components of hemoglobin.) Although the majority of mammalian promoters are CpG islands,[61] most of the associated genes are expressed in multiple tissues and few if any are expressed at such a high level as the α-globin gene. Thus the presence of a CpG island in the promoter for a globin gene is curious, and it leads to several unanswered questions about the α-globin gene promoters. What prevents their expression in nonerythroid tissues? What sequences in addition to the CpG island lead to very high-level expression in erythroid cells? No GATA-1-binding site is found in the α-globin gene promoters of most placental mammals (the mouse α-globin genes is a notable exception), so sequence-directed binding of this protein to the proximal sequences is not the answer. Several studies have shown that the CpG island is a key component of the *cis*-regulatory elements for the α-globin gene of humans and rabbits, possibly through its effects on chromatin structure.[78,79]

The differences in the arrays of proteins functioning at ε-, γ-, β-, and α-globin genes indicate that a distinct battery of proteins functions in the promoter for each type of gene. Indeed, this is consistent with the observation that *cis*-acting sequences needed for stage-specific regulation of expression map close to the genes.[80]

Proximal Enhancers

Enhancers are DNA sequences that increase the activity of promoters; they can be located on either side of a gene or internal to it, and they can act at considerable distances from genes.[81] Two enhancers have been found close to genes in the β-globin gene cluster, one that is 3′ to *HBB* and one that is 3′ to *HBG1* (Fig. 3.3.A). In both cases the enhancers are less than 1 kb downstream of the polyA additional signal for the respective genes. The *HBB* enhancer was discovered by its effect on developmental timing of expression of globin transgenes when introduced into mice. High-level expression of human γ- or β-globin transgene constructs in fetal erythroid cells (the normal onset of expression of mouse β-globin genes) is dependent on the presence of the enhancer.[74,82–84] The *HBG1* enhancer was discovered as the only DNA segment in a 22-kb region surrounding the γ-globin genes that boosted expression of a reporter gene driven by a γ-globin gene promoter in transfected erythroid cells.[85] Deletion of this enhancer from a large construct containing the human LCR and β-like

A. 3′ enhancer for *HBG1*

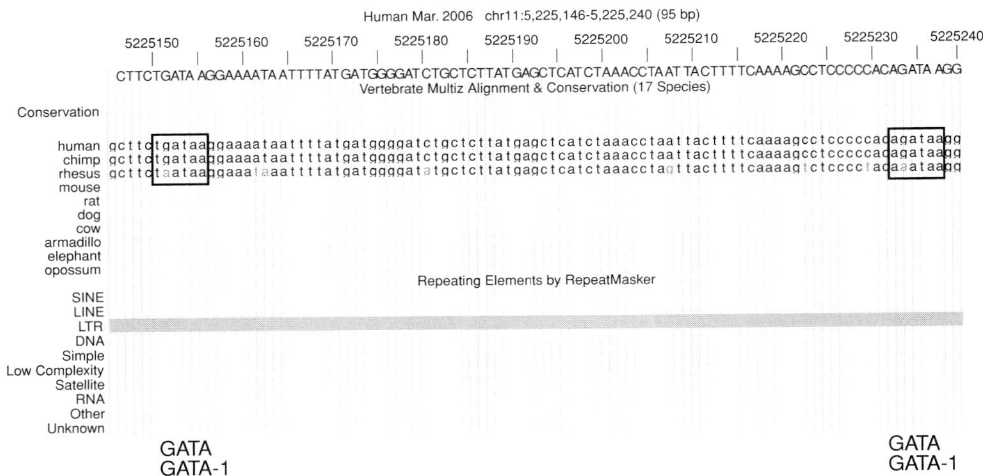

B. Distal enhancer for *HBA*

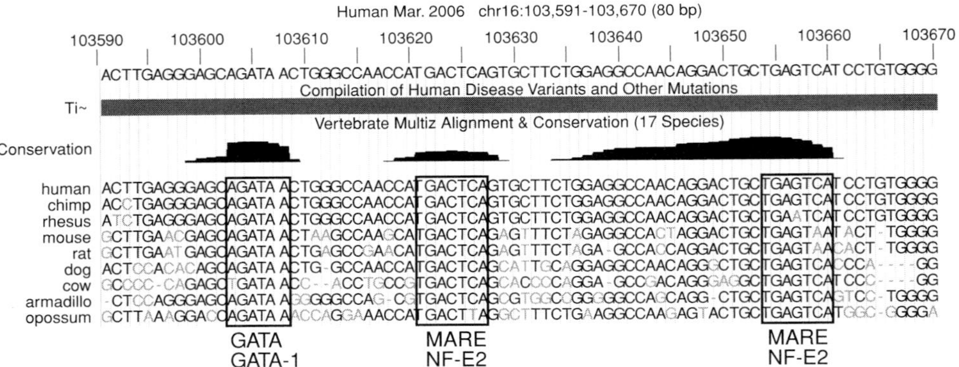

Figure 3.6. Wide range of conservation in globin gene enhancers. (**A**) Proximal enhancer for *HBG1*, showing the sequence of part of the 3′ enhancer, alignments with sequences of other anthropoid primates, the encompassing repetitive element, and binding motifs. (**B**) Distal enhancer for the α-globin gene cluster, HS-40. The panel shows an 80-bp segment of the enhancer, along with the Ti∼α thalassemia deletion that removes this DNA and more, the conservation track and alignments with several eutherian mammals and the marsupial opossum. Binding sites are boxed and labeled by name and proteins binding to them.

globin genes had no effect on expression levels in transgenic mice,[86] which could mean that it actually has no function, or that other sequences compensate for its loss, or that its function is not apparent in mice.

Indeed, comparative sequence analysis of these proximal enhancers strongly supports the conclusion that both play roles in higher primates but not in other species. As illustrated in Figure 3.4.C, both enhancers contain binding sites for GATA-1,[87,88] and the *HBG1* enhancer also binds to the γPE protein.[75] The DNA homologous to the *HBB* enhancer in other mammals is not strongly conserved, even in the GATA motifs. Furthermore, two of the GATA-1–binding sites in the *HBG1* enhancer were introduced via an LTR-type transposable element that is present only in higher primates (Fig. 3.6.A). Thus the presence of the *HBG1* proximal enhancer correlates with the fetal recruitment of γ-globin gene expression in anthropoids, and its function may not be observed in transgenic mice. Likewise, the presence of GATA-1–binding sites only in higher primates suggests that the function of the *HBB* proximal enhancer may also be lineage-specific, perhaps related to the delay in expression of *HBB* in higher primates. In this case, an effect on developmental timing is readily demonstrable in transgenic mice, but because of the differences in timing of *HBB* expression in humans (the source of the transgene) and mouse (the host species), it is difficult to understand fully this function.

Distal Enhancers

In addition to the proximal promoters and enhancers, both the α-like and β-like globin gene clusters are regulated by distal control regions. The β-like globin cluster is regulated by the distal LCR (reviewed in refs. 89, 90), and the α-like globin gene cluster is regulated by HS-40.[91] In both cases, deletion of the distal control region is associated with thalassemia (Fig. 3.3). Addition of the distal control regions has profound effects on expression of linked genes in transgenic mice. Without the LCR, erythroid expression of a β-globin transgene is not seen in all mouse lines,[92] presumably because of integration in a repressive region of a chromosome (a position effect). With the LCR, the β-globin transgene is expressed at a high level in erythroid cells in almost all mouse lines, indicating strong enhancement and a reduction in position effects.[93] HS-40 of the α-globin gene complex is a strong enhancer of globin gene expression, both in transgenic mice[91,94] and in transfected cells.[95]

The β-globin LCR is a very large regulatory region, containing at least five DNase hypersensitive sites in humans spread over approximately 17 kb[96–98] between *HBE1* and an *OR* gene (Fig. 3.3.A). This region is highly conserved in mammals, with highly similar sequences indicative of constraint found both in the hypersensitive sites and between them.[50,90] This can be seen in Figure 3.3.A as the string of peaks of conservation and RP in this region.

The distal enhancer for the α-globin gene, HS-40, is much smaller than the LCR. It is approximately 250 bp in length,[99] located in a widely expressed gene called *C16orf35* (Fig. 3.3.B). Additional erythroid DNase hypersensitive sites are present in this large gene, but none has been shown to play a role in regulation of globin genes.[26] HS-40 is sufficient for strong enhancement and high activity in erythroid cells of transgenic mice, especially during embryonic and fetal development.[91] It is very strongly conserved in mammals, with obvious matches to species as distant as opossum (Figs. 3.3.B and 3.6.B). Functional tests have shown that the homologous regions of chicken and fish also have enhancer activity, despite considerable divergence outside the protein-binding sites.[44]

Regulatory activities in addition to tissue-specific enhancement have been attributed to the β-globin LCR, but they are not seen consistently in multiple lines of investigation.[100] Examination of chromatin structure after deletion of the LCR led to the inference that the LCR is needed for tissue-specific chromosomal domain opening.[101] Chromosome 11 from a patient with the Hispanic (εγδβ)^0 thalassemia (missing most of the LCR and some adjacent sequences, but leaving all of the β-like globin genes intact) (Fig. 3.3A) was transferred through multiple somatic cells to generate a hybrid murine erythroleukemia cell line containing the mutant human chromosome. The β-globin gene cluster in this hybrid cell line is inactive and is insensitive to DNase, indicating that the LCR is needed for opening a chromosomal domain.[101] An engineered mouse line carrying a deletion of the mouse β-globin LCR and the sequences homologous to those lost in the Hispanic deletion retains an open chromatin conformation (accessible to DNase) in the mouse β-globin gene.[102] Although expression of the mouse β-globin genes is reduced substantially, the locus is not silenced. Thus the repressive heterochromatin seen in the hybrid murine erythroleukemia cells carrying human chromosome 11 with the Hispanic deletion may have been produced during the chromosome transfers between cell lines. Currently, the DNA sequence determinants of chromatin opening have still not been discovered. The β-globin LCR has also been implicated in overcoming position effects in transgenic mice,[103] in keeping with the inferred effect on opening a chromatin domain. Transgene constructs containing the β-globin can still show position effect variegation.[104] Both the β-globin LCR and the α-globin HS-40 are very strong, erythroid-specific enhancers needed for the expression of any of the linked globin genes. They also can overcome some but not all repressive effects after integration at a variety of chromosomal locations. This could be a consequence of the strong enhancement.

Three transcription factor–binding motifs are present in almost all DNase hypersensitive sites that have a strong function in the distal enhancers (Fig. 3.4.D). All contain Maf-response elements (MAREs) to which transcriptional activator proteins of the basic leucine zipper class can bind.[105] A subfamily of proteins related to AP1, such as NF-E2, LCRF1/Nrf1, and Bach1, bind to this element (reviewed in refs. 106, 107). All are heterodimers containing a Maf protein as one subunit, which is the basis for the name of the response element. All the hypersensitive sites have GATA motifs, to which GATA-1 and its relatives bind.[108] The third common motif is CACC, to which a family of Zinc-finger proteins including erythroid Krüppel-like factor can bind.[64] At HS3 in the β-globin LCR, there is evidence that motifs related to CACC are bound by additional KLFs, such as Sp1.[109] HS2 of the β-globin LCR also has three E-boxes, which are the binding sites for TAL-1 and its heterodimeric partners.[47] This protein has been implicated in regulation of hematopoiesis, and it appears to also play a role in enhancement by HS2.

Initial studies of protein binding at these and other CRMs used various in vitro methods and in vivo footprinting.[99,110–112] Recent experiments using chromatin immunoprecipitation have demonstrated occupancy of the CRMs by several of these proteins in erythroid cells.[113–116] Many of the sites have been implicated directly in activity by mutagenesis and gene transfer.[47,117–119]

The protein binding sites in the distal positive regulators show some common patterns (Fig. 3.4.D). A MARE plus two GATA motifs is present in most of the CRMs, and this arrangement has been shown to be needed for formation of a hypersensitive site at HS4.[120] The strongest enhancers (as assayed by gene transfer in somatic cells) are HS2 and HS-40. Both of these have two MAREs, and mutation of those MAREs removes much of the enhancing activity.[117,119] Thus the MAREs and proteins binding to them are critical for high-level enhancement, but the other binding sites contribute to function as well.

The CRMs marked by these hypersensitive sites in the distal positive regulators are conserved across almost all mammals.[26,90] The portion of the alignments for HS-40 shown in Figure 3.6.B indicates the very strong constraint seen in the known binding sites and additional short segments both for this enhancer and for HS2. Most of the binding sites in HS3 are also highly conserved, but some are not, likely reflecting both common and lineage-specific functions. HS4, with the MARE and two GATA motifs, is conserved across a wide span of placental mammals, but this DNA sequence is part of an LTR-type repeat, a member of the ERV1 repeat family. This appears to be an old transposable element (predating most of the mammalian radiation), but one that continues to provide a regulatory function.

CONCLUDING REMARKS

Molecular clones containing mammalian globin gene clusters were isolated approximately 30 years ago. Intense study since then has revealed much about their structure, evolution, and regulation; however, understanding sufficient to lead to clinical applications continues to elude us. The myriad levels of regulation and function that operate within these gene clusters certainly confound attempts to find simplifying conclusions. Despite these challenges, studies of the globin gene clusters have consistently provided new insights into function, regulation, and evolution. The lessons being learned as we try to integrate information from classic molecular biology and genetics, new high-through-put biochemical assays, and extensive interspecies sequence comparisons are paving the way for applying these approaches genome wide. The globin gene clusters illustrate the need to distinguish common from lineage-specific regulation. Although simple generalizations are rare, the extensive information that one needs for interpreting data in the context of comparative genomics is readily accessible. Throughout this chapter, we have illustrated points using output from the UCSC Genome Browser (http://genome.ucsc.edu), with special emphasis on the tracks showing Conservation, Regulatory Potential, and Locus Variants. Deeper information on the variants associated with disorders of the hemoglobins can be obtained from HbVar (http://www.bx.psu.edu). We hope that the examples presented here will be helpful in guiding interpretation of the multitude of data available to the readers now and in the future.

ACKNOWLEDGMENTS

RH was supported by NIH grant R01 DK065806 and BGF was supported by NIH grants R01 DK19482 and P01 HL63357.

REFERENCES

1. Weatherall DJ, Clegg JB. *Thalassemia Syndromes.* 3rd ed. Oxford: Blackwell Scientific; 1981.
2. Baglioni C. The fusion of two peptide chains in hemoglobin Lepore and its interpretation as a genetic deletion. *Proc Natl Acad Sci USA.* 1962;48:1880–1886.
3. Kendall AG, Ojwang PJ, Schroeder WA, Huisman TH. Hemoglobin Kenya, the product of a gamma-beta fusion gene: studies of the family. *Am J Hum Genet.* 1973;25:548–563.
4. Deisseroth A, Nienhuis A, Turner P, et al. Localization of the human alpha globin structural gene to chromosome 16 in somatic cell hybrids by molecular hybridization assay. *Cell.* 1977;12:205–218.
5. Deisseroth A, Nienhuis AW, Lawrence J, Giles RE, Turner P, Ruddle FH. Chromosomal localization of the human beta globin gene to human chromosome 11 in somatic cell hybrids. *Proc Natl Acad Sci USA.* 1978;75:1456–1460.
6. Tilghman SM, Tiemeier DC, Seidman JG, et al. Intervening sequence of DNA identified in the structural portion of a mouse beta-globin gene. *Proc Natl Acad Sci USA.* 1978;75:725–729.
7. Goodman M, Czelusniak J, Koop B, Tagle D, Slightom J. Globins: a case study in molecular phylogeny. *Cold Spring Harbor Symp Quant Biol.* 1987;52:875–890.
8. Proudfoot NJ, Gil A, Maniatis T. The structure of the human zeta-globin gene and a closely linked, nearly identical pseudogene. *Cell.* 1982;31:553–563.
9. Tilghman SM, Curtis PJ, Tiemeier DC, Leder P, Weissmann C. The intervening sequence of a mouse beta-globin gene is transcribed within the 15S beta-globin mRNA precursor. *Proc Natl Acad Sci USA.* 1978;75:1309–1313.
10. Krainer AR, Maniatis T, Ruskin B, Green MR. Normal and mutant human beta-globin pre-mRNAs are faithfully and efficiently spliced in vitro. *Cell.* 1984;36:993–1005.
11. Mount SM. A catalogue of splice junction sequences. *Nucl Acids Res.* 1982;10:459–472.
12. Padgett RA, Grabowski PJ, Konarska MM, Seiler S, Sharp PA. Splicing of messenger RNA precursors. *Annu Rev Biochem.* 1986;55:1119–50.
13. Patrinos GP, Giardine B, Riemer C, et al. Improvements in the HbVar database of human hemoglobin variants and thalassemia mutations for population and sequence variation studies. *Nucl Acids Res.* 2004;32 Database issue:D537–D541.
14. Giardine B, Riemer C, Hefferon T, et al. PhenCode: connecting ENCODE data with mutations and phenotype. *Hum Mutat.* 2007;28:554–562.
15. Jeffreys AJ, Flavell RA. The rabbit beta-globin gene contains a large large insert in the coding sequence. *Cell.* 1977;12:1097–1108.
16. Tuan D, Biro PA, deRiel JK, Lazarus H, Forget BG. Restriction endonuclease mapping of the human gamma globin gene loci. *Nucl Acids Res.* 1979;6:2519–2544.
17. Southern EM. Detection of specific sequences among DNA fragments separated by gel electrophoresis. *J Mol Biol.* 1975; 98:503–517.
18. Fritsch E, Lawn R, Maniatis T. Molecular cloning and characterization of the human beta-like globin gene cluster. *Cell.* 1980;19:959–972.
19. Zhang Z, Gerstein M. Large-scale analysis of pseudogenes in the human genome. *Curr Opin Genet Dev.* 2004;14:328–335.
20. Hsu S, Marks J, Shaw J, et al. Structure and expression of the human theta 1 globin gene. *Nature.* 1988;331:94–96.
21. Ley TJ, Maloney KA, Gordon JI, Schwartz AL. Globin gene expression in erythroid human fetal liver cells. *J Clin Invest.* 1989;83:1032–1038.

22. Albitar M, Peschle C, Liebhaber SA. Theta, zeta and epsilon globin messenger RNA are expressed in adults. *Blood.* 1989; 74:629–637.
23. Goh SH, Lee YT, Bhanu NV, et al. A newly discovered human alpha-globin gene. *Blood.* 2005;106:1466–1472.
24. Cooper SJ, Wheeler D, De Leo A, et al. The mammalian alphaD-globin gene lineage and a new model for the molecular evolution of alpha-globin gene clusters at the stem of the mammalian radiation. *Mol Phylogenet Evol.* 2006;38:439–448.
25. Hardison RC, Sawada I, Cheng J-F, Shen C-KJ, Schmid CW. A previously undetected pseudogene in the human alpha globin gene cluster. *Nucl Acids Res.* 1986;14:1903–1911.
26. Hughes JR, Cheng JF, Ventress N, et al. Annotation of cis-regulatory elements by identification, subclassification, and functional assessment of multispecies conserved sequences. *Proc Natl Acad Sci USA.* 2005;102:9830–9835.
27. Clegg JB. Can the product of the theta gene be a real globin? *Nature.* 1987;329:465–466.
28. Craddock CF, Vyas P, Sharpe JA, Ayyub H, Wood WG, Higgs DR. Contrasting effects of alpha and beta globin regulatory elements on chromatin structure may be related to their different chromosomal environments. *EMBO J.* 1995;14:1718–1726.
29. Lander ES, Linton LM, Birren B, et al. Initial sequencing and analysis of the human genome. *Nature.* 2001;409:860–921.
30. Bird AP. CpG-rich islands and the function of DNA methylation. *Nature.* 1986;321:209–213.
31. Collins FS, Weissman SM. The molecular genetics of human hemoglobin. *Prog Nucl Acids Res Mol Biol.* 1984;31: 315–462.
32. Fischel-Ghodsian N, Nicholls RD, Higgs DR. Unusual features of CpG-rich (HTF) islands in the human α-globin complex: association with nonfunctional pseudogenes and presence within the 3′ portion of the ζ genes. *Nucl Acids Res.* 1987;15:9215–9225.
33. Groudine M, Kohwi-Shigematsu T, Gelinas R, Stamatoyannopoylos G, Papyannopoulou T. Human fetal to adult hemoglobin switching: changes in chromatin structure of the β-globin gene locus. *Proc Natl Acad Sci USA.* 1983;80: 7551–7555.
34. Van Der Ploeg LHT, Flavell RA. DNA methylation in the human g-d-b globin locus in erythroid and nonerythroid tissues. *Cell.* 1980;19:947–958.
35. Bird A, Taggart M, Nicholls R, Higgs D. Non-methylated CpG-rich islands at the human α-globin locus: implications for evolution of the α-globin pseudogene. *EMBO J.* 1987;6:999–1004.
36. Epner E, Rifkind RA, Marks PA. Replication of alpha and beta globin DNA sequences occurs during early S phase in murine erythroleukemia cells. *Proc Natl Acad Sci USA.* 1981;78:3058–3062.
37. Goldman MA, Holmquist GP, Gray MC, Caston LA, Nag A. Replication timing of genes and middle repetitive sequences. *Science.* 1984;224:686–692.
38. Dhar V, Mager D, Iqbal A, Schildkraut CL. The co-ordinate replication of the human b-globin gene domain reflects its transcriptional activity and nuclease hypersensitivity. *Mol Cell Biol.* 1988;8:4958–4965.
39. Bulger M, Bender MA, von Doorninck JH, et al. Comparative structural and functional analysis of the olfactory receptor genes flanking the human and mouse β-globin gene clusters. *Proc Natl Acad Sci USA.* 2000;97:14560–14565.
40. Feingold EA, Forget BG. The breakpoint of a large deletion causing hereditary persistence of fetal hemoglobin occurs within an erythroid DNA domain remote from the beta-globin gene cluster. *Blood.* 1989;74:2178–2186.
41. Anagnou NP, Perez-Stable C, Gelinas R, et al. Sequences located 3′ to the breakpoint of the hereditary persistence of fetal hemoglobin-3 deletion exhibit enhancer activity and can modify the developmental expression of the human fetal A gamma-globin gene in transgenic mice. *J Biol Chem.* 1995;270:10256–10263.
42. Flint J, Thomas K, Micklem G, et al. The relationship between chromosome structure and function at a human telomeric region. *Nat Genet.* 1997;15:252–257.
43. Anguita E, Johnson CA, Wood WG, Turner BM, Higgs DR. Identification of a conserved erythroid specific domain of histone acetylation across the alpha-globin gene cluster. *Proc Natl Acad Sci USA.* 2001;98:12114–12119.
44. Flint J, Tufarelli C, Peden J, et al. Comparative genome analysis delimits a chromosomal domain and identifies key regulatory elements in the alpha globin cluster. *Hum Mol Genet.* 2001;10:371–382.
45. Gumucio DL, Heilstedt-Williamson H, Gray TA, et al. Phylogenetic footprinting reveals a nuclear protein which binds to silencer sequences in the human γ and ε globin genes. *Mol Cell Biol.* 1992;12:4919–4929.
46. Gumucio D, Shelton D, Zhu W, et al. Evolutionary strategies for the elucidation of *cis* and *trans* factors that regulate the developmental switching programs of the beta-like globin genes. *Mol Phylog Evol.* 1996;5:18–32.
47. Elnitski L. Conserved E boxes in the locus control region contribute to enhanced expression of beta-globin genes via TAL1 and other basic helix-loop-helix proteins. The Pennsylvania State University; 1998.
48. Tagle DA, Koop BF, Goodman M, Slightom J, Hess DL, Jones RT. Embryonic ε and γ globin genes of a prosimian primate (*Galago crassicaudatus*): Nucleotide and amino acid sequences, developmental regulation and phylogenetic footprints. *J Mol Biol.* 1988;203:7469–7480.
49. Gumucio DL, Shelton DA, Blanchard-McQuate K, et al. Differential phylogenetic footprinting as a means to identify base changes responsible for recruitment of the anthropoid γ gene to a fetal expression pattern. *J Biol Chem.* 1994;269:15371–15380.
50. Hardison R, Miller W. Use of long sequence alignments to study the evolution and regulation of mammalian globin gene clusters. *Mol Biol Evol.* 1993;10:73–102.
51. Margot JB, Demers GW, Hardison RC. Complete nucleotide sequence of the rabbit beta-like globin gene cluster: Analysis of intergenic sequences and comparison with the human beta-like globin gene cluster. *J Mol Biol.* 1989;205:15–40.
52. Shehee R, Loeb DD, Adey NB, et al. Nucleotide sequence of the BALB/c mouse β-globin complex. *J Mol Biol.* 1989; 205:41–62.
53. Hardison R, Krane D, Vandenbergh D, et al. Sequence and comparative analysis of the rabbit alpha-like globin gene cluster reveals a rapid mode of evolution in a G+C-rich region of mammalian genomes. *J Mol Biol.* 1991;222:233–249.
54. Hardison RC. The nucleotide sequence of the rabbit embryonic globin gene β4. *J Biol Chem.* 1983;258:8739–8744.

55. Cooper GM, Brudno M, Stone EA, Dubchak I, Batzoglou S, Sidow A. Characterization of evolutionary rates and constraints in three Mammalian genomes. *Genome Res.* 2004;14:539–548.
56. Siepel A, Bejerano G, Pedersen JS, et al. Evolutionarily conserved elements in vertebrate, insect, worm, and yeast genomes. *Genome Res.* 2005;15:1034–1050.
57. Taylor J, Tyekucheva S, King DC, Hardison RC, Miller W, Chiaromonte F. ESPERR: Learning strong and weak signals in genomic sequence alignments to identify functional elements. *Genome Res.* 2006;16:1596–1604.
58. Maston GA, Evans SK, Green MR. Transcriptional regulatory elements in the human genome. *Annu Rev Genomics Hum Genet.* 2006;7:29–59.
59. Efstratiadis A, Posakony JW, Maniatis T, et al. The structure and evolution of the human β-globin gene family. *Cell.* 1980;21:653–668.
60. Stuve LL, Myers RM. A directly repeated sequence in the β-globin promoter regulates transcription in murine erythroleukemia cells. *Mol Cell Biol.* 1990;10:972–981.
61. Carninci P, Sandelin A, Lenhard B, et al. Genome-wide analysis of mammalian promoter architecture and evolution. *Nat Genet.* 2006;38:626–635.
62. Cohen RB, Sheffery M, Kim CG. Partial purification of a nuclear protein that binds to the CCAAT box of the mouse α1-globin gene. *Mol Cell Biol.* 1986;6:821–832.
63. deBoer E, Antoniou M, Mignotte V, Wall L, Grosveld F. The human β-globin promoter; nuclear protein factors and erythroid specific induction of transcription. *EMBO J.* 1988;7:4203–4212.
64. Miller IJ, Bieker JJ. A novel, erythroid cell-specific murine transcription factor that binds to the CACCC element and is related to the *Kruppel* family of nuclear factors. *Mol Cell Biol.* 1993;13:2776–2786.
65. Perkins AC, Sharpe AH, Orkin SH. Lethal β-thalassaemia in mice lacking the erythroid CACCC-transcription factor EKLF. *Nature.* 1995;375:318–322.
66. Asano H, Li XS, Stamatoyannopoulos G. FKLF, a novel Kruppel-like factor that activates human embryonic and fetal beta-like globin genes. *Mol Cell Biol.* 1999;19:3571–3579.
67. Pevny L, Simon MC, Robertson E, et al. Erythroid differentiation in chimaeric mice blocked by a targeted mutation in the gene for transcription factor GATA-1. *Nature.* 1991;349:257–60.
68. Simon MC, Pevny L, Wiles MV, Keller G, Costantini F, Orkin SH. Rescue of erythroid development in gene targeted GATA-1-mouse embryonic stem cells. *Nat Genet.* 1992;1:92–98.
69. Welch JJ, Watts JA, Vakoc CR, et al. Global regulation of erythroid gene expression by transcription factor GATA-1. *Blood.* 2004;104:3136–3147.
70. Martin D, Orkin S. Transcriptional activation and DNA binding by the erythroid factor GF-1/NF-E1/Eryf 1. *Genes Dev.* 1990;4:1886–1898.
71. Gong Q-H, Dean A. Enhancer-dependent transcripion of the ε-globin promoter requires promoter-bound GATA-1 and enhancer-bound AP-1/NF-E2. *Mol Cell Biol.* 1993;13:911–917.
72. Macleod K, Plumb M. Derepression of mouse β-major-globin gene transcription during erythroid differentiation. *Mol Cell Biol.* 1991;11:4324–4332.
73. Hardison R, Chao K-M, Schwartz S, Stojanovic N, Ganetsky M, Miller W. Globin gene server: A prototype E-mail database server featuring extensive multiple alignments and data compilation. *Genomics.* 1994;21:344–353.
74. Antoniou M, deBoer E, Habets G, Grosveld F. The human β–globin gene contains multiple regulatory regions: Identification of one promoter and two downstream enhancers. *EMBO J.* 1988;7:377–384.
75. Lloyd JA, Case SS, Ponce E, Lingrel JB. Positive transcriptional regulation of the human γ-globin gene: γPE is a novel nuclear factor with multiple binding sites near the gene. *J Biol Chem.* 1994;269:26–34.
76. TomHon C, Zhu W, Millinoff D, et al. Evolution of a fetal expression pattern via *cis*-changes near the γ-globin gene. *J Biol Chem.* 1997;272:14062–14066.
77. Jane SM, Ney PA, Vanin EF, Gumucio DL, Nienhuis AW. Identification of a stage selector element in the human γ-globin gene promoter that fosters preferential interaction with the 5′ HS2 enhancer when in competition with the β-promoter. *EMBO J.* 1992;11:2961–2969.
78. Pondel M, Murphy S, Pearson L, Craddock C, Proudfoot N. Sp1 functions in a chromatin-dependent manner to augment human alpha-globin promoter activity. *Proc Natl Acad Sci USA.* 1995;92:7237–7241.
79. Shewchuk BM, Hardison RC. CpG islands from the α-globin gene cluster increase gene expression in an integration-dependent manner. *Mol Cell Biol.* 1997;17:5856–5866.
80. Trudel M, Magram J, Bruckner L, Costantini F. Upstream G gamma-globin and downstream beta-globin sequences required for stage-specific expression in transgenic mice. *Mol Cell Biol.* 1987;7:4024–4029.
81. Tjian R, Maniatis T. Transcriptional activation: A complex puzzle with few easy pieces. *Cell.* 1994;77:5–8.
82. Trudel M, Costantini F. A 3′ enhancer contributes to the stage-specific expression of the human β-globin gene. *Genes Dev.* 1987;1:954–961.
83. Behringer RR, Hammer RE, Brinster RL, Palmiter RD, Townes TM. Two 3′ sequences direct adult erythroid-specific expression of human beta-globin genes in transgenic mice. *Proc Natl Acad Sci USA.* 1987;84:7056–7060.
84. Liu Q, Bungert J, Engel JD. Mutation of gene-proximal regulatory elements disrupts human epsilon-, gamma-, and beta-globin expression in yeast artificial chromosome transgenic mice. *Proc Natl Acad Sci USA.* 1997;94:169–174.
85. Bodine D, Ley T. An enhancer element lies 3′ to the human A gamma globin gene. *EMBO J.* 1987;6:2997–3004.
86. Liu Q, Tanimoto K, Bungert J, Engel JD. The A gamma-globin 3′ element provides no unique function(s) for human beta-globin locus gene regulation. *Proc Natl Acad Sci USA.* 1998;95:9944–9949.
87. Wall L, deBoer E, Grosveld F. The human β-globin gene 3′ enhancer contains multiple binding sites for an erythroid-specific protein. *Genes Dev.* 1988;2:1089–1100.
88. Puruker M, Bodine D, Lin H, McDonagh K, Nienhuis AW. Structure and function of the enhancer 3′ to the human Aγ-globin gene. *Nucl Acids Res.* 1990;18:7407–7415.
89. Grosveld F, Antoniou M, Berry M, et al. The regulation of human globin gene switching. *Philos Trans R Soc Lond.* 1993;339:183–191.
90. Hardison R, Slightom JL, Gumucio DL, Goodman M, Stojanovic N, Miller W. Locus control regions of mammalian β-globin gene clusters: combining phylogenetic analyses and experimental results to gain functional insights. *Gene.* 1997;205:73–94.

91. Higgs D, Wood W, Jarman A, et al. A major positive regulatory region located far upstream of the human α-globin gene locus. *Genes Dev.* 1990;4:1588–1601.
92. Chada K, Magram J, Costantini F. Tissue- and stage-specific expression of a cloned adult beta globin gene in transgenic mice. *Prog Clin Biol Res.* 1985;191:305–319.
93. Grosveld F, van Assendelft GB, Greaves D, Kollias G. Position-independent, high-level expression of the human β-globin gene in transgenic mice. *Cell.* 1987;51:975–985.
94. Sharpe JA, Chan-Thomas PS, Lida J, Ayyub H, Wood WG, Higgs DR. Analysis of the human α-globin upstream regulatory element (HS-40) in transgenic mice. *EMBO J.* 1992;11:4565–4572.
95. Ren S, Luo X-n, Atweh G. The major regulatory element upstream of the α-globin gene has classical and inducible enhancer activity. *Blood.* 1993;81:1058–1066.
96. Tuan D, Abelovich A, Lee-Oldham M, Lee D. Identification of regulatory elements of human b-like globin genes. In: Stamatoyannopoulos G, Nienhuis AW, eds. *Developmental Control of Globin Gene Expression.* New York: A.R. Liss; 1987:211–220.
97. Forrester W, Takegawa S, Papayannopoulou T, Stamatoyannopoulos G, Groudine M. Evidence for a locus activating region: The formation of developmentally stable hypersensitive sites in globin-expressing hybrids. *Nucl Acids Res.* 1987;15:10159–10177.
98. Dhar V, Nandi A, Schildkraut CL, Skoultchi AI. Erythroid-specific nuclease-hypersensitive sites flanking the human b-globin gene cluster. *Mol Cell Biol.* 1990;10:4324–4333.
99. Jarman A, Wood W, Sharpe J, Gourdon G, Ayyub H, Higgs D. Characterization of the major regulatory element upstream of the human α-globin gene cluster. *Mol Cell Biol.* 1991;11:4679–4689.
100. Higgs DR. Do LCRs open chromatin domains? *Cell.* 1998;95: 299–302.
101. Forrester WC, Epner E, Driscoll MC, et al. A deletion of the human b-globin locus activation region causes a major alteration in chromatin structure and replication across the entire b-globin locus. *Genes Dev.* 1990;4:1637–1649.
102. Bender MA, Byron R, Ragoczy T, Telling A, Bulger M, Groudine M. Flanking HS-62.5 and 3′ HS1, and regions upstream of the LCR, are not required for beta-globin transcription. *Blood.* 2006;108:1395–1401.
103. Fraser P, Hurst J, Collis P, Grosveld F. DNase I hypersensitive sites 1, 2 and 3 of the human b-globin dominant control region direct position-independent expression. *Nucl Acids Res.* 1990;18:3503–3508.
104. Alami R, Greally JM, Tanimoto K, et al. beta-globin YAC transgenes exhibit uniform expression levels but position effect variegation in mice. *Hum Mol Genet.* 2000;9:631–636.
105. Motohashi H, Shavit JA, Igarashi K, Yamamoto M, Engel JD. The world according to Maf. *Nucl. Acids Res.* 1997;25:2953–2959.
106. Orkin S. Regulation of globin gene expression in erythroid cells. *Eur J Biochem.* 1995;231:271–281.
107. Baron MH. Transcriptional control of globin gene switching during vertebrate development. *Biochim Biophys Acta.* 1997;1351:51–72.
108. Evans T, Felsenfeld G, Reitman M. Control of globin gene transcription. *Annu Rev Cell Biol.* 1990;6:95–124.
109. Shelton DA, Stegman L, Hardison R, et al. Phylogenetic footprinting of hypersensitive site 3 of the β-globin locus control region. *Blood.* 1997;89:3457–3469.
110. Talbot D, Philipsen S, Fraser P, Grosveld F. Detailed analysis of the site 3 region of the human β-globin dominant control region. *EMBO J.* 1990;9:2169–2178.
111. Strauss EC, Andrews NC, Higgs DR, Orkin SH. In vivo footprinting of the human α-globin locus upstream regulatory element by guanine and adenine ligation-mediated polymerase chain reaction. *Mol Cell Biol.* 1992;12:2135–2142.
112. Reddy PMS, Stamatoyannopoulos G, Papayannopoulou T, Shen C-KJ. Genomic footprinting and sequencing of human β-globin locus: Tissue specificity and cell line artifact. *J Biol Chem.* 1994;269:8287–8295.
113. Forsberg EC, Downs KM, Bresnick EH. Direct interaction of NF-E2 with hypersensitive site 2 of the beta-globin locus control region in living cells. *Blood.* 2000;96:334–339.
114. Sawado T, Igarashi K, Groudine M. Activation of beta-major globin gene transcription is associated with recruitment of NF-E2 to the beta-globin LCR and gene promoter. *Proc Natl Acad Sci USA.* 2001;98:10226–10231.
115. Letting DL, Rakowski C, Weiss MJ, Blobel GA. Formation of a tissue-specific histone acetylation pattern by the hematopoietic transcription factor GATA-1. *Mol Cell Biol.* 2003;23:1334–1340.
116. Anguita E, Hughes J, Heyworth C, Blobel GA, Wood WG, Higgs DR. Globin gene activation during haemopoiesis is driven by protein complexes nucleated by GATA-1 and GATA-2. *EMBO J.* 2004;23:2841–2852.
117. Ney P, Sorrentino B, McDonagh K, Nienhuis A. Tandem AP-1-binding sites within the human β-globin dominant control region function as an inducible enhancer in erythroid cells. *Genes Dev.* 1990;4:993–1006.
118. Caterina JJ, Ciavatta DJ, Donze D, Behringer RR, Townes TM. Multiple elements in human β-globin locus control region 5′ HS2 are involved in enhancer activity and position-independent transgene expression. *Nucl Acids Res.* 1994;22:1006–1011.
119. Gong Q, McDowell JC, Dean A. Essential role of NF-E2 in remodeling of chromatin structure and transcriptional activation of the ε-globin gene in vivo by 5′ hypersensitive site 2 of the β-globin locus control region. *Mol Cell Biol.* 1996; 16:6055–6064.
120. Stamatoyannopoulos JA, Goodwin A, Joyce T, Lowrey CH. NFE2 and GATA binding motifs are required for the formation of DNase I hypersensitive site 4 of the human β-globin locus control region. *EMBO J.* 1995;14:106–116.
121. Kent WJ, Sugnet CW, Furey TS, et al. The human genome browser at UCSC. *Genome Res.* 2002;12:996–1006.
122. Hsu F, Kent WJ, Clawson H, Kuhn RM, Diekhans M, Haussler D. The UCSC known genes. *Bioinformatics.* 2006;22:1036–1046.
123. Montgomery SB, Griffith OL, Sleumer MC, et al. ORegAnno: an open access database and curation system for literature-derived promoters, transcription factor binding sites and regulatory variation. *Bioinformatics.* 2006;22:637–640.

4

Nuclear Factors That Regulate Erythropoiesis

Gerd A. Blobel and Mitchell J. Weiss

INTRODUCTION

Studies of erythroid transcription factors originate from efforts to identify and characterize the numerous tissue-specific and ubiquitous proteins that bind *cis*-regulatory motifs within the globin gene loci (Chapters 3 and 5). In addition to elucidating mechanisms of globin gene regulation and erythroid development, this approach has led to the discovery of nuclear proteins that function in a wide range of developmental processes. Experimental approaches and insights gained through studies of the globin loci have broad implications for understanding how transcription factors regulate the expression of individual genes and work together to coordinate cellular differentiation.

Erythrocyte formation in the vertebrate embryo occurs in several distinct waves[1,2] (see also Chapter 1). The first erythrocytes, termed primitive (EryP), arise in the extraembryonic yolk sac at mouse embryonic day 7.5 (E7.5) and weeks 3–4 in the human embryo. Later, erythropoiesis shifts to the fetal liver where adult-type (EryD, definitive) erythrocytes are produced. Finally, at birth, blood formation shifts to the bone marrow, and also the spleen in mice. EryPs and EryDs are distinguished by their unique cellular morphology, cytokine responsiveness, transcription factor requirements, and patterns of gene expression.[3–10] Most notably, the expression of individual globin genes is developmentally regulated (Chapter 3). Understanding how transcription factors regulate the temporal control of β-like globin genes during mammalian development is of general interest to the study of gene regulation in higher eukaryotes and could eventually lead to new approaches to reactivate the human fetal γ-globin genes in patients with β chain hemoglobinopathies, such as sickle cell anemia and β thalassemia.

The primary *cis*-acting determinants of individual globin gene expression reside in the promoter regions immediately upstream of each gene and act in concert with more distant regulatory elements (Chapters 3 and 5). For example, the β-globin locus control region (β–LCR) encompasses approximately 20 kb of DNA situated upstream of the β-globin gene cluster. Originally identified as a set of erythroid-specific DNase hypersensitive sites (HS), the β-LCR is now known to be essential for high-level erythroid expression of β-globin genes.[11–14] Detailed analysis of globin gene promoters and the β-LCR has revealed a number of conserved DNA motifs important for globin expression. Among these motifs, the best studied are the "GATA," "CACCC," and "TGA(C/G)TCA" (NF-E2/AP-1-like) elements (Fig. 4.1). Not surprisingly, identical motifs also function in the promoters and enhancers of many other erythroid genes such as heme biosynthetic enzymes, red cell membrane proteins, and α-globin. One or more transcription factors has been discovered to bind each of these *cis* elements in erythroid cells.

GENERAL PRINCIPLES

General studies of transcription factors have conveyed several important concepts and experimental approaches applicable to studies of erythroid nuclear proteins.

1) Transcription factors are modular proteins with distinct domains mediating DNA binding, transcriptional activation, repression, and protein interactions.[15] However, a single domain may have more than one function. For example, GATA and Krüppel zinc fingers mediate both DNA binding and protein interactions. Typically, domains are analyzed by determining the effects of various mutations and "domain swaps" on the ability to activate or repress synthetic promoter–reporter constructs in transient transfection assays using heterologous cells, such as 3T3 or COS. Such studies are useful but fail to provide the native chromosomal and cellular contexts in which a lineage-specific factor normally operates. In this regard, the availability of more biologically relevant cellular and in vivo models complements the use of conventional promoter–reporter studies.
2) Transcription factors function within multiprotein complexes.[16,17] Defining these complexes in erythroid cells is critical to understanding the mechanisms that underlie globin gene expression and erythroid differentiation. Several approaches, including yeast two-hybrid screening, classic biochemical purification, and affinity purification with molecular tags are commonly used to identify interacting proteins and delineate higher order transcription factor networks in erythroid cells.
3) Posttranslational alterations, such as phosphorylation, acetylation, ubiquitination, and sumoylation, can modulate transcription factor function. These chemical modifications establish additional levels of

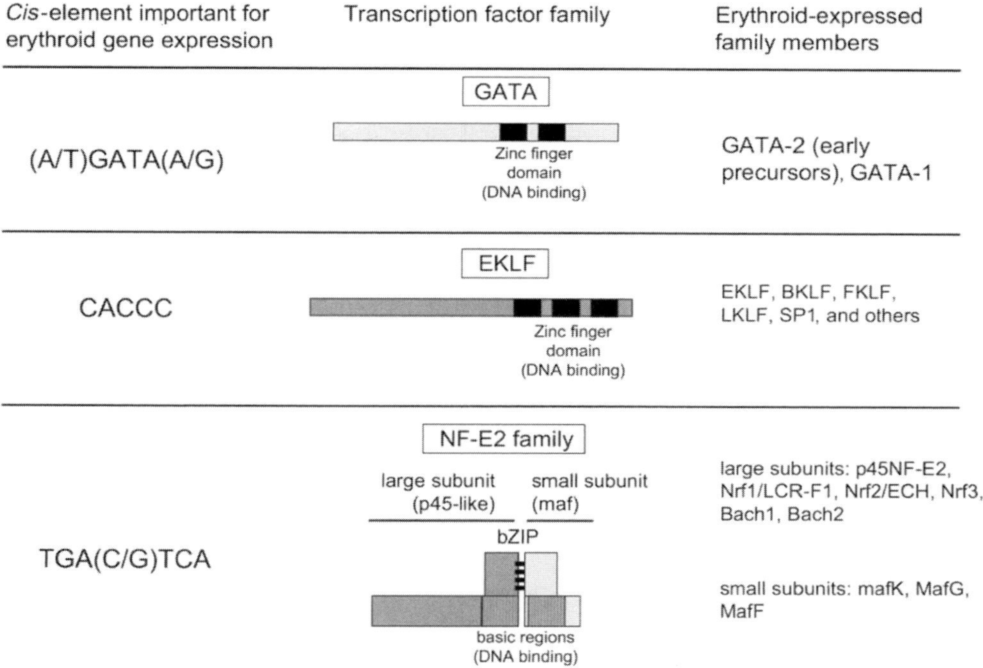

Figure 4.1. *Cis*-acting elements and corresponding transcription factor families important for erythroid gene expression.

control through which gene expression may be regulated rapidly in response to changes in the nuclear environment and/or extracellular signals. Examples relevant to erythroid biology are discussed later in this chapter.

4) Most transcription factors can both activate and repress gene expression. Among erythroid transcription factors, GATA-1, EKLF, and SCL/TAL-1 all have the capacity to activate and repress gene expression. These dual functions enhance the utility of transcription factors in several key stages of tissue development. For example, during terminal maturation, a single nuclear protein can simultaneously activate genes associated with the differentiated phenotype and silence those associated with the immature state. In addition, tissue-restricted transcription factors may participate in cell fate decisions of multipotent progenitors by activating genes for one lineage and silencing those of alternative lineages.

5) Cellular environment and target promoter context influence transcription factor activities by regulating the assembly of specific multiprotein complexes at individual genes. For example, the megakaryocyte-specific α-IIb gene contains a promoter that is activated by GATA-1 alone, but inhibited by GATA-1 bound to its cofactor FOG-1.[18,19] Binding of megakaryocyte-expressed Ets transcription factor, such as Fli1, to an adjacent DNA element converts FOG-1 into a coactivator. This identifies a mechanism by which GATA-1 and FOG-1 regulate the same gene differently in separate lineages.

6) As discussed in more detail later, transcription factors exert their functions in part by modifying chromatin, either directly or by assembling multiprotein complexes to establish and maintain active or repressive chromatin states. Many erythroid transcription factors associate with histone acetyltransferases. Hyperacetylation is typically found at sites of open chromatin that surround active genes. More recent work shows that erythroid nuclear factors facilitate the formation of long-range chromatin loops that bring critical regulatory elements into physical proximity.[20,21] How erythroid transcription factors regulate chromatin and DNA accessibility is an active area of research.

EXPERIMENTAL APPROACHES FOR STUDYING TRANSCRIPTION FACTORS

Several recently developed technologies have revolutionized the study of transcription factor function. Some of the technologies that have accelerated our understanding of erythropoiesis and globin gene expression are reviewed here.

Biochemical Purification

Transcription factors invariably interact chemically with cofactor complexes to modify histone proteins, to remodel nucleosomes, and to recruit basal transcription factors. Thus, one fruitful approach to define the functions of individual nuclear factors is to identify interacting proteins. In particular, yeast two-hybrid screens and in vitro purification of transcription factor complexes by using conventional biochemistry have elucidated gene regulation by defining higher order regulatory networks. Such studies are greatly facilitated by recent advances in mass spectrometry that permit identification of small amounts of proteins in complex mixtures.

Tissue Culture Models for Erythroid Differentiation

Numerous tissue culture models recapitulate selected aspects of erythroid maturation of multiple species, including chicken, mouse, and human. These include murine erythroleukemia (MEL) cells, which represent definitive (adult-type) erythroid precursors and K562, a human erythroleukemia line that expresses embryonic and fetal globins. A variety of chemical agents can be used to induce erythroid maturation of K562 and MEL cells.[23,24] Mouse G1E cells are arrested at the proerythroblast stage due to a lack of transcription factor GATA-1.[25] Conditional expression of GATA-1 in these cells induces synchronous erythroid maturation. Numerous avian cell lines have also provided useful models for erythropoiesis.[26,27] Established erythroid cell lines provide unlimited quantities of material for biochemical purification studies and frequently allow for synchronous differentiation on exposure to chemical compounds. Moreover, in established cell lines it is relatively simple to manipulate the expression of key transcription factors via overexpression or siRNA silencing and determine the effects on erythroid maturation and/or gene expression. Biological studies in cell lines are confounded by the effects of immortalization or outright transformation necessitating the use of primary cells for some studies. In mice and humans, primary erythroid progenitors can be purified from yolk sac, fetal liver, spleen, or bone marrow and expanded or differentiated in short-term cultures by using appropriate growth and differentiation factors.[28–32] It is also possible to generate primary erythroid cultures from in vitro differentiation of embryonic stem cells (ESCs).[33,34]

Chromatin Immunoprecipitation

Historically, interactions between DNA-binding proteins and their target sequences were demonstrated by electrophoretic mobility shift assay, in which binding of a transcription factor retards the migration of an oligonucleotide during polyacrylamide gel electrophoresis (see Fig. 4.6 for an example). This assay does not, however, assess transcription factor binding to chromatinized DNA in live cells. Chromatin immunoprecipitation (ChIP) is used to determine whether a nuclear factor is physically associated with a specific region of DNA sequence in vivo. The topic is described by Orlando and Paro[35] and experimental protocols are outlined by Boyd et al.[36] To perform ChIP, cells are treated with a crosslinking reagent that covalently attaches DNA to its associated proteins. Then, the cells are lysed and chromatin is purified and fragmented into defined sizes (typically 0.5–1 kb) by sonication or partial nuclease digestion. The resulting material is immunoprecipitated with antibodies against the nuclear protein of interest or control antibodies. Protein–DNA crosslinks are reversed and the protein-associated DNA is purified and analyzed by quantitative polymerase chain reaction (PCR) using specific primer pairs that flank putative transcription factor binding sites or control regions where binding is not expected to occur (Fig. 4.2). Global analysis of ChIP products can be performed by hybridizing them to DNA-based microarrays (see later) or by using high throughput DNA sequencing technologies.[37,38]

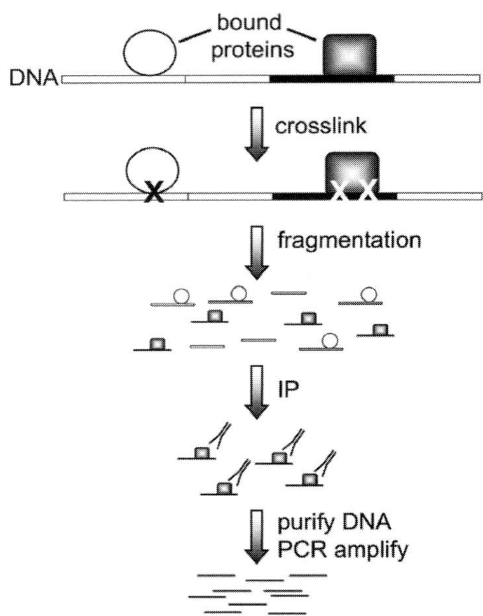

Figure 4.2. ChIP analysis. ChIP can identify histone and nonhistone proteins and protein modifications associated with genomic regions of interest. The first step of ChIP is to cross link proteins to DNA or other proteins. Following lysis of cells, extracts are sonicated to shear the DNA. Micrococcal nuclease can also be used to fragment the DNA. Proteins are immunoprecipitated with specific or control antibodies. Cross links are reversed; DNA is purified and amplified by PCR. For quantification, the amounts of PCR product are compared with those of unprecipitated PCR-amplified DNA (input). PCR reactions with primers against regions not bound by protein are used as additional controls.

In addition to determining transcription factor binding to specific genes, ChIP can be used to examine whether histone proteins or transcription factors are acetylated, methylated, or phosphorylated at specific chromosomal positions. Currently, ChIP analysis is the gold standard to determine transcription factor binding and posttranslational protein modifications at gene loci in vivo and has been used extensively at the globin loci to examine erythroid development.

MICROARRAY ANALYSIS TO IDENTIFY TRANSCRIPTION FACTOR TARGET GENES

In microarray or "gene chip" analysis, genomic DNA or cDNA derived from cells of interest is labeled with fluorescent probes and incubated with nucleic acids specifying

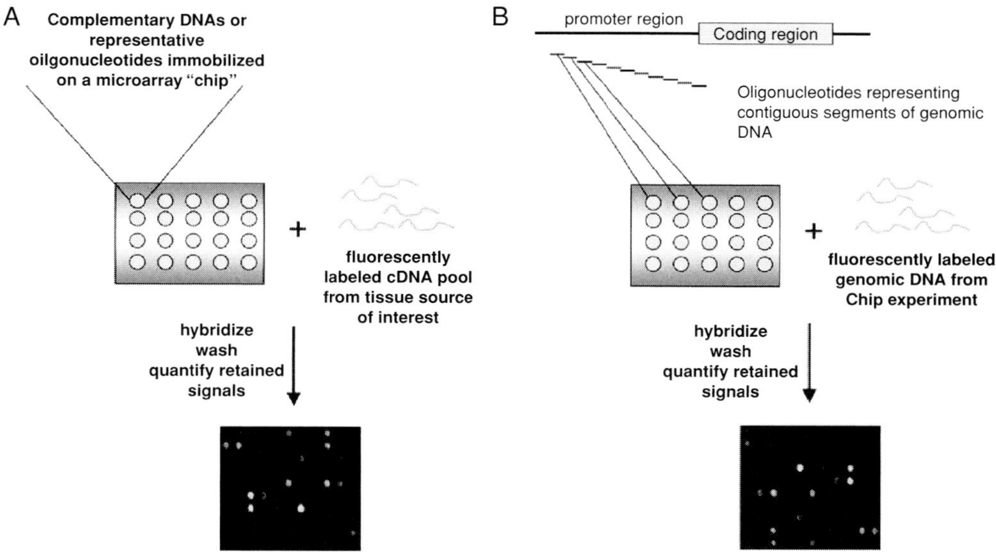

Figure 4.3. Microarray analysis. **(A)** Messenger RNA profiling. Complementary DNAs from a tissue source of interest are prepared, labeled with a fluorescent tag, and incubated with a slide or "chip" containing immobilized oligonucleotides or DNA segments that hybridize to specific cDNAs. The retained fluorescent signal at a fixed position or "address" on the chip reflects the relative expression level of a specific mRNA transcript. **(B)** ChIP–chip analysis. DNA from ChIP (Fig. 4.2) is amplified, labeled with a fluorescent tag, and incubated with a "tiled" microarray chip containing oligonucleotides that hybridize to contiguous segments of genomic DNA. Microarray chips representing all known promoter regions or even entire genomes are available commercially. In addition, it is possible to prepare microarray chips that specifically interrogate smaller genomic regions of interest.

unique chromosomal loci or mRNA transcripts that are immobilized on a solid surface (Fig. 4.3). Hybridization of the labeled cellular nucleic acids to sequences at specific locations on the chip is quantified and studied by optical scanning and computational analysis. This technology has advanced to a point where many thousands of different sequences can be examined in a single experiment.

Microarrays are used in two general approaches to identify transcription factor targets. First, transcriptome analysis can identify mRNAs that are up- or down-regulated in response to altered transcription factor activities (Fig. 4.3A). For example, it is possible to manipulate specific transcription factors in biologically relevant cells through gene targeting (discussed later in this chapter), viral transduction, dominant negative mutants, and by creating conditional alleles that are activated or silenced by drugs. Then, microarray studies can be used to compare mRNA expression patterns between identical cells in which the transcription factor function is specifically altered. Remarkably, commercially available microarray platforms can interrogate most or all expressed genes in many species including mice and humans. Using this approach, it is possible to define the actions of any transcription factor on global gene expression in biologically relevant contexts. Follow-up studies using ChIP can investigate whether effects on the expression of specific genes are direct or indirect consequences of transcription factor activities. Examples of mRNA profiling using microarrays or other methods to identify erythroid transcription factor targets are described.[39–42]

Another approach to identify transcription factor targets combines ChIP with microarrays (ChIP–Chip) (Fig. 4.3B). DNA derived from ChIP using a transcription factor specific antibody is labeled to generate probes for microarrays containing genomic DNA. For this purpose, microarrays containing promoter regions of most expressed genes are available. In addition, it is possible to represent large chromosomal regions of interest, or even the entire genome, in "tiling arrays" that contain contiguous segments of genomic DNA. In this fashion, it is possible to screen for regions of genomic DNA in which the transcription factor binds in vivo. Currently, these experiments, particularly those that survey the entire genome, are expensive and technologically challenging, but the field is advancing rapidly. One limitation of this assay is that occupancy of a genomic sequence by a transcription factor does not necessarily reflect function – a transcription factor bound to DNA in vivo can activate, repress, or have no effect. An example of ChIP–chip analysis using a tiled microarray representing the α-globin locus is described by De Gobbi et al.[43]

DEFINING PHYSICAL INTERACTIONS BETWEEN DISTANT DNA ELEMENTS

Several models are invoked to explain how transcription factors enhance or inhibit gene expression over substantial genomic distances. Tracking models propose that transcription factors bound at distant regulatory sites recruit RNA polymerase and/or basal transcription factors, which then move along the chromatin fiber until a promoter

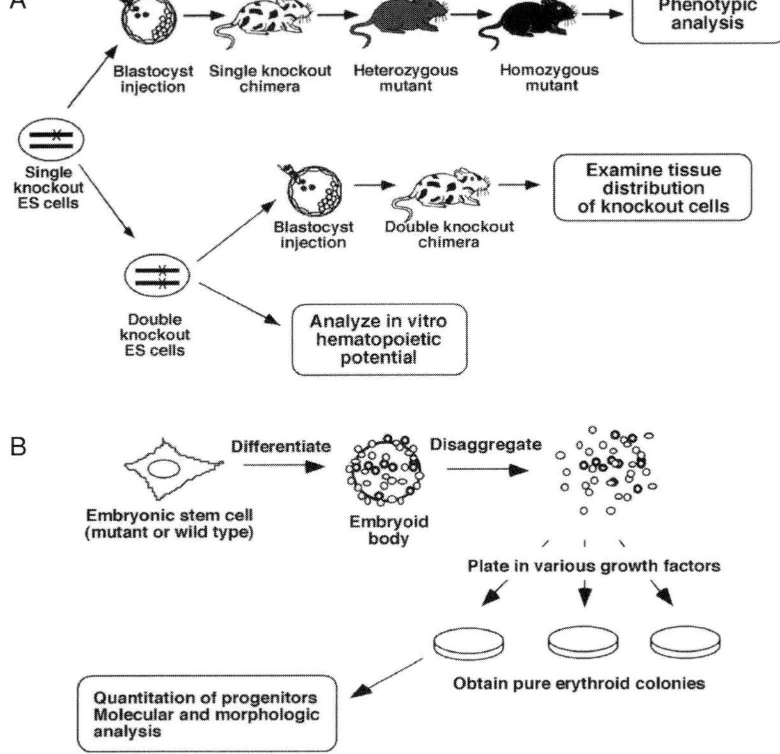

Figure 4.4. **(A)** Experimental strategies for studying gene knockouts. **(B)** In vitro differentiation of ESCs to obtain pure hematopoietic colonies. Reprinted from Weiss and Orkin[100] with permission from Elsevier Science, Copyright 1995.

is reached. Looping models posit that distal elements are brought in physical proximity with their dedicated promoters through the formation of chromatin loops. Although the latter model clearly applies to the α and β-globin gene loci,[44–46] tracking intermediates that precede loop formation remain a distinct possibility. Evidence to support this is found at the human ε-globin gene.[47] The most commonly used method to detect physical interactions among chromosomal fragments is called chromosome conformation capture ([3C] or nuclear ligation assay).[48,49] If performed with the appropriate controls, it can be used to demonstrate interactions among chromosomal fragments located in *cis* and on different chromosomes. 3C analysis has demonstrated that transcription factors GATA-1 and EKLF both promote folding of the β-globin locus to ensure physical proximity between the LCR and the active globin gene promoters.[20,21,50] 3C has also been used in the context of transgenic mice carrying versions of the human β-globin locus to delineate *cis*-acting sequences that organize the β-globin locus.[51]

ELUCIDATING GENE FUNCTION BY TARGETED MUTAGENESIS

Transcription factor functions identified in vitro must be examined in the context of primary cells and whole organisms. The advent of targeted gene disruption using homologous recombination in ESCs and mice has been instrumental in assessing transcription factor function by providing a means to inactivate (knockout) genes of interest or to modify them (knockin) and examine the biological consequences. Murine embryonic stem ESCs derived from the inner cell mass of blastocyst stage mouse embryos provide the basis for gene targeting.[52–54] ESCs can be maintained in a pluripotent state in culture and contribute to somatic and germ line tissues when introduced into blastocysts by microinjection. The first step toward studying a gene of interest is to disrupt a single allele by homologous recombination in ESCs to create a heterozygous, or "single knockout" state.[55,56] Several complementary experimental approaches are then available for further study (Fig. 4.4).

First, genetically altered ESCs may be injected into host blastocysts to produce chimeric mice, which may transmit the mutant allele to progeny. Through interbreeding of heterozygous offspring, homozygous null animals can be created for analysis. One limitation of this approach is that mutations causing early embryonic death can obscure the analysis of later developmental events. For example, direct examination of definitive hematopoiesis is difficult to assess in embryos that die prior to development of the fetal liver. Another potential problem in interpreting the phenotypes of knockout animals is failure to distinguish whether observed defects are cell autonomous or an indirect consequence of lesions in other cell types (noncell-autonomous). Both of these problems may be circumvented through chimera analysis or in vitro ESC differentiation assays (see later). In addition, more recent technology now permits developmental stage and tissue-specific gene targeting by expressing specific recombinases to excise or modify the target gene in a controlled spatiotemporal fashion.[57–60]

Second, heterozygous mutant ESCs can be converted to a homozygous-null state.[61–63] These mutant ESCs may be injected into wild-type host blastocysts to create chimeric animals in which the ability of the mutant donor ESCs to contribute to various tissues is assessed using polymorphic markers. For loci that are X-linked, such as *Gata1*, a single targeting event renders male ESCs null for the gene of interest. Failure of homozygous or hemizygous null ESCs to contribute to a specific cell type or tissue indicates a cell-autonomous requirement for the disrupted gene in the formation of that tissue.

Finally, the hematopoietic potential of genetically modified ESCs may be examined by in vitro techniques (Fig. 4.4). Under appropriate conditions, ESCs form embryoid bodies, spherical aggregates containing numerous differentiated cell types, including mature hematopoietic cells that can be studied directly.[64] Embryoid bodies may be disaggregated into a single cell suspension and analyzed for hematopoietic progenitors by using standard methylcellulose-based colony assays.[33] Wild-type and genetically manipulated ESCs can also be induced to form hematopoietic lineages by cocultivation on the stromal line OP9.[65,66] More recently, in vitro differentiation techniques have been used to generate hematopoietic cells from human ESCs.[67–72] Of note, human ESC-derived definitive erythroid cells produced by current methods express mainly embryonic and fetal globins, but not adult globins. In the future, this experimental system may provide a useful tool to study the mechanisms of globin gene switching.

SPECIFIC ERYTHROID TRANSCRIPTION FACTORS

GATA-1 and Related Proteins

The abundant erythroid nuclear protein GATA-1 was identified through its ability to bind the (T/A)GATA(A/G) consensus motif found in regulatory regions of virtually all erythroid-specific genes including α- and β-globins, heme biosynthetic enzymes, red cell membrane proteins, and transcription factors.[73,74] GATA-1 recognizes DNA through two related, tandemly arranged zinc fingers of the configuration Cys-X2-Cys-X17-Cys-X2-Cys. The carboxyl (C) finger is necessary and sufficient for DNA binding, whereas the amino (N) finger stabilizes protein–DNA interactions at a subset of sites, in particular those that contain two GATA motifs arranged as direct or inverted repeats.[75–78] In addition, both zinc fingers serve as docking sites for various protein interaction partners.[79,80]

GATA-1 is Required for Terminal Erythroid Maturation and Platelet Formation

Gene targeting studies demonstrate that GATA-1 is essential for the production of mature erythrocytes. In chimeric mice, *Gata1*-donor ESCs contribute to all tissues examined except red blood cells; reintroduction of GATA-1 cDNA into the mutant ESCs restores their ability to contribute circulating red blood cells.[81,82] *Gata1* embryos die of anemia between E10.5 and E11.5 (Fig. 4.5A).[83] Examination of these embryos, combined with in vitro differentiation of *Gata1*-ESCs revealed a block to erythroid maturation and apoptosis at the proerythroblast stage (Fig. 4.4B).[84,85] Together, these experiments demonstrated an essential, cell-autonomous role for GATA-1 in the production of mature erythrocytes. Subsequently, additional studies showed that GATA-1 is also important for the formation and/or function of platelets,[86–88] eosinophils,[89] mast cells,[90] and dendritic cells.[91]

The GATA Protein Family

The discovery of GATA-1 led to the identification of several related proteins with highly conserved zinc finger

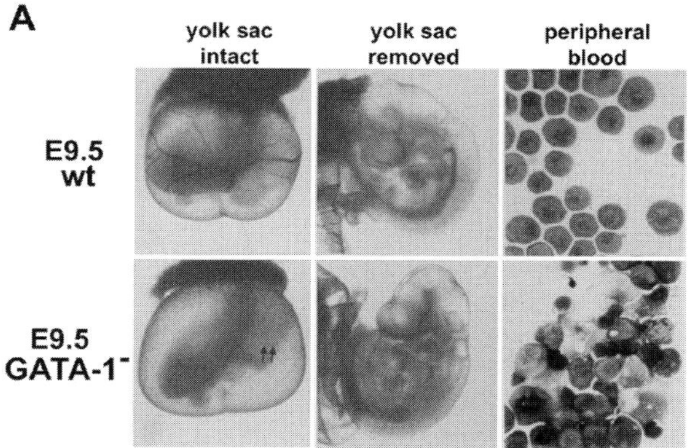

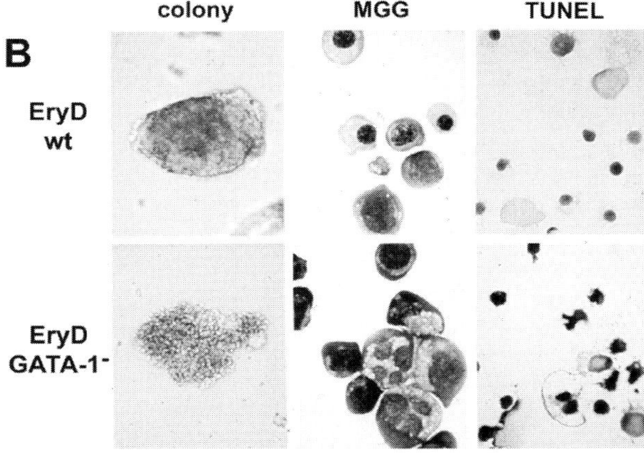

Figure 4.5. Loss of GATA-1 blocks erythroid maturation. **(A)** Impaired primitive erythropoiesis in *Gata1*-embryos. **(B)** Developmental arrest and apoptosis of cells within definitive erythroid (EryD) colonies generated by in vitro differentiation of *Gata1*-ESCs. Modified from Weiss et al.[84] and Fujiwara et al.[83] Copyright 1995 and 1996, National Academy of Sciences, U.S.A. Photographs in panel A provided by Yuko Fujiwara and Stuart Orkin. (See color plate 4.5.)

domains but little similarity outside of this region.[92–98] (for reviewed see refs. 99–102). Six vertebrate GATA proteins, named in the order of their discovery, function in the development of various tissues. GATA-1 and GATA-2 are most relevant for erythroid maturation and appear to act sequentially and coordinately during this process. Both are expressed in hematopoietic stem cells and multipotential progenitors, although GATA-2 function predominates at these early stages.[103–105] Concurrent with erythroid differentiation, GATA-2 expression declines as that of GATA-1 increases. Most likely, GATA-2 initiates the erythroid program in early progenitors and subsequently becomes replaced by GATA-1 during terminal maturation.[100,106] Presumably, these two transcription factors have both unique and overlapping functions at different stages of erythropoiesis. In this regard, GATA-2 probably activates its own gene by binding to an upstream enhancer.[107] GATA-1 displaces GATA-2 at this position to repress GATA-2 transcription.[107] These studies highlight molecular crosstalk between the GATA factors during erythropoiesis and illustrate one target gene (*Gata2*) where GATA-1 and GATA-2 have opposing functions.

GATA-1 Represses Transcription

GATA-1 was originally viewed as a positive regulator of erythroid gene expression. As noted earlier, GATA-1 also functions as a transcriptional repressor. For example, GATA-1 negatively regulates human ε-globin expression by interacting with one or more silencer elements within the 5′ flanking region of the ε gene.[108,109] Interestingly, GATA-1 binding to a region upstream of the Gγ-globin gene is required for developmental silencing of fetal globin synthesis. Although there is no obvious GATA consensus site in this region, patients with a mutation that abrogates GATA-1 binding display hereditary persistence of fetal hemoglobin.[110] Transcriptome analysis in erythroid cells indicates that the repertoire of GATA-1 repressed target genes may be quite extensive.[39] Among these targets are *Gata2, Kit, Myc,* and *Myb,* which mark early progenitors.[107,111–113] The latter three are all protooncogenes that stimulate proliferation and their repression likely reflects a mechanism through which GATA-1 coordinates division arrest with terminal maturation.

Structure–Function Analysis of GATA-1

GATA-1 acts as a potent transcriptional activator when cotransfected into heterologous cells (such as COS or 3T3) with a reporter gene containing a promoter with one or more GATA motifs.[75,114] In this assay, several domains of murine GATA-1 are required for activity.[75] In particular, the amino terminus contains an acidic domain that is required for transactivation of reporter constructs, and functions as an independent activator when fused to a heterologous GAL4 DNA binding domain. This domain is a target for somatic mutations associated with megakaryoblastic leukemias in patients with Down syndrome (discussed later in this chapter). The GATA-1 C-finger, which is required for DNA binding, is also essential for reporter gene activation.

A strikingly different view emerges from structure-function analyses that exploit GATA-1's ability to influence hematopoietic lineage selection or maturation. Remarkably, the GATA-1 zinc finger region alone is sufficient to induce megakaryocytic differentiation of 416B myeloid cells[115] and restore erythropoiesis in GATA-1–embryoid bodies.[116] Hence, the amino terminal activation domain that is critical for activity in promotor–reporter assays is dispensable for at least some functions in hematopoietic cells. These findings demonstrate that structure–function relationships within the GATA-1 protein are context-dependent, and reveal potent biological activity within the zinc finger region. Further dissection of the GATA-1 DNA binding domain revealed that the N-finger is essential for activity in erythroid cells.[25,117] One critical role of the N-finger is to mediate the interaction between GATA-1 and FOG-1.[118] The N-finger also functions through its ability to stabilize in vivo DNA interactions at a subset of bipartite GATA-1 motifs.[75–78,119]

Posttranslational Modifications of GATA-1

Murine GATA-1 is phosphorylated constitutively on six serine residues within the amino terminus. An additional serine, at position 310, which lies in a conserved region near the carboxyl boundary of the DNA binding domain, is phosphorylated upon chemically induced differentiation of MEL cells. Extensive mutagenesis experiments have shown that phosphorylation at these sites does not significantly influence DNA binding, DNA bending, or transcriptional activation by GATA-1.[120] Phosphorylation of GATA-1 has been reported to influence DNA binding in human K562 cells.[121] GATA-1 is also phosphorylated through erythropoietin-mediated activation of AKT in erythroid cells,[122–124] although mutation of the target serine residues in mice has minimal effects on erythroid development.[125]

GATA-1 is acetylated in vivo at two highly conserved, lysine-rich motifs at the C-terminal tails of both fingers, adjacent to regions that contact DNA. Acetylation within these regions is mediated by interaction with the ubiquitous transcriptional cofactors CREB-binding protein (CBP) and its relative, P300.[126,127] These modifications appear to be functionally important as mutation of the acetylated lysine motifs reduces the ability of GATA-1 to rescue erythroid maturation in a tissue culture model.[127] It has been proposed that acetylation augments the affinity of GATA-1 for DNA,[126] although this was not confirmed by another study.[127] Rather, acetylation of GATA-1 might be required for its stable association with chromatin.[128] Finally, ubiquitination and sumoylation of GATA-1 are reported, although it remains uncertain to what extent these modifications affect GATA-1 function in vivo.[129,130]

GATA-1–Interacting Proteins

GATA-1 participates in erythroid gene activation and repression through interactions with numerous erythroid specific and ubiquitous nuclear factors (for review see ref. 80). For instance, GATA-1 physically interacts with zinc finger proteins such as GATA-1 itself, other GATA factors, EKLF, and SP1.[131–134] In each case, protein interactions occur through the zinc finger regions of the respective proteins and potentiate GATA-1 transcriptional activity at defined promoters. Unique combinations of interacting transcription factors might establish target gene specificity by synergistically enhancing transcription at erythroid enhancers. It is also possible that they mediate physical interactions between erythroid gene promoters and more distant regulatory regions (Chapter 3). For example, promoters of genes within the β-globin locus and the core elements of the LCR each contain CACCC and GATA motifs. Interactions between proteins bound to these elements appear to facilitate direct communication via looping between the LCR and specific globin genes.[20,21]

Interaction between the N-terminal finger of GATA-1 and FOG-1 (Zfpm1) particularly important for erythroid and megakaryocytic development.[118,135] Disruption of the *Fog1/2fpm1* gene produces an erythroid defect similar to that of GATA-1 loss, albeit not as severe, suggesting the possibility of both FOG-1-dependent and-independent functions of GATA-1 in red blood cells. In contrast, *Fog1/2fpm1*$^{-/-}$ mice and ESCs exhibit a complete block to megakaryocytopoiesis, indicating that GATA-1-independent functions for FOG-1 exist in megakaryocytes.[135]

The mechanisms of FOG-1 actions are likely to be complex; for example, FOG-1 can either activate or repress transcription, depending on promoter and cell context.[118,136] FOG-1 itself participates in several important protein interactions that help to assemble higher order complexes at GATA-1 target sites. For example, different regions of FOG-1 interact with the corepressor CtBP2 and the NuRD corepressor complex.[136–138] NuRD is present at GATA-1-repressed genes and is required for efficient repression of the GATA-1 target gene *Kit*.[138,139] Point mutations that abrogate the FOG–CtBP2 interaction have no obvious erythroid effects in mice, indicating the possibility of functional redundancy with other repressors, including NuRD.[140] Preliminary gene targeting studies indicate that the FOG-1–NuRD interaction is essential for normal erythroid and megakaryocytic development (Blobel GA, unpublished data).

Tissue-restricted nuclear factors must communicate with the general transcriptional machinery. For GATA-1, a direct and functionally important interaction with TRAP220, a component of the basal transcription factor complex called "mediator," has been described.[141] Moreover, GATA-1 interacts with the highly related general coactivators CBP and p300, which both interact with numerous basal transcription factors.[126,142–144] In addition, CBP and p300 possess intrinsic and associated histone acetyltransferase activities. Histone acetylation is associated with an "open" chromatin configuration characteristic of the β-globin locus in erythroid cells. Indeed, GATA-1 may stimulate histone acetylation at this locus and other active genes by recruiting CBP.[144,145] As noted earlier, CBP-mediated acetylation of GATA-1 itself is also of functional importance in erythroid cells. Moreover, CBP interacts with additional erythroid transcription factors (see later) and may therefore participate in the formation of large multiprotein complexes.

GATA-1 also physically interacts with the Ets family transcription factor PU.1, which is normally expressed in multipotential progenitors, myeloid cells, and B lymphocytes and is required for normal myelopoiesis and lymphopoiesis (for review see ref. 146). Inappropriate expression of PU.1 by retroviral insertion and transgenesis causes erythroleukemia[147–149] and forced expression of PU.1 blocks differentiation in erythroid cell lines and primary progenitors.[150–153] Hence, it has been postulated that downregulation of PU.1 is essential for normal erythropoiesis. One underlying mechanism stems from recent observations that PU.1 and GATA-1 cross antagonize each other through direct physical interaction.[154,155] In support, overexpression of GATA-1 relieves the PU.1-induced block to chemical-induced maturation of erythroleukemia cells. It is proposed that inhibition of PU.1 inhibits GATA-1 via formation of a RB-containing corepressor complex.[156,157] PU.1 has also been shown to inhibit CBP-mediated GATA-1 acetylation.[158] Conversely, GATA-1 (and GATA-2) inhibit PU.1 transactivation activity, in part by displacing the PU.1 coactivator, c-Jun.[159] Together, these data suggest that GATA-1 and PU.1 oppose each other's actions and that their relative stoichiometry may influence differentiation decisions in multipotent myelo–erythroid progenitors.

The SCL protein complex binds DNA directly, but can also associate with genes indirectly through interaction with GATA-1.[160] This complex, which contains numerous proteins including LMO2, Ldb, and E2A is recruited to GATA-1-regulated genes via the LMO2 subunit. These proteins were also shown to cooccupy some erythroid regulatory elements in vivo.[106,161] It is likely that SCL and associated proteins function as activators of GATA-1-dependent transcription, likely by recruiting additional coregulators. The role of SCL in erythroid development is discussed in greater detail later in this chapter.

GATA-1 and Human Disease

Two major classes of human disease are caused by mutations in the X-linked *GATA1* gene. A comprehensive review can be found at the following URL: http://www.ncbi.nlm.nih.gov/books/bv.fcgi?rid=gene.chapter.gata1. First, germline *GATA1* missense mutations cause various cytopenias.[119,162–167] Most commonly, these mutations occur in the N-finger, either at the FOG-1-interaction surface or at the region involved in DNA binding. Affected patients usually exhibit anemia and/or thrombocytopenia of variable severity. Interestingly, the nature of the phenotype varies considerably depending on the exact mutation, presumably reflecting varying structural requirements for GATA-1 at different target genes. For example, some mutations spare the erythroid lineage and affect platelet function and production more prominently. One interesting mutation, R216W, causes congenital erythropoietic porphyria due to reduced production of the GATA-1 target gene uroporphyrinogen III synthase.[168] The same patient was also noted to have very high levels of fetal hemoglobin, consistent with the possibility that GATA-1 may be involved in the γ- to β-globin gene switch.

Second, somatic mutations in the *GATA1* are associated with transient myeloproliferative disorder and acute megakaryoblastic leukemia in patients with trisomy 21 (Down syndrome).[169–175] All of these mutations occur in the first coding exon (exon 2) and cause splicing abnormalities or premature termination of translation that interferes with the production of full-length protein. In these cases, translation initiation at an internal methionine results in the production of a GATA-1 variant (termed "GATA-1 short" or "GATA-1s") that is truncated at the amino terminus. Because the *GATA1* gene is X-linked, a single mutation leads to exclusive production of GATA-1s in male cells and in female cells with unfavorable Lyonization. Of note, one extended pedigree with a similar exon 2 mutation in the germline has been described.[176] Affected males, who do not have trisomy 21, exhibit anemia and neutropenia, but do not develop leukemias. This suggests that altered GATA-1 somehow synergizes with trisomy 21 to cause leukemia through unknown mechanisms. One interesting problem relates to the cellular functions of the amino terminus of GATA-1, which is absent in the short form. In gene-targeted mice this domain is dispensable for erythropoiesis, but is required to restrain the proliferation of embryonic megakaryocytic precursors.

Stem Cell Leukemia (SCL, TAL1, TCL5)

The *SCL/TAL1* gene was originally identified via chromosomal rearrangements involving 11p13 in acute T-cell leukemias (for review see ref. 177) SCL, a member of the basic helix-loop-helix class of transcription factors, functions as a heterodimer in association with a variety of widely expressed partner proteins including E2A, E2-2, or HEB (for review see ref. 178). The SCL complex recognizes a cognate DNA element termed E box (consensus CANNTG). Gene-targeting studies have demonstrated that SCL is critical for the establishment of all primitive and definitive blood lineages and for organization of the yolk sac vasculature in early embryos.[179–183] These studies indicate that SCL functions at the onset of hematopoiesis, possibly within the hemangioblast, a bipotential hematopoietic endothelial cell precursor (Chapter 2). Genetic studies indicate that SCL is dispensable for formation of hemangioblasts, but required for their subsequent maturation.[184–186] Interestingly, although SCL is required for the onset of hematopoiesis in the embryo, conditional gene-targeting studies indicate that SCL is dispensable for the maintenance of adult hematopoietic stem cells.[187–189]

The role of SCL in erythroid development is supported by numerous lines of investigation. First, SCL is expressed at a relatively high level in erythroid precursors and erythroid cell lines.[190–192] Second, overexpression of SCL stimulates erythroid differentiation of murine erythroleukemia cells and the multipotential myeloid cell line, TF-1.[193,194] Moreover, forced expression of SCL in human CD34+ cells stimulates formation of erythroid and megakaryocyte progenitors and an increase in the size of erythroid colonies.[195,196] Third, ablation of the SCL gene in adult hematopoietic stem cells causes erythroid and megakaryocytic defects.[183,188,189] Notably, the erythroid defects resemble that of GATA-1 or FOG-1 loss, consistent with physical and functional interactions between GATA-1, SCL, and associated proteins. Fourth, conserved, functionally important E box motifs are present at numerous erythroid genes including *EKLF/KLF1*, the HS2 core of the β-*globin* LCR, Band 3/*SLC4A*1, Band 4.2/*EPB42*, Glycophorin A/*GYPA* and the *GATA1* gene itself.[106,197–202] In some cases these E boxes are juxtaposed to GATA sites, and binding of both factors is thought to facilitate assembly of a larger complex containing GATA-1 (or GATA-2), SCL, E2A, and two non-DNA-binding nuclear proteins, Lmo-2 and Ldb-1.[160,203]

SCL complexes can activate and repress transcription in part through recruitment of coactivators such as p300/CBP or corepressors such as Sin3A or Eto-2.[204–209] How these activities are controlled is unclear, although acetylation of SCL by PCAF, which reduces binding to Sin3A, might play a role in this process.[206] Moreover, Eto-2 binding to SCL diminishes during erythroid differentiation, thus changing the composition of SCL-associated complexes, perhaps tipping the balance in favor of transcriptional activation.[207,208] Transcriptional activation by SCL–GATA complexes also appears to be enhanced by single-stranded DNA-binding proteins, which bind and protect Lmo2 and Lbd1 from proteosomal degradation.[209] Given the combinatorial complexity of SCL- and GATA-1-associated proteins, understanding the exact functional interplay among all of these subunits in vivo remains a long-term challenge.

EKLF and Other CACCC Box-binding Proteins

Functionally important GC-rich elements, also referred to as CACCC boxes, are found in many erythroid gene regulatory elements including several globin gene promoters and the LCR (Chapter 3). The importance of an intact CACCC box in the β-globin gene promoter is underscored by the observation that certain thalassemias are associated with mutations in these elements.[210–212] CACCC boxes, which vary somewhat in their sequence, are recognized by a diverse set of transcription factors that share a related DNA-binding domain composed of three zinc fingers with homology to the *Drosophila melanogaster* Krüppel protein (for reviews see refs. 213–215). These factors include the Sp1 family and proteins related to EKLF (Fig. 4.6).

EKLF is of particular interest to studies of globin gene regulation because its expression is restricted mainly to erythroid cells, with low-level expression in mast cells.[216,217] EKLF binds to the β-globin CACCC box with high affinity and mutations found in CACCC boxes of β thalassemia patients abrogate EKLF binding.[218]

EKLF is Required for β-globin Gene Expression

The presence of numerous erythroid factors that bind the same CACCC elements suggested considerable functional redundancy at a given promoter or enhancer in vivo. Therefore, it was surprising to discover that targeted disruption of the *Eklf* (*Klf1*) gene leads to significant loss of adult-type β-globin expression with resultant anemia

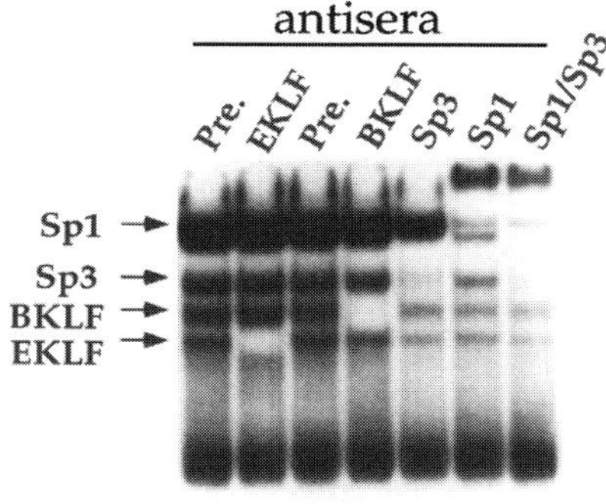

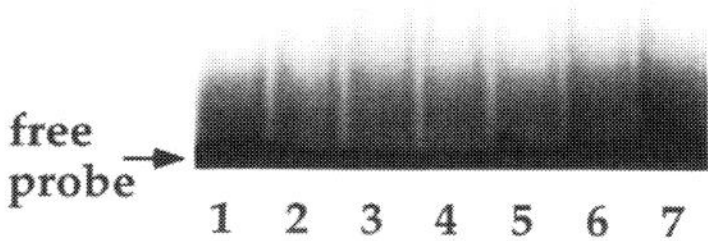

Figure 4.6. Gel mobility shift experiment showing multiple CACCC box–binding proteins in erythroid cells. In this assay, CACCC binding proteins present in nuclear extracts of murine erythroleukemia cells bind a radiolabeled oligonucleotide containing a single CACCC box, retarding its electrophoretic mobility. Migration of individual protein–DNA complexes is altered by incubation with specific antisera, as shown (Pre, preimmune serum). Note the presence of four major complexes, the most prominent one being Sp1. Despite the low abundance of EKLF in this assay, loss of EKLF function leads to a pronounced defect in β-globin gene transcription, which cannot be compensated for by other CACCC box–binding factors (see text). Although gel mobility shift experiments such as this identify factors that can bind to a CACCC box in vitro, they do not permit conclusions as to which factor(s) binds to a given CACCC box–containing promoter in vivo. Photograph provided by Merlin Crossley.

and embryonic lethality of homozygous null animals at E14–E16.[219,220] *Klf1*$^{-/-}$ definitive erythrocytes exhibit molecular and morphological features typical of severe β thalassemia including hypochromia, poikilocytosis and markedly elevated α/β globin ratio with Heinz body formation and ineffective erythropoiesis. Although EKLF can be detected at the embryonic β-like globin genes β*H1* (*Hbb-hh1*) and *Epsilon (Hbb-y)* by ChIP,[221] their expression is unaffected by the loss of EKLF, and primitive erythropoiesis appears to be normal in the mutant mice. Notably, there is a loss of the low, but detectable, levels of adult-type β-globin (beta adult major, Hbb-b1) in E11 yolk sac.[220] Hence, EKLF appears to be selectively required for high-level expression of adult β-globin. One mechanism may be to facilitate the formation of a DNA loop that brings the β-globin gene into contact with LCR.[20] Recently, EKLF has been found to occupy the α-globin locus and participate in its expression, although to a lesser extent than for β-globin.[222]

A Role for EKLF in β-Globin Switching

Selective loss of adult β-globin gene expression in mutant embryos suggested that EKLF might participate in the switch from γ- to β-globin in humans. Indeed, when transgenic mice bearing an extended human β-globin gene cluster were crossed with *Klf1*$^{-/-}$ mice, the resulting EKLF-deficient fetal liver cells displayed dramatically reduced human β-globin levels with a concomitant increase in the levels of γ-globin.[223,224] In addition, human γ- to β-globin switching was delayed in *Klf1*$^{-/+}$ heterozygous mice[224] and accelerated by transgenic overexpression of EKLF.[225] These studies are consistent with a model in which the γ- and β-globin gene promoters compete for the action of the LCR. Hence, EKLF might contribute to a more stable interaction between the LCR and the β-globin promoter to accelerate shutoff of γ-globin. γ-Globin gene silencing can also occur independent of a competing β promoter.[226]

Loss of EKLF also leads to reduced DNaseI hypersensitivity at HS3 and the β-globin promoter of both transgenic human and endogenous globin loci.[224] This suggests that EKLF might contribute to changes in the chromatin configuration at selected sites at the β-globin gene locus. These alterations might facilitate binding of transcription factors to DNA or increase the interaction between the β-globin promoter and the LCR. Alternatively, they might merely be a secondary consequence of promoter–LCR interactions and transcriptional activity. The former possibility is supported by observations that EKLF associates with factors that have chromatin remodeling activity (see later).

Broader Roles for EKLF in Erythroid Development

Initially, it was believed that EKLF might only regulate adult-type β-globin gene expression. Subsequent studies, however, demonstrated that EKLF controls numerous other erythroid genes. This possibility was raised initially by experiments showing that enforced expression of γ-globin fails to rescue the defects in survival and maturation of *Klf1*$^{-/-}$ erythroid precursors.[227,228] Subsequently, microarray-based studies examining mRNA expression in *Klf1*$^{-/-}$ erythroblasts identified numerous potential EKLF targets with important roles in erythropoiesis. These include genes encoding α-hemoglobin stabilizing protein AHSP (*Eraf*), the erythroid membrane skeletal protein band 4.9, ankyrin, and heme biosynthetic enzymes.[40,228] In follow-up studies, ChIP experiments demonstrated that EKLF directly occupies its regulatory regions of *Ahsp/Eraf* and Band 4.9 genes in erythroid cells.[41,42,229,230] Of note, microarray studies suggested that EKLF functions predominantly as an activator of gene expression. However, EKLF interacts with corepressor proteins and has been shown to repress transcription in several experimental contexts.

Recent overexpression and loss of function studies raised the possibility that EKLF not only promotes erythropoiesis, but also suppresses megakaryocyte formation.[231] This indicates that EKLF might play a role in the developmental bifurcation between these two lineages from common bipotential megakaryocyte–erythroid progenitors. One mechanism may be through EKLF-mediated repression of the gene encoding the megakaryocyte Ets nuclear factor Fli1, the first candidate target for biologically relevant EKLF-mediated transcriptional repression.[231]

An interesting question remains as to why some erythroid genes containing CACC boxes are more sensitive to the loss of EKLF than others. In particular, adult-type globin genes require EKLF but the embryonic ones do not, despite findings that EKLF binds to these genes in primitive erythroid cells in vivo.[221] This cannot simply be explained by general loss of EKLF function in a primitive environment because adult β-globin expression is selectively impaired in *Klf1*$^{-/-}$ primitive erythroid cells.[220] Early biochemical studies suggest that this selectivity might be explained by the higher affinity of EKLF for the β-globin CACCC box when compared with the γ-globin CACCC box.[232] In GAL4 fusion constructs, however, the activation domain of EKLF, but not that of Sp1, can activate a β-globin–containing reporter construct in erythroid cells, suggesting that DNA binding affinity is not the sole determinant of EKLF specificity.[233] In agreement with this interpretation, when the β- and γ-globin CACCC boxes are switched, EKLF still only activates the β- but not γ-globin gene promoter. Hence, the specificity of EKLF depends, at least in part, on the surrounding DNA and protein context of its binding site. It is also noteworthy that the activation domains of EKLF and other Krüppel proteins such as Sp1 share no obvious homology, the former being proline rich and the latter being glutamine rich, suggesting that they interact with different coactivator/adaptor molecules.

Posttranslational Modifications of ELKF

Terminal differentiation of MEL cells is accompanied by dramatic increases in α- and β-globin gene expression, whereas EKLF protein levels remain largely unchanged.[233] This raises the possibility that EKLF activity might be subject to regulation by posttranslational modifications. Indeed, EKLF is phosphorylated at its N-terminal activation domain, and mutation of the phosphorylation site leads to reduced activity.[234] Furthermore, EKLF is also acetylated by CBP and p300. CBP and p300 bind to EKLF and stimulate its activity in transient transfection assays.[235] Although acetylation does not alter EKLF DNA binding it does regulate its interaction with SWI/SNF, an adenosine triphosphate–dependent chromatin-remodeling complex.[236] EKLF is also sumoylated, and this modification appears to be important for its function as transcriptional repressor, which may relate to inhibition of megakaryopoiesis.[237]

EKLF Remodels Chromatin Structure

ELKF interacts with the mammalian SWI/SNF chromatin-remodeling complex (also referred to as EKLF coactivator-remodeling complex 1, E-RC1).[238] E-RC1 is required for EKLF-dependent formation of a DNaseI hypersensitive, transcriptionally active, chromatinized β-globin promoter template in vitro. Another mechanism by which EKLF could modify chromatin structure is by recruiting the acetyltransferases CBP and p300, similar to what has been described for GATA-1 (as described previously) and NF-E2 (see later).

EKLF-related Transcription Factors

If EKLF acts at the β-globin gene promoter to participate in its stage-specific activation, what are the factors that control expression of the embryonic and fetal globin genes at their respective CACCC boxes? Candidates include fetal Krüppel-like factors (FKLFs), which share homology to EKLF.[239,240] FKLFs activate the ε-, γ-, and β-globin gene promoters in transient transfection assays with the embryonic and fetal gene promoters showing the strongest response. This suggests that FKLFs might be important for embryonic/fetal globin gene expression in vivo. In contrast to the globin genes, regulatory regions of several other erythroid-expressed genes that contain functional CACCC boxes are not activated by FKLF.[239]

Another major CACCC box–binding activity found in embryonic yolk sac and fetal liver erythroid cells is basic Krüppel-like factor (BKLF).[240] BKLF is a widely expressed protein that activates or represses transcription depending on cell and promoter context. Repression by BKLF is mediated through the association with a corepressor, CtBP2.[137] Of note, EKLF-deficient erythroid cells display dramatically reduced BKLF levels,[220,240] and EKLF directly activates BKLF expression.[241] In light of the complexity of proteins bound to the β-globin CACCC box, this finding underscores the difficulty in directly linking a transcription factor to a specific target gene in vivo and in interpreting the phenotype of a gene knockout experiment on a molecular level. Targeted mutation of BKLF does not dramatically alter globin gene expression, suggesting that the ELKF null phenotype is not solely attributable to secondary loss of BLKF.[242] The role of BKLF, if any, in regulating β-globin gene expression remains to be determined.

Sp1, which was the first CACCC binding factor to be cloned, is expressed in a wide variety of cell types. Mice lacking Sp1 die approximately day 10 of embryogenesis with a multitude of defects.[243] Embryonic α- and β-like globin genes are expressed normally in the mutant mice, which was somewhat surprising considering the relative abundance of Sp1 in erythroid cells. Mouse embryos that are heterozygous for null mutations in Sp1 and Sp3, a related Krüppel protein, exhibit multiple defects in organogenesis, including anemia.[244] This underscores the complex functional interactions and redundancy of CACC binding factors for global tissue development, including erythropoiesis.

It is clear from these previously noted studies that a formidable effort is required to establish which transcription factor operates at any given CACCC box. Combined gene knockouts are one approach to address this issue.

Of equal importance will be to investigate further the mechanisms by which CACCC factors regulate transcription. The identification of novel interacting proteins and their analysis in vivo and in vitro will contribute to the understanding of the function of CACCC box binding proteins.

NF-E2 and Related Proteins

AP-1-like motifs [(T/C)GCTGA(G/C)TCA(T/C)], now called maf recognition elements (MAREs), are functionally important cis elements within HS2 and HS3 of the *β-globin* LCR (Chapters XX). Although GATA elements are mostly associated with the position independence conferred by the LCR, MAREs contribute to LCR-mediated enhancer activity.[245] Factors binding to MAREs contribute to the formation of DNase1 hypersensitivity, suggesting that these proteins modify chromatin.[246–249] MAREs are also found in some nonglobin genes such as those encoding porphobilinogen deaminase and ferrochelatase.[250,251] Careful analysis of these elements led to the realization that they are bound by an erythroid-specific transcription factor, called NF-E2.[250,252] Affinity purification of NF-E2 from erythroleukemia cells identified a simple heterodimer with subunits named according to their molecular weights: p45 and p18 (now referred to as MafK).[253–255] Both subunits contain a basic-zipper (b-Zip) domain, which mediates dimerization and DNA binding. p45 is expressed predominantly in erythroid cells and megakaryocytes, whereas p18 is found in a variety of cell types. It is now appreciated that both p45 and p18 belong to multiprotein families that are expressed in distinct but overlapping patterns, generating a large number of possible combinations of NF-E2–related protein–DNA complexes in different cell types.

The p45 Family of Proteins

p45 is the founding member of a family of proteins that contain a region of similarity to the Drosophila Cap'n'collar (CNC) protein. This family includes Nrf-1 (LCRF1, TCF11), Nrf-2 (ECH), Nrf-3, Bach1 and Bach2. These proteins bind DNA as obligate heterodimers with Maf proteins (see later) (for reviews see refs. 256, 257).

Expression of p45 is restricted to the hematopoietic system.[253,255] Erythroid cells and megakaryocytes express high levels of p45 mRNA whereas little or no p45 mRNA is found in macrophages and B and T cells. This expression pattern suggests that p45 is a critical regulator of globin gene expression. Consistent with this idea, the murine erythroleukemia cell line CB3, which lacks both functional alleles of p45, expresses very low levels of α- and β-globin. Upon introduction of an intact p45 gene, globin gene expression is restored.[258,259] Surprisingly, however, targeted inactivation of the p45 gene in mice has little effect on erythropoiesis or globin gene expression. In contrast p45 null mice exhibit a profound defect in megakaryocyte maturation resulting in severe thrombocytopenia and frequent fatal hemorrhage.[260,261]

Given the large body of evidence implicating MARE elements in globin gene transcription, the minimal effect of p45 gene disruption on erythropoiesis suggested the potential for compensation by other CNC family members; however, homozygous disruption of the *Nfe2l2/Nrf2* gene does not reduce globin gene expression in mice,[262] and the combined loss of Nrf-2 and p45 is no more severe than the p45 knock out alone.[263,264] Disruption of the *Nrf1* gene causes anemia and embryonic lethality, but the defect in erythropoiesis is not cell autonomous.[265,266] Thus, the exact contribution of each CNC-b-Zip protein to globin gene expression in vivo remains to be determined.

Bach1 and Bach2 are additional p45-related molecules that bind MAREs as heterodimers with Maf family members.[267] Bach1 is expressed in hematopoietic cells starting at the earliest progenitor stages.[267,268] Bach-Maf complexes are transcriptional repressors that bind MARE elements in a heme-regulated fashion.[269] Heme binding to Bach–Maf complexes stimulates their release from DNA, export from the nucleus, ubiquitination, and subsequent proteolysis.[270,271] In this fashion, Bach transcription factors provide an elegant mechanism to coordinate heme availability with gene expression in numerous tissues. For example, in erythroid cells depleted of heme, Bach1–Maf complexes bind MARE elements in the α- and *β-globin* genes to repress their transcription.[272,273]

The Maf Family

The small subunit of NF-E2 (p18, MafK) belongs to the Maf family of proteins, which share homology with the c-Maf protooncoprotein. The small Maf proteins (MafF, MafG, and MafK) heterodimerize with CNC-b-Zip family and exhibit distinct temporal and spatial expression patterns. MafG and MafK are highly expressed in megakaryocytes and erythroid cells with a predominance of MafG in megakaryocytes and MafK in erythroid cells.[256,257] Small Maf proteins lack an activation domain and are thought to stimulate transcription as heterodimers with CNC-b-Zip (p45-like) molecules. Small Maf proteins can also form homodimers on DNA and repress transcription, presumably by competing with activating transcription factor complexes.[274]

Surprisingly, *MafK*$^{-/-}$ mice develop normally and display no obvious defects in erythroid maturation, globin gene expression, or platelet formation,[275] and NF-E2-like DNA binding activity is still detected in fetal liver erythroid cells, consistent with the presence of other compensating Maf family members. Moreover, *MafK*$^{-/-}$ *p45/Nfe2*$^{-/-}$ compound mutant mice exhibit minimal defects in erythropoiesis.[275] Presumably, other members of the *p45/Nfe2* and *MafK* gene families can provide sufficient NF-E2-like activity to support globin production in vivo. Targeting of the *MafG* gene produces no obvious defects in erythropoiesis, but impairs megakaryocytic differentiation, although to a lesser extent than in p45 knockout mice.[276]

The exchange of partners for Maf proteins is critical for the control of MARE activity (see later). It has also been observed that MafG is sumoylated. Mutation of the critical N-terminal sumoylation sites impairs the ability of MafG to repress transcription in megakaryocytes but leaves intact its ability to interact with p45 NF-E2 and activate gene expression.[277]

Mechanisms of NF-E2 Action

Structure–function analysis of p45 in transient transfection experiments and in gene complementation assays using p45 null CB3 cells revealed that full NF-E2 activity requires an intact N-terminal activation domain and CNC domain.[259,278] The N terminus of p45 interacts with numerous proteins including CBP/p300,[279] ubiquitin ligase,[280,281] and the TBP-associated factor TAFII130.[282]

As is the case for GATA-1 and EKLF (noted previously), the implications for NF-E2 interactions with CBP/p300 are twofold: First, CBP and p300 might link NF-E2 with basal transcription factors (for review see ref. 283). p45 may also communicate with basal transcription machinery via interactions with TAFII130.[282] Second, recruitment of CBP/p300 and associated histone acetyltransferase activity to the LCR and other erythroid gene regulatory elements could promote the formation of "open" chromatin structure through histone acetylation. An additional role for NF-E2 in chromatin modification is indicated by the finding that NF-E2 can disrupt chromatin structure on in vitro assembled chromatinized templates containing the β-globin LCR HS2 site.[284] This adenosine triphosphate–dependent chromatin opening activity facilitates binding of GATA-1 to its nearby *cis* elements. It is not known whether this activity also contains histone acetyltransferases.

The N terminus of p45 harbors two PPXY motifs that mediate interactions with several ubiquitin ligases.[280,281] Mutations in these motifs reduce transcriptional activity of NF-E2,[281] raising the possibility that ubiquitin ligases might modify nearby histones to regulate chromatin structure. In addition, NF-E2 interacts with the MLL2 methyltransferase complex.[285] This complex is related to the MLL1 complex and methylates lysine 4 of histone H3, a chromatin mark that is found at most active genes. Thus, NF-E2 is linked with several histone-modifying enzymes, similar to other transcriptional regulators.

In an erythroid cell line, MafK associates with Bach1 in the immature state and with p45 NF-E2 after chemical-induced erythroid maturation. Notably, the exchange of MafK partner proteins was accompanied by redistribution of coregulator complexes.[286] Thus, components of the NuRD and SIN3A repressor complexes copurified with Bach1 in immature cells, whereas the p45 NF-E2–containing complex associated with a transcriptional activators including CBP/p300. This suggests that MARE binding proteins not only function during transcriptional activation but might also be involved in actively suppressing the expression of globin genes and perhaps other erythroid-specific genes in immature cells, consistent with findings that Bach1 binds and represses globin synthesis in low heme states.[272,273]

The onset of high level globin gene expression is coordinated with cellular differentiation and proliferation arrest, suggesting that these pathways may be mechanistically linked. Consistent with this idea is that NF-E2 is regulated by the MAP kinase pathway. In MEL cells, activation of MAP kinase potentiates NF-E2 DNA binding and transcriptional activation.[287] In addition, NF-E2 binding sites are required for MAP kinase inducibility of the HS2 region within the LCR.[288] The p45 subunit of NF-E2 is also phosphorylated by protein kinase A, but the physiological significance of this modification is unclear.[289]

It is interesting to consider that signals which trigger erythroid maturation might act in part by facilitating the exchange of partners for the small Maf proteins and their coregulator complexes. In addition, posttranslational modifications can modulate the activity of MARE binding proteins. For example, similar to certain Maf proteins, p45 NF-E2 is also subject to sumoylation, which reduces transcriptional activation by impairing the association of NF-E2 with its target sites in vivo.[290] Whether sumoylation of Maf and p45 NF-E2 can occur simultaneously within the same complex or whether it is targeted to distinct complexes is unknown. It is possible that cellular signaling events influence the targeting of the SUMO modification to the appropriate subunit.

In summary, MARE-associating factors are a heterogeneous group of proteins with distinct but overlapping functions and expression patterns. As an additional complexity, MARE factors activate transcription as heterodimers, leading to increased diversity through combinatorial associations. The major future challenge is to determine which combinations of MARE binding proteins act at a given gene regulatory element in vivo. In particular for erythroid biology, it will be important to learn the full complement of NF-E2-like proteins that activate the β-globin locus during normal erythropoiesis and in the background of various targeted mutations of MARE binding protein subunits.

Candidate Nuclear Factors Involved in Globin Switching

One model to account for developmental regulation of gene expression within the β-globin locus is based on the principle that individual globin genes compete for β-LCR enhancer activity, which is available only to a single gene at any given time.[291–293] These competitive interactions are believed to be influenced by variations in the relative concentrations and/or posttranslational modifications of transcription factors that are expressed at all developmental stages.[294,295]

In addition to EKLF and GATA-1, other protein complexes have been invoked to play direct roles in hemoglobin switching. One example is human stage selector protein (SSP), which recognizes a DNA motif, termed stage selector element (SSE), found in the proximal γ-globin gene promoter. SSE was identified through its ability to allow the γ-promoter to function in preference to a linked β-globin gene in plasmid constructs containing the HS-2 portion of the β-LCR.[296] SSP DNA binding activity appears to be relatively restricted to fetal erythroid cells. Thus, it is believed that γ-globin synthesis is stimulated in part by expression of SSP, which binds SSE to impart a competitive advantage for recruitment of the LCR to the γ-promoter. This is supported by recent studies showing that transgenic overexpression of the p22 NF-E4 SSP subunit can increase the ratio of γ-globin to β-globin gene expression in mice carrying the human β-globin locus.[297] The SSE, however, is neither necessary nor sufficient for competitive inhibition of β-globin gene expression in immortalized erythroid cell lines.[296,298,299] Therefore, it is particularly important to determine the extent to which this *cis*-acting element influences γ gene expression in vivo.

Another protein complex with potential roles in β-globin gene switching is direct repeat erythroid definitive (DRED). DRED was isolated through its affinity for direct repeat (DR) elements that cluster near the ε-globin and γ-globin promoters and contains the orphan nuclear receptors TR2 and TR4.[300] Notably, another nuclear receptor, COUP-TFII also binds the DR elements.[301] DR sequences are of interest because mutations in this region are associated with several cases of hereditary persistence of fetal hemoglobin.[302] Gain- and loss-of-function studies support a model in which DRED subunits TR2 and TR4 cooperate to silence directly endogenous embryonic mouse β-globin genes and transgenic human embryonic and γ-globin genes. As is the case for studies on SSP, the effects of altered transcription factor levels on globin gene expression are gradual but not absolute, suggesting that multiple protein complexes operate in concert to modulate hemoglobin switching.

Summary and Perspective

Studies of globin gene regulation are paradigms for investigating tissue-specific and developmental control of eukaryotic gene expression. Therefore, it is no surprise that pursuit of nuclear factors that coordinate globin gene transcription has produced a complexity of information with important implications for a variety of developmental processes. For example, GATA-1 regulates many aspects of terminal erythropoiesis and megakaryocyte maturation, presumably by controlling a number of as yet unidentified target genes. Moreover, discovery of GATA-1 led to the identification of several related proteins important for the formation of hematopoietic stem cells, T lymphocytes, heart, nervous system, and endodermally derived tissues. NF-E2, originally believed to be red blood cell specific, was shown by knockout studies to be largely dispensable for globin synthesis and erythroid development, yet critical for platelet formation. In addition, studies of NF-E2 have focused attention on the large family of MARE binding proteins that participate in numerous processes including cognitive development and formation of early embryonic mesoderm. Likewise, the discovery and characterization of several Krüppel-related proteins with diverse functions was initiated largely by studies of globin regulation.

Discovery of numerous tissue-restricted and widely expressed transcription factors that function in red blood cells provides a solid foundation for understanding globin gene expression and erythroid differentiation. The current challenge is to better understand the mechanistic basis for transcription factor function in intact organisms. Presumably, insights will be gained through continued investigation of the dynamic developmental stage and tissue-specific regulatory networks that exist among erythroid nuclear factors, basal transcription machinery, and chromatin.

In addition, it is important to examine the hierarchical order by which transcription factors regulate each other's expression. For example, GATA-1 activates its own expression but represses GATA-2, which may be prerequisite for terminal erythroid maturation.[100] Prior to repression by GATA-1, GATA-2 appears to autoregulate.[107] Moreover, GATA-1 positively regulates expression of the EKLF gene,[303] and EKLF is required for full expression of BKLF.[220,240] Such cross-regulation imposes a tissue-restricted and developmental order on the erythroid gene expression program. Analysis of *cis*-acting regulatory regions of erythroid transcription factor genes is beginning to explore how their expression is regulated.

One ultimate goal is to exploit basic knowledge of transcription factor function for manipulating gene expression in the treatment of human diseases. In this regard, pharmacological alteration of transcription factor–DNA interactions may be difficult because these usually occur over extended surfaces and the affinities are usually high. Transcription cofactor complexes, however, typically contain one or more enzymatically active subunits (adenosine triphosphatases, deacetylases, acetyltransferases, and methyltransferases etc.) that might lend themselves to pharmacological intervention. For example the drug butyrate, which is used to activate fetal globin gene expression in patients with sickle cell anemia or β thalassemia (Chapter 3) inhibits histone deacetylases.[304] More potent agents with similar activity are now under study.[305,306] Histone deacetylase inhibitors have also been shown to reactivate silenced globin transgenes delivered by retroviral vectors designed for gene therapy.[307] Together, these results define an interface through which basic studies of gene regulation might ultimately impinge on clinical management of hematological disorders.

Recent genetic association studies indicate that polymorphisms in the *BCL11A* gene influence fetal hemoglobin levels significantly. *BCL11A* encodes a zinc finger nuclear protein that binds to DNA but can also associate with other erythroid nuclear factors such GATA-1 and FOG-1. Using a knock-down approach in human erythroid cells, it was shown that depletion of BCL11A leads to a significant up-regulation of gamma-globin expression. These levels could be therapetatic if achieved in hemoglobinopathy patients. How BCL11A regulates gamma globin expression in still nuclear. Thus, BCL11A represents a newly discovered target protein for better understanding and manipulating fetal hemoglobin expression.[308–312]

REFERENCES

1. Brotherton TW, Chui DHK, Gauldie J, Patterson M. Hemoglobin ontogeny during normal mouse fetal development. *Proc Natl Acad Sci USA.* 1979;76:2853–2857.
2. Wood WG. Erythropoiesis and haemoglobin production during development. In: Jones CT, ed. *Biochemical Development of the Fetus and Neonate.* New York: Elsevier Biomedical Press; 1982:127–162.
3. Mucenski ML, McLain K, Kier AB, et al. A functional c-myb gene is required for normal fetal hematopoiesis. *Cell.* 1991;65:677–689.
4. Ogawa M, Nishikawa S, Yoshinaga K, et al. Expression and function of c-Kit in fetal hemopoietic progenitor cells: transition from the early c-Kit-independent to the late c-Kit-dependent wave of hemopoiesis in the murine embryo. *Development.* 1993;117:1089–1098.
5. Wu H, Liu X, Jaenisch R, Lodish HF. Generation of committed erythroid BFU-E and CFU-E progenitors does not require erythropoietin or the erythropoietin receptor. *Cell.* 1995;83:59–67.
6. Chyuan-Sheng L, Lim S-K, D'Agati V, Costantini F. Differential effects of an erythropoietin receptor gene disruption on primitive and definitive erythropoiesis. *Genes Dev.* 1996;10:154–164.
7. Okuda T, van Deursen J, Hiebert SW, Grosveld G, Downing JR. AML 1, the target of multiple chromosomal translocations in human leukemia, is essential for normal fetal liver hematopoiesis. *Cell.* 1996;84:321–330.
8. Wang Q, Stacy T, Binder M, Marin-Padilla M, Sharpe AH, Speck N. Disruption of the Cbfa2 gene causes necrosis and hemorrhaging in the central nervous system and blocks definitive hematopoiesis. *Proc Natl Acad Sci USA.* 1996;93:3444–3449.
9. Kingsley PD, Malik J, Fantauzzo KA, Palis J. Yolk sac-derived primitive erythroblasts enucleate during mammalian embryogenesis. *Blood.* 2004;104(1):19–25.
10. Kingsley PD, Malik J, Emerson RL. "Maturational" globin switching in primary primitive erythroid cells. *Blood.* 2006;107(4):1665–1672.
11. Tuan D, Solomon W, Li Q, London IM. The "beta-like-globin" gene domain in human erythroid cells. *Proc Natl Acad Sci USA.* 1985;82(19):6384–6388.
12. Forrester WC, Takegawa S, Papayannopoulou T, Stamatoyannopoulos G, Groudine M. Evidence for a locus activation region: the formation of developmentally stable hypersensitive sites in globin-expressing hybrids. *Nucl Acids Res.* 1987;15(24):10159–10177.
13. Grosveld F, van Assendelft GB, Greaves DR, Kollias G. Position-independent, high-level expression of the human beta-globin gene in transgenic mice. *Cell.* 1987;51(6):975–985.
14. Tuan DY, Solomon WB, London IM, Lee DP. An erythroid-specific, developmental-stage-independent enhancer far upstream of the human "beta-like globin" genes. *Proc Natl Acad Sci USA.* 1989;86(8):2554–2558.
15. Mitchell PJ, Tjian R. Transcriptional regulation in mammalian cells by sequence-specific DNA binding proteins. *Science.* 1989;245(4916):371–378.
16. Ptashne M, Gann A. Transcriptional activation by recruitment. *Nature.* 1997;386(6625):569–577.
17. Kadonaga JT. Eukaryotic transcription: an interlaced network of transcription factors and chromatin-modifying machines. *Cell.* 1998;92(3):307–313.
18. Wang X, Crispino JD, Letting DL, Nakazawa M, Poncz M, Blobel GA. Control of megakaryocyte-specific gene expression by GATA-1 and FOG-1: role of Ets transcription factors. *EMBO J.* 2002;21(19):5225–5234.
19. Pang L, Xue HH, Szalai G, et al. Maturation stage-specific regulation of megakaryopoiesis by pointed-domain Ets proteins. *Blood.* 2006;108(7):2198–2206.
20. Drissen R, Palstra RJ, Gillemans N, et al. The active spatial organization of the beta-globin locus requires the transcription factor EKLF. *Genes Dev.* 2004;18(20):2485–2490.
21. Vakoc CR, Letting, DL, Gheldof N, et al. Proximity among distant regulatory elements at the beta-globin locus requires GATA-1 and FOG-1. *Mol Cell.* 2005;17(3):453–462.
22. Friend C, Scher W, Holland JG, Sato T. Hemoglobin synthesis in murine virus-induced leukemic cells in vitro: stimulation of erythroid differentiation by dimethyl sulfoxide. *Proc Natl Acad Sci USA.* 1971;68(2):378–382.
23. Friend C, Scher W, Holland JG, Sato T. Hemoglobin synthesis in murine virus-induced leukemic cells in vitro: stimulation of erythroid differentiation by dimethyl sulfoxide. *Proc Natl Acad Sci USA.* 1971;68:378–382.
24. Rutherford TR, Clegg JB, Weatherall DJ. K562 human leukaemic cells synthesise embryonic haemoglobin in response to haemin. *Nature.* 1979;280(5718):164–165.
25. Weiss MJ, Yu C, Orkin SH. Erythroid-cell-specific properties of transcription factor GATA-1 revealed by phenotypic rescue of a gene targeted cell line. *Mol Cell Biol.* 1997;17:1642–1651.
26. Beug H, Doederlein G, Freudenstein C, Graf T. Erythroblast cell lines transformed by a temperature-sensitive mutant of avian erythroblastosis virus: a model system to study erythroid differentiation in vitro. *J Cell Physiol.* 1982;Suppl 1:195–207.
27. Metz T, Graf T. v-myb and v-ets transform chicken erythroid cells and cooperate both in trans and in cis to induce distinct differentiation phenotypes. *Genes Dev.* 1991;5(3):369–380.
28. Fibach E, Manor D, Oppenheim A, Rachmilewitz EA. Proliferation and maturation of human erythroid progenitors in liquid culture. *Blood.* 1989;73(1):100–103.
29. von Lindern, M, Zauner, W, Mellitzer, G, et al. The glucocorticoid receptor cooperates with the erythropoietin receptor and c-Kit to enhance and sustain proliferation of erythroid progenitors in vitro. *Blood.* 1999;94(2):550–559.
30. Pope SH, Fibach E, Sun J, Chin K, Rodgers GP. Two-phase liquid culture system models normal human adult erythropoiesis at the molecular level. *Eur J Haematol.* 2000;64(5):292–303.

31. von Lindern M, Deiner EM, Dolznig H, et al. Leukemic transformation of normal murine erythroid progenitors: v- and c-ErbB act through signaling pathways activated by the EpoR and c-Kit in stress erythropoiesis. *Oncogene.* 2001;20(28):3651–3664.
32. Wojda U, Leigh KR, Njoroge JM, et al. Fetal hemoglobin modulation during human erythropoiesis: stem cell factor has "late" effects related to the expression pattern of CD117. *Blood.* 2003;101(2):492–497.
33. Keller G, Kennedy M, Papayannopoulou T, Wiles MV. Hematopoietic differentiation during embryonic stem cell differentiation in culture. *Mol Cell Biol.* 1993;13(1):472–486.
34. Carotta S, Pilat S, Mairhofer A, et al. Directed differentiation and mass cultivation of pure erythroid progenitors from mouse embryonic stem cells. *Blood.* 2004;104(6):1873–1880.
35. Orlando V, Paro R. Mapping Polycomb-repressed domains in the bithorax complex using in vivo formaldehyde cross-linked chromatin. *Cell.* 1993;75(6):1187–1198.
36. Boyd KE, Wells J, Gutman J, Bartley SM, Farnham PJ. c-Myc target gene specificity is determined by a post-DNA binding mechanism. *Proc Natl Acad Sci USA.* 1998;95(23):3887–13892.
37. Metzker ML. Emerging technologies in DNA sequencing. *Genome Res.* 2005;15(12):1767–1776.
38. Bentley DR. Whole-genome re-sequencing. *Curr Opin Genet Dev.* 2006;16(6):545–552.
39. Welch JJ, Watts JA, Vakoc CR, et al. Global regulation of erythroid gene expression by transcription factor GATA-1. *Blood.* 2004;104(10):3136–3147.
40. Drissen R, von Lindern M, Kolbus A, et al. The erythroid phenotype of EKLF-null mice: defects in hemoglobin metabolism and membrane stability. *Mol Cell Biol.* 2005;25(12):5205–5214.
41. Hodge D, Coghill E, Keys J, et al. A global role for EKLF in definitive and primitive erythropoiesis. *Blood.* 2005.
42. Pilon AM, Nilson DG, Zhou D, et al. Alterations in expression and chromatin configuration of the alpha hemoglobin-stabilizing protein gene in erythroid Kruppel-like factor-deficient mice. *Mol Cell Biol.* 2006;26(11):4368–4377.
43. De Gobbi M, Anguita E, Hughes J, et al. Tissue-specific histone modification and transcription factor binding in {alpha} globin gene expression. *Blood.* 2007;110:4503–4510.
44. Carter D, Chakalova L, Osborne CS, Dai YF, Fraser P. Long-range chromatin regulatory interactions in vivo. *Nat Genet.* 2002;32(4):623–626.
45. Tolhuis B, Palstra RJ, Splinter E, Grosveld F, de Laat W. Looping and interaction between hypersensitive sites in the active beta-globin locus. *Mol Cell.* 2002;10(6):1453–1465.
46. Vernimmen D, De Gobbi M, Sloane-Stanley JA, Wood WG, Higgs DR. Long-range chromosomal interactions regulate the timing of the transition between poised and active gene expression. *EMBO J.* 2007;26(8):2041–2051.
47. Kim A, Dean A. Developmental stage differences in chromatin subdomains of the beta-globin locus. *Proc Natl Acad Sci USA.* 2004;101(18):7028–7033.
48. Cullen KE, Kladde MP, Seyfred MA. Interaction between transcription regulatory regions of prolactin chromatin. *Science.* 1993;261(5118):203–206.
49. Dekker J, Rippe K, Dekker M, Kleckner N. Capturing chromosome conformation. *Science.* 2002;295(5558):1306–1311.
50. Kooren J, Palstra RJ, Klous P, et al. Beta-globin active chromatin Hub formation in differentiating erythroid cells and in p45 NF-E2 knock-out mice. *J Biol Chem.* 2007;282(22):16544–16552.
51. Patrinos GP, de Krom M, de Boer E, et al. Multiple interactions between regulatory regions are required to stabilize an active chromatin hub. *Genes Dev.* 2004;18(12):1495–1509.
52. Evans MJ, Kaufman MH. Establishment in culture of pluripotent cells from mouse embryos. *Nature.* 1981;292:154–156.
53. Martin GR. Isolation of a pluripotent cell line from early mouse embryos cultured in medium conditioned by teratocarcinoma cells. *Proc Natl Acad Sci USA.* 1981;78:7634–7638.
54. Robertson E. Pluripotential stem cell lines as a route into the mouse germ line. *Trends Genet.* 1986;2:9–13.
55. Smithies O, Gregg RG, Boggs SS, Kordewski MA, Kucherlapati RS. Insertion of DNA sequences into the human chromosomal beta-globin locus by homologous recombination. *Nature.* 1985;317:230–234.
56. Capecchi MR. Altering the genome by homologous recombination. *Science.* 1989;244:1288–1292.
57. Gu H, Marth JD, Orban PC, Mossman H, Rajewsky K. Deletion of a DNA polymerase ß gene segment in T cells using cell type-specific gene targeting. *Science.* 1994;265:103–106.
58. Rossant J, McMahon A. "Cre"-ating mouse mutants – a meeting review on conditional mouse genetics. *Genes Dev.* 1999;13(2):142–145.
59. Glaser S, Anastassiadis K, Stewart AF. Current issues in mouse genome engineering. *Nat Genet.* 2005;37(11):1187–1193.
60. Garcia-Otin AL, Guillou F. Mammalian genome targeting using site-specific recombinases. *Front Biosci.* 2006;11:1108–1136.
61. te Riele H, Maandag ER, Clarke A, Hooper M, Berns A. Consecutive inactivation of both alleles of the pim-1 proto-oncogene by homologous recombination in embryonic stem cells. *Nature.* 1990;348:649–651.
62. Mortensen RM, Conner DA, Chao S, Geisterfer-Lowrance AAT, Seidman JG. Production of homozygous mutant ES cells with a single targeting construct. *Mol Cell Biol.* 1992;12:2391–2395.
63. Donahue SL, Lin Q, Cao S, Ruley HE. Carcinogens induce genome-wide loss of heterozygosity in normal stem cells without persistent chromosomal instability. *Proc Natl Acad Sci USA.* 2006;103(31):11642–11646.
64. Doetschman TC, Eistetter H, Katz M, Schmidt W, Kemler R. The in vitro development of blastocyst-derived embryonic stem cell lines: formation of visceral yolk sac, blood islands, and myocardium. *J Embryol Exp Morphol.* 1985;87:27–45.
65. Nakano,T, Kodama H, Honjo T. Generation of lymphohematopoietic cells from embryonic stem cells in culture. *Science.* 1994;265:1098–1101.
66. Suwabe N, Takahashi S, Nakano T, Yamamoto M. GATA-1 regulates growth and differentiation of definitive erythroid lineage cells during in vitro ES cell differentiation. *Blood.* 1998;92(11):4108–4118.
67. Kaufman DS, Hanson ET, Lewis RL, Auerbach R, Thomson JA. Hematopoietic colony-forming cells derived from human embryonic stem cells. *Proc Natl Acad Sci USA.* 2001;98(19):10716–10721.
68. Qiu C, Hanson E, Olivier E, et al. Differentiation of human embryonic stem cells into hematopoietic cells by coculture with human fetal liver cells recapitulates the globin switch that occurs early in development. *Exp Hematol.* 2005;33(12):1450–1458.

69. Vodyanik MA, Bork JA, Thomson JA, Slukvin II. Human embryonic stem cell-derived CD34 +cells: efficient production in the coculture with OP9 stromal cells and analysis of lymphohematopoietic potential. *Blood.* 2005;105(2):617–626.
70. Zambidis ET, Peault B, Park TS, Bunz F, Civin CI. Hematopoietic differentiation of human embryonic stem cells progresses through sequential hematoendothelial, primitive, and definitive stages resembling human yolk sac development. *Blood.* 2005;106(3):860–870.
71. Olivier EN, Qiu C, Velho M, Hirsch RE, Bouhassira EE. Large-scale production of embryonic red blood cells from human embryonic stem cells. *Exp Hematol.* 2006;34(12):1635–1642.
72. Kennedy M, D'Souza SL, Lynch-Kattman M, Schwantz S, Keller G. Development of the hemangioblast defines the onset of hematopoiesis in human ES cell differentiation cultures. *Blood.* 2007;109(7):2679–2687.
73. Evans T, Felsenfeld G. The erythroid-specific transcription factor Eryf1: a new finger protein. *Cell.* 1989;58:877–885.
74. Tsai SF, Martin DIK, Zon LI, D'Andrea AD, Wong GG, Orkin SH. Cloning of cDNA for the major DNA-binding protein of the erythroid lineage through expression in mammalian cells. *Nature.* 1989;339:446–451.
75. Martin DIK, Orkin SH. Transcriptional activation and DNA binding by the erythroid factor GF-1/NF-E1/Eryf 1. *Genes Dev.* 1990;4:1886–1898.
76. Yang H-Y, Evans T. Distinct roles for the two cGATA-1 finger domains. *Mol Cell Biol.* 1992;12:4562–4570.
77. Whyatt DJ, deBoer E, Grosveld F. The two zinc finger-like domains of GATA-1 have different DNA binding specifties. *EMBO J.* 1993;12:4993–5005.
78. Trainor CD, Omichinski JG, Vandergon TL, Gronenborn AM, Clore GM, Felsenfeld G. A Palindromic regulatory site within vertebrate GATA-1 promoters requires both zinc fingers of the GATA-1 DNA-binding domain for high-affinity interaction. *Mol Cell Biol.* 1996;16:2238–2247.
79. Cantor AB, Orkin SH. Transcriptional regulation of erythropoiesis: an affair involving multiple partners. *Oncogene.* 2002;21(21):3368–3376.
80. Ferreira R, Ohneda K, Yamamoto M, Philipsen S. GATA1 function, a paradigm for transcription factors in hematopoiesis. *Mol Cell Biol.* 2005;25(4):1215–1227.
81. Pevny L, Simon MC, Robertson E, et al. Erythroid differentiation in chimaeric mice blocked by a targeted mutation in the gene for transcription factor GATA-1. *Nature.* 1991;349:257–260.
82. Simon MC, Pevny L, Wiles M, Keller G, Costantini F, Orkin SH. Rescue of erythroid development in gene targeted GATA-1-mouse embryonic stem cells. *Nat Genet.* 1992;1:92–98.
83. Fujiwara Y, Browne CP, Cunniff K, Goff SC, Orkin SH. Arrested development of embryonic red cell precursors in mouse embryos lacking transcription factor GATA-1. *Proc Natl Acad Sci USA.* 1996;93(22):12355–12358.
84. Weiss MJ, Keller G, Orkin SH. Novel insights into erythroid development revealed through in vitro differentiation of GATA-1 embryonic stem cells. *Genes Dev.* 1994;8:1184–1197.
85. Weiss MJ, Orkin SH. Transcription factor GATA-1 permits survival and maturation of erythroid precursors by preventing apoptosis. *Proc Natl Acad Sci USA.* 1995;92:9623–9627.
86. Pevny L, Chyuan-Sheng L, D'Agati V, Simon MC, Orkin SH, Costantini F. Development of hematopoietic cells lacking transcription factor GATA-1. *Development.* 1994;121:163–172.
87. Shivdasani RA, Fujiwara Y, McDevitt MA, Orkin SH. A lineage-selective knockout establishes the critical role of transcription factor GATA-1 in megakaryocyte growth and platelet development. *EMBO J.* 1997;16(13):3965–3973.
88. Vyas P, Ault K, Jackson CW, Orkin S.H, Shivdasani RA. Consequences of GATA-1 deficiency in megakaryocytes and platelets. *Blood.* 1999;93(9):2867–2875.
89. Yu C, Cantor AB, Yang H, et al. Targeted deletion of a high-affinity GATA-binding site in the GATA-1 promoter leads to selective loss of the eosinophil lineage in vivo. *J Exp Med.* 2002;195(11):1387–1395.
90. Migliaccio AR, Rana RA, Sanchez M, et al. GATA-1 as a regulator of mast cell differentiation revealed by the phenotype of the GATA-1 low mouse mutant. *J Exp Med.* 2003;197(3):281–296.
91. Gutierrez L, Nikolic T, van Dijk TB, et al. Gata1 regulates dendritic-cell development and survival. *Blood.* 2007;110(6):1933–1941.
92. Yamamoto M, Ko LJ, Leonard MW, Beug H, Orkin S, Engel JD. Activity and tissue-specific expression of the transcription factor NF-E1 mutligene family. *Genes Dev.* 1990;4:1650–1662.
93. Zon LI, Mather C, Burgess S, Bolce ME, Harland RM, Orkin SH. Expression of GATA-binding proteins during embryonic development in *Xenopus laevis. Proc Natl Acad Sci USA.* 1991;88:10642–10646.
94. Arceci RJ, King AAJ, Simon MC, Orkin SH, Wilson DB. Mouse GATA-4: a retinoic acid-inducible GATA-binding transcription factor expressed in endodermally derived tissues and heart. *Mol Cell Biol.* 1993;13(4):2235–2246.
95. Kelley C, Blumberg H, Zon LI, Evans T. GATA-4 is a novel transcription factor expressed in endocardium of the developing heart. *Development.* 1993;118(3):817–827.
96. Laverriere AC, MacNeill C, Mueller C, Poelman RE, Burch JBE, Evans T. GATA-4/5/6, a subfamily of three transcription factors transcribed in developing heart and gut. *J Biol Chem.* 1994;269:23177–23184.
97. Detrich HW, Kieran MW, Chan FY, et al. Intraembryonic hematopoietic cell migration during vertebrate development. *Proc Natl Acad Sci USA.* 1995;92(23):10713–10717.
98. Jiang Y, Evans T. The Xenopus GATA-4/5/6 genes are associated with cardiac specification and can regulate cardiac-specific transcription during embryogenesis. *Dev Biol.* 1996;174(2):258–270.
99. Orkin SH. GATA-binding transcription factors in hematopoietic cells. *Blood.* 1992;80(3):575–581.
100. Weiss MJ, Orkin SH. GATA transcription factors: Key regulators of hematopoiesis. *Exp Hematol.* 1995;23:99–107.
101. Molkentin JD. The zinc finger-containing transcription factors GATA-4, -5, and -6. Ubiquitously expressed regulators of tissue-specific gene expression. *J Biol Chem.* 2000;275(50):38949–38952.
102. Patient RK, McGhee JD. The GATA family (vertebrates and invertebrates). *Curr Opin Genet Dev.* 2002;12(4):416–422.
103. Sposi NM, Zon LI, Care A, et al. Cycle-dependent initiation and lineage-dependent abrogation of GATA-1 expression

in pure differentiating hematopoietic progenitors. *Proc Natl Acad Sci USA.* 1992;89:6353–6357.
104. Leonard M, Brice M, Engel JD, Papayannopoulou T. Dynamics of GATA transcription factor expression during erythroid differentiation. *Blood.* 1993;82(4):1071–1079.
105. Tsai F-Y, Keller G, Kuo FC, et al. An early hematopoietic defect in mice lacking the transcription factor GATA-2. *Nature.* 1994;371:221–226.
106. Anguita E, Hughes J, Heyworth C, Blobel GA, Wood WG, Higgs DR. Globin gene activation during haemopoiesis is driven by protein complexes nucleated by GATA-1 and GATA-2. *EMBO J.* 2004;23(14):2841–2852.
107. Grass JA, Boyer ME, Pal S, Wu J, Weiss MJ, Bresnick EH. GATA-1-dependent transcriptional repression of GATA-2 via disruption of positive autoregulation and domain-wide chromatin remodeling. *Proc Natl Acad Sci USA.* 2003;100(15):8811–8816.
108. Raich N, Clegg CH, Grofti J, Romeo PH, Stamatoyannopoulos G. GATA1 and YY1 are developmental repressors of the human epsilon-globin gene. *EMBO J.* 1995;14(4):801–809.
109. Li J, Noguchi CT, Miller W, Hardison, R, Schechter AN. Multiple regulatory elements in the 5′-flanking sequence of the human epsilon-globin gene. *J Biol Chem.* 1998;273(17): 10202–10209.
110. Berry M, Grosveld F, Dillon N. A single point mutation is the cause of the Greek form of hereditary persistence of fetal haemoglobin. *Nature.* 1992;358(6386):499–502.
111. Bartunek P, Kralova J, Blendinger G, Dvorak M, Zenke M. GATA-1 and c-myb crosstalk during red blood cell differentiation through GATA-1 binding sites in the c-myb promoter. *Oncogene.* 2003;22(13):1927–1935.
112. Rylski M, Welch JJ, Chen YY, et al. GATA-1-mediated proliferation arrest during erythroid maturation. *Mol Cell Biol.* 2003;23(14):5031–5042.
113. Munugalavadla V, Dore LC, Tan BL, et al. Repression of c-kit and its downstream substrates by GATA-1 inhibits cell proliferation during erythroid maturation. *Mol Cell Biol.* 2005;25(15):6747–6759.
114. Evans T, Felsenfeld G. *trans*-Activation of a globin promoter in nonerythroid cells. *Mol Cell Biol.* 1991;11:843–853.
115. Visvader JE, Crossley M, Hill J, Orkin SH, Adams JM. The C-terminal zinc finger of GATA-1 or GATA-2 is sufficient to induce megakaryocytic differentiation of an early myeloid cell line. *Mol Cell Biol.* 1995;15:634–641.
116. Blobel GA, Simon MC, Orkin SH. Rescue of GATA-1-deficient embryonic stem cells by heterologous GATA-binding proteins. *Mol Cell Biol.* 1995;15:626–633.
117. Shimizu R, Takahashi S, Ohneda K, Engel JD, Yamamoto M. In vivo requirements for GATA-1 functional domains during primitive and definitive erythropoiesis. *EMBO J.* 2001;20(18):5250–5260.
118. Tsang AP, Visvader JE, Turner CA, Fujiwara Y, et al. FOG, a multitype zinc finger protein, acts as a cofactor for transcription factor GATA-1 in erythroid and megakaryocytic differentiation. *Cell.* 1997;90:109–119.
119. Yu C, Niakan KK, Matsushita M, Stamatoyannopoulos G, Orkin SH, Raskind WH. X-linked thrombocytopenia with thalassemia from a mutation in the amino finger of GATA-1 affecting DNA binding rather than FOG-1 interaction. *Blood.* 2002;100(6):2040–2045.
120. Crossley M, Orkin SH. Phosphorylation of the erythroid transcription factor GATA-1. *J Biol Chem.* 1994;269(24):16589–16596.
121. Partington GA, Patient RK. Phosphorylation of GATA-1 increases its DNAbinding affinity and is correlated with induction of human K562 erythroleukaemia cells. *Nucl Acids Res.* 1999;27(4):1168–1175.
122. Ghaffari S, Kitidis C, Zhao W, et al. AKT induces erythroid cell maturation of JAK2-deficient fetal liver progenitor cells and is required for epo regulation of erythroid cell differentiation. *Blood.* 2006;107:1888–1891.
123. Kadri Z, Maouche-Chretien L, Rooke HM, et al. Phosphatidylinositol 3–kinase/Akt induced by erythropoietin renders the erythroid differentiation factor GATA-1 competent for TIMP-1 gene transactivation. *Mol Cell Biol.* 2005;25(17):7412–7422.
124. Zhao W, Kitidis C, Fleming MD, Lodish HF, Ghaffari S. Erythropoietin stimulates phosphorylation and activation of GATA-1 via the PI3-kinase-AKT signaling pathway. *Blood.* 2005;107:907–915.
125. Rooke HM, Orkin SH. Phosphorylation of Gata1 at serine residues 72, 142, and 310 is not essential for hematopoiesis in vivo. *Blood.* 2006;107(9):3527–3530.
126. Boyes J, Byfield P, Nakatani Y, Ogryzko V. Regulation of activity of the transcription factor GATA-1 by acetylation. *Nature.* 1998;396(6711):594–598.
127. Hung HL, Lau J, Kim AY, Weiss MJ, Blobel GA. CREB-Binding protein acetylates hematopoietic transcription factor GATA-1 at functionally important sites. *Mol Cell Biol.* 1999;19(5):3496–3505.
128. Lamonica JM, Vakoc CR, Blobel GA. Acetylation of GATA-1 is required for chromatin occupancy. *Blood.* 2006;108(12): 3736–3738.
129. Collavin L, Gostissa M, Avolio F, et al. Modification of the erythroid transcription factor GATA-1 by SUMO-1. *Proc Natl Acad Sci USA.* 2004;101(24):8870–8875.
130. Hernandez-Hernandez A, Ray P, Litos G, et al. Acetylation and MAPK phosphorylation cooperate to regulate the degradation of active GATA-1. *EMBO J.* 2006;25(14):3264–3274.
131. Fischer K-D, Haese A, Nowock J. Cooperation of GATA-1 and Sp1 can result in synergistic transcriptional activation or interference. *J Biol Chem.* 1993;268(32):23915–23923.
132. Crossley M, Merika M, Orkin SH. Self association of the erythroid transcription factor GATA-1 mediated by its zinc finger domains. *Mol Cell Biol.* 1995;15:2448–2456.
133. Merika M, Orkin SH. Functional synergy and physical interactions of the erythroid transcription factor GATA-1 with the *Krüppel* family proteins Sp1 and EKLF. *Mol Cell Biol.* 1995;15:2437–2447.
134. Gregory RC, Taxman DJ, Seshasayee D, Kensinger MH, Bieker JJ, Wojchowski DM. Functional interaction of GATA1 with erythroid Kruppel-like factor and Sp1 at defined erythroid promoters. *Blood.* 1996;87(5):1793–1801.
135. Tsang AP, Fujiwara Y, Hom DB, Orkin SH. Failure of megakaryopoiesis and arrested erythropoiesis in mice lacking the GATA-1 transcriptional cofactor FOG. *Genes Dev.* 1998;12(8):1176–1188.
136. Fox AH, Liew C, Holmes M, Kowalski K, Mackay J, Crossley M. Transcriptional cofactors of the FOG family interact with GATA proteins by means of multiple zinc fingers. *EMBO J.* 1999;18(10):2812–2822.

137. Turner J, Crossley M. Cloning and characterization of mCtBP2, a corepressor that associates with basic Kruppel-like factor and other mammalian transcriptional regulators. *EMBO J.* 1998;17:5129–5140.
138. Hong W, Nakazawa M, Chen YY, et al. FOG-1 recruits the NuRD repressor complex to mediate transcriptional repression by GATA-1. *EMBO J.* 2005;24(13):2367–2378.
139. Rodriguez P, Bonte, E, Krijgsveld, J, et al. GATA-1 forms distinct activating and repressive complexes in erythroid cells. *EMBO J.* 2005;24(13):2354–2366.
140. Katz SG, Cantor AB, Orkin SH. Interaction between FOG-1 and the corepressor C-terminal binding protein is dispensable for normal erythropoiesis in vivo. *Mol Cell Biol.* 2002;22(9):3121–3128.
141. Stumpf M, Waskow C, Krotschel M, et al. The mediator complex functions as a coactivator for GATA-1 in erythropoiesis via subunit Med1/TRAP220. *Proc Natl Acad Sci USA.* 2006;103(49):18504–18509.
142. Blobel GA, Nakajima T, Eckner R, Montminy M, Orkin SH. CREB binding protein (CBP) cooperates with transcription factor GATA-1 and is required for erythroid differentiation. *Proc Natl Acad Sci USA.* 1998;95:2061–2066.
143. Blobel GA. CBP/p300: molecular integrators of hematopoietic transcription. *Blood.* 2000;95:745–755.
144. Letting DL, Rakowski C, Weiss MJ, Blobel GA. Formation of a tissue-specific histone acetylation pattern by the hematopoietic transcription factor GATA-1. *Mol Cell Biol.* 2003;23(4):1334–1340.
145. Kiekhaefer CM, Grass JA, Johnson KD, Boyer ME, Bresnick EH. Hematopoietic-specific activators establish an overlapping pattern of histone acetylation and methylation within a mammalian chromatin domain. *Proc Natl Acad Sci USA.* 2002;99(22):14309–14314.
146. Koschmieder S, Rosenbauer F, Steidl U, Owens BM, Tenen DG. Role of transcription factors C/EBPalpha and PU.1 in normal hematopoiesis and leukemia. *Int J Hematol.* 2005;81(5):368–377.
147. Moreau-Gachelin F, Ray D, Mattei MG, Tambourin P, Tavitian A. The putative oncogene Spi-1: murine chromosomal localization and transcriptional activation in murine acute erythroleukemias [published erratum appears in *Oncogene.* 1990;5(6):941]. *Oncogene.* 1989;4(12):1449–1456.
148. Moreau-Gachelin F, Tavitian A, Tambourin P. Spi-1 is a putative oncogene in virally induced murine erythroleukaemias. *Nature.* 1988;331(6153):277–280.
149. Moreau-Gachelin F, Wendling F, Molina T, et al. Spi-1/PU.1 transgenic mice develop multistep erythroleukemias. *Mol Cell Biol.* 1996;16(5):2453–2463.
150. Quang CT, Pironin M, von Lindern M, Beug H, Ghysdael J. Spi-1 and mutant p53 regulate different aspects of the proliferation and differentiation control of primary erythroid progenitors. *Oncogene.* 1995;11(7):1229–1239.
151. Rao G, Rekhtman N, Cheng G, Krasikov T, Skoultchi AI. Deregulated expression of the PU.1 transcription factor blocks murine erythroleukemia cell terminal differentiation. *Oncogene.* 1997;14(1):123–131.
152. Yamada T, Kondoh N, Matsumoto M, Yoshida M, Maekawa A, Oikawa T. Overexpression of PU.1 induces growth and differentiation inhibition and apoptotic cell death in murine erythroleukemia cells. *Blood.* 1997;89(4):1383–1393.
153. Delgado MD, Gutierrez P, Richard C, Cuadrado MA, Moreau-Gachelin F, Leon J. Spi-1/PU.1 proto-oncogene induces opposite effects on monocytic and erythroid differentiation of K562 cells. *Biochem Biophys Res Commun.* 1998;252(2):383–391.
154. Yamada T, Kihara-Negishi F, Yamamoto H, Yamamoto M, Hashimoto Y, Oikawa T. Reduction of DNA binding activity of the GATA-1 transcription factor in the apoptotic process induced by overexpression of PU.1 in murine erythroleukemia cells. *Exp Cell Res.* 1998;245(1):186–194.
155. Rekhtman N, Radparvar F, Evans T, Skoultchi AI. Direct interaction of hematopoietic transcription factors PU.1 and GATA- 1: functional antagonism in erythroid cells. *Genes Dev.* 1999;13(11):1398–1411.
156. Rekhtman N, Choe KS, Matushansky I, Murray S, Stopka T, Skoultchi AI. PU.1 and pRB interact and cooperate to repress GATA-1 and block erythroid differentiation. *Mol Cell Biol.* 2003;23(21):7460–7474.
157. Stopka T, Amanatullah DF, Papetti M, Skoultchi AI. PU.1 inhibits the erythroid program by binding to GATA-1on DNA and creating a repressive chromatin structure. *EMBO J.* 2005;24(21):3712–3723.
158. Hong W, Kim AY, Ky S, et al. Inhibition of CBP-mediated protein acetylation by the Ets family oncoprotein PU.1. *Mol Cell Biol.* 2002;22(11):3729–3743.
159. Zhang P, Behre G, Pan J, et al. Negative cross-talk between hematopoietic regulators:GATA proteins repress PU.1. *Proc Natl Acad Sci USA.* 1999;96(15):8705–8710.
160. Wadman IA, Osada H, Grutz GG, et al. The LIM-only protein Lmo2 is a bridging molecule assembling an erythroid, DNA-binding complex which includes the TAL1, E47, GATA-1 and Ldb1/NLI proteins. *EMBO J.* 1997;16(11):3145–3157.
161. Lecuyer E, Herblot S, Saint-Denis M, et al. The SCL complex regulates c-kit expression in hematopoietic cells through functional interaction with Sp1. *Blood.* 2002;100(7):2430–2440.
162. Nichols K, Crispino JD, Poncz M, et al. Familial dyserythropoietic anemia and thrombocytopenia due to an inherited mutation in GATA1. *Nat Genet.* 2000;24:266–270.
163. Freson, K, Devriendt, K, Matthijs, G, et al.Platelet characteristics in patients with X-linked macrothrombocytopenia because of a novel GATA1 mutation. *Blood.* 2001;98(1):85–92.
164. Mehaffey MG, Newton AL, Gandhi MJ, Crossley M, Drachman JG. X-linked thrombocytopenia caused by a novel mutation of GATA-1. *Blood.* 2001;98(9):2681–2688.
165. Freson K, Matthijs G, Thys C, et al. Different substitutions at residue D218 of the X-linked transcription factor GATA1 lead to altered clinical severity of macrothrombocytopenia and anemia and are associated with variable skewed X inactivation. *Hum Mol Genet.* 2002;11(2):147–152.
166. Balduini CL, Pecci A, Loffredo G, et al. Effects of the R216Q mutation of GATA-1 on erythropoiesis and megakaryocytopoiesis. *Thromb Haemost.* 2004;91(1):129–140.
167. Del Vecchio GC, Giordani L, De Santis A, De Mattia D. Dyserythropoietic anemia and thrombocytopenia due to a novel mutation in GATA-1. *Acta Haematol.* 2005;114(2):113–116.
168. Phillips JD, Steensma DP, Pulsipher MA, Spangrude GJ, Kushner JP. Congenital erythropoietic porphyria due to a mutation in GATA1: the first transacting mutation causative for a human porphyria. *Blood.* 2007;109(6):2618–2621.
169. Wechsler J, Greene M, McDevitt MA, et al. Acquired mutations in GATA1 in the megakaryoblastic leukemia of Down syndrome. *Nat Genet.* 2002;32(1):148–152.

170. Greene ME, Mundschau G, Wechsler J, et al. Mutations in GATA1 in both transient myeloproliferative disorder and acute megakaryoblastic leukemia of Down syndrome. *Blood Cells Mol Dis.* 2003;31(3):351–356.
171. Hitzler JK, Cheung J, Li Y, Scherer SW, Zipursky A. GATA1 mutations in transient leukemia and acute megakaryoblastic leukemia of Down syndrome. *Blood.* 2003;101:4301–4304.
172. Mundschau G, Gurbuxani S, Gamis AS, Greene ME, Arceci RJ, Crispino JD. Mutagenesis of GATA1 is an initiating event in Down syndrome leukemogenesis. *Blood.* 2003;101(11):4298–4300.
173. Rainis L, Bercovich D, Strehl S, et al. Mutations in exon 2 of GATA1 are early events in megakaryocytic malignancies associated with trisomy 21. *Blood.* 2003;102(3):981–986.
174. Xu G, Nagano M, Kanezaki R, et al. Frequent mutations in the GATA-1 gene in the transient myeloproliferative disorder of Down syndrome. *Blood.* 2003;102(8):2960–2968.
175. Taub JW, Mundschau G, Ge Y, et al. Prenatal origin of GATA1 mutations may be an initiating step in the development of megakaryocytic leukemia in Down syndrome. *Blood.* 2004;104(5):1588–1589.
176. Hollanda LM, Lima CS, Cunha AF, et al.An inherited mutation leading to production of only the short isoform of GATA-1 is associated with impaired erythropoiesis. *Nat Genet.* 2006;38(7):807–812.
177. Begley CG, Green AR. The SCL gene: from case report to critical hematopoietic regulator. *Blood.* 1999;93(9):2760–2770.
178. Lecuyer E, Hoang T. SCL: from the origin of hematopoiesis to stem cells and leukemia. *Exp Hematol.* 2004;32(1):11–24.
179. Robb L, Lyons I, Li R, et al. Absence of yolk sac hematopoiesis from mice with a targeted disruption of the scl gene. *Proc Natl Acad Sci USA.* 1995;92:7075–7079.
180. Shivdasani RA, Mayer EL, Orkin SH. Absence of blood formation in mice lacking the T-cell leukemia oncoprotein tal-1/SCL. *Nature.* 1995;373:432–434.
181. Porcher C, Swat W, Rockwell K, Fujiwara Y, Alt F, Orkin SH. The T cell leukemia oncoprotein SCL/tal-1 is essential for development of all hematopoietic lineages. *Cell.* 1996;86:47–57.
182. Robb L, Elwood NJ, Elefanty AG, et al. The scl gene is required for the generation of all hematopoietic lineages in the adult mouse. *EMBO J.* 1996;15:4123–4129.
183. Hall MA, Curtis DJ, Metcalf D, et al. The critical regulator of embryonic hematopoiesis, SCL, is vital in the adult for megakaryopoiesis, erythropoiesis, and lineage choice in CFU-S12. *Proc Natl Acad Sci USA.* 2003;100(3):992–997.
184. D'Souza SL, Elefanty AG, Keller G. SCL/Tal-1 is essential for hematopoietic commitment of the hemangioblast but not for its development. *Blood.* 2005;105(10):3862–3870.
185. Dooley KA, Davidson AJ, Zon LI. Zebrafish scl functions independently in hematopoietic and endothelial development. *Dev Biol.* 2005;277(2):522–536.
186. Patterson LJ, Gering M, Patient R. Scl is required for dorsal aorta as well as blood formation in zebrafish embryos. *Blood.* 2005;105(9):3502–3511.
187. Visvader JE, Crossley M, Hill J, Orkin SH, Adams JM. The C-terminal zinc finger of GATA-1 or GATA-2 is sufficient to induce megakaryocytic differentiation of an early myeloid cell line. *Mol Cell Biol.* 1995;15:634–641.
188. Mikkola HK, Klintman J, Yang, H, et al. Haematopoietic stem cells retain long-term repopulating activity and multipotency in the absence of stem-cell leukaemia SCL/tal-1 gene. *Nature.* 2003;421(6922):547–551.
189. Curtis DJ, Hall MA, Van Stekelenburg LJ, Robb L, Jane SM, Begley CG. SCL is required for normal function of short-term repopulating hematopoietic stem cells. *Blood.* 2004;103(9):3342–3348.
190. Green AR, Salvaris E, Begley CG. Erythroid expression of the helix-loophelix gene, SCL. *Oncogene.* 1991;6:475–479.
191. Visvader J, Begley CG, Adams JM. Differential expression of the Lyl, SCL, E2a helix-loop-helix genes within the hemopoietic system. *Oncogene.* 1991;6:187–194.
192. Mouthon M-A, Bernard O, Mitjavila M-T, Romeo PH, Vainchenker W, Mathieu-Mahul D. Expression of tal-1 and GATA-binding proteins during human hematopoiesis. *Blood.* 1993;81:647–655.
193. Aplan PD, Nakahara K, Orkin SHO, Kirsch IR. The SCL gene product: a positive regulator of erythroid differentiation. *EMBO J.* 1992;11(11):4073–4081.
194. Hoang T, Paradis E, Brady G, et al. Opposing effects of the basic helix-loop-helix transcription factor SCL on erythroid and monocytic differentiation. *Blood.* 1996;87(1):102–111.
195. Elwood NJ, Zogos H, Pereira DS, Dick JE, Begley CG. Enhanced megakaryocyte and erythroid development from normal human CD34(+) cells: consequence of enforced expression of SCL. *Blood.* 1998;91(10):3756–3765.
196. Valtieri M, Tocci A, Gabbianelli M, et al. Enforced TAL-1 expression stimulates primitive, erythroid and megakaryocytic progenitors but blocks the granulopoietic differentiation program. *Cancer Res.* 1998;58(3):562–569.
197. Elnitski L, Miller W, Hardison R. Conserved E boxes function as part of the enhancer in hypersensitive site 2 of the beta-globin locus control region. Role of basic helix- loop-helix proteins. *J Biol Chem.* 1997;272(1):369–378.
198. Anderson KP, Crable SC, Lingrel JB. Multiple proteins binding to a GATA-E box-GATA motif regulate the erythroid Kruppel-like factor (EKLF) gene. *J Biol Chem.* 1998;273(23):14347–14354.
199. Vyas P, McDevitt MA, Cantor AB, Katz SG, Fujiwara Y, Orkin SH. Different sequence requirements for expression in erythroid and megakaryocytic cells within a regulatory element upstream of the GATA-1 gene. *Development.* 1999;126(12):2799–2811.
200. Anderson KP, Crable, SC, Lingrel JB. The GATA-E box-GATA motif in the EKLF promoter is required for in vivo expression. *Blood.* 2000;95(5):1652–1655.
201. Xu Z, Huang S, Chang LS, Agulnick AD, Brandt SJ. Identification of a TAL1 target gene reveals a positive role for the LIM domain-binding protein Ldb1 in erythroid gene expression and differentiation. *Mol Cell Biol.* 2003;23(21):7585–7599.
202. Lahlil R, Lecuyer E, Herblot S, Hoang T. SCL assembles a multifactorial complex that determines glycophorin A expression. *Mol Cell Biol.* 2004;24(4):1439–1452.
203. Cohen-Kaminsky S, Maouche-Chretien L, Vitelli L, et al. Chromatin immunoselection defines a TAL-1 target gene. *EMBO J.* 1998;17(17):5151–5160.
204. Huang S, Qiu Y, Stein RW, Brandt SJ. p300 functions as a transcriptional coactivator for the TAL1/SCL oncoprotein. *Oncogene.* 1999;18(35):4958–4967.
205. Huang S, Brandt SJ. mSin3A regulates murine erythroleukemia cell differentiation through association with the

TAL1 (or SCL) transcription factor. *Mol Cell Biol.* 2000; 20(6):2248–2259.
206. Huang S, Qiu Y, Shi Y, Xu Z, Brandt SJ. P/CAF-mediated acetylation regulates the function of the basic helix- loop-helix transcription factor TAL1/SCL. *EMBO J.* 2000;19(24): 6792–6803.
207. Schuh AH, Tipping AJ, Clark AJ, et al. ETO-2 associates with SCL in erythroid cells and megakaryocytes and provides repressor functions in erythropoiesis. *Mol Cell Biol.* 2005;25(23):10235–10250.
208. Goardon N, Lambert JA, Rodriguez P, et al. ETO2 coordinates cellular proliferation and differentiation during erythropoiesis. *EMBO J.* 2006;25(2):357–366.
209. Meier N, Krpic S, Rodriguez P, et al. Novel binding partners of Ldb1 are required for haematopoietic development. *Development.* 2006;133(24):4913–4923.
210. Orkin SH, Kazazian HHJ, Antonarakis SE, et al. Linkage of beta-thalassaemia mutations and beta-globin gene polymorphisms with DNA polymorphisms in human beta-globin gene cluster. *Nature.* 1982;296:627–631.
211. Orkin SH, Antonarakis SE, Kazazian HHJ. Base substitution at position -88 in a beta-thalassemic globin gene. Further evidence for the role of distal promoter element ACACCC. *J Biol Chem.* 1984;259:8679–8681.
212. Kulozik AE, Bellan-Koch A, Bail S, Kohne E, Kleihauer E. Thalassemia intermedia: moderate reduction of beta globin gene transcriptional activity by a novel mutation of the proximal CACCC promoter element. *Blood.* 1991;77:2054–2058.
213. Cook T, Gebelein B, Urrutia R. Sp1 and its likes: biochemical and functional predictions for a growing family of zinc finger transcription factors. *Ann NY Acad Sci.* 1999;880:94–102.
214. Philipsen S, Suske G. Survey and summary. A tale of three fingers: the family of mammalian Sp/XKLF transcription factors. *Nucl Acids Res.* 1999;27:2991–3000.
215. Turner J, Crossley M. Mammalian Kruppel-like transcription factors: more than just a pretty finger. *Trends Biochem Sci.* 1999;24:236–240.
216. Miller IJ, Bieker JJ. A novel, erythroid cell-specific murine transcription factor that binds to the CACCC element and is related to the Kruppel family of nuclear proteins. *Mol Cell Biol.* 1993;13(5):2776–2786.
217. Southwood CM, Downs KM, Bieker JJ. Erythroid Kruppel-like factor exhibits an early and sequentially localized pattern of expression during mammalian erythroid ontogeny. *Dev Dyn.* 1996;206(3):248–259.
218. Feng WC, Southwood CM, Bieker JJ. Analyses of beta-thalassemia mutant DNA interactions with erythroid Kruppel-like factor (EKLF), an erythroid cell-specific transcription factor. *J Biol Chem.* 1994;269(2):1493–1500.
219. Nuez B, Michalovich D, Bygrave A, Ploemacher R, Grosveld F. Defective haematopoiesis in fetal liver resulting from inactivation of the EKLF gene. *Nature.* 1995;375:316–318.
220. Perkins AC, Sharpe AH, Orkin SH. Lethal b-thalassaemia in mice lacking the erythroid CACCC-transcription factor EKLF. *Nature.* 1995;375:318–322.
221. Zhou D, Pawlik KM, Ren J, Sun CW, Townes TM. Differential binding of erythroid Krupple-like factor to embryonic/fetal globin gene promoters during development. *J Biol Chem.* 2006;281(23):16052–16057.
222. Shyu YC, Wen SC, Lee TL, et al. Chromatin-binding in vivo of the erythroid kruppellike factor, EKLF, in the murine globin loci. *Cell Res.* 2006;16(4):347–355.
223. Perkins AC, Gaensler KM, Orkin SH. Silencing of human fetal globin expression is impaired in the absence of the adult beta-globin gene activator protein EKLF. *Proc Natl Acad Sci USA.* 1996;93(22):12267–12271.
224. Wijgerde M, Gribnau J, Trimborn T, et al. The role of EKLF in human b-globin gene competition. *Genes Dev.* 1996;10:2894–2902.
225. Tewari R, Gillemans N, Wijgerde M, et al. Erythroid Kruppel-like factor (EKLF) is active in primitive and definitive erythroid cells and is required for the function of 5′HS3 of the betaglobin locus control region. *EMBO J.* 1998;8:2334–2341.
226. Dillon N, Grosveld F. Human gamma-globin genes silenced independently of other genes in the beta-globin locus. *Nature.* 1991;350(6315):252–254.
227. Lim SK, Bieker JJ, Lin CS, Costantini F. A shortened life span of EKLF−/− adult erythrocytes, due to a deficiency of beta-globin chains, is ameliorated by human gamma-globin chains. *Blood.* 1997;90(3):1291–1299.
228. Gallagher PG, Pilon AM, Arcasoy MO, Bodine DM. Multiple defects in erythroid gene expression in erythroid Kruppel-like factor (EKLF) target genes in EKLF-deficient mice. *Blood.* 2004;104(11):446a.
229. Nilson DG, Sabatino DE, Bodine DM, Gallagher PG. Major erythrocyte membrane protein genes in EKLF-deficient mice. *Exp Hematol.* 2006;34(6):705–712.
230. Keys JR, Tallack M.R, Hodge DJ, Cridland SO, David R, Perkins AC. Genomic organisation and regulation of murine alpha haemoglobin stabilising protein by erythroid Kruppel-like factor. *Br J Haematol.* 2007;136(1):150–157.
231. Frontelo, P, Manwani, D, Galdass, M, et al. 2007. Novel role for EKLF in megakaryocyte lineage commitment. *Blood.* 2007;110:3871–3880.
232. Donze D, Townes TM, Bieker JJ. Role of erythroid Kruppel-like factor in human gamma- to beta-globin gene switching. *J Biol Chem.* 1995;270(4):1955–1959.
233. Bieker JJ, Southwood CM. The erythroid Kruppel-like factor transactivation domain is a critical component for cell-specific inducibility of a beta-globin promoter. *Mol Cell Biol.* 1995;15(2):852–860.
234. Ouyang L, Chen X, Bieker JJ. Regulation of erythroid Kruppel-like factor (EKLF) transcriptional activity by phosphorylation of a protein kinase casein kinase II site within its interaction domain. *J Biol Chem.* 1998;273(36):23019–23025.
235. Zhang W, Bieker JJ. Acetylation and modulation of erythroid Kruppel-like factor (EKLF) activity by interaction with histone acetyltransferases. *Proc Natl Acad Sci USA.* 1998;95(17):9855–9860.
236. Zhang W, Kadam S, Emerson BM, Bieker JJ. Site-specific acetylation by p300 or CREB binding protein regulates erythroid Kruppel-like factor transcriptional activity via its interaction with the SWI-SNF complex. *Mol Cell Biol.* 2001;21(7):2413–2422.
237. Siatecka M, Xue L, Bieker JJ. Sumoylation of EKLF promotes transcriptional repression and is involved in inhibition of megakaryopoiesis. *Mol Cell Biol.* 2007;27(24):8547–8560.
238. Armstrong J.A, Bieker J.J, Emerson BM. A SWI/SNF-related chromatin remodeling complex, E-RC1, is required for tissue-specific transcriptional regulation by EKLF in vitro. *Cell.* 1998;95(1):93–104.
239. Asano H, Li XS, Stamatoyannopoulos G. FKLF, a novel Kruppel-like factor that activates human embryonic and fetal beta-like globin genes. *Mol Cell Biol.* 1999;19(5):3571–3579.

240. Asano H, Li XS, Stamatoyannopoulos G. FKLF-2: a novel Kruppel-like transcriptional factor that activates globin and other erythroid lineage genes. *Blood.* 2000;95(11):3578–3584.
241. Funnell AP, Maloney CA, Thompson LJ, et al. Erythroid Kruppel-like factor directly activates the basic Kruppel-like factor gene in erythroid cells. *Mol Cell Biol.* 2007;27(7):2777–2790.
242. Perkins AC, Yang H, Crossley PM, Fujiwara Y, Orkin SH. Deficiency of the CACC-element binding protein BKLF leads to a progressive myeloproliferative disease and impaired expression of SHP-1. *Blood.* 1997;90(Suppl 1):575a.
243. Marin M, Karis A, Visser P, Grosveld F, Philipsen S. Transcription factor Sp1 is essential for early embryonic development but dispensable for cell growth and differentiation. *Cell.* 1997;89:619–628.
244. Kruger I, Vollmer M, Simmons D, Elsasser HP, Philipsen S, Suske G. Sp1/Sp3 compound heterozygous mice are not viable: impaired erythropoiesis and severe placental defects. *Dev Dyn.* 2007;236(8):2235–2244.
245. Talbot D, Grosveld F. The 5′HS2 of the globin locus control region enhances transcription through the interaction of a multimeric complex binding at two functionally distinct NF-E2 binding sites. *EMBO J.* 1991;10(6):1391–1398.
246. Stamatoyannopoulos JA, Goodwin A, Joyce T, Lowrey CH. NF-E2 and GATA binding motifs are required for the formation of DNase I hypersensitive site 4 of the human b-globin locus control region. *EMBO J.* 1995;14:106–116.
247. Boyes J, Felsenfeld G. Tissue-specific factors additively increase the probability of the all-or-none formation of a hypersensitive site. *EMBO J.* 1996;15: 2496–2507.
248. Gong QH, McDowell JC, Dean A. Essential role of NF-E2 in remodeling of chromatin structure and transcriptional activation of the epsilon-globin gene in vivo by 5′ hypersensitive site 2 of the beta-globin locus control region. *Mol Cell Biol.* 1996;16(11):6055–6064.
249. Pomerantz O, Goodwin AJ, Joyce T, Lowrey CH. Conserved elements containing NF-E2 and tandem GATA binding sites are required for erythroid-specific chromatin structure reorganization within the human b-globin locus control region. *Nucl Acid Res.* 1998;26:5684–5691.
250. Mignotte V, Eleouet JF, Raich N, Romeo P-H. Cis- and trans-acting elements involved in the regulation of the erythroid promoter of the human porphobilinogen deaminase gene. *Proc Natl Acad Sci USA.* 1989;86:6548–6552.
251. Taketani S, Inazawa J, Nakahashi Y, Abe T, Tokunaga R. Structure of the human ferrochelatase gene. Exon/intron gene organization and location of the gene to chromosome 18. *Eur J Biochem.* 1992;205:217–222.
252. Mignotte V, Wall L, deBoer E, Grosveld F, Romeo P-H. Two tissuespecific factors bind the erythroid promoter of the human porphobilinogen deaminase gene. *Nucl Acids Res.* 1989;17(1):37–54.
253. Andrews NC, Erdjument-Bromage H, Davidson M, Tempst P, Orkin SH. Erythroid transcription factor NF-E2 is a haematopoietic-specific basic leucine zipper protein. *Nature.* 1993;362:722–728.
254. Andrews NC, Kotkow KJ, Ney PA, Erdjument-Bromage H, Tempst P, Orkin SH. The ubiquitous subunit of erythroid transcription factor NF-E2 is a small basic-leucine zipper protein related to the v-maf oncogene. *Proc Natl Acad Sci USA.* 1993;90:11488–11492.
255. Ney PA, Andrews NC, Jane SM, et al. Purification of the human NF-E2 complex: cDNA cloning of the hematopoietic cell-specific subunit and evidence for an associated partner. *Mol Cell Biol.* 1993;13:5604–5612.
256. Blank V, Andrews NC. The Maf transcription factors: regulators of differentiation. *Trends Biochem Sci.* 1997;22(11):437–441.
257. Motohashi H, Shavit JA, Igarashi K, Yamamoto M, Engel JD. The world according to Maf. *Nucl Acids Res.* 1997;25(15): 2953–2959.
258. Lu SJ, Rowan S, Bani MR, Ben-David Y. Retroviral integration within the Fli-2 locus results in inactivation of the erythroid transcription factor NF-E2 in Friend erythroleukemias: evidence that NF-E2 is essential for globin gene expression. *Proc Natl Acad Sci USA.* 1994;91:8398–8402.
259. Kotkow K, Orkin SH. Dependence of globin gene expression in mouse erythroleukemia cells on the NF-E2 heterodimer. *Mol Cell Biol.* 1995;15:4640–4647.
260. Shivdasani RA, Orkin SH. Erythropoiesis and globin gene expression in mice lacking the transcription factor NF-E2. *Proc Natl Acad Sci USA.* 1995;92:8690–8694.
261. Shivdasani RA, Rosenblatt MF, Zucker-Franklin DC, et al. Transcription factor NF-E2 is required for platelet formation independent of the actions of thrombopoieitin/MGDF in megakaryocyte development. *Cell.* 1995;81:695–701.
262. Chan K, LuR, Chang JC, Kan YW. NRF2, a member of the NFE2 family of transcription factors, is not essential for murine erythropoiesis, growth, and development. *Proc Natl Acad Sci USA.* 1996;93:13943–13948.
263. Kuroha T, Takahashi S, Komeno T, Itoh K, Nagasawa T, Yamamoto M. Ablation of Nrf2 function does not increase the erythroid or megakaryocytic cell lineage dysfunction caused by p45 NF-E2 gene disruption. *J Biochem.* 1998;123:376–379.
264. Martin F, van Deursen JM, Shivdasani RA, Jackson CW, Troutman AG, Ney PA. Erythroid maturation and globin gene expression in mice with combined deficiency of NF-E2 and nrf-2. *Blood.* 1998;91:3459–3466.
265. Farmer SC, Sun CW, Winnier GE, Hogan BL, Townes TM. The bZIP transcription factor LCR-F1 is essential for mesoderm formation in mouse development. *Genes Dev.* 1997;11:786–798.
266. Chan JY, Kwong M, Lu R, et al. Targeted disruption of the ubiquitous CNC-bZIP transcription factor, Nrf-1, results in anemia and embryonic lethality in mice. *EMBO J.* 1998;17:1779–1787.
267. Oyake T, Itoh K, Motohashi H, et al. Bach proteins belong to a novel family of BTB-basic leucine zipper transcription factors that interact with MafK and regulate transcription through the NF-E2 site. *Mol Cell Biol.* 1996;16:6083–6095.
268. Igarashi K, Hoshino H, Muto A, et al. Multivalent DNA binding complex generated by small Maf and Bach1 as a possible biochemical basis for beta-globin locus control region complex. *J Biol Chem.* 1998;273:11783–11790.
269. Ogawa K, Sun J, Taketani S, Nakajima O, et al. Heme mediates derepression of Maf recognition element through direct binding to transcription repressor Bach1. *EMBO J.* 2001;20(11):2835–2843.
270. Suzuki H, Tashiro S, Hira S, et al. Heme regulates gene expression by triggering Crm1-dependent nuclear export of Bach1. *EMBO J.* 2004;23(13):2544–2553.

271. Zenke-Kawasaki Y, Dohi Y, Katoh, Y, et al. Heme induces ubiquitination and degradation of the transcription factor Bach1. *Mol Cell Biol.* 2007;27(19):6962–6971.
272. Tahara T, Sun J, Igarashi K, Taketani S. Heme-dependent up-regulation of the alpha-globin gene expression by transcriptional repressor Bach1 in erythroid cells. *Biochem Biophys Res Commun.* 2004;324(1):77–85.
273. Tahara T, Sun J, Nakanishi K, et al. Heme positively regulates the expression of b-globin at the locus control region via the transcriptional factor Bach1 in erythroid cells. *J Biol Chem.* 2004;279:5480–5487.
274. Igarashi K, Kataoka K, Itoh K, Hayashi N, Nishizawa M, Yamamoto M. Regulation of transcription by dimerization of erythroid factor NF-E2 p45 with small Maf proteins. *Nature.* 1994;367:568–572.
275. Kotkow KJ, Orkin SH. Complexity of the erythroid transcription factor NFE2 as revealed by gene targeting of the mouse p18 NF-E2 locus. *Proc Natl Acad Sci USA.* 1996;93:3514–3518.
276. Shavit JA, Motohashi H, Onodera K, Akasaka J-E, Yamamoto M, Engel JD. Impaired megakaryopoiesis and behavioral defects in mafG-null mutant mice. *Genes Dev.* 1998;12:2164–2174.
277. Motohashi H, Katsuoka F, Miyoshi C, et al. MafG sumoylation is required for active transcriptional repression. *Mol Cell Biol.* 2006;26(12):4652–4663.
278. Bean TL, Ney PA. Multiple regions of p45 NF-E2 are required for b-globin gene expression in erythroid cells. *Nucl Acids Res.* 1997;25:2509–2515.
279. Cheng X, Reginato MJ, Andrews NC, Lazar MA. The Transcriptional Integrator CREB- binding protein mediates positive cross talk between nuclear hormone receptors and the hematopoietic bZip protein p45/NF-E2. *Mol Cell Biol.* 1997;1:1407–1416.
280. Gavva NR, Gavva R, Ermekova K, Sudol M, Shen CJ. Interaction of WW domains with hematopoietic transcription factor p45/NF-E2 and RNA polymerase II. *J Biol Chem.* 1997;272:24105–24108.
281. Mosser EA, Kasanov JD, Forsberg EC, Kay BK, Ney PA, Bresnick EH. Physical and functional interactions between the transactivation domain of the hematopoietic transcription factor NF-E2 and WW domains. *Biochemistry.* 1998;37:13686–13695.
282. Amrolia PJ, Ramamurthy L, Saluja D, Tanese N, Jane SM, Cunningham JM. The activation domain of the enhancer binding protein p45NF-E2 interacts with TAFII130 and mediates long-range activation of the alpha- and beta-globin gene loci in an erythroid cell line. *Proc Natl Acad Sci USA.* 1997;94:10051–10056.
283. Shikama N, Lyon J, LaThangue NB. The p300/CBP family: integrating signals with transcription factors and chromatin. *Trends Cell Biol.* 1997;7:230–236.
284. Armstrong JA, Emerson BM. NF-E2 disrupts chromatin structure at human beta-globin locus control region hypersensitive site 2 in vitro. *Mol Cell Biol.* 1996;16(10):5634–5644.
285. Demers C, Chaturvedi CP, Ranish JA, et al. Activator-mediated recruitment of the MLL2 methyltransferase complex to the beta-globin locus. *Mol Cell.* 2007;27(4):573–584.
286. Brand M, Ranish JA, Kummer NT, et al. Dynamic changes in transcription factor complexes during erythroid differentiation revealed by quantitative proteomics. *Nat Struct Mol Biol.* 2004;11(1):73–80.
287. Nagai T, Igarashi K, Akasaka J, et al. Regulation of NF-E2 activity in erythroleukemia cell differentiation. *J Biol Chem.* 1998;273:5358–5365.
288. Versaw WK, Blank V, Andrews NM, Bresnick EH. Mitogen-activated protein kinases enhance long-range activation by the beta-globin locus control region. *Proc Natl Acad Sci USA.* 1998;95:8756–8760.
289. Casteel D, Suhasini M, Gudi T, Naima R, Pilz RB. Regulation of the erythroid transcription factor NF-E2 by cyclic adenosine monophosphate dependent protein kinase. *Blood.* 1998;91(9):3193–3201.
290. Shyu YC, Lee TL, Ting CY, et al. Sumoylation of p45/NF-E2: nuclear positioning and transcriptional activation of the mammalian beta-like globin gene locus. *Mol Cell Biol.* 2005;25(23):10365–10378.
291. Choi O-RB, Engel JD. Developmental regulation of b-globin gene switching. *Cell.* 1988;56:17–26.
292. Wijgerde M, Grosveld F, Fraser P. Transcription complex stability and chromatin dynamics in vivo. *Nature.* 1995; 377(6546):209–213.
293. Trimborn T, Gribnau J, Grosveld F, Fraser P. Mechanisms of developmental control of transcription in the murine alpha- and beta-globin loci. *Genes Dev.* 1999;13(1):112–124.
294. Minie ME, Kimura T, Felsenfeld G. The developmental switch in embryonic rho-globin expression is correlated with erythroid lineage–specific differences in transcription factor levels. *Development.* 1992;115(4):1149–1164.
295. Knezetic JA, Felsenfeld G. Mechanism of developmental regulation of alpha pi, the chicken embryonic alpha-globin gene. *Mol Cell Biol.* 1993;13(8):4632–4639.
296. Jane SM, Ney PA, Vanin EF, Gumucio DL, Nienhuis AW. Identification of a stage selector element in the human gamma-globin gene promoter that fosters preferential interaction with the 5′ HS2 enhancer when in competition with the beta-promoter. *EMBO J.* 1992;11(8):2961–2969.
297. Zhou W, Zhao Q, Sutton R, et al. The role of p22 NF-E4 in human globin gene switching. *J Biol Chem.* 2004; 279(25):26227–26232.
298. Sargent TG, Buller AM, Teachey DT, McCanna KS, Lloyd JA. The gamma-globin promoter has a major role in competitive inhibition of beta-globin gene expression in early erythroid development. *DNA Cell Biol.* 1999;18(4):293–303.
299. Sargent TG, DuBois CC, Buller AM, Lloyd JA. The roles of 5′-HS2, 5′-HS3, and the gamma-globin TATA, CACCC, and stage selector elements in suppression of beta-globin expression in early development. *J Biol Chem.* 1999;274(16):11229–11236.
300. Tanabe O, Katsuoka F, Campbell AD, et al. An embryonic/fetal beta-type globin gene repressor contains a nuclear receptor TR2/TR4 heterodimer. *EMBO J.* 2002;21(13):3434–3442.
301. Filipe A, Li Q, Deveaux S, Godin I, et al. Regulation of embryonic/fetal globin genes by nuclear hormone receptors: a novel perspective on hemoglobin switching. *EMBO J.* 1999;18(3):687–697.
302. Huisman THJ, Carver MFH, Baysal E. *A Syllabus of Thalassemia Mutations.* Augusta, GA: The Sickle Cell Anemia Foundation; 1997.
303. Crossley M, Tsang AP, Bieker JJ, Orkin SH. Regulation of the erythroid Kruppel-like factor (EKLF) gene promoter by the erythroid transcription factor GATA-1. *J Biol Chem.* 1994;269(22):15440–15444.

304. Candido EP, Reeves R, Davie JR. Sodium butyrate inhibits histone deacetylation in cultured cells. *Cell.* 1978;14(1):105–113.
305. McCaffrey PG, Newsome DA, Fibach E, Yoshida M, Su MS. Induction of gamma-globin by histone deacetylase inhibitors. *Blood.* 1997;90(5):2075–2083.
306. Cao H, Stamatoyannopoulos G, Jung M. Induction of human gamma globin gene expression by histone deacetylase inhibitors. *Blood.* 2004;103(2):701–709.
307. Chen WY, Bailey EC, McCune SL, Dong JY, Townes TM. Reactivation of silenced, virally transduced genes by inhibitors of histone deacetylase. *Proc Natl Acad Sci USA.* 1997;94(11):5798–5803.
308. Sankaran VG, Menns TF, Xe J. et al. Human fetal hemoglobin expression is regulated by the developmental stage-specific repressorr BCL11A. Science. 2008;322:1839–1842.
309. Uda M, Galanello R, Sanna S, et al. Genome-wide association study shows BCL11A associated with persistent fetal hemoglobin and amelioration of the phenotype of beta-thalassemia. Proc Nati Acad Sci USA. 2008;105:1620–1625.
310. Lettre G, Sankaran VG, Bezerra MA, et al. DNA polymorphisms at the BCL11A, HBSIL-MYB, and beta-globin loci associate with fetal hemoglobin levels and pain crises in sickle cell disease. Proc Nati Acad Sci USA. 2008;105:11869–11874.
311. Sedgewick AE, Timofeev N, Sebastiani P, et al. BCL11A is a major HbF quantitative trait locus in three different populations with beta-hemoglobinopathies. Blood Cells Mol Dis. 2008;41:255–258.
312. Manzel S, Garner C, Gut I, et al. A QTL, influencing F cell production maps to a gene recoding a zinc-finger protein on chromosome 2p15. Nat Genet. 2007;39:1197–1199.

5

Molecular and Cellular Basis of Hemoglobin Switching

George Stamatoyannopoulos, Patrick A. Navas, and Qiliang Li

INTRODUCTION

Hemoglobin switching is characteristic of all animal species that use hemoglobin for oxygen transport. Most species have only one switch, from embryonic to adult globin formation. Humans and a few other mammals have two globin gene switches, from embryonic to fetal globin coinciding with the transition from embryonic (yolk sac) to definitive (fetal liver) hematopoiesis and from fetal to adult globin formation, occurring around the perinatal period (Fig. 5.1; see Chapters 1 and 2). The switch from ε- to γ-globin production begins very early in gestation, as fetal hemoglobin (HbF) is readily detected in 5-week-old human embryos,[1,2] and it is completed well before the 10th week of gestation.[1,3] β-globin expression starts early in human development, and small amounts of adult hemoglobin (HbA) have been detected by biosynthetic or immunochemical methods even in the smallest human fetuses studied. In these fetuses γ- and β-globins are present in the same fetal red cells.[4] β-chain synthesis increases to approximately 10% of total hemoglobin by 30–35 weeks of gestation. At birth, HbF comprises 60%–80% of the total hemoglobin. It takes approximately 2 years to reach the level of 0.5%–1% HbF that is characteristic of adult red cells. HbF in the adult is restricted to a few erythrocytes called "F cells" (see chapter 7).[5,6] Approximately 3%–7% of erythrocytes are F cells[6] and each contains approximately 4–8 pg of HbF.[5]

Hemoglobin switching has been the target of intensive investigation for two reasons. First, it provides an excellent model for studying the control of gene activity during development. Indeed, until the late 1970s, hemoglobin switching was the only developmental system that could be investigated in detail at the protein level. Second, understanding of the control of switching is expected to lead to the development of treatments of hemoglobinopathies. The β-chain hemoglobinopathies, sickle cell disease, and thalassemia are unique among genetic disorders in that nature has shown an effective means of treatment: the production of HbF that can compensate for the loss of β-chain activity or can decrease the propensity for sickling. Research on the cell and molecular control of switching is expected to lead to discoveries that will cure these disorders through abundant production of HbF in the patient's red cells.

CELLULAR CONTROL OF SWITCHING

Before the era of molecular biology, insights on the cellular mechanisms of hemoglobin switching were obtained through phenomenological observations in human and animal models and from cell biological studies. The observation that human fetuses have different hemoglobin than adults was made more than 100 years ago when it was discovered that the hemoglobin of neonates is alkali resistant. The observation that amphibia have different hemoglobins in the embryonic and the adult stages was made in the 1930s when the oxygen affinity of frog and tadpole blood was examined. The two types of hemoglobin were actually separated by Svedberg while he was developing the ultracentrifuge. Hemoglobin switching was more intensely investigated when the introduction of electrophoretic techniques allowed detailed studies of hemoglobin during the development of many species. Several questions on the cellular control of switching were asked during that time and, amazingly, clonal models of switching (see later) were proposed even before it became possible to analyze hemoglobin switching at the protein level. Systematic investigation of the cellular control of switching, however, started only when modern methods of cell biology became available in the 1970s.

Models of Cellular Control

The first models of hemoglobin switching assumed that it represents an epiphenomenon due to replacement of hematopoietic stem cell lineages. The model was eloquently formulated by the late Vernon Ingram.[7] To explain hemoglobin switching in the mouse or in the chicken, it was postulated that there is an embryonic stem cell lineage that is committed to embryonic globin gene formation and this is replaced by an adult stem cell lineage committed to expression of the adult globin genes. In the case of the human hemoglobin switching, three lineages were thought to exist: an embryonic, a fetal, and an adult stem cell lineage. The fetal (γ-) to adult (β-) switch was attributed to the replacement of the fetal stem cell lineage by the adult stem cell lineage.[8–12] The transitions in major erythropoietic sites during ontogeny (see Chapter 1) seemed to support the clonal hypothesis of switching. The clonal hypothesis was also appealing because of the restriction of HbF in few red cells, the F cells, in the adult blood. When, in adult individuals, HbF was elevated, the number of F cells was elevated. Hence it was thought that F cells and A cells (i.e., cells that did not contain HbF) were derived from two distinct stem cell lineages.[9]

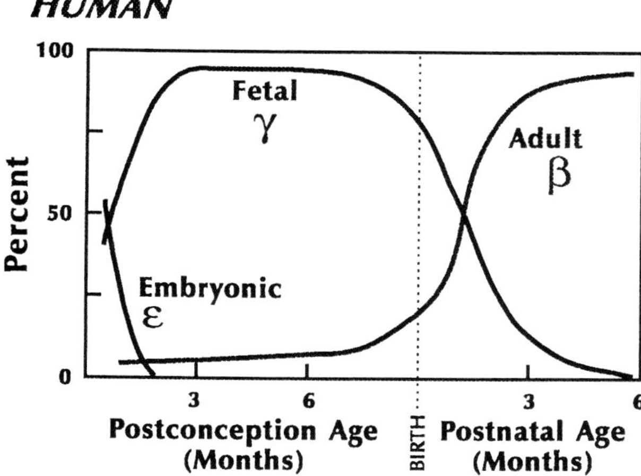

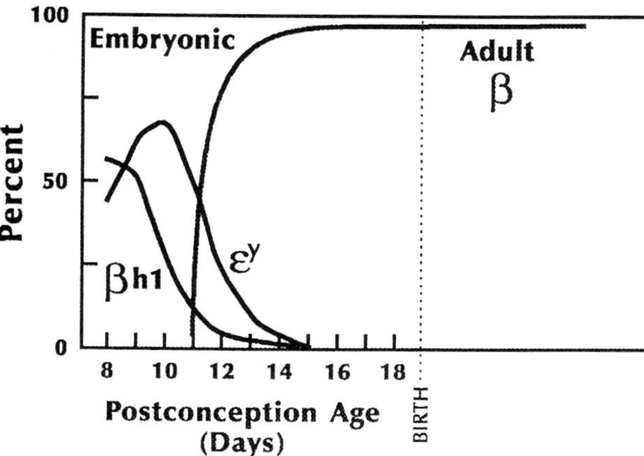

Figure 5.1. Hemoglobin switching in humans and mice. The human ε gene is homologous to murine εy. The γ-globin gene is homologous to βh1 whereas the β-globin gene is homologous to murine βminor and βmajor.

An alternative model was elaborated in the mid-1970s.[13] It proposed that fetal to adult globin gene switching is not due to changes in stem cell populations but to changes in programs of gene expression that occur in the progeny of a single stem cell population. A fetal program is activated in the progenitor cells of the fetus and an adult program in the progenitor cells of the adult.

Finding out which of the two models (i.e., changes in stem cell populations or changes in programs) is correct was important from the theoretical and the therapeutic point of view. In the 1970s it was thought that it was difficult to manipulate stem cell populations; on the other hand, it was possible that manipulation of gene expression programs could be achieved with pharmacological means. Therefore, a systematic investigation of the two models was conducted.

The lineage models assume an absolute restriction of embryonic globins to primitive cells and of adult globins to definitive cells. During switching in chickens,[14] in the mouse,[15] and in quail–chick chimeras,[16,17] there are cell populations coexpressing both embryonic and adult hemoglobins. The hematopoietic cells of human embryos can be used to produce erythroid colonies, each of which originates from a single progenitor cell; typically, these colonies coexpress ε- and γ-globins.[18,19] Thus, a single progenitor cell can form progeny producing adult and embryonic globins, contrary to the expectations of the lineage models.

Three types of experiments provided evidence against the model of replacement of stem cell lineages as an explanation of the γ- to β-switch. First, studies of individuals with clonal hemopoietic stem cell disorders (polycythemia vera, chronic myelogenous leukemia, or paroxysmal nocturnal hemoglobinuria) clearly showed that both F cells and A cells are produced by a single stem cell clone (summarized in Stamatoyannopoulos and Grosveld[20]). Second, studies in culture showed that erythroid colonies derived from single progenitor cells of fetuses, neonates, or adults, contain both fetal and adult globins.[20] Third, direct evidence came from analyses of somatic cell hybrids produced by fusion of mouse erythroleukemia (MEL) cells with human cells. These hybrids initially synthesize only (or predominantly) fetal human globin, and after 20–40 weeks in culture they switch to β-globin chain formation. Since each hybrid originated from a single cell, these results provided direct evidence that γ- to β-switching can occur in cells of a single lineage.[21]

It is thus clear that the fetal to adult hemoglobin switching takes place in the progeny of a single stem cell lineage. It represents changes in transcriptional environments at the level of committed cells rather than changes in stem cell populations "frozen" in a single gene expression program. It is of interest that despite the extensive evidence, even today the cellular phenotypes of HbF elevations in the adult are attributed by some authors to the presence of a fetal stem cell population in the adult marrow!

The Question of Developmental Clock of Switching

If switching takes place in the cells of a single lineage, how do these cells know when to switch their globin gene expression program? Many changes occur during development and there is ample evidence that the cell's microenvironment can determine the fate of a cell. Initially, inductive mechanisms were thought to trigger hemoglobin switching, and several experiments have been done to test whether changes in the environment of the developing fetus, especially hormonal changes, are responsible for the γ- to β-switch. The summary of this work indicates that there is no evidence that there exists a specific environmental signal that is responsible for the switch. On the other hand, there is evidence that the environment can influence the rate of the γ- to β-switching. Thus, in sheep, removal of the adrenals abolishes the increase in plasma cortisol that precedes birth.[22] The γ- to β-switch in such adrenalectomized animals is delayed, although the animals are normal with respect to developmental progression. Administration of cortisol allows the switch to progress with normal kinetics. Also, external factors can influence the rate of the γ- to β-switch in MEL/fetal erythroid hybrids: serum deprivation or addition of dexamethasone in the culture media strikingly accelerates, while addition of butyrate inhibits, the γ- to β-switch.[23,24]

Considerable evidence suggests that the rate and the timing of switching is inherently controlled, perhaps through the action of a developmental clock type of mechanism. Three arguments in favor of a clock-type of mechanism will be mentioned here. First, in vivo observations in humans indicate that the level of HbF in newborns is related to their developmental age from conception rather than to the time of birth itself.[25,26] Thus, the switch is independent of the intrauterine or extrauterine status of the individual; rather, the degree of developmental maturity of the fetus determines the rate as well as the timing of the γ- to β-switch. Second, the rate of γ- to β-switching of the MEL/human fetal erythroid hybrids correlates with the age of the fetus from which the human erythroblasts were derived.[21] Thus, hybrids produced using cells of younger fetuses switch more slowly than do hybrids produced using cells of older fetuses, as if the human fetal erythroid cells "know" whether they belong to an early or to a late developmental stage, and transmit this information to the hybrid cells. Third, transplantation experiments of hematopoietic stem cells have been done in sheep to determine whether the hematopoietic environment can influence the rate of the switch in transplanted cells. Adult stem cells were transplanted into fetuses and fetal stem cells into adult animals, and hemoglobin production in the engrafted donor cells was monitored. The adult cells transplanted into fetuses continued to produce adult globin, suggesting that the fetal environment cannot change the program of the adult cells.[27] Transplantation of fetal sheep stem cells into lethally irradiated adult recipients showed that the donor cells switch.[28] The rate of switching of the transplanted fetal cells, however, depended on the gestational age of the donor fetus, suggesting that switching reflects the action of a mechanism that in some fashion can count developmental time.

Presumably, a clock determining the rate of switching is set sometime during embryogenesis and proceeds to execute a preset program as development advances. It has been difficult to test experimentally the molecular basis of this phenomenon. There are several examples of developmental clocks in drosophila, but these are usually associated with circadian rhythms. It is difficult to conceive how a "clock" that can operate for several months (as in the case of human γ- to β-globin gene switching) is controlled; although hypotheses on how cells can count developmental time have been proposed.[29] The available evidence suggests that the clock of human γ- to β-switching is located on chromosome 11.[30] It acts in *cis* and certain findings,[31] although interpreted differently by these authors, suggest that the clock may be controlled through sequences located in the β-globin gene cluster.

MOLECULAR CONTROL OF SWITCHING

The last 20 years have witnessed considerable progress in the understanding of the molecular control of globin gene switching. Several tools have been used. Transgenic mice have provided information on the sequences of the locus that are responsible for developmental control and on the mechanisms that control switching in vivo. Traditional biochemistry and gene cloning techniques have led to the discovery of *trans* factors that interact with motifs of globin gene promoters and the locus control region (LCR). Essentially, we know today, in very broad terms, the mechanisms that regulate globin gene activity during development. There is, however, a vast amount of specific information that still needs to be learned until the phenomenon is completely understood at the molecular level.

Regulatory Elements of the ε-Globin Gene

In vitro experiments indicate that the CACCC and CCAAT boxes in conjunction with the GATA sites of the ε-globin gene promoter are required for expression expression.[32–35] However, it is not known which factors interact with these sequences in vivo. The CACCC box binds the ubiquitous factor Sp1,[36] but inactivation of Sp1 in vivo[37] does not result in defective ε-gene expression. Two factors belonging to the erythroid Krüppel-like factor (EKLF)/Sp1 family, designated fetal Krüppel-like factor (FKLF)[38] and FKLF-2,[39] have been shown to interact with the ε-gene CACCC box and activate gene transcription in transient expression assays and in stably transfected red cells. The CAAT box of the ε gene binds CP1; binding of CP1 activates in vitro gene expression. In the region of the CCAAT box of the embryonic and fetal, but not of adult, globin-gene promoters there exist direct repeats of a short motif that is analogous to DR-1 binding sites for nonsteroid nuclear hormone receptors.[35] In vitro experiments and studies in transgenic mice have demonstrated that COUP-TF, an orphan nuclear receptor, binds to the DR-1 element of the gene promoter and acts as a developmental repressor.[35] The role of the DR-1 element in ε-gene silencing was confirmed in a study performed in βYAC transgenic mice.[40] Furthermore, this study demonstrated that the DR-1 element binds a 540-kD complex named DRED (direct repeat erythroid-definitive), which contains nuclear orphan receptors TR2 and TR4.[40,41] TR2 and TR4 form a heterodimer and are able to bind to the ε- and γ-globin gene promoters. In TR2 and TR4 null mutant mice, silencing of both the ε- and γ-globin genes is delayed in definitive erythroid cells. In transgenic mice expressing a dominant-negative TR4, the ε gene is activated in primitive and definitive erythroid cells.[42] Forced expression of wild-type TR2 and TR4 leads to precocious repression of the ε-globin gene; however, γ-globin expression is increased in definitive erythroid cells.[42] The ε-globin gene promoter also contains a number of GATA sites. Studies in transgenic mice suggest that when GATA-1 binds at the −163 or −269 site it acts as a gene activator, but when it binds to the −208 site it acts as a repressor.[43] Several binding sites for factors that can act either as repressors or activators in vitro have been identified in the upstream ε-gene promoter.[44,45] Sox6, a member of the Sox transcription factor family, is able to bind at the proximal promoter of the mouse εy-globin gene and to silence directly expression of the gene in definitive erythroid cells.[46,47] It remains to be seen whether Sox6 is involved in the autonomous silencing of the human ε-globin gene in adult erythropoiesis.

Regulatory Elements of the γ-Globin Genes

Evidence that the γ-globin gene promoter contains elements important for developmental control is provided by the point mutations that produce phenotypes of hereditary persistence of fetal hemoglobin (HPFH) (see Chapter 16). Most of these HPFH mutations occur in transcription factor binding motifs. Between the CAAT box and the TATA box of the γ-gene promoter there exists a G-rich sequence designated as stage selector element. This sequence is conserved in species that express the γ gene in the fetal stage, but diverges in species in which the γ-gene homolog is expressed in embryonic cells.[48] A binding activity, called stage selector protein,[49,50] binds to this sequence. Stage selector protein is composed of the ubiquitously expressed factor CP2 and a recently cloned protein, NF-E4, which is erythroid specific and activates γ-gene expression in transfection experiments in vitro.[51,52]

Several proteins bind to the CAAT box region of the promoter.[53–58] CP1, a ubiquitously expressed protein, acts as a positive transcriptional activator in vitro. CAAT displacement protein (CDP) binds to both CAAT boxes, competitively displacing CP1 and, in vitro, acts as a transcriptional repressor.[59] NF-E3 and GATA-1 bind in the CAAT box region[53,54,58,60] and are considered to act as gene suppressors, but this hypothesis is not supported by experiments in transgenic mice.[61] Studies in transgenic mice indicate that the CACCC box plays an important role in gene expression at the fetal stage of definitive hematopoiesis when the major synthesis of fetal hemoglobin takes place in humans.[62] FKLF[38] and FKLF-2[39] bind to the γ-globin gene CACCC box in vitro but their in vivo role has not yet been determined. As mentioned previously, a DR-1 element is also identified in the γ-globin gene promoter.[35,40] The DR-1 binding site is disrupted by the HPFH-117 mutation in support of the hypothesis that the DR-1 element is implicated in γ-gene silencing.

Other developmentally important sites have been revealed in the upstream promoter by HPFH mutants. GATA and octamer 1 sites are located near position −175. The −175 HPFH mutation alters the interaction with GATA-1 and removes the binding site for octamer 1,[63,64] but the relevance of these in vitro effects to the HPFH phenotype remains unknown. Several HPFH mutations are located in the −200 region. This region of the promoter is capable of forming a triple-stranded structure, which is thought to be the binding site for a repressor complex that is displaced by the transcription factors that bind to the novel sequences created by the HPFH mutations mutations.[65,66] Other potential binding sites are located further upstream in the promoter promoter.[48,67] Transgenic mouse experiments have localized a potential silencer element in the −382 to −730 region.[68] Also, this region contains a butyrate response element element.[69] That the −382 to −730 region may contain a silencer has also been shown by the finding of an HPFH mutation at position −567. This mutation alters a GATA site and in vitro experiments showed a complete loss of GATA-1 binding,[70] a phenotype recapitulated in transgenic mice.[71] Chromatin immunoprecipitation experiments using fetal liver tissue from βYAC transgenic mice showed a recruitment of GATA-1, FOG-1, and Mi2 to the −567 GATA site late in fetal development when γ-gene expression is silenced.[71] Mi2 is a member of the NuRD complex whose functions include nucleosome remodeling and histone deacetylase activities resulting in transcription repression.[72–74]

An "enhancer" has been located downstream from the $^{A}\gamma$ gene on the basis of transient transfection experiments.[75] This element contains binding sites for various transcription factors,[76,77] but it appears to have no effect on γ-globin gene expression in vivo.[78] In transgenic mice, presence of this 3′ element protects the γ gene from position effects,[79,80] suggesting that its likely role is stabilization of the interaction between the γ-globin gene and the LCR.

The effects of the three basic *cis* elements of the γ-globin gene promoter, CACCC, CCAAT, and TATA, on the transcriptional potentials of the promoter at different developmental stages have been studied in transgenic mice. Mutations in each box disrupt γ-gene expression in adult erythropoiesis, but have no effect on γ-gene expression in embryonic erythropoiesis.[62,81–83] These results imply that the transcriptional machinery in embryonic and adult erythroid cells may differ; thus, an intact promoter is required for highly effective transcription in adult erythroid cells whereas a partially defective γ-globin promoter can initiate high levels of transcription in embryonic erythroid cells.

Regulatory Elements of the β-Globin Gene

Several factors have been shown to bind in the CAAT box region of the β-globin gene;[84–86] CP1 behaves as a positive regulator of the CAAT box in vitro. The CACCC box binds several factors in vitro[87] but the protein that appears to be the most important in vivo is EKLF.[88,89] The β-globin CACC box has a higher binding affinity for EKLF than the ε- or γ-globin CACC boxes.[90]

Studies using transgenic mice have identified two regions that could enhance β-globin gene expression.[84,91–93] An enhancer is located downstream from the poly A site of the β-globin gene.[84,91–93] Its deletion markedly decreases β-gene expression in transgenic mice,[94] indicating that this element plays an important role in β-globin gene expression. Another enhancer is located in intron 2 of the β gene.[95,96]

The β-Globin Locus Control Region

This region is described in Chapter 3 of this book. It is located 6–25 kb upstream from the ε-globin gene and contains a series of developmentally stable DNase I hypersensitive sites.[97,98] A large body of data indicates that the activities of the LCR are mostly localized to the core elements of the hypersensitive sites, which are approximately 300 bp long. The regions flanking the hypersensitive site core elements of the LCR are also important for function. The current concept is that the LCR functions as a complex formed by interaction of the transcriptional factors that bind to the individual hypersensitive site elements.

The unique property of the LCR is its activating function, which "opens" the chromatin domain and provides the possibility for gene transcription. In transgenic mice, the LCR is recognized by its capacity to confer integration site- or position-independent expression of a linked gene.[99,100] Position effects are always overcome by the LCR in a dominant manner.[101,100] Experiments in knockout mice have been recently interpreted to indicate that the LCR is not required for opening the chromatin domain.[102–104] In ε-γ-δ-β thalassemia mutants due to LCR deletions,[105–109] there is total inactivation of the β-locus chromatin and total absence of transcription of the β-cluster genes in *cis*. However, when the LCR is deleted from the endogenous murine locus by homologous recombination, the globin genes continue to show some low levels of expression, and the chromatin of the β locus remains in the open configuration.[102,104,110] Why the phenotypes of the LCR deletions in humans and the LCR knockouts in mice differ is still unknown.[111,112] Among the possible reasons are differences in the composition and organization of the murine and the human LCRs. Alternatively, the total silencing of the β locus in the human LCR deletions might not be due to the deletion of the LCR per se, but the juxtaposition to the locus of heterochromatic regions, located upstream, that silence the genes of the locus.

The DNase I hypersensitive sites of the LCR have developmental specificity.[113] This was unequivocally shown in the studies of transgenic mice carrying β locus yeast artificial chromosomes (YAC mice). Deletion of the core element of HS3 in the context of a β locus YAC results in total absence of ε-globin gene expression in day-9 embryonic cells,[114] suggesting that sequences of the core element of HS3 are necessary for activation of ε-globin gene transcription. γ-Gene expression in embryonic cells is normal, suggesting that a hypersensitive site other than HS3 interacts with the γ promoter in embryonic cells. However, γ-globin gene expression, is totally absent in fetal liver cells, indicating that the core of HS3 is necessary for γ-gene transcription in the fetal stage of definitive erythropoiesis. These results are also compatible with the possibility that the LCR changes conformation during the course of development.[114]

Molecular Control of Switching

Major insights on the molecular control of switching have been obtained through studies of transgenic mice. As mentioned earlier, in the mouse there is only one switch during development – the switch from embryonic to definitive globin gene expression, which coincides with the transition from yolk sac to definitive, fetal liver, erythropoiesis. The murine εy and βh1 genes are expressed exclusively in the yolk sac and they are silenced in the fetal liver where βmajor- and βminor-globin gene expression occurs. The εy gene is homologous to human ε whereas the βh1 is homologous to human γ. Studies of transgenic mice carrying human γ- or β-globin transgenes, performed before the discovery of the LCR, have shown that the human γ and β transgenes are regulated similarly to their murine homologous genes (references in Stamatoyannopoulos and Grosveld[20]). Thus, the γ genes, like the murine βh1, are expressed only in the yolk sac cells whereas the β genes are expressed only in the definitive cells, indicating that all the elements required for correct developmental regulation are included in the sequences of the genes or their flanking sequences.

With the discovery of the LCR, questions arose about how the globin genes are developmentally regulated in the presence of this powerful regulatory element. Studies in transgenic mice revealed that two mechanisms, gene silencing and gene competition, control hemoglobin switching.

Globin Gene Silencing

The studies of *cis* elements and *trans* factors involved in turning off the embryonic globin gene provide a good example of the complexity of the control of gene silencing during development. ε-Globin gene expression is totally restricted in the embryonic yolk sac cells and its developmental control is autonomous, that is, all the sequences required for silencing of the ε gene in definitive erythropoietic cells are contained in the sequences flanking the gene.[115,116] Regulatory sequences mediating this autonomous silencing have been mapped to the distal and proximal ε-gene promoter.[40,43,44,117,118]

Controversy has been generated with the studies of a putative negative regulatory element initially identified in the upstream gene promoter by using transient transfection assays.[119] This element is located between −182 and

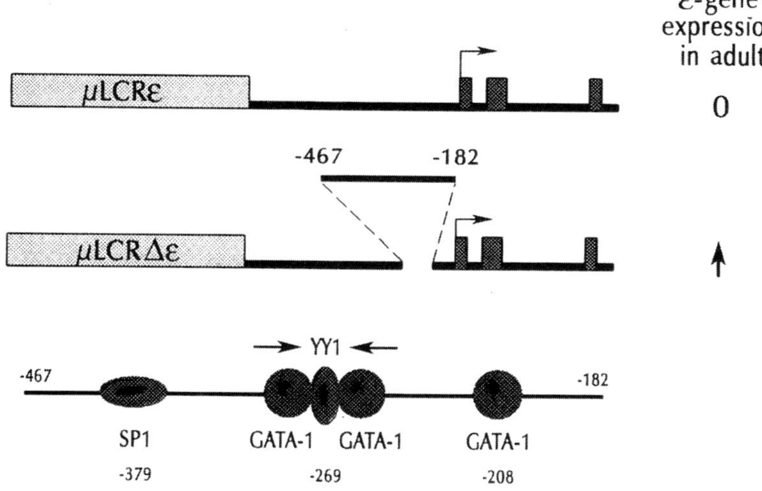

Figure 5.2. Globin gene silencing. The middle diagram shows the sequence of the upstream gene promoter, which when deleted results in continuation of γ-gene expression in the adult. The lower diagram shows the binding sites for transcriptional factors contained in this silencer.

−467 bp from the initiation site and contains three binding motifs: a GATA site at −208, a YY1 site at −269, and a CACC motif at −379[43,120] (Fig. 5.2). Deletion of the element resulted in ε gene expression in the red cells of adult transgenic mice carrying an ε gene with an upstream micro LCR.[121] Disruption of either the −208 GATA-1 or the −269 YY1 binding site also resulted in ε-gene expression in adult transgenic mice.[43] Presumably, several transcriptional factors interact to form the silencing complex and disruption of any of these factors results in inhibition of silencing. ε-Gene silencing, therefore, is probably combinatorial (Fig. 5.3). The fact that GATA-1 binding at −208 results in ε-gene suppression was subsequently shown using a binary transgenic mouse system: Overexpression of GATA-1 in transgenic mice carrying a human β locus YAC resulted in a specific decrease of human ε-globin expression.[122] The function of this ε-gene silencer was, however, questioned by studies in transgenic mice containing an intact human β-globin locus. Thus, deletion of a portion (125 bp) of the sequence of the ε silencer in a βYAC construct did not lead to expression of the ε gene in definitive erythropoietic cells.[94] In contrast, the deletion resulted in a significant decrease of ε-gene expression in the yolk sac, suggesting that the deleted sequence could harbor a cryptic activity that is required for stimulation of ε-globin RNA synthesis. Transgenic mice carrying a βYAC construct harboring a slightly larger (224 bp vs. 125 bp) deletion of the silencer[123] had no abnormalities in ε-gene expression in either embryonic or in definitive erythropoietic cells, and there was no continuation of ε-gene expression in fetal or adult erythroid cells. The function of this sequence of the ε-gene promoter is thus still unclear. As mentioned earlier, COUP-TF and/or DRED binding in the DR repeats near the CAAT box has suppressive effects and there is evidence that sequences having silencing properties are located further upstream in the ε-gene promoter.

The mechanism that turns off the γ-globin gene has been more difficult to determine. Initially, the silencing of the γ gene was attributed solely to gene competition.[124,125] Other experiments in transgenic mice suggested that the gene turns off solely through an autonomous silencing mechanism.[126] It seems that autonomous silencing is the main mechanism whereby the γ genes are turned off during development. Evidence was provided by two types of experiments. First, in transgenic mice carrying βYAC constructs from which the β gene has been deleted,[127] the γ genes turn off after birth, even though the β genes are absent, thus arguing against the hypothesis that γ-gene silencing is solely the result of competition for *trans* factors and/or the LCR by the β gene. Second, when the β-globin gene is placed close to the LCR, it is expressed throughout development.[128,129] When the γ gene is placed in the same position, it is expressed in the embryonic and the early fetal liver cells, but it is turned off postnatally, as expected if γ-gene silencing is autonomous.[129] However, the story is not that simple: other transgenic studies[130] as well as the increase in γ-globin gene expression in patients with β thalassemia due to β-gene promoter deletions,[20] suggest that competition by the β-gene promoter, in addition to autonomous silencing, contributes to the turning off of the γ-globin gene.

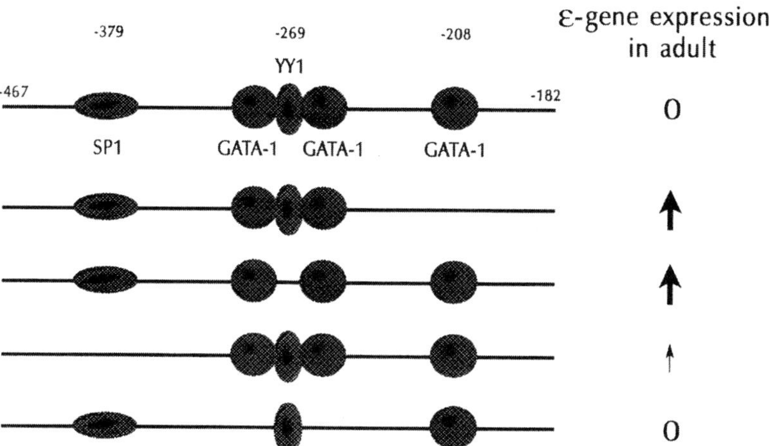

Figure 5.3. Evidence that the silencing of the ε gene is combinatorial. Mutations that affect binding of GATA-1 at −208 or YY1 at −269 or a CACCC binding protein at −379 result in continuation of ε-globin gene expression in the adult. Other transcriptional factors involved in silencing include COUP-TF that binds to the DR-1 element near the gene's CAAT box.

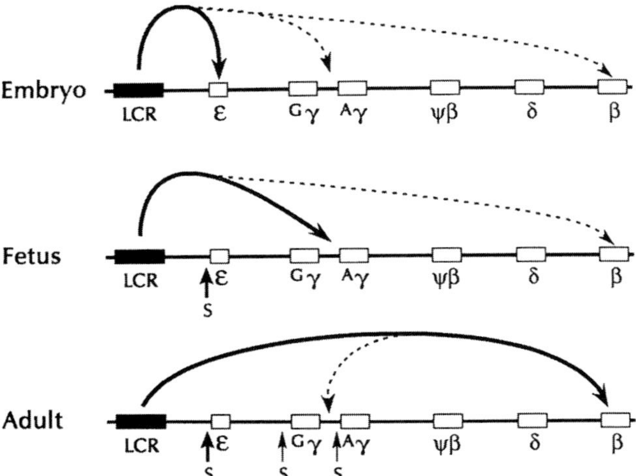

Figure 5.4. Model of the competitive control of hemoglobin switching. "S" indicates the activity of a silencer element.

Gene Competition

The initial observation that led to the formulation of the competition model was made in transgenic mice carrying either the γ- or the β-globin gene or both genes linked to the LCR. When the genes were alone, developmental control was lost. When the genes were linked together, developmental control was restored. Such findings led to the proposal that the γ-globin gene is regulated through competition with the β-globin gene and vice versa.[124,125] The hypothesis is that in the embryonic stage, the LCR interacts with the ε-globin gene; the downstream genes are being turned off competitively. In the fetus, the ε gene is silenced, and the LCR interacts with the $^{G}\gamma$ and $^{A}\gamma$ genes. In the adult, the γ genes are silenced, and the LCR now interacts with the β-globin gene, the last gene of the locus (Fig. 5.4).

Two conditions influence the probability of interaction of a gene with the LCR: the prevailing transcriptional environment and the distance from the LCR. Among the *trans*-acting factors that are likely to facilitate the interaction of the LCR with the γ- or β-gene promoters is EKLF and perhaps other factors of the KLF/SP1 family. In addition to the *trans*-acting factors, gene order and proximity to the LCR are important in determining a gene's competitive advantage for interaction with the LCR.[131,132] The closer the gene, the higher is the advantage. Its placement at the 3′ end of the locus might explain why the β gene is totally shut off in embryonic cells when it is located in its normal chromosomal position, whereas it is always expressed in the embryo if it is placed next to the LCR.

In situ hybridization methods have allowed the visualization of the interaction of globin genes with the LCR.[100,133] This element interacts with only one promoter of the locus at a given time, and switching essentially represents a change in frequency of interaction of the LCR with either the γ- or the β-gene promoter. Results from newly developed technologies, such as 3C[134] and RNA trap assays, demonstrate that actively transcribed globin genes are located in proximity to the LCR, suggesting that a chromatin loop is formed when a globin gene is enhanced by the LCR.[135–137] The formation of the loop between the LCR and the β-globin gene requires erythroid-specific *trans*-acting factors EKLF, GATA-1, and its cofactor FOG-1, but not NF-E2.[138–140] Binding of these factors to their cognate *cis* elements is not sufficient for loop formation,[140] and binding of *trans*-acting factors represents an independent event that occurs prior to loop formation.[139] Thus, although EKLF, GATA-1, and FOG are indispensable for loop formation, they use a complex pathway to regulate the process.

Control of HbF in the Adult

One of the most interesting characteristics of human γ- to β-switching is its leakiness and the continuation of synthesis of small amounts of HbF in the adult. This has been known since the time the alkali denaturation method was used for HbF quantitation, but its significance was only realized when immunofluorescent methods were used to stain peripheral blood smears. These methods were first applied in the mid-1960s and they were rediscovered in the 1970s. It was then realized that this residual γ-globin expression is restricted to a minority of cells, the F cells. The question was then raised about how these F cells are formed. Initially, clonal hypotheses (reviewed earlier in this chapter) were proposed to explain the origin of F cells: They could be the progeny of fetal stem cell clones. Major insights into the understanding of the control of HbF in the adult were obtained through analyses of HbF expression in erythroid cultures and through observations in patients with activated erythropoiesis.

The first clue on mechanisms came from studies in erythroid cultures, which showed that high levels of HbF are characteristic of colonies produced by erythroid burst-forming units (BFU-E) of adult origin.[13,141] In erythroid cells of these colonies, HbF was not uniformly distributed but the colonies were usually composed of erythroblasts that contained both HbF and HbA, and erythroblasts that contained only HbA. These observations were interpreted to indicate that the production of F cells was related to the phenomenon of erythroid cell differentiation.[13]

The second clue on mechanisms came from studies showing that rapid regeneration of the erythroid marrow induces F-cell production (reviewed in Stamatoyannopoulos et al.[142]). For example, increased F-cell production is characteristic of bone marrow regeneration following bone marrow transplantation,[10] or following recovery from the aplastic phase of erythroblastopenia of childhood,[143] or following chemotherapeutic ablation of the bone marrow,[144] and following acute hemolysis.[143] Experimental acute bleeding in baboons activated γ-globin production.[145,146] Acute phlebotomy and decrease of hematocrit in humans stimulated F-cell production.[143] Proof that acute erythropoietic stress can induce HbF production was obtained when baboons were treated with high doses of recombinant erythropoietin: These animals responded with striking elevation of F-cell production.[147,148]

It should be mentioned that in contrast to the consistent activation of HbF in acute erythropoietic expansion, with the exception of hemoglobinopathies and congenital hypoplastic anemias, there is no elevation of HbF in most patients with chronic anemias.[149] Administration of low doses of erythropoietin to baboons increases the hematocrit but fails to induce HbF.[147] Following acute bleeding, there is a surge of F-reticulocyte production, but when chronic anemia is instituted, the number of F-reticulocytes falls.[142,146] The difference in the rates of F-cell formation between acute and chronic erythropoietic stress provided strong evidence that the kinetics of erythroid regeneration determine whether a cell will become an F cell or an A cell.

The mechanism proposed to explain the induction of HbF in response to erythropoietic stress assumes that early progenitors encode a program allowing expression of fetal globin genes, but this program is changed to one allowing only adult globin expression during the downstream differentiation of erythroid progenitor cells (Fig. 5.5).[13,150] Presumably, the earlier progenitor cells contain a combination of *trans*-acting factors that favors γ-globin gene expression, whereas the late progenitors have a combination of *trans*-acting factors that favors β-globin gene expression. F cells are produced when earlier progenitors become committed to terminal differentiation prematurely.[150] In acute erythropoietic stress, the accelerated erythropoiesis increases the chance of premature commitment of early progenitors, resulting in increased production of F cells. Experimental evidence in support of this hypothesis was obtained by daily measurements of erythroid progenitor pools in baboons treated with high doses of recombinant erythropoietin.[148] The major effect of erythropoietin in vivo is an acute expansion of colony-forming unit (CFU-E) and a mobilization of BFU-E. Umemura et al.[148] showed that following the administration of high doses of erythropoietin, an increase in F-programmed CFU-E accounts for almost all of the expansion of CFU-E. The increase in these F-programmed CFU-E is followed by a striking increase in F-positive early erythroblasts, which precedes the appearance of F reticulocytes in the circulation.[148]

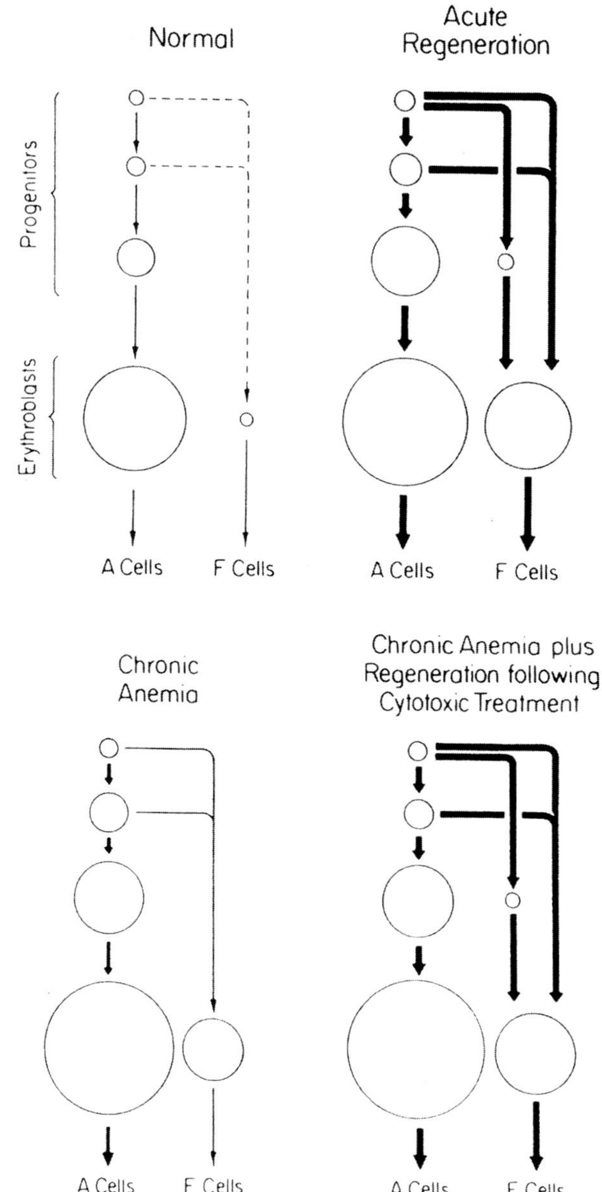

Figure 5.5. Model of regulation of fetal hemoglobin and F-cell production in the adult following acute erythroid regeneration or treatment with cytotoxic drugs such as hydroxyurea.

THE CONCEPTUAL BASIS OF PHARMACOLOGICAL INDUCTION OF FETAL HEMOGLOBIN SYNTHESIS

The pharmacological induction of HbF synthesis was a direct consequence of the studies on the cellular control of HbF production in the adult. Cytotoxic drugs were initially used to test, in primates, whether acute regeneration will induce HbF synthesis in the adult. The use of cytotoxic drugs in patients with sickle cell disease or with β thalassemia followed.

The origin of the use of cytotoxic drugs for HbF induction can be traced to the debate about the mechanism whereby 5-azacytidine stimulates HbF production. To test the hypothesis that DNA demethylation can activate γ-globin gene expression, DeSimone et al.[151] treated anemic juvenile baboons with escalating doses of 5-azacytidine; a striking augmentation of HbF production was observed. Induction of HbF synthesis was subsequently demonstrated in β thalassemia patients treated with 5-azacytidine.[152] At this stage, a debate about the mechanism of this phenomenon started. 5-azacytidine, a cytotoxic compound, is expected to kill the most actively cycling erythroid cells. The resulting decrease in late erythroid progenitor cells could trigger rapid erythroid regeneration and induce F-cell formation. Therefore, it was argued that the induction of HbF was not simply due to the demethylating effect of 5-azacytidine but to its cytotoxicity that triggers secondary erythroid regeneration. Measurements of erythroid progenitor cell pools in baboons treated with 5-azacytidine supported this hypothesis.[153]

To test whether cytoreduction and the ensuing secondary erythroid regeneration were the cause of HbF induction by 5-azacytidine, Papayannopoulou et al.[154] asked whether other cytotoxic compounds producing erythroid regeneration but not DNA demethylation would also induce F-cell formation. Baboons were treated with cytotoxic doses of ara-C and responded with striking elevations of F reticulocytes, with kinetics indistinguishable from those elicited by 5-azacytidine.[154] Induction of γ-globin gene expression was also observed in monkeys or baboons treated with hydroxyurea.[154,155] Vinblastine, a cell cycle–specific agent that arrests cells in mitosis, also produces secondary erythroid regeneration and stimulates HbF synthesis in baboons.[156] Following these studies, hydroxyurea was used for induction of HbF production in humans (see Chapter 30). Although other hypotheses for the mechanisms of action of hydroxyurea have been proposed, its activation of HbF synthesis through stimulation of erythroid regeneration is broadly accepted, although the initial rational for using cytotoxic drugs for stimulation of HbF production has been forgotten.[157–159]

Short-Chain Fatty Acids

The seminal observation that eventually led to the discovery that short-chain fatty acids induce the synthesis of HbF was the finding by Perrine et al.[160] that the γ- to β-switch is delayed in infants of diabetic mothers. Perrine and coworkers hypothesized that a metabolite in the blood of diabetic mothers was responsible for this finding and, using experiments in clonal erythroid cell cultures, they showed that γ-aminobutyric acid, which is elevated in the blood of diabetic mothers, is an inducer of HbF production.[161] Subsequent studies showed that butyrate stimulated γ-globin chain production in adult baboons,[162] and it induced γ-globin gene expression in erythroid progenitors of adult animals or of patients with sickle cell anemia.[162,163] Several other short-chain fatty acids were found to increase HbF in adult BFU-E cultures and in baboons.[164,165] Derivatives of short-chain fatty acids such as phenylbutyrate[166] and valproic acid[165,167] induce HbF production in vivo. Increased levels of HbF were also recorded in patients with metabolic disorders resulting in accumulation of short-chain fatty acids.[168,169] Butyrate and various short chain fatty acid derivatives have been used in a number of clinical trials (see Chapter 30).

The induction of HbF production by short-chain fatty acids is very interesting from the practical and biological points of view. The practical significance lies in the fact that there are very large numbers of short-chain fatty acid derivatives that are potential inducers of HbF synthesis.[170,171] Therefore, there are ample opportunities for discovering HbF inducers that can be administered orally and are more potent than butyrate.

The prevailing hypothesis is that short-chain fatty acids activate γ-globin gene expression through inhibition of histone deacetylases. Histone acetyltransferases catalyze histone acetylation through the transfer of acetyl groups to lysine residues of the core histones.[172–174] It is believed that histone acetylation leads to gene activation by weakening the binding of histones to nucleosomal DNA, which makes the DNA subsequently accessible to transcription factors.[175] Conversely, histone deacetylases are believed to largely mediate gene repression, as deacetylation of histones would allow the histone to bind more tightly to the nucleosomal DNA and displace transcription factors. Thus, histone deacetylase inhibitors may induce γ-globin gene activity by increasing the accessibility of chromatin around the γ-globin gene promoter to activating transcription factors. The exact mechanism whereby the short-chain fatty acids affect gene transcription remains unknown. Studies in transgenic mice are compatible with the assumption that the stimulation of HbF synthesis reflects inhibition of silencing rather than activation of transcription,[176] but the evidence is indirect. It is obvious that the delineation of the mechanisms of stimulation of HbF synthesis by short-chain fatty acids will provide new insights into the control of silencing or activation of γ-globin gene expression.

Role of the BCL11A Locus

Recent studies have identified the BCL11A locus as a major locus regulating the levels of fetal hemoglobin in β-thalassemia or sickle cell disease. A SNP located in the second intron of the BCL11A gene was found to be correlated with HbF levels in patients with β-thalassemia suggesting that this genetic polymorphism is an important indicator of disease severity.[177,178] The BCL11A gene encodes three isoforms of a multi-zinc finger transcription factor and is developmentally regulated such that only the two largest isoforms (X and XL) are exclusively expressed during adult erythropoiesis.[179] BCL11A binds to GG-rich motifs and has been shown to function as a transcription repressor.[180,181] BCL11A knockdown experiments in adult erythroid progenitor cells resulted in a dramatic increase in F-cells numbers and HbF levels suggesting that BCL11A is involved in γ-globin gene silencing.[179] Chromatin immunoprecipitation experiments showed that BCL11A directly binds to several locations of the β-globin locus in adult erythroid progenitor cells.[179] Electromobility shift assays using extracts from BCL11A over expressing K562 cells showed BCL11A binding to a GGCCGG motif at position −56 to −51 of the $^{G}\gamma$ gene promoter.[182] Collectively the studies of patients and the biochemical investigations strongly suggest that BCL11A acts as a stage specific repressor of γ-globin expression. Thus, BCL11A has emerged as an attractive target for reactivation of HbF in patients with β-thalassemia or sickle cell disease.

REFERENCES

1. Huehns ER, Dance N, Beaven GH, Keil JV, Hecht F, Motulsky AG. Human embryonic haemoglobins. *Nature.* 1964;201:1095–1097.
2. Hecht F, Motulsky AG, Lemire RJ, Shepard TE. Predominance of hemoglobin Gower 1 in early human embryonic development. *Science.* 1966;152:91–92.
3. Gale RE, Clegg JB, Huehns ER. Human embryonic haemoglobins Gower 1 and Gower 2. *Nature.* 1979;280:162–164.
4. Papayannopoulou T, Shepard TH, Stamatoyannopoulos G. Studies of hemoglobin expression in erythroid cells of early human fetuses using antiγ- and anti-β-globin chain fluorescent antibodies. *Prog Clin Biol Res.* 1983;134:421–430.
5. Boyer SH, Belding TK, Margolet L, Noyes AN. Fetal hemoglobin restriction to a few erythrocytes (F cells) in normal human adults. *Science.* 1975;188:361–363.
6. Wood WG, Stamatoyannopoulos G, Lim G, Nute PE. F-cells in the adult: normal values and levels in individuals with hereditary and acquired elevations of Hb F. *Blood.* 1975;46:671–682.
7. Ingram VM. Embryonic red blood cell formation. *Nature.* 1972;235:338–339.
8. Weatherall DJ, Edwards JA, Donohoe WT. Haemoglobin and red cell enzyme changes in juvenile myeloid leukaemia. *Br Med J.* 1968;1:679–681.
9. Weatherall DJ, Clegg JB, Wood WG. A model for the persistence or reactivation of fetal haemoglobin production. *Lancet.* 1976;2:660–663.
10. Alter BP, Rappeport JM, Huisman TH, Schroeder WA, Nathan DG. Fetal erythropoiesis following bone marrow transplantation. *Blood.* 1976;48:843–853.
11. Alter BP, Jackson BT, Lipton JM, et al. Control of the simian fetal hemoglobin switch at the progenitor cell level. *J Clin Invest.* 1981;67:458–466.
12. Alter BP, Jackson BT, Lipton JM, et al. Three classes of erythroid progenitors that regulate hemoglobin synthesis during ontogeny in the primate. In: Stamatoyannopoulos G, Nienhuis AW, eds. *Hemoglobins in Development and Differentiation.* New York: Alan R. Liss; 1981:331–340.
13. Papayannopoulou T, Brice M, Stamatoyannopoulos G. Hemoglobin F synthesis in vitro: evidence for control at the level of primitive erythroid stem cells. *Proc Natl Acad Sci USA.*1977;74:2923–2927.
14. Chapman BS, Tobin AJ. Distribution of developmentally regulated hemoglobins in embryonic erythroid populations. *Dev Biol.* 1979;69:375–387.
15. Brotherton TW, Chui DH, Gauldie J, Patterson M. Hemoglobin ontogeny during normal mouse fetal development. *Proc Natl Acad Sci USA.* 1979;76:2853–2857.
16. Le Douarin N. Ontogeny of hematopoietic organs studied in avian embryo interspecific chimeras. In: Clarkson B, Marks P, Till J, eds. *Differentiation in Normal and Neoplastic Hemopoietic Cells.* New York: Cold Spring Harbor; 1978:5–31.
17. Beaupain D, Martin C, Dieterlen-Lievre F. Origin and evolution of hemopoietic stem cells in the avian embryo. In: Stamatoyannopoulos G, Nienhuis AW, eds. *Hemoglobins in Development and Differentiation.* New York: Alan R. Liss; 1981: 161–169.
18. Peschle C, Migliaccio AR, Migliaccio G, et al. Embryonic–Fetal Hb switch in humans: studies on erythroid bursts generated by embryonic progenitors from yolk sac and liver. *Proc Natl Acad Sci USA.* 1984;81:2416–2420.
19. Stamatoyannopoulos G, Constantoulakis P, Brice M, Kurachi S, Papayannopoulou T. Coexpression of embryonic, fetal, and adult globins in erythroid cells of human embryos: relevance to the cell-lineage models of globin switching. *Dev Biol.* 1987;123:191–197.
20. Stamatoyannopoulos G, Grosveld F. Hemoglobin switching. In: Stamatoyannopoulos G, Majerus P, Perlmutter R, Varmus H, eds. *The Molecular Basis of Blood Diseases.* 3rd ed. Philadelphia: W.B. Saunders Co.; 2001:135–182.
21. Papayannopoulou T, Brice M, Stamatoyannopoulos G. Analysis of human hemoglobin switching in MEL × human fetal erythroid cell hybrids. *Cell.* 1986;46:469–476.
22. Wintour EM, Smith MB, Bell RJ, McDougall JG, Cauchi MN. The role of fetal adrenal hormones in the switch from fetal to adult globin synthesis in the sheep. *J Endocrinol.* 1985;104:165–170.
23. Zitnik G, Li Q, Stamatoyannopoulos G, Papayannopoulou T. Serum factors can modulate the developmental clock of γ- to β-globin gene switching in somatic cell hybrids. *Mol Cell Biol.* 1993;13:4844–4851.
24. Zitnik G, Peterson K, Stamatoyannopoulos G, Papayannopoulou T. Effects of butyrate and glucocorticoids on γ- to β-globin gene switching in somatic cell hybrids. *Mol Cell Biol.* 1995;15:790–795.
25. Della Torre L, Meroni P. [Studies of fetal blood. I. Fetal and adult hemoglobin levels in normal pregnancy. Relation to fetal maturity]. *Ann Ostet Ginecol Med Perinat.* 1969;91:148–157.
26. Bard H, Makowski EL, Meschia G, Battaglia FC. The relative rates of synthesis of hemoglobins A and F in immature red cells of newborn infants. *Pediatrics.* 1970;45:766–772.
27. Zanjani ED, Lim G, McGlave PB, et al. Adult haematopoietic cells transplanted to sheep fetuses continue to produce adult globins. *Nature.* 1982;295:244–246.
28. Wood WG, Bunch C, Kelly S, Gunn Y, Breckon G. Control of haemoglobin switching by a developmental clock? *Nature.* 1985;313:320–323.
29. Holliday R, Pugh JE. DNA modification mechanisms and gene activity during development. *Science.* 1975;187:226–232.
30. Melis M, Demopulos G, Najfeld V, et al. A chromosome 11-linked determinant controls fetal globin expression and the fetal-to-adult globin switch. *Proc Natl Acad Sci USA.* 1987;84:8105–8109.
31. Stanworth SJ, Roberts NA, Sharpe JA, Sloane-Stanley JA, Wood WG. Established epigenetic modifications determine the expression of developmentally regulated globin genes in somatic cell hybrids. *Mol Cell Biol.* 1995;15:3969–3978.
32. Gong Q, Dean A. Enhancer-dependent transcription of the ε-globin promoter requires promoter-bound GATA-1 and enhancer-bound AP-1/NF-E2. *Mol Cell Biol.* 1993;13: 911–917.
33. Gong QH, Stern J, Dean A. Transcriptional role of a conserved GATA-1 site in the human ε-globin gene promoter. *Mol Cell Biol.* 1991;11:2558–2566.
34. Walters M, Martin DI. Functional erythroid promoters created by interaction of the transcription factor GATA-1 with CACCC and AP-1/NFE-2 elements. *Proc Natl Acad Sci USA.* 1992;89:10444–10448.
35. Filipe A, Li Q, Deveaux S, et al. Regulation of embryonic/fetal globin genes by nuclear hormone receptors: a novel perspective on hemoglobin switching. *EMBO J.* 1999;18:687–697.

36. Yu CY, Motamed K, Chen J, Bailey AD, Shen CK. The CACC box upstream of human embryonic ε globin gene binds Sp1 and is a functional promoter element in vitro and in vivo. *J Biol Chem.* 1991;266:8907–8915.
37. Marin M, Karis A, Visser P, Grosveld F, Philipsen S. Transcription factor Sp1 is essential for early embryonic development but dispensable for cell growth and differentiation. *Cell.* 1997;89:619–628.
38. Asano H, Li XS, Stamatoyannopoulos G. FKLF, a novel Kruppel-like factor that activates human embryonic and fetal β-like globin genes. *Mol Cell Biol.* 1999;19:3571–3579.
39. Asano H, Li XS, Stamatoyannopoulos G. FKLF-2: a novel Kruppel-like transcriptional factor that activates globin and other erythroid lineage genes. *Blood.* 2000;95:3578–3584.
40. Tanimoto K, Liu Q, Grosveld F, Bungert J, Engel JD. Context-dependent EKLF responsiveness defines the developmental specificity of the human ε-globin gene in erythroid cells of YAC transgenic mice. *Genes Dev.* 2000;14:2778–2794.
41. Tanabe O, Katsuoka F, Campbell AD, et al. An embryonic/fetal β-type globin gene repressor contains a nuclear receptor TR2/TR4 heterodimer. *EMBO J.* 2002;21:3434–3442.
42. Tanabe O, McPhee D, Kobayashi S, et al. Embryonic and fetal β-globin gene repression by the orphan nuclear receptors, TR2 and TR4. *EMBO J.* 2007;26:2295–2306.
43. Raich N, Clegg CH, Grofti J, Romeo PH, Stamatoyannopoulos G. GATA1 and YY1 are developmental repressors of the human ε-globin gene. *EMBO J.* 1995;14:801–809.
44. Li J, Noguchi CT, Miller W, Hardison R, Schechter AN. Multiple regulatory elements in the 5′-flanking sequence of the human ε-globin gene. *J Biol Chem.* 1998;273:10202–10209.
45. Trepicchio WL, Dyer MA, Baron MH. Developmental regulation of the human embryonic β-like globin gene is mediated by synergistic interactions among multiple tissue- and stage-specific elements. *Mol Cell Biol.* 1993;13:7457–7468.
46. Yi Z, Cohen-Barak O, Hagiwara N, et al. Sox6 directly silences ε globin expression in definitive erythropoiesis. *PLoS Genet.* 2006;2:e14.
47. Cohen-Barak O, Erickson DT, Badowski MS, et al. Stem cell transplantation demonstrates that Sox6 represses εy globin expression in definitive erythropoiesis of adult mice. *Exp Hematol.* 2007;35:358–367.
48. Gumucio DL, Heilstedt-Williamson H, Gray TA, et al. Phylogenetic footprinting reveals a nuclear protein which binds to silencer sequences in the human γ and ε globin genes. *Mol Cell Biol.* 1992;12:4919–4929
49. Jane SM, Ney PA, Vanin EF, Gumucio DL, Nienhuis AW. Identification of a stage selector element in the human γ-globin gene promoter that fosters preferential interaction with the 5′ HS2 enhancer when in competition with the β-promoter. *EMBO J.* 1992;11:2961–2969.
50. Jane SM, Gumucio DL, Ney PA, Cunningham JM, Nienhuis AW. Methylation-enhanced binding of Sp1 to the stage selector element of the human γ-globin gene promoter may regulate development specificity of expression. *Mol Cell Biol.* 1993;13:3272–3281.
51. Jane SM, Nienhuis AW, Cunningham JM. Hemoglobin switching in man and chicken is mediated by a heteromeric complex between the ubiquitous transcription factor CP2 and a developmentally specific protein. *EMBO J.* 1995;14:97–105.
52. Zhou WL, Clouston X, Wang L, Cerruti J, Cunningham JM, Jane SM. Isolation and characteriztion of human NF-E4, the tissue restricted component of the stage selector protein complex. *Blood.* 1999;94(Suppl 1):614a.
53. Gumucio DL, Rood KL, Gray TA, Riordan MF, Sartor CI, Collins FS. Nuclear proteins that bind the human γ-globin gene promoter: alterations in binding produced by point mutations associated with hereditary persistence of fetal hemoglobin. *Mol Cell Biol.* 1988;8:5310–5322.
54. Mantovani R, Malgaretti N, Nicolis S, Ronchi A, Giglioni B, Ottolenghi S. The effects of HPFH mutations in the human γ-globin promoter on binding of ubiquitous and erythroid specific nuclear factors. *Nucl Acids Res.* 1988;16:7783–7797.
55. Mantovani R, Superti-Furga G, Gilman J, Ottolenghi S. The deletion of the distal CCAAT box region of the A γ-globin gene in black HPFH abolishes the binding of the erythroid specific protein NFE3 and of the CCAAT displacement protein. *Nucl Acids Res.* 1989;17:6681–6691.
56. Fucharoen S, Shimizu K, Fukumaki Y. A novel C-T transition within the distal CCAAT motif of the G γ-globin gene in the Japanese HPFH: implication of factor binding in elevated fetal globin expression. *Nucl Acids Res.* 1990;18:5245–5253.
57. McDonagh K, Nienhuis AW. Induction of the human γ-globin gene promoter in K562 cells by sodium butyrate: Reversal of repression by CCAAT displacement protein. *Blood.* 1991;78:255a.
58. Berry M, Grosveld F, Dillon N. A single point mutation is the cause of the Greek form of hereditary persistence of fetal haemoglobin. *Nature.* 1992;358:499–502.
59. Skalnik DG, Strauss EC, Orkin SH. CCAAT displacement protein as a repressor of the myelomonocytic-specific gp91-phox gene promoter. *J Biol Chem.* 1991;266:16736–16744.
60. Ronchi AE, Bottardi S, Mazzucchelli C, Ottolenghi S, Santoro C. Differential binding of the NFE3 and CP1/NFY transcription factors to the human γ- and ε-globin CCAAT boxes. *J Biol Chem.* 1995;270:21934–21941.
61. Ronchi A, Berry M, Raguz S, et al. Role of the duplicated CCAAT box region in γ-globin gene regulation and hereditary persistence of fetal haemoglobin. *EMBO J.* 1996;15:143–149.
62. Li Q, Fang X, Olave I, et al. Transcriptional potential of the γ-globin gene is dependent on the CACCC box in a developmental stage-specific manner. *Nucl Acids Res.* 2006;34:3909–3916.
63. McDonagh KT, Lin HJ, Lowrey CH, Bodine DM, Nienhuis AW. The upstream region of the human γ-globin gene promoter. Identification and functional analysis of nuclear protein binding sites. *J Biol Chem.* 1991;266:11965–11974.
64. Magis W, Martin DI. HMG-I binds to GATA motifs: implications for an HPFH syndrome. *Biochem Biophys Res Commun.* 1995;214:927–933.
65. Ulrich MJ, Gray WJ, Ley TJ. An intramolecular DNA triplex is disrupted by point mutations associated with hereditary persistence of fetal hemoglobin. *J Biol Chem.* 1992;267:18649–18658.
66. Bacolla A, Ulrich MJ, Larson JE, Ley TJ, Wells RD. An intramolecular triplex in the human γ-globin 5′-flanking region is altered by point mutations associated with hereditary persistence of fetal hemoglobin. *J Biol Chem.* 1995;270:24556–24563.

67. Ponce E, Lloyd JA, Pierani A, Roeder RG, Lingrel JB. Transcription factor OTF-1 interacts with two distinct DNA elements in the A γ-globin gene promoter. *Biochemistry.* 1991;30:2961–2967.
68. Stamatoyannopoulos G, Josephson B, Zhang JW, Li Q. Developmental regulation of human γ-globin genes in transgenic mice. *Mol Cell Biol.* 1993;13:7636–7644.
69. Pace BS, Li Q, Stamatoyannopoulos G. In vivo search for butyrate responsive sequences using transgenic mice carrying A γ gene promoter mutants. *Blood.* 1996;88:1079–1083.
70. Luo HY, Mang D, Patrinos GP, et al. A mutation in a GATA-1 binding site 5' to the Gγ-globin gene (nt -567, T>G) may be associated with increased levels of fetal hemoglobin. *Blood.* 2004;104:500.
71. Peterson KR, Costa FC, Harju-Baker S. Silencing of γ-globin gene expression during adult definitive erythropoiesis is mediated by a GATA-1 repressor complex. *Blood.* 2007;110:271.
72. Ahringer J. NuRD and SIN3 histone deacetylase complexes in development. *Trends Genet.* 2000;16:351–356.
73. Bowen NJ, Fujita N, Kajita M, Wade PA. Mi-2/NuRD: multiple complexes for many purposes. *Biochim Biophys Acta.* 2004;1677:52–57.
74. Le Guezennec X, Vermeulen M, Brinkman AB, et al. MBD2/NuRD and MBD3/NuRD, two distinct complexes with different biochemical and functional properties. *Mol Cell Biol.* 2006;26:843–851.
75. Bodine DM, Ley TJ. An enhancer element lies 3′ to the human A γ globin gene. *EMBO J.* 1987;6:2997–3004.
76. Purucker M, Bodine D, Lin H, McDonagh K, Nienhuis AW. Structure and function of the enhancer 3′ to the human A γ globin gene. *Nucl Acids Res.* 1990;18:7407–7415.
77. Dickinson LA, Joh T, Kohwi Y, Kohwi-Shigematsu T. A tissue-specific MAR/SAR DNA-binding protein with unusual binding site recognition. *Cell.* 1992;70:631–645.
78. Liu Q, Tanimoto K, Bungert J, Engel JD. The A γ-globin 3′ element provides no unique function(s) for human β-globin locus gene regulation. *Proc Natl Acad Sci USA.* 1998;95:9944–9949.
79. Li Q, Stamatoyannopoulos JA. Position independence and proper developmental control of γ-globin gene expression require both a 5′ locus control region and a downstream sequence element. *Mol Cell Biol.* 1994;14:6087–6096.
80. Stamatoyannopoulos JA, Clegg CH, Li Q. Sheltering of γ-globin expression from position effects requires both an upstream locus control region and a regulatory element 3' to the A g-globin gene. *Mol Cell Biol.* 1997;17:240–247.
81. Duan ZJ, Fang X, Rohde A, Han H, Stamatoyannopoulos G, Li Q. Developmental specificity of recruitment of TBP to the TATA box of the human γ-globin gene. *Proc Natl Acad Sci USA.* 2002;99:5509–5514.
82. Fang X, Han H, Stamatoyannopoulos G, Li Q. Developmentally specific role of the CCAAT box in regulation of human γ-globin gene expression. *J Biol Chem.* 2004;279:5444–5449.
83. Li Q, Han H, Ye X, Stafford M, Barkess G, Stamatoyannopoulos G. Transcriptional potentials of the β-like globin genes at different developmental stages in transgenic mice and hemoglobin switching. *Blood Cells Mol Dis.* 2004;33:318–325.
84. Antoniou M, deBoer E, Habets G, Grosveld F. The human β-globin gene contains multiple regulatory regions: identification of one promoter and two downstream enhancers. *EMBO J.* 1988;7:377–384.
85. deBoer E, Antoniou M, Mignotte V, Wall L, Grosveld F. The human β-globin promoter; nuclear protein factors and erythroid specific induction of transcription. *EMBO J.* 1988;7:4203–4212.
86. Wall L, Destroismaisons N, Delvoye N, Guy LG. CAAT/enhancer-binding proteins are involved in β-globin gene expression and are differentially expressed in murine erythroleukemia and K562 cells. *J Biol Chem.* 1996;271:16477–16484.
87. Hartzog GA, Myers RM. Discrimination among potential activators of the β-globin CACCC element by correlation of binding and transcriptional properties. *Mol Cell Biol.* 1993;13:44–56.
88. Miller IJ, Bieker JJ. A novel, erythroid cell-specific murine transcription factor that binds to the CACCC element and is related to the Kruppel family of nuclear proteins. *Mol Cell Biol.* 1993;13:2776–2786.
89. Feng WC, Southwood CM, Bieker JJ. Analyses of β-thalassemia mutant DNA interactions with erythroid Kruppel-like factor (EKLF), an erythroid cell-specific transcription factor. *J Biol Chem.* 1994;269:1493–1500.
90. Donze D, Townes TM, Bieker JJ. Role of erythroid Kruppel-like factor in human γ- to β-globin gene switching. *J Biol Chem.* 1995;270:1955–1959.
91. Behringer RR, Hammer RE, Brinster RL, Palmiter RD, Townes TM. Two 3′ sequences direct adult erythroid-specific expression of human β-globin genes in transgenic mice. *Proc Natl Acad Sci USA.* 1987;84:7056–7060.
92. Kollias G, Hurst J, deBoer E, Grosveld F. The human β-globin gene contains a downstream developmental specific enhancer. *Nucl Acids Res.* 1987;15:5739–5747.
93. Trudel M, Costantini F. A 3′ enhancer contributes to the stage-specific expression of the human β-globin gene. *Genes Dev.* 1987;1:954–961.
94. Liu Q, Bungert J, Engel JD. Mutation of gene-proximal regulatory elements disrupts human ε-, γ-, and β-globin expression in yeast artificial chromosome transgenic mice. *Proc Natl Acad Sci USA.* 1997;94:169–174.
95. Rubin JE, Pasceri P, Wu X, Leboulch P, Ellis J. Locus control region activity by 5'HS3 requires a functional interaction with β-globin gene regulatory elements: expression of novel β/γ-globin hybrid transgenes. *Blood.* 2000;95:3242–3249.
96. Bharadwaj RR, Trainor CD, Pasceri P, Ellis J. LCR-regulated transgene expression levels depend on the Oct-1 site in the AT-rich region of β-globin intron-2. *Blood.* 2003;101:1603–1610.
97. Tuan D, Solomon W, Li Q, London IM. The "β-like-globin" gene domain in human erythroid cells. *Proc Natl Acad Sci USA.* 1985;82:6384–6388.
98. Forrester WC, Thompson C, Elder JT, Groudine M. A developmentally stable chromatin structure in the human β-globin gene cluster. *Proc Natl Acad Sci USA.* 1986;83:1359–1363.
99. Grosveld F, van Assendelft GB, Greaves DR, Kollias G. Position-independent, high-level expression of the human β-globin gene in transgenic mice. *Cell.* 1987;51:975–985.
100. Fraser P, Grosveld F. Locus control regions, chromatin activation and transcription. *Curr Opin Cell Biol.* 1998;10:361–365.

101. Milot E, Strouboulis J, Trimborn T, et al. Heterochromatin effects on the frequency and duration of LCR-mediated gene transcription. *Cell.* 1996;87:105–114.
102. Epner E, Reik A, Cimbora D, et al. The β-globin LCR is not necessary for an open chromatin structure or developmentally regulated transcription of the native mouse β-globin locus. *Mol Cell.* 1998;2:447–455.
103. Reik A, Telling A, Zitnik G, Cimbora D, Epner E, Groudine M. The locus control region is necessary for gene expression in the human β-globin locus but not the maintenance of an open chromatin structure in erythroid cells. *Mol Cell Biol.* 1998;18:5992–6000.
104. Bender MA, Bulger M, Close J, Groudine M. β-globin gene switching and DNase I sensitivity of the endogenous β-globin locus in mice do not require the locus control region. *Mol Cell.* 2000;5:387–393.
105. Van Der Ploeg LH, Konings A, Oort M, Roos D, Bernini L, Flavell RA. γ-β-Thalassaemia studies showing that deletion of the γ- and δ-genes influences β-globin gene expression in man. *Nature.* 1980;283:637–642.
106. Vanin EF, Henthorn PS, Kioussis D, Grosveld F, Smithies O. Unexpected relationships between four large deletions in the human β-globin gene cluster. *Cell.* 1983;35:701–709.
107. Curtin P, Pirastu M, Kan YW, Gobert-Jones JA, Stephens AD, Lehmann H. A distant gene deletion affects β-globin gene function in an atypical γ δ β-thalassemia. *J Clin Invest.* 1985;76:1554–1558.
108. Driscoll MC, Dobkin CS, Alter BP. γ δ β-thalassemia due to a de novo mutation deleting the 5′ β-globin gene activation-region hypersensitive sites. *Proc Natl Acad Sci USA.* 1989; 86:7470–7474.
109. Forrester WC, Epner E, Driscoll MC, et al. A deletion of the human β-globin locus activation region causes a major alteration in chromatin structure and replication across the entire β-globin locus. *Genes Dev.* 1990;4:1637–1649.
110. Bender MA, Byron R, Ragoczy T, Telling A, Bulger M, Groudine M. Flanking HS-62.5 and 3′ HS1, and regions upstream of the LCR, are not required for β-globin transcription. *Blood.* 2006;108:1395–1401.
111. Higgs DR. Do LCRs open chromatin domains? *Cell.* 1998; 95:299–302.
112. Grosveld F. Activation by locus control regions? *Curr Opin Genet Dev.* 1999;9:152–157.
113. Fraser P, Pruzina S, Antoniou M, Grosveld F. Each hypersensitive site of the human β-globin locus control region confers a different developmental pattern of expression on the globin genes. *Genes Dev.* 1993;7:106–113.
114. Navas PA, Peterson KR, Li Q, et al. Developmental specificity of the interaction between the locus control region and embryonic or fetal globin genes in transgenic mice with an HS3 core deletion. *Mol Cell Biol.* 1998;18:4188–4196.
115. Raich N, Enver T, Nakamoto B, Josephson B, Papayannopoulou T, Stamatoyannopoulos G. Autonomous developmental control of human embryonic globin gene switching in transgenic mice. *Science.* 1990;250:1147–1149.
116. Shih DM, Wall RJ, Shapiro SG. Developmentally regulated and erythroid-specific expression of the human embryonic β-globin gene in transgenic mice. *Nucl Acids Res.* 1990;18:5465–5472.
117. Wada-Kiyama Y, Peters B, Noguchi CT. The ε-globin gene silencer. Characterization by in vitro transcription. *J Biol Chem.* 1992;267:11532–11538.
118. Li Q, Blau CA, Clegg CH, Rohde A, Stamatoyannopoulos G Multiple ε-promoter elements participate in the developmental control of ε-globin genes in transgenic mice. *J Biol Chem.* 1998;273:17361–17367.
119. Cao SX, Gutman PD, Dave HP, Schechter AN. Negative control of the human ε-globin gene. *Prog Clin Biol Res.* 1989;316A:279–289.
120. Peters B, Merezhinskaya N, Diffley JF, Noguchi CT. Protein-DNA interactions in the ε-globin gene silencer. *J Biol Chem.* 1993;268:3430–3437.
121. Raich N, Papayannopoulou T, Stamatoyannopoulos G, Enver T. Demonstration of a human ε-globin gene silencer with studies in transgenic mice. *Blood.* 1992;79:861–864.
122. Li Q, Clegg C, Peterson K, Shaw S, Raich N, Stamatoyannopoulos G. Binary transgenic mouse model for studying the trans control of globin gene switching: evidence that GATA-1 is an in vivo repressor of human ε gene expression. *Proc Natl Acad Sci USA.* 1997;94:2444–2448.
123. Navas PA, Li Q, Peterson KR, Stamatoyannopoulos G. Investigations of a human embryonic globin gene silencing element using YAC transgenic mice. *Exp Biol Med (Maywood).* 2006;231:328–334.
124. Behringer RR, Ryan TM, Palmiter RD, Brinster RL, Townes TM. Human γ- to β-globin gene switching in transgenic mice. *Genes Dev.* 1990;4:380–389.
125. Enver T, Raich N, Ebens AJ, Papayannopoulou T, Costantini F, Stamatoyannopoulos G. Developmental regulation of human fetal–to-adult globin gene switching in transgenic mice. *Nature.* 1990;344:309–313.
126. Dillon N, Grosveld F. Human γ-globin genes silenced independently of other genes in the β-globin locus. *Nature.* 1991;350:252–254.
127. Peterson KR, Li QL, Clegg CH, et al. Use of yeast artificial chromosomes (YACs) in studies of mammalian development: production of β-globin locus YAC mice carrying human globin developmental mutants. *Proc Natl Acad Sci USA.* 1995;92:5655–5659.
128. Dillon N, Trimborn T, Strouboulis J, Fraser P, Grosveld F. The effect of distance on long-range chromatin interactions. *Mol Cell.* 1997;1:131–139.
129. Harju S, Navas PA, Stamatoyannopoulos G, Peterson KR. Genome architecture of the human β-globin locus affects developmental regulation of gene expression. *Mol Cell Biol.* 2005;25:8765–8778.
130. Yu M, Han H, Xiang P, Li Q, Stamatoyannopoulos G. Autonomous silencing as well as competition controls γ-globin gene expression during development. *Mol Cell Biol.* 2006;26:4775–4781.
131. Hanscombe O, Whyatt D, Fraser P, et al. Importance of globin gene order for correct developmental expression. *Genes Dev.* 1991;5:1387–1394.
132. Peterson KR, Stamatoyannopoulos G. Role of gene order in developmental control of human γ- and β-globin gene expression. *Mol Cell Biol.* 1993;13:4836–4843.
133. Wijgerde M, Grosveld F, Fraser P. Transcription complex stability and chromatin dynamics in vivo. *Nature.* 1995;377:209–213.
134. Dekker J, Rippe K, Dekker M, Kleckner N. Capturing chromosome conformation. *Science.* 2002;295:1306–1311.
135. Tolhuis B, Palstra RJ, Splinter E, Grosveld F, de Laat W. Looping and interaction between hypersensitive sites in the active β-globin locus. *Mol Cell.* 2002;10:1453–1465.

136. Palstra RJ, Tolhuis B, Splinter E, Nijmeijer R, Grosveld F, de Laat W. The β-globin nuclear compartment in development and erythroid differentiation. *Nat Genet.* 2003;35:190–194.
137. Carter D, Chakalova L, Osborne CS, Dai YF, Fraser P. Long-range chromatin regulatory interactions in vivo. *Nat Genet.* 2002;32:623–626.
138. Drissen R, Palstra RJ, Gillemans N, et al. The active spatial organization of the β-globin locus requires the transcription factor EKLF. *Genes Dev.* 2004;18:2485–2490.
139. Vakoc CR, Letting DL, Gheldof N, et al. Proximity among distant regulatory elements at the β-globin locus requires GATA-1 and FOG-1. *Mol Cell.* 2005;17:453–462.
140. Kooren J, Palstra RJ, Klous P, et al. B-globin active chromatin Hub formation in differentiating erythroid cells and in p45 NF-E2 knock-out mice. *J Biol Chem.* 2007;282:16544–16552.
141. Papayannopoulou TH, Brice M, Stamatoyannopoulos G. Stimulation of fetal hemoglobin synthesis in bone marrow cultures from adult individuals. *Proc Natl Acad Sci USA.* 1976;73:2033–2037.
142. Stamatoyannopoulos G, Veith R, Galanello R, Papayannopoulou T. Hb F production in stressed erythropoiesis: observations and kinetic models. *Ann NY Acad Sci.* 1985; 445:188–197.
143. Papayannopoulou T, Vichinsky E, Stamatoyannopoulos G. Fetal Hb production during acute erythroid expansion. I. Observations in patients with transient erythroblastopenia and post-phlebotomy. *Br J Haematol.* 1980;44:535–546.
144. Sheridan BL, Weatherall DJ, Clegg JB, et al. The patterns of fetal haemoglobin production in leukaemia. *Br J Haematol.* 1976;32:487–506.
145. DeSimone J, Biel SI, Heller P. Stimulation of fetal hemoglobin synthesis in baboons by hemolysis and hypoxia. *Proc Natl Acad Sci USA.* 1978;75:2937–2940.
146. Nute PE, Papayannopoulou T, Chen P, Stamatoyannopoulos G. Acceleration of F-cell production in response to experimentally induced anemia in adult baboons (Papio cynocephalus). *Am J Hematol.* 1980;8:157–168.
147. Al-Khatti A, Veith RW, Papayannopoulou T, Fritsch EF, Goldwasser E, Stamatoyannopoulos G. Stimulation of fetal hemoglobin synthesis by erythropoietin in baboons. *N Engl J Med.* 1987;317:415–420.
148. Umemura T, Al-Khatti A, Papayannopoulou T, Stamatoyannopoulos G. Fetal hemoglobin synthesis in vivo: direct evidence for control at the level of erythroid progenitors. *Proc Natl Acad Sci USA.* 1988;85:9278–9282.
149. Beaven GH, Ellis MJ, White JC. Studies on human foetal haemoglobin. II. Foetal haemoglobin levels in healthy children and adults and in certain haematological disorders. *Br J Haematol.* 1960;6:201–222.
150. Stamatoyannopoulos G, Papayannopoulou T. Fetal hemoglobin and the erythroid stem cell differentiation process. In: Stamatoyannopoulos G, Nienhuis AW, eds. *Cellular and Molecular Regulation of Hemoglobin Switching.* New York: Grune & Stratton; 1979:323–349.
151. DeSimone J, Heller P, Hall L, Zwiers D. 5-Azacytidine stimulates fetal hemoglobin synthesis in anemic baboons. *Proc Natl Acad Sci USA.* 1982;79:4428–4431.
152. Ley TJ, DeSimone J, Anagnou NP, et al. 5-azacytidine selectively increases γ-globin synthesis in a patient with b+thalassemia. *N Engl J Med.* 1982;307:1469–1475.
153. Torrealba de Ron AT, Papayannopoulou T, Knapp MS, Fu MF, Knitter G, Stamatoyannopoulos G. Perturbations in the erythroid marrow progenitor cell pools may play a role in the augmentation of HbF by 5-azacytidine. *Blood.* 1984;63:201–210.
154. Papayannopoulou T, Torrealba de Ron A, Veith R, Knitter G, Stamatoyannopoulos G. Arabinosylcytosine induces fetal hemoglobin in baboons by perturbing erythroid cell differentiation kinetics. *Science.* 1984;224:617–619.
155. Letvin NL, Linch DC, Beardsley GP, McIntyre KW, Nathan DG. Augmentation of fetal-hemoglobin production in anemic monkeys by hydroxyurea. *N Engl J Med.* 1984;310:869–873.
156. Veith R, Papayannopoulou T, Kurachi S, Stamatoyannopoulos G. Treatment of baboon with vinblastine: insights into the mechanisms of pharmacologic stimulation of Hb F in the adult. *Blood.* 1985;66:456–459.
157. Fibach E, Burke LP, Schechter AN, Noguchi CT, Rodgers GP. Hydroxyurea increases fetal hemoglobin in cultured erythroid cells derived from normal individuals and patients with sickle cell anemia or β-thalassemia. *Blood.* 1993;81: 1630–1635.
158. Platt OS, Falcone JF. Membrane protein interactions in sickle red blood cells: evidence of abnormal protein 3 function. *Blood.* 1995;86:1992–1998.
159. Steinberg MH, Lu ZH, Barton FB, Terrin ML, Charache S, Dover GJ. Fetal hemoglobin in sickle cell anemia: determinants of response to hydroxyurea. Multicenter study of hydroxyurea. *Blood.* 1997;89:1078–1088.
160. Perrine SP, Greene MF, Faller DV. Delay in the fetal globin switch in infants of diabetic mothers. *N Engl J Med.* 1985; 312:334–338.
161. Perrine SP, Miller BA, Greene MF, et al. Butryic acid analogues augment γ globin gene expression in neonatal erythroid progenitors. *Biochem Biophys Res Commun.* 1987;148: 694–700.
162. Constantoulakis P, Papayannopoulou T, Stamatoyannopoulos G. α-Amino-N-butyric acid stimulates fetal hemoglobin in the adult. *Blood.* 1988;72:1961–1967.
163. Perrine SP, Miller BA, Faller DV, et al. Sodium butyrate enhances fetal globin gene expression in erythroid progenitors of patients with Hb SS and b thalassemia. *Blood.* 1989;74:454–459.
164. Stamatoyannopoulos G, Nienhuis AW. Hemoglobin switching. In: Stamatoyannopoulos G, Nienhuis AW, Majerus P, Varmus H, eds. *Molecular Basis of Blood Diseases.* 2nd ed. Philadelphia: W.B. Saunders Co.; 1994:107–154.
165. Liakopoulou E, Blau CA, Li Q, et al. Stimulation of fetal hemoglobin production by short chain fatty acids. *Blood.* 1995;86:3227–3235.
166. Dover GJ, Brusilow S, Charache S. Induction of fetal hemoglobin production in subjects with sickle cell anemia by oral sodium phenylbutyrate. *Blood.* 1994;84:339–343.
167. Collins AF, Dover GJ, Luban NL. Increased fetal hemoglobin production in patients receiving valproic acid for epilepsy. *Blood.* 1994;84:1690–1691.
168. Little JA, Dempsey NJ, Tuchman M, Ginder GD. Metabolic persistence of fetal hemoglobin. *Blood.* 1995;85:1712–1718.
169. Peters A, Rohlloff D, Kohlmann T, et al. Fetal hemoglobin in starvation ketosis of young women. *Blood.* 1998;91:691–694.
170. Cao H, Stamatoyannopoulos G, Jung M. Induction of human γ globin gene expression by histone deacetylase inhibitors. *Blood.* 2004;103:701–709.

171. Pace BS, White GL, Dover GJ, Boosalis MS, Faller DV, Perrine SP. Short-chain fatty acid derivatives induce fetal globin expression and erythropoiesis in vivo. *Blood.* 2002;100:4640–4648.
172. Kuo MH, Brownell JE, Sobel RE, et al. Transcription-linked acetylation by Gcn5p of histones H3 and H4 at specific lysines. *Nature.* 1996;383:269–272.
173. Mizzen CA, Yang XJ, Kokubo T, et al. The TAF(II)250 subunit of TFIID has histone acetyltransferase activity. *Cell.* 1996;87:1261–1270.
174. Ogryzko VV, Schiltz RL, Russanova V, Howard BH, Nakatani Y. The transcriptional coactivators p300 and CBP are histone acetyltransferases. *Cell.* 1996;87:953–959.
175. Vettese-Dadey M, Grant PA, Hebbes TR, Crane- Robinson C, Allis CD, Workman JL. Acetylation of histone H4 plays a primary role in enhancing transcription factor binding to nucleosomal DNA in vitro. *EMBO J.* 1996;15:2508–2518.
176. Pace B, Li Q, Peterson K, Stamatoyannopoulos G. α-Amino butyric acid cannot reactivate the silenced γ gene of the β locus YAC transgenic mouse. *Blood.* 1994;84:4344–4353.
177. Uda M, Galanello R, Sanna S, et al. Genome-wide association study shows BCL11A associated with persistent fetal hemoglobin and amelioration of the phenotype of β-thalassemia. *Proc Natl Acad Sci USA.* 2008;105:1620–1625.
178. Lettre G, Sankaran VG, Bezerra MA, et al. DNA polymorphisms at the BCL11A, HBS1L-MYB, and β-globin loci associate with fetal hemoglobin levels and pain crises in sickle cell disease. *Proc Natl Acad Sci USA.* 2008;105:11869–11874.
179. Sankaran VG, Menne TF, Xu J, et al. Human fetal hemoglobin expression is regulated by the developmental stage-specific repressor BCL11A. *Science.* 2008;322:1839–1842.
180. Senawong T, Peterson VJ, Leid M. BCL11A-dependent recruitment of SIRT1 to a promoter template in mammalian cells results in histone deacetylation and transcriptional repression. *Arch Biochem Biophys.* 2005;434:316–325.
181. Liu H, Ippolito GC, Wall JK, et al. Functional studies of BCL11A: characterization of the conserved BCL11A-XL splice variant and its interaction with BCL6 in nuclear paraspeckles of germinal center B cells. *Mol cancer.* 2006;5:18–34.
182. Chen, Z, Luo, HY, Steinberg, MH, Chui DH. BCL11A represses HBG transcription in K562 cells. *Blood Cells Mol Dis.* 2009;42:144–149.

6

Structure and Function of Hemoglobin and Its Dysfunction in Sickle Cell Disease

Daniel B. Kim-Shapiro

INTRODUCTION

Hemoglobin has evolved to be an efficient oxygen (O_2) transporter. Its function, understood in terms of a two-state model of allostery, serves as a paradigm for many other proteins. A single β-globin gene (*HBB* glu6val) point mutation resulting in sickle hemoglobin (HbS) is the proximate cause of sickle cell disease (Chapter 19). The primary cause of the disease is HbS polymerization that injures and deforms the sickle erythrocyte, causing many pathological consequences discussed elsewhere in this book.

STRUCTURAL ASPECTS OF HEMOGLOBIN

Hemoglobin is a 64-kD, nearly spherical protein with a diameter of approximately 5.5 nm. Its three-dimensional structure was solved by Max F. Perutz who discussed the molecular anatomy and physiology of hemoglobin in the first edition of this book.[1] It is a dimer of dimers, with two α subunits and two β subunits (Fig. 6.1). The α chains have 141 amino acid residues and the β chains have 146 residues. Each of the α and β chains resemble each other closely in both secondary (α helical) and tertiary structure. Moreover, even though the primary amino acid sequence is different, each subunit also resembles myoglobin, a heme-containing globin having only one subunit in both secondary and tertiary structure. Generally, nonpolar groups are found in the interior of the subunits and polar residues are found on the surface. The SH group of the cysteine at position 93 of the β chain is exposed to solvent in the oxygenated form of hemoglobin, but it is partially hidden when hemoglobin is deoxygenated. This is due to the change in quaternary structure of the protein when hemoglobin binds O_2. One αβ dimer rotates approximately 12^0 with respect to the other and moves approximately 0.1 nm along the rotation axis.

Each of the subunits of the tetramer contains a heme prosthetic group (Figs. 6.1 and 6.2). Hemes are attached to the globin protein via a histidine side chain (Fig. 6.2). Heme is an iron-containing protoporphyrin IX, a tetrapyrrole with an iron atom at its center. The iron is usually ferrous, having a valency of +2. It can be oxidized to the ferric form (+3) and is then commonly referred to as methemoglobin. In the ferrous form, the heme group can bind to gaseous ligands including O_2, CO, and NO and can also bind alkylisocyanides.[2] In the ferric form, hemoglobin does not bind to O_2 or CO. It binds to NO, but with a much lower affinity than ferrous heme. Ferric hemoglobin also reversibly binds nitrite, nitrate, azide, and binds to cyanide very tightly, forming cyanomethemoglobin.

In addition to the heme group, there are several other sites within hemoglobin through which it interacts with small molecules. Bisphosphoglycerate (BPG) and inositol hexaphosphate (IHP) bind in the central cavity of hemoglobin, crosslinking the four subunits. The β-93 cysteine binds N-ethylmaleimide, iodoacetamide, and nitrosonium ion (NO^+), the latter forming S-nitrosated hemoglobin or SNO–hemoglobin. Carbon dioxide binds to the terminal amino groups.

NORMAL HEMOGLOBIN FUNCTION

Oxygen Transport

The primary function of hemoglobin is to transport O_2 from the lungs to the tissues. The pressure and solubility of O_2 in liquids make it such that only 200 μmol/L, at most, could be carried by blood in the absence of an O_2-carrying protein such as hemoglobin. Whole blood contains approximately 10 mmol/L hemoglobin (in heme), thus greatly increasing the O_2-carrying capacity of blood. The ability of hemoglobin to transport O_2 effectively is illustrated by plotting its fractional O_2 saturation (hemoglobin bound to O_2/total hemoglobin) against O_2 pressure (Fig. 6.3). Hemoglobin binds O_2 cooperatively, a phenomenon discovered by Christian Bohr, the father of the famous physicist Niels Bohr.[3] Cooperative binding means that the affinity of a hemoglobin tetramer for O_2 increases as more O_2 is bound. Myoglobin binds O_2 noncooperatively. In Figure 6.3, we see that at pressure of 20 mm Hg (close to that of metabolically active tissue), myoglobin is almost completely saturated with O_2, whereas hemoglobin is less than 40% saturated. Thus, hemoglobin has a lower affinity for O_2 at this pressure. As the O_2 pressure is raised to 90 mm Hg, which is close to that in the lungs, both hemoglobin and myoglobin are fully saturated with O_2 so that the hemoglobin–O_2 affinity has caught up to that of myoglobin. If myoglobin were contained in red blood cells instead of hemoglobin, then the red blood cells would be fully O_2

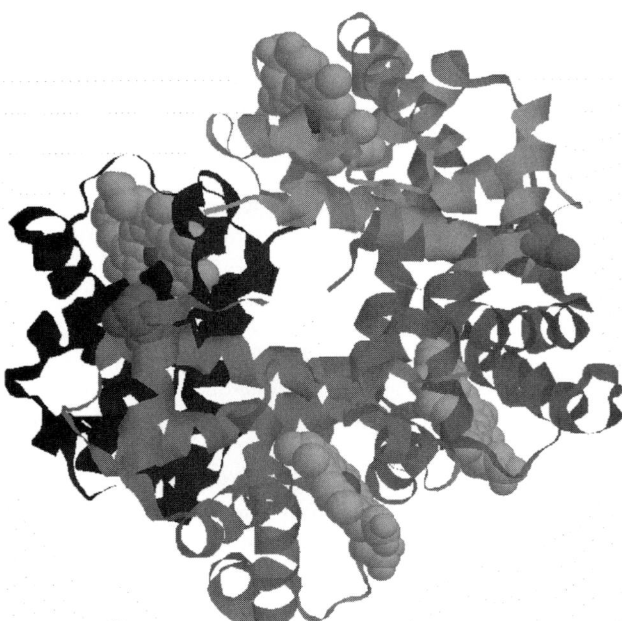

Figure 6.1. Ribbon diagram of a sickle cell hemoglobin tetramer. Each of the four subunits is shown in a different color. Four heme groups (yellow-orange) are shown with an iron (red) atom in the middle. The valine residues resulting from the single point mutation causing sickle cell disease are shown at the β6 position on each β subunit (purple). The molecule is shown looking down the axis where 2,3 bisphosphoglycerate binds. Except for the substitution of valine for glutamate, normal HbA would appear the same as the molecule shown. (The illustration was derived from the Protein Explorer (http://www.umass.edu/microbio/rasmol/) and data from the Protein Data Bank.) (See color plate 6.1.)

loaded in the lungs, but they would not release sufficient O_2 in the tissues. By combining four myoglobin-like chains into a single tetramer, hemoglobin is able to function as an efficient O_2 transporter.

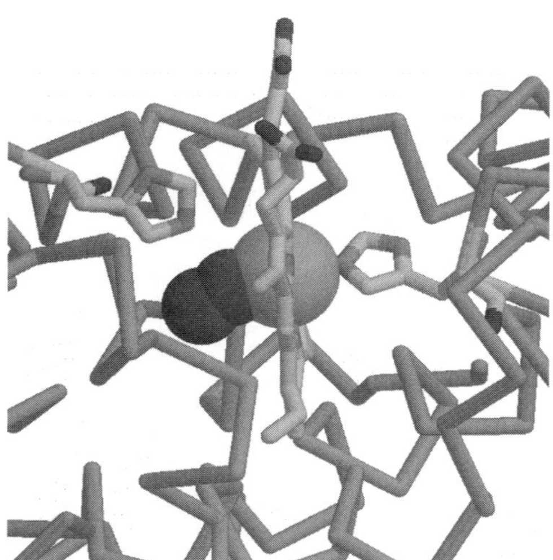

Figure 6.2. Close up of oxygen bound to the heme. Looking down the heme, the iron atom (yellow-orange) is shown bound to an oxygen molecule (red). The proximal histidine side chain is also shown bound to the iron and the distal histidine is also clearly visible on the other side of the proximal one. (The illustration derived from the Protein Explorer (http://www.umass.edu/microbio/rasmol/) and data from the Protein Data Bank.) (See color plate 6.2.)

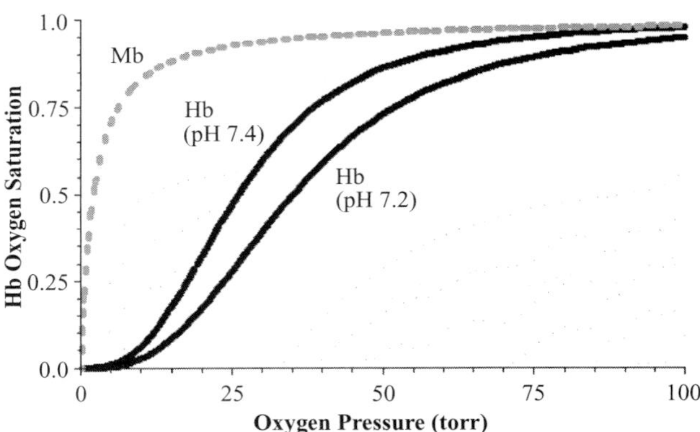

Figure 6.3. Hemoglobin and myoglobin oxygen binding curves. The myoglobin oxygen binding curve was drawn according to Equation 6.1 with P_{50} taken as 2 mm Hg. The hemoglobin oxygen binding curves were drawn using Equation 6.2 with $n = 2.8$ and P_{50} taken as 26 mm Hg at pH 7.4 and as 35 mm Hg for pH 7.2. (See color plate 6.3.)

The myoglobin O_2 saturation, Y, as a function of O_2 pressure can be described by the simple relation

$$Y = \frac{MbO_2}{MbO_2 + Mb} = \frac{pO_2}{pO_2 + P_{50}}, \tag{6.1}$$

where pO_2 is the O_2 pressure and P_{50} is the O_2 pressure where $Y = 0.5$ (the myoglobin is half saturated with O_2). The hemoglobin O_2 saturation dependence on O_2 pressure is more complicated and can be described by

$$Y = \frac{HbO_2}{HbO_2 + Hb} = \frac{(pO_2)^n}{(pO_2)^n + (P_{50})^n}, \tag{6.2}$$

where the exponent n is called the Hill coefficient. The Hill coefficient describes the degree of cooperativity in O_2 binding. For myoglobin, where there is no cooperativity, $n = 1$. For hemoglobin, several factors could affect the value of n, but it is usually found to be approximately 2.8 under normal conditions.

The ability of hemoglobin to bind O_2 cooperatively is well-described in terms of a two-state model developed by Monod, Wyman, and Changeux (MWC).[4] According to the model, there are two states of hemoglobin defined by the quaternary structure: the relaxed, high-O_2 affinity R-state and the tense, low-O_2 affinity T-state. When hemoglobin is completely deoxygenated, it is essentially all in the T-state and thereby has a low affinity. As O_2 binds, a hemoglobin tetramer that has 2–3 O_2 molecules bound will be likely to undergo the allosteric transition to the R-state, gaining a higher affinity for O_2. Thus, the allostery, whereby binding at one heme site affects binding at another site, explains the cooperative O_2 binding of hemoglobin.

One of the beautiful aspects of the MWC model is its simplicity. It is assumed that the affinity of a particular subunit heme group is only a function of the quaternary state (R or T) of the tetramer. Only three parameters are needed to apply the model. These are K_R, the R-state association constant; K_T, the T-state association constant; and L, the quaternary equilibrium constant between unligated tetramers (how much T-state there is vs. R-state in the absence of O_2 or

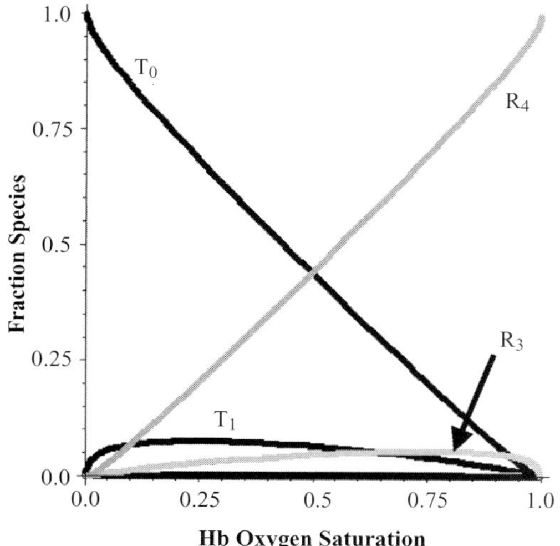

Figure 6.4. Fraction of hemoglobin states. The fraction of each state is plotted vs. hemoglobin oxygen saturation. Only the species T_0, T_1, R_3, and R_4 are present at large enough fractions to be visible. At zero oxygen saturation the hemoglobin is virtually all in the T_0 state and at 100% oxygen saturation it is all in the R_4 state. The parameters used were $L = 2 \times 10^6$, $c = 0.001$, and $K_T = 1/(75\text{ mm Hg})$. (See color plate 6.4.)

other ligands). The equilibrium constants between R_x and T_x are determined by Lc^x, where x represents the number of ligands bound (so R_3 is a hemoglobin molecule with three ligands bound in the R quaternary state) and $c = K_T/K_R$. As hemes in R-state hemoglobin have a much higher affinity than T-state hemes, the only species that are effectively present at any O_2 tension are T_0, R_4, T_1, and R_3 (Fig. 6.4).

The phenomenon of allostery, action at a distance, whereby binding at one heme site affects the affinity at another is explained by motions of the heme iron coupled to the globin and communicated to other subunits via salt bridges and other interactions.[5,6] When O_2 binds to the heme iron, the iron moves approximately 0.05 nm into the plane of the heme, pulling along the proximal histidine. This movement is transmitted to the subunit interfaces and leads to disruption of the salt links. Binding of the first O_2 molecule to hemoglobin is the most difficult because the many salt links must be broken. As these salt links break, the (tense) tetramer relaxes so that there are fewer salt links. At this point, binding of O_2 to the R-state molecule is easier. This relative "relaxed" nature of R-state hemoglobin is evidenced by the fact that the dissociation constant for ligated hemoglobin tetramers into dimers is approximately 1 mM but deoxygenated (T-state) hemoglobin has an extremely low tendency for dimer formation.

The MWC–Perutz model is supported by a large amount of theoretical and experimental evidence.[7] One of the key elements comes from kinetics studies showing that the rate of ligand binding by a heme depends on the quaternary state of the hemoglobin and not on the number of ligands bound.[8] The equilibrium constant describing the ligand affinity, such as that plotted for O_2 in Figure 6.3, depends on the rate of association and dissociation, $K = k_{on}/k_{off}$. The cooperativity in equilibrium binding of O_2 to hemoglobin is mainly due to the differences in the rate of O_2 dissociation, that is approximately 100 times slower for R-state than T-state, rather than differences in the rate of O_2 association, that is approximately 10 times faster for R-state than T-state.[9,10]

Several compounds greatly affect the ligand-binding properties of hemoglobin. These are classified as homotropic effectors (those that effect like ligands) and heterotrophic effectors, such as BPG, protons, chloride, and phosphate. Without BPG, the P_{50} of hemoglobin (partial pressure of O_2 at which the hemoglobin molecule is half saturated) for O_2 binding would be approximately 2 mm Hg, rather than approximately 25 mm Hg. According to the MWC–Perutz model, effectors alter the ligand binding by affecting L. BPG binding in the central cavity stabilizes the T-state. N-ethylmaleimide or NO^+ binding at the β93 cysteine stabilizes the R-state. Thus, SNO–hemoglobin has a higher O_2 affinity than hemoglobin that is not nitrosated.[11] Lowering the pH also stabilizes the T-state, so that more O_2 can be given off under acidic conditions (Fig. 6.3).

The two-state MWC–Perutz model is capable of explaining many of the phenomena associated with ligand binding. When applied with more rigor to a variety of phenomenon, however, the need for modification is clear. This should not be a surprise as hemoglobin is not a homotetramer. Thus, a clearly necessary modification of the MWC–Perutz model is to account for chain differences.[12,13] The α subunits have a higher equilibrium affinity for O_2 than the β subunits, mainly due to faster dissociation rates from β subunits.[10,14] These differences in chain affinities are not consistent with a strict interpretation of a two-state model in which the ligand affinity is only a function of quaternary state (T or R). A further, commonly accepted modification involves a slight cooperativity within αβ dimers in the T quaternary state.[15,16] This modified two-state model is sufficient to explain a large variety of quantitative equilibrium and kinetic data. Exceptions to these have lead to further extended or alternative models.[16–18]

The effect of hemoglobin binding of gaseous ligands on O_2 affinity is particularly interesting. CO_2 reduces the ligand affinity of hemoglobin, similarly to protons. This combination leads to effective O_2 delivery to metabolically active tissue. When NO is bound to the α subunits forming α nitrosyl hemoglobin, it acts as a negative allosteric effector, lowering the O_2 affinity of the β subunits.[19] This is an example of how, in some cases, hemoglobin function at vacant hemes is dependent on the subunits to which ligand is bound and the type of ligand. Thus, α nitrosyl hemoglobin function is not consistent with the MWC–Perutz model.

The two-state model is formulated in terms of two structures obtained from x-ray crystallography. In 1992, a new crystal structure of liganded hemoglobin was discovered called R2.[20] More recently, other liganded crystal structures have been determined.[21] One might wonder which of these is the one present in solution and how this information relates to the two-state model.[22,23] Using multidimensional and multinuclear nuclear magnetic resonance, it has been found that the solution structure of liganded hemoglobin is actually a dynamic ensemble of states that include those determined by x-ray crystallography.[23–25] Similarly, the structure of deoxyhemoglobin in solution is likely to comprise several quaternary states that include the many ones found by x-ray crystallography.[26] Thus, the actual picture of how hemoglobin functions is significantly more complicated than that described by a two-state model. For many applications, however, a two-state MWC–Perutz model is sufficient to explain biological phenomena. Nevertheless, it should be kept in mind that, like all models, especially simple ones that are applied to many complex behaviors, it has limitations.

Transport of Other Gases

Hemoglobin also transports CO_2, which binds more tightly to deoxyhemoglobin than to oxyhemoglobin, so it is taken up in the tissues and given off in the lungs. In addition, deoxyhemoglobin uptake of protons helps transport CO_2 as bicarbonate, HCO_3^-, which is more soluble than CO_2.

$$CO_2 + H_2O \leftrightarrow HCO_3^- + H^+ \tag{6.3}$$

Without uptake of protons by deoxyhemoglobin, the equilibrium in Equation 6.3, would shift to the left, limiting bicarbonate formation. Thus, cooperative binding of O_2 links to that of CO_2 so that hemoglobin is an effective transporter of both molecules.

CO is produced by heme oxygenase during heme metabolism. The equilibrium affinity of hemoglobin for CO is approximately 200 times higher than that for O_2. This is due to the slow dissociation rate of CO from hemoglobin; O_2 actually binds to hemoglobin faster than does CO. Due to its high O_2 affinity and slow dissociation rate, CO has been recognized as a poison that disturbs O_2 delivery (Chapter 24); however, potential beneficial effects of CO have recently been recognized.[27–30] CO has been shown to have antiinflammatory effects and diminish apoptosis.[28–30] Recently, infusion of red cells saturated with CO at 25% of blood volume was shown to be effective in hemorrhagic shock resuscitation.[27] These beneficial effects of CO and hemoglobin's role in transporting such activity demand more study.

The ability of hemoglobin to destroy NO activity was an important element in the identification of NO as the endothelial-derived relaxing factor.[31,32] This is due to the rapid dioxygenation of NO with oxyhemoglobin to form nitrate (Chapter 10). NO can also bind to the heme, and the degree to which this reaction preserves biological activity has been debated. One certainty is that the equilibrium binding affinity of hemoglobin for NO is extremely high, approximately 1,500 times stronger than CO and 500,000 times stronger than O_2.[2]

Because of its high affinity, little knowledge about NO binding to deoxyhemoglobin can be obtained from equilibrium studies. Virtually any NO added to molar excess hemoglobin will bind the heme – there will be essentially none left in solution. Thus, binding studies have focused on kinetics. Early studies showed that the rate of dissociation of NO from T-state hemoglobin is 100-fold faster than from R-state hemoglobin, with the T-state rate being approximately 10^{-3}/s.[9,33,34] A difference in the dissociation rates from different subunits was also recognized.[33,34] A unique feature of NO binding to the α subunits is that when the α nitrosyl hemoglobin is in the T-state, a proportion of iron–proximal histidine bonds break, resulting in a characteristic triplet hyperfine structure in electron paramagnetic resonance spectra.[19,34–38] Recently, the dissociation rate of NO from this pentacoordinate α nitrosyl hemoglobin was measured to be 4×10^{-4}/s.[39] Thus, the rate of dissociation of NO from hemoglobin is faster for T-state hemoglobin and faster for β subunits than α subunits.

Early stopped-flow absorption experiments mixing NO and deoxyhemoglobin found that the association rate of NO with hemoglobin is noncooperative and occurs at a rate of 3×10^7 M/s.[40] Experiments examining the rate of release of a fluorescent BPG analog and the rate that partially NO-ligated hemoglobin binds CO indicated that a T- to R-state transition does take place after two–three NO molecules bind a tetramer.[40] The rate of NO binding to α and β chains was also found to be identical.[41] One study has suggested that although NO binds to R-state hemoglobin at the same rate as T-state hemoglobin, when the R-state transition has been caused by binding of two–three NO molecules, the rate of R-state association of NO is 100 times faster when the R-state transition has been invoked by O_2 binding.[42] In other words, NO would bind R_3 at the same rate as T_0 when the three ligands on R-state are NO but it would bind 100 times faster if they were O_2. Such a phenomenon would violate the tenet of the two-state model whereby binding properties at one heme only depends on the quaternary state of the protein. Subsequent studies have challenged the idea that the binding rate of NO to R-state oxyhemoglobin is faster than to R-state NO hemoglobin.[43,44] In addition, photolysis studies using a commonly accepted model of CO bound hemoglobin for oxyhemoglobin have also found that R-state hemoglobin binds NO at the same rate as T-state hemoglobin.[45,46] Thus, the preponderance of evidence indicates that the association rate of NO to hemoglobin is independent of the quaternary state. This is likely to be because once in the heme pocket, NO binds the heme extremely quickly in both cases so that the rate-limiting step in NO binding is diffusion of the ligand through the protein to the heme pocket.

Examination of both association and dissociation rates of NO shows that hemoglobin binds NO cooperatively, with all of the cooperativity being manifest in the dissociation rates. This is similar to O_2 where most of the cooperativity is in the dissociation rates. Due to the faster dissociation rate from β subunits, α nitrosyl hemoglobin is the primary form found in equilibrium. The association rate of NO to hemoglobin is only approximately 1.5-fold slower than the rate of the dioxygenation reaction.[47] Thus, even at high O_2 tensions, some NO will escape destruction via the dioxygention reaction to form NO bound hemoglobin. Another mechanism of potential preservation of NO activity via the formation of SNO–hemoglobin is discussed in Chapter 10, as it is a mechanism whereby NO activity is created via hemoglobin reduction of nitrite. Simple binding of NO to the heme is unlikely to constitute a mechanism of transport due to the very slow dissociation rate. However, a recent study suggests that NO-bound hemoglobin might be dislodged more quickly because of oxidation of the heme due to concurrent reactions of nitrite with oxyhemoglobin.[48] The potential of hemoglobin to transport NO, discussed in more depth in Chapter 10, is an area of current intense study.

Methemoglobin

In normal physiology, approximately 0.25% of hemes contain ferric iron (methemoglobin). Free heme oxidizes rapidly and aggregates. Incorporation of the heme into hemoglobin prevents aggregation and greatly slows autooxidation, facilitating O_2 transport, as methemoglobin does not bind O_2. Low levels of methemoglobin are also maintained by reducing systems within the red blood cell.[49–51] Although excessive formation of methemoglobin has been viewed strictly in terms of pathology (Chapter 24), some potential positive roles for methemoglobin have been discussed.

Two studies have suggested a role of NO bound to methemoglobin (methemoglobin–NO) in potential transport or delivery of NO activity.[52,53] It is likely that methemoglobin–NO forms transiently in the reaction of nitrite with deoxyhemoglobin, in analogy to some bacterial nitrite reductases.[54] The dissociation rate of NO from methemoglobin is, however, relatively fast ($\sim$1 s^{-1})[55] and methemoglobin also undergoes reductive nitrosylation to form ferrous iron nitrosyl hemoglobin.[56] The overall affinity of ferrous hemoglobin for NO is approximately 1 million times higher than that of ferric hemoglobin for NO.[55] Given that more than 99% of hemoglobin in the red blood cell is ferrous hemoglobin and that NO in the red cell is quickly destroyed via the dioxygenation reaction, it is extremely unlikely that there is any stable methemoglobin–NO in a red cell. The contention that NO is transported in the red cell bound to methemoglobin is untenable due to the relative stability of this species, as demonstrated recently.[57]

Some ligands bind methemoglobin more tightly than ferrous hemoglobin. Given recent evidence for a role of nitrite in physiology, disease, and therapeutics[58] and the potential involvement of hemoglobin (see Chapter 10), the role of nitrite-bound methemoglobin might be worth exploring. At the very least, this could be one way that nitrite is stored in a red blood cell because, even though oxyhemoglobin and deoxyhemoglobin are in great excess to methemoglobin, nitrite will preferentially bind to methemoglobin given the relative affinities.

SICKLE CELL HEMOGLOBIN

HbS differs from normal adult hemoglobin (HbA) by a single amino acid residue (Fig. 6.1). A variety of physical methods including x-ray diffraction, nuclear magnetic resonance, and circular dichroism all indicate that the protein conformation of a HbS tetramer in solution is the same or at least very similar to that to that of HbA.[59] Some evidence exists for subtle changes in the structure of central cavity BPG binding site.[60] Similar structure in solution phase HbS and HbA is supported by similar function. The equilibrium binding of solution phase HbS is the same as HbA.[61] The bimolecular ligand rebinding rates of solution phase HbS are also the same as those of HbA.[62,63] Finally, tertiary and quaternary changes that are induced on CO photolysis of solution phase HbS–CO exhibit the same kinetics as HbA–CO.[64]

The pathological consequences typical of sickle cell disease must derive, in part, due to a difference in function of HbS compared with HbA. Only one notable exception to the notion that, in the solution phase, HbS tetramers have very similar function as HbA exists: the propensity for HbS autooxidation.[65–68] Although increased propensity to form methemoglobin and associated oxidative damage could contribute to several aspects of the disease, this propensity is not likely to be of primary importance in sickle cell disease and HbS polymerization seems paramount.

HbS Polymer

The HbS polymer is made of seven twisted double stands (Fig. 6.5).[59,69–71] It has a diameter of 21 nm and a mean helical pitch length of 270 nm.[59] Each of the double strands is believed to be similar to ones formed by deoxyHbS when it crystallizes (Fig. 6.6). Having the structure of the double strand at 0.2 nm resolution greatly aids in understanding the structure of the 21 nm fiber because information on these larger structures cannot be obtained directly at the atomic level. A variety of techniques including mutational analysis, linear dichroism spectroscopy, resonance Raman spectroscopy, and x-ray diffraction support the idea that the basic building block of the polymer is the double strand with each of these twisted around one another.[59,72]

Contact sites between tetramers within double strands are known in the most detail.[70] Valine at the β6 position makes a lateral contact with a hydrophobic pocket formed by Leu β88, Phe β85, and the heme of tetramer on the other strand within the double strand. Only one of the two Val β6 residues per tetramer is involved in the double strand formation. In addition to these hydrophobic interactions, there are some neighboring hydrophilic ones and bridging water contacts that have been recently observed.[70] Lateral

A

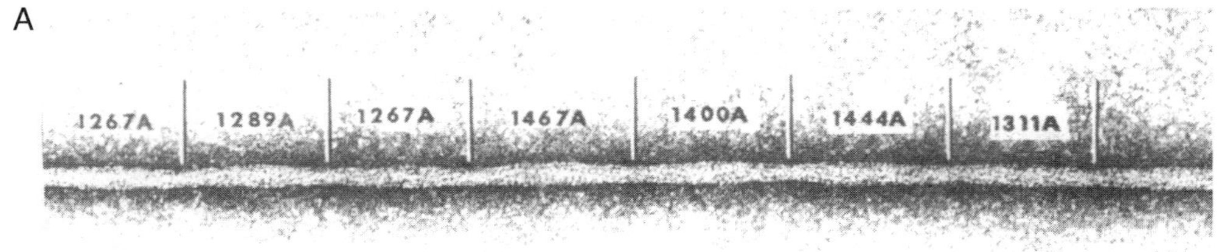

B

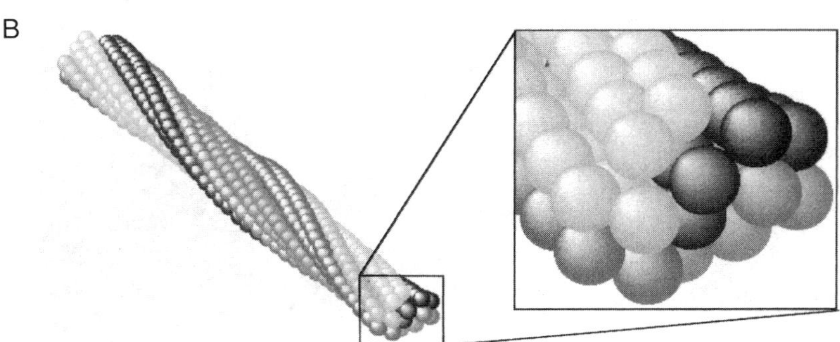

Figure 6.5. **(A)** Electron micrograph of a fiber. The pitch of the fiber is not fixed, but varies as indicated by the different distances between the minimum diameter points. **(B)** Fiber model with double strands. The model is built according to the description of Watowich et al.[75] This 14-strand model (whose end is shown in the inset) was first proposed by Dykes et al. (1978) and is now universally accepted as the basic fiber description.[17] Note the double strands that are a basic structural element of the fiber and are based on a structure determined by crystallography (see Fig. 6.6). The wrapping of the 14 strands leads to a structure that gently varies from narrow to wide along the fiber.

and axial contacts are mostly between β subunits. Nonpolar interactions involving Pro α114 and Ala α115 of one tetramer form an axial contact with His β116, His β117, and Phe β118 of a second tetramer.

In deoxy Hbs crystals, the double strands are linear. How these double strands twist around each other to make up the 21-nm fiber is incompletely understood. Interdouble strand contacts are believed to mainly involve α subunits,[59] but the second Val β6 has also recently been proposed to play a role.[73] Electron microscopy has provided useful information that has lead to two detailed models that agree on overall architecture.[74,75] but differ in some details, including overall density and water content.[76]

Recent theoretical calculations show that the twist in the HbS polymer plays an important role in its stabilization.[77] Confirmed by experimental observations, the torsional rigidity of HbS fibers is found to be approximately 100-fold less than the bending rigidity.[77,78] The resistance to twisting compared with bending is usually approximately the same for isotropic materials. Linear double strands are the lowest equilibrium form and the relative ease for these to twist is proposed as an explanation for the metastability of the 21-nm fibers.[78]

Higher Order Aggregation of HbS

Further aggregation of the 21-nm fibers can take several forms. Understanding the nature of these aggregates has been aided recently by novel applications of differential interference (DIC) microscopy.[79–81] Analysis of DIC microscopy data collected on two 21-nm fibers zippering up has allowed estimations of the interaction energies between two fibers. Two such fibers can be strongly bonded to each other.[81] As described in detail later, HbS polymerization involves both de novo fiber formation through homogeneous nucleation and fiber formation on the surface of a second one through heterogeneous nucleation.[82,83] It has been proposed that the same intermolecular mutation contact sites that are involved within a fiber are available in 4 of 10 HbS surface tetramers in each layer of the 21-nm fiber.[84] This proposal has recently been confirmed by studying cross-linked hybrid molecules.[85]

HbS polymer formation deforms the red cell, decreases its deformability, and increases its fragility. Aggregation of fibers into fascicles or bundles is of great interest because these are likely to exacerbate these phenomena. The fascicles are composed of twisted 21-nm fibers as shown in Figure 6.7.[86] These fascicles form crystals in vitro, probably through release of twist in the double strands with concomitant loss of polarity.[86] The fascicles always form first. The system of aligned fibers and HbS tetramers is referred to as a gel and this is thought to be what is formed inside of red blood cells. Crystals are not formed even though they are the lowest energy state. The gel is highly viscous and semisolid and, due to alignment of the polymers, it is birefringent. Because the hemes of hemoglobin are largely parallel to each other, and the hemoglobin tetramers are arranged so that the hemes are nearly perpendicular to the

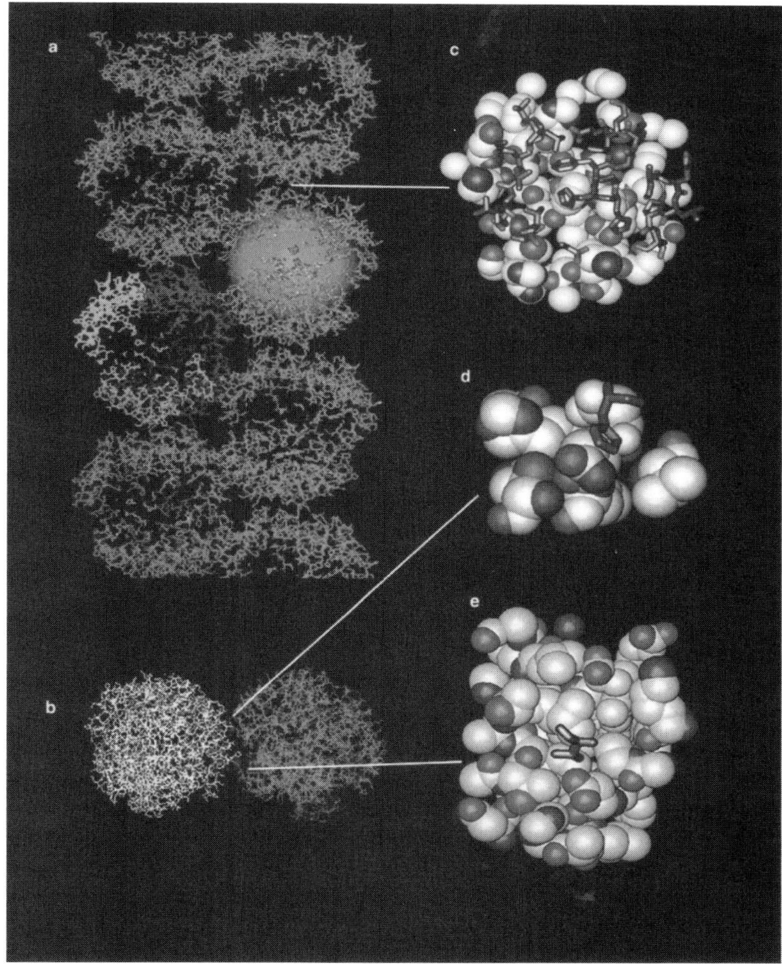

Figure 6.6. **(a)** The double strand of deoxyHbS, based on the crystal structure of Harrington et al.[70] The tetramers of HbS have been drawn with the central region excluded for clarity; one tetramer illustrates the exclusion region as a solid green sphere in the center of the molecule. Another tetramer is shown with the four subunits colored differently to differentiate them. Red and purple are β-globin chains; blue and orange are α-globin chains. Contacts along the axis of the double strand (vertical here) are denoted as axial, whereas those that connect diagonally are denoted as lateral. The β6 mutation site is in a lateral contact. Note that both the axial and the lateral contacts are dominated by interactions between the beta chains. **(b)** An end view of the double strand. The two molecules, with all amino acids now showing, are colored differently to aid the eye. The β6 contact is shown on the bottom (expanded view in **(E)**), and the salt bridge between αHis50 and βAsp79 is above (expanded view in **(d)**). **(c).** The axial contact region in **A** has been enlarged to allow a better view. Unlike the lateral contact, no single amino acid dominates the geometry. Carbon atoms that are filled to van der Waals radii are yellow, oxygen atoms are red, and nitrogen atoms are blue. **(d)** The salt bridge between Asp β79 and His α50 in the lateral contact area viewed from the α-globin chain. The His is shown as a green licorice stick drawing in the foreground. **(e)** The lateral contact region showing the β6 Val (green stick figure, foreground) in the receptor pocket on its complementary chain. (Note that in the crystal there are two such regions.) β88Leu is just forward and above Val; β85Phe is then just below β88 Leu and behind the Val. (See color plate 6.6.)

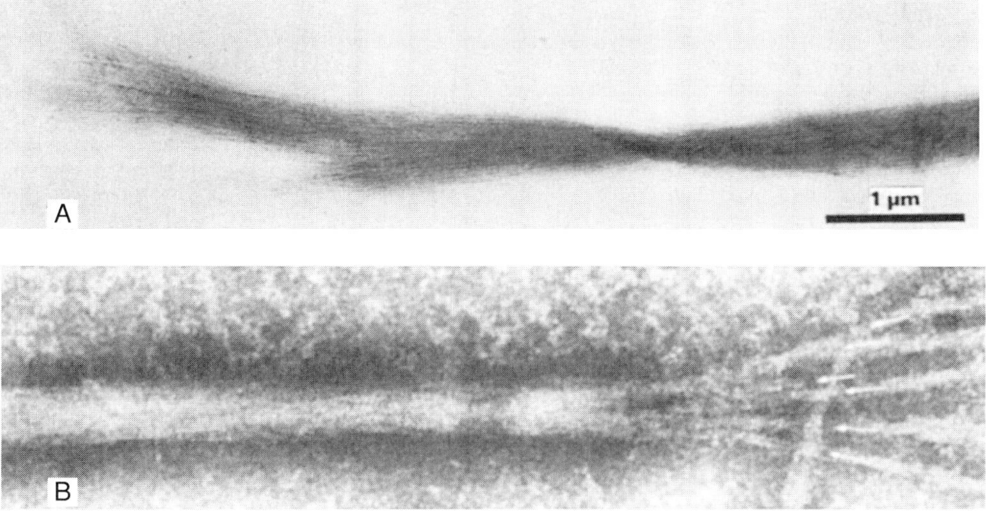

Figure 6.7. Sickle hemoglobin assembly creates structures larger than the fibers shown in Fig. 6.5. **(A)** Fibers can associate in bundles or fascicles.[86] Fascicles ultimately form into crystals. The fascicle shown here has a twist, which also appears in crystals. **(B)** A macrofiber with six fibers extending from the end. Macrofibers are composed of double strands in antiparallel rows, and such structures appear at low pH (below 6.7 in 0.05 mol/L phosphate buffer). (This macrofiber is from the unpublished work of Wellems and Josephs.)

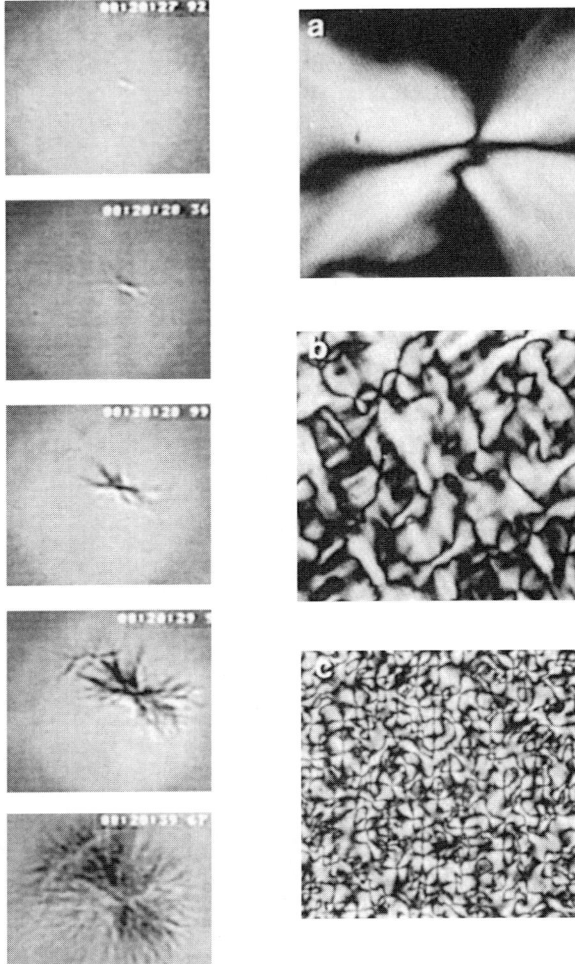

Figure 6.8. Polymer domains. As seen in the DIC images in the left sequence of panels, polymerization produces fibers in attached arrays called domains. In these pictures laser photolysis (as evidenced by the light-colored circles, of approximately 15 μm diameter) creates deoxyHb, which generates fibers.[80] The attached fibers form twofold symmetrical patterns that spread to form larger structures with nearly radial symmetry. These patterns are also visible in birefringence seen as transmission of light when the sample is placed between crossed polarizers and is shown in panels **a** through **c** on the right. Each cross or bow-tie defines a polymer domain. Each domain is formed from a single homogeneous nucleation event. The size of the polymer domains is inversely related to the speed of their formation, and speed of formation in turn is related to concentration. The concentrations were 23.4 g/dL, 25.7 g/dL and 27.4 g/dL, respectively. Samples were gelled by temperature jump from 3°C to 23°C.

fiber, the index of refraction is greater perpendicular to the fiber axis than parallel, resulting in birefringence and linear dichroism (where light is more strongly absorbed when polarized perpendicular to the fiber axis than parallel). The result is that, as observed both in solution and in red cells, gels are visible when viewed through crossed polarizers. Because of the way that clusters of polymers or domains form, they can have a large degree of radial symmetry, which produces a Maltese cross pattern when viewed through crossed polarizers (Fig. 6.8). The formation of radially symmetrical polymer domains has been confirmed using DIC microscopy (Fig. 6.9).

HbS Polymer Rheology

As rigidification of the red blood cell is probably the most important immediate affect of polymerization, it is useful to understand the rheology of the gel. A full understanding of the mechanical properties of the gel begins with understanding those of single fibers. Recently, DIC microscopy was used to determine the intrinsic Young modulus as well the persistence lengths of individual fibers and bundles.[87] The Young modulus (a measure of stiffness) was found to be approximately 0.1 GPa, much less than structural proteins like actin fibers and microtubules but greater than fibers that are meant to bend, like elastin. The persistence length was found to vary from 0.24 to 13 mm, increasing as the radius of bundles increased. These values are much larger than the length of a red blood cell so that one can conclude that the fibers are stiff on the scale of a red blood cell.

Macroscopic measurements of gel rheology are difficult due to the fact that shear applied in the measurement can disturb the mechanical properties of the gel itself. The rheology of the gel will depend on the number of cross links, which will be different for a few long fibers compared with many short ones. Breaking fibers, followed by additional growth, changes rigidity.[88–90] In the absence of shear, the gel behaves like a solid and at low shear it behaves like an elastic solid in which all deformations are reversible.[59] At higher shear, the gel can become irreversibly deformed. The rheological properties of sickle cell gels and their understanding in terms of single-fiber rheology, gel architecture, and quantitative contribution to vasoocclusion events remains an area in need of investigation.

HbS Thermodynamics

It has been widely accepted that the gel is made of two phases: a polymer phase and a solution phase where the

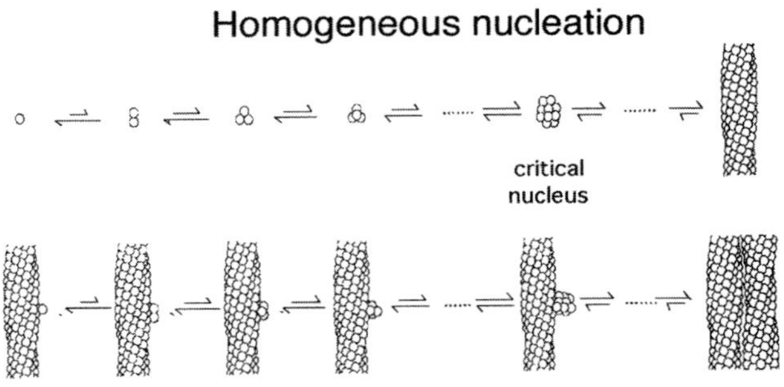

Figure 6.9. The double nucleation mechanism.[83] Polymers may form by homogeneous nucleation or heterogeneous nucleation onto other polymers. In either case, the initial steps are unfavorable, as indicated by the arrows, until a critical nucleus is formed. The critical nucleus is the first aggregrate that is equally likely to add monomers or to lose them. No special structure is assumed for the nuclei.

solution phase contains HbS tetramers (which can be referred to as monomers in the context of single building blocks of the polymer). In equilibrium, no intermediate aggregates are generally observed.[59,91] The thermodynamics of polymerization can be understood within this two-phase model in terms of the solubility of HbS known as c_s or c_{sat}. When the total concentration of HbS, c_0, is below the solubility, there will be no polymers. In equilibrium, when $c_0 > c_s$, the concentration of HbS tetramers in the solution phase is c_s, and the concentration of HbS tetramers in the polymer phase is equal to the total concentration of HbS minus the solubility ($c_0 - c_s$). Although individual tetramers might exchange between the two phases, once equilibrium is reached, the concentration in each phase will not change unless environmental conditions that affect the solubility (discussed later) are altered. The solubility is easily measured by sedimenting the polymers in an ultracentrifuge, for example, at 150,000 g for 2 hours, and taking the concentration of HbS in the supernatant as the solubility.

Recently, evidence from light scattering and DIC microscopy has been presented that suggests the existence of a third phase prior to and during HbS gelation.[92–96] This phase consists of metastable clusters of liquid phase molecules or dense liquid droplets that have been implicated in the initial formation of homogeneous nuclei discussed further later.[94] The clusters form within a few seconds of solution formation and are several hundred nm in diameter.[94,95] These clusters also form in solutions of HbA and oxygenated HbS but do not lead to polymer nucleation as in HbS.[94,95]

A major factor that must be taken into account when evaluating polymerization is crowding.[97] In most biochemical experiments, protein solutions are dilute enough so that they can be considered to be ideal, that is, when interactions between the molecules can be ignored, like in an ideal gas. The concentration of hemoglobin in a red cell is so high, however, ($\sim$ 20 mmol/L in heme which is 32 g/dL or 0.32 g/cm^3) that the solution is nonideal and interactions need to be accounted for. Theoretical treatments of nonideality in sickle cell hemoglobin polymerization have been worked out and agree very well with experiments.[59,97] Generally, one needs to include the activity coefficient, γ, when evaluating the potential for HbS to polymerize so that $c_0 \rightarrow \gamma c_0$ and $c_s \rightarrow \gamma_s c_s$, where γ_s is the activity coefficient at the solubility concentration. These activity coefficients are close to one in dilute solutions. For hemoglobin concentrations found in red blood cells, γ is quite large, equal to 70 for 0.35 g/cm^3.[59] For HbS concentrations found in very dense cells with 0.45 g/cm^3, γ is 900! The relevance of these crowding effects to sickle cell hemoglobin polymerization thermodynamics and kinetics cannot be overstated (for a fuller discussion see references 59, 97, 98). Increased crowding leads to increased polymerization, so that dehydration of red cells can have a dramatic effect where by γc_0 increases much faster than c_0. Any other solutes that take up significant volume also increase γ. Thus, replacing HbS with hemoglobin molecules that do not polymerize can reduce c_s but γ remains unchanged, diminishing the effect of the substitution.

Effectors of Polymerization

Generally, only T-state HbS molecules will polymerize.[99,100] Because only T-state hemoglobin polymerizes, any effectors that stabilize the T-state tend to decrease HbS solubility or increase polymerization.[59] Thus, BPG and IHP increase polymerization. In the physiological pH range, increasing proton concentration increases polymerization, but as the pH is lowered below 6.5, the solubility increases. The solubility is lowest around body temperature. This fact has been used extensively to prepare HbS gel samples where the solutions are prepared at 0°C and then temperature-jumped to 37°C.

The effect of phosphate on solubility is quite interesting and useful. The solubility of HbS decreases dramatically in concentrated phosphate buffers.[101–105] In 1.8 M phosphate the solubility is 0.04 g/dL (4×10^{-4} g/cm^3 or 0.025 mmol/L) at 30°C.[103] The effect of phosphate is likely to be due largely to increasing the activity by volume exclusion but there are also likely to be electrostatic interactions.[106] The ability to study polymerization at such low concentrations is beneficial as the volume of HbS is required for studies under physiological conditions is large and this requirement is very restrictive when studying new modified hemoglobins and those from mouse models. Another method to study polymerization with lower total hemoglobin concentrations is to use dextran to exclude volume and decrease the solubility.[106] With 12 g/dL of dextran, the solubility can be decreased approximately 5-fold.[106] This is a much smaller effect than using 1.8 M phosphate but some differences in polymerization in high phosphate and physiological phosphate have been reported.[106–111] It has recently been noted that a small amount of protein aggregates form in high phosphate that are not due to polymerization so that care is warranted in making sure that these are not misconstrued as HbS polymers.[111] In general, use of high phosphate can be recommended as an excellent initial screening method for effects on polymerization with subsequent experiments with dextran being more likely to provide physiologically relevant data. Finally, all such effects should be confirmed using physiological conditions.

The most important physiologically relevant variable involved in HbS polymerization is the O_2 pressure. As O_2 binding promotes R-state hemoglobin, it decreases polymerization. The effect of CO on polymerization is very similar to that of O_2 – the solubility as a function of solution phase hemoglobin ligand saturation is the same for O_2 as it is for CO.[99] This is consistent both with the idea that only T-state HbS polymerizes and the MWC–Perutz model of hemoglobin cooperativity. To understand fully the effect of O_2 saturation on solubility, the affinity of polymer phase HbS for O_2 must be determined. Using linear dichroism spectroscopy, because the linear dichroism of solution phase HbS averages out, it was found that polymer phase HbS has approximately one third the O_2 affinity as solution phase T-state hemoglobin.[99] Using data for the solubility of HbS at a variety of temperatures and ligand saturations, Eaton and Hofrichter[59] derived an empirical equation for the solubility as a function of these variables,

$$c_s\,(\mathrm{g/cm^3}) = 0.321 - 0.00883\,T + 0.000125\,T^2 + 0.0924\,Y_s + 0.098\,Y_s^3 + 0.235\,Y_s^{15}, \qquad (6.4)$$

where T is the temperature in degrees Celsius and Y_s is the fractional hemoglobin O_2 saturation of the solution phase HbS. In the absence of O_2 ($Y_s = 0$), the solubility is calculated to be 0.17 g/cm^3 (10 mmol/L in heme) at 37°C, and 0.32 g/cm^3 (20 mmol/L in heme) at 0°C. When the solution phase O_2 saturation is 0.7, the solubility is 0.26 g/cm^3 (17 mmol/L in heme) at 37°C.

The effects of NO on polymerization have been controversial. NO inhalation therapy is being studied as treatment for sickle cell disease. One of the main ways of benefiting patients is likely to be by reducing the NO scavenging ability of cell-free hemoglobin that results from intravascular hemolysis (Chapter 11)[112] and possibly due to induction of fetal hemoglobin (HbF) production.[113,114] It has also been proposed that NO binding to the heme would reduce HbS polymerization, like O_2 does.[115] In early work, Briehl and Salhany showed that tetranitrosyl hemoglobin (where all four hemes have NO bound) polymerizes in the presence of IHP but does not polymerize when the hemoglobin is stripped of organic phosphates. More recently, it was shown that when HbS polymerization is studied in conditions mimicking those in vivo (with BPG present), the solubilizing or sparing effect of NO binding to the heme is much less than that of O_2.[38] The minimal effects of iron nitrosylation can be understood in terms of the ability of NO compared with that of O_2, to convert T-state hemoglobin to R-state hemoglobin, because R-state hemoglobin has a much higher affinity for O_2 than T-state hemoglobin, and 25% oxygenated hemoglobin will be nearly 25% R-state (Fig. 6.3). On the other hand, NO tends to favor binding to the α subunits and α nitrosyl hemoglobin has properties like T-state hemoglobin. Thus, a given amount of NO will tend to reduce polymerization less than the same amount of O_2.

Another important factor to consider is that iron nitrosylation of hemoglobin through NO inhalation or other means is not likely to ever yield a significant fraction of the total hemoglobin bound to NO (<0.02%[116]). The best effect of any direct antipolymerizing agent would be to make HbS molecules disappear in the red cell. When an antisickling/antipolymerization agent binds to a hemoglobin molecule and converts it from one that enters the polymer phase (like T-state HbS) to one that does not or is less likely to (like R-state HbS), that HbS molecule still contributes to polymerization by its affects on crowding – increasing the activity coefficient. The fact that there is so much hemoglobin in the red blood cell (~10 mmol/L) and that one needs to achieve a conversion of so much HbS to a type that does not polymerize (at least a few percent to have any effect) has been a great challenge for the development of antisickling agents. Because so little iron nitrosylation can be achieved and that it does not have a great sparing effect provide very strong arguments against the idea that NO binding to the heme will benefit patients by reducing polymerization.

Controversy over the effect on polymerization of S-nitrosation of the β-93 cysteine by nitrosonium (one electron oxidation of NO) is also present. Several studies have shown that ligands that bind the β-93 cysteine stabilize the R-state and thereby increase O_2 affinity and increase HbS solubility or reduce polymerization.[117,118] In particular, Bonaventura and colleagues reported that incubation of S-nitrosated cysteine with HbS, which forms SNO–hemoglobin, decreases polymerization.[118] This result has been challenged in studies, using NEM as a model for NO^+. A single modification at the β-93 cysteine, as in SNO-hemoglobin, actually enhanced polymerization and modification at α-104 cysteine stabilized the R-state and decreased polymerization.[119] It was argued that previous studies in which higher O_2 affinities and reduced polymerization were observed actually involved modifications both at the β-93 and the α-104 cysteines.[119] Nevertheless, the work by Bonaventura and colleagues included careful analysis of the sites of modification by using mass spectrometry[118] and the sites of modification were also examined in other studies of polymerization.[117] They did find that an excess of CysNO (10:1) leads to some modification of the α-104 residue in addition to β-93, but their examinations of effects on polymerization did not include these samples. The effect of chemical modification at the β-93 cysteine was also studied using hemoglobin mutations and the increase in O_2 affinity was confirmed[120] Exposure of HbCO crystals to NO gas leads to S-nitrosation, probably via the intermediacy of N_2O_3, and x-ray diffraction has shown that only the β-93 cysteines are nitrosated.[121] Although the recent study stating otherwise calls for further investigation,[119] the preponderance of data at this time suggest that nitrosation occurs primarily at the β-93 cysteine unless the protein is denatured, or has formed a large percentage of dimers, and that SNO–HbS is more soluble than unmodified HbS. That being said, as in the case of HbS with NO bound at the heme, the small amounts of SNO–hemoglobin achievable in vivo (without deleterious effects), combined with the null effect on crowding, makes SNO–hemoglobin formation an unlikely means to effectively reduce polymerization in vivo.

Copolymerization of HbS with Other Hemoglobins

Individuals with sickle cell trait (HbAS) are rarely ill (chapter 22) and very high levels of HbF benefit individuals with sickle cell anemia.[122–126] The sparing effect of HbA and

HbF and the degree to which they reduce polymerization depend on the extent to which they enter the polymer phase or copolymerize with HbS.[59,127,128] Tetramers of HbF, HbA_2 ($\alpha_2\delta_2$), and HbA do not enter the polymer phase. The sparing effects of HbF and HbA_2 are enhanced by their ability to form hybrids with HbS. Hybrids form by the dimerization of hemoglobin wherein the tetramer, particularly when in the R-state, breaks into two $\alpha\beta$ dimers. The dissociation constant for dimerization is low when compared with the concentration of hemoglobin under physiological conditions (~1 μmol/L) but because the tetramers are constantly dimerizing and coming back together, an equilibrium mixture consisting of a binomial distribution of hybrids is obtained in less than a minute when different hemoglobins are mixed.[59] Hybrids of HbS with HbF and HbA_2, in which one dimer is from HbS and one is from HbF or HbA_2, do not enter the polymer phase so that replacing one HbS tetramer in a mixture with one HbF or HbA_2 tetramer can result in more than one hemoglobin tetramer being excluded from the polymer phase.[129–131] Hybrids of HbS and HbA enter the polymer phase with approximately half the frequency of HbS tetramers.[132–134] Thus, HbF and HbA_2 are more effective than HbA at decreasing polymerization.

Patients with HbAS have approximately 40% HbS and 60% HbA. In the absence of ligand like O_2 or CO used as a model for O_2, the solubility of 70% HbS and 30% HbF or HbA_2 was found to be equivalent to the solubility of a hemoglobin mixture from patients with HbAS.[128] It was also found that as hemoglobin saturation with CO increased, less HbF or HbA_2 was necessary to achieve the solubility of HbAS blood.[128] These data suggest that if one were to achieve 30% HbF or HbA_2 uniformly among erythrocytes, it would essentially alleviate all the symptoms of sickle cell anemia; however, HbA_2, because of its positive charge, could have deleterious affects (Chapter 7).

Kinetics of Polymerization

The kinetics of polymerization has been studied by taking a solution of HbS and rapidly changing the conditions so that the solubility is decreased. For example, the sample can be temperature jumped from 0°C to 37°C or HbCO can be converted to deoxyhemoglobin by photolysis. When this is done, observations of the kinetics of polymerization present an astounding result, whether by examining light scattering, calorimetry, birefringence or other indicators of polymer content. There is a long period of time when no polymer is detected, followed by relatively rapid growth in detected polymer.[59] This delay time before polymerization is detected has been described by an empirical equation,[59,135,136]

$$\frac{1}{t_d} = \lambda \left(\frac{c_0}{c_s}\right)^n, \qquad (6.5)$$

where t_d is the delay time, λ is a proportionality factor, and the exponent, n is found to be approximately as high as 30–40, but is significantly lower (15 or lower) when the hemoglobin concentration is very high. For studies in conditions where $n = 35$, and t_d is 1 minute, increasing the solubility by just 10% would increase the delay time to 28 minutes. This extreme dependence of the delay time on the supersaturation ratio, c_0/c_s or, more accurately, $\gamma_0 c_0/\gamma_s c_s$, is not only fascinating from a biophysical perspective, but also of great interest for its potential for treatment strategies whereby the delay time is increased by changing the solubility.[59]

Most phenomenon associated with polymerization kinetics can be understood in terms of the double nucleation theory (Fig. 6.9[82,83,137]). This mechanism is based on the idea that the aggregation of HbS monomers (a hemoglobin tetramer) into a polymer is initially thermodynamically unfavorable but becomes more favorable as the aggregate grows. The smallest aggregate for which growth is thermodynamically favorable is called the critical nucleus. After the critical nucleus has formed, the polymer grows, most likely at its ends,[79,80] and heterogeneous nucleation can occur. Heterogeneous nucleation involves the formation of additional polymer on the surface of an existing one. As the polymerization reaction proceeds, more surface area becomes available for heterogeneous nucleation to occur and the polymer phase grows exponentially. Because homogeneous nucleation is a rare event compared with heterogeneous nucleation, a network of polymers or a domain forms from each critical nucleus. The accuracy of the double-nucleation theory has been dramatically confirmed by observations of polymerization using DIC microscopy (Fig. 6.8).[80]

The interpretation of the delay time for polymerization seen in many in vitro experiments has often been misconstrued as the time necessary for formation of the critical nucleus.[138] Both homogeneous and heterogeneous nucleation occur during the time period when no polymers are detected, but the amount of polymer is too small to be observed. Processes that grow exponentially can appear to have taken much longer to begin than they actually do (Fig. 6.10). The beginning of polymerization can be approximately described by the relation[138]

$$\text{Polymerization} \sim \frac{A}{2}\exp(Bt), \qquad (6.6)$$

where A and B are constants that depend on solution conditions. Figure 6.10 shows approximate progress curves based on this equation for two different HbS concentrations. Note that each curve appears to have a long period in which there is no polymer, but polymers are actually present throughout the entire time period plotted but the amounts are simply too small to observe. The delay time actually depends mostly on the constant B, which is dominated by the rate of heterogeneous nucleation.[138]

In microscopic situations, including red cells, where only a few if any nucleation events occur, the time before homogeneous nucleation does constitute part of the delay time.[138] The formation of an individual critical nucleus is a random event; an empirical equation like Equation 6.6

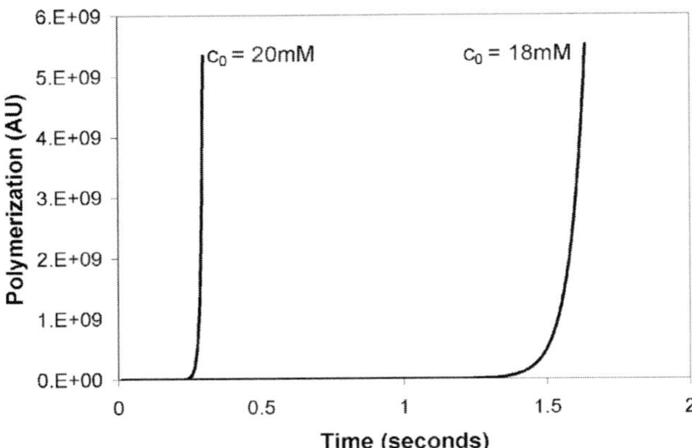

Figure 6.10. Polymerization progress curves. Each curve represents an estimation of the relative amount of polymer (in arbitrary units (AU)) vs. time for two concentrations of hemoglobin, 18 mM and 20 mM in heme. The amount of polymerization is plotted as $\frac{A}{2}$ exp(Bt) (138) where A and B were obtained by visual inspection of previously determined values (Figure 8 of (138)). Note that each curve displays a delay time, but there is polymer present throughout the time courses plotted. In addition, a small change in the total hemoglobin concentration, c_0, results in a large change in the delay time. Note that this figure is shown for pedagogical purposes to demonstrate the nature of exponential processes and it fails in quantitative aspects.

could only predict the average time for the formation of a critical nucleus. In these cases, the observed delay time will depend both on the time to form the critical nucleus and on the time for there to be enough polymer to give a large enough signal, for example, by light scattering. For a single set of conditions, the observed delay time can vary by almost an order of magnitude, from approximately 1–10 seconds, due to the stochastic nature of homogeneous nucleation.[138,139]

The rate of homogeneous nucleation was greatly enhanced by the presence of membranes from sickle erythrocytes, but much less so, if at all, from normal red cell membranes, but the cause of this is still unclear.[140] In a radical new development, it has been proposed that homogeneous nucleation is a two-step process involving dense metastable liquid clusters that serve as precursors for ordered HbS homogeneous nuclei.[94] It was further suggested that the formation of these dense liquid clusters is the rate-limiting step in homogeneous nucleation so that new treatment strategies might be developed around delaying or preventing their formation.[94]

Additional progress has been made in understanding the kinetics of heterogeneous nucleation, particularly with respect to the effects of crowding.[97,141] Improvements in the theory of how crowding affects heterogeneous nucleation have made it possible to predict kinetics in mixtures of nonpolymerizing hemoglobins.[141] The effect of crowding on the rates of polymer growth are great, where addition of 50% crowding agent increases exponential growth by a factor of 10,000–100,000.[97]

Crowding has also recently been found to play an unexpected role in reducing the effects of HbF on polymerization kinetics.[142] Generally, factors that reduce the solubility are expected to reduce the rate of polymerization as well, consistent with the empirical relation relating the delay time to the supersaturation ratio (Equation 6.5). As discussed in the context of NO binding to hemoglobin, however, one needs to account for the fact that a nonpolymerizing hemoglobin tetramer, whether it is R-state HbS or a T-state HbF/HbS hybrid, still contributes to polymerization by increasing the activity coefficient due to crowding. It has recently been determined that HbF/HbS exchange does not affect HbS polymerization kinetics as much as previously thought due to the fact that the HbF contributes to crowding.[142] Given that there is no reason to doubt the experiments on the sparing effect of HbF on solubility, these data suggest that the empirical relation given in Equation 6.4 needs to take activities into account and the exponential factor, n, gets significantly smaller in crowded solutions. The therapeutic goal of 30% HbF, based on its effects on solubility, remains reasonable. Interestingly, when examining the amounts of HbF formed by hydroxyurea treatment (Chapter 30) and the measured intracellular delay times,[143] an unknown effect of hydroxyurea on polymerization kinetics other than increased HbF production is implicated.[142]

HbS Polymer Melting

Less effort has gone into the study of HbS depolymerization, or melting, than has gone into the study of polymerization, but recent progress has been made. The mechanism and kinetics of HbS polymer melting are important in determining how much polymer, if any, persists in tissues after sickle erythrocytes are reoxygenated. As only T-state or deoxygenated HbS polymerizes, the delay time might prevent some or many red cells from causing vasoocclusion if it is long enough for significant polymerization to be delayed until the cells reach large veins and/or the lungs. If melting is slow, however, a significant amount of polymer present in the lungs could enter hypoxic tissues and any benefit from a delay time would be lost or diminished. Most early studies have found that when the solubility of HbS is quickly raised above the concentration of HbS by lowering the temperature or introducing O_2 or CO quickly, polymer melting proceeds without a delay time and is rather slow, on the order of seconds–minutes.[135,144–146]

Recent studies have done much to define the kinetics and mechanism of polymer melting.[80,147–152] Polymer melting can occur at both the sides and the ends of the polymer (Fig. 6.11).[148] On the ends, HbS tetramers constantly come on and off the polymer. During melting, the rate of tetramer dissociation is faster than the rate of association, so the fibers get shorter. The rate of dissociation or association depends on the quaternary state and hence ligation state. If tetramers on the fiber ends bind CO or O_2 (dark spheres in Fig. 6.11) they are likely to dissociate faster. Several studies have provided evidence for direct binding of CO to the polymers during melting.[148,150–152] R-state tetramers do not

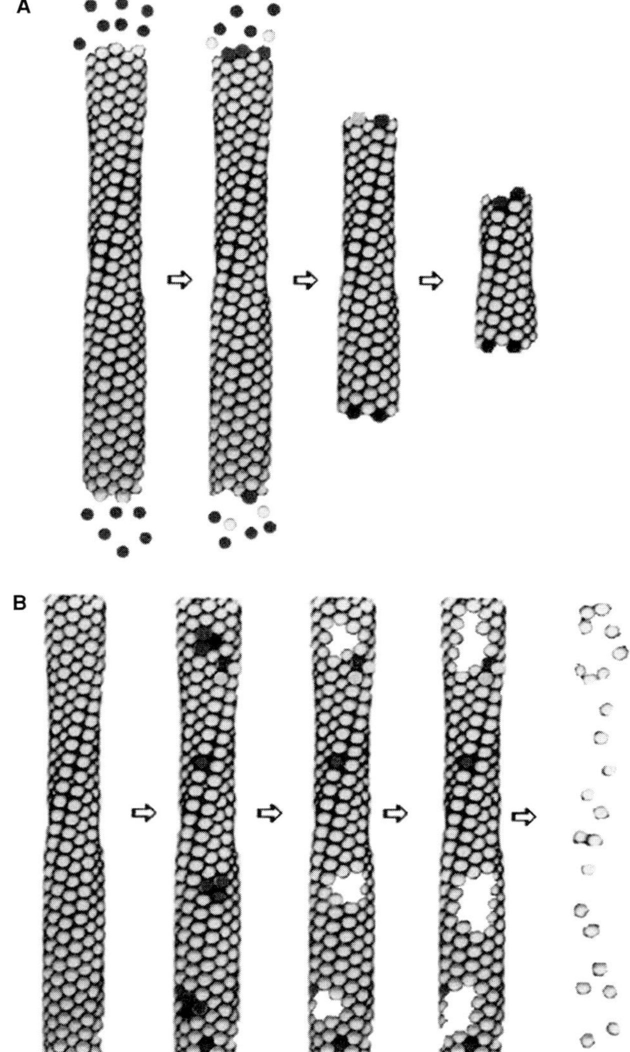

Figure 6.11. Mechanisms of HbS polymer melting. **(a)** Ends melting. Polymers get shorter at the ends through unligated (T-state) tetramers (open spheres) coming off the polymer and becoming ligated (binding CO or O_2, filled spheres) or by enhanced dissociation of ligated HbS tetramers on the fiber. **(b)** Side melting. Ligation of HbS tetramers on the sides of polymers can nucleate holes, which leads to rapid depolymerization. (From Figure 10 of ref. 148.)

effectively enter the polymer phase so that polymer melting at the ends can occur either through CO binding directly to tetramers at the fiber ends and expediting their dissociation or through binding to solution phase HbS tetramers and preventing their association.[148,150] When ligand pressure of CO, or presumably O_2, is higher, rapid melting can also occur at the sides of fibers (Fig. 6.11).[148] Here, it is believed that ligand binding to HbS tetramers at the surface of fibers can nucleate a hole in the fiber that leads to breaking it up and increases the rate of melting through increasing the number of polymer ends.[147,148] The rate of polymer melting has recently been addressed by examination of changes in red cell deformability upon oxygenation.[149] This rate is likely to be limited by the rate of HbS polymer melting because polymer content is related to poor deformability. It was concluded that the rate is sometimes likely to be too small for all existing polymers to melt upon reoxygenation in the lungs so that there will be some persistence of polymer during circulation.[149]

HbS Polymerization in Red Blood Cells

Polymerization of HbS in sickle erythrocytes is likely to have the same structure, thermodynamics, and kinetics as in solution, and except for modulation of ion content and hydration, which can have a large effect on polymerization as it greatly affects c_0, the red blood cell can be viewed as a "flexible microcuvette."[59] Using CO photolysis, it was determined that polymerization progresses with characteristic delay times and, based on theoretical analysis, it was proposed that most cells never contain polymer, because the delay time is long enough to allow cells to complete a cycle in the circulation, returning to the lungs before polymerization begins.[144] The relative importance of the delay time has been questioned based on careful studies using nuclear magnetic resonance to determine intracellular polymerization at various O_2 tensions.[127,153–156] In these studies, polymers were detected even when the hemoglobin O_2 saturation was above 90%.[154] Crowding of hemoglobin in the red blood cell is responsible for polymerization at these high O_2 tensions. In this model, the amount of polymer present in vivo for most cells is determined by the intracellular hemoglobin content and the O_2 tension along the circulation and is not rate limited by polymerization kinetics.[127,155]

The relative importance to pathology of the polymerization kinetics compared with polymer content defined by equilibrium conditions has been the subject of some controversy. It is currently not clear how much polymer needs to persist through the pulmonary circulation for a measurable delay time to be observed. In addition, although early work reported well-defined transit times through various parts of the circulation, more recent work has found that such times vary a great deal; 0.03–14.5 seconds was measured for the transit time in the pulmonary capillaries.[157] Importantly, it is also not known how much polymer is necessary to cause red cell damage or to contribute to microvascular occlusion. As polymerization is the primary cause of sickle cell disease, it must eventually lead to increased fragility and hemolysis, increased vascular adherence, disturbed hemostasis and all the other pathology associated with sickle cell disease. The degree of polymerization necessary to lead to these pathological consequences is not known. This author believes that polymerization kinetics (involving a delay time) plays a role in determining polymer content in some cells, whereas in others the amount of polymer for a given cell is defined by the oxygen tension at each point in the circulation. In any case, reducing polymerization by increasing HbS solubility is sure to effectively treat patients.

REFERENCES

1. Perutz MF. Structure and mechanism of hemoglobin. *Br Med Bull.* 1976;32(3):195–208.
2. Antonini E, Brunori M. Hemoglobin and Myoglobin in their Reactions with Ligands. Amsterdam, North Holland Publishing Co.; 1971.
3. Bohr C, Hasselbalch K, Krogh A. Ueber einen in biologischer Beziehung wichtigen Einfluss, den die Kohlensaeurespannung des Blutes auf dessen Sauerstoffbindung ubt. *Skand Arch Physiol.* 1904;16:402–412.
4. Monod J, Wyman J, Changeux J-P. On the nature of allosteric transitions: a plausible model. *J Mol Biol.* 1965;12:88–112.
5. Perutz MF. Stereochemistry of cooperative effects in haemoglobin. *Nature.* 1970;228:726–739.
6. Perutz MF, Wilkinson AJ, Paoli M, Dodson GG. The stereochemical mechanism of the cooperative effects in hemoglobin revisited. *Ann Rev Biophys Biomolec Struct.* 1998;27: 1–34.
7. Eaton WA, Henry ER, Hofrichter J, Mozzarelli A. Is cooperative oxygen binding by hemoglobin really understood? *Nat Struct Biol.* 1999;6(4):351–358.
8. Gibson QH. The photochemical formation of a quickly reacting form of haemoglobin. *Biochem J.* 1959;71:293–303.
9. Moore EG, Gibson QH. Cooperativity in dissociation of nitric-oxide from hemoglobin. *J Biol Chem.* 1976;251(9): 2788–2794.
10. Ivano Bertini HBG, Stiefel EI, Valentine JS. *Biological Inorganic Chemistry Structure and Reactivity.* Sausalito, CA: University Science Books; 2007.
11. Patel RP, Hogg N, Spencer NY, Kalyanaraman B, Matalon S, Darley-Usmar VM. Biochemical characterization of human S-nitrosohemoglobin – Effects on oxygen binding and transnitrosation. *J Biol Chem.* 1999;274(22):15487–15492.
12. Edelstein SJ. Cooperative interactions of hemoglobin. *Annu Rev Biochem.* 1975;44:209–232.
13. Mathews AJ, Olson JS. Assignment of rate constants for O2 and CO binding to alpha-subunit and beta-subunit within R-state and T-state human hemoglobin. *Methods Enzymol.* 1994;232:363–386.
14. Fetler BK, Simplaceanu V, Ho C. H-1-Nmr investigation of the oxygenation of hemoglobin in intact human red-blood-cells. *Biophys J.* 1995;68(2):681–693.
15. Brunori M, Coletta M, Dicera E. A cooperative model for ligand-binding to biological macromolecules as applied to oxygen carriers. *Biophys Chem.* 1986;23(3–4):215–222.
16. Henry ER, Bettati S, Hofrichter J, Eaton WA. A tertiary two-state allosteric model for hemoglobin. *Biophys Chem.* 2002;98(1–2):149–164.
17. Yonetani T, Park S, Tsuneshige A, Imai K, Kanaori K. Global allostery model of hemoglobin – Modulation of O-2 affinity, cooperativity, and Bohr effect by heterotropic allosteric effectors. *J Biol Chem.* 2002;277(37):34508–34520.
18. Ackers GK, Holt JM, Huang YW, Grinkova Y, Klinger AL, Denisov I. Confirmation of a unique intra-dimer cooperativity in the human hemoglobin alpha(1)beta(1) half-oxygenated intermediate supports the symmetry rule model of allosteric regulation. *Proteins.* Suppl. 4, 2000:23–43.
19. Yonetani T, Tsuneshige A, Zhou YX, Chen XS. Electron paramagnetic resonance and oxygen binding studies of alpha-nitrosyl hemoglobin – A novel oxygen carrier having no-assisted allosteric functions. *J Biol Chem.* 1998;273(32): 20323–20333.
20. Silva MM, Rogers PH, Arnone A. A 3rd quaternary structure of human hemoglobin-a at 1.7-a-angstrom resolution. *J Biol Chem.* 1992;267(24):17248–17256.
21. Safo MK, Abraham DJ. The enigma of the liganded hemoglobin end state: a novel quaternary structure of human carbonmonoxy hemoglobin. *Biochemistry.* 2005;44(23): 8347–8359.
22. Tame H. JR. What is the true structure of liganded haemoglobin? *Trends Biochem Sci.* 1999;24(10):372–377.
23. Lukin JA, Ho C. The structure-function relationship of hemoglobin in solution at atomic resolution. *Chem Rev.* 2004;104(3):1219–1230.
24. Lukin JA, Kontaxis G, Simplaceanu V, Yuan Y, Bax A, Ho C. Quaternary structure of hemoglobin in solution. *Proc Natl Acad Sci USA.* 2003;100(2):517–520.
25. Gong QG, Simplaceanu V, Lukin JA, Giovannelli JL, Ho NT, Ho C. Quaternary structure of carbonmonoxyhemoglobins in solution: structural changes induced by the allosteric effector inositol hexaphosphate. *Biochemistry.* 2006;45(16):5140–5148.
26. Sahu SC, Simplaceanu V, Gong Q, et al. Insights into the Solution Structure of Human Deoxyhemoglobin in Absence and Presence of an Allosteric Effector. *Biochem Cell Biol.* 2007;46(35):9973–9980.
27. Cabrales P, Tsai AG, Intaglietta M. Hemorrhagic shock resuscitation with carbon monoxide saturated blood. *Resuscitation.* 2007;72(2):306–318.
28. Mannaioni PF, Vannacci A, Masini E. Carbon monoxide: the bad and the good side of the coin, from neuronal death to anti-inflammatory activity. *Inflamm Res.* 2006;55(7):261–273.
29. Ryter SW, Choi AMK. Therapeutic applications of carbon monoxide in lung disease. *Curr Opin Pharmacol.* 2006;6(3): 257–262.
30. Morse D, Choi AMK. Heme oxygenase-1 – From bench to bedside. *Am J Resp Crit Care.* 2005;172(6):660–670.
31. Ignarro LJ, Buga GM, Wood KS, Byrns RE, Chaudhuri G. Endothelium-derived relaxing factor produced and released from artery and vein is nitric-oxide. *Proc Natl Acad Sci USA.* 1987;84(24):9265–9269.
32. Ignarro LJ. *Nitric Oxide Biology and Pathobiology.* San Diego: Academic Press; 2000.
33. Sharma VS, Ranney HM. Dissociation of NO from nitrosylhemoglobin. *J Biol Chem.* 1978;253(18):6467–6472.
34. Hille R, Olson JS, Palmer G. Spectral transitions of nitrosyl hemes during ligand-binding to hemoglobin. *J Biol Chem.* 1979;254(23):2110–2120.
35. Kon H. Paramagnetic resonance study of nitric oxide hemoglobin. *J Biol Chem.* 1968;243:4350–4357.
36. Szabo A, Perutz MF. Equilibrium between 6-coordinated and 5-coordinated hemes in nitrosylhemoglobin – Interpretation of electron-spin resonance-spectra. *Biochemistry.* 1976;15(20):4427–4428.
37. Huang TH. Nmr-studies of the quaternary structure and heterogeneity of nitrosylhemoglobin and methemoglobin. *J Biol Chem.* 1979;254(22):1467–74.
38. Xu XL, Lockamy VL, Chen KJ, et al. Effects of iron nitrosylation on sickle cell hemoglobin solubility. *J Biol Chem.* 2002;277(39):36787–36792.

39. Azizi F, Kielbasa JE, Adeyiga AM, et al. Rates of nitric oxide dissociation from hemoglobin. *Free Rad Biol Med.* 2005;39: 145–151.
40. Cassoly R, Gibson QH. Conformation, co-operativity and ligand-binding in human hemoglobin. *J Mol Biol.* 1975; 91(3):301–313.
41. Hille R, Palmer G, Olson JS. Chain equivalence in reaction of nitric-oxide with hemoglobin. *J Biol Chem.* 1977;252(1):403–405.
42. Gow AJ, Luchsinger BP, Pawloski JR, Singel DJ, Stamler JS. The oxyhemoglobin reaction of nitric oxide. *Proc Natl Acad Sci USA.* 1999;96(16):9027–9032.
43. Huang Z, Louderback JG, Goyal M, Azizi F, King SB, Kim-Shapiro DB. Nitric oxide binding to oxygenated hemoglobin under physiological conditions. *Biochim Biophys Acta.* 2001;1568(3):252–260.
44. Joshi MS, Ferguson TB, Han TH, et al. Nitric oxide is consumed, rather than conserved, by reaction with oxyhemoglobin under physiological conditions. *Proc Natl Acad Sci USA.* 2002;99(16):10341–10346.
45. Morris RJ, Gibson QH. The role of diffusion in limiting the rate of ligand-binding to hemoglobin. *J Biol Chem.* 1980; 255(17):8050–8053.
46. Huang Z, Ucer KB, Murphy T, Williams RT, King SB, Kim-Shapiro DB. Kinetics of nitric oxide binding to R-state hemoglobin. *Biochem Biophys Res Commun.* 2002;292(4): 812–818.
47. Huang KT, Huang Z, Kim-Shapiro DB. Nitric oxide red blood cell membrane permeability at high and low oxygen tension. *Nitric Oxide.* 2006;16:209–216.
48. Grubina R, Huang Z, Shiva S, et al. Concerted nitric oxide formation and release from the simultaneous reactions of nitrite with deoxy- and oxyhemoglobin. *J Biol Chem.* 2007; 282(17):12916–12927.
49. Kinoshita A, Nakayama Y, Kitayama T, Tomita M. Simulation study of methemoglobin reduction in erythrocytes – Differential contributions of two pathways to tolerance to oxidative stress. *FEBS J.* 2007;274(6):1449–1458.
50. Mansouri A, Lurie AA. Concise review – Methemoglobinemia. *Am J Hematol.* 1993;42(1):7–12.
51. Jaffe ER. Methemoglobinemia. *Clin Hematol.* 1981;10(1):99–122.
52. Nagababu E, Ramasamy S, Abernethy DR, Rifkind JM. Active nitric oxide produced in the red cell under hypoxic conditions by deoxyhemoglobin-mediated nitrite reduction. *J Biol Chem.* 2003;278(47):46349–46356.
53. Angelo M, Singel DJ, Stamler JS. An S-nitrosothiol (SNO) synthase function of hemoglobin that utilizes nitrite as a substrate. *Proc Natl Acad Sci USA.* 2006;103(22):8366–8371.
54. Marti MA, Crespo A, Bari SE, Doctorovich FA, Estrin DA. QM-MM study of nitrite reduction by nitrite reductase of Pseudomonas aeruginosa. *J Phys Chem B.* 2004;108(46):18073–18080.
55. Cooper CE. Nitric oxide and iron proteins. *Biochim Biophys Acta.* 1999;1411(2–3):290–309.
56. Fernandez BO, Ford PC. Nitrite catalyzes ferriheme protein reductive nitrosylation. *J Am Chem Soc.* 2003;125(35):10510–10511.
57. Huang KT, Keszler A, Patel N, et al. The reaction between nitrite and deoxyhemoglobin: reassessment of reaction kinetics and stoichiometry. *J Biol Chem.* 2005;280:31126–31131.
58. Gladwin MT, Schechter AN, Kim-Shapiro DB, et al. The emerging biology of the nitrite anion. *Nat Chem Biol.* 2005; 1:308–314.
59. Eaton WA, Hofrichter J. Sickle cell hemoglobin polymerization. *Adv Protein Chem.* 1990;40:63–279.
60. Hirsch RE, Juszczak LJ, Fataliev NA, Friedman JM, Nagel RL. Solution-active structural alterations in liganded hemoglobins C (beta 6 Glu right-arrow Lys) and S (beta 6 Glu right-arrow Val). *J Biol Chem.* 1999;274(20):13777–13782.
61. Allen DW, Wyman J. Equilibre de l'hémoglobine de drépanoctose avec l'oxygène. *Rev Hematol.* 1954;9:155–157.
62. Penneley RR, Noble RW. Functional identity of hemoglobin S and A in the absence of polymerization. In: Caughey WS, ed. *Biochemical and Chemical Aspects of Hemoglobin Abnormalities.* New York: Academic Press; 1978:401–411.
63. Deyoung A, Noble RW. Oxygen binding to sickle cell hemoglobin. *Methods Enzymol.* 1981;76:792–805.
64. Shapiro DB, Paquette SJ, Esquerra RM, et al. Nanosecond absorption study of kinetics associated with carbonmonoxide rebinding to hemoglobin-S and hemoglobin-C following ligand photolysis. *Biochem Biophys Res Commun.* 1994;205(1):154–160.
65. Eaton WA, Hofrichter J. Hemoglobin S gelation and sickle cell disease. *Blood.* 1987;70(5):1245–1266.
66. Eaton WA, Hofrichter J. Sickle cell hemoglobin polymerization. *Adv Protein Chem.* 1990;40:63–279.
67. Harrington JP. Alteration of redox stability of hemoglobins A and S by biological buffers. *Comp Biochem Physiol B Biochem Mol Biol.* 1998;119(2):305–309.
68. Hebbel RP, Morgan WT, Eaton JW, Hedlund BE. Accelerated autooxidation and heme loss due to instability of sickle hemoglobin. *Proc Natl Acad Sci USA.* 1988;85(1):237–241.
69. Dykes GW, Crepeau RH, Edelstein SJ. Three-dimensional reconstruction of 14-filament fibers of hemoglobin S. *J Mol Biol.* 1979;130:451–472.
70. Harrington DL, Adachi K, Royer, WE. The high resolution crystal structure of deoxyhemoglobin S. *J Mol Biol.* 1997;272:398–407.
71. Dykes GW, Crepeau RH, Edelstein SJ. Three dimensional reconstruction of the fibers of sickle cell hemoglobin. *Nature.* 1978;272:506–510.
72. Sokolov L, Mukerji I. Structure of sickle cell hemoglobin fibers probed with UV resonance Raman spectroscopy. *J Phys Chem B.* 2000;104(46):10835–10843.
73. Roufberg A, Ferrone FA. A model for the sickle hemoglobin fiber using both mutation sites. *Protein Sci.* 2000;9(5):1031–1034.
74. Cretegny I, Edelstein SJ. Double strand packing in hemoglobin-S fibers. *J Mol Biol.* 1993;230(3):733–738.
75. Watowich SJ, Gross LJ, Josephs R. Analysis of the intermolecular contacts within sickle hemoglobin fibers – Effect of site-specific substitutions, fiber pitch, and double-strand disorder. *J Struct Biol.* 1993;111(3):161–179.
76. Mu XQ, Makowski L, Magdoff-Fairchild B. Analysis of the stability of hemoglobin S double strands. *Biophys J.* 1998;74(1): 655–668.
77. Turner MS, Briehl RW, Ferrone FA, Josephs R. Twisted protein aggregates and disease: The stability of sickle hemoglobin fibers. *Phys Rev Lett.* 2003;90(12).

78. Turner MS, Briehl RW, Wang JC, Ferrone FA, Josephs R. Anisotropy in sickle hemoglobin fibers from variations in bending and twist. *J Mol Biol.* 2006;357(5):1422–1427.
79. Samuel RE, Salmon ED, Briehl RW. Nucleation and growth of fibers and gel formation in sickle-cell hemoglobin. *Nature.* 1990;345(6278):833–835.
80. Briehl RW. Nucleation, fiber growth and melting, and domain formation and structure in sickle-cell hemoglobin gels. *J Mol Biol.* 1995;245(5):710–723.
81. Jones CW, Wang JC, Ferrone FA, Briehl RW, Turner MS. Interactions between sickle hemoglobin fibers. *Faraday Discuss.* 2003;123:221–236.
82. Ferrone FA, Hofrichter J, Eaton WA. Kinetics of sickle hemoglobin polymerization. 1. Studies using temperature-jump and laser photolysis techniques. *J Mol Biol.* 1985;183(4): 591–610.
83. Ferrone FA, Hofrichter J, Eaton WA. Kinetics of sickle hemoglobin polymerization. 2. A double nucleation mechanism. *J Mol Biol.* 1985;183(4):611–631.
84. Mirchev R, Ferrone FA. The structural link between polymerization and sickle cell disease. *J Mol Biol.* 1997;265(5):475–479.
85. Rotter MA, Kwong S, Briehl RW, Ferrone FA. Heterogeneous nucleation in sickle hemoglobin: experimental validation of a structural mechanism. *Biophys J.* 2005;89(4):2677–2684.
86. McDade WA, Carragher B, Miller CA, Josephs R. On the assembly of sickle hemoglobin fascicles. *J Mol Biol.* 1989; 206(4):637–649.
87. Wang JC, Turner MS, Agarwal G, et al. Micromechanics of isolated sickle cell hemoglobin fibers: bending moduli and persistence lengths. *J Mol Biol.* 2002;315(4):601–612.
88. Briehl RW, Guzman AE. Fragility and structure of hemoglobin S fibers and gels and their consequences for gelation kinetics and rheology. *Blood.* 1994;83(2):573–579.
89. Samuel RE, Guzman AE, Briehl RW. Hemoglobin-S polymerization and gelation under shear. 2. The joint concentration and shear dependence of kinetics. *Blood.* 1993;82(11):3474–3481.
90. Briehl RW, Nikolopoulou P. Kinetics of hemoglobin S polymerization and gelation under shear. 1. Shape of the viscosity progress curve and dependence of delay time and reaction-rate on shear rate and temperature. *Blood.* 1993;81(9):2420–2428.
91. Kam Z, Hofrichter J. Quasi-elastic laser-light scattering from solutions and gels of hemoglobin-S. *Biophys J.* 1986;50(5): 1015–1020.
92. Galkin O, Nagel RL, Vekilov PG. The kinetics of nucleation and growth of sickle cell hemoglobin fibers. *J Mol Biol.* 2007; 365(2):425–439.
93. Galkin O, Chen K, Nagel RL, Hirsch RE, Vekilov PG. Liquid-liquid separation in solutions of normal and sickle cell hemoglobin. *Proc Natl Acad Sci USA.* 2002;99(13):8479–8483.
94. Galkin O, Pan W, Filobelo L, Hirsch R, Nagel R, Vekilov PG. Two-step mechanism of homogeneous nucleation of sickle cell hemoglobin polymers. *Biophys J.* 2007;93:902–913.
95. Pan WC, Galkin O, Filobelo L, Nagel RL, Vekilov PG. Metastable mesoscopic clusters in solutions of sickle-cell hemoglobin. *Biophys J.* 2007;92(1):267–277.
96. San Biagio PL, Palma MU. Solvent-induced forces and fluctuations: a novel comparison of human hemoglobin S and A. *Comm Theoretic Biol.* 1992;2:453–470.
97. Ferrone FA, Rotter MA. Crowding and the polymerization of sickle hemoglobin. *J Mol Recogn.* 2004;17(5):497–504.
98. Minton AP. Molecular crowding: Analysis of effects of high concentrations of inert cosolutes on biochemical equilibria and rates in terms of volume exclusion. *Methods Enzymol.* 1998;295:127–149.
99. Sunshine HR, Hofrichter J, Ferrone FA, Eaton WA. Oxygen binding by sickle-cell hemoglobin polymers. *J Mol Biol.* 1982;158(2):251–273.
100. Padlan EA, Love WE. Refined crystal-structure of deoxy-hemoglobin-S. 2. Molecular-interactions in the crystal. *J Biol Chem.* 1985;260(14):8280–82891.
101. Itano HA. Solubilities of naturally occurring mixtures of human hemoglobin. *Arch Biochem Biophys.* 1953;47:148–159.
102. Adachi K, Asakura T. Demonstration of a delay time during aggregation of diluted solutions of deoxyhemoglobin-S and hemoglobin charlem in concentrated phosphate buffer. *J Biol Chem.* 1978;253(19):6641–6643.
103. Adachi K, Asakura T. Nucleation-controlled aggregation of deoxyhemoglobin-S – possible difference in the size of nuclei in different phosphate concentrations. *J Biol Chem.* 1979;254(16):7765–7771.
104. Adachi K, Asakura T. Kinetics of the polymerization of hemoglobin in high and low phosphate buffers. *Blood Cells.* 1982;8(2):213–224.
105. Adachi K, Asakura T. Multiple nature of polymers of deoxyhemoglobin-S prepared by different methods. *J Biol Chem.* 1983;258(5):3045–3050.
106. Bookchin RM, Balazs T. Polymer structure and solubility of deoxyhemoglobin S in the presence of high concentrations of volume-excluding 70-kDa dextran – Effects of non-S hemoglobins and inhibitors. *J Biol Chem.* 1999;274(10):6689–6697.
107. Yohe ME, Sheffield KM, Mukerji I. Solubility of fluoromethemoglobin S: effect of phosphate and temperature on polymerization. *Biophys J.* 2000;78(6):3218–3226.
108. Fabry ME, Desrosiers L, Suzuka SM. Direct intracellular measurement of deoxygenated hemoglobin S solubility. *Blood.* 2001;98(3):883–884.
109. Roth EF, Bookchin RM, Nagel RL. Deoxyhemoglobin S gelation and insolubility at high ionic-strength are distinct phenomena. *J Lab Clin Med.* 1979;93(5):867–871.
110. Poillon WN, Bertles JF. Effects of ethanol and 3,4,-dihydro-2,2-dimethyl-2h-1-benzopyran-6-butyric acid on solubility of sickle hemoglobin. *Biochem Biophys Res Commun.* 1977;75(3):636–642.
111. Chen KJ, Ballas SK, Hantgan RR, Kim-Shapiro DB. Aggregation of normal and sickle hemoglobin in high concentration phosphate buffer. *Biophys J.* 2004;87(6):4113–4121.
112. Reiter CD, Wang XD, Tanus-Santos JE, et al. Cell-free hemoglobin limits nitric oxide bioavailability in sickle-cell disease. *Nat Med.* 2002;8(12):1383–1389.
113. Cokic VP, Smith RD, Beleslin-Cokic BB, Gladwin MT, Schechter AN. Nitric oxide donors induce fetal hemoglobin in human erythroid cells by a mechanism involving cGMP. *Blood Cell Mol Dis.* 2003;31(1):164–164.

114. Cokic VP, Smith RD, Beleslin-Cokic BB, et al. Hydroxyurea induces fetal hemoglobin by the nitric oxide-dependent activation of soluble guanylyl cyclase. *J Clin Invest.* 2003;111(2): 231–239.
115. Head CA, Brugnara C, MartinezRuiz R, et al. Low concentrations of nitric oxide increase oxygen affinity of sickle erythrocytes in vitro and in vivo. *J Clin Invest.* 1997;100(5):1193–1198.
116. Gladwin MT, Ognibene FP, Pannell LK, et al. Relative role of heme nitrosylation and beta-cysteine 93 nitrosation in the transport and metabolism of nitric oxide by hemoglobin in the human circulation. *Proc Natl Acad Sci USA.* 2000;97(18):9943–9948.
117. Garel MC, Domenget C, Caburimartin J, Prehu C, Galacteros F, Beuzard Y. Covalent binding of glutathione to hemoglobin. 1. Inhibition of hemoglobin S polymerization. *J Biol Chem.* 1986;261(31):4704–4709.
118. Bonaventura C, Godette G, Ferruzzi G, Tesh S, Stevens RD, Henkens R. Responses of normal and sickle cell hemoglobin to S-nitroscysteine: implications for therapeutic applications of NO in treatment of sickle cell disease. *Biophys Chem.* 2002;98(1–2):165–181.
119. Knee KM, Roden CK, Flory MR, Mukerji I. The role of beta 93 Cys in the inhibition of Hb S fiber formation. *Biophys Chem.* 2007;127(3):181–193.
120. Cheng Y, Shen TJ, Simplaceanu V, Ho C. Ligand binding properties and structural studies of recombinant and chemically modified hemoglobins altered at beta 93 cysteine. *Biochemistry.* 2002;41(39):11901–11913.
121. Chan NL, Rogers PH, Arnone A. Crystal structure of the S-nitroso form of liganded human hemoglobin. *Biochemistry.* 1998;37(47):16459–16464.
122. Brittenham GM, Schechter AN, Noguchi CT. Hemoglobin-S polymerization – primary determinant of the hemolytic and clinical severity of the sickling syndromes. *Blood.* 1985; 65(1):183–189.
123. Trabuchet G, Elion J, Baudot G, et al. Origin and spread of beta-globin gene-mutations in India, Africa, and Mediterranean – analysis of the 5′ flanking and intragenic sequences of beta-S and beta-C genes. *Hum Biol.* 1991;63(3):241–252.
124. Brittenham G, Lozoff B, Harris JW, Mayson SM, Miller A, Huisman THJ. Sickle-cell anemia and trait in southern India – further-studies. *Am J Hematol.* 1979;6(2):107–123.
125. Perrine RP, Pembrey ME, John P, Perrine S, Shoup F. Natural history of sickle-cell anemia in Saudi Arabs – study of 270 subjects. *Ann Intern Med.* 1978;88(1):1–6.
126. Brittenham G, Lozoff B, Harris JW, Sharma VS, Narasimhan S. Sickle-cell anemia and trait in a population of southern India. *Am J Hematol.* 1977;2(1):25–32.
127. Noguchi CT, Schechter AN. Sickle hemoglobin polymerization in solution and in cells. *Annu Rev Biophys Bio.* 1985; 14:239–263.
128. Poillon WN, Kim BC, Rodgers GP, Noguchi CT, Schechter AN. Sparing effect of hemoglobin-F and hemoglobin-A2 on the polymerization of hemoglobin-S at physiological ligand saturations. *Proc Natl Acad Sci USA.* 1993;90(11):5039–5043.
129. Goldberg MA, Husson MA, Bunn HF. Participation of hemoglobins A and F in polymerization of sickle hemoglobin. *J Biol Chem.* 1977;252(10):3414–3421.
130. Benesch RE, Edalji R, Benesch R, Kwong S. Solubilization of hemoglobin-S by other hemoglobins. *Proc Natl Acad Sci USA.* 1980;77(9):5130–5134.
131. Bertles JF, Rabinowitz R, Dobler J. Hemoglobin interaction: modification of solid phase composition in sickling phenomenon. *Science.* 1970;169:375–377.
132. Bunn HF, Noguchi CT, Hofrichter J, Schechter GP, Schechter AN, Eaton WA. Molecular and cellular pathogenesis of hemoglobin-Sc disease. *Proc Natl Acad Sci USA.* 1982;79(23): 7527–7531.
133. Sunshine HR, Hofrichter J, Eaton WA. Gelation of sickle-cell hemoglobin in mixtures with normal adult and fetal hemoglobins. *J Mol Biol.* 1979;133(4):435–467.
134. Cheetham RC, Huehns ER, Rosemeyer MA. Participation of hemoglobin-A, hemoglobin-F, hemoglobin-A2 and hemoglobin-C in polymerization of hemoglobin-S. *J Mol Biol.* 1979;129(1):45–61.
135. Hofrichter J. Kinetics and mechanism of deoxyhemoglobin-S gelation – new approach to understanding sickle-cell disease. *Proc Natl Acad Sci USA.* 1974;71:4864–4848.
136. Hofrichter J, Ross PD, Eaton WA. Supersaturation in sickle cell hemoglobin solutions. *Proc Natl Acad Sci USA.* 1976; 73(9):3035–3039.
137. Ferrone FA, Hofrichter J, Sunshine HR, Eaton WA. Kinetic studies on photolysis-induced gelation of sickle-cell hemoglobin suggest a new mechanism. *Biophys J.* 1980;32(1):361–380.
138. Ferrone FA. Polymerization and sickle cell disease: a molecular view. *Microcirculation.* 2004;11(2):115–128.
139. Cao ZQ, Ferrone FA. Homogeneous nucleation in sickle hemoglobin: stochastic measurements with a parallel method. *Biophys J.* 1997;72(1):343–52.
140. Aprelev A, Rotter MA, Etzion Z, Bookchin RM, Briehl RW, Ferrone FA. The effects of erythrocyte membranes on the nucleation of sickle hemoglobin. *Biophys J.* 2005;88(4):2815–2822.
141. Ferrone FA, Ivanova M, Jasuja R. Heterogeneous nucleation and crowding in sickle hemoglobin: an analytic approach. *Biophys J.* 2002;82(1):399–406.
142. Rotter M, Aprelev A, Adachi K, Ferrone FA. Molecular crowding limits the role of fetal hemoglobin in therapy for sickle cell disease. *J Mol Biol.* 2005;347(5):1015–1023.
143. Bridges KR, Barabino GD, Brugnara C, et al. A multiparameter analysis of sickle erythrocytes in patients undergoing hydroxyurea therapy. *Blood.* 1996;88(12):4701–4710.
144. Mozzarelli A, Hofrichter J, Eaton WA. Delay time of hemoglobin-S polymerization prevents most cells from sickling in vivo. *Science.* 1987;237(4814):500–506.
145. Moffat K, Gibson QH. The rates of polymerization and depolymerization of sickle cell hemoglobin. *Biochem Biophys Res Commun.* 1974;61:237–242.
146. Messer MJ, Hahn JA, Bradley TB. The kinetics of sickling and unsickling of red cells under physiological conditions: rheologic and ultrastructural correlations. In: Hercules JI, Cottam MR, Waterman MR, Schechter AN, eds. *Proceedings of the Symposium on Molecular and Cellular Aspects of Sickle Cell Disease.* Bethesda: National Institutes of Health; 1976:225–234.
147. Turner MS, Agarwal G, Jones CW, et al. Fiber depolymerization. *Biophys J.* 2006;91(3):1008–1013.

148. Agarwal G, Wang JC, Kwong S, et al. Sickle hemoglobin fibers: mechanisms of depolymerization. *J Mol Biol.* 2002;322(2): 395–412.
149. Huang Z, Hearne L, Irby CE, King SB, Ballas SK, Kim-Shapiro DB. Kinetics of increased deformability of deoxygenated sickle cells upon oxygenation. *Biophys J.* 2003;85(4):2374–2383.
150. Louderback JG, Ballas SK, Kim-Shapiro DB. Sickle hemoglobin polymer melting in high concentration phosphate buffer. *Biophys J.* 1999;76(4):2216–2222.
151. Louderback JG, Aroutiounian SK, Kerr WC, Ballas SK, Kim-Shapiro DB. Temperature and domain size dependence of sickle cell hemoglobin polymer melting in high concentration phosphate buffer. *Biophys Chem.* 1999;80(1):21–30.
152. Aroutiounian SK, Louderback JG, Ballas SK, Kim-Shapiro DB. Evidence for carbon monoxide binding to sickle cell polymers during melting. *Biophys Chem.* 2001;91(2):167–181.
153. Noguchi CT, Torchia DA, Schechter AN. C-13-Nmr quantitation of polymer in deoxyhemoglobin-S gels. *Proc Natl Acad Sci USA.* 1979;76(10):4936–4940.
154. Noguchi CT, Torchia DA, Schechter AN. Determination of deoxyhemoglobin-S polymer in sickle erythrocytes upon deoxygenation. *Proc Natl Acad Sci USA.* 1980;77(9):5487–5491.
155. Noguchi CT, Schechter AN. The intracellular polymerization of sickle hemoglobin and its relevance to sickle-cell disease. *Blood.* 1981;58(6):1057–1068.
156. Noguchi CT, Rodgers GP, Schechter AN. Intracellular polymerization – disease severity and therapeutic predictions. *Ann NY Acad Sci.* 1989;565:75–82.
157. Hogg JC, Coxson HO, Brumwell ML, et al. Erythrocyte and polymorphonuclear cell transit-time and concentration in human pulmonary capillaries. *J Appl Physiol.* 1994;77(4): 1795–1800.

7

Hemoglobins of the Embryo, Fetus, and Adult

Martin H. Steinberg and Ronald L. Nagel

INTRODUCTION

During development, humans express six different hemoglobin types, the products of eight different globin genes (Fig. 3.1, Chapter 3). Hb Gower I ($\zeta_2\varepsilon_2$), Gower II ($\alpha_2\varepsilon_2$), and Portland ($\zeta_2\gamma_2$) are found in the embryo, fetal hemoglobin (HbF; $\alpha_2\gamma_2$) is present mainly in the fetus but also in the embryo and adult, whereas HbA ($\alpha_2\beta_2$) and HbA_2 ($\alpha_2\delta_2$) are seen primarily in adults. All hemoglobins undergo posttranslational modifications forming minor hemoglobins. Globin genes are discussed in Chapter 3, hemoglobin switching in Chapter 5, and the structure and function of hemoglobin in Chapter 6 and. In this chapter we discuss the clinical and physiological attributes of HbF, HbA_2, embryonic hemoglobins, and their posttranslational modifications.

HEMOGLOBIN F

The observation that hemoglobin in newborns' erythrocytes was resistant to alkaline denaturation provided the first suggestion that a hemoglobin existed that differed from normal HbA.[1]

Structure of the γ-Globin Genes and γ-Globin

γ-Globin chains differ from β-globin chains in either 39 or 40 amino acid residues, depending on whether a glycine or alanine residue is present at γ136.[2] γ-Globin is the product of two nearly identical γ-globin genes. A glycine codon is present in the 5′ or $^G\gamma$ gene (*HBG2*) and an alanine codon characterizes the 3′, or $^A\gamma$ gene (*HBG1*). Also, a common polymorphism is found in the $^A\gamma$ gene, where threonine ($^A\gamma^T$) replaces isoleucine ($^A\gamma^I$) at codon γ75 (HbF-Sardinia). This striking similarity in protein sequence and structure of the γ-globin genes reflect their concerted evolution from gene duplication and gene conversion.[3] Gene conversion of the γ-globin genes might be an ongoing process during evolution as suggested by the analysis of chromosomes in which the Bantu haplotype is linked to the sickle cell (β^S) gene; a subgroup of these chromosomes has undergone a recent gene conversion, eliminating several sequence differences between the two γ-globin genes.[4] Selection could maintain the sequence of γ-globin chains and the structure of HbF. Because HbF is present throughout fetal life and functionally critical sequence abnormalities could affect fetal development, maintaining the normal gene sequence could be vitally important.

Protein Conformation: Of the 39–amino acid residue differences between γ- and β-globin chains, 22 are on the molecule's surface. Four critical differences are present in the $\alpha_1\beta_1$ area of contact (the packing contact) that dissociates only under extreme conditions. Two differences, γ112 thr (β112 cys) and γ130 trp (β130 tyr), in the $\alpha_1\gamma_1$ interface could contribute to HbF's resistance to alkaline and acid compared with HbA and provide the structural basis for measuring HbF by alkali denaturation. Sequence differences are not present in the $\alpha_1\beta_2$ area of contact (the sliding contact) that is the center of ligand-dependent conformational changes (Chapter 6). At position 116 in the $\alpha_1\beta_1$ interface, the γ-globin chain contains isoleucine and the β-globin chain contains histidine. Using recombinant β chains with γ chain substitutions, it was suggested that amino acid hydrophobicity at the G-18 position in non-α chains plays a key role in homotetramer, dimer, and monomer formation, which in turn plays a critical role in assembly of HbA and HbF tetramers. It was also suggested that stable dimer formation of γ-globin chains must not occur in vivo because this would inhibit association with α chains to form HbF.[5] The increased tetramer strength of HbF compared with HbA is only partially caused by the amino acid differences at the αβ interfaces and tetramer strengthening is also contributed to by the 18–amino acid N-terminal A helix of the γ-globin chain. Greater tetramer strength permits HbF to obtain O_2 from maternal HbA and might account for the resistance of fetal red cells to the malaria parasite, as it less readily dissociates into digestible dimers. Three amino acid differences at positions 1, 5, and 7 of the γ-globin chain account for practically all of the tetramer strength of HbF.[6]

Crystallographic studies of HbF at 2.5-Å resolution showed almost complete isomorphism between HbA and HbF with the sole difference in the N-terminal portion of the γ-globin chain.[7] This change increases the distance from 2,3 bisphosphoglycerate (2,3 BPG) inserted in the central cavity of the hemoglobin molecule to the γ2 histidine, possibly a secondary contributor to the reduction in 2,3 BPG effect exhibited by HbF.

Functional Properties

Erythrocytes of newborns have higher O_2 affinity than adult red cells, but in hemolysates, the O_2 affinity of HbF and HbA are identical. This suggests that HbF and HbA have

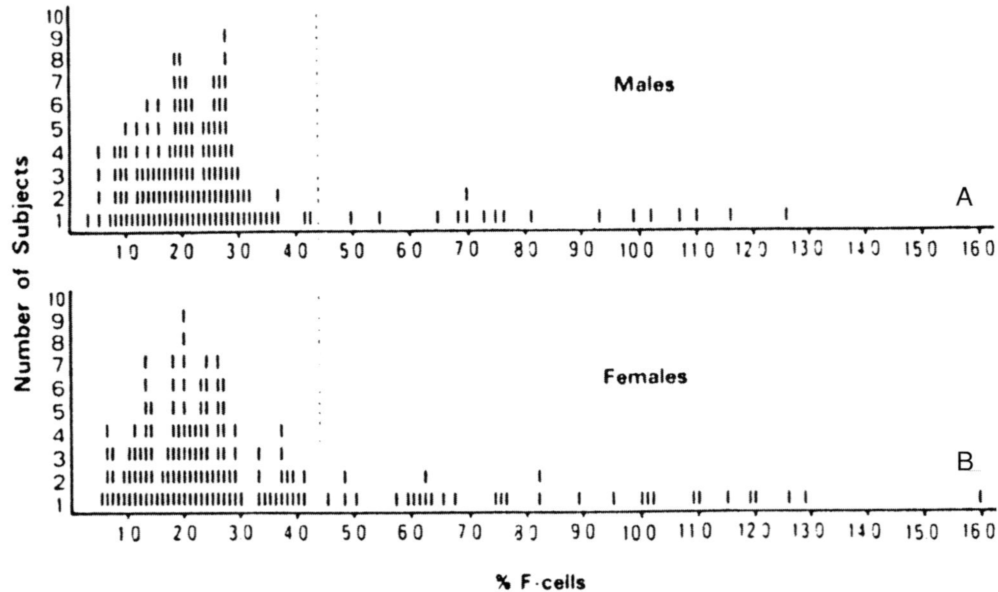

Figure 7.1. Distribution of F cells in 150 normal men and 150 normal women. The vertical broken lines are at 4.4% F cells.[12]

the same intrinsic O_2-binding properties but interact differentially with heterotopic modifiers of hemoglobin function. 2,3 BPG has decreased binding to HbF due to the replacement of β143 histidine, a phosphate-binding site in the central cavity, with a serine residue at γ143. Displacement of the N-terminal portion of the γ-globin chain alters phosphate binding with γ2 his; acetylation at the N terminus of the γ-globin chain also inhibits 2,3 BPG binding.

HbF-containing erythrocytes have an impaired Cl^- effect. Chloride binds at the 2,3 BPG binding site in the central cavity. At low NaCl concentrations, HbF has a lower affinity for O_2 than HbA. At higher Cl^- concentrations this difference disappears. This effect might be due to the diminution of positive charges in the central cavity with a reduction in the binding affinity for anions and destabilization of the T-state. Increased stability of the T-state induced by the absence of anion neutralizing positive charges would favor low ligand affinity.

CO_2 binding by HbF is drastically decreased. Fewer carbamates are formed at the N terminus at a wide range of pCO_2. The γ chain N terminus has a higher pKa than the β chain, making 90% of the site protonated at physiological conditions and unable to bind CO_2.

The alkaline Bohr effect (relation between high pH and ligand affinity) is increased 20% in HbF-containing red cells. This might be a Cl^- effect because at low anion concentration HbF and HbA have an identical Bohr effect, whereas the Bohr effect of HbF increases with the Cl^- concentration. A plausible explanation is that the binding of Cl^- at low pH at the β143 histidine stabilizes the R-state. The absence of this Cl^- site would reduce the low-pH Bohr effect because this condition favors the T-state. Consequently, the alkaline Bohr effect is favored in HbF.

When HbS was made "HbF-like" by substituting the four differences between HbA and HbF in the $\alpha_1\beta_1$ interface, the hybrid molecule had decreased binding with 2,3 BPG, much like HbF, although the central cavity was entirely HbA and dissociation into dimers was intermediate between HbA and HbF.[8] These results suggested that 2,3 BPG binding and dimerization are not simply dependent on the so-called critical residues, but that other long-range interactions could be important.

Physiology of HbF-containing Erythrocytes

O_2 loading in the fetal circulation is done via a liquid–liquid interface compared with the gas–liquid interface found postnatally. As fetal tissue has a high metabolic rate, O_2 loading rather than O_2 delivery might be limiting because it is likely that a blood/tissue pO_2 gradient exists. The high O_2 affinity of fetal erythrocytes promotes uptake of O_2 in the placenta. Despite the increased P_{50} and reduced 2,3 BPG response of HbF, O_2 delivery is compensated for by an increased Bohr effect. The pH of HbF increases when red cells pass through the intravillous spaces of the placenta because HbF releases CO_2. Fifty percent of O_2 delivery to tissues is accounted for by the increased Bohr effect. An increased Bohr effect also could explain the paradox of mothers with high-O_2 affinity hemoglobin variants who have neither pregnancy-related complications nor increased fetal morbidity (Chapter 24).[9] Heat release could also be an important function of HbF in the fetus.[10,11]

Modulation of HbF Levels

In healthy Japanese adults, the range of HbF and F cells was affected by sex and had a dominant X-linked pattern of inheritance (Fig. 7.1).[12] In sickle cell anemia, males had HbF of 6.1% ± 4.3% compared with 8.6% ± 7.5% in females,

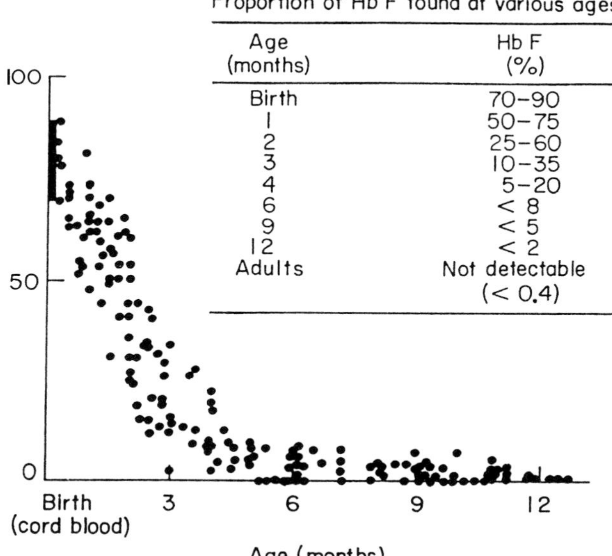

Proportion of Hb F found at various ages

Age (months)	Hb F (%)
Birth	70–90
1	50–75
2	25–60
3	10–35
4	5–20
6	< 8
9	< 5
12	< 2
Adults	Not detectable (< 0.4)

Figure 7.2. Fall in HbF concentration in normal infants from birth to age 1 year.

a result confirmed in other studies.[13–15] These observations were among the first to suggest that the modulation of HbF levels could occur from *trans*-acting factors and *cis*-acting elements. Many factors modulate the final concentration of HbF and these are discussed in detail in Chapters 5 and 27.[16,17]

Hemoglobin Switching

In normal newborns, it takes approximately 1 year for HbF to fall from 55% to 85% at birth to less than 1%, the HbF concentration that is present in most adults (Fig. 7.2). In early life a switch occurs in the expression of the $^{G}\gamma$- and $^{A}\gamma$-globin genes (Fig. 7.3). Most individuals have a decline in $^{G}\gamma$-globin chains in the first 3 months of life with a reciprocal rise in $^{A}\gamma$-globin chains, but a minority of infants maintains the neonatal pattern of γ-globin chain expression, especially when the *HBG2* −158 C-T SNP is present (Fig. 7.3).

Fetal cells decrease in number rapidly after birth as shown by the decrease in mean cell volume (MCV), an event followed by the progressive decrease in the number of F cells. Sickle cell anemia patients have a much-delayed switch from γ-globin gene expression to β^{S}-globin gene expression and from HbF to HbS. A stable HbF level in these patients might not be reached for 20 years.[18] A delay in the decline of γ-globin gene expression could be due to anemia because thalassemia trait individuals with very slight anemia also exhibit a delay in HbF switching, albeit much more moderate, than sickle cell anemia patients (Fig. 7.4).

Cellular Heterogeneity of HbF

Fetal Cells: HbF makes up close to 100% of the hemoglobin in fetal erythrocytes. During the first 10 days of life, hemoglobin synthesis decreases 10-fold from antenatal levels, and the bulk of this fall occurs in the first 2–3 postnatal days. Characteristics of neonatal erythrocytes are shown in Table 7.1.

F Cells: HbF is distributed unevenly among nonfetal or "adult" erythrocytes. The elution of HbF at low pH, leaving HbA that can be stained with acid hematoxylin, forms the basis for the acid–elution or "Betke" test for HbF. Boyer and coworkers[19,20] delineated the origins, genetics, and physiology of F cells.

By definition F cells contain measurable HbF, implying that the sensitivity of the method used for detecting HbF, of which there are many, will determine the number of F cells.[21] Relatively insensitive, the acid–elution method can detect a minimum of 5–6 pg of HbF per cell; radial immunoprecipitation methods can detect 3 pg of HbF per cell; flow cytometry, the most commonly used means of enumerating F cells, can detect cells with a HbF content of 6 pg.

Depending on the methodology used, Caucasian adult blood contained 1.7% ± 2.2% to 2.6% ± 1.6% F cells and normal African Americans had 2.8% ± 1.6% F cells. Establishing precisely the average concentration of HbF per F cell has been difficult because cells with HbF levels below the limits of detection will not be counted. Mature F cells contained an average of 4.4 ± 0.3 pg HbF. In African Americans with sickle cell anemia, the range of F cells was between 2% and 80% and the average HbF per F cell was 6.4 ± 1.6 pg. Patients with β thalassemia also have increased numbers of F cells.[22] In one study of sickle cell trait, in which the mean HbF level was 1.4% as determined by high-performance liquid chromatography (HPLC), F cells were 14.1% ± 7.5% (normal 4.5%).[23]

Rare, apparently normal individuals have more than 8% F cells in their blood. In most of these cases, one parent of the proband had similar numbers of F cells. Many of these high–F cell individuals have a form of nongene deletion hereditary persistence of fetal hemoglobin ([HPFH]; discussed later). F cell numbers are affected by age, although

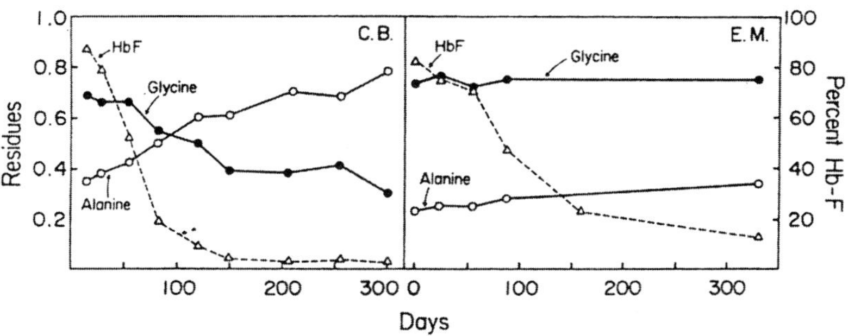

Figure 7.3 $^{G}\gamma$-globin chains are approximately 70% at birth and fall to approximately 40% at age 150 days when $^{A}\gamma$-globin chains become predominant (left panel). A decline in $^{G}\gamma$-globin gene expression might not always happen. This is associated with the presence of a −158 C → T mutation 5′ to the $^{G}\gamma$-globin gene, and its linked to the Senegal haplotype and the Arab–India haplotype.

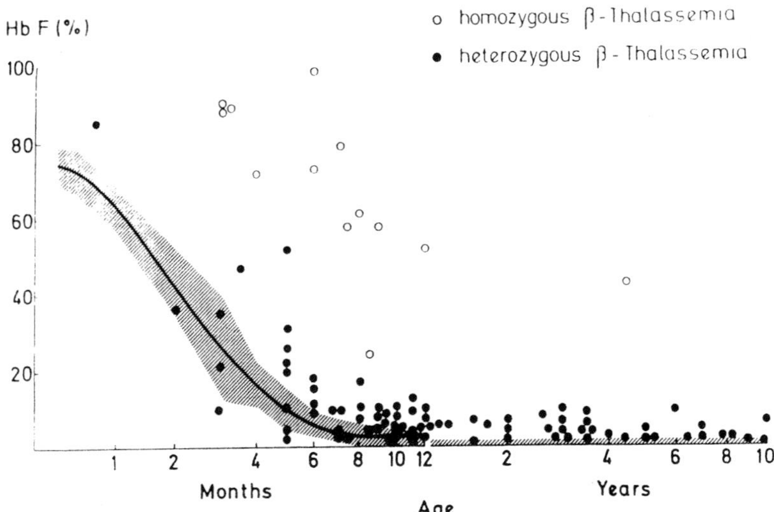

Figure 7.4. Decline in HbF concentration in normal individuals and patients with homozygous (○) and heterozygous (•) β thalassemia. Shaded area is the range for normal controls.

this has been incompletely studied, and acutely increased erythropoiesis can cause transient increases in HbF and F cells.

For any level of HbF in the hemolysate, the distribution and concentration of HbF in F cells can differ. Patients with sickle cell anemia have individually characteristic distributions of HbF per F cell.[24] This variance has pathophysiological implications, as concentrations of HbF in some cells sufficient to retard HbS polymerization could affect the disease differently than concentrations of HbF insufficient to retard HbS polymerization in many cells. When autologous sickle erythrocytes were labeled with biotin and reinfused, F cells survived longer in all individuals and non-F cell survival correlated inversely with the percentage of F cells. As labeled cells aged in the circulation, the HbF content of surviving cells increased, suggesting that high HbF content was related to cell survival.[25]

Table 7.1. Characteristics of neonatal erythrocytes

Increased MCV (approximately 120–130 fl at birth)
Erythrocyte lifespan of 60–70 d (Premature babies have fetal red cell lifespans of 35–55 d
Decreased osmotic fragility
Increased numbers of abnormally shaped cells
Increased numbers of "pocked" cells
Increased membrane total lipid, phospholipid, and cholesterol (perhaps a result of macrocytosis)
Excess membrane sphingomyelin and decreased lecithin
Enhanced tendency toward lipid peroxidation
Antigenic differences from adult cells in the Lewis and ABO systems – A and B antigens are weakly expressed – reduced or absent I antigen and presence of i antigen
Increased glucose consumption and activity of many glycolytic enzymes
Tendency toward methemoglobin formation, probably reflecting decreased activity of methemoglobin reductase and increased glutathione stability
Decreased deformability
Low S-nitrosohemoglobin levels

Most evidence suggests that F cells are not clonal but acquire their particular characteristics stochastically during development. In clonal disorders, including polycythemia vera, paroxysmal nocturnal hemoglobinuria, and Philadelphia chromosome–positive chronic granulocytic leukemia, F cells are present in the same proportion as in normal individuals. In adult red cells, no relationship exists between F cells and i-antigen, a maker for fetal like cells.

F Reticulocytes: Using a double-labeling technique that detects both HbF and reticulocytes (F reticulocytes), F reticulocytes in sickle cell anemia numbered 10.6% ± 7.0%. These observations raised the question of preferential survival of F cells in sickle cell anemia. Preferential survival was suggested by finding more F cells than F reticulocytes in most, but not all patients. Increased F cell survival could be the result of inhibition of HbS polymerization by HbF and differential susceptibility of F cells and non-F cells to phagocytosis and endothelial cell adherence.

Laboratory Detection of HbF

Different methods of measuring HbF can give different results on the same blood sample, and the most precise method for determining HbF varies according to the blood HbF concentration. Currently, the most prevalent means of measuring HbF is by HPLC. In normal adults, HbF concentrations measured by cation-exchange HPLC were between 0.1% and 0.4%.[26] Sex, polymorphisms in the β-globin gene like cluster, γ-globin gene duplications, and γ-globin gene promoter mutation can all increase HbF in otherwise normal individuals.

Medical Conditions Associated with Increased HbF

HPFH is a condition in which increased HbF levels persist into adult life. Several large deletions affecting the β- and δ-globin genes lead to pancellular HPFH syndromes with HbF levels of 20%–30% and to the closely related δβ thalassemias (Chapter 16). Point mutations within the promoters of the γ-globin genes lead to a heterocellular or a pancellular form of HPFH with increased HbF and F cell levels. In these conditions, the HbF concentration varies from slightly elevated to nearly 40% in heterozygotes (Table 7.2). These mutations could increase the promoter activity by effecting transcription factor binding.[27]

Pregnancy is associated with a modest increase in HbF in the second trimester. Hydatidiform moles are associated with up to 6% HbF. Although hormones secreted during

Table 7.2. Point mutations in the promoters of the γ-globin genes associated with an HPFH phenotype

Gene	Mutation	Percent $^{A}\gamma$ Globin	Percent HbF	Notes
HBG1 ($^{A}\gamma$)	C-202T	89–96	1.6–3.9	Seen with HbS
	T-198C	90–100	2–13	20% in homozygote
	C-201T		10.2	
	C-196T	80	12–16	also positive for $^{G}\gamma$-158 C-T
	C-195G	85	4–7	
	T-175G	60–80	38	in HbAS, 41% HbF, 17% HbS; also 40% HbF with HbC trait
	C-158T	51	3–5	
	G-117A	~90	7–19	25% in homozygote
	C-114T	~90	~5	
HBG2 ($^{G}\gamma$)	C-202G	100	14–21	with HbAS 18%–24% HbF, 25%–35% HbA
	T-175C	100	22	with HbAS 30% HbF, 28% HbA
	C-196T		8.6	also positive for $^{G}\gamma$-158 C-T
	C-114A	90	0.6–3.5	4%–11% HbF with associated with β thalassemia
	C-114G	90	8.6	
	C-114T	~90	11–14	also homozygous for $^{G}\gamma$-158 C-T
	A-110C	97	0.8	

Some of these mutations are also associated with β thalassemia. References to these polymorphisms can be found at http://globin.cse.psu.edu/.

pregnancy have been implicated in these effects, the mechanism of HbF elevation is not clear.

Premature infants and infants of diabetic mothers have a delayed γ→β switch and higher HbF levels than other neonates. This switch is accelerated in Down syndrome and other chromosomal translocations. Controversy exists regarding the relationship of HbF to sudden infant death syndrome (SIDS). In most studies carefully controlled for the postconceptual or gestational age, the prime determinant of neonatal HbF level, infants dying with SIDS aged between 8 and 16 weeks, had significantly higher levels of HbF than controls.[28] HbF, measured by different techniques, was between 28% and 65% in SIDS infants, whereas controls had HbF concentrations between 12% and 41%. HbF synthesis was increased in infants considered at risk for SIDS.[29] Perhaps the high O_2 affinity of HbF contributes to chronic hypoxia, a common finding in these patients. A recent study of SIDS and control cases found that they were not different with respect to mean age, sex, gestational age, method of delivery, birth weight, or mean autopsy interval and that the percentage of HbF levels in SIDS cases and control were not significantly different.[30]

HbF elevations can be seen in different cancers. HbF was detected immunohistologically in metastatic germ cell tumors such as embryonal carcinomas and teratomas, lymphoma, colorectal carcinoma, myelodysplastic syndrome, and myeloma.[31,32] Juvenile chronic myeloid leukemia and Fanconi anemia are often accompanied by HbF levels of up to 30% and levels are highest in patients with the C-T SNP at −158 5′ to the $^{G}\gamma$-globin gene. Kala-Azar and paroxysmal nocturnal hemoglobinuria, particularly when hemolysis is present, can have HbF levels of 5%–10%. The highest levels are found in DiGuglielmo disease and juvenile myeloid leukemia in which levels more than 50% have been reported.

Mutations of the γ-Globin Genes (*HBG2, HBG1*)

Nearly 100 mutations have been described in the $^{G}\gamma$-globin gene, the $^{A}\gamma$-globin gene, and the $^{A}\gamma^{T}$-globin gene. γ-Globin chain variants will alter a single major hemoglobin during fetal and neonatal life but, after the first year of life, will alter only the trace of HbF usually present and are therefore rarely detected. Mutations can be present in γ-globin loci of the usual $^{G}\gamma$-$^{A}\gamma$ arrangement, on chromosomes with $^{G}\gamma$-$^{G}\gamma$ loci and in *cis* or *trans* to the $^{A}\gamma^{T}$-globin gene. Depending on the chromosomal arrangement of the γ-globin genes, and many other factors, the levels of $^{G}\gamma$-globin gene variants can range from 5% to 30% of total hemoglobin present in neonates, with most accounting for approximately 25% of all hemoglobin. Levels of most $^{A}\gamma$-globin gene variants are approximately half this amount. This difference is due to the greater expression of the $^{G}\gamma$-globin gene in fetal erythroid cells. Very few γ-globin gene variants have been subjected to functional studies so that the numbers of mutants reported to have altered properties might be underestimated. A listing of variant γ-globin genes and γ thalassemia and the properties of the variants can be found at (http://globin.cse.psu.edu). These variants can be unstable, have high or low O_2 affinity and can be subject to oxidation and cause methemoglobinemia and neonatal "cyanosis" that disappears with maturation.

HbF-Sardinia (*HBG1* (E19) ile75thr) present in the $^{A}\gamma^{T}$ gene is a frequent polymorphism without functional or clinical abnormalities. Although present at high frequency in many populations, it has a low frequency among Africans and individuals of African descent, except among carriers of the Cameroon haplotype. A reason for the high frequency of this variant has not been established, but its low frequency in most of Africa and high frequency elsewhere suggest that it occurred after man left Africa, or that its advantage, if any, is related to selective pressure not existent in Africa. Mutants of HbF-Sardinia have been described.

γ *Thalassemia:* γ Thalassemia that results from the types of point mutations that typify β thalassemia, has not yet been described. Most instances of γ thalassemia are due to gene deletion and are better classified as γδβ thalassemias or εγδβ thalassemia. Their phenotypes and pathophysiology are discussed in Chapters 16 and 17. A γ^{+} thalassemia phenotype was proposed to result from an IVS II-115 A-G substitution in both the $^{A}\gamma$- and $^{G}\gamma$-globin genes and the deletion of an A at position -6 relative to the $^{G}\gamma$-globin gene polyadenylation site. Yet, the IVS II substitutions appear to have gene frequencies of 0.73 for the $^{A}\gamma$-globin gene and 0.86 for the $^{G}\gamma$-globin gene suggesting that they are common polymorphisms. One γ thalassemia resulted from an unequal crossover between the $^{G}\gamma$ and $^{A}\gamma$-globin genes, deleting one γ-globin gene from the affected chromosome, and leaving a hybrid γ-globin gene, akin to the Hb Lepore-type genes. Found in heterozygotes and in two homozygotes, newborns homozygous for this deletion had only 50% HbF, all of the $^{A}\gamma$ type.

HEMOGLOBIN A_2

HbA_2 ($\alpha_2\delta_2$) is a hemoglobin without an obvious physiological function. In normal hemolysates, HbA_2 represents between 2% and 3% of all hemoglobin.

Evolution of the δ-Globin Gene (*HBD*)

HbA_2 is present in humans, apes, and New World monkeys, but not Old World monkeys, a finding at variance with the evolutionary data that suggested that humans and Old World monkeys diverged after the divergence of New World monkeys. This inconsistency was resolved with the observation that δ-globin genes are present in Old World monkeys but have been inactivated by mutation.

Comparisons of δ-globin genes among mammals have shown that this locus has not evolved independently but has done so in concert with the β-globin gene and is the product of gene conversion. Three variants of the δ-globin gene could have arisen by gene conversion. HbA_2 Flatbush (*HBD* ala22glu), HbA_2 Coburg (*HBD* arg116his) and Hb Parchman (*HBD* ala22glu, ser50thr).[33,34]

It has been suggested that the δ-globin gene is a pseudogene in evolution, destined for the biological scrap heap of history. This presupposes that the sole functional role of all hemoglobins is O_2 transport but this is clearly not true. Increased binding of HbA_2 to the membrane might mask another functional role for this hemoglobin. The presence of a variant HbA_2 at polymorphic frequencies in the Dogon region of Mali at least hints at possible selection of this hemoglobin.

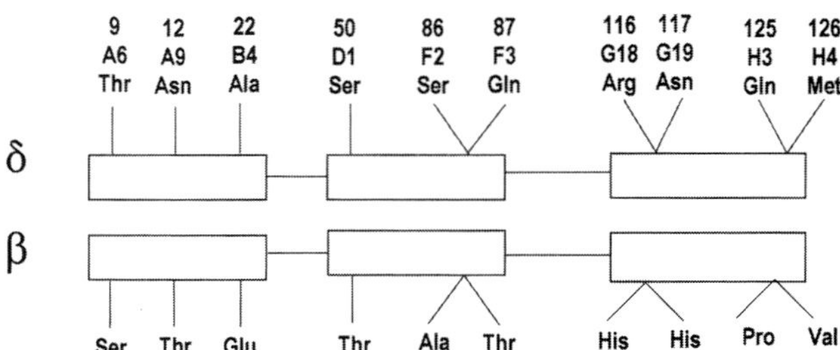

Figure 7.5. Amino acid differences in the δ- and β-globin genes.

The δ-Globin Gene and δ Globin

Linked to the β-globin gene on chromosome 11, the structure of the δ-globin gene is identical to all other expressed globin genes. δ-Globin chains of HbA_2 differ from β-globin chains of HbA by 10 amino acid residues, and 31 nucleotide differences are found between the coding regions of the β- and δ-globin genes (Fig. 7.5, Table 7.3). A high level of homology persists until 70 bp 5′ to the mRNA capping site. Greater sequence differences in the 5′ noncoding portion are found beyond this point, accounting, in part for the diminished transcription of the δ-compared with the β-globin gene.

The crystal structure of HbA_2 at 2.20 A in the R2-state has been solved and used to provide the probable explanations of its thermal stability. The structure of the T-state has also been modeled allowing the structural basis of the antisickling property of HbA_2 to be studied.[35]

Table 7.3. Nucleotide differences in the coding regions of the δ- and β-globin genes

	2 His	10 Ala	11 Val	30 Arg	31 Leu	66 Lys	68 Leu
β	CAC	GCC	GTT	AGG	CTG	AAA	CTC
δ	CAT	GCT	GTC	AGA	TTA	AAG	CTA
	84 Thr	106 Leu	108 Asn	111 Val	120 Lys	132 Lys	142 Ala
β	ACC	CTG	AAC	GTC	AAA	AAA	GCC
δ	ACT	TTG	AAT	GTG	AAG	AAG	GCT
	145 Tyr	146 His					
β	TAT	CAC					
δ	TAC	CAT					

Codon usage in the β- and the δ-globin genes. Codons of the amino acid that differ between the β- and the δ-globin chains are not included. Two of the codons that specify amino acid differences between the β- and the δ-globin chain contain two base pair differences and one codon contains three differences. Codon 31 Leu has a two base change.

δ-Globin Chain Synthesis: Quantitatively, the expression of the δ- and β-globin genes is strikingly different and the sequences responsible for this have been studied. Although HbA_2 comprises only 2%–3% of the hemolysate, it is synthesized in all erythroid progenitors and has a pancellular distribution in distinction to the heterocellular distribution of HbF. In bone marrow, δ-globin chains are synthesized at a reduced rate compared with β chains; δ-globin is not synthesized in reticulocytes and reticulocytes contain almost no δ-globin mRNA. Maturity-fractionated bone marrow erythroblasts showed a progressive decline of δ- in relation to β-globin chain synthesis as the maturity of the erythroid cell increased.

Relative instability of δ-globin mRNA was postulated to be responsible for the premature decline in δ-globin synthesis. The half-life of δ-globin mRNA was less than one third that of β-globin mRNA. Instability of δ mRNA might depend on the sequence of its 3′ untranslated region. Instability alone does not account for the vast reduction of HbA_2 compared with HbA concentration.

In vitro transcription of the δ-globin gene was 50 times less efficient than that of the β-globin gene. Studies of hybrid genes suggested that the δ-globin gene promoter was faulty. In the δ-globin gene promoter, the conserved CCAAT box is replaced by CCAAC. CCAAC binds the ubiquitous CCAAT-binding protein, CP1, less avidly than CCAAT and forms unstable complexes with other possible CCAAT binding proteins, reducing β-globin gene promoter activation by the locus control region (LCR). Another major difference between the β- and δ-globin gene promoters is the absence of the proximal CACC in the δ-globin gene. This sequence forms the binding site for the β-globin gene-specific transcription factor, erythroid Krüppel-like factor.

The transcriptional defect of the δ-globin gene was partially normalized when both the CCAAC and CACC sequences were "corrected" by substituting the CCAAT sequence of the β-globin gene promoter for the δ gene CCAAC motif. Introducing EKLF binding sites into the δ-globin gene promoter, increased expression 6.5- to 26.8-fold to 35% of the total δ and β chains produced.[36,37]

Mutations in the gene promoter do not totally explain the reduced accumulation of δ-globin mRNA suggesting that additional sites in the δ-globin gene could account for its reduced expression. IVS-II of the δ-globin gene also has been shown to reduce the δ-globin gene transcription but the mechanism of this effect is unclear. Further insight might come from the example of the Lepore hemoglobins, products of δβ fusion genes (Chapter 16) that contain δ-globin gene sequences in their 5′ portion that might explain their characteristically reduced rate of synthesis. Nevertheless, the Lepore δβ-globin chain is synthesized at a higher rate than the δ-globin chain, perhaps because of the presence of a β-globin-like IVS-II. A βδ chain variant, β-like through IVS-1 and then δ-like, was expressed at levels that were greater than the δ-globin gene, but less than the β-globin gene, again suggesting that δ IVS-II and 3′ sequences influence gene expression. The δ-globin gene IVS-II contains only a single GATA-I binding site, whereas β IVS-II has two GATA-I sites and an Oct-I site, perhaps accounting for the effects of δ IVS-II.

Functional Aspects of HbA_2: HbA_2 has functional properties nearly identical to HbA; ligand-binding curves are similar although HbA_2 has higher O_2 affinity, however Bohr effect, cooperativity, and response to 2,3 BPG are identical to HbA. Greater thermal stability of HbA_2 might be due to the δ116 arginine that can form a salt bridge with α114 proline, increasing even further the stability of the $\alpha_1\delta_1$ contact. HbA_2 has slightly increased autoxidation to methemoglobin and its hemichrome had increased stability. These differences could explain its increased membrane binding. The positive charge of HbA_2 could endow it with properties similar to other positively charged hemoglobins, like HbC, in its interaction with the erythrocyte membrane. HbA_2 has a higher affinity for erythrocyte membrane band 3 than HbA. Although the interaction of HbC with the membrane is believed to determine the red cell phenotype of HbC trait and HbC disease (Chapter 21), the very low concentration of HbA_2 makes it doubtful that it meaningfully affects cation transport and mean corpuscular hemoglobin concentration.

HbA_2 inhibits the polymerization of HbS and δ22 ala and δ87 gln might be the important inhibitory sites.[38] When HbA_2 levels are exceptionally high and in the presence of elevated HbF levels, the combination of these two hemoglobins could modulate the phenotype of HbS-β^0 thalassemia (Chapter 23). A δ6 valine mutation introduced into the δ-globin chain in the presence or absence of either or both δ22 glutamic acid and δ87 threonine, causes the deoxy molecule to polymerize without a delay time in the simple δ6 val variant and with delay times when other mutations are present.[39]

Mutations of the δ-Globin Gene: Far fewer than expected number of δ thalassemia–causing mutations and δ-globin chain variants have been described. Detecting δ-globin chain hemoglobinopathies is difficult because of the low concentration of δ-globin gene variants and the few clinical or hematological abnormalities that are expected with δ thalassemia. The inconsequential hematological changes of δ thalassemia appear to be an insufficient basis for natural selection to protect the carrier from *Falciparum* malaria

Approximately 60 variants of the δ-globin gene have been described (http://globin.cse.psu.edu). In individuals heterozygous for stable δ-globin chain variants, the concentration of the HbA_2 variant is equivalent to approximately half the usual HbA_2 concentration, and the sum of normal and variant HbA_2 is equal to the normal HbA_2 level. Homozygotes for these HbA_2 variants, unless they are unstable, have normal HbA_2 levels. δ-globin gene variants can also have increased O_2 affinity.

HbA_2' (*HBD* gly16arg), sometimes called HbB_2, is the most common variant of the δ-globin gene. Among more than 5,500 hemoglobin HPLC studies, 57 instances of

HbA_2' trait were found, making it the third most prevalent hemoglobin variant detected after HbS and HbC. The mean HbA_2 level was 1.7% and the mean HbA_2' level was 1.3%.[40] Present in approximately 1% of African Americans, both homozygotes and heterozygotes are found. In Africa, it has been described in samples from different geographical locations and has been described in *cis* and in *trans* to HbS and HbC. More recently, it has been found at polymorphic frequencies in one cast in the Dogon region of the Republic of Mali. Although haplotype analysis of the β-like globin gene cluster in individuals from Mali with HbA_2' showed that all unrelated individuals carried this mutation on the same haplotype, samples from unrelated African Americans with this mutation displayed haplotype heterogeneity. It is therefore possible that this mutation arose in Africa unicentrically and distributed itself to other regions of Africa by gene flow. HbA_2' is easily detectable by HPLC in the absence of HbS, C, or G.[40] It migrates cathodic to normal HbA_2 on alkaline electrophoresis.

Measurement of HbA_2

Separation of HbA_2 from HbA is simplified by the presence of two additional positive charges in the δ-globin chain compared with the β-globin chain. Different methods of measurement, including new and traditional methods of electrophoresis and spectrophotometric measurement of eluted fractions, HPLC, column chromatography, immunological detection, and enzyme-linked immunosorbent assay are available. HPLC hemoglobin separation is the preferred means of measuring HbA_2 but the results must be interpreted cautiously in the presence of HbS because the coelution of minor HbS species falsely elevates the HbA_2 fraction.[41,42] Newer HPLC analytical methods can reduce this inaccuracy.

Clinical Aspects of HbA_2

Developmental Changes in HbA_2 Level: Little δ-globin chain synthesis occurs in utero so that HbA_2 does not become easily measurable until late in gestation. In normal newborns, HbA_2 concentration is 0.27% ± 0.02%. HbA_2 levels vary with gestational age and are lowest in the least mature infants. HbA_2 levels do not rise synchronously with HbA, but lag behind; the HbA/HbA_2 ratio is approximately 100 by 32 weeks gestation, 75 by 45 weeks and "adult" ratios of approximately 40:1 are not reached until at least age 6 months. This sluggish response of HbA_2 during maturation can reduce its value for the diagnosis of β thalassemia in young infants. In the presence of an α-globin variant, such as $HbG^{Philadelphia}$, the variant α-chain combines with the δ-chain to form a hemoglobin tetramer with the structure, $\alpha^{Variant}{}_2\,\delta_2$. This tetramer, often called HbG_2, usually comprises less than one half the total amount of HbA_2. HbG_2 is more positively charged than HbA_2 because of the positive charge of the α^G chain and is easily separated from HbA_2.

Table 7.4. Low HbA_2 levels

Iron deficiency	lowest with increasing severity
G-6-PD deficiency	reports are conflicting – levels probably not reduced
α Thalassemia	related to severity of the thalassemia
Myelodysplastic syndromes	only in a minority of cases
Hb Lepore	half normal in heterozygotes
Gene deletion hereditary persistence of HbF	half normal in heterozygotes
δβ Thalassemia	half normal in heterozygotes
δ Thalassemia	usually approximately half normal
HbA_2 variants	variant can be poorly expressed
Sideroblastic anemia	due to impaired α-globin synthesis
Juvenile chronic granulocytic leukemia with increased HbF	only in a minority of cases
Acute myelocytic leukemia	minor reduction
α-Globin gene variants	hybrid HbA_2 might not separate

Extra HbA_2 bands are a valuable clue to the presence of variant α-globin chains, although, depending on the charge of the α-globin variant, they might or might not separate from the major hemoglobin bands (Chapter 23).

Low HbA_2 (Table 7.4): Low HbA_2 values are usually the result of either posttranslational modifications in the assembly of the HbA_2 tetramer, reduced synthesis of the δ-globin chain secondary to δ thalassemia or δ-globin chain mutants.

Among Greek Cypriots with an HbA_2 of less than 1.6%, all had of δ-globin mutants. Five of the 11 mutations were amino acid substitutions and the others were more typical thalassemia mutations. When HbA_2 was 1.7%–1.8%, 91% of subjects had a δ-globin variant and this percentage fell to 53% if the HbA_2 was 1.9%. Based on their screening, it was estimated that 1.26% of Greek Cypriots had a δ-globin gene mutation.[43] In 29 patients with a low HbA_2 level, 20 δ-globin gene mutations, including those causing δ thalassemia and structural abnormalities of the δ-globin gene, were found.[44]

Posttranslational Causes of Reduced HbA_2: Posttranslational causes of reduced HbA_2 can result from either acquired or genetic disorders. In either case, the underlying cause of the low HbA_2 level is insufficient synthesis of α-globin chains. Assembly of hemoglobin tetramers is dependent on charge differences of α- and non-α-globin chains (Chapter 22). Normal α- and β-globin monomers have nearly equivalent positive and negative charges, respectively, and are united by electrostatic attraction to form αβ dimers. δ-Globin chains are more positively charged than the β-globin chains (or γ-globin chains). Under normal conditions of α chain sufficiency or slight excess, HbA is formed in preference to HbA_2 because αβ dimers assemble more readily than αδ dimers. When the supply of α-globin chain is limited, this effect of monomer charge on dimer formation is exaggerated, as β chains (and γ-chains) compete more effectively than δ chains for scarce α-globin.[45–47]

Acquired conditions that reduce α-globin chain synthesis appear to work through the common mechanism of absolute or functional iron deficiency. Lacking sufficient iron, a repressor of initiation of protein synthesis is formed that preferentially effects α-, rather than non-α-globin chain initiation, resulting in a relative deficiency of α chains. Patients with iron deficiency anemia have reduced levels of HbA_2. This reduction is greatest in individuals with the most severe iron deficiency.[48 49] Individuals with anemia, microcytosis, and low levels of HbA_2 from iron deficiency might be mistaken for carriers of α thalassemia. When iron deficiency and β thalassemia coexist, the HbA_2 level has been occasionally reported to fall, although it can remain within the range expected for thalassemia heterozygotes. The iron utilization defect associated with sideroblastic anemias can also reduce HbA_2 levels.

In the α thalassemia/myelodysplasia syndrome (Chapter 15), inhibition of α-globin chain synthesis is associated with low HbA_2 levels. With acute myeloid leukemia, HbA_2 is lower than in acute lymphocytic leukemias, suggesting that the leukemic clone involves the erythroid lineage. Patients with juvenile chronic granulocytic leukemia can have a hemoglobin pattern very similar to fetal erythropoiesis, and high HbF is accompanied by low HbA_2 recapitulating normal neonatal findings. Erythroleukemia has also been associated with very low levels of HbA_2 without HbH. These acquired "α thalassemias" bridge the gap between reduced HbA_2 secondary to acquired diseases and low HbA_2 associated with genetic abnormalities of α-globin synthesis.

α Thalassemia is the common cause of a genetically determined reduction in HbA_2 level due to posttranslational mechanisms. HbA_2 concentration varies commensurately with the deficit in α-globin chain synthesis. With the mildest types of α thalassemia, HbA_2 values might be indistinguishable from normal. When α-globin production is impaired significantly, the reduction in HbA_2 is dramatic. In 21 patients with HbH disease, the HbA_2 ranged from 0.5% to 1.8% and averaged 0.8%.[50] Homotetramers of δ chains have been reported in α thalassemia hydrops fetalis.

δ *Thalassemia:* Approximately 20 different δ thalassemias due to the usual types of thalassemia-causing mutations have been described and cause either δ^+ or δ^0 thalassemia (http://globin.cse.psu.edu). Uncomplicated δ thalassemia has no clinical repercussions other than complicating the diagnosis of β thalassemia trait. By decreasing the level of HbA_2, δ thalassemia makes the use of HbA_2 levels less reliable. Homozygosity for δ^0 thalassemia causes absence of HbA_2.

Early descriptions of δ thalassemia were based on hematological and family studies and are often error prone. δ Thalassemias have been reported most often in Japanese, Italian, and Greek populations. Whether this represents their true distribution is not known because extensive surveys have not been done. In Italians and potentially in other ethnic groups in which β thalassemia is common, the coexistence of δ thalassemia and β thalassemia might cause the HbA_2 to be normal and complicate β thalassemia screening programs. In Greece, approximately 5% of individuals with β thalassemia can have borderline or normal HbA_2 concentrations and most of these cases also have δ thalassemia due to point mutations or the 7.2-kb Corfu deletion.[51] Interactions between α thalassemia and β thalassemia can also result in normal HbA_2 values. β Thalassemia can escape detection if the sole basis of diagnosis is the level of HbA_2.

In the Corfu 7.2-kb deletion, most of the δ-globin gene is absent. Although the initial molecular characterization of this deletion suggested that it inactivated the β-globin gene, subsequent studies revealed a β^+ thalassemia mutation that was responsible for the reduced expression of the β-globin gene in *cis* to this deletion.

Heterozygotes for δβ thalassemia, Hb Lepore, and gene-deletion HPFH have half-normal HbA_2 levels and homozygotes have no HbA_2. Although the percentage of HbA_2 might be low when δ-globin gene expression is abolished, the absolute level, expressed as pg HbA_2 per cell, is elevated, reflecting increased synthesis of HbA_2 from the chromosome in *trans* to the deleted gene.

High HbA_2 (Table 7.5): Heterozygous β thalassemia is the cause of at least 95% of the cases of high HbA_2 levels (Table 7.5). Only a few of the point mutations causing β thalassemia are not associated with a raised HbA_2 level. "Normal" or borderline HbA_2 thalassemias have multiple causes including triplicated α-globin loci, β thalassemia with α-globin gene deletion, and δ plus β thalassemia, usually in *trans* but rarely in *cis*.[52] Mean HbA_2 levels in 879 carriers of β thalassemia of diverse ethnic backgrounds were 5.08% ± 0.39%.[53] The highest observed value was 6.8%. In 184 African American patients with β thalassemia trait, the mean HbA_2 level was 4.97% ± 1.07%.[53] With the few exceptions mentioned previously, an elevated level of HbA_2, in the presence of microcytic erythrocytes, identifies patients

Table 7.5. Increased HbA_2

Proven Cases	
β Thalassemia	4%–6%, rarely up to 12%, microcytosis
Sickle cell anemia–α thalassemia	4%–5%, microcytosis, similar to HbS–β^0 thalassemia
Megaloblastic anemia	modest increases
Unstable hemoglobinopathies	not uniformly found
Zidovudine-treated HIV patients	HbA_2 lower than in β thalassemia, macrocytosis
CDA, Type I	HbA_2 lower than in β thalassemia, macrocytosis
Hyperthyroidism	HbA_2 lower than in β thalassemia,
Normal individuals	rare, normal red blood cell indices, no thalassemia
Doubtful Cases	
Malaria	
Sickle cell trait	
Sickle cell anemia	
Hereditary spherocytosis	

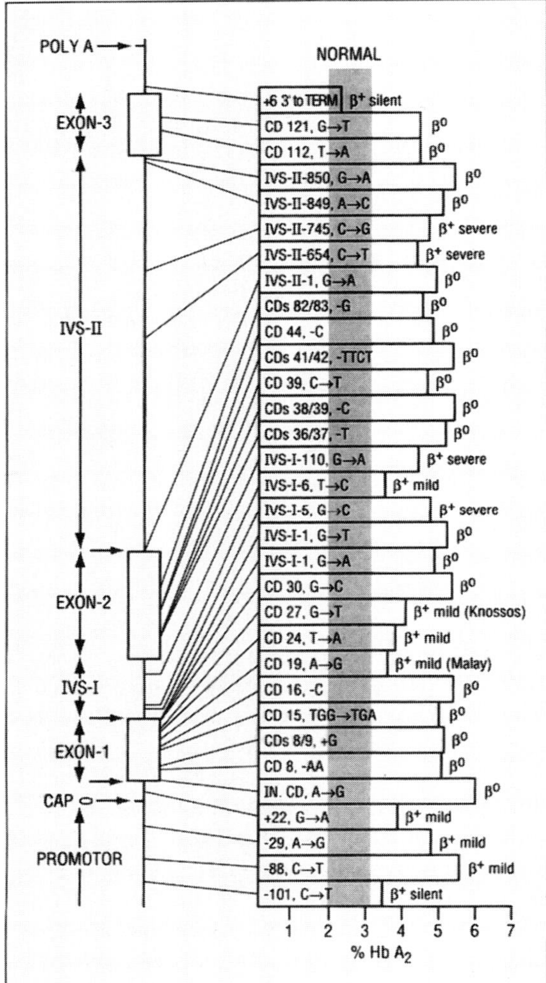

Figure 7.6. HbA_2 concentrations according to the β thalassemia mutation in more than 600 patients.[55]

with heterozygous β thalassemia. HbA_2 levels could be higher in heterozygous β^0 thalassemia and severe β^+ thalassemia than in mild β^+ thalassemia because of their greater impairment of β-globin chain synthesis.[54] Average levels of HbA_2 in heterozygotes for 32 different β alleles are shown in Figure 7.6.[55] In mild β thalassemia mutations, a nominal suppression of β chain synthesis and a minor excess of α-globin chains can lead to less αδ–dimer formation. It possible, however, that point mutations in the β-globin gene promoter might alter binding of transcription factors and augment δ-globin gene transcription in *cis* to the mutation. Nevertheless, in 10 heterozygotes with the -88 C→T β^+ thalassemia mutation, HbA_2 was 5.4% ± 0.4%; in another six heterozygotes HbA_2 was 4.9%; in a patient with the -88 C→T β^+ thalassemia and HbA_2' in *trans*, the total HbA_2 level was approximately 7%.

Because of the striking increases of HbF that typify the severe β thalassemias, HbA_2 levels in homozygous β thalassemia are variable and of little diagnostic value. The level of HbA_2 in homozygotes for the promoter mutations -88C→T and -29 A→G averaged 6.6% (4.0%–9.7%).[55] Transcription of the δ-globin gene appears to vary reciprocally with that of the γ-globin gene. This reciprocity is evident as HbF levels fall rapidly during the last trimester of gestation and is also observed in the β thalassemia syndromes. In homozygous β thalassemia, cells with the highest HbF levels have the lowest HbA_2 concentrations. One example of the relationship between HbA_2 and HbF was seen when chemotherapy for Hodgkin disease appeared to reactivate HbF synthesis in a patient with β thalassemia trait and the Swiss-type HPFH. HbF level rose from 4.5% to 26%, accompanied by a fall in HbA_2 from 4.5% to 2.4%. The mechanism of this effect has not been studied but could be a result of competition for the LCR and transcription factors.

Increased HbA_2 in heterozygous β thalassemia appears to result from both transcriptional and posttranslational mechanisms.[56] Both the percentage and absolute amount of HbA_2 are increased with the former approximately twice as great as the latter. Reduced production of β-globin chains, with a relative excess of α-globin chains, favors the formation of αδ dimers and the assembly of HbA_2 tetramers. Posttranslational effects occur in *cis* and in *trans* to the thalassemia mutation as suggested by studies in which a δ-globin variant was in *trans* to the β thalassemia mutation. Increased δ-globin gene transcription might be expected to occur only in *cis* to the thalassemia mutation.

Exceptionally High HbA_2: Some individuals with β thalassemia trait have HbA_2 concentrations much higher than usual. These exceptionally high HbA_2 levels are usually the result of a unique class of small deletions of DNA that usually begin within the β-globin gene and extend 5′, removing the gene promoter (Chapter 16). Removing the β-globin gene promoter sequences by the 5′ deletion might increase the likelihood that transcription factors bind the remaining δ- and γ-globin gene promoters, enhancing the transcription of these genes. Alternatively, deletion-induced disruption of higher-order DNA or chromatin structure could make γ- and δ-globin promoters more accessible to the LCR. The absence of a functional β promoter might permit the LCR to interact with the δ-globin gene in *cis*, enhancing its expression.

HbA_2 levels in heterozygotes for these 5′ β-gene deletion thalassemias have been reported to range from approximately 7%–12%. HbA_2 levels that exceed the top of this range have not been reported. Laboratory reports of HbA_2 values more than 15% or 20% are usually spurious or represent instances of HbC or HbE heterozygosity complicated by α thalassemia or iron deficiency.

Miscellaneous Causes of High HbA_2: Patients with either sickle cell anemia–α thalassemia or HbS–β^0 thalassemia have high HbA_2 concentrations (Chapter 23). In the former group of patients, the δ-globin chain competes more effectively than the β^S-globin chain for the limited quantities of α-globin chain.

HbA_2 levels are consistently elevated in hyperthyroidism, although not as markedly as in β thalassemia. Both the percentage and absolute amount of HbA_2 are increased, suggesting increased synthesis of the δ-globin chain and an effect of thyroid hormone on δ-globin gene transcription. The combination of high HbA_2 and low MCV can be confused with β thalassemia. Euthyroidism following treatment is accompanied by a fall in HbA_2 and rise in MCV. In untreated, nonanemic, hypothyroidism, HbA_2 levels cluster toward the low end of normal.[57]

Megaloblastic anemias have been associated with HbA_2 concentrations that exceed normal. The most severely anemic patients have the highest HbA_2 values. The incidence of this finding seems low, however, the amount of the increase above normal is slight, and in one study the mean HbA_2 levels in the normal and megaloblastic anemia groups were similar. Perhaps the high HbA_2 of megaloblastic anemia is a result of more hemoglobin synthesis occurring in less mature erythroid precursors.

Seventy-eight human immunodeficiency virus (HIV)–infected patients taking zidovudine had HbA_2 levels of 3.2% ± 0.5% compared with 2.7% ± 0.4% in HIV-positive controls not exposed to this drug. The MCV was higher in zidovudine-treated patients but evidence of folic acid or vitamin B_{12} deficiency was lacking. It was speculated that increased HbA_2 levels of the treated patients was secondary to drug-induced megaloblastic erythropoiesis.

In 14 Israeli Bedouins with congenital dyserythropoietic anemia, type I, the mean HbA_2 was 3.5% ± 0.5%. MCV was 98 ± 5 fl but biosynthesis studies showed a deficit of β-globin chain synthesis with a mean α/β synthesis ratio of 1.27, suggesting β thalassemia trait. The sequence of the β-globin gene in four individuals was normal however.

HbA_2 levels are increased in some examples of unstable hemoglobin. An unstable β-globin chain might have difficulty forming αβ dimers, increasing αδ dimer assembly.

In one report, 20% of individuals with pseudoxanthoma elasticum had increased HbA_2.[58]

Malaria infestation and elevated HbA_2 levels have been linked in some reports but not others. The best-controlled study casts doubt on such an association. An association of hereditary spherocytosis and very high HbA_2 levels has also not been proven.

EMBRYONIC HEMOGLOBINS (*HBE1, HBZ*)

Between 4 and 14 weeks gestation, the human embryo synthesizes three distinct hemoglobins in yolk sac–derived primitive nucleated erythroid cells: Hb Gower I ($\zeta_2\varepsilon_2$), Hb Gower II ($\alpha_2\varepsilon_2$), and Hb Portland ($\zeta_2\gamma_2$). ζ- and ε-globin are expressed before γ- and α-globin. By 14 days of development, after the establishment of the placenta, embryonic hemoglobins start to be replaced by HbF but some ζ- and ε-globin chains can be found in definitive and primitive erythrocytes.[59] At 15–22 weeks of gestation, 53% of fetal cells contained ζ-globin chains and 5% had ε-globin chains. At term, cord blood contained 34% ζ- and 0.6% ε-globin chain–positive cells. Erythrocytes from normal adults did not contain embryonic globins.

Recombinant technology using plasmid-based expression systems in yeast and transgenic mice have provided sufficient amounts of functional embryonic hemoglobin tetramer to permit studies of their structural and functional properties (reviewed in [11]).[60]

Presently, embryonic hemoglobins have little apparent clinical importance. Detection of the ζ-globin chain in blood provides a means of diagnosing α thalassemia due to the Southeast Asian mutation.[61–64] Hb Gower II can inhibit polymerization of HbS, suggesting that the reactivation of the gene could be therapeutically useful in sickle cell disease.[65]

Function

Embryonic hemoglobins exhibit cooperative O_2 binding with P_{50} values of 4, 12, and 6 mm Hg for Hb Gower I, Gower II, and Portland, compared with a P_{50} of 26 for HbA. Cooperativity of embryonic hemoglobins is less than that of HbF and HbA. The higher O_2 affinity of embryonic hemoglobins is likely to be a result of reduced relative stability of the T-state ascribed to the substitution of several residues that stabilize the T-state in HbA. The presence of the ζ 38 glycine has major significance in producing high O_2 affinity within the ζ chain–containing human embryonic hemoglobins.

In the presence of organic phosphates, the O_2 affinities of $\zeta_2\varepsilon_2$ and $\alpha_2\varepsilon_2$ suggest that whereas the ζ- and ε-globin chains bind 2,3-BPG, differences from binding to β-globin are present. Hb Portland, because its central cavity is formed by γ-globin chains and because of the N-terminal ζ-chain acetylation, binds organic phosphates poorly. The N-terminal acetylation of the ζ-globin chain makes it incapable of combining directly with CO_2 and accounts for its reduced Bohr effect. The rates of O_2 dissociation from the embryonic hemoglobins seem responsible for their high O_2-binding affinity compared with HbA. The pH dependence of the O_2 dissociation rate constants also accounts for the unusual Bohr effects of embryonic hemoglobins.[66–69] These differences and the difference in O_2 affinity among the embryonic hemoglobins are accounted for by differences in specific amino acids in the ε-, ζ-, and γ-globin chains.

Nuclear magnetic resonance studies show that the embryonic globins bind heme rapidly.[70] They also bind heme more tightly than HbA.[71,72] At pH 9.0, both embryonic hemoglobin and HbA dissociate into dimers with associated equilibrium constants in the micromolar range. At low pH, Hb Portland shows a high degree of globin dissociation and Hb Barts can be found in equilibrium with dimeric and monomeric globin chains.[73,74]

Embryonic hemoglobins show a similar pattern of O_2 dissociation to HbA, but with the ζ chains losing O_2 at approximately twice the rate of the α chains. The rate of conversion of deoxy dimers to tetramers is very similar for HbA and embryonic hemoglobins. Hb Portland has a lower rate of dissociation.

Structure

Only Hb Gower II and Portland have been crystallized and only the Gower II structure has been solved to 2.9-A resolution.[75] The quaternary structure of the CO form of hemoglobin Gower II lies between that reported for the R- and R2-states, lying closer to the R2 structure. The structure of the heme pocket of the α subunit of Gower II is, within experimental error, identical to that reported for the adult protein. The tertiary structure of the ε subunit is similar to that reported for the β chain. Some amino acid substitutions between the ε and β chains are within the internal core of the molecule but appear to have no major structural effects. The overall structure of the ε chain heme pocket is essentially identical to that of the β chain. Differences from the β chain include a position ala70ser substitution within the heme pocket and a gly83pro substitution at the beginning of the F helix that might reduce the flexibility of the EF loop and contribute to the destabilization of the T-state, causing an increase in O_2 affinity of hemoglobin Gower II. Compared with HbA, Gower II contains three amino acid substitutions at the $\alpha_2\beta_1$ interface, but the $\alpha_1\beta_2$ interface is more strongly conserved.

The crystal structure of Hb Portland has not yet been solved. The structure of Hb Barts has been solved at 1.7-A resolution in both the azide and CO state. The γ-globin chain has a structure similar to the β chain with a closer correspondence to the β structure in HbH than that in HbA. The major difference between the γ- and β-globin tertiary structure is in the N-terminal region of the protein, which is implicated in the greater stability of HbF.

In a chimeric ζ(human)$_2$ β(mouse)$_2$ protein, the ζ chain showed structural differences from the human α chain.[73]

Thalassemias and Hemoglobinopathies of the Embryonic Globin Genes

Thalassemic or structural variants of the embryonic ε- and ζ-globin chains due to point mutations have not been described at the DNA or protein level. Mutations in the ε-globin gene have yet to be found.[76] Some large deletions that affect the β- and the α-globin gene clusters remove embryonic genes. The phenotypes of these conditions, when expressed postnatally, derive from loss of the β- or the α-globin genes rather than the embryonic genes. Deletion of the ζ- and α-globin genes cause early embryonic loss, presumably because a functional hemoglobin tetramer cannot be synthesized.

POSTTRANSLATIONAL MODIFICATION OF NORMAL ADULT, FETAL, AND EMBRYONIC HEMOGLOBINS: THE "MINOR" HEMOGLOBINS

So-called "minor" components of normal hemoglobins are the result of posttranslational hemoglobin modifications that include nonenzymatic glycation (glycosylation), acetylation, pyruvatization, S-glutathionylation, and acetaldehyde adduct formation. Using ever more sensitive methods of mass spectrometry it seems likely that other modified hemoglobins will be found.

Modified HbA variants are termed HbA1a1, A1a2, A1b, A1c, and A1d (and its subtypes, A1d1, 2, and 3). HbS, HbF, HbC and other variant hemoglobins also have minor components. Separation of minor hemoglobins in neonates and in patients with sickle cell anemia, HbSC disease, HbC disease, and sickle cell trait by HPLC is shown in Figure 7.7. HbA1c is the best-studied minor hemoglobin and its clinical importance dwarfs that of other minor components whose major clinical significance is the confusion and uncertainty they cause in the interpretation of isoelectric focusing gel patterns, HPLC columns, and hemoglobin electrophoresis. Although the impact of glycated hemoglobin in diabetology is outside the purview of this book, we will describe some functional properties of HbA1c and provide a brief description of other minor normal hemoglobins components.

Minor hemoglobins can vary in quantity according to whether diseases such as diabetes or uremia are present and if an individual is exposed to external agents such as penicillin and aspirin. Minor components of normal hemoglobin have been suggested to be "reporters" of physiological and pathophysiological events. HbA1c levels in patients with acquired immunodeficiency syndrome and with normal glucose concentrations might be increased when compared with normal controls ($9.1\% \pm 0.5\%$ vs. $7.4\% \pm 0.2\%$); however a mechanism for this observation is not obvious. An inverse relationship existed between glycohemoglobin concentrations and the CD4 cell count and acquired immunodeficiency syndrome patients with the most advanced disease and lowest CD4 counts had glycohemoglobin levels of approximately 8%.[77]

Matrix-assisted laser desorption/ionization time-of-flight mass spectrometry identified pyruvatization, glycation, acetylation, carbamylation, and acetaldehyde adduct formation in all hemoglobins and found that a minor hemoglobin containing the carbamylated α- and β^S globin eluted with HbA_2 accounting for the falsely increased HbA_2 values in patients with HbS when blood is analyzed by HPLC.[42]

Glycated Hemoglobins

HbA1c: HbA1c is a result of posttranslational and nonenzymatic glycation of HbA. The most abundant minor hemoglobin component in human red cells, HbA1c is

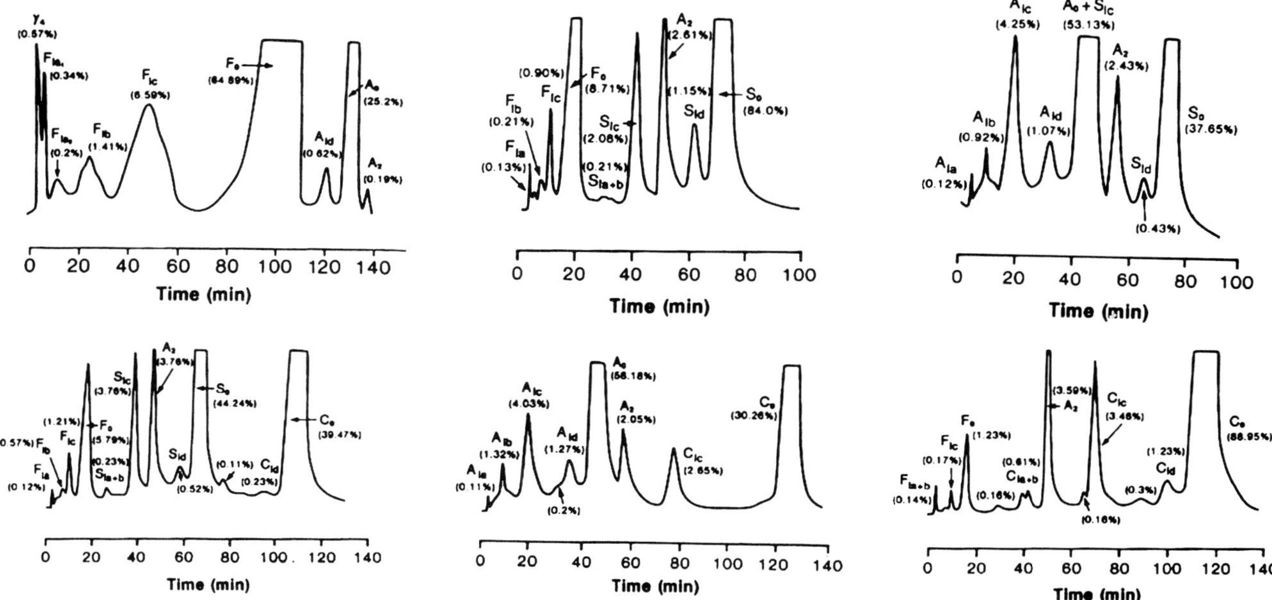

Figure 7.7. Separation by HPLC of the minor hemoglobins from neonates (top left), adults with sickle cell anemia (top center), adults with sickle cell trait (top right), HbSC disease (bottom left), HbC trait (bottom center), and HbC disease (bottom right).[85,86] These examples illustrate the complexity of patterns caused by the presence of minor hemoglobins on HPLC separation (and by isoelectrical focusing) and the difficulty of knowing, without DNA analysis or protein sequencing, whether one of these minor peaks represents or contains a genetically encoded hemoglobin variant that can be present in trace amounts.

formed by the rapid nonenzymatic condensation of glucose with the N terminus of the β-globin chain to form a Schiff base that undergoes a slow Amadori rearrangement to a stable ketoamine linkage (Fig. 7.8). This adduct is increased in patients with diabetes mellitus and its measurement is a useful index of diabetic glycemic control. Glucose also forms covalent attachments with the ε-amino groups of lysine residues of both the α- and the β-globin chain, although these adducts are not readily resolved by electrophoretic and chromatographic techniques. Nonenzymatic glycation also occurs in proteins with long turnover times exposed to high glucose concentrations. Examples are proteins of the red cell membrane, albumin, and lens crystallins. Nonenzymatic glycation of other proteins with the generation of advanced glycation endproducts (AGEs) could contribute significantly to the long-term complications of diabetes and other vascular diseases. Using AGE-specific antibodies, an AGE-modified form of human hemoglobin has also been identified. Hemoglobin-AGE (Hb-AGE) accounts for 0.42% of circulating hemoglobin in normal individuals but increases to 0.75% in patients with diabetes-induced hyperglycemia. Hemoglobin-AGE measurements might provide an index of long-term tissue modification by AGEs and prove useful in assessing the contribution of advanced glycosylation to a variety of diabetic, vascular, and age-related complications.[78]

Glycohemoglobin levels can be measured by ion-exchange column chromatography on Bio-Rex 70, affinity chromatography, HPLC, by electrophoresis, and colorimetrically. Electrospray ionization mass spectrometry to detect glycation of samples separated by boronate affinity and cation exchange chromatography has provided additional

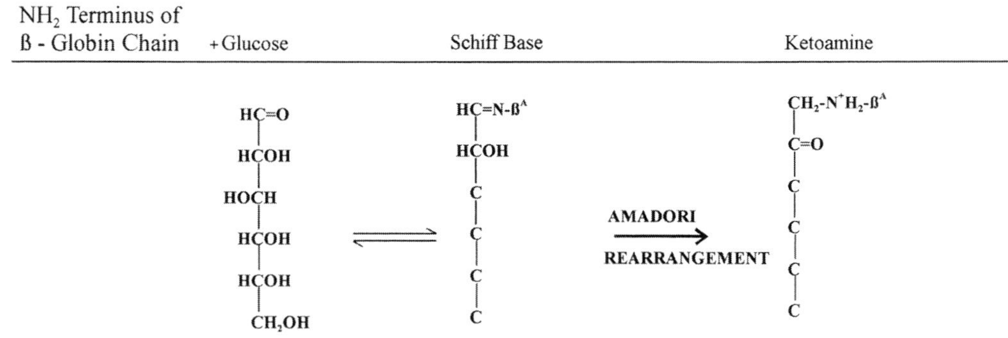

Figure 7.8. Mechanism of HbA1c formation.

insights.[79] Analyses of clinical samples were consistent with the curvilinear relationship between serum glucose and HbA1c. As glycation increased, the ratio of β- to α-globin chain glycation increased and the number of glycated sites on the β chain increased, although these were minor components. Several glycated species that cochromatographed with HbA1c on cation exchange chromatography, including species with both glycated α- and β-globin chains, nonglycated α- and glycated β-globin chains, and multiply glycated β-globin chains.

The P_{50} of stripped HbA and HbA1c is similar but as HbA1c has blocked N-terminal, it has reduced interaction with 2,3-BPG and a decreased P_{50}. The low-affinity conformation T-state of HbA1c is destabilized by the chemical modification per se and the Bohr effect is reduced compared with nonglycated HbA. The affinity of the T-state of HbA1c for 2,3-BPG is approximately 2.6-times lower than that of HbA, whereas the R-state is approximately 1.7-times lower.[80]

At the structural level, computer modeling studies showed that the two sugar moieties are asymmetrically disposed within the 2,3-BPG binding site. Calculations concerning the interaction with 2,3-BPG show that although in HbA the effector can assume two different stable orientations, in glycated hemoglobin only one orientation is possible. Together, these results show that glycation of the valine 1 residues of both β-globin chains do not impair the binding of 2,3-BPG but impose a different mode of binding by changing the internal geometry of the complex and the surface distribution of the positive electrostatic potential within the binding pocket.

When used to assess diabetic control, HbA1c levels can be affected by variant hemoglobins including elevated HbF.[81] Therefore, it has been suggested that in individual heterozygous for hemoglobin variants, laboratories either choose not to report HbA1c and propose another strategy for monitoring blood sugar levels or report HbA1c with the needed cautions.[82]

Other Glycated Hemoglobins: Like Hb A1c, components HbA1a1, HbA1a2, and HbA1b also contain a sugar moiety linked to the N terminus of the β-globin chain. Bio-Rex 70 chromatography in normal and diabetic patients detects the following minor hemoglobins: A1a1, A1a2, A1b1, A1b2, A1b3, A1d1, A1d2, and A1d3. Based on colorimetric assay, protein-bound ketoamine was present in all the minor hemoglobins, which was confirmed by chromatographic separation of hemoglobins after reduction with NaB_3H_4. All the minor hemoglobins, except HbA1a1, Hba2, and HbA1b1, were increased twofold in diabetics. HbA1d3, measures approximately 1.9% in normal individuals and approximately 3.2% in diabetics and has reduced O_2 affinity in the presence of 2,3-BPG. Glycation of hemoglobin with [^{14}C]glucose followed by separation of hemoglobins by two Bio-Rex 70 chromatographic methods indicated that the minor hemoglobin formed by glycation of the α-globin chain amino terminus was separable from HbA, whereas the minor hemoglobins formed by the glycation of ε-amino groups chromatographed with HbA.

Cord blood samples from women with preterm fetuses of gestational ages 30–36 weeks and from a control group of term fetuses of 40 weeks gestational age were analyzed for total glycated hemoglobin and the percentages of the minor hemoglobins F1a+b and F1c. The absolute levels and the increase due to red cell aging of glycohemoglobins F1a+b and Hb F1c were significantly reduced in the preterm samples compared with the term samples, suggesting decreased hemoglobin glycation in preterm fetus. The acetylated form of HbFIc also showed an increase with red cell aging indicating posttranslational enzymatic or nonenzymatic acetylation of HbF during the entire lifespan of red cells. As with glycohemoglobins, the acetylated HbF was also decreased in the preterm newborns. Both erythrocyte age and the time of gestation are factors that influence hemoglobin glycation. Minor components of Hb Barts are also acetylated and glycated.

The structure of HbA1b that forms less than 0.5% of total hemoglobin has been established and shown to be consistent with a ketoamine-linked pyruvic acid at the amino end of the β chain.[83]

Hemoglobin variants also have glycated minor components and those of HbS have been best studied. HbS1c and HbSo, a component formed by glycation of the ε-amino groups of lysine, made up 33% and 42%, respectively, of the total glycohemoglobin in individuals with sickle cell anemia, the remainder being glycated HbF and HbA_2. These modified HbS fractions had higher minimum gelling concentrations, suggesting that HbS polymerization was inhibited, perhaps because of interference with contact points in the polymer by glycated amino acid residues. Diabetics with sickle cell anemia had a twofold increase in glycohemoglobin but this increase is less than the increase in HbA1c seen in diabetics without sickle cell anemia, perhaps a result of the very short lifespan of sickle cells. A direct relationship is present between HbF concentration and the level of glycated hemoglobin in patients with sickle cell anemia, presumably due to the longer lifespan of cells containing high concentrations of HbF that permits additional time for the slow process of nonenzymatic glycation.

Other Minor Hemoglobins

Hemoglobin acetylation, in contrast to glycation, is usually an enzymatically driven process, although, at least in vitro, nonenzymatic acetylation has been reported. Additional discussion of hemoglobin and protein acetylation is provided in Chapter 24 in which acetylated mutant hemoglobins are discussed. Acetylation is more common in proteins where the N-terminal amino acid is alanine, serine, and to a lesser extent, glycine. Hemoglobin requires an unblocked N terminus to function normally, so that blocked N-terminal residues have been largely excluded by selection. A blocked N-terminal glycine in HbF contributes to its decreased 2,3-BPG binding. Acetylation occurs early in the posttranslational period and involves the acetyltransferase-mediated catalytic transfer of the acetyl moiety from acetyl–coenzyme A to the hemoglobin. Acetylated HbF is called HbF_1. Whether or not there is any functional advantage or disadvantage of HbF_1 is unknown. Feline hemoglobin, in which the β1 residue is serine, is also acetylated and binds 2,3-BPG poorly.

Acetaldehyde, a metabolic product of ethanol, forms nonenzymatically mediated adducts with hemoglobin and approximately 15%–25% of the adducts are stable to dialysis. No current assay systems are available to detect acetaldehyde adducts in the blood of humans consuming alcohol. Acetaldehyde adducts separate chromatographically with HbA1a and HbA1b. The amount of stable hemoglobin adducts formed is proportional to the amount of acetaldehyde. Acetaldehyde adducts with hemoglobin involve primarily three different amino acid residues of the β-globin chain. The acetaldehyde possibly reacts with the ε-amino group of lysine and α-amino group of valine probably through an initial Schiff base. The secondary amines of glycated valine or glycated lysine residues are also proposed to be at the sites of reaction with acetaldehyde. Acetaldehyde adduct formation with tyrosine residues is not as well understood.

Urea is in equilibrium with cyanate, and when urea concentrations are high, as in uremia, irreversible covalent adducts of cyanate with the N-terminal amino groups of both α- and β-globin chains are present. Carbamylated hemoglobin levels of up to 4% have been found in individuals with untreated uremia but are unlikely to be functionally significant.

Hemoglobin can also be glutathionylated via S-glutathionylation of reactive cysteine residues. The levels of this minor hemoglobin, which has a high O_2 affinity and reduced cooperativity, are markedly increased in diabetic individuals with microangiopathy, perhaps reflecting oxidative tissue damage.[84]

REFERENCES

1. Singer K, Chernoff AI, Singer L. Studies on abnormal hemoglobins. I. Their demonstration in sickle cell anemia and other hematologic disorders by means of alkali denaturation. *Blood.* 1951;6:413–428.
2. Schroeder WA, Shelton JR, Shelton JB, Cormick J, Jones RT. The amino acid sequence of the gamma chain of human fetal hemoglobin. *Biochemistry.* 1963;2:992–1008.
3. Slightom JL, Blechl AE, Smithies O. Human fetal G-gamma and A-gamma globin genes: complete nucleotide sequences suggest that DNA can be exchanged between these duplicated genes. *Cell.* 1980;21:627–638.
4. Bouhassira EE, Lachman H, Krishnamoorthy R, Labie D, Nagel RL. A gene conversion located 5′ to the A gamma gene in linkage disequilibrium with the Bantu haplotype in sickle cell anemia. *J Clin Invest.* 1989;83:2070–2073.
5. Adachi K, Yang Y, Lakka V, Wehrli S, Reddy KS, Surrey S. Significance of β116 His (G18) at α1β1 contact sites for αβ assembly and autoxidation of hemoglobin. *Biochemistry.* 2003;42(34):10252–10259.
6. Yagami T, Ballard BT, Padovan JC, Chait BT, Popowicz AM, Manning JM. N-terminal contributions of the gamma-subunit of fetal hemoglobin to its tetramer strength: remote effects at subunit contacts. *Protein Sci.* 2002;11(1):27–35.
7. Frier JA, Perutz MF. Structure of human foetal deoxyhaemoglobin. *J Mol Biol.* 1977;112(1):97–112.
8. Dumoulin A, Manning LR, Jenkins WT, Winslow RM, Manning JM. Exchange of subunit interfaces between recombinant adult and fetal hemoglobins. Evidence for a functional inter-relationship among regions of the tetramer. *J Biol Chem.* 1997;272(50):31326–31332.
9. Charache S, Catalano P, Burns S, et al. Pregnancy in carriers of high-affinity hemoglobins. *Blood.* 1985;65(3):713–718.
10. Giardina B, Messana I, Scatena R, Castagnola M. The multiple functions of hemoglobin. *Crit Rev Biochem Mol Biol.* 1995;30(3):165–196.
11. Brittain T. Molecular aspects of embryonic hemoglobin function. *Mol Aspects Med.* 2002;23(4):293–342.
12. Miyoshi K, Kaneto Y, Kawai H, et al. X-linked dominant control of F-cells in normal adult life: characterization of the Swiss type as hereditary persistence of fetal hemoglobin regulated dominantly by gene(s) on X chromosome. *Blood.* 1988;72:1854–1860.
13. Nagel RL. Severity, pathobiology, epistatic effects, and genetic markers in sickle cell anemia. *Semin Hematol.* 1991; 28(3):180–201.
14. Morris J, Dunn D, Beckford M, et al. The haematology of homozygous sickle cell disease after the age of 40 years. *Br J Haematol.* 1991;77:382.
15. Steinberg MH, Hsu H, Nagel RL, et al. Gender and haplotype effects upon hematological manifestations of adult sickle cell anemia. *Am J Hematol.* 1995;48(3):175–181.
16. Stamatoyannopoulos G. Control of globin gene expression during development and erythroid differentiation. *Exp Hematol.* 2005;33(3):259–271.
17. Bank A. Regulation of human fetal hemoglobin: new players, new complexities. *Blood.* 2006;107(2):435–443.
18. Sebastiani P, Wang L, Nolan VG, et al. Fetal hemoglobin in sickle cell anemia: Bayesian modeling of genetic associations. *Am J Hematol.* 2008;83:189–195.
19. Boyer SH, Belding TK, Margolet L, Noyes AN. Fetal hemoglobin restriction to a few erythrocytes (F cells) in normal human adults. *Science.* 1975;188(4186):361–363.
20. Dover GJ, Boyer SH, Pembrey ME. F cell production in sickle cell anemia: regulation by genes linked to beta-hemoglobin locus. *Science.* 1981;211(4489):1441–1444.
21. Tsantes A, Androutsos G, Bonovas S, et al. Assessment of a new immunocytochemical technique in HbF-cell counting by a novel objective evaluation method. *Br J Haematol.* 2003;123(5):948–951.
22. Amoyal I, Fibach E. Flow cytometric analysis of fetal hemoglobin in erythroid precursors of beta-thalassemia. *Clin Lab Haematol.* 2004;26(3):187–193.
23. Italia KY, Colah R, Mohanty D. Evaluation of F cells in sickle cell disorders by flow cytometry – comparison with the Kleihauer-Betke's slide method. *Intl J Lab Hematol.* 2007; 29(6):409–414.

24. Horiuchi K, Osterhout ML, Kamma H, Bekoe NA, Hirokawa KJ. Estimation of fetal hemoglobin levels in individual red cells via fluorescence image cytometry. *Cytometry.* 1995; 20:261–267.
25. Franco RS, Yasin Z, Palascak MB, Ciraolo P, Joiner CH, Rucknagel DL. The effect of fetal hemoglobin on the survival characteristics of sickle cells. *Blood.* 2006;108(3):1073–1076.
26. Leonova JY, Kazanetz EG, Smetanina NS, Adekile AD, Efremov GD, Huisman THJ. Variability in the fetal hemoglobin level of the normal adult. *Am J Hematol.* 1996;53:59–65.
27. Wood WG. Hereditary persistence of fetal hemoglobin and δ thalassemia. In: Steinberg MH, Forget BG, Higgs DR, Nagel RL, eds. *Disorders of Hemoglobin: Genetics, Pathophysiology, and Clinical Management.* 1st ed. Cambridge: Cambridge University Press; 2001:356–388.
28. Perry GW, Vargas-Cuba R, Vertes RP. Fetal hemoglobin levels in sudden infant death syndrome. *Arch Pathol Lab Med.* 1997;121:1084–1054.
29. Bard H, Cote A, Praud JP, Infante-Rivard C, Gagnon C. Fetal hemoglobin synthesis determined by gamma-mRNA/gamma-mRNA + beta-mRNA quantitation in infants at risk for sudden infant death syndrome being monitored at home for apnea. *Pediatrics.* 2003;112(4):e285.
30. Krous HF, Haas EA, Chadwick AE, Masoumi H, Stanley C, Perry GW. Hemoglobin F in sudden infant death syndrome: a San Diego SIDS/SUDC Research Project report. *J Forensic Leg Med.* 2007;14(8):456–460.
31. Wolk M, Martin JE, Constantin R. Blood cells with fetal haemoglobin (F cells) detected by immunohistochemistry as indicators of solid tumours. *J Clin Pathol.* 2004;57(7):740–745.
32. Wolk M, Martin JE, Reinus C. Development of fetal haemoglobin-blood cells (F cells) within colorectal tumour tissues. *J Clin Pathol.* 2006;59(6):598–602.
33. Adams JG, Morrison WT, Steinberg MH. Hemoglobin Parchman: double crossover within a single human gene. *Science.* 1982;218:291–293.
34. Petes TD. Evidence that structural variants within the human δ-globin protein may reflect genetic inteactions between the δ- and β-globin genes. *Am J Hum Genet.* 1982;34:820–823.
35. Sen U, Dasgupta J, Choudhury D, et al. Crystal structures of HbA2 and HbE and modeling of hemoglobin delta 4: interpretation of the thermal stability and the antisickling effect of HbA2 and identification of the ferrocyanide binding site in Hb. *Biochemistry.* 2004;43(39):12477–12488.
36. Donze D, Jeancake PH, Townes TM. Activation of d-globin gene expression by erythroid Krupple-like factor: a potential approach for gene therapy of sickle cell disease. *Blood.* 1996;88:4051–4057.
37. Tang DC, Ebb D, Hardison RC, Rodgers GP. Restoration of the CCAAT box or insertion of the CACCC motif activate d-globin gene expression. *Blood.* 1997;90:421–427.
38. Nagel RL, Bookchin RM, Labie D, Wajcman H, Isaac-Sadeye WA, Honig GR. Structural basis for the inhibitory effects of hemoglobin F and hemoglobin A2 on the polymerization of hemoglobin S. *Proc Natl Acad Sci USA.* 1979;76:670–672.
39. Adachi K, Pang JA, Reddy LR, et al. Polymerization of three hemoglobin A2 variants containing Val<6< and inhibition of hemoglobin S polymerization by hemoglobin A2. *J Biol Chem.* 1996;271:24557–24563.
40. Van Kirk R, Sandhaus LM, Hoyer JD. The detection and diagnosis of hemoglobin A2′ by high-performance liquid chromatography. *Am J Clin Pathol.* 2005;123(5):657–661.
41. Head CE, Conroy M, Jarvis M, Phelan L, Bain BJ. Some observations on the measurement of haemoglobin A2 and S percentages by high performance liquid chromatography in the presence and absence of alpha thalassaemia. *J Clin Pathol.* 2004;57(3):276–280.
42. Zurbriggen K, Schmugge M, Schmid M, et al. Analysis of minor hemoglobins by matrix-assisted laser desorption/ionization time-of-flight mass spectrometry. *Clin Chem.* 2005;51(6):989–996.
43. Pavlou E, Phylactides M, Kyrri A, et al. delta-Thalassemia in Cyprus. *Hemoglobin.* 2006;30(4):455–462.
44. Bouva MJ, Harteveld CL, van DP, Giordano PC. Known and new delta globin gene mutations and their diagnostic significance. *Haematologica.* 2006;91(1):129–132.
45. Bunn HF. Subunit assembly of hemoglobin: an important determinant of hematologic phenotype. *Blood.* 1987;69:1–6.
46. Mrabet NT, McDonald MJ, Turci S, Sarkar R, Szabo A, Bunn HF. Electrostatic attraction governs the dimer assembly of human hemoglobin. *J Biol Chem.* 1986;261:5222–5228.
47. McDonald MJ, Turci SM, Mrabet NT, Himelstein BP, Bunn HF. The kinetics of assembly of normal and variant human oxyhemoglobins. *J Biol Chem.* 1987;262:5951–5956.
48. Harthoorn-Lasthuizen EJ, Lindemans J, Langenhuijsen MMAC. Influence of iron deficiency anaemia on haemoglobin A2 levels: possible consequences for b-thalassaemia screening. *Scand J Clin Lab Invest.* 1999;59(1):65–70.
49. El-Agouza I, Abu SA, Sirdah M. The effect of iron deficiency anaemia on the levels of haemoglobin subtypes: possible consequences for clinical diagnosis. *Clin Lab Haematol.* 2002;24(5):285–289.
50. Kutlar F, Gonzalez-Redondo JM, Kutlar A, et al. The levels of zand d chains in patients with Hb H disease. *Hum Genet.* 1989;82:179–186.
51. Loudianos G, Cao A, Ristaldi MS, et al. Molecular basis of delta beta-thalassemia with normal fetal hemoglobin level. *Blood.* 1990;75:526–528. [Letter].
52. Oggiano L, Guiso L, Frogheri L, et al. A novel Mediterranean "δ-thalassemia" determinant containing the δ+27 and $\beta^0$39 point mutations in cis. *Am J Hematol.* 1994;45:81–84.
53. Steinberg MH, Coleman MB, Adams JG. Beta-thalassemia with exceptionally high hemoglobin A2. Differential expression of the delta-globin gene in the presence of beta-thalassemia. *J Lab Clin Med.* 1982;100:548–557.
54. Weatherall DJ, Clegg JB. *The Thalassaemia Syndromes.* 4th ed. Oxford: Blackwell Science; 2001.
55. Huisman TH. Levels of Hb A2 in heterozygotes and homozygotes for beta-thalassemia mutations: Influence of mutations in the CACCC and ATAAA motifs of the beta-globin gene promoter. *Acta Haematol.* 1997;98(4):187–194.
56. Codrington JF, Li HW, Kutlar F, Gu LH, Ramachandran M, Huisman TH. Observations on the levels of Hb A2 in patients with different b-thalassemia mutations and a d chain variant. *Blood.* 1990;76:1246–1249.
57. Kendall AG, Bastomsky CH. Hemoglobin A2 in hyperthyroidism. *Hemoglobin.* 1981;5:571–577.
58. Martin L, Pissard S, Blanc P, et al. [Increased haemoglobin A2 levels in pseudoxanthoma elasticum]. *Ann Dermatol Venereol.* 2006;133(8–9 Pt 1):645–651.

59. Luo HY, Liang XL, Frye C, et al. Embryonic hemoglobins are expressed in definitive cells. *Blood.* 1999;94(1):359–361.
60. He Z, Russell JE. Expression, purification, and characterization of human hemoglobins Gower-1 (zeta(2) epsilon(2)), Gower-2 (alpha(2)epsilon(2)), and Portland-2 (zeta(2)beta(2)) assembled in complex transgenic-knockout mice. *Blood.* 2001;97(4):1099–1105.
61. Chui DH, Wong SC, Chung SW, Patterson M, Bhargava S, Poon MC. Embryonic zeta-globin chains in adults: a marker for alpha- thalassemia-1 haplotype due to a greater than 17.5-kb deletion. *N Engl J Med.* 1986;314:76–79.
62. Chui DH, Mentzer WC, Patterson M, et al. Human embryonic zeta-globin chains in fetal and newborn blood. *Blood.* 1989;74:1409–1414.
63. Lafferty JD, Crowther MA, Waye JS, Chui DHK. A reliable screening test to identify adult carriers of the (–SEA) alpha^0-thalassemia deletion – Detection of embryonic zeta-globin chains by enzyme-linked immunosorbent assay. *Am J Clin Pathol.* 2000;114(6):927–931.
64. Ma SK, Ma V, Chan AY, Chan LC, Chui DH. Routine screening of (–(SEA)) alpha-thalassemia deletion by an enzyme-linked immunosorbent assay for embryonic zeta-globin chains. *Acta Haematol.* 2002;108(1):8–12.
65. He Z, Russell JE. A human embryonic hemoglobin inhibits Hb S polymerization in vitro and restores a normal phenotype to mouse models of sickle cell disease. *Proc Natl Acad Sci USA.* 2002;99(16):10635–10640.
66. Hofmann OM, Brittain T, Wells RM. The control of oxygen affinity in the three human embryonic haemoglobins by respiration linked metabolites. *Biochem Mol Biol Int.* 1997;42(3):553–566.
67. Hofmann O, Brittain T. Ligand binding kinetics and dissociation of the human embryonic haemoglobins. *Biochem J.* 1996;315(Pt 1):65–70.
68. Hofmann O, Carrucan G, Robson N, Brittain T. The chloride effect in the human embryonic haemoglobins. *Biochem J.* 1995;309(Pt 3):959–962.
69. Hofmann O, Mould R, Brittain T. Allosteric modulation of oxygen binding to the three human embryonic haemoglobins. *Biochem J.* 1995;306(Pt 2):367–370.
70. Mathews AJ, Brittain T. Haem disorder in recombinant- and reticulocyte-derived haemoglobins: evidence for stereoselective haem insertion in eukaryotes. *Biochem J.* 2001;357 (Pt 1):305–311.
71. Robson N, Brittain T. Heme stability in the human embryonic hemoglobins. *J Inorg Biochem.* 1996;64(3):137–147.
72. Robson N, Brittain T. Conformational relaxation and ligand binding to singly reduced human embryonic haemoglobins. *Biochem Mol Biol Int.* 1996;38(6):1245–1253.
73. Kidd RD, Baker HM, Mathews AJ, Brittain T, Baker EN. Oligomerization and ligand binding in a homotetrameric hemoglobin: two high-resolution crystal structures of hemoglobin Bart's (gamma(4)), a marker for alpha-thalassemia. *Protein Sci.* 2001;10(9):1739–1749.
74. Kidd RD, Mathews A, Baker HM, Brittain T, Baker EN. Subunit dissociation and reassociation leads to preferential crystallization of haemoglobin Bart's ($\gamma 4$) from solutions of human embryonic haemoglobin Portland ($\zeta 2 \gamma 2$) at low pH. *Acta Crystallogr D Biol Crystallogr.* 2001;57(Pt 6):921–924.
75. Sutherland-Smith AJ, Baker HM, Hofmann OM, Brittain T, Baker EN. Crystal structure of a human embryonic haemoglobin: the carbonmonoxy form of Gower II ($\alpha 2 \varepsilon 2$) haemoglobin at 2.9 A resolution. *J Mol Biol.* 1998;280(3):475–484.
76. Papachatzopoulou A, Menounos PG, Kolonelou C, Patrinos GP. Mutation screening in the human epsilon-globin gene using single-strand conformation polymorphism analysis. *Am J Hematol.* 2006;81(2):136–138.
77. Kabadi UM, Gopal V, Hood L, Kabadi MU, Platt K. Elevated glycosylated hemoglobin concentrations in AIDS. *AIDS.* 1992;6(2):236–238.
78. Wautier JL, Schmidt AM. Protein glycation: a firm link to endothelial cell dysfunction. *Circ Res.* 2004;95(3):233–238.
79. Peterson KP, Pavlovich JG, Goldstein D, Little R, England J, Peterson CM. What is hemoglobin A1C? An analysis of glycated hemoglobins by electrospray ionization mass spectrometry. *Clin Chem.* 1998;44(9):1951–1958.
80. De Rosa MC, Sanna MT, Messana I, et al. Glycated human hemoglobin (HbA1C): functional characteristics and molecular modeling studies. *Biophys Chem.* 1998;72(3):323–335.
81. Bry L, Chen PC, Sacks DB. Effects of hemoglobin variants and chemically modified derivatives on assays for glycohemoglobin. *Clin Chem.* 2001;47(2):153–163.
82. Manley SE, Round RA, Smith JM. Calibration of HbA1C and its measurement in the presence of variant haemoglobins: report on questionnaire to manufacturers. *Ann Clin Biochem.* 2006;43(Pt 2):135–145.
83. Prome D, Blouquit Y, Ponthus C, Prome JC, Rosa J. Structure of the human adult hemoglobin minor fraction A1b by electrospray and secondary ion mass spectrometry. Pyruvic acid as amino-terminal blocking group. *J Biol Chem.* 1991; 266(20):13050–13054.
84. Sampathkumar R, Balasubramanyam M, Sudarslal S, Rema M, Mohan V, Balaram P. Increased glutathionylated hemoglobin (HbSSG) in type 2 diabetes subjects with microangiopathy. *Clin Biochem.* 2005;38(10):892–899.
85. Abraham EC, Abraham A, Stallings M. High-pressure liquid chromatographic separation of glycosylated and acetylated minor hemoglobins in newborn infants and in patients with sickle cell disease. *J Lab Clin Med.* 1984;104(6):1027–1034.
86. Abraham EC, Cameron BF, Abraham A, Stallings M. Glycosylated hemoglobins in heterozygotes and homozygotes for hemoglobin C with or without diabetes. *J Lab Clin Med.* 1984;104(4):602–609.

SECTION TWO

PATHOPHYSIOLOGY OF HEMOGLOBIN AND ITS DISORDERS

Martin H. Steinberg

One convenient classification of hemoglobin disorders dichotomizes these conditions into mutations that either change the primary structure of globin, called hemoglobinopathies, or reduce the expression of globin genes, called thalassemia. Rarely, a single mutation affects both the structure and expression level of the affected gene, and these have been called thalassemic hemoglobinopathies. Although at the level of the abnormal erythrocyte, many hemoglobinopathies and thalassemias can have similar pathophysiological effects, and result in similar clinical features, such generalizations do not apply to all hemoglobin disorders. For example, only sickle hemoglobin (HbS) polymerizes, triggering many features of sickle cell disease, and extreme ineffective erythropoiesis is characteristic of β thalassemia major.

The next four chapters consider how hemoglobin disorders can perturb vascular biology, the erythrocyte membrane, nitric oxide biology, and the lifespan of the affected red cell. A final chapter brings up to date the animal models that permit certain detailed study of this pathobiology. All these chapters are new to this edition.

In sickle cell disease and thalassemia, chronic hypoxia and hemolysis require vascular tone and flow adaptations. In sickle cell disease, red cell deformability is sensitive to intravascular oxygen tension as deoxygenation results in HbS polymerization, erythrocyte sickling, and vasoocclusion. Vasoocclusive events in sickle cell disease result in reperfusion injury characterized by excessive oxidant generation, endothelial activation and dysfunction, and inflammation. Similarly, in thalassemia, red cell abnormalities caused by precipitation of excess globin chains and oxidative stress lead to hemolysis and reduced red cell deformability and contribute to vascular pathobiology. In Chapter 8, Kaul discusses factors that contribute to the vascular pathobiology of sickle cell disease and thalassemia, with special emphasis on blood rheology, its sensitivity to oxygen saturation, and cell heterogeneity in sickle cell disease and the adhesive interactions between sickle erythrocytes and the endothelium that mediate sickle vasoocclusion.

The erythrocyte membrane is a complex dynamic structure with multiple regulated functions. Cytoskeletal proteins maintain its structural integrity, which must simultaneously be flexible enough to deform in the microcirculation and sufficiently durable to resist high shear stresses in large vessels. Multiple ligands and receptors interact with the external surface of the membrane. Specific proteins maintain a highly ordered lipid structure, which in turn might modulate other membrane protein functions or cellular interactions. Multiple regulated transport systems control solute and water flux across the membrane to facilitate the transport of respiratory gases, provide metabolic substrates, and regulate cell volume.

Given the physiological interactions of hemoglobin with the erythrocyte membrane, it is perhaps not surprising that abnormal hemoglobins can elicit significant pathological effects on membrane structure and function. A significant source of membrane damage in hemoglobinopathies is the increased level of oxidant species produced by reactive sulfhydryls on unstable or denatured hemoglobin molecules, membrane bound heme, or free iron. Oxidation affects cytoskeletal function, increases membrane rigidity and fragility, and perturbs cation transport and volume regulation.

HbS polymerization produces major damage to the membrane. Polymer formation, in addition to increasing cellular rigidity and blood viscosity, results in formation of membrane spicules in which the cytoskeleton is dissociated from its membrane connections. Associated with this membrane disruption is externalization of phosphatidyl serine and an increase in cation permeability. Calcium influx results in activation of the Gardos pathway, which mediates selective potassium loss that results in cation depletion. Potassium-chloride cotransport is excessively active in the red cells of HbSC disease and sickle cell anemia and in other hemoglobinopathies and thalassemias, and leads to dehydrated, dense cells with high hemoglobin concentrations. In sickle erythrocytes, elevated hemoglobin concentration greatly potentiates the rate and extent of HbS polymer formation. Gallagher and Joiner, in Chapter 9, discuss structural and functional abnormalities of the erythrocyte membrane and their contributions to the pathophysiology of hemoglobin disorders.

One of the most notable advances in the field since the first edition of this book has been the greater understanding of the role of dysregulated nitric oxide biology in the vasculopathy associated with hemolytic anemia. Two new chapters address this issue. In Chapter 10, Leopold and Loscalzo discuss the role of nitric oxide as the key mediator of endothelial function and vascular tone, its modulation of the integrity of the endothelium, and interactions between circulating blood components and the vessel wall. In this paradigm, endothelium-derived nitric oxide is released to the vascular smooth muscle cells where it activates soluble guanylyl cyclase to generate cyclic guanine monophosphate and modulate cation flux that in turn induces vasodilation and adjusts vascular tone.

Anemia is the most basic clinical characteristic of sickle cell disease and thalassemia. The lifespan of the erythrocyte in sickle cell disease is shortened to less than one-tenth of normal, and in severe β thalassemia, it can be even shorter. In Chapter 11, Kato and Gladwin discuss the mechanisms that give rise to the accelerated hemolysis characteristic of these disorders. Emerging data suggest that chronic intravascular hemolysis produces endothelial dysfunction and progressive vasculopathy due to nitric oxide scavenging and reduced bioavailability of this key vasodilator and antiinflammatory molecule. This in turn contributes to complications shared by many chronic hemolytic anemias that include pulmonary arterial hypertension and cutaneous leg ulceration. Understanding this pathophysiology also suggests new treatment approaches.

Transgenic mice are important adjuncts for the study of the pathophysiology and treatment of human hemoglobin disorders. Insights into human gene therapy, new therapeutics, and disease pathophysiology have come from studies of transgenic and knockout mice, more so for sickle cell disease than thalassemia. Many inbred strains with spontaneous and induced mutations, and engineered knockout and knockin lines are available. Transgenic mice provide both advantages and disadvantages for studying human disease. Different inbred mouse strains can have different physiological characteristics, complicating the interpretation of some experiments and making it wise to examine more than one transgenic line before drawing conclusions about the relevance of a result to the human disease. State-of-the-art animal models for the study of hemoglobin disorders are discussed by Fabry in Chapter 12.

8

Rheology and Vascular Pathobiology in Sickle Cell Disease and Thalassemia

Dhananjay K. Kaul

INTRODUCTION

Oxygen delivery and metabolite transfer occur in the exchange compartment of the microcirculation, processes affected by erythrocyte abnormalities and alterations in components of the vascular wall, with the latter influencing flow regulation at the arteriolar level. In sickle cell disease and thalassemia, red cell rheology is abnormal; there is hemolysis, anemia, and red cell and tissue oxidative stress. Chronic hypoxia and hemolysis, common to both conditions, necessitate vascular tone and flow adaptations. In sickle cell disease, red cell deformability is sensitive to intravascular O_2 tension as deoxygenation results in hemoglobin S (HbS) polymerization, erythrocyte sickling, and vasoocclusion. Vasoocclusive events in sickle cell disease result in reperfusion injury characterized by excessive oxidant generation, endothelial activation and dysfunction, and inflammation. Similarly, in thalassemia, red cell abnormalities caused by precipitation of excess globin chains and oxidative stress lead to hemolysis and reduced red cell deformability and contribute to vascular pathobiology. Therefore, the heterozygote advantage seen in carriers of both these diseases (Chapter 26) is balanced by the vasculopathy characteristic of the homozygote.[1] This chapter addresses the role of blood components and other factors that contribute to the vascular pathobiology of sickle cell disease and thalassemia.

SICKLE CELL DISEASE

Red Cell Rheology

Red cell rheology is the study of the cellular deformation under shear forces as encountered in the blood circulation. Pliability, or deformability, is a prominent feature of normal red cells, which enables them to traverse the microcirculation. The average diameter of normal human erythrocytes is approximately 8 μm. Their biconcave discoid shape provides a high surface area/volume ratio enabling their extensive deformation during passage through narrow-diameter capillaries. Red cell deformability is indispensable for it to perform its basic functions. Cell deformability is a major determining factor of microvascular flow, as it affects the rate of erythrocyte entry into capillaries, which influences the pressure drop across small vessels and pressure distribution in the vascular bed, impacting microcirculatory vascular resistance.

In sickle cell disease, under deoxygenated conditions, HbS polymerization (Chapter 6) results in the formation of rigid sickled cells that have markedly reduced deformability accompanied by increases in whole blood viscosity. Ham and Castle[2] propounded the hypothesis of deoxygenation-induced increased blood viscosity resulting in a "vicious circle" of sickling. Using ektacytometry, micropipettes, the rheoscope, and nucleopore filtration, reduced red cell deformability and membrane fragility have been shown to be major determinants of the blood rheological abnormalities and hemolysis in sickle cell disease.

Oxygen Tension: In the oxygenated state, rheological and hemodynamic abnormalities of sickle red cells are attributed to higher than normal mean corpuscular hemoglobin concentration (MCHC) and the presence of irreversibly sickled cells (ISCs).[3–6] Micropipette studies have revealed that oxygenated sickle erythrocytes show an increase in both static (extensional deformation) and dynamic (rate of recovery following extensional deformation) rigidities.[7] Bulk viscosity of whole sickle cell disease blood and the rigidity of individual sickle cells are significantly influenced by their state of dehydration or increased MCHC. The static rigidity of individual sickle cells increases with decreasing O_2 tension (pO_2).[8,9] Intravital studies have shown that the hemodynamic behavior of deoxygenated sickle cell blood is dependent on pO_2 and perfusion pressure.[10–12] A decline in microvascular red blood cell velocities (Vrbc) and wall shear rates occurs at a relatively high pO_2 level of 60 mm Hg. When pO_2 is lowered to 40 mm Hg, it induces sufficient rigidity and some sickling to account for the drastic reduction in Vrbc and wall shear rates at low perfusion pressure.[12] Deoxygenation might induce arteriolar dilation, which is insufficient to overcome increased capillary resistance to deoxygenated sickle cells.[13] An issue of potential physiological importance concerns the rate of deoxygenation of sickle erythrocytes cells and how this affects HbS polymer characteristics and rheology. When subjected to gradual deoxygenation, most sickle red cells assume typical sickle shapes. This is accompanied by a steady increase in the bulk viscosity of sickle red cell suspensions during deoxygenation.[14] In contrast, rapid deoxygenation causes a high rate of homogeneous nucleation and formation of independent polymer domains resulting in granular morphology, regardless of MCHC differences among heterogeneous sickle red cells.

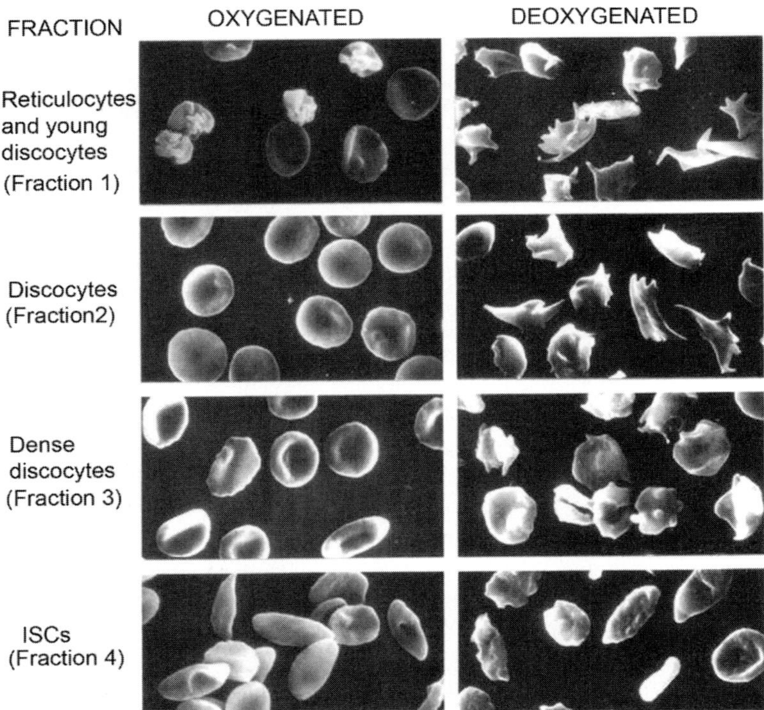

Figure 8.1. Density gradient separation of sickle cell blood reveals marked heterogeneity of red cells. Four distinct sickle red cell populations are identified. Fraction 1 is characterized by the presence of mostly reticulocytes; immature reticulocytes appear multilobulated. Fraction 2 consists of mainly discocytes that form the largest component of sickle blood and transform to typical sickled forms upon deoxygenation. Dense sickle red cells (e.g., dense discocytes and ISCs) seen in fractions 3 and 4 show minimal transformation with deoxygenation. (Modified from ref. 17.) (See color plate 8.1.)

The viscosity of rapidly deoxygenated sickle cell suspensions shows two distinct phases,[14] Following an initial rapid rise in viscosity to a peak value, in the second phase there is a significant time-dependent decrease in bulk viscosity. This phase is characterized by the appearance of elongated cells that are unlike typical sickled cells. Transmission electron microscopy shows that these cells develop long processes after prolonged deoxygenation that contain regions of aligned polymers in addition to regions of very small polymer domains or hemoglobin aggregates. This is in accordance with earlier kinetic, morphological, and ultrastructural analyses of rapidly deoxygenated sickle cells.[15] Prolonged deoxygenation would then result in elongated shape caused by growth of the aligned domains. The viscosity decrease is probably due to alignment of the elongated cells along the direction of the flow. Another study[16] concluded that it is the polymer fraction but not the cell shape that determines the filterability of deoxygenated sickle cells. This study, however, did not subject the cells to different rates of deoxygenation to produce distinct polymer domains. Thus, HbS polymer characteristics, as determined by the rate and duration of deoxygenation, could affect the microvascular flow dynamics of sickle red cells.

Sickle Red Cell Heterogeneity: Density gradient separation of sickle cell blood reveals marked heterogeneity. Red cell density is determined by MCHC. Sickle erythrocytes are bimodally distributed when centrifuged on density gradients. One major population comprised discocytic red cells with MCHC similar to normal red cells (fraction 2); the other major population was very dense (fraction 4) sickle cells and contained mainly rigid ISCs (Fig. 8.1). Light Fraction 1 cells contained a high percentage of reticulocytes. Fraction 3 was characterized by very dense and somewhat irregular shaped discocytes with high MCHC. In the gradient, the range of MCHC varied from approximately 30 g/dL for fraction 1 to more than 45 g/dL for fraction 4. Gradual deoxygenation of fraction 1 and 2 cells with low MCHC resulted in the formation of typical sickled cells and holly leaf forms; under the same deoxy conditions, hemoglobin in fraction 3 and 4 cells with high MCHC polymerized more rapidly but the cells had minimal shape changes.[17] The generation of dense sickle cells is mainly attributed to cell dehydration caused by abnormal membrane cation and water transport (Chapter 9). Homodynamic behavior of density-defined sickle erythrocytes populations, examined in an ex vivo microcirculatory preparation, showed that deoxygenation caused approximately a 10-fold increase in the vascular resistance of very dense sickle discocytes compared with oxygenated cells. The hemodynamic results indicated profound vasoocclusive behavior of dense sickle cells with deoxygenation. The observed differences in the hemodynamic behavior of deoxygenated sickle cell subpopulations reflect differences not only in the polymer characteristics but also in the extent of intracellular polymer. The abnormal viscoelastic behavior of individual deoxygenated sickle red cells correlates with the amount of intracellular polymer that is determined by MCHC.[9] Therefore, the microvascular flow of sickle cell blood will be determined by contributions from the distinct hemodynamic characteristics of heterogeneous sickle erythrocyte populations.

Factors Affecting Vascular Biology

Adhesion of sickle erythrocytes to vascular endothelial cells led to the recognition that vascular factors played an important role in the pathophysiology of sickle cell disease.[18,19] The study of vascular dysfunction in sickle cell disease has been facilitated by the discoveries of endothelial vasoactive molecules, especially nitric oxide (NO), elucidation of the role of oxidative stress, and identification of adhesion molecules expressed by activated endothelium that mediate increased red cell adhesion and inflammatory responses.

Oxidative Stress: Reperfusion injury and cell-free plasma heme are major elements in intravascular and endothelial oxidant generation (Chapter 11). The initiation, progression, and resolution of a vasoocclusive episode (Chapter 20) have features of reperfusion injury. Subclinical transient vasoocclusive events, caused by intravascular sickling and abnormal adhesion of red cells, are likely to be even more frequent than acute events recognized clinically. These "microcrises"[20] could inflict organ damage by chronic generation of reactive oxygen species (ROS). Reperfusion with the resupply of O_2 after a vasoocclusive event has a deleterious effect on vascular endothelium resulting in increased levels of superoxide ($O_2^{\cdot -}$) generated by xanthine oxidase (XO), nicotinamide adenine dinucleotide phosphate oxidase (NADPH oxidase)[21,22] and "uncoupling" of endothelial nitric oxide synthase (eNOS).[23] Uncoupling is likely due to depletion of the substrate arginine and cofactor tetrahydrobiopterin (BH_4).[24] Thus, endothelium is an early and prominent, but not exclusive, target of reperfusion injury. Increased oxidant generation causes endothelial activation and dysfunction, altered responses of resistance vessels, and inflammatory effects in postcapillary venules, the site of blood cell–endothelium interactions.

Increased lipid peroxidation, and hydroxyl ($^{\cdot}OH^-$) radical generation in transgenic sickle mice (NY1DD model; mild pathology) suggested an inflammatory state.[25] Elevated leukocyte and neutrophil counts in the peripheral circulation in transgenic sickle mice was consistent with the pro-inflammatory condition in human sickle cell disease.[26,27] Increased oxidative stress was later confirmed[28] in sickle cell disease patients and transgenic-knockout BERK mice (expressing exclusively human α- and β^{S-}-globins; severe pathology; Chapter 12), where increased vascular $O_2^{\cdot -}$ production and elevated plasma XO activity was observed. Hypoxia/reoxygenation in NY1DD mice enhanced endothelial oxidant generation and heightened leukocyte-endothelium interactions compared with control mice. Because NY1DD mice have little hemolysis, these studies indicated that hypoxia-induced sickling was preceded by reoxygenation-induced endothelial activation, oxidant production, and leukocyte recruitment.[26,29,30]

Oxidative stress in sickle cell disease is not limited to vascular endothelium and erythrocytes. Although increased leukocyte counts in sickle cell disease and sickle transgenic mice models suggest a systemic effect of oxidative stress, direct evidence of oxidative stress in can be found in mice.[31] Homozygous sickle mice have peroxidation of membrane lipids and a depletion of antioxidants, including reduced glutathione (GSH), superoxide dismutase (SOD), catalase and glutathione peroxidase (GPx).[31] Lipid peroxidation is perhaps the most recognized biological effect of O_2 radicals that occurs when free radicals attack double bonds of unsaturated fatty acids producing peroxides. In sickle cell disease, depleted levels of antioxidants likely cause increased susceptibility to lipid peroxidation.[32,33] Lipid peroxidation causes damage to the cell membrane and membranes of cellular organelles like mitochondria. Among the best-characterized enzymatic pathways are SOD, catalase, and GPx. H_2O_2 is a potential source of $^{\cdot}OH$, and two enzymatic oxidants, catalase and GPx, transform it to water. GPx is specific for GSH as a hydrogen donor but accepts peroxides as well as H_2O_2. During reperfusion, these endogenous defenses are likely to be ineffective as a result of overproduction of O_2 radicals. Additionally, during reperfusion, degradation and consumption of antioxidants by the release of ROS has been documented.[34] Failure to replenish antioxidants might exacerbate oxidative stress and contribute to hemolysis and multiple organ damage in sickle cell disease.

GSH levels in muscle, kidney, and liver are higher in BERK mice compared with NY1DD mice but are significantly lower when compared with wild-type controls.[31] This could represent a protective response to a greater oxidative stress caused by recurring ischemia-reperfusion events, increased amounts of inflammatory cytokines, and higher levels of protein nitration.[35] Induction of mitochondrial peroxynitrite ($ONOO^-$) can also induce GSH synthesis[36] and BERK mice have increased nitrotyrosine (nitration of tyrosine residues by $ONOO^-$) levels.[35] This might be a result of the initial higher production of NO followed by consumption of NO by O_2 radicals and plasma heme that leads to increased depletion of arginine.[37,38] In idiopathic pulmonary arterial hypertension, GSH content in bronchoalveolar lavage fluid is increased, probably as an adaptive response to increased oxidant generation in the inflamed lungs.[39] The reported reduction in cellular GSH in sickle cell disease could be in response to oxidative stress, vasoocclusion, and hemolysis.[40,41] Decreased GSH and glutamine have been associated with compromised red cell integrity, hemolysis, and reduced NO bioavailability, all factors that might contribute to the pathogenesis of pulmonary hypertension in sickle cell disease.[23,42] Arginine supplementation of BERK mice significantly elevated NO metabolites accompanied by enhanced GSH and reduced lipid peroxidation,[31] further suggesting a role for NO bioavailability in modulating oxidative stress.

Endothelial Activation: Endothelial injury and activation is a prominent feature of sickle cell disease.[43,118] This is likely to be the result of reperfusion injury and oxidative stress (Chapter 11). Even under normoxic conditions, transgenic sickle mice show endothelial expression of P-selectin[44] and greater leukocyte rolling compared with wild-type mice, indicating activated endothelium.[26] Greater leukocyte recruitment caused by transient reperfusion injury in transgenic sickle mice is ameliorated by antibodies to P-selectin.[26] Similarly, P-selectin knockout mice transplanted with bone marrow from BERK mice showed absence of an inflammatory response.[45]

Endothelial oxidant generation can lead to increased peroxidation and up-regulation of the redox-sensitive transcription factor nuclear factor (NF)-κB that can activate genes for intercellular adhesion molecule-1 (ICAM-1), vascular cell adhesion molecule-1 (VCAM-1), and E-selectin.[46] Similarly, transgenic sickle mouse models show up-regulation of these markers of endothelial activation.[29,47,48] Another source of endothelial injury is ROS generated by sickle erythrocytes due to the presence of unstable HbS and spontaneous autoxidation of heme iron.[49] Furthermore, elevated levels of inflammatory cytokines such as tumor necrosis factor-α (TNFα), interleukin-1β, and platelet-activating factor (PAF) induce up-regulation of endothelial adhesion molecules like VCAM-1, E-selectin, and ICAM-1, probably via endothelial oxidant generation and activation of NF-κB.[50,51]

Sickle cell disease patients have increased numbers of circulating endothelial cells.[52,53] Endothelial damage and detachment are also present following reperfusion injury in other ischemic diseases.[54] The activated phenotype of circulating endothelial cells in sickle cell disease is suggested by increased expression of cell adhesion markers and up-regulation of αVβ3 integrin[53] that have a pivotal role in sickle cell–endothelium adhesion. These data suggest the endothelium in sickle cell disease is likely to be in a perpetually activated state. Inflammatory cytokines, oxidant generation, and up-regulation of endothelial adhesive molecules might influence not only adhesion of leukocytes and sickle red cells but also potentially influence platelet activation and aggregation.

Sickle Red Cell Adhesion

Among multiple pathologies, sickle erythrocyte–endothelial interaction has been implicated as a potential initiating mechanism in vasoocclusion. In the microcirculation, sickle red cell adhesion can potentially prolong capillary transit time, promote hypoxia, and initiate sickling as suggested by higher peripheral resistance following enhanced sickle red cell adhesion.[55] Sickle red cell adhesion involves contributions from erythrocyte, plasma, and microvascular elements. These include red cell heterogeneity, deformability and adhesion molecules, oxidant radical generation, endothelial activation, and multiple vascular adhesion molecules.

Static incubation assays showed that sickle red cells adhere abnormally to endothelial monolayers and suggests that this mechanism contributes to vasoocclusion.[18,56] Studies using a parallel plate flow chamber showed sickle cell adhesion under controlled flow conditions at a low shear stress (1 dyne/cm^2).[57] In contrast to greatest adhesion of most dense sickle cells in static assays, flow studies showed that the greatest adhesion was exhibited by cells from the least dense fraction, the reticulocytes. Similar results were found with respect to adhesion of ISCs, but irregular, deformable dense discocytes were more adhesive.[58] The reduced adhesivity of dense sickle red cells in shear flow conditions could be due in part to their inability to deform to establish sufficient areas of contact with endothelial cell surface. Controlled dehydration of deformable discocytes, using Nystatin-sucrose to increase their density, rendered them less adherent; rehydration of dense red cells increased their adhesivity.[59] Cell dehydration might also alter the conformation of the red cell surface receptors.

Using a more physiological ex vivo microcirculatory preparation, postcapillary venules were identified as the exclusive sites of sickle cell adhesion in the microcirculation (Fig. 8.2A-D)[60] Adhesion was inversely correlated with vessel diameter (Fig. 8.2D) where smaller-diameter immediate postcapillary venules showed maximal adhesion[60] and were frequent sites of vasoocclusion when a pro-adhesive stimulus was applied.[61] Maximal adhesion was observed at vessel bending and vascular junctions (Fig. 8.2C). The relationship between sickle red cell adhesion and the venular diameter was recently confirmed.[62] In the ex vivo experiments, selective fluorescent labeling allowed identification of a given density sickle red cell class in a defined mixture of two cell classes. When a bolus of defined mixture was infused, the resulting adhesion of sickle red cells was density-class dependent in the following order; reticulocytes and young discocytes > discocytes > dense discocytes and ISCs. Dense sickle red cells contributed maximally to microvascular obstruction, as shown by their selective trapping in postcapillary venules in which deformable light-density sickle red cells preferentially adhered.

Sickle cell adhesion has been confirmed using a variety of assay systems.[58,60,63,64] Studies using the cremaster muscle microcirculation of transgenic sickle mice expressing HbS and HbS-Antilles (S+S-Antilles) confirmed venules as the exclusive sites of red cell adhesion in vivo.[65] In contrast to S+S-Antilles mice, red cell adhesion is less obvious in BERK mice. In studies of C57BL mice transplanted with BERK marrow, adhesion was not observed, although transient interactions between leukocytes and red cells were noted.[45] In contrast to S+S-Antilles mice, BERK mice have fewer dense red cells and have erythrocyte features of β thalassemia, with microcytic red cells having reduced mean cell hemoglobin.[66] BERK mice, however, have erythrocytes that sickle, hemolyse and undergo oxidative stress. These mice are more suitable for studying the role of hemolysis and inflammation than sickle cell adhesion and illustrate the imperfection of sickle mice and that different sickle mouse strains must be used for understanding different features of this disease (Chapter 12).

Mechanisms of Sickle Red Cell Adhesion

Sickle erythrocytes adhere to endothelium by multiple mechanisms via adhesion molecules expressed on both sickle red cells and endothelium. Although repeated sickling–unsickling cycles result in red cell membrane damage and exposure of red cell membrane components like sulfated glycolipids and phosphatidylserine (PS) that might mediate adhesion, increased red cell destruction results

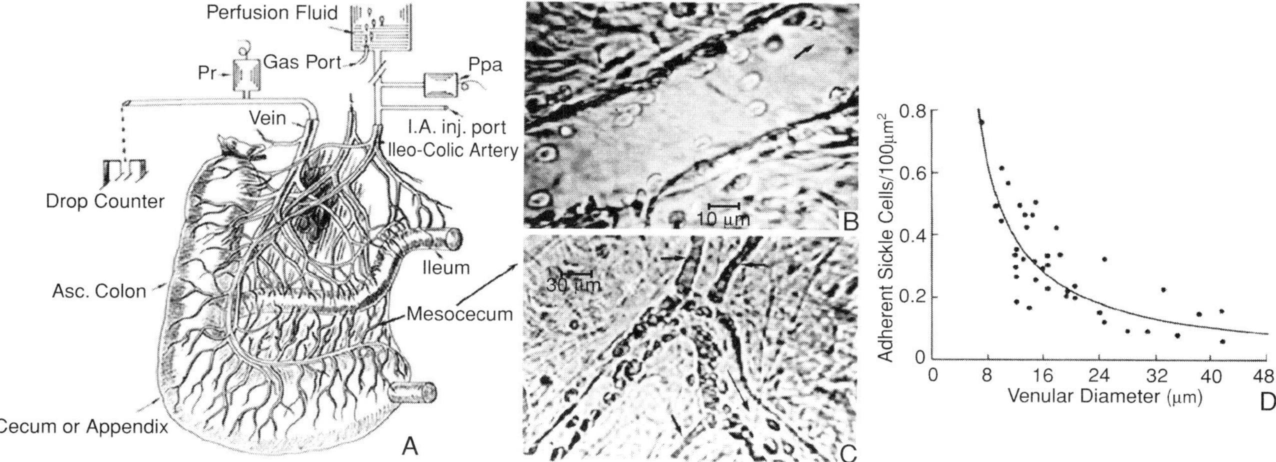

Figure 8.2. Adhesion of sickle red cells in venules of the ex vivo mesocecum vasculature infused with a bolus of human sickle red cells during perfusion with Ringers albumin. **(A)** Artificially perfused mesocecum preparation of the rat (Asc. Colon, ascending colon; I.A. inj. port, arterial injection port; Ppa, arterial perfusion pressure; and Pv, venous outflow pressure). **(B)** Adherent sickle red cells of discocyte morphology are seen deformed in the direction of the flow (arrow). **(C)** Increased adhesion of sickle red cells at venular bending and at junctions of small-diameter immediate postcapillary venules. In this instance, the immediate postcapillary venules are completely blocked (arrows). **(D)** The inverse relationship between vessel diameter and sickle red cell adhesion in venules of the ex vivo mesocecum vasculature. The regression fits the equation $y = aX^{-b}$, $r = -0.81$, $P < 0.001$). (Modified from ref. 60.) (See color plate 8.2.)

in excessive production of stress reticulocytes that display adhesion molecules.

The adhesion molecules implicated in sickle red cell adhesion are broadly categorized as 1) red cell receptors; 2) adhesive bridging proteins; 3) endothelial adhesion molecules; 4) extracellular matrix adhesion molecules (Fig. 8.3).

Red Cell Receptors: Two subcategories of receptors have been recognized in sickle erythrocytes. The first consists of receptors that are expressed on stress sickle reticulocytes. Two well-characterized receptors on reticulocytes are very-late-activation-antigen-4 (VLA-4/$\alpha_4\beta_1$) and CD36.[63,67,68] The integrin $\alpha_4\beta_1$ binds its endothelial ligand VCAM-1.

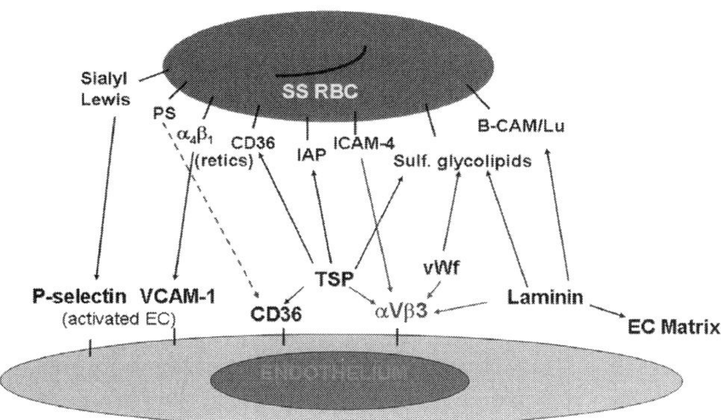

Figure 8.3. Schematic representation of adhesion molecules involved in sickle red cell–endothelium interactions. B-CAM/Lu = basal cell adhesion molecule/Lutheran; EC matrix = extracellular (subendothelial) matrix; IAP = integrin-associated protein; ICAM-4 = intercellular adhesion molecule-4; and Sulf. Glycolipids = sulfated glycolipids.

VCAM-1 is not constitutively expressed on endothelium but can be induced by cytokines or hypoxia.[67,69] Importantly, VCAM-1 interactions with $\alpha_4\beta_1$ are enhanced under hypoxic conditions, and this interaction might play an important role in sickle acute chest syndrome, which is characterized by infiltration and retention of sickle red cells into the lung microcirculation.[70,71] CD36 interacts with soluble thrombospondin (TSP), an adhesive bridging protein.[68] Plausibly, CD36-expressing reticulocytes could also interact with endothelial $\alpha V\beta 3$ integrin receptor via soluble TSP. Exposed membrane sulfated glycolipids could facilitate sickle red cell interaction with von Willebrand factor (vWF), an endothelial ultra-large-molecular weight protein and TSP, contributing to sickle cell–endothelium adhesion.[72,73]

The second subcategory of receptors includes more recently described molecules that are activated by signal transduction. Activation of integrin-associated protein (IAP/CD47) on sickle erythrocytes can induce signal transduction to activate still unidentified red cell receptors for TSP.[74] A receptor, intercellular adhesion molecule-4 (ICAM-4 (Landsteiner–Weiner protein or CD 242) has been identified on sickle erythrocytes, which can mediate adhesion by binding endothelial $\alpha v\beta 3$ integrin.[75] Activation of ICAM-4 by the physiological stress mediator epinephrine enhances sickle red cell adhesion. The epinephrine-induced activation of ICAM-4 involves a cyclic adenosine monophosphate–dependent signaling pathway, probably via stimulation of the red cell β-adrenergic receptor.[75] Previous studies have ascribed a role of cyclic adenosine monophosphate–dependent pathways in sickle

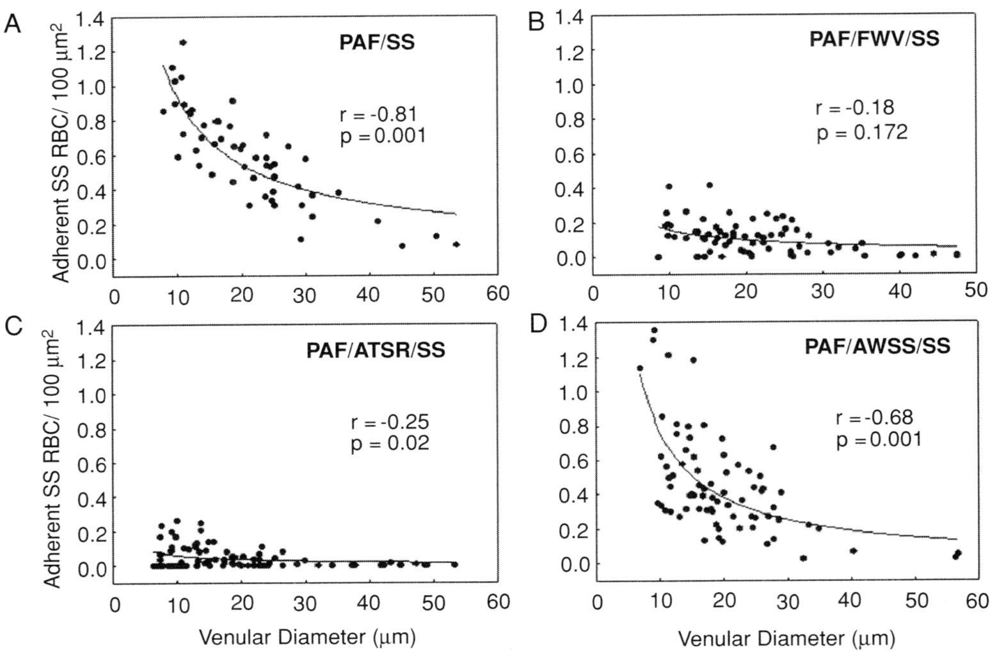

Figure 8.4. Regression plots for the number of adherent sickle red cells (SS RBC)/100 μm^2 relative to venular diameters in ex vivo preparations treated as follows: **(A)** PAF alone, **(B)** PAF and peptide FWV, **(C)** PAF and peptide ATSR, and **(D)** PAF and control peptide AWSS. The regression lines represent the multiplicative equation of the form $Y = aX^{-b}$ for the best fit. In preparations treated with PAF alone, adhesion of sickle erythrocytes showed a strong correlation with the venular diameter. Preparations treated with peptide FWV or ATSR showed a marked inhibition of sickle erythrocyte adhesion in venules of all diameters, with ATSR having the maximal inhibitory effect, especially in small-diameter venules, the sites of frequent blockage. In contrast, in the presence of the control peptide AWSS, the resulting adhesion was essentially similar to that observed in PAF-treated preparations. (Modified from ref. 61.)

red cell adhesion wherein epinephrine-induced activation of basal cell adhesion molecule/Lutheran (B-CAM/Lu) increased adhesion to immobilized laminin, an extracellular matrix molecule.[76] Although epinephrine can activate both B-CAM/Lu and ICAM-4 in sickle red cells, the latter is specifically involved in adhesion to endothelial cells, as antibodies to B-CAM/Lu and laminin are ineffective in the ICAM-4–mediated interactions.[75] Epinephrine enhances sickle cell adhesion to the extracellular matrix via B-CAM/LU and laminin and to endothelium via ICAM-4 and αVβ3, suggesting a role for physiological stress in vasoocclusion. Among the ICAM-4 family of adhesive proteins, ICAM-4 is unique in its expression on erythroid cells. ICAM-4 can bind diverse arrays of integrins including several αV integrins, β2 integrins expressed on leukocytes and α4β1 integrin,[77,78] suggesting multiple functions of this adhesion molecule. Although exposed PS might mediate adhesion,[79] the tenacity of this interaction has not been evaluated.

Adhesive Bridging Proteins: Adhesive proteins released by platelet and vascular endothelium are implicated in sickle red cell adhesion. Unusually large molecular weight forms of vWf and soluble TSP are known to enhance adhesion of sickle red cells to endothelium.[80,81] Soluble TSP is likely to contribute to adhesion of sickle red cells via its C-terminal cell-binding domain.[82] TSP and vWf, both present in platelets and endothelial cells, can be released into the local environment under appropriate stimulation.[83] Elevated levels of both these adhesive bridging proteins have been identified in the plasma of patients with sickle cell disease.[68,84,85] vWf and TSP can act as bridging proteins because they can bind specific red cell receptors and endothelial αVβ3 integrin. Inhibition of sickle erythrocyte adhesion to TSP by vWf involved the use of plasma vWf that lacked the extra-large molecular weight forms of vWf released by endothelial cells and were implicated in sickle red cell adhesion.[86]

Endothelial Adhesion Molecules: Among the most prominent endothelial adhesion molecules, in addition to TSP and vWf, are P-selectin, CD36, and integrin αVβ3. P-selectin is expressed in activated endothelial cells in transgenic mouse models of sickle cell disease. P-selectin might facilitate a weak adhesion via interaction with red cell sialyl Lewis moieties.[87] P-selectin–mediated transient interaction could affect local wall shear rates followed by a more tenacious adhesion via high affinity adhesion mechanisms. Antibodies to P-selectin can partially inhibit sickle red cell adhesion to human endothelial cells in a flow system.[88] Moreover, P-selectin–mediated sickle red cell adhesion was inhibited by unfractionated heparin. Heparin and other anionic polysaccharides can inhibit TSP-mediated adhesion of sickle cells in the ex vivo mesocecum preparation, and in human endothelial cells under flow conditions,[72] suggesting that an inhibitory effect of anionic polysaccharides is not limited to P-selectin–mediated adhesion. An agonist peptide for murine protease–activated receptor-1 (PARS-1), which selectively activates mouse endothelial cells, but not platelets, resulted in flow stoppage of infused BERK sickle red cells in the microcirculation, an effect not observed in P-selectin knockout mice.[89] The contribution of leukocytes, however, was not confirmed. Moreover, the endothelial activation by murine protease–activated receptor-1 could concomitantly release vWF as both P-selectin and vWf are stored in endothelial Weibel–Palade bodies. Additional studies are needed to clarify the relative roles of P-selectin and extra-large forms of endothelial vWF in sickle red cell adhesion.

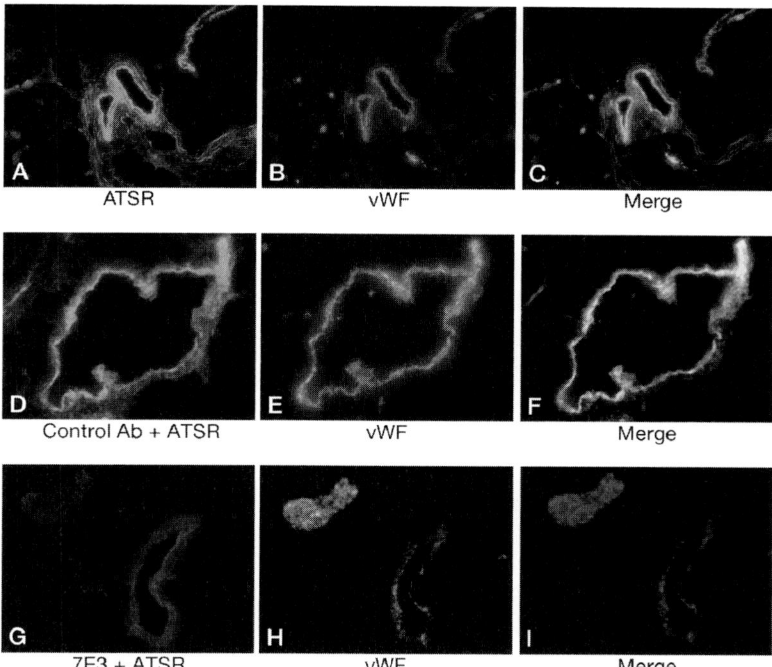

Figure 8.5. Top panel: Colocalization of fluoresceinated ATSR peptide with vascular endothelium of the ex vivo mesocecum preparation pretreated with PAF **(A–C)**. **(A)** The presence of the fluorescent peptide is shown in green. **(B)** Blood vessels were identified by a polyclonal primary antibody to vWF and a secondary TRITC-conjugated antibody (red). **(C)** Merged image signals showed colocalization (yellow) of ATSR with the endothelial lining. Middle panel: The effect of a control antibody OC125 **(D–F)** on the colocalization of fluoresceinated ATSR peptide with vascular endothelium of PAF-treated ex vivo preparation. **(D)** The presence of the fluorescent peptide is shown in green. **(E)** Blood vessels were identified by a polyclonal antibody to vWF as in **B** (red). **(F)** Merged image signals showed colocalization (yellow) of ATSR with the vessel wall. Bottom panel: The effect of 7E3 antibody to $\alpha V\beta 3$ **(G–I)** on the colocalization of fluoresceinated ATSR peptide with vascular endothelium in PAF-treated ex vivo preparation. **(G)** In the presence of 7E3 antibody, there was a marked decrease in ATSR localization with the vessel wall. ATSR infusion resulted in weak green staining likely attributable to autofluorescence or a low level of binding of ATSR peptide. **(H)** Vessel was identified by immunofluorescent staining for vWF (red). **(I)** No colocalization of ATSR with vessel wall in the presence of 7E3. (Modified from ref. 61.) (See color plate 8.5.)

CD36, an 88-kD protein, is expressed by microvascular endothelial cells[90] in addition to platelets and sickle reticulocytes. CD36 has been implicated as a ligand to the exposed PS on sickle red cells.[79] Moreover, endothelial CD36 can interact with soluble TSP to promote TSP-mediated adhesion.

The vitronectin receptor, $\alpha V\beta 3$ integrin, expressed on activated endothelium, is likely to play an important role in stable sickle red cell adhesion. $\alpha V\beta 3$ integrin can interact with several adhesive bridging proteins (TSP, vWf, and possibly soluble laminin),[85,91,92] and also with ICAM-4 (a receptor for $\alpha V\beta 3$) on sickle red cells.[75] Antibodies directed against this integrin can dramatically inhibit sickle red cell adhesion in the ex vivo mesocecum preparation[83] and to human endothelial cells.[75] Peptides (ATSR and FWV) based on αV-binding domains of ICAM-4 markedly decreased sickle cell adhesion and vasoocclusion in the PAF-treated ex vivo mesocecum vasculature under shear flow conditions[61] (Fig. 8.4A-D). PAF is a potent endothelial activating and inflammatory agent that is elevated in sickle cell disease.[93] The infused fluoresceinated ATSR peptide is colocalized with vascular endothelium and pretreatment with function-blocking antibody (7E3) to $\alpha V\beta 3$ markedly inhibited this interaction (Fig. 8.5). These studies show that ICAM-4 on sickle red cells binds endothelium via $\alpha V\beta 3$ and that this interaction contributes to vasoocclusion, suggesting that peptides or small molecules based on αV-binding domains of ICAM-4 might have a therapeutic potential. Moreover, small-molecule cyclic $\alpha V\beta 3$ antagonists containing the integrin recognition motif RGD are potent inhibitors of sickle cell adhesion.[94] Because of its ability to bind several adhesive proteins, $\alpha V\beta 3$ is a potential target in designing antiadhesive therapies.[95] In addition to direct interaction between red cell ICAM-4 and endothelial $\alpha V\beta 3$ integrin, possible formation of tripartite complexes involving the red cell receptor, adhesive protein, and endothelial receptor with $\alpha V\beta 3$ might contribute to sickle red cell adhesion (Fig. 8.6),

Endothelial $\alpha V\beta 3$ in sickle red cell adhesion

Red cell receptor	Bridging protein	Endothelial receptor
• CD36	TSP	$\alpha V\beta 3$
• Sulfated glycolipids	TSP	$\alpha V\beta 3$
• Sulfated glycolipids	vWf	$\alpha V\beta 3$
• IAP	TSP	$\alpha V\beta 3$
• ICAM-4	⟵⟶	$\alpha V\beta 3$

Figure 8.6. Endothelial $\alpha V\beta 3$ integrin in sickle red cell adhesion.

for example, CD36-TSP-$\alpha V\beta 3$, IAP-TSP-$\alpha V\beta 3$, sulfated glycolipids-TSP-$\alpha V\beta 3$, and sulfated glycolipids-vWF-$\alpha V\beta 3$.

Endothelial oxidant generation induced by elevated inflammatory stimuli and intermittent vasoocclusion events will cause endothelial activation and up-regulation of adhesion molecules, particularly $\alpha V\beta 3$. PAF-induced endothelial oxidant generation resulted in markedly enhanced sickle red cell adhesion to vascular endothelium, which was abrogated by SOD and catalase.[55]

The Effect of Hydroxyurea and NO on Adhesion: One therapeutic approach to treat sickle cell disease is to increase fetal hemoglobin (HbF) concentration (Chapter 30).[96,97] An inverse relationship exists between CD36-positive reticulocytes and F cells[98] and patients with higher levels of F cells have fewer adherent cells. Hydroxyurea decreases red cell adhesion and down-regulates endothelial adhesion molecules such as sVCAM-1 and sICAM-1.[99,100] Hydroxyurea is an NO donor and by the activation of soluble guanylate cyclase (cGMP) might induce HbF expression.[101] NO generation by hydroxyurea could be a critical factor for its reported antiinflammatory action and down-regulation of endothelial adhesion molecules such as sVCAM-1 and sICAM-1.[99] Sickle cell adhesion to TNFα-treated endothelial monolayers is markedly inhibited by the NO donor DETA-NO.[102] The relative roles of HbF and NO in the therapeutic efficacy of hydroxyurea have yet to be clarified.

Extracellular Matrix Adhesion Molecules: Indirect evidence indicates the potential exposure of subendothelial matrix of the vascular intima where endothelial cell damage and detachment occurs, probably due to rheological insult and adhesion of sickle cells. Endothelial detachment is probably exemplified by the presence of circulating endothelial cells.[52,53] Matrix proteins, including TSP, vWf, and laminin have been implicated in sickle cell adhesion (Fig. 8.7). Such interactions could be relevant to the pathophysiology of this disease but might not represent a generalized phenomenon.

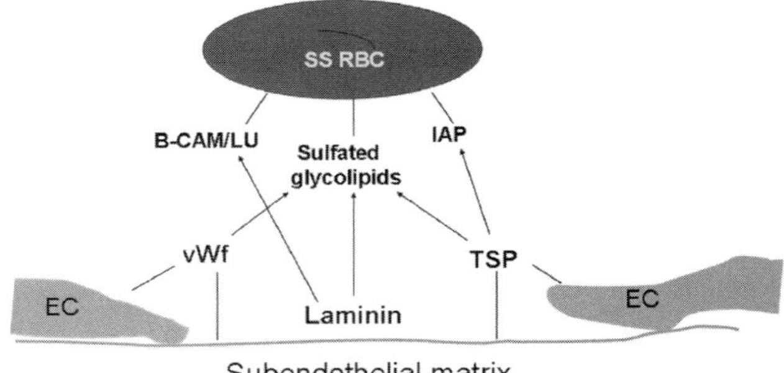

Figure 8.7. Schematic representation of matrix adhesive proteins involved in potential adhesion of sickle red cells to extracellular (subendothelial) matrix.

Pathophysiological Implications of Sickle Erythrocyte Adhesive Interactions

Sickle red cell adhesion in postcapillary venules increases microvascular transit times, induces hypoxia, and promotes HbS polymerization in the adherent and trapped cells, as shown by direct intravital microscopy and by increased peripheral resistance caused by sickle red cell adhesion.[55,61] It was proposed that sickle red cell adhesion–induced vasoocclusion is a two-step process in which preferential adhesion of deformable, light-density cells in postcapillary venules is followed by reduced effective lumen diameter and selective trapping of dense cells causing vessel blockage.[60,103] Dense cell trapping permits rapid HbS polymerization due to the high MCHC of these cells. Postcapillary obstruction might proceed to involve whole feeding capillary networks in a retrograde fashion.[104–107] The obstructive behavior of dense sickle red cells has also been shown in a perfused rat leg model[108] corroborating findings in the ex vivo mesocecum. That obstruction results in a disproportionate trapping of dense sickle red cells was suggested by the analysis of cells eluted in venous effluents under high perfusion pressure.[109] Selective trapping of dense cells might occur during the evolution of the acute painful episode (Chapter 20). Following an initial increase in the circulating dense cells at the onset of the acute painful event,[111] an observation explained by the sequestration of deformable light-density sickle red cells as they interact with endothelium, the highest density fraction of sickle erythrocytes disappears from the peripheral circulation during the course of the event. Together, these observations support the proposed two-step model of sickle vasoocclusion.[110]

Sickle Red Cell Adhesion and the Endothelial Response

Sickle cell adhesion and intravascular sickling are likely to contribute not only to endothelial damage and up-regulation of vasoactive molecules such as prostaglandins and endothelin-1 (ET-1)[112] but also to up-regulation of adhesion molecules involved in blood cell–endothelium interactions.[27] In vitro studies have shown that sickle cell contact and adhesion to cultured endothelial cells can inhibit endothelial DNA synthesis, increase ET-1 mRNA,[113] impair NO synthesis,[114] and stimulate arachidonic acid metabolism and prostacyclin release[115,116] and up-regulate expression of endothelial adhesion molecules.[46] Adhesion might promote release of hemoglobin and adenosine diphosphate. Damaged endothelium also releases adenosine diphosphate,[117] a potent platelet activator that causes aggregation. Although of potential importance, the significance of these observations remains to be validated in the context of pathophysiology of sickle cell disease.[46,118,119]

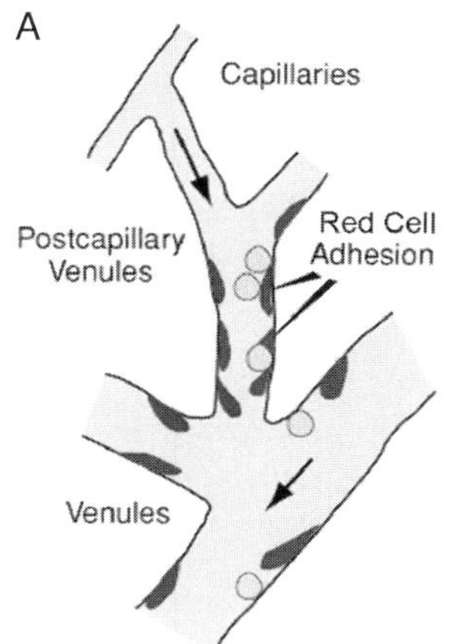

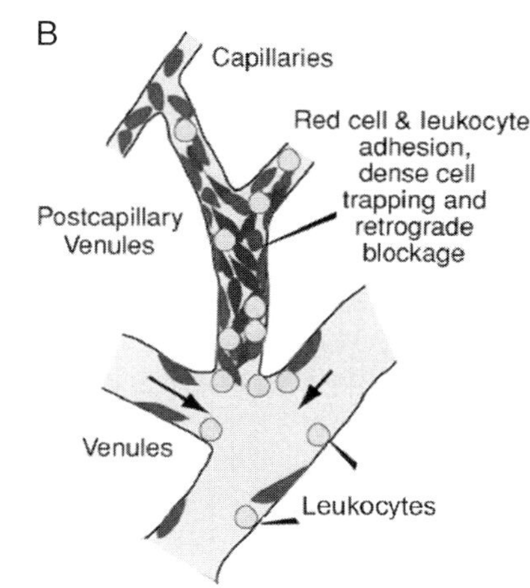

Figure 8.8. A model for vasoocclusion in sickle cell disease. **(A)** Adhesion of deformable sickle red cells and leukocytes (light colored) in postcapillary venules. **(B)** Adhesion of these cells is followed by reduction in local wall shear rates and selective trapping of dense sickle red cells, which could result in HbS polymerization in the trapped (dark red) and adhered sickle cells and obstruction of the affected vessels. (See color plate 8.8.)

Leukocytes and Vasoocclusion

Neutrophils are increased in the peripheral circulation of most patients with sickle cell anemia and could be an important factor modulating microvascular flow.[120,121] Because neutrophils are relatively large and less deformable than erythrocytes, an increase in their numbers, activation and recruitment to sites of injury will increase intravascular resistance and adversely affect microvascular flow.[122,123] Increases numbers of neutrophils might increase red cell transit time and impair O_2 delivery. In vivo studies have shown that microcirculatory flow is significantly influenced not only by sickle erythrocytes but also by increased leukocyte recruitment due to reperfusion injury and oxidant generation. In transgenic sickle mice, hypoxia/reoxygenation generated by transient occlusion might induce an inflammatory endothelial phenotype resulting in increased leukocyte–endothelium interactions.[26] When bone marrow from BERK mice was transplanted into C57BL mice, adherent leukocytes facilitated mechanical trapping of elongated sickled red cells in venules.[45] This log jamming of sickled red cells among adherent leukocytes was similar to the pattern of dense cell and ISC trapping among adherent sickle erythrocytes.[60] These observations suggest that both erythrocyte and leukocyte adhesion to endothelium can help entrap sickled or dense red cells, potentially initiating vasoocclusion (Fig. 8.8).

The results from C57BL mice that underwent BERK mouse bone marrow transplantation were used to further address the role of leukocytes in sickle vasoocclusion.[124] Pretreatment with intravenous human gamma globulin (IVIG) followed by an inflammatory stimulus by using TNFα caused a significant reduction in leukocyte recruitment and associated red cell trapping in recipient mice. Pretreating the BERK marrow recipient C57BL mice with TNFα followed by IVIG administration reversed TNFα-induced vasoocclusion.[125] These studies suggested a role for IVIG for treatment of acute painful episode, nevertheless, the underlying mechanism(s) of IVIG action are unresolved.

Vascular Function

Vascular tone adaptations in sickle cell disease are a response to hemolytic anemia, intravascular sickling, and vasoocclusive events, all of which can contribute to tissue hypoxia. Subclinical transient vasoocclusive events or "microcrises" triggered by intravascular sickling and cell adhesion not only contribute to an inflammatory state and local tissue hypoxia, but are likely to cause endothelial dysfunction as reported for other inflammatory diseases.[35] Chronic anemia is compensated for by hyperperfusion to maintain O_2 delivery.[126,127] Hyperperfusion is not limited to large conduit arteries but is also observed in the microcirculation of transgenic knockout sickle mice as a consequence of arteriolar dilation.[35] In sickle cell disease and transgenic knockout sickle mice, relatively reduced systemic blood pressure[35,128] is a likely consequence of the dilation of resistance arterioles. In patients, vasodilation and reduced blood pressure are associated with a 50%–60% decrease in the peripheral resistance.[126]

Vascular Tone Response to Red Cell Rheology: Abnormal rheology of sickle red cells might require appropriate adjustments in the vascular tone to facilitate their capillary passage. Increased intravascular pressure caused by less deformable sickle red cells could potentially trigger an oscillatory vasomotion pattern, or intermittent periodic flow, to facilitate microvascular passage of rheologically abnormal sickle cell blood.[129,130] Vasomotor response is depressed following postocclusive hyperemia.[130]

The effect of red cell rheology on vascular tone was studied in transgenic sickle mice exposed to different levels of oxygenation.[65] Experiments performed to determine the effect of local, transient hyperoxia revealed striking differences in the microvascular responses in control and transgenic sickle mice. In S+S-Antilles transgenic sickle mice, Vrbc was significantly reduced under hypoxic conditions with pO_2 of 15–20 mm Hg, consistent with increased viscosity due to in vivo HbS polymer formation. During transient hyperoxia, an altered microvascular tone and response was observed. In control animals, O_2 caused approximately 70% arteriolar constriction, accompanied by 75% reduction in Vrbc. In contrast, in transgenic sickle mice, hyperoxia resulted in only an 8% decrease in the arteriolar diameter and a 70% increase in Vrbc. The altered response in transgenic mice to hyperoxia was probably due to an improved flow behavior of red cells as a consequence of HbS depolymerization and cell unsickling, although possibly intrinsic or acquired differences in the endothelial/vascular smooth muscle might also contribute to this response. This attenuated response to O_2 was later validated in patients who showed a considerably smaller decrease in the brachial artery diameter when exposed to 100% O_2.[127]

NO Bioavailability, Non-NO Vasodilators and Vascular Reactivity: Vascular function in sickle cell disease has been facilitated by recent studies of NO bioavailability.[23,26,28,38,131] Reduced NO bioavailability in patients and in transgenic sickle mice,[35,132,133] results in vascular tone adaptations and attenuated vascular responses to NO-mediated stimuli.

The biological functions of NO are discussed in detail in Chapters 10 and 11. NO has diverse biological functions and its altered metabolism is a feature of many diseases.[31,131,134–136] NO consumption by plasma hemoglobin and O_2 radicals potentially results in excess consumption of arginine substrate by eNOS to compensate for reduced NO availability. In both patients and sickle mouse models, the evidence shows depleted levels of L-arginine and NO metabolites (NOx).[37,137–142]

NO depletion attenuates vascular reactivity to NO-mediated vasodilators and NOS antagonists in transgenic sickle mice[35,143,144] and in patients with high plasma hemoglobin levels.[145,146] Impaired NO bioavailability is suggested by attenuated vascular reactivity in sickle mouse models to endothelium-dependent vasodilators like acetylcholine (ACh), and in particular to sodium nitroprusside (SNP), a NO donor.[28,35,143,144] Reduced flow-mediated vasodilation in sickle cell disease patients also suggests reduced bioavailability of NO.[133,146] Nevertheless, plethysmographic measurements of the forearm flow in patients show an increased blood flow greater or an enhanced vasodilatory response to ACh compared with normal individuals.[127,146] This response to ACh might imply up-regulation of non-NO vasodilators because ACh augments the release of NO, prostaglandins and endothelium hyperpolarizing factors.[146] Interestingly, responses to both ACh and SNP are reduced in men but not women with sickle cell disease,[146] suggesting sex differences in NO bioavailability.

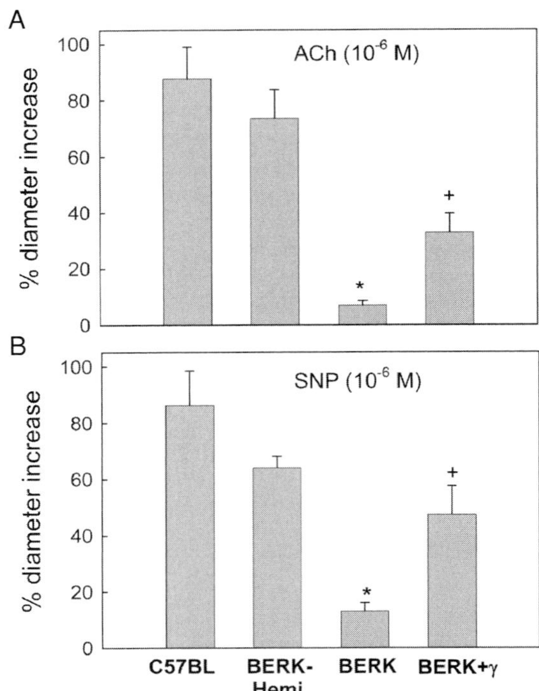

Figure 8.9. Arteriolar diameter (percentage of increase) responses to topical application of acetylcholine (ACh, 10^{-6} M) and sodium nitroprusside (SNP, 10^{-6} M) in C57BL, BERK-trait, BERK, and BERK+γ mice. Note the blunted response of arterioles in BERK mice to ACh **(A)** and SNP **(B)**. ACh and SNP caused significant increases in arteriolar diameters of BERK+γ mice as compared with that in BERK mice (~33% and ~50% increases, respectively). $^*P <$ 0.005–0.000001 compared with C57BL and BERK-trait mice. $^+P <$ 0.00–0.002 compared with the diameter increase in BERK mice. (Reproduced with permission from ref. 35.)

Because vascular resistance to blood flow is determined mainly by the vascular tone of arterioles, BERK mice were used to determine the role of NO and non-NO-related mechanisms in affecting the arteriolar tone.[35] Arteriolar responses to NO-mediated vasoactive stimuli such as ACh and SNP were attenuated in BERK mice compared with C57BL and hemizygous BERK (BERK-Hemi) controls (Fig. 8.9). N^G-nitro-L-arginine methyl ester (L-NAME) had no appreciable effect on blood pressure in these mice. Almost complete attenuation of arteriolar dilation to SNP, reflected inactivation and/or destruction of NO. As shown in Figure 8.10B, the arteriolar diameter response to SNP is strongly correlated with hemolytic rate. This observation is consistent with the ability of plasma heme to consume NO (Fig. 8.10A).[38] The greater plasma heme level in BERK mice caused blunted vessel diameter response. In contrast, the low plasma heme levels in control mice were associated with maximal arteriolar dilation. BERK-Hemi and BERK mice expressing 20% HbF that had intermediate levels of plasma heme showed improved vessel diameter response to SNP. Sickle cell disease patients have a diminished response to SNP.[38] The BERK model differs markedly from ischemic coronary artery disease, which is

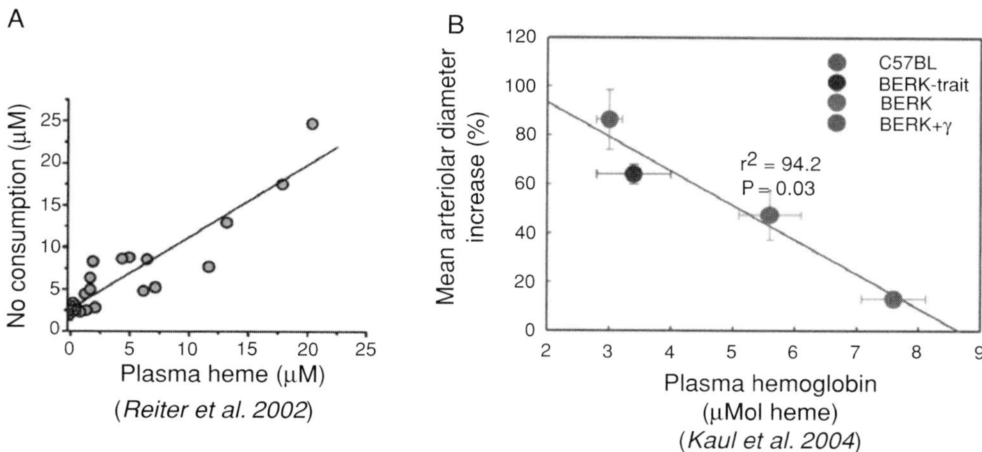

Figure 8.10. Plasma heme and its effect on NO consumption and microvascular response to sodium nitroprusside (SNP). **(A)** Heme concentration within plasma of sickle cell disease patients shows a significant correlation with NO consumption ($r = 0.9$, $P < 0.0001$). **(B)** Relationship between plasma heme levels and the arteriolar diameter response to SNP in the cremaster microcirculation of C57BL (control), BERK, BERK-trait, and BERK+γ mice. A strong correlation is observed between the percent arteriolar diameter increase in response to SNP and the extent of hemolysis (plasma heme). With a greater hemolysis in sickle (BERK) mice the diameter response was blunted. Low plasma heme levels in controls were associated with maximal arteriolar dilation, whereas BERK mice expressing 20% HbF showed a lower plasma heme and an improved diameter response compared with BERK mice. (**A** is reproduced from ref. 38 by permission, and **B** is based on the published data in ref. 61.)

characterized by blunted responses to L-N^G-monomethyl arginine but normal responses to SNP.[54]

BERK mice have more than a 2.5-fold increase in the plasma hemoglobin compared with control mice.[35] They have an increase in the endothelial-bound XO,[28] which might catalyze the increased generation of $O_2^{\cdot -}$ and H_2O_2, altering the vascular response to NO-mediated vasodilators. Increased $O_2^{\cdot -}$ generation will consume NO forming $ONOO^-$, resulting in the increased formation of nitrotyrosine.[35] Additional studies are needed to differentiate the relative contributions of oxidative stress and cell-free plasma hemoglobin in NO consumption and sickle vasculopathy.

With chronic hypoxia and hemolysis, induction of non-NO vasodilators such as prostaglandins and heme oxygenase-1 (HO-1) could compensate for reduced NO bioavailability.[131,146] HO-1, also a marker of hemolysis, catalyzes degradation of excess heme to produce carbon monoxide, a vasodilator. Also, elevated levels of cyclic guanosine monophosphate caused by HO-1 induction[144] in response to excess plasma heme could contribute to the blunted effect of SNP in BERK mice. The second non-NO vasodilator enzyme, cyclooxygenase-2 (COX-2), is induced under the conditions of chronic hypoxia and oxidative stress. $ONOO^-$ has been implicated in the induction of COX-2.[147] In BERK mice, reduced NO bioavailability and increased nitrotyrosine formation are associated with COX-2 induction in microvascular endothelium,[35] suggesting that the reported increase in prostaglandin E_2 levels in sickle cell disease[112] might be due to COX-2 activity. Moreover, COX-2 induction in BERK mice is associated with dilation of arteriolar resistance vessels, hyperperfusion, and hypotension as reported in sickle patients.[35,26,127] Activation of non-NO vasodilator mechanisms in the BERK model might compensate for NO deficiency and help maintain optimal O_2 delivery in the face of chronic anemia.

Depletion of the substrate arginine and cofactor BH_4 results in uncoupling of electron flow from L-arginine oxidation and NO production.[148] This uncoupling of eNOS leads to its inactivation and O_2 radical generation.[149,150] Increased inflammatory effects were seen when bone marrow from transgenic sickle mice was transplanted into eNOS overexpressing mice.[151] This was likely an effect caused by excessive $ONOO^-$ formation and BH_4 depletion. Enhanced nitrotyrosine formation in transgenic sickle mice (Fig. 8.11A)[35] has been supported by recent studies[23] that showed increased $ONOO^-$ formation was associated with impaired eNOS activity with a loss of eNOS dimerization (Fig. 8.11B and C). The role of BH_4 supplementation in microvascular tone and reactivity has not been examined, except for its role in leukocyte adhesion.[151] NO depletion also up-regulates endothelin-1, a potent vasoconstrictor whose levels are increased in sickle cell disease.

Altered Vascular Responses to Vasoconstrictors: Enhanced oxidative stress, particularly the formation of nitrotyrosine, might cause chronic vascular injury and impaired vascular reactivity. Nitrotyrosine infusion in rats attenuated the hemodynamic responses to epinephrine, norepinephrine, and angiotensin II,[152,153] which is comparable to the blunted blood pressure response to norepinephrine

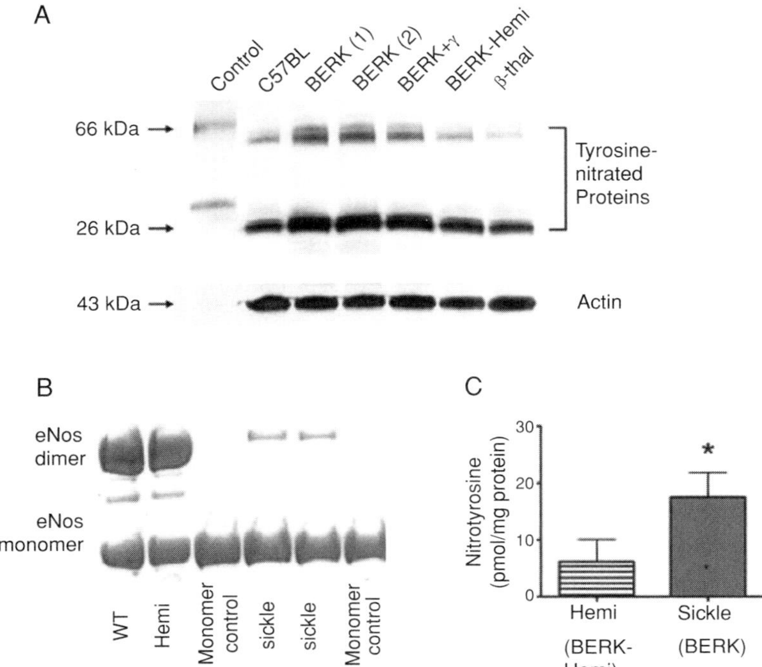

Figure 8.11. Elevated nitrotyrosine levels and endothelial nitric oxide synthase (eNOS) monomerization in BERK mice. **(A)** Western blot analysis of cremaster muscle lysates for the expression of nitrotyrosine. Two prominent bands of nitrated proteins (66 and 26 kD) were detected by the antibody to nitrotyrosine. BERK mice showed increased tyrosine nitration of both 66- and 26-kD proteins (i.e., average increase: fivefold and ~twofold, respectively), whereas the BERK+γ mouse showed a smaller increase compared with C57BL controls. The nitrotyrosine levels in BERK-trait and β thalassemia mice showed no increase as compared with C57BL controls. Control lane depicts positive nitrotyrosine controls provided by the antibody manufacturer. **(B)** Western blots of lung homogenates under nondenaturing conditions demonstrate 280-kD dimer (active form) and 140-kD eNOS monomer. Wild-type (WT) and hemizygous (Hemi) sickle mice had more eNOS dimer than monomer, but sickle mice show almost a complete lack of dimerized eNOS. Positive monomer controls show eNOS dissociated completely to monomeric form by boiling. **(C)** Lung nitrotyrosine, evidence of NO scavenging by superoxide, was elevated in sickle mice. (Figure **A** is reproduced with permission from ref. 61. Figures **B** and **C** are reproduced from ref. 23 by permission.)

in BERK mice.[35] An attenuated hemodynamic response to angiotensin II[154] in sickle patients could also involve a similar mechanism.

Hypercoagulability

Under normal conditions, vascular endothelium exerts a potent anticoagulant effect. Inhibition of coagulation by endothelium involves the expression of thrombomodulin that activates protein C; heparan sulfate that activates antithrombin III; annexin V that prevents binding of procoagulation factors such as PS; NO that has inhibitory effect on platelet activation and leukocyte adhesion; and prostacyclin, a vasodilator and an inhibitor of platelet aggregation. In sickle cell disease, inflammatory cytokines, hypoxia, sickle red cell–endothelium interaction, and perhaps apoptosis of injured endothelial cells can shift endothelium to a prothrombotic state. During acute painful episodes, there is excessive thrombin generation, platelet activation, and plasma fibrinolytic activity.[27] The expression of tissue factor, a trigger of coagulation, is abnormally increased in sickle monocytes and circulating endothelial cells.[27] Furthermore, procoagulant properties of sickle red cells are linked to externalization of PS, which is a consequence of repeated cycles of sickling and unsickling. PS exposure and thrombin generation are correlated in sickle patients.[155] Thrombotic events in large vessels of the brain are implicated in sickle cell strokes[156] and thrombi in the pulmonary vessels might be associated with acute chest syndrome and are often found in postmortem.

THALASSEMIA

Red Cell Rheology

An imbalance in globin chain synthesis is the major cause of red cell abnormalities in thalassemia and affects cell survival and deformability.[157,158] In α and β thalassemia, the relative excess of unpaired β- and α-globin chains, respectively, result in accumulation of excessive amounts of unpaired globin chains that precipitate, and by different mechanisms, damage the cell membrane and cause their premature destruction (Chapters 14 and 17). Globin chain inclusion bodies are "pitted" from erythrocytes by reticuloendothelial cells. Erythrocytes in β-thalassemia major are less deformable than normal cells.[159]

Analysis of cellular and membrane deformability characteristics has shown that red cells of both α and β thalassemia have excess surface area in relation to cell volume, increased membrane dynamic rigidity, and a decreased ability to undergo cellular deformation under hypertonic osmotic stress.[160] Nevertheless, when blood from thalassemia is analyzed on density gradients, erythrocytes of HbH disease, characterized by the presence of β_4 tetramers, appeared less dense than normal red cells. In contrast, erythrocytes from β thalassemia intermedia and major showed a much broader range of density distribution with cell populations showing both lower and higher densities than that observed for normal red cells.[160] Therefore, the presence of dense cells in β thalassemia indicates cellular dehydration owing to abnormal membrane transport. The membrane rigidity of β thalassemia cells from nonsplenectomized and splenectomized patients showed a progressive increase with increasing cell density. The greater membrane rigidity in splenectomized patients is associated with increased pathological interactions of hemichromes with the membrane protein band 3,[161] and with ankyrin, spectrin, and protein 4.1 of the membrane skeleton.[162] Overall, the mechanical stability of α-thalassemia red cell membranes is normal or slightly decreased, and that of β thalassemia membranes is markedly decreased.[160] The membrane instability in β thalassemia was attributed to decreased binding of spectrin to protein 4.1.

The coexistence of α thalassemia with sickle cell disease has a salutary effect on MCHC, dense cell numbers and the erythrocyte deformability (Chapter 23).[163,164] The deformability of sickle cell anemia α thalassemia erythrocytes is inversely correlated with the number of α-globin genes.[164] Introduction of a β^S-globin gene into β thalassemic mice was associated with a significant improvement in red cell deformabilities.[165] This improvement, however, is probably due to a slight excess synthesis of α-globin chains in these mice, suggesting that a mild decrement in β-globin synthesis might have a beneficial effect on hemoglobin concentration in sickle cell anemia by normalizing red cell density distribution profiles; however, reduced anemia might promote the viscosity/vasoocclusion features of sickle cell anemia (Chapters 11 and 19).

Hypercoagulation

Hemostatic changes have been reported in patients with β thalassemia major and β thalassemia intermedia and HbH disease. An increased incidence of thromboembolic events, mainly in β thalassemia intermedia, and the occurrence of prothrombotic hemostatic anomalies in the majority of the patients suggest the existence of a hypercoagulable state.[166] Thalassemia is associated enhanced platelet and endothelial and monocyte activation.[158] Thalassemia red cells show increased expression of PS as in sickle cell disease[167] and patients have decreased levels of proteins C, S, and antithrombin III.[166]

Vascular Pathobiology

Pulmonary Hypertension: Pulmonary hypertension is a feature of β thalassemia and the same risk factors as in sickle cell disease are involved. These include platelet activation, hypercoagulability, and chronic hemolysis and reduced NO bioavailability.[168–170] Chronic hypoxia and lung injury caused by infections and iron deposition could also contribute to this complication.[171,172] In β thalassemia, the incidence of pulmonary hypertension is increased following splenectomy,[170] probably due to increased hypercoagulability consequent to erythrocyte PS exposure.[167] Plausibly, reduced NO bioavailability, chronic hypoxia, and hypercoagulability might act in concert or independently to cause elevation of pulmonary artery pressure. Pulmonary hypertension in hemolytic anemia is discussed in detail in Chapter 11.

Cardiac and Arterial Abnormalities: Chronic hemolysis, the release of iron from lysed red cells, blood transfusions, and the resulting iron overload in thalassemia leads to the formation of O_2 free radicals. Increased oxidative stress and lipid peroxidation can have detrimental effects on cell membranes. Moreover, in thalassemia, the iron-transport protein transferrin becomes saturated, causing a marked increase in nonheme- and non-transferrin-bound iron in the plasma (Chapter 29).[158] In β thalassemia major, iron overload constitutes the major cause of heart disease because unbound iron is readily taken up by cardiac monocytes, causing heart failure, structural alterations of arteries, and deleterious effects on endothelial function.[173,174] Iron overload might result in left ventricular systolic and diastolic dysfunction.[174] Alterations of arterial components with disruption of elastic tissue and calcification also occur in β thalassemia major. These arterial changes could translate functionally into altered arterial stiffness in vivo.[175] Arterial stiffness is related to vascular impedance and, in turn, to the afterload that is presented to left ventricle, resulting in decreased mechanical efficiency of the heart. Endothelial dysfunction and vasoconstriction might be promoted by reduced NO bioavailability, leading to diffuse elastic tissue injury.[174,176] Although right ventricular dysfunction is a prominent feature in β thalassemia intermedia, left ventricular impairment also develops consequent to an increased state of volume and pressure overload needed to maintain high cardiac output through a dilated and yet rigid vascular bed.[174] A uniform feature of β thalassemia intermedia patients is high cardiac output. Echocardiographic measurements in these patients show an almost two-fold increase in the cardiac output levels when compared with normal individuals.[176] β Thalassemia mice have significantly increased peripheral vascular resistance, suggesting that altered arteriolar diameters, endothelial dysfunction and abnormal rheology of red cells contribute significantly to the increased resistance.[177]

CONCLUSIONS

The presence of HbS in the sickle cell makes this disorder unique. Nevertheless, sickle cell disease and thalassemia share certain vascular abnormalities, although the majority of experimental work has focused on sickle cell disease. Some common features are a result of hemolysis and diminished NO bioavailability, reduced or absent splenic function, and damage to the erythrocyte membrane. The commonality of certain vascular abnormalities suggests that common approaches to treatment, for example, restoration of NO bioavailability or antiinflammatory agents, might be useful. These approaches are discussed in disease-specific chapters and in Chapter 31.

REFERENCES

1. Clegg JB, Weatherall DJ. Thalassemia and malaria: new insights into an old problem. *Proc Assoc Am Physicians.* 1999;111(4):278–282.
2. Ham TH, Castle WB. Relationship of increased hyotonic fragility to rythrostasis in certain anemias. *Trans Assoc Am Physicians.* 1940;55:127–132.
3. Chien S, Usami S, Bertles JF. Abnormal rheology of oxygenated blood in sickle cell anemia. *J Clin Invest.* 1970;49(4):623–634.
4. Clark MR, Mohandas N, Shohet SB. Deformability of oxygenated irreversibly sickled cells. *J Clin Invest.* 1980;65(1):189–196.
5. Self F, McIntire LV, Zanger B. Rheological evaluation of hemoglobin S and hemoglobin C hemoglobinopathies. *J Lab Clin Med.* 1977;89(3):488–497.
6. Kaul DK, Baez S, Nagel RL. Flow properties of oxygenated HbS and HbC erythrocytes in the isolated microvasculature of the rat. A contribution to the hemorheology of hemoglobinopathies. *Clin Hemorheol.* 1981;1:73–86.
7. Evans E, Mohandas N, Leung A. Static and dynamic rigidities of normal and sickle erythrocytes. Major influence of cell hemoglobin concentration. *J Clin Invest.* 1984;73(2):477–488.
8. Usami S, Chien S, Scholtz PM, Bertles JF. Effect of deoxygenation on blood rheology in sickle cell disease. *Microvasc Res.* 1975;9(3):324–334.
9. Nash GB, Johnson CS, Meiselman HJ. Influence of oxygen tension on the viscoelastic behavior of red blood cells in sickle cell disease. *Blood.* 1986;67(1):110–118.
10. Lacelle PL. Oxygen delivery to muscle cells during capillary vascular occlusion by sickle erythrocytes. *Blood Cells.* 1977;3:273–281.
11. Baez S, Kaul DK, Nagel RL. Microvascular determinants of blood flow behavior and HbSS erythrocyte plugging in microcirculation. *Blood Cells.* 1982;8(1):127–137.
12. Kaul DK, Nagel RL, Baez S. Pressure effects on the flow behavior of sickle (HbSS) red cells in isolated (ex-vivo) microvascular system. *Microvasc Res.* 1983;26(2):170–181.
13. Lipowsky HH, Usami S, Chien S. Human SS red cell rheological behavior in the microcirculation of cremaster muscle. *Blood Cells.* 1982;8(1):113–126.
14. Kaul DK, Xue H. Rate of deoxygenation and rheologic behavior of blood in sickle cell anemia. *Blood.* 1991;77(6):1353–1361.
15. Eaton WA, Hofrichter J. Hemoglobin S gelation and sickle cell disease. *Blood.* 1987;70(5):1245–1266.
16. Hiruma H, Noguchi CT, Uyesaka N, et al. Sickle cell rheology is determined by polymer fraction – not cell morphology. *Am J Hematol.* 1995;48(1):19–28.
17. Kaul DK, Fabry ME, Windisch P, Baez S, Nagel RL. Erythrocytes in sickle cell anemia are heterogeneous in their rheological and hemodynamic characteristics. *J Clin Invest.* 1983;72(1):22–31.
18. Hoover R, Rubin R, Wise G, Warren R. Adhesion of normal and sickle erythrocytes to endothelial monolayer cultures. *Blood.* 1979;54(4):872–876.
19. Hebbel RP, Boogaerts MA, Eaton JW, Steinberg MH. Erythrocyte adherence to endothelium in sickle-cell anemia. A possible determinant of disease severity. *N Engl J Med.* 1980;302(18):992–995.
20. Ferrone FA. Kinetic models and the pathophysiology of sickle cell disease. *Ann NY Acad Sci.* 1989;565:63–74.
21. Griendling KK, Sorescu D, Ushio-Fukai M. NAD(P)H oxidase: role in cardiovascular biology and disease. *Circ Res.* 2000;86(5):494–501.
22. Wood KC, Hebbel RP, Granger DN. Endothelial cell NADPH oxidase mediates the cerebral microvascular dysfunction in sickle cell transgenic mice. *FASEB J.* 2005;19(8):989–991.
23. Hsu LL, Champion HC, Campbell-Lee SA, et al. Hemolysis in sickle cell mice causes pulmonary hypertension due to global impairment in nitric oxide bioavailability. *Blood.* 2007;109(7):3088–3098.
24. Vasquez-Vivar J, Kalyanaraman B, Martasek P, et al. Superoxide generation by endothelial nitric oxide synthase: the influence of cofactors. *Proc Natl Acad Sci USA.* 1998;95(16):9220–9225.
25. Osarogiagbon UR, Choong S, Belcher JD, Vercellotti GM, Paller MS, Hebbel RP. Reperfusion injury pathophysiology in sickle transgenic mice. *Blood.* 2000;96:314–320.
26. Kaul DK, Hebbel RP. Hypoxia/reoxygenation causes inflammatory response in transgenic sickle mice but not in normal mice [see comments]. *J Clin Invest.* 2000;106(3):411–420.
27. Hebbel RP, Osarogiagbon R, Kaul D. The endothelial biology of sickle cell disease: inflammation and a chronic vasculopathy. *Microcirculation.* 2004;11(2):129–151.
28. Aslan M, Ryan TM, Adler B, et al. Oxygen radical inhibition of nitric oxide-dependent vascular function in sickle cell disease. *Proc Natl Acad Sci USA.* 2001;98(26):15215–15220.
29. Kaul DK, Liu XD, Choong S, Belcher JD, Vercellotti GM, Hebbel RP. Anti-inflammatory therapy ameliorates leukocyte adhesion and microvascular flow abnormalities in transgenic sickle mice. *Am J Physiol Heart Circ Physiol.* 2004;287(1):H293–H301.
30. Kalambur VS, Mahaseth H, Bischof JC, et al. Microvascular blood flow and stasis in transgenic sickle mice: utility of a dorsal skin fold chamber for intravital microscopy. *Am J Hematol.* 2004;77(2):117–125.
31. Dasgupta T, Hebbel RP, Kaul DK. Protective effect of arginine on oxidative stress in transgenic sickle mouse models. *Free Rad Biol Med.* 2006;41(12):1771–1780.
32. Chiu D, Lubin B. Abnormal vitamin E and glutathione peroxidase levels in sickle cell anemia: evidence for increased susceptibility to lipid peroxidation in vivo. *J Lab Clin Med.* 1979;94(4):542–548.
33. Das SK, Nair RC. Superoxide dismutase, glutathione peroxidase, catalase and lipid peroxidation of normal and sickled erythrocytes. *Br J Haematol.* 1980;44(1):87–92.
34. Nita DA, Nita V, Spulber S, et al. Oxidative damage following cerebral ischemia depends on reperfusion – a biochemical study in rat. *J Cell Mol Med.* 2001;5(2):163–170.
35. Kaul DK, Liu XD, Chang HY, Nagel RL, Fabry ME. Effect of fetal hemoglobin on microvascular regulation in sickle transgenic-knockout mice. *J Clin Invest.* 2004;114(8):1136–1145.
36. Kurozumi R, Takahashi M, Kojima S. Involvement of mitochondrial peroxynitrite in nitric oxide-induced glutathione synthesis. *Biol Pharm Bull.* 2005;28(5):779–785.
37. Morris CR, Kuypers FA, Larkin S, et al. Arginine therapy: a novel strategy to induce nitric oxide production in sickle cell disease. *Br J Haematol.* 2000;111(2):498–500.

38. Reiter CD, Wang X, Tanus-Santos JE, et al. Cell-free hemoglobin limits nitric oxide bioavailability in sickle-cell disease. *Nat Med.* 2002;8(12):1383–1389.
39. Kaneko FT, Arroliga AC, Dweik RA, et al. Biochemical reaction products of nitric oxide as quantitative markers of primary pulmonary hypertension. *Am J Respir Crit Care Med.* 1998;158(3):917–923.
40. Wetterstroem N, Brewer GJ, Warth JA, Mitchinson A, Near K. Relationship of glutathione levels and Heinz body formation to irreversibly sickled cells in sickle cell anemia. *J Lab Clin Med.* 1984;103(4):589–596.
41. Reid M, Badaloo A, Forrester T, Jahoor F. In vivo rates of erythrocyte glutathione synthesis in adults with sickle cell disease. *Am J Physiol Endocrinol Metab.* 2006;291(1):E73–E79.
42. Morris CR, Suh JH, Hagar W, et al. Erythrocyte glutamine depletion, altered redox environment, and pulmonary hypertension in sickle cell disease. *Blood.* 2008;111(1):402–410.
43. Klug PP, Kaye N, Jensen WN. Endothelial cell and vascular damage in the sickle cell disorders. *Blood Cells.* 1982;8(1):175–184.
44. Wood KC, Hebbel RP, Granger DN. Endothelial cell P-selectin mediates a proinflammatory and prothrombogenic phenotype in cerebral venules of sickle cell transgenic mice. *Am J Physiol Heart Circ Physiol.* 2004;286(5):H1608–H1614.
45. Turhan A, Weiss LA, Mohandas N, Coller BS, Frenette PS. Primary role for adherent leukocytes in sickle cell vascular occlusion: a new paradigm. *Proc Natl Acad Sci USA.* 2002;99(5):3047–3051.
46. Sultana C, Shen Y, Rattan V, Johnson C, Kalra VK. Interaction of sickle erythrocytes with endothelial cells in the presence of endothelial cell conditioned medium induces oxidant stress leading to transendothelial migration of monocytes. *Blood.* 1998;92(10):3924–3935.
47. Belcher JD, Bryant CJ, Nguyen J, et al. Transgenic sickle mice have vascular inflammation. *Blood.* 2003;101(10):3953–3959.
48. Wood K, Russell J, Hebbel RP, Granger DN. Differential expression of E- and P-selectin in the microvasculature of sickle cell transgenic mice. *Microcirculation.* 2004;11(4):377–385.
49. Hebbel RP, Eaton JW, Balasingam M, Steinberg MH. Spontaneous oxygen radical generation by sickle erythrocytes. *J Clin Invest.* 1982;70(6):1253–1259.
50. Das KC, Lewis-Molock Y, White CW. Thiol modulation of TNF alpha and IL-1 induced MnSOD gene expression and activation of NF-kappa B. *Mol Cell Biochem.* 1995;148(1):45–57.
51. Haddad JJ. Science review: Redox and oxygen-sensitive transcription factors in the regulation of oxidant-mediated lung injury: role for nuclear factor-kappaB. *Crit Care.* 2002;6(6):481–490.
52. Sowemimo-Coker SO, Meiselman HJ, Francis RB, Jr. Increased circulating endothelial cells in sickle cell crisis. *Am J Hematol.* 1989;31(4):263–265.
53. Solovey A, Lin Y, Browne P, Choong S, Wayner E, Hebbel RP. Circulating activated endothelial cells in sickle cell anemia [see comments]. *N Engl J Med.* 1997;337(22):1584–1590.
54. Conger JD, Weil JV. Abnormal vascular function following ischemia-reperfusion injury. *J Invest Med.* 1995;43(5):431–442.
55. Kaul DK, Liu XD, Zhang X, Ma L, Hsia CJ, Nagel RL. Inhibition of sickle red cell adhesion and vasoocclusion in the microcirculation by antioxidants. *Am J Physiol Heart Circ Physiol.* 2006;291(1):H167–H175.
56. Hebbel RP, Yamada O, Moldow CF, Jacob HS, White JG, Eaton JW. Abnormal adherence of sickle erythrocytes to cultured vascular endothelium: possible mechanism for microvascular occlusion in sickle cell disease. *J Clin Invest.* 1980;65(1):154–160.
57. Barabino GA, McIntire LV, Eskin SG, Sears DA, Udden M. Endothelial cell interactions with sickle cell, sickle trait, mechanically injured, and normal erythrocytes under controlled flow. *Blood.* 1987;70(1):152–157.
58. Mohandas N, Evans E. Sickle erythrocyte adherence to vascular endothelium. Morphologic correlates and the requirement for divalent cations and collagen-binding plasma proteins. *J Clin Invest.* 1985;76(4):1605–1612.
59. Kaul DK, Chen D, Zhan J. Adhesion of sickle cells to vascular endothelium is critically dependent on changes in density and shape of the cells. *Blood.* 1994;83(10):3006–3017.
60. Kaul DK, Fabry ME, Nagel RL. Microvascular sites and characteristics of sickle cell adhesion to vascular endothelium in shear flow conditions: pathophysiological implications. *Proc Natl Acad Sci USA.* 1989;86(9):3356–3360.
61. Kaul DK, Liu XD, Zhang X, et al. Peptides based on {alpha}V-binding domains of erythrocyte ICAM-4 inhibit sickle red cell-endothelial interactions and vaso-occlusion in the microcirculation. *Am J Physiol Cell Physiol.* 2006;291(5):C922–C930.
62. Zennadi R, Moeller BJ, Whalen EJ, et al. Epinephrine-induced activation of LW-mediated sickle cell adhesion and vaso-occlusion in vivo. *Blood.* 2007;110(7):2708–2717.
63. Brittain HA, Eckman JR, Swerlick RA, Howard RJ, Wick TM. Thrombospondin from activated platelets promotes sickle erythrocyte adherence to human microvascular endothelium under physiologic flow: a potential role for platelet activation in sickle cell vaso-occlusion. *Blood.* 1993;81(8):2137–2143.
64. Wick TM, Moake JL, Udden MM, Eskin SG, Sears DA, McIntire LV. Unusually large von Willebrand factor multimers increase adhesion of sickle erythrocytes to human endothelial cells under controlled flow. *J Clin Invest.* 1987;80(3):905–910.
65. Kaul DK, Fabry ME, Costantini F, Rubin EM, Nagel RL. In vivo demonstration of red cell-endothelial interaction, sickling and altered microvascular response to oxygen in the sickle transgenic mouse. *J Clin Invest.* 1995;96(6):2845–2853.
66. Fabry ME, Suzuka SM, Weinberg RS, et al. Second generation knockout sickle mice: the effect of HbF. *Blood.* 2001;97(2):410–418.
67. Swerlick RA, Eckman JR, Kumar A, Jeitler M, Wick TM. Alpha 4 beta 1-integrin expression on sickle reticulocytes: vascular cell adhesion molecule-1-dependent binding to endothelium. *Blood.* 1993;82(6):1891–1899.
68. Sugihara K, Sugihara T, Mohandas N, Hebbel RP. Thrombospondin mediates adherence of CD36+ sickle reticulocytes to endothelial cells. *Blood.* 1992;80(10):2634–2642.
69. Setty BN, Stuart MJ. Vascular cell adhesion molecule-1 is involved in mediating hypoxia-induced sickle red blood cell adherence to endothelium: potential role in sickle cell disease. *Blood.* 1996;88(6):2311–2320.
70. Stuart MJ, Setty BN. Acute chest syndrome of sickle cell disease: new light on an old problem. *Curr Opin Hematol.* 2001;8(2):111–122.

71. Vichinsky EP, Styles LA, Colangelo LH, Wright EC, Castro O, Nickerson B. Acute chest syndrome in sickle cell disease: clinical presentation and course. Cooperative Study of Sickle Cell Disease. *Blood.* 1997;89(5):1787–1792.
72. Barabino GA, Liu XD, Ewenstein BM, Kaul DK. Anionic polysaccharides inhibit adhesion of sickle erythrocytes to the vascular endothelium and result in improved hemodynamic behavior. *Blood.* 1999;93(4):1422–1429.
73. Hillery CA, Du MC, Montgomery RR, Scott JP. Increased adhesion of erythrocytes to components of the extracellular matrix: isolation and characterization of a red blood cell lipid that binds thrombospondin and laminin. *Blood.* 1996;87(11):4879–4886.
74. Brittain JE, Mlinar KJ, Anderson CS, Orringer EP, Parise LV. Activation of sickle red blood cell adhesion via integrin-associated protein/CD47-induced signal transduction. *J Clin Invest.* 2001;107(12):1555–1562.
75. Zennadi R, Hines PC, De Castro LM, Cartron JP, Parise LV, Telen MJ. Epinephrine acts through erythroid signaling pathways to activate sickle cell adhesion to endothelium via LW-alphavbeta3 interactions. *Blood.* 2004;104(12):3774–3781.
76. Hines PC, Zen Q, Burney SN, et al. Novel epinephrine and cyclic AMP-mediated activation of BCAM/Lu-dependent sickle (SS) RBC adhesion. *Blood.* 2003;101(8):3281–3287.
77. Hermand P, Gane P, Callebaut I, Kieffer N, Cartron JP, Bailly P. Integrin receptor specificity for human red cell ICAM-4 ligand. Critical residues for alphaIIbeta3 binding. *Eur J Biochem.* 2004;271(18):3729–3740.
78. Spring FA, Parsons SF, Ortlepp S, et al. Intercellular adhesion molecule-4 binds alpha(4)beta(1) and alpha(V)-family integrins through novel integrin-binding mechanisms. *Blood.* 2001;98(2):458–466.
79. Setty BN, Kulkarni S, Stuart MJ. Role of erythrocyte phosphatidylserine in sickle red cell-endothelial adhesion. *Blood.* 2002;99(5):1564–1571.
80. Wick TM, Moake JL, Udden MM, McIntire LV. Unusually large von Willebrand factor multimers preferentially promote young sickle and nonsickle erythrocyte adhesion to endothelial cells. *Am J Hematol.* 1993;42(3):284–292.
81. Kaul DK, Nagel RL, Chen D, Tsai HM. Sickle erythrocyte-endothelial interactions in microcirculation: the role of von Willebrand factor and implications for vasoocclusion. *Blood.* 1993;81(9):2429–2438.
82. Hillery CA, Scott JP, Ming cD. The carboxy-terminal cell-binding domain of thrombospondin is essential for sickle red cell adhesion. *Blood.* 1999;94(1):302–309.
83. Kaul DK, Tsai HM, Liu XD, Nakada MT, Nagel RL, Coller BS. Monoclonal antibodies to alphaVbeta3 (7E3 and LM609) inhibit sickle red blood cell-endothelium interactions induced by platelet-activating factor [see comments]. *Blood.* 2000;95(2):368–374.
84. Richardson SG, Matthews KB, Stuart J, Geddes AM, Wilcox RM. Serial changes in coagulation and viscosity during sickle-cell crisis. *Br J Haematol.* 1979;41(1):95–103.
85. Felding-Habermann B, Cheresh DA. Vitronectin and its receptors. *Curr Opin Cell Biol.* 1993;5(5):864–868.
86. Barabino GA, Wise RJ, Woodbury VA, et al. Inhibition of sickle erythrocyte adhesion to immobilized thrombospondin by von Willebrand factor under dynamic flow conditions. *Blood.* 1997;89(7):2560–2567.
87. Matsui NM, Borsig L, Rosen SD, Yaghmai M, Varki A, Embury SH. P-selectin mediates the adhesion of sickle erythrocytes to the endothelium. *Blood.* 2001;98(6):1955–1962.
88. Matsui NM, Varki A, Embury SH. Heparin inhibits the flow adhesion of sickle red blood cells to P-selectin. *Blood.* 2002;100(10):3790–3796.
89. Embury SH, Matsui NM, Ramanujam S, et al. The contribution of endothelial cell P-selectin to the microvascular flow of mouse sickle erythrocytes in vivo. *Blood.* 2004;104(10):3378–3385.
90. Swerlick RA, Lee KH, Wick TM, Lawley TJ. Human dermal microvascular endothelial but not human umbilical vein endothelial cells express CD36 in vivo and in vitro. *J Immunol.* 1992;148(1):78–83.
91. Cheresh DA. Human endothelial cells synthesize and express an Arg-Gly-Asp-directed adhesion receptor involved in attachment to fibrinogen and von Willebrand factor. *Proc Natl Acad Sci USA.* 1987;84(18):6471–6475.
92. Kramer RH, Cheng YF, Clyman R. Human microvascular endothelial cells use beta 1 and beta 3 integrin receptor complexes to attach to laminin. *J Cell Biol.* 1990;111(3):1233–1243.
93. Oh SO, Ibe BO, Johnson C, Kurantsin-Mills J, Raj JU. Platelet-activating factor in plasma of patients with sickle cell disease in steady state. *J Lab Clin Med.* 1997;130(2):191–196.
94. Finnegan EM, Barabino GA, Liu XD, Chang HY, Jonczyk A, Kaul DK. Small-molecule cyclic {alpha}Vbeta3 antagonists inhibit sickle red cell adhesion to vascular endothelium and vasoocclusion. *Am J Physiol Heart Circ Physiol.* 2007; 293(2):H1038–H1045.
95. Hebbel RP. Blockade of adhesion of sickle cells to endothelium by monoclonal antibodies. *N Engl J Med.* 2000; 342(25):1910–1912.
96. Charache S, Barton FB, Moore RD, et al. Hydroxyurea and sickle cell anemia. Clinical utility of a myelosuppressive "switching" agent. The Multicenter Study of Hydroxyurea in Sickle Cell Anemia. *Medicine.* 1996;75(6):300–326.
97. Steinberg MH, Lu ZH, Barton FB, Terrin ML, Charache S, Dover GJ. Fetal hemoglobin in sickle cell anemia: determinants of response to hydroxyurea. Multicenter Study of Hydroxyurea. *Blood.* 1997;89(3):1078–1088.
98. Setty BN, Kulkarni S, Dampier CD, Stuart MJ. Fetal hemoglobin in sickle cell anemia: relationship to erythrocyte adhesion markers and adhesion. *Blood.* 2001;97(9):2568–2573.
99. Saleh AW, Duits AJ, Gerbers A, de Vries C, Hillen HF. Cytokines and soluble adhesion molecules in sickle cell anemia patients during hydroxyurea therapy. *Acta Haematol.* 1998;100(1):26–31.
100. Bridges KR, Barabino GD, Brugnara C, et al. A multiparameter analysis of sickle erythrocytes in patients undergoing hydroxyurea therapy. *Blood.* 1996;88(12):4701–4710.
101. Cokic VP, Smith RD, Beleslin-Cokic BB, et al. Hydroxyurea induces fetal hemoglobin by the nitric oxide-dependent activation of soluble guanylyl cyclase. *J Clin Invest.* 2003; 111(2):231–239.
102. Space SL, Lane PA, Pickett CK, Weil JV. Nitric oxide attenuates normal and sickle red blood cell adherence to pulmonary endothelium. *Am J Hematol.* 2000;63(4):200–204.

103. Kaul DK, Fabry ME, Nagel RL. Erythrocytic and vascular factors influencing the microcirculatory behavior of blood in sickle cell anemia. *Ann NY Acad Sci.* 1989;565:316–326.
104. Kaul DK, Fabry ME, Nagel RL. The pathophysiology of vascular obstruction in the sickle syndromes. *Blood Rev.* 1996;10(1):29–44.
105. Kaul DK. Flow properties and endothelial adhesion of sickle erythrocytes in an ex vivo microvascular preparation. In: Ohnishi ST, Ohnishi T, eds. *Membrane Abnormalities in Sickle Cell Disease and in Other Red Blood Cell Disorders.* Boca Raton, FL: CRC Press; 1994:217–241.
106. Embury SH. The not-so-simple process of sickle cell vasoocclusion. *Microcirculation.* 2004;11(2):101–113.
107. Fabry ME, Fine E, Rajanayagam V, et al. Demonstration of endothelial adhesion of sickle cells in vivo: a distinct role for deformable sickle cell discocytes. *Blood.* 1992;79(6):1602–1611.
108. Fabry ME, Rajanayagam V, Fine E, et al. Modeling sickle cell vasoocclusion in the rat leg: quantification of trapped sickle cells and correlation with 31P metabolic and 1H magnetic resonance imaging changes. *Proc Natl Acad Sci USA.* 1989;86(10):3808–3812.
109. Kaul DK, Fabry ME, Nagel RL. Vaso-occlusion by sickle cells: evidence for selective trapping of dense red cells. *Blood.* 1986;68(5):1162–1166.
110. Fabry ME, Benjamin L, Lawrence C, Nagel RL. An objective sign in painful crisis in sickle cell anemia: the concomitant reduction of high density red cells. *Blood.* 1984;64(2):559–563.
111. Ballas SK, Smith ED. Red blood cell changes during the evolution of the sickle cell painful crisis. *Blood.* 1992;79(8):2154–2163.
112. Graido-Gonzalez E, Doherty JC, Bergreen EW, Organ G, Telfer M, McMillen MA. Plasma endothelin-1, cytokine, and prostaglandin E2 levels in sickle cell disease and acute vaso-occlusive sickle crisis. *Blood.* 1998;92(7):2551–2555.
113. Weinstein R, Zhou MA, Bartlett-Pandite A, Wenc K. Sickle erythrocytes inhibit human endothelial cell DNA synthesis. *Blood.* 1990;76(10):2146–2152.
114. Phelan M, Perrine SP, Brauer M, Faller DV. Sickle erythrocytes, after sickling, regulate the expression of the endothelin-1 gene and protein in human endothelial cells in culture. *J Clin Invest.* 1995;96(2):1145–1151.
115. Setty BN, Chen D, Stuart MJ. Sickle red blood cells stimulate endothelial cell production of eicosanoids and diacylglycerol. *J Lab Clin Med.* 1996;128(3):313–321.
116. Sowemimo-Coker SO, Haywood LJ, Meiselman HJ, Francis RB Jr. Effects of normal and sickle erythrocytes on prostacyclin release by perfused human umbilical cord veins. *Am J Hematol.* 1992;40(4):276–282.
117. Hollopeter G, Jantzen HM, Vincent D, et al. Identification of the platelet ADP receptor targeted by antithrombotic drugs. *Nature.* 2001;409(6817):202–207.
118. Hebbel RP, Vercellotti GM. The endothelial biology of sickle cell disease. *J Lab Clin Med.* 1997;129(3):288–293.
119. Villagra J, Shiva S, Hunter LA, Machado RF, Gladwin MT, Kato GJ. Platelet activation in patients with sickle disease, hemolysis-associated pulmonary hypertension and nitric oxide scavenging by cell-free hemoglobin. *Blood.* 2007;110:2166–2172.
120. Boggs DR, Hyde F, Srodes C. An unusual pattern of neutrophil kinetics in sickle cell anemia. *Blood.* 1973;41(1):59–65.
121. Platt OS. Sickle cell anemia as an inflammatory disease. *J Clin Invest.* 2000;106(3):337–338.
122. Helmke BP, Bremner SN, Zweifach BW, Skalak R, Schmid-Schonbein GW. Mechanisms for increased blood flow resistance due to leukocytes. *Am J Physiol.* 1997;273(6 Pt 2): H2884–H2890.
123. Lipowsky HH, Scott DA, Cartmell JS. Leukocyte rolling velocity and its relation to leukocyte-endothelium adhesion and cell deformability. *Am J Physiol.* 1996;270(4 Pt 2):H1371–H1380.
124. Turhan A, Jenab P, Bruhns P, Ravetch JV, Coller BS, Frenette PS. Intravenous immune globulin prevents venular vaso-occlusion in sickle cell mice by inhibiting leukocyte adhesion and the interactions between sickle erythrocytes and adherent leukocytes. *Blood.* 2004;103(6):2397–2400.
125. Chang J, Shi PA, Chiang EY, Frenette PS. Intravenous immunoglobulins reverse acute vaso-occlusive crises in sickle cell mice through rapid inhibition of neutrophil adhesion. *Blood.* 2008;111(2):915–923.
126. Lonsdorfer J, Bogui P, Otayeck A, Bursaux E, Poyart C, Cabannes R. Cardiorespiratory adjustments in chronic sickle cell anemia. *Bull Eur Physiopathol Respir.* 1983;19(4):339–344.
127. Belhassen L, Pelle G, Sediame S, et al. Endothelial dysfunction in patients with sickle cell disease is related to selective impairment of shear stress-mediated vasodilation. *Blood.* 2001;97(6):1584–1589.
128. Johnson CS, Giorgio AJ. Arterial blood pressure in adults with sickle cell disease. *Arch Intern Med.* 1981;141(7):891–893.
129. Rodgers GP, Schechter AN, Noguchi CT et al. Periodic microcirculatory flow in patients with sickle-cell disease. *N Engl J Med.* 1984;311(24):1534–1538.
130. Lipowsky HH, Sheikh NU, Katz DM. Intravital microscopy of capillary hemodynamics in sickle cell disease. *J Clin Invest.* 1987;80(1):117–127.
131. Nath KA, Katusic ZS, Gladwin MT. The perfusion paradox and vascular instability in sickle cell disease. *Microcirculation.* 2004;11(2):179–193.
132. Gladwin MT, Kato GJ. Cardiopulmonary complications of sickle cell disease: role of nitric oxide and hemolytic anemia. *Hematol Am Soc Hematol Educ Program.* 2005;51–57.
133. Eberhardt RT, McMahon L, Duffy SJ, et al. Sickle cell anemia is associated with reduced nitric oxide bioactivity in peripheral conduit and resistance vessels. *Am J Hematol.* 2003;74(2):104–111.
134. Kubes P, Suzuki M, Granger DN. Nitric oxide: an endogenous modulator of leukocyte adhesion. *Proc Natl Acad Sci USA.* 1991;88(11):4651–4655.
135. Moncada S, Palmer RM, Higgs EA. Nitric oxide: physiology, pathophysiology, and pharmacology. *Pharmacol Rev.* 1991;43(2):109–142.
136. Ogawa T, Nussler AK, Tuzuner E, et al. Contribution of nitric oxide to the protective effects of ischemic preconditioning in ischemia-reperfused rat kidneys. *J Lab Clin Med.* 2001;138(1):50–58.

137. Morris CR, Morris SM Jr, Hagar W, et al. Arginine therapy: a new treatment for pulmonary hypertension in sickle cell disease? *Am J Respir Crit Care Med.* 2003;168(1):63–69.
138. Romero JR, Suzuka SM, Nagel RL, Fabry ME. Arginine supplementation of sickle transgenic mice reduces red cell density and Gardos channel activity. *Blood.* 2002;99(4):1103–1108.
139. Enwonwu CO. Increased metabolic demand for arginine in sickle cell anemia. *Med Sci Res.* 1989;17:997–998.
140. Morris CR, Kato GJ, Poljakovic M, et al. Dysregulated arginine metabolism, hemolysis-associated pulmonary hypertension, and mortality in sickle cell disease. *JAMA.* 2005;294(1):81–90.
141. Harrison DG. Cellular and molecular mechanisms of endothelial cell dysfunction. *J Clin Invest.* 1997;100(9):2153–2157.
142. Gladwin MT, Lancaster JR Jr, Freeman BA, Schechter AN. Nitric oxide's reactions with hemoglobin: a view through the SNO-storm. *Nat Med.* 2003;9(5):496–500.
143. Kaul DK, Liu XD, Fabry ME, Nagel RL. Impaired nitric oxide-mediated vasodilation in transgenic sickle mouse. *Am J Physiol Heart Circ Physiol.* 2000;278(6):H1799–H1806.
144. Nath KA, Shah V, Haggard JJ, et al. Mechanisms of vascular instability in a transgenic mouse model of sickle cell disease. *Am J Physiol Regul Integr Comp Physiol.* 2000;279(6):R1949–R1955.
145. Gladwin MT, Kato GJ. Cardiopulmonary complications of sickle cell disease: role of nitric oxide and hemolytic anemia. *Hematol. Am Soc Hematol Educ Program.* 2005;51–57.
146. Gladwin MT, Schechter AN, Ognibene FP, et al. Divergent nitric oxide bioavailability in men and women with sickle cell disease. *Circulation.* 2003;107(2):271–278.
147. Landino LM, Crews BC, Timmons MD, Morrow JD, Marnett LJ. Peroxynitrite, the coupling product of nitric oxide and superoxide, activates prostaglandin biosynthesis. *Proc Natl Acad Sci USA.* 1996;93(26):15069–15074.
148. Alp NJ, Channon KM. Regulation of endothelial nitric oxide synthase by tetrahydrobiopterin in vascular disease. *Arterioscler Thromb Vasc Biol.* 2004;24(3):413–420.
149. Landmesser U, Dikalov S, Price SR, et al. Oxidation of tetrahydrobiopterin leads to uncoupling of endothelial cell nitric oxide synthase in hypertension. *J Clin Invest.* 2003;111(8):1201–1209.
150. Katusic ZS, d'Uscio LV. Tetrahydrobiopterin: mediator of endothelial protection. *Arterioscler Thromb Vasc Biol.* 2004;24(3):397–398.
151. Wood KC, Hebbel RP, Lefer DJ, Granger DN. Critical role of endothelial cell-derived nitric oxide synthase in sickle cell disease-induced microvascular dysfunction. *Free Rad Biol Med.* 2006;40(8):1443–1453.
152. Kooy NW, Lewis SJ. Nitrotyrosine attenuates the hemodynamic effects of adrenoceptor agonists in vivo: relevance to the pathophysiology of peroxynitrite. *Eur J Pharmacol.* 1996;310(2–3):155–161.
153. Kooy NW, Lewis SJ. The peroxynitrite product 3-nitro-L-tyrosine attenuates the hemodynamic responses to angiotensin II in vivo. *Eur J Pharmacol.* 1996;315(2):165–170.
154. Hatch FE, Crowe LR, Miles DE, Young JP, Portner ME. Altered vascular reactivity in sickle hemoglobinopathy. A possible protective factor from hypertension. *Am J Hyperten.* 1989;2(1):2–8.
155. Setty BNY, Rao AK, Stuart MJ. Thrombophilia in sickle cell disease: the red cell connection. *Blood.* 2001;98(12):3228–3233.
156. Ataga KI, Orringer EP. Hypercoagulability in sickle cell disease: a curious paradox. *Am J Med.* 2003;115(9):721–728.
157. Weatherall DJ. The thalassemias. In: Stamatoyannopoulos G, ed. *Molecular Basis of Blood Diseases.* Philadelphia: WB Saunders; 1994:157–205.
158. Urbinati F, Madigan C, Malik P. Pathophysiology and therapy for haemoglobinopathies. Part II: thalassaemias. *Expert Rev Mol Med.* 2006;8(10):1–26.
159. Lacelle PL. Behavior of abnormal erythrocytes in capillaries. In: Cokelet GR, Meiselman HJ, Brooks DF, eds. *Erythrocyte Mechanics and Blood Flow.* New York: Alan R. Liss; 1980:195–211.
160. Schrier SL, Rachmilewitz E, Mohandas N. Cellular and membrane properties of alpha and beta thalassemic erythrocytes are different: implication for differences in clinical manifestations. *Blood.* 1989;74(6):2194–2202.
161. Waugh SM, Low PS. Hemichrome binding to band 3: nucleation of Heinz bodies on the erythrocyte membrane. *Biochemistry.* 1985;24(1):34–39.
162. Shinar E, Rachmilewitz EA, Lux SE. Differing erythrocyte membrane skeletal protein defects in alpha and beta thalassemia. *J Clin Invest.* 1989;83(2):404–410.
163. Noguchi CT, Dover GJ, Rodgers GP, et al. Alpha thalassemia changes erythrocyte heterogeneity in sickle cell disease. *J Clin Invest.* 1985;75(5):1632–1637.
164. Embury SH, Clark MR, Monroy G, Mohandas N. Concurrent sickle cell anemia and alpha-thalassemia. Effect on pathological properties of sickle erythrocytes. *J Clin Invest.* 1984;73(1):116–123.
165. Rubin EM, Kan YW, Mohandas N. Effect of human beta (s)-globin chains on cellular properties of red cells from beta-thalassemic mice. *J Clin Invest.* 1988;82(3):1129–1133.
166. Eldor A, Rachmilewitz EA. The hypercoagulable state in thalassemia. *Blood.* 2002;99(1):36–43.
167. Borenstain-Ben Y, V, Barenholz Y, Hy-Am E, Rachmilewitz EA, Eldor A. Phosphatidylserine in the outer leaflet of red blood cells from beta-thalassemia patients may explain the chronic hypercoagulable state and thrombotic episodes. *Am J Hematol.* 1993;44(1):63–65.
168. Singer ST, Kuypers FA, Styles L, Vichinsky EP, Foote D, Rosenfeld H. Pulmonary hypertension in thalassemia: association with platelet activation and hypercoagulable state. *Am J Hematol.* 2006;81(9):670–675.
169. Morris CR, Kuypers FA, Kato GJ, et al. Hemolysis-associated pulmonary hypertension in thalassemia. *Ann NY Acad Sci.* 2005;1054:481–485.
170. Aessopos A, Farmakis D. Pulmonary hypertension in beta-thalassemia. *Ann NY Acad Sci.* 2005;1054:342–349.
171. Factor JM, Pottipati SR, Rappoport I, Rosner IK, Lesser ML, Giardina PJ. Pulmonary function abnormalities in thalassemia major and the role of iron overload. *Am J Respir Crit Care Med.* 1994;149(6):1570–1574.
172. Zakynthinos E, Vassilakopoulos T, Kaltsas P, et al. Pulmonary hypertension, interstitial lung fibrosis, and lung iron deposition in thalassaemia major. *Thorax.* 2001;56(9):737–739.

173. Link G, Pinson A, Hershko C. Heart cells in culture: a model of myocardial iron overload and chelation. *J Lab Clin Med.* 1985;106(2):147–153.
174. Aessopos A, Kati M, Farmakis D. Heart disease in thalassemia intermedia: a review of the underlying pathophysiology. *Haematologica.* 2007;92(5):658–665.
175. Cheung YF, Chan GC, Ha SY. Arterial stiffness and endothelial function in patients with beta-thalassemia major. *Circulation.* 2002;106(20):2561–2566.
176. Aessopos A, Farmakis D, Karagiorga M, et al. Cardiac involvement in thalassemia intermedia: a multicenter study. *Blood.* 2001;97(11):3411–3416.
177. Stoyanova E, Trudel M, Felfly H, Garcia D, Cloutier G. Characterization of circulatory disorders in beta-thalassemic mice by noninvasive ultrasound biomicroscopy. *Physiol Genom.* 2007;29(1):84–90.

9

The Erythrocyte Membrane

Patrick G. Gallagher and Clinton H. Joiner

INTRODUCTION

Hemoglobinopathies, including the thalassemia syndromes and sickle cell disease, are complex disorders with protean manifestations. Their pathophysiology is influenced by environmental and genetic factors in addition to the pleiotropic effects of the globin gene mutations themselves. The erythrocyte membrane plays a critical role in these disorders because of the effects of its structural and functional perturbations and alterations in ion and water homeostasis regulated by membrane proteins.[1] The first portion of this chapter reviews the structural and functional characteristics of the erythrocyte membrane; this is followed by a review of the alterations in ion and water homeostasis observed in the erythrocytes of sickle cell disease and thalassemia.

MEMBRANE STRUCTURE AND FUNCTION

The erythrocyte membrane is a complex, multifunctional structure. Although providing a protective layer between hemoglobin and other intracellular components and the external environment, it provides the erythrocyte with the deformability and stability required to withstand its travels through the circulation. The erythrocyte is subjected to high sheer stress in the arterial system, dramatic changes in size in the microcirculation, and wide variations in tonicity, pH, and pO_2 as it travels throughout the body. It facilitates the transport of cations, anions, urea, water and other small molecules in and out of the cell, but denies entry to larger molecules, particularly if charged. A unique anucleate cell, the erythrocyte has a limited capacity for self-repair.

Membrane Structure

The erythrocyte membrane is composed of a lipid bilayer linked to an underlying cortical membrane skeleton.[2] Membrane proteins are classified as integral, penetrating or crossing the lipid bilayer and interacting with the hydrophobic lipid core, or peripheral, interacting with integral proteins or lipids at the membrane surface, but not penetrating the bilayer core. Integral membrane proteins of the erythrocyte include the glycophorins, the Rh proteins, transport proteins such as band 3, the sodium pump, Ca^{2+}–adenosine triphosphatase (ATPase) and Mg^{2+}-ATPase. Peripheral membrane proteins include the structural proteins of the spectrin-actin–based membrane skeleton.

Membrane Pathobiology

The membrane is in intimate contact with excess unpaired globin chains found in the thalassemia syndromes and sickle hemoglobin (HbS) in sickle cell disease, leading to membrane distortion by physical effects. Membrane proteins are also subjected to the toxic byproducts of the oxidative stress induced by the presence of excess unpaired globin, and hemoglobin, particularly that induced by the decompartmentalization of erythrocyte iron.[3]

Oxidant Stress. The normal erythrocyte is under continuous oxidative stress, with cyclic hemoglobin oxygenation and deoxygenation constantly generating oxidants in the form of reactive oxygen species. Because the mature, anucleate erythrocyte lacks the ability to synthesize proteins or lipids damaged by reactive oxygen species, it has many antioxidants, including superoxide dismutase, catalase, thiol species such as glutathione and peroxyredoxin, and vitamin E, to combat this ongoing oxidant stress.

Thalassemic and sickle erythrocyte are especially challenged by oxidants. The instability of reactive, heme-containing α- or β-globin chains and HbS, which is relatively unstable compared with normal HbA, leads to autooxidation,[4–7] generating additional peroxide and oxygen radicals. As a result, the erythrocyte's normal defenses against reactive oxidant species begins to be overwhelmed, and irreversible oxidative damage of both membrane and cytoplasmic proteins and lipids occurs.[8,9]

Excess globin chains and HbS precipitate on the inner membrane surface. This most likely is mediated by the formation of insoluble hemichromes that are oxidation products of methemoglobin. They prompt formation of reactive oxygen species and lead to the release of iron from heme in the form of highly reactive free, or molecular iron.[10] The interaction between HbS and phosphatidylserine (PS) present on the inner leaflet of the lipid bilayer also promotes the formation of methemoglobin, hemichromes, and the release of heme into the lipid phase.[11,12] In the presence of peroxidation byproducts, this process liberates free iron and causes additional lipid peroxidation. The rate of HbS oxidation becomes 3.4-fold faster in the presence of lipids, which corresponds to a doubling rate for the oxidation rate for HbS in solution (1.7-fold greater for HbS than HbA).[11]

Thalassemia and sickle erythrocytes constantly generate excessive amounts of superoxide, peroxide, and hydroxyl radicals. Furthermore, levels or activities of scavengers and enzymes involved in antioxidant defenses are perturbed, with decreased levels of glutathione, vitamin C, glutathione reductase, possibly glutathione peroxidase and catalase,[13] decreased levels of plasma and erythrocyte vitamin E,[14] variable levels of superoxide dismutase,[13,15] and increased levels of glucose-6-phosphate dehydrogenase. Sickle erythrocytes also demonstrate decreased NADH redox potential, decreased hexose monophosphate shunt activity, and increased ATP catabolism, attributed to the ongoing need to regenerate intracellular glutathione.

Membrane-associated Iron. In living cells, iron is typically separated from lipids. Thus, the association of iron with the lipid bilayer would be expected to lead to significant pathological effects, particularly by iron-catalyzed lipid oxidation. In the hemoglobinopathies, membrane-associated iron plays a major role in erythrocyte pathobiology by its damaging oxidative effects.[12,16–18] On the cytoplasmic face of thalassemic and sickle erythrocyte membranes, abnormal membrane association of iron is compartmentalized into heme-derived iron, as heme-protein or as free heme, or non-heme-derived iron, as molecular free iron or as ferritin iron. Quantitatively, these erythrocyte membranes contain approximately three times more total heme (heme proteins plus free heme) than normal erythrocytes.[19]

The deposition of heme proteins is primarily in the form of hemichromes.[20,21] These heme proteins are associated with integral or membrane skeletal proteins, partially through disulfide bonding, with a fraction nonrandomly associated with membrane aggregates of the protein, band 3.[22–24] Normal erythrocytes exposed to oxidant stress also develop clusters of denatured hemoglobin and band 3.[25] Sickle membranes also contain free heme, at approximately 5% of total membrane heme.[26]

Nonheme-derived iron associates with the erythrocyte membrane as ferritin iron or as molecular iron (nonheme, nonferritin iron). Ferritin iron is present in small amounts and its significance is unknown. Molecular iron, which reacts rapidly with ferrozone and is removed from ghost membranes by high-affinity free iron chelators, is present in larger amounts than heme iron.[21,27] Membrane affinity for molecular iron is extremely high, predicting that binding sites on the membrane are able to maintain cytosolic free iron at a concentration below 10^{-20}.[16,28] Molecular iron is bioactive and accounts for most of the ability of these variant erythrocyte to generate highly reactive hydroxyl radicals.[29] It is likely that molecular iron plays an important role in promoting oxidation of hemoglobin to methemoglobin and deposition of denatured hemoglobin onto the red cell membrane. Thus, catalytic iron associated with the membrane can valence cycle between ferric and ferrous states, allowing it to participate in redox reactions.

Molecular iron is associated with the membrane either as a chelate with bilayer phospholipids, particularly PS, or nonrandomly associated with clusters of hemichrome and band 3 aggregates. The specific amounts of molecular iron associated with phospholipids or hemichromes are unknown. Interestingly, denatured hemoglobin on sickle erythrocyte membranes can be coated with phospholipids, suggesting that some membrane-associated molecular iron is associated with hemichromes because of the phospholipids that cover them.[30]

The amount of membrane-associated molecular iron is unrelated to systemic iron status; however, the removal of iron from the sickle membrane has several potential benefits for the erythrocyte and might have potential therapeutic benefit. The iron chelator deferiprone (L1) is effective in removing free iron from sickle and thalassemic erythrocytes (Chapter 29).[31,32] This has been attributed to the neutral charge of L1, allowing it to penetrate erythrocyte membranes. In contrast, the chelator deferoxime, which is charged, does not penetrate the membrane.[33] L1 therapy has also been associated with a significant reduction in the activity of the potassium-chloride (KCl) cotransporter (KCC), whose activity is abnormally increased as the result of oxidative damage present in homozygous β thalassemia erythrocytes.[34] Development of a safe, effective, and high-affinity iron chelator would be useful to reduce the membrane damage associated with the deposition of free iron in sickle erythrocytes.

The Membrane Skeleton

The membrane skeleton (Fig. 9.1) is composed of an intricately interwoven meshwork of proteins that interact with the lipid bilayer and integral membrane proteins. The major proteins of the membrane skeleton include spectrin, actin, ankyrin, protein 4.1R, and protein 4.2. Spectrin is the primary structural component of the membrane skeleton and its most abundant protein. Spectrin functions include provision of structural support for the lipid bilayer, maintenance of cellular shape, and regulation of lateral movement of integral membrane proteins. αβ-Spectrin heterodimers self-associate with other αβ-spectrin heterodimers to form tetramers, the functional spectrin subunit in the erythrocyte. Tetramers provide significant flexibility and structural support for the lipid bilayer, helping maintain cellular shape. Spectrin heterodimer–tetramer interconversion is a moderate affinity, temperature-dependent association that favors tetramer formation.

The membrane skeleton is linked to the plasma membrane by several interactions. These include binding of spectrin tetramers to ankyrin, which in turn binds to the integral protein band 3 and binding of spectrin to the "junctional complex," a multiprotein complex that includes actin, adducin, protein 4.1R, tropomyosin, tropomodulin, and dematin. Another membrane skeleton linkage to the plasma membrane is mediated via binding of a multiprotein complex containing the Rh proteins, the RH-associated glycoproteins, CD47, LW, glycophorin B, and protein 4.2 to ankyrin. Finally, direct interactions of several skeletal proteins with the anionic phospholipids provides another linkage of the membrane skeleton to the lipid bilayer.

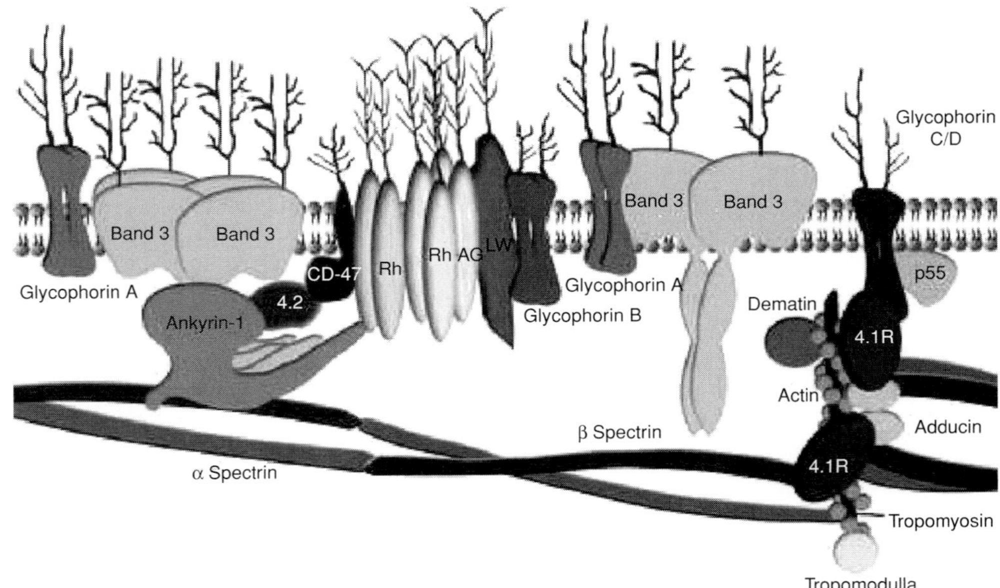

Figure 9.1. Schematic model of the red cell membrane. (Reprinted with permission from ref. 2.)

Membrane Skeleton in Thalassemia and in Sickle Erythrocytes. Numerous alterations in the membrane skeleton have been described in thalassemic and sickle erythrocytes. In thalassemic erythrocytes, alterations in the membrane skeleton vary depending on the type of thalassemia.[35–39] α Thalassemia erythrocyte membranes, isolated from patients with HbH disease (Chapter 14), have approximately a 50% decrease in high-affinity spectrin-binding sites, thought to be due to perturbed or aggregated ankyrin. β Thalassemia membranes, isolated from patients with β thalassemia intermedia, have abnormal protein 4.1R.[35,38] These findings are highly selective; protein 4.1R function is normal in α- thalassemia erythrocytes and spectrin binding is normal in β thalassemia erythrocytes. In both types of erythrocytes, spectrin function is normal.[40]

In normal erythrocytes, hemoglobin binds to the cytoplasmic surface of band 3, which is linked to the membrane skeleton via ankyrin,[41–44] HbS, especially its deoxy form, binds more avidly than HbA.[45–48] The precipitation of byproducts derived from excessive α- or β-globin chains or HbS on the inner surface of the membrane, followed by the associated oxidative damage leads to the formation of Heinz bodies. Denatured hemoglobin, the major constituent of Heinz bodies, binds to the cytoplasmic surface of band 3 with extremely high avidity, leading to aggregation of band 3 into clusters followed by binding of autologous immunoglobulin G and erythrocyte removal.[22–24,30,49,50] Sickle erythrocytes lack the typical large Heinz bodies associated with HbH molecules in α thalassemia or oxidant-challenged glucose-6-phosphate dehydrogenase–deficient erythrocytes. Instead there are smaller inclusions composed of hemichrome,[20] called by some "micro-Heinz bodies."

In the regions of sickle erythrocyte membrane associated with micro-Heinz bodies, protein topography and distribution are drastically altered, with aggregation and clustering of band 3, glycophorin and ankyrin.[22] As sickle erythrocytes dehydrate, there is progressive membrane protein redistribution, particularly near micro-Heinz bodies, leading to irregular, negatively charged clumps on the membrane surface. A similar process of band 3 aggregation and altered topography occurs in thalassemic red cell membranes.

Continuous polymerization of HbS with formation of long spicules can physically dissociate fragments of the lipid bilayer from the membrane skeleton.[51] This uncoupling of membrane from skeleton is most likely due to the growth of the sickle polymer though gaps in the membrane skeletal network. The membrane that comprises the spicule contains band 3, but not spectrin, which is limited to the body of the cell and the base of the spicule. The detachment of the lipid bilayer containing band 3 and possibly other integral membrane proteins from the skeleton likely facilitates membrane release from the erythrocyte as spectrin-poor vesicles (see later).

Other changes have been observed in membrane proteins in sickle cell disease. The lateral mobility of band 3 and glycophorin is abnormal, becoming increasingly and progressively more aggregated in erythrocytes of increasing density.[52] Ankyrin exhibits abnormal binding properties in sickle erythrocytes, both in binding band 3 and binding spectrin,[53,54] similar to defects observed in erythrocytes containing Heinz bodies due to unstable

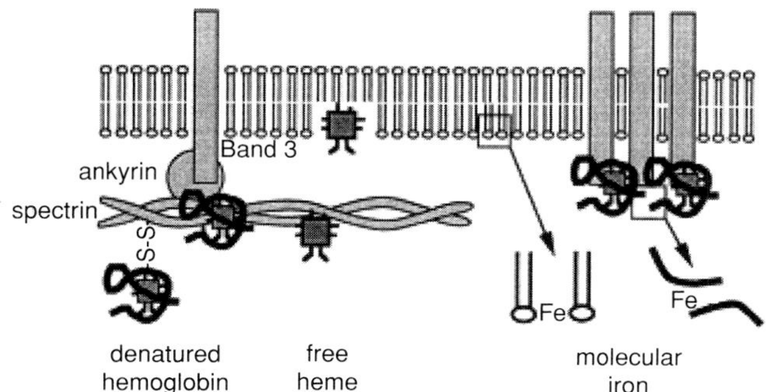

Figure 9.2. Pathological iron compartments on sickle red cell membranes. These compartments include (left to right): denatured hemoglobin associated by disulfide bonding or noncovalently, free heme associated with protein or lipid, and molecular iron associated with membrane aminophospholipid and with denatured hemoglobin. (Reprinted with permission from ref. 16.)

hemoglobinopathies (Chapter 24).[55] These changes could be induced by changes brought about by oxidation, for example the thiol redox status of spectrin, ankyrin, and protein 4.1R is abnormal in sickle erythrocytes,[56] or by direct deposition of denatured hemoglobin on the inner membrane. Functional abnormalities of protein 4.1R have been reported in sickle erythrocytes on one study[57] but are unconfirmed.[53] Oxidative changes of skeletal proteins might lead to loss of membrane flexibility.[58]

Membrane Loss and Vesiculation

Sickle erythrocytes shed part of their membrane as spectrin-deficient vesicles during cyclic oxygenation and deoxygenation.[59,60] These vesicles are likely derived from spicules that are apparently completely uncoupled from the underlying membrane skeleton.[51] This vesicular shedding is viewed by some as the ultimate stage in membrane deformation induced by erythrocyte sickling.

Some vesicles contain phosphoinositol-anchored membrane proteins,[60–62] leading to depletion in the residual erythrocytes of the complement regulatory proteins acetylcholinesterase and decay accelerating factor (CD55). It has been hypothesized that this leaves the erythrocyte susceptible to complement-mediated intravascular hemolysis,[63,64] facilitating erythrocyte recognition and removal by macrophages.[65]

Vesicles are also thought to play a role in the hypercoagulability of sickle cell disease.[66] Vesicles produced by erythrocyte shedding shorten in vitro clotting times[67,68] dramatically enhance generation of thrombin from the prothrombinase complex in vitro,[69] and bind protein S in vitro, possibly accounting for decreased protein S levels in vivo.[70]

Irreversibly Sickled Cells. Irreversibly sickled cells (ISCs) are elongated, pointed erythrocytes that are found in the well-oxygenated peripheral blood smears of most patients with sickle cell disease, especially individuals with sickle cell anemia (Chapter 19; Fig. 19.1). These dense, HbF-poor cells contain virtually no polymerized hemoglobin when they are fully oxygenated; they survive only a few days. ISCs maintain a deformed shape when exposed to oxygen or other factors that result in reversal of HbS polymerization;[71,72] they were one of the first indicators of membrane perturbation in sickle erythrocytes. The number of ISCs is greatest in the dense, dehydrated cell population and correlates well with hemolysis and spleen size, but not with the prevalence of vasoocclusive complications.[73,74] ISCs can be produced by ATP depletion, calcium accumulation, and oxy-deoxy cycling.[75–78]

The abnormal morphology of the ISC is maintained by irreversible deformation of the spectrin–actin membrane skeleton.[79] Spectrin dimer–tetramer self-association could play a role in this permanent deformation, by the dissociation of spectrin tetramers into dimers, which then reassociate into tetramers in a permanently deformed configuration.[80] It has also been proposed that the rigidity of the ISC is due to a defect in β-actin, which is brought about by oxidative changes that lead to formation of a disulfide bridge between two cysteine residues critical for actin function.[81,82] Diminished content of reduced glutathione and other crucial antioxidants in ISCs might play a role in facilitating oxidant damage and posttranslational modification of β-actin in sickle erythrocytes.[13,83,84]

Membrane Lipids

The human erythrocyte contains approximately 455 million lipid molecules within the lipid bilayer, where they comprise approximately half the weight of the plasma membrane. This bilayer is composed predominantly of phospholipids intercalated with unesterified cholesterol in nearly equimolar concentrations, and small amounts of glycolipids. The major membrane phospholipids are phosphatidyl choline (PC), phosphatidyl ethanolamine (PE), sphingomyelin (SM), and PS. Small quantities of phosphatidic acid, phosphatidyl inositol (PI) and lysophosphatidyl choline (lysoPC) are also found. Cholesterol is distributed unequally between the inner and outer monolayers,[85] and

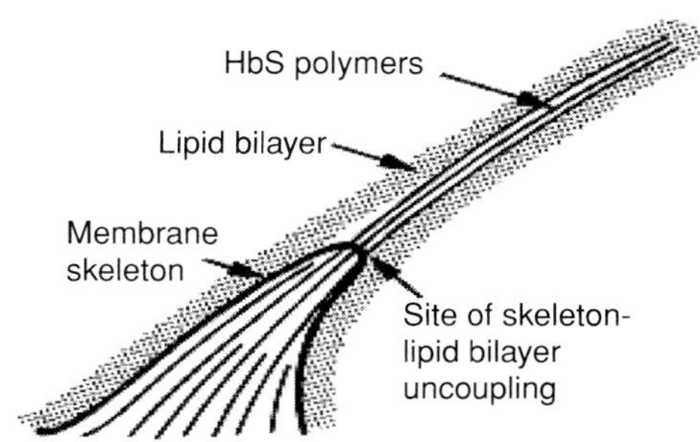

Figure 9.3. Model of the long spicule in the deoxygenated sickled cell. Hemoglobin S polymers penetrate the membrane skeleton, and uncouple the lipid bilayer from the skeleton. (Reprinted with permission from ref. 51.)

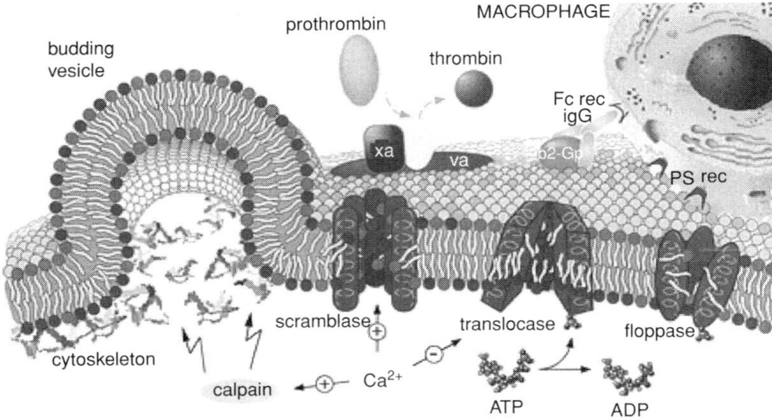

Figure 9.4. The regulation and physiology of membrane phospholipids asymmetry. This model describes how membrane phospholipids asymmetry is generated, maintained, and perturbed as a prerequisite to various PS-related pathophysiologies. Membrane lipid asymmetry is regulated by the cooperative activities of three transporters: 1) the ATP-dependent aminophospholipid-specific translocase, which rapidly transports PS and PE from the cell's outer-to-inner leaflet; 2) the ATP-dependent nonspecific lipid floppase, which slowly transports lipids from the cell's inner-to-outer leaflet; and 3) the Ca^{2+}-dependent nonspecific lipid scramblase, which allows lipids to move randomly between both leaflets. The model predicts that the translocases are targets for Ca^{2+} that directly regulates the transporter's activities. Elevated intracellular Ca^{2+} induces PS randomization across the cell's plasma membrane by providing a stimulus that positively and negatively regulates scramblase and translocase activities, respectively. At physiological Ca^{2+} concentrations, PS asymmetry is promoted because of an active translocase and floppase by inactive scramblase. Depending on the type of cell, elevated intracellular Ca^{2+} levels can be achieved by cellular stores. Increased cytosolic Ca^{2+} can also result in calpain activation, which facilitates membrane blebbing and the release of PS-expressing procoagulant microvesicles. The appearance of PS at the cell's outer leaflet promotes coagulation and thrombosis by providing a catalytic surface for the assembly of the prothrombinase and tenase (not shown) complexes and marks the cell as a pathological target for elimination by phagocytes. Recognition of the PS-expressing targets can occur by both antibody-dependent and direct receptor-mediated pathways. (Amino phospholipids are shown with dark polar head groups and choline phospholipids with lights polar head groups b2-Gp, B2-glycoprotein-1; rec, receptor). (Reprinted with permission from ref. 106.)

the phospholipids are also asymmetrically organized, with PC and SM, the choline phospholipids, primarily in the outer monolayer, with most of PE, all of PS, the amino phospholipids, and the phosphoinositides, in the inner monolayer.

Maintenance of Phospholipid Asymmetry. The asymmetrical distribution of membrane bilayer phospholipids, first recognized in erythrocytes,[86] is universal in eukaryotic cells. This asymmetrical distribution of phospholipids is a dynamic system involving a constant exchange between phospholipids of the two bilayer leaflets. Generated primarily by selective synthesis of lipids on one side of the membrane, a number of proteins participate in the maintenance or dissipation of this lipid gradient.[87,88] "Flippases," or aminophospholipid translocases, move phospholipids, particularly PS, from the outer to the inner monolayer using Mg^{++}-ATP, keeping them sequestered from the cell surface, and "floppases" do the opposite against a concentration gradient in an energy-dependent manner. "Scramblases" are bidirectional, ATP-independent transporters that move phospholipids bidirectionally down their concentration gradients in an energy-independent manner. The precise identity of all the proteins maintaining phospholipid asymmetry in the erythrocyte is still unclear.[87] Moreover, despite exhaustive searching, the identity of the PS receptor has not yet been discovered in any biological system.[89] A recent study demonstrated the existence of a novel functional adhesion receptor for PS on the microendothelium upregulated by hypoxia, cytokines, and heme.[90]

Membrane Lipid Alterations. Mature erythrocytes are unable to synthesize fatty acids, phospholipids or cholesterol; thus exchange pathways account for lipid modifications. Cholesterol is rapidly exchanged with unesterified cholesterol from plasma lipoproteins in the circulation. PC and SM are slowly exchanged with plasma lipids, whereas PS and PE do not participate in lipid exchange. Another potential lipid renewal pathway, fatty acid acylation, is an ATP-dependent process in which fatty acids combine with lysophosphatides to remake the native phospholipids, renewing damaged or lost fatty acid side chains. The composition of red cell phospholipids is quite distinct from that of plasma phospholipids, suggesting that specific pathways exist in red cells to remodel phospholipids to optimize their function. Dietary changes have only a minimal effect on the composition of erythrocyte membrane phospholipids. The inability of the erythrocyte from individuals with sickle cell disease and thalassemia to maintain normal lipid composition and repair or renew oxidized lipids, particularly fatty acids, during periods of oxidative stress, a process essential for erythrocyte survival, leads to a variety of changes in membrane structure and function.[91]

Loss of Phospholipid Asymmetry. Maintenance of phospholipid asymmetry, particularly localization of PS and phosphoinositides to the inner monolayer, has important functional consequences.[92] Typically, PS is exposed when a signal for activation of a specific biological process, such as blood clotting or cell recognition and removal, is required. In thalassemia and sickle cell disease,[93–97] outward exposure of PS in subpopulations of erythrocytes leads to activation of blood clotting, increased cellular destruction, increased adhesion to endothelial and mononuclear phagocytic cells[1,98,99] and other effects. In sickle cell disease, morphological sickling upon deoxygenation results in exposure of external PS, especially in membrane spicules.[94] In some cells, PS exposure persists after reoxygenation. These PS-exposing cells are in the densest and very lightest or reticulocyte-rich erythrocyte fractions[100–102] with the number of PS-exposing cells varying among patients, changing during time in individual patients, and decreasing after transfusion.[95] Normal and sickle reticulocytes both exhibit a moderate degree of externalized PS, and the reticulocytosis of sickle cell disease complicates so some degree the interpretation of studies on PS exposure. Unlike mature erythrocytes, however, some "mature" sickle erythrocytes have moderate PS exposure, and a subset of the dense, ISC-rich population shows much higher degrees of PS exposure than that seen in reticulocytes.[101]

PS-exposing surfaces propagate the proteolytic reactions that result in thrombin formation and activation of fibrinolysis by conversion of prothrombin to thrombin by providing docking sites for assembly of coagulation factors on their surfaces.[103,104] Exposure of PS also participates in feedback inhibition of thrombin formation via activation of the protein C pathway. These PS-exposing surfaces also can promote anticoagulation by providing a catalytic surface for factor Va inactivation by activated protein C.[105,106]

In sickle cell disease, the number of circulating erythrocytes with exposed PS has been correlated with the risk of stroke.[107] It has been suggested that other coagulation abnormalities observed in thalassemia and sickle cell disease, including decreased protein C and S activity and increased anti-PS antibodies, might be caused by circulation of PS-exposing erythrocytes.[108–110] In support of this hypothesis, the number of PS-exposing sickle erythrocytes correlated with plasma 1.2 (F1.2), d-dimer, and plasmin–antiplasmin complexes, but not the number of PS-positive platelets in pediatric sickle cell disease patients, suggesting that sickle erythrocytes and not platelets are responsible for the hemostatic activation.[111] High levels of HbF are associated with decreased erythrocyte PS exposure and decreased levels of thrombin generation and microvesicle formation.[112] Splenectomized HbE–β thalassemia patients exhibit significant levels of circulating plasma thrombin–antithrombin III complex associated with increased numbers of PS-exposing erythrocytes (Chapter 18).[113]

PS-exposure has been thought to be a signal for recognition by and attachment of these cells by macrophages of the reticuloendothelial system, marking them for destruction.[114,115] This mechanism of erythrocyte removal, shown in a murine model of sickle cell disease, is thought by some to contribute to the reduced red blood cell survival observed in sickle cell disease and the thalassemias.[91,108] In vivo studies using autologous, biotin-labeled sickle cells are not consistent with rapid removal of PS-exposing erythrocytes.[101]

PS exposure has other effects on sickle erythrocytes. Increased PS and PE exposure has been associated with activation of the alternative complement pathway.[116] Highly PS-positive sickle erythrocytes, including the densest sickle cells, cause an increase in endothelial cell tissue factor expression in vitro, not due to erythrocyte–endothelial interactions, but rather to increased levels of cell-free hemoglobin due to hemolysis (Chapter 11). Finally, PS-exposing erythrocytes can become targets for phospholipases. For example, secretory phospholipase A_2 ($sPLA_2$) will hydrolyze lipids of PS-exposing but not normal erythrocytes,[117] generating lysophospholipids and free fatty acids. In the presence of sPLA2, PS-exposing erythrocytes generate lysophosphatidic acid, which effects vascular integrity.[117] sPLA2 levels appear to predict impeding acute chest syndrome in sickle cell disease,[118] which would potentially allow intervention to prevent or ameliorate this devastating condition.[119] Strategies to bind PS or inhibit sPLA2 activity could prove to be therapeutic targets in sickle cell and other diseases.[91]

Although initially attributed to oxidative damage to the membrane, oxidative damage per se is not the cause of increased PS-exposure in sickle erythrocytes.[120] Repeated cycles of sickling and unsickling associated with HbS polymerization and depolymerization with resulting changes to the erythrocyte membrane likely contributes to the production of terminal spicules and vesicles with increased PS exposure.[60] In normal erythrocytes, neither "flippase" nor "floppase" activity is influenced by cellular oxygenation. Deoxygenation of sickle erythrocytes, however, is associated with increased PS and PE exposure and decrease in "flippase" activity,[121] particularly in PS-exposing erythrocytes.[100] Decreased "flippase" activity has been attributed to oxidative stress and sulfhydryl modifications. Deoxygenation of sickle cells results in both exposure of PS and the disruption of the membrane skeleton in membrane spicules, suggesting a role of skeletal proteins in the maintenance of phospholipid asymmetry.

"Flippase" inactivation alone, however, will not precipitate PS exposure. Activation of the "scramblase" is also required via increased levels of cytosolic calcium and/or enhanced calcium influx.[120] Not surprisingly, sulfhydryl modifications of the "scramblase" leads to increased PS exposure and a lower calcium requirement for scrambling,[122] leading to the suggestion that oxidative modifications of sulfhydryl groups in both the "flippase" and "scramblase" contribute to increased PS exposure by sickle erythrocytes.

Phosphoinositides. Phospholipids with a phosphoinositol-containing polar head group, which may be mono- (PIP or PI-4-monophosphate) or biphosphorylated (PIP2 or PI-4,5-biphosphate), make up the phosphoinositides. Comprising only approximately 2.5% of membrane phospholipids, they have significant biological activity, including a role in maintenance of erythrocyte red cell shape and deformability. Some membrane proteins, including proteins involved in complement regulation, are anchored to the red cell membrane through a phosphoinositol lipid domain.[123] This allows these proteins to move laterally in the membrane, preventing complement-mediated membrane damage. Phosphoinositol-anchored proteins are lost through the release of lipid-enriched vesicles from the cell during the membrane remodeling that accompanies reticulocyte maturation or cell aging. This process of vesiculation and loss of complement regulatory proteins is accelerated in sickle cell anemia by repeated cycles of

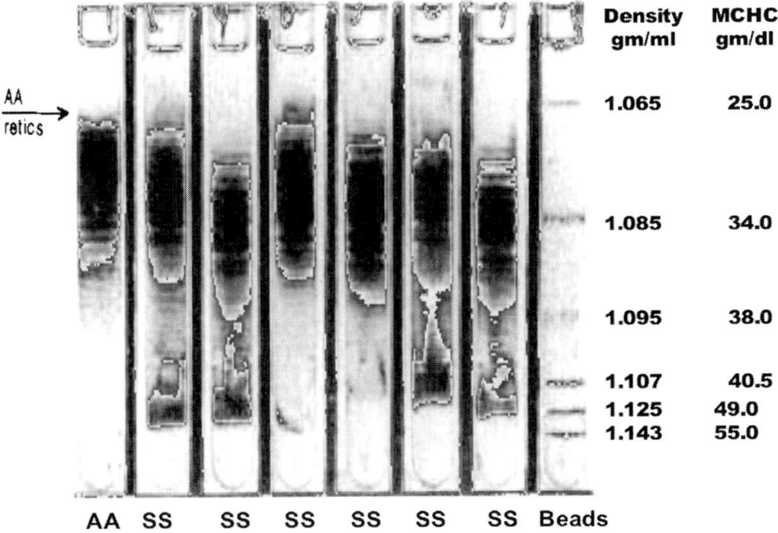

Figure 9.5. Dense erythrocytes in sickle cell blood. Whole blood samples on continuous density gradients reveal a range of densities for normal blood (AA). Sickle cell anemia (SS) blood contains a broader distribution with more low-density cells, mostly reticulocytes, and variable numbers of dehydrated cells with extremely high hemoglobin. (From ref. 148.)

sickling, making these cells sensitive to complement-mediated lysis.[64]

ALTERATIONS IN CATION CONTENT AND CELLULAR HYDRATION

The critical cellular function of maintaining cell volume is accomplished by regulation of water content. Because water is at osmotic equilibrium in most cells, cellular hydration state is a function of the content of cations (Na^+, K^+, Ca^{2+}, and Mg^{2+}) and anions (Cl^-, HCO_3^-, 2,3-BPG, hemoglobin). In red cells, hemoglobin content, which is similar in sickle and normal cells, is determined by synthesis during erythroid differentiation, and monovalent anion content is fixed by Donnan effects. Thus, cation content is the major variable determinant of cell volume and is subject to regulation by several specialized transport systems. Substantial volume reduction occurs after release of normal reticulocytes from the marrow: within approximately 2 days, cell volume drops from 115 to 85 fL and cell hemoglobin concentration (CHC) increases from 26–28 to 32–34 g/dL. Thereafter, cell volume and hemoglobin concentration remain remarkably stable over the cell's 100–120 day lifespan.

In sickle cells, dysregulation of cell volume is evident in the presence of dehydrated cells with high CHC. This abnormal hydration state is an important factor in the pathogenesis of sickle cell disease, because the polymerization of HbS is exquisitely dependent on its cellular concentration (Chapter 6).[124] Increased CHC resulting from erythrocyte dehydration markedly enhances the tendency of HbS to polymerize, reducing delay time for polymerization and resulting in the persistence of the polymer in the oxygenated state.[124–126] Dehydrated sickle cells also exhibit increased adhesion to endothelial cells, leukocytes, and other sickle erythrocytes, promoting endothelial damage and facilitating vasoocclusion.[98,127–129] Experimental evidence for enhanced adherence of dense cells to endothelium is dependent on assay conditions, particularly shear stress (Chapter 8) In addition, dehydration directly impairs the rheological integrity of sickle cells, reducing deformability and increasing fragility.[130–133]

A distinguishing feature of sickle cell disease is the heterogeneity in the volume and water content of erythrocytes (Fig. 9.5).[72,134] In addition to large numbers of reticulocytes and young red cells with increased volume and normal to low CHC, the blood of patients with sickle cell disease contains dense, dehydrated erythrocytes and reticulocytes. The number of dehydrated cells with high CHC can be estimated by flow cytometry as the number or percentage of cells with CHC more than 41 g/dL or by centrifugation on density gradients (density $>$ 1.1100).[134–137] This dense cell population is rich in ISCs. Early work established that the cation content of sickle erythrocytes was abnormal and was perturbed by deoxygenation.[138–140] Later studies established that the dense, ISC-rich fraction of sickle cells was due to severe potassium depletion, with a lesser variable degree of sodium loading.[141,142] More recently, the presence of overhydrated, sodium-loaded cells has been found in sickle cell disease.[143–145] These low-density cells with low CHC are older than most other sickle erythrocytes, appear to be derived from dehydrated cells, exhibit greater oxidative damage than other sickle cells or normal cells, and have very short in vivo survival.[143,145–147] High cation permeability of these cells[144] supports the idea that they represent a population of end-stage cells with damaged membranes undergoing swelling that culminates in intravascular hemolysis. Such osmotic lysis may be a source of free plasma hemoglobin contributing to the perturbations of nitric oxide metabolism that foster endothelial cell dysfunction and inflammation (Chapter 11).

The fraction of dense, dehydrated sickle cell ranges from 0% to 40% and varies among patients and over time in each patient. The number of dense cells decreases during pain episodes,[148–151] suggesting their selective removal during vasoocclusion. Dense cells are more susceptible to hemolysis,[130] and dense cell numbers correlate with the degree of hemolysis.[74] Coincident α thalassemia is associated with reduced numbers of dense sickle cells and milder hemolytic disease.[152–154] Individuals with the greatest numbers of dense cells appear to have the fewest pain episodes,[134,152–157] a paradox that might be explained by the selective destruction of dense cells during vasoocclusive episodes.

Because of the importance of cellular dehydration in sickle cell disease pathophysiology, understanding the mechanisms of dehydration has potential for stimulating new therapeutic approaches to the disease. Proof of principle of this approach has been provided by several studies in humans and mouse models using specific inhibitors for cation transport pathways involved in sickle cell dehydration (Chapter 31).[158–163] Four major transport mechanisms have been implicated in the dehydration of sickle erythrocytes.

Deoxygenation-induced Cation Leak, Sodium–Potassium ATPase, Cell Sodium, and Sodium/Hydrogen Exchange in Sickle Erythrocytes

Deoxygenation-induced Cation Permeability. Seminal studies established that deoxygenation of sickle cells was associated with potassium loss and sodium gain and that increased permeability took place through a diffusional pathway and was accompanied by stimulation of the sodium–potassium pump.[138–140] The deoxygenation-induced increase in cation permeability of sickle cells has been amply confirmed[75,164–166] and extensively characterized.[167–172] Deoxy sodium influx and potassium efflux are activated when oxygen tension drops below 40–50 mm Hg (Fig. 9.6), correlating with deoxygenation of HbS and cell sickling.[171,173] Cation flux via the activated deoxygenation-induced pathway is dependent on external and internal pH, reaching maximal values at pH 6.9–7.0.[171] The deoxygenation-induced pathway is not selective among the alkali metal cations lithium, sodium, potassium, rubidium or cesium, and also permits passage of calcium and magnesium.[174–176] Deoxygenation does not, however, increase membrane permeability to organic cations such as tetramethyl- or tetraethyl-ammonium,[171,177] or sugars such as erythritol, arabinose, or mannitol,[177] reflecting a selectivity for metal cations. The basal permeability of the erythrocyte membrane to anions is roughly three orders of magnitude higher than that for cations, so that the permeability of the deoxygenation-induced pathway to anions cannot be assessed with accuracy.[170] These properties are suggestive of ion movement via a diffusion pathway, with restriction to monovalent or divalent cations. Under conditions of very low osmotic strength, deoxygenation induces an increase in sucrose permeability,[178] but its relationship to the sickling-induced cation pathway is not clear.

Inward transport of sodium and outward transport of potassium are balanced in deoxygenated sickle cells and do not lead directly to cell dehydration (Fig. 9.6);[166–168,179] however, the presence of external calcium and other divalent cations inhibits sodium influx more that potassium efflux, resulting in an imbalance between the two fluxes and a net potassium loss.[172,179] No evidence of Gardos channel activation was found in these experiments, indicating that the net potassium loss was indeed mediated by the deoxygenation-induced pathway. Interestingly, this effect was enhanced by the presence of heparin, suggesting modulation by a receptor–ligand interaction.[179]

The sodium–potassium pump might also play a role in sickle cell dehydration. Early work in normal human red cells indicated that activation of the pump in conditions of high sodium content lead to cell dehydration.[180] In vitro evidence for erythrocyte dehydration mediated by activation of the sodium–potassium pump has been provided for deoxygenated sickle cells and for red cells in hereditary xerocytosis that exhibit a balanced cation leak.[167] In deoxygenated sickle cells, increased cell sodium, even though initially balanced by potassium loss, stimulates the sodium–potassium pump to effect net cation loss due to its 3 $Na_{out}/2\ K_{in}$ stoichiometry. The integrated red cell model, discussed later, predicts that this mechanism cannot fully account for the extreme potassium depletion of sickle cells[181] because its contribution diminishes as the potassium gradient dissipates.

The activation of deoxygenation-induced permeability pathway is associated with morphological sickling[171,173] and can be impeded by agents that interfere with HbS polymerization.[182,183] High cation fluxes are associated with deoxygenation under conditions producing marked morphological changes and extensive spicule formation, such as gradual deoxygenation, alkaline pH, low hemoglobin concentrations, and reticulocyte deoxygenation.[171,173,179] This suggests that activation of this pathway is triggered by spicule formation, which is associated with disruption of spectrin–band 3 associations and perturbation of phospholipid and cholesterol domains.[51,69,184] A relationship between deoxygenation-induced cation pathway and the nonselective cation leak induced by shear stress and membrane deformation is suggested by their similar physiological and pharmacological characteristics.[185] The nature of these associations and the identification of the deoxygenation-induced pathway deserve further study.

Deoxygenation-induced fluxes of sodium, potassium, and calcium are reduced by the anion exchange inhibitor diisothiocyanostilbene disulfonate (DIDS) without affected morphological sickling.[169,175,177] Dipyridamole, an anion transport inhibitor, also blocks deoxygenation-induced cations fluxes in vitro, although other anion transport blockers are ineffective.[176] DIDS-sensitive cation fluxes, presumably mediated by the anion exchanger, can be elicited in normal red cells by incubation in low chloride media.[186] Single amino acid substitution in the anion exchange protein associated with stomatocytosis syndromes has been shown to be associated with increased erythrocyte cation permeability, sensitive to DIDS and dipyridamole; expression of these mutant anion exchangers in xenopus oocytes conferred increased cation permeability with similar inhibitor sensitivity.[187] These findings

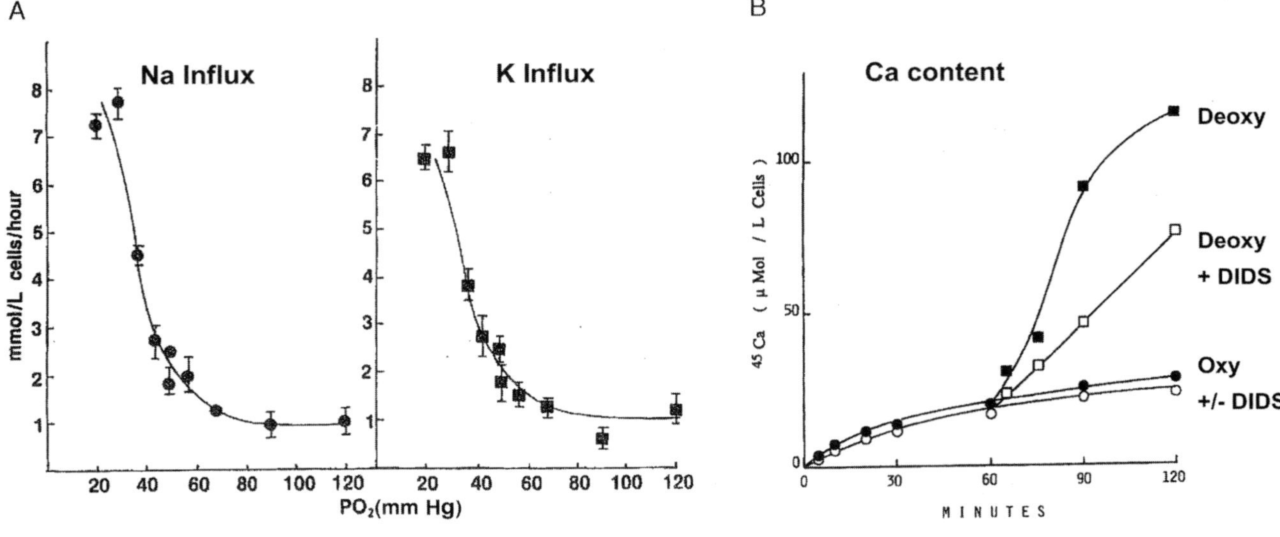

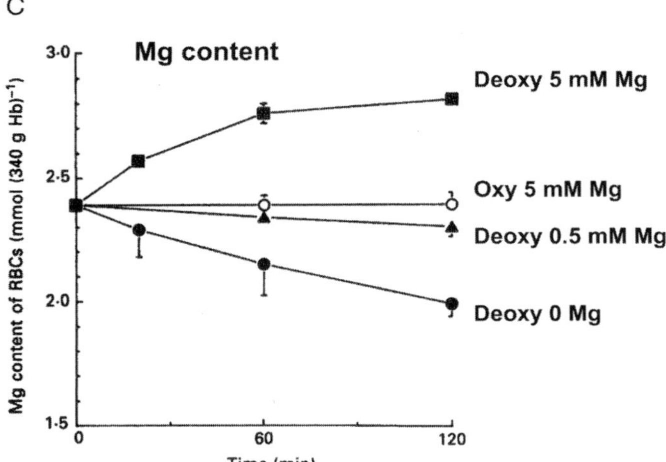

Figure 9.6. Deoxygenation-induced permeability increase to mono- and divalent cations in sickle red cells. **(A)** Sodium and potassium influx as a function of pO_2. Increased permeability below 40 mm Hg corresponds to morphological sickling. (from ref. 168, used with permission) **(B)** Ca permeability, assessed as ^{45}Ca content of cells containing the chelator quin2 to minimize efflux. Increased cellular calcium uptake in deoxygenated sickle cells (■) compared with oxygenated cells (●); DIDS partially inhibits calcium uptake in deoxygenated (□), but not oxygenated cells (○). (from ref. 175, used with permission) **(C)**. Changes in cellular magnesium content upon deoxygenation in sickle cell incubated in high external Mg (5 mmol ■), normal Mg (0.5 mmol ▲) or no Mg (5 mmol EDTA ●). Oxygenated cells (○) had stable Mg contents under all conditions. (Used with permission from ref. 174.). Normal red cells exhibit minimal changes in cation permeability upon deoxygenation.

support the notion that the anion exchange protein, at least in some altered states, could mediate deoxygenation-induced fluxes in sickle erythrocytes. Regardless of the mechanism, pharmacological inhibition of deoxygenation-induced cation movements provides a potential avenue for therapeutic intervention to improve sickle cell hydration (see Chapter 31).

Alterations in Cation Permeability by Shear Stress and Oxidation in Sickle Erythrocytes. Marked mechanical deformation of normal cells leads to a reversible increase in cation permeability.[188–191] In the absence of external calcium, the pathway mediates equivalent sodium and potassium movement,[189,190] but in the presence of calcium, potassium loss is accelerated by activation of the calcium-dependent Gardos pathway,[192] suggesting that the pathway also mediates calcium influx. Cation fluxes induced by mechanical stress are chloride-independent. The pathway is activated in sickle erythrocytes at lower shear stress than normal cells,[193] perhaps as a consequence of the oxidant damage to the membrane. When normal cells are mildly oxidized with t-butyl hydroperoxide, the leak is increased and activated at lower shear stress.[188,189] Under hypotonic conditions that induce cell swelling, the deformation-induced leak is increased, with potassium loss in excess of sodium gain, and is partially inhibited by bromide.[185] Interestingly, deoxygenation-induced cation leaks in sickle cells was also reduced by bromide.[185] Mechanically induced cation fluxes are partially blocked by DIDS, independently from the drug's effect on anion permeability.[185,194] Thus, the mechanically induced cation leak and the deoxygenation-induced pathway share a number of physiological and pharmacological characteristics, including an apparent origin in membrane deformation. It is conceivable that they represent the same mechanism and that the abnormal oxidation state of the sickle membrane increases the deoxygenation-induced cation leak in sickle erythrocytes.

Sodium Permeability and Cell Sodium Content in Sickle Erythrocytes. The potassium depletion responsible for sickle erythrocyte dehydration is associated with variable degrees of sodium loading, especially marked in high-density cell populations rich in ISCs,[195] which could result from increased sodium permeability or decreased activity of the sodium–potassium pump. Pump activity is abnormally decreased in dehydrated sickle cells, although ATPase activity in membranes derived from these cells is not,[142] suggesting that there is abnormal downregulation of sodium–potassium pump activity in dense cells. One possible inhibitory factor might be the increased magnesium to phosphate ratio in these cells; when this ratio was normalized in vitro, the activity of the sodium–potassium pump was restored to normal.[174]

Increase sodium permeability could also contribute to high cell sodium content of dense cells. Several sodium influx pathways have been identified, including Na/H exchange,[196] NaKCl cotransport,[197] Na/Mg exchange,[198] but assessment of their activities and contribution to net sodium influx has been variable. Earlier estimates of very high Na/H exchange rates in sickle erythrocytes[196] have not been reproduced,[199] and the sodium permeability in the dense cell population does not appear abnormally elevated. Sodium/hydrogen exchange is not stimulated by deoxygenation, indicating that the increase in intracellular calcium associated with deoxygenation is not sufficient to activate phosphokinase C and stimulate the Na/H exchanger. Likewise, there are no data to suggest that reduction in a sodium influx pathway contributes to dehydration in any sickle cell population.

The presence of a subpopulation of extremely sodium loaded cells in the least dense fraction of sickle blood was revealed by the failure of these cells to undergo dehydration upon exposure to the potassium ionophore valinomycin.[143] These cells are older sickle cells that arise from the dense cell population[145,146] and might represent a terminal stage on their way to osmotic lysis (see below). Some of the sodium loading apparent in both the high- and low-density population of sickle cells could be due to this subpopulation of sodium loaded cells.

Cell Calcium and Calcium-activated Potassium Channel (Gardos Pathway) in Sickle Erythrocytes

Cell Calcium and Calcium Pump Activity. Early studies indicated very high cell calcium in sickle cells, ranging from 110 to 300 μmol/L cells,[200,201] two orders of magnitude higher than in normal cells (0.9–2.8 μmol/L cells).[202] Free ionized cytoplasmic calcium measured by a variety of techniques, such as ionophore-induced equilibration of intracellular chelator and ^{45}Ca, calcium-sensitive fluorescent dyes, fura-2 or benz-2, and nuclear magnetic resonance, ranges from 11 to 30 nmol/L and is similar in sickle and normal erythrocytes.[175,203–205] This apparent discrepancy was explained by the demonstration of compartmentation of calcium in sickle erythrocytes into cytoplasmic vesicles, first demonstrated by electron probe x-ray analysis of cryosections.[206–208] These vesicles are derived from the plasma membrane and contain integral membrane proteins, including the Ca-ATPase, in an inside-out configuration. The Ca-ATPase pumps calcium from the cytoplasm into these vesicles, creating a very high intravesicular calcium concentration.[206,207] Most of the calcium contained in sickle erythrocytes is sequestered into vesicles.

Deoxygenation of sickle, but not normal, red cells increases the permeability of the membrane to calcium, resulting in enhanced calcium influx (Fig. 9.6).[175,176,209,210] The effects on cellular ionized calcium are complex and heterogeneous within a population of cells, depending on the balance between the influx rate in an individual cell and its capacity to extrude calcium via the Ca–ATPase pump. Deoxygenation enhanced calcium influx rate in sickle cells is increased five fold, and reduced calcium pump activity by as much as 28%.[210] The net effect produced a threefold increase in cellular ionized calcium level from 10 to 30 nmol in the discocyte fraction. Although these levels do not rise to the 40-nmol concentration estimated as the threshold for activation of the Gardos channel,[211] it was suggested that cellular heterogeneity could account for higher calcium levels in certain cell populations. Indeed, sickling-induced permeability changes were greatest in reticulocytes,[179] which are known to exhibit the most dramatic morphological changes upon deoxygenation and to deform at higher oxygen tensions, despite their relatively low CHC.[212] It was later shown that the deoxygenation-induced permeability change occurred in a subset of cells (see later).[213] The deoxygenation-induced fluxes of calcium, sodium and potassium have similar pharmacological sensitivity to DIDS and dipyridamole, suggesting mediation by a common pathway.[169,175,176]

Calcium-activated Potassium Channel (Gardos Pathway). In 1958, the Hungarian physiologist, Gyorgy Gárdos, described calcium-dependent potassium efflux from ATP-depleted red cells.[214] These fluxes are now known to be mediated by a specific type of potassium channel activated by increased cytoplasmic calcium and known by several designations. Small (or intermediate) conductance

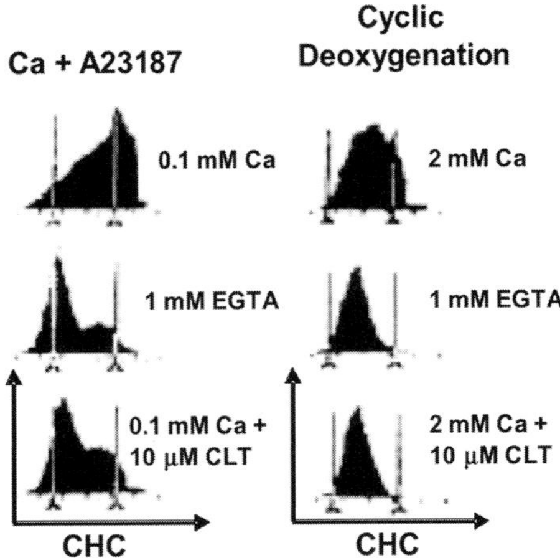

Figure 9.7. Dehydration of sickle cells via the Gardos pathway. Frequency distributions of cellular hemoglobin concentrations (CHC) were measured by Bayer Advia automated cell counter; normal range of 28–41 g/dL is shown vertical markers. In vitro activation of the Gardos pathway by incubation of sickle cells in the presence of external calcium plus ionophore A23187 induces shift to higher CHC (upper left), which is blocked by chelation of calcium or by the Gardos channel inhibitor, clotrimazole (CLT). Cyclic deoxygenation (3 hours, 1 min O_2, 4 min N_2) also produces a calcium-dependent (upper right) shift to higher CHC, absent in EGTA and inhibited by CLT. (Modified from ref. 239.)

calcium-activated potassium channel, IK1, SK4, all describe the product of the *KCCN4* gene,[215–217] which codes for a protein of 428 amino acids with six transmembrane domains and a pore region with the canonical GYGD sequence that determines K^+ selectivity in numerous potassium channels.[218] mRNA for *KCNN4*, but not *KCNN3*, increases during erythroid differentiation and is present in reticulocytes; protein is detected by *KCNN4* protein antibodies in mature erythrocyte membranes.[215] The peptide toxin charbydotoxin (ChTx) is a specific inhibitor of the human red cell Gardos channel.[219,220] Binding studies with ^{125}I-ChTx demonstrated that normal human erythrocytes possess approximately 150 of these channels per cell.[221] Upon uniform, maximal activation of Gardos channels via controlled ionophore-induced permeabilization of red cells to calcium, rapid, but remarkably uniform dehydration of both sickle and normal erythrocytes occurs.[222] These results suggest a uniform distribution of channels among erythrocytes and are consistent with estimates of several hundred channels per cell.

Generation of dense ISCs under conditions of ATP depletion was dependent on external calcium and an outwardly directed potassium gradient.[75] When sickle cells are deoxygenated under conditions in which ATP levels are maintained, calcium-dependent formation of dense, dehydrated cells was observed (Fig. 9.7).[76,158,223–226] Sickle erythrocyte dehydration produced by rapid in vitro deoxygenation–oxygenation cycles that mimicked in vivo circulatory times was predominantly calcium dependent, suggesting it was predominantly mediated by the Gardos channel.[227] The integrated red cell model[181,228] has examined the different modalities of dehydration for reticulocytes and provided theoretical and indirect experimental evidence for a calcium dependent process based on transient activation of the Gardos pathway upon deoxygenation.[179] Nevertheless, although Gardos channel potassium fluxes can be readily elicited in red cells in vitro, calcium-dependent potassium fluxes blocked by the specific Gardos channel inhibitors have been difficult to demonstrate directly upon deoxygenation of sickle cells.

An elegant set of experiments helps to explain this apparent paradox. When sickle discocytes were deoxygenated, only 10%–40% became dense, and thus had evidence for calcium permeabilization and Gardos channel activation upon deoxygenation. The process was rapid and transient, and the resultant dense cell fraction did not increase with prolonged deoxygenation. If those dehydrated cells were removed, however, and the procedure was repeated, a similar fraction of cells became dense. These studies suggest that the activation of the sickling-induced permeability pathway that permits calcium influx in deoxygenated sickle cell is a stochastic process affecting a small fraction of cells during each deoxygenation event. Thus Gardos-mediated potassium efflux is rapid and transient in only a few cells upon a given deoxygenation. This explains why oxy–deoxy cycling has generally been more effective than continuous deoxygenation in eliciting calcium-dependent density shifts in sickle cells and why Gardos potassium fluxes have been difficult to measure directly in vitro.

Modulation of Gardos Channel Activity in Sickle Cell Disease. Gardos channel activity is subject to regulation in vitro by cytokines and lipid mediators of inflammation known to be elevated in persons with sickle cell disease as a result of the inflammatory vasculopathy associated with oxidative stress, endothelial cell damage and leukocyte activation (Chapters 8, 10, and 11). In murine erythrocytes, endothelin-1 (ET-1), a cytokine released from endothelial cells under oxidative or other stresses, increases both the internal calcium affinity and the V_{max} of the Gardos channel. Pharmacological studies indicated that this effect was mediated by the ET-1 receptor B and involved activation of protein kinase C.[229] Treatment of SAD sickle mice (Chapter 12) with a specific inhibitor of the ET-1 receptor B but not A, reduced sickle cell dehydration in vivo and Gardos channel fluxes measured ex vivo.[161] The ability of ET-1 to augment Gardos channel activity was also demonstrated in human sickle cells in vitro. The increase in sickle cell density produced by oxy/deoxy cycling in vitro was enhanced by ET-1,[230] indicating increased activation of the Gardos channel via sickling-induced calcium influx. In addition, two inflammatory cytokines – interleukin-10 and RANTES (Regulated upon Activation, Normal T lymphocyte Expressed and Secreted) – and the inflammatory phospholipid mediator, platelet activating factor, had similar effects on Gardos channel activity in sickle cells.

Other lipid mediators could augment Gardos channel activity by enhancing calcium influx. Treatment of normal erythrocytes with subnanomolar concentrations of prostaglandin E2 (PGE_2) activated the Gardos channel in vitro in approximately 15% of cells, producing reduced cell volume and osmotic resistance,[231] apparently as a result of an increase in calcium uptake by PGE_2, which has been demonstrated independently.[232] Lysophosphatidic acid, a lipid mediator released from activated platelets, stimulates calcium uptake, detected by fluorescent dyes, in approximately 25% of red cells, as does activation of protein kinase C by phorbol esters and diacylglycerol. Calcium influx stimulated by lysophosphatidic and protein kinase C are both inhibited by ω-agatoxin-TK, suggesting mediation by a P-type calcium channel and are modulated by inhibitors of tyrosine kinases (TK), but in subtly different ways, indicating that multiple signaling pathways might be involved.[233,234]

The modulation of Gardos channel activity by inflammatory cytokines and other mediators could be particularly relevant in sickle cell disease. Endothelial cells are stimulated to produce endothelin by interactions with sickle cells and activated leukocytes. Plasma levels of ET-1 and PGE_2 are abnormally elevated in patients with sickle cell disease in the "steady state"[235–237] and increase further with acute chest syndrome or other vasoocclusive events.[236,238] It is possible that local levels of ET-1 and/or PGE_2 in the microcirculation are even higher and potentiate Gardos channel activity of sickle cells during vasoocclusive or adhesive interactions. Such receptor ligand interactions could be exploited pharmacologically, as several specific blockers, such as ET-1 receptor antagonists, have been found to have clinical benefit in other disorders.

Direct blockade of the Gardos channel is possible using the imidazole antimycotic clotrimazole and its derivatives, which acts by binding to the external pore of the channel (Chapter 31).[239] Early studies indicated the ability of clotrimazole to reduce the number of dense cells in sickle cell patients.[158] More recently, compounds lacking the imidazole ring have been shown to be effective Gardos channel blockers.[240] One of these, senicapoc, has been tested in phase II and phase III clinical trials in sickle cell disease. Patients treated with a daily oral dose of senicapoc exhibited fewer dense cells, increased hemoglobin levels, reduced reticulocyte counts, lower bilirubin and lactate dehydrogenase levels, which was consistent with reduced hemolysis,[163] and a predictable outcome of the mitigation of cellular dehydration. A phase III (ClinTrials.gov/, NCT00102791) study of senicapoc was recently terminated, as it was unlikely that its chosen endpoint, a reduction in pain episodes, could be reached. Nevertheless, given that vasoocclusion and hemolysis represent different aspects of sickle cell pathology, that dense cell numbers are most closely associated with hemolysis, and that hemolysis appears to be associated with long-term complications, such as pulmonary hypertension, a drug such as senicapoc that reduces hemolysis might ultimately have important long-term benefit in sickle cell disease.

In summary, the ionized calcium level in red cells in vivo is a dynamic balance between calcium influx and the compensatory capacity of the calcium pump and is normally maintained well below the threshold for activation of the Gardos pathway. Calcium influx can increase, especially in sickle cells, by a variety of mechanisms – triggering of the deoxygenation-induced pathway by sickling, modulation of calcium channels by cytokines or inflammatory mediators, or activation of stretch-induced cation channels by circulatory shear stress. Such influx events appear to produce calcium transients in red cells sufficient to activate the Gardos pathway. Compromise of the capacity of the calcium pump by physiological regulation or pathological damage would make such calcium transients greater in magnitude and/or more prolonged, increasing the probability of potassium channel activation and enhancing its adverse effects on cell volume. Modulation of the kinetic properties of the Gardos channel by inflammatory mediators might also enhance potassium loss in some cells. A substantial body of data now exists to support the occurrence of such events in vivo, at least in some populations of sickle erythrocytes. The quantitative integration of these events and their pathophysiological modulation in vivo remains a fruitful area of study.

Potassium Chloride Cotransport in Sickle Erythrocytes

KCC was first described in red cells as a chloride-dependent potassium efflux stimulated by the sulfhydryl alkylating agent N-ethylmaleimide.[241,242] Other activators of KCC in vitro include cell swelling, acid pH, urea, sulfhydryl oxidation, reduced cellular magnesium, and hyperbaric conditions.[243–246] The activity of KCC is maximal in normal reticulocytes and young cells and is progressively reduced to negligible values in mature and dense normal red cells.[197,247–250] Early reports established that sickle cell disease blood samples had high KCC activity (Fig. 9.8),[197,251,252] although the quantitative comparison to normal cells is complicated by the presence of large number of reticulocytes and young cells in patient blood.

KCC activity is highest in the least dense sickle cells, which contain most of the reticulocytes, and is least active in the dense cell fractions.[197,252,253] The relative importance of activating stimuli for KCC and volume regulation in vivo is not known. Even reticulocyte rich fractions of sickle erythrocytes have minimal KCC activity in the absence of stimulation, and reticulocyte volume and CHC are stable upon in vitro incubation under these conditions.[254] KCC fluxes are inversely proportional to whole blood MCHC over the range from 24 to 34 g/dL, but the relative activation of KCC in sickle and normal cells is indistinguishable

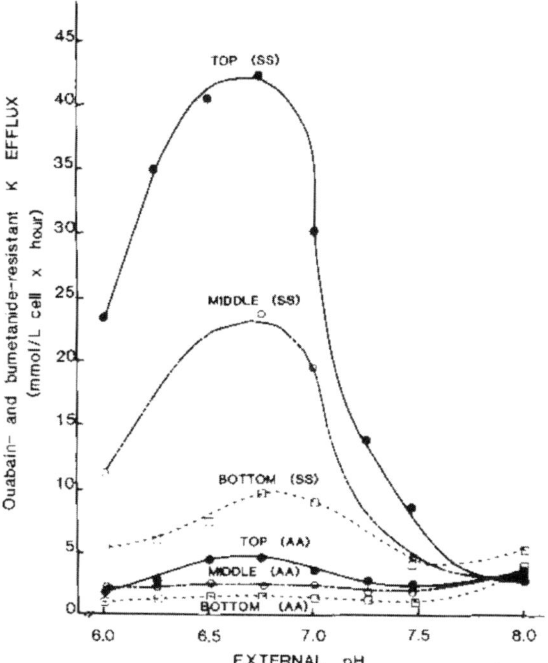

Figure 9.8. High levels KCl cotransport activity in sickle cells. High rate of acid-stimulated potassium efflux in various density fractions reflects high activity of KCC in sickle cell disease blood. The highest activity is in the "top" density fraction containing the most reticulocytes, but other density fractions contain more reticulocytes than normal blood. Given that KCC activity declines with reticulocyte maturation, higher reticulocyte counts in sickle cell blood and the absence of older sickle cells means that cell age must be taken into account in any comparison of flux rates between sickle and normal erythrocytes, even in density fractionated cells. (From ref. 252.)

(Fig. 9.9). KCC activation by acid pH is exaggerated in sickle cells compared with normal cells (Fig. 9.9), so that if acidic conditions occur in the circulation, sickle cells would be more vulnerable to KCC-mediation dehydration than normal cells. Likewise, sickle cells are more sensitive to KCC activation by urea than normal cells (Fig. 9.9), showing activation at lower concentrations, well within those found in the medulla of the kidney. The heightened sensitivity of KCC in sickle cells to activation by acid pH and urea is due at least in part to reversible sulfhydryl oxidation, as suggested by its normalization on treatment by the sulfhydryl agent dithiothreitol. This raises the possibility of the therapeutic potential of reducing agents, such as N-acetyl cysteine, which has been shown to block in vitro dehydration of sickle cells,[255] and, in a limited trial, to improve sickle cell hydration.[256]

Activation of KCC results in potassium, chloride and water loss, with reduction in cell volume and increase in CHC.[252–254,257–260] This can be demonstrated in the phthalate density profile of sickle cell disease blood,[257] but changes in normal erythrocytes with low reticulocyte counts are minimal. Measurement of the rapid reduction in reticulocyte CHC upon activation of KCC permits direct comparison of sickle and normal cells, as shown in Figure 9.9. Whether activated by swelling, acid pH, or urea, sickle cells exhibit more extensive volume reduction than normal cells, achieving in each case a higher CHC. Swelling-induced volume regulation is not altered by sulfhydryl-reducing agents, but abnormal sickle cell volume reduction triggered by acid pH and urea is partially normalized by dithiothreitol.[254,261] Thus the CHC 'set point' for KCC-mediated volume regulation appears to be abnormal in sickle cells and could result in part from their abnormal oxidation state.[3,262,263]

Deoxygenation of sickle erythrocytes produces complex changes in KCC activity. In normal human cells, and in fish and horse cells, KCC activity stimulated by urea, acid pH, or cell swelling is inhibited as pO_2 falls.[264,265] In sickle cells, activity initially declines with deoxygenation, but begins to increase again at approximately 40 mm Hg, with the onset of sickling; blockade of sickling with dimethyl adipimidate abolishes this effect.[182] Nevertheless, activated KCC fluxes in fully deoxygenated cells are lower than in oxygenated cells, so that the overall effect of deoxygenation on activated KCC in sickle cells appears inhibitory. Part of this inhibition, although probably not all, results from the increase in cellular free magnesium concentration associated with binding of 2,3-BPG to deoxyhemoglobin.[249] In sickle cells suspended in isotonic media at normal pH, in which KCC activity is minimal at high pO_2, deoxygenation activates KCC, especially if deoxygenation-induced increase in ionized magnesium is prevented by use of divalent cation ionophores.[266] This behavior might explain other observations that cycles of oxygenation and deoxygenation produced chloride-dependent potassium loss and shifts toward higher density in sickle cells, especially reticulocytes. It has been suggested that on deoxygenation, changes in phosphorylation activate KCC, but the activity is masked by the increase in cellular magnesium, which is known to inhibit KCC. On reoxygenation, magnesium levels are restored to normal more rapidly than the changes in phosphorylation are reversed, providing a brief pulse of KCC activity that produces cumulative dehydration upon repeated cycling. If this mechanism occurs in vivo, cyclic deoxygenation in the circulation might be responsible for activation of KCC and dehydration of sickle cells, especially in reticulocytes which can linger in the venous circulation due to abnormal adhesive interactions.[127]

Cellular Magnesium and KCC in Sickle Cells. Although total erythrocyte magnesium content is reduced, especially in dense sickle cells, during deoxygenation the binding of 2,3-BPG, a major chelator of magnesium, to deoxy hemoglobin results in a large increase in free magnesium concentration. Cell sickling increases membrane permeability to magnesium and the transient outwardly directed magnesium gradient during deoxygenation produces magnesium efflux, resulting in reduced total magnesium content in sickle erythrocytes.[174] Human erythrocytes also

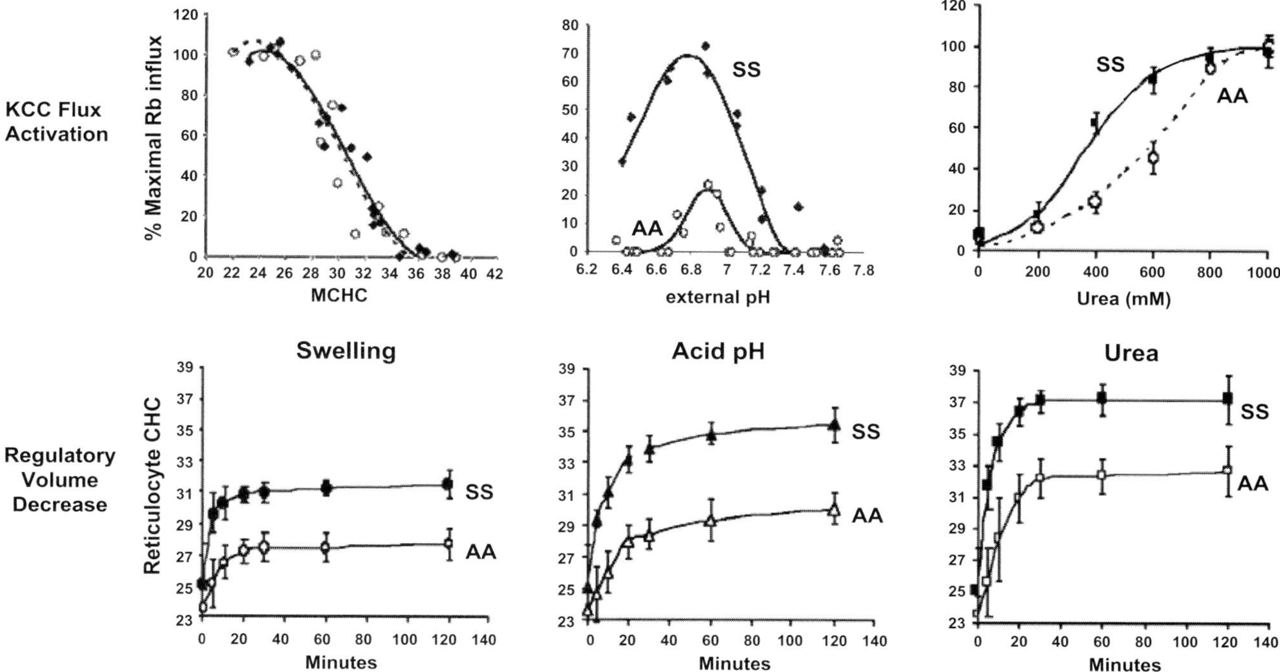

Figure 9.9. Abnormal regulation of KCC in sickle reticulocytes. Upper panels show activation of KCC-mediated fluxes as a function of initial MCHC (cell swelling), external pH, and urea concentration in normal (AA; open symbols) and sickle (SS; filled symbols) red cells. Fluxes are expressed as a percentage of the maximal volume stimulated flux to normalize for differences in the age distribution of the cells. Although SS proportionate activation by cell swelling is "normal," response to acid pH is exaggerated, and activation by urea occurs at lower concentrations than in AA cells. (From refs. 254, 260.) Lower panels depict regulatory volume decrease, reflected as an increase in reticulocyte CHC with time upon activation of KCC. Reticulocyte CHC was measured by Advia cell counter. Regardless of how KCC is activated, the final MCHC achieved is higher in SS than in AA reticulocytes (From CH Joiner, unpublished data.)

possess a specific sodium–magnesium exchanges system, whose activity produces slow loss of magnesium from the erythrocyte.[267] Sickle erythrocytes exhibit markedly increased activity of the sodium–magnesium exchanger, which could theoretically contribute to their reduced total magnesium content.

Magnesium depletion of sickle cells is pathophysiologically relevant in view of the sensitivity of KCC to cellular magnesium. KCC is stimulated by the reduced levels of cellular magnesium found in sickle erythrocytes.[159,174,268,269] The inhibition of KCC by increasing cellular magnesium content provides a new potential opportunity for preventing dehydration in thalassemic[270,271] and sickle erythrocytes.[160,272] Oral magnesium supplementation corrects the deficit in cellular magnesium in sickle cells, inhibits KCC cotransport, and reduces cell dehydration.[160,272] Small pilot studies of magnesium supplementation demonstrate that oral magnesium supplementation can improve sickle cell hydration and decrease dense cell numbers, and phase I and II trials are in progress in sickle cell anemia and in HbSC disease (NCT00143572, NCT00532883). Large-scale trials have not been reported. Interestingly, magnesium supplements also reduced the activity of the sodium–magnesium exchanger in sickle cells (Chapter 31).[160]

Molecular Basis for KCC. KCC is mediated by members of the cation-chloride cotransporter (SLC12) family,[273,274] which includes the thiazide-sensitive NaCl cotransporters, the bumetanide-sensitive Na-K-Cl cotransporter and the volume-sensitive KCCs. These electroneutral transporters play three important physiological roles: transepithelial movement of solute, maintenance of intracellular ion concentrations (especially chloride) in electrically excitable cells, and regulation of cell volume. In erythrocytes, the KCC mediates the volume reduction and resultant increase in CHC that accompanies reticulocyte maturation.[244,245,275,276]

The prototype KCC (KCC1, *SLC12A4*)[277] is expressed in most tissues. Three other KCC genes code for additional isoforms with more limited tissue distributions. The neuronal-specific KCC2 (*SLC12A5*) appears to function primarily as a regulator of chloride concentrations in neurons.[278,279] KCC3 (*SLC12A6*) is expressed predominantly in kidney, lung, skeletal muscle, and brain, with a unique splicing isoform present in kidney.[280–283] KCC4 (*SLC12A7*) is highly expressed in heart, kidney, and pancreas.[282,284]

The functional characteristics of the four isoforms are generally similar, although anion selective is subtly different and KCC1, KCC3, and KCC4 respond to hypotonic stimuli, whereas KCC2 does not.

Human, sheep, and mouse red cell membranes contain both KCC1 and KCC3.[285–288] In mouse cells, deletion of the KCC1 gene has little effect on KCC activity or cell volume; deletion of KCC3 results in a reduction of KCC activity, associated with an increase in KCC1 expression. Dual deletion abolishes KCC activity and results in overhydration of red cells with normal hemoglobin and mitigation of the dehydrated red cell phenotype found in the SAD mouse (Chapter 12).[287] These data suggest that KCC3 is the predominant KCC transporter in mouse red cells. Human erythroid cells also express KCC4[288,289] in addition to KCC1 and KCC3. The relative contribution of each of these transporters to KCC activity in human cells is unknown. It is possible that they interact with each other to modulate activity, as has been shown with artificially truncated KCC constructs,[290] naturally occurring splicing isoforms of the sodium-potassium-chloride cotransporter (NKCC),[291] and interactions between KCC and NKCC.[292]

Recent reports reveal that KCC isoforms interact differently with various regulatory kinases.[293,294] Differences in the relative expression of KCC isoforms between sickle and normal red cells could conceivably produce increased KCC activity and/or abnormal regulation of KCC activity in sickle cells (Fig. 9.9). Interindividual differences in KCC isoform expression could also be a source of genetic variation that affects the phenotype of sickle cell disease (Chapter 27).

Activation of KCC is associated with a serine/threonine dephosphorylation event, as protein phosphatase inhibitors such as okadaic acid and calyculin A block activation. Membrane stretch or shape change is not a signal transduction mechanism for KCC activation.[295] Rather, studies of activation/inactivation kinetics in response to volume changes have suggested that cell swelling inhibits the putative inactivating protein kinase, shifting the kinase/phosphatase equilibrium toward dephosphorylation and activating the transporter.[296–299] Perhaps changes in cellular hemoglobin concentration associated with swelling produce dramatic alteration in the activity of cellular enzymes through macromolecular crowding effects in the nonideal thermodynamic conditions of concentrated protein solutions as present in erythrocytes (Chapter 6).[300]

The ubiquitous and promiscuous protein phosphatases 1 and 2A (PP1, PP2A) activate KCC and might function redundantly.[269,301–304] Neither the phosphorylation sites on KCC nor the inhibitory kinase in red cells have been identified. In KCC1, threonine phosphorylation sites on the N terminus have been shown to be altered in response to changes in cell volume and to modulate the activity of the transporter.[305] Several ST kinases have been shown to interact with NKCC1, including the stress-related kinase SPAK (STE20-related-proline-alanine-rich kinase, also known as PASK), OSR1 (oxidative stress response kinase), and the WNK (with-no-lysine) kinases. Using a yeast two-hybrid system, SPAK and OSR1 have been shown to interact with KCC3, but not KCC1 or KCC4,[293] although SPAK was unable to modulate KCC3 activity[294] when coexpressed in xenopus oocytes. Coexpression of WNK 4 with KCC1, KCC3, or KCC4 resulted in inhibition of hypotonic activation of these transporters, whereas coexpression of a kinase-inactive mutant WNK4 activated KCC3 although not KCC1 and KCC4, under isotonic conditions. Interestingly, although inactivated SPAK was not able to activate KCC3 alone, it enhanced the activation of KCC3 by inactivated WNK4, suggesting interaction of these kinases, as has been shown in the regulation of NKCC1.[306] The behavior of the WNK4 kinase in these in vitro systems is consistent with that expected from the putative swelling-inhibited kinase responsible for modulating KCC activity in red cells, but this identity remains to be demonstrated. Identification of the regulatory sites of KCC and the associated kinases would be an important step in delineating its dysregulation in sickle cell disease.

The activities of PP1 and PP2A are themselves regulated by TKs. TK inhibitors such as staurosporine and celerythine activate KCC, probably by maintaining PP1/PP2A in the dephosphorylated, active state. Mice with genetic knockout of two src tyrosine kinases, fgr and hck, have constitutively activated KCC and exhibit dehydrated erythrocytes,[307] elimination of either kinase alone was not sufficient to produce this phenotype, suggesting redundant function of the src kinases. Interestingly these animals do not show the normal decline in KCC activity with red cell aging, which could be explained by age-associated reduction in the paired TK. Deoxygenation alters protein phosphorylation state of the erythrocyte membrane, decreasing phosphorylation of several high abundance membrane proteins.[308] Deoxygenation increased the activity of the syk kinase, and inhibitors of *syk* blocked the stimulation of KCC that accompanied deoxygenation. Activity of the src kinase expressed in human cells (lyn) was not changed by deoxygenation and lyn inhibitors did not alter the deoxy-stimulation of KCC.[309] Thus, src-family TKs are negative regulators of KCC activity, probably via effects on the activating phosphatases, and syk-family TKs appear to be positive regulators. This complex pattern of regulation probably explains why some TK inhibitors stimulate and others inhibit KCC.[310,311]

MULTITRACK MODEL OF SICKLE CELL VOLUME REGULATION PATHOBIOLOGY

Cell heterogeneity is a hallmark of sickle cell disease,[134] with high numbers of dense cells and many low-density reticulocytes. In general, low-density sickle cells have high KCC activity and dehydrated cells exhibit low activity.[249,252] Even if fractionated by age or density, sickle cells exhibit considerable heterogeneity. Some reticulocytes are found in the dense cell fraction, suggest very rapid dehydration in the circulation, or, fast-track dehydration. Within the low-density fraction containing most of the sickle reticulocytes is a pool of cells exhibiting enhanced capacity to dehydrate via KCC.[179] A similar fraction of reticulocytes/young cells was found with decreased F cell content.[258] Transferrin receptor–positive sickle reticulocytes present in the dense cell fraction had greater KCC activity than sickle reticulocytes which had normal hydration in vivo;[253] both studies demonstrated that KCC activity did not correlate with HbF content.[259]

Sickle erythrocyte maturation and density changes have been followed in vivo by using biotin-labeled erythrocytes.[146,312,313] After ex vivo labeling and reinfusion, biotin-labeled cells exhibit increased density and dehydration within the first week, with loss of the least dense fractions and relative increases in high-density populations. This suggests that density changes in vivo occur soon after release of young cells into the circulation, supporting the notion of rapid dehydration. Sickle cells surviving longer than 1 week in the circulation, which account for 50%–66% of the population, are all strikingly dehydrated, with densities exceeding the densest normal cells.[312]

The low HbF content of dense reticulocytes suggests a sickling-induced mechanism for fast-track dehydration.[179,181] This model envisions initial dehydration of a population of reticulocytes via activation of the Gardos channel by calcium influx through the sickling-induced pathway. Incremental dehydration would result in a slight intracellular acidification, which in turn would activate KCC in susceptible cells. Mathematical modeling of this mechanism predicts rapid volume collapse after cycles of deoxygenation.[181] Reticulocyte heterogeneity in susceptibility to KCC activation by intracellular acidification could account for a subset of rapidly dehydrating cells. This notion is supported by the increased susceptibility of KCC activation to acid pH in sickle cells compared with normal cells.[179,254] An alternative model for fast-track dehydration is that reticulocytes reach a state of intermediate dehydration via KCC activity, with heterogeneity derived from cellular differences in KCC capacity, function, or regulation. Reticulocytes with CHC thus increased would be "set up" for sickling, calcium permeabilization via the sickling-induced pathway, Gardos channel activation and subsequent severe dehydration.[226] This model is supported by the finding that formation of transferrin receptor–positive cells of intermediate density, which are dehydrated compared with normal reticulocytes, is not dependent on HbF concentration.[259] Presently, the data do distinguish between these two models of initial dehydration through sickling-induced Gardos activation followed by KCC activation compared with dehydration by abnormal KCC activation potentiating sickling-induced Gardos activation.

The lifespan of sickle erythrocytes that contain little or no HbF is approximately 2 weeks, compared with 6–8 weeks for F cells,[312] confirming the selective survival of F cells inferred from the number of F cells and F reticulocytes in the circulation (Chapter 7).[314] Unexpectedly high levels of HbF, either naturally occurring or induced by hydroxyurea, were found to be associated with shortened survival times of non-F cells.[313] The survival of dense sickle cells in vivo is extremely short, with 50% survival times ranging from 40 to 60 hours for dehydrated non-F cells and 120–330 hours for dense F cells.[146] Their fragility and selective involvement in vascular occlusion and hemolysis, plus their rapid clearance during vasoocclusive episodes, supported the notion that dense sickle cells represented an end-stage in the life of sickle cells. That model has recently expanded to accommodate the existence of significant numbers of low-density, potassium-depleted, and sodium-loaded sickle erythrocytes resistant to dehydration by in vitro treatment with valinomycin, as discussed previously. The majority of low-density sickle cells that were older as assessed by biotin labeling were in fact, valinomycin-resistant, sodium-loaded cells. Such low-density cells arose spontaneously in vitro upon incubation of dense sickle erythrocytes under oxygenated conditions, and this process was accelerated by cyclic deoxygenation.[145] The steady-state in vivo levels of valinomycin-resistant cells in sickle blood is approximately 3%–10%.[143] Together with their short survival, this suggests that a significant proportion of sickle cells pass through this phase of sodium loading and over hydration prior to their destruction.

A new model of the sickle cell "hydration" cycle thus includes pathological rehydration following pathological dehydration. The potassium loss that produces initial dense cell production deprives the cell of the ability to offset cation uptake driven by Donnan forces. Progressive sodium loading would then ensue, by virtue either of the deoxygenation-induced permeability increase or in response to dehydration, as has been shown experimentally under other conditions. Provided that the combination of sodium influx and potassium efflux exceeded the capacity for compensation by the sodium pump, the cell would be destined to swell to the point of osmotic lysis. This process of osmotic volume regulatory failure could contribute to intravascular hemolysis in sickle cell disease, now appreciated as an important aspect of the pathophysiology in light of the perturbations in nitric oxide metabolism brought about by free hemoglobin in the plasma (Chapter 11).[315]

Pharmacological Inhibition of Sickle Cell Dehydration

The pathological dehydration of sickle cells and its contribution to hemolysis and vasoocclusion raised the possibility of a therapeutic benefit from improving sickle cell hydration.[316] Attempts to rehydrate cells by infusions of hypotonic fluids or treatment with antidiuretic hormone proved impractical.[317] More recently, drugs targeting specific pathways contributing to dehydration have undergone preliminary testing and some are discussed in Chapter 31. A trial of dipyridamole, an inhibitor of the deoxygenation-induced cation leak,[176] is currently underway (NCT00276146).

Cation Transport and Volume Regulation in Other Hemoglobinopathies and Thalassemia

Specific and nonspecific interactions of hemoglobin with components of the red cell membrane can have important functional effects, which can be pathological when abnormal hemoglobins are involved. HbC is capable of powerful stimulation of KCC, resulting in excessive volume reduction of erythrocytes to produce elevated MCHC.[252,318–321] The pathological consequences of elevated MCHC could contribute to crystal formation in the case of HbC disease (Chapter 21). Dehydration is particularly significant in HbSC disease, in which cellular dehydration produces conditions that permit sickling, even thought the participation of HbC in polymer formation is no greater than HbA.[319] An argument has been made that KCC stimulation is specifically related to mutations around the sixth amino acid position of *HBB*, as HbS and HbC. Hb Siriraj (*HBB* glu7lys) and Hb San Jose (*HBB* glu7gly) produce slight elevations in KCC activity in heterozygotes, which were not observed in heterozygotes with HbO Arab or HbD (Chapter 23).[320] Other studies, however, showed marked KCC stimulation and dehydration of both mature red cells and reticulocytes in homozygotes with HbO Arab and compound heterozygote with HbS and HbO Arab.[322]

In thalassemia, both hemoglobin content and abnormal cation transport affect cell volume. Although the responsible mechanisms are poorly understood, total hemoglobin content is an important determinant of cell volume so any condition that reduces hemoglobin synthesis produces microcytic, hypochromic erythrocytes. Indeed, the red cell "phenotype" in α thalassemia, where one or two α-globin genes are deleted (Chapters 13 and 14) is virtually indistinguishable from that in iron deficiency. MCHC in these conditions and in HbH disease is slightly less than in normal erythrocytes.

In contrast, despite their reduced hemoglobin content, β-thalassemia erythrocytes, especially those of β-thalassemia intermedia (Chapter 17), exhibit a substantial population of dense erythrocytes (Fig. 9.10).[36] This elevated hemoglobin concentration results in increased cellular viscosity, which contributes to increased dynamic rigidity. KCC is increased in both β and α thalassemia erythrocytes, in proportion to the severity of disease. Swelling-induced KCC activity is substantially increased in both types of thalassemia.[323] Although high reticulocyte counts might contribute to some of the elevation of KCC activity in these samples, several lines of evidence suggest that pathological activation might also occur. In vitro treatment of thalassemia red cells with dithiothreitol markedly reduced KCC activity, suggesting KCC activation by oxidative stress, consistent with the presence of hemichromes and other oxidant products in membrane. This connection is strengthened by the finding that treatment of patients with the iron chelator L1, which reduced iron content of red cell membranes, also lowered KCC activity and improved cellular potassium content.[324] Like sickle cells,

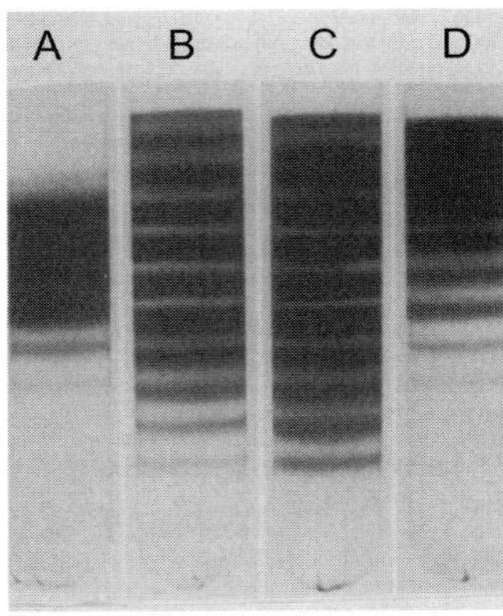

Figure 9.10. Density gradient analysis of thalassemic erythrocytes on discontinuous Stractan gradients. Density range 1.065–1.130 g/mL in 0.0045 g/mL increments. **(A)** Normal red blood cells. **(B)** β thalassemia intermedia, unsplenectomized. **(C)** β thalassemia intermedia, splenectomized. **(D)** HbH disease. (From ref. 36.)

β thalassemia red cells are depleted of cellular magnesium, and oral supplementation with magnesium pidolate has been shown to restore cellular magnesium, reduce KCC activity, and improve cellular potassium content.[271] Although these findings support a link between abnormal KCC regulation and cellular dehydration in thalassemia, erythrocytes, especially in HbH disease, show quantitatively similar increases in KCC activity, with no increase in cellular hemoglobin concentration (Fig. 9.10).

Whether mechanisms other than KCC contribute to dehydration of β thalassemia red cells is unknown. Calcium content of β thalassemia red cells is elevated, but most is sequestered in intracellular vesicles or retained organelles, and cytoplasmic calcium levels appear to be normal, as do active and passive calcium fluxes.[325,326] In contrast, in a mouse model of β thalassemia, treatment of animals with the Gardos channel blocker, clotrimazole, resulted in fewer dense cells, higher MCHC, and higher potassium content, but no change in hemoglobin or reticulocyte count.[327] This suggested that the Gardos pathway plays a role in cellular dehydration in β thalassemia red cells, but that dehydration does not shorten red cell survival. As yet there are no experimental data to support the hypothetical possibility of K channel activation via increase calcium influx due to shear stress on the mechanically unstable thalassemic membrane.

SUMMARY

The erythrocyte membrane is a complex dynamic structure with multiple regulated functions. Cytoskeletal proteins maintain the structural integrity of a membrane that must simultaneously be flexible enough to deform in the microcirculation and durable enough to resist high shear stresses in large vessels. Multiple ligands and receptors interact with the external surface of the membrane, and some of these interactions trigger signaling cascades that regulate cell function. Specific proteins maintain a highly ordered lipid structure, which in turn, might modulate other membrane protein functions or cellular interactions. Multiple regulated transport systems control solute and water fluxes across the membrane to facilitate the transport of respiratory gases, provide metabolic substrates, and regulate cell volume. Substantial energy is required to detoxify oxidant molecules that arise as an occupational hazard of the erythrocyte's major tasks, the transport of oxygen.

Given the physiological interactions of hemoglobin with the erythrocyte membrane, it is perhaps not surprising that abnormal hemoglobins can elicit significant pathological effects on membrane structure and function. A significant source of membrane damage in hemoglobinopathies is the increased level of oxidant species produced by reactive sulfhydryl on unstable or denatured hemoglobin molecules, membrane bound heme, or free iron. Oxidation affects cytoskeletal function, leads to externalization of PS, increases membrane rigidity and fragility, and perturbs cation transport and volume regulation.

HbS polymerization elicits major perturbations of membrane structure and function. Polymer formation, in addition to increasing cellular rigidity and blood viscosity, results in formation of membrane spicules in which the cytoskeleton is dissociated from its membrane connections. Associated with this membrane disruption is externalization of PS and an increase in cation permeability via a nonselective cation pathway. Calcium influx via this deoxygenation-induced pathway results in activation of the Gardos pathway, which mediates selective potassium loss that results in cation depletion. KCC, normally involved in establishing reticulocyte hemoglobin concentration, is excessively active in the red cells of certain hemoglobinopathies and thalassemias, and leads to dehydrated, dense cells with high hemoglobin concentrations. In cells containing HbS, elevated hemoglobin concentrations greatly potentiates the rate and extent of polymer formation.

The pleiotropic effects of abnormal hemoglobins on erythrocyte membrane structure and function contribute to the pathophysiology of sickle cell disease and thalassemia. Strategies targeting specific membrane pathology offer novel avenues to develop new therapy for these diseases.

REFERENCES

1. Hebbel RP. Beyond hemoglobin polymerization: the red blood cell membrane and sickle disease pathophysiology. *Blood.* 1991;77(2):214–237.
2. Perrotta S, Gallagher PG, Mohandas N. Hereditary spherocytosis. *Lancet.* 2008;372:1411–1426.
3. Hebbel RP. The sickle erythrocyte in double jeopardy: autooxidation and iron decompartmentalization. *Semin Hematol.* 1990;27(1):51–69.
4. Asakura T, Agarwal PL, Relman DA, et al. Mechanical instability of the oxy-form of sickle haemoglobin. *Nature.* 1973;244(5416):437–438.
5. MacDonald VW, Charache S. Drug-induced oxidation and precipitation of hemoglobins A, S and C. *Biochim Biophys Acta.* 1982;701(1):39–44.
6. Schrier SL. Thalassemia: pathophysiology of red cell changes. *Annu Rev Med.* 1994;45:211–218.
7. Shinar E, Rachmilewitz EA. Haemoglobinopathies and red cell membrane function. *Baillieres Clin Haematol.* 1993; 6(2):357–369.
8. Chiu D, Lubin B. Oxidative hemoglobin denaturation and RBC destruction: the effect of heme on red cell membranes. *Semin Hematol.* 1989;26(2):128–135.
9. Hebbel RP, Eaton JW. Pathobiology of heme interaction with the erythrocyte membrane. *Semin Hematol.* 1989;26(2):136–149.
10. Rice-Evans C, Omorphos SC, Baysal E. Sickle cell membranes and oxidative damage. *Biochem J.* 1986;237(1):265–269.
11. Marva E, Hebbel RP. Denaturing interaction between sickle hemoglobin and phosphatidylserine liposomes. *Blood.* 1994; 83(1):242–249.
12. Sugihara T, Repka T, Hebbel RP. Detection, characterization, and bioavailability of membrane-associated iron in the intact sickle red cell. *J Clin Invest.* 1992;90(6):2327–2332.
13. Das SK, Nair RC. Superoxide dismutase, glutathione peroxidase, catalase and lipid peroxidation of normal and sickled erythrocytes. *Br J Haematol.* 1980;44(1):87–92.
14. Chiu D, Lubin B. Abnormal vitamin E and glutathione peroxidase levels in sickle cell anemia: evidence for increased susceptibility to lipid peroxidation in vivo. *J Lab Clin Med.* 1979;94(4):542–548.
15. Schacter LP, DelVillano BC, Gordon EM, Klein BL. Red cell superoxide dismutase and sickle cell anemia symptom severity. *Am J Hematol.* 1985;19(2):137–144.
16. Browne P, Shalev O, Hebbel RP. The molecular pathobiology of cell membrane iron: the sickle red cell as a model. *Free Radic Biol Med.* 1998;24(6):1040–1048.
17. Scott MD, Eaton JW. Thalassaemic erythrocytes: cellular suicide arising from iron and glutathione-dependent oxidation reactions? *Br J Haematol.* 1995;91(4):811–819.
18. Tavazzi D, Duca L, Graziadei G, Comino A, Fiorelli G, Cappellini MD. Membrane-bound iron contributes to oxidative damage of beta-thalassaemia intermedia erythrocytes. *Br J Haematol.* 2001;112(1):48–50.
19. Repka T, Shalev O, Reddy R, et al. Nonrandom association of free iron with membranes of sickle and beta-thalassemic erythrocytes. *Blood.* 1993;82(10):3204–3210.
20. Asakura T, Minakata K, Adachi K, Russell MO, Schwartz E. Denatured hemoglobin in sickle erythrocytes. *J Clin Invest.* 1977;59(4):633–640.
21. Kuross SA, Hebbel RP. Nonheme iron in sickle erythrocyte membranes: association with phospholipids and potential role in lipid peroxidation. *Blood.* 1988;72(4):1278–1285.
22. Waugh SM, Willardson BM, Kannan R, Labotka RJ, Low PS. Heinz bodies induce clustering of band 3, glycophorin, and ankyrin in sickle cell erythrocytes. *J Clin Invest.* 1986; 78(5):1155–1160.
23. Cappellini MD, Tavazzi D, Duca L, et al. Metabolic indicators of oxidative stress correlate with haemichrome attachment to membrane, band 3 aggregation and erythrophagocytosis in beta-thalassaemia intermedia. *Br J Haematol.* 1999;104(3):504–512.
24. Mannu F, Arese P, Cappellini MD, et al. Role of hemichrome binding to erythrocyte membrane in the generation of band-3 alterations in beta-thalassemia intermedia erythrocytes. *Blood.* 1995;86(5):2014–2020.

25. Low PS, Waugh SM, Zinke K, Drenckhahn D. The role of hemoglobin denaturation and band 3 clustering in red blood cell aging. *Science.* 1985;227(4686):531–533.
26. Kuross SA, Rank BH, Hebbel RP. Excess heme in sickle erythrocyte inside-out membranes: possible role in thiol oxidation. *Blood.* 1988;71(4):876–882.
27. Hartley A, Davies MJ, Rice-Evans C. Desferrioxamine and membrane oxidation: radical scavenger or iron chelator? *Biochem Soc Trans.* 1989;17(6):1002–1003.
28. Shalev O, Hebbel RP. Extremely high avidity association of Fe(III) with the sickle red cell membrane. *Blood.* 1996; 88(1):349–352.
29. Repka T, Hebbel RP. Hydroxyl radical formation by sickle erythrocyte membranes: role of pathologic iron deposits and cytoplasmic reducing agents. *Blood.* 1991;78(10):2753–2758.
30. Liu SC, Yi SJ, Mehta JR, et al. Red cell membrane remodeling in sickle cell anemia. Sequestration of membrane lipids and proteins in Heinz bodies. *J Clin Invest.* 1996;97(1):29–36.
31. Shalev O, Repka T, Goldfarb A, et al. Deferiprone (L1) chelates pathologic iron deposits from membranes of intact thalassemic and sickle red blood cells both in vitro and in vivo. *Blood.* 1995;86(5):2008–2013.
32. Browne PV, Shalev O, Kuypers FA, et al. Removal of erythrocyte membrane iron in vivo ameliorates the pathobiology of murine thalassemia. *J Clin Invest.* 1997;100(6):1459–1464.
33. Shalev O, Hebbel RP. Catalysis of soluble hemoglobin oxidation by free iron on sickle red cell membranes. *Blood.* 1996;87(9):3948–3952.
34. de Franceschi L, Shalev O, Piga A, et al. Deferiprone therapy in homozygous human beta-thalassemia removes erythrocyte membrane free iron and reduces KCl cotransport activity. *J Lab Clin Med.* 1999;133(1):64–69.
35. Advani R, Sorenson S, Shinar E, Lande W, Rachmilewitz E, Schrier SL. Characterization and comparison of the red blood cell membrane damage in severe human alpha- and beta-thalassemia. *Blood.* 1992;79(4):1058–1063.
36. Schrier SL, Rachmilewitz E, Mohandas N. Cellular and membrane properties of alpha and beta thalassemic erythrocytes are different: implication for differences in clinical manifestations. *Blood.* 1989;74(6):2194–2202.
37. Scott MD, Van Den Berg JJ, Repka T, et al. Effect of excess alpha-hemoglobin chains on cellular and membrane oxidation in model beta-thalassemic erythrocytes. *J Clin Invest.* 1993;91(4):1706–1712.
38. Shinar E, Rachmilewitz EA, Lux SE. Differing erythrocyte membrane skeletal protein defects in alpha and beta thalassemia. *J Clin Invest.* 1989;83(2):404–410.
39. Yuan J, Bunyaratvej A, Fucharoen S, Fung C, Shinar E, Schrier SL. The instability of the membrane skeleton in thalassemic red blood cells. *Blood.* 1995;86(10):3945–3950.
40. Shinar E, Shalev O, Rachmilewitz EA, Schrier SL. Erythrocyte membrane skeleton abnormalities in severe beta-thalassemia. *Blood.* 1987;70(1):158–164.
41. Eisinger J, Flores J, Salhany JM. Association of cytosol hemoglobin with the membrane in intact erythrocytes. *Proc Natl Acad Sci USA.* 1982;79(2):408–412.
42. Salhany JM, Cordes KA, Gaines ED. Light-scattering measurements of hemoglobin binding to the erythrocyte membrane. Evidence for transmembrane effects related to a disulfonic stilbene binding to band 3. *Biochemistry.* 1980;19(7):1447–1454.
43. Shaklai N, Yguerabide J, Ranney HM. Classification and localization of hemoglobin binding sites on the red blood cell membrane. *Biochemistry.* 1977;16(25):5593–5597.
44. Shaklai N, Yguerabide J, Ranney HM. Interaction of hemoglobin with red blood cell membranes as shown by a fluorescent chromophore. *Biochemistry.* 1977;16(25):5585–5592.
45. Bank A, Mears G, Weiss R, O'Donnell JV, Natta C. Preferential binding of beta s globin chains associated with stroma in sickle cell disorders. *J Clin Invest.* 1974;54(4):805–809.
46. Fischer S, Nagel RL, Bookchin RM, Roth EF, Jr., Tellez-Nagel I. The binding of hemoglobin to membranes of normal and sickle erythrocytes. *Biochim Biophys Acta.* 1975;375(3):422–433.
47. Shaklai N, Sharma VS, Ranney HM. Interaction of sickle cell hemoglobin with erythrocyte membranes. *Proc Natl Acad Sci USA.* 1981;78(1):65–68.
48. Klipstein FA, Ranney HM. Electrophoretic components of the hemoglobin of red cell membranes. *J Clin Invest.* 1960;39:1894–1899.
49. Schluter K, Drenckhahn D. Co-clustering of denatured hemoglobin with band 3: its role in binding of autoantibodies against band 3 to abnormal and aged erythrocytes. *Proc Natl Acad Sci USA.* 1986;83(16):6137–6141.
50. Yuan J, Kannan R, Shinar E, Rachmilewitz EA, Low PS. Isolation, characterization, and immunoprecipitation studies of immune complexes from membranes of beta-thalassemic erythrocytes. *Blood.* 1992;79(11):3007–3013.
51. Liu SC, Derick LH, Zhai S, Palek J. Uncoupling of the spectrin-based skeleton from the lipid bilayer in sickled red cells. *Science.* 1991;252(5005):574–576.
52. Corbett JD, Golan DE. Band 3 and glycophorin are progressively aggregated in density-fractionated sickle and normal red blood cells. Evidence from rotational and lateral mobility studies. *J Clin Invest.* 1993;91(1):208–217.
53. Platt OS, Falcone JF. Membrane protein interactions in sickle red blood cells: evidence of abnormal protein 3 function. *Blood.* 1995;86(5):1992–1998.
54. Platt OS, Falcone JF, Lux SE. Molecular defect in the sickle erythrocyte skeleton. Abnormal spectrin binding to sickle inside-our vesicles. *J Clin Invest.* 1985;75(1):266–271.
55. Platt OS, Falcone JF. Membrane protein lesions in erythrocytes with Heinz bodies. *J Clin Invest.* 1988;82(3):1051–1058.
56. Rank BH, Carlsson J, Hebbel RP. Abnormal redox status of membrane-protein thiols in sickle erythrocytes. *J Clin Invest.* 1985;75(5):1531–1537.
57. Schwartz RS, Rybicki AC, Heath RH, Lubin BH. Protein 4.1 in sickle erythrocytes. Evidence for oxidative damage. *J Biol Chem.* 1987;262(32):15666–15672.
58. Shaklai N, Frayman B, Fortier N, Snyder M. Crosslinking of isolated cytoskeletal proteins with hemoglobin: a possible damage inflicted to the red cell membrane. *Biochim Biophys Acta.* 1987;915(3):406–414.
59. Allan D, Limbrick AR, Thomas P, Westerman MP. Microvesicles from sickle erythrocytes and their relation to irreversible sickling. *Br J Haematol.* 1981;47(3):383–390.
60. Allan D, Limbrick AR, Thomas P, Westerman MP. Release of spectrin-free spicules on reoxygenation of sickled erythrocytes. *Nature.* 1982;295(5850):612–613.
61. Butikofer P, Kuypers FA, Xu CM, Chiu DT, Lubin B. Enrichment of two glycosyl-phosphatidylinositol-anchored proteins, acetylcholinesterase and decay accelerating factor,

in vesicles released from human red blood cells. *Blood.* 1989;74(5):1481–1485.

62. Padilla F, Bromberg PA, Jensen WN. The sickle-unsickle cycle: a cause of cell fragmentation leading to permanently deformed cells. *Blood.* 1973;41(5):653–660.
63. Test ST, Butikofer P, Yee MC, Kuypers FA, Lubin B. Characterization of the complement sensitivity of calcium loaded human erythrocytes. *Blood.* 1991;78(11):3056–3065.
64. Test ST, Woolworth VS. Defective regulation of complement by the sickle erythrocyte: evidence for a defect in control of membrane attack complex formation. *Blood.* 1994;83(3):842–852.
65. Turrini F, Arese P, Yuan J, Low PS. Clustering of integral membrane proteins of the human erythrocyte membrane stimulates autologous IgG binding, complement deposition, and phagocytosis. *J Biol Chem.* 1991;266(35):23611–23617.
66. Ataga KI, Key NS. Hypercoagulability in sickle cell disease: new approaches to an old problem. *Hematology Am Soc Hematol Educ Program.* 2007;2007:91–96.
67. Wagner GM, Chiu DT, Yee MC, Lubin BH. Red cell vesiculation – a common membrane physiologic event. *J Lab Clin Med.* 1986;108(4):315–324.
68. Westerman MP, Cole ER, Wu K. The effect of spicules obtained from sickle red cells on clotting activity. *Br J Haematol.* 1984;56(4):557–562.
69. Franck PF, Bevers EM, Lubin BH, et al. Uncoupling of the membrane skeleton from the lipid bilayer. The cause of accelerated phospholipid flip-flop leading to an enhanced procoagulant activity of sickled cells. *J Clin Invest.* 1985;75(1):183–190.
70. Lane PA, O'Connell JL, Marlar RA. Erythrocyte membrane vesicles and irreversibly sickled cells bind protein S. *Am J Hematol.* 1994;47(4):295–300.
71. Bertles JF, Dobler J. Reversible and irreversible sickling: a distinction by electron microscopy. *Blood.* 1969;33(6):884–898.
72. Bertles JF, Milner PF. Irreversibly sickled erythrocytes: a consequence of the heterogeneous distribution of hemoglobin types in sickle-cell anemia. *J Clin Invest.* 1968;47(8):1731–1741.
73. Serjeant GR. Irreversibly sickled cells and splenomegaly in sickle-cell anaemia. *Br J Haematol.* 1970;19(5):635–641.
74. Serjeant GR, Serjeant BE, Milner PF. The irreversibly sickled cell; a determinant of haemolysis in sickle cell anaemia. *Br J Haematol.* 1969;17(6):527–533.
75. Glader BE, Nathan DG. Cation permeability alterations during sickling: relationship to cation composition and cellular hydration of irreversibly sickled cells. *Blood.* 1978;51(5):983–989.
76. Horiuchi K, Ballas SK, Asakura T. The effect of deoxygenation rate on the formation of irreversibly sickled cells. *Blood.* 1988;71(1):46–51.
77. Jensen M, Shohet SB, Nathan DG. The role of red cell energy metabolism in the generation of irreversibly sickled cells in vitro. *Blood.* 1973;42(6):835–842.
78. Nash GB, Johnson CS, Meiselman HJ. Rheologic impairment of sickle RBCs induced by repetitive cycles of deoxygenation-reoxygenation. *Blood.* 1988;72(2):539–545.
79. Lux SE, John KM, Karnovsky MJ. Irreversible deformation of the spectrin-actin lattice in irreversibly sickled cells. *J Clin Invest.* 1976;58(4):955–963.
80. Liu SC, Derick LH, Palek J. Dependence of the permanent deformation of red blood cell membranes on spectrin dimer-tetramer equilibrium: implication for permanent membrane deformation of irreversibly sickled cells. *Blood.* 1993;81(2):522–528.
81. Bencsath FA, Shartava A, Monteiro CA, Goodman SR. Identification of the disulfide-linked peptide in irreversibly sickled cell beta-actin. *Biochemistry.* 1996;35(14):4403–4408.
82. Shartava A, Monteiro CA, Bencsath FA, et al. A posttranslational modification of beta-actin contributes to the slow dissociation of the spectrin-protein 4.1-actin complex of irreversibly sickled cells. *J Cell Biol.* 1995;128(5):805–818.
83. Chiu D, Lubin B, Shohet SB. Erythrocyte membrane lipid reorganization during the sickling process. *Br J Haematol.* 1979;41(2):223–234.
84. Wetterstroem N, Brewer GJ, Warth JA, Mitchinson A, Near K. Relationship of glutathione levels and Heinz body formation to irreversibly sickled cells in sickle cell anemia. *J Lab Clin Med.* 1984;103(4):589–596.
85. Schroeder F, Woodford JK, Kavecansky J, Wood WG, Joiner C. Cholesterol domains in biological membranes. *Mol Membr Biol.* 1995;12(1):113–119.
86. Daleke DL. Phospholipid flippases. *J Biol Chem.* 2007; 282(2):821–825.
87. Daleke DL. Regulation of phospholipid asymmetry in the erythrocyte membrane. *Curr Opin Hematol.* 2008;15(3):191–195.
88. Sims PJ, Wiedmer T. Unraveling the mysteries of phospholipid scrambling. *Thromb Haemost.* 2001;86(1):266–275.
89. Schlegel RA, Williamson P. P.S. to PS (phosphatidylserine)–pertinent proteins in apoptotic cell clearance. *SciSTK.* 2007; 2007(408):pe57.
90. Setty BN, Betal SG. Microvascular endothelial cells express a phosphatidylserine receptor: a functionally active receptor for phosphatidylserine-positive erythrocytes. *Blood.* 2008;111(2):905–914.
91. Kuypers FA. Membrane lipid alterations in hemoglobinopathies. *Hematology Am Soc Hematol Educ Program.* 2007;2007:68–73.
92. Yeung T, Gilbert GE, Shi J, Silvius J, Kapus A, Grinstein S. Membrane phosphatidylserine regulates surface charge and protein localization. *Science.* 2008;319(5860):210–213.
93. Kuypers FA, Lewis RA, Hua M, et al. Detection of altered membrane phospholipid asymmetry in subpopulations of human red blood cells using fluorescently labeled annexin V. *Blood.* 1996;87(3):1179–1187.
94. Lubin B, Chiu D, Bastacky J, Roelofsen B, Van Deenen LL. Abnormalities in membrane phospholipid organization in sickled erythrocytes. *J Clin Invest.* 1981;67(6):1643–1649.
95. Wood BL, Gibson DF, Tait JF. Increased erythrocyte phosphatidylserine exposure in sickle cell disease: flow-cytometric measurement and clinical associations. *Blood.* 1996;88(5):1873–1880.
96. Kuypers FA, Schott MA, Scott MD. Phospholipid composition and organization in model beta-thalassemic erythrocytes. *Am J Hematol.* 1996;51(1):45–54.
97. Kuypers FA, Yuan J, Lewis RA, et al. Membrane phospholipid asymmetry in human thalassemia. *Blood.* 1998;91(8):3044–3051.

98. Hebbel RP, Schwartz RS, Mohandas N. The adhesive sickle erythrocyte: cause and consequence of abnormal interactions with endothelium, monocytes/macrophages and model membranes. *Clin Haematol.* 1985;14(1):141–161.
99. Schwartz RS, Tanaka Y, Fidler IJ, Chiu DT, Lubin B, Schroit AJ. Increased adherence of sickled and phosphatidylserine-enriched human erythrocytes to cultured human peripheral blood monocytes. *J Clin Invest.* 1985;75(6):1965–1972.
100. de Jong K, Larkin SK, Styles LA, Bookchin RM, Kuypers FA. Characterization of the phosphatidylserine-exposing subpopulation of sickle cells. *Blood.* 2001;98(3):860–867.
101. Yasin Z, Witting S, Palascak MB, Joiner CH, Rucknagel DL, Franco RS. Phosphatidylserine externalization in sickle red blood cells: associations with cell age, density, and hemoglobin F. *Blood.* 2003;102(1):365–370.
102. Basu S, Banerjee D, Chandra S, Chakrabarti A. Loss of phospholipid membrane asymmetry and sialylated glycoconjugates from erythrocyte surface in haemoglobin E beta-thalassaemia. *Br J Haematol.* 2008;141(1):92–99.
103. Horne MK 3rd, Cullinane AM, Merryman PK, Hoddeson EK. The effect of red blood cells on thrombin generation. *Br J Haematol.* 2006;133(4):403–408.
104. Stuart MJ, Setty BN. Hemostatic alterations in sickle cell disease: relationships to disease pathophysiology. *Pediatr Pathol Mol Med.* 2001;20(1):27–46.
105. Bezeaud A, Venisse L, Helley D, Trichet C, Girot R, Guillin MC. Red blood cells from patients with homozygous sickle cell disease provide a catalytic surface for factor Va inactivation by activated protein C. *Br J Haematol.* 2002;117(2):409–413.
106. Zwaal RF, Schroit AJ. Pathophysiologic implications of membrane phospholipid asymmetry in blood cells. *Blood.* 1997;89(4):1121–1132.
107. Styles L, De Jong K, Vichinsky E, Lubin B, Adams R, Kuypers FA. Increased RBC phosphatidylserine exposure in sickle cell disease patients at risk for stroke by transcranial Doppler screening. *Blood.* 1997;90:604a.
108. de Jong K, Emerson RK, Butler J, Bastacky J, Mohandas N, Kuypers FA. Short survival of phosphatidylserine-exposing red blood cells in murine sickle cell anemia. *Blood.* 2001;98(5):1577–1584.
109. Ataga KI, Cappellini MD, Rachmilewitz EA. Beta-thalassaemia and sickle cell anaemia as paradigms of hypercoagulability. *Br J Haematol.* 2007;139(1):3–13.
110. Panigrahi I, Agarwal S. Thromboembolic complications in beta-thalassemia: Beyond the horizon. *Thromb Res.* 2007; 120(6):783–789.
111. Setty BN, Rao AK, Stuart MJ. Thrombophilia in sickle cell disease: the red cell connection. *Blood.* 2001;98(12):3228–3233.
112. Setty BN, Kulkarni S, Rao AK, Stuart MJ. Fetal hemoglobin in sickle cell disease: relationship to erythrocyte phosphatidylserine exposure and coagulation activation. *Blood.* 2000;96(3):1119–1124.
113. Atichartakarn V, Angchaisuksiri P, Aryurachai K, et al. Relationship between hypercoagulable state and erythrocyte phosphatidylserine exposure in splenectomized haemoglobin E/beta-thalassaemic patients. *Br J Haematol.* 2002;118(3):893–898.
114. Lang F, Lang KS, Lang PA, Huber SM, Wieder T. Mechanisms and significance of eryptosis. *Antioxid Redox Signal.* 2006;8(7–8):1183–1192.
115. Vance JE, Steenbergen R. Metabolism and functions of phosphatidylserine. *Prog Lipid Res.* 2005;44(4):207–234.
116. Wang RH, Phillips G Jr, Medof ME, Mold C. Activation of the alternative complement pathway by exposure of phosphatidylethanolamine and phosphatidylserine on erythrocytes from sickle cell disease patients. *J Clin Invest.* 1993;92(3):1326–1335.
117. Neidlinger NA, Larkin SK, Bhagat A, Victorino GP, Kuypers FA. Hydrolysis of phosphatidylserine-exposing red blood cells by secretory phospholipase A2 generates lysophosphatidic acid and results in vascular dysfunction. *J Biol Chem.* 2006;281(2):775–781.
118. Styles LA, Aarsman AJ, Vichinsky EP, Kuypers FA. Secretory phospholipase A(2) predicts impending acute chest syndrome in sickle cell disease. *Blood.* 2000;96(9):3276–3278.
119. Styles LA, Abboud M, Larkin S, Lo M, Kuypers FA. Transfusion prevents acute chest syndrome predicted by elevated secretory phospholipase A2. *Br J Haematol.* 2007;136(2):343–344.
120. de Jong K, Geldwerth D, Kuypers FA. Oxidative damage does not alter membrane phospholipid asymmetry in human erythrocytes. *Biochemistry.* 1997;36(22):6768–6776.
121. Blumenfeld N, Zachowski A, Galacteros F, Beuzard Y, Devaux PF. Transmembrane mobility of phospholipids in sickle erythrocytes: effect of deoxygenation on diffusion and asymmetry. *Blood.* 1991;77(4):849–854.
122. de Jong K, Kuypers FA. Sulphydryl modifications alter scramblase activity in murine sickle cell disease. *Br J Haematol.* May 2006;133(4):427–432.
123. Devaux PF, Morris R. Transmembrane asymmetry and lateral domains in biological membranes. *Traffic.* 2004;5(4):241–246.
124. Eaton WA, Hofrichter J. Hemoglobin S gelation and sickle cell disease. *Blood.* 1987;70(5):1245–1266.
125. Eaton WA, Hofrichter J. Sickle cell hemoglobin polymerization. *Adv Protein Chem.* 1990;40:63–279.
126. Noguchi CT, Rodgers GP, Schechter AN. Intracellular polymerization. Disease severity and therapeutic predictions. *Ann NY Acad Sci.* 1989;565:75–82.
127. Kaul DK, Fabry ME, Nagel RL. Microvascular sites and characteristics of sickle cell adhesion to vascular endothelium in shear flow conditions: pathophysiological implications. *Proc Natl Acad Sci USA.* 1989;86(9):3356–3360.
128. Kaul DK, Chen D, Zhan J. Adhesion of sickle cells to vascular endothelium is critically dependent on changes in density and shape of the cells. *Blood.* 1994;83(10):3006–3017.
129. Morris CL, Rucknagel DL, Joiner CH. Deoxygenation-induced changes in sickle cell-sickle cell adhesion. *Blood.* 1993;81(11):3138–3145.
130. Platt OS. Exercise-induced hemolysis in sickle cell anemia: shear sensitivity and erythrocyte dehydration. *Blood.* 1982;59(5):1055–1060.
131. Hiruma H, Noguchi CT, Uyesaka N, Schechter AN, Rodgers GP. Contributions of sickle hemoglobin polymer and sickle cell membranes to impaired filterability. *Am J Physiol.* 1995;268(5 Pt 2):H2003–2008.
132. Hasegawa S, Hiruma H, Uyesaka N, Noguchi CT, Schechter AN, Rodgers GP. Filterability of mixtures of sickle and normal erythrocytes. *Am J Hematol.* 1995;50(2):91–97.
133. Dong C, Chadwick RS, Schechter AN. Influence of sickle hemoglobin polymerization and membrane properties on deformability of sickle erythrocytes in the microcirculation. *Biophys J.* 1992;63(3):774–783.

134. Fabry ME, Nagel RL. Heterogeneity of red cells in the sickler: a characteristic with practical clinical and pathophysiological implications. *Blood Cells.* 1982;8(1):9–15.
135. Mohandas N, Ballas S. Erythrocyte density and heterogeneity. In: Embury S, Hebbel RP, Mohandas N, Steinberg MH, eds. *Sickle Cell Disease: Basic Principles and Clinical Practice.* New York: Raven Press; 1994.
136. Mohandas N, Johnson A, Wyatt J, et al. Automated quantitation of cell density distribution and hyperdense cell fraction in RBC disorders. *Blood.* 1989;74(1):442–447.
137. Mohandas N, Kim YR, Tycko DH, Orlik J, Wyatt J, Groner W. Accurate and independent measurement of volume and hemoglobin concentration of individual red cells by laser light scattering. *Blood.* 1986;68(2):506–513.
138. Tosteson D, Carlen, E, Dunham, ET. The effects of sickling on ion transport I. Effect of sickling on potassium transport. *J. Gen. Physiol.* 1955;39:31–54.
139. Tosteson D, E Shea et al. The efftects of sickling on ion transport II. The effects of sickling on sodium and cesium transport. *J. Gen. Physiol.* 1955;39:55–67.
140. Tosteson D, E Shea et al. Potassium and sodium in red blood cells in sickle cell anemia. *J Clin Invest.* 1952;48:406–411.
141. Glader BE, Lux SE, Muller-Soyano A, Platt OS, Propper RD, Nathan DG. Energy reserve and cation composition of irreversibly sickled cells in vivo. *Br J Haematol.* 1978;40(4):527–532.
142. Clark MR, Morrison CE, Shohet SB. Monovalent cation transport in irreversibly sickled cells. *J Clin Invest.* 1978;62(2): 329–337.
143. Bookchin RM, Etzion Z, Sorette M, Mohandas N, Skepper JN, Lew VL. Identification and characterization of a newly recognized population of high-Na+, low-K+, low-density sickle and normal red cells. *Proc Natl Acad Sci USA.* 2000;97(14):8045–8050.
144. Etzion Z, Lew VL, Bookchin RM. K(86Rb) transport heterogeneity in the low-density fraction of sickle cell anemia red blood cells. *Am J Physiol.* 1996;271(4 Pt 1):C1111–1121.
145. Holtzclaw JD, Jiang M, Yasin Z, Joiner CH, Franco RS. Rehydration of high-density sickle erythrocytes in vitro. *Blood.* 2002;100(8):3017–3025.
146. Franco RS, Yasin Z, Lohmann JM, et al. The survival characteristics of dense sickle cells. *Blood.* 2000;96(10):3610–3617.
147. Amer J, Etzion Z, Bookchin RM, Fibach E. Oxidative status of valinomycin–resistant normal, beta-thalassemia and sickle red blood cells. *Biochim Biophys Acta.* 2006;1760(5):793–799.
148. Fabry ME, Benjamin L, Lawrence C, Nagel RL. An objective sign in painful crisis in sickle cell anemia: the concomitant reduction of high density red cells. *Blood.* 1984;64(2):559–563.
149. Lawrence C, Fabry ME, Nagel RL. Red cell distribution width parallels dense red cell disappearance during painful crises in sickle cell anemia. *J Lab Clin Med.* 1985;105(6):706–710.
150. Lawrence C, Fabry ME. Objective indices of sickle cell painful crisis: decrease in RDW and percent dense cells and increase in ESR and fibrinogen. *Prog Clin Biol Res.* 1987;240:329–336.
151. Ballas SK, Smith ED. Red blood cell changes during the evolution of the sickle cell painful crisis. *Blood.* 1992;79(8):2154–2163.
152. Fabry ME, Mears JG, Patel P, et al. Dense cells in sickle cell anemia: the effects of gene interaction. *Blood.* 1984;64(5): 1042–1046.
153. Embury SH, Clark MR, Monroy G, Mohandas N. Concurrent sickle cell anemia and alpha-thalassemia. Effect on pathological properties of sickle erythrocytes. *J Clin Invest.* 1984;73(1):116–123.
154. Ballas SK. Sickle cell anemia with few painful crises is characterized by decreased red cell deformability and increased number of dense cells. *Am J Hematol.* 1991;36(2):122–130.
155. Lande WM, Andrews DL, Clark MR, et al. The incidence of painful crisis in homozygous sickle cell disease: correlation with red cell deformability. *Blood.* 1988;72(6):2056–2059.
156. Ballas SK, Larner J, Smith ED, Surrey S, Schwartz E, Rappaport EF. Rheologic predictors of the severity of the painful sickle cell crisis. *Blood.* 1988;72(4):1216–1223.
157. Billett HH, Kim K, Fabry ME, Nagel RL. The percentage of dense red cells does not predict incidence of sickle cell painful crisis. *Blood.* 1986;68(1):301–303.
158. Brugnara C, Gee B, Armsby CC, et al. Therapy with oral clotrimazole induces inhibition of the Gardos channel and reduction of erythrocyte dehydration in patients with sickle cell disease. *J Clin Invest.* 1996;97(5):1227–1234.
159. De Franceschi L, Beuzard Y, Jouault H, Brugnara C. Modulation of erythrocyte potassium chloride cotransport, potassium content, and density by dietary magnesium intake in transgenic SAD mouse. *Blood.* 1996;88(7):2738–2744.
160. De Franceschi L, Bachir D, Galacteros F, et al. Oral magnesium pidolate: effects of long-term administration in patients with sickle cell disease. *Br J Haematol.* 2000;108(2):284–289.
161. Rivera A. Reduced sickle erythrocyte dehydration in vivo by endothelin-1 receptor antagonists. *Am J Physiol Cell Physiol.* 2007;293:in press.
162. Stocker JW, De Franceschi L, McNaughton-Smith GA, Corrocher R, Beuzard Y, Brugnara C. ICA-17043, a novel Gardos channel blocker, prevents sickled red blood cell dehydration in vitro and in vivo in SAD mice. *Blood.* 2003;101(6):2412–2418.
163. Ataga KI, Smith WR, De Castro LM et al. Efficacy and safety of the Gardos channel blocker, senicapoc (ICA-17043), in patients with sickle cell anemia. *Blood.* 2008;111(8):3991–3997.
164. Bookchin RM, Lew VL. Effects of a 'sickling pulse' on the calcium and potassium permeabilities of intact, sickle trait red cells [proceedings]. *J Physiol.* 1978;284:93P–94P.
165. Roth EF, Jr, Nagel RL, Bookchin RM. pH dependency of potassium efflux from sickled red cells. *Am J Hematol.* 1981;11(1):19–27.
166. Berkowitz LR, Orringer EP. Passive sodium and potassium movements in sickle erythrocytes. *Am J Physiol.* 1985;249(3 Pt 1):C208–214.
167. Joiner CH, Platt OS, Lux SE. Cation depletion by the sodium pump in red cells with pathologic cation leaks. Sickle cells and xerocytes. *J Clin Invest.* 1986;78(6):1487–1496.
168. Joiner CH, Dew A, Ge DL. Deoxygenation-induced cation fluxes in sickle cells: relationship between net potassium efflux and net sodium influx. *Blood Cells.* 1988;13(3):339–358.
169. Joiner CH. Deoxygenation-induced cation fluxes in sickle cells: *II.* Inhibition by stilbene disulfonates. *Blood.* 1990; 76(1):212–220.
170. Joiner CH, Gunn RB, Frohlich O. Anion transport in sickle red blood cells. *Pediatr Res.* 1990;28(6):587–590.
171. Joiner CH, Morris CL, Cooper ES. Deoxygenation-induced cation fluxes in sickle cells. III. Cation selectivity and

response to pH and membrane potential. *Am J Physiol.* 1993;264(3 Pt 1):C734–744.

172. Joiner CH, Jiang M, Franco RS. Deoxygenation-induced cation fluxes in sickle cells. IV. Modulation by external calcium. *Am J Physiol.* 1995;269(2 Pt 1):C403–409.
173. Mohandas N, Rossi ME, Clark MR. Association between morphologic distortion of sickle cells and deoxygenation-induced cation permeability increase. *Blood.* 1986;68(2):450–454.
174. Ortiz OE, Lew VL, Bookchin RM. Deoxygenation permeabilizes sickle cell anaemia red cells to magnesium and reverses its gradient in the dense cells. *J Physiol.* 1990;427:211–226.
175. Rhoda MD, Apovo M, Beuzard Y, Giraud F. Ca2+ permeability in deoxygenated sickle cells. *Blood.* 1990;75(12):2453–2458.
176. Joiner CH, Jiang M, Claussen WJ, Roszell NJ, Yasin Z, Franco RS. Dipyridamole inhibits sickling-induced cation fluxes in sickle red blood cells. *Blood.* 2001;97(12):3976–3983.
177. Clark MR, Rossi ME. Permeability characteristics of deoxygenated sickle cells. *Blood.* 1990;76(10):2139–2145.
178. Browning JA, Robinson HC, Ellory JC, Gibson JS. Deoxygenation-induced non-electrolyte pathway in red cells from sickle cell patients. *Cell Physiol Biochem.* 2007;19(1–4):165–174.
179. Bookchin RM, Ortiz OE, Lew VL. Evidence for a direct reticulocyte origin of dense red cells in sickle cell anemia. *J Clin Invest.* 1991;87(1):113–124.
180. Clark MR, Guatelli JC, White AT, Shohet SB. Study on the dehydrating effect of the red cell Na+/K+-pump in nystatin-treated cells with varying Na+ and water contents. *Biochim Biophys Acta.* 1981;646(3):422–432.
181. Lew VL, Freeman CJ, Ortiz OE, Bookchin RM. A mathematical model of the volume, pH, and ion content regulation in reticulocytes. Application to the pathophysiology of sickle cell dehydration. *J Clin Invest.* 1991;87(1):100–112.
182. Gibson JS, Stewart GW, Ellory JC. Effect of dimethyl adipimidate on K+ transport and shape change in red blood cells from sickle cell patients. *FEBS Letters.* 2000;480(2–3):179–183.
183. Lubin BH, Pena V, Mentzer WC, Bymun E, Bradley TB, Packer L. Dimethyl adipimidate: a new antisickling agent. *Proc Natl Acad Sci USA.* 1975;72(1):43–46.
184. Kavecansky J, Schroeder F, Joiner CH. Deoxygenation-induced alterations in sickle cell membrane cholesterol exchange. *Am J Physiol.* 1995;269(5 Pt 1):C1105–1111.
185. Sugihara T, Yawata Y, Hebbel RP. Deformation of swollen erythrocytes provides a model of sickling-induced leak pathways, including a novel bromide-sensitive component. *Blood.* 1994;83(9):2684–2691.
186. Jones GS, Knauf PA. Mechanism of the increase in cation permeability of human erythrocytes in low-chloride media. Involvement of the anion transport protein capnophorin. *J Gen Physiol.* 1985;86(5):721–738.
187. Bruce LJ, Robinson HC, Guizouarn H, et al. Monovalent cation leaks in human red cells caused by single amino-acid substitutions in the transport domain of the band 3 chloride-bicarbonate exchanger, AE1. *Nat Genet.* 2005;37(11):1258–1263.
188. Hebbel RP, Mohandas N. Reversible deformation-dependent erythrocyte cation leak. Extreme sensitivity conferred by minimal peroxidation. *Biophys J.* 1991;60(3):712–715.
189. Ney PA, Christopher MM, Hebbel RP. Synergistic effects of oxidation and deformation on erythrocyte monovalent cation leak. *Blood.* 1990;75(5):1192–1198.
190. Johnson RM, Gannon SA. Erythrocyte cation permeability induced by mechanical stress: a model for sickle cell cation loss. *Am J Physiol.* 1990;259(5 Pt 1):C746–751.
191. Johnson RM. Membrane stress increases cation permeability in red cells. *Biophys J.* 1994;67(5):1876–1881.
192. Johnson RM, Tang K. Induction of a Ca(2+)-activated K+ channel in human erythrocytes by mechanical stress. *Biochim Biophys Acta.* 1992;1107(2):314–318.
193. Sugihara T, Hebbel RP. Exaggerated cation leak from oxygenated sickle red blood cells during deformation: evidence for a unique leak pathway. *Blood.* 1992;80(9):2374–2378.
194. Johnson RM, Tang K. DIDS inhibition of deformation-induced cation flux in human erythrocytes. *Biochim Biophys Acta.* 1993;1148(1):7–14.
195. Clark MR, Unger RC, Shohet SB. Monovalent cation composition and ATP and lipid content of irreversibly sickled cells. *Blood.* 1978;51:1169–1178.
196. Canessa M, Fabry ME, Suzuka SM, Morgan K, Nagel RL. Na+/H+ exchange is increased in sickle cell anemia and young normal red cells. *J Membr Biol.* 1990;116(2):107–115.
197. Canessa M, Fabry ME, Blumenfeld N, Nagel RL. Volume-stimulated, Cl(-)-dependent K+ efflux is highly expressed in young human red cells containing normal hemoglobin or HbS. *J Membr Biol.* 1987;97(2):97–105.
198. Rivera A, Ferreira A, Bertoni D, Romero JR, Brugnara C. Abnormal regulation of Mg2+ transport via Na/Mg exchanger in sickle erythrocytes. *Blood.* 2005;105(1):382–386.
199. Joiner CH, Jiang M, Fathallah H, Giraud F, Franco RS. Deoxygenation of sickle red blood cells stimulates KCl cotransport without affecting Na+/H+ exchange. *Am J Physiol.* 1998;274(6 Pt 1):C1466–1475.
200. Eaton JW, Skelton TD, Swofford HS, Kolpin CE, Jacob HS. Elevated erythrocyte calcium in sickle cell disease. *Nature.* 1973;246(5428):105–106.
201. Palek J, Thomae M, Ozog D. Red cell calcium content and transmembrane calcium movements in sickle cell anemia. *J Lab Clin Med.* 1977;89(6):1365–1374.
202. Engelmann B, Duhm J. Intracellular calcium content of human erythrocytes: relation to sodium transport systems. *J Membr Biol.* 1987;98(1):79–87.
203. Lew VL, Tsien RY, Miner C, Bookchin RM. Physiological [Ca2+]i level and pump-leak turnover in intact red cells measured using an incorporated Ca chelator. *Nature.* 1982;298(5873):478–481.
204. Murphy E, Berkowitz LR, Orringer E, Levy L, Gabel SA, London RE. Cytosolic free calcium levels in sickle red blood cells. *Blood.* 1987;69(5):1469–1474.
205. Bookchin RM, Ortiz OE, Somlyo AV, et al. Calcium-accumulating inside-out vesicles in sickle cell anemia red cells. *Trans Assoc Am Physicians.* 1985;98:10–20.
206. Lew VL, Hockaday A, Sepulveda MI, et al. Compartmentalization of sickle-cell calcium in endocytic inside-out vesicles. *Nature.* 1985;315(6020):586–589.
207. Williamson P, Puchulu E, Penniston JT, Westerman MP, Schlegel RA. Ca2+ accumulation and loss by aberrant endocytic vesicles in sickle erythrocytes. *J Cell Physiol.* 1992;152(1):1–9.

208. Westerman MP, Puchulu E, Schlegel RA, Salameh M, Williamson P. Intracellular Ca(2+)-containing vesicles in sickle cell disorders. *J Lab Clin Med.* 1994;124(3):416–420.
209. Bookchin RM, Lew VL. Effect of a 'sickling pulse' on calcium and potassium transport in sickle cell trait red cells. *J Physiol.* 1981;312:265–280.
210. Etzion Z, Tiffert T, Bookchin RM, Lew VL. Effects of deoxygenation on active and passive Ca2+ transport and on the cytoplasmic Ca2+ levels of sickle cell anemia red cells. *J Clin Invest.* 1993;92(5):2489–2498.
211. Tiffert T, Spivak JL, Lew VL. Magnitude of calcium influx required to induce dehydration of normal human red cells. *Biochim Biophys Acta.* 1988;943(2):157–165.
212. Horiuchi K, Onyike AE, Osterhout ML. Sickling in vitro of reticulocytes from patients with sickle cell disease at venous oxygen tension. *Exp Hematol.* 1996;24(1):68–76.
213. Lew VL, Ortiz OE, Bookchin RM. Stochastic nature and red cell population distribution of the sickling-induced Ca2+ permeability. *J Clin Invest.* 1997;99(11):2727–2735.
214. Gardos G. The function of calcium in the potassium permeability of human erythrocytes. *Biochim Biophys Acta.* 1958;30:653–654.
215. Hoffman JF, Joiner W, Nehrke K, Potapova O, Foye K, Wickrema A. The hSK4 (KCNN4) isoform is the Ca2+-activated K+ channel (Gardos channel) in human red blood cells. *Proc Natl Acad Sci USA.* 2003;100(12):7366–7371.
216. Vandorpe DH, Shmukler BE, Jiang L, et al. cDNA cloning and functional characterization of the mouse Ca2+-gated K+ channel, mIK1. Roles in regulatory volume decrease and erythroid differentiation. *J Biol Chem.* 1998;273(34):21542–21553.
217. Ishii TM, Silvia C, Hirschberg B, Bond CT, Adelman JP, Maylie J. A human intermediate conductance calcium-activated potassium channel. *Proc Natl Acad Sci USA.* 1997;94(21):11651–11656.
218. Heginbotham L, Lu Z, Abramson T, MacKinnon R. Mutations in the K+ channel signature sequence. *Biophys J.* 1994;66(4):1061–1067.
219. Wolff D, Cecchi X, Spalvins A, Canessa M. Charybdotoxin blocks with high affinity the Ca-activated K+ channel of Hb A and Hb S red cells: individual differences in the number of channels. *J Membr Biol.* 1988;106(3):243–252.
220. Brugnara C, Armsby CC, De Franceschi L, Crest M, Euclaire MF, Alper SL. Ca(2+)-activated K+ channels of human and rabbit erythrocytes display distinctive patterns of inhibition by venom peptide toxins. *J Membr Biol.* 1995;147(1):71–82.
221. Brugnara C, De Franceschi L, Alper SL. Ca(2+)-activated K+ transport in erythrocytes. Comparison of binding and transport inhibition by scorpion toxins. *J Biol Chem.* 1993;268(12):8760–8768.
222. Lew VL, Etzion Z, Bookchin RM. Dehydration response of sickle cells to sickling-induced Ca(++) permeabilization. *Blood.* 2002;99(7):2578–2585.
223. Ohnishi ST, Katagi H, Katagi C. Inhibition of the in vitro formation of dense cells and of irreversibly sickled cells by charybdotoxin, a specific inhibitor of calcium-activated potassium efflux. *Biochim Biophys Acta.* 1989;1010(2):199–203.
224. Ohnishi ST, Horiuchi KY, Horiuchi K. The mechanism of in vitro formation of irreversibly sickled cells and modes of action of its inhibitors. *Biochim Biophys Acta.* 1986;886(1):119–129.
225. Horiuchi K, Asakura T. Formation of light irreversibly sickled cells during deoxygenation-oxygenation cycles. *J Lab Clin Med.* 1987;110(5):653–660.
226. Franco RS, Palascak M, Thompson H, Rucknagel DL, Joiner CH. Dehydration of transferrin receptor-positive sickle reticulocytes during continuous or cyclic deoxygenation: role of KCl cotransport and extracellular calcium. *Blood.* 1996;88(11):4359–4365.
227. McGoron AJ, Joiner CH, Palascak MB, Claussen WJ, Franco RS. Dehydration of mature and immature sickle red blood cells during fast oxygenation/deoxygenation cycles: role of KCl cotransport and extracellular calcium. *Blood.* 2000; 95(6):2164–2168.
228. Lew VL, Bookchin RM. Volume, pH, and ion-content regulation in human red cells: analysis of transient behavior with an integrated model. *J Membr Biol.* 1986;92(1):57–74.
229. Rivera A, Rotter MA, Brugnara C. Endothelins activate Ca(2+)-gated K(+) channels via endothelin B receptors in CD-1 mouse erythrocytes. *Am J Physiol.* 1999;277(4 Pt 1): C746–754.
230. Rivera A, Jarolim P, Brugnara C. Modulation of Gardos channel activity by cytokines in sickle erythrocytes. *Blood.* 2002;99(1):357–603.
231. Li Q, Jungmann V, Kiyatkin A, Low PS. Prostaglandin E2 stimulates a Ca2+-dependent K+ channel in human erythrocytes and alters cell volume and filterability. *J Biol Chem.* 1996;271(31):18651–18656.
232. Lang PA, Kempe DS, Myssina S, et al. PGE(2) in the regulation of programmed erythrocyte death. *Cell Death Differ.* 2005;12(5):415–428.
233. Andrews DA, Yang L, Low PS. Phorbol ester stimulates a protein kinase C-mediated agatoxin-TK-sensitive calcium permeability pathway in human red blood cells. *Blood.* 2002;100(9):3392–3399.
234. Yang L, Andrews DA, Low PS. Lysophosphatidic acid opens a Ca(++) channel in human erythrocytes. *Blood.* 2000;95(7):2420–2425.
235. Werdehoff SG, Moore RB, Hoff CJ, Fillingim E, Hackman AM. Elevated plasma endothelin-1 levels in sickle cell anemia: relationships to oxygen saturation and left ventricular hypertrophy. *Am J Hematol.* 1998;58(3):195–199.
236. Graido-Gonzalez E, Doherty JC, Bergreen EW, Organ G, Telfer M, McMillen MA. Plasma endothelin-1, cytokine, and prostaglandin E2 levels in sickle cell disease and acute vaso-occlusive sickle crisis. *Blood.* 1998;92(7):2551–2555.
237. Rybicki AC, Benjamin LJ. Increased levels of endothelin-1 in plasma of sickle cell anemia patients. *Blood.* 1998;92(7):2594–2596.
238. Hammerman SI, Kourembanas S, Conca TJ, Tucci M, Brauer M, Farber HW. Endothelin-1 production during the acute chest syndrome in sickle cell disease. *Am J RespirCrit Care Med.* 1997;156(1):280–285.
239. Brugnara C, de Franceschi L, Alper SL. Inhibition of Ca(2+)-dependent K+ transport and cell dehydration in sickle erythrocytes by clotrimazole and other imidazole derivatives. *J Clin Invest.* 1993;92(1):520–526.
240. Brugnara C, Armsby CC, Sakamoto M, Rifai N, Alper SL, Platt O. Oral administration of clotrimazole and blockade of

human erythrocyte Ca(++)-activated K+ channel: the imidazole ring is not required for inhibitory activity. *J Pharmacol Exp Ther.* 1995;273(1):266–272.

241. Lauf PK, Theg BE. A chloride dependent K+ flux induced by N-ethylmaleimide in genetically low K+ sheep and goat erythrocytes. *Biochem Biophys Res Commun.* 1980;92(4):1422–1428.

242. Dunham PB, Stewart GW, Ellory JC. Chloride-activated passive potassium transport in human erythrocytes. *Proc Natl Acad Sci USA.* 1980;77(3):1711–1715.

243. Brugnara C. Sickle cell disease: from membrane pathophysiology to novel therapies for prevention of erythrocyte dehydration. *J Pediatr Hematol Oncol.* 2003;25(12):927–933.

244. Adragna NC, Fulvio MD, Lauf PK. Regulation of K-Cl cotransport: from function to genes. [*erratum appears in J Membr Biol.* 2006 Apr;210(3):213]. *J Membr Biol.* 2004;201(3):109–137.

245. Lauf PK, Adragna NC. K-Cl cotransport: properties and molecular mechanism. *Cell Physiol Biochem.* 2000;10(5–6):341–354.

246. Joiner CH. Cation transport and volume regulation in sickle red blood cells. *Am J Physiol.* 1993;264(2 Pt 1):C251–270.

247. Brugnara C, Tosteson DC. Cell volume, K transport, and cell density in human erythrocytes. *Am J Physiol.* 1987;252(3 Pt 1): C269–276.

248. Hall AC, Ellory JC. Evidence for the presence of volume-sensitive KCl transport in 'young' human red cells. *Biochim Biophys Acta.* 1986;858(2):317–320.

249. Canessa M, Fabry ME, Nagel RL. Deoxygenation inhibits the volume-stimulated, Cl(-)-dependent K+ efflux in SS and young AA cells: a cytosolic Mg2+ modulation. *Blood.* 1987;70(6):1861–1866.

250. Ellory JC, Hall AC, Ody SA. Factors affecting the activation and inactivation of KCl cotransport in 'young' human red cells. *Biomed Biochim Acta.* 1990;49(2–3):S64–69.

251. Canessa M, Spalvins A, Nagel RL. Volume-dependent and NEM-stimulated K+,Cl- transport is elevated in oxygenated SS, SC and CC human red cells. *FEBS Letters.* 1986;200(1):197–202.

252. Brugnara C, Bunn HF, Tosteson DC. Regulation of erythrocyte cation and water content in sickle cell anemia. *Science.* 1986;232(4748):388–390.

253. Franco RS, Palascak M, Thompson H, Joiner CH. KCl cotransport activity in light versus dense transferrin receptor-positive sickle reticulocytes. *J Clin Invest.* 1995;95(6):2573–2580.

254. Joiner CH, Rettig RK, Jiang M, Franco RS. KCl cotransport mediates abnormal sulfhydryl-dependent volume regulation in sickle reticulocytes. *Blood.* 2004;104(9):2954–2960.

255. Gibson XA, Shartava A, McIntyre J, et al. The efficacy of reducing agents or antioxidants in blocking the formation of dense cells and irreversibly sickled cells in vitro. *Blood.* 1998;91(11):4373–4378.

256. Pace BS, Shartava A, Pack-Mabien A, Mulekar M, Ardia A, Goodman SR. Effects of N-acetylcysteine on dense cell formation in sickle cell disease. *Am J Hematol.* 2003;73(1):26–32.

257. Brugnara C, Van Ha T, Tosteson DC. Acid pH induces formation of dense cells in sickle erythrocytes. *Blood.* 1989;74(1):487–495.

258. Fabry ME, Romero JR, Buchanan ID, et al. Rapid increase in red blood cell density driven by K:Cl cotransport in a subset of sickle cell anemia reticulocytes and discocytes. *Blood.* 1991;78(1):217–225.

259. Franco RS, Thompson H, Palascak M, Joiner CH. The formation of transferrin receptor-positive sickle reticulocytes with intermediate density is not determined by fetal hemoglobin content. *Blood.* 1997;90(8):3195–3203.

260. Joiner CH, Rettig RK, Jiang M, Risinger M, Franco RS. Urea stimulation of KCl cotransport induces abnormal volume reduction in sickle reticulocytes. [erratum appears in *Blood.* 2007;109(7):2735]. *Blood.* 2007;109(4):1728–1735.

261. Joiner CH, Rettig RK, Jiang M, Risinger M, Franco RS. Urea stimulation of KCl cotransport induces abnormal volume reduction in sickle reticulocytes. *Blood.* 2007;109(4):1728–1735.

262. Hebbel RP, Ney PA, Foker W. Autoxidation, dehydration, and adhesivity may be related abnormalities of sickle erythrocytes. *Am J Physiol.* 1989;256(3 Pt 1):C579–583.

263. De Franceschi L, Beuzard Y, Brugnara C. Sulfhydryl oxidation and activation of red cell K(+)-Cl- cotransport in the transgenic SAD mouse. *Am J Physiol.* 1995;269(4 Pt 1):C899–906.

264. Gibson JS, Speake PF, Ellory JC. Differential oxygen sensitivity of the K+-Cl- cotransporter in normal and sickle human red blood cells. [see comment]. *J Physiol.* 1998;511(Pt 1):225–234.

265. Gibson JS, Khan A, Speake PF, Ellory JC. O2 dependence of K+ transport in sickle cells: the effect of different cell populations and the substituted benzaldehyde 12C79. *FASEB J.* 2001;15(3):823–832.

266. Joiner CH, Franco RS. The activation of KCL cotransport by deoxygenation and its role in sickle cell dehydration. *Blood Cell Mol Dis.* 2001;27(1):158–164.

267. Feray JC, Garay R. An Na+-stimulated Mg2+-transport system in human red blood cells. *Biochim Biophys Acta.* 1986;856(1):76–84.

268. Olukoga AO, Adewoye HO, Erasmus RT, Adedoyin MA. Erythrocyte and plasma magnesium in sickle-cell anaemia. *East African Med J.* 1990;67(5):348–354.

269. De Franceschi L, Villa-Moruzzi E, Fumagalli L, et al. K-Cl cotransport modulation by intracellular Mg in erythrocytes from mice bred for low and high Mg levels. *Am J Physiol Cell Physiol.* 2001;281(4):C1385–1395.

270. De Franceschi L, Brugnara C, Beuzard Y. Dietary magnesium supplementation ameliorates anemia in a mouse model of beta-thalassemia. *Blood.* 1997;90(3):1283–1290.

271. De Franceschi L, Cappellini MD, Graziadei G, et al. The effect of dietary magnesium supplementation on the cellular abnormalities of erythrocytes in patients with beta thalassemia intermedia. *Haematologica.* 1998;83(2):118–125.

272. De Franceschi L, Bachir D, Galacteros F, et al. Oral magnesium supplements reduce erythrocyte dehydration in patients with sickle cell disease. *J Clin Invest.* 1997; 100(7):1847–1852.

273. Gamba G. Molecular physiology and pathophysiology of electroneutral cation-chloride cotransporters. *Physiol Rev.* 2005;85(2):423–493.

274. Hebert SC, Mount DB, Gamba G. Molecular physiology of cation-coupled Cl- cotransport: the SLC12 family. *Eur J Physiol.* 2004;447(5):580–593.

275. Haas M, Forbush B 3rd. The Na-K-Cl cotransporter of secretory epithelia. *Annu Rev Physiol.* 2000;62:515–534.

276. Haas M, Forbush B 3rd. The Na-K-Cl cotransporters. *J Bioenerg Biomembr.* 1998;30(2):161–172.

277. Gillen CM, Brill S, Payne JA, Forbush B 3rd. Molecular cloning and functional expression of the K-Cl cotransporter from rabbit, rat, and human. A new member of the cation-chloride cotransporter family. *J Biol Chem.* 1996;271(27):16237–16244.

278. Payne JA, Stevenson TJ, Donaldson LF. Molecular characterization of a putative K-Cl cotransporter in rat brain. A neuronal-specific isoform. *J Biol Chem.* 1996;271(27):16245–16252.

279. Song L, Mercado A, Vazquez N, et al. Molecular, functional, and genomic characterization of human KCC2, the neuronal K-Cl cotransporter. *Brain Res Mol Brain Res.* 2002;103(1–2):91–105.

280. Race JE, Makhlouf FN, Logue PJ, Wilson FH, Dunham PB, Holtzman EJ. Molecular cloning and functional characterization of KCC3, a new K-Cl cotransporter. *Am J Physiol.* 1999;277(6 Pt 1):C1210–1219.

281. Hiki K, D'Andrea RJ, Furze J, et al. Cloning, characterization, and chromosomal location of a novel human K+-Cl- cotransporter. *J Biol Chem.* 1999;274(15):10661–10667.

282. Mount DB, Mercado A, Song L, et al. Cloning and characterization of KCC3 and KCC4, new members of the cation-chloride cotransporter gene family. *J Biol Chem.* 1999;274(23):16355–16362.

283. Mercado A, Vazquez N, Song L, et al. NH2-terminal heterogeneity in the KCC3 K+-Cl- cotransporter. *Am J Physiol Renal Physiol.* 2005;289(6):F1246–1261.

284. Boettger T, Hubner CA, Maier H, Rust MB, Beck FX, Jentsch TJ. Deafness and renal tubular acidosis in mice lacking the K-Cl co-transporter Kcc4. *Nature.* 2002;416(6883):874–878.

285. Pellegrino CM, Rybicki AC, Musto S, Nagel RL, Schwartz RS. Molecular identification and expression of erythroid K:Cl cotransporter in human and mouse erythroleukemic cells. *Blood Cell Mol Dis.* 1998;24(1):31–40.

286. Lauf PK, Zhang J, Delpire E, Fyffe RE, Mount DB, Adragna NC. K-Cl co-transport: immunocytochemical and functional evidence for more than one KCC isoform in high K and low K sheep erythrocytes. *Comp Biochem Physiol.* 2001;130(3):499–509.

287. Rust MB, Alper SL, Rudhard Y, et al. Disruption of erythroid K-Cl cotransporters alters erythrocyte volume and partially rescues erythrocyte dehydration in SAD mice. *J Clin Invest.* 2007;117(6):1708–1717.

288. Crable SC, Hammond SM, Papes R, et al. Multiple isoforms of the KC1 cotransporter are expressed in sickle and normal erythroid cells. *Exp Hematol.* 2005;33(6):624–631.

289. Joiner C, Papes R, Crable S, Pan D, Mount DB. Functional Comparison of Red Cell KCl Cotransporter isoforms, KCC1, KCC3, and KCC4. *Blood.* 2006;108:a.

290. Casula S, Shmukler BE, Wilhelm S, et al. A dominant negative mutant of the KCC1 K-Cl cotransporter: both N- and C-terminal cytoplasmic domains are required for K-Cl cotransport activity. *J Biol Chem.* 2001;276(45):41870–41878.

291. Plata C, Mount DB, Rubio V, Hebert SC, Gamba G. Isoforms of the Na-K-2Cl cotransporter in murine TAL II. Functional characterization and activation by cAMP. *Am J Physiol.* 1999;276(3 Pt 2):F359–366.

292. Gillen CM, Forbush B, 3rd. Functional interaction of the K-Cl cotransporter (KCC1) with the Na-K-Cl cotransporter in HEK-293 cells. *Am J Physiol.* 1999;276(2 Pt 1):C328–336.

293. Piechotta K, Lu J, Delpire E. Cation chloride cotransporters interact with the stress-related kinases Ste20-related proline-alanine-rich kinase (SPAK) and oxidative stress response 1 (OSR1). *J Biol Chem.* 2002;277(52):50812–50819.

294. Garzon-Muvdi T, Pacheco-Alvarez D, Gagnon KB, et al. WNK4 kinase is a negative regulator of K+-Cl- cotransporters. *Am J Physiol Renal Physiol.* 2007;292(4):F1197–1207.

295. Jennings ML, Schulz RK. Swelling-activated KCl cotransport in rabbit red cells: flux is determined mainly by cell volume rather than shape. *Am J Physiol.* 1990;259(6 Pt 1):C960–967.

296. Jennings ML, al-Rohil N. Kinetics of activation and inactivation of swelling-stimulated K+/Cl- transport. The volume-sensitive parameter is the rate constant for inactivation. *J Gen Physiol.* 1990;95(6):1021–1040.

297. Jennings ML, Schulz RK. Okadaic acid inhibition of KCl cotransport. Evidence that protein dephosphorylation is necessary for activation of transport by either cell swelling or N-ethylmaleimide. *J Gen Physiol.* 1991;97(4):799–817.

298. Kaji DM, Tsukitani Y. Role of protein phosphatase in activation of KCl cotransport in human erythrocytes. *Am J Physiol.* 1991;260(1 Pt 1):C176–180.

299. Colclasure GC, Parker JC. Cytosolic protein concentration is the primary volume signal for swelling-induced [K-Cl] cotransport in dog red cells. *J Gen Physiol.* 1992;100(1):1–10.

300. Parker JC, Colclasure GC. Macromolecular crowding and volume perception in dog red cells. *Mol Cell Biochem.* 1992;114(1–2):9–11.

301. Mallozzi C, De Franceschi L, Brugnara C, Di Stasi AM. Protein phosphatase 1alpha is tyrosine-phosphorylated and inactivated by peroxynitrite in erythrocytes through the src family kinase fgr. *Free Radic Biol Med.* 2005;38(12):1625–1636.

302. Bize I, Taher S, Brugnara C. Regulation of K-Cl cotransport during reticulocyte maturation and erythrocyte aging in normal and sickle erythrocytes. *Am J Physiol Cell Physiol.* 2003;285(1):C31–38.

303. Bize I, Guvenc B, Buchbinder G, Brugnara C. Stimulation of human erythrocyte K-Cl cotransport and protein phosphatase type 2A by n-ethylmaleimide: role of intracellular Mg++. *J Membr Biol.* 2000;177(2):159–168.

304. Bize I, Guvenc B, Robb A, Buchbinder G, Brugnara C. Serine/threonine protein phosphatases and regulation of K-Cl cotransport in human erythrocytes. *Am J Physiol.* 1999;277(5 Pt 1):C926–936.

305. Lytle C, Forbush B 3rd. The Na-K-Cl cotransport protein of shark rectal gland. II. Regulation by direct phosphorylation. *J Biol Chem.* 1992;267(35):25438–25443.

306. Dowd BF, Forbush B. PASK (proline-alanine-rich STE20-related kinase), a regulatory kinase of the Na-K-Cl cotransporter (NKCC1). *J Biol Chem.* 2003;278(30):27347–27353.

307. De Franceschi L, Fumagalli L, Olivieri O, Corrocher R, Lowell CA, Berton G. Deficiency of Src family kinases Fgr and Hck results in activation of erythrocyte K/Cl cotransport. *J Clin Invest.* 1997;99(2):220–227.

308. Fathallah H, Coezy E, de Neef RS, Hardy-Dessources MD, Giraud F. Inhibition of deoxygenation-induced membrane protein dephosphorylation and cell dehydration by phorbol esters and okadaic acid in sickle cells. *Blood.* 1995;86(5):1999–2007.

309. Merciris P, Claussen WJ, Joiner CH, Giraud F. Regulation of K-Cl cotransport by Syk and Src protein tyrosine kinases

in deoxygenated sickle cells. *Pflugers Archiv – Eur J Physiol.* 2003;446(2):232–238.

310. Flatman PW, Adragna NC, Lauf PK. Role of protein kinases in regulating sheep erythrocyte K-Cl cotransport. *Am J Physiol.* 1996;271(1 Pt 1):C255–263.
311. Bize I, Dunham PB. Staurosporine, a protein kinase inhibitor, activates K-Cl cotransport in LK sheep erythrocytes. *Am J Physiol.* 1994;266(3 Pt 1):C759–770.
312. Franco RS, Lohmann J, Silberstein EB, et al. Time-dependent changes in the density and hemoglobin F content of biotin-labeled sickle cells. *J Clin Invest.* 1998;101(12):2730–2740.
313. Franco RS, Yasin Z, Palascak MB, Ciraolo P, Joiner CH, Rucknagel DL. The effect of fetal hemoglobin on the survival characteristics of sickle cells. *Blood.* 2006;108(3):1073–1076.
314. Dover GJ, Boyer SH, Charache S, Heintzelman K. Individual variation in the production and survival of F cells in sickle–cell disease. *N Engl J Med.* 1978;299(26):1428–1435.
315. Reiter CD, Gladwin MT. An emerging role for nitric oxide in sickle cell disease vascular homeostasis and therapy. *Curr Opin Hematol.* 2003;10(2):99–107.
316. Bookchin R, Tieffert JT, Daives SC, Vichinsky E, Lew, VL. Magnesium therapy for sickle cell anemia: a new rationale. In: Beuzard Y, Lubin, B, Rosa, J, eds. *Sickle Cell Disease and Thalasssaemias: New Trends in Therapy.* Paris, London: John Libby; 1995.
317. Rosa RM, Bierer BE, Thomas R, et al. A study of induced hyponatremia in the prevention and treatment of sickle-cell crisis. *N Engl J Med.* 1980;303(20):1138–1143.
318. Lawrence C, Fabry ME, Nagel RL. The unique red cell heterogeneity of SC disease: crystal formation, dense reticulocytes, and unusual morphology. *Blood.* 1991;78(8):2104–2112.
319. Nagel RL, Fabry ME, Steinberg MH. The paradox of hemoglobin SC disease. *Blood Rev.* 2003;17(3):167–178.
320. Olivieri O, Vitoux D, Galacteros F, et al. Hemoglobin variants and activity of the (K+Cl-) cotransport system in human erythrocytes. *Blood.* 1992;79(3):793–797.
321. Brugnara C, Kopin AS, Bunn HF, Tosteson DC. Regulation of cation content and cell volume in hemoglobin erythrocytes from patients with homozygous hemoglobin C disease. *J Clin Invest.* 1985;75(5):1608–1617.
322. Nagel RL, Krishnamoorthy R, Fattoum S, et al. The erythrocyte effects of haemoglobin O(ARAB). *Br J Haematol.* 1999;107(3):516–521.
323. Olivieri O, De Franceschi L, Capellini MD, Girelli D, Corrocher R, Brugnara C. Oxidative damage and erythrocyte membrane transport abnormalities in thalassemias. *Blood.* 1994;84(1):315–320.
324. de Franceschi L, Shalev O, Piga A, et al. Deferiprone therapy in homozygous human beta-thalassemia removes erythrocyte membrane free iron and reduces KCl cotransport activity. *J Lab Clin Med.* 1999;133(1):64–69.
325. Bookchin RM, Ortiz OE, Shalev O, et al. Calcium transport and ultrastructure of red cells in beta-thalassemia intermedia. *Blood.* 1988;72(5):1602–1607.
326. Rhoda MD, Galacteros F, Beuzard Y, Giraud F. Ca2+ permeability and cytosolic Ca2+ concentration are not impaired in beta-thalassemic and hemoglobin C erythrocytes. *Blood.* 1987;70(3):804–808.
327. de Franceschi L, Rouyer-Fessard P, Alper SL, Jouault H, Brugnara C, Beuzard Y. Combination therapy of erythropoietin, hydroxyurea, and clotrimazole in a beta thalassemic mouse: a model for human therapy. *Blood.* 1996;87(3):1188–1195.

10

The Biology of Vascular Nitric Oxide

Jane A. Leopold and Joseph Loscalzo

The role of nitric oxide (NO) as the key mediator of endothelial function and vascular tone was initially recognized by Furchgott and Zawadski[1] over two decades ago when they discovered that an intact endothelium was required for acetylcholine-stimulated vasodilation. From these studies, they determined that the endothelium released a potent vasodilator substance that they termed endothelium-derived relaxing factor;[1] several years later, this factor was identified as NO.[2,3] Since that time, NO has been shown to modulate a host of functions that maintain the integrity of the endothelium as well as regulate interactions between circulating blood components and the vessel wall. Through its chemical reactions with a variety of species, including heme iron, NO is uniquely positioned to regulate these vascular homeostatic processes.

Endothelium-derived NO serves as a paracrine regulator of vascular function. NO is released to the vascular smooth muscle cells where it activates soluble guanylyl cyclase to generate cyclic guanosine monophosphate (cGMP) and modulate cation flux which, in turn, induce vasodilation and adjust vascular tone accordingly.[4,5] NO is also released to the bloodstream where it encounters erythrocytes, platelets, and plasma components. Here, the metabolic fate of NO is determined by a complex series of reactions that both consume and preserve stores of bioavailable NO. Owing to the relative abundance of erythrocytes compared with other circulating cell types, interactions between NO and redox-active hemoglobin achieve biological significance. In this chapter, we will discuss NO synthesis and biological chemistry, with particular focus on NO reactions with hemoglobin as well as the physiological relevance of NO-hemoglobin derivatives. In addition, we will detail the importance of NO for endothelial, vascular smooth muscle, and platelet homeostatic functions.

THE BIOCHEMISTRY, GENETICS, AND VASCULAR CELL BIOLOGY OF NITRIC OXIDE

Nitric Oxide Synthesis

NO is synthesized in numerous cell types and tissues by NO synthases (NOS). NOSs exists as two main isoform classes: the constitutive enzyme identified in the endothelium (eNOS or NOS3) and neuronal cells (nNOS or NOS1) and the inducible enzyme (iNOS or NOS2) found in smooth muscle cells, neutrophils, and macrophages (as well as many other cell types) following exposure to inflammatory cytokines or bacterial endotoxin.[6] NO is generated via the five-electron oxidation of L-arginine to form L-citrulline and stoichiometric amounts of NO.[3] This reaction requires molecular O_2 and nicotinamide adenine dinucleotide phosphate as cosubstrates and flavin adenine dinucleotide, flavin mononucleotide, and tetrahydrobiopterin as cofactors to facilitate electron transfer to the NOS heme moiety.[7] Each of the NOS isoforms possesses specific structural and functional characteristics that determine the degree to which cofactors regulate enzyme activity and NO production. Comparison of the amino acid sequences reveals that there is 50%–55% homology among NOS isoforms with the greatest conservation between sequences for the two main catalytic domains.[8]

All NOS isoforms are under the regulatory control of Ca^{2+} and calmodulin for effective electron transfer between the reductase and oxygenase domains of the enzyme; however, the affinity of NOS for the Ca^{2+}–calmodulin complex differs among isoforms and accounts, in part, for the difference in regulation of NO production. In endothelial cells, eNOS is membrane-bound within caveoli and binds calmodulin in a strongly Ca^{2+}-dependent manner that is reversible.[9] Following stimulation with agonists such as acetylcholine or bradykinin, inositol 1,4,5-trisphosphate production is increased to promote the release of intracellular Ca^{2+} stores.[10] This transient increase in intracellular Ca^{2+} enhances the formation of a Ca^{2+}–calmodulin complex, which, in turn, activates eNOS to facilitate dissociation from caveolin-1.[11] Once activated, eNOS generates continuously low levels of NO until Ca^{2+} stores are depleted.[9,12] Although eNOS is constitutively expressed, it is now recognized that expression may be differentially regulated under physiological and pathophysiological conditions and is subject to both posttranscriptional and posttranslational modification.[6] In contrast, iNOS binds calmodulin in states of low intracellular Ca^{2+}, is regulated at the transcriptional level, and, therefore, requires several hours to effect a physiological response.[13] Concentrations of NO (per mole of enzyme per minute) generated by iNOS are substantially greater than those achieved by eNOS,[14] are potentially cytotoxic, and indicate that iNOS may play an integral role in both the immune response and apoptosis.[15,16]

In the vascular endothelium, a number of signaling molecules as well as hemodynamic forces modulate eNOS expression to influence NO production. For example, transforming growth factor-β1, lysophosphatidylcholine, hydrogen peroxide, tumor necrosis factor–α (TNFα), oxidized low-density lipoprotein, laminar shear stress, and hypoxia all mediate eNOS expression by regulating gene transcription. In addition, TNFα, lipopolysaccharide, oxidized low-density lipoprotein, hydroxymethylglutaryl coenzyme A reductase inhibitors (statins), thrombin, and hydrogen peroxide have been shown to regulate eNOS expression by influencing mRNA degradation.[17]

NO production may be influenced further by a number of polymorphisms of the eNOS gene that have been identified and evaluated to determine the consequences for eNOS activity and association with vascular disease. Among these polymorphisms, a single nucleotide polymorphism in the promoter region (−786T/C) and in exon 7 resulting in the conversion of glutamate to aspartate at position 298 (Glu298Asp) and a variable number of tandem repeats in intron 4 (b/a) have been the most extensively studied. In a meta-analysis of 26 studies that examined these three polymorphisms, homozygosity for the Asp298 (odds ratio = 1.31; 95% confidence interval = 1.13−1.51) or the intron-4a allele (odds ratio = 1.34; 95% confidence interval = 1.03−1.75) was associated with an increased risk of ischemic heart disease, whereas no association was demonstrated for the −786C allele.[18]

Despite these findings, individual studies examining the functional significance of the Glu298Asp polymorphism have yielded conflicting results. Select studies of subjects homozygous for Asp298 demonstrate impaired endothelium-dependent brachial artery flow–mediated dilation, suggesting decreased bioavailable NO,[19] whereas other studies fail to make this association.[20–22] Although direct measures of eNOS activity and NO production were not determined in these studies, in vitro studies performed in primary human endothelial cells with the Glu298Asp polymorphism revealed enhanced eNOS protein cleavage, implying that this polymorphism should be associated with decreased NO production.[23]

A second polymorphism that has been studied is located in the promoter region and results from a T-to-C substitution, which may influence eNOS transcriptional activity, although this effect has not yet been confirmed in vivo. In contrast to what was found in the meta-analysis,[18] individuals with the −786C promoter polymorphism had impaired endothelium-dependent vascular reactivity[24] that was associated with a significant increase in death from cardiovascular causes at the end of a 2,000-day follow-up period.[25]

Interestingly, among the hemoglobinopathies, eNOS polymorphisms have been associated with disease status only in individuals with sickle cell disease.[26] In African-American women with sickle cell disease, the presence of the −786C promoter polymorphism was significantly associated with acute chest syndrome (relative risk = 8.7; 95% confidence interval = 1.76–42.92).[27] A mechanism to explain this association has not yet been elucidated; however, the −786T/C polymorphism adversely influences erythrocyte deformability.[28]

Bioreactivity of Nitric Oxide

NO, as a free radical, is only modestly reactive compared with other biological free radicals (i.e., it can diffuse over micron rather than Ångstrom distances before encountering another coreactant). NO may exist in one of three closely related redox forms, each with discrete properties and reactivities: $NO^{\bullet}$, NO^+ (nitrosonium, formed by single-electron oxidation of $NO^{\bullet}$), and NO^- (nitroxyl, formed by single-electron reduction of $NO^{\bullet}$).[29] These NO species react further with O_2-derived free radicals, redox metals, and thiols to generate NO compounds that have unique biological effects (Fig. 10.1).[30] For example, the reaction of NO with the heme iron of guanylyl cyclase results in enzyme activation, whereas the reaction of NO derivatives (NO^+, N_2O_3, or $ONOO^-$) with –SH (or $–S^-$ derivatives)-containing low-molecular-weight molecules and proteins generates *S*-nitrosothiols, a stable reservoir of bioavailable NO.[31] In plasma, *S*-nitroso-albumin serves as an NO adduct and limits the inactivation of NO by reactive oxygen species.[29] NO also forms *N*-nitroso adducts with amine moieties and nitrosyl adducts with heme groups to yield *N*-nitrosamines and nitrosylheme, respectively.[32,33] Human plasma contains an approximately fivefold higher concentration of *N*-nitrosamine species (32.3 +/− 5.0 nmol/L) than *S*-nitrosothiols (7.2 +/− 1.1 nmol/L);[34] however, functional studies in animal models studies suggest that *S*-nitrosothiols are biologically more active by an order of magnitude compared to *N*-nitrosamine species.[35] Dinitrosyl iron complexes also possess biological activity, inhibiting platelet aggregation and decreasing vascular tone in experimental models.[36,37]

In an O_2-rich environment, NO can be oxidized to nitrite (NO_2^-) and nitrate (NO_3^-), stable end products of its metabolism.[30] Although nitrite has been reported to have no intrinsic vasodilator activity,[38] nitrite does serve as a physiologically important source of NO, which is released in the circulation through the nitrite reductase activity of hemoglobin (*vide infra*).[39] Under ischemic conditions, where the pH is in the acidic range, nitrite may be reduced directly to NO through a nonenzymatic mechanism.[40] NO may also interact with reactive oxygen species, including superoxide, hydrogen peroxide, and lipid peroxyl radicals, formed during normal cellular metabolism or states of increased oxidant stress. In this manner, bioavailable NO is inactivated through the formation of peroxynitrite ($ONOO^-$), nitrous acid (HNO_2), and lipid peroxynitrites (LOONO), respectively.[30]

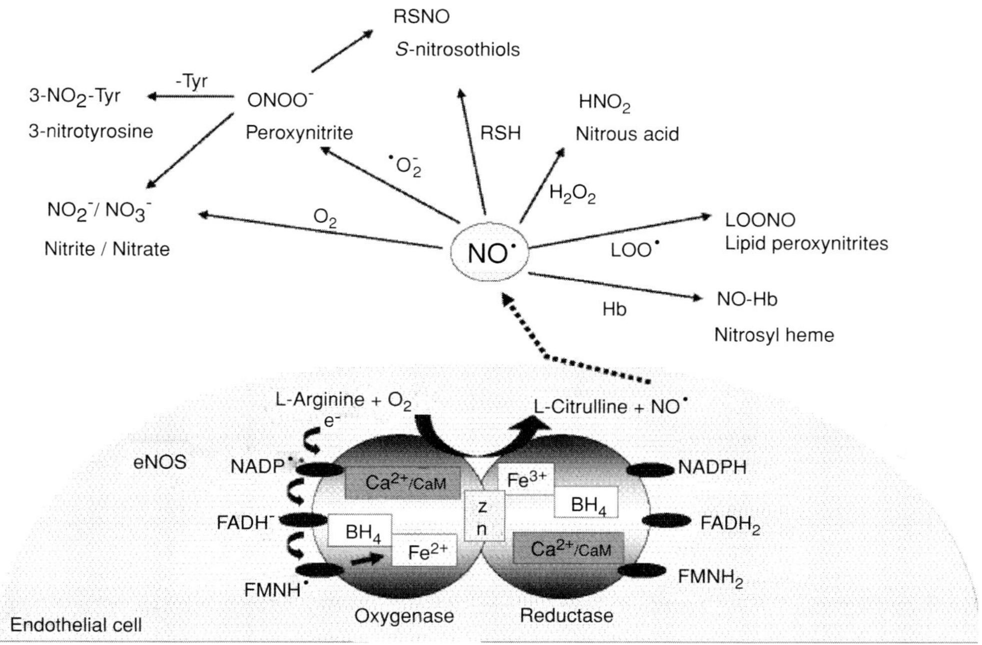

Figure 10.1. Biological source and reactions of nitric oxide. Nitric oxide ($NO^{\bullet}$) is synthesized in endothelial cells by the endothelial isoform of nitric oxide synthase (eNOS) via the five-electron oxidation reaction of L-arginine to L-citrulline. eNOS is activated by Ca^{2+}/calmodulin (Ca^{2+}/CaM) and the reaction requires molecular O_2 and NADPH as cosubstrates and flavin adenine dinucleotide ($FADH^+$), flavin mononucleotide ($FMNH^+$), and tetrahydrobiopterin (BH_4) as cofactors to facilitate electron transfer to the NOS heme moiety. Once generated, $NO^{\bullet}$ diffuses into the interstitium and the bloodstream where it reacts with molecular O_2, superoxide anion ($^{\bullet}O_2^-$), R-SH groups, hydrogen peroxide (H_2O_2), lipid oxides ($LOO^{\bullet}$), and hemoglobin (Hb) to generate NO species – some of which have biological activity. (See color plate 10.1.)

Bioreactivity of Nitric Oxide with Hemoglobin

NO can also bind to transition metals within heme groups, including myoglobin and hemoglobin itself. Endothelial-derived NO diffuses readily from the endothelial cell into the blood pool, where it first encounters platelets, which are enriched in the blood lamina nearest to the endothelial monolayer, and then erythrocytes, in which it can react with hemoglobin (Fig. 10.2). The reaction of NO with hemoglobin was first carefully characterized by Drabkin and Austin,[41] who recorded the absorption spectrum of nitrosyl-hemoglobin under anaerobic (i.e., deoxygenated) conditions:

$$Hb(II) + NO \rightarrow Hb(II)NO \qquad (10.1)$$

This reaction occurs with a second-order rate constant of $2\text{–}6 \times 10^7$ M/s,[42,43] and an extremely slow off-rate of approximately 10^{-3}–10^{-5} s.[44,45] This slow off-rate renders the bound NO effectively irreversibly complexed to deoxygenated hemoglobin. Under normal conditions in circulating whole blood, there is a large pool of oxyhemoglobin with which NO also readily reacts to form methemoglobin [Hb(III)] and nitrate:

$$Hb(II)O_2 + NO \rightarrow Hb(III) + NO_3^- \qquad (10.2)$$

The second-order rate constant for this reaction is $6\text{–}8 \times 10^7$ M/s,[46,47] leading to an estimated half-life in the erythrocyte of approximately 0.5 μs. The kinetics of the reaction of NO with deoxyhemoglobin and with oxyhemoglobin suggests that the erythrocyte should serve as an highly efficient sink for NO; however, if this were the case, erythrocytic hemoglobin would significantly limit NO's bioavailability for vascular smooth muscle cell and platelet homeostatic functions. This is best explained by the finding that erythrocytic hemoglobin is far less efficient than cell-free hemoglobin at scavenging NO, owing to the time required for NO to diffuse from the endothelial cell to the erythrocyte (accounted for by the erythrocyte-free zone nearest the endothelial monolayer and by the unstirred fluid layer surrounding the erythrocyte).[48] Furthermore, the erythrocyte membrane provides a physical diffusion barrier that effectively compartmentalizes hemoglobin and limits its access to the endothelial monolayer or vascular interstitium.[49,50] As shown in ex vivo studies performed in the absence of flow, 1,000 times more erythrocyte-encapsulated hemoglobin is required to inactivate NO compared with cell-free hemoglobin.[51]

Nitrite has recently been recognized as a reservoir of bioactive NO in mammals. Under ischemic or acidic conditions, nitrite can be reduced to NO directly or enzymatically via xanthine oxidase.[52,53] Recent data suggest that nitrite is

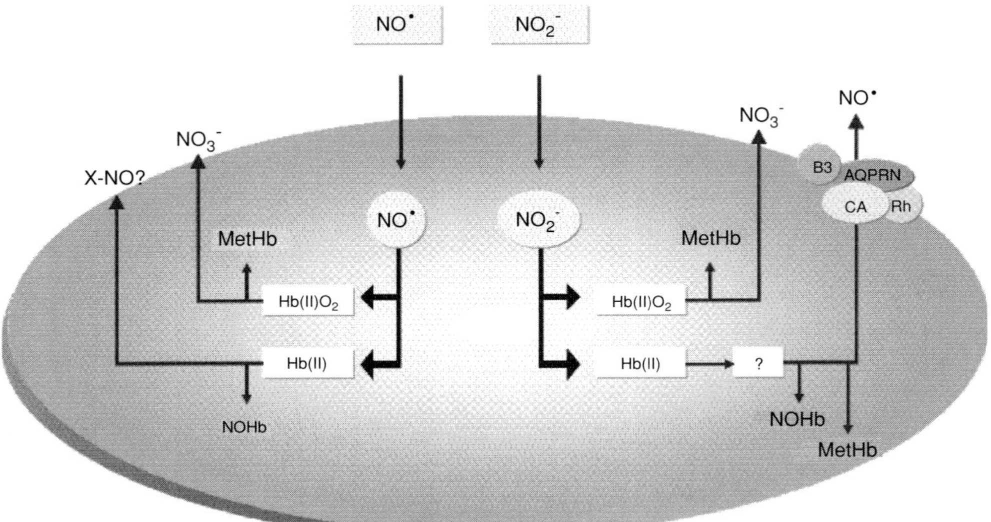

Figure 10.2. Reactions between NO and hemoglobin in erythrocytes. Nitric oxide (NO•), synthesized by the endothelium, or nitrite (NO_2^-) circulating in plasma, diffuses into the erythrocyte where it reacts with oxyhemoglobin [$Hb(II)O_2$] to yield methemoglobin (MetHb) and nitrate (NO_3^-), or with deoxyhemoglobin [Hb(II)] to generate nitrosylhemoglobin (NOHb) and NO adducts (X-NO). Nitrite also diffuses into the erythrocyte and reacts with deoxyhemoglobin and, via a possible intermediate species (?), produces nitrosylhemoglobin and methemoglobin. Once formed, NO• and NO• adducts are thought to exit the cell through a functional metabolon that is composed of oxy- and deoxyhemoglobin, Rh channels (Rh), aquaporin (AQPRN), band-3 complex (B3), and carbonic anhydrase (CA). These channels theoretically may transport NO• through the erythrocyte membrane. (See color plate 10.2.)

reduced by deoxygenated hemoglobin and that this reaction yields bioactive NO and methemoglobin.[39,54] In this construct, hemoglobin can be viewed as a nitrite reductase that mediates hypoxic vasodilation and in this way contributes to homeostatic regulation of tissue perfusion and O_2 delivery.[50] The reactions involved in this process are:

$$HONO + 2Hb(II) \rightarrow Hb(III) + Hb(II)NO + OH^- \quad (10.3)$$

$$Hb(II)NO \rightarrow Hb(II) + NO \quad (10.4)$$

Hb(II)NO can also transfer NO to glutathione to yield *S*-nitrosoglutathione. These reactions are further complicated by hemoglobin allostery, as indicated by their sigmoidal (rather than pseudo-first-order) kinetics when nitrite is in excess over hemoglobin,[55] and derives from the fact that the relaxed- (R-) state hemoglobin reduces nitrite faster than does tense- (T-) state hemoglobin. This allosteric dependence of the reaction coupled with its stoichiometry leads to accelerated kinetics as hemoglobin is converted from the R- to T-state during the reaction.[56] Consistent with an allosteric mechanism, hemoglobin-mediated nitrite reduction proceeds most rapidly at the hemoglobin P_{50} (where only half the hemoglobin is O_2 bound). At the P_{50}, the reduced rate of the reaction caused by fewer deoxygenated hemes being present than at zero O_2 is compensated for by the presence of more deoxygenated hemes in R-state hemoglobin tetramers.[56] Recent data suggest that NO dissociation from hemoglobin (Eq. 10.4) alone cannot account for an exportable pool of NO within the erythrocyte that can manifest bioactivity.[57] Either compartmentalization or a reaction intermediate (an S-nitrosothiol?) may provide a physiological explanation for the phenomenon, but neither mechanism has been proven to date.

Another hypothesis that has been advanced to explain the role of erythrocytic hemoglobin in NO bioactivity is that of *S*-nitrosation of its β-93 cysteinyl residue to form *S*-nitrosohemoglobin (SNO-Hb).[58] According to this view, NO binds allosterically to a deoxyheme moiety on a partially oxygenated hemoglobin tetramer, and is then transferred to the cysteinyl residue upon transition from the T- to the R-state with reoxygenation. Upon deoxygenation, the process is reversed with release of NO (possibly transferred to a protein or thiol-carrier), according to the following reaction mechanism:

$$Hb(II)NO + O_2 \rightarrow Hb(II)O_2^{cys93}SNO \quad (10.5)$$

$$Hb(II)O_2^{cys93}SNO \rightarrow Hb(II) + O_2 + NO \quad (10.6)$$

or

$$Hb(II)O_2^{cys93}SNO + GSH \rightarrow Hb(II) + O_2 + GSNO \quad (10.7)$$

Based on this hypothesis, NO is then exported from the cell as an "X-NO." The identity of the X-NO species and the mechanism of export have not been elucidated. Although this hypothesis received much attention when first proposed, it remains controversial, owing largely to published experimental data that reveal the preferential (if not exclusive) binding of NO to deoxygenated heme groups on

R-state hemoglobin,[59,60] an inability to detect cyclic transfer of NO from the heme group to the β-93 cysteinyl residue and vice versa,[61] and failure to determine the O_2 dependency of SNO-Hb instability in the presence of erythrocyte concentrations of glutathione (i.e., the S-NO linkage decays independent of O_2 tension in the presence of millimolar concentrations of glutathione). Most important, the high intracellular concentration of glutathione would limit the stability of the β-93 S-NO bond.[62] Thus, it is our opinion that the preponderance of data support the nitrite reductase hypothesis as the principal mechanism for the generation of bioactive NO by erythrocytes.

Nitrite Reductase Activity of Hemoglobin

Nitrite, a stable end-product formed by the oxidation of NO, is generated and/or accumulates in the blood, measurements of which in human plasma isolated from healthy volunteers demonstrate levels of approximately 0.20 ± 0.02 μmol/L.[34] Although nitrite itself does not possess intrinsic vasodilator properties at physiological concentrations, it may be considered an important vasodilator substance via its reduction to NO by the nitrite reductase activity of hemoglobin.

Evidence to support the role of hemoglobin-mediated nitrite reduction as a physiological source of NO was first demonstrated when Gladwin and colleagues[59] observed a plasma gradient of nitrite across vascular beds of human subjects under basal conditions and following the inhalation of NO gas. They next infused nitrite into the forearm brachial artery at near physiological levels (0.9–2.5 μmol/L) and noted an increase in blood flow as measured by strain gauge plethysmography.[39] When subjects were pretreated with L-N^G-monomethyl arginine citrate to inhibit eNOS and endogenous NO synthesis, infusion of near physiological levels of nitrite resulted in an increase in forearm blood flow during exercise. Nitrite infusion was associated with a detectable increase in erythrocyte Hb(II)NO that formed rapidly indicating that nitrite was being reduced to NO during one artery-to-vein transit in a manner that was inversely proportional to oxyhemoglobin saturation.[39] When NO gas production was measured by chemiluminescence, the rate of NO production following the addition of nitrite to erythrocytes was significantly greater when hemoglobin was in a deoxygenated than oxygenated state. The ability to measure NO gas production in this system demonstrated further that some fraction of the released NO escaped autocapture by free heme groups and that NO generation is augmented under anaerobic conditions, consistent with a nitrite–deoxyhemoglobin reaction.[39]

The bioactivity of NO generated by the reaction between nitrite and hemoglobin was confirmed in a rat aortic ring bioassay where it was demonstrated that this reaction was, indeed, responsible for the observed vasodilation. In these studies, the aortic rings were found to relax spontaneously only at very low O_2 tensions (10–15 mm Hg); however, in the presence of nitrite (0.5–2 μmol/L) and erythrocytes, the vessel tension–O_2 threshold curve was left-shifted to higher O_2 tensions (~40 mm Hg). This effect was mediated by the nitrite reductase activity of deoxygenated hemoglobin as oxygenated hemoglobin had no effect on vasodilation, even in the presence of excess nitrite. Together, these studies demonstrate that hemoglobin serves as a nitrite reductase under hypoxic conditions to release NO from nitrite and effect vasodilation.[50]

Nitric Oxide Export from Erythrocytes

Although the aforementioned studies convincingly demonstrate a role for hemoglobin as an effective nitrite reductase to generate bioavailable NO from nitrite, the mechanism by which NO is exported from the erythrocyte remains to be determined. As noted, the half-life of NO in the erythrocyte is estimated to be approximately 5 μs, suggesting that it is unlikely that NO itself freely diffuses across the erythrocyte membrane.[63] One proposed mechanism for NO export suggests that erythrocyte membrane proteins comprise a potential nitrite reductase metabolon containing deoxyhemoglobin and methemoglobin, anion exchange protein, carbonic anhydrase, aquaporin, and Rh channels that reside within the erythrocyte lipid raft, a caveola homolog. This metabolon would facilitate NO export by localizing nitrite, proton, and deoxyheme with highly hydrophobic channels at the membrane complex. Another proposed mechanism suggests that the reaction of nitrite with deoxyhemoglobin yields an intermediate species that could be stabilized by and transported through the red blood cell membrane (via lipid raft, Rh channels, or aquaporin); candidate species include *S*-nitrosothiols, nitrogen dioxide, peroxynitrite, and nitrated lipids.[63,64] Measurements obtained in simulation studies support the existence of a NO intermediate species. Here, when the rate of NO formation was as high as 100 nM/s, the maximal NO concentration in blood was less than 0.012 nM in the setting of erythrocyte membrane permeability to NO of 4.5 cm/s at a hematocrit of 45%. Thus, it is unlikely that NO is exported directly from the erythrocyte because the resident plasma concentration would be too low to have physiological effects.[65] At present, it remains to be determined which systems of export and candidate intermediate signaling molecule(s) are operative.

NITRIC OXIDE–DEPENDENT REGULATION OF TISSUE OXYGEN LEVELS

Nitric Oxide and Hemoglobin–Oxygen Affinity

By virtue of its reaction(s) with hemoglobin, it has been suggested that NO directly influences hemoglobin–O_2 affinity; however, it is difficult to predict a priori the effect of NO binding on net hemoglobin–O_2 affinity owing to the different hemoglobin species present at any given time that react with NO. For example, NO oxidizes oxyhemoglobin to form methemoglobin, which increases O_2 affinity,[66] although the reaction of NO with deoxyhemoglobin yields nitrosylhemoglobin, which has a markedly decreased affinity for O_2.[67] It has also been reported that when NO reacts with the β-Cys93 residue to form SNO-Hb, its O_2 affinity increases compared to underivatized hemoglobin.[68] As such, the overall net effect of NO on hemoglobin–O_2 affinity may result, in part, from the relative abundance of each of these NO-hemoglobin derivatives.

Despite the recognized differences in hemoglobin–O_2 affinity of these NO-hemoglobin products, evidence indicates that the reaction of NO and hemoglobin may not, in fact, significantly influence hemoglobin–O_2 affinity by a mechanism other than by increasing methemoglobin formation. In a study that examined the effect of NO gas (80 ppm) inhalation for 2 hours on hemoglobin–O_2 affinity, inhaled NO did not alter hemoglobin–O_2 affinity in normal subjects, and methemoglobin levels rose to only 1%, suggesting that the level of NO bound to hemoglobin was too low to influence overall O_2 affinity.[69] In vitro studies that exposed erythrocytes to NO gas (80 ppm) or the NO donors diethylamine NONOate and *S*-nitrosocysteine reported similar findings. Here, exposure to NO did not affect hemoglobin–O_2 affinity per se, but a significant rise in methemoglobin formation was detected that was associated with a leftward shift in the P_{50}.[70] These observations, therefore, imply that low concentrations of NO do not alter the hemoglobin–O_2 affinity of erythrocytes directly, and perceived changes likely result from an increase in methemoglobin formation and loss of cooperativity (Hill coefficient).[70,71]

Tissue Oxygen Consumption

The interaction between NO and O_2 is of physiological importance: NO has been shown to regulate tissue O_2 consumption and, conversely, O_2 levels may determine the rate of NO catabolism. Endothelium-derived NO limits tissue O_2 consumption, an effect that is independent of the rate of O_2 delivery and associated with a decrease in both intravascular and tissue pO_2 as well as a rightward shift in the hemoglobin–O_2 dissociation curve.[72]

Other studies have confirmed that endothelium-derived NO modulates tissue oxygenation by decreasing vessel wall O_2 consumption. Although it has been shown that the pO_2 drops in arterioles, the observed decreases were too great to be explained by diffusion alone suggesting active consumption of O_2 by the vessel wall. In a series of studies performed in vivo to examine the O_2 consumption rate of arteriolar walls in rat cremaster muscle, inhibition of NO synthesis with N^G-nitro-L-arginine methyl ester (L-NAME) resulted in a 42% increase in vessel wall O_2 consumption. In contrast, enhancement of flow-mediated NO release resulted in a 34% decrease in O_2 consumption by the vessel wall.[73] One explanation for these findings is that O_2 consumption by the arteriole wall is, in part, dependent upon vascular tone; vasoconstriction increases vessel wall O_2 consumption whereas vasodilation has the opposite effect.[74,75] Further study of this model during NO-dependent and NO-independent vasodilation revealed that the NO-mediated reduction in O_2 consumption resulted principally from a decrease in the mechanical work of vascular smooth muscle cells.[76]

Although the aforementioned studies demonstrate that NO regulates tissue and vessel wall O_2 consumption, it has also been demonstrated that O_2 determines vascular NO catabolism. Under normoxic conditions, rat aortas incubated in a solution injected with NO at constant O_2 tension demonstrated a 50% increase in NO consumption as compared to what was observed in the absence of the vessel. Furthermore, aorta NO consumption declined as the O_2 concentration was decreased to mimic hypoxic conditions, suggesting that mitochondria may be involved in the vessel wall interaction between O_2 and NO. This may result from the direct reaction of NO with O_2 in the mitochondrial membrane or with cytochrome *c* oxidase. In support of this theory, increased aorta NO consumption under anaerobic conditions was inhibited by the cytochrome *c* oxidase inhibitor sodium cyanide. These studies imply that decreased aorta NO catabolism that occurs under low O_2 concentrations may preserve bioavailable NO levels to promote vasodilation. In contrast, increased NO consumption observed under anaerobic conditions suggests that this phenomenon may limit formation or accumulation of toxic NO metabolites in the vessel wall.[77]

HYPOXIC VASODILATION

NO plays an integral role in hypoxic vasodilation, a physiological response that regulates blood flow to deliver O_2 and meet tissue metabolic demands. It has been hypothesized that this response results from a feedback mechanism that signals alterations in O_2 or pH levels resulting from a discordance between the basal delivery rate of O_2 and tissue O_2 consumption.[78] To ensure tissue O_2 demands in the setting of perceived hypoxia, vasodilator substances such as NO are released to increase blood flow and, thereby, maintain tissue oxygenation. In mammalian systems, hypoxic vasodilation occurs concomitant with the desaturation of hemoglobin from 60% to 40% corresponding to partial pressures of O_2 from 40 to 20 mm Hg.[64]

Interestingly, in skeletal muscle tissue O_2 extraction occurs mainly in resistance arterioles implying that hypoxic sensing takes place in the vasculature at a location proximal to the arterioles and arteriolar capillaries.[79] In this vascular bed, erythrocytes, which traverse the artery-to-arteriole-to-capillary in approximately 10 s, form a column of moving blood such that the hemoglobin and O_2 concentrations remain relatively constant at any given location within an arteriole.[64] As such, it is likely that there is one anatomical site within the microcirculation that contains the greatest number of R_3 tetramers with maximal nitrite reductase activity. It is at this anatomical location that hemoglobin-mediated nitrite reduction to release NO will be maximal in response to tissue O_2 consumption and metabolic demands, and hypoxic vasodilation will ensue.[64] In contrast, in the heart and brain, tissue O_2 is delivered via the capillary bed through a mechanism that involves retrograde signaling. Here, it is believed that the capillaries or venous circulation provide the vasodilator signal.[80,81] One proposed mechanism to explain vasodilation in these vascular beds involves the diffusional shunting of NO from veins to an adjacent arteriole. In fact, when cotransport of NO and O_2 in a paired arteriole-venule surrounded by capillary-perfused tissue was modeled, it was found that the capillary bed connecting the arteriole and venule facilitates the release of O_2 from the vessel pair to the surrounding tissue. In this model, decreasing the distance between the arteriole and venule resulted in a higher local NO concentration in the venule than in the arteriole wall, suggesting that transvalvular diffusional shunting of NO is plausible.[82]

Although the identity of the O_2 sensor and released vasodilator has not yet been confirmed definitively, evidence suggests that hemoglobin serves as the O_2 sensor and, owing to its nitrite reductase properties, reduces nitrite to release NO, the vasodilator. Hemoglobin is well poised to serve as the O_2 sensor; the O_2-linked allosteric structural transition from the R-state to the T-state may function to signal for release of NO from the erythrocyte.[83] NO as the candidate vasodilator agent to regulate hypoxic vasodilation is intuitively sound. NO is a paracrine-signaling molecule synthesized by the endothelium and released into the bloodstream where it reacts at a nearly diffusion-limited rate (10^7 M/s) with both oxy- and deoxyhemoglobin to yield methemoglobin/nitrite and iron-nitrosyl-hemoglobin, respectively. Although these reactions limit the half-life of NO in blood ($\sim$5 μs half-life in blood) as well as the diffusion distance ($<$2 μs in lysed blood),[50,84] from a biochemical perspective, the pool of circulating NO may be stabilized in blood by the formation of NO-modified proteins, peptides, and lipids or by oxidation to nitrite.[64] Nitrite, in turn, serves as a source of bioavailable NO under hypoxic or ischemic conditions.[85–88]

HOMEOSTATIC FUNCTIONS OF NO IN THE VASCULATURE

In addition to its reaction with erythrocytes, NO released to the vessel wall diffuses readily across biological membranes to modulate endothelial and vascular smooth muscle physiological functions. In this manner, NO is a key determinant of vascular tone, vascular permeability, and cell proliferation. Moreover, NO released to the erythrocyte-free zone nearest the endothelial monolayer encounters platelets and, as such, modulates platelet activation, adhesion, and aggregation. The key mechanisms by which NO regulates these processes to maintain normal endothelial cell and vessel wall phenotype are discussed later.

Vascular Tone

Continuous, low levels of NO released by the endothelium initiate relaxation of the underlying vascular smooth muscle cells and, thereby, determine vascular tone. The importance of NO in maintaining vascular tone is demonstrated in disease states characterized by decreased or increased bioavailable NO; inhibition of vascular NO synthesis by pharmacological agents or targeted gene disruption promotes vasoconstriction and hypertension, whereas overproduction of NO, as occurs in septic shock, leads to profound vasodilation and hypotension.[89–92]

Under basal conditions, endothelium-derived NO production is stimulated in response to a number of physiological biochemical factors including thrombin, adenosine diphosphate, serotonin, acetylcholine, and bradykinin, as well as physical forces, such as shear stress and cyclic strain. In addition, NO is generated in response to changes in O_2 tension (as discussed previously) and, thereby, autoregulates blood flow in both large vessels and the microcirculation. In this manner, NO is a determinant of both the state of vascular relaxation and the distribution of blood flow among multiple vascular beds concurrently.[93,94]

NO diffuses readily from the endothelium to adjacent vascular smooth muscle cells and binds to the heme-containing enzyme soluble guanylyl cyclase (Fig. 10.3).[95] Among heme-containing proteins, guanylyl cyclase is of interest because it selectively binds NO in preference to O_2, despite a greater affinity of heme for O_2 and higher concentrations of O_2 than NO in eukaryotic cells. This phenomenon has been resolved by the recent discovery that guanylyl cyclase lacks a distal pocket tyrosine or alternative hydrogen donor to bind O_2 and, therefore, selectively binds NO to activate the enzyme.[96] Once NO activates soluble guanylyl cyclase in vascular smooth muscle cells, there is an increase in cytosolic cGMP, and several signaling pathways converge to decrease intracellular Ca^{2+} stores and initiate vascular smooth muscle relaxation. For example, voltage-gated Ca^{2+} channels are inhibited to decrease intracellular Ca^{2+} flux, whereas protein kinase G I, which phosphorylates Ca^{2+}-dependent potassium channels, 1,4,5 inositol triphosphate receptor–associated cGMP kinase substrate, and phospholamban, is activated.[5,97,98] Phospholamban, in turn, activates sarcoplasmic reticulum adenosine triphosphatase to sequester Ca^{2+} in the sarcoplasmic reticulum and decrease further intracellular Ca^{2+} flux and limit formation of the Ca^{2+}-calmodulin-myosin light chain complex.[4] Activation of protein kinase G I also regulates myosin light chain phosphorylation state. Phosphorylation of myosin light chain at Ser19 by myosin light

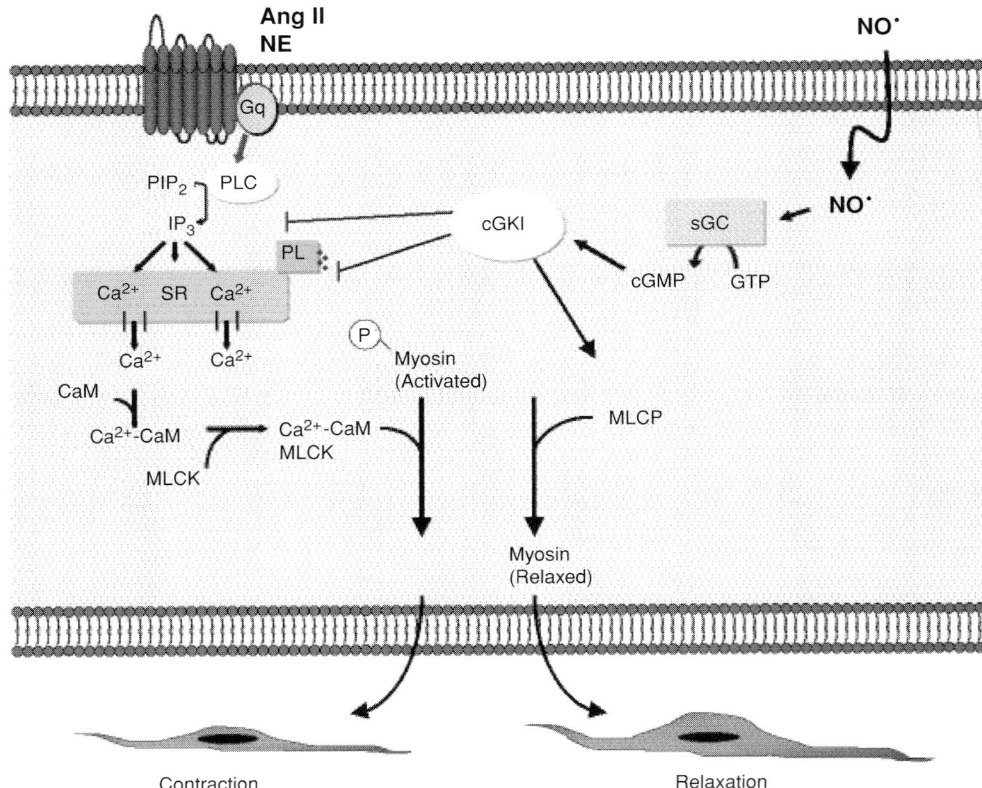

Figure 10.3. NO and vascular smooth muscle relaxation. NO•, synthesized by the endothelium, diffuses into the vascular smooth muscle cytosol and reacts with the heme iron of soluble guanylyl cyclase (sGC). This activates the enzyme, which in turn generates cGMP. As cGMP levels rise, cGMP-dependent kinase I (cGKI) is activated to inhibit inositol 1,4,5, trisphosphate (IP_3)-mediated release of Ca^{2+} from the sarcoplasmic reticulum (SR). cGKI activates phospholamban (PL), which facilitates this process by stimulating Ca^{2+} sequestration by the SR. This effect in turn also limits the ability of the Ca^{2+}-calmodulin (CaM)-myosin-light chain kinase (MLCK) complex to phosphorylate myosin and initiate contraction. cGKI also promotes vascular smooth muscle relaxation by stimulating myosin-light chain phosphatase (MLCP) to dephosphorylate myosin. (See color plate 10.3.)

chain kinase is required for actin activation of actomyosin ATPase and cross-bridge cycling.[99] Although there is no definitive evidence that protein kinase G I phosphorylates myosin light chain kinase directly to modulate its activity, protein kinase G I stimulates myosin light chain phosphatase, which dephosphorylates myosin and initiates vascular smooth muscle relaxation.[100]

Vascular Permeability

Traditionally, it is believed that NO is necessary to maintain endothelial barrier function and limit vascular permeability; however, a number of studies have challenged this tenet and provided compelling evidence to demonstrate that physiological levels of NO may actually increase microvascular permeability. The concept that NO is required to maintain endothelial barrier integrity is supported by electron microscopy analysis of vascular beds that demonstrated interendothelial junction opening and increased transendothelial transport of albumin in the setting of eNOS inhibition.[101] Moreover, when eNOS knockout mice were studied, open interendothelial junctions were observed in capillaries and venules, and there was enhanced leakage of a tracer agent indicating increased vascular permeability.[102] Conversely, other studies suggested that endothelium-derived NO is permissive for increased vascular permeability. NO donors have been shown to facilitate leakage of water and macromolecules across the endothelium, whereas eNOS inhibitors limit the edemagenic response to carrageenan and inflammatory mediators, including histamine, platelet-activating factor (PAF), and cytokines.[101,103] A number of theories have been advanced to explain these conflicting results, including differences in the agonists and models studied, methodology used to asses vascular permeability, heterogeneity of the microvascular beds, and the concomitant effect of NO as a vasodilator to increase local blood flow and, therefore, hydrostatic pressure.[101]

One potentially unifying explanation for these seemingly discordant observations suggests that vascular permeability and vasodilator agents differentially influence intracellular eNOS trafficking. This hypothesis was validated in ECV-304 (an immortalized endothelial cell line) cells stimulated with acetylcholine, which induces vasodilation with minimal effect on vascular permeability, or PAF, which promotes interendothelial junction opening with limited effect on vasodilation. In unstimulated cells, eNOS resides in association with caveolae and lipid rafts in the plasma membrane, where caveolin-1 binds eNOS to inhibit its activity.[103] In ECV-304 cells that were stably transfected with eNOS-GFP, acetylcholine stimulated translocation of eNOS from the caveolae to the Golgi network. In contrast, PAF administration resulted in translocation of eNOS to the cell cytosol. In the cytosol, eNOS was localized near mitogen-activated protein kinase, myosin light chain kinase, protein kinase C, and protein kinase G, all signaling molecules that are modulated by NO to enhance cytoskeletal contraction and cell junction disassembly.[104] A second mechanism by which eNOS translocation may influence endothelial cell permeability is by directly destabilizing the structural integrity of the endothelium.[105] As such, these findings suggest that PAF initiates an edemagenic response by trafficking eNOS to the cell cytosol to induce cytoskeletal conformational changes, whereas acetylcholine-mediated translocation to the Golgi apparatus localizes eNOS to a signaling cascade that favors vasodilation.

Endothelial Cell Proliferation, Migration, and Angiogenesis

Angiogenesis, a form of postnatal neovascularization in which new vessels are derived from preexisting blood vessels in response to tissue ischemia, is dependent on the coordinated processes of endothelial cell proliferation, migration, and tube formation. Experimental evidence confirms the central role of NO in these angiogenic processes. For example, augmentation of eNOS-generated NO production improved neovascularization in a rabbit hind limb ischemia model, whereas, in contrast, eNOS knockout mice demonstrate a limited angiogenic response to surgically induced hind limb ischemia compared with wild-type mice.[106] Furthermore, a number of proangiogenic factors, including vascular endothelial growth factor(s), platelet-derived growth factor(s), angiopoietins, and sphingosine-1-phosphate, all stimulate angiogenesis by increasing NO production.[107]

NO facilitates angiogenesis, in part, by enhancing endothelial cell proliferation. eNOS expression and activity are increased in proliferating cell cultures and reach a peak level at confluence, whereas gene transfer of eNOS promotes endothelial cell proliferation.[108,109] Other studies have shown that eNOS mRNA levels are fourfold higher and eNOS mRNA half-life is three times longer in proliferating compared with quiescent cells.[110] NO also stimulates endothelial cell migration, an effect that may be due to activation of podokinesis.[107] NO increases dissolution of the extracellular matrix via upregulation of urokinase-type plasminogen activator to initiate matrix metalloproteinase activation and dissolution of the extracellular matrix.[111] NO generated by the NO donor diethylamine NONOate has been shown to increase endothelial cell chemotaxis in a cGMP-dependent manner. Interestingly, the effect of NO on chemotaxis was found to be dependent upon the presence of a spatial NO subnanomolar gradient as well as the absolute magnitude of NO exposure per unit time to increase endothelial cell mobilization.[112]

Vascular endothelial growth factor (VEGF), one of the most potent angiogenic factors known, stimulates angiogenesis by increasing eNOS activity and NO production via PI3-kinase-Akt–mediated phosphorylation of eNOS, induction of Ca^{2+} flux, and the recruitment of heat shock protein 90.[113] VEGF has also been shown to increase eNOS expression and NO synthesis in endothelial cells and isolated rabbit thoracic aortic strips. In a tube formation assay, endothelial cells stimulated with VEGF transform from a monolayer to capillary tube–like structures concomitant with an increase in NO production. In contrast, when VEGF-stimulated cells are pretreated with L-NAME, capillary tube formation does not occur.[107]

Evidence suggests that soluble guanylyl cyclase may be an important downstream mediator of NO in angiogenic processes. In a chick chorioallantoic membrane angiogenesis assay, inhibition of endogenous guanylyl cyclase limited angiogenesis, whereas activation of guanylyl cyclase increased neovascularization. In cultured endothelial cells, pharmacologic activation, or gene transfer, of guanylyl cyclase increased endothelial cell proliferation, migration, and tube formation that was associated with extracellular signal–regulated kinase 1/2 and p38 MAPK signaling.[114] Interestingly, sildenafil, which inhibits cGMP-specific phosphodiesterase 5 to increase cGMP levels, also promotes endothelial cell proliferation, migration, and endothelial tube formation in a similar manner.[114]

Apoptosis

As an adjunct to angiogenesis, NO has been shown to have opposing, dose-dependent effects on endothelial cell apoptosis: low physiological concentrations of NO are cytoprotective, whereas markedly elevated levels of NO induce apoptosis.[115] Physiological levels of NO prevent endothelial cell apoptosis by the cGMP-dependent inhibition of cytochrome *c* release from mitochondria and downstream caspase activation, the cGMP-independent increase of bcl-2 expression, and the inactivation of caspases through *S*-nitrosation reactions.[116] The apoptosis-inducing effects of pathophysiologically elevated levels of NO in endothelial cells are cGMP-independent and include direct DNA damage by NO or peroxynitrite, activation of JNK/SAPK signaling pathways to stimulate caspases, and increased intracellular ceramide levels that induce the release of cytochrome *c*.[116]

Statins, which have been shown to promote angiogenesis via activation of eNOS, were also reported to initiate endothelial cell apoptosis owing to a concentration-dependent effect of these agents. For example, low doses of atorvastatin (0.01–0.1 μmol/L) were shown to enhance endothelial cell migration and tube formation, whereas higher concentrations (>0.1 μmol/L) stimulated endothelial cell apoptosis. These findings were attributed to the influence of statins on eNOS expression; low doses of statins did not influence eNOS expression whereas higher doses markedly increased eNOS expression and NO generation.[117]

NO has also been shown to modulate endothelial cell senescence, recognized as the limited ability of cells to proliferate in vitro accompanied by phenotypic changes in morphology, gene expression, and function. As such, cellular senescence is believed to contribute to the pathogenesis of vascular disease. Endothelial cell senescence, measured as senescence-associated β-galactosidase and telomerase activity, is inhibited in cells treated with the NO donor diethylamine NONOate or gene transfer of eNOS. In contrast, in cells treated with L-NAME, transfection with eNOS had no effect, indicating that endothelium-derived NO was essential to maintain the proliferating phenotype.[118]

Vascular Smooth Muscle Cell Proliferation

In contrast to its stimulatory effects on endothelial cell proliferation, endothelium-derived NO inhibits vascular smooth muscle cell proliferation to maintain the normal architecture of the vascular wall and preserve the vessel lumen. When the endothelium is injured, as occurs in vascular disease states such as atherosclerosis or mechanical disruption by angioplasty, the resultant decrease in bioavailable NO is permissive for vascular smooth muscle cell phenotype transition from a contractile state to a dedifferentiated synthetic phenotype. Once this phenotype transition occurs, vascular smooth muscle cells proliferate, migrate, and elaborate extracellular matrix proteins to fashion the neointima and thereby narrow the vessel lumen.

NO maintains a constant inhibition of vascular smooth muscle cell proliferation via cGMP-dependent and -independent signaling pathways. NO increases cAMP levels in a cGMP-dependent manner to activate protein kinase A and decrease intracellular Ca^{2+} stores; increased levels of intracellular Ca^{2+} have been shown to promote vascular smooth muscle proliferation.[119] Protein kinase A activation limits cell proliferation further by inhibiting Raf-1 activation of mitogen-activated protein kinase signaling cascades to decrease DNA synthesis, and studies performed in eNOS-transfected vascular smooth muscle cells demonstrate increased expression of the cyclin-dependent kinase inhibitor $p21^{waf1/Cip1}$, which inhibits proliferation.[120,121] Recently, it has been shown that cyclic nucleotide phosphodiesterases (PDE), which catalyze the hydrolysis of cGMP to 5′GMP, participate in the regulation of vascular smooth muscle cell proliferation. In quiescent cells in the contractile state, PDE1A is primarily localized in the cytoplasm of the cell, whereas in synthetic vascular smooth muscle cells PDE1A is translocated to the nucleus. The functional significance of PDE1A nuclear translocation was elucidated using siRNA to decrease PDE1A expression; increased cGMP levels were associated with $p27^{kip1}$ upregulation, cyclin D1 downregulation, and p53 activation to decrease proliferation and promote apoptosis.[122]

Similarly, NO inhibits vascular smooth muscle cell proliferation via a number of mechanisms that are cGMP-independent. For example, NO mediates two distinct cell cycle arrests; an immediate cGMP-independent block in S-phase followed by a shift back in the cell cycle from G_1–S to a quiescent G_0-like state.[123] NO also decreases the activity of arginase and ornithine decarboxylases, resulting in reduced formation of polyamines that are required for DNA synthesis and increased expression of $p21^{waf1/Cip1}$.[124,125] NO further increases $p21^{waf1/Cip1}$ expression by inhibition of the small GTPase RhoA by *S*-nitrosation.[126] Together, the divergent signaling pathways regulated by NO that converge to inhibit vascular smooth muscle cell proliferation highlight the importance of NO in maintaining the vascular smooth muscle cell contractile phenotype.

Platelet Adhesion and Aggregation

NO synthesized by the endothelium as well as by platelets importantly limits platelet adhesion, aggregation, and recruitment (Fig. 10.4). Although the formation of a hemostatic plug by platelets is a physiological response to vessel wall damage, platelet hyperreactivity, as occurs in NO-deficient states, results in pathophysiological arterial thrombosis. Under basal conditions, platelets remain in an inactive state that is regulated by NO, prostacyclin, and ecto-AD(T)Pase (CD39).[127] In the bloodstream, platelets circulate in the erythrocyte-free low-shear boundary near the endothelial surface and are in optimal position to be affected by endothelium-derived NO.[128] Platelets are also exposed to NO via a circulating pool of *S*-nitrosothiols; however, here, NO uptake is in part dependent on protein disulfide isomerase activity for *S*-nitrosothiol metabolism and transmembrane NO transfer.[129]

Once NO reaches the platelet cytosol, it activates soluble guanylyl cyclase to increase cGMP levels resulting in a decrease in intracellular Ca^{2+} flux and inhibition of platelet activation.[130] In resting platelets, intracellular Ca^{2+} levels are maintained between 50 and 100 nM by the collaborative actions of the cGMP-responsive sarcoplasmic reticulum ATPase and plasma membrane Ca^{2+} ATPase pumps.[131,132] NO also inhibits inositol-1,4,5-trisphosphate–induced intracellular Ca^{2+} release by stimulating cyclic GMP-dependent kinase to phosphorylate the inositol-1,4,5-trisphosphate receptor-associated cGMP kinase substrate (IRAG). IRAG is expressed in platelets and phosphorylated at Ser664 and Ser677 to negatively regulate inositol-1,4,5-trisphosphate-induced intracellular Ca^{2+} flux.[133] NO-dependent regulation of the intracellular Ca^{2+} flux limits the conformational change to the active state of the heterodimeric fibrinogen-binding integrin glycoprotein IIb/IIIa as well as decreases the number (by 50%) and

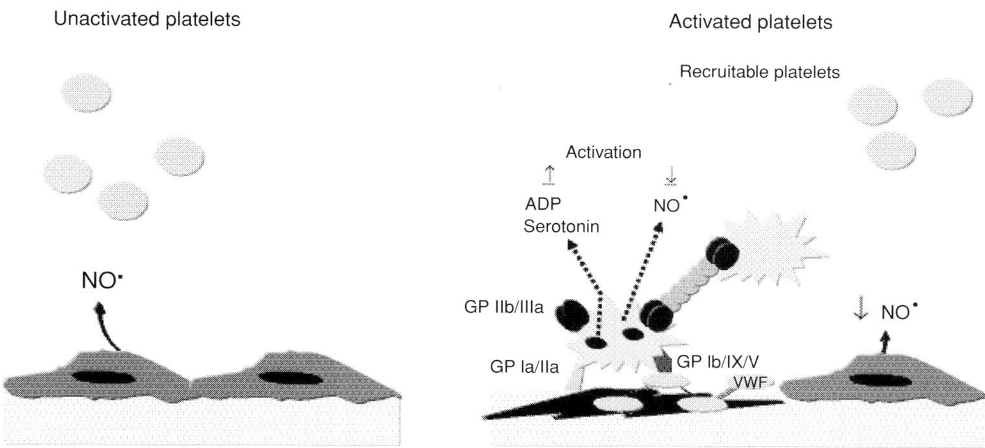

Figure 10.4. NO and platelet activation. Under basal conditions, the vascular endothelium elaborates NO• to maintain a nonthrombogenic surface. In contrast, when the endothelium is disrupted and NO• levels are decreased, platelets become activated and adhere to collagen via the cell surface receptor glycoprotein Ib/IIa (GP Ia/IIa) and glycoprotein Ib/IX/V (GP Ib/IX/V) that binds to the interstitium by von Willebrand factor (VWF). These activated platelets undergo shape change and release adenosine diphosphate (ADP) and serotonin to recruit and activate additional circulating platelets to the growing thrombus, and increase expression of the conformationally active fibrinogen receptor, glycoprotein IIb/IIIa (GP IIb/IIIa) to increase platelet aggregation and thrombus formation; the concomitant release of NO limits platelet aggregation. Platelet-derived NO limits recruitment of platelets to the growing platelet-rich hemostatic plug (or thrombus). (See color plate 10.4.)

the affinity (2.7-fold increase in K_d) of fibrinogen binding sites on the platelet surface.[134,135]

Another key component of platelet activation that is inhibited by NO is the exocytosis of platelet granules, which release mediators that modulate platelet interactions with the endothelium. Exocytosis is regulated, in part, by N-ethylmaleimide-sensitive factor (NSF), an ATPase that promotes disassembly of soluble NSF attachment protein–receptor complexes. In human platelets, it has been shown that NO inhibits exocytosis of dense, lysosomal, and α-granules by *S*-nitrosation of NSF. Furthermore, platelets isolated from an eNOS$^{-/-}$ mouse model demonstrate increased exocytosis in vivo.[136] In fact, it is this mechanism that may explain the observation that eNOS-deficient mice do not demonstrate enhanced thrombosis in vivo. In these mice, it was shown that fibrinolysis is enhanced owing to the lack of NO-dependent inhibition of the release of endothelial Weibel–Palade body storage granule contents, which include von Willebrand factor, P-selectin, and tissue plasminogen activator.[137,138]

NO donors have also been shown to inhibit platelet adhesion by interfering with the interaction between von Willebrand factor and glycoprotein IIb/IIIa.[139] In fact, an *S*-nitrosated derivative of the recombinant von Willebrand factor fragment, AR545C, has been shown to decrease platelet adhesion in both in vitro and in vivo studies. Furthermore, poly-*S*-nitrosated bovine serum albumin, an NO-releasing protein that increases platelet cGMP levels, has also been shown to limit platelet adhesion to collagen.[140]

In addition to the effects of endothelium-derived NO on platelet function, human platelets and megakaryoblastic cells express eNOS and synthesize NO.[141,142] NO release has been measured in resting platelets and reported to be approximately 11.2 pmol NO min/10^8 cells, suggesting that the amount of NO generated and released by platelets approaches that of endothelial cells.[143] Based on these observations, it is therefore important to note the relative contribution of endothelium-derived as compared to platelet-derived NO to platelet activation and aggregation. To examine this phenomenon, platelets were isolated from eNOS knockout mice or wild-type mice, and transfused into a thrombocytopenic eNOS knockout mouse model. In mice transfused with eNOS knockout platelets, bleeding time was decreased significantly compared to what was observed in mice transfused with wild-type platelets (Δ bleeding time $= 24.6 \pm 9$ s vs. 3.4 ± 5 s; $P < 0.04$), indicating that platelet-derived NO contributes significantly to limit platelet recruitment and thrombus formation.[144]

The importance of platelet-generated NO has also demonstrated in studies of patients with clinical atherothrombotic vascular disease. In 87 patients with symptomatic coronary artery disease referred for coronary angiography, platelets isolated from patients with acute coronary syndromes generated significantly less NO than those isolated from patients with stable angina (0.26 ± 0.05 pmol/10^8 platelets vs. 1.78 ± 0.36 pmol/10^8 platelets, $P = 0.0001$).[144] This finding suggests that platelet-derived NO, in addition to endothelium-derived NO, importantly modulates platelet function and thereby affects vascular disease risk.

Leukocyte Adhesion

Endothelium-derived NO also prevents leukocyte adhesion to the endothelium and transmigration into the vessel wall. NO donors, or endogenous NO, limit(s) leukocyte adherence to the endothelium, whereas inhibition of eNOS results in increased adhesion and emigration from the bloodstream.[145] Following exposure to cytokines such as interleukin (IL)-1β or TNFα, the endothelium is activated and expresses endothelial-leukocyte adhesion molecules including vascular cell adhesion molecule-1, E-selectin, P-selectin, and intercellular adhesion molecule-1.[146] In addition, activated endothelial cells produce leukocyte chemoattractants (chemokines), such as IL-8 and monocyte chemotactic protein-1. In this manner, activated endothelium both recruits and traps circulating leukocytes. NO regulates leukocyte chemotaxis by inhibiting expression of adhesion molecules and synthesis of chemoattractant proteins.[146,147] NO also inhibits exocytosis of Weibel–Palade bodies and release of P-selectin through *S*-nitrosylation of NSF.[148] NO limits leukocyte recruitment and adhesion further by decreasing the synthesis of IL-1β, TNFα, IL-6, and interferon-γ in lymphocytes and monocytes. These effects are mediated, in part, by *S*-nitrosation of transcription factors, including NF-KB/IkB and JAK/STAT, to inhibit upregulation of adhesion molecule expression.[149]

CONCLUSION

NO, a paracrine mediator of vascular homeostasis, is synthesized by the endothelium and released continuously to the vascular interstitium to regulate basal vascular tone. NO also diffuses into the bloodstream where it undergoes a complex series of reactions and may be oxidized to nitrite and nitrate, or react with redox metals and thiols to yield NO compounds, including dinitrosyl iron, *N*-nitrosamines, and *S*-nitrosothiols that have unique biological effects. Notably, NO also reacts with erythrocyte deoxy- and oxyhemoglobin to generate nitrosyl-hemoglobin or methemoglobin and nitrite, respectively. Moreover, owing to the nitrite reductase activity of hemoglobin, NO is released in the vasculature response to tissue ischemia and, thereby, modulates tissue O_2 consumption and hypoxic vasodilation. Endothelium-derived NO is also a key determinant of vascular permeability, endothelial and vascular smooth muscle cell proliferation and apoptosis, platelet adhesion and aggregation, as well as leukocyte recruitment and adhesion. As such, NO serves as an integral mediator of vessel wall integrity and vascular homoeostasis.

REFERENCES

1. Furchgott RF, Zawadzki JV. The obligatory role of endothelial cells in the relaxation of arterial smooth muscle by acetylcholine. *Nature.* 1980;288(5789):3736.
2. Ignarro LJ, Buga GM, Wood KS, Byrns RE, Chaudhuri G. Endothelium-derived relaxing factor produced and released from artery and vein is nitric oxide. *Proc Natl Acad Sci USA.* 1987;84(24):9265–9269.
3. Palmer RM, Ashton DS, Moncada S. Vascular endothelial cells synthesize nitric oxide from L-arginine. *Nature.* 1988;333(6174):664–666.
4. Cohen RA, Weisbrod RM, Gericke M, Yaghoubi M, Bierl C, Bolotina VM. Mechanism of nitric oxide-induced vasodilatation: refilling of intracellular stores by sarcoplasmic reticulum Ca2+ ATPase and inhibition of store-operated Ca2+ influx. *Circ Res.* 1999;84(2):210–219.
5. Bolotina VM, Najibi S, Palacino JJ, Pagano PJ, Cohen RA. Nitric oxide directly activates calcium-dependent potassium channels in vascular smooth muscle. *Nature.* 1994;368(6474): 850–853.
6. Feron O, Michel T. Cell and molecular biology of nitric oxide synthases. In: Loscalzo J, Vita JA, eds. *Nitric Oxide and the Cardiovascular System.* Totowa, NJ: Humana; 2000:11–31.
7. Bredt DS, Snyder SH. Nitric oxide: a physiologic messenger molecule. *Annu Rev Biochem.* 1994;63:175–195.
8. Michel T, Xie QW, Nathan C. Molecular biological analysis of nitric oxide synthases. In: Feelisch M, Stamler JS, eds. *Methods in Nitric Oxide Research.* Chichester, UK: Wiley; 1995:161–175.
9. Bredt DS, Snyder SH. Isolation of nitric oxide synthetase, a calmodulin-requiring enzyme. *Proc Natl Acad Sci USA.* 1990;87(2):682–685.
10. Dinerman JL, Lowenstein CJ, Snyder SH. Molecular mechanisms of nitric oxide regulation. Potential relevance to cardiovascular disease. *Circ Res.* 1993;73(2):217–222.
11. Minshall RD, Sessa WC, Stan RV, Anderson RG, Malik AB. Caveolin regulation of endothelial function. *Am J Physiol.* 2003;285(6):L1179–L1183.
12. Busse R, Mulsch A. Induction of nitric oxide synthase by cytokines in vascular smooth muscle cells. *FEBS Lett.* 1990; 275(1–2):87–90.
13. Xie QW, Cho HJ, Calaycay J, et al. Cloning and characterization of inducible nitric oxide synthase from mouse macrophages. *Science.* 1992;256(5054):225–228.
14. Welch G, Loscalzo J. Nitric oxide and the cardiovascular system. *J Cardiac Surg.* 1994;9(3):361–371.
15. Nathan CF, Hibbs JB Jr. Role of nitric oxide synthesis in macrophage antimicrobial activity. *Curr Opin Immunol.* 1991;3(1):65–70.
16. Wang BY, Ho HK, Lin PS, et al. Regression of atherosclerosis: role of nitric oxide and apoptosis. *Circulation.* 1999; 99(9):1236–1241.
17. Searles CD. Transcriptional and posttranscriptional regulation of endothelial nitric oxide synthase expression. *Am J Physiol Cell Physiol.* 2006;291(5):C803–C816.
18. Casas JP, Bautista LE, Humphries SE, Hingorani AD. Endothelial nitric oxide synthase genotype and ischemic heart disease: meta-analysis of 26 studies involving 23028 subjects. *Circulation.* 2004;109(11):1359–1365.
19. Paradossi U, Ciofini E, Clerico A, Botto N, Biagini A, Colombo MG. Endothelial function and carotid intima-media thickness in young healthy subjects among endothelial nitric oxide synthase Glu298–>Asp and T-786–>C polymorphisms. *Stroke.* 2004;35(6):1305–1309.
20. Rossi GP, Taddei S, Virdis A, et al. The T-786C and Glu298Asp polymorphisms of the endothelial nitric oxide gene affect the forearm blood flow responses of Caucasian hypertensive patients. *J Am Coll Cardiol.* 2003;41(6):938–945.

21. Chen W, Srinivasan SR, Elkasabany A, Ellsworth DL, Boerwinkle E, Berenson GS. Combined effects of endothelial nitric oxide synthase gene polymorphism (G894T) and insulin resistance status on blood pressure and familial risk of hypertension in young adults: the Bogalusa Heart Study. *Am J Hypertens.* 2001;14(10):1046–1052.
22. Chen W, Srinivasan SR, Bond MG, et al. Nitric oxide synthase gene polymorphism (G894T) influences arterial stiffness in adults: The Bogalusa Heart Study. *Am J Hypertens.* 2004;17(7):553–559.
23. Tesauro M, Thompson WC, Rogliani P, Qi L, Chaudhary PP, Moss J. Intracellular processing of endothelial nitric oxide synthase isoforms associated with differences in severity of cardiopulmonary diseases: cleavage of proteins with aspartate vs. glutamate at position 298. *Proc Natl Acad Sci USA.* 2000;97(6):2832–2835.
24. Rossi GP, Cesari M, Zanchetta M, et al. The T-786C endothelial nitric oxide synthase genotype is a novel risk factor for coronary artery disease in Caucasian patients of the GENICA study. *J Am Coll Cardiol.* 2003;41(6):930–937.
25. Rossi GP, Maiolino G, Zanchetta M, et al. The T(-786)C endothelial nitric oxide synthase genotype predicts cardiovascular mortality in high-risk patients. *J Am Coll Cardiol.* 2006;48(6):1166–1174.
26. Vargas AE, da Silva MA, Silla L, Chies JA. Polymorphisms of chemokine receptors and eNOS in Brazilian patients with sickle cell disease. *Tissue Antigens.* 2005;66(6):683–690.
27. Sharan K, Surrey S, Ballas S, et al. Association of T-786C eNOS gene polymorphism with increased susceptibility to acute chest syndrome in females with sickle cell disease. *Br J Haematol.* 2004;124(2):240–243.
28. Fatini C, Mannini L, Sticchi E, et al. eNOS gene affects red cell deformability: role of T-786C, G894T, and 4a/4b polymorphisms. *Clin Appl Thromb Hemostat.* 2005;11(4):481–488.
29. Stamler JS, Jaraki O, Osborne J, et al. Nitric oxide circulates in mammalian plasma primarily as an S-nitroso adduct of serum albumin. *Proc Natl Acad Sci USA.* 1992;89(16):7674–7677.
30. Loscalzo J. The biological chemistry of nitric oxide. In: Loscalzo J, Vita J, eds. *Nitric Oxide in the Cardiovascular System.* Totowa, NJ: Humana; 2000:3–10.
31. Rassaf T, Kleinbongard P, Preik M, et al. Plasma nitrosothiols contribute to the systemic vasodilator effects of intravenously applied NO: experimental and clinical Study on the fate of NO in human blood. *Circ Res.* 2002;91(6):470–477.
32. Feelisch M, Rassaf T, Mnaimneh S, et al. Concomitant S-, N-, and heme-nitros(yl)ation in biological tissues and fluids: implications for the fate of NO in vivo. *FASEB J.* 2002;16(13):1775–1785.
33. Butler AR, Flitney FW, Williams DL. NO, nitrosonium ions, nitroxide ions, nitrosothiols and iron-nitrosyls in biology: a chemist's perspective. *Trends Pharmacol Sci.* 1995;16(1):18–22.
34. Rassaf T, Bryan NS, Kelm M, Feelisch M. Concomitant presence of N-nitroso and S-nitroso proteins in human plasma. *Free Rad Biol Med.* 2002;33(11):1590–1596.
35. Rodriguez J, Maloney RE, Rassaf T, Bryan NS, Feelisch M. Chemical nature of nitric oxide storage forms in rat vascular tissue. *Proc Natl Acad Sci USA.* 2003;100(1):336–341.
36. Mordvintstev PI, Putintsev MD, Glalgan ME, Oranovskaia EV, Medvedov OS. Hypotensive activity of dinitrosyl complexes of iron and proteins in anesthetized animals. *Biull Vsesoiunzogo Kardiol Nauchn Tsentra AMN SSSR.* 1988;11:46–51
37. Kuznetsov VA, Mordvintstev PI, Dank EK, Iurkiv VA, Vanin AF. Low molecular weight and protein dinitrosyl complexes of non-heme iron as inhibitors of platelet aggregation. *Vopr Med Khim.* 1988;34:43–46.
38. Lauer T, Preik M, Rassaf T, et al. Plasma nitrite rather than nitrate reflects regional endothelial nitric oxide synthase activity but lacks intrinsic vasodilator action. *Proc Natl Acad Sci USA.* 2001;98(22):12814–12819.
39. Cosby K, Partovi KS, Crawford JH, et al. Nitrite reduction to nitric oxide by deoxyhemoglobin vasodilates the human circulation. *Nat Med.* 2003;9(12):1498–1505.
40. Zweier JL, Wang P, Samouilov A, Kuppusamy P. Enzyme-independent formation of nitric oxide in biological tissues. *Nat Med.* 1995;1(8):804–809.
41. Drabkin DR, Austin JH. Spectrophotometric studies. II. Preparations from washed blood cells/nitric oxide hemoglobin and sulfhemoglobin. *J Biol Chem.* 1935;112:51–65.
42. Cassoly R, Gibson Q. Conformation, co-operativity and ligand binding in human hemoglobin. *J Mol Biol.* 1975;91(3):301–313.
43. Kim-Shapiro DB. Hemoglobin-nitric oxide cooperativity: is NO the third respiratory ligand? *Free Rad Biol Med.* 2004;36(4):402–412.
44. Moore EG, Gibson QH. Cooperativity in the dissociation of nitric oxide from hemoglobin. *J Biol Chem.* 1976;251(9):2788–2794.
45. Sharma VS, Ranney HM. The dissociation of NO from nitrosylhemoglobin. *J Biol Chem.* 1978;253(18):6467–6472.
46. Doyle MP, Hoekstra JW. Oxidation of nitrogen oxides by bound dioxygen in hemoproteins. *J Organic Biochem.* 1981;14(4):351–358.
47. Herold S, Exner M, Nauser T. Kinetic and mechanistic studies of the NO*-mediated oxidation of oxymyoglobin and oxyhemoglobin. *Biochemistry.* 2001;40(11):3385–3395.
48. Liu X, Samouilov A, Lancaster JR Jr, Zweier JL. Nitric oxide uptake by erythrocytes is primarily limited by extracellular diffusion not membrane resistance. *J Biol Chem.* 2002;277(29):26194–26199.
49. Vaughn MW, Huang KT, Kuo L, Liao JC. Erythrocytes possess an intrinsic barrier to nitric oxide consumption. *J Biol Chem.* 2000;275(4):2342–2348.
50. Kim-Shapiro DB, Schechter AN, Gladwin MT. Unraveling the reactions of nitric oxide, nitrite, and hemoglobin in physiology and therapeutics. *Arterioscler Thromb Vasc Biol.* 2006;26(4):697–705.
51. Liao JC, Hein TW, Vaughn MW, Huang KT, Kuo L. Intravascular flow decreases erythrocyte consumption of nitric oxide. *Proc Natl Acad Sci USA.* 1999;96(15):8757–8761.
52. Li H, Samouilov A, Liu X, Zweier JL. Characterization of the magnitude and kinetics of xanthine oxidase-catalyzed nitrite reduction. Evaluation of its role in nitric oxide generation in anoxic tissues. *J Biol Chem.* 2001;276(27):24482–24489.
53. Lundberg JO, Weitzberg E. NO generation from nitrite and its role in vascular control. *Arterioscler Thromb Vasc Biol.* 2005;25(5):915–922.

54. Nagababu E, Ramasamy S, Abernethy DR, Rifkind JM. Active nitric oxide produced in the red cell under hypoxic conditions by deoxyhemoglobin-mediated nitrite reduction. *J Biol Chem.* 2003;278(47):46349–46356.
55. Huang KT, Keszler A, Patel N, et al. The reaction between nitrite and deoxyhemoglobin. Reassessment of reaction kinetics and stoichiometry. *J Biol Chem.* 2005;280(35):31126–31131.
56. Huang Z, Shiva S, Kim-Shapiro DB, et al. Enzymatic function of hemoglobin as a nitrite reductase that produces NO under allosteric control. *J Clin Invest.* 2005;115(8):2099–2107.
57. Jeffers A, Xu X, Huang KT, et al. Hemoglobin mediated nitrite activation of soluble guanylyl cyclase. *Comp Biochem Physiol.* 2005;142(2):130–135.
58. Stamler JS, Jia L, Eu JP, et al. Blood flow regulation by S-nitrosohemoglobin in the physiological oxygen gradient. *Science.* 1997;276(5321):2034–2037.
59. Gladwin MT, Ognibene FP, Pannell LK, et al. Relative role of heme nitrosylation and beta-cysteine 93 nitrosation in the transport and metabolism of nitric oxide by hemoglobin in the human circulation. *Proc Natl Acad Sci USA.* 2000;97(18):9943–9948.
60. Joshi MS, Ferguson TB Jr, Han TH, et al. Nitric oxide is consumed, rather than conserved, by reaction with oxyhemoglobin under physiological conditions. *Proc Natl Acad Sci USA.* 2002;99(16):10341–10346.
61. Huang KT, Azarov I, Basu S, Huang J, Kim-Shapiro DB. Lack of allosterically controlled intramolecular transfer of nitric oxide from the heme to cysteine in the beta subunit of hemoglobin. *Blood.* 2006;107(7):2602–2604.
62. Crawford JH, White CR, Patel RP. Vasoactivity of S-nitrosohemoglobin: role of oxygen, heme, and NO oxidation states. *Blood.* 2003;101(11):4408–4415.
63. Gladwin MT, Schechter AN, Kim-Shapiro DB, et al. The emerging biology of the nitrite anion. *Nat Chem Biol.* 2005;1(6):308–314.
64. Gladwin MT, Raat NJ, Shiva S, et al. Nitrite as a vascular endocrine nitric oxide reservoir that contributes to hypoxic signaling, cytoprotection, and vasodilation. *Am J Physiol Heart Circ Physiol.* 2006;291(5):H2026–H2035.
65. Liu X, Yan Q, Baskerville KL, Zweier JL. Estimation of nitric oxide concentration in blood for different rates of generation: evidence that intravascular nitric oxide levels are too low to exert physiological effects. *J Biol Chem.* 2007;282(12):8831–8833
66. Darling RC, Roughton FJW. The effect of methemoglobin on the equilibrium between oxygen and hemoglobin. *Am J Physiol.* 1942;137:56–68.
67. Yonetani T, Tsuneshige A, Zhou Y, Chen X. Electron paramagnetic resonance and oxygen binding studies of alpha-Nitrosyl hemoglobin. A novel oxygen carrier having no-assisted allosteric functions. *J Biol Chem.* 1998;273(32):20323–20333.
68. Bonaventura C, Ferruzzi G, Tesh S, Stevens RD. Effects of S-nitrosation on oxygen binding by normal and sickle cell hemoglobin. *J Biol Chem.* 1999;274(35):24742–24748.
69. Gladwin MT, Schechter AN, Shelhamer JH, et al. Inhaled nitric oxide augments nitric oxide transport on sickle cell hemoglobin without affecting oxygen affinity. *J Clin Invest.* 1999;104(7):937–945.
70. Hrinczenko BW, Alayash AI, Wink DA, Gladwin MT, Rodgers GP, Schechter AN. Effect of nitric oxide and nitric oxide donors on red blood cell oxygen transport. *Br J Haematol.* 2000;110(2):412–419.
71. Hrinczenko BW, Schechter AN, Wojtkowski TL, Pannell LK, Cashon RE, Alayash AI. Nitric oxide-mediated heme oxidation and selective beta-globin nitrosation of hemoglobin from normal and sickle erythrocytes. *Biochem Biophys Res Commun.* 2000;275(3):962–967.
72. Cabrales P, Tsai AG, Frangos JA, Intaglietta M. Role of endothelial nitric oxide in microvascular oxygen delivery and consumption. *Free Rad Biol Med.* 2005;39(9):1229–1237.
73. Shibata M, Ichioka S, Kamiya A. Nitric oxide modulates oxygen consumption by arteriolar walls in rat skeletal muscle. *Am J Physiol Heart Circ Physiol.* 2005;289(6):H2673–H2679.
74. Friesenecker B, Tsai AG, Dunser MW, et al. Oxygen distribution in microcirculation after arginine vasopressin-induced arteriolar vasoconstriction. *Am J Physiol Heart Circ Physiol.* 2004;287(4):H1792–H1800.
75. Hangai-Hoger N, Tsai AG, Friesenecker B, Cabrales P, Intaglietta M. Microvascular oxygen delivery and consumption following treatment with verapamil. *Am J Physiol Heart Circ Physiol.* 2005;288(4):H1515–H1520.
76. Shibata M, Qin K, Ichioka S, Kamiya A. Vascular wall energetics in arterioles during nitric oxide-dependent and -independent vasodilation. *J Appl Physiol.* 2006;100(6):1793–1798.
77. Liu X, Cheng C, Zorko N, Cronin S, Chen YR, Zweier JL. Biphasic modulation of vascular nitric oxide catabolism by oxygen. *Am J Physiol Heart Circ Physiol.* 2004;287(6):H2421–H2426.
78. Tune JD, Gorman MW, Feigl EO. Matching coronary blood flow to myocardial oxygen consumption. *J Appl Physiol.* 2004;97(1):404–415.
79. Tsai AG, Johnson PC, Intaglietta M. Oxygen gradients in the microcirculation. *Physiol Rev.* 2003;83(3):933–963.
80. Segal SS, Duling BR. Flow control among microvessels coordinated by intercellular conduction. *Science.* 1986;234(4778):868–870.
81. Segal SS, Duling BR. Communication between feed arteries and microvessels in hamster striated muscle: segmental vascular responses are functionally coordinated. *Circ Res.* 1986;59(3):283–290.
82. Chen X, Buerk DG, Barbee KA, Jaron D. A Model of NO/O(2) Transport in Capillary-perfused Tissue Containing an Arteriole and Venule Pair. *Ann Biomed Eng.* 2007;35(4):517–529.
83. Ellsworth ML, Forrester T, Ellis CG, Dietrich HH. The erythrocyte as a regulator of vascular tone. *Am J Physiol.* 1995;269(6 Pt 2):H2155–H2161.
84. Azarov I, Huang KT, Basu S, Gladwin MT, Hogg N, Kim-Shapiro DB. Nitric oxide scavenging by red blood cells as a function of hematocrit and oxygenation. *J Biol Chem.* 2005;280(47):39024–39032.
85. Webb A, Bond R, McLean P, Uppal R, Benjamin N, Ahluwalia A. Reduction of nitrite to nitric oxide during ischemia protects against myocardial ischemia-reperfusion damage. *Proc Natl Acad Sci USA.* 2004;101(37):13683–13688.
86. Duranski MR, Greer JJ, Dejam A, et al. Cytoprotective effects of nitrite during in vivo ischemia-reperfusion of the heart and liver. *J Clin Invest.* 2005;115(5):1232–1240.
87. Ng ES, Jourd'heuil D, McCord JM, et al. Enhanced S-nitroso-albumin formation from inhaled NO during ischemia/reperfusion. *Circ Res.* 2004;94(4):559–565.

88. Hataishi R, Rodrigues AC, Neilan TG, et al. Inhaled nitric oxide decreases infarction size and improves left ventricular function in a murine model of myocardial ischemia-reperfusion injury. *Am J Physiol Heart Circ Physiol.* 2006; 291(1):H379–H384.
89. Stamler JS, Loh E, Roddy MA, Currie KE, Creager MA. Nitric oxide regulates basal systemic and pulmonary vascular resistance in healthy humans. *Circulation.* 1994;89(5):2035–2040.
90. Huang PL, Huang Z, Mashimo H, et al. Hypertension in mice lacking the gene for endothelial nitric oxide synthase. *Nature.* 1995;377(6546):239–242.
91. Panza JA, Quyyumi AA, Brush JE Jr, Epstein SE. Abnormal endothelium-dependent vascular relaxation in patients with essential hypertension. *N Engl J Med.* 1990;323(1):22–27.
92. Kilbourn RG, Jubran A, Gross SS, et al. Reversal of endotoxin-mediated shock by NG-methyl-L-arginine, an inhibitor of nitric oxide synthesis. *Biochem Biophys Res Commun.* 1990;172(3):1132–1138.
93. Just A. Nitric oxide and renal autoregulation. *Kidney Blood Press Res.* 1997;20(3):201–204.
94. White RP, Vallance P, Markus HS. Effect of inhibition of nitric oxide synthase on dynamic cerebral autoregulation in humans. *Clin Sci (Lond).* 2000;99(6):555–560.
95. Horowitz A, Menice CB, Laporte R, Morgan KG. Mechanisms of smooth muscle contraction. *Physiol Rev.* 1996;76(4):967–1003.
96. Boon EM, Huang SH, Marletta MA. A molecular basis for NO selectivity in soluble guanylate cyclase. *Nat Chem Biol.* 2005;1(1):53–59.
97. Schlossmann J, Ammendola A, Ashman K, et al. Regulation of intracellular calcium by a signalling complex of IRAG, IP3 receptor and cGMP kinase Ibeta. *Nature.* 2000;404(6774): 197–201.
98. Cornwell TL, Pryzwansky KB, Wyatt TA, Lincoln TM. Regulation of sarcoplasmic reticulum protein phosphorylation by localized cyclic GMP-dependent protein kinase in vascular smooth muscle cells. *Mol Pharmacol.* 1991;40(6):923–931.
99. Somlyo AP, Somlyo AV. Signal transduction and regulation in smooth muscle. *Nature.* 1994;372(6503):231–236.
100. Surks HK, Mochizuki N, Kasai Y, et al. Regulation of myosin phosphatase by a specific interaction with cGMP-dependent protein kinase Ialpha. *Science.* 1999;286(5444):1583–1587.
101. Yuan SY. New insights into eNOS signaling in microvascular permeability. *Am J Physiol Heart Circ Physiol.* 2006; 291(3):H1029–H1031.
102. Predescu D, Predescu S, Shimizu J, Miyawaki-Shimizu K, Malik AB. Constitutive eNOS-derived nitric oxide is a determinant of endothelial junctional integrity. *Am J Physiol.* 2005;289(3):L371–L381.
103. Bucci M, Roviezzo F, Posadas I, et al. Endothelial nitric oxide synthase activation is critical for vascular leakage during acute inflammation in vivo. *Proc Natl Acad Sci USA.* 2005;102(3):904–908.
104. Sanchez FA, Savalia NB, Duran RG, Lal BK, Boric MP, Duran WN. Functional significance of differential eNOS translocation. *Am J Physiol Heart Circ Physiol.* 2006;291(3):H1058–H1064.
105. Schubert W, Frank PG, Woodman SE, et al. Microvascular hyperpermeability in caveolin-1 (-/-) knock-out mice. Treatment with a specific nitric-oxide synthase inhibitor, L-NAME, restores normal microvascular permeability in Cav-1 null mice. *J Biol Chem.* 2002;277(42):40091–40098.
106. Murohara T, Asahara T, Silver M, et al. Nitric oxide synthase modulates angiogenesis in response to tissue ischemia. *J Clin Invest.* 1998;101(11):2567–2578.
107. Cooke JP. NO and angiogenesis. *Atherosclerosis.* 2003;4(4):53–60.
108. Zollner S, Aberle S, Harvey SE, Polokoff MA, Rubanyi GM. Changes of endothelial nitric oxide synthase level and activity during endothelial cell proliferation. *Endothelium.* 2000;7(3):169–184.
109. Cooney R, Hynes SO, Sharif F, Howard L, O'Brien T. Effect of gene delivery of NOS isoforms on intimal hyperplasia and endothelial regeneration after balloon injury. *Gene Ther.* 2007:14:396–404.
110. Searles CD, Miwa Y, Harrison DG, Ramasamy S. Posttranscriptional regulation of endothelial nitric oxide synthase during cell growth. *Circ Res.* 1999;85(7):588–595.
111. Ziche M, Parenti A, Ledda F, et al. Nitric oxide promotes proliferation and plasminogen activator production by coronary venular endothelium through endogenous bFGF. *Circ Res.* 1997;80(6):845–852.
112. Isenberg JS, Ridnour LA, Thomas DD, Wink DA, Roberts DD, Espey MG. Guanylyl cyclase-dependent chemotaxis of endothelial cells in response to nitric oxide gradients. *Free Rad Biol Med.* 2006;40(6):1028–1033.
113. Brouet A, Sonveaux P, Dessy C, Balligand JL, Feron O. Hsp90 ensures the transition from the early Ca2+-dependent to the late phosphorylation-dependent activation of the endothelial nitric-oxide synthase in vascular endothelial growth factor-exposed endothelial cells. *J Biol Chem.* 2001; 276(35):32663–32669.
114. Pyriochou A, Zhou Z, Koika V, et al. The phosphodiesterase 5 inhibitor sildenafil stimulates angiogenesis through a protein kinase G/MAPK pathway. *J Cell Physiol.* 2007;211(1):197–204.
115. Shen YH, Wang XL, Wilcken DE. Nitric oxide induces and inhibits apoptosis through different pathways. *FEBS Lett.* 1998;433(1–2):125–131.
116. Walford G, Loscalzo J. Nitric oxide in vascular biology. *J Thromb Haemostat.* 2003;1(10):2112–2118.
117. Urbich C, Dernbach E, Zeiher AM, Dimmeler S. Double-edged role of statins in angiogenesis signaling. *Circ Res.* 2002;90(6):737–744.
118. Hayashi T, Matsui-Hirai H, Miyazaki-Akita A, et al. Endothelial cellular senescence is inhibited by nitric oxide: implications in atherosclerosis associated with menopause and diabetes. *Proc Natl Acad Sci USA.* 2006;103(45):17018–17023.
119. Cornwell TL, Arnold E, Boerth NJ, Lincoln TM. Inhibition of smooth muscle cell growth by nitric oxide and activation of cAMP-dependent protein kinase by cGMP. *Am J Physiol.* 1994;267(5 Pt 1):C1405–C1413.
120. Ciullo I, Diez-Roux G, Di Domenico M, Migliaccio A, Avvedimento EV. cAMP signaling selectively influences Ras effectors pathways. *Oncogene.* 2001;20(10):1186–1192.
121. D'Souza FM, Sparks RL, Chen H, Kadowitz PJ, Jeter JR Jr. Mechanism of eNOS gene transfer inhibition of vascular smooth muscle cell proliferation. *Am J Physiol Cell Physiol.* 2003;284(1):C191–C199.
122. Nagel DJ, Aizawa T, Jeon KI, et al. Role of nuclear Ca2+/calmodulin-stimulated phosphodiesterase 1A in vascular

smooth muscle cell growth and survival. *Circ Res.* 2006;98(6): 777–784.

123. Sarkar R, Gordon D, Stanley JC, Webb RC. Cell cycle effects of nitric oxide on vascular smooth muscle cells. *Am J Physiol.* 1997;272(4 Pt 2):H1810–H1818.
124. Ignarro LJ, Buga GM, Wei LH, Bauer PM, Wu G, del Soldato P. Role of the arginine-nitric oxide pathway in the regulation of vascular smooth muscle cell proliferation. *Proc Natl Acad Sci USA.* 2001;98(7):4202–4208.
125. Bauer PM, Buga GM, Ignarro LJ. Role of p42/p44 mitogen-activated-protein kinase and p21waf1/cip1 in the regulation of vascular smooth muscle cell proliferation by nitric oxide. *Proc Natl Acad Sci USA.* 2001;98(22):12802–12807.
126. Zuckerbraun BS, Stoyanovsky DA, Sengupta R, et al. Nitric oxide-induced inhibition of smooth muscle cell proliferation involves S-nitrosation and inactivation of RhoA. *Am J Physiol Cell Physiol.* 2007;292(2):C824–C831.
127. Battinelli EM, Loscalzo J. Nitric oxide and platelet-mediated hemostasis. In: Loscalzo J, Vita JA, eds. *Nitric Oxide and the Cardiovascular System.* Totowa, NJ: Humana; 2000:123–138.
128. Loscalzo J. Nitric oxide insufficiency, platelet activation, and arterial thrombosis. *Circ Res.* 2001;88(8):756–762.
129. Bell SE, Shah CM, Gordge MP. Protein disulphide-isomerase mediates delivery of nitric oxide redox derivatives into platelets. *Biochem J.* 2006;403(Pt 2):283–288.
130. Nakashima S, Tohmatsu T, Hattori H, Okano Y, Nozawa Y. Inhibitory action of cyclic GMP on secretion, polyphosphoinositide hydrolysis and calcium mobilization in thrombin-stimulated human platelets. *Biochem Biophys Res Commun.* 1986;135(3):1099–1104.
131. Redondo PC, Rosado JA, Pariente JA, Salido GM. Collaborative effect of SERCA and PMCA in cytosolic calcium homeostasis in human platelets. *J Physiol Biochem.* 2005;61(4):507–516.
132. Kroll MH, Schafer AI. Biochemical mechanisms of platelet activation. *Blood.* 1989;74(4):1181–1195.
133. Antl M, von Bruhl ML, Eiglsperger C, et al. IRAG mediates NO/cGMP-dependent inhibition of platelet aggregation and thrombus formation. *Blood.* 2007;109(2):552–559.
134. Michelson AD, Benoit SE, Furman MI, et al. Effects of nitric oxide/EDRF on platelet surface glycoproteins. *Am J Physiol.* 1996;270(5 Pt 2):H1640–H1648.
135. Mendelsohn ME, O'Neill S, George D, Loscalzo J. Inhibition of fibrinogen binding to human platelets by S-nitroso-N-acetylcysteine. *J Biol Chem.* 1990;265(31):19028–190234.
136. Morrell CN, Matsushita K, Chiles K, et al. Regulation of platelet granule exocytosis by S-nitrosylation. *Proc Natl Acad Sci USA.* 2005;102(10):3782–3787.
137. Iafrati MD, Vitseva O, Tanriverdi K, et al. Compensatory mechanisms influence hemostasis in setting of eNOS deficiency. *Am J Physiol Heart Circ Physiol.* 2005;288(4):H1627–H1632.
138. Matsushita K, Morrell CN, Cambien B, et al. Nitric oxide regulates exocytosis by S-nitrosylation of N-ethylmaleimide-sensitive factor. *Cell.* 2003;115(2):139–150.
139. Inbal A, Gurevitz O, Tamarin I, et al. Unique antiplatelet effects of a novel S-nitroso derivative of a recombinant fragment of von Willebrand factor, AR545C: in vitro and ex vivo inhibition of platelet function. *Blood.* 1999;94(5):1693–1700.
140. Marks DS, Vita JA, Folts JD, Keaney JF Jr, Welch GN, Loscalzo J. Inhibition of neointimal proliferation in rabbits after vascular injury by a single treatment with a protein adduct of nitric oxide. *J Clin Invest.* 1995;96(6):2630–2638.
141. Mehta JL, Chen LY, Kone BC, Mehta P, Turner P. Identification of constitutive and inducible forms of nitric oxide synthase in human platelets. *J Lab Clin Med.* 1995;125(3):370–377.
142. Sase K, Michel T. Expression of constitutive endothelial nitric oxide synthase in human blood platelets. *Life Sci.* 1995; 57(22):2049–2055.
143. Zhou Q, Hellermann GR, Solomonson LP. Nitric oxide release from resting human platelets. *Thromb Res.* 1995;77(1):87–96.
144. Freedman JE, Sauter R, Battinelli EM, et al. Deficient platelet-derived nitric oxide and enhanced hemostasis in mice lacking the NOSIII gene. *Circ Res.* 1999;84(12):1416–14121.
145. Kubes P, Suzuki M, Granger DN. Nitric oxide: an endogenous modulator of leukocyte adhesion. *Proc Natl Acad Sci USA.* 1991;88(11):4651–4655.
146. Tailor A, Granger DN. Role of adhesion molecules in vascular regulation and damage. *Curr Hypertens Rep.* 2000;2(1):78–83.
147. Hickey MJ, Kubes P. Role of nitric oxide in regulation of leucocyte-endothelial cell interactions. *Exp Physiol.* 1997; 82(2):339–348.
148. Wallace JL. Nitric oxide as a regulator of inflammatory processes. *Memorias do Instituto Oswaldo Cruz.* 2005;100 (Suppl 1):5–9.
149. Guzik TJ, Korbut R, Adamek-Guzik T. Nitric oxide and superoxide in inflammation and immune regulation. *J Physiol Pharmacol.* 2003;54(4):469–487.

11

Mechanisms and Clinical Complications of Hemolysis in Sickle Cell Disease and Thalassemia

Gregory J. Kato and Mark T. Gladwin

OVERVIEW OF HEMOLYSIS IN SICKLE CELL DISEASE AND THALASSEMIA

Anemia is the most basic clinical characteristic of sickle cell disease and thalassemia. In sickle cell disease, the polymerization of sickle hemoglobin (HbS) causes profound changes in the integrity and viability of the erythrocyte, leading to both extravascular and intravascular hemolysis. The lifespan of the erythrocyte in sickle cell disease is often shortened to less than one-tenth of normal. In β-thalassemia intermedia and major, but not in sickle cell disease, a substantial portion of the hemolysis occurs in the intramedullary space before the developing erythrocytes can even exit the bone marrow, referred to as ineffective erythropoiesis. In either case, erythropoiesis is markedly increased, but insufficient to compensate completely for the accelerated hemolysis, resulting in chronic anemia. This chapter examines the mechanisms that give rise to the accelerated hemolysis characteristic of these hemoglobinopathies and considers emerging data suggesting that chronic intravascular hemolysis produces endothelial dysfunction and a progressive vasculopathy. The latter mechanism of disease contributes to a clinical subphenotype of complications shared by many of the hemolytic anemias, including pulmonary arterial hypertension, cutaneous leg ulceration, priapism, and perhaps stroke. The mechanisms and consequences of hemolysis differ by two main anatomical compartments: extravascular hemolysis, which primarily involves phagocytosis by macrophages in the reticuloendothelial system, and intravascular hemolysis, which occurs within the blood vessel lumen.

Approximately two-thirds of hemolysis in sickle cell disease is extravascular and one-third intravascular.[1] Extravascular hemolysis occurs primarily through mechanisms involving cell surface phosphatidylserine exposure, adherent immunoglobulin G (IgG) and splenic entrapment of rigid red cells. Intravascular hemolysis decompartmentalizes the red cell contents into blood plasma, releasing hemoglobin, arginase-1, erythroid isoforms of lactate dehydrogenase (LDH), and other intraerythrocytic enzymes. In sickle cell disease, the development of irreversibly sickled cells (ISCs), and oxidative injury to red cell membrane proteins and lipids are believed to contribute to intravascular hemolysis (Chapter 9).

Irreversibly Sickled Cells

Aging sickle erythrocytes become increasingly dense and noncompliant.[2] Dehydration of the red cell (Chapter 9) involves leakage of intracellular potassium and sodium, and dysfunction of K:Cl cotransport and calcium-dependent potassium transport. This loss of solute and water increases the mean corpuscular hemoglobin concentration (MCHC), which promotes HbS polymerization (Chapter 6) (Fig. 11.1).[3] This effect can be inhibited by the coinheritance of α thalassemia which decreases the MCHC, or increased fetal hemoglobin (HbF) levels, which inhibits HbS polymerization.[4] Cycles of polymerization and depolymerization give rise to ISCs.[5]

ISCs cells are rigid and prone to being removed from the circulation by physical entrapment in the microvasculature, including peripheral blood vessels and the spleen, where presumably the lysis occurs.[6] The ISC has a short survival and its numbers reflect the hemolytic rate.[7,8] In fact, the severity of hemolysis correlates with the extent of HbS polymerization, as estimated from the MCHC and the relative proportion of hemoglobin fractions.[9,10] Following red cell dehydration and polymerization of HbS, the formation of ISCs involves oxidation of erythrocyte components, and loss of aminophospholipid asymmetry, with subsequent binding of IgG or complement.

Oxidation of Erythrocyte Proteins and Lipids

In sickle erythrocytes, oxygen radicals are formed at rates twice that of control erythrocytes, and membrane-bound hemichrome (oxidized hemoglobin precipitates) greatly enhances superoxide and peroxide-driven hydroxyl radical generation (Fig. 11.1).[11] Data from many laboratories suggest that in sickle cell disease the red cell is exposed to high levels of superoxide produced by intravascular enzymes such as xanthine oxidase,[12] nicotinamide adenine dinucleotide phosphate (NADPH) oxidase[13] and uncoupled nitric oxide (NO) synthase.[14] Signs of oxidative injury are seen in the cytoplasm and membrane of the red cell, in association with membrane bound iron.[15,16] The sickle erythrocyte membrane has reduced abundance of reduced sulfhydryl groups and increased lipid peroxidation.[17–21] Cytoskeletal proteins, particularly protein 4.1, are also oxidized.[22,23] These oxidative changes in the red cell cytoskeleton appear to contribute to the development of ISCs

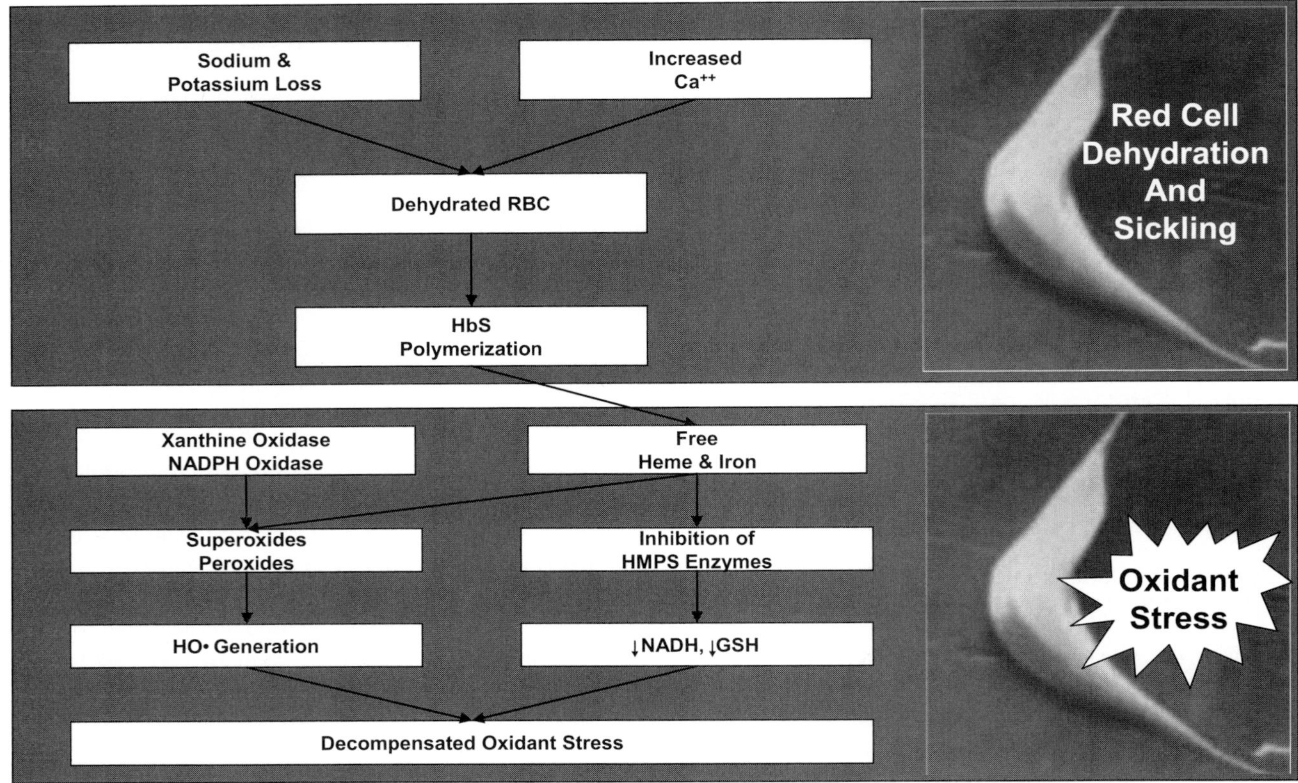

Figure 11.1. Factors leading to sickling and oxidant stress in erythrocytes in sickle cell disease. Solute loss and increased intracellular calcium promote red cell dehydration, which raises the intracellular concentration of sickle hemoglobin. This promotes polymerization of sickle hemoglobin, which is associated with generation of increased levels of oxidant species and depletion of cellular antioxidants, leading to a heightened state of oxidative stress. Each of these steps is described in the text, although the exact sequence of these events is somewhat speculative. (See color plate 11.1.)

(Fig. 11.2),[24] as the red cell membrane ghosts and the cytoskeletons of ISCs remain deformed after removal of hemoglobin.[24,25] Oxidation-induced defects in β-actin and spectrin appear to slow the dissociation of their ternary complex with protein 4.1. In ISCs, formation of a disulfide bridge is favored in β-actin involving cysteines at the 284 and 373 positions.[24]

The intense oxidative stress places high demands on metabolic pathways that provide compensatory reducing capacity in the red cell, such as the hexose monophosphate shunt, which produces NADH and reduced glutathione (Fig. 11.1).[26,27] The enzymes in these pathways are inhibited by the excess free heme present in sickle[11] and thalassemic red cells.[28] As glutathione becomes oxidized, identified by a high ratio of oxidized to reduced glutathione or as a low level of total glutathione,[11,29–31] cysteine residues in α-spectrin become glutathiolated.[24] This blocks the normal ubiquitin-conjugating and ligating activity of α-spectrin, impairing its autoubiquitination in sickle erythrocytes.[32,33] The lack of ubiquitination prevents normal dissociation of α-spectrin and protein 4.1, diminishing erythrocyte cytoskeletal flexibility and contributing to the rigid shape of the ISC.[34]

Consistent with a role for oxidative stress in ISC formation, the reducing agent N-acetylcysteine in vitro can convert ISCs into biconcave discs.[35] A pilot trial of N-acetylcysteine in 16 patients with sickle cell disease did not, however, produce a significant change in the hemoglobin level or reticulocyte count, despite achieving higher erythrocyte glutathione levels and a lower percentage of ISCs at the highest dose tested.[36] This suggests that the mechanisms of hemolysis are not solely related to erythrocyte shape. Some investigators have found deficiency of the naturally occurring antioxidant vitamin E in patients with sickle cell disease or thalassemia,[37–39] although this has been inconsistent.[40] Pilot studies have suggested that vitamin E supplementation may reduce hemolysis in sickle cell disease.[41,42] Future approaches will likely attempt to inhibit extracellular sources of reactive oxygen species, including xanthine oxidase, NADPH oxidase, and uncoupled endothelial NO synthase.

Membrane Phospholipid Asymmetry

In erythrocytes and other cell types, active mechanisms maintain asymmetry of membrane phospholipids. Over

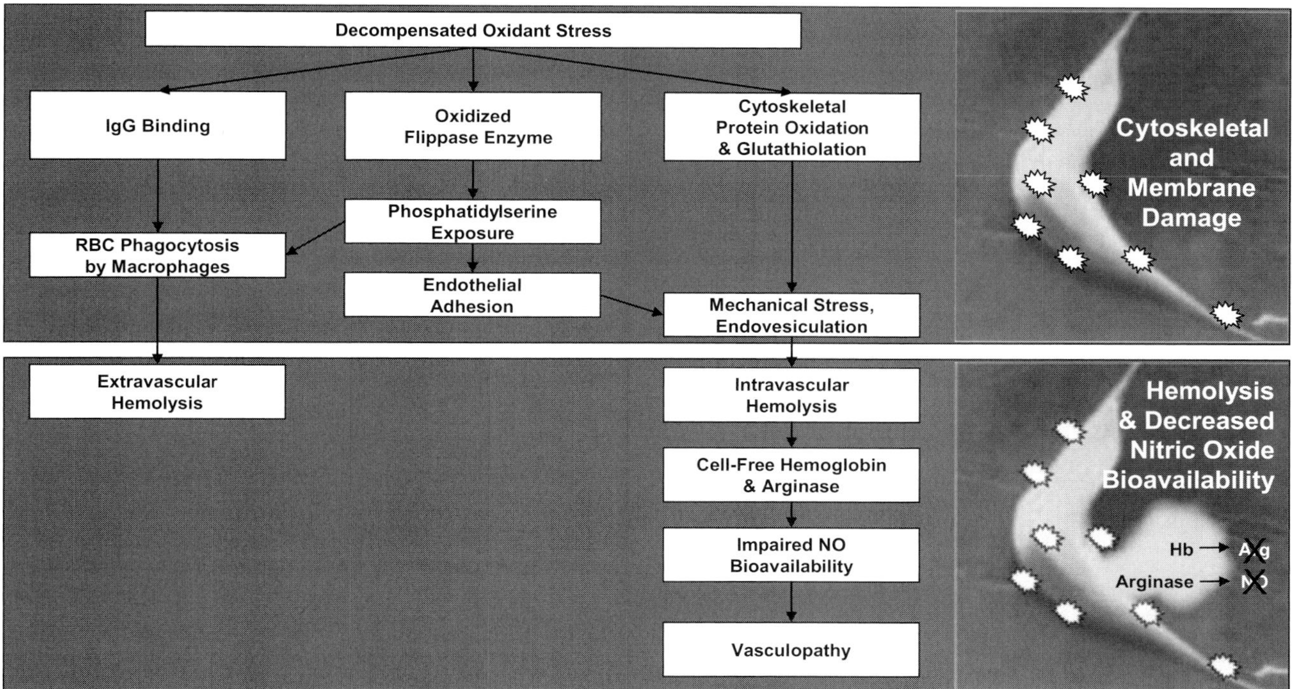

Figure 11.2. Factors promoting hemolysis in sickle cell disease. Decompensated oxidative stress in the sickle erythrocyte is associated with multiple lesions in its cytoskeleton and membrane. These lesions are responsible for binding of immunoglobulin to the membrane, promoting Fc receptor–mediated endocytosis of the damaged red cell by reticuloendothelial macrophages, considered extravascular hemolysis. Oxidative damage to the flippase enzyme is proposed to cause externalization of phosphatidylserine and phosphatidylethanolamine that also stimulate uptake of the red cell by macrophages, in addition to adhesion to endothelium. Oxidative damage and glutathiolation of the cytoskeleton can trigger endovesiculation of the membrane and release of membrane microparticles, and mechanical fragility of the damaged red cell. These latter events tend to produce intravascular hemolysis, resulting in the decompartmentalization of erythrocyte contents into plasma. (See color plate 11.2.)

75% of cellular phosphatidylcholine and sphingomyelin normally are maintained in the outer leaflet of the red cell membrane, whereas more than 80% of total phosphatidylserine and phosphatidylethanolamine are maintained in the inner leaflet (Chapter 9). This is accomplished by adenosinetriphosphate (ATP)–dependent aminophospholipid translocase, or flipase, which actively transports phosphatidylserine and phosphatidylethanolamine from the outer to the inner monolayer. Flippase can become dysfunctional with hypoxia-induced sickling (Fig. 11.2).[43,44] The mechanism of flippase inactivation in murine sickle cells involves its oxidation,[45] although this has not been confirmed in human sickle cells.[46] Inactivation of flipase permits phosphatidylserine exposure on the outer leaflet of the red cell membrane.[47]

Phosphatidylserine and phosphatidylethanolamine also are transported actively to the outer leaflet by activation of a Ca^{2+}-dependent scramblase. With increased Ca^{2+} flux, this scramblase can become activated, resulting in abundant phosphatidylserine exposure on the red cell surface in sickle cell disease and β thalassemia.[48] Thus Ca^{2+} flux and accumulated oxidant stress may both play a role in red cell aging and destruction, mediated though phosphatidylserine exposure.[49]

Cytoskeletal abnormalities in sickled cells, particularly spiculation, also appear to promote localized membrane phospholipid asymmetry.[50–52] Similar localized phospholipid asymmetry occurs at sites of Heinz bodies.[53] Reticuloendothelial system macrophages bind to and engulf these phosphatidylserine-externalized red cells, contributing to extravascular hemolysis (Fig. 11.2).[45,54] Phosphatidylserine exposure also induces binding of red cells to endothelial cells,[55–57] likely leading to sequestration of phosphatidylserine-exposing cells in peripheral blood vessels. Other mechanisms also induce adhesion of young sickled cells to endothelial cells. Immobilization of ISCs in flowing blood onto vascular endothelium may lead to increased shear stress and intravascular hemolysis (Chapter 8).

Fragility of ISCs to Mechanical and Shear Stress

The numbers of circulating ISCs decreases during the latter stages of vasoocclusive crisis, suggesting that the rigid, adhesive red cells might become sequestered in the microvasculature.[58,59] ISCs are also implicated in intravascular hemolysis during mechanical membrane fragmentation. Repeated cycles of sickling in vitro generate dehydrated red cells with membrane spiculation apparent on electron microscopy, which appear to give rise to spectrin-free, hemoglobin-containing microparticles.[60,61] Increased mechanical fragility of sickle erythrocytes has been documented in vitro by increased lysis with application of shear stress, and confirmed in vivo with the increased shear stress due to exercise-induced increase in blood flow.[62] Cell fractionation experiments indicate that the dense, dehydrated sickle erythrocytes are the most sensitive to mechanical or shear-induced hemolysis[62–66] and that rehydration restores resistance to shear stress, except in the densest red cells.[62] The membrane structure of ISCs is weakened and may contribute to intravascular fragmentation (Fig. 11.2).[67] Mechanical stress also induces hemoglobin denaturation and loss of hemin, which contributes to oxidative stress.[68] ISCs may be the most sensitive circulating red cells to this mechanical lysis induced by shear stress.

Adherent Immunoglobulin G

A subpopulation of erythrocytes in sickle cell disease binds IgG.[20,69–71] Cyclic oxygenation-deoxygenation, or oxidant stress in sickle cell disease, indicated by malondialdehyde production stimulates binding of IgG to the red cell surface.[20,72] Part or all of this effect may be related to Heinz bodies, oxidatively denatured hemoglobin, which generates a hemichrome that cross-links the major red cell membrane spanning protein, band-3.[73] A cryptic antigen exposed on the clustered band-3 complexes on the erythrocyte surface is recognized and bound by specific IgG antibodies, which in turn bind avidly to the Fc receptors on reticuloendothelial system macrophages.[74,75] This culminates in phagocytosis and lysis of the antibody-coated sickle erythrocytes by macrophages, a normal consequence of aging of red cells that is accelerated in sickle cells (Fig. 11.2).[72] This Fc receptor–mediated mechanism is a second significant contributor to oxidant stress-related, extravascular hemolysis in sickle cell disease.

Complement-mediated Hemolysis

Sickle cells are particularly sensitive to attack by complement-inducing intravascular hemolysis. Similar to erythrocytes in paroxysmal nocturnal hemoglobinuria, sickle cells show a defect in activity of the membrane attack complex, C5b-9.[76] This occurs due to increased binding of complement C5b-7 and C9 to sickle cells, particularly to the densest cells. This binding leads to C5b-9-mediated lysis initiated by C5b-6, especially on ISCs. Because it has been found that anionic lipids on the surface of the red cell can induce binding of C5b-6,[77] it is possible this binding occurs via the increased phosphatidylserine exposure that has been described on the outer membrane of the sickle and thalassemic erythrocyte.[45,78–84]

Clinical Consequences of Extravascular Hemolysis

Chronic extravascular hemolytic anemias in general are associated with the gradual development of splenomegaly that occurs frequently in patients with β-thalassemia intermedia and major. Although most adults and older children with sickle cell anemia have functional asplenia and splenic atrophy due to chronic subclinical splenic infarction, there are cases of sickle cell disease in which splenomegaly is present. These include young children homozygous for the HbS gene and patients with clinically milder sickling syndromes such as HbSC disease and HbS-β^+ thalassemia.[85,86] Patients with splenomegaly and sickle cell disease or β thalassemia often are more anemic than similar patients without splenomegaly, presumably due to chronic hypersplenism.[87,88] In some of these cases, chronic hypersplenism has been documented by improvement in anemia following splenectomy.[89,90]

CLEARANCE OF HEMOGLOBIN

Extracellular hemoglobin is toxic to vascular health, and humans have developed multiple redundant pathways to facilitate its rapid clearance.[91] During intravascular hemolysis, large amounts of hemoglobin are released from the lysed red cells into plasma. During extravascular hemolysis, the red cell is engulfed by a reticuloendothelial macrophage, and hemoglobin is degraded directly in the macrophage, releasing small amounts of hemoglobin into plasma. Upon its dilution into plasma, the hemoglobin tetramers decompose into αβ dimers. Dimeric hemoglobin rapidly forms complexes with the soluble plasma protein haptoglobin, the principal hemoglobin scavenging protein, which prevents hemoglobin from crossing the glomerular membrane. Upon formation of the complex, haptoglobin displays a previously hidden binding site for its cognate receptor on macrophages, CD163, the hemoglobin scavenger receptor (Fig. 11.3).[92] This high-affinity binding promotes endocytosis of the CD163-haptoglobin-hemoglobin complex, where it is degraded, disposing of the hemoglobin and along with it, haptoglobin, which is not recycled. Even with the lower-grade hemolysis seen in HbSC disease, serum haptoglobin levels are low. During the robust hemolysis of sickle cell anemia or β-thalassemia intermedia, haptoglobin is completely depleted from plasma. Thus, an undetectable plasma haptoglobin clinically signifies high-level hemolysis and pathophysiologically indicates that the primary, rapid mechanism for hemoglobin clearance has become saturated. The binding capacity of haptoglobin to hemoglobin is reported to be 0.07–0.15 g/dL, depending on different genetic variants of haptoglobin.

Hemopexin plays a complementary role, clearing plasma of free heme. Plasma hemoglobin that becomes oxidized to methemoglobin is prone to lose the oxidized heme

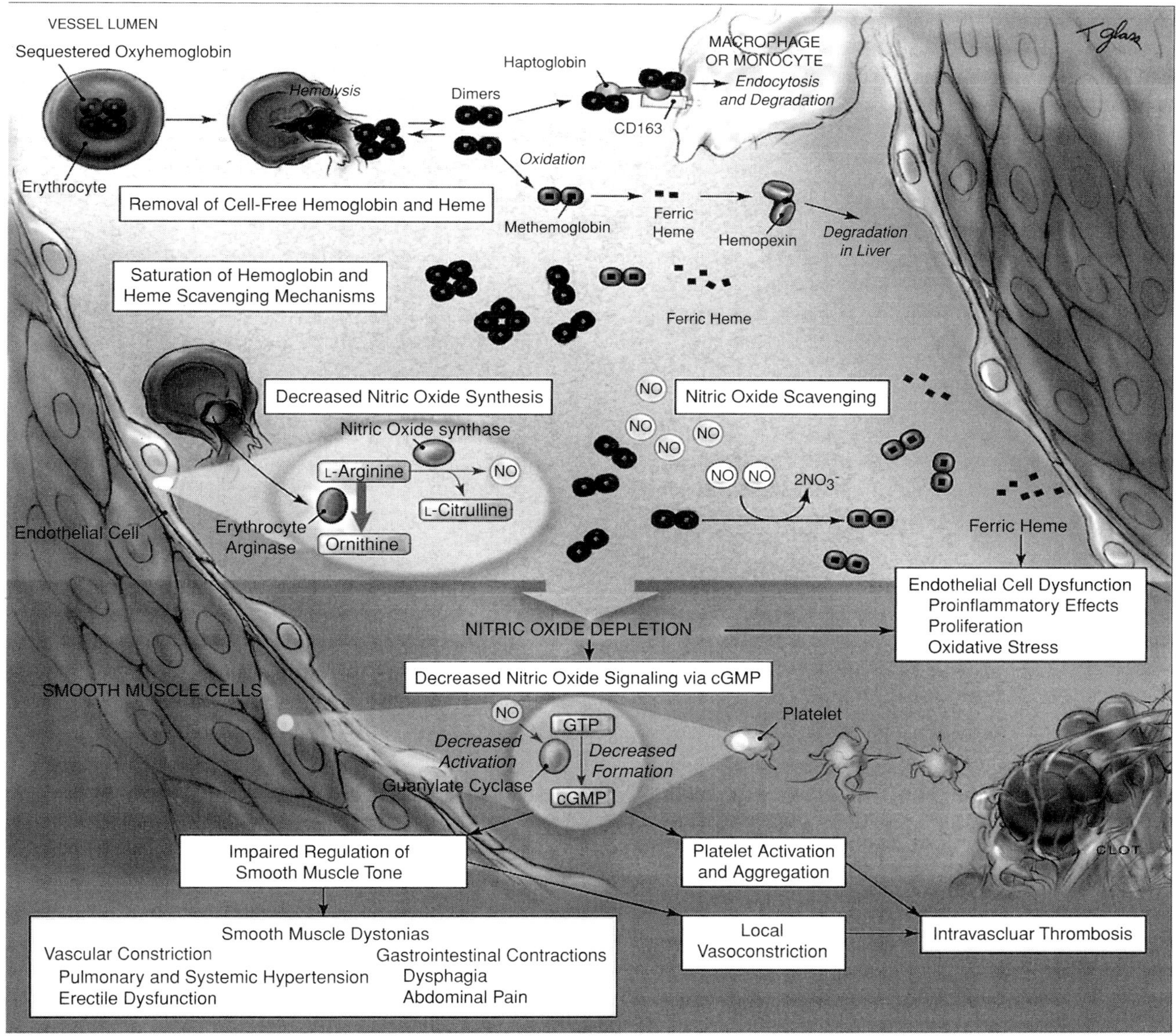

Figure 11.3. Pathophysiological consequences of intravascular hemolysis. Decompartmentalization of red cell contents results in ectopic localization of hemoglobin and arginase into plasma. Hemoglobin is rapidly bound to haptoglobin, and this complex binds to CD163 on macrophages, resulting in endocytosis and clearance of the whole complex. If the utilization of haptoglobin exceeds its replacement by hepatic synthesis, plasma cell–free hemoglobin accumulates, which stoichiometrically inactivates NO. Plasma cell–free arginase converts plasma arginine to ornithine, reducing availability of arginine, the obligate substrate for NOS. Depletion of NO results in pulmonary vasoconstriction, platelet activation, smooth muscle dystonias, and reduced antioxidant capacity. (Reproduced with permission of the publisher from ref. 110.)

porphyrin ring, known as hemin. Free heme is capable of inserting into cell membranes and producing hydroxyl and nitrogen dioxide radicals via Fenton and peroxidase chemistry, respectively, and a specific clearance pathway exists to avoid this oxidative insult. Hemin is bound by another β-globulin plasma glycoprotein, hemopexin, and the complex is slowly cleared by hepatic parenchymal cells. After saturation of hemopexin, free hemin is adsorbed to albumin as the brown pigment methemalbumin. Depletion of plasma hemopexin is another indicator of hemolysis.

Disposal of plasma hemoglobin via the haptoglobin–CD163 pathway activates a program that helps to counteract the adverse effects of plasma hemoglobin on vascular homeostasis. Binding of hemoglobin-haptoglobin to CD163 activates the antiinflammatory cytokine interleukin-10 and the heme oxygenase-1 heme catabolic enzyme, which also has antioxidant activities (Fig. 11.3).[93]

Heme oxygenase-1 breaks down heme into biliverdin, free iron, and carbon monoxide. Carbon monoxide induces vasodilatory, antioxidant, antiinflammatory, and antiproliferative responses.[94–96] Biliverdin is converted by biliverdin reductase to bilirubin, which also has antioxidant properties.[97] Carbon monoxide, produced in the body solely through the heme oxygenase reaction and eliminated via the lungs, may be monitored in exhaled breath as an indicator of the rate of heme turnover.[98]

The hemoglobin scavenging activity of haptoglobin is supplemented by the haptoglobin-related protein (Hpr). This plasma protein also binds to plasma hemoglobin with high affinity, but this complex does not bind to CD163. Instead, the hemoglobin–Hpr complex is directed to specialized high-density lipoprotein particles called HDL3 OR TLF-1, which contain apolipoprotein A-I, L-I, and others.[99] Whether this sequestration protects the vascular system against the toxic effects of plasma hemoglobin is unknown. Unlike haptoglobin, Hpr is not depleted from plasma of patients with sickle cell disease or other forms of intravascular hemolysis.[100] It is not known whether hemoglobin–Hpr complexes in HDL particles are capable of scavenging NO.

High-grade intravascular hemolysis may saturate the capacity of the haptoglobin-hemopexin-Hpr system, forcing hemoglobin clearance through alternative mechanisms. The relatively small size of $\alpha\beta$ globin dimers allows their penetration of the glomerulus into filtrate.[91] Hemoglobinuria results when the maximal tubular reabsorption rate of 1.4 mg/min is exceeded.[101] Hemoglobin reabsorbed into renal tubular cells is degraded, generating bilirubin and iron. Iron stored in ferritin in the renal tubular cells can accumulate to high levels, generating insoluble hemosiderin.[102,103] The hemosiderin-laden renal epithelial cells are eventually sloughed into urine, where they may be identified in urinary sediment by Prussian blue staining and are indicative of high-grade chronic intravascular hemolysis. Such hemolytic rates are common in paroxysmal nocturnal hemoglobinuria, and may occur in sickle cell disease. In states of haptoglobin depletion, plasma hemoglobin also undergoes endocytosis by hepatic macrophages via direct binding to CD163.[92] There is also indirect evidence of similar activity in macrophages of neovascularized atherosclerotic lesions. This might suggest a protective role for this pathway in the development of proliferative vasculopathy related to cases of chronic intravascular hemolysis or to intraplaque hemorrhage.

CLINICAL CONSEQUENCES OF INTRAVASCULAR HEMOLYSIS

When the rate of intravascular hemolysis exceeds the capacity of the hemoglobin scavenging mechanisms, hemoglobin and other red cell constituents accumulate in plasma compartment. Several of these constituents are toxic to vascular health, and a clinical vasculopathy syndrome has been identified in sickle cell disease, thalassemia, and other hemolytic anemias.

Hemolysis-associated Vascular Dysfunction: A Unique State of NO Resistance in Hemolytic Diseases

NO is a free radical molecule produced in endothelium by the endothelial NO synthase enzyme, via the oxygen-dependent five-electron oxidation of L-arginine to citrulline.[104–106] Once produced, NO diffuses as a paracrine-signaling molecule to adjacent smooth muscle where it binds avidly to the heme moiety of soluble guanylate cyclase. This activates the enzyme which in turn converts guanosine triphosphate (GTP) to cyclic guanosine monophosphate (cGMP), activating cGMP-dependent protein kinases, which ultimately leads to Ca^{2+} sequestration and relaxation of the perivascular smooth muscle to produce vasodilation (Chapter 10).

NO-dependent vasodilation can be stimulated by shear stress and direct activation of muscarinic receptors by agonists such as acetylcholine. Vascular NO production is also tonic and controls approximately 25% of our resting blood flow.[107,108] This steady-state vascular NO flux promotes general vascular homeostasis and health. NO tonically down-regulates transcription of endothelial adhesion molecules such as VCAM-1, ICAM-1, P-selectin and E-selectin[109] and inhibits platelet activation, tissue factor expression and thrombin generation.[110] NO modulates the expression of endothelin receptors (promoting a vasodilator effect by increasing endothelial endothelin receptor B expression) and decreases expression of endothelin-1, a potent mitogen and vasoconstrictor.[111,112] Finally, NO reacts in a nearly diffusion limited reaction with the superoxide radical, critically modulating vascular redox balance. All these pathways, normally inhibited by NO, are pathologically activated in sickle cell disease and perhaps other hemolytic anemias.

The concentration of NO available for the activation of soluble guanylate cyclase depends on the rate of production from endothelial NO synthase and the extent of scavenging reactions with superoxide and hemoglobin (or other high affinity heme-globins such as myoglobin).[113] NO reacts with oxy- and deoxy-hemoglobin at the near diffusion limit (10^7 Ms) to produce methemoglobin and nitrate or iron-nitrosyl-hemoglobin, respectively (Equations 11.1 and 11.2).[114,115] NO will react even faster with superoxide (at the diffusion limit, 10^{9-10} Ms), formed by the enzymes xanthine oxidase, NADPH oxidase, uncoupled NO synthase, as well as by hemoglobin autooxidation ($HbFe^{+2}\text{-}O_2 \rightarrow HbFe^{+3} + O_2{\cdot}^-$), to form peroxynitrite (Equation 11.3).[106] Although the reaction of NO with superoxide is approximately 100 times faster than that with hemoglobin, the concentration of hemoglobin in the plasma of patients with sickle cell disease (approximate mean concentrations of 4 μM[116]) is approximately more than 100 times that of superoxide, suggesting that both pathways have the potential to limit NO bioavailability in vivo.

$$NO + HbFe^{+2}\text{-}O_2 \text{ [oxyhemoglobin]} \rightarrow HbFe^{+3} \text{ [methemoglobin]} + NO_3^- \text{ [nitrate]} \quad (11.1)$$

$$NO + HbFe^{+2} \text{ [deoxyhemoglobin]} \rightarrow HbFe^{+2}\text{-}NO \text{ [iron-nitrosyl-hemoglobin]} \quad (11.2)$$

$$NO + O_2^{\bullet -} \text{[superoxide]} \rightarrow ONOO^- \text{ [peroxynitrite]} \quad (11.3)$$

Because mammals do not possess nitrate reductase enzymes and the off-rate of NO from iron-nitrosyl-hemoglobin is so slow, these three reactions represent irreversible scavenging reactions. Indeed, the half-life of NO in a free (i.e., not encapsulated by a red cell membrane) solution of 10 mM oxyhemoglobin (the concentration of hemoglobin in whole blood) is estimated to be 1 μs and this NO could only diffuse 1 μm.[117] Based on the kinetics of these reactions (nearly diffusion limited) and the concentration of intravascular hemoglobin in red blood cells (10 mM concentration in heme in whole blood), theoretical calculations suggest that the diffusion radius of NO from endothelium would be severely limited.[117] This effect is only slightly diminished by the fact that the smooth muscle cells are on one side of the endothelium and the blood is on the other.[105] Because the net flux of NO is always defined by the three dimensional spatial gradient in its concentration, the presence of hemoglobin on one side of the endothelium decreases the concentration on the other side. Conceptually, one can appreciate that NO diffusion is random from its source of production, so that a particular NO molecule can diffuse luminally and then back abluminally; if a trap is present on one side, any molecule that diffuses in that direction is eliminated and the concentration of NO on the other side will thus diminish. Indeed, recent modeling studies reveal that as little as one micromolar cell-free intraluminal hemoglobin in plasma will dramatically reduce NO concentrations that reach smooth muscle.[118] This effect is magnified in hemolytic anemia, where the total level of NO scavenging by the red cells is reduced as the red cell mass decreases, so that the relative contribution of NO scavenging by the plasma hemoglobin compartment increases.[118]

These chemical reactions create a paradox in vascular biology: How can NO be the endothelium derived relaxing factor if the massive concentrations of intravascular hemoglobin should scavenge it and limit its ability to diffuse from endothelium to smooth muscle? This paradox has been largely solved by the understanding that there are major diffusional barriers for NO between the source of production, endothelial NO synthases, and hemoglobin in the red blood cell (Fig. 11.4).[113] There exist several major diffusional barriers for NO in the unstirred layer around the erythrocyte,[119,120] in the cell free zone that forms along the endothelium in laminar flowing blood,[121–123] and possibly in the red cell submembrane, formed from the protein lattice of actin, spectrin, methemoglobin, hemichromes, band-3, and other components of the inner membrane scaffolding.[124–126] These three major diffusional barriers reduce the reaction of NO with intracellular hemoglobin by approximately 300–1,000 fold and allow sufficient NO diffusion for paracrine signaling from endothelium to smooth muscle. For example, with a cell-free zone of 5 micrometers, the lifetime of NO would increase from 1 microsecond to approximately 7.5 ms before it reached the red cell rich zone and would be scavenged; thus the lifetime of NO increases by a factor of almost 10,000 in this situation.[117]

Understanding this balance between NO production, diffusion to smooth muscle, and scavenging reactions with intracellular hemoglobin helps explain the clear toxicity observed in the clinical development of the stroma-free hemoglobin-based blood substitutes (recently reviewed[110] and illustrated in Figure 11.4). The infusion of cell free hemoglobin solutions into normal volunteers and patients immediately disrupts the NO diffusion barriers and produces dose-dependent vasoconstriction (systemic and pulmonary hypertension),[127–136] smooth muscle dystonias (gastroparesis, esophageal spasm and abdominal and chest pain),[127,128,130,133,137] platelet activation,[138–141] and death.[142,143] The toxicity of cell free hemoglobin solutions has resulted in serious morbidity (myocardial infarction) and excess mortality in most clinical trials of blood substitutes in at-risk patients.[110]

In sickle cell disease, thalassemia, malaria and other acquired, iatrogenic, infectious and hereditary hemolytic conditions, intravascular hemolysis similarly disrupts the NO diffusional barriers created by the red cell membrane that limit NO reactions with hemoglobin, and the cell-free plasma hemoglobin destroys NO at a rate 1,000-fold faster than intraerythrocytic hemoglobin.[110,113,116,144] As a result of hemolysis, hemoglobin is released into plasma where it reacts with and destroys NO, resulting in abnormally high rates of NO consumption and produces a state of resistance to NO bioactivity. Consequently, smooth muscle guanylyl cyclase is not activated and vasodilation is impaired. In support of this mechanism, plasma from patients with sickle cell disease contains cell-free ferrous oxyhemoglobin, which stoichiometrically consumes micromolar quantities of NO and abrogates forearm blood flow responses to NO donor infusions.[116]

This NO resistance syndrome is a unique form of vascular dysfunction. In coronary artery disease and its risk factors, diabetes, obesity, hypertension, smoking, increasing age, and hyperlipidemia, NO production is reduced. This is clinically characterized by the demonstration that infusions of the competitive NO synthase inhibitor, L-NMMA, into the brachial artery or coronary arteries exhibits a blunted vasoconstrictor response, suggesting that tonic NO synthase activity is impaired.[107,145] However, in these patients with the metabolic syndrome, the infusion of sodium

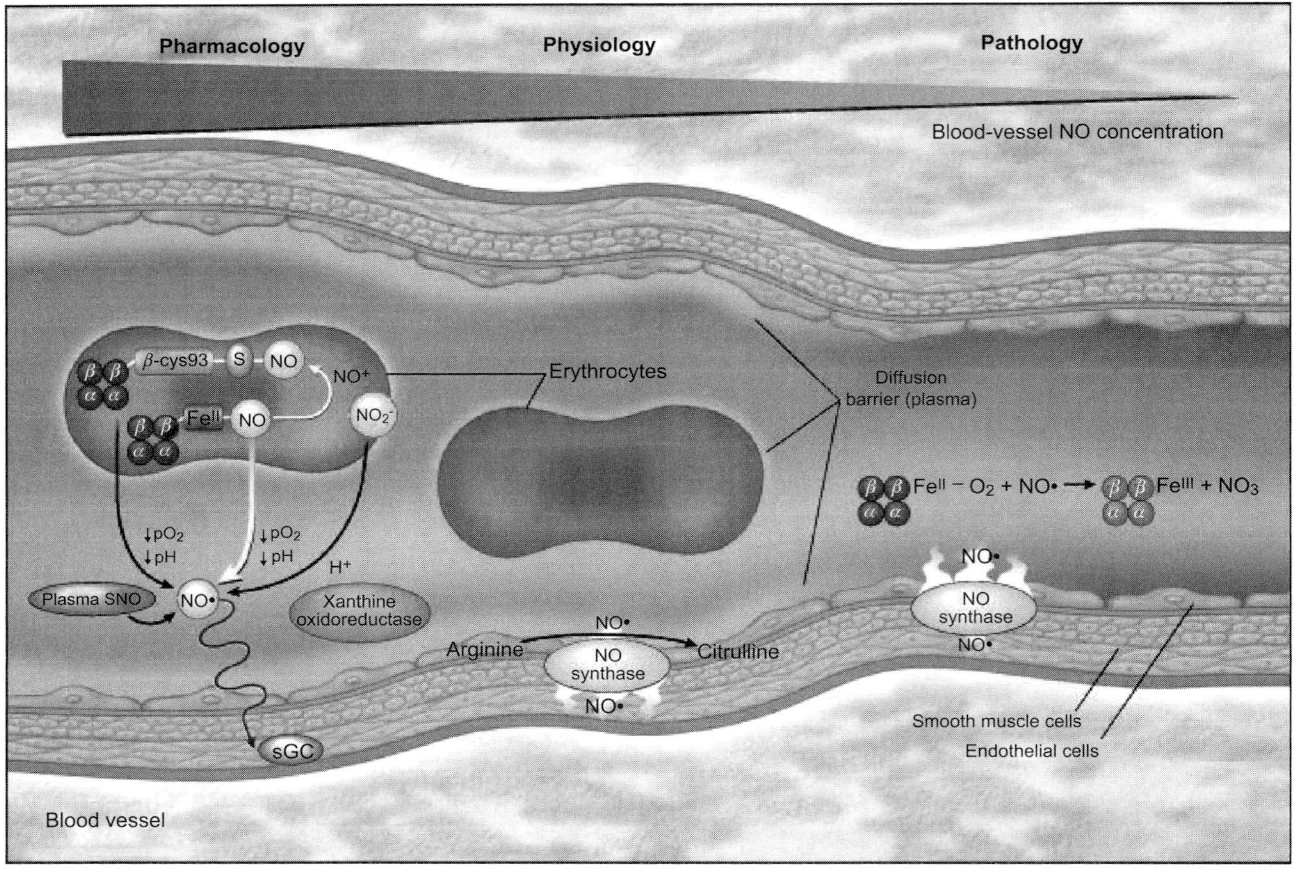

Figure 11.4. Role of diffusion barriers in intact red cells and plasma cell–free hemoglobin. Intact red cells carry a reservoir of NO in the form of nitrite. Nitrite can be reduced by deoxyhemoglobin to NO, although it remains to be determined how NO escapes from the erythrocyte. Xanthine oxidoreductase may also have the potential to perform this reaction. S-nitroso-hemoglobin has also been proposed as another erythrocyte storage form of NO. NO is produced principally by NOS from arginine and binds to soluble guanylyl cyclase in vascular smooth muscle cells, producing tonic vasodilation. Diffusion barriers to consumption of NO by intact erythrocyte hemoglobin are provided by the cell-free zone along the endothelium associated with laminar flow of blood, and by the unstirred layer surrounding the red cell. (Reproduced with permission from ref. 113.)

nitroprusside or nitroglycerin, NO donor medications, produces normal vasodilation effects and are used as controls to show that the vessels are capable of vasodilation. In striking contrast, in patients with sickle cell disease with high hemolytic rates and high plasma hemoglobin levels, the vasodilatory effect to L-NMMA and the NO donor sodium nitroprusside are both blunted. This unique state of resistance to NO-dependent vasodilation[146] has been recapitulated in numerous mouse and human studies (Fig. 11.5).

- In patients with sickle cell disease and high plasma hemoglobin concentrations the blood flow responses to infusions of the NO synthase inhibitor L-NMMA are blunted and blood flow responses to the NO donor sodium nitroprusside are nearly abolished.[116,147] This effect appears to be more pronounced in males, consistent with estrogenic effects on NO synthase expression and activity.
- Endothelium-dependent, NO-dependent blood flow is impaired in patients with sickle cell disease, when measured by flow-mediated vasodilation. The responses to the exogenous NO donor, nitroglycerin are impaired, compared with control subjects with non-hemolytic anemia.[148]
- A similar state of resistance to exogenous NO (the NO donor NONOate or sodium nitroprusside) in different transgenic mouse models of sickle cell disease has also been described.[149,150] NO resistance was highly correlated with plasma hemoglobin levels suggesting that NO resistance in this model was linked to hemolytic rate and oxidant stress.[151]
- NO is inhibited in the vasculature of transgenic sickle cell mice with sickle cell disease by a diffusion-limited reaction with superoxide produced from xanthine oxidase on endothelium.[12,152] Increased xanthine oxidase expression in the lung of the transgenic mouse has also been reported to scavenge NO in this vascular system.[153]

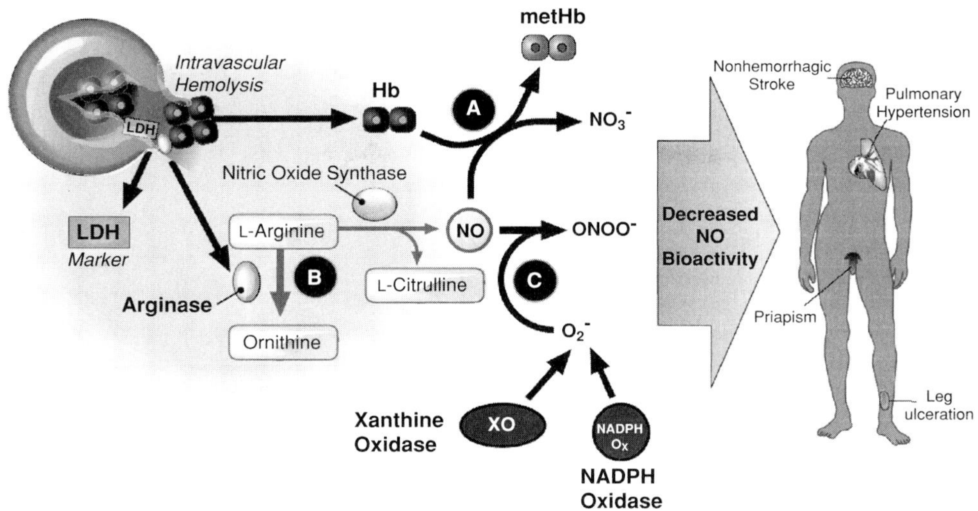

Figure 11.5. Intravascular hemolysis and decreased NO bioactivity. Arginine is converted by NOS to NO plus citrulline. Intravascular hemolysis releases cell-free hemoglobin into blood plasma, where it stoichiometrically can react with NO (reaction A), producing methemoglobin and inert nitrate. In addition, erythrocyte arginase released into plasma catabolizes plasma arginine (reaction B), reducing its availability to NOS. In reactions not directly related to hemolysis, increased xanthine oxidase and NADPH oxidase activities found in sickle cell disease produce oxygen radicals, which can react with and further deplete NO, producing highly oxidative peroxynitrites (reaction C). Consequent decreased NO bioactivity contributes to the clinical risk of pulmonary hypertension, nonhemorrhagic stroke, priapism, and leg ulceration. (Reproduced with permission of the publisher from ref. 183.)

Recent studies have suggested a role for vascular NADPH oxidase in enhanced superoxide mediated NO scavenging in the sickle cell cerebral vasculature.[154]

- Sickle cell transgenic mice develop spontaneous pulmonary hypertension associated with a global impairment in both the production of NO (from uncoupled eNOS) and from NO inactivation by plasma hemoglobin and superoxide.[155] Both pulmonary and systemic impairment in the vasodilatory responses to inhaled NO, sodium nitroprusside, NONOates and even phosphodiesterase-5 inhibitors were observed. A similar state of NO resistance developed in an alloimmunized intravascular hemolysis mouse model.[156]
- In a canine model of acute intravascular hypotonic water hemolysis,[157] pulmonary and systemic vasoconstriction was associated with the degree of hemoglobinemia and the development of resistance to the NO donor sodium nitroprusside.

Similar effects of hemolysis on NO bioavailability and endothelial function have been considered in paroxysmal nocturnal hemoglobinuria,[110] in primate models of thrombotic thrombocytopenic purpura,[158] and have recently been described in animal models of malaria.[159,160] In the latter malaria studies, the degree of hemoglobinemia, which reduced systemic NO bioavailability, was even more closely linked to risk of death than the severity of parasitemia.

Arginasemia Limitations on NOS Substrate Bioavailability

In addition to release of hemoglobin from the red cell into plasma, hemolysis releases erythrocyte arginase, which converts L-arginine, the substrate for NO synthesis, to ornithine (Figs. 11.4 and 11.5).[161–163] Arginase activities in the plasma of patients correlated significantly with cell-free plasma hemoglobin and was increased in the plasma and red cells of patients with sickle cell disease (Fig. 11.6). Consistent with this observation, the arginine:ornithine ratio decreased significantly as plasma arginase activity rose. Low arginine:ornithine ratios were found in patients with sickle cell disease and comorbid pulmonary hypertension and were associated with increasing mortality.[163,164]

Hemolysis, Coagulation and the Spleen

Intravascular hemolysis has the potential to drive a procoagulant state. Platelet activation is profoundly inhibited by NO and such NO-dependent inhibition may in turn be blocked by plasma hemoglobin-mediated NO scavenging.[139,141,165,166] Activation of platelets in sickle cell disease correlated with pulmonary artery pressures and indices of hemolysis. In vitro experiments suggested that cell-free hemoglobin could directly activate platelets and inhibit the modulatory effects of NO on platelet activation.[141] High hemolytic rate, reflected by reticulocytosis, was also associated with hemoglobin desaturation (ventilation/perfusion inhomogeneity) and adhesion molecule

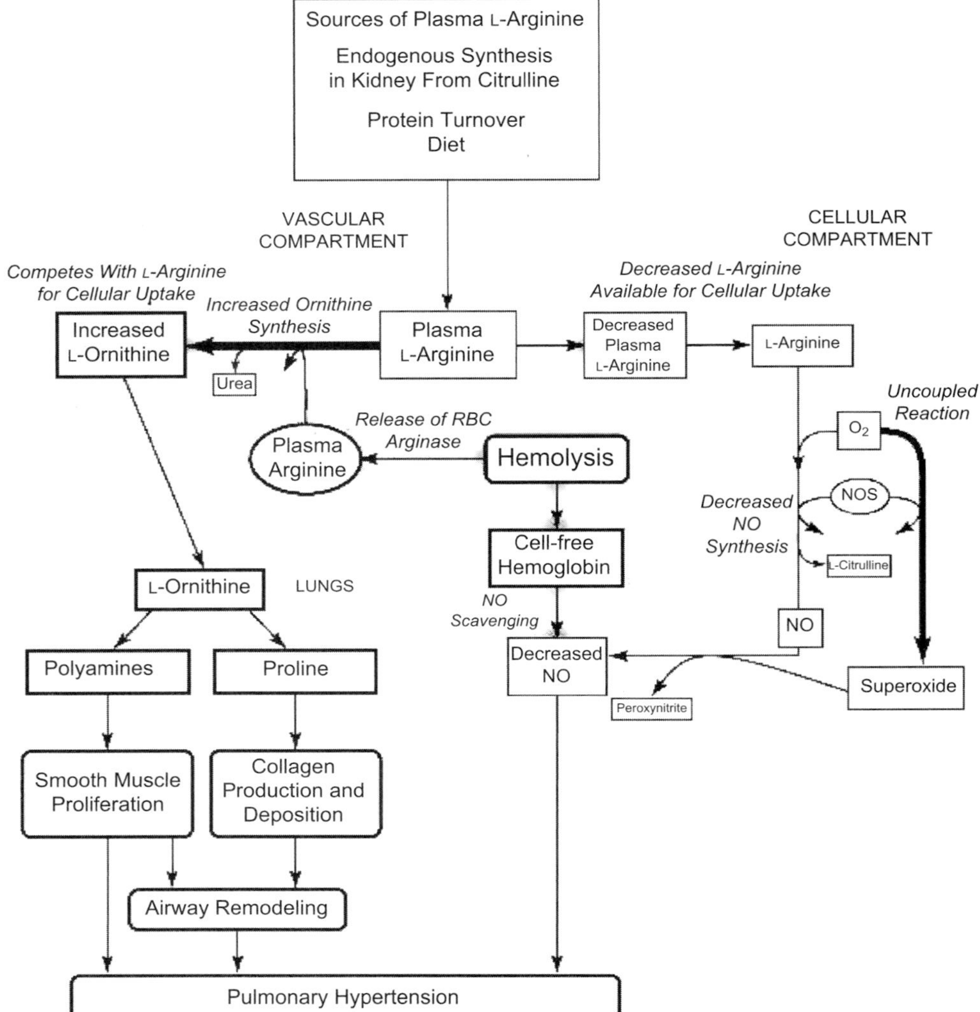

Figure 11.6. Alterations in arginine metabolism in sickle cell disease and thalassemia. Plasma L-arginine is derived from synthesis in the kidney, from protein turnover, and from dietary sources. Intravascular hemolysis results in ectopic localization of erythrocyte arginase into blood plasma, where it can convert L-arginine into L-ornithine, reducing the availability of L-arginine as a substrate for NO synthesis. Under such conditions of limiting substrate, the subunits of NO synthase can become uncoupled, producing superoxides that can react with NO to form peroxynitrites. Excess production of ornithine has been proposed to provide substrate for production of polyamines and proline. Polyamines can fuel DNA production and cell proliferation, and proline can stimulate collagen production. These processes are proposed along with decreased NO bioavailability to contribute to pulmonary hypertension in patients with chronic intravascular hemolysis. (Reproduced with permission of the publisher from ref. 163.)

expression;[167,168] it is possible that such a hypoxic state can induce hypoxia-inducing factor-1 (HIF-1) dependent factors such as erythropoietin, vascular endothelial growth factor (VEGF), and endothelin-1.

Splenectomy has been reported to be a risk factor for the development of pulmonary hypertension, particularly in patients with hemolytic disorders.[169–173] Perhaps the loss of splenic function increases the circulation of platelet derived mediators and that senescent and abnormal erythrocytes in the circulation trigger platelet activation, promoting pulmonary microthrombosis and red cell adhesion to the endothelium.[169] A role for intensification of intravascular hemolysis by splenectomy has also been suggested by the demonstration of significantly higher plasma hemoglobin and erythrocyte-derived microvesicles levels patients with β-thalassemia intermedia who have undergone splenectomy, compared with those who have not.[174] It is likely that splenic reticuloendothelial cells subserve a critical function in the removal of senescent and damaged erythrocytes and that following surgical or autosplenectomy, the rate of intravascular hemolysis increases, resulting in increased plasma hemoglobin and NO scavenging, and increased circulating red cells with phosphatidylserine exposed on their membranes. Consistent with such a mechanism, the

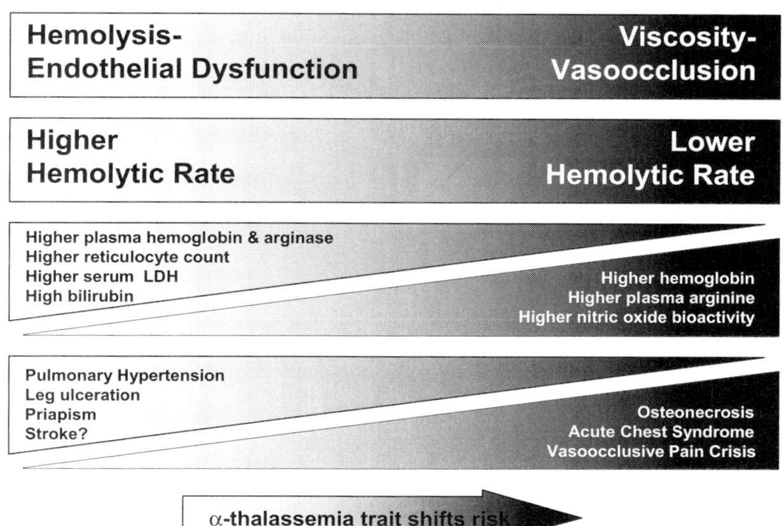

Figure 11.7. Spectrum of sickle cell subphenotypes affected by hemolytic rate. The viscosity-vasoocclusion subphenotype is associated with a lower hemolytic rate, marked by a higher hemoglobin level, and low plasma hemoglobin, lactate dehydrogenase, bilirubin, and arginase levels. Patients with these features have a higher incidence of vasoocclusive pain crisis, the acute chest syndrome, and osteonecrosis. In contrast, patients with the hemolysis-endothelial dysfunction subphenotype exhibit markers of high hemolytic rate, including low hemoglobin level, high plasma hemoglobin, LDH, bilirubin, and arginase, culminating in low NO bioavailability and high prevalence of pulmonary hypertension, leg ulceration, priapism, and stroke. Coinheritance of α thalassemia trait with sickle cell disease reduces the hemolytic rate, reducing the risk of hemolysis-associated complications and increasing the risk of viscosity-related complications. (Adapted with permission from ref. 183.)

experimental intravenous injection of hemolysate promotes the formation of platelet-rich thrombi in the pulmonary vascular bed of rabbits after ligation of the splenic artery, without any thrombus formation in the animals without splenic artery ligation.[175,176]

HEMOLYTIC ANEMIA-ASSOCIATED CLINICAL SUBPHENOTYPES

Recent epidemiological reexamination of the clinical complications of sickle cell disease suggests that the clinical manifestations of sickle cell disease may fall into two partially overlapping subphenotypes (Fig. 11.7). The first subphenotype encompasses the more classic manifestations of the disease: vasoocclusive crisis, acute chest syndrome and osteonecrosis. These morbidities are epidemiologically associated with high steady-state white blood cell counts, high steady-state hemoglobin levels and low HbF concentrations.[177] These complications are largely mediated by microvascular obstruction by sickle erythrocytes and the pathogenesis characterized by ischemia-reperfusion injury, adhesion, infarction and inflammation.[178,179] The second subphenotype encompasses clinical complications shared by other hemolytic anemias and includes pulmonary arterial hypertension, systemic systolic arterial hypertension, cutaneous leg ulceration, priapism, sudden death and possibly stroke.[116,164,180–182] Consistent with this formulation, coinheritance of α thalassemia, which reduces hemolytic rate in sickle cell disease, reduces the risk of leg ulceration, priapism and stroke, and increases the risk of vasoocclusive pain crisis, acute chest syndrome, and osteonecrosis as hemolysis is reduced and blood viscosity increases.[183]

Pulmonary hypertension is an increasingly recognized complication of chronic hereditary and acquired hemolytic anemias, including sickle cell disease,[164,184–192] β thalassemia (in particular β-thalassemia intermedia and inadequately transfused and chelated patients with β-thalassemia major),[169,193–201] paroxysmal nocturnal hemoglobinuria,[202–204] hereditary spherocytosis and stomatocytosis,[205–211] microangiopathic hemolytic anemias,[212,212–218] pyruvate kinase deficiency,[219] red cell alloimmune–mediated hemolytic anemia,[220] unstable hemoglobin variants,[221] and possibly malaria.[222–224] Additionally, certain conditions are associated with both intravascular hemolysis and risk of pulmonary hypertension, such as schistosomiasis,[225,226] iatrogenic hemolysis from mechanical heart valves,[227,228] left ventricular assist devices, and cardiopulmonary bypass procedures.[93,229–232] These studies are consistent with growing appreciation for a distinct syndrome of hemolysis-associated pulmonary hypertension.

Priapism and Hemolytic Anemia

Priapism has been reported in patients with sickle cell disease, β-thalassemia intermedia, red cell enzymopathy, unstable hemoglobin disorders, and other hemolytic anemias.[233–241] In one study, patients with a history of priapism had evidence of increased hemolytic rate and were five-fold more likely to have pulmonary hypertension, supporting a mechanistic and epidemiological link between these complications.[164] Further analysis of this cohort based on stratum of hemolysis defined by relative levels of LDH confirmed an association between the intensity of hemolysis and the prevalence of priapism, cutaneous leg ulceration, and pulmonary hypertension.[181] In a case-control analysis of data from the Comprehensive Study of Sickle Cell Disease (CSSCD), priapism was associated with laboratory markers of high hemolytic rate and

Table 11.1. Laboratory characteristics of cases with priapism and controls in a population of patients with sickle cell disease

	Case subjects n = 273	Control subjects n = 979	*P*
Age at last follow-up, y ± SD	26.2 ± 12.28	22.8 ± 12.72	.001
Hemoglobin, g/dL	8.64 ± 0.13	9.51 ± 0.07	<.001
HbF, g/dL	0.44 ± 0.04	0.50 ± 0.02	.309
Bilirubin, mg/dL	3.52 ± 0.13	2.92 ± 0.07	<.001
Urea nitrogen (BUN), mg/dL	9.49 ± 0.39	10.09 ± 0.20	.178
Mean corpuscular volume, μm^3	89.82 ± 0.48	87.18 ± 0.25	<.001
LDH, U/L	526.19 ± 13.08	459.23 ± 6.92	<.001
Reticulocytes	11.67 ± 0.35	9.37 ± 0.18	<.001
AST, U/L	50.34 ± 1.44	45.78 ± 0.76	.005
ALT, U/L	36.70 ± 2.96	35.18 ± 1.55	.649
WBC count, $\times 10^9$/L	11.62 ± 0.20	10.18 ± 0.10	<.0001

With the exception of age at last follow-up (presented as mean ± SD), the means shown in the table are age-adjusted and presented as mean ± standard error. HbF indicates fetal hemoglobin; BUN, blood urea nitrogen; LDH, lactic dehydrogenase; RBC, red blood cell; AST, aspartate aminotransferase; ALT, alanine aminotransferase; and WBC, white blood cell. (Adapted from ref. 258.)

leukocytosis (Table 11.1).[180,242] Genetic polymorphism in Klotho (*KL*), a gene that regulates NO bioavailability, was also linked to priapism.[242] Additionally, priapism is less common in patients with HbSC disease and HbS-β^+-thalassemia, and is less prevalent among ethnically distinct subpopulations of sickle cell disease characterized by high expression of HbF and lower hemolytic rates.[243]

From a mechanistic standpoint, recent transgenic and knock out mouse studies have revealed increased priapic activity in the double *nos3* and *nos1* null mouse and in the sickle cell mouse,[244] consistent with a paradoxical role for NO deficiency in the mechanism of priapism. NO deficiency in these models produced a secondary severe downregulation of phosphodiesterase-5, resulting in episodic surges in vascular smooth muscle cGMP and dysregulated penile blood flow.

Cutaneous Leg Ulceration and Hemolytic Anemia

Cutaneous leg ulceration has also been associated with hemolytic anemias including sickle cell disease, thalassemia, and spherocytosis.[245–257] Consistent with this shared complication of hemolytic anemias, patients with a history of leg ulcers had the highest rates of hemolysis (Table 11.2).[181,258]

Stroke and Hemolytic Anemia

Although less clearly linked to hemolytic rate, there are a number of pathological and clinical features of stroke in children with sickle cell disease that suggest a parallel pathobiology with the vasculopathy of pulmonary hypertension.[259] Stroke and pulmonary hypertension have many epidemiological risk factors in common, including history of prior stroke, systolic hypertension, low transcutaneous oxygen saturation, and severe anemia.[177,260–263] Both have histopathological evidence of large vessel arterial disease, featuring smooth muscle hyperplasia with overlying endothelial damage, fibrosis, and thrombosis in situ. HbF expression has not proven protective in either condition. Although the potential role of NO resistance and hemolysis in cerebrovascular disease remains to be investigated in sickle cell disease and thalassemia, recent studies suggest that chronic transfusion reduces plasma cell-free hemoglobin levels and stroke incidence in children with sickle cell disease at risk for stroke[264] and LDH has been associated with increased transcranial Doppler blood flow, a predictor of stroke.

Pulmonary Arterial Hypertension in Sickle Cell Disease and Thalassemia

Echocardiographic studies have reported that approximately 30% of screened adult patients with sickle cell

Table 11.2. Association of sickle cell leg ulcers with hemolysis

	Cases (n = 243)	Controls (n = 516)	*P*
Age at last follow-up (yr)	34.8 ±12.5	30.7 ± 9.4	<0.0001
Hemoglobin (g/dL)	7.91	8.52	0.0001
Fetal hemoglobin (%)	5.05	6.12	0.021
Bilirubin (μmol/L)	62.75	54.09	0.0012
Lactate dehydrogenase (U/L)	530	454	<0.0001
Reticulocytes (%)	12	12	0.29
AST (U/L)	48.61	44.43	0.02

Values present as n (%) or age-adjusted means, n = 759. This table includes only patients with sickle cell anemia and genotype data. (Adapted from ref. 258.)

21. Jain SK, Shohet SB. A novel phospholipid in irreversibly sickled cells: evidence for in vivo peroxidative membrane damage in sickle cell disease. *Blood.* 1984;63:362–367.
22. Platt OS, Falcone JF, Lux SE. Molecular defect in the sickle erythrocyte skeleton. Abnormal spectrin binding to sickle inside-our vesicles. *J Clin Invest.* 1985;75:266–271.
23. Schwartz RS, Rybicki AC, Heath RH, Lubin BH. Protein 4.1 in sickle erythrocytes. Evidence for oxidative damage. *J Biol Chem.* 1987;262:15666–15672.
24. Goodman SR. The irreversibly sickled cell: a perspective. *Cell Mol Biol.* 2004;50:53–58.
25. Lux SE, John KM, Karnovsky MJ. Irreversible deformation of the spectrin-actin lattice in irreversibly sickled cells. *J Clin Invest.* 1976;58:955–963.
26. Lachant NA, Davidson WD, Tanaka KR. Impaired pentose phosphate shunt function in sickle cell disease: a potential mechanism for increased Heinz body formation and membrane lipid peroxidation. *Am J Hematol.* 1983;15:1–13.
27. Schrader MC, Simplaceanu V, Ho C. Measurement of fluxes through the pentose phosphate pathway in erythrocytes from individuals with sickle cell anemia by carbon-13 nuclear magnetic resonance spectroscopy. *Biochim Biophys Acta.* 1993;1182:179–188.
28. Schrier SL. Pathophysiology of thalassemia. *Curr Opin Hematol.* 2002;9:123–126.
29. Amer J, Ghoti H, Rachmilewitz E, et al. Red blood cells, platelets and polymorphonuclear neutrophils of patients with sickle cell disease exhibit oxidative stress that can be ameliorated by antioxidants. *Br J Haematol.* 2006;132:108–113.
30. Wetterstroem N, Brewer GJ, Warth JA, Mitchinson A, Near K. Relationship of glutathione levels and Heinz body formation to irreversibly sickled cells in sickle cell anemia. *J Lab Clin Med.* 1984;103:589–596.
31. Morris CR, Suh JH, Hagar W, et al. Erythrocyte glutamine depletion, altered redox environment, and pulmonary hypertension in sickle cell disease. *Blood.* 2008;111:402–410.
32. Chang TL, Kakhniashvili DG, Goodman SR. Spectrin's E2/E3 ubiquitin conjugating/ligating activity is diminished in sickle cells. *Am J Hematol.* 2005;79:89–96.
33. Hsu YJ, Zimmer WE, Goodman SR. Erythrocyte spectrin's chimeric E2/E3 ubiquitin conjugating/ligating activity. *Cell Mol Biol.* 2005;51:187–193.
34. Ghatpande SS, Goodman SR. Ubiquitination of spectrin regulates the erythrocyte spectrin-protein-4.1-actin ternary complex dissociation: implications for the sickle cell membrane skeleton. *Cell Mol Biol.* 2004;50:67–74.
35. Gibson XA, Shartava A, McIntyre J, et al. The efficacy of reducing agents or antioxidants in blocking the formation of dense cells and irreversibly sickled cells in vitro. *Blood.* 1998;91:4373–4378.
36. Pace BS, Shartava A, Pack-Mabien A, et al. Effects of N-acetylcysteine on dense cell formation in sickle cell disease. *Am J Hematol.* 2003;73:26–32.
37. Jaja SI, Aigbe PE, Gbenebitse S, Temiye EO. Changes in erythrocytes following supplementation with alpha-tocopherol in children suffering from sickle cell anaemia. *Niger Postgrad Med J.* 2005;12:110–114.
38. Natta C, Machlin L. Plasma levels of tocopherol in sickle cell anemia subjects. *Am J Clin Nutr.* 1979;32:1359–1362.
39. Hasanato RM. Zinc and antioxidant vitamin deficiency in patients with severe sickle cell anemia. *Ann Saudi Med.* 2006;26:17–21.
40. Walter PB, Fung EB, Killilea DW, et al. Oxidative stress and inflammation in iron-overloaded patients with beta-thalassaemia or sickle cell disease. *Br J Haematol.* 2006;135: 254–263.
41. Gbenebitse S, Jaja SI, Kehinde MO. Effect of changes in plasma vitamin E level of vascular responses and lipid peroxidation in sickle cell anaemia subjects. *Niger Postgrad Med J.* 2005;12:81–84.
42. Ray D, Deshmukh P, Goswami K, Garg N. Antioxidant vitamin levels in sickle cell disorders. *Natl Med J India.* 2007;20:11–13.
43. Middelkoop E, Lubin BH, Bevers EM, et al. Studies on sickled erythrocytes provide evidence that the asymmetric distribution of phosphatidylserine in the red cell membrane is maintained by both ATP-dependent translocation and interaction with membrane skeletal proteins. *Biochim Biophys Acta.* 1988;937:281–288.
44. Blumenfeld N, Zachowski A, Galacteros F, Beuzard Y, Devaux PF. Transmembrane mobility of phospholipids in sickle erythrocytes: effect of deoxygenation on diffusion and asymmetry. *Blood.* 1991;77:849–854.
45. Kuypers FA, de Jong K. The role of phosphatidylserine in recognition and removal of erythrocytes. *Cell Mol Biol.* 2004;50:147–158.
46. de Jong K, Geldwerth D, Kuypers FA. Oxidative damage does not alter membrane phospholipid asymmetry in human erythrocytes. *Biochemistry.* 1997;36:6768–6776.
47. Lang KS, Roll B, Myssina S, et al. Enhanced erythrocyte apoptosis in sickle cell anemia, thalassemia and glucose-6-phosphate dehydrogenase deficiency. *Cell Physiol Biochem.* 2002;12:365–372.
48. Kuypers FA, Yuan J, Lewis RA, et al. Membrane phospholipid asymmetry in human thalassemia. *Blood.* 1998;91:3044–3051.
49. Westerman MP, Diloy-Puray M, Streczyn M. Membrane components in the red cells of patients with sickle cell anemia. Relationship to cell aging and to irreversibility of sickling. *Biochim Biophys Acta.* 1979;557:149–155.
50. Franck PF, Bevers EM, Lubin BH, et al. Uncoupling of the membrane skeleton from the lipid bilayer. The cause of accelerated phospholipid flip-flop leading to an enhanced procoagulant activity of sickled cells. *J Clin Invest.* 1985;75:183–190.
51. Liu SC, Derick LH, Zhai S, Palek J. Uncoupling of the spectrin-based skeleton from the lipid bilayer in sickled red cells. *Science.* 1991;252:574–576.
52. Choe HR, Schlegel RA, Rubin E, Williamson P, Westerman MP. Alteration of red cell membrane organization in sickle cell anaemia. *Br J Haematol.* 1986;63:761–773.
53. Liu SC, Yi SJ, Mehta JR, et al. Red cell membrane remodeling in sickle cell anemia. *Sequestration of membrane lipids and proteins in Heinz bodies. J Clin Invest.* 1996;97:29–36.
54. Connor J, Pak CC, Schroit AJ. Exposure of phosphatidylserine in the outer leaflet of human red blood cells. Relationship to cell density, cell age, and clearance by mononuclear cells. *J Biol Chem.* 1994;269:2399–2404.
55. Closse C, chary-Prigent J, Boisseau MR. Phosphatidylserine-related adhesion of human erythrocytes to vascular endothelium. *Br J Haematol.* 1999;107:300–302.

56. Setty BN, Kulkarni S, Stuart MJ. Role of erythrocyte phosphatidylserine in sickle red cell-endothelial adhesion. *Blood.* 2002;99:1564–1571.
57. Manodori AB, Barabino GA, Lubin BH, Kuypers FA. Adherence of phosphatidylserine-exposing erythrocytes to endothelial matrix thrombospondin. *Blood.* 2000;95:1293–1300.
58. Ballas SK, Smith ED. Red blood cell changes during the evolution of the sickle cell painful crisis. *Blood.* 1992;79:2154–2163.
59. Fabry ME, Benjamin L, Lawrence C, Nagel RL. An objective sign in painful crisis in sickle cell anemia: the concomitant reduction of high density red cells. *Blood.* 1984;64:559–563.
60. Allan D, Limbrick AR, Thomas P, Westerman MP. Release of spectrin-free spicules on reoxygenation of sickled erythrocytes. *Nature.* 1982;295:612–613.
61. Padilla F, Bromberg PA, Jensen WN. The sickle-unsickle cycle: a cause of cell fragmentation leading to permanently deformed cells. *Blood.* 1973;41:653–660.
62. Platt OS. Exercise-induced hemolysis in sickle cell anemia: shear sensitivity and erythrocyte dehydration. *Blood.* 1982;59:1055–1060.
63. Diggs LW, Bibb J. The erythrocyte in sickle cell anemia: Morphology, size, hemoglobin content, fragility and sedimentation rate. *JAMA.* 1939;112:695–701.
64. Lange RD, Minnich V, Moore CV. Effects of oxygen tension and of pH of the sickling and mechanical fragility of erythrocytes from patients with sickle cell anemia and the sickle cell trait. *J Lab Clin Med.* 1951;37:789–802.
65. Shen SC, Fleming EM. Experimental and clinical observations on increased mechanical fragility of erythrocytes. *Science.* 1944;100:387–389.
66. Harris JW, Brewster HH, Ham TH, Castle WB. Studies on the destruction of red blood cells. X. The biophysics and biology of sickle-cell disease. *AMA Arch Intern Med.* 1956;97:145–168.
67. Messmann R, Gannon S, Sarnaik S, Johnson RM. Mechanical properties of sickle cell membranes. *Blood.* 1990;75:1711–1717.
68. Liu SC, Zhai S, Palek J. Detection of hemin release during hemoglobin S denaturation. *Blood.* 1988;71:1755–1758.
69. Petz LD, Yam P, Wilkinson L, et al. Increased IgG molecules bound to the surface of red blood cells of patients with sickle cell anemia. *Blood.* 1984;64:301–304.
70. Bosman GJ. Erythrocyte aging in sickle cell disease. *Cell Mol Biol.* 2004;50:81–86.
71. Galili U, Clark MR, Shohet SB. Excessive binding of natural anti-alpha-galactosyl immunoglobin G to sickle erythrocytes may contribute to extravascular cell destruction. *J Clin Invest.* 1986;77:27–33.
72. Hebbel RP, Miller WJ. Unique promotion of erythrophagocytosis by malondialdehyde. *Am J Hematol.* 1988;29:222–225.
73. Low PS, Waugh SM, Zinke K, Drenckhahn D. The role of hemoglobin denaturation and band 3 clustering in red blood cell aging. *Science.* 1985;227:531–533.
74. Schluter K, Drenckhahn D. Co-clustering of denatured hemoglobin with band 3: its role in binding of autoantibodies against band 3 to abnormal and aged erythrocytes. *Proc Natl Acad Sci USA.* 1986;83:6137–6141.
75. Green GA, Kalra VK. Sickling-induced binding of immunoglobulin to sickle erythrocytes. *Blood.* 1988;71:636–639.
76. Test ST, Woolworth VS. Defective regulation of complement by the sickle erythrocyte: evidence for a defect in control of membrane attack complex formation. *Blood.* 1994;83:842–852.
77. Liu C, Marshall P, Schreibman I, et al. Interaction between terminal complement proteins C5b-7 and anionic phospholipids. *Blood.* 1999;93:2297–2301.
78. Schroit AJ, Tanaka Y, Madsen J, Fidler IJ. The recognition of red blood cells by macrophages: role of phosphatidylserine and possible implications of membrane phospholipid asymmetry. *Biol Cell.* 1984;51:227–238.
79. Boas FE, Forman L, Beutler E. Phosphatidylserine exposure and red cell viability in red cell aging and in hemolytic anemia. *Proc Natl Acad Sci USA.* 1998;95:3077–3081.
80. Kean LS, Brown LE, Nichols JW, et al. Comparison of mechanisms of anemia in mice with sickle cell disease and beta-thalassemia: peripheral destruction, ineffective erythropoiesis, and phospholipid scramblase-mediated phosphatidylserine exposure. *Exp Hematol.* 2002;30:394–402.
81. Wood BL, Gibson DF, Tait JF. Increased erythrocyte phosphatidylserine exposure in sickle cell disease: flow-cytometric measurement and clinical associations. *Blood.* 1996;88:1873–1880.
82. Atichartakarn V, Angchaisuksiri P, Aryurachai K, et al. Relationship between hypercoagulable state and erythrocyte phosphatidylserine exposure in splenectomized haemoglobin E/beta-thalassaemic patients. *Br J Haematol.* 2002;118:893–898.
83. Borenstain-Ben Y, Barenholz Y, Hy-Am E, Rachmilewitz EA, Eldor A. Phosphatidylserine in the outer leaflet of red blood cells from beta-thalassemia patients may explain the chronic hypercoagulable state and thrombotic episodes. *Am J Hematol.* 1993;44:63–65.
84. Wang RH, Phillips G Jr, Medof ME, Mold C. Activation of the alternative complement pathway by exposure of phosphatidylethanolamine and phosphatidylserine on erythrocytes from sickle cell disease patients. *J Clin Invest.* 1993;92:1326–1335.
85. Pearson HA, Spencer RP, Cornelius EA. Functional asplenia in sickle-cell anemia. *N Engl J Med.* 1969;281:923–926.
86. Powars DR, Pegelow CH. The spleen in sickle cell disease and thalassemia. *Am J Pediatr Hematol Oncol.* 1979;1:343–353.
87. Zimmerman SA, Ware RE. Palpable splenomegaly in children with haemoglobin SC disease: haematological and clinical manifestations. *Clin Lab Haematol.* 2000;22:145–150.
88. Wright JG, Hambleton IR, Thomas PW, et al. Postsplenectomy course in homozygous sickle cell disease. *J Pediatr.* 1999;134:304–309.
89. Al Salem AH, Qaisaruddin S, Nasserallah Z, al Dabbous, I, al Jam'a A. Splenectomy in patients with sickle-cell disease. *Am J Surg.* 1996;172:254–258.
90. Badaloo A, Emond A, Venugopal S, Serjeant G, Jackson AA. The effect of splenectomy on whole body protein turnover in homozygous sickle cell disease. *Acta Paediatr Scand.* 1991;80:103–105.
91. Robinson SH. Degradation of hemoglobin. In: Williams WJ, Beutler E, Erslev AJ, Lichtman MA, eds. *Hematology.* New York: McGraw-Hill; 1983:388–395.

92. Schaer DJ, Alayash AI, Buehler PW. Gating the radical hemoglobin to macrophages: the anti-inflammatory role of CD163, a Scavenger Receptor. *Antioxid Redox Signal.* 2007;9:991–999.
93. Philippidis P, Mason JC, Evans BJ, et al. Hemoglobin scavenger receptor CD163 mediates interleukin-10 release and heme oxygenase-1 synthesis: antiinflammatory monocyte-macrophage responses in vitro, in resolving skin blisters in vivo, and after cardiopulmonary bypass surgery. *Circ Res.* 2004;94:119–126.
94. Jison ML, Munson PJ, Barb JJ, et al. Blood mononuclear cell gene expression profiles characterize the oxidant, hemolytic, and inflammatory stress of sickle cell disease. *Blood.* 2004;104:270–280.
95. Ryter SW, Otterbein LE, Morse D, Choi AM. Heme oxygenase/carbon monoxide signaling pathways: regulation and functional significance. *Mol Cell Biochem.* 2002;234–235:249–263.
96. Belcher JD, Mahaseth H, Welch TE, et al. Heme oxygenase-1 is a modulator of inflammation and vaso-occlusion in transgenic sickle mice. *J Clin Invest.* 2006;116:808–816.
97. Sedlak TW, Snyder SH. Bilirubin benefits: cellular protection by a biliverdin reductase antioxidant cycle. *Pediatrics.* 2004;113:1776–1782.
98. Giblett ER, Coleman DH, Pirzio-Biroli G, et al. Erythrokinetics: quantitative measurements of red cell production and destruction in normal subjects and patients with anemia. *Blood.* 1956;11:291–309.
99. Nielsen MJ, Petersen SV, Jacobsen C, et al. Haptoglobin-related protein is a high-affinity hemoglobin-binding plasma protein. *Blood.* 2006.
100. Removed in press.
101. Tizianello A, Pannacciulli I. The effect of splenomegaly on dilution curves of tagged erythrocytes and red blood cell volume. Coparative studies on normal, anaemic and splenomegalic patients. *Acta Haematol.* 1959;21:346–359.
102. Nomof N, Hopper J, Jr., Brown E, Scott K, Wennesland R. Simultaneous determinations of the total volume of red blood cells by use of carbon monoxide and chromium in healthy and diseased human subjects. *J Clin Invest.* 1954;33:1382–1387.
103. Huff RL, Feller DD. Relation of circulating red cell volume to body density and obesity. *J Clin Invest.* 1956;35:1–10.
104. Palmer RM, Ashton DS, Moncada S. Vascular endothelial cells synthesize nitric oxide from L-arginine. *Nature.* 1988;333:664–666.
105. Lancaster JR Jr. A tutorial on the diffusibility and reactivity of free nitric oxide. *Nitric Oxide.* 1997;1:18–30.
106. Wink DA, Mitchell JB. Chemical biology of nitric oxide: Insights into regulatory, cytotoxic, and cytoprotective mechanisms of nitric oxide. *Free Radic Biol Med.* 1998;25:434–456.
107. Quyyumi AA, Dakak N, Andrews NP, et al. Nitric oxide activity in the human coronary circulation. Impact of risk factors for coronary atherosclerosis. *J Clin Invest.* 1995;95:1747–1755.
108. Cannon RO, III, Schechter AN, Panza JA, et al. Effects of inhaled nitric oxide on regional blood flow are consistent with intravascular nitric oxide delivery. *J Clin Invest.* 2001;108:279–287.
109. De CR, Libby P, Peng HB, et al. Nitric oxide decreases cytokine-induced endothelial activation. Nitric oxide selectively reduces endothelial expression of adhesion molecules and proinflammatory cytokines. *J Clin Invest.* 1995;96:60–68.
110. Rother RP, Bell L, Hillmen P, Gladwin MT. The clinical sequelae of intravascular hemolysis and extracellular plasma hemoglobin: a novel mechanism of human disease. *JAMA.* 2005;293:1653–1662.
111. Wong J, Fineman JR, Heymann MA. The role of endothelin and endothelin receptor subtypes in regulation of fetal pulmonary vascular tone. *Pediatr Res.* 1994;35:664–670.
112. Black SM, Mata-Greenwood E, Dettman RW, et al. Emergence of smooth muscle cell endothelin B-mediated vasoconstriction in lambs with experimental congenital heart disease and increased pulmonary blood flow. *Circulation.* 2003;108:1646–1654.
113. Schechter AN, Gladwin MT. Hemoglobin and the paracrine and endocrine functions of nitric oxide. *N Engl J Med.* 2003;348:1483–1485.
114. Doherty DH, Doyle MP, Curry SR, et al. Rate of reaction with nitric oxide determines the hypertensive effect of cell-free hemoglobin. *Nat Biotechnol.* 1998;16:672–676.
115. Dou Y, Maillett DH, Eich RF, Olson JS. Myoglobin as a model system for designing heme protein based blood substitutes. *Biophys Chem.* 2002;98:127–148.
116. Reiter CD, Wang X, Tanus-Santos JE, et al. Cell-free hemoglobin limits nitric oxide bioavailability in sickle-cell disease. *Nat Med.* 2002;8:1383–1389.
117. Kim-Shapiro DB, Schechter AN, Gladwin MT. Unraveling the reactions of nitric oxide, nitrite, and hemoglobin in physiology and therapeutics. *Arterioscler Thromb Vasc Biol.* 2006;26:697–705.
118. Jeffers A, Gladwin MT, Kim-Shapiro DB. Computation of plasma hemoglobin nitric oxide scavenging in hemolytic anemias. *Free Radic Biol Med.* 2006;41:1557–1565.
119. Coin JT, Olson JS. The rate of oxygen uptake by human red blood cells. *J Biol Chem.* 1979;254:1178–1190.
120. Liu X, Miller MJ, Joshi MS, et al. Diffusion-limited reaction of free nitric oxide with erythrocytes. *J Biol Chem.* 1998;273:18709–18713.
121. Butler AR, Megson IL, Wright PG. Diffusion of nitric oxide and scavenging by blood in the vasculature. *Biochim Biophys Acta.* 1998;1425:168–176.
122. Liao JC, Hein TW, Vaughn MW, Huang KT, Kuo L. Intravascular flow decreases erythrocyte consumption of nitric oxide. *Proc Natl Acad Sci USA.* 1999;96:8757–8761.
123. Vaughn MW, Kuo L, Liao JC. Effective diffusion distance of nitric oxide in the microcirculation. *Am J Physiol.* 1998;274:H1705–H1714.
124. Han TH, Hyduke DR, Vaughn MW, Fukuto JM, Liao JC. Nitric oxide reaction with red blood cells and hemoglobin under heterogeneous conditions. *Proc Natl Acad Sci USA.* 2002;99:7763–7768.
125. Huang KT, Han TH, Hyduke DR, et al. Modulation of nitric oxide bioavailability by erythrocytes. *Proc Natl Acad Sci USA.* 2001;98:11771–11776.
126. Vaughn MW, Huang KT, Kuo L, Liao JC. Erythrocytes possess an intrinsic barrier to nitric oxide consumption. *J Biol Chem.* 2000;275:2342–2348.
127. Savitsky JP, Doczi J, Black J, Arnold JD. A clinical safety trial of stroma-free hemoglobin. *Clin Pharmacol Ther.* 1978;23:73–80.

128. Carmichael FJ, Ali AC, Campbell JA, et al. A phase I study of oxidized raffinose cross-linked human hemoglobin. *Crit Care Med.* 2000;28:2283–2292.
129. Lamy ML, Daily EK, Brichant JF, et al. Randomized trial of diaspirin cross-linked hemoglobin solution as an alternative to blood transfusion after cardiac surgery. The DCLHb Cardiac Surgery Trial Collaborative Group. *Anesthesiology.* 2000;92:646–656.
130. Viele MK, Weiskopf RB, Fisher D. Recombinant human hemoglobin does not affect renal function in humans: analysis of safety and pharmacokinetics. *Anesthesiology.* 1997;86:848–858.
131. Saxena R, Wijnhoud AD, Carton H, et al. Controlled safety study of a hemoglobin-based oxygen carrier, DCLHb, in acute ischemic stroke. *Stroke.* 1999;30:993–996.
132. Saxena R, Wijnhoud AD, Man in 't Veld AJ, et al. Effect of diaspirin cross-linked hemoglobin on endothelin-1 and blood pressure in acute ischemic stroke in man. *J Hypertens.* 1998;16:1459–1465.
133. Przybelski RJ, Daily EK, Kisicki JC, et al. Phase I study of the safety and pharmacologic effects of diaspirin cross-linked hemoglobin solution. *Crit Care Med.* 1996;24:1993–2000.
134. Reah G, Bodenham AR, Mallick A, Daily EK, Przybelski RJ. Initial evaluation of diaspirin cross-linked hemoglobin (DCLHb) as a vasopressor in critically ill patients. *Crit Care Med.* 1997;25:1480–1488.
135. Lamuraglia GM, O'Hara PJ, Baker WH, et al. The reduction of the allogenic transfusion requirement in aortic surgery with a hemoglobin-based solution. *J Vasc Surg.* 2000;31:299–308.
136. Olson JS, Foley EW, Rogge C, et al. No scavenging and the hypertensive effect of hemoglobin-based blood substitutes. *Free Radic Biol Med.* 2004;36:685–697.
137. Murray JA, Ledlow A, Launspach J, et al. The effects of recombinant human hemoglobin on esophageal motor functions in humans. *Gastroenterology.* 1995;109:1241–1248.
138. Olsen SB, Tang DB, Jackson MR, et al. Enhancement of platelet deposition by cross-linked hemoglobin in a rat carotid endarterectomy model. *Circulation.* 1996;93:327–332.
139. Schafer A, Wiesmann F, Neubauer S, et al. Rapid regulation of platelet activation in vivo by nitric oxide. *Circulation.* 2004;109:1819–1822.
140. Simionatto CS, Cabal R, Jones RL, Galbraith RA. Thrombophlebitis and disturbed hemostasis following administration of intravenous hematin in normal volunteers. *Am J Med.* 1988;85:538–540.
141. Villagra J, Shiva S, Hunter LA, et al. Platelet activation in patients with sickle disease, hemolysis-associated pulmonary hypertension and nitric oxide scavenging by cell-free hemoglobin. *Blood.* 2007;110:2166–2172.
142. Sloan EP, Koenigsberg M, Brunett PH, et al. Post hoc mortality analysis of the efficacy trial of diaspirin cross-linked hemoglobin in the treatment of severe traumatic hemorrhagic shock. *J Trauma.* 2002;52:887–895.
143. Sloan EP, Koenigsberg M, Gens D, et al. Diaspirin cross-linked hemoglobin (DCLHb) in the treatment of severe traumatic hemorrhagic shock: a randomized controlled efficacy trial. *JAMA.* 1999;282:1857–1864.
144. Gladwin MT, Lancaster JR Jr, Freeman BA, Schechter AN. Nitric oxide's reactions with hemoglobin: a view through the SNO-storm. *Nat Med.* 2003;9:496–500.
145. Panza JA, Casino PR, Kilcoyne CM, Quyyumi AA. Role of endothelium-derived nitric oxide in the abnormal endothelium-dependent vascular relaxation of patients with essential hypertension. *Circulation.* 1993;87:1468–1474.
146. Gladwin MT. Deconstructing endothelial dysfunction: soluble guanylyl cyclase oxidation and the NO resistance syndrome. *J Clin Invest.* 2006;116:2330–2332.
147. Gladwin MT, Schechter AN, Ognibene FP, et al. Divergent nitric oxide bioavailability in men and women with sickle cell disease. *Circulation.* 2003;107:271–278.
148. Eberhardt RT, McMahon L, Duffy SJ, et al. Sickle cell anemia is associated with reduced nitric oxide bioactivity in peripheral conduit and resistance vessels. *Am J Hematol.* 2003;74:104–111.
149. Nath KA, Shah V, Haggard JJ, et al. Mechanisms of vascular instability in a transgenic mouse model of sickle cell disease. *Am J Physiol Regul Integr Comp Physiol.* 2000;279:R1949–R1955.
150. Kaul DK, Liu XD, Fabry ME, Nagel RL. Impaired nitric oxide-mediated vasodilation in transgenic sickle mouse. *Am J Physiol Heart Circ Physiol.* 2000;278:H1799–H1806.
151. Kaul DK, Liu XD, Chang HY, Nagel RL, Fabry ME. Effect of fetal hemoglobin on microvascular regulation in sickle transgenic-knockout mice. *J Clin Invest.* 2004;114:1136–1145.
152. Aslan M, Ryan TM, Townes TM, et al. Nitric oxide-dependent generation of reactive species in sickle cell disease. Actin tyrosine induces defective cytoskeletal polymerization. *J Biol Chem.* 2003;278:4194–4204.
153. Pritchard KA, Jr., Ou J, Ou Z, et al. Hypoxia-induced acute lung injury in murine models of sickle cell disease. *Am J Physiol Lung Cell Mol Physiol.* 2004;286:L705–L714.
154. Wood KC, Hebbel RP, Granger DN. Endothelial cell NADPH oxidase mediates the cerebral microvascular dysfunction in sickle cell transgenic mice. *FASEB J.* 2005;19:989–991.
155. Removed in press.
156. Hsu LL, Champion HC, Campbell-Lee SA, et al. Hemolysis in sickle cell mice causes pulmonary hypertension due to global impairment in nitric oxide bioavailability. *Blood.* 2007;109:3088–3098.
157. Minneci PC, Deans KJ, Zhi H, et al. Hemolysis-associated endothelial dysfunction mediated by accelerated NO inactivation by decompartmentalized oxyhemoglobin. *J Clin Invest.* 2005;115:3409–3417.
158. Siegler RL, Pysher TJ, Tesh VL, et al. Reduced nitric oxide bioavailability in a baboon model of Shiga toxin mediated hemolytic uremic syndrome (HUS). *Renal Fail.* 2005;27:635–641.
159. Gramaglia I, Sobolewski P, Meays D, et al. Low nitric oxide bioavailability contributes to the genesis of experimental cerebral malaria. *Nat Med.* 2006;12:1417–1422.
160. Sobolewski P, Gramaglia I, Frangos J, Intaglietta M, van der Heyde HC. Nitric oxide bioavailability in malaria. *Trends Parasitol.* 2005;21:415–422.
161. Azizi E, Dror Y, Wallis K. Arginase activity in erythrocytes of healthy and ill children. *Clin Chim Acta.* 1970;28:391–396.
162. Morris CR, Morris SM, Jr., Hagar W, et al. Arginine therapy: a new treatment for pulmonary hypertension in sickle cell disease? *Am J Respir Crit Care Med.* 2003;168:63–69.

163. Morris CR, Kato GJ, Poljakovic M, et al. Dysregulated Arginine Metabolism, Hemolysis-Associated Pulmonary Hypertension and Mortality in Sickle Cell Disease. *JAMA.* 2005;294:81–90.
164. Gladwin MT, Sachdev V, Jison ML, et al. Pulmonary hypertension as a risk factor for death in patients with sickle cell disease. *N Engl J Med.* 2004;350:886–895.
165. Radomski MW, Palmer RM, Moncada S. Endogenous nitric oxide inhibits human platelet adhesion to vascular endothelium. *Lancet.* 1987;2:1057–1058.
166. Radomski MW, Palmer RM, Moncada S. Comparative pharmacology of endothelium-derived relaxing factor, nitric oxide and prostacyclin in platelets. *Br J Pharmacol.* 1987;92: 181–187.
167. Setty BN, Stuart MJ, Dampier C, Brodecki D, Allen JL. Hypoxaemia in sickle cell disease: biomarker modulation and relevance to pathophysiology. *Lancet.* 2003;362:1450–1455.
168. Quinn CT, Ahmad N. Clinical correlates of steady-state oxyhaemoglobin desaturation in children who have sickle cell disease. *Br J Haematol.* 2005;131:129–134.
169. Atichartakarn V, Likittanasombat K, Chuncharunee S, et al. Pulmonary arterial hypertension in previously splenectomized patients with beta-thalassemic disorders. *Int J Hematol.* 2003;78:139–145.
170. Chou R, DeLoughery TG. Recurrent thromboembolic disease following splenectomy for pyruvate kinase deficiency. *Am J Hematol.* 2001;67:197–199.
171. Hayag-Barin JE, Smith RE, Tucker FC, Jr. Hereditary spherocytosis, thrombocytosis, and chronic pulmonary emboli: a case report and review of the literature. *Am J Hematol.* 1998;57:82–84.
172. Aessopos A, Farmakis D, Deftereos S, et al. Cardiovascular effects of splenomegaly and splenectomy in beta-thalassemia. *Ann Hematol.* 2005;84:353–357.
173. Vichinsky EP. Pulmonary hypertension in sickle cell disease. *N Engl J Med.* 2004;350:857–859.
174. Westerman MP, Pizzey A, Hirschmann JV, et al. Plasma 'free' HB is related to red cell derived vesicle numbers in sickle cell anemia and thalassemia intermedia: implications for nitric oxide (NO) scavenging and pulmonary hypertension [abstract]. *Blood.* 2004;104:465a.
175. Kisanuki A, Kietthubthew S, Asada Y, et al. Intravenous injection of sonicated blood induces pulmonary microthromboembolism in rabbits with ligation of the splenic artery. *Thromb Res.* 1997;85:95–103.
176. Kietthubthew S, Kisanuki A, Asada Y, et al. Pulmonary microthromboembolism by injection of sonicated autologous blood in rabbits with splenic artery ligations. *Southeast Asian J Trop Med Public Health.* 1997;28(Suppl 3):138–140.
177. Platt OS, Brambilla DJ, Rosse WF, et al. Mortality in sickle cell disease. Life expectancy and risk factors for early death. *N Engl J Med.* 1994;330:1639–1644.
178. Platt OS. Sickle cell anemia as an inflammatory disease. *J Clin Invest.* 2000;106:337–338.
179. Kaul DK, Hebbel RP. Hypoxia/reoxygenation causes inflammatory response in transgenic sickle mice but not in normal mice. *J Clin Invest.* 2000;106:411–420.
180. Nolan VG, Wyszynski DF, Farrer LA, Steinberg MH. Hemolysis-associated priapism in sickle cell disease. *Blood.* 2005;106:3264–3267.
181. Kato GJ, McGowan VR, Machado RF, et al. Lactate dehydrogenase as a biomarker of hemolysis-associated nitric oxide resistance, priapism, leg ulceration, pulmonary hypertension and death in patients with sickle cell disease. *Blood.* 2006;107:2279–2285.
182. Kato GJ, Hsieh M, Machado R, et al. Cerebrovascular disease associated with sickle cell pulmonary hypertension. *Am J Hematol.* 2006;81:503–510.
183. Kato GJ, Gladwin MT, Steinberg MH. Deconstructing sickle cell disease: reappraisal of the role of hemolysis in the development of clinical subphenotypes. *Blood Rev.* 2007;21:37–47.
184. Collins FS, Orringer EP. Pulmonary hypertension and cor pulmonale in the sickle hemoglobinopathies. *Am J Med.* 1982;73:814–821.
185. Powars D, Weidman JA, Odom-Maryon T, Niland JC, Johnson C. Sickle cell chronic lung disease: prior morbidity and the risk of pulmonary failure. *Medicine (Baltimore).* 1988;67:66–76.
186. Sutton LL, Castro O, Cross DJ, Spencer JE, Lewis JF. Pulmonary hypertension in sickle cell disease. *Am J Cardiol.* 1994;74:626–628.
187. Castro O. Systemic fat embolism and pulmonary hypertension in sickle cell disease. *Hematol Oncol Clin North Am.* 1996;10:1289–1303.
188. Simmons BE, Santhanam V, Castaner A, et al. Sickle cell heart disease. Two-dimensional echo and Doppler ultrasonographic findings in the hearts of adult patients with sickle cell anemia. *Arch Intern Med.* 1988;148:1526–1528.
189. Haque AK, Gokhale S, Rampy BA, et al. Pulmonary hypertension in sickle cell hemoglobinopathy: a clinicopathologic study of 20 cases. *Hum Pathol.* 2002;33:1037–1043.
190. Castro O, Hoque M, Brown BD. Pulmonary hypertension in sickle cell disease: cardiac catheterization results and survival. *Blood.* 2003;101:1257–1261.
191. Boussaada R, Boubaker K, Mourali S, et al. [Pulmonary hypertension in sickle cell anemia. A case report]. *Tunis Med.* 2004;82(Suppl 1):180–184.
192. Ataga KI, Sood N, De GG, et al. Pulmonary hypertension in sickle cell disease. *Am J Med.* 2004;117:665–669.
193. Wu TJ, Tseng CD, Tseng YZ, et al. [A case of beta-thalassemia major with mediastinal hematopoietic tumor and pulmonary hypertension]. *Taiwan Yi Xue Hui Za Zhi.* 1986;85:315–320.
194. Aessopos A, Stamatelos G, Skoumas V, et al. Pulmonary hypertension and right heart failure in patients with beta-thalassemia intermedia. *Chest.* 1995;107:50–53.
195. Jootar P, Fucharoen S. Cardiac involvement in beta-thalassemia/hemoglobin E disease: clinical and hemodynamic findings. *Southeast Asian J Trop Med Public Health.* 1990;21:269–273.
196. Grisaru D, Rachmilewitz EA, Mosseri M, et al. Cardiopulmonary assessment in beta-thalassemia major. *Chest.* 1990; 98:1138–1142.
197. Finazzo M, Midiri M, D'Angelo P, et al. [The heart of the patient with beta thalassemia major. Study with magnetic resonance]. *Radiol Med (Torino).* 1998;96:462–465.
198. Derchi G, Fonti A, Forni GL, et al. Pulmonary hypertension in patients with thalassemia major. *Am Heart J.* 1999;138:384.
199. Aessopos A, Farmakis D, Karagiorga M, et al. Cardiac involvement in thalassemia intermedia: a multicenter study. *Blood.* 2001;97:3411–3416.

200. Zakynthinos E, Vassilakopoulos T, Kaltsas P, et al. Pulmonary hypertension, interstitial lung fibrosis, and lung iron deposition in thalassaemia major. *Thorax.* 2001;56:737–739.
201. Morris CR, Kuypers FA, Kato GJ, et al. Hemolysis-associated pulmonary hypertension in thalassemia. *Ann NY Acad Sci.* 2005;1054:481–485.
202. Uchida T, Miyake T, Matsuno M, et al. [Fatal pulmonary thromboembolism in a patient with paroxysmal nocturnal hemoglobinuria]. *Rinsho Ketsueki.* 1998;39:150–152.
203. Heller PG, Grinberg AR, Lencioni M, Molina MM, Roncoroni AJ. Pulmonary hypertension in paroxysmal nocturnal hemoglobinuria. *Chest.* 1992;102:642–643.
204. Hill A, Richards SJ, Hillmen P. Recent developments in the understanding and management of paroxysmal nocturnal haemoglobinuria. *Br J Haematol.* 2007;137:181–192.
205. Hayag-Barin JE, Smith RE, Tucker FC, Jr. Hereditary spherocytosis, thrombocytosis, and chronic pulmonary emboli: a case report and review of the literature. *Am J Hematol.* 1998;57:82–84.
206. Verresen D, De Backer W, Van Meerbeeck J, et al. Spherocytosis and pulmonary hypertension coincidental occurrence or causal relationship? *Eur Respir J.* 1991;4:629–631.
207. Stewart GW, Amess JA, Eber SW, et al. Thrombo-embolic disease after splenectomy for hereditary stomatocytosis. *Br J Haematol.* 1996;93:303–310.
208. Jais X, Till SJ, Cynober T, et al. An extreme consequence of splenectomy in dehydrated hereditary stomatocytosis: gradual thrombo-embolic pulmonary hypertension and lung-heart transplantation. *Hemoglobin.* 2003;27:139–147.
209. Murali B, Drain A, Seller D, Dunning J, Vuylsteke A. Pulmonary thromboendarterectomy in a case of hereditary stomatocytosis. *Br J Anaesth.* 2003;91:739–741.
210. Jardine DL, Laing AD. Delayed pulmonary hypertension following splenectomy for congenital spherocytosis. *Intern Med J.* 2004;34:214–216.
211. Smedema JP, Louw VJ. Pulmonary arterial hypertension after splenectomy for hereditary spherocytosis. *Cardiovasc J S Afr.* 2007;18:84–89.
212. Alvarez NR, Marin R. [Severe maternal complications associated with pre-eclampsia: an almost forgotten pathology?]. *Nefrologia.* 2001;21:565–573.
213. Stuard ID, Heusinkveld RS, Moss AJ. Microangiopathic hemolytic anemia and thrombocytopenia in primary pulmonary hypertension. *N Engl J Med.* 1972;287:869–870.
214. McCarthy JT, Staats BA. Pulmonary hypertension, hemolytic anemia, and renal failure. A mitomycin-associated syndrome. *Chest.* 1986;89:608–611.
215. Jubelirer SJ. Primary pulmonary hypertension. Its association with microangiopathic hemolytic anemia and thrombocytopenia. *Arch Intern Med.* 1991;151:1221–1223.
216. Suzuki H, Nakasato M, Sato S, et al. Microangiopathic hemolytic anemia and thrombocytopenia in a child with atrial septal defect and pulmonary hypertension. *Tohoku J Exp Med.* 1997;181:379–384.
217. Labrune P, Zittoun J, Duvaltier I, et al. Haemolytic uraemic syndrome and pulmonary hypertension in a patient with methionine synthase deficiency. *Eur J Pediatr.* 1999;158:734–739.
218. Fischer EG, Marek JM, Morris A, Nashelsky MB. Cholesterol granulomas of the lungs associated with microangiopathic hemolytic anemia and thrombocytopenia in pulmonary hypertension. *Arch Pathol Lab Med.* 2000;124:1813–1815.
219. Chou R, DeLoughery TG. Recurrent thromboembolic disease following splenectomy for pyruvate kinase deficiency. *Am J Hematol.* 2001;67:197–199.
220. Zhang Y, Qui Y, Zhu J, Gao D. Pulmonary hypertension associated with autoimmune hemolytic anemia: a case report. *Int J Cardiol.* 2007;115:e1–e2.
221. Lode HN, Krings G, Schulze-Neick I, et al. Pulmonary hypertension in a case of Hb-Mainz hemolytic anemia. *J Pediatr Hematol Oncol.* 2007;29:173–177.
222. Huchzermeyer FW. Avian pulmonary hypertension syndrome. IV. Increased right ventricular mass in turkeys experimentally infected with Plasmodium durae. *Onderstepoort J Vet Res.* 1988;55:107–108.
223. Saissy JM, Rouvin B, Koulmann P. [Severe malaria in intensive care units in 2003]. *Med Trop (Mars.).* 2003;63:258–266.
224. Ehrhardt S, Mockenhaupt FP, Anemana SD, et al. High levels of circulating cardiac proteins indicate cardiac impairment in African children with severe Plasmodium falciparum malaria. *Microbes Infect.* 2005;7:1204–1210.
225. Strauss E, Da Costa Gayotto LC, Antonelli R, et al. Systemic surgical shunts and splenomegaly as causes of haemolysis in portal hypertension in mansonic schistosomiasis. Evaluation through serum levels of haptoglobin, hemopexin and bilirubins. *J Hepatol.* 1986;2:340–350.
226. de CR, Herman P, Pugliese V, et al. Prevalence of pulmonary hypertension in patients with hepatosplenic Mansonic schistosomiasis–prospective study. *Hepatogastroenterology.* 2003;50:2028–2030.
227. Kyllonen K, Mattila T, Hartikainen M, Tala P. Mitral valve replacement with ball and tilting disc valve prosthesis. A clinical and haemodynamic study. *Scand J Thorac Cardiovasc Surg.* 1976;10:15–20.
228. Iwaki H, Kuraoka S, Tatebe S. [Hemolytic anemia due to aortic valve regurgitation after mitral valve replacement]. *Kyobu Geka.* 2003;56:124–128.
229. Chukwuemeka AO, Turtle MR, Trivedi UH, Venn GE, Chambers DJ. A clinical evaluation of platelet function, haemolysis and oxygen transfer during cardiopulmonary bypass comparing the Quantum HF-6700 to the HF-5700 hollow fibre membrane oxygenator. *Perfusion.* 2000;15:479–484.
230. Pierangeli A, Masieri V, Bruzzi F, et al. Haemolysis during cardiopulmonary bypass: how to reduce the free haemoglobin by managing the suctioned blood separately. *Perfusion.* 2001;16:519–524.
231. Gerrah R, Shargal Y, Elami A. Impaired oxygenation and increased hemolysis after cardiopulmonary bypass in patients with glucose-6-phosphate dehydrogenase deficiency. *Ann Thorac Surg.* 2003;76:523–527.
232. Takami Y, Makinouchi K, Nakazawa T, et al. Hemolytic characteristics of a pivot bearing supported Gyro centrifugal pump (C1E3) simulating various clinical applications. *Artif Organs.* 1996;20:1042–1049.
233. Jackson N, Franklin IM, Hughes MA. Recurrent priapism following splenectomy for thalassaemia intermedia. *Br J Surg.* 1986;73:678.
234. Rao KR, Patel AR. Priapism and thalassaemia intermedia. *Br J Surg.* 1986;73:1048.

235. Macchia P, Massei F, Nardi M, et al. Thalassemia intermedia and recurrent priapism following splenectomy. *Haematologica.* 1990;75:486–487.
236. Dore F, Bonfigli S, Pardini S, Pirozzi F, Longinotti M. Priapism in thalassemia intermedia. *Haematologica.* 1991;76: 523.
237. Andrieu V, Dumonceau O, Grange MJ. Priapism in a patient with unstable hemoglobin: hemoglobin Koln. *Am J Hematol.* 2003;74:73–74.
298. Gyan E, Darre S, Jude B, et al. Acute priapism in a patient with unstable hemoglobin Perth and Factor V Leiden under effective oral anticoagulant therapy. *Hematol J.* 2001;2:210–211.
239. Thuret I, Bardakdjian J, Badens C, et al. Priapism following splenectomy in an unstable hemoglobin: hemoglobin Olmsted beta 141 (H19) Leu–>Arg. *Am J Hematol.* 1996;51:133–136.
240. Goulding FJ. Priapism caused by glucose phosphate isomerase deficiency. *J Urol.* 1976;116:819–820.
241. Edney MT, Schned AR, Cendron M, Chaffee S, Ellsworth PI. Priapism in a 15-year-old boy with congenital dyserythropoietic anemia type II (hereditary erythroblastic multinuclearity with positive acidified serum lysis test). *J Urol.* 2002;167:309–310.
242. Nolan VG, Baldwin C, Ma Q, et al. Association of single nucleotide polymorphisms in klotho with priapism in sickle cell anaemia. *Br J Haematol.* 2005;128:266–272.
243. Christakis J, Vavatsi N, Hassapopoulou H, et al. Comparison of homozygous sickle cell disease in northern Greece and Jamaica. *Lancet.* 1990;335:637–640.
244. Champion HC, Bivalacqua TJ, Takimoto E, Kass DA, Burnett AL. Phosphodiesterase-5A dysregulation in penile erectile tissue is a mechanism of priapism. *Proc Natl Acad Sci USA.* 2005;102:1661–1666.
245. Sawhney H, Weedon J, Gillette P, Solomon W, Braverman A. Predilection of hemolytic anemia-associated leg ulcers for the medial malleolus. *Vasa.* 2002;31:191–193.
246. Fucharoen S, Ketvichit P, Pootrakul P, et al. Clinical manifestation of beta-thalassemia/hemoglobin E disease. *J Pediatr Hematol Oncol.* 2000;22:552–557.
247. Eckman JR. Leg ulcers in sickle cell disease. *Hematol Oncol Clin North Am.* 1996;10:1333–1344.
248. Koshy M, Entsuah R, Koranda A, et al. Leg ulcers in patients with sickle cell disease. *Blood.* 1989;74:1403–1408.
249. Levy LA. Foot and ankle ulcers associated with hematologic disorders. *Clin Podiatry.* 1985;2:631–637.
250. Gimmon Z, Wexler MR, Rachmilewitz EA. Juvenile leg ulceration in beta-thalassemia major and intermedia. *Plast Reconstr Surg.* 1982;69:320–325.
251. Daneshmend TK, Peachey RD. Leg ulcers in alpha-thalassaemia (haemoglobin H disease). *Br J Dermatol.* 1978; 98:233–235.
252. Stevens DM, Shupack JL, Javid J, Silber R. Ulcers of the leg in thalassemia. *Arch Dermatol.* 1977;113:1558–1560.
253. Leverkus M, Schwaaf A, Brocker EB, Runger TM. Recurrent hemolysis-associated pseudoerysipelas of the lower legs in a patient with congenital spherocytosis. *J Am Acad Dermatol.* 2004;51:1019–1023.
254. Giraldi S, Abbage KT, Marinoni LP, et al. Leg ulcer in hereditary spherocytosis. *Pediatr Dermatol.* 2003;20:427–428.
255. Lawrence P, Aronson I, Saxe N, Jacobs P. Leg ulcers in hereditary spherocytosis. *Clin Exp Dermatol.* 1991;16:28–30.
256. Vanscheidt W, Leder O, Vanscheidt E, et al. Leg ulcers in a patient with spherocytosis: a clinicopathological report. *Dermatologica.* 1990;181:56–59.
257. Rivera-Biaschoechea ZA. Hereditary spherocytosis with leg ulcer and unaffected parents or siblings. Report of one case. *Bol Asoc Med P R.* 1964;56:109–114.
258. Nolan VG, Adewoye A, Baldwin C, et al. Sickle cell leg ulcers: associations with haemolysis and SNPs in Klotho, TEK and genes of the TGF-beta/BMP pathway. *Br J Haematol.* 2006;133:570–578.
259. Kato GJ, Hsieh M, Machado R, et al. Cerebrovascular disease associated with sickle cell pulmonary hypertension. *Am J Hematol.* 2006;81:503–510.
260. Pegelow CH, Colangelo L, Steinberg M, et al. Natural history of blood pressure in sickle cell disease: risks for stroke and death associated with relative hypertension in sickle cell anemia. *Am J Med.* 1997;102:171–177.
261. Buchanan GR, DeBaun MR, Quinn CT, Steinberg MH. Sickle cell disease. *Hematology Am Soc Hematol Educ Program.* 200:435–447.
262. Steinberg MH. Predicting clinical severity in sickle cell anaemia. *Br J Haematol.* 2005;129:465–481.
263. Ohene-Frempong K, Weiner SJ, Sleeper LA, et al. Cerebrovascular accidents in sickle cell disease: rates and risk factors. *Blood.* 1998;91:288–294.
264. Lezcano NE, Odo N, Kutlar A, Brambilla D, Adams RJ. Regular transfusion lowers plasma free hemoglobin in children with sickle-cell disease at risk for stroke. *Stroke.* 2006;37:1424–1426.
265. Gladwin MT, Sachdev V, Jison ML, et al. Pulmonary hypertension as a risk factor for death in patients with sickle cell disease. *N Engl J Med.* 2004;350:886–895.
266. Graham JK, Mosunjac M, Hanzlick RL, Mosunjac M. Sickle cell lung disease and sudden death: a retrospective/prospective study of 21 autopsy cases and literature review. *Am J Forensic Med Pathol.* 2007;28:168–172.
267. Aessopos A, Stamatelos G, Skoumas V, et al. Pulmonary hypertension and right heart failure in patients with beta-thalassemia intermedia. *Chest.* 1995;107:50–53.
268. Wu KH, Chang JS, Su BH, Peng CT. Tricuspid regurgitation in patients with beta-thalassemia major. *Ann Hematol.* 2004;83:779–783.
269. Singer ST, Kuypers FA, Styles L, et al. Pulmonary hypertension in thalassemia: Association with platelet activation and hypercoagulable state. *Am J Hematol.* 2006;81:670–675.
270. Aessopos A, Farmakis D, Deftereos S, et al. Thalassemia heart disease: a comparative evaluation of thalassemia major and thalassemia intermedia. *Chest.* 2005;127:1523–1530.
271. Aessopos A, Farmakis D, Hatziliami A, et al. Cardiac status in well-treated patients with thalassemia major. *Eur J Haematol.* 2004;73:359–366.
272. Ataga KI, Sood N, De GG, et al. Pulmonary hypertension in sickle cell disease. *Am J Med.* 2004;117:665–669.
273. De Castro LM, Jonassaint JC, Graham FL, Ashley-Koch A, Telen MJ. Pulmonary hypertension associated with sickle cell disease: Clinical and laboratory endpoints and disease outcomes. *Am J Hematol.* 2008;83:19–25.

274. Ataga KI, Sood N, De GG, et al. Pulmonary hypertension in sickle cell disease. *Am J Med.* 2004;117:665–669.
275. Ataga KI, Moore CG, Jones S, et al. Pulmonary hypertension in patients with sickle cell disease: a longitudinal study. *Br J Haematol.* 2006;134:109–115.
276. Taylor JG, Woods GM, Machado R, Kato GJ, Gladwin MT. Severe pulmonary hypertension in an adolescent with sickle cell disease. *Am J Hematol.* 2007;83:71–72.
277. Kato GJ, Onyekwere OC, Gladwin MT. Pulmonary hypertension in sickle cell disease: relevance to children. *Pediatr Hematol Oncol.* 2007;24:159–170.
278. Young EM, Zilberman MV, Du W, Sarnaik SA. Pulmonary hypertension in pediatric patients with sickle cell disease: a retrospective study. *Blood.* 2004;104:23b.
279. Onyekwere OC, Campbell AD, Teshome M, et al. Pulmonary hypertension in sickle cell disease children and adolescents. *Pediatr Cardiol.* 2007;24:159–170.
280. Ambrusko SJ, Gunawardena S, Sakara A, et al. Elevation of tricuspid regurgitant jet velocity, a marker for pulmonary hypertension in children with sickle cell disease. *Pediatr Blood Cancer.* 2006;47:907–913.
281. Liem RI, Young LT, Thompson AA. Tricuspid regurgitant jet velocity is associated with hemolysis in children and young adults with sickle cell disease evaluated for pulmonary hypertension. *Haematologica.* 2007;92:1549–1552.
282. Minniti CP, Sable C, Campbell A, et al. Elevated tricuspid regurgitant jet velocity in children and adolescents with sickle cell disease: association with hemolysis and hemoglobin oxygen desaturation. *Br J Haematol.* In press.
283. Sedrak A, Rao SP, Miller ST, Hekmet V, Rao M. Pulmonary hypertension in children and adolescents with sickle cell disease. *Blood.* 2006;108:21b–22b.
284. Deem S, Kim SS, Min JH, et al. Pulmonary vascular effects of red blood cells containing S-nitrosated hemoglobin. *Am J Physiol Heart Circ Physiol.* 2004;287:H2561–H2568.
285. Sachdev V, Machado RF, Shizukuda Y, et al. Diastolic dysfunction is an independent risk factor for death in patients with sickle cell disease. *J Am Coll Cardiol.* 2007;49:472–479.
286. Anthi A, Machado RF, Jison ML, et al. Hemodynamic and functional assessment of patients with sickle cell disease and pulmonary hypertension. *Am J Respir Crit Care Med.* 2007;175:1272–1279.
287. Machado RF, Mack AK, Martyr S, et al. Severity of pulmonary hypertension during vaso-occlusive pain crisis and exercise in patients with sickle cell disease. *Br J Haematol.* 2007;136:319–325.
288. Bossone E, Rubenfire M, Bach DS, Ricciardi M, Armstrong WF. Range of tricuspid regurgitation velocity at rest and during exercise in normal adult men: implications for the diagnosis of pulmonary hypertension. *J Am Coll Cardiol.* 1999;33:1662–1666.
289. Little JA, McGowan VR, Kato GJ, et al. Combination erythropoietin-hydroxyurea therapy in sickle cell disease: experience from the National Institutes of Health and a literature review. *Haematologica.* 2006;91:1076–1083.
290. Machado RF, Martyr S, Kato GJ, et al. Sildenafil therapy in patients with sickle cell disease and pulmonary hypertension. *Br J Haematol.* 2005;130:445–453.
291. Machado RF, Gladwin MT. Chronic sickle cell lung disease: new insights into the diagnosis, pathogenesis and treatment of pulmonary hypertension. *Br J Haematol.* 2005;129:449–464.
292. Lin EE, Rodgers GP, Gladwin MT. Hemolytic anemia-associated pulmonary hypertension in sickle cell disease. *Curr Hematol Rep.* 2005;4:117–125.

12

Animal Models of Hemoglobinopathies and Thalassemia

Mary Fabry

INTRODUCTION

Transgenic mice are important adjuncts for the study of the pathophysiology and treatment of human hemoglobin disorders. Many inbred strains with spontaneous and induced mutations and engineered knockout and knockin lines are available (Table 12.1). Transgenic mice have both advantages and disadvantages for studying human disease. Most available mice are of mixed or poorly characterized genetic backgrounds and must be bred onto another inbred strain to obtain sustainable lines and consistent physiology. The choice of genetic background or the presence of a mixed background can affect both hematology and physiology.

Different inbred mouse strains, and male and female mice, can have different physiological characteristics, complicating the interpretation of some experiments. Mice have a higher plasma osmolarity than man[1] and the 2,3-BPG content of mouse red cells is twice that of human erythrocytes. Inbred strains have five common α-globin chains and three common β-globin chains.[2] The common C57BL/6 strain has only a single α- and β-globin chain; other strains can have two α- or two β-globin chains. When these are combined with human globin transgenes, many homotetramers due to the presence of interspecies αβ dimers result, some of which form tetramers with low oxygen affinity that will affect polymer formation and pathophysiology.[3] These are some examples of factors likely to alter sickle cell mouse pathophysiology when compared with human.

THE TECHNOLOGY OF TRANSGENIC AND KNOCKOUT MICE

In the early 1980s cloned DNA was introduced into fertilized mouse embryos. Following the discovery of a locus control region (LCR) 5′ to the β-globin gene cluster (Chapter 5), investigators linked the LCR to various globin gene constructs and achieved erythroid expression in transgenic animals.[4–9] The process of producing transgenic mice from constructs injected into fertilized mouse embryos is illustrated in Figure 12.1.[10]

Knockout or knockin technology is a means of deleting endogenous genes or introducing new genes into a genome by homologous recombination (Fig. 12.2). Homologous sequences flanking the gene of interest are isolated and inserted into a targeting construct that contains selectable markers, in the illustration, neomycin resistance and herpes virus thymidine kinase, driven by a promoter. This targeting vector is transfected into a line of embryonic stem cells (ESCs) that are selected by exposure to neomycin and ganciclovir. Colonies are picked, expanded, and analyzed by Southern blot analysis for fragments of the predicted size. Cells with the mutated β-globin gene are then injected into blastocysts to generate chimeric animals that are screened for the mutation and bred to detect animals with germ line mutations (Fig. 12.3).

THALASSEMIC MICE

Mouse models of thalassemia with either deletions or knockouts of the α- and β-globin genes have been studied. A nonlethal deletion of the β^{major}-globin gene ($Hbb^{th\text{-}1}$) in a mouse with so-called diffuse hemoglobin, which can be bred to homozygosity, was detected by electrophoretic screening.[11] The excess of mouse β^{minor} in this model might be a general response to anemia or a more specific response to the deletion that generated the thalassemia. Mice homozygous for the β^{major} deletion have a high reticulocyte count, anemia, microcytosis, low mean corpuscular hemoglobin (MCH) and a low mean corpuscular hemoglobin concentration (MCHC). Their broad distribution of red cell densities looks much like the density distribution obtained for human patients with β-thalassemia intermedia.

Three different deletions in the α-globin chain have been described that lead to α thalassemia.[12] These deletions are sufficiently large so that they are lethal when homozygous, even in the presence of a rescuing human transgene. In the heterozygotes, the α:β globin chain synthesis chain ratio is approximately 0.75, and hence the induced thalassemia is relatively mild. If a single α-globin gene deletion is bred into mice homozygous for the β^{major} deletion, much of the red cell pathology is corrected; reticulocyte counts decrease from approximately 20% to 5% and red cell density is normalized, an observation akin to that observed when human β and α thalassemia coexist (Chapters 13, 14, 16, and 17). This is due to correction of the imbalance of α and β globin chains that is responsible for thalassemia pathology.

Mouse models have been advocated as models for human thalassemia[11,13–17] and mice with deletional thalassemia have been used to study treatments with erythropoietin, clotrimazole, and hydroxyurea.[18]

Table 12.1. Nomenclature of transgenic mice

Nickname	γ-Globin gene	αβ-Globin gene	Mouse α-knockout	Mouse β-deletion or knockout
C57BL/6	–	–	+//+	+//+
Thal	–	–	+//+	Hbb^{th-1}/Hbb^{th-1} ±
NY1DD	–	NY1 #	+//+	Hbb^{th-1}/Hbb^{th-1}
SAD	–	SAD &	+//+	+//+
S-Antilles-thal	–	S-Antilles $	+//+	Hbb^{th-1}/Hbb^{th-1}
S+S-Antilles	–	NY1 and S-Antilles %	+//+	Hbb^{th-1}/Hbb^{th-1}
NY1KO-yL	F1352 &	NY1	Hba^{0}//Hba^{0} ¶	Hbb$^{\circ}$//Hbb^{0} †
NY1KO-yM	G203 §	NY1	Hba$^{\circ}$//Hba$^{\circ}$	Hbb$^{\circ}$//Hbb$^{\circ}$
NY1KO-yH	G100 ¥	NY1	Hba$^{\circ}$//Hba$^{\circ}$	Hbb$^{\circ}$//Hbb$^{\circ}$
β^{S}-Ryan et al, six lines	Mixed £	β^{S}-Ryan et al	Hba$^{\circ}$//Hba$^{\circ}$	Hbb$^{\circ}$//Hbb$^{\circ}$
BERK β-hemi L		BERK ‡ 1 copy	Hba$^{\circ}$//Hba$^{\circ}$	Hbb$^{\circ}$//+
BERK β-hemi H		BERK 2 copies	Hba$^{\circ}$//Hba$^{\circ}$	Hbb$^{\circ}$//+
BERK		BERK 1 copy	Hba$^{\circ}$//Hba$^{\circ}$	Hbb$^{\circ}$//Hbb$^{\circ}$
BERK-γM	G203	BERK 1 copy	Hba$^{\circ}$//Hba$^{\circ}$	Hbb$^{\circ}$//Hbb$^{\circ}$
BERK-γH	G100	BERK 1 copy	Hba$^{\circ}$//Hba$^{\circ}$	Hbb$^{\circ}$//Hbb$^{\circ}$
β^{S}-YAC		β^{S}-YAC €	Hba$^{\circ}$//Hba$^{\circ}$	Hbb$^{\circ}$//Hbb$^{\circ}$
β^{S}-Knockin		β^{S}-knockin ₤	+//+	+//+

Symbols refer to separate references pertaining to this table only. ± (1), # (2), & (3), $ (4), % (5), & (6), ¶ (7), † (8,9), § (10,11), ¥ (10,12), £ (13), ‡ (14), € (15), ₤ (16).

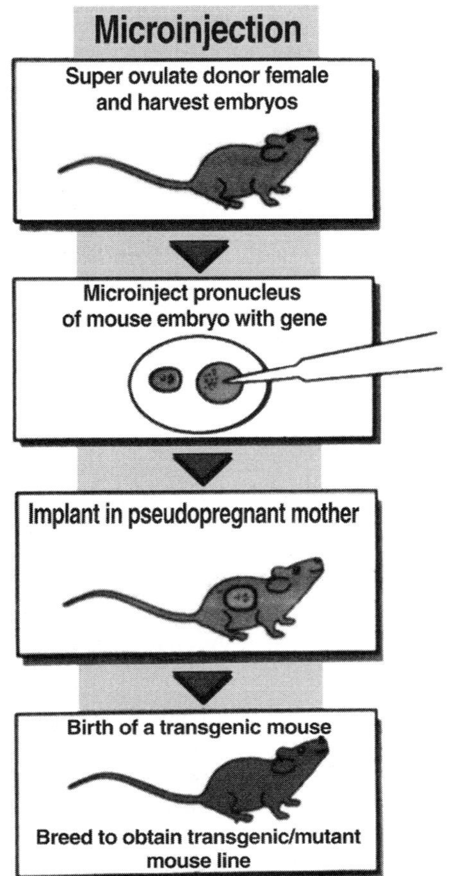

Figure 12.1. Creation of a transgenic mouse by injection of a construct into the pronucleus of a fertilized mouse egg. The injected eggs are then implanted into pseudopregnant females and the resulting pups are screened for the presence of the transgene. Pups positive for the transgene are bred to determine if the transgene is present in the germ line.

A disruption of the β^{major}-chain was generated by inserting a bacterial gene into the second exon of the mouse β^{major} gene.[19] This resulted in a more severe form of thalassemia than the previously described β^{major}deletion and is lethal in homozygotes despite the continued production of β^{minor}-globin. When bred into mice expressing the human β-globin gene, the percentage of human β-globin chain is higher than that obtained with the β^{major} deletion.[20] The reduced severity of the deletion model when compared with the disruption model might be due to the ability of the remaining β^{minor} gene to interact directly with the LCR without competition from the missing β^{major} gene. In contrast to the deletion, with a disrupted gene, not only is the β^{major} promoter intact, but, the inserted *tk* promoter

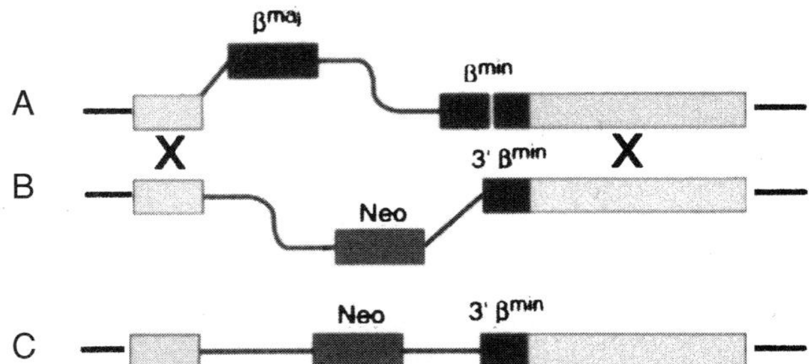

Figure 12.2. Targeted insertional deletion of the mouse β-globin genes. Line A is a simplified representation of the β-globin locus in the diffuse mouse, which makes two β-globins: β^{major} and β^{minor}. Line B represents the replacement vector, which has an area of homology on the 5′ side, a Neo fragment capable of conferring resistance to G418, which also contains thymidine kinase genes driven by a promoter, and another area of homology corresponding to a portion of the β^{minor} gene and extending beyond it. Line C shows the result of a crossover that contains the Neo fragment and an inactive remnant of the β^{minor} gene.

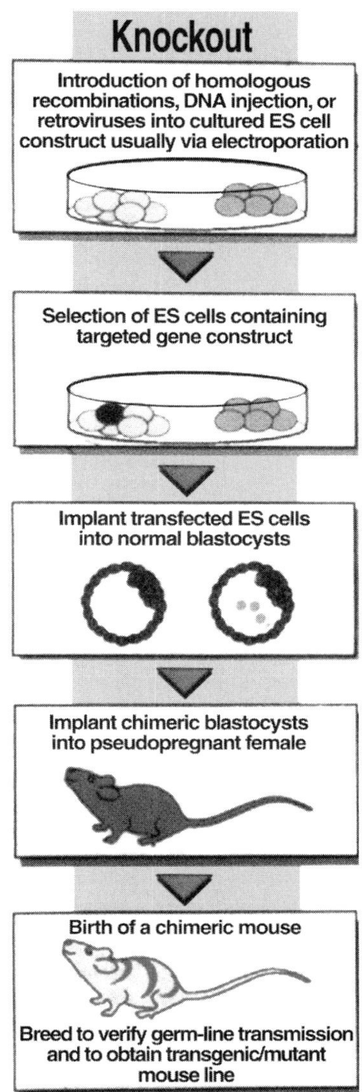

Figure 12.3. Creation of a knockout mouse by using ESC technology. The targeting vector is introduced into ESCs, which are then selected by exposure to neomycin and ganciclovir. The selected cells are implanted into normal blastocysts that are then implanted into pseudopregnant females. The resulting pups are then screened and bred to verify transmission of the mutated genes into the germ line.

driving the *neo* gene is present possibly resulting in further competition for the LCR and reduced transcription of the β^{minor} globin gene. A similar hypothesis has been proposed to account for the higher levels of HbA_2 and HbF when the β-globin gene promoter is deleted in some types of human β thalassemia (Chapters 16 and 17). Full β-globin gene knockout mice are available.[20–22] Full knockout of the α-globin gene cluster has also been generated[23] making possible transgenic mice with exclusively human hemoglobins. The knockouts are lethal in the homozygous state unless rescued by a transgene. In homozygotes, without a rescuing transgene, the α knockout mouse has a condition similar to human hydrops fetalis.[23]

MODELS FOR SICKLE CELL DISEASE

The complex pathophysiology of sickle cell disease (Chapters 8–11) and its modulation by many genetic, epistatic, and environmental elements (Chapter 27) make it unlikely that a single animal model will adequately represent all aspects of the disease; nonetheless, animal models have already made significant contributions to sickle cell pathophysiology and treatment.

Sickle Transgenic Mice

Early transgenic models of sickle cell disease had little pathology and the first models expressing moderately high levels of both human α- and β^S-globin chains were reported in 1990.[24–28] Subsequently, many different lines of mice with variable degrees of severity became available allowing more detailed studies of pathology (Tables 12.1 and 12.2). These strains included: mice expressing the "super β^S" HbS-Antilles (Chapters 22 and 23), which failed to exhibit the expected level of pathology in part because of low human α-globin expression;[29] the SAD mouse expressing the β^S mutation and two additional "super" β^S mutations, HbS-Antilles and HbD-Punjab (Chapter 23).[30] The enhanced effects on polymer formation of mice expressing the "super" β^S globins are due to reduction in oxygen affinity, which shifts the conformation of the hemoglobin to the T-state and favors polymer formation, and reduced solubility, which suggests that new contact sites in the polymer have been created.

The first report of the SAD mouse described mice with no deletions and a mouse with a single β^{major} deletion. The former had 19% of all β-globin as β-SAD and is used most often for study. Expression of HbS was increased in mice expressing both human α- and β^S-globins by breeding in a homozygous mouse β-globin gene deletion and, in some cases, addition of a heterozygous α-globin gene deletion.[29,31,32] Another model still in use is mice expressing human α-, β^S-, and $\beta^{S\text{-Antilles}}$, which balanced the high human α-globin gene expression of the β^S line against the low human α-globin gene expression of the $\beta^{S\text{-Antilles}}$ line; these mice are known as S+S-Antilles mice. A further model contains mouse high oxygen affinity globins and HbS-Antilles. Deoxygenation produced sickled cells and intracellular polymer formation.[33–38]

Many transgenic sickle cell mice have no anemia or very mild anemia. Hematological findings in sickle mice are shown in Table 12.2. The SAD mouse and the S+S-Antilles mouse have a modest reduction of packed cell volume, most evident neonatally. As sickle vasoocclusion appears to have association with high PCV, the absence of anemia in these models might be pathophysiologically important.

The most recent stage of creating mouse models of human sickle cell disease has been the creation of mice expressing exclusively human hemoglobins.[39,40] Available

Table 12.2. Hematological characteristics of transgenic mice

Nickname	β^S %	α^H %	γ % 9 Weeks	MCH pg/cell	% Retics	Hct
C57BL/6	–	–	–	14.5	2.2	48
Thal	–	–	–	12.7	24.6	32.3
NY1DD	75	56	–	14.1	3.2	47.0
SAD	19	58	–	15.1	3.6	44.0
S-Antilles-Thal	49	17	–	–	10.8	28.8
S+S-Antilles	80	58	–	14.3	11.1	44.5
NY1KO-γL	97	100	<3	14.2	63.2	22.4
NY1KO-γM	80	100	20	13.7	30.1	34.0
NY1KO-γH	60	100	40	14.4	12.9	41.1
β^S-Ryan et al, six lines	92–97	100	3.2–7.7	–	56–82	13–27
BERK hemiL	15–26	100	–	11.3	7.8	41.0
BERK hemiH	30–42	100	–	12.4	–	43.5
BERK	99	100	<1	9.3	36.5	28.7
BERK-γM	79	100	21	10.8	22.9	41.6
BERK-γH	55	100	45	12.9	5.0	42.2
β^S-YAC	>99	100	<1	10.4	20	22.4
β^S-Knockin	>99	100	<1	10.6	75.4	35.1

lines incorporate the mouse α-globin gene knockout and the mouse β-globin gene knockout and transgenes expressing human α-, β-, and γ-globin genes.[21,23] Six different lines expressing HbS and varying levels of human HbF have been described. One of the most frequently utilized models is the BERK mouse. Although these mice have many useful similarities to human sickle cell disease including anemia, reticulocytosis, loss of urine concentrating ability, and tissue damage, many of these mice had features of β thalassemia, with a very low MCH and low MCHC. Most of the transgenic sickle mice previously described had elevated MCHC, a feature attributed to deoxygenation-induced potassium efflux.[41] Very low MCHC in these full knockout mice is coupled with low MCH. This combination will reduce both the rate and extent of HbS polymer formation and be protective against sickling-related pathology. It will also confound attempts to evaluate the effect of introducing antisickling globins into these mice because their introduction will correct the low MCH and raise the MCHC, which will have a strong propolymerization effect due to the increase in hemoglobin concentration; at the same time, the antisickling globin will interfere with polymer formation making evaluation of efficacy in treatment studies difficult.[42]

NY1KO mice express exclusively human hemoglobins and incorporate three different human γ-globin gene–expressing lines that express different levels of HbF.[43–46] Mice with the least adult HbF expression (more than 3%, NY1KO-γL) were the most severe; those with intermediate HbF (20%, NY1KO-γM) were less severe; and those with the highest HbF (40%, NY1KO-γH) were least severe.[44] The increase in HbF was correlated with progressive increase in PCV (from 22% to 34% to 40%) and progressive decrease in reticulocyte count (from 60% to 30% to 13%). Lifespan was also strongly correlated with HbF levels and increased as HbF increased.[45] These results suggest that pathology in NY1KO mice is strongly driven by HbS polymerization. The γ-globin gene–expressing lines have much higher expression of HbF expression during the fetal and neonatal period.[46]

All of the knockout sickle mice described are the product of hundreds of matings and once a successful line has been established it has been possible to propagate it. In contrast, a recently described line expressing exclusively HbC[47] was fully knocked-out in a relatively small number of matings, which implies that mouse red cells tolerate the presence of exclusively human hemoglobins relatively well. One possible explanation for this contrast is that the many matings of the HbS mice are required to find an epistatic ameliorating feature that allows each line to survive. This speculation can only be validated by extensive analysis of the existing lines.

Because mice expressing a sickle transgene with a full knockout of both mouse α- and β-globins are difficult to breed and are physiologically fragile, mice that are hemizygous for the mouse β-globin knockout are used for both breeding and sometimes experimentation, either as controls or as experimental animals. These mice are sometimes called BERK trait or sickle trait mice, but they are better referred to as BERK hemi or some other neutral appellation. These mice segregate into two populations, those with one copy of the BERK transgene (that expresses human α and human β^S) and those with two copies of the BERK transgene.[48] As expected those with two copies of the BERK transgene had higher expression of β^S (~30% vs. 15% for a single copy), but unexpectedly the pathophysiology of mice with a single transgene was more severe. Perhaps this was due to the abnormally high P_{50} of approximately 60 mm Hg compared with 40 mm Hg for a C57BL/6 control.

The BERK β-hemizygous mouse and the SAD mouse share the properties of a relatively low level of polymerizing hemoglobin and a very low oxygen affinity. Red cells from the BERK β-hemizygous mouse were used to induce endothelial inflammation in lung by producing reactive oxygen species leading to cytosolic Ca^{2+} increase and P-selectin-dependent leukocyte recruitment.[49] Adding catalase to the infusion blocked the effects of red cell released reactive oxygen species. The rationale for using red cells from these mice was that hypoxia dramatically increases the rate of hemoglobin autoxidation[50,51] and results in increased production of superoxide and hydrogen peroxide that can leak from erythrocytes.[52] Low oxygen affinity and presence of unstable HbS would be expected to increase these effects in BERK β-hemizygous red cells; therefore, one would predict that these mice would have a stronger oxidative stress component in their pathology than that attributable to hemoglobin polymerization alone.[53]

Two other lines of mice expressing exclusively human hemoglobins have been described.[54,55] Mice created with a β-globin YAC (yeast artificial chromosome) also exhibited β thalassemic characteristics; however, the percentage of live births was increased from less than 2% to approximately 35% by placing the mothers in a high oxygen environment after day 10 of gestation and keeping the pups in this environment until weaning. A knockin mouse has been used to demonstrate correction of sickle cell disease by homologous recombination.[56]

Erythrocytes of Transgenic Mice

Human erythrocytes live approximately 120 days whereas mouse red cells live approximately 40 days. Therefore, the baseline reticulocyte count in human blood is much lower than in mice. The oxygen affinity of murine hemoglobins is lower than that of human hemoglobins. Human red cells with HbA have a P_{50} of approximately 25 mm Hg, whereas C57BL/6 mouse red cells have a P_{50} of approximately 40 mm Hg. Mice do not have a high oxygen affinity HbF to cope with the low oxygen fetal environment. Instead, the red cells of fetal mice do not upregulate 2,3-BPG levels, which decreases oxygen affinity, until after birth and adult levels are not reached until approximately age 3 weeks.[57] Adult mouse red cells have much higher levels of 2,3-BPG than human red cells and mouse red cells that express exclusively human hemoglobin have even more elevated levels of 2,3-BPG, which reduces the P_{50} from that found in humans. For example the P_{50} of HbA in a fully knocked-out line expressing only human globins is 33 mm Hg due to the high level of 2,3-BPG. Polymer formation is enhanced by elevated levels of 2,3-BPG and the severity of pathology induced by HbS in mice might be due in part to 2,3-BPG elevation.[58]

MCHC plays a crucial role in the pathophysiology of sickle cell disease because the delay time for polymer formation is inversely proportional to the 30th power of the concentration of deoxyHbS and the extent of polymer formation is directly proportional to the concentration of HbS. Two features of mouse erythrocytes would be expected to increase the pathology caused by introduced HbS: elevated MCHC due to the higher plasma osmolarity of mice and elevated red cell 2,3-BPG content.

Transgenic mice offered a unique opportunity to study the mechanisms of cation transport in sickle cell disease. Deoxy potassium efflux, unique to human sickle cells, is also found in the red cells of transgenic mice expressing high levels of HbS.[41,59] The calcium-stimulated potassium channel (Gardos channel) is similar in mouse and the human red cells.[60] This property has been used to demonstrate the beneficial effects on red cell density of inhibition of the potassium channel by clotrimazole. Hypoxia leads to the formation of dense cells in both NY1DD[31] and SAD[61] mice due to the deoxy-stimulated potassium efflux of potassium via the Gardos channel, and dense cell formation was used to evaluate the use of clotrimazole and its derivatives as inhibitors.[62,63] Arginine supplementation of NY1DD mice and S+S-Antilles mice reduced red cell density by reduction of Gardos channel activity[64] that is in part coupled to the observed reduction of endothelin.[65–67] Endothelin receptor antagonists also reduce erythrocyte dehydration in the SAD mouse (Chapters 9 and 31).[68]

The characteristics of K-Cl cotransport in the mouse red cell are more controversial with differences in mouse and human red cells.[69] These include, lack of inhibition by NO_3^-,[70] lack of sensitivity to [(dihydroindenyl)oxy] alkanoic acid (DIOA), a long delay time for activation, lack of volume-sensitive activation, and a large isotonic flux.[69] These differences imply that the mouse erythrocyte may be an imperfect model for cation transport in sickle cell disease.

When the mice expressing exclusively human HbC, HbS and HbF were tested, sensitivity to NO_3^- and DIOA were restored, strongly suggesting interaction of the K-Cl cotransporter or its modulators with both human and murine hemoglobin.[71] The SAD mouse has been used to show that Mg^{2+} supplementation inhibits K-Cl cotransport.[72] The mouse K-Cl cotransporter is similar to that of human.[73–75] Three *KCC* genes were found to be expressed in normal and sickle human red cells and splicing variants were also evident.[77] In SAD mice *kcc1* and *kcc3* were knocked out and *kcc1* (−/−) mice had normal transport, *kcc3* (−/−) mice had reduced transport but only in the double knockout *kcc1:kcc3* mice was K-Cl cotransport completely abolished and erythrocyte properties normalized.[77]

Signs of oxidative damage have also been noted in erythrocytes of transgenic sickle mice and might also contribute to mouse red cell pathology.[78,79] Alterations in phosphatidylserine exposure are associated with shortened red cell survival.[80] Red cell characteristics of sickle transgenic mice and the utility of these models for developing therapies for prevention of dehydration of sickle cells has been reviewed.[81–84]

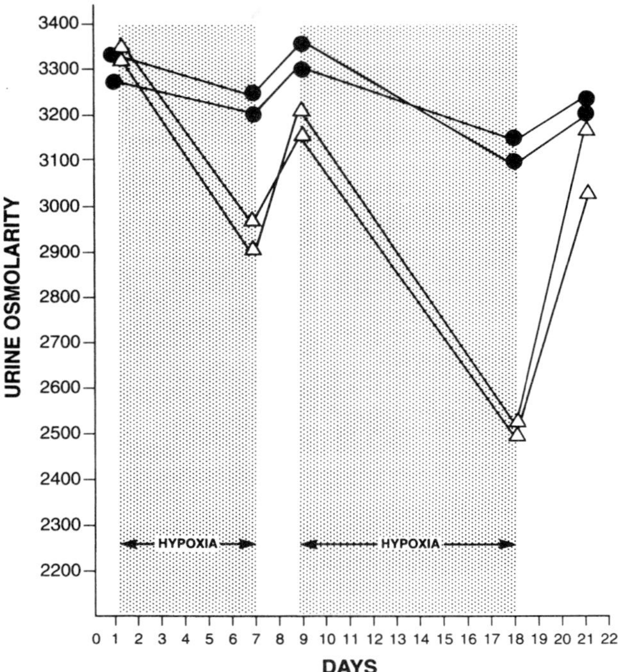

Figure 12.4. Urine-concentrating ability of mice expressing the $\alpha^H\beta^S$ transgene that are homozygous for the mouse β^{major} deletion. The mice were maintained under hypoxic conditions during the periods indicated and urine-concentrating ability was measured after 24 hours of water deprivation. Transgenic animals are indicated by open triangles and control C57BL/6 mice by filled circles. Note that significant but incomplete recovery occurred after 2 days at room air.

Organ Pathology in Sickle Mice

Kidney. The kidney in sickle transgenic mice has several abnormalities including glomerular sclerosis, increased blood urea nitrogen, and proteinuria in the SAD mouse.[30,85] Mice expressing human α- and β^S-globin on a homozygous deletional background (NY1DD) have an enhanced glomerular filtration rate and a urine-concentrating defect when exposed to hypoxia[31] (Fig. 12.4); S+S-Antilles mice have a severe and spontaneous urine-concentrating defect[86] and elevated levels of the nitric oxide synthases (NOSs) eNOS and iNOS that increase further with hypoxia. This might explain their elevated glomerular filtration rate.

When L-arginine is depleted, the production of nitric oxide (NO) from NOS falls, accompanied by increased production of O_2^- and peroxynitrite. A cytotoxic effect of peroxynitrite on tubular cells was evident by nitrotyrosine staining and release of lactate dehydrogenase.[87] In studies of control and sickle mice, using an antibody directed against nitrotyrosine, elevated levels colocalized with elevated iNOS in renal tubular epithelial cells. Moderate degrees of renal tubular cell apoptosis was also seen in transgenic sickle mice exposed to hypoxia.[88] Arginine, the precursor of NO, is depleted in the plasma of sickle cell disease patients[89] and other possible symptoms of dysregulated NOS activity such as low systemic blood pressure have been found in both human sickle cell disease patients[90–92] and in transgenic mice expressing HbS and HbS-Antilles (Chapters 10 and 11).[93] Magnetic resonance imaging of two sickle transgenic mouse models showed the presence of high levels of deoxyhemoglobin in the renal medulla of sickle mice under room air conditions.[94] The medulla is generally regarded as the most hypoxic region of the kidney[95] and polymer formation in this area would be expected to result in a urine-concentrating defect. Micromagnetic resonance imaging has also been used to detect renal cysts in a mouse model of sickle cell disease.[96] Inhibition of NOS was found to ameliorate renal damage in sickle transgenic mice,[97] as expected if elevated levels of NOS resulted in superoxide and peroxynitrite production. S+S-Antilles mice also have evidence of oxidative stress, increased plasma creatinine, and elevated heme oxygenase activity.[98] Gene expression studies using kidneys of S+S-Antilles mice showed up-regulation of the genes for arginase II, Na/K adenosine triphosphatase, renin-1, and alkaline phosphatase-2.[99] Up-regulation of arginase II could contribute to arginine depletion.[64] These mice were sensitive to ischemia/reperfusion injury after clamping the renal artery. Animals had 28% mortality after 22.5 minutes of clamping, and increase in the murine homolog of C-reactive protein,[100] and caspase-3 with congestion of lungs and heart.[101] The observation of increased caspase-3 activity is consistent with apoptosis in the kidneys of these mice.[88]

Renal function in BERK hemizygous mice showed that approximately half had mild to moderate abnormalities including glomerulonephritis, and elevated levels of iNOS, nitrotyrosine, and vascular cell adhesion molecule–1.[102] This could be due to the presence of sickle hemoglobin and/or the low oxygen affinity of this model and the naturally low pO_2 of the kidney. When SAD mice were exposed to 8% oxygen for 18 hours, ultrasound imaging revealed decreased renal blood flow velocity; histology showed congestion in peritubular capillaries and glomerular abnormalities with trapped sickle red cells that the authors suggested caused reduced flow.[103]

Retina. NY1DD sickle transgenic mice display preretinal neovascularization with many of the features of the retina in sickle cell disease (Chapters 19 and 21). Found in approximately 30% of transgenic mice aged more than 1 year, the abnormalities include drop-out of retinal vessels, structures reminiscent of black sunbursts that are due to invasion of pigmented epithelial cells from the choroid, and loss of photoreceptors in regions where the underlying choroid has been destroyed, forecasting the subsequent observations in human sickle retinopathy (Fig. 12.5).[104–106]

Microcirculation. In vivo adhesion of sickle cells to the endothelium[107,108] (Chapter 8) was first observed in the cremaster muscle preparation of the S+S-Antilles mouse.[109] Reduced red cell velocity and blood flow in the S+S-Antilles mouse was present when the cremaster muscle was suffused with a solution equilibrated with room air. When the gas used to equilibrate the suffusate contained increased oxygen, red cell velocity increased, blood flow

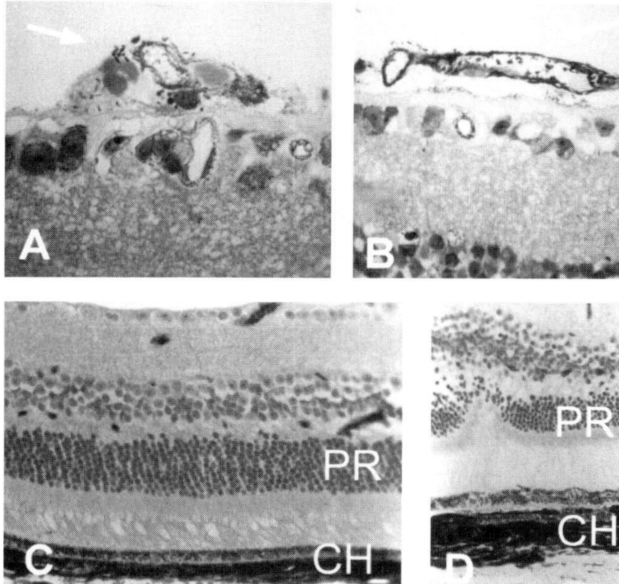

Figure 12.5. Examples of retinopathy in sickle transgenic mice expressing the $\alpha^H\beta^S$ transgene and homozygous for the β^{major} deletion. **(A** and **B)** Preretinal neovascularization indicated by arrows. **(C)** Normal retina indicating choroid (CH) and photoreceptor (PR) layers. **(D)** Pathological retina showing dilated obstructed CH with a disrupted PR layer above it. (See color plate 12.5.)

increased, and the vessel diameter was maintained. In contrast, in C57BL/6 mice, a change to suffusion with oxygen-equilibrated solutions resulted in decreased flow and vasoconstriction. Perhaps in the transgenic mouse, with equilibration with room air, there is HbS polymer formation that increases viscosity and reduces flow; oxygenation reverses this condition. This does not explain the failure to observe vasoconstriction under these conditions and has lead to the speculation that vascular response is blunted in sickle transgenic mice, a condition long suspected in humans with sickle cell disease and supported in studies outlined in Chapter 11. This observation lead to examination of other aspects of the vascular response in the S+S-Antilles mouse and it was found that these mice had constitutively low blood pressure and that vessel diameter did not respond to administration of acetylcholine, an endothelium-dependent vasodilator, or sodium nitroprusside, an NO donor. Nevertheless, N^G-nitro-L-arginine-methyl-ester, a nonselective inhibitor of NOS did cause a significant increase in blood pressure in both sickle and control mice.[110] It was concluded that increased NOS/NO activity resulted in hypotension and altered microvascular response to NO-mediated vasodilators in the S+S-Antilles mouse. Loss of vascular tone probably has both advantages and disadvantages. Vasodilation or lack of vasoconstriction might minimize the chance for blockage by nondeformable cells, but at the cost of over-exposure of tissues to oxygen with the consequent risk of oxidative damage. Intravital microscopy studies of the BERK knockout mouse showed that hyperoxia increased flow in contrast to the decreased flow observed in controls.[111] Hypoxia/reoxygenation of NY1DD mice resulted in elevated peroxide production in sickle transgenic animals but not controls with increased adherent and emigrated leukocytes, an effect blocked by P-selectin infusion.[112] In one sickle knockout line[40] oxygen radical inhibition of NO-dependent vascular function was due to increased vessel wall xanthine oxidase.[113] In C57BL/6 mice transplanted with BERK and BERK hemizygous bone marrow, adherent leukocytes recruited sickle cells.[114] Transplanted double-knockout mice for P- and E-selectins were protected from sickle vasoocclusion, leading to the suggestion that drugs targeting sickle erythrocyte–leukocyte or leukocyte–endothelial interactions might have a role in treating sickle cell disease. In BERK mice and C57BL/6 mice transplanted with BERK bone marrow, administration of tumor necrosis factor–α to simulate a sickle cell vasoocclusive event was rescued by commercial intravenous immunoglobulin.[115] Two criteria were used to evaluate outcome: survival time and the number of adherent leukocytes. The authors concluded that immunoglobulin was protective, and this agent is presently being evaluated in a clinical trial (ClinicalTrials.gov, NCT00644865).

Bone marrow from BERK β-hemizygous mice was transplanted into eNOS-overproducing and eNOS-deficient mice to study the effect of superoxide on leukocyte and platelet adhesion in cerebral venules. It was observed that eNOS overexpression enhanced and eNOS deficiency decreased adhesion. Sepiapterin, which enhances production of the cofactor of eNOS, tetrahydrobiopterin, and polyethylene glycol–superoxide dismutase had similar effects.[116] It was concluded that an imbalance of NO and superoxide contribute to the proinflammatory and prothrombogenic phenotype of these mice. Arginine significantly reduced expression of non-NO vasodilators COX-2 and heme oxygenase in BERK mice.[117] Reduced COX-2 expression correlated with reduced PGE2 levels. Response to the NO donor sodium nitroprusside was strongly correlated with the hemolytic rate and nitrotyrosine formation suggesting that improved microvascular function was a response to reduced hemolysis.

Liver. The liver in sickle mice shows infarcts that increase when mice are hypoxic[118] and occur with a greater frequency, as judged by both histology[34] and elevated levels of the serum enzyme alanine transaminase, in the more severe mouse models. Liver pathology has also been described in full knockout mice[39,40] and might be a source of arginase that results in arginine depletion in S+S-Antilles mice.[64] Elevated levels of iNOS and eNOS have been found in livers of transgenic sickle mice and have been attributed to hypoxic damage or the effect of shear stress due to the effectively higher viscosity of sickle blood and possibly damage by adhesion of red cells.[118] Extramedullary hematopoiesis has been detected in the liver of knockout transgenic sickle mice[40] and in mice expressing exclusively HbC.[119] Opioid metabolism was found to be altered in the hepatic microsomal fraction of BERK hemizygous mice and it was proposed that similar changes in sickle cell disease patients might alter clearance of this drug.[120]

Spleen. Splenic enlargement, fibrosis, and expansion of the erythropoietic red pulp was noted even in sickle transgenic mice with a relatively mild phenotype and was more pronounced in more severe strains.[30,32,34] A significant proportion of the total red cell mass is found in the spleen in these animals and might be partially responsible for their low hematocrit. Reduced spleen size has been used as an end point in gene therapy proof-of-principle using transgenic mouse models.[121–124]

Lung. The lung in transgenic and knock-out sickle mice with more severe pathology shows congestion, thickened septa fibrosis, and thrombosis.[39,42,44,85] Inhaled NO protected the SAD mouse from hypoxia/reoxygenation damage;[125] the mechanism of NO protection might be conversion of plasma free hemoglobin that can scavenge NO to inactive methemoglobin.[126] When hypoxia was used to induce acute lung injury in BERK sickle transgenic mice and BERK hemizygous mice,[127] under normoxic conditions xanthine oxidase, nitrotyrosine, and cyclic guanosine monophosphate were elevated in the sickle mice and hypoxia increased xanthine oxidase and nitrotyrosine and decreased cGMP. BERK mice challenged with endotoxin[128] had a higher increase in mortality and increased airway tone with cytokines found in serum and bronchoalveolar lavage. It was suggested that a subclinical proinflammatory state existed that resulted in an enhanced response to a proinflammatory challenge.

Polynitroxyl albumin has been proposed as an antioxidant and scavenger of reactive oxygen species and has been used to attenuate lung capillary leak.[129] A similar compound, S-nitrosoalbumin, was studied[130] in an acute hypoxia, SAD transgenic model to see if it protected against lung injury. Treatment resulted in reduced levels of interleukin (IL)-6 and IL-1β and hypoxia-induced increased granulocytosis.

Pulmonary hypertension is present in BERK mice and C57BL/6 mice transplanted with BERK bone marrow.[131] Mice expressing exclusively HbS suffered from pulmonary hypertension, pulmonary, and systemic endothelial dysfunction that was the result of reduced response to NO, NO donors, and impaired NOS activity. Similar effects were found in mice with immune-mediated hemolysis. In SAD mice used[132] to study the effect of peritonitis on lung NO production, control C57BL/6 mice, but not SAD mice, had an increase in eNOS and iNOS mRNA and proteins and an increase in exhaled NO leading to the conclusion that SAD mice have a defect in lung NO production and bioavailability that results in acute systemic and lung complications.

More severe pulmonary pathology was induced in SAD mice by exposure to 8% oxygen for 7 days.[133] Hypoxia increased neutrophils in bronchoalveolar lavage fluid and peripheral circulation, increased IL-1β, IL-6, and tumor necrosis factor–α, and upregulated genes for endothelin-1, cyclooxygenase-2, angiotensin-converting enzyme, and IL-1β. Hypoxia also increased *pde4* gene expression. A phosphodiesterase inhibitor prevented hypoxia-induced *pde4* up-regulation and prevented pulmonary arterial hypertension. In another publication, hypoxic erythrocytes from control C57BL/6 and BERK and hemizygous knockout mice induced endothelial inflammation in lung by producing reactive oxygen species leading to cytosolic Ca^{2+} increase, and P-selectin-dependent leukocyte recruitment.[49] Catalase blocked the effects of red cell–released oxidant radicals.

Brain. The brain in transgenic sickle mice is relatively unexplored. Occasional red neurons and rare pyknotic neurons were observed in S+S-Antilles mice.[34] The red neurons may be indicative of hypoxic episodes secondary to vasoocclusion. When perfusion and oxygenation in the brains of C57BL/6, S+S-Antilles, and BERK mice was studied, increased deoxyhemoglobin was correlated with reduced perfusion.[134] Although hyperoxia caused cerebral blood flow to decrease in control C57BL/6 mice, this resulted in increased blood flow in sickle transgenic mice, perhaps an effect of melting of sickle polymer found under room air conditions and/or loss of brain autoregulation.

Cerebral venules were studied in BERK β-hemizygous mice transplanted onto P-selectin knockout mice. Platelet and leukocyte adhesion was elevated in both unstimulated and posthypoxic sickle mice, suggesting both an inflammatory and prothrombogenic phenotype. In BERK β-hemizygous mice transplanted onto gp91phox NADPH-deficient mice and onto superoxide dismutase–overexpressing mice, strong platelet–endothelial and leukocyte–endothelial adhesion that was blunted by the iron chelator desferrioxamine, but not by the xanthine oxidase inhibitor allopurinol, was found. It was concluded that superoxide and catalytically active iron contributed to the proinflammatory and prothrombogenic responses.[135,136]

Other Hemoglobinopathies

Other nonsickle, human globin transgenes have been introduced into the mouse. These include *HBA*,[7,137] *HBG*,[43,138] *HBD* and the β^C-globin gene.[119] Some have been bred onto full knockout backgrounds. For example, a mouse expressing human α- and β^A-globin chains was bred onto a full knockout background.[137] This mouse has features of β thalassemia with a low MCHC that can be corrected by introducing the γ-globin gene. A mouse expressing exclusively human HbC has many features of human HbC disease (Chapter 21) including dehydrated, high MCHC red cells, high K-Cl cotransport, circulating intracellular crystals of HbC, which increase when the mice are splenectomized and folded red cells. More recently a mouse expressing HbE has been generated that has many of the features of HbE disease, without thalassemia.[140]

SUMMARY

Sickle cell transgenic mice, however imperfect as models, have made significant contributions to understanding the pathophysiology of sickle cell disease. Yet, the quest for a more perfect mouse is reasonable, as animal models allow the possibility of detecting early results of new therapies and understanding complex physiological interactions that cannot be confidently predicted or verified in human studies. Mouse physiology has some features mentioned previously that might make the physiological consequences of sickle cell disease even more severe than they are in humans and it might not be possible to make a viable mouse with exclusively HbS, low levels of HbF in adults, and a normal MCHC.

Some hematological features of transgenic mice confound analysis in terms of disease severity, the ameliorating effects of natural human γ-globin chains or other antisickling hemoglobins and the applicability of results to gene therapy in humans. Although many transgenic lines have high expression of human HbF during the fetal period, 2,3-BPG production is delayed until just after birth. Many lines of transgenic mice express their human hemoglobins in a pancellular mode. F cells do occur in some mouse lines, which can both enhance the verisimilitude of the model and complicate data analysis because the percentage of γ-globin chains in whole blood is a balance between the synthesis of γ-globin and selective destruction of non-F cells. The amount of hemoglobin in whole blood due to transgene expression might not be constant during the lifetime of the mouse. Gene expression, the site of erythropoiesis, hemoglobin assembly, and selective red cell destruction can all play roles in this outcome. It is important to be aware of these features and transgene expression should be measured as a function of mouse age. Production of human hemoglobin in mouse red cells appears to require extremely high levels of mRNA and globin chain synthesis and the concentration of globin protein from the transgene should be measured before reaching conclusions about hemoglobin gene expression in transgenic mice.[141] Currently, the best way to demonstrate that the effect of antisickling globin chains in a sickle cell mouse model is due to inhibition of HbS polymer formation is by producing a similar mouse that expresses β^A-globin chains at a comparable level. The β^A chains will dilute the concentration of HbS but will not reduce polymer formation as effectively as HbF (Chapters 5–7). Similarly, antisickling hemoglobins intended for use in gene therapy need to be compared with γ-globin chains expressed at a similar level to validate their antisickling properties. A major obstacle to comparing the "same" mouse with β^A- or γ-globin chains is that every transgene is inserted in a different location in the chromosome and with a different copy number and potentially with a different level of expression at different ages in the mouse. This limitation can now be overcome with new technology based on site-specific recombination that eliminates position and variable copy number effects.[142,143]

Hematological severity might not equate to physiological severity. The full knockout HbC mouse has nearly the same level of hematological severity as some of the full sickle knockout mice. That is, the hematocrit and reticulocyte counts are nearly the same; however, homozygous HbC disease in human is trivial clinically (Chapter 21). The physiological impact of HbC is much milder in mice than suggested by the hematology alone, as these mice were bred to a full knockout with a very small number of matings and both male and female HbC mice can breed. Many matings are required to produce full knockout mice with HbS both with and without human γ-globin gene expression and female mice with high levels of β^S-globin uncommonly survive pregnancy and give birth to viable pups. In evaluating antisickling hemoglobins physiological parameters should be evaluated along with strictly hematological parameters.

The current generation of mice expressing exclusively human hemoglobin is technologically state of the art, and yet they too have imperfections. Most of the full knockouts have low MCHC, a condition not associated with human sickle cell disease. Low MCHC might be a necessary compensation to ameliorate the induced pathology and allow survival. Regulation of globin chain synthesis balance is imperfectly understood and in most transgenic lines chain balance is the result of chance as the mechanisms responsible for balanced globin synthesis are probably circumvented by transgene insertion. When chain balance is not achieved in mice expressing HbS, and the mice suffer from a thalassemic phenotype, the pathology observed will be a combination of HbS polymer–related damage and oxidative damage. Even in the absence of globin chain imbalance, low MCHC can confound the interpretation of results in experiments where breeding in an anti-sickling hemoglobin might alter red cell MCHC by ameliorating β thalassemia and affecting polymer formation or other MCHC-related pathology.

A single model does not "fit all," and it is wise to examine more than one transgenic line before drawing conclusions about the relevance of a result to the human disease. One might look for features that are consistent over several different mouse models. Recent reviews of transgenic sickle mice are available and deal with such issues as their roles in evaluating gene therapy, drug discovery and sickle vasculopathy.[146–153]

Reference Resources

A number of useful Internet sites can be accessed to find characteristics of mutant hemoglobins, inbred mouse strains, and associated literature.

Useful Internet Sites

Name	Site	Contents
Globin database	http://globin.cse.psu.edu	mutant hemoglobins and their properties
Swiss protein database	www.expasy.ch	protein sequences, molecular weights
Protein Data Bank	www.rcsb.org/pdb	protein sequences, crystallographic coordinates
JAX phenome	www.jax.org/phenome	Phenotypes of inbred mouse strains

References for the Tables

1. Skow LC, Burkhart BA, Johnson FM, et al. A mouse model for beta-thalassemia. *Cell.* 1983;34:1043–1052.
2. Fabry ME, Costantini F, Pachnis A, et al. High expression of human b^S- and a-globins in transgenic mice: erythrocyte abnormalities, organ damage, and the effect of hypoxia. *Proc Natl Acad Sci USA.* 1992;89:12155–12159.
3. Trudel M, Garel MC, Saadane N, et al. Towards a mouse model for sickle cell disease: HB SAD. *Nouv Rev Fr Hematol.* 1990;32:407–408.
4. Rubin EM, Witkowska HE, Spangler E, et al. Hypoxia-induced in vivo sickling of transgenic mouse red cells. *J Clin Invest.* 1991;87:639–647.
5. Fabry ME, Sengupta A, Suzuka SM, et al. A second generation transgenic mouse model expressing both hemoglobin S (HbS) and HbS-Antilles results in increased phenotypic severity. *Blood.* 1995;86:2419–2428.
6. Arcasoy MO, Romana M, Fabry ME, et al. High levels of human gamma-globin gene expression in adult mice carrying a transgene of deletion-type hereditary persistence of fetal hemoglobin. *Mol Cell Biol.* 1997;17:2076–2089.
7. Paszty C, Mohandas N, Stevens ME, et al. Lethal alpha-thalassaemia created by gene targeting in mice and its genetic rescue. *Nat Genet.* 1995;11:33–39.
8. Yang B, Kirby S, Lewis J, et al. A mouse model for beta 0-thalassemia. *Proc Natl Acad Sci USA.* 1995;92:11608–11612.
9. Ciavatta DJ, Ryan TM, Farmer SC, Townes TM. Mouse model of human beta zero thalassemia: targeted deletion of the mouse beta maj- and beta min-globin genes in embryonic stem cells. *Proc Natl Acad Sci USA.* 1995;92:9259–9263.
10. Gilman JG. Developmental changes of human ^{G}g and ^{A}g and mouse embryonic e^{y1}, e^{y2}, and b^{h1} in transgenic mice with HS4-^{G}g-^{A}g. *Blood.* 1995;86:648a.
11. Shear HL, Grinberg L, Gilman J, et al. Transgenic mice expressing human fetal globin are protected from malaria by a novel mechanism. *Blood.* 1998;92:2520–2526.
12. Fabry ME, Suzuka SM, Weinberg RS, et al. Second generation knockout sickle mice: the effect of HbF. *Blood.* 2001;97:410–418.
13. Ryan TM, Ciavatta DJ, Townes TM. Knockout-transgenic mouse model of sickle cell disease. *Science.* 1997;278:873–876.
14. Paszty C, Brion CM, Manci E, et al. Transgenic knockout mice with exclusively human sickle hemoglobin and sickle cell disease. *Science.* 1997;278:876–878.
15. Chang JC, Lu R, Lin C, et al. Transgenic knockout mice exclusively expressing human hemoglobin S after transfer of a 240-kb betas-globin yeast artificial chromosome: A mouse model of sickle cell anemia. *Proc Natl Acad Sci USA.* 1998;95:14886–14890.
16. Wu LC, Sun CW, Ryan TM, et al. Correction of sickle cell disease by homologous recombination in embryonic stem cells. *Blood.* 2006;108:1183–1188.

REFERENCES

1. Crispins CG. *Handbook on the Laboratory Mouse.* Springfield, IL: Charles C Thomas; 1975.
2. Whitney JB III. Mouse hemoglobinopathies: detection and characterization of thalassemias and globin-structure mutations. *Prog Clin Biol Res.* 1982;94:133–142.
3. Roy RP, Nacharaju P, Nagel RL, Acharya AS. Symmetric inter-species hybrids of mouse and human hemoglobin: molecular basis of their abnormal oxygen affinity. *J Protein Chem.* 1995;14:81–88.
4. Gordon JW, Scangos GA, Plotkin DJ, Barbosa JA, Ruddle FH. Genetic transformation of mouse embryos by microinjection of purified DNA. *Proc Natl Acad Sci USA.* 1980;77:7380–7384.
5. Costantini F, Lacy E. Introduction of a rabbit beta-globin gene into the mouse germ line. *Nature.* 1981;294:92–94.
6. Tuan D, Solomon W, Li Q, London IM. The "beta-like-globin" gene domain in human erythroid cells. *Proc Natl Acad Sci USA.* 1985;82:6384–6388.
7. Chada K, Magram J, Raphael K, et al. Specific expression of a foreign beta-globin gene in erythroid cells of transgenic mice. *Nature.* 1985;314:377–380.
8. Kollias G, Wrighton N, Hurst J, Grosveld F. Regulated expression of human A gamma-, beta-, and hybrid gamma beta-globin genes in transgenic mice: manipulation of the developmental expression patterns. *Cell.* 1986;46:89–94.
9. Townes TM, Lingrel JB, Chen HY, Brinster RL, Palmiter RD. Erythroid-specific expression of human beta-globin genes in transgenic mice. *EMBO J.* 1985;4:1715–1723.
10. Hogan BLM, Costantini F, Lacy E. *Manipulating the Mouse Embryo: A Laboratory Manual.* Cold Spring Harbor: Cold Spring Harbor Laboratory; 1986.
11. Skow LC, Burkhart BA, Johnson FM, et al. A mouse model for beta-thalassemia. *Cell.* 1983;34:1043–1052.
12. Whitney JB, Martinell J, Popp RA, Russell LB, Anderson WF. Deletions in the alpha-globin gene complex in alpha-thalassemic mice. *Proc Natl Acad Sci USA.* 1981;78:7644–7647.
13. Martinell J, Whitney JB, III, Popp RA, Russell LB, Anderson WF. Three mouse models of human thalassemia. *Proc Natl Acad Sci USA.* 1981;78:5056–5060.
14. Rouyer Fessard P, Scott MD, Leroy Viard K, et al. Fate of alpha-hemoglobin chains and erythrocyte defects in beta-thalassemia. *Ann NY Acad Sci.* 1990;612:106–117.
15. Rivella S, May C, Chadburn A, Riviere I, Sadelain M. A novel murine model of Cooley anemia and its rescue by lentiviral-mediated human beta-globin gene transfer. *Blood.* 2003;101:2932–2939.
16. Rouyer Fessard P, Leroy Viard K, Domenget C, Mrad A, Beuzard Y. Mouse beta thalassemia, a model for the membrane defects of erythrocytes in the human disease. *J Biol Chem.* 1990;265:20247–20251.
17. Whitney JB, III, Popp RA. Animal model of human disease: thalassemia: alpha-thalassemia in laboratory mice. *Am J Pathol.* 1984;116:523–525.
18. de Franceschi L, Rouyer-Fessard P, Alper SL, et al. Combination therapy of erythropoietin, hydroxyurea, and clotrimazole in a beta thalassemic mouse: a model for human therapy. *Blood.* 1996;87:1188–1195.
19. Shehee WR, Oliver P, Smithies O. Lethal thalassemia after insertional disruption of the mouse major adult beta-globin gene. *Proc Natl Acad Sci USA.* 1993;90:3177–3181.
20. Fabry ME, Suzuka SM, Rubin EM, Costantini F, Gilman J, Nagel RL. Strategies for amelioration of sickle cell disease:

Use of transgenic mice for validation of anti-sickling strategies. In: Beuzard Y, Lubin B, Rosa J, eds. *Sickle Cell Disease and Thalassemias: New Trends in Therapy.* London: John Libbey Eurotext Ltd; 1995:253–262.

21. Ciavatta DJ, Ryan TM, Farmer SC, Townes TM. Mouse model of human beta zero thalassemia: targeted deletion of the mouse beta maj- and beta min-globin genes in embryonic stem cells. *Proc Natl Acad Sci USA.* 1995;92:9259–9263.
22. Yang B, Kirby S, Lewis J, et al. A mouse model for beta 0-thalassemia. *Proc Natl Acad Sci USA.* 1995;92:11608–11612.
23. Paszty C, Mohandas N, Stevens ME, et al. Lethal alpha-thalassaemia created by gene targeting in mice and its genetic rescue. *Nat Genet.* 1995;11:33–39.
24. Costantini F, Chada K, Magram J. Correction of murine beta-thalassemia by gene transfer into the germ line. *Science.* 1986;233:1192–1194.
25. Rubin EM, Lu RH, Cooper S, Mohandas N, Kan YW. Introduction and expression of the human βs-globin gene in transgenic mice. *Am J Hum Genet.* 1988;42:585–591.
26. Rhoda MD, Domenget C, Vidaud M, et al. Mouse α-chains inhibit polymerization of hemoglobin induced by human β^{S} or $\beta^{S\text{-Antilles}}$ chains. *Biochim Biophys Acta.* 1988;952:208–212.
27. Greaves DR, Fraser P, Vidal MA, et al. A transgenic mouse model of sickle cell disorder. *Nature.* 1990;343:183–185.
28. Ryan TM, Townes TM, Reilly MP, et al. Human sickle hemoglobin in transgenic mice. *Science.* 1990;247:566–568.
29. Rubin EM, Witkowska HE, Spangler E, et al. Hypoxia-induced in vivo sickling of transgenic mouse red cells. *J Clin Invest.* 1991;87:639–647.
30. Trudel M, Saadane N, Garel M-C, et al. Towards a transgenic mouse model of sickle cell disease: hemoglobin SAD. *EMBO J.* 1991;10:3157–3168.
31. Fabry ME, Costantini F, Pachnis A, et al. High expression of human β^{S}- and α-globins in transgenic mice: erythrocyte abnormalities, organ damage, and the effect of hypoxia. *Proc Natl Acad Sci USA.* 1992;89:12155–12159.
32. Fabry ME, Nagel RL, Pachnis A, Suzuka SM, Costantini F. High expression of human β^{S}- and α-globins in transgenic mice: hemoglobin composition and hematological consequences. *Proc Natl Acad Sci USA.* 1992;89:12150–12154.
33. Reilly MP, Chomo MJ, Obata K, Asakura T. Red blood cell membrane and density changes under ambient and hypoxic conditions in transgenic mice producing human sickle hemoglobin. *Exp Hematol.* 1994;22:501–509.
34. Fabry ME, Sengupta A, Suzuka SM, et al. A second generation transgenic mouse model expressing both hemoglobin S (HbS) and HbS-Antilles results in increased phenotypic severity. *Blood.* 1995;86:2419–2428.
35. Popp RA, Popp DM, Shinpock SG, et al. A transgenic mouse model of hemoglobin S Antilles disease. *Blood.* 1997;89:4204–4212.
36. Monplaisir N, Merault G, Poyart C, et al. Hemoglobin S Antilles: a variant with lower solubility than hemoglobin S and producing sickle cell disease in heterozygotes. *Proc Natl Acad Sci USA.* 1986;83:9363–9367.
37. Monplaisir N, Galacteros F, Arous N, et al. [Abnormal hemoglobins identified in Martinique]. *Nouv Rev Fr Hematol.* 1985;27:11–14.
38. Li X, Mirza UA, Chait BT, Manning JM. Systematic enhancement of polymerization of recombinant sickle hemoglobin mutants: implications for transgenic mouse model for sickle cell anemia. *Blood.* 1997;90:4620–4627.
39. Paszty C, Brion CM, Manci E, et al. Transgenic knockout mice with exclusively human sickle hemoglobin and sickle cell disease. *Science.* 1997;278:876–878.
40. Ryan TM, Ciavatta DJ, Townes TM. Knockout-transgenic mouse model of sickle cell disease. *Science.* 1997;278:873–876.
41. Romero J, Fabry ME, Suzuka SM, Nagel RL, Canessa M. Red blood cells of a transgenic mouse expressing high levels of human hemoglobin S exhibit deoxy-stimulated cation flux. *J Membr Biol.* 1997;159:187–196.
42. Manci EA, Hillery CA, Bodian CA, et al. Pathology of Berkeley sickle cell mice: similarities and differences with human sickle cell disease. *Blood.* 2006;107:1651–1658.
43. Gilman JG, Fabry ME, Suzuka SM, Nagel RL. Human G-gamma:A-gamma globin ratios switch during prenatal development in a transgenic mouse with HS4-G-gamma(-158T)-A-gamma. *Blood.* 1995;86:648a.
44. Fabry ME, Suzuka SM, Weinberg RS, et al. Second generation knockout sickle mice: the effect of HbF. *Blood.* 2001;97:410–418.
45. Fabry ME, Witt WM, Suzuka SM, Nagel RL. Impact of HbF and gender on mean survival time of NY1KO sickle transgenic ice expressing exclusively human hemoglobins. *Blood.* 2001;98:750aa.
46. Gilman JG. Developmental changes of human $^{G}\gamma$ and $^{A}\gamma$ and mouse embryonic ε^{y1}, ε^{y2}, and β^{h1} in transgenic mice with HS4-$^{G}\gamma$-$^{A}\gamma$. *Blood.* 1995;86:648a.
47. Fabry ME, Romero JR, Suzuka SM, et al. Hemoglobin C in transgenic mice: effect of HbC expression from founders to full mouse globin knockouts. *Blood Cell Mol Dis.* 2000;26:331–347.
48. Noguchi CT, Gladwin M, Diwan B, et al. Pathophysiology of a sickle cell trait mouse model: human alpha(beta)(S) transgenes with one mouse beta-globin allele. *Blood Cell Mol Dis.* 2001;27:971–977.
49. Kiefmann R, Rifkind JM, Nagababu E, Bhattacharya J. Red blood cells induce hypoxic lung inflammation. *Blood.* 2008;111:5205–5214.
50. Rifkind JM, Nagababu E, Ramasamy S, Ravi LB. Hemoglobin redox reactions and oxidative stress. *Redox Rep.* 2003;8:234–237.
51. Abugo OO, Rifkind JM. Oxidation of hemoglobin and the enhancement produced by nitroblue tetrazolium. *J Biol Chem.* 1994;269:24845–24853.
52. Rifkind JM, Zhang L, Heim JM, Levy A. The role of hemoglobin in generating oxyradicals. *Basic Life Sci.* 1988;49:157–162.
53. Ieremia J, Blau CA. Limitations of a mouse model of sickle cell anemia. *Blood Cell Mol Dis.* 2002;28:146–151.
54. Chang JC, Lu R, Lin C, et al. Transgenic knockout mice exclusively expressing human hemoglobin S after transfer of a 240-kb betas-globin yeast artificial chromosome: A mouse model of sickle cell anemia. *Proc Natl Acad Sci USA.* 1998;95:14886–14890.
55. Ye L, Chang JC, Lu R, Kan YW. High oxygen environment during pregnancy rescues sickle cell anemia mice from prenatal death. *Blood Cell Mol Dis.* 2008;41:67–72.

56. Wu LC, Sun CW, Ryan TM, et al. Correction of sickle cell disease by homologous recombination in embryonic stem cells. *Blood*. 2006;108:1183–1188.
57. Scott AF, Bunn HF, Brush AH. Functional aspects of hemoglobin evolution in the mammals. *J Mol Evol*. 1976;8:311–316.
58. Swerdlow PH, Bryan RA, Bertles JF, et al. Effect of 2, 3-diphosphoglycerate on the solubility of deoxy-sickle hemoglobin. *Hemoglobin*. 1977;1:527–537.
59. Tosteson DC, Carlsen E, Dunham ET. The effect of sickling on ion transport. I. The effect of sickling on potassium transport. *J Gen Physiol*. 1955;39:31–53.
60. Vandorpe DH, Shmukler BE, Jiang L, et al. cDNA cloning and functional characterization of the mouse Ca2+-gated K+ channel, mIK1. Roles in regulatory volume decrease and erythroid differentiation. *J Biol Chem*. 1998;273;21542–21553.
61. de Franceschi L, Brugnara C, Rouyer-Fessard P, Jouault H, Beuzard Y. Formation of dense erythrocytes in SAD mice exposed to chronic hypoxia: evaluation of different therapeutic regimens and of a combination of oral clotrimazole and magnesium therapies. *Blood*. 1999;94:4307–4313.
62. de Franceschi L, Saadane N, Trudel M, et al. Treatment with oral clotrimazole blocks Ca(2+)-activated K+ transport and reverses erythrocyte dehydration in transgenic SAD mice. A model for therapy of sickle cell disease. *J Clin Invest*. 1994;93:1670–1676.
63. Stocker JW, de Franceschi L, McNaughton-Smith GA, et al. ICA-17043, a novel Gardos channel blocker, prevents sickled red blood cell dehydration in vitro and in vivo in SAD mice. *Blood*. 2003;101:2412–2418.
64. Romero JR, Suzuka SM, Nagel RL, Fabry ME. Arginine supplementation of sickle transgenic mice reduces red cell density and Gardos channel activity. *Blood*. 2002;99:1103–1108.
65. Rivera A, Rotter MA, Brugnara C. Endothelins activate Ca(2+)-gated K(+) channels via endothelin B receptors in CD-1 mouse erythrocytes. *Am J Physiol*. 1999;277:C746–C754.
66. Rivera A, Jarolim P, Brugnara C. Modulation of Gardos channel activity by cytokines in sickle erythrocytes. *Blood*. 2002;99:357–603.
67. Romero JR, Rivera A, Muniz A, Suzuka SM, Nagel RL, Fabry ME. Effect of arginine diet for sickle transgenic mice on plasma cytokine levels and the mechanism of reduction of Gardos channel activity. *Blood*. 2003;102:260a.
68. Rivera A. Reduced sickle erythrocyte dehydration in vivo by endothelin-1 receptor antagonists. *Am J Physiol Cell Physiol*. 2007;293:C960–966.
69. Romero JR, Fabry ME, Suzuka SM, et al. K:Cl cotransport in red cells of transgenic mice expressing high levels of human hemoglobin S. *Am J Hematol*. 1997;55:112–114.
70. Armsby CC, Brugnara C, Alper SL. Cation transport in mouse erythrocytes: role of K(+)-Cl- cotransport in regulatory volume decrease. *Am J Physiol*. 1995;268(Pt 1):C894–902.
71. Romero JR, Suzuka SM, Nagel RL, Fabry ME. Expression of HbC and HbS, but not HbA, results in activation of K-Cl cotransport activity in transgenic mouse red cells. *Blood*. 2004;103:2384–2390.
72. de Franceschi L, Beuzard Y, Jouault H, Brugnara C. Modulation of erythrocyte potassium chloride cotransport, potassium content, and density by dietary magnesium intake in transgenic SAD mouse. *Blood*. 1996;88:2738–2744.
73. Su W, Shmukler BE, Chernova MN, et al. Mouse K-Cl cotransporter KCC1: cloning, mapping, pathological expression, and functional regulation. *Am J Physiol*. 1999;277:C899–C912.
74. Pellegrino CM, Rybicki AC, Musto S, Nagel RL, Schwartz RS. Molecular identification and expression of erythroid K:Cl cotransporter in human and mouse erythroleukemic cells. *Blood Cell Mol Dis*. 1998;24:31–40.
75. Gillen CM, Brill S, Payne JA, Forbush B III. Molecular cloning and functional expression of the K-Cl cotransporter from rabbit, rat, and human. A new member of the cation-chloride cotransporter family. *J Biol Chem*. 1996;271:16237–16244.
76. Crable SC, Hammond SM, Papes R, et al. Multiple isoforms of the KC1 cotransporter are expressed in sickle and normal erythroid cells. *Exp Hematol*. 2005;33:624–631.
77. Rust MB, Alper SL, Rudhard Y, et al. Disruption of erythroid K-Cl cotransporters alters erythrocyte volume and partially rescues erythrocyte dehydration in SAD mice. *J Clin Invest*. 2007;117:1708–1717.
78. Reilly MP, Obata K, Chomo M, Asakura T. Red blood cell membrane alterations and dense cell formation in transgenic mice expressing different levels of human sickle hemoglobin. National Sickle Cell Disease Program 18th, 1a. 1993.
79. de Franceschi L, Beuzard Y, Brugnara C. Sulfhydryl oxidation and activation of red cell K(+)-Cl- cotransport in the transgenic SAD mouse. *Am J Physiol*. 1995;269(Pt 1):C899–906.
80. de Jong K, Emerson RK, Butler J, et al. Short survival of phosphatidylserine-exposing red blood cells in murine sickle cell anemia. *Blood*. 2001;98:1577–1584.
81. Brugnara C. Therapeutic strategies for prevention of sickle cell dehydration. *Blood Cell Mol Dis*. 2001;27:71–80.
82. Brugnara C. Sickle cell disease: from membrane pathophysiology to novel therapies for prevention of erythrocyte dehydration. *J Pediatr Hematol Oncol*. 2003;25:927–933.
83. Lew VL, Bookchin RM. Ion transport pathology in the mechanism of sickle cell dehydration. *Physiol Rev*. 2005;85:179–200.
84. Wulff H, Kolski-Andreaco A, Sankaranarayanan A, Sabatier JM, Shakkottai V. Modulators of small- and intermediate-conductance calcium-activated potassium channels and their therapeutic indications. *Curr Med Chem*. 2007;14:1437–1457.
85. Trudel M, De Paepe ME, Chretien N, et al. Sickle cell disease of transgenic SAD mice. *Blood*. 1994;84:3189–3197.
86. Bank N, Aynedjian HS, Qiu JH, et al. Renal nitric oxide synthases in transgenic sickle cell mice. *Kidney Int*. 1996;50:184–189.
87. Xia Y, Dawson VL, Dawson TM, Snyder SH, Zweier JL. Nitric oxide synthase generates superoxide and nitric oxide in arginine-depleted cells leading to peroxynitrite-mediated cellular injury. *Proc Natl Acad Sci USA*. 1996;93:6770–6774.
88. Bank N, Kiroycheva M, Ahmed F, et al. Peroxynitrite formation and apoptosis in transgenic sickle cell mouse kidneys. *Kidney Int*. 1998;54:1520–1528.
89. Enwonwu CO. Increased metabolic demand for arginine in sickle cell anemia. *Med Sci Res*. 1989;17:997–998.
90. Lipowsky HL, Sheikh NU, Katz DM. Intravital microscopy of capillary hemodynamics in sickle cell disease. *J Clin Invest*. 1987;80:117–127.
91. Rodgers GP, Walker EC, Podgor MJ. Is "relative" hypertension a risk factor for vaso-occlusive complications in sickle cell disease? *Am J Med Sci*. 1993;305:150–156.

92. Pegelow CH, Colangelo L, Steinberg M, et al. Natural history of blood pressure in sickle cell disease: risks for stroke and death associated with relative hypertension in sickle cell anemia. *Am J Med.* 1997;102:171–177.
93. Kaul DK, Liu XD, Fabry ME, Nagel RL. Increased nitric oxide synthase expression in transgenic sickle mice is associated with relative hypotension and altered microvascular response. *Blood.* 1998;92:330a.
94. Fabry ME, Kennan RP, Paszty C, et al. Magnetic resonance evidence of hypoxia in a homozygous a-knockout of a transgenic mouse model for sickle cell disease. *J Clin Invest.* 1996;98:2450–2455.
95. Brezis M, Rosen S. Hypoxia of the renal medulla – its implications for disease. *N Engl J Med.* 1995;332:647–655.
96. Kobayashi H, Kawamoto S, Brechbiel MW, et al. Micro-MRI methods to detect renal cysts in mice. *Kidney Int.* 2004;65:1511–1516.
97. Bank N, Kiroycheva M, Singhal PC, et al. Inhibition of nitric oxide synthase ameliorates cellular injury in sickle cell mouse kidneys. *Kidney Int.* 2000;58:82–89.
98. Nath KA, Grande JP, Haggard JJ, et al. Oxidative stress and induction of heme oxygenase-1 in the kidney in sickle cell disease. *Am J Pathol.* 2001;158:893–903.
99. Rybicki AC, Fabry ME, Does MD, Kaul DK, Nagel RL. Differential gene expression in the kidney of sickle cell transgenic mice: upregulated genes. *Blood Cell Mol Dis.* 2003;31:370–380.
100. Belcher JD, Bryant CJ, Nguyen J, et al. Transgenic sickle mice have vascular inflammation. *Blood.* 2003;101:3953–3959.
101. Nath KA, Grande JP, Croatt AJ, et al. Transgenic sickle mice are markedly sensitive to renal ischemia-reperfusion injury. *Am J Pathol.* 2005;166:963–972.
102. Diwan BA, Gladwin MT, Noguchi CT, et al. Renal pathology in hemizygous sickle cell mice. *Toxicol Pathol.* 2002;30:254–262.
103. Bonnin P, Sabaa N, Flamant M, Debbabi H, Tharaux PL. Ultrasound imaging of renal vaso-occlusive events in transgenic sickle mice exposed to hypoxic stress. *Ultrasound Med Biol.* 2008;34:1076–1084.
104. Lutty GA, McLeod DS, Pachnis A, et al. Retinal and choroidal neovascularization in a transgenic mouse model of sickle cell disease. *Am J Pathol.* 1994;145:490–497.
105. Lutty GA, Merges C, McLeod DS, et al. Nonperfusion of retina and choroid in transgenic mouse models of sickle cell disease. *Curr Eye Res.* 1998;17:438–444.
106. McLeod DS, Merges C, Fukushima A, Goldberg MF, Lutty GA. Histopathologic features of neovascularization in sickle cell retinopathy. *Am J Ophthalmol.* 1997;124:455–472.
107. Hebbel RP, Yamada O, Moldow CF, et al. Abnormal adherence of sickle erythrocytes to cultured vascular endothelium: possible mechanism for microvascular occlusion in sickle cell disease. *J Clin Invest.* 1980;65:154–160.
108. Hebbel RP, Boogaerts MAB, Eaton JW, Steinberg MH. Erythrocyte adherence in sickle cell disorders. *N Engl J Med.* 1980;302:992.
109. Kaul DK, Fabry ME, Costantini F, Rubin EM, Nagel RL. In vivo demonstration of red cell-endothelial interaction, sickling and altered microvascular response to oxygen in the sickle transgenic mouse. *J Clin Invest.* 1995;96:2845–2853.
110. Kaul DK, Liu XD, Fabry ME, Nagel RL. Impaired nitric oxide-mediated vasodilation in transgenic sickle mouse. *Am J Physiol Heart Circ Physiol.* 2000;278:H1799–H1806.
111. Embury SH, Mohandas N, Paszty C, Cooper P, Cheung AT. In vivo blood flow abnormalities in the transgenic knockout sickle cell mouse. *J Clin Invest.* 1999;103:915–920.
112. Kaul DK, Hebbel RP. Hypoxia/reoxygenation causes inflammatory response in transgenic sickle mice but not in normal mice. *J Clin Invest.* 2000;106:411–420.
113. Aslan M, Ryan TM, Adler B, et al. Oxygen radical inhibition of nitric oxide-dependent vascular function in sickle cell disease. *Proc Natl Acad Sci USA.* 2001;98:15215–15220.
114. Turhan A, Weiss LA, Mohandas N, Coller BS, Frenette PS. Primary role for adherent leukocytes in sickle cell vascular occlusion: a new paradigm. *Proc Natl Acad Sci USA.* 2002;99:3047–3051.
115. Chang J, Shi PA, Chiang EY, Frenette PS. Intravenous immunoglobulins reverse acute vaso-occlusive crises in sickle cell mice through rapid inhibition of neutrophil adhesion. *Blood.* 2008;111:915–923.
116. Wood KC, Hebbel RP, Lefer DJ, Granger DN. Critical role of endothelial cell-derived nitric oxide synthase in sickle cell disease-induced microvascular dysfunction. *Free Radic Biol Med.* 2006;40:1443–1453.
117. Kaul DK, Zhang X, Dasgupta T, Fabry ME. Arginine therapy of transgenic-knockout sickle mice improves microvascular function by reducing non-nitric oxide vasodilators, hemolysis and oxidative stress. *Am J Physiol Heart Circ Physiol.* 2008;295:H39–47.
118. Osei SY, Ahima RS, Fabry ME, Nagel RL, Bank N. Immunohistochemical localization of hepatic nitric oxide synthase in normal and transgenic sickle cell mice: the effect of hypoxia. *Blood.* 1996;88:3583–3588.
119. Fabry ME, Romero JR, Suzuka SM, et al. Hemoglobin C in transgenic mice: effect of HbC expression from founders to full mouse globin knockouts. *Blood Cell Mol Dis.* 2000;26:331–347.
120. Nagar S, Remmel RP, Hebbel RP, Zimmerman CL. Metabolism of opioids is altered in liver microsomes of sickle cell transgenic mice. *Drug Metab Dispos.* 2004;32:98–104.
121. May C, Rivella S, Callegari J, et al. Therapeutic haemoglobin synthesis in beta-thalassaemic mice expressing lentivirus-encoded human beta-globin. *Nature.* 2000;406:82–86.
122. Pawliuk R, Westerman KA, Fabry ME, et al. Correction of sickle cell disease in transgenic mouse models by gene therapy. *Science.* 2001;294:2368–2371.
123. Levasseur DN, Ryan TM, Pawlik KM, Townes TM. Correction of a mouse model of sickle cell disease: lentiviral/antisickling beta-globin gene transduction of unmobilized, purified hematopoietic stem cells. *Blood.* 2003;102:4312–4319.
124. Imren S, Payen E, Westerman KA, et al. Permanent and panerythroid correction of murine beta thalassemia by multiple lentiviral integration in hematopoietic stem cells. *Proc Natl Acad Sci USA.* 2002;99:14380–14385.
125. de Franceschi L, Baron A, Scarpa A et al. Inhaled nitric oxide protects transgenic SAD mice from sickle cell disease-specific lung injury induced by hypoxia/reoxygenation. *Blood.* 2003;102:1087–1096.
126. Minneci PC, Deans KJ, Zhi H, et al. Hemolysis-associated endothelial dysfunction mediated by accelerated NO

inactivation by decompartmentalized oxyhemoglobin. *J Clin Invest.* 2005;115:3409–3417.

127. Pritchard KA Jr, Ou J, Ou Z, et al. Hypoxia-induced acute lung injury in murine models of sickle cell disease. *Am J Physiol Lung Cell Mol Physiol.* 2004;286:L705–L714.

128. Holtzclaw JD, Jack D, Aguayo SM, et al. Enhanced pulmonary and systemic response to endotoxin in transgenic sickle mice. *Am J Respir Crit Care Med.* 2004;169:687–695.

129. Zhang S, Li H, Ma L, et al. Polynitroxyl-albumin (PNA) plus tempol attenuate lung capillary leak elicited by prolonged intestinal ischemia and reperfusion. *Free Radic Biol Med.* 2000;29:42–50.

130. de Franceschi L, Malpeli G, Scarpa A, et al. Protective effects of S-nitrosoalbumin on lung injury induced by hypoxia-reoxygenation in mouse model of sickle cell disease. *Am J Physiol Lung Cell Mol Physiol.* 2006;291:L457–L465.

131. Hsu LL, Champion HC, Campbell-Lee SA, et al. Hemolysis in sickle cell mice causes pulmonary hypertension due to global impairment in nitric oxide bioavailability. *Blood.* 2007;109:3088–3098.

132. Bartolucci P, Ngo MT, Beuzard Y, et al. Decrease in lung nitric oxide production after peritonitis in mice with sickle cell disease. *Crit Care Med.* 2007;35:502–509.

133. de Franceschi L, Platt OS, Malpeli G, et al. Protective effects of phosphodiesterase-4 (PDE-4) inhibition in the early phase of pulmonary arterial hypertension in transgenic sickle cell mice. *FASEB J.* 2008;22:1849–1860.

134. Kennan RP, Suzuka SM, Nagel RL, Fabry ME. Decreased cerebral perfusion correlates with increased BOLD hyperoxia response in transgenic mouse models of sickle cell disease. *Magn Reson Med.* 2004;51:525–532.

135. Wood KC, Hebbel RP, Granger DN. Endothelial cell P-selectin mediates a proinflammatory and prothrombogenic phenotype in cerebral venules of sickle cell transgenic mice. *Am J Physiol Heart Circ Physiol.* 2004;286:H1608–H1614.

136. Wood KC, Hebbel RP, Granger DN. Endothelial cell NADPH oxidase mediates the cerebral microvascular dysfunction in sickle cell transgenic mice. *FASEB J.* 2005;19:989–991.

137. White SP, Birch P, Kumar R. Interactions at the alpha 1 beta 1 interface in hemoglobin: a single amino acid change affects dimer ratio in transgenic mice expressing human hemoglobin. *Hemoglobin.* 1994;18:413–426.

138. Arcasoy MO, Romana M, Fabry ME, et al. High levels of human gamma-globin gene expression in adult mice carrying a transgene of deletion-type hereditary persistence of fetal hemoglobin. *Mol Cell Biol.* 1997;17:2076–2089.

139. Nagel RL, Sharma A, Kumar R, Fabry ME. Severe red cell abnormalities in transgenic mice expressing high levels of normal human delta chains. *Blood.* 1995;86(10):990A.

140. Chen Q, Bouhassira EE, Besse A, et al. Generation of transgenic mice expressing human hemoglobin E. *Blood Cell Mol Dis.* 2004;33:303–307.

141. Alami R, Gilman JG, Feng YQ, et al. Anti-b^S-ribozyme reduces b^S mRNA levels in transgenic mice: potential application to the gene therapy of sickle cell anemia. *Blood Cell Mol Dis.* 1999;25:110–119.

142. Seibler J, Schubeler D, Fiering S, Groudine M, Bode J. DNA cassette exchange in ES cells mediated by Flp recombinase: an efficient strategy for repeated modification of tagged loci by marker-free constructs. *Biochemistry.* 1998;37:6229–6234.

143. Bouhassira EE, Westerman K, Leboulch P. Transcriptional behavior of LCR enhancer elements integrated at the same chromosomal locus by recombinase-mediated cassette exchange. *Blood.* 1997;90:3332–3344.

144. Aird WC. Phenotypic heterogeneity of the endothelium: I. Structure, function, and mechanisms. *Circ Res.* 2007;100:158–173.

145. Aird WC. Phenotypic heterogeneity of the endothelium: II. Representative vascular beds. *Circ Res.* 2007;100:174–190.

146. Nagel RL, Fabry ME. The panoply of animal models for sickle cell anaemia. *Br J Haematol.* 2001;112:19–25.

147. Beuzard Y. Mouse models of sickle cell disease. *Transfus Clin Biol.* 2008;15:7–11.

148. Sadelain M. Recent advances in globin gene transfer for the treatment of beta-thalassemia and sickle cell anemia. *Curr Opin Hematol.* 2006;13:142–148.

149. Pei D. The magic continues for the iPS strategy. *Cell Res.* 2008;18:221–223.

150. Brugnara C, de Franceschi L. Clinical trials of new therapeutic pharmacology for sickle cell disease. *Sante.* 2006;16:263–268.

151. Wood KC, Granger DN. Sickle cell disease: role of reactive oxygen and nitrogen metabolites. *Clin Exp Pharmacol Physiol.* 2007;34:926–932.

152. Wood KC, Hsu LL, Gladwin MT. Sickle cell disease vasculopathy: A state of nitric oxide resistance. *Free Radic Biol Med.* 2008;44:1506–1528.

153. Kaul DK. Sickle red cell adhesion: many issues and some answers. *Transfus Clin Biol.* 2008;15:51–55.

SECTION THREE

α THALASSEMIA

Douglas R. Higgs

At all stages of development, human hemoglobin is made up of two α-like and two β-like globin chains. In embryonic life the ζ and ε genes are fully active, producing embryonic hemoglobin ($\zeta_2\epsilon_2$). Between 6 and 8 weeks of gestation there is a switch in expression so that the α- and γ-globin genes become fully expressed, producing fetal hemoglobin ($\alpha_2\gamma_2$). Finally, at around the time of birth there is a further switch from γ- to β-globin expression so that in adult red cells HbA ($\alpha_2\beta_2$) predominates.

In α thalassemia, the synthesis of α-globin chains is downregulated so that in fetal life there is anemia and the excess γ-globin chains form soluble tetramers (γ_4) called Hb Bart's. In adult life, α thalassemia also causes anemia but, because by this time the γ to β switch is complete, the excess non–α chains assemble into β_4 tetramers, called HbH. The degree of anemia and the amounts of the abnormal hemoglobins (Bart's and H) produced broadly reflect the degree to which α-globin synthesis has been downregulated.

We now know that normal individuals have four α-globin genes, arranged as linked pairs of genes at the tip of each copy of chromosome 16, written in shorthand as αα/αα. α Thalassemia most commonly results from the deletion of one (-α) or both (--) α genes from chromosome 16. Carriers of α thalassemia (-α/αα and --/αα) have mild hypochromic microcytic anemia and may produce detectable amounts of Hb Bart's at birth. In addition, occasional cells containing HbH may be detected in adults with the --/αα genotype, although hemoglobin electrophoresis is unremarkable. In all other respects carriers of α thalassemia are entirely normal and the most important consideration, from a clinical and hematological point of view, is to ensure that such patients do not become misdiagnosed and inappropriately treated for iron-deficiency anemia.

α Thalassemia is probably the most common disease-causing mutation affecting humankind. There is good circumstantial evidence that α thalassemia has attained such high frequencies by virtue of its selective advantage in areas where Falciparum malaria is or has been endemic. In tropical and subtropical regions of the world the carrier frequency of the mildest type of α thalassemia (-α) is very high and may be present in more than 90% of individuals in such populations. In southeast Asia and the Mediterranean basin the more severe defect (--) is also present at high frequencies (up to 10%). In these areas various combinations of alleles are seen. Homozygotes for the -α/ haplotype (-α/-α) have a mild hypochromic microcytic anemia. Compound heterozygotes (--/-α) have a hemolytic anemia producing large amounts of Hb Bart's at birth and similar levels of HbH in adult life, a condition known as HbH disease. Homozygotes for the --/ haplotype (--/--) have a lethal condition referred to as the Hb Bart's hydrops fetalis syndrome. As predicted from the distribution of the --/ haplotype, HbH disease and the Hb Bart's Hydrops Fetalis syndrome are mainly found in individuals of southeast Asian and Mediterranean origins.

Within the "malaria belt" there has been selection for a very wide range of hemoglobin variants and different types of α and β thalassemia. The major hemoglobinopathies include the HbS mutation and HbE. Coinheritance of α thalassemia has an important influence on the hematology and clinical manifestations of these common β-chain abnormalities and β thalassemia.

The molecular basis of α thalassemia is now understood in great detail. Normally, the α-like genes are arranged along chromosome 16 in the order in which they are expressed in development (telomere-ζ2-α2-α1-centromere). Furthermore, we now know that the cluster lies in a telomeric, gene-rich region of the genome, surrounded by widely expressed genes. Full expression of the α-like genes is critically dependent on the presence of a regulatory element (called HS-40), which lies 40 kb upstream of the cluster (toward the telomere). As many as 50 deletions removing one (-α/) or both (--) genes have been characterized and of these six ($-\alpha^{3.7}$/, $-\alpha^{4.2}$/, $--^{SEA}$/, $--^{MED}$/, $-(\alpha)^{20.5}$/ and $--^{FIL}$/) represent by far the most common causes of α thalassemia worldwide. In addition, many different point mutations affecting the structural genes have been identified, these cause the less common nondeletional forms of α thalassemia ($\alpha^T\alpha$/). This information has allowed researchers and hematologists to establish logical and robust screening programs for identifying patients with α thalassemia. This in turn allows clinicians to provide accurate genetic counseling and prenatal diagnosis for the severe syndromes of α thalassemia, including Hb Bart's Hydrops Fetalis and transfusion-dependent forms of HbH disease.

In addition to these common forms of α thalassemia there are many rare and unusual molecular defects that have been identified. These are important because they provide an explanation for patients with hitherto undiagnosed anemia, and they help us to understand how the α cluster is normally regulated in vivo. Rarely, α thalassemia is caused by deletions that remove the α-globin regulatory element (HS-40). In general these mutations have been observed outside of the "malaria belt," indicating that they are sporadic genetic events that have not been selected during evolution. These natural deletions first indicated the existence of this unexpected form of long-range control of α-globin expression.

There are also two rare forms of α thalassemia that are found in association with a variety of developmental abnormalities, and in particular with mental retardation (so-called α thalassemia with mental retardation, ATR syndromes). The first group of patients has large (>1 Mb) deletions from the tip of chromosome 16 including the α-globin genes (ATR-16). These usually result from chromosome truncations or translocations and in fact this syndrome provided the first examples in human genetics of subcytogenetic chromosomal translocations, which are now known to underlie many cases of unexplained mental retardation. The second group of patients is now known to have mutations in a *trans*-acting factor (called ATRX) encoded on the X-chromosome (ATR-X syndrome). These patients have α thalassemia with profound mental retardation, facial abnormalities, and urogenital anomalies. In this case it is thought that the X-encoded factor regulates expression of many genes, the α genes being but one target.

Finally, there is a rare and unexplained form of α thalassemia that is seen as an acquired mutation in patients with myelodysplasia, hence called the ATMDS syndrome. These patients inherit a normal complement of α genes (αα/αα) but later in life develop myelodysplasia and presumably acquire a clonal genetic abnormality during the course of their disease. It is interesting that the majority of these patients are elderly males who at some stage of their disease have abnormal erythropoiesis. It has recently been shown that these patients have acquired mutations in the *ATRX* gene.

In the following chapters we will review the epidemiology, molecular pathology, pathophysiology, and clinical syndromes of α thalassemia in detail.

13

The Molecular Basis of α Thalassemia

Douglas R. Higgs

INTRODUCTION

Before describing the various ways in which α-globin expression may be downregulated in patients with α thalassemia, it is worth briefly reviewing the normal structure of the human α-globin cluster and how the genes are expressed throughout erythroid differentiation and development.

The α-globin cluster is located in a gene dense region of the genome close to the telomere of chromosome 16 (16p13.3). The genes are arranged along the chromosome in the order, telomere-ζ-$\psi\zeta$-α^D-$\psi\alpha1$-$\alpha2$-$\alpha1$-θ-centromere (Fig. 13.1). Upstream of the α cluster there are four highly conserved, noncoding sequences multispecies conserved sequences called MCS-R1–R4[1] that are thought to be important in the regulation of the α-like globin genes. They correspond to previously identified erythroid-specific DNase I hypersensitive sites (DHS) referred to as HS-48, HS-40, HS-33, and HS-10,[2] the coordinates referring to their positions (kb) with respect to the ζ-globin mRNA cap site. Of these elements, only MCS-R2 (HS-40) has been shown to be essential for α globin expression (summarized in Higgs et al.[3]). The role(s) of the other MCS sequences are as yet unclear.

It has been shown that as progenitors commit to the erythroid lineage and differentiate to form mature red cells, a subset of the key erythroid transcription factors and cofactors (Chapter 4) progressively bind the upstream elements and the promoters of the α-like globin genes.[4–6] Finally, RNA polymerase II is recruited to both the upstream regions and the globin promoters as transcription starts in early and intermediate erythroblasts.[4,5] At the same time, it has been shown[5] that the upstream elements and promoters of the globin genes physically interact, forming a chromatin loop (Fig. 13.2).

Both ζ- and α-globins are expressed in primitive erythroblasts[7] emanating from the yolk sac (up to 6–7 weeks of gestation in human). It has been shown in mouse that as such cells mature there is a switch from ζ– to α-globin expression[8] and it seems likely that a similar maturational switch occurs in human[9] (E. E. Bouhassira, personal communication, 2006). Definitive line erythroblasts in the liver almost exclusively synthesize α-globin (from 6 weeks onward)[7] Very small amounts of ζ-mRNA are present throughout fetal life (for example, see ref. 10) and ζ-globin (as Hb Portland) can be detected in the cord bloods of nonthalassemic newborn (for example, see ref. 11). Using sensitive mRNA assays, low levels of θ-transcripts are detected in yolk sac, fetal liver,[12] adult blood,[13] and bone marrow[14] Similarly, very low levels of α^D (also called μ) mRNA can be detected in cord blood, adult blood and bone marrow[15] but proteins corresponding to θ and α^D have not yet been identified.

α–Globin transcription starts in basophilic erythroblasts and reaches a maximum in intermediate (polychromatophilic) erythroblasts and subsequently switches off as the erythroid cell matures.[16] Despite this, translation of globin mRNA continues for 2–3 days in reticulocytes from which the nucleus has been extruded. Continued globin synthesis, in these transcriptionally inert red cells, is critical for normal red cell production and is made possible by the long half life (>24 hours) of globin mRNA. This in turn depends on an RNA binding complex called the α-globin poly(C) binding protein (αCP). This is thought to stabilize α-globin mRNA by controlling deadenylation of its polyA tail and protecting the RNA from an erythroid enriched endoribonuclease (ErEN[17]).

Although the protein products of the $\alpha2$- and $\alpha1$-genes are identical, two methods exploiting the sequence divergence in their 3′ noncoding regions have enabled the relative amounts of $\alpha2$- and $\alpha1$-mRNA to be determined in reticulocytes.[18–20] This shows that in fetal and adult life the steady-state level of $\alpha2$-mRNA predominates over $\alpha1$-mRNA by approximately 3:1, probably as a result of differences at the level of transcription of the two genes. This may result from a competition between the $\alpha2$ and $\alpha1$ gene for access to the upstream MCS elements, which the $\alpha2$ gene wins because of its relative proximity to HS-40. It is also possible, but less likely, that the $\alpha2$ and $\alpha1$ mRNAs may be made in similar amounts but have different stabilities.

It is still not clear whether the protein resulting from $\alpha2$mRNA translation outweighs that from $\alpha1$mRNA translation. Assessment of the ribosome loading of $\alpha2$- and $\alpha1$-mRNA has shown that they have identical translational profiles and therefore should be produced with equal efficiencies predicting a dominant role for the $\alpha2$-globin locus.[21] It follows that, in heterozygotes, naturally occurring structural mutations of the $\alpha2$ gene should represent approximately 37% of the peripheral blood hemoglobin and $\alpha1$ mutants approximately 13%. Two studies addressing this point come to different conclusions. In the first,[22] it was found that $\alpha2$ variants represented 24%–40% whereas $\alpha1$ variants represented 11%–23%, suggesting a predominant role for the $\alpha2$ gene at both mRNA and protein levels.

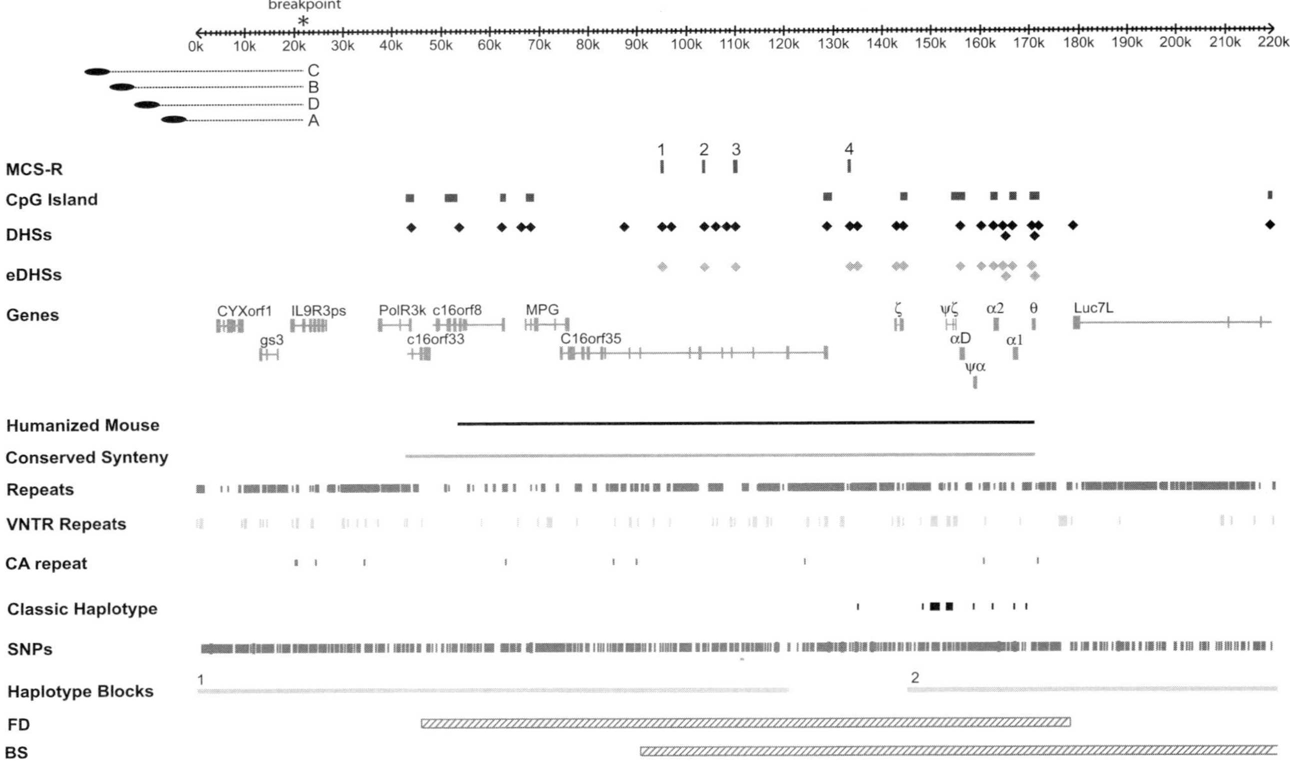

Figure 13.1. The normal α-cluster located at 16p13.3. The annotated genes extending from the 16p telomere (left) are shown. The polymorphic subtelomeric regions (A, B, C, and D) are shown, and the point of divergence between different subtelomeric regions is marked with an asterisk (breakpoint). Below the scale, the positions of multispecies conserved sequences (MCS-R1–4), CpG islands, all DNase I hypersensitive sites (DHSs) and erythroid specific sites (eDHS) are shown. Below the genes are shown the segment of DNA replaced in the "humanized mouse,"[27] the region of conserved synteny[1] and various repeat sequences (including VNTRs and CA repeats). Below this, the positions of the polymorphisms used to score the "classic haplotype"[48] SNPs and extended haplotype blocks (1 and 2) are shown. At the bottom are the two duplications of the α cluster described in ref. 26.

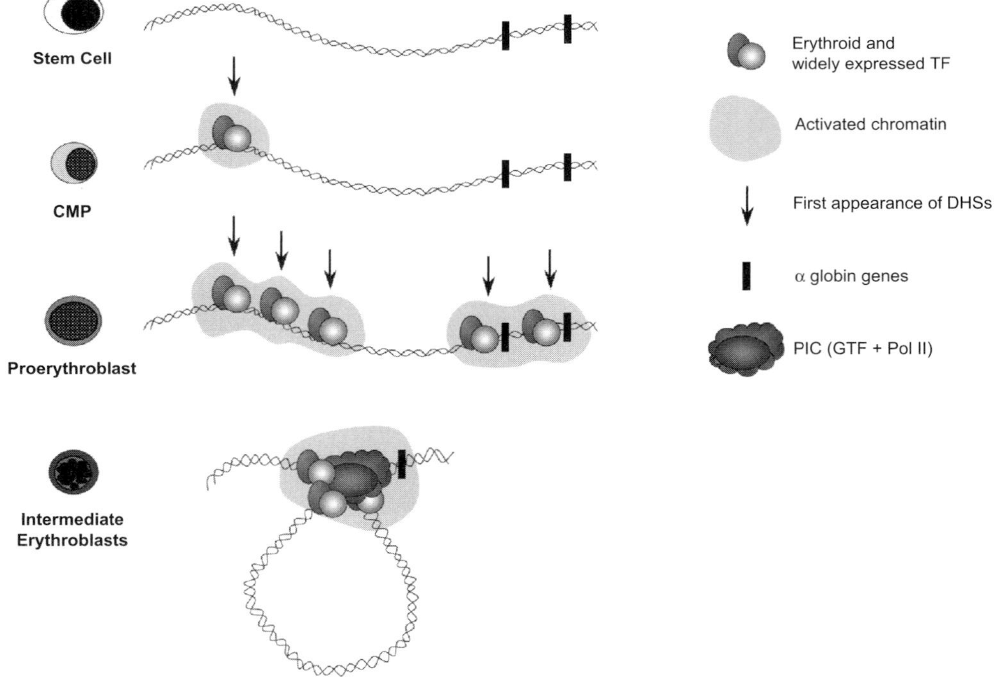

Figure 13.2. A summary of the events leading to α-globin gene activation during erythropoiesis with a key to the events (on the right). At the time the preinitiation complex (PIC) is recruited, the upstream elements form a loop via their interaction with the globin gene promoters.

Table 13.1. α-Globin variants associated with deletional forms of α-thalassemia

Variant		Haplotype	Population(s)	Reference
Hb Evanston	α^{14} Trp→Arg	$-\alpha^{3.7}$	Black	166, 167
Hb Hasharon	α^{47} Asp→His	$-\alpha^{3.7}$ and αα	Mediterranean, Ashkenazi Jews	22, 168–172
Hb G Philadelphia	α^{68} Asn→Lys	$-\alpha^{3.7}$ and αα	Algerian, Mediterranean, Black, Melanesian	22, 168, 173–177
Hb Q (Mahidol)	α^{74} Asp→His	$-\alpha^{4.2}$	Southeast Asian	178, 179
Hb Duan	α^{75} Asp→Ala	$-\alpha^{4.2}$	Chinese	180
Hb Stanleyville II	α^{78} Asn→Lys	$-\alpha^{3.7}$	Black	181
Hb Nigeria	α^{81} Ser→Lys	Not determined	Black	182
Hb J Capetown	α^{92} Arg→Gln	$-\alpha^{3.7I}$	South African	183
Hb J Tongariki	α^{115} Ala→Asp	$-\alpha^{3.7II}$	Melanesian	77, 184

In contrast, a more extensive survey of α globin variants by Molchanova et al.[20] found that in heterozygotes the average proportion of stable variants resulting from α2 mutants (23.5%) was only slightly higher than from α1 mutations (19.7%), suggesting a less efficient translation of the α2 mRNA and a more equal contribution from the two genes at the protein level. Further work is still needed to resolve this issue because it is of importance for understanding the pathophysiology of the nondeletional forms of α thalassemia (see later).

VARIANTS OF THE GLOBIN CLUSTER THAT DO NOT CAUSE THALASSEMIA

Before considering mutations of the α cluster that cause α thalassemia we will briefly review variants that occur in the nonthalassemic population. Some of these are relatively common and provide useful genetic markers for the α cluster and the 16p telomere. In addition, they illustrate some of the chromosomal rearrangements and DNA sequence changes that have taken place during the evolution of this multigene family. Furthermore, some mutants help to differentiate between regions of the gene cluster that are important for expression in vivo and those that may be irrelevant.

Chromosomal Rearrangements Involving 16p13.3

Rarely, chromosomal translocations involving 16p13.3 place the α-globin locus at the tip of another chromosome, as seen, for example, in some relatives of patients with the ATR-16 syndrome (see Chapter 15). To date we know of 16 individuals with such balanced translocations and none of them has α thalassemia. Fifteen were summarized in Table 13.1 in the previous edition of this book (see web site) and one additional case (EW) also has a balanced rearrangement 46,XX,-16.+der(16) (16;20)(p13.3;q13.3) and normal hematological indices (Hb 11.5 g/dL, mean corpuscular volume [MCV] 87 fL, and mean corpuscular hemoglobin [MCH] 27.9 pg). Because the closest centromeric breakpoint of these chromosomal translocations lies only 1.2 Mb from the α-globin genes, these findings demonstrate that the *cis*-acting sequences required for full α-globin regulation are contained within this region and expression is not perturbed by rearrangements on this scale. In two individuals with unbalanced translocations, and three copies of 16p13.3, the α/β globin chain synthesis ratios were 1.5 and 1.6,[23,24] (and unpublished data) again indicating that the additional, mislocalized copy of the α complex is expressed even though its genomic position has been altered.

Two large duplications of the terminal region have also been described in patients with β thalassemia intermedia (see Chapter 16). Because these patients are simply heterozygotes for the β thalassemia mutations it implies that their relatively severe phenotype results from the production of excess α-globin chains from the α genes in the duplicated regions. In one pedigree, three α clusters (αα:αα:αα) are present on one copy of chromosome 16[25] (and unpublished data). Provisional data suggest that at least two and possibly all three clusters in the duplicated region are fully active. A carrier for this abnormal chromosome (αα:αα:αα/αα), with a total of 8 α genes, has an α/β-globin chain synthesis ratio of 2.7.[25] A recent study has more fully characterized what appears to be a very similar rearrangement in another Italian family with β thalassemia intermedia[26] revealing a duplication of approximately 260 kb (BS in Fig. 13.1). These authors also characterized another duplication of approximately 175 kb of chromosome 16 lying between the end of the α cluster and the telomere (FD in Fig 13.1). Again the phenotype of a compound heterozygote for this rearrangement (αα:αα/αα) and β thalassemia trait suggested that the additional α clusters in the duplicated segment are fully active indicating that all sequences required for fully regulated α globin expression lie in this duplicated segment of chromosome 16.

More recently, these observations, based on "experiments of nature," have been refined by evolutionary studies and experimental observations. Hughes et al[1] cloned and sequenced the α-globin cluster and the surrounding region in 22 vertebrate species spanning 500 million years of evolution. The most informative comparison was with the mouse in which the orthologous α-globin cluster has translocated from its normal telomeric location (seen in most species) to an interstitial position (on mouse chromosome 11). Presumably this translocation, which

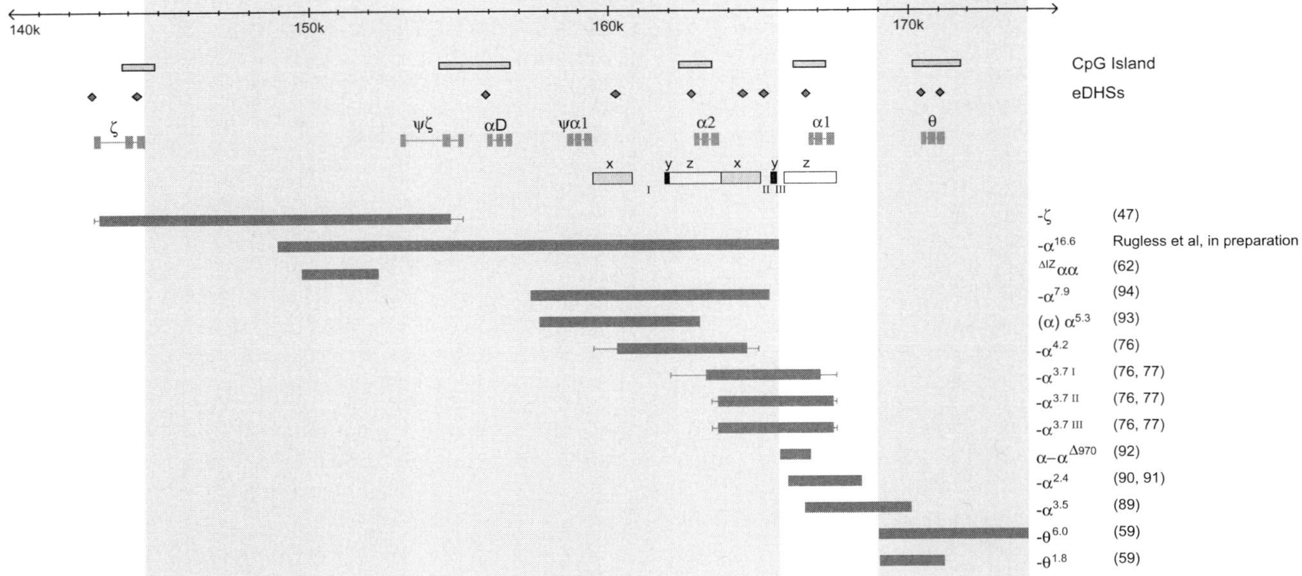

Figure 13.3. Deletions that cause α^+ thalassemia. Above the α-like globin genes, CpG island, and erythroid specific DHS as in Figure 13.1. Below this are shown the duplication units divided into X, Y, and Z boxes with regions of nonhomology (I, II, III). Below the extent of each deletion is represented by a black bar. The thin bars at the end of each thick bar denote the regions of uncertainty for the deletion breakpoints. Primary references for the characterization of these deletions are shown on the right hand side of the diagram. It is interesting to note that based on the observed phenotypes of some of these mutations (discussed in the text), it may be possible to conclude that there are no *cis*-acting sequences critical to the α cluster (other than the α2 gene itself) lying between coordinates approximately 145,000–165,000 (indicated by shaded boxes).

involves approximately 135 kb including the α cluster and its regulatory elements (region of conserved synteny, Fig. 13.1), includes all of the *cis*-acting sequences required to maintain fully regulated tissue- and developmental-stage specific expression of the α globin cluster. To test this, Wallace and colleagues[27] replaced the endogenous mouse α-globin cluster with the syntenic region of the human cluster (humanized mouse in Fig. 13.1) by using homologous recombination and showed that this segment of DNA was sufficient to recapitulate the normal pattern of human α-globin expression in a mouse background. Together these observations have helped to define the region of chromosome 16, which directs fully regulated expression of the human α globin locus.

Variation at the 16p Telomere

The human α globin locus lies very close to the telomere of the short arm of chromosome 16 (Fig. 13.1). There are four alleles in which the α-globin genes lie 170 kb (A), 245 kb (D), 350 kb (B), or 430 kb (C) from the 16p telomeric repeats[28,29] (see Fig. 13.1). Detailed analysis has shown that these polymorphic, subtelomeric alleles are structurally quite different. For example, beyond the region of divergence (*breakpoint in Fig. 13.1), the A and B alleles are more closely related to nonhomologous chromosomes than to each other. The A allele is related to the subtelomeric regions of Xqter and Yqter whereas the B allele is more like Xqter, 10pter and 18pter. Similar long-range polymorphisms have been identified at several other human telomeres.[30] Despite these major structural differences at the 16p telomere, the hematological indices of individuals with A and B alleles are indistinguishable.

Variation in the Number of Globin Genes

As a result of unequal genetic exchange (see later) hematologically normal individuals may have 4, 5 or 6 α genes.[31–35] A recently described individual with 7 α (ααααα/αα) genes had a minor degree of microcytosis.[36] A curiously high frequency of the ααα chromosome (gene frequency ~0.01–0.08) is found in most populations that have been studied although the reasons for this are not yet clear. Although there appears to be an excess of α-mRNA[18,34] and α-globin[34,37–41] produced from the ααα arrangement, homozygotes (ααα/ααα) still appear to be hematologically normal.[31,42] Although it has not been formally analyzed in human, in sheep it has been shown that the efficiency with which multiple α genes are expressed decreases from the 5′ to 3′ position on the chromosome.[43] In this case, as more α genes are added to the cluster (αα to ααα to αααα), any increase in α-globin expression may be less than expected from the addition of fully expressed extra genes.

In addition to these variations in the number of α genes, normal individuals may also have variations (from two to six) in the number of ζ-like genes.[44–47] Chromosomes bearing a single ζ gene (ζ2 rather than the normal ζ2-ψζ1 arrangement see Fig. 13.3) are relatively common (gene frequency ~0.05) in West Africans[44,47–49] (and unpublished data) and occur sporadically in other populations. There is no discernible phenotype associated with the -ζ/ζζ genotype[44,46,47] and unpublished data) although, to date, only one homozygote (-ζ/-ζ) has been identified who appears hematologically normal.

The triplicated ζ-gene arrangement (ζζζ) has the structure ζ2-ψζ1-ψζ1[10] and was originally identified in Southeast Asia where its frequency is 0.09–0.20;[47,48,50] it is also particularly common throughout Melanesia, Micronesia, and Polynesia where phenotypically normal homozygotes (ζζζ/ζζζ) have been described.[46,48,51] Elsewhere ζζζ is uncommon. Structural analysis of the ζζζ arrangement shows that it has arisen by an unusual interchromosomal recombination event[10,51] between Ia and IId haplotypes (the common α-globin haplotypes are described in Higgs et al.[48] (also see Fig. 13.1, classic haplotype). All of the ζζζ chromosomes studied from Southeast Asia and the Pacific have this unusual structure,[51] suggesting that they have a common, single origin. Some of these chromosomes appear to have been subsequently modified, as indicated by the presence of a Bgl II polymorphism in 8%–15% of cases[51] and the occasional presence of the Hb-CS (Constant Spring). mutation on the linked α2 gene.[47] A single example of a chromosome with four ζ genes (ζζζζ) was described by Titus et al.[45]

Gene Conversion in the Globin Cluster

The DNA strand exchanges involved in misaligned but reciprocal recombination (see later) may resolve with nonreciprocal genetic exchange, known also as gene conversions; reviewed in Strachan and Read.[52] During the process of gene conversion genetic information may be exchanged between allelic (homologous) or nonallelic (paralogous) sequences without any crossovers or chromosomal rearrangements occurring. Gene conversion events between both the α1/α2 pair and the ζ2/ψζ1 pair may occur quite frequently. DNA sequence analysis suggests that gene conversion events have taken place, during evolution, between α1 and α2[53] and ζ2 and ψζ1 genes[10,54] maintaining the sequence identity of the non-allelic duplicated genes (concerted evolution). A likely example of such a conversion event between α2 and α1 has been documented in individuals expressing an unexpectedly high level of Hb-l, an α-variant ($\alpha^{16\text{Lys}\rightarrow\text{Glu}}$), in which the same mutation is present on both α2 and α1 genes in *cis*[55] (Chapter 24). Further possible examples of nonreciprocal exchange were described by Molchanova et al.[20] who observed identical sequence mutations affecting the α1 and α2 genes on independent chromosomes; one possibility is that these arise by conversion from one gene to another. Additional evidence, consistent with gene conversion, comes from the identification of "patchwork" α genes in which the α2 gene contains sequences characteristic of the α1 gene and vice versa.[33,56] These and other[57] patchwork-like genes have now been found in many, diverse populations suggesting that genetic information is passed between the duplicated regions containing the α genes relatively frequently.

Analysis of the downstream ζ-like gene in several populations has shown that it exists in two distinct forms.[10] In one its structure is clearly that of a pseudogene (ψζ1) and in the other (ζ1) the ψζ1 gene has undergone a gene conversion by the ζ2 gene such that it becomes more similar to the functional ζ gene although it still appears not to be expressed in vivo. The frequency of the ζ2-ζ1 chromosome varies from one population to another (0.14–0.57), and phenotypically normal individuals homozygous for either ζ2-ψζ1 or ζ2-ζ1 chromosomes have been observed.[10] Conversions of the ζ2 gene by ψζ1 have not yet been described although several candidate chromosomes have been identified.

In addition to these examples of gene conversion it seems likely that, as in other mammalian multigene families[58] short segmental conversions may also be responsible for transferring thalassemic and nonthalassemic variants within and between different chromosomal backgrounds.

Deletions and Insertions Within the α-Complex

Two uncommon deletions involving the θ1 gene remove either 1.8 kb or 6.0 kb from between the intact α1 gene and the α-globin 3′HVR[59] (Fig. 13.3). Neither variant was associated with any phenotypic abnormalities in the neonatal period and an adult, heterozygous for the 1.8 kb deletion also appears normal. The reported individual with the 6.0-kb deletion also had a -ζ chromosome.[59] We have also studied an individual who apparently has the same 6.0-kb deletion and in this case the -ζ arrangement is present in *cis* to the θ1 deletion.[60] Similarly, Ballas et al.[61] found that both of these rearrangements may exist on the same chromosome. Thus these individuals have deletions at both the 5′ (10 kb) and 3′ (6 kb) ends of the cluster with no discernible effect on α-gene expression. In a large survey of newborn babies,[62] a small (2.5-kb) deletion (see Fig. 13.3) between the ζ and ψζ genes was observed in two hematologically normal babies from Sardinia.

Phenotypically silent insertions are also recognized in the α-complex. An insertion of 0.5–0.7 kb between the α2 and α1 genes was identified in the nonthalassemic chromosome of a Chinese individual.[63] This most probably arose from a reciprocal crossover between a normal chromosome (αα) and the common α-thalassemia determinant (-$\alpha^{3.7}$, see later). In addition we have observed an insertion/deletion polymorphism in the 5′ flanking region of the α-complex that appears to involve members of the *Alu* family of repeats[60]

Restriction Site Polymorphisms

It is now known that single nucleotide polymorphisms (SNPs) are found, on average, once every 2 kb[64] in normal individuals and some of these changes were originally identified as restriction fragment length polymorphisms

(RFLPs) within and flanking the α-cluster.[48] SNPs identified in this way were divided into common (the frequency of the rarer allele in most populations being 0.05–0.50) and uncommon (<0.05) variants; the latter were frequently found to be race or population-specific. Analysis of nine common polymorphisms (including the ψζ1/ζ1 polymorphism and the interzeta hypervariable region, IZHVR) showed that linkage disequilibrium exists between these genetic markers and some common α-globin haplotypes (non-random linkage groups) could be derived (classic haplotype[48] [Fig. 13.1]). Although a large number of haplotypes are now recognized, in each population only one or two are common and several others are present at low frequencies. There is, as yet, no evidence that α-globin expression differs between the common α-globin haplotypes.

More recently this type of analysis has been expanded using 80 validated SNPs located in the terminal region of 16p13.3 (coordinates ~20,000–320,000) to study 7 diverse populations and thereby to extend the haplotypes and define regions of linkage disequilibrium (LD) across this segment of the genome (Viprakasit et al. unpublished). From this we have defined two blocks of LD located between the telomere and coordinate approximately 120,000, and approximately 150,000–260,000 (LD blocks 1 and 2 in Fig. 13.1). In theory, the chromatin between these blocks should contain a region of relatively high recombination although, at present, this area does not clearly correlate with any of the other structural or functional features associated with the α globin cluster.

Within block 1, DNA sequence analysis has revealed six minor variants of the HS -40 regulatory element.[65] Again, these polymorphic subhaplotypes are found in normal, nonthalassemic individuals and provide informative examples of in vivo mutagenesis, which allows one to relate the structure of this important regulatory region to its function.

Variable Number of Tandem Repeats

Preliminary Southern blot analysis identified several variable number tandem repeats (VNTRs) in and around the α-globin locus.[66,67] The number of repeats in such arrays may be altered at mitosis or meiosis[68] producing highly polymorphic segments of the cluster. Further DNA sequence analysis of the terminal 300-kb region of 16p[69] identified at least ten VNTRs in this region consistent with the view that such sequences tend to cluster at the ends of human chromosomes.[70] At present we have identified more than 100 tandem repeats but only a few have been tested to establish whether or not they vary in normal human populations. In the α-complex, when analyzed, there appears to be no relationship between the structure of such regions and the associated phenotype. Whatever their function, if any, they are of great value as genetic markers throughout the genome and have been used to produce individual-specific genetic fingerprints.[71,72]

VARIANTS THAT CAUSE THALASSEMIA

As set out previously, analysis of the human α-globin cluster has revealed a remarkable degree of polymorphism due to point mutations, deletions and insertions of DNA. These polymorphisms are found in all populations. Variants that cause α thalassemia are largely limited to tropical and subtropical regions of the world where malaria is, or has been, endemic (see Chapter 26). Some rare and very informative mutations have been found in individuals outside of these regions. In contrast to β thalassemia, in which mutations are frequently due to point mutations in the structural genes (Chapter 16), α thalassemia is most often due to deletions involving one or both of the α genes. Less frequently, deletions removing the α-globin regulatory element (HS-40) are seen. This difference in molecular pathology (deletions rather than point mutations) represents another contrast between the α and β clusters, which may also reflect their different chromosomal environments (see Chapter 3).

α Thalassemia due to Deletions

DNA sequence analysis has shown that the α-globin genes are embedded within two highly homologous, 4-kb duplication units whose sequence identity appears to have been maintained throughout evolution by gene conversion and unequal crossover events.[53,73–75] These regions are divided into homologous subsegments (X, Y, and Z) by nonhomologous elements (I, II, and III, Figs. 13.3 and 13.4). Reciprocal recombination between Z segments (Fig. 13.4), which are 3.7 kb apart, produces chromosomes with only one α-gene ($-\alpha^{3.7}$, rightward deletion, Figs. 13.3 and 13.4)[76] that cause α thalassemia and others with three α-genes ($\alpha\alpha\alpha^{anti3.7}$).[32,34] These events can be further subdivided, depending on exactly where within the Z box the crossover took place into $-\alpha^{3.7I}$, $-\alpha^{3.7II}$ and $-\alpha^{3.7III}$ (Fig. 13.3).[77] These subregions are defined by sequence differences in the Zα2 and Zα1 boxes that can be detected by Southern blot hybridization. Recombination between homologous X boxes, which are 4.2 kb apart, also gives rise to an α thalassemia determinant ($-\alpha^{4.2}$, leftward deletion, Figs. 13.3 and 13.4)[76] and a $\alpha\alpha\alpha^{anti4.2}$ chromosome.[78] Further recombination events between the resulting chromosomes (α, αα, ααα) may give rise to quadruplicated α-genes ($\alpha\alpha\alpha\alpha^{anti3.7}$, $\alpha\alpha\alpha\alpha^{anti4.2}$),[78,79] quintuplicated ($\alpha\alpha\alpha\alpha\alpha^{anti3.7}$),[36] or other unusual patchwork rearrangements[56,57]

The variety of independent recombination events giving rise to -α and ααα and other, related arrangements identified in extant human populations suggests that recombination between the homologous X and Z boxes is relatively frequent and several indirect observations support this notion. Both -α and ααα chromosomes are present in most population groups. Moreover, the -α determinant is associated with many different hemoglobin variants (e.g., see Higgs et al.[60] and Table 17.1) HVR alleles and α-globin

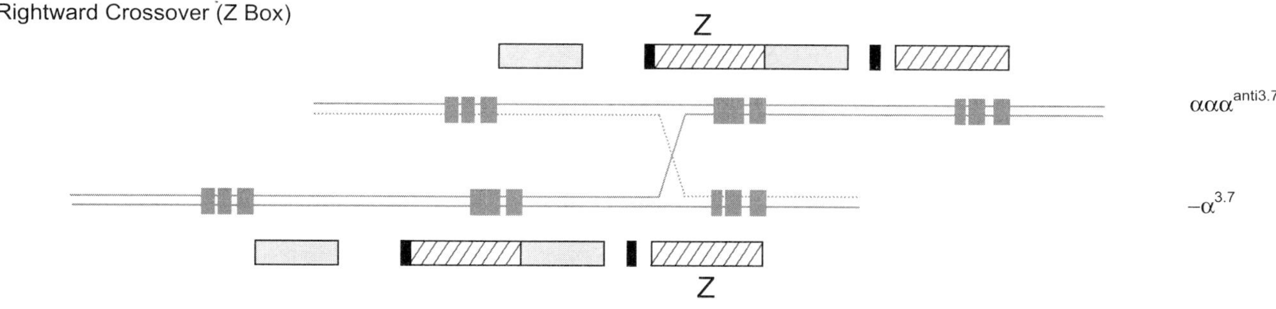

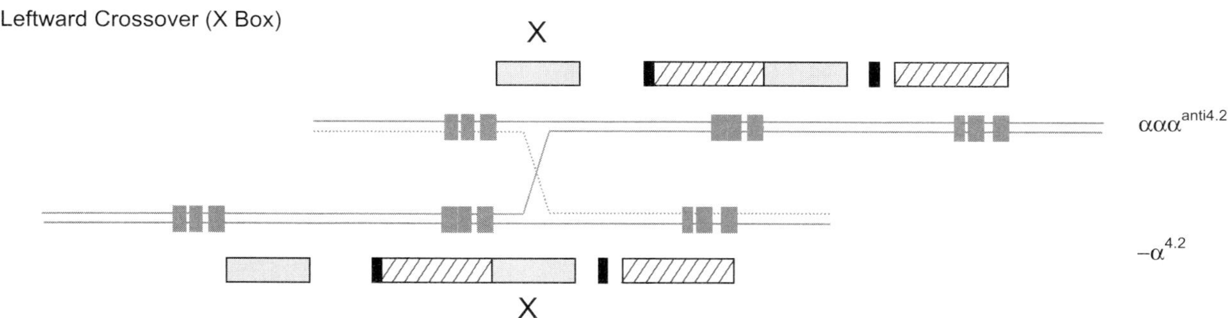

Figure 13.4. The mechanism by which the common deletions underlying α^+ thalassemia occur. Crossovers between misaligned Z boxes give rise to the -$\alpha^{3.7}$ and $\alpha\alpha\alpha^{\text{anti }3.7}$ chromosomes. Crossovers between misaligned X boxes give rise to -$\alpha^{4.2}$ and $\alpha\alpha\alpha^{\text{anti }4.2}$ chromosomes.

haplotypes.[66,80,81] Furthermore, in population isolates such as Papua New Guinea and Vanuatu the -α determinants are only found on the common α-globin haplotypes for that population suggesting that they have arisen *de novo* in each population group[80] rather than having been "imported" from other populations and selected. Moreover, some α-globin variants (e.g. Hb-G Philadelphia, $\alpha^{68\ \text{Asn}\rightarrow\text{Lys}}$) are found on both normal (αα) chromosomes and chromosomes bearing an α thalassemia determinant (-α), suggesting a connection between the two through recombination and/or gene conversion. Similar observations have been made for the poly(A) signal mutation found in Saudi Arabia (see later), which is present on both αα and ααα chromosomes.[82]

It is interesting that recombination hotspots in duplicated elements (such as the X and Z boxes) often show patchy gene conversion at the site of crossover,[83–85] emphasizing the connection between these two processes. It has also been noted that the relative frequencies of the various types of α thalassemia observed throughout the world correlate with the length of the homologous segments (X, Y and Z) that serve as target areas for the crossovers involved (-$\alpha^{3.7\text{I}}$ [1436 bp] > -$\alpha^{4.2}$ [1339 bp] > -$\alpha^{3.7\text{II}}$ [171 bp] > -$\alpha^{3.7\text{III}}$ [46 bp]). Correlations between frequency of recombination and target size have been noted in other systems;[86] however, because the α-thalassemia determinants are highly selected for in many areas[80] these observations may not truly reflect recombination rates.

Although these long standing observations have pointed to the mechanism by which -α and ααα chromosomes arise it has only recently been shown (using single DNA molecule polyermase chain reaction [PCR]) how they may occur *in vivo*.[87,88] From this work, the overall picture is one of reciprocal recombination (and unequal exchange) occurring in mitosis (premeiotic) in the germ line. The estimated frequencies of -α and ααα arrangements in sperm are in the order of $1–5 \times 10^{-5}$. Deletions and duplications may also occur in somatic tissues by related mechanisms although deletions detected in blood occur by intrachromosomal rather than interchromosomal recombination.[87] Consistent with the observations in human populations, recombination was found to be associated with patchy gene conversion and the position of crossover was, to some extent, governed by the length of high sequence identity, with the -$\alpha^{3.7}$ chromosome arising more frequently than -$\alpha^{4.2}$.[87] Given the high frequency with which these chromosomes are generated, the authors argue that in populations in which there is no α thalassemia, there must be selection against -α/-α and ααα/ααα homozygotes.[87,88]

In addition to the common -α chromosomes, seven rare deletions that produce α^+ thalassemia have been described (Fig. 13.3). One that removes the entire α1 gene and its flanking DNA (-$\alpha^{3.5}$) has been observed in two Asian Indian patients.[89] The breakpoints of this deletion have not been examined in detail. Another rare α^+ thalassemia deletion (called -$\alpha^{2.7}$) removing the α1 gene and its flanking DNA was originally described in a Chinese patient with HbH disease.[90] A subsequent report[91] of a Canadian/Chinese patient with HbH disease (in whom the breakpoints were sequenced) identified a deletion, accurately assessed as 2.4 kb (-$\alpha^{2.4}$). It seems likely that these two deletions (-$\alpha^{2.4}$ and -$\alpha^{2.7}$) are the same mutation and hence we have grouped them in Figure 13.3. Recently Poodt et al.[92] described a small deletion (970 bp) removing the entire promoter of the α1 gene and DNA-encoding 26 bp of the 5′ end of the mRNA, which completely inactivates the α1 gene. In all three of these deletions it appears that the remaining α2 gene is fully active.

Three large deletions remove the α2 gene and a variable amount of the α globin cluster lying upstream. The first, referred to as (α)$\alpha^{5.3}$, was observed in a family from Italy.[93] It removes the 5′ end of the α2-globin gene; the 5′ breakpoint lies 822 bp upstream of the mRNA cap site of the $\psi\alpha$1-gene, the 3′ breakpoint is located in IVS1 of the α2 gene. Sequence analysis indicates that this deletion has arisen by an illegitimate recombination event. The second is a deletion of 7.9 kb (-$\alpha^{7.9}$), which was found in two unrelated individuals of Surinam/Indian origins.[94] This deletion removes the $\psi\alpha$1 and α2 genes by non-homologous recombination. The third is a 16.6-kb deletion (-$\alpha^{16.6}$) found in a family of Vietnamese origin (M. Rugless et al., in preparation). The deletion removes the $\psi\zeta$, α^D, $\psi\alpha$1, and α2 genes by non-homologous recombination and the junction is filled with approximately 360 bp of orphan sequence derived from the intron of the ζ or $\psi\zeta$ gene.

Analyzing the hematological indices, globin synthesis ratios, and genetic interactions involving these three deletions ((α)$\alpha^{5.3}$, -$\alpha^{7.9}$, -$\alpha^{16.6}$) it appears that the remaining α1 gene on each of these chromosomes is expressed at normal or near normal levels. This is of interest when considering regulation of the normal cluster because it implies that, other than the α2 gene itself, no other important, *cis*-regulatory elements are removed by these deletions. When all of the data from the α^+ thalassemias are considered alongside the observations from nonthalassemic variants, it appears that large segments of the α-globin cluster (Fig. 13.3 and legend) are not essential for α-globin expression.

Expression from the α^+ Chromosomes

Although the relative expression of mRNA from the α2 and α1 genes on a normal chromosome is approximately 3:1, there are several lines of evidence indicating that the α-gene in the various -α chromosomes behaves like neither α1 nor α2. For example, homozygotes for the -$\alpha^{4.2}$ determinant who essentially have two α1 genes (-$\alpha^{4.2}$/-$\alpha^{4.2}$) appear to express more α-globin than the predicted 25% of normal[95] and homozygotes for -$\alpha^{3.7III}$, with the equivalent of two α2 genes (-$\alpha^{3.7}$/-$\alpha^{3.7}$), express less than the predicted 75% of normal.[95] Direct measurements of α-mRNA levels in patients with the -$\alpha^{3.7}$ determinant also suggest that the remaining α gene is expressed at a level roughly half way between that of a normal α2 and normal α1 gene.[96] Because the transcriptional units of all the recombined genes (-$\alpha^{3.7I}$, -$\alpha^{3.7II}$, -$\alpha^{3.7III}$, -$\alpha^{4.2}$) are virtually identical to either the native α1 or α2 gene, the alteration in expression most likely results from a change in the rate of transcription of the gene. Assuming that this is a *cis* effect, it could be brought about by the new combinations of flanking sequences, a release of transcriptional interference from the upstream gene,[97] or by the change in chromosome conformation as a result of the deletions.

Another possibility (Fig. 13.2) is that the promoters of the α2 and α1 genes normally compete for interaction with the single α-globin regulatory element (MCS-R2, HS-40) in a similar way to which the γ and β genes are thought to compete for the β-globin LCR (see Chapters 4 and 5). In this case a single promoter in the -α chromosome would have unchallenged access to HS-40 and might consequently be expressed more efficiently than when competing with a second ($\alpha\alpha$) or third ($\alpha\alpha\alpha$) promoter. As discussed previously such competition might also help explain the progressively inefficient expression of duplicated genes in the α clusters.

Although there is no a priori reason to anticipate changes in ζ-globin expression in patients with the -α haplotype, it is useful to know that none of the -α mutations is associated with any significant change in ζ-globin expression.[98]

α^0-Thalassemia due to Deletions of the Structural α-Globin Genes

All of the deletions described in this section either completely or partially (e.g., -(α)$^{5.2}$ and -(α)$^{20.5}$) delete both α-globin genes (Figs. 13.5 and 13.6), and therefore no α chain synthesis is directed by these chromosomes in vivo (hence the term α^0 thalassemia). Homozygotes for such chromosomes have the Hb Bart's hydrops fetalis syndrome (see Chapter 14).

Many deletions remove both ζ genes and the α-globin genes (Figs. 13.5 and 13.6). Although heterozygotes for these variants survive and appear to develop normally, homozygotes do not survive even the early stages of gestation because neither embryonic ($\zeta_2\gamma_2$, $\zeta_2\varepsilon_2$, $\alpha_2\varepsilon_2$) nor fetal ($\alpha_2\gamma_2$) hemoglobin (HbF) can be made (see Chapter 7). Some, but not all, heterozygotes for deletions in which the embryonic gene remains intact have continued expression of very small amounts of ζ-globin in both fetal[11] and adult life[99,100] This may be analogous to the persistent γ-globin production documented in patients with similar downstream deletions of the β-complex (see Chapter 16). The amount of ζ-globin present in adults with these types of α thalassemia is considerably less than the level of γ-globin present in individuals with comparable deletions of the

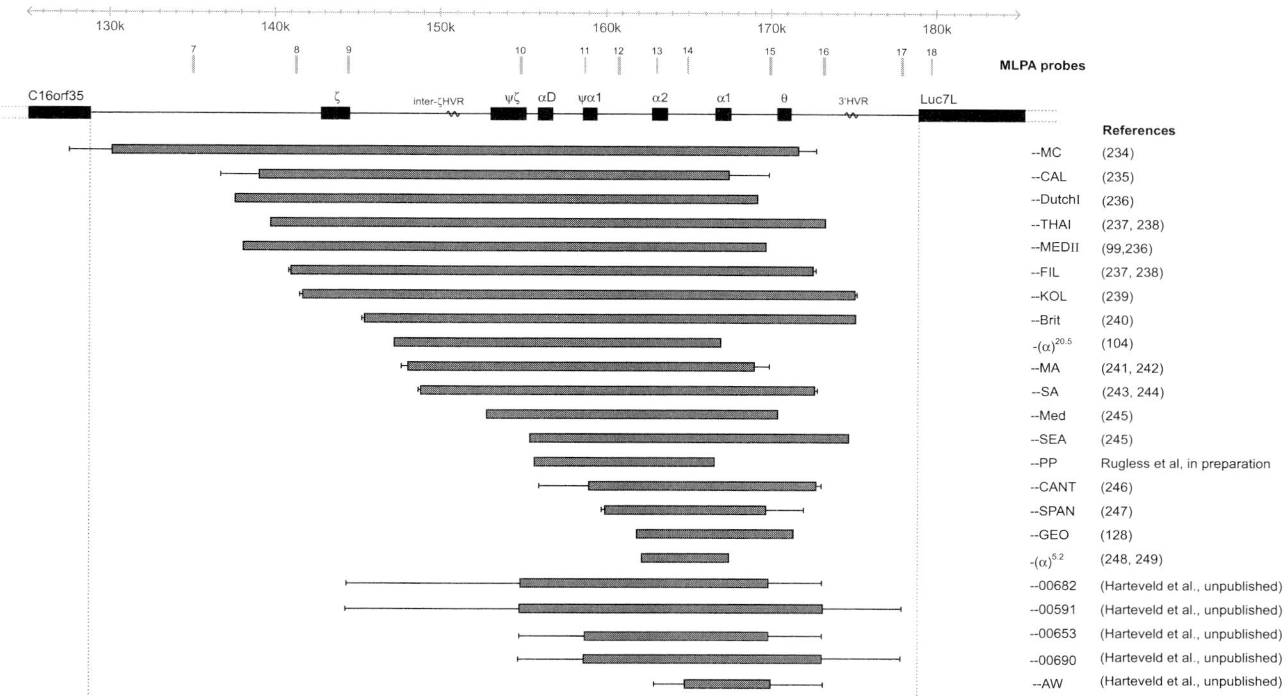

Figure 13.5. Deletions that cause α^0 thalassemia with breakpoints lying within the α-globin cluster. Above, the α-like globin genes are shown (scale in kilobases) and the cluster is delimited by two flanking genes (c16orf35 and Luc7L). The positions of MLPA probes currently used to characterize large deletions from the α-globin cluster[162] are shown. Below, the extent of each deletion is shown by a black bar. Regions of uncertainty for each breakpoint are shown by thin black lines. To the right are the shorthand notations and primary references for the characterization and examples of PCR analysis for each deletion. The --^{BRIT} deletion is probably the same mutation as the rare α^0 thalassemia defect described in a black patient.[164]

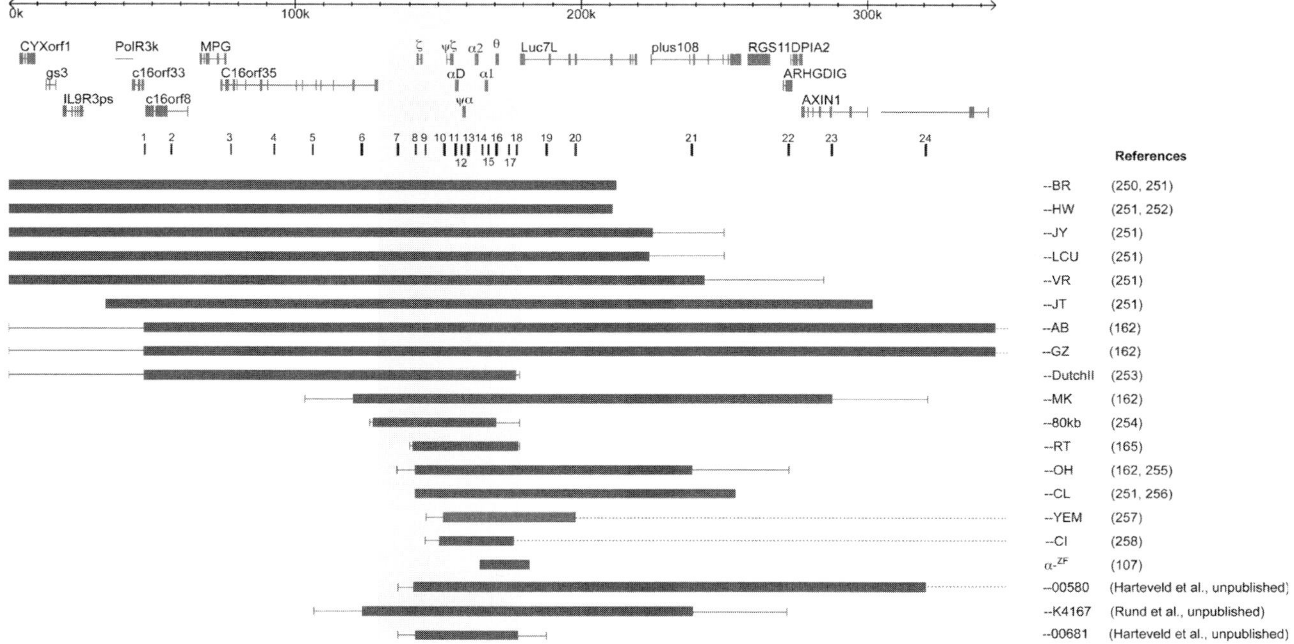

Figure 13.6. Rare, large deletions extending beyond the α cluster that cause α thalassemia but no other associated abnormalities. Above, the terminal 340 kb of chromosome 16p as described in the legend to Figure 13.1 (scale in kilobases). The positions of MLPA probes currently used to characterize large deletions from the α-globin cluster[162] are shown. Below, black bars indicate the extent of each deletion. Regions of uncertainty for the breakpoints are shown by thin black lines. Dashed lines indicate that the 3′ end of two deletions (YEM and CI) has not yet been investigated. To the right, are the shorthand notations and primary references for each deletion.

β-complex. It seems that this increase of embryonic globin expression is not simply due to the increased erythropoiesis because, in one study, no ε- or ζ-globin transcripts were detected in several patients with erythroid hyperplasia.[14]

At the 3′ end of the complex many of these deletions include the θ1-gene whose function is unknown. In individuals, homozygous for --^{SEA}, who have been treated with blood transfusion, both θ1-genes are deleted and yet these children may develop normally despite the complete absence of θ-gene expression (Chapter 14).[101]

With completion of the DNA sequence of 16p13.3[102] and beyond[103] it has been possible to define the full extent of many of the α globin deletions. They can be grouped into those that lie entirely within the α globin cluster (Fig. 13.5) and deletions that extend beyond the α-cluster to include the flanking genes (Fig. 13.6). Although these deletions remove other genes, affected heterozygotes appear phenotypically normal, apart from their α thalassemia; in some patients α thalassemia trait (--/αα) and in others HbH disease (--/-α). In patients with more extensive deletions with monosomy for a large segment of 16p13.3, α thalassemia is associated with developmental abnormalities and mental retardation (see Chapter 15). It is interesting to note that all of the α^0 thalassemia deletions that occur at polymorphic frequencies in human populations are limited to the α-cluster and do not extend into the surrounding genes suggesting that deletion of these genes (even in heterozygotes) may result in a selective disadvantage.

Detailed analysis of several determinants of α^0 thalassemia indicates that they often result from illegitimate or nonhomologous recombination events.[104] Such events may involve short regions of partial sequence homology at the breakpoints of the molecules that are rejoined but they do not involve the extensive sequence matching required for homologous recombination as described in the previous section.

Sequence analysis has shown that members of the dispersed family of Alu repeats are frequently found at or near the breakpoints of these deletions. Alu family repeats occur frequently in the genome (3×10^5 copies) and seem to be particularly common in and around the α-globin cluster where they make up approximately 25% of the entire sequence.[69] These repeats may simply provide partially homologous sequences that promote DNA strand exchanges during replication, or possibly a subset of Alu sequences may be more actively involved in the process. Detailed sequence analysis of the junctions of the α-globin deletions has revealed a number of interesting features including palindromes, direct repeats, regions of weak homology and frequent occurrence of the motif GAGG. Some deletions (e.g., --^{MED}) involve more complex rearrangements that introduce new pieces of DNA bridging the two breakpoints of the deletion. In the --^{MED} deletion this inserted DNA originates from upstream of the α-cluster and appears to have been incorporated into the junction in a manner that suggests that the upstream segment lies close to the breakpoint regions during replication.[104] Orphan sequences from unknown regions of the genome are frequently found bridging the sequence breakpoints of other α^0 thalassemia deletions.

At least two of the deletions (--^{HW} and --^{BR}, Fig. 13.6) result from chromosomal breaks in the 16p telomeric region that have been "healed" by the direct addition of telomeric repeats $(TTAGGG)_n$. This mechanism is described in further detail later.

α^0 THALASSEMIA DUE TO A DELETION OF THE α2-GLOBIN GENE THAT ALSO INACTIVATES THE α1-GLOBIN PROMOTER

We have recently characterized a deletion of approximately 11 kb (called --^{PP}) in a single patient with the phenotype of severe α thalassemia trait (Hb 12.3 g/dL, MCV 71 fL, MCH 21.7 pg and rare HbH inclusions). This deletion (Fig. 13.5) completely removes the α2 gene and the 3′ breakpoint lies within the promoter of the linked α1 gene that is otherwise intact. The phenotype of the patient combined with detailed biochemical analyses (M. Rugless et al., in preparation) has shown that the α1 gene *in cis* is inactivated by this mutation so that there is no α-globin synthesis directed by this chromosome (hence α^0 thalassemia).

α^0 THALASSEMIA DUE TO A DELETION OF THE α1-GLOBIN GENE THAT ALSO INACTIVATES THE α2-GLOBIN GENE

During a study to identify thalassemia in families from the Czech Republic, Indrak et al.[105] reported a novel deletion (>18 kb) involving the α1 and θ gene, α-^{ZF} (Fig. 13.6). Heterozygotes for this deletion have a mild hypochromic microcytic anemia (Hb 12.6 g/dL, MCH 22 pg, MCV 68 fL) with a reduced α/β-globin chain biosynthesis ratio (0.62–0.66) and HbH inclusions. These findings suggested that although the α2 gene appeared to be intact it had been inactivated by the novel deletion.

Barbour et al.[106] and Tufarelli et al.[107] further characterized this mutation and showed that the deletion juxtaposes a downstream gene (Luc7L) next to the structurally normal α2-globin gene. Although this α2 gene retains all of its local (e.g., promoter) and remote (e.g., MCS-R2 or HS-40) *cis*-acting elements, its expression is silenced and its associated CpG island (see Fig. 13.1) becomes completely methylated during early development and the chromatin associated with the promoter remains inactive and inaccessible, even in erythroid cells. From the analysis of experimental models recapitulating this deletion and from further characterization of the affected individual,[107] it was shown that transcription of antisense mRNA from Luc7L, through the α2-globin gene was responsible for methylation of the associated CpG island and silencing of α-globin expression. The mutation is not only important for understanding the molecular basis for this rare form of thalassemia but also

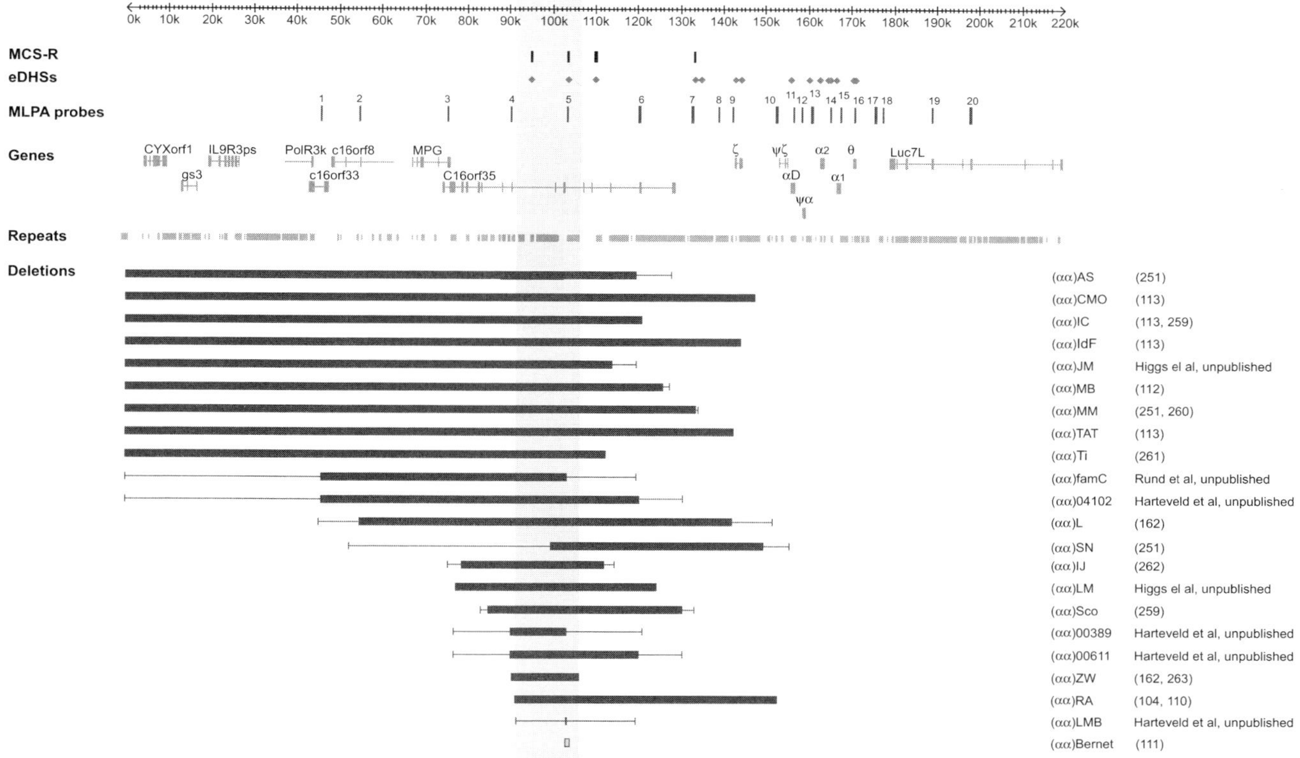

Figure 13.7. Deletions extending upstream of the α-cluster that cause α thalassemia by removing the α-globin regulatory element (HS-40) and a variable amount of flanking DNA. Above, the α-cluster (scale in kilobases) showing the α-like genes, the flanking genes, MLPA probes[162] together with the erythroid-specific DHS and positions of conserved regulatory sequences (MCS-R). The extent of each deletion is indicated by black bars and the uncertainty of breakpoints is shown by thin black lines. The stippled box represents the shortest region of overlap between all deletions, including HS-40 (MCS-R2) and HS-48 (MCS-R1). Primary references and shorthand notations are shown on the right.

illustrated a new mechanism underlying human genetic disease.

α THALASSEMIA DUE TO DELETIONS OF THE α-GLOBIN REGULATORY ELEMENT

As discussed previously, expression of the α genes is critically dependent on a multispecies conserved, noncoding regulatory sequence (MCS-R) that lies 40 kb upstream of the ζ2-globin gene.[2] This region (called MCS-R2[1]) is associated with an erythroid-specific DNase I hypersensitive site, referred to as HS-40. Detailed analysis of MCS-R2 has shown that it contains multiple binding sites for the erythroid-restricted *trans*-acting factors GATA-1 and NF-E2.[1,108,109] The role(s) of other upstream MCS elements (MCS-R1, R3, and R4) are not yet clear (see introduction).

The first indication that remote regulatory sequences might exist came from observations on a patient with α thalassemia.[110] Analysis of the abnormal chromosome $(\alpha\alpha)^{RA}$ from this patient demonstrated a 62-kb deletion from upstream of the α-complex (Fig. 13.7), which includes HS-40. Although both α genes on this chromosome are intact and entirely normal they appear to be nonfunctional. Since this original observation, 20 more patients with α thalassemia due to a deletion of HS-40 and a variable amount of the flanking DNA have been described (see Fig. 13.7). An approximately 15-kb segment of DNA containing both MCS-R1 (HS-48) and MCS-R2 (HS-40) is deleted in all of these chromosomes, and all of these mutations give rise to the phenotype associated with α^0 thalassemia: some patients have the severe form of α thalassemia trait αα/(αα), others have HbH disease -α/(αα).

Interspecific hybrids each containing an abnormal copy of chromosome 16 from such patients have been made by fusing EBV cell lines with mouse erythroleukemia cells (MEL). In contrast to normal copies of chromosome 16, the abnormal chromosomes produce severely reduced (often $<1\%$ of normal) levels of human α-globin mRNA, indicating that these deletions severely downregulate expression of the α genes and are responsible for the associated α thalassemia. A specific knockout of MCS-R2 (HS-40) alone[111] from such a chromosome (Fig. 13.7) together with many experiments in transgenic mice[3] strongly suggests that MCS-R2 is the major active element deleted by these arrangements. More recently this observation was further strengthened by showing that removal of just MCS-R2 from a mouse model which recapitulates human α globin expression (see introduction and humanized mouse in Fig. 13.1) severely reduces α-globin expression.[27]

The mechanisms by which these natural mutations have arisen are quite diverse. In the $(\alpha\alpha)^{RA}$ chromosome the deletion resulted from a recombination event between partially homologous Alu repeats that are normally 62 kb apart.[110] In the $(\alpha\alpha)^{MB}$ chromosome[112] the deletion arose via a subtelomeric rearrangement. The chromosomal breakpoint was found in an Alu element located approximately 105 kb from the 16p subtelomeric region. The broken chromosome was stabilized with a new telomere acquired by recombination between this Alu element and a subtelomeric Alu repeat associated with the newly acquired chromosome end. In at least five cases $(\alpha\alpha)^{CMO}$, $(\alpha\alpha)^{IdF}$, $(\alpha\alpha)^{TAT}$, $(\alpha\alpha)^{IC}$ and $(\alpha\alpha)^{TI}$ the chromosomes appear to have been broken and then stabilized by the direct addition of telomeric repeats to nontelomeric DNA.[113] Sequence analysis suggests that these chromosomes are "healed" via the action of telomerase, an enzyme that is normally involved in maintaining the integrity of telomeres.[113,114]

In the remaining cases the mechanism has not yet been established. It is interesting that some (e.g., $(\alpha\alpha)^{IJ}$, $(\alpha\alpha)^{Sco}$), but not all, of these mutations appear to have arisen *de novo* because neither parent has the abnormal chromosome.

NONDELETION TYPES OF α THALASSEMIA

In all surveys reported so far, α thalassemia is much more frequently due to deletions, as described in previous sections, than single point mutations or oligonucleotide insertions and deletions involving the canonical sequences that control gene expression (so called nondeletion variants, in which the affected gene is denoted α^T). This is in contrast to the situation in β thalassemia in which point mutations affecting almost every stage of gene expression are known (see Chapter 16) and deletions are less frequent.

Nondeletion types of α thalassemia were first described in 1977[115] and shown to result from a variety of mechanisms.[116] At present we know of 69 well-defined causes of nondeletion α thalassemia (Table 13.2). Forty-six of these occur in the α2 gene ($\alpha^T\alpha$), 17 in the α1 gene ($\alpha\alpha^T$) and 5 occur on a -α chromosome ($-\alpha^T$). In 1 case the mutation has not yet been assigned to the α1 or α2 gene.

As a group, the nondeletion α thalassemia determinants ($\alpha^T\alpha$ and $\alpha\alpha^T$) appear to have a more severe effect on α globin expression and hematological phenotype than simple deletions that remove one or other of the α genes (-α) (see Chapter 14). This may be explained by the majority of mutations affecting the α2 gene, whose expression may predominate over the α1 gene (see previous section); this may also lead to a bias in ascertainment. In addition, unlike when one α gene is deleted (see previous section), there appears to be no compensatory increase in expression of the remaining functional α gene when the other is inactivated by a point mutation. Furthermore, some highly unstable variants may have multiple secondary effects on red cell interactions that produce a more severe phenotype than predicted from the anticipated decrease in α gene expression. At present these general assertions are based on a relatively small number of observations and further evaluation of the pathophysiology of each mutation will be needed in the future.

Mutants that Affect RNA Splicing

Eight nondeletion α thalassemia variants affect RNA splicing. With one exception ($\alpha^{Cd22;C\rightarrow T}\alpha$, see below) they all involve either the donor (GT) or acceptor (AG) consensus splice sites of either IVSI or IVSII. Four affect the dominant α2 globin gene and three mutate the α1 gene (Table 17.2). In general, it is now clear that mutations affecting the consensus donor (GT) and acceptor (AG) splice sites severely down regulate expression of the associated gene. The principles are illustrated by one of the first nondeletion determinants described. This splicing mutation ($\alpha^{IVSI;\ del5bp}\alpha$) results from a pentanucleotide deletion at the 5′ donor site of IVS 1 of the α2-globin gene. This affects the invariant GT sequence and eliminates splicing from the normal donor site while activating a cryptic donor consensus that lies in exon l. Aberrantly spliced mRNA was detected in a transient expression system and in bone marrow from an affected patient. By contrast, in peripheral blood very little if any mRNA from the mutated α2 gene was detected, suggesting that the aberrantly spliced RNA is unstable.[19,117] Very often in these types of mutation any aberrantly spliced mRNA transcripts are not only unstable but they also alter the translational frame so that an abnormal truncated protein is produced as seen in the mutation of the acceptor site of IVS1 of the α2 gene ($\alpha^{IIVS1-116A\rightarrow G}\alpha$) described by Harteveld et al.[118]

A different type of splicing defect ($\alpha^{Cd22;C\rightarrow T}\alpha$) was observed in patient of Surinamese–Hindustani origin. Sequence analysis revealed a silent mutation at codon 22 of the α2 globin gene that creates a splice donor consensus. Abnormally spliced mRNA leads to a premature termination between codons 48 and 49 and probably nonsense mediated decay of the abnormal RNA product. The only patient described with this mutation had a moderate hypochromic microcytic anemia.[119]

Of these eight splicing mutations, five affect the dominant α2-globin gene and three mutate the α1 gene. Many but not all of the heterozygotes for these mutations ($\alpha^T\alpha/\alpha\alpha$ and $\alpha\alpha^T/\alpha\alpha$) have readily detectable changes in their red cell indices. Furthermore, where documented, these alleles most frequently interact with α^0 thalassemia to produce HbH disease (e.g. $--/\alpha^T\alpha$ and $--/\alpha\alpha^T$).[120,121]

Mutations Affecting the Poly(A) Addition Signal

The highly conserved sequence motif AATAAA is present 10–30 bp upstream of most poly(A) addition sites and forms

Table 13.2. Summary of nondeletional mutations that cause α thalassemia*

Affected sequence	Affected gene	Mutation(s)	Distribution	Phenotype	Reference
		mRNA Processing			
Cryptic splicing	α2	Cd22; C→T	Surinamese	α^+	119
IVS (donor)	α2	IVS I; del 5bp	Mediterranean	α^+	117
	α1	IVS I; (G→A)	Thai	α	120
	α2	IVS II; 2(T→A)	North European	α^+ - α^0	185
IVS (acceptor)	α2	IVS I; 116 (A→G)	Dutch	α^+	118
	α1	IVS I; 117 (G→A)	Asian Indian	α^+	187
	α2	IVS II; 142 (G→A)	Argentinian	α^+ - α^0	121
	α1	IVS II; 148 (A→G)	Iranian	α^+	140
Poly A signal	α2	PA; del 16bp	Arab	α^+ - α^0	127
	α2	PA6; A→G	Middle east Mediterranean	α^+ - α^0	126, 188
	α2	PA4; A→G	Mediterranean Chinese	α^+ - α^0	129, 189
	α2	PA; del 2bp	Asian Indian Thai	α^+ - α^0	130, 190, 191
		mRNA Translation			
Initiation codon	$-\alpha^{3.7}$	IN; ATG→GTG	African	α^0	132
	$-\alpha^{3.7II}$	IN; del 2bp	North African Mediterranean	α^+ - α^0	133, 134, 192
	α2	IN; ATG→ACG	Mediterranean	α^+	193
	α2	IN; ATG→A-G	Vietnam	α^+	194
	α1	IN; ATG→GTG	Mediterranean	α^+	138, 195
	α2	IN; ATG→-TG	Southeast Asian		139
Exon I	α1	cd 14; G→A	Iranian	α^0	140
	α2	cd 19; del G	Iranian	α^+	140
	α2	Cd22; del C	African		145
	α2	Cd 23; G→T	Tunisian	α^0	142
	-α	Cd 30/31; del 2bp	African	α^0	147
Exon II	α2	Cd 39/41; del/ins	Yemenite-Jewish	α^+	196
	α1	Cd51–55; del 13bp	Spanish	α^+	148
	α1	Cd62; del G	African		144
	α1	Cd 78; del C	Black/Chinese		139
	α2	Cd 90; A→T	Middle Eastern	α^+	143
Exon III	α1	Cd108; delC	Jewish	α^+ - α^0	197
	α2	Cd113/114; delC	Unknown		139
	α2	Cd 113–1 16; del 12 bp (Leida)	Spanish	α^+ - α^0	149
	α2	Cd116; G→T	African	α^+	141
	α1	Cd131; ins T (Pak Num Po)	Thai	α^0	146
Termination codon	α2	TER; TAA→CAA (Constant Spring)	Southeast Asian	α^+	198
	α2	TER; TAA→AAA (Icaria)	Mediterranean	α^+	199, 200
	α2	TER; TAA→TCA (Koya Dora)	Indian	α^+	201
	α2	TER;TAA→GAA (Seal Rock)	African	α^+	202, 203
	α2	TER; TAA→TAT (Paksé)	Laotian Thai	α^+	204, 205
		Posttranslational			
Exon I	-α	Cd 14;T→G (Evanston)	African	α^+	166
	α2	Cd21; G→T (Zoetermeer)	Dutch	α^+	206
	α2	Cd29; T→C (Agrinio)	Mediterranean	α^+	207
	α2	Cd30; 3bpdel (del Q)	Chinese	α^+ - α^0	160
	α2	Cd 31; G→A (R-L)	Chinese	α^+ - α^0	208
Exon II	α2	Cd 32; G→A (Amsterdam, M-I)	Surinamese-Black	α^+ - α^0	209
	α2	Cd 35; T→C (Evora, S-P)	Filipino Portuguese	α^+ - α^0	210, 211
	α2	Cd 35; T→C (Chartres, F-S)	French	α^+	212
	α1	Cd 37; del 3bp (Heraklion, del P)	Greece	α^+ - α^0	213
	α2	Cd 59; G→A (Adana, G-D)	Chinese	α^+ - α^0	160
	α1	Cd 60/61; del 3bp (Clinic, del K)	Spanish	α^+ - α^0	214
	α1	Cd 62; del 3bp (Aghia Sophia, del V)	Greece	α^0	215
	α1	Cd 64–74; del 33bp	Greece	α^0	216
	α2	Cd 66; T→C (Dartmouth, L-P)	Caucasian	α^+ - α^0	217
	α2	Cd 93; T→G (Bronte, V-G)	Italian	α^+	218
	α1	Cd 93–99; dupl 22bp	Iranian	α^+ - α^0	216

(continued)

Table 13.2 *(continued)*

Affected sequence	Affected gene	Mutation(s)	Distribution	Phenotype	Reference
Exon III	α2	Cd103; A→T (Hb Bronovo, H-L)	Turkish	α^+	219
	α2	Cd104; G→A (Sallanches, C-Y)	French Pakistanis	α^+	220, 221
	α1	Cd104; T→A (Hb Oegstgeest, C-S)	Surinamese	α^+	222
	α2	Cd108; C→A (Hb Bleuland, T-N)	Surinamese	α^+	223
	α2	Cd109; T→G (Suan Dok, L-R)	Thai	α^+	224
	α	Cd110; C→A (Petah Tikva, A-D)	Middle east	α^+	225
	α1	Cd119; C→T (Groene Hart or Bemalda P)	Moroccan	α^+	226, 227
	α2	Cd 125; T→C (Quong Sze, L-P)	Chinese	α^+	228
	$-\alpha^{3.7}$	Cd125; T→A (L-G)	Jewish	α^0	197
	α1	Cd129; T→C (Tunis-Bizerte, L- P)	Tunisian	α^+	229
	α2	Cd 129; T→C (Utrecht, L-P)	Dutch	a	186
	α2	Cd 130; G→C (Sun Prairie, A-P)	Asian Indian	α^+	230
	α2	Cd131; T→C (Questembert, S-W)	French Yugoslavian	α^+	231
	α2	Cd132; T→G (Caen, V-G)	Caucasian	α^+	232
	α2	Cd 136; T→C (Bibba, L-P)	Caucasian	α^+	233

del; deletion, ins; insertion, dupl; duplication, Cd; codon, PA; poly(A) signal, UTR; untranslated region.

part of the signal for mRNA cleavage and polyadenylation of primary transcripts (see Chapter 3). This sequence is required for transcriptional termination and some evidence suggests that, when mutated, transcription may proceed into neighboring genes and "interfere" with their expression.[122]

At present there are four known mutations of the α2 gene polyadenylation signal (Table 13.2). The first to be identified (AATAAA → AATAAG) was found in the Saudi Arabian population. Heterozygotes have the hematological phenotype of severe carriers of α thalassemia trait but homozygotes have HbH disease.[123] The mechanisms by which this mutation causes such a severe phenotype are not fully understood.

Homozygotes for other nondeletion mutations that inactivate the α2 gene do not always have HbH disease and when present it is often mild with low levels of HbH (see later). By contrast homozygotes for the $\alpha^{PA6:A\rightarrow G}\alpha$ haplotype always have HbH disease with relatively high levels of HbH. It is interesting that in these individuals α2 mRNA is reduced but not absent and therefore, if the α1 gene were fully active, one would expect to see a severe form of α thalassemia trait rather than HbH disease. The implication of these findings is that the poly(A) site mutation down regulates both α2 and α1 genes on the same chromosome. In some rare individuals, the $\alpha^{PA6:A\rightarrow G}$ α mutation is duplicated producing a chromosome with three α genes $\alpha^{PA6:A\rightarrow G}\alpha^{PA6:A\rightarrow G}\alpha$ that still interacts with the $\alpha^{PA6:A\rightarrow G}\alpha$ chromosome to produce HbH disease.[82]

Analysis of the $\alpha^{PA6:A\rightarrow G}$ mutation has shown that it has at least two effects. It reduces the amount of α2 mRNA that accumulates and, in a transient assay, readthrough transcripts extending beyond the mutated poly(A) addition site are detected. Extended transcripts were also detected in reticulocytes of patients with this defect using reverse transcription (RT) –PCR.[124] It seems possible that transcription extending through the normal termination point could run on and interfere with expression of the linked α1 gene. Given the reduction in α chain synthesis associated with the $\alpha^{PA6:A\rightarrow G}\alpha$ haplotype one would predict that compound heterozygotes for this mutation and a common α^0 thalassemia determinant should be severely affected. Although this is not always the case in two families, compound heterozygotes ($--^{MED}/\alpha^{PA6:A\rightarrow G}\alpha$) had severe HbH disease with hydrops fetalis.[125,126]

Since the original description of the $\alpha^{PA6:A\rightarrow G}$ allele, three other poly(A) signal mutations have been described (Table 13.2), including one that results from a 16bp deletion removing sequences from the 3′ untranslated mRNA and the first base of the PolyA site.[127]

At present there are insufficient data to know whether these more recently described mutations down regulate α gene expression in a similar way to the $\alpha^{PA6:A\rightarrow G}\alpha$ allele. Compound heterozygotes for these mutations and α^0 thalassemia have HbH disease as expected[128,129] (unpublished) and homozygotes for the $\alpha^{PA4:A\rightarrow G}\alpha$ or $\alpha^{PA4;del2bp}\alpha$ alleles have HbH disease.[130] Homozygotes for the $\alpha^{PA;del2bp}\alpha$ allele may have severe HbH disease with hydrops fetalis.[131]

Mutations Affecting Initiation of mRNA Translation

Several nondeletion mutations affect mRNA translation and six of them disrupt the initiation consensus sequence CCRCCATG (Table 13.2). Two mutations occur on chromosomes with a single α gene. In one ($-\alpha^{IN;ATG\rightarrow GTG}$) the mutation abolishes translation of mRNA from the gene. It was identified via its interaction with a second α thalassemia chromosome ($-\alpha^{IN;ATG\rightarrow GTG}/-\alpha$); affected patients had the typical hematological features of HbH disease with 2.4 and 7.2% HbH.[132] In another case ($-\alpha^{IN;del2bp}$) a 2-bp deletion from the consensus sequence reduces the level of mRNA translation by 30%–50%.[133,134] This mutation produces HbH disease in homozygotes ($-\alpha^{IN;del2bp}/-\alpha^{IN;del2bp}$) who have a mild hypochromic microcytic anemia (Hb 9.7–9.9, MCV 63, MCH 18–20) with 4.5%–5.6% HbH.[135]

Two mutations ($\alpha^{IN;ATG\rightarrow ACG}\alpha$ and $\alpha^{IN:ATG\rightarrow A\text{-}G}\alpha$) abolish translation of mRNA from the α2 gene. Six of seven homozygotes for the $\alpha^{IN;T\rightarrow C}\alpha$ haplotype have a severe form of α thalassemia trait but one had a mild form of HbH disease with 2.6% HbH[136,137] (unpublished). Compound heterozygotes for this mutation with common α^0 thalassemia defects have HbH disease with substantial amounts of HbH (~8%–24%) in the peripheral blood.

One mutation $\alpha\alpha^{IN;ATG\rightarrow GTG}$ abolishes translation of mRNA from the α1 globin gene.[138] In the single family reported with this mutation compound heterozygotes ($--/\alpha\alpha^{IN;ATG\rightarrow GTG}$) had relatively low levels of HbH (1.5% and 3%) suggesting that mutation of the α1 gene causes a less severe degree of α chain deficit than a similar mutation of the α2 gene. This mutation adds weight to the argument that the α2 gene is expressed at a higher level than the α1 gene.

Finally, Eng et al.[139] reported a single nucleotide deletion from the initiation codon ($\alpha^{IN;\ ATG\rightarrow TG}\alpha$) in a newborn infant who also carried the $--^{SEA}$ mutation. More than 25% Hb Bart's was present at birth, consistent with HbH disease.

Inframe Deletions, Frameshifts, and Nonsense Mutations

Inframe deletions, insertions and nonsense mutations all affect the frame of translation and either cause premature termination of translation (with or without nonsense-mediated decay of the mRNA) or lead to the production of an abnormal protein, which is often unstable.

Four of the mutations described in this section result simply from single base changes in a coding triplet creating a premature stop codon thereby causing premature termination of translation.[140–143] Seven result from single base insertions and deletions that alter the triplet code and give rise to premature termination or the production of an abnormal α-globin.[139,140,144–146] Although some of these may be a relatively frequent cause of α thalassemia in some populations (e.g., $\alpha^{cd19;delG}\alpha$ in Iran), most are rare mutations which either cause α thalassemia trait ($\alpha\alpha^T/\alpha\alpha$ or $\alpha^T\alpha/\alpha\alpha$) or interact with α^0 thalassemia to produce HbH disease ($--/\alpha\alpha^T$ or $--/\alpha^T\alpha$), which in some cases can be clinically severe.

Other mutations are more complex. In 1988 Safaya and Rieder[147] described a Black American with HbH disease and HbG Philadelphia who synthesized only α^G and no α^A chains. The patient was shown to have the genotype $-\alpha/-\alpha^G$ and they therefore concluded that the -α chromosome was inactivated by a further mutation. Sequence analysis showed that this single α gene has a dinucleotide deletion from one or other of the Glu (GAG) or Arg (AGG) codons (30 and 31). The loss of two nucleotides leads to a frameshift and a novel protein sequence in exon II from codons 31–54 followed by a new, in-phase termination codon (TAA) at position 55. Hence the $-\alpha^{cd30/31;del2bp}$ haplotype is an inactive α^0 thalassemia determinant.

A single Spanish family with a frameshift mutation in the α1-globin gene has been described by Ayala et al.[148] Two affected individuals ($\alpha\alpha^{cd51-55;13bpdel}/\alpha\alpha$) have α thalassemia trait. Direct sequence analysis of the α1 gene revealed a 13-bp deletion, between codons 51 and 55. This mutation results in a mRNA reading frameshift that introduces a new stop signal at codon 62.

In another patient a 12-bp deletion of the α2 gene results in the loss of four amino acids (codons 113–116) from the α-chain, which is reduced from its normal length of 141 amino acids to 137. It is thought that this produces an unstable α chain which is rapidly broken down and unable to form a Hb tetramer, like some mutants described later. In a heterozygote this mutation produced the phenotype of α thalassemia trait (Hb Lleida,[149]).

All of these complex rearrangements appear to be relatively uncommon and have been observed sporadically in families with α thalassemia trait and HbH disease.

Chain Termination Mutants

There are potentially nine single nucleotide variants of the natural termination codon (TAA) of the α2-globin gene. Two (TGA and TAG) encode stop (nonsense) mutations; the others encode amino acids.[150] When mutations change the stop codon to one of these amino acids they allow mRNA translation to continue to the next in-phase termination codon (UAA) located within the polyadenylation signal (AAUAAA); in each case extending the α-chain by 31 amino acids from the natural C-terminal arginine (codon 141). Of the six predicted α2 variants, five have been described, each with a unique amino acid at α142. These are Hb Constant Spring (α142 Gin), Hb Icaria (α142 Lys), Hb Koya Dora (α142 Ser), Hb Seal Rock (α142 Glu), and Hb Paksé (α142 Tyr) (Table 17.2). An extended α-globin variant with leucine at position 142 is predicted but has not yet been described.

The mechanism by which chain termination mutants cause α thalassemia has been difficult to elucidate although there are now sufficient observations to provide a plausible explanation. Nevertheless, we still do not fully understand how the unusual hematological phenotype associated with these mutations arises. Heterozygotes clearly have α thalassemia, but the MCV is higher than normally seen (for examples see refs. 150, 151). Homozygotes for the HbCS mutation have an unexpectedly severe form of thalassemia considering that only two of the four α genes are inactive[152,153] and compound heterozygotes for HbCS and an α^0 thalassemia determinant have an unusually severe form of HbH disease (for example see refs. 154, 155 and see Chapter 14).

HbCS is the most extensively studied of this group. Heterozygotes for this mutation $\alpha^{TER;TAA\rightarrow CAA}\alpha/\alpha\alpha$ have approximately 1% Hb-CS in their red cells rather than the approximately 25% usually found in carriers of α-chain variants.[150] It seems likely that the α2 gene affected by this mutation is transcribed normally, although this has not been formally demonstrated. Substantial amounts of the abnormal α^{CS} mRNA are found in erythroid precursors from the bone marrow but the level decreases during erythroid maturation and is virtually absent from reticulocytes.[18,156] The synthesis of α^{CS}-globin chains follows the same pattern, decreasing from bone marrow to reticulocytes.[150,157] From these findings it was suggested that α^{CS} mRNA is unstable, possibly due to disruption of a sequence(s) in the 3′ noncoding region that is translated inappropriately as a result of the chain termination mutant.[156] Subsequent experimental data support this interpretation. Weiss and Liebhaber[158] showed that translational readthrough disrupts an RNA–protein complex associated with the α2-globin 3′ UTR which is required for mRNA stability in erythroid cells (summarized in introduction and in ref. 17).

Unstable β-Chain Variants Associated with α Thalassemia

It is well established that some globin variants alter the tertiary structure of the hemoglobin molecule making the dimer (αβ) or tetramer ($\alpha_2\beta_2$) unstable. Such molecules may precipitate within the red cell forming insoluble inclusions (Heinz bodies) which damage the red cell membrane. This situation classically causes a chronic hemolytic anemia with equal loss of α- and β-like globin chains from the red cell (see Chapter 24).

Over the past few years it has become apparent that some α globin variants are so unstable that they undergo very rapid, postsynthetic degradation. In this case, because the α chains probably do not form dimers or tetramers, there is no associated loss of normal β chains which remain, in excess, within the red cell: Such patients, by definition, have α thalassemia. Many of these α globin variants are so unstable, that they cannot be detected by conventional protein analysis. Therefore affected patients often present with nondeletional α thalassemia that can only be explained when the mutation is identified by DNA sequence analysis.

The hematological findings in this group of patients are complex because the defects may involve the α1 or α2 gene, may cause different degrees of instability and may be greatly influenced by interacting alleles. For example, some mutants may be fully or temporarily stabilized when incorporated into a dimer or tetramer; the coinheritance of α thalassemia will reduce the normal pool of free α chains and drive abnormal α chains into dimers or tetramers. In this case, subsequent instability may cause loss of both α-like and β-like chains changing the pathophysiology from α thalassemia to a hemolytic anemia. This is discussed further in Chapter 16. The simplest way to look at the effect of these mutations is to consider simple heterozygotes. They usually have the phenotype of α thalassemia trait with low or undetectable amounts of the α-globin variant.

To date, 31 unstable α variants have been shown to produce this phenotype to a greater or lesser extent (Table 17.2). The mutations most frequently affect the heme pocket, internal hydrophobic regions of the molecule that normally maintain its conformation or hydrophobic residues involved in the formation of α1 β1 contacts.

α THALASSEMIA CAUSED BY A MUTATION THAT CREATES A NEW TRANSCRIPTIONAL PROMOTER

α Thalassemia is common throughout Melanesia and is frequently caused by the known $-\alpha^{3.7}$ and $-\alpha^{4.2}$ mutations. It is also documented that in some Melanesian patients (from Papua New Guinea and Vanuatu) with α thalassemia (α thalassemia trait and HbH disease) the α-globin genes are intact,[51] suggesting a nondeletional form of α thalassemia ($\alpha^T\alpha/\alpha\alpha$ or $\alpha^T\alpha/\alpha^T\alpha$). In these patients detailed mapping and DNA sequence analysis of the α genes and all of the upstream MCS elements was normal and yet further studies showed that this form of α thalassemia is linked to the α-globin cluster at 16p13.3.[159] To identify the mutation responsible for this unusual form of α thalassemia, De Gobbi et al.[159] cloned this region from an affected homozygote and resequenced approximately 213 kb of DNA containing and flanking the α-globin cluster, identifying 283 SNPs. The SNP responsible for the mutation was identified when the SNPs were aligned with a tiled microarray analyzed using labeled RNA from the patient's erythroid cells. This revealed a new peak of mRNA expression (located between the ζ and ψζ genes) that coincides with a SNP that creates a GATA-1 binding site. In association studies this SNP is always linked to the phenotype of α thalassemia. Like the MCS elements, this new GATA site binds erythroid transcription factors *in vivo* and becomes activated in erythroid cells. Since the first report of this SNP, we have subsequently identified a second family in which a compound heterozygote for this mutation and the codon 59 mutation described by Chan et al.[160] has HbH disease (Iswari et al., personal communication, 2006).

Why should creating a new promoter-like sequence between the α genes and their regulatory elements cause α thalassemia? Perhaps the most likely explanation is that, because it lies closer to the MCS elements, this new promoter "steals" the activity of the upstream regulatory elements away from the natural α-globin promoters, and down regulates their expression. The details of this mechanism are currently under investigation.

MOLECULAR DIAGNOSIS OF α THALASSEMIA

Patients with well-defined phenotypes of α thalassemia (Chapter 14) have inherited one or more of the determinants described in this chapter. Most common deletional forms of α thalassemia can be diagnosed by analyzing both α globin–specific *Bam*H1 fragments and ζ globin–specific *Bgl*II fragments using conventional Southern blot analyses.[161] When both the α and ζ globin genes have been deleted (e.g., --^{FIL}, --^{THAI}; Fig. 13.5), breakpoints can only be identified using probes located outside of the α-complex. Over the past few years an increasing number of large deletions extending beyond the α globin cluster have been identified. The use of multiplex ligation-dependent probe amplification (MLPA) analysis[162] has enabled all of the common and rare deletions to be detected and this currently represents the most efficient way to screen for such deletions of the α-globin cluster in an unbiased way.

In addition, many PCR based analyses have been developed to diagnose the common forms of α^+ and α^0 thalassemia in single and multiplex assays (summarized in ref. 163). Now that the entire sequence of the human α globin cluster is available[69,102,103] it is a simple matter to design primers to amplify any of the currently known α globin deletions that have been described. One should bear in mind, however, that although PCR-based assays will identify the deletions for which they are designed they will not identify unexpected mutations that can often be suspected and confirmed by Southern blot and MLPA analysis.

It is more difficult to screen for the nondeletional forms of α thalassemia. Because the α1 and α2 genes can be amplified independently, those that cause a restriction site change can be readily identified. In the remaining cases for which one strongly suspects a nondeletion mutation the simplest procedure is to screen by DNA sequence analysis (Chapter 28).

CONCLUSIONS

This chapter has reviewed all of the natural sequence and structural variants that have been observed in and around the human α-globin gene cluster. These mutations have been of great value in pointing to regions of the chromosome that are important in the regulation of α-globin gene expression. Equally, some have ruled out other segments of the cluster as being important in this respect. From a clinical and hematological point of view it is important to remember that the mutations that cause α thalassemia are among the most frequently encountered human genetic abnormalities and in some areas of the world give rise to severe genetic diseases. The careful definition of these mutants has therefore underpinned the development of logical and comprehensive screening programs (see Chapters 26 and 28) to prevent the most severe forms of α thalassemia.

REFERENCES

1. Hughes JR, Cheng JF, Ventress N, et al. Annotation of *cis*-regulatory elements by identification, subclassification, and functional assessment of multispecies conserved sequences. *Proc Natl Acad Sci USA.* 2005;102(28):9830–9835.
2. Higgs DR, Wood WG, Jarman AP, et al. A major positive regulatory region located far upstream of the human α-globin gene locus. *Genes Dev.* 1990;4(9): 1588–1601.
3. Higgs DR, Sharpe JA, Wood WG. Understanding αglobin gene expression: a step towards effective gene therapy. *Semin Hematol.* 1998;35(2):93–104.
4. Anguita E, Hughes J, Heyworth C, Blobel GA, Wood WG, Higgs DR. Globin gene activation during haemopoiesis is driven by protein complexes nucleated by GATA-1 and GATA-2. *EMBO J.* 2004;23(14):2841–2852.
5. Vernimmen D, De Gobbi M, Sloane-Stanley JA, Wood WG, Higgs DR. Long-range chromosomal interactions regulate the timing of the transition between poised and active gene expression. *EMBO J.* 2007;26(8):2041–2051.
6. De Gobbi M, Anguita E, Hughes J, et al. Tissue-specific histone modification and transcription factor binding in α globin gene expression. *Blood.* 2007;110(13): 4503–4510.
7. Peschle C, Mavilio F, Care A, et al. Haemoglobin switching in human embryos: asynchrony of ζ–α and ε–γ-globin switches in primitive and definite erythropoietic lineage. *Nature.* 1985;313(5999):235–238.
8. Kingsley PD, Malik J, Emerson RL, et al. "Maturational" globin switching in primary primitive erythroid cells. *Blood.* 2006;107(4):1665–1672.
9. Olivier EN, Qiu C, Velho M, Hirsch RE, Bouhassira EE. Large-scale production of embryonic red blood cells from human embryonic stem cells. *Exp Hematol.* 34(12):1635–1642.
10. Hill AV, Nicholls RD, Thein SL, Higgs DR. Recombination within the human embryonic ζ-globin locus: a common ζ-ζ chromosome produced by gene conversion of the ψζ gene. *Cell.* 1985;42(3):809–819.
11. Chui DH, Mentzer WC, Patterson M, et al. Human embryonic ζ-globin chains in fetal and newborn blood. *Blood.* 1989;74(4):1409–1414.
12. Leung S, Proudfoot NJ, Whitelaw E. The gene for θ-globin is transcribed in human fetal erythroid tissues. *Nature.* 1987;329(6139):551–554.
13. Albitar M, Peschle C, Liebhaber SA. θ, ζ, and ε globin messenger RNAs are expressed in adults. *Blood.* 1989;74(2):629–637.
14. Ley TJ, Maloney KA, Gordon JI, Schwartz AL. Globin gene expression in erythroid human fetal liver cells. *J Clin Invest.* 1989;83(3):1032–1038.
15. Goh SH, Lee YT, Bhanu NV, et al. A newly discovered human α-globin gene. *Blood.* 2005;106(4):1466–72.
16. Brown JM, Leach J, Reittie JE, et al. Coregulated human globin genes are frequently in spatial proximity when active. *J Cell Biol.* 2006;172(2):177–187.
17. Waggoner SA, Liebhaber SA. Regulation of α-globin mRNA stability. *Exp Biol Med (Maywood).* 2003;228(4):387–395.
18. Liebhaber SA, Kan YW. Differentiation of the mRNA transcripts originating from the α1- and α2-globin loci in normals and α-thalassemics. *J Clin Invest.* 1981;68(2):439–446.
19. Orkin SH, Goff SC. The duplicated human α-globin genes: their relative expression as measured by RNA analysis. *Cell.* 1981;24(2):345–351.
20. Molchanova TP, Pobedimskaya DD, Huisman TH. The differences in quantities of α2- and α1-globin gene variants in heterozygotes. *Br J Haematol.* 1994;88(2):300–306.
21. Shakin SH, Liebhaber SA. Translational profiles of α1-, α2-, and β-globin messenger ribonucleic acids in human reticulocytes. *J Clin Invest.* 1986;78(4):1125–1129.

22. Liebhaber SA, Cash FE, Ballas SK. Human α-globin gene expression. The dominant role of the α2-locus in mRNA and protein synthesis. *J Biol Chem.* 1986;261(32):15327–15333.
23. Buckle VJ, Higgs DR, Wilkie AO, Super M, Weatherall DJ. Localisation of human α globin to 16p13.3 -- -pter. *J Med Genet.* 1988;25(12):847–849.
24. Wainscoat JS, Kanavakis E, Weatherall DJ, et al. Regional localisation of the human α-globin genes. *Lancet.* 1981;2 (8241):301–302.
25. Fichera M, Rappazzo G, Spalletta A, et al. Triplicated α-globin gene locus with translocation of the whole telomeric end in association with β-thalassemia trait, results in a severe syndrome. *Blood.* 1994;84:260a.
26. Harteveld CL, Refaldi C, Cassinerio E, Cappellini MD, Giordano PC. Segmental duplications involving the α-globin gene cluster are causing β-thalassemia intermedia phenotypes in β-thalassemia heterozygous patients. *Blood Cell Mol Dis.* 2008;40:312–316.
27. Wallace HA, Marques-Kranc F, Richardson M, et al. Manipulating the mouse genome to engineer precise functional syntenic replacements with human sequence. *Cell.* 2007 12;128(1):197–209.
28. Higgs DR, Wilkie AOM, Vyas P, Vickers MA, Buckle VJ, Harris PC. Characterization of the telomeric region of human chromosome 16p. *Chromosomes Today.* 1993;11:35–47.
29. Wilkie AO, Higgs DR, Rack KA, et al. Stable length polymorphism of up to 260 kb at the tip of the short arm of human chromosome 16. *Cell.* 1991;64(3):595–606.
30. Riethman H, Ambrosini A, Paul S. Human subtelomere structure and variation. *Chromosome Res.* 2005;13(5):505–515.
31. Galanello R, Ruggeri R, Paglietti E, Addis M, Melis MA, Cao A. A family with segregating triplicated α globin loci and β thalassemia. *Blood.* 1983;62(5):1035–1040.
32. Goossens M, Dozy AM, Embury SH, et al. Triplicated α-globin loci in humans. *Proc Natl Acad Sci USA.* 1980;77(1):518–521.
33. Gu YC, Landman H, Huisman TH. Two different quadruplicated α globin gene arrangements. *Br J Haematol.* 1987;66(2):245–250.
34. Higgs DR, Old JM, Pressley L, Clegg JB, Weatherall DJ. A novel α-globin gene arrangement in man. *Nature.* 1980; 284(5757):632–635.
35. Premawardhena A, Fisher CA, Olivieri NF, et al. A novel molecular basis for β thalassemia intermedia poses new questions about its pathophysiology. *Blood.* 2005;106(9): 3251–3255.
36. Cook RJ, Hoyer JD, Highsmith WE. Quintuple α-globin gene: a novel allele in a Sudanese man. *Hemoglobin.* 2006;30(1):51–55.
37. Camaschella C, Bertero MT, Serra A, et al. A benign form of thalassaemia intermedia may be determined by the interaction of triplicated α locus and heterozygous β-thalassaemia. *Br J Haematol.* 1987;66(1):103–107.
38. Henni T, Belhani M, Morle F, et al. α globin gene triplication in severe heterozygous β thalassemia. *Acta Haematol.* 1985;74(4):236–239.
39. Higgs DR, Clegg JB, Weatherall DJ, Serjeant BE, Serjeant GR. Interaction of the ααα globin gene haplotype and sickle haemoglobin. *Br J Haematol.* 1984;57(4):671–678.
40. Kulozik AE, Thein SL, Wainscoat JS, Gale R, Kay LA, Wood JK, et al. Thalassaemia intermedia: interaction of the triple α-globin gene arrangement and heterozygous β-thalassaemia. *Br J Haematol.* 1987;66(1):109–112.
41. Sampietro M, Cazzola M, Cappellini MD, Fiorelli G. The triplicated α-gene locus and heterozygous β thalassaemia: a case of thalassaemia intermedia. *Br J Haematol.* 1983;55(4):709–710.
42. Trent RJ, Mickleson KN, Wilkinson T, et al. α globin gene rearrangements in Polynesians are not associated with malaria. *Am J Hematol.* 1985;18(4):431–433.
43. Ristaldi MS, Casula S, Rando A, Vestri R. Sheep α-globin gene sequences: implications for their concerted evolution and for the down-regulation of the 3′ genes. *J Mol Evol.* 1995;40(4):349–353.
44. Felice AE, Cleek MP, Marino EM, et al. Different ζ globin gene deletions among black Americans. *Hum Genet.* 1986;73(3):221–224.
45. Titus EA, Hsia YE, Hunt JA. α-thalassemia screening reveals quadruple ζ-globin genes in a Laotian family. *Hemoglobin.* 1988;12(5–6):539–550.
46. Trent RJ, Mickleson KN, Wilkinson T, et al. Globin genes in Polynesians have many rearrangements including a recently described γγγγ. *Am J Hum Genet.* 1986;39(3):350–360.
47. Winichagoon P, Higgs DR, Goodbourn SE, Lamb J, Clegg JB, Weatherall DJ. Multiple arrangements of the human embryonic ζ globin genes. *Nucl Acids Res.* 1982;10(19):5853–5868.
48. Higgs DR, Wainscoat JS, Flint J, et al. Analysis of the human α-globin gene cluster reveals a highly informative genetic locus. *Proc Natl Acad Sci USA.* 1986;83(14):5165–5169.
49. Rappaport EF, Schwartz E, Poncz M, Surrey S. Frequent occurrence of a ζ-globin-region deletion in American blacks accounts for a previously-described restriction site polymorphism. *Biochem Biophys Res Commun.* 1984;125(2):817–823.
50. Chan V, Chan TK, Cheng MY, Kan YW, Todd D. Organization of the ζ-α genes in Chinese. *Br J Haematol.* 1986;64(1):97–105.
51. Hill AV, Thein SL, Mavo B, Weatherall DJ, Clegg JB. Non-deletion haemoglobin H disease in Papua New Guinea. *J Med Genet.* 1987;24(12):767–771.
52. Strachan T, Read AP. *Human Molecular Genetics 2.* 2nd ed. Oxford: BIOS Scientific Publishers Ltd.; 1999.
53. Michelson AM, Orkin SH. Boundaries of gene conversion within the duplicated human α-globin genes. Concerted evolution by segmental recombination. *J Biol Chem.* 1983;258(24):15245–15254.
54. Proudfoot NJ, Gil A, Maniatis T. The structure of the human ζ-globin gene and a closely linked, nearly identical pseudogene. *Cell.* 1982;31(3 Pt 2):553–563.
55. Liebhaber SA, Rappaport EF, Cash FE, Ballas SK, Schwartz E, Surrey S. Hemoglobin I mutation encoded at both α-globin loci on the same chromosome: concerted evolution in the human genome. *Science.* 1984;226(4681):1449–1451.
56. Law HY, Luo HY, Wang W, et al. Determining the cause of patchwork HBA1 and HBA2 genes: recurrent gene conversion or crossing over fixation events. *Haematologica.* 2006;91(3):297–302.
57. Wang W, Chan AY, Chan LC, Ma ES, Chong SS. Unusual rearrangement of the α-globin gene cluster containing both the -α3.7 and αααanti-4.2 crossover junctions: clinical diagnostic implications and possible mechanisms. *Clin Chem.* 2005;51(11):2167–2170.
58. Collier S, Tassabehji M, Sinnott P, Strachan T. A *de novo* pathological point mutation at the 21-hydroxylase locus: implications for gene conversion in the human genome. *Nat Genet.* 1993;3(3):260–265.

59. Fei YJ, Fujita S, Huisman TH. Two different θ globin gene deletions observed among black newborn babies. *Br J Haematol.* 1988;68(2):249–53.
60. Higgs DR, Vickers MA, Wilkie AO, Pretorius IM, Jarman AP, Weatherall DJ. A review of the molecular genetics of the human α-globin gene cluster. *Blood.* 1989;73(5):1081–1104.
61. Ballas SK, Fei YJ, Huisman TH. ζ and θ1-globin gene deletions located on the same chromosome. *Br J Haematol.* 1989;73(3):429.
62. Fei YJ, Kutlar F, Harris HF 2nd, et al. A search for anomalies in the ζ, α, β and γ globin gene arrangements in normal black, Italian, Turkish, and Spanish newborns. *Hemoglobin.* 1989;13(1):45–65.
63. Nakatsuji T, Landman H, Huisman TH. An elongated segment of DNA observed between two human α globin genes. *Hum Genet.* 1986;74(4):368–371.
64. Sachidanandam R, Weissman D, Schmidt SC, et al. A map of human genome sequence variation containing 1.42 million single nucleotide polymorphisms. *Nature.* 2001; 409(6822):928–933.
65. Harteveld CL, Muglia M, Passarino G, Kielman MF, Bernini LF. Genetic polymorphism of the major regulatory element HS-40 upstream of the human α-globin gene cluster. *Br J Haematol.* 2002;119(3):848–854.
66. Goodbourn SE, Higgs DR, Clegg JB, Weatherall DJ. Molecular basis of length polymorphism in the human ζ-globin gene complex. *Proc Natl Acad Sci USA.* 1983;80(16):5022–5026.
67. Higgs DR, Goodbourn SE, Wainscoat JS, Clegg JB, Weatherall DJ. Highly variable regions of DMA flank the human α globin genes. *Nucl Acids Res.* 1981;9(17):4213–4224.
68. Jeffreys AJ, Barber R, Bois P, et al. Human minisatellites, repeat DNA instability and meiotic recombination. *Electrophoresis.* 1999;20(8):1665–1675.
69. Flint J, Thomas K, Micklem G, et al. The relationship between chromosome structure and function at a human telomeric region. *Nat Genet.* 1997;15(3):252–257.
70. Royle NJ, Clarkson RE, Wong Z, Jeffreys AJ. Clustering of hypervariable minisatellites in the proterminal regions of human autosomes. *Genomics.* 1988;3(4):352–360.
71. Fowler SJ, Gill P, Werrett DJ, Higgs DR. Individual specific DNA fingerprints from a hypervariable region probe: α-globin 3′HVR. *Hum Genet.* 1988;79(2):142–146.
72. Jeffreys AJ. Highly variable minisatellites and DNA fingerprints. *Biochem Soc Trans.* 1987;15(3):309–317.
73. Hess JF, Schmid CW, Shen CK. A gradient of sequence divergence in the human adult α-globin duplication units. *Science.* 1984;226(4670):67–70.
74. Lauer J, Shen CK, Maniatis T. The chromosomal arrangement of human α-like globin genes: sequence homology and α-globin gene deletions. *Cell.* 1980;20(1):119–130.
75. Zimmer EA, Martin SL, Beverley SM, Kan YW, Wilson AC. Rapid duplication and loss of genes coding for the α chains of hemoglobin. *Proc Natl Acad Sci USA.* 1980;77(4):2158–2162.
76. Embury SH, Miller JA, Dozy AM, Kan YW, Chan V, Todd D. Two different molecular organizations account for the single α-globin gene of the α-thalassemia-2 genotype. *J Clin Invest.* 1980;66(6):1319–1325.
77. Higgs DR, Hill AV, Bowden DK, Weatherall DJ, Clegg JB. Independent recombination events between the duplicated human α globin genes; implications for their concerted evolution. *Nucl Acids Res.* 1984;12(18):6965–6977.
78. Trent RJ, Higgs DR, Clegg JB, Weatherall DJ. A new triplicated α-globin gene arrangement in man. *Br J Haematol.* 1981;49(1):149–152.
79. De Angioletti M, Lacerra G, Castaldo C, et al. $\alpha\alpha\alpha\alpha^{\text{anti-3.7 type II}}$: a new α-globin gene rearrangement suggesting that the α-globin gene duplication could be caused by intrachromosomal recombination. *Hum Genet.* 1992;89(1):37–41.
80. Flint J, Hill AV, Bowden DK, et al. High frequencies of α-thalassaemia are the result of natural selection by malaria. *Nature.* 1986;321(6072):744–750.
81. Winichagoon P, Higgs DR, Goodbourn SE, Clegg JB, Weatherall DJ, Wasi P. The molecular basis of α-thalassaemia in Thailand. *EMBO J.* 1984;3(8):1813–1818.
82. Thein SL, Wallace RB, Pressley L, Clegg JB, Weatherall DJ, Higgs DR. The polyadenylation site mutation in the α-globin gene cluster. *Blood.* 1988;71(2):313–319.
83. Han LL, Keller MP, Navidi W, Chance PF, Arnheim N. Unequal exchange at the Charcot-Marie-Tooth disease type 1A recombination hot-spot is not elevated above the genome average rate. *Hum Mol Genet.* 2000;9(12):1881–1889.
84. Lopes J, Tardieu S, Silander K, et al. Homologous DNA exchanges in humans can be explained by the yeast double-strand break repair model: a study of 17p11.2 rearrangements associated with CMT1A and HNPP. *Hum Mol Genet.* 1999;8(12):2285–2292.
85. Reiter LT, Hastings PJ, Nelis E, De Jonghe P, Van Broeckhoven C, Lupski JR. Human meiotic recombination products revealed by sequencing a hotspot for homologous strand exchange in multiple HNPP deletion patients. *Am J Hum Genet.* 1998;62(5):1023–1033.
86. Jinks-Robertson S, Michelitch M, Ramcharan S. Substrate length requirements for efficient mitotic recombination in Saccharomyces cerevisiae. *Mol Cell Biol.* 1993;13(7):3937–3950.
87. Lam KW, Jeffreys AJ. Processes of copy-number change in human DNA: the dynamics of α-globin gene deletion. *Proc Natl Acad Sci USA.* 2006;103(24):8921–8927.
88. Lam KW, Jeffreys AJ. Processes of *de novo* duplication of human α-globin genes. *Proc Natl Acad Sci USA.* 2007; 104(26):10950–10955.
89. Kulozik AE, Kar BC, Serjeant GR, Serjeant BE, Weatherall DJ. The molecular basis of α thalassemia in India. Its interaction with the sickle cell gene. *Blood.* 1988;71(2):467–472.
90. Zhao JB, Zhao L, Fei YJ, Liu JC, Huisman TH. A novel α-thalassemia-2 (-2.7-kb) observed in a Chinese patient with Hb H disease. *Am J Hematol.* 1991;38(3):248–249.
91. Eng B, Walsh R, Walker L, Patterson M, Waye JS. Characterization of a rare single α-globin gene deletion in a Chinese woman with Hb H disease. *Hemoglobin.* 2005;29(4):297–299.
92. Poodt J, Martens HA, Walsh IB, Felix-Schollaart B, Hermans MH. A newly identified deletion of 970 bp at the α-globin locus that removes the promoter region of the α1gene. *Hemoglobin.* 2006;30(4):471–477.
93. Lacerra G, Fioretti G, De Angioletti M, et al. (α)α 5.3: a novel α^+-thalassemia deletion with the breakpoints in the α2-globin gene and in close proximity to an Alu family repeat between the ψα2- and ψα1-globin genes. *Blood.* 1991;78(10):2740–2746.
94. Harteveld CL, van Delft P, Wijermans PW, et al. A novel 7.9 kb deletion causing α^+-thalassaemia in two independent families of Indian origin. *Br J Haematol.* 2003;120(2):364–366.

95. Bowden DK, Hill AV, Higgs DR, Oppenheimer SJ, Weatherall DJ, Clegg JB. Different hematologic phenotypes are associated with the leftward (-$\alpha^{4.2}$) and rightward (-$\alpha^{3.7}$) α^{+}-thalassemia deletions. *J Clin Invest.* 1987;79(1):39–43.
96. Liebhaber SA, Cash FE, Main DM. Compensatory increase in α1-globin gene expression in individuals heterozygous for the α-thalassemia-2 deletion. *J Clin Invest.* 1985;76(3):1057–1064.
97. Proudfoot NJ. Transcriptional interference and termination between duplicated α-globin gene constructs suggests a novel mechanism for gene regulation. *Nature.* 1986; 322(6079):562–565.
98. Chui DH, Wong SC, Chung SW, Patterson M, Bhargava S, Poon MC. Embryonic ζ-globin chains in adults: a marker for α-thalassemia-1 haplotype due to a greater than 17.5-kb deletion. *N Engl J Med.* 1986;314(2):76–79.
99. Kutlar F, Gonzalez-Redondo JM, Kutlar A, et al. The levels of ζ, γ and δ chains in patients with Hb H disease. *Hum Genet.* 1989;82(2):179–186.
100. Tang W, Luo HY, Albitar M, et al. Human embryonic ζ-globin chain expression in deletional α-thalassemias. *Blood.* 1992;80(2):517–522.
101. Fischel-Ghodsian N, Higgs DR, Beyer EC. Function of a new globin gene. *Nature.* 1987;329(6138):397.
102. Daniels RJ, Peden JF, Lloyd C, et al. Sequence, structure and pathology of the fully annotated terminal 2 Mb of the short arm of human chromosome 16. *Hum Mol Genet.* 2001;10(4):339–352.
103. International Human Genome Sequencing Consortium. Finishing the euchromatic sequence of the human genome. *Nature.* 2004;431(7011):931–945.
104. Nicholls RD, Fischel-Ghodsian N, Higgs DR. Recombination at the human α-globin gene cluster: sequence features and topological constraints. *Cell.* 1987;49(3):369–378.
105. Indrak K, Gu YC, Novotny J, Huisman TH. A new α-thalassemia-2 deletion resulting in microcytosis and hypochromia and *in vitro* chain imbalance in the heterozygote. *Am J Hematol.* 1993;43(2):144–145.
106. Barbour VM, Tufarelli C, Sharpe JA, et al. α-thalassemia resulting from a negative chromosomal position effect. *Blood.* 2000;96(3):800–807.
107. Tufarelli C, Stanley JA, Garrick D, et al. Transcription of antisense RNA leading to gene silencing and methylation as a novel cause of human genetic disease. *Nat Genet.* 2003;34(2): 157–165.
108. Jarman AP, Wood WG, Sharpe JA, Gourdon G, Ayyub H, Higgs DR. Characterization of the major regulatory element upstream of the human α-globin gene cluster. *Mol Cell Biol.* 1991;11(9):4679–4689.
109. Strauss EC, Andrews NC, Higgs DR, Orkin SH. *In vivo* footprinting of the human α-globin locus upstream regulatory element by guanine and adenine ligation-mediated polymerase chain reaction. *Mol Cell Biol.* 1992;12(5):2135–2142.
110. Hatton CS, Wilkie AO, Drysdale HC, et al. α-thalassemia caused by a large (62 kb) deletion upstream of the human α globin gene cluster. *Blood.* 1990;76(1):221–227.
111. Bernet A, Sabatier S, Picketts DJ, Ouazana R, Morle F, Higgs DR, et al. Targeted inactivation of the major positive regulatory element (HS-40) of the human α–globin gene locus. *Blood.* 1995;86(3):1202–1211.
112. Flint J, Rochette J, Craddock CF, et al. Chromosomal stabilisation by a subtelomeric rearrangement involving two closely related Alu elements. *Hum Mol Genet.* 1996;5(8):1163–1169.
113. Flint J, Craddock CF, Villegas A, et al. Healing of broken human chromosomes by the addition of telomeric repeats. *Am J Hum Genet.* 1994;55(3):505–512.
114. Chan SR, Blackburn EH. Telomeres and telomerase. *Philos Trans R Soc Lond B Biol Sci.* 2004;359(1441):109–121.
115. Kan YW, Dozy AM, Trecartin R, Todd D. Identification of a nondeletion defect in α-thalassemia. *N Engl J Med.* 1977;297(20):1081–1084.
116. Higgs DR, Pressley L, Aldridge B, et al. Genetic and molecular diversity in nondeletion Hb H disease. *Proc Natl Acad Sci USA.* 1981;78(9):5833–5837.
117. Felber BK, Orkin SH, Hamer DH. Abnormal RNA splicing causes one form of α thalassemia. *Cell.* 1982;29(3):895–902.
118. Harteveld CL, Heister JG, Giordano PC, et al. An IVS1-116 (A→G) acceptor splice site mutation in the α2 globin gene causing α^{+} thalassaemia in two Dutch families. *Br J Haematol.* 1996;95(3):461–466.
119. Harteveld CL, Wijermans PW, van Delft P, Rasp E, Haak HL, Giordano PC. An α-thalassemia phenotype in a Dutch Hindustani, caused by a new point mutation that creates an alternative splice donor site in the first exon of the α2-globin gene. *Hemoglobin.* 2004;28(3):255–259.
120. Harteveld CL, Beijer C, van Delft P, Zanardini R, Bernini LF, Giordano PC. α-thalassaemia as a result of a novel splice donor site mutation of the αl-globin gene. *Br J Haematol.* 2000;110(3):694–698.
121. Noguera Nl, Gonzalez FA, Davoli RA, Milani AC, Villegas A. A novel splice acceptor site mutation of the α2-globin gene causing α-thalassemia. *Hemoglobin.* 2001;25(3):311–315.
122. Whitelaw E, Proudfoot N. α-thalassaemia caused by a poly(A) site mutation reveals that transcriptional termination is linked to 3′ end processing in the human α2 globin gene. *EMBO J.* 1986;5(11):2915–2922.
123. Pressley L, Higgs DR, Clegg JB, Perrine RP, Pembrey ME, Weatherall DJ. A new genetic basis for hemoglobin-H disease. *N Engl J Med.* 1980;303(24):1383–1388.
124. Molchanova TP, Smetanina NS, Huisman TH. A second, elongated, α2-globin mRNA is present in reticulocytes from normal persons and subjects with terminating codon or poly A mutations. *Biochem Biophys Res Commun.* 1995;214(3):1184–1190.
125. Traeger-Synodinos J, Papassotiriou I, Karagiorga M, Premetis E, Kanavakis E, Stamoulakatou A. Unusual phenotypic observations associated with a rare HbH disease genotype (--Med/$\alpha^{TSaudi}\alpha$): implications for clinical management. *Br J Haematol.* 2002;119(1):265–267.
126. Viprakasit V, Green S, Height S, Ayyub H, Higgs DR. Hb H hydrops fetalis syndrome associated with the interaction of two common determinants of α thalassaemia (--MED/$\alpha^{TSaudi}\alpha$). *Br J Haematol.* 2002;117(3):759–762.
127. Tamary H, Klinger G, Shalmon L, et al. α-thalassemia caused by a 16 bp deletion in the 3′ untranslated region of the α2-globin gene including the first nucleotide of the poly A signal sequence. *Hemoglobin.* 1997;21(2):121–130.
128. Fei YJ, Liu JC, Walker EL 3rd, Huisman TH. A new gene deletion involving the α2-, α1-, and θ1-globin genes in a black family with Hb H disease. *Am J Hematol.* 1992;39(4):299–300.
129. Yuregir GT, Aksoy K, Curuk MA, et al. Hb H disease in a Turkish family resulting from the interaction of a deletional

α-thalassaemia-1 and a newly discovered poly A mutation. *Br J Haematol.* 1992;80(4):527–532.

130. Harteveld CL, Losekoot M, Haak H, Heister GA, Giordano PC, Bernini LF. A novel polyadenylation signal mutation in the α2-globin gene causing α thalassaemia. *Br J Haematol.* 1994;87(1):139–143.
131. Henderson S, Chappie M, Rugless M, Fisher C, Kinsey S, Old J. Haemoglobin H hydrops fetalis syndrome associated with homozygosity for the α2-globin gene polyadenylation signal mutation AATAAA→AATA. *Br J Haematol.* 2006;135(5):743–745.
132. Olivieri NF, Chang LS, Poon AO, Michelson AM, Orkin SH. An α-globin gene initiation codon mutation in a black family with HbH disease. *Blood.* 1987;70(3):729–732.
133. Morle F, Lopez B, Henni T, Godet J. α-Thalassaemia associated with the deletion of two nucleotides at position -2 and -3 preceding the AUG codon. *EMBO J.* 1985;4(5):1245–1250.
134. Morle F, Starck J, Godet J. α-thalassemia due to the deletion of nucleotides -2 and -3 preceding the AUG initiation codon affects translation efficiency both *in vitro* and *in vivo*. *Nucl Acids Res.* 1986;14(8):3279–3292.
135. Tabone P, Henni T, Belhani M, Colonna P, Verdier G, Godet J. Hemoglobin H disease from Algeria: genetic and molecular characterization. *Acta Haematol.* 1981;65(1):26–31.
136. Cao A, Rosatelli C, Pirastu M, Galanello R. Thalassemias in Sardinia: molecular pathology, phenotype-genotype correlation, and prevention. *Am J Pediatr Hematol Oncol.* 1991;13(2):179–188.
137. Galanello R, Aru B, Dessi C, et al. HbH disease in Sardinia: molecular, hematological and clinical aspects. *Acta Haematol.* 1992;88(1):1–6.
138. Moi P, Cash FE, Liebhaber SA, Cao A, Pirastu M. An initiation codon mutation (AUG→GUG) of the human α1-globin gene. Structural characterization and evidence for a mild thalassemic phenotype. *J Clin Invest.* 1987;80(5):1416–1421.
139. Eng B, Patterson M, Walker L, et al. Three new α-thalassemia point mutations ascertained through newborn screening. *Hemoglobin.* 2006;30(2):149–153.
140. Harteveld CL, Yavarian M, Zorai A, Quakkelaar ED, van Delft P, Giordano PC. Molecular spectrum of α-thalassemia in the Iranian population of Hormozgan: three novel point mutation defects. *Am J Hematol.* 2003;74(2):99–103.
141. Liebhaber SA, Coleman MB, Adams JG 3rd, Cash FE, Steinberg MH. Molecular basis for nondeletion α-thalassemia in American blacks. *Alpha* 2(116GAG→DAG). *J Clin Invest.* 1987;80(1):154–159.
142. Siala H, Fattoum S, Messaoud T, Ouali F, Gerard N, Krishnamoorthy R. A novel α-thalassemia nonsense mutation in codon 23 of the α2-globin gene (GAG→TAG) in a Tunisian family. *Hemoglobin.* 2004;28(3):249–254.
143. Twomey AP, Brasch JM, Betheras FR, Bowden DK. A new α2-globin gene codon 90 (AAG→TAG) nonsense mutation. *Hemoglobin.* 2003;27(4):261–265.
144. Luo HY, Adewoye AH, Pilichowska M, Li MY, Basran RK, Steinberg MH, et al. Two new α-thalassemia frameshift mutations. *Hemoglobin.* 2007;31(2):135–139.
145. Pereira FJ, do Ceu Silva M, Picanco I, et al. Human α2-globin nonsense-mediated mRNA decay induced by a novel α-thalassaemia frameshift mutation at codon 22. *Br J Haematol.* 2006;133(1):98–102.
146. Viprakasit V, Tanphaichitr VS, Veerakul G, et al. Coinheritance of Hb Pak Num Po, a novel α1 gene mutation, and α^{O} thalassemia associated with transfusion-dependent Hb H disease. *Am J Hematol.* 2004;75(3):157–163.
147. Safaya S, Rieder RF. Dysfunctional α-globin gene in hemoglobin H disease in blacks. A dinucleotide deletion produces a frameshift and a termination codon. *J Biol Chem.* 1988;263(9):4328–4332.
148. Ayala S, Colomer D, Aymerich M, Abella E, Vives Corrons JL. First description of a frameshift mutation in the α1-globin gene associated with α-thalassaemia. *Br J Haematol.* 1997;98(1):47–50.
149. Ayala S, Colomer D, Pujades A, Aymerich M, Vives Corrons JL. Haemoglobin Lleida: a new α2-globin variant (12 bp deletion) with mild thalassaemic phenotype. *Br J Haematol.* 1996;94(4):639–644.
150. Weatherall DJ, Clegg JB. The α-chain-termination mutants and their relation to the alpha-thalassaemias. *Philos Trans R Soc Lond B Biol Sci.* 1975;271(913):411–455.
151. Schrier SL, Bunyaratvej A, Khuhapinant A, et al. The unusual pathobiology of hemoglobin constant spring red blood cells. *Blood.* 1997;89(5):1762–1769.
152. Lie-lnjo LE, Ganesan J, Clegg JB, Weatherall DJ. Homozygous state for Hb Constant Spring (slow-moving Hb X components). *Blood.* 1974;43(2):251–259.
153. Pootrakul P, Winichagoon P, Fucharoen S, Pravatmuang P, Piankijagum A, Wasi P. Homozygous haemoglobin Constant Spring: a need for revision of concept. *Hum Genet.* 1981;59(3):250–255.
154. Fucharoen S, Winichagoon P, Pootrakul P, Piankijagum A, Wasi P. Differences between two types of Hb H disease, α-thalassemia 1/α-thalassemia 2 and α-thalassemia 1/Hb constant spring. *Birth Defects Orig Artic Ser.* 1987;23(5A):309–315.
155. Vichinsky EP, MacKlin EA, Waye JS, Lorey F, Olivieri NF. Changes in the epidemiology of thalassemia in North America: a new minority disease. *Pediatrics.* 2005;116(6):e818–825.
156. Hunt DM, Higgs DR, Winichagoon P, Clegg JB, Weatherall DJ. Haemoglobin Constant Spring has an unstable alpha chain messenger RNA. *Br J Haematol.* 1982;51(3):405–413.
157. Kan YW, Todd D, Dozy AM. Haemoglobin Constant Spring synthesis in red cell precursors. *Br J Haematol.* 1974;28(1):103–107.
158. Weiss IM, Liebhaber SA. Erythroid cell-specific determinants of α-globin mRNA stability. *Mol Cell Biol.* 1994;14(12):8123–8132.
159. De Gobbi M, Viprakasit V, Hughes JR, et al. A regulatory SNP causes a human genetic disease by creating a new transcriptional promoter. *Science.* 2006;312(5777):1215–1217.
160. Chan V, Chan VW, Tang M, Lau K, Todd D, Chan TK. Molecular defects in Hb H hydrops fetalis. *Br J Haematol.* 1997;96(2):224–228.
161. Old JM, Higgs DR. Gene analysis. In: Weatherall DJ, ed. *The Thalassemias, Methods in Hematology.* Edinburgh: Churchill Livingstone; 1983:74–102.
162. Harteveld CL, Voskamp A, Phylipsen M, et al. Nine unknown rearrangements in 16p13.3 and 11p15.4 causing α- and β-thalassaemia characterised by high resolution multiplex ligation-dependent probe amplification. *J Med Genet.* 2005;42(12):922–931.

163. Chong SS, Boehm CD, Higgs DR, Cutting GR. Single-tube multiplex-PCR screen for common deletional determinants of α-thalassemia. *Blood.* 2000;95(1):360–362.

164. Steinberg MH, Coleman MB, Adams JG 3rd, Hartmann RC, Saba H, Anagnou NP. A new gene deletion in the α-like globin gene cluster as the molecular basis for the rare α-thalassemia-1 (--/αα) in blacks: HbH disease in sickle cell trait. *Blood.* 1986;67(2):469–473.

165. Sabath DE, Detter JC, Tait JF. A novel deletion of the entire α globin locus causing α-thalassemia-1 in a northern European family. *Am J Clin Pathol.* 1994;102(5):650–654.

166. Honig GR, Shamsuddin M, Vida LN, et al. Hemoglobin Evanston (α14 Trp→Arg). An unstable α-chain variant expressed as α -thalassemia. *J Clin Invest.* 1984;73(6):1740–1749.

167. Moo-Penn WF, Baine RM, Jue DL, et al. Hemoglobin Evanston: α14(A12) Trp leads to Arg. A variant hemoglobin associated with α-thalassemia-2. *Biochim Biophys Acta.* 1983;747:65–70.

168. Liebhaber SA, Cash FE. Locus assignment of α-globin structural mutations by hybrid-selected translation. *J Clin Invest.* 1985;75(1):64–70.

169. del Senno L, Bernard F, Marchetti G, et al. Organization of α-globin genes and mRNA translation in subjects carrying haemoglobin Hasharon (α47 Asp replaced by His) from the Ferrara Region (Northern Italy). *Eur J Biochem.* 1980;111(1):125–130.

170. Giglioni B, Comi P, Taramelli R, et al. Organization of α-globin genes in Hb Hasharon (α47 Asp replaced by His) carriers. *Blood.* 1980;56(6):1145–1149.

171. Mavilio F, Marinucci M, Massa A, Fontanarosa PP, Tentori L, Cappellozza G. Hemoglobin Hasharon [α247 (CD5)Asp leads to His β2] linked to α-thalassemia in northern Italian carriers. Hematological and biosynthetic studies. *Acta Haematol.* 1980;63(6):305–311.

172. Pich PG, Gallo E, Mazza U, Ricco G. [Study on a case of double heterozygosis between Hb-C and β-thalassemia]. *Boll Soc Ital Biol Sper.* 1973;49(9):507–512.

173. Bruzdzinski CJ, Sisco KL, Ferrucci SJ, Rucknagel DL. The occurrence of the $\alpha^{\text{G-Philadelphia}}$-globin allele on a double-locus chromosome. *Am J Hum Genet.* 1984;36(1):101–109.

174. Hill AV, Bowden DK, Trent RJ, et al. Melanesians and Polynesians share a unique α-thalassemia mutation. *Am J Hum Genet.* 1985;37(3):571–580.

175. Sancar GB, Tatsis B, Cedeno MM, Rieder RF. Proportion of hemoglobin G Philadelphia (α268 Asn leads to Lys β2) in heterozygotes is determined by α-globin gene deletions. *Proc Natl Acad Sci USA.* 1980;77(11):6874–6878.

176. Sciarratta GV, Sansone G, Ivaldi G, Felice AE, Huisman TH. Alternate organization of $\alpha^{\text{G-Philadelphia}}$ globin genes among U.S. black and Italian Caucasian heterozygotes. *Hemoglobin.* 1984;8(6):537–547.

177. Surrey S, Ohene-Frempong K, Rappaport E, Atwater J, Schwartz E. Linkage of $\alpha^{\text{G-Philadelphia}}$ to α-thalassemia in African-Americans. *Proc Natl Acad Sci USA.* 1980;77(8):4885–4889.

178. Higgs DR, Hunt DM, Drysdale HC, Clegg JB, Pressley L, Weatherall DJ. The genetic basis of Hb Q-H disease. *Br J Haematol.* 1980;46(3):387–400.

179. Lie-lnjo LE, Dozy AM, Kan YW, Lopes M, Todd D. The α-globin gene adjacent to the gene for HbQ-α74 Asp replaced by His is deleted, but not that adjacent to the gene for HbG-α30 Glu replaced by Gln; three-fourths of the α-globin genes are deleted in HbQ-α-thalassemia. *Blood.* 1979 Dec;54(6):1407–1416.

180. Liang S, Tang Z, Su C, et al. Hb Duan α75(EF4)Asp – -Ala], Hb Westmead[α122(H5)His -- -Gln], and α-thalassemia-2 (-4.2 Kb deletion) in a Chinese family. *Hemoglobin.* 1988;12(1):13–21.

181. Costa FF, Sonati MF, Zago MA. Hemoglobin Stanleyville II (α78 Asn→Lys) is associated with a 3.7-kb α-globin gene deletion. *Hum Genet.* 1991;86(3):319–320.

182. Honig GR, Shamsuddin M, Mason RG, Vida LN, Tremaine LM, Tarr GE, et al. Hemoglobin Nigeria (α-81 Ser replaced by Lys): a new variant associated with α-thalassemia. *Blood.* 1980;55(1):131–137.

183. Lambridis AJ, Ramsay M, Jenkins T. The haematological puzzle of Hb J Cape Town is partly solved. *Br J Haematol.* 1986;63(2):363–367.

184. Old JM, Clegg JB, Weatherall DJ, Booth PB. Haemoglobin J Tongariki is associated with α thalassaemia. *Nature.* 1978;273(5660):319–320.

185. Harteveld CL, Jebbink MC, Van Der Lely N, et al. α-thalassemia phenotype induced by the new IVS-ll-2 (T→A) splice donor site mutation on the α2-globin gene. *Hemoglobin.* 2006;30(1):3–7.

186. Harteveld CL, Giordano PC, Losekoot M, Heister JG, Batelaan D, van Delft P, et al. Hb Utrecht [α2 129(H12)Leu→Pro], a new unstable α2-chain variant associated with a mild α-thalassaemic phenotype. *Br J Haematol.* 1996;94(3):483–485.

187. Curuk MA, Baysal E, Gupta RB, Sharma S, Huisman TH. An IVS-l-117 (G→A) acceptor splice site mutation in the α1-globin gene is a nondeletional α-thalassaemia-2 determinant in an Indian population. *Br J Haematol.* 1993;85(1):148–152.

188. Higgs DR, Goodbourn SE, Lamb J, Clegg JB, Weatherall DJ, Proudfoot NJ. α-thalassaemia caused by a polyadenylation signal mutation. *Nature.* 1983;306(5941):398–400.

189. Ma ES, Chow EY, Chan AY, Chan LC. Interaction between ($--^{\text{SEA}}$) α-thalassemia deletion and uncommon non-deletional α-globin gene mutations in Chinese patients. *Haematologica.* 2001;86(5):539–540.

190. Hall GW, Higgs DR, Murphy P, Villegas A, de Miguel A. A mutation in the polyadenylation signal of the α2 globin gene (AATAAA→AATA--) as a cause of α thalassaemia in Asian Indians. *Br J Haematol.* 1994;88(1):225–227.

191. Laosombat V, Fucharoen S, Wiriyasateinkul A. Interaction of the α2 polyadenylation signal mutation (AATAAA→AATA--) and α^{0}-thalassemia ($-^{\text{SEA}}$), resulting in Hb H disease in a Thai patient. *Hemoglobin.* 2001;25(4):383–389.

192. Viprakasit V, Ayyub H, May A. Dinucleotide deletion in $-\alpha^{3.7}$ allele causes a severe form of α^{+} thalassaemia. *Eur J Haematol.* 2003;71(2):133–136.

193. Pirastu M, Saglio G, Chang JC, Cao A, Kan YW. Initiation codon mutation as a cause of α thalassemia. *J Biol Chem.* 1984;259(20):12315–12317.

194. Waye JS, Eng B, Patterson M, et al. Novel mutation of the α2-globin gene intiation codon (ATG→A-G) in a Vietnamese girl with HbH disease. *Blood.* 1996;88:28b.

195. Paglietti E, Galanello R, Moi P, Pirastu M, Cao A. Molecular pathology of haemoglobin H disease in Sardinians. *Br J Haematol.* 1986;63(3):485–496.

196. Oron-Karni V, Filon D, Rund D, Oppenheim A. A novel mechanism generating short deletion/insertions following slippage is suggested by a mutation in the human α2-globin gene. *Hum Mol Genet.* 1997;6(6):881–885.
197. Oron-Karni V, Filon D, Shifrin Y, et al. Diversity of α-globin mutations and clinical presentation of α-thalassemia in Israel. *Am J Hematol.* 2000;65(3):196–203.
198. Clegg JB, Weatherall DJ, Milner PF. Haemoglobin Constant Spring–a chain termination mutant? *Nature.* 1971; 234(5328):337–340.
199. Clegg JB, Weatherall DJ, Contopolou-Griva I, Caroutsos K, Poungouras P, Tsevrenis H. Haemoglobin Icaria, a new chain-termination mutant with causes α thalassaemia. *Nature.* 1974;251(5472):245–247.
200. Efremov GD, Josifovska O, Nikolov N, et al. Hb Icaria-Hb H disease: identification of the Hb Icaria mutation through analysis of amplified DNA. *Br J Haematol.* 1990 Jun;75(2):250–253.
201. De Jong WW, Meera Khan P, Bernini LF. Hemoglobin Koya Dora: high frequency of a chain termination mutant. *Am J Hum Genet.* 1975;27(1):81–90.
202. Bradley TB, Wohl RC, Smith GJ. Elongation of the α-globin chain in a Black family: interaction with HbG Philadelphia. *Clin Res.* 1975;23:131A.
203. Merritt D, Jones RT, Head C, et al. Hb Seal Rock [(α2)142 term→Glu, codon 142 TAA→GAA]: an extended α chain variant associated with anemia, microcytosis, and α-thalassemia-2 (-3.7 Kb). *Hemoglobin.* 1997;21(4):331–344.
204. Viprakasit V, Tanphaichitr VS, Pung-Amritt P, et al. Clinical phenotypes and molecular characterization of Hb H-Pakse disease. *Haematologica.* 2002;87(2):117–125.
205. Waye JS, Eng B, Patterson M, Chui DH, Olivieri NF. Identification of a novel termination codon mutation (TAA→TAT, Term→Tyr) in the α2 globin gene of a Laotian girl with hemoglobin H disease. *Blood.* 1994;83(11):3418–3420.
206. Harteveld CL, van Helden WC, Boxma GL, et al. Hb Zoetermeer: a new mutation on the α2gene inducing an Ala→Ser substitution at codon 21 is possibly associated with a mild thalassemic phenotype. *Hemoglobin.* 2007;31(3):325–332.
207. Hall GW, Thein SL, Newland AC, et al. A base substitution (T→C) in codon 29 of the α2-globin gene causes α thalassaemia. *Br J Haematol.* 1993;85(3):546–552.
208. Chen FE, Ooi C, Ha SY, et al. Genetic and clinical features of hemoglobin H disease in Chinese patients. *N Engl J Med.* 2000;343(8):544–550.
209. Harteveld CL, Vervloet M, Zweegman S, et al. Hb Amsterdam [α32(B13)Met-lle (α2)]: a new unstable variant associated with an α-thalassemia phenotype and a new African polymorphism. *Hemoglobin.* 2005;29(4):257–262.
210. Gomes S, Picanco I, Miranda A, et al. Hb Evora [α2–35 (B16), Ser→Pro], a novel hemoglobin variant associated with an α-thalassemia phenotype. *Haematologica.* 2007;92(2):252–253.
211. Lorey F, Charoenkwan P, Witkowska HE, et al. Hb H hydrops foetalis syndrome: a case report and review of literature. *Br J Haematol.* 2001;115(1):72–78.
212. Prehu C, Mazurier E, Riou J, et al. A new unstable α2-globin gene variant: Hb Chartres [α33(B14)Phe→Ser]. *Hemoglobin.* 2003;27(2):111–115.
213. Traeger-Synodinos J, Papassotiriou I, Metaxotou-Mavrommati A, Vrettou C, Stamoulakatou A, Kanavakis E. Distinct phenotypic expression associated with a new hyperunstable alpha globin variant (Hb Heraklion, α1cd37(C2)Pro>0): comparison to other α-thalassemic hemoglobinopathies. *Blood Cells Mol Dis.* 2000;26(4):276–284.
214. Ayala S, Colomer D, Gelpi JL, Corrons JL. α-thalassaemia due to a single codon deletion in the α1-globin gene. Computational structural analysis of the new α-chain variant. Mutations in brief no. 132. *Hum Mutat.* 1999;11(5).
215. Traeger-Synodinos J, Harteveld CL, Kanavakis E, Giordano PC, Kattamis C, Bernini LF. Hb Aghia Sophia [α62(E11)Val→0 (α1)], an "in-frame" deletion causing α-thalassemia. *Hemoglobin.* 1999;23(4):317–324.
216. Waye JS, Eng B, Patterson M, et al. Identification of two new α-thalassemia mutations in exon 2 of the αl -globin gene. *Hemoglobin.* 2001;25(4):391–396.
217. McBride KL, Snow K, Kubik KS, et al. Hb Dartmouth [α66(E15)Leu→Pro (α2) (CTG→CCG)]: a novel α2-globin gene mutation associated with severe neonatal anemia when inherited in trans with Southeast Asian α-thalassemia-1. *Hemoglobin.* 2001;25(4):375–382.
218. Lacerra G, Testa R, De Angioletti M, Schiliro G, Carestia C. Hb Bronte or α93(FG5)Val→Gly: a new unstable variant of the α2-globin gene, associated with a mild α^+-thalassemia phenotype. *Hemoglobin.* 2003;27(3):149–159.
219. Harteveld CL, Steen G, Vlasveld LT, van Delft P, Giordano PC. Hb Bronovo, a new globin gene mutation at α2 103 (His→Leu) associated with an α thalassemia phenotype. *Haematologica.* 2006;91(4):570–571.
220. Khan SN, Butt Fl, Riazuddin S, Galanello R. Hb Sallanches [α104(G11)Cys→Tyr]: a rare α2-globin chain variant found in the homozygous state in three members of a Pakistani family. *Hemoglobin.* 2000;24(1):31–35.
221. Morle F, Francina A, Ducrocq R, et al. A new α chain variant Hb Sallanches [α2 104(G11) Cys→Tyr] associated with HbH disease in one homozygous patient. *Br J Haematol.* 1995;91(3):608–611.
222. Harteveld CL, Rozendaal L, Blom NA, et al. Hb Oegstgeest [α104(G11)Cys→Ser (α1)]. A new hemoglobin variant associated with a mild α-thalassemia phenotype. *Hemoglobin.* 2005;29(3):165–169.
223. Harteveld CL, Versteegh FG, Kok PJ, van Rooijen-Nijdam IH, van Delft P, Giordano PC. Hb Bleuland [αl08(G15)Thr→Asn, ACC→AAC (α2)]: a new abnormal hemoglobin associated with a mild α-thalassemia phenotype. *Hemoglobin.* 2006;30(3):349–354.
224. Sanguansermsri T, Matragoon S, Changloah L, Flatz G. Hemoglobin Suan-Dok (α2 109 (G16) Leu replaced by Arg β2): an unstable variant associated with α-thalassemia. *Hemoglobin.* 1979;3(2–3):161–174.
225. Honig GR, Shamsuddin M, Zaizov R, Steinherz M, Solar I, Kirschmann C. Hemoglobin Petah Tikva (α110 ala replaced by asp): a new unstable variant with α-thalassemia-like expression. *Blood.* 1981;57(4):705–711.
226. Harteveld CL, van Delft P, Plug R, et al. Hb Groene Hart: a new Pro→Ser amino acid substitution at position 119 of the α1-globin chain is associated with a mild α-thalassemia phenotype. *Hemoglobin.* 2002;26(3):255–260.
227. Giordano PC, Zweegman S, Akkermans N, et al. The first case of Hb Groene Hart [α119(H2)Pro→Ser, CCT→TCT

(α1)] homozygosity confirms that a thalassemia phenotype is associated with this abnormal hemoglobin variant. *Hemoglobin.* 2007;31(2):179–182.

228. Goossens M, Lee KY, Liebhaber SA, Kan YW. Globin structural mutant α125Leu leads to Pro is a novel cause of α-thalassaemia. *Nature.* 1982;296(5860):864–865.

229. Darbellay R, Mach-Pascual S, Rose K, Graf J, Beris P. Haemoglobin Tunis-Bizerte: a new α1 globin 129 Leu→Pro unstable variant with thalassaemic phenotype. *Br J Haematol.* 1995;90(1):71–76.

230. Harkness M, Harkness DR, Kutlar F, Kutlar A, Wilson JB, Webber BB, et al. Hb Sun Prairie or α(2)130(H13)Ala – Pro beta 2, a new unstable variant occurring in low quantities. *Hemoglobin.* 1990;14(5):479–489.

231. Rochette J, Barnetson R, Thein SL, Varet B, Valensi F. Hb Questembert is due to a base substitution (T→C) in codon 131 of the α2-globin gene and has an α-thalassemia biosynthetic ratio. *Am J Hematol.* 1995;48(4):289–290.

232. Wajcman H, Vasseur C, Blouquit Y, et al. Unstable α-chain hemoglobin variants with factitious β-thalassemia biosynthetic ratio: Hb Questembert (α131[H14]Ser→Pro) and Hb Caen (α132[H15]Val→Gly). *Am J Hematol.* 1993;42(4):367–374.

233. Prchal JT, Adler B, Wilson JB, et al. Hb Bibba or α2 136(H19)Leu→Pro β2 in a Caucasian family from Alabama. *Hemoglobin.* 1995;19(3–4):151–164.

234. Vickers MA, Higgs DR. A novel deletion of the entire α-globin gene cluster in a British individual. *Br J Haematol.* 1989;72(3):471–473.

235. Fortina P, Dianzani I, Serra A, Gottardi E, Saglio G, Farinasso L, et al. A newly-characterized α-thalassaemia-1 deletion removes the entire α-like globin gene cluster in an Italian family. *Br J Haematol.* 1991;78(4):529–534.

236. Harteveld KL, Losekoot M, Fodde R, Giordano PC, Bernini LF. The involvement of Alu repeats in recombination events at the α-globin gene cluster: characterization of two α^0-thalassaemia deletion breakpoints. *Hum Genet.* 1997;99(4):528–534.

237. Eng B, Patterson M, Borys S, Chui DH, Waye JS. PCR-based diagnosis of the Filipino (--^{FIL}) and Thai (--^{THAI}) α-thalassemia-1 deletions. *Am J Hematol.* 2000;63(1):54–56.

238. Fischel-Ghodsian N, Vickers MA, Seip M, Winichagoon P, Higgs DR. Characterization of two deletions that remove the entire human ζ-α globin gene complex (--^{THAI} and --^{FIL}). *Br J Haematol.* 1988;70(2):233–238.

239. Sarkar AA, Banerjee S, Chandra S, et al. A novel 33.3 kb deletion (--^{KOL}) in the α-globin gene cluster: a brief report on deletional α-thalassaemia in the heterogeneous eastern Indian population. *Br J Haematol.* 2005;130(3):454–457.

240. Higgs DR, Ayyub H, Clegg JB, et al. Alpha thalassaemia in British people. *Br Med J.* 1985;290(6478):1303–1306.

241. Gonzalez-Redondo JM, Gilsanz F, Ricard P. Characterization of a new α-thalassemia-1 deletion in a Spanish family. *Hemoglobin.* 1989;13(2):103–116.

242. Villegas A, Sanchez J, Carreno DL, Ropero P, Gonzalez FA, Espinos D, et al. Molecular characterization of a new family with α-thalassemia-1 (--^{MA} mutation). *Am J Hematol.* 1995;49(4):294–298.

243. Shaji RV, Eunice SE, Baidya S, Srivastava A, Chandy M. Determination of the breakpoint and molecular diagnosis of a common α-thalassaemia-1 deletion in the Indian population. *Br J Haematol.* 2003;123(5):942–947.

244. Vandenplas S, Higgs DR, Nicholls RD, Bester AJ, Mathew CG. Characterization of a new α^0 thalassaemia defect in the South African population. *Br J Haematol.* 1987;66(4):539–542.

245. Pressley L, Higgs DR, Clegg JB, Weatherall DJ. Gene deletions in α thalassemia prove that the 5′ ζ locus is functional. *Proc Natl Acad Sci USA.* 1980;77(6):3586–3589.

246. Villegas A, Sanchez J, Ricard P, et al. Characterization of a new α-thalassemia-1 mutation in a Spanish family. *Hemoglobin.* 1994;18(1):29–37.

247. Villegas A, Calero F, Vickers MA, Ayyub H, Higgs DR. Alpha thalassaemia in two Spanish families. *Eur J Haematol.* 1990;44(2):109–115.

248. Fortina P, Parrella T, Sartore M, et al. Interaction of rare illegitimate recombination event and a poly A addition site mutation resulting in a severe form of α thalassemia. *Blood.* 1994;83(11):3356–3362.

249. Pressley L, Higgs DR, Aldridge B, Metaxatou-Mavromati A, Clegg JB, Weatherall DJ. Characterisation of a new α thalassemia 1 defect due to a partial deletion of the α globin gene complex. *Nucl Acids Res.* 1980;8(21):4889–4898.

250. Harris PC, Barton NJ, Higgs DR, Reeders ST, Wilkie AO. A long-range restriction map between the α-globin complex and a marker closely linked to the polycystic kidney disease 1 (PKD1) locus. *Genomics.* 1990;7(2):195–206.

251. Horsley SW, Daniels RJ, Anguita E, et al. Monosomy for the most telomeric, gene-rich region of the short arm of human chromosome 16 causes minimal phenotypic effects. *Eur J Hum Genet.* 2001;9(3):217–225.

252. Waye JS, Eng B, Chui DH. Identification of an extensive ζ-α globin gene deletion in a Chinese individual. *Br J Haematol.* 1992;80(3):378–380.

253. Harteveld KL, Losekoot M, Heister AJ, Van Der Wielen M, Giordano PC, Bernini LF. α-Thalassemia in The Netherlands: a heterogeneous spectrum of both deletions and point mutations. *Hum Genet.* 1997;100(3–4):465–471.

254. Huisman TH, Gu LH, Liu JC, Fei YJ, Walker EL 3rd. Black α-thalassemia-1: partial characterization of an approximately 80 kb deletion which includes the ζ- and α-globin genes. *Hemoglobin.* 1993;17(4):345–353.

255. Nooitgedagt JE, Harteveld CL, Starreveld JS, Versteegh FG, Giordano PC. A new deletion defect leading to α-thalassaemia in a large Dutch Caucasian family. *Br J Haematol.* 2007;136(4):662–665.

256. Lamb J, Wilkie AO, Harris PC, Buckle VJ, Lindenbaum RH, Barton NJ, et al. Detection of breakpoints in submicroscopic chromosomal translocation, illustrating an important mechanism for genetic disease. *Lancet.* 1989;2(8667):819–824.

257. Shalmon L, Kirschmann C, Zaizov R. A new deletional α-thalassemia detected in Yemenites with hemoglobin H disease. *Am J Hematol.* 1994;45(3):201–204.

258. Gonzalez-Redondo JM, Diaz-Chico JC, Malcorra-Azpiazu JJ, Balda-Aguirre MI, Huisman TH. Characterization of a newly discovered α-thalassaemia-1 in two Spanish patients with Hb H disease. *Br J Haematol.* 1988;70(4):459–463.

259. Viprakasit V, Kidd AM, Ayyub H, Horsley S, Hughes J, Higgs DR. *De novo* deletion within the telomeric region flanking the human α globin locus as a cause of α thalassaemia. *Br J Haematol.* 2003;120(5):867–875.

260. Romao L, Osorio-Almeida L, Higgs DR, Lavinha J, Liebhaber SA. Alpha-thalassemia resulting from deletion of regulatory sequences far upstream of the α-globin structural genes. *Blood.* 1991;78(6):1589–1595.

261. Wilkie AO, Lamb J, Harris PC, Finney RD, Higgs DR. A truncated human chromosome 16 associated with α thalassaemia is stabilized by addition of telomeric repeat (TTAGGG)n. *Nature.* 1990;346(6287):868–871.

262. Liebhaber SA, Griese EU, Weiss I, et al. Inactivation of human α-globin gene expression by a *de novo* deletion located upstream of the α-globin gene cluster. *Proc Natl Acad Sci USA.* 1990;87(23):9431–9435.

263. Viprakasit V, Harteveld CL, Ayyub H, et al. A novel deletion causing α thalassemia clarifies the importance of the major human α globin regulatory element. *Blood.* 2006;107(9): 3811–3812.

14

The Pathophysiology and Clinical Features of α Thalassemia

Douglas R. Higgs

INTRODUCTION

The primary abnormality in patients with α thalassemia is the underproduction of α-globin chains. Important secondary effects occur because of the continued production of excess γ chains in fetal life, which form the $\gamma 4$ tetramer (Hb Bart's) and excess β-chains in adult life producing a $\beta 4$ tetramer (HbH). Excess, unmatched non-α-globin chains damage the developing erythroid precursors, giving rise to intramedullary hemolysis or ineffective erythropoiesis. In addition, the presence of Hb Bart's and HbH cause premature destruction of mature red cells, giving rise to the predominant pathophysiology of α thalassemia that involves extravascular hemolysis.[1]

As set out in Chapter 13 and http://globin.bx.psu.edu/hbvar/[2] we currently know of approximately 80 mutations associated with α^+ thalassemia and approximately 40 that cause α^0 thalassemia. There are potentially several hundred different interactions that could take place between the large numbers of determinants described. Phenotypically, these interactions result in one of three broad categories; α thalassemia trait, in which there are mild hematological changes but no major clinical abnormalities, HbH disease, and the Hb Bart's hydrops fetalis syndrome. We shall consider each of these in this chapter.

The information set out in Chapter 13 suggests that the α thalassemia determinants can be arranged in the order of their severity (from $\alpha\alpha$ to --) as shown in Table 14.1. In general the phenotypes resulting from their interactions correlate well with the reduction in α-chain synthesis predicted for each mutation. Although this scheme accurately predicts the outcome of interactions between chromosomes in which α-chain synthesis is abolished (α^0 thalassemia) or reduced (α^+ thalassemia) by a simple deletion, the pathophysiology and consequent hematological effects appear more complex and less predictable when nondeletional defects are involved. One might expect that nondeletional defects affecting the $\alpha 2$ gene would cause a greater reduction in α-globin synthesis than those affecting the $\alpha 1$ gene (see Chapter 13) and in general this appears to be so. Aberrantly processed mRNA or structurally abnormal globin chains may, however, have additional deleterious effects on erythropoiesis and red cell metabolism, producing a more severe effect on phenotype than would be predicted simply from the associated reduction in normal α-globin chain synthesis.

α THALASSEMIA TRAIT

The term α thalassemia trait describes a spectrum of phenotypes spanning the clinical and hematological gap between normal individuals and those with HbH disease (discussed later). Such individuals usually originate from tropical or subtropical regions of the world (see Chapter 26) and have a hypochromic, microcytic blood picture with a normal or slightly reduced level of HbF and HbA_2. The main differential diagnosis is from iron deficiency, the anemia of chronic disorders, the "low HbA_2" types of β thalassemia trait (see Chapter 16) and, rarely, sideroblastic anemia. In addition to the hypochromic microcytic red cell indices,[3] characteristic, diagnostic features of α thalassemia trait include a raised level of Hb Bart's ($\gamma 4$) at birth,[4,5] the presence of HbH ($\beta 4$) inclusions in adults (first reported in ref. 6, 7) and the demonstration of a reduced α/β-globin chain synthesis ratio.[8] Unfortunately, these diagnostic parameters fail to identify a significant proportion of carriers for α thalassemia and discriminate poorly between carriers with different molecular defects. Before the application of molecular biology to this problem (around 1980) these 'blunt' diagnostic tools produced a huge amount of confusing literature on the distribution, frequency and genetics of α thalassemia reviewed in Weatherall and Clegg.[9]

The geographical distribution and frequency of α thalassemia are now well documented (Chapter 26) and knowing the ethnic origin of any individual under investigation provides an important initial guide to the potential types of α thalassemia that may be present. We know that α thalassemia trait most frequently results from interactions between a normal haplotype, $\alpha\alpha$, and one of the α^0 or α^+ thalassemia defects.[10] α Thalassemia trait also occurs in some homozygotes and compound heterozygotes for α^+ thalassemia (e.g., $-\alpha/-\alpha$, $-\alpha/\alpha^T\alpha$ and some $\alpha^T\alpha/\alpha^T\alpha$).

α/β-Globin mRNA and Globin Synthesis Ratios in α Thalassemia Trait

Experiments using heterologous cell-free assays consistently show that mRNA from the reticulocytes of patients with α thalassemia direct the synthesis of less α- than β-globin.[11–14] Subsequently, it has been shown that this results from under representation of accumulated mRNA in most determinants of α thalassemia.[15–18] Hunt et al.[19] were the first to analyze the α/β-globin mRNA ratios in carriers of α thalassemia and although the precise genotypes of the

Table 14.1. Ineractions producing the phenotype of α thalassemia

			α^+				α^0	
		αα	$\alpha\alpha^T$	-α	$\alpha^T\alpha$	$-\alpha^T$	(αα)	--
α^0	--	T	H	H	H,Hy			Hy
	(αα)	T		H				
α^+	$-\alpha^T$	T		H	T	H		
	$\alpha^T\alpha$	T		T	H, Hy			
	-α	T		T				
	$\alpha\alpha^T$	T						
	αα	N						

N = nonthalassemic; T = α thalassemia trait; H = HbH disease; Hy = Bart's hydrops fetails syndrome.

patients studied were not known, they demonstrated clear differences between normal individuals and obligate carriers of α thalassemia (Fig. 14.1).

Subsequently studies using reverse transcription polymerase chain reaction (PCR)–based quantitation of α- and β-globin mRNA in patients with accurately known genotypes have confirmed these observations.[20,21] Although Hunt et al.[19] showed no overlap in the α/β-globin mRNA ratios of normal individuals and those with α thalassemia

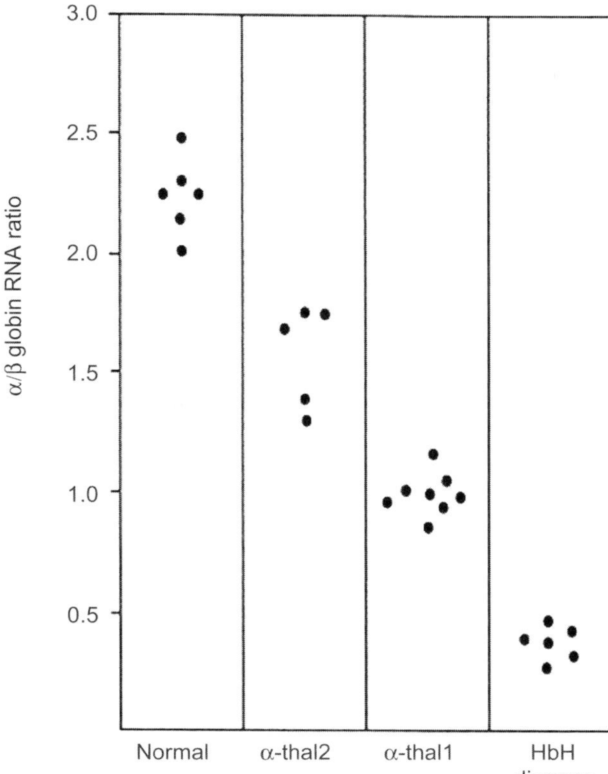

Figure 14.1. α/β-Globin-specific RNA ratios determined by cDNA hybridization with total RNA prepared from the peripheral blood of nonthalassemic individuals or obligate carriers with mild (α^+ thalassemia) or severe (α^0 thalassemia) α thalassemia trait or HbH disease. (The data are redrawn from ref. 19.)

trait, other studies demonstrated wider variation.[20,21] Nevertheless, Smetanina et al.[21] confirmed that the α/β-globin mRNA ratios of patients with two functional α genes (-α/-α and --/αα) are quite distinct from those of nonthalassemic individuals (αα/αα).

The α/β-globin chain biosynthesis ratios in patients with well-defined α-globin genotypes, measured by *in vitro* hemoglobin synthesis[8,22–24] broadly reflect the α/β-globin mRNA ratios (Fig. 14.2 and Table 14.2). Again carriers of α thalassemia with two functional α genes (-α/-α and --/αα) can be clearly distinguished from normal individuals (αα/αα).

It is interesting that the same trends in α/β-globin mRNA, globin synthesis, and hematological indices (see later) are seen when comparing individuals with four, three, or two functional α genes. In each case individuals with two α genes can be clearly distinguished from those with four genes. The values in those with three genes (-α/αα) overlap the two groups but are more closely related to those with four genes (αα/αα).

At present mRNA and globin synthesis ratios have been evaluated in relatively few patients with nondeletional determinants of α thalassemia. Nevertheless, one would predict that α/β mRNA ratios might be a poor way to evaluate such patients because, in some instances, the red cell precursors will contain nonfunctional mRNA and in many cases structurally abnormal mRNA and globin chains may be metabolized in quite complex ways during erythroid maturation.

All of these observations highlight the absolute necessity for accurate genotype analysis (see Chapter 13) when evaluating and counseling individuals with α thalassemia trait.

Red Cell Indices and Hematological Findings in α Thalassemia Trait

In the following discussion we will first consider the effect of α-globin deletions on red cell indices, comparing normal individuals (αα/αα) and those with α thalassemia trait (-α/αα, -α/-α and -/αα). As discussed in Ganczakowski et al.[25] and Williams et al.[26] we make no distinction between the $-\alpha^{3.7}$ and $-\alpha^{4.2}$ defects. Although the hematological effects of such deletions will be illustrated by reference to specific studies, it is important to remember that these measurements can vary from one normal (αα/αα) population to another,[27] and, in practice, slight variations may also be obtained even in healthy, nonthalassemic individuals.[28]

Unbalanced globin synthesis in α thalassemia leads to a deficiency in the amount of Hb per cell and because Hb accounts for 30%–35% of the red cell content the red cell volume is also reduced producing hypochromic, microcytic cells with an increased surface area to volume ratio (hence target cells). In general, individuals with α thalassemia trait

Table 14.2. Hematological data for Mendelian a thalassemia

α Globin Genotype	Age (y)		Hemoglobin (g/dL)			RBC ($\times 10^{12}$/L)			MCV (fL)	MCH (pg)	% HbH	α/β ratio
			M		F	M		F				
αα/αα	1–4	N		–			–		–	–	–	
		μ		12.6			4.55		79	27.5	0	
		SD		0.8			0.35		4	2.0	–	
	5–9	N		–			–		–	–	–	
		μ		13.2			4.6		81.5	28.5	0	
		SD		0.8			0.3		4	2.0	–	
	10–15	N		–			–		–	–	–	
		μ		13.9			4.7		84	29.5	0	
		SD		1.0			0.3		4.5	2.0	–	
	≥16	N	–		–	–		–	–	–	–	27
		μ	15.5		14.0	5.2		4.6	90	30	0	1.06
		SD	1.0		1.0	0.35		0.3	5	2.0	–	0.11
--α/αα	1–4	N		55			52		55	52	–	
		μ		10.9			4.74		73.0	23.2	0	
		SD		1.2			0.53		6.4	2.5	–	
	5–9	N		49			49		49	49	–	
		μ		11.8			4.87		76.4	24.5	0	
		SD		0.86			0.50		5.6	2.2	–	
	10–15	N		42			42		42	42	–	
		μ		12.5			5.00		80.2	25.2	0	
		SD		1.2			0.48		6.1	1.8	–	
	≥16	N	81		106	77		102	191	184	–	29
		μ	14.3		12.6	5.42		4.88	81.2	26.2	0	0.87
		SD	1.4		1.2	0.58		0.53	6.9	2.3	–	0.12
$\alpha^T\alpha$/αα	10–15	N		4			4		4	4	–	
		μ		12.8			5.3		71.7	24.2	0	
		SD		0.2			0.26		2.4	1.3	–	
	≥16	N	22		17	21		17	39	38	–	12
		μ	14.5		12.5	5.76		5.21	75.5	24.8	0	0.75
		SD	0.9		0.6	0.49		0.50	4.68	1.7	–	0.12
-α/-α	1–4	N		10			10		10	10	–	
		μ		10.1			5.08		63.0	19.9	0	
		SD		1.7			0.30		6.1	6.1	–	
	5–9	N		7			7		7	7	–	
		μ		10.8			5.0		66.2	21.5	0	
		SD		1.4			0.5		3.0	0.9	–	
	10–15	N		14			14		14	14	–	
		μ		12.0			5.47		72.1	22.1	0	
		SD		0.9			0.49		8.7	2.3	–	
	≥16	N	31		45	30		45	77	75	–	8
		μ	13.9		12.0	5.98		5.30	71.6	22.9	0	0.72
		SD	1.7		1.0	0.81		0.49	4.1	1.3	–	0.12
--/αα	1–4	N		6			5		6	5	–	
		μ		11.2			5.79		60.7	19.6	0	
		SD		0.6			0.58		4.9	1.2	–	
	5–9	N		8			7		8	7	–	
		μ		11.0			5.47		62.5	20.3	0	
		SD		0.8			0.48		3.4	0.8	–	
	10–15	N		13			14		14	13	–	
		μ		12.2			5.83		67.5	21.4	0	
		SD		1.0			0.70		3.4	1.8	–	

α Globin Genotype	Age (y)		Hemoglobin (g/dL) M	Hemoglobin (g/dL) F	RBC (× 10^{12}/L) M	RBC (× 10^{12}/L) F	MCV (fL)	MCH (pg)	% HbH	α/β ratio
	≥16	N	63	83	54	71	145	130	–	31
		μ	13.7	12.1	6.28	5.65	69.1	21.7	0	0.65
		SD	1.1	1.1	0.63	0.49	4.4	1.7	–	0.12
$\alpha^T\alpha$/-α	1–4	N	1		1		1	1	–	
		μ	10.8		5.78		59	18.7	0	
		SD	–		–		–	–	–	
	5–9	N	1		1		1	1	–	
		μ	11.4		5.79		60.2	19.7	0	
		SD	–		–		–	–	–	
	≥16	N	6	6	5	6	12	12	–	4
		μ	12.3	10.6	5.78	5.10	66.1	21.0	0	0.8
		SD	1.05	0.65	0.80	0.37	3.3	1.5	–	0.06
$\alpha^T\alpha/\alpha^T\alpha$	1–4	N	2		2		2	2	2	
		μ	7.9		4.25		63.3	18.9	14.2	
		SD	3.2		2.30		2.9	2.8	5.3	
	5–9	N	1		1		1	1	1	
		μ	6.9		3.5		68	19.7	8.4	
		SD	–		–		–	–	–	
	10–15	N	3		3		3	3	3	
		μ	10.7		5.97		58.3	17.8	7.6	
		SD	2.8		0.82		5.7	2.8	8.0	
	≥16	N	2	3	2	3	6	6	5	5
		μ	11.2	9.9	5.82	5.21	60.5	18.9	10.5	0.47
		SD	0.5	1.4	0.35	0.56	4.77	1.2	7.6	0.18
-α/--	1–4	N	17		16		17	16	13	
		μ	9.6		5.77		57.7	17.0	5.7	
		SD	0.8		0.66		8.5	2.2	3.4	
	5–9	N	11		11		11	11	10	
		μ	9.6		5.52		58.7	17.7	4.8	
		SD	0.8		0.86		6.4	2.5	4.0	
	10–15	N	19		18		19	18	15	
		μ	9.5		5.47		59.3	17.7	5.1	
		SD	0.8		0.76		5.6	1.3	2.4	
	≥16	N	28	59	24	58	121	120	110	32
		μ	11.1	9.4	6.10	5.14	64.8	19.1	7.0	0.44
		SD	1.1	1.2	0.82	0.78	7.2	2.3	4.8	0.20
$\alpha^T\alpha$/--	1–4	N	4		3		4	3	3	
		μ	7.8		5.16		67.4	16.6	19.6	
		SD	1.4		1.13		16.7	5.3	2.1	
	5–9	N	8		8		8	8	8	
		μ	8.8		4.69		66.6	19.3	13.4	
		SD	1.9		1.23		7.7	2.5	7.2	
	10–15	N	8		8		8	8	8	
		μ	9.2		5.03		66.1	17.8	22.8	
		SD	0.9		0.49		3.4	1.5	3.5	
	≥16	N	6	5	3	5	14	14	13	17
		μ	10.5	8.5	5.10	4.68	68.0	18.7	22.3	0.32
		SD	1.0	0.7	0.31	0.66	5.9	1.5	6.5	0.15

The number of samples (N), mean (μ), and unbiased estimate of the standard deviation (SD) are shown for the nine possible combinations of the αα, -α, α^T α and -- genotypes (excluding --/--), in increasing order of severity, for the age groups (years) 1–4, 5–9, 10–15, and ≥16 (adult). (The normal data are derived from refs. 240–242; the principal sources for the α thalassemia data are described in the text. In addition to the unpublished datasets acknowledged in ref. 10 further valuable series were contributed by CC Thompson (Hamilton, Ontario) and T Sophocleous (Nicosia).) Because of significant sex differences, the hemoglobin and RBC counts are tabulated separately for adult men and women; although both MCV and MCH tend to be slightly higher in males than females, the relative differences are much smaller (~1 fL and ~0.5 pg, respectively), so these data are pooled, as are the α/β-globin chain synthesis ratios for all ages.

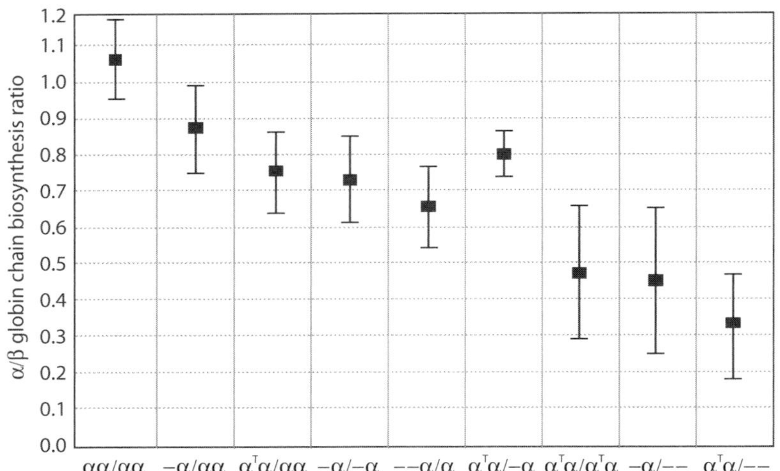

Figure 14.2. The α/β-globin chain biosynthesis ratios in individuals with well-defined α-globin genotypes. (Data derived from the references in the legend to Table 14.2.)

due to simple gene deletions (-α/αα, -α/-α and --/αα) have lower levels of total hemoglobin, mean corpuscular hemoglobin concentration (MCHC), mean corpuscular volume (MCV), and mean corpuscular hemoglobin (MCH) but higher red blood cell (RBC) counts than nonthalassemic (αα/αα) individuals (Table 14.2 and Fig. 14.3).

The degree of abnormality varies from one parameter to another. The greatest differences are seen in MCH (Figs. 14.3 and 14.4); individuals with α thalassemia clearly make less hemoglobin per cell than normal individuals. Despite this, patients with α thalassemia trait maintain adequate hemoglobin levels (within ~1.0–1.5 g/dL of normal) at all stages of development (Figs. 14.3 and 14.4). It appears that the main compensatory mechanism for the underproduction of hemoglobin in each red cell occurs via an increase in the concentration of red cells (RBC count) maintained in the peripheral blood.

Developmental changes in the hematological indices of individuals with α thalassemia trait follow the same patterns as those of normal individuals (αα/αα). Hemoglobin, hematocrit, MCH, and MCV fall rapidly after birth and begin to rise slowly in the second year. The RBC count is relatively low at birth and then rises slowly. Throughout development one can clearly distinguish the hematological indices found in patients with the αα/αα, -α/αα, and -α/-α genotypes. For all parameters there is a greater difference between those with the -α/-α and -α/αα genotypes and those with the -α/αα and αα/αα genotypes. The smaller data set for individuals with the --/αα genotype most closely resembles those with -α/-α genotype. Few differences are seen between males and females prior to puberty after which there are significant sex-dependent differences in both hemoglobin and RBC count in all genotypic groups (Fig. 14.4).

At present there are insufficient developmental data to extend these conclusions to all determinants of α thalassemia. There is now, however, adequate information to compare hematological indices in adults with various interactions that produce α thalassemia trait (Fig. 14.3). Although there is a good correlation between the predicted reduction in α-chain synthesis and hemoglobin, MCV, and MCH, there is considerable overlap. Therefore these indices are of only limited value in distinguishing one genotype from another. It is clear that with the exception of the -α/αα genotype and some carriers of nondeletional mutations[29] most carriers of deletional types of α thalassemia can be distinguished from normal individuals on the basis of their MCH, which is usually less than 26 pg and always below 27 pg (refs. 10, 30, 31 and Table 14.2).

The peripheral blood film in patients with α thalassemia trait is quite variable from one genotype to another but often shows hypochromasia, with occasional poikilocytes and target cells (Fig 14.5). The reticulocyte count is usually raised to 2%–3% in patients with the severe forms of α thalassemia trait. Rees et al.[32] have shown that the levels of soluble serum transferrin receptors (sTfR), which reflect the erythroid cell mass, are raised in individuals with α thalassemia trait (-α/αα and -α/-α). They concluded that even patients with minimal globin chain imbalance have significant ineffective erythropoiesis and/or hemolysis. Red cell survival and erythrokinetic studies have not been performed in many cases of α thalassemia trait. In general, ^{51}Cr-labeled red cells from patients with α thalassemia have a shortened red cell half-life in the circulation,[33] and specifically, red cell ^{51}Cr half-life estimates in two cases of α thalassemia trait reported by Wasi et al.[34] were 25 days and 29.5 days (normal range 25–30 d).

Hemoglobin Analysis in α Thalassemia Trait

The patterns of hemoglobin seen in adult individuals with α thalassemia trait are indistinguishable from those seen in normal individuals, although as a group they may have slightly lower levels of HbA_2. Based on a small survey,[35] there appeared to be no significant differences throughout development in the levels of HbA_2 and HbF between individuals with the αα/αα, -α/αα, and -α/-α genotypes (Fig. 14.6a).

Prior to the application of molecular genetic methods to the diagnosis of α thalassemia there was good evidence that a raised level of Hb Bart's (γ4) in the neonatal period (Fig. 14.7) indicated the presence of α thalassemia;[5] this was reviewed in Wasi et al.[34] It was not clear, however, if normal individuals (αα/αα) produced Hb Bart's at birth or if all individuals with α thalassemia had a raised level of Hb Bart's at birth. Furthermore, the relationship between the amount of Hb Bart's and the underlying molecular defect was not known. These issues have now been evaluated in

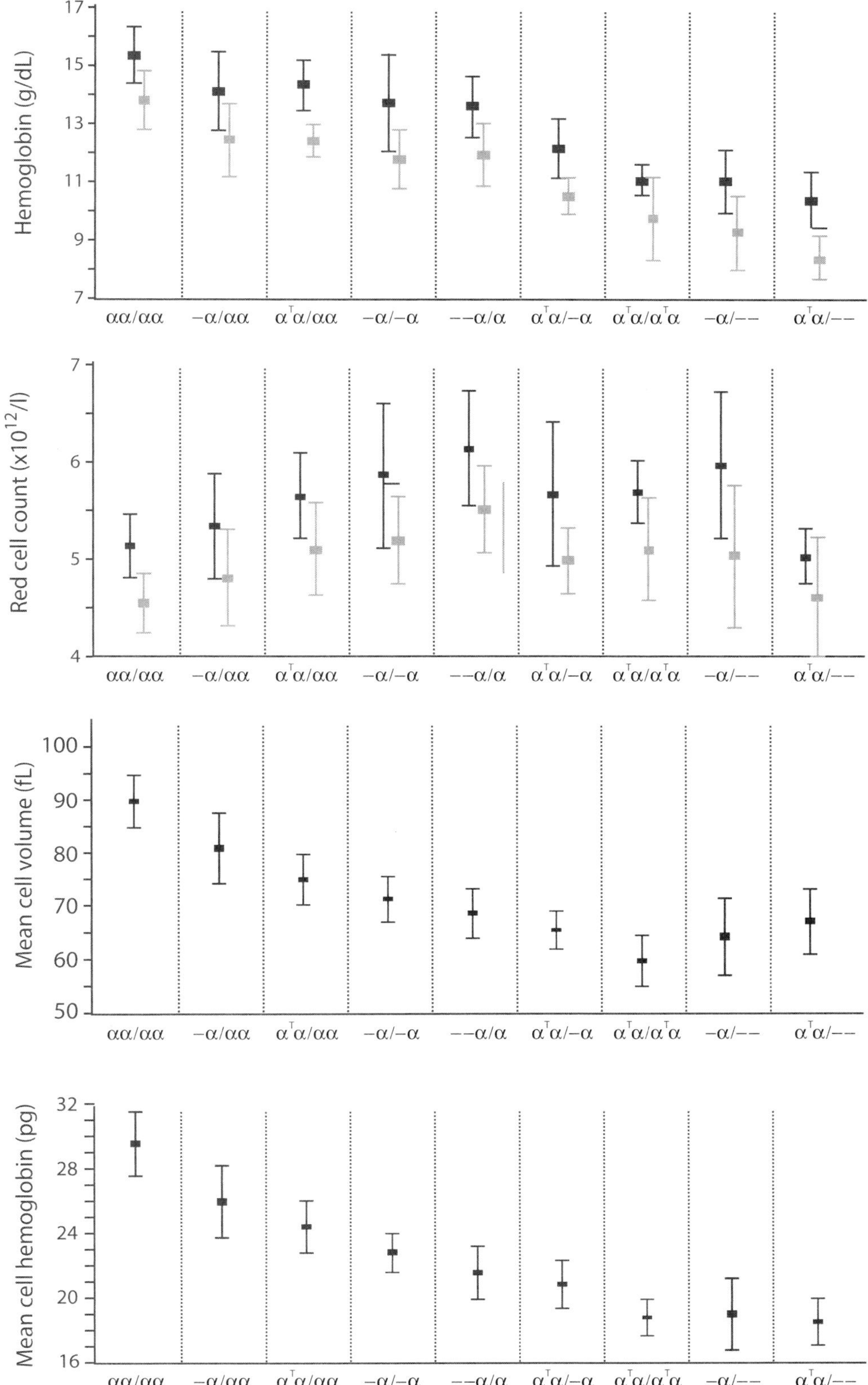

Figure 14.3. The RBC indices in patients with various genotypes associated with α thalassemia. For each set of data the mean and 1 SD is shown. For the level of hemoglobin and estimates of RBC count, differences between males (solid lines) and females (gray lines) are shown. (Data are from ref. 239.)

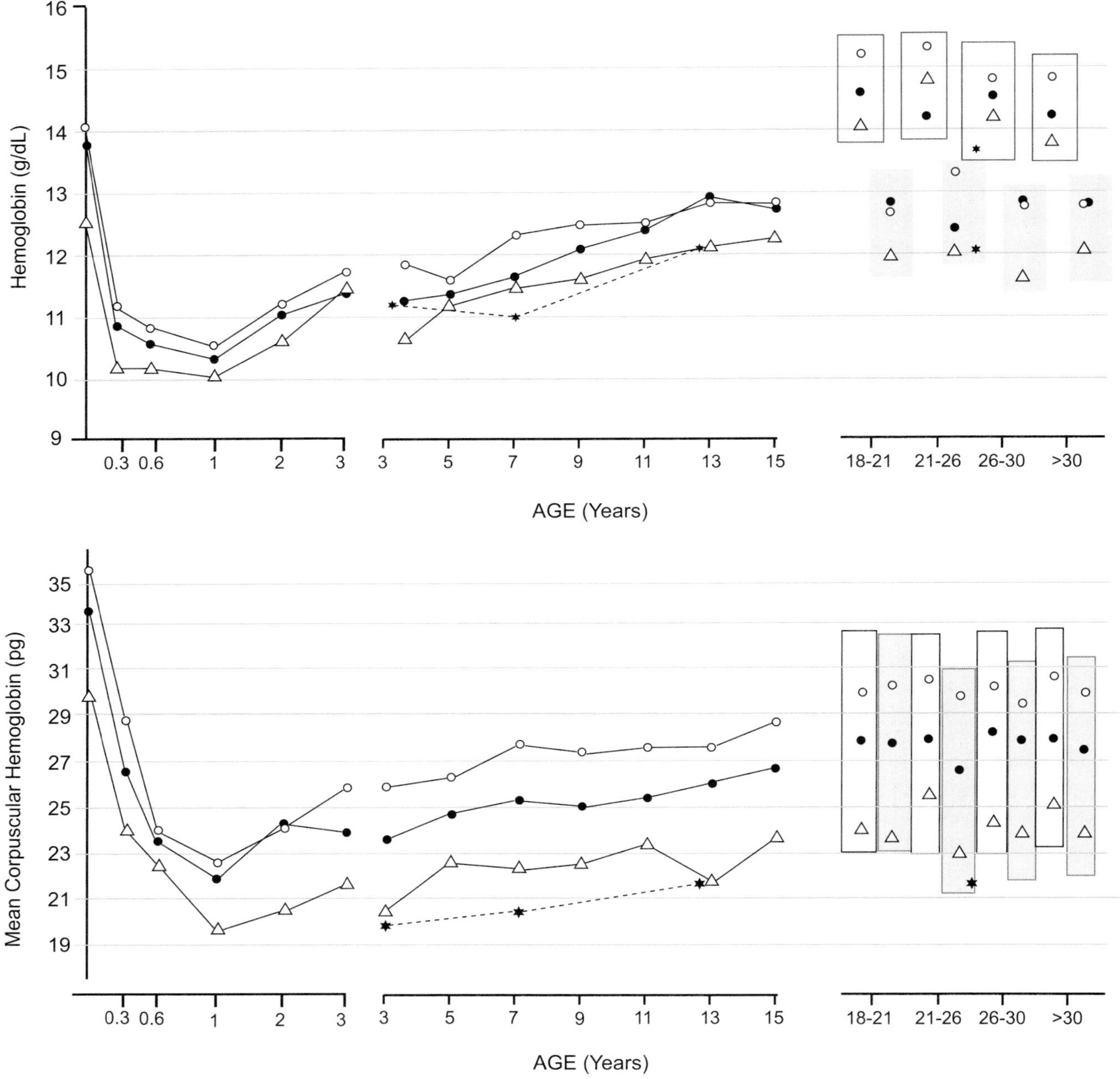

Figure 14.4. Developmental changes in the level of hemoglobin (above) and MCH (below) in individuals with the αα/αα (○), -α/αα (•), -α/-α (△), and –/αα (∗) genotypes. Beyond the age of 15 years results are grouped into males (hatched surround) and females (stippled background).

many surveys correlating the level of Hb Bart's with the α-globin genotype. Most surveys using assays that are sufficiently sensitive to detect a minimum of 0.5%–1% Hb Bart's at birth, detect a large proportion of neonates with α thalassemia but may not detect all cases with the mild -α/αα interaction.[36] Therefore, surveys based solely on the presence of Hb Bart's in the cord blood may underestimate the frequency of α thalassemia. More recent surveys have confirmed that the level of Hb Bart's correlates well with the α globin genotype and that this provides a useful screening tool for α thalassemia.[37,38] Although the levels of Hb Bart's are generally related to the degree of α-chain deficit they do not accurately distinguish the various α genotypes.

During the first 6 months after birth, the level of Hb Bart's in individuals with α thalassemia declines (Fig. 14.6b) and eventually becomes undetectable by conventional assays,[5] although minute amounts may be detected in adults with α thalassemia by using an immunological assay.[39] Similarly small amounts of embryonic ζ-globin chains can be detected (using an enzyme-linked

(a)

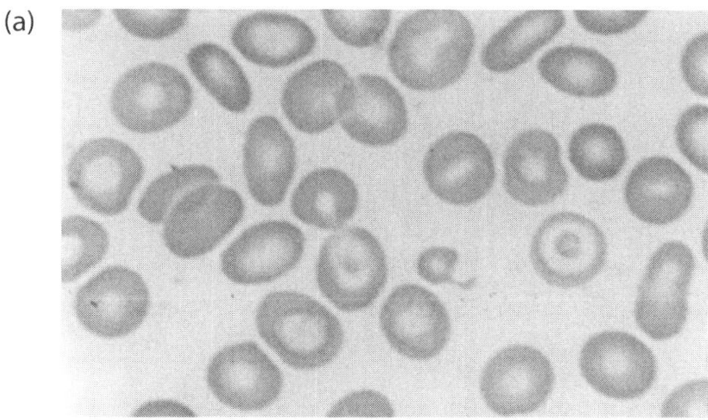

(b)

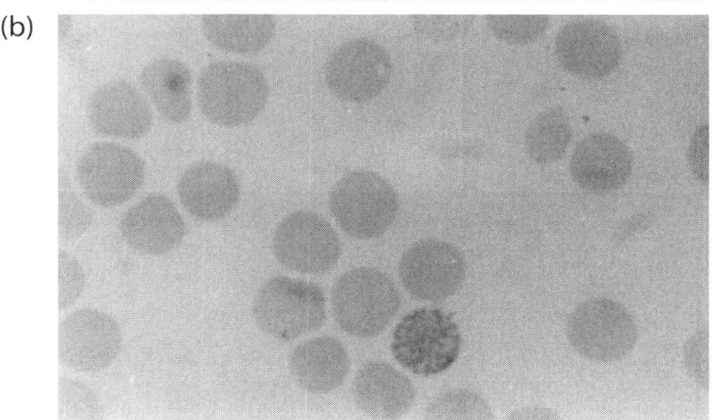

(c)

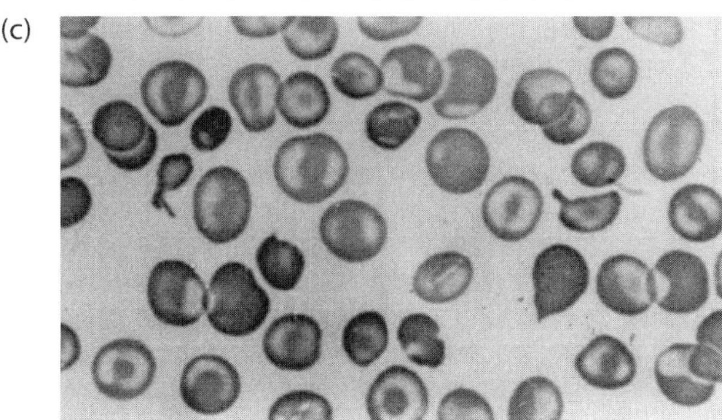

(d)

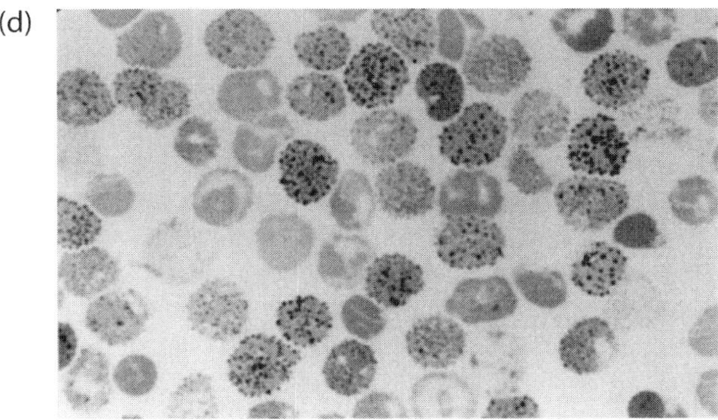

Figure 14.5. Typical hematological findings in patients with α thalassemia trait **(a)** and HbH disease **(c)**. Rare HbH inclusions may be found in patients with α thalassemia trait **(b)**, whereas they are commonly found in patients with HbH disease **(d)**.

immunosorbent assay) in some adults with α thalassemia.[40] It is now clear that this detects a significant proportion of individuals with the - ^{SEA}/αα genotype and could be used as a simple way of detecting carriers of this specific mutation (but no others).[41]

Unfortunately, from a diagnostic point of view, Hb Bart's is not replaced by an equivalent amount of HbH in adults; however, occasional cells containing HbH can be detected (Fig. 14.5) in up to 65% of individuals with α thalassemia trait.[42] In our experience using the standard HbH preparations,[43] inclusions are usually found in individuals with α thalassemia trait due to the --/αα, $\alpha^T\alpha$/αα, -α/$\alpha^T\alpha$, $\alpha^T\alpha$/$\alpha^T\alpha$, and (αα)/αα genotypes but very rarely in those with the -α/αα and -α/-α genotypes (for example see Lafferty et al.[41] and unpublished). Various modifications of the standard HbH preparation may significantly increase the sensitivity of this assay. This is fully discussed in Sabath et al.[44]

α Thalassemia commonly occurs in areas where β-globin variants (e.g., HbS, HbC, and HbE) are also found at a high frequency. The presence of α thalassemia can alter the proportion of variant hemoglobin found in the peripheral blood and therefore, when α thalassemia coexists with β variants the proportion of hemoglobin variant can be a sensitive guide to the presence of α thalassemia (see Chapter 26 and later). In regions where both β thalassemia and α thalassemia are common some individuals with microcytosis and a raised level of HbA_2 may concomitantly harbor α thalassemia.[45] Without correct diagnosis the risk of these individuals producing offspring with HbH disease or Bart's hydrops fetalis (see later) may be overlooked.[30]

Management and Genetic Counseling of α Thalassemia Trait

Individuals with α thalassemia trait are clinically normal and require no specific treatment. Nevertheless, it is important to recognize this condition to avoid unnecessary investigation of the hypochromic microcytic indices and to ensure that the patient does not receive inappropriate treatment with hematinics, which may be harmful.

A diagnosis of α thalassemia trait should be considered in any individual from tropical or subtropical areas of the world (see Chapter 26) who has a reduced MCH but a normal level of HbA_2 ($<3.5\%$) and a normal iron status: Such patients with MCH of 26 pg or less almost always have α thalassemia trait. The geographical and ethnic origin of the patient may provide an important guide to the underlying molecular defect (Chapter 13). In some patients there may be a family history of HbH disease or Hb Bart's hydrops fetalis (see later). In most (at least $>70\%$[41]) patients with α^0 thalassemia and some with α^+ thalassemia, the diagnosis can be confirmed by demonstrating HbH inclusions in the peripheral blood. In most clinical situations there is no need to pursue investigations beyond this stage because a definitive diagnosis can only be made by DNA

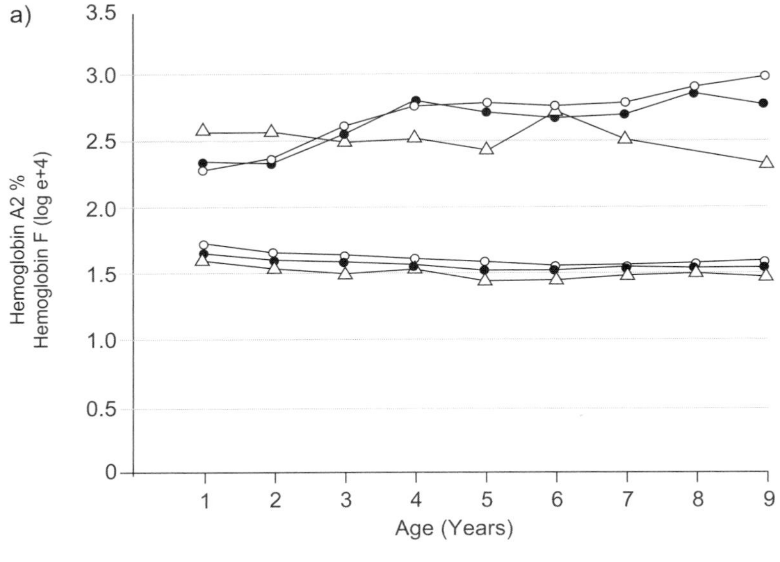

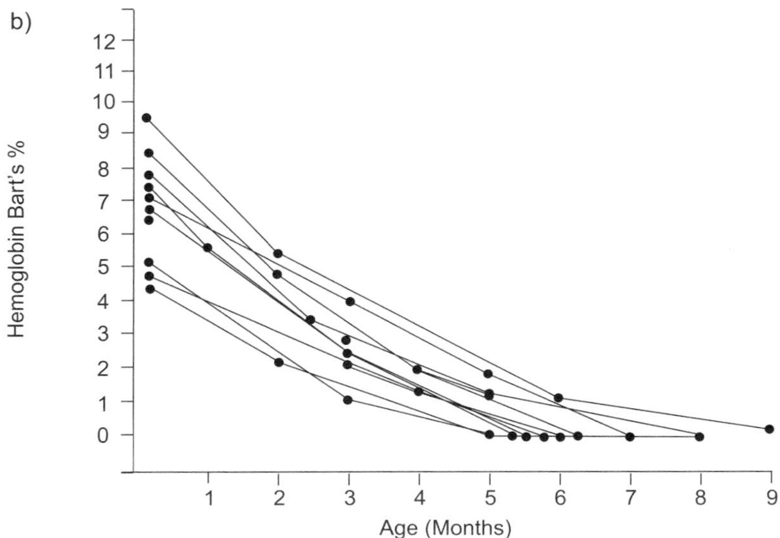

Figure 14.6. Above, developmental changes in the levels of HbA_2 (above in **a**) and HbF (below in **b**) in patients with the αα/αα (○), -α/αα (•), and -α/-α (△) genotypes (data from ref. 35). Below, developmental changes in the level of Hb Bart's in individuals with α thalassemia during the first few months of life. (Redrawn from ref. 5.)

analysis, using one or other of the PCR- and multiplex ligation–dependent probe ammplification–based protocols described in Chapter 13.

The main indication for further investigation occurs when a potential carrier of α thalassemia requires genetic counselling to avoid the Hb Bart's hydrops fetalis syndrome or, rarely, severe transfusion dependent forms of HbH disease (see later). Because resources for genetic screening are limited, efforts should be concentrated on individuals most at risk of producing infants with the Hb Bart's hydrops fetalis syndrome. Ideally, one should identify all southeast Asian women with an MCH of 26 pg or less before or soon after they become pregnant (most carriers of the common α^0 thalassemia defects will have an MCH of between 20 and 26 pg). The partners of such individuals should be screened and if they too have α thalassemia trait, with an MCH of 26 pg or less, the couple should be offered counseling and genotype analysis (see later). If resources are available this approach should be extended to individuals of Mediterranean or mixed ethnic origins who are much less commonly at risk.

α Thalassemia Trait and Pregnancy

The physiological changes of pregnancy result in an increase in plasma volume (~40%–45%) and red cell mass (20%–30%), which by the third trimester results in a variable fall in hemoglobin concentration (10.5–14.5 g/dL) even in normal women.[46] In addition increased maternal and fetal demands for hematinics (iron and folic acid) may lead to a further drop in hemoglobin if there is no supplementation. It is not surprising therefore that pregnant women with HbH disease, and to a lesser extent α thalassemia trait, may become anemic.

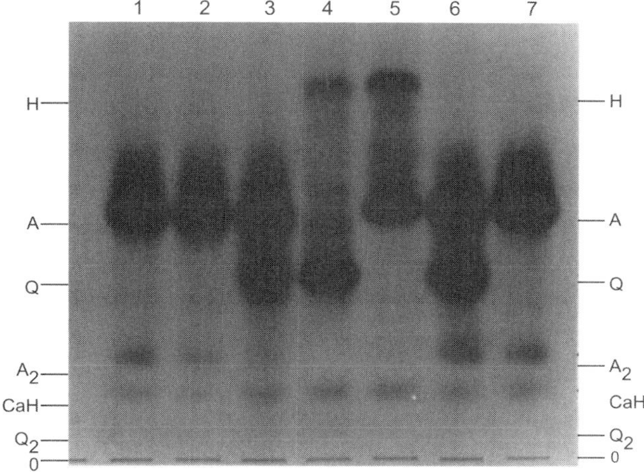

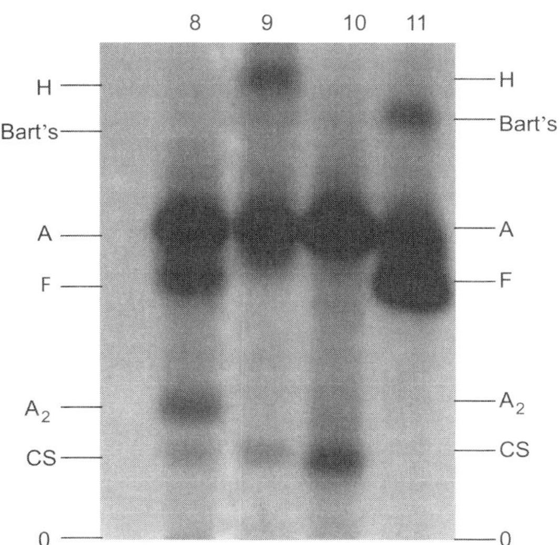

Figure 14.7. Hemoglobin electrophoresis (stained with Coomassie blue) in normal individuals (1, 2, and 7), a heterozygote for hemoglobin Q (3), hemoglobin Q-H disease (4), hemoglobin H disease (5 and 9), a heterozygote for hemoglobin S (6), a homozygote for hemoglobin Constant Spring (CS) (10), and cord blood with an elevated level of hemoglobin Bart's (11). o denotes the origin and CaH indicates the position of carbonic anhydrase.

In a prospective study of 987 pregnancies O'Donnell et al.[47] found that the median Hb concentration (and red cell indices) was significantly lower in women homozygous for α^+ thalassemia than those with a normal α-globin genotype. Similar results have been obtained by others.[48,49] M. Ganczakowski and D.K. Bowden (unpublished) studied 515 pregnant women in Vanuatu with the αα/αα (53%), -α/αα (34%), and -α/-α (13%) genotypes. The changes in hemoglobin (Fig. 14.8) and red cell indices were similar in all three groups: the greatest fall in hemoglobin (~1.4 g/dL) occurring around 30 weeks of pregnancy. Only a small proportion (6%) of women with the -α/-α genotype developed an Hb of less than 9 g/dL, which was not significantly different from those in the αα/αα group, of whom 5% developed

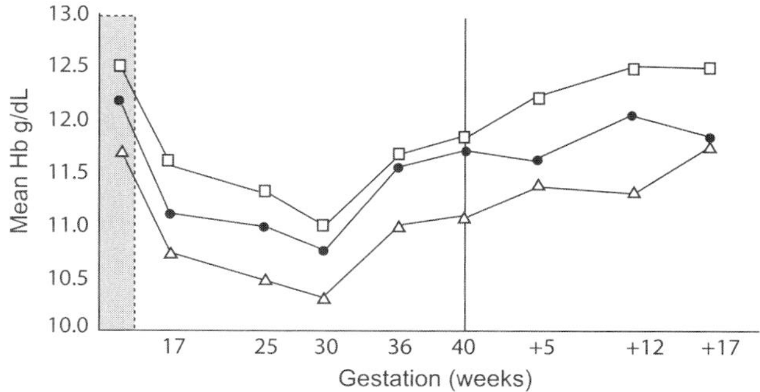

Figure 14.8. Changes in the level of hemoglobin in pregnant women with the αα/αα (□), -α/αα (•), and -α/-α (△) genotypes. Results in shaded area indicate normal values prior to pregnancy. The thick black vertical line denotes the usual time of birth (From M. Ganczakowski and D.K. Bowden, personal communication.)

an Hb below 9 g/dL. The red cell indices (MCV and MCH) showed a small increase (5%–7% of nonpregnant value) in pregnant women with α thalassemia (-α/αα and -α/-α). In none of these studies were the minor changes in hematological indices and Hb levels associated with any adverse effects on the outcome or course of pregnancy.

α THALASSEMIA CAUSING MILD HEMOLYTIC ANEMIA

As set out previously, carriers for both deletional and nondeletional forms of α thalassemia trait have hypochromic microcytic red cell indices but are asymptomatic. Some homozygotes for nondeletional α^+ thalassemia have more severely affected indices[50] but nevertheless have the phenotype of α thalassemia trait. Homozygotes for other nondeletional mutations (e.g., $\alpha^{T\ Saudi}\alpha/\alpha^{T\ Saudi}\alpha$) may have HbH disease[51] and rarely hydrops fetalis[52,53] (see Table 14.1 and later). Patients homozygous for some nondeletional mutations have a phenotype intermediate between α thalssemia trait and HbH disease with a mild hemolytic anemia; this situation has been particularly well documented in patients homozygous for the Hb Constant Spring mutation ($\alpha^{cs}\alpha/\alpha^{cs}\alpha$).

The homozygous state for Hb Constant Spring was first described by Lie-lnjo et al.[54] Since that time several homozygotes have been described[55,56] with a large survey of 22 patients presented by Pootrakul et al.[57] In this report, all of the patients had mild anemia (hemoglobin 10.3 ± 1.4 g/dL) and the majority of cases had mild jaundice with total serum bilirubin levels elevated in 8 of 14 cases examined. Splenomegaly was detectable in most cases and mild hepatomegaly was present in approximately half.

The hematological indices were very unusual for patients with α thalassemia. The RBC count was low (3.9 ± 0.9 × 10^{12}/L) with a normal mean corpuscular volume (MCV 88 ± 6 fL) and only slightly reduced MCH (26 ± 3 pg). The peripheral blood films showed mild anisocytosis and hypochromia with a few fragmented cells. Approximately 6% of the cells showed basophilic stippling and reticulocyte counts were consistently raised (6.0% ± 3.3%). Chromium-51 RBC count survival was reduced (17.3 and 20.5 days) in the two patients studied. In 6 of 15 patients studied transferrin iron saturation was greater than 50%. All of these findings suggest that these patients have a mild hemolytic anemia resulting from the attachment of partially oxidized α^{cs} chains on the red cell membrane and its cytoskeleton, which cause increased membrane rigidity and stability. Hemolysis in patients with homozygous Hb Constant Spring may be exacerbated during intercurrent infections or oxidative stress.[58]

Starch gel electrophoresis (for example see Fig. 14.7) provided conclusive evidence that these patients have α thalassemia. One newborn infant had 14.2% Hb Bart's that fell to 4.6% at 8 months.[55] In the study of Pootrakul et al.[57] seven adults had raised levels (1.8%–3.6%) of Hb Bart's and similarly raised levels have been seen in adults in other studies. The levels of Hb Constant Spring varied from 2.6% to 11.6%.

Another surprising aspect of this condition is that prolonged incubation of reticulocytes for *in vitro* globin chain synthesis revealed an α/β-globin synthesis ratio of 1.5 ± 0.16 rather than a reduced ratio as one would expect. This appears to result from the fact that globin synthesis only remains linear in the cells of $\alpha^{cs}\alpha/\alpha^{cs}\alpha$ homozygotes for approximately 30 minutes, an unexpectedly short time for samples with such a high reticulocyte count. This together with the rapid removal of excess β-globin chains accounts for the high α/β ratios observed in 2–3 hour incubations.[59] It remains to be seen if other patients, homozygous for some nondeletional forms of α thalassemia have similar findings to those with Hb Constant Spring.

HEMOGLOBIN H DISEASE

Interactions between the many determinants of α thalassemia (Table 14.1) lead to a spectrum of clinical and hematological phenotypes ranging from normal individuals to infants with the lethal, Hb Bart's hydrops fetalis syndrome. Young children (>6–12 months) and adults with sufficient globin chain imbalance to produce readily detectable levels of HbH (>1%–2%) in the peripheral blood on routine hemoglobin electrophoresis (Fig. 14.7) are said to have HbH disease. HbH inclusions are always detectable in the peripheral blood of such individuals (Fig. 14.5).

Not surprisingly, patients defined in this ad hoc way span a wide range of clinical and hematological phenotypes. The majority are clinically well and in these the epithet HbH "disease" may be inappropriate. Some have thalassemia intermedia. The most severe forms of HbH disease may be lethal late in gestation or in the perinatal period, causing a condition referred to as HbH hydrops fetalis (see later).

Extensive surveys have demonstrated that most cases of HbH disease occur in patients from southeast Asia, the Mediterranean basin, and the middle East (see Chapter 26). This geographical distribution is easily explained now that we understand the molecular basis of this disorder (Table 14.1). HbH disease most commonly results from the interaction of α^0 and α^+ thalassemia. Although α thalassemia is common throughout all tropical and subtropical regions, α^0 determinants (and hence HbH disease) are predominantly found in the Mediterranean and southeast Asia. In southeast Asia the most common genotype associated with HbH disease is $--^{SEA}/-\alpha$ whereas in the Mediterranean $--^{MED}/-\alpha$ and $-(\alpha)^{20.5}/-\alpha$ are the most frequent (reviewed in Chui et al.[1]). Less often HbH disease results from the interaction of α^0 thalassemia with nondeletional forms of α^+ thalassemia (genotype $--/\alpha^T\alpha$) or in homozygotes for some nondeletional forms of α^+ thalassemia (genotype $\alpha^T\alpha/\alpha^T\alpha$).[51,60–67] Again these molecular interactions are most frequently seen in southeast Asia and the Mediterranean but also occur at high frequencies in some areas of the middle East (see Chapter 26).

Despite these useful geographical "rules of thumb," one should be aware that patients with α thalassemia trait and HbH disease have been described in almost every racial group. On detailed examination, patients originating from regions where α thalassemia is otherwise rare are often found to have unusual and biologically interesting molecular defects.

The Pathophysiology of HbH Disease

In HbH disease there is a moderately severe reduction in α globin RNA and α globin chain synthesis (see later). During fetal life excess γ chains form γ_4 tetramers (Hb Bart's). Similarly, in adults (after the γ to β switch, Chapter 5) excess β-globin chains form $\beta 4$ tetramers (HbH). Both of these homotetramers have high oxygen affinity, lack heme–heme interaction, and do not exhibit any Bohr shift.[68] Therefore, neither of these hemoglobins contributes to oxygen transport and their presence compounds the effects of anemia in patients with HbH disease. The reduced synthesis of HbA together with the production of nonfunctional Hb thus cause anemia and provoke an appropriate response of an increased level of erythropoietin.[62,69]

A second component of the pathophysiology arises from the fact that HbH is unstable and when oxidized forms intracellular precipitates, which cause cell death in a proportion of erythroblasts leading to ineffective erythropoiesis. This is reflected in an increase in the level of serum transferrin receptors (sTfR) reflecting the increased number of erythroid precursors in the bone marrow.[62,69] Thirdly, and most importantly, when HbH precipitates it attaches to the cell membrane in circulating red cells as they age. This in turn causes local oxidative damage and membrane dysfunction. Thus the erythrocytes in HbH disease are rigid and their membrane is more stable than normal.[70,71] Loss of normal membrane phospholipid asymmetry, exposure of phosphatidylserine, and the presence of increased amounts of Immunoglobulin G on the cell surface may also enhance the engulfment of abnormal, ageing red cells by macrophages. Together these properties are thought to slow the passage of red cells through the microvasculature and promote erythrophagocytosis causing extravascular hemolysis, which is reflected in an increase in the reticulocyte count.[62,69,72,73]

The red cell survival, as judged by ^{51}Cr studies is reduced in patients with HbH disease; reported figures range from 8–17 days.[74–77] External scanning indicates that most of the red cell destruction occurs in the spleen.[76,77] Srichaikul et al.[78] performed full erythrokinetic studies on nine, nonsplenectomized patients with HbH disease. They demonstrated a reduced red cell volume, increased plasma volume, and a reduced red cell survival of 6–19.5 days (normal range 25–32 days) with sequestration of ^{51}Cr-labeled red cells in the liver and spleen. In addition they showed that patients with HbH disease have a rapid clearance of ^{59}Fe with relatively good ^{59}Fe incorporation into red cells compared with patients with β thalassemia. They also found that the patient's hematocrit was correlated to the red cell survival. Together these findings suggest that both hemolysis and ineffective erythropoiesis contribute to anemia in HbH disease but most studies have concluded that the predominant mechanism is extravascular hemolysis.

α/β mRNA and Globin Synthesis Ratios in Patients with HbH Disease

As one would expect from the studies of α/β mRNA ratios in carriers of α thalassemia (see previously), the red cell precursors of patients with HbH disease contain approximately one half to one quarter of the amount of α-globin mRNA present in normal red cell precursors[11,16,19,21] as demonstrated in Figure 14.1. Again this is generally reflected in the α/β-globin chain synthesis ratios of patients with the deletional forms of HbH disease (average of 0.44, standard deviation 0.2, see Table 14.2 and Fig. 14.2. Also see Kanavakis et al.[62]). Excess β-globin chains synthesized during erythroid maturation mainly form β4 tetramers but in addition supply a small intracellular pool of β-chains that combine with newly synthesized α chains as they become available. Nevertheless, it is clear that HbH is not present in the peripheral blood in amounts reflecting the rate at which it is synthesized indicating that it must be lost from the red cells while they are in the circulation consistent with the pathophysiology set out previously.

Red Cell Indices and Hematological Findings in HbH Disease

As before, we will first consider the effect of α-globin deletions on red cell indices, comparing individuals with one functional α gene (--/-α) with normal individuals (αα/αα). Those who inherit only a single α gene have lower levels of total hemoglobin, MCH and MCV but higher RBC counts than nonthalassemic (αα/αα) individuals (Table 14.2 and Fig. 14.3). Similar trends have been shown by others.[1,62,73] These differences in hematological indices are seen at all stages of development (see Table 14.2) although at present there are only anecdotal data on infants with HbH disease in the perinatal period or during the early months of life.[73,79] Perhaps the most important hematological finding is that, using data accumulated from a variety of surveys (see Table 14.2) patients with HbH disease are anemic with, on average, approximately 2-g/dL less hemoglobin than age and sex matched normal individuals. It has been noted in some surveys that there may be striking fluctuations in the level of hemoglobin measured sequentially in the same individual over the course of 1–2 years,[34,80] although in our experience, and that of others[73] this is not common.

The peripheral blood film shows hypochromia and polychromasia with variable anisopoikilocytosis and target cells (Fig. 14.5). The reticulocyte count is usually raised to approximately 3%–6%, although higher counts may be observed.[72,73,81] Nucleated red cells and basophilic stippling may be present[34] but in our more limited experience this is quite rare.

Although bone marrow examination is rarely necessary in the investigation of patients with HbH disease, when analyzed it shows erythroid hyperplasia with only slight or absent deposition of hemosiderin.[34] The erythroid hyperplasia is reflected increased levels of sTfR in the peripheral blood.[62,69]

Over the past 10–15 years the precise genotype of many patients with HbH disease has been established. In addition to the common deletional forms (--/-α) discussed previously, HbH disease may also result from interactions involving nondeletional determinants (--/$\alpha^T\alpha$ and $\alpha^T\alpha/\alpha^T\alpha$). Using data from several studies (Table 14.2 and Fig. 14.3), patients with nondeletional HbH disease and the $\alpha^T\alpha/\alpha^T\alpha$ genotype have hematological indices that are similar to those with the deletional type of HbH disease (--/-α), whereas those with the --/$\alpha^T\alpha$ are slightly more anemic with lower RBC counts and higher MCVs (Table 14.2 and refs. 1, 72, 73, 82). Limited data (Table 14.2) indicate that these differences are present throughout development.

Several studies have compared the hematological findings in patients with deletional forms of HbH disease (--/-α) and those with specific nondeletional defects including [--/$\alpha^{CS}\alpha$] (HbH-Constant Spring),[72,79,83] [--/$\alpha^{Nco}\alpha$] and [--/$\alpha^{Hph}\alpha$][61,73,84] and anecdotally many other rarer mutations (reviewed in refs. 1, 73). In all of these nondeletional genotypes one finds lower levels of hemoglobin and RBC counts but higher MCVs than in patients with the pure deletional types of HbH disease.

Hemoglobin Analysis in HbH Disease

Infants who go on to develop HbH disease later in life produce large amounts (19%–27%) of Hb Bart's (γ4) at birth.[34,85,86] During the first few months of development Hb Bart's falls and is replaced by variable amounts of HbH in adult life. The level of Hb Bart's at birth often exceeds that of HbH in adult life. This is consistent with other observations[87] showing that HbH (β_4) is less stable than Hb Bart's ($\gamma 4$). Adults with HbH disease have 0.8–40% HbH in the peripheral blood. It has been consistently noted that patients with the nondeletional type of HbH disease (--/$\alpha^T\alpha$) produce larger amounts of HbH.[1,61,62,72,73,88,89] Hb Bart's may still be detected in some adults with HbH disease but HbH usually predominates; occasionally the fetal pattern, with an excess of Hb Bart's, persists.[90] The reasons why some patients with HbH disease produce significant amounts of Hb Bart's are not clear. It is possible that some have co-inherited β-globin clusters with point mutations that are associated with increased γ globin synthesis (see ref. 91 and Chapters 5 and 16).

HbH and Hb Bart's are easily detected as fast migrating bands on hemoglobin electrophoresis (Fig. 14.7). In addition HbH can be precipitated from peripheral blood red cells after incubation for 3 hours at room temperature (see ref. 43 for details). These characteristic inclusions are artefacts produced by the redox action of the dye (Fig. 14.5). The proportion of cells containing HbH inclusions is directly related to the level of HbH detected in the peripheral blood. Again patients with nondeletional α thalassemia have a higher proportion of HbH cells than those with the deletional types of HbH disease.[92] Even after prolonged incubation it is unusual to find inclusions in every cell; the reason for this heterogeneity is not clear. Splenectomized patients have large numbers of preformed inclusions in the red cells that can be detected by methyl violet staining.

Other minor changes in the hemoglobin composition found in patients with HbH disease include a tendency to low levels of HbA_2 (1%–2%) probably due to the lower affinity of α-chains for δ- than β-chains; when the supply of α chains is limited less HbA_2 is formed (Chapter 7). In addition, variant chains creating abnormal hemoglobins may be detected in patients with chain termination mutants (for example see ref. 93) and some unstable mutants associated with α thalassemia (e.g., Hb QuongSze and Hb Agrinio, see Chapter 13). Finally some α chain variants, such as Hb J Tongariki and Hb G Philadelphia may be linked *in cis* to α thalassemia variants (see Table 13.2 in Chapter 13).

Clinical Features of HbH Disease

Although HbH disease is quite a common genetic disorder in the Mediterranean, Middle East, and southeast Asia, there have been relatively few systematic studies addressing the natural history of this condition or the relationship between genotype and phenotype. Most physicians caring for such patients agree that there is a remarkably wide clinical spectrum but often comment on the mild nature of this condition. Even from the biased perspective of hospital-based studies, the majority of patients with HbH disease appear to have little disability.[1,9,61,62,72,73,94–97] However, it has emerged over the past 10 years or so that a minority of patients with HbH disease may be severely affected, requiring regular blood transfusion and rare cases may present as hydropic, newborn infants (see later).

The largest clinical experience of HbH disease, including data from 500 adults and 502 children, was summarized over 30 years ago by Wasi et al.[34] More recent studies have reviewed relatively large numbers patients whose molecular defects have been accurately defined,[1,62,72,73,79,82,98] allowing us to make some predictions about the severity of HbH disease based on genotype. The following discussion is largely based on these reviews.

Presentation

At birth, infants destined to develop HbH disease may have near-normal levels of hemoglobin with no hepatosplenomegaly,[34] whereas other newborn infants may already show evidence of hemolytic anemia.[73,79] In many infants, the clinical features of HbH disease (see later) develop in the first year of life. The age at which patients with HbH disease first present varies from birth to older than 70 years and in more than half of the patients the finding of HbH disease is incidental (e.g., associated with health checks or prenatal screening) or found during investigation for an unrelated illness. Some patients may first present at the time of an acute fall in the level of Hb,[62,72] as will be discussed. Anecdotally, survival of patients with HbH disease into adult life appears to be the rule but there are no actuarial data to quantify this assertion.

Episodes of Severe Anemia

The level of Hb in most patients appears to be relatively stable and above approximately 8 g/dL; however, the Hb level may fall (2–3 g/dL) quite dramatically,[34] causing episodes of profound weakness and pallor requiring hospital admission and blood transfusion. The cause of such events is not always understood; they may recur and may vary from one environment to another. They are often thought to arise from increased hemolysis associated with pregnancy intercurrent infection/pyrexia or administration of oxidant drugs such as sulphonamides[76] or transient aplasia due to B19 parvovirus infection.[73] Such events may also occur in patients with hypersplenism.

Blood Transfusion

Blood transfusion is often used in the management of patients who have an acute fall in the level of Hb (see previous discussion). In many studies up to 50% of patients with HbH disease have had a few transfusions during such episodes. In general, those with the lowest steady state levels of Hb (with nondeletional HbH disease) more frequently require such transfusions. It is unusual for patients with HbH disease to require regular blood transfusion and even in cases in which this has been thought necessary, it is not always clear what criteria have been used to make such a decision. Nevertheless, nearly all such examples occur in patients with nondeletional types of HbH disease.

Hepatosplenomegaly and Jaundice

In addition to pallor and jaundice most patients with HbH disease have enlarged livers and spleens, although clinically significant hepatomegaly is unusual in patients with uncomplicated HbH disease unless they have iron loading. Liver enlargement and spleen enlargement are both more common in patients with nondeletional types of HbH disease. Hypersplenism, which can significantly aggravate the anemia and lead to reduced platelet and white blood cell counts, occurs in approximately 10% of patients;[34] splenectomy may be of benefit to such patients with persistent anemia. Severe liver disease has occasionally been reported in patients with HbH disease but it is not clear that this was directly attributable to thalassemia. Gallstones are quite frequent (up to ~40%) in patients with HbH disease their frequency increasing with age and possibly modified by the co-inheritance of predisposing alleles of the uridine diphosphate glucuronosyl transferase locus.[73,99] Complications of gallstones appear relatively infrequent; for example, in 95 patients followed by Piankijagum et al.[80] for 2 years, there were four episodes of cholecystitis.

Growth and Bone Changes

Approximately one third of patients with HbH disease were said to have bone changes associated with thalassemia.[86] In general these are mild but may affect the facial features. In one study from Thailand 17% of children with deletional HbH disease and almost half of patients with HbH/CS disease had thalassemic facies.[79] In the latter group half of the patients had moderately severe changes with maxillary overgrowth. Approximately 13% of children with HbH disease in Hong Kong and Sardinia had growth rates below the third percentile.[72,73] A study from Thailand found more than half of children with HbH disease had growth impairment.[79] Clinically significant extramedullary hemopoiesis rarely occurs in HbH disease.[9,34,100]

Hemoglobin H Disease and Pregnancy

The normal physiological changes associated with pregnancy are even more challenging in patients with HbH disease than those with α thalassemia trait (see previous discussion). In patients with HbH disease, there is usually an increasing severity of anemia and the level of Hb may fall to approximately 6.0 g/dL[1,73,101] or even less.[34,102] Some patients with the most severe anemias may also be iron deficient.[34] In patients with severe anemia (<6.0 g/dL), blood transfusion may be necessary to maintain the health of the mother and the developing fetus.[34,73,101,103] Even in the absence of specific treatment, the level of the mother's Hb usually returns to 8–10 g/dL a few months after delivery.

Vaeusorn et al.[101] described 34 pregnancies in 29 Thai women. Preeclampsia occurred in 18% of cases, and there were 2 miscarriages and 3 premature births. In a study of 127 pregnancies in Thai women 38 of 111 required caesarean section.[102] In a more recent study Origa et al.[73] described the outcome of 82 pregnancies in 31 Sardinian women with HbH disease. Nine (11%) resulted in miscarriage. Four (5.5%) had preeclampsia. Six children (8.2%) were born prematurely and 22 children were delivered by caesarean section. Therefore, although many women with HbH disease experience no adverse effects during pregnancy, special care is required to ensure that the reduced levels of Hb do not deleteriously affect the mother or developing fetus.

Iron Status in Patients with HbH Disease

The issue of iron overloading, even in normal individuals, is complex and is influenced by genetic background, environment, and diet (Chapter 29). The complexity is even greater in patients with chronic hemolysis and dyserythropoiesis. Ferrokinetic studies have suggested that although iron absorption is increased in HbH disease,[104] iron utilization appears normal, consistent with this being primarily a hemolytic anemia,[78,104] in contrast to β thalassemia, which is predominantly dyserythropoietic. In general, the severe clinical manifestations of iron overload frequently encountered in patients with β thalassemia intermedia and major (Chapter 29) are rarely seen in HbH disease,[9,96,105,106] and Sonakul et al.[107] noticed less tissue hemosiderosis at autopsy in patients with HbH disease than those with homozygous β thalassemia.

Nevertheless, in southeast Asia, some degree of iron overload (as judged by markedly elevated serum ferritin) is present in approximately 70% of adults with HbH,[106,108,109] and the level of ferritin is related to age.[72] In Hong Kong, 51 of 60 patients (85%) evaluated by computed tomography scanning of the liver showed evidence of iron overload.[72,110] In a few patients liver biopsy revealed increased liver iron content and hepatic fibrosis without evidence of hepatitis B or C.[72,111] Rare patients with HbH disease have been reported to have clinically significant cardiac and endocrine complications associated with iron overload.[72,105]

In a large study in Sardinia[73] approximately 20% children, 26% of adult females, and 50% of adult males with HbH disease had serum ferritin levels greater than normal. Again there was a clear age-related correlation and a small number of patients had liver disease, which may or may not have been related simply to iron overload. Clearly the risk of iron overload will be increased in patients with HbH disease who undergo regular transfusion and such patients require appropriate chelation therapy. Whether nontransfused patients with high levels of ferritin will benefit from chelation is currently being assessed.[112] One should be aware that HbH disease may coexist with the common form of hereditary hemochromatosis,[113] which may account for unexplained, clinically significant iron overload in occasional patients with HbH disease.[61,109]

Rare Complications

Other complications of HbH disease include leg ulcers,[114] which are rare,[34] an increased susceptibility to certain infections,[34,80,115] retinopathy,[116] and risk of thromboembolic disease.[117]

The Relationship Between Genotype and Phenotype in HbH Disease

The numbers of patients studied in detail are too small to draw firm conclusions. Nevertheless, several studies now agree that, in general, patients with nondeletional forms of HbH disease are more anemic and jaundiced with higher levels of HbH than patients with deletional forms of HbH disease. Patients with nondeletion HbH disease also have higher levels of sTfR and serum erythropoietin and greater degrees of hepatosplenomegaly, more severe bone changes, and more episodes of infection than patients with deletional forms of HbH disease. Some studies suggest that patients with nondeletional HbH disease present earlier in life than those with deletional types of HbH disease. These findings are consistent with the more severe hematological phenotype reported in patients with nondeletional HbH disease (as stated previously). They more frequently require blood transfusion and nearly all patients requiring regular blood transfusion have the nondeletional forms of HbH disease (see later). Patients with nondeletional HbH disease most frequently require and benefit from splenectomy.[1,31,61,62,72,73,83,88,89,94,95,118]

Treatment of Patients with HbH Disease

The overwhelming impression is that the majority of patients with HbH disease are clinically well; they are often unaware of their condition and may go on to have families of their own. Therefore, the major point to make about the management of patients with HbH disease is that no specific treatment other than folic acid supplements should be offered unless there are well-defined reasons for doing so.

Oral iron is not required routinely for patients with HbH disease and may be deleterious due to the potential for iron overload (as noted previously). Nevertheless when appropriate, one should suspect and investigate iron, folate, and B12 deficiency in patients with HbH disease and treat just as for nonthalassemic patients. Most clinicians recommend that all patients with chronic hemolytic anemias should be given regular folic acid supplements.[119,120] Women with HbH disease who are not iron overloaded should be given the same supplements in the management of pregnancy as nonthalassemic women according to local obstetrical practices.

Occasional blood transfusions may be required when the level of hemoglobin suddenly dips. Hemolytic episodes occur most commonly in children who should therefore be examined at least every 12 months to determine steady-state levels of hemoglobin (many adult patients are so well that they neglect to come for review). Occasionally both hemolytic and aplastic episodes can result in rapid falls in the hemoglobin level to the point at which transfusion is potentially life saving. Hence education is a very important part of management. Any episodes of profound weakness and pallor should prompt individuals or families to take the patient to the hospital as a matter of urgency. Aplastic episodes usually last only a week or so with rapid recovery, and transfusion is not necessarily required. It is important to exclude the coexistence of glucose-6-phosphate dehydrogenase deficiency in males, which is common in many communities and may cause hemolysis in individuals with HbH disease. Naphthalene, antimalarials, and sulphas are the most common causes of hemolytic episodes in glucose-6-phosphate dehydrogenase–deficient children. In many cases the cause of sudden severe anemia in HbH disease remains unknown. Particular care must be taken to monitor pregnant women with HbH disease who may have especially low levels of hemoglobin. In all of these situations it is reasonable to provide temporary support with blood transfusion.

Chronic blood transfusion should be avoided for all but the most carefully considered cases. Once instituted, the patients will require all the long-term care, including iron chelation, used for patients with homozygous β thalassemia (see Chapter 29). The clearest examples in which this should be considered are 1) patients who are unable to maintain normal cardiovascular function with the given level of hemoglobin; and 2) patients who would otherwise develop the chronic problems associated with erythroid expansion (thalassemic facies, extramedullary tumors, etc.). In most hematologists' experience these criteria rarely apply to patients with HbH disease and when transfusions are required they are usually in patients with nondeletional forms of HbH disease.

Splenomegaly is one of the commonest complications of HbH disease and may be accompanied by hypersplenism. Wasi et al.[86] reported that splenectomy in 50 patients with HbH disease increased the level of hemoglobin by 2–3 g/dL (other reports are reviewed in refs. 118, 121, 122). Although splenectomy may be indicated in some cases to ameliorate the problems associated with splenomegaly or hypersplenism, this should be very carefully balanced against the potential complication of venous thrombosis, which has been reported in some patients with HbH disease following splenectomy.[123–125]

Based on the discussion of iron status, ferritin or iron estimations should be performed at least annually. Iron loading may be caused by regular blood transfusion, inappropriate iron therapy or abnormal absorption: in many patients several mechanisms contribute. Based on preliminary evaluation it may be necessary to assess iron loading by liver biopsy to determine the need for chelation. Alternatively liver iron storage can be evaluated by noninvasive methods such as dual energy computed tomography[72,126] or magnetic resonance imaging,[127] thus avoiding the need for liver biopsy (the detection of iron overloading is discussed further in Chapter 29). At present we do not know whether iron loading in HbH disease can ever be severe enough to cause cirrhosis and liver failure.

Other complications such as leg ulcers have been reported in patients with HbH disease and require the general medical or surgical treatment appropriate for the clinical situation. Gallstones occur commonly and routine ultrasound should be performed at some stage during late teens. When present, gallstones should be managed conservatively; few patients require cholecystectomy.

Genetic Counseling of Patients with HbH Disease

The presence of HbH disease in one or both partners is not known to impair their ability to have children although there are no data to evaluate fertility in such individuals.

Once a diagnosis has been made in any patient of reproductive age it is important to offer them advice about the potential problems of producing children with the Hb Bart's hydrops fetalis syndrome and their partner should be tested to see if they are at risk of producing such a pregnancy. Because there are so many potential interactions (see Table 14.1) it will be necessary to obtain a full genotype analysis from both partners to evaluate the relative risks of all possible outcomes.

In each case the primary aim is to avoid pregnancies leading to Hb Bart's hydrops fetalis or the uncommon, severe forms of HbH hydrops fetalis and transfusion-dependent HbH disease.

HEMOGLOBIN BART'S HYDROPS FETALIS SYNDROME

The combination of generalized edema, ascites, and pleural and pericardial effusions in a developing fetus (hydrops fetalis) may occur in a wide variety of fetal and maternal disorders.[128–132] The predominant causes vary from one population to another. In the West, rhesus immunization used to be the major cause, but with the widespread introduction of immunoprophylaxis and the decline in rhesus isoimmunization[133] "nonimmune" causes (intrauterine infection, chromosomal abnormalities, and congenital cardiac and renal defects) now account for 75% of cases.[131,134] In Southeast Asia, up to 90% of all cases are caused by α thalassemia, giving rise to the Hb Bart's hydrops fetalis syndrome.[132,135–139]

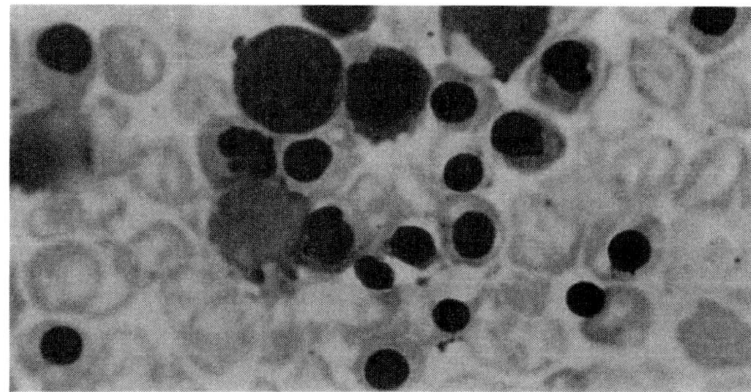

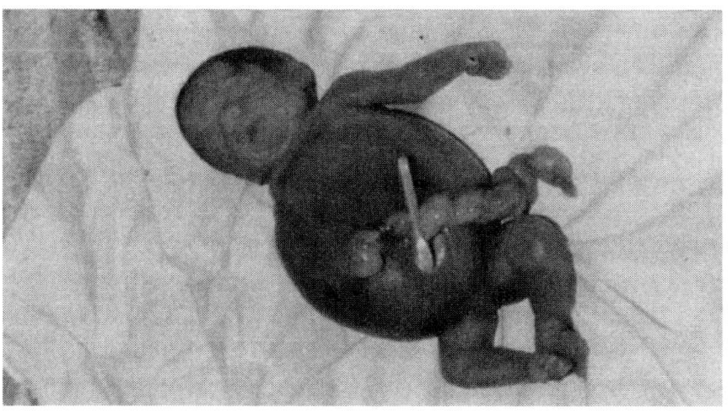

Figure 14.9. Upper the typical peripheral blood films of an infant with the Hb Bart's hydrops fetalis syndrome, showing many immature red cell precursors and hypochromic, microcytic, and anisopoikiolytic red cells. Lower the typical clinical features of a hydropic infant at birth (see text). (See color plate 14.9.)

Throughout southeast Asia where the frequency of α^0 thalassemia trait (--/$\alpha\alpha$) is high (4%–14%, see Chapter 26), up to 1:200 infants may inherit no functional α genes (--/--) from their parents.[140–142] Because α-globin chains are normally produced throughout development, contributing to embryonic ($\alpha_2\varepsilon_2$), fetal ($\alpha_2\gamma_2$) and adult ($\alpha_2\beta_2$) hemoglobins, affected fetuses suffer from severe hypochromic anemia in utero, which causes hypoxia, heart failure and consequently hydrops fetalis (Fig. 14.9). Such infants produce large amounts of nonfunctional Hb Bart's ($\gamma4$) and small amounts of functional, embryonic hemoglobin (Hb Portland $\zeta_2\gamma_2$), which allows sufficient tissue oxygenation for them to survive until the third trimester of pregnancy when they are usually born prematurely and die (see later).

The Hb Bart's hydrops fetalis syndrome nearly always results from the coinheritance of two α^0 thalassemia defects (Table 14.1). In southeast Asia, $--^{SEA}/--^{SEA}$ is the most common genotype but in areas where the $--^{FIL}$ [143] and $--^{THAI}$ [143] determinants occur some hydropic babies may be compound heterozygotes ($--^{FIL}/--^{SEA}$ and $--^{THAI}/--^{SEA}$). These two less common defects ($--^{FIL}$ and $--^{THAI}$) remove both fetal/adult (α) and embryonic (ζ) genes. Because homozygotes (e.g. $--^{FIL}/--^{FIL}$) do not produce any normal embryonic hemoglobins (Portland $\zeta_2\gamma_2$, Gower 1 $\zeta_2\varepsilon_2$ and

Table 14.3. Hematology in the normal developing fetus and those with the Hb Bart's hydrops fetalis syndrome

Age (wk)	RBC ($\times 10^{12}$/L)	Hb g/dL	Hct %	MCV fL	MCH pg	Retic. %	Hb Bart's %	Hb Portland %	Reference
					Nonthalassemic				
30–31	4.79 ± 0.74	19.1 ± 2.2	60 ± 8	127 ± 12.7	38*	5.8 ± 2			[119]
~40	5.14 ± 0.7	19.3 ± 2.2	61 ± 7.4	119 ± 9.4	34*	3.2 ± 1.4	<1		[119]
~40	4.7 ± 0.8	16.5 ± 3.0	51 ± 9	108 ± 10	34 ± 3	–			[240]
					Hydrops fetalis				
28–43	2.2 ± 0.8	6.5 ± 2.3	30.4 ± 13.8	136 ± 23	31.9 ± 9	–	86.9 ± 5.1	13.1 ± 5.8	[152]
30–40	–	6.7	–	100–190	–	variable may be >60%	70–80	–	[34]
28–38	–	4.9 (3–8.5)	21.3	–	–	–	–	–	[139]

Mean values ± SD.
* Calculated MCH.

Gower 2 $\alpha_2\varepsilon_2$) they die very early in gestation and do not produce the classic hydrops fetalis syndrome.[143] α^0-thalassemia is much less common in other regions of the world. Nevertheless, rare cases of Hb Bart's hydrops fetalis have been reported in individuals of Greek ($--^{MED}/--^{MED}$),[144–147] Cypriot ($--^{MED}/--^{MED}$, $--^{MED}/-(\alpha)^{20.5}$, $-(\alpha)^{20.5}/-(\alpha)^{20.5}$),[148,149] Sardinian ($--^{MED}/--^{MED}$),[150] Turkish ($-(\alpha)^{20.5}/-(\alpha)^{20.5}$),[151] and Asian Indian (J.M. Old, personal communication, 2000) origins. Many of these cases occur in restricted population groups or, in some cases, result from consanguineous marriages. Given the large number of α^0 thalassemia mutations that have been described (Chapter 13) one should be aware of potential, rare interactions in such situations.

Very rarely, severe fetal anemia with or without overt hydrops fetalis may also result from the co-inheritance of α° and nondeletional α^+ thalassemia (Table 14.1), an interaction that normally causes HbH disease (noted previously). There are now several examples of HbH hydrops fetalis and these are described below.

mRNA and Globin Synthesis Studies in Infants with the Hb Bart's Hydrops Fetalis Syndrome

Using complementary cDNA probes Kan et al.[17] were first to demonstrate that there is no detectable α mRNA in patients with the Hb Bart's hydrops fetalis syndrome. This has subsequently been confirmed in several studies (for example see ref. 19). Consequently, no α-globin chain synthesis is detected in the peripheral blood of such infants,[24] although β-globin synthesis appears entirely unaffected, underscoring the fact that there appears to be no regulatory feedback at any level between α- and β-globin chain synthesis.

The Red Cell Indices and Hematological Findings in the Hb Bart's Hydrops Fetalis Syndrome

The peripheral blood of infants with the Hb Bart's hydrops fetalis syndrome contains large, hypochromic red cells and shows considerable anisopoikilocytosis (Fig. 14.9). Some elongated cells are said to have the appearance of "sickle cells".[34] The typical hematological findings in infants with the hydrops fetalis syndrome are summarized in Table 14.3, the most striking abnormality being the severe degree of anemia with a mean hemoglobin of 6.5 g/dL.[152]

The reticulocyte count is high[34] and the blood contains many nucleated red cells (Fig. 14.9). The bone marrow is hyperplastic and there are many sites (liver, spleen, kidney, and adrenals) of extramedullary hemopoiesis, predominantly erythropoietic, with widespread deposition of hemosiderin.

The cause of the anemia is poorly understood and is probably multifactorial, involving underproduction of hemoglobin, hemolysis, and ineffective erythropoiesis. The role of Hb Bart's in the hemolysis and/or ineffective erythropoiesis is not clear; unlike HbH, Hb Bart's is soluble and appears relatively stable. Factors other than anemia (e.g., plasma protein concentration, umbilical blood flow) may contribute to the development of hydrops fetalis.[34,153]

Developmental Changes in Hemoglobin Composition

We now know that the Hb Bart's hydrops fetalis syndrome most commonly results from deletion of all four α genes; α mRNA is undetectable[17] and therefore the primary abnormality is an inability to synthesize the α-globin chains of hemoglobin.

In affected individuals, the embryonic hemoglobins Gower 1 ($\zeta_2\varepsilon_2$) and Portland I ($\zeta_2\gamma_2$) are expressed normally, in the first few weeks of life, although there is no Hb Gower 2 ($\alpha_2\varepsilon_2$). Severe anemia probably develops at approximately 6–7 weeks of gestation when the switch from embryonic (ζ and ε) to fetal (α and γ) gene expression occurs.[154] In the absence of α-chain synthesis no Hb F ($\alpha_2\gamma_2$) can be made and excess γ chains form soluble tetramers (γ4, Hb Bart's), which makes up to approximately 90% of the total hemoglobin. Toward the end of gestation, as the fetal (γ) to adult (β) switch occurs, small amounts of HbH (β_4) appear in the fetal blood. Neither Hb Bart's nor HbH display any heme–heme interaction[68,155] or Bohr effect and both bind oxygen very highly, as in the R-state of normal hemoglobin (see Chapter 6). Consequently, oxygen delivery to the fetus is severely impaired throughout most of development and it is remarkable that the fetus survives at all.

It appears that viability depends on the persistent synthesis of embryonic ζ globin chains. In affected individuals Hb Portland I ($\zeta_2\gamma_2$) and to a lesser extent Portland II ($\zeta_2\beta_2$) make up approximately 10%–20% of the fetal blood. Hb Portland displays a normal pattern of oxygen dissociation[156] and can therefore deliver oxygen to the developing fetus.

The molecular and cellular basis for persistent ζ globin expression is not understood. A very small increase in ζ globin chains[40,157–160] is seen in some carriers of deletions that cause α^0 thalassemia and, superficially, this resembles the persistent γ-globin expression that accompanies some deletions that remove the β-globin genes (hereditary persistence of fetal hemoglobin [HPFH], see Chapter 16). The levels of ζ-globin observed in carriers of α^0 thalassemia (<1%) are much lower than levels of γ-globin in HPFH. It seems likely that mechanisms other than increased ζ-globin gene transcription (e.g., cell selection or alterations in ζ-globin mRNA stability) must be operating to allow such high levels of Hb Portland to accumulate. It is interesting, however, that the embryonic Hb Gower 1 ($\zeta_2\varepsilon_2$) does not persist in this condition, suggesting that the effect specifically acts on ζ-globin expression rather than a general effect on embryonic (ζ and ε) globin expression.

Clinical and Autopsy Findings

Following a gestation of approximately 33 weeks (range 23–43) infants with the Hb Bart's hydrops fetalis syndrome usually die in utero, during delivery, or within 1–2 hours of birth.[136,139,152,153,161] Occasionally even without specific treatment, some babies survive for a few days.[161,162] Typically, affected infants are pale, slightly jaundiced, growth retarded, and edematous with a massive, friable placenta (see Fig. 14.9). The skin may be affected by a "blueberry muffin" rash caused by subcutaneous nodules of extramedullary hemopoiesis.[163] In one study the placenta/fetal weight ratio ranged from 0.37 to 1.16 (mean 0.68) compared with the normal ratio of 0.15–0.25.[136] Sometimes the abdomen is distended with ascites but not all cases are grossly hydropic (e.g., ref. 153). Developmental abnormalities have been reported in up to 17% of cases.[136,161,164] These include hydrocephaly,[136] microcephaly,[136] abnormal limb development,[136,165–170] and urogenital abnormalities, including undescended testes, variable degrees of hypospadias, ambiguous genitalia, and even male pseudohermaphroditism (reviewed in refs. 34, 86, 136, 162, 165, 171–173). The cause of these common genital abnormalities associated with Bart's hydrops is unexplained and of interest.

At autopsy ascites is usually pronounced and there are often pleural and pericardial effusions. Organ weights are usually reported with respect to gestational age, body weight, and body length (Fig. 14.10). The combination of edema and disturbed growth in hydropic babies can severely distort these relationships. With this caveat, enlargement of the heart, liver, and to a lesser degree the spleen are usually observed, whereas retarded development of the lung, thymus, adrenals, and kidney are often reported.[34,86,152,161] Of particular interest there is a progressive decrease in brain weight relative to that expected for gestational age from approximately 8 weeks of gestation (Fig. 14.10). Again, many congenital abnormalities have been noted postmortem including cardiac defects,[136,152] pulmonary hypoplasia,[152] and undescended and intraabdominal testes[161] (reviewed in ref. 165).

Histologically, interstitial edema is noted in all tissues. There are multiple sites of extramedullary erythropoiesis. Up to 60%–70% of the liver parenchyma may consist of developing red cells. The placenta is vascular and edematous, containing many nucleated red cells. It has been speculated that hematological changes in this condition may cause occlusion of small blood vessels with subsequent disruption of end organs (e.g., as in abnormal limb development).[166,168]

It is interesting that even though the vast majority of infants with hydrops fetalis have an identical genotype ($--^{SEA}/--^{SEA}$) there is considerable variation in the pace and extent of abnormal development in each fetus.

Maternal Complications

Mothers of infants with this disorder often have a history of stillbirths or neonatal deaths; early miscarriages are probably uncommon. All reports point to an increased incidence of serious maternal complications (see Table 14.4 and refs. 136, 152, 161).

In the antenatal period most problems arise in the third trimester when some mothers note a cessation of fetal movements. Common complications include anemia, preeclampsia (hypertension, fluid retention with or without proteinuria), polyhydramnios (excessive accumulation of amniotic fluid), oligohydramnios (decreased amniotic fluid), antepartum hemorrhage, and the premature onset of labor (Table 14.4). Less common general medical and obstetric complications have also been reported.[136,152,161,164]

Labor and delivery may be particularly difficult and assistance (in the form of embryotomy, breech, forceps, and caesarean section) is required in approximately 50% of cases. Postpartum complications include retained placenta, hemorrhage, eclampsia (fits and coma), sepsis, and anemia.

It has been suggested that, without medical care, up to 50% of women carrying affected fetuses would die as a result of such pregnancies.[152] To date, however, there have

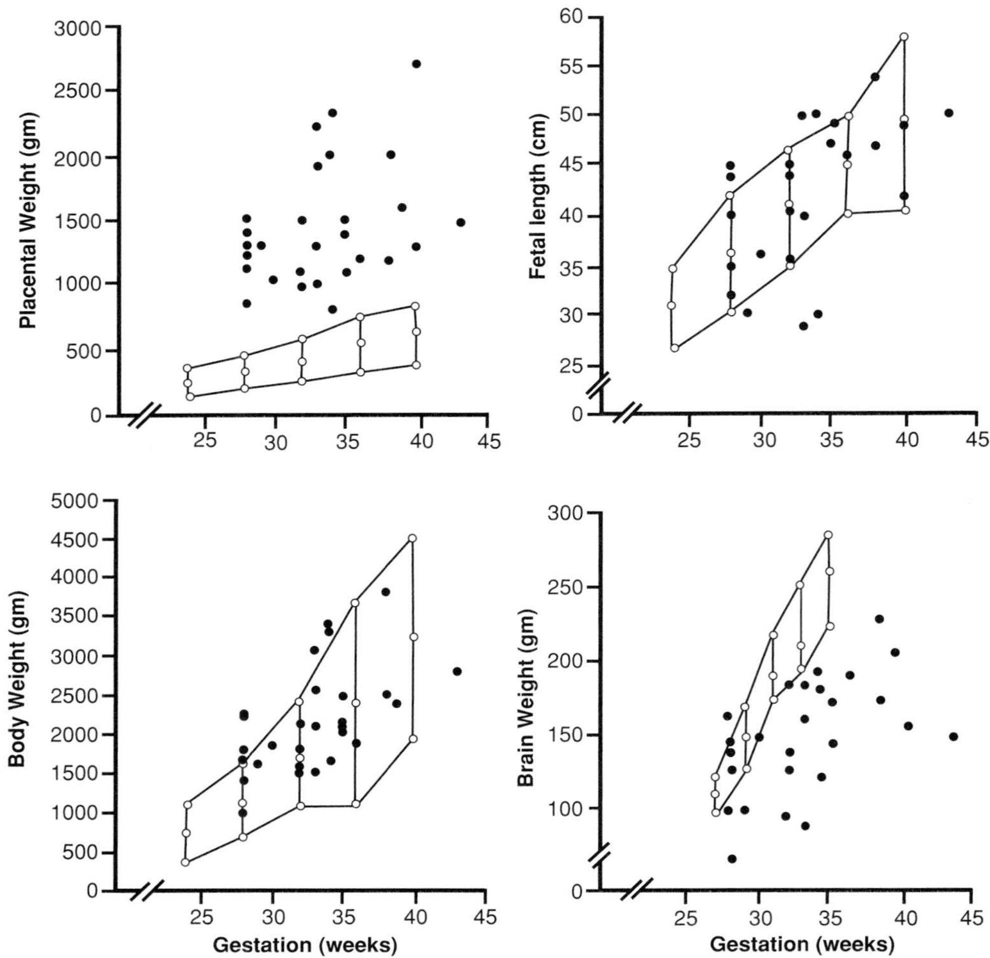

Figure 14.10. The placental weight, body weight, fetal length, and brain weight of a series of infants with the Hb Bart's hydrops fetalis syndrome. The open circles represent the mean normal values and 95% confidence limits. (Redrawn with permission from S. Fucharoen in ref. 152.)

been no retrospective studies of maternal mortality rates in communities where medical assistance is unavailable.

Hemoglobin H Hydrops Fetalis

Nearly all babies with the Hb Bart's hydrops fetalis syndrome inherit no α genes from their parents (genotype --/--). There are, however, several reports describing rare neonates with severe anemia and various changes associated with hydrops fetalis due to the coinheritance of α^0 and α^+ thalassemia. These infants are distinguished from the common forms of Bart's hydrops in that they do make some α-globin chains and they are referred to as having HbH hydrops fetalis. Many of the molecular interactions underlying this condition have been fully characterized.

The first involves the common α° mutations and nondeletional α thalassemia determinants ($--/\alpha^T\alpha$) that result from highly unstable α-globin variants including Hb Adana,[98,174] the $\alpha^{CD30}\alpha$ mutation,[174–176] Hb Dartmouth,[177] Hb Evora,[98] and Hb Quong Sze.[178] HbH hydrops was also seen in a homozygote for Hb Taybe.[52] A second class of interaction involves the chain termination mutant Hb Constant Spring and involves a homozygote ($\alpha^{cs}\alpha/\alpha^{cs}\alpha$,[53]), whereas this interaction normally causes a moderately severe hemolytic anemia. The third type of interaction ($--/\alpha^{PA}\alpha$) occurs between α^0 thalassemia and the polyA addition signal mutations,[179,180] including a homozygote ($\alpha^{PA}\alpha/\alpha^{PA}\alpha$) for the Indian polyA signal mutation.[181] In addition there are several less well characterized examples of HbH hydrops.[135,171,182]

At birth all affected infants were anemic (hemoglobin, 3.4–9.7 g/dL) with large amounts of Hb Bart's (17%–66%). Although approximately 50% of the affected infants died at birth, others survived following intrauterine blood transfusion but have remained transfusion dependent (e.g., ref. 174). Some have developed normally and require no further transfusions after the perinatal period (e.g., refs. 52, 53).

These cases thus represent the transition between severe, transfusion-dependent HbH disease and Hb Bart's hydrops fetalis and some of these patients have been

Table 14.4. Maternal complications in the Hb Bart's hydrops fetalis syndrome

	Hydrops %			Nonhydrops** %
Antepartum				
Anemia	65			17
Preeclampsia	61	78	35	7
Eclampsia	0	1.5		<1
Polyhydramnios	59	3	17.5	<1
Antepartum hemorrhage	6.5	11*		3
Placenta praevia	4.3			
Abruptio placenta	+		10	
Premature delivery	93		35	5–10
Delivery and Postpartum				
Malpresentation	37			<5
Assisted vaginal delivery	35	34		5
Caesarian section	17	14		2–3
Retained placenta	+			+
Postpartum hemorrhage		11*		5
Anemia	46			+
Reference	[136]	[152]	[161]	[136; 243]

+ recorded but figures not given.
* includes ante- and postpartum hemorrhage.
** These figures are only a guide because they will vary greatly depending on the population studied and the level of antenatal care provided.

included as examples of infants surviving with the Hb Bart's hydrops fetalis syndrome (e.g., ref. 173). As accurate molecular diagnosis becomes more common we would expect to identify further similar cases of HbH hydrops fetalis. Mothers of these children often have a history of neonatal deaths due to anemia and in some cases, siblings with the same interactions have severe HbH disease. Nevertheless some siblings with identical interactions have not experienced the same degree of anemia. It is not clear why some patients with $\alpha^{\circ}/\alpha^{+}$ interactions should be so severely affected whereas others with an identical interaction may survive normally.

Long-Term Survival of α^0 Thalassemia Homozygotes

As noted above, there is considerable variability in the clinical course of infants with the Hb Bart's hydrops fetalis syndrome. Although most die *in utero*, during delivery, or within 1 or 2 hours of birth, others may survive for several days:[162,183,184] In some cases the diagnosis may not be immediately obvious in a newborn infant. It is therefore not surprising that during the last 20 years, as neonatal care (e.g., ventilator therapy, and the use of nitric oxide, and surfactant) has continued to improve, several homozygotes for α^0 thalassemia have survived either as a result of treatment prior to confirmation of the diagnosis or as a result of preplanned intervention. This has generated a great deal of interest in how best to counsel and manage parents when the mother carries an affected fetus (reviewed in ref. 185).

In a recent review Lee et al.[186] usefully approached this problem by collating data from live, newborn infants with the Hb Bart's hydrops fetalis syndrome who had received no prior treatment in utero. All of these had naturally survived until delivery and then, some were treated with intensive neonatal care and blood transfusion. One group (11 fetuses) died in the first few hours after delivery[186] or lived for only a few days,[183,184] in keeping with the conventional descriptions of this condition. By contrast, the second group (10 fetuses) have all survived for months or years.[171,186–193] Half of these long-term survivors have abnormal neurodevelopment, variously affecting speech, hearing, and motor function. In addition, these patients have a wide variety of other developmental abnormalities including genital abnormalities and limb deformities. Therefore, despite modern neonatal intensive care, based on these observations, the chance of survival with Bart's hydrops fetalis remains small and at least half of the survivors have abnormal development.

Lee et al.[186] also reviewed the outcome in 16 fetuses that had received early prenatal diagnosis followed by intrauterine therapy, thus correcting the effects of α thalassemia earlier in development.[167,173,185,194–203] Intrauterine therapy included blood transfusion, exchange transfusion, and in two cases[197,203] intrauterine hematopoietic stem cell transplantation. It seems that intrauterine therapy combined with neonatal intensive care results in a relatively low mortality and morbidity. Nevertheless, serious complications and developmental abnormalities still occur in this group (e.g., refs. 194, 195, 200) and even when these are avoided, the affected child and the family may still be committed to lifelong blood transfusion and chelation therapy unless the child undergoes successful transplantation.[173,185]

Prevention and Management

Ideally one should screen and identify couples at risk of conceiving a fetus with the Hb Bart's hydrops fetalis syndrome before or early in pregnancy, as set out in the section on management of patients with α thalassemia trait. The majority of these patients will be of southeast Asian origin but less commonly individuals of Mediterranean or mixed origins may be at risk.[204]

For accurate genetic counselling and prenatal diagnosis, it is essential to determine precisely the parental genotypes by Southern blot or PCR-based strategies (see Chapter 13). If both parents carry one or other of the known α^0 thalassemia defects there will be a one in four chance that they will conceive a fetus with the Hb Bart's hydrops fetalis syndrome. If *both* parents have α^0 thalassemia haplotypes in which both α and ζ genes are deleted (e.g., $--^{FIL}/--^{THAI}$) then they will not produce hydropic infants because homozygotes (e.g., $--^{FIL}/--^{FIL}$) and compound heterozygotes (e.g. $--^{FIL}/--^{THAI}$) for these defects will be lost soon after conception.[143] Compound heterozygotes for the $--^{SEA}/--^{FIL}$ mutations may have the common form of hydrops fetalis.

If at risk couples request prenatal testing, fetal DNA can be obtained from chorionic villi or fetal cells obtained by amniocentesis. DNA and hemoglobin analysis can be performed on blood samples obtained by cordocentesis in the second trimester of pregnancy. These techniques are discussed in Chapter 28.

Ultrasonography can also be useful in the management of at risk pregnancies for the Hb Bart's hydrops fetalis syndrome.[141,164,205–208] In most cases placental thickness is more than two standard deviations above normal[141] after 12 weeks of gestation; by 18 weeks it is abnormal in all cases.[205,209] Similarly, the cardiothoracic ratio is increased (>0.5 between the 12th and 17th week and 0.52 between the 18th and 21st weeks) in most, if not all, affected fetuses by 13–14 weeks gestation.[141,210,211] Other features including subcutaneous edema, hepatomegaly, pleural effusion, pericardial effusion, enlarged umbilical vessels, oligohydramnios, and ascites appear with increasing frequency from approximately 12 weeks onward[210] but are not consistently detected by ultrasonography until 22–28 weeks of gestation.[208]

These findings can be of help in two situations. First they may alert an obstetrician to the diagnosis if this has not been considered earlier in pregnancy. Second, in areas where DNA analysis is currently unavailable, it provides a reasonable way to monitor and select at risk pregnancies for further investigation by hemoglobin electrophoresis of samples obtained by cordocentesis.[210,211] This approach has been used increasingly over the past few years.[212]

At present there is no suitable treatment for the Hb Bart's hydrops fetalis syndrome. Early intervention with intrauterine transfusions (reviewed in ref. 186) are difficult to justify because even when successful the child is committed to lifelong blood transfusion and iron chelation. To address this, there have been three unsuccessful attempts to perform *in utero* hematopoietic stem cell transplantation.[203,213,214] Again survivors of such unsuccessful procedures[203] require life-long transfusion. In addition, we do not yet understand when or why other congenital abnormalities arise in this condition; therefore, current attempts to treat this condition are associated with an unknown risk of rescuing infants with multiple, often severe developmental abnormalities. Until these problems have been adequately addressed and solved (e.g., by using the excellent mouse model developed by Paszty and coworkers,[215,216]) further human experimentation should be avoided. Given the serious obstetrical risk to the mother of an affected fetus it seems most prudent to advise early termination of pregnancy in all cases.

INTERACTIONS BETWEEN α THALASSEMIA AND STRUCTURAL GLOBIN VARIANTS

Historically, interactions between α thalassemia and structural variants of the α- and β-globin chains were of considerable importance in developing our understanding of the genetics of hemoglobin synthesis (Chapter 3). Now that we have a more detailed knowledge, one of the main reasons for considering these interactions is to provide a framework for interpreting the many different patterns they produce on routine hemoglobin electrophoresis. The coinheritance of α thalassemia with some clinically important hemoglobinopathies is discussed in Chapters 16–19.

Interactions Between α Thalassemia and α-Globin Structural Variants

When a patient inherits an entirely normal β-globin genotype (β^A/β^A) and a full complement of α genes with one structural variant ($\alpha\alpha/\alpha^v\alpha$: β^A/β^A or $\alpha\alpha/\alpha\alpha^v$:$\beta^A/\beta^A$) the amount of variant hemoglobin produced will depend on the rate at which it is synthesized, its stability, its affinity for β^A chains (see later) and on whether the mutation affects the α_2 or α_1 gene. As discussed in Chapter 13, although the ratio of α_2/α_1 mRNA is 3:1 there is still some disagreement about the relative contributions of these two genes to hemoglobin synthesis. In addition there is considerable methodological variation in the quantitation of hemoglobin variants. Not surprisingly the reported proportions of α-globin variants range from 0% (e.g., Hb Quong Sze) to approximately 35% (e.g., Hb J Toronto) with an average value of approximately 25% (Chapter 13). Even if one excludes highly unstable α mutants there is still considerable variation, but in general, mutations affecting the α2 gene are present at higher levels than those affecting the α1 gene[217] (data available via http://globin.cse.psu.edu). Hematologically most α-globin variants are quite innocuous, although some give rise to high oxygen affinity (e.g., Hb Luton), congenital cyanosis (e.g., Hb M Boston), or hemolytic anemias (Chapter 25). Some heterozygotes for highly unstable mutants (e.g., Hb Quong Sze) may have the phenotype of α thalassemia trait and these are best considered as determinants of nondeletional α thalassemia (see Chapter 13).

The effect of coinheriting α thalassemia with α-globin variants is to increase the proportion of the variant and to reinforce any associated clinical phenotype (Table 14.5). This principle is best demonstrated by the variant G-Philadelphia (α68(E17)Asn$\rightarrow$Lys) (Chapter 13). Individuals with HbG-Philadelphia may have a full complement of four α genes ($\alpha^G\alpha/\alpha\alpha$) and 20%–25% of the variant hemoglobin with no hematological abnormalities.[218,219] In some individuals the HbG-Philadelphia variant is present on an -$\alpha^{3.7}$ haplotype (-α^G) giving rise to the -$\alpha^G/\alpha\alpha$, -α^G/-α and -α^G/-α^G genotypes that produce 30%–35%, approximately 45% and 100% G Philadelphia, respectively:[220–222] Such patients have the hematological phenotype of α thalassemia trait. Rarely the -α^G haplotype may interact with α^0 thalassemia to produce HbH disease (--/-α^G). Such patients produce only HbH and HbG and have the classic clinical and hematological phenotypes associated with HbH disease. The condition is referred to as HbG-H disease.[222,223] A list of

Table 14.5. Interactions between α-globin variants and α thalassemia

		Predicted + % of variant Hb	Hematological phenotype
$\alpha\alpha/\alpha^v\alpha$	β^A/β^A	25*–37.5**	normal
$\alpha\alpha/\alpha\alpha^v$	β^A/β^A	12.5*–25**	normal
$\alpha\alpha/\alpha^v\alpha^v$	β^A/β^A	50	normal
$-\alpha/\alpha^v\alpha$	β^A/β^A	30*–50**	α thalassemia trait
$-\alpha/\alpha\alpha^v$	β^A/β^A	16.6**–30*	α thalassemia trait
$-\alpha/\alpha^v\alpha^v$	β^A/β^A	66	α thalassemia trait
$--/\alpha\alpha^v$	β^A/β^A	30*–50**	α thalassemia trait
$-\alpha^v/\alpha\alpha$	β^A/β^A	50	α thalassemia trait
$-\alpha^v/-\alpha$	β^A/β^A	50	α thalassemia trait
$--/\alpha^v\alpha$	β^A/β^A	50*–70**	α thalassemia trait
$-\alpha^v/-\alpha^v$	β^A/β^A	100	α thalassemia trait
$--/-\alpha^v$	β^A/β^A	100	HbH disease

+ Assuming that the α^v variant is synthesized efficiently, completely stable, and associates with β^A-chains with the same kinetics α^A-chains.
* Assuming that the relative contribution of α2 and α1 is 1:1.
** Assuming that the contribution of α2 and α1 is 3:1.
As shown in ref. 217, all of these assumptions almost never apply to any known variant and estimated values often differ greatly from these predicted values.

all mutations directly linked to an α thalassemia determinant is given in Table 13.2 in Chapter 13; their interactions with other α-globin haplotypes are very similar to those described for HbG Philadelphia (also see Table 14.5).

The interaction between HbI (α^{16}Lys-Glu) and α thalassemia was initially very puzzling.[224] Most often this variant accounts for 24%–28% of the total hemoglobin.[217] In one family that also had α thalassemia, however, the level was 70%. It is now known that rarely the mutation may occur on both the α2 and α1 genes on the same chromosome, presumably as a result of gene conversion.[225] Thus the patient with the $-\alpha/\alpha^I\alpha^I$ genotype had approximately 70% HbI as we would now predict (Table 14.5).

The interactions between α thalassemia and highly unstable α-globin variants have been described previously and in Chapter 13. In general, the $-\alpha/\alpha^v\alpha$ and $-\alpha/\alpha\alpha^v$ genotypes in these cases give rise to α thalassemia trait and the $--/\alpha^v\alpha$ genotype is associated with HbH disease. There is a tendency for such individuals to fall at the severe end of the clinical spectrum of patients with HbH disease, including patients with HbH hydrops.

Interactions Between α Thalassemia and β-Globin Structural Variants

When a patient inherits an entirely normal α-globin genotype (αα/αα) and two β genes, one of which encodes a structural variant (β^A/β^V), the amount of variant hemoglobin produced will depend on its rate of synthesis, its stability, and the pattern of subunit assembly to form αβ dimers.[226,227] Ideally one would predict that equal amounts of HbA and variant hemoglobin would be present in the red cell, but in reality, as for α-globin mutants, considerable variation is observed.[217] Some β-globin variants (e.g., HbE and Hb Knossos) are synthesized less efficiently than β^A and represent less than 50% in heterozygotes. Others (e.g., Hb Köln) are unstable and may represent 30% or less of the hemoglobin. The third factor, differences in the rates of αβ subunit assembly, may influence the accumulated levels of many stable hemoglobin variants.

The formation of αβ dimers is a rate-limiting step in the assembly of hemoglobin. This process is thought to be facilitated by the electrostatic attraction between positively charged α-globin subunits and negatively charged β-globin subunits. Many commonly encountered β-globin variants acquire positive charge (e.g., β^S Glu→Val), thereby reducing their ability to compete with β^A-chains for hemoglobin assembly. In such cases less variant hemoglobin accumulates than HbA. The opposite is seen with negatively charged β-globin variants (Fig. 14.11). These observations are supported by *in vitro* subunit competition assays using

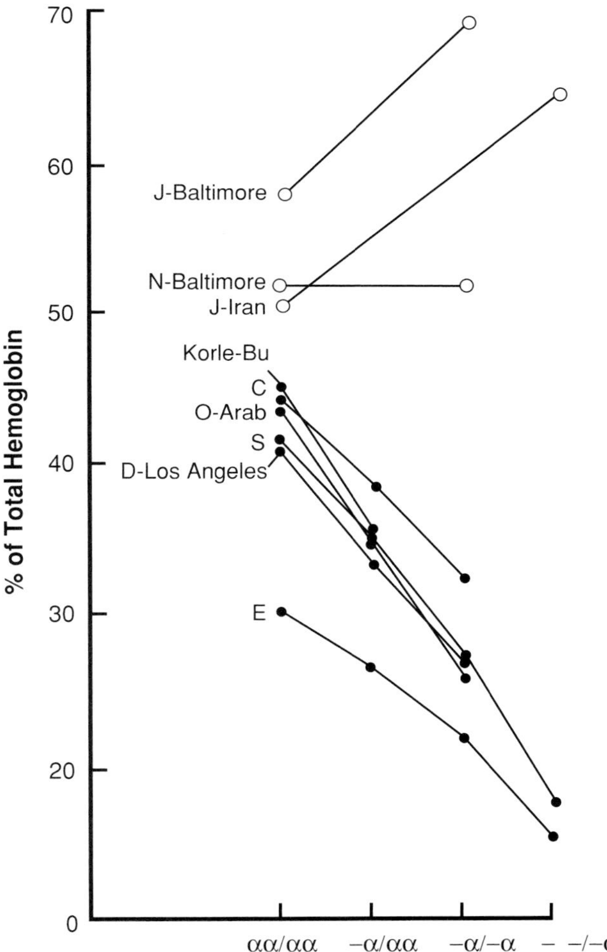

Figure 14.11. Effect of α-thalassemia on the proportion of negatively charged (○) and positively charged (•) β-globin variants in heterozygotes. In all cases HbA constitutes the majority of the remaining Hb. In three-gene deletion α thalassemia (--/-α), a small amount of Hb H (β_4) is present. (Redrawn from ref. 227.)

mixtures of normal (β^A) and variant (e.g., β^S and β^C) subunits.[226,227]

In the presence of α thalassemia, in which limiting amounts of α-chains are synthesized in the red cell, these effects are exaggerated. The accumulated levels of positively charged β variants (e.g., β^C, β^O, β^E, β^S) are further decreased in proportion to the deficit in α-globin chains.[226,227] By contrast the levels of negatively charged variants may increase (Fig. 14.11). This is a good rule of thumb although there are exceptions (e.g., HbN-Baltimore) and the situation becomes complex when more than one β variant is involved (e.g., HbS and HbC) or if α-globin variants are also present.

The presence of α thalassemia may influence the levels of HbA_2 in the presence of β-globin variants. The δ-globin subunit is considerably more positively charged than the β-globin subunit. In α thalassemia one would therefore expect the amount of HbA_2 to decrease, and, in general, this is what one sees.[34,86] In the presence of a variant, positively charged β subunit that has less affinity for α subunits, there may be sufficient free α-chains to interact with all δ subunits thereby increasing the level of HbA_2. Such increases have been observed in individuals with sickle cell trait[228] and sickle cell disease.

The presence of α thalassemia may also influence the levels of HbF ($\alpha_2\gamma_2$) and Hb Bart's ($\gamma 4$) in some interactions. Several observations suggest that αγ dimers form less readily than αβ dimers. As discussed before there is more Hb Bart's in newborns with α thalassemia than HbH in adults with the same genotype. There is some preliminary evidence that the proportion of HbF in newborns is lower in those with α thalassemia than those with four α genes.[229] Evidence also comes from the study by Chui et al.[91] who described an Italian boy who coinherited HbH disease (--/-α) and the -117 $^A\gamma$ globin HPFH mutation. They found that approximately 90% of the α-chains combined with β-globin chains to form HbA (~78%) and 10% of the α-chains associated with γ to form HbF (9.5%). Although there were sufficient free γ-chains to produce approximately 11% Hb Bart's, there were insufficient free β-chains remaining to detect HbH on electrophoresis, although HbH inclusions were detected. Taken together these findings support the hypothesis that α-globin has a higher affinity for β- than γ-globin. The interpretation of these complex interactions is by no means certain because there are other patients with similar interactions who produce different patterns of hemoglobin expression (e.g. see ref. 230).

Hematological Phenotype of Patients with α Thalassemia and β-Globin Variants

The hematological phenotype of patients with α thalassemia and stable β-globin variants is usually determined by the α-globin status giving rise to α thalassemia trait (-α/αα, -α/-α -/αα) or HbH disease (--/-α) (see Table 14.6). Interactions between nondeletional forms of α thalassemia and β-globin variants follow these same principles.

Table 14.6. Proportion of hemoglobin variant and hematological phenotypes in patients with positively charged β-globin variants

		Predicted level of variant	Hemoglobin hematological phenotype
αα/αα	β^A/β^v	50%*	Normal
-α/αα	β^A/β^v	↓	α thalassemia trait
-α/-α	β^A/β^v	↓↓	α thalassemia trait
--/αα	β^A/β^v	↓↓↓	α thalassemia trait
--/-α	β^A/β^v	↓↓↓↓	HbH disease

* Assuming that the variant is synthesized efficiently, completely stable, and associates with α^A-chains with the same kinetics as β^A-chains.

When a patient inherits only one functional α gene (or its equivalent) and a β-globin variant (β^C, β^S, β^E) they usually have the clinical and hematological phenotype of HbH disease. Splenomegaly is particularly prominent in some patients.[231] Such interactions have been described with HbC,[231] HbE,[232] HbS,[233] and Hb Hope.[234] Hemoglobin analysis usually demonstrates HbA with a very reduced amount (10%–20%) of the variant hemoglobin. The reported levels of HbH are quite variable in this interaction and sometimes undetectable by routine hemoglobin electrophoresis. Nevertheless, HbH inclusions can usually be demonstrated following incubation with brilliant cresyl blue. Hb Bart's may be detectable in some patients and is characteristically present (1%–6%) in carriers for HbE with HbH disease, a condition referred to as AE-Bart's disease (--/-α, β^A/β^E or --/$\alpha^{CS}\alpha$, β^A/β^E)[232,235] (see Chapter 18).

Rare interactions between HbH disease and β-globin variants support the electrostatic model for hemoglobin subunit assembly. Su et al.[236] reported HbH disease in a Chinese patient with the benign β mutant Hb Hamilton, which has the same charge as β^A and it appeared that the level of this mutant was not significantly reduced. Rahbar and Bunn[237] described an Iranian female with HbH disease and HbJ-lran (β77 His→Asp), a negatively charged subunit. In this case the interaction with α thalassemia produced an increased level (65%) of the variant hemoglobin.

Finally, Chan et al.[238] described a Chinese female with a severe transfusion-dependent hemolytic anemia (hemoglobin 3.4–6.8 g/dL) resulting from the interaction of HbH disease with Hb New York (β113 Val→Glu acid), an unstable negatively charged β-globin variant. In this case the coinheritance of α thalassemia increased the formation of Hb New York and thus exacerbated the hemolytic anemia.

α Thalassemia in Homozygotes and Compound Heterozygotes for β-Chain Abnormalities

α Thalassemia is common wherever β thalassemia occurs. Similarly α thalassemia is found wherever β^E and β^S reach polymorphic frequencies (see Chapter 26). Consequently, there are many potential interactions between the determinants of α thalassemia and these β-chain abnormalities.

In some cases the coinheritance of α thalassemia may significantly alter the phenotype of patients with β-chain hemoglobinopathies. The interactions between α thalassemia and β thalassemia are discussed in Chapters 16 and 17. Interactions between α thalassemia and homozygotes for β^E are set out in Chapter 18 and interactions with homozygotes for β^S in Chapters 19 and 20.

SUMMARY

Given the ever-increasing number of natural mutations affecting the α-globin cluster, the number of potential interactions increases in a corresponding manner and this review provides an update of these interactions. Despite the large number of interactions, there are limited numbers of clinical phenotypes observed in patients with α thalassemia, ranging from the innocuous thalassemia trait, through mild to severe hemolytic anemia in adults and finally to the most severe anemias associated with hydrops fetalis in neonates. The main issues in management are how to counsel and prevent the most severe anemias and how to treat those patients who, despite prenatal counseling and testing, are born and survive with the most severe anemias.

REFERENCES

1. Chui DH, Fucharoen S, Chan V. Hemoglobin H disease: not necessarily a benign disorder. *Blood.* 2003;101:791–800.
2. Giardine B, van Baal S, Kaimakis P, et al. HbVar database of human hemoglobin variants and thalassemia mutations: 2007 update. *Hum Mutat.* 2007;28:206.
3. Pornpatkul M, Wasi P, Na-Nakorn S. Hematologic parameters in obligatory alpha-thalassemia. *J Med Assoc Thai.* 1969;52:801.
4. Hunt JA, Lehmann H. Abnormal human haemoglobins. Haemoglobin 'Bart's: a foetal haemoglobin without a chains. *Nature.* 1959;184:872–873.
5. Weatherall DJ. Abnormal haemoglobins in the neonatal period and their relationship to thalassaemia. *Br J Haematol.* 1963;9:265.
6. McNiel JR. The inheritance of hemoglobin H disease. Abstracts of the Simultaneous Sessions. Paper presented at XII Congress International and National Society of Hematology. New York, 1968.
7. Pornpatkul M, Pootrakul S-N, Muangsrup W, Wasi P. Intraerythrocytic inclusion bodies in obligatory alpha thalassemia traits. *J Med Assoc Thai.* 1978;61:63.
8. Kan YW, Schwartz E, Nathan DG. Globin chain synthesis in alpha thalassemia syndromes. *J Clin Invest.* 1968;47:2515–2522.
9. Weatherall DJ, Clegg JB. *The Thalassemia Syndromes.* 4th ed. Oxford: Blackwell Science; 2001.
10. Higgs DR, Vickers MA, Wilkie AO, Pretorius IM, Jarman AP, Weatherall DJ. A review of the molecular genetics of the human alpha-globin gene cluster. *Blood.* 1989;73:1081–1104.
11. Benz EJ Jr, Swerdlow PS, Forget BG. Globin messenger RNA in hemoglobin H disease. *Blood.* 1973;42:825–833.
12. Gambino R, Kacian DL, Ramirez F, et al. Decreased globin messenger RNA in thalassemia by hydridization and biologic activity assays. *Ann NY Acad Sci.* 1974;232:6–14.
13. Grossbard E, Terada M, Dow LW, Bank A. Decreased globin messenger RNA activity associated with polyribosomes in. *Nat New Biol.* 1973;241:209–211.
14. Pritchard J, Clegg JB, Weatherall DJ, Longley J. Proceedings: The translation of human globin messenger RNA in heterologous assay systems. *Br J Haematol.* 1974;28:141–142.
15. Housman D, Forget BG, Skoultchi A, Benz EJ Jr. Quantitative deficiency of chain-specific globin messenger ribonucleic acids in the thalassemia syndromes. *Proc Natl Acad Sci USA.* 1973;70:1809–1813.
16. Kacian DL, Gambino R, Dow LW, et al. Decreased globin messenger RNA in thalassemia detected by molecular hybridization. *Proc Natl Acad Sci USA.* 1973;70:1886–1890.
17. Kan YW, Todd D, Holland J, Dozy A. Absence of a globin mRNA in homozygous α-thalassemia. *J Clin Invest.* 1974;53:37a.
18. Natta CL, Ramirez F, Wolff JA, Bank A. Decreased alpha globin mRNA in nucleated red cell precursors in alpha thalassemia. *Blood.* 1976;47:899–907.
19. Hunt DM, Higgs DR, Clegg JB, Weatherall DJ, Marsh GW. Determination of alpha thalassaemia phenotypes by messenger RNA analysis. *Br J Haematol.* 1980;45:53–64.
20. Lin SF, Liu TC, Chen TP, Chiou SS, Liu HW, Chang JG. Diagnosis of thalassaemia by non-isotope detection of alpha/beta and zeta/alpha mRNA ratios. *Br J Haematol.* 1994;87:133–138.
21. Smetanina NS, Leonova JY, Levy N, Huisman TH. The alpha/beta and alpha 2/alpha 1-globin mRNA ratios in different forms of alpha-thalassemia. *Biochim Biophys Acta.* 1996; 1315:188–192.
22. Clegg JB, Weatherall DJ. Haemoglobin synthesis in alpha-thalassaemia (haemoglobin H disease). *Nature.* 1967;215: 1241–1243.
23. Pootrakul S, Sapprapa S, Wasi P, Na-Nakorn S, Suwanik R. Hemoglobin synthesis in 28 obligatory cases for alpha-thalassemia traits. *Humangenetik.* 1975;29:121–126.
24. Weatherall DJ, Clegg JB, Boon WH. The haemoglobin constitution of infants with the haemoglobin Bart's hydrops foetalis syndrome. *Br J Haematol.* 1970;18:357–367.
25. Ganczakowski M, Bowden DK, Maitland K, et al. Thalassaemia in Vanuatu, south-west Pacific: frequency and haematological phenotypes of young children. *Br J Haematol.* 1995;89:485–495.
26. Williams TN, Maitland K, Ganczakowski M, et al. Red blood cell phenotypes in the alpha + thalassaemias from early childhood to maturity. *Br J Haematol.* 1996;95:266–272.
27. Owen GM, Yanochik-Owen A. Should there be a different definition of anemia in black and white children? *Am J Public Health.* 1977;67:865–866.
28. Ross DW, Ayscue LH, Watson J, Bentley SA. Stability of hematologic arameters in healthy subjects. Intraindividual versus interindividual ariation. *Am J Clin Pathol.* 1988;90:262–267.
29. Chan LC, Ma SK, Chan AY, et al. Should we screen for globin gene mutations in blood samples with mean corpuscular volume (MCV) greater than 80 fL in areas with a high relevance of thalassaemia? *J Clin Pathol.* 2001;54:317–320.
30. Chui DH. Alpha-thalassaemia and population health in southeast Asia. *Ann Hum Biol.* 2005;32:123–130.

31. Higgs DR. alpha-Thalassaemia. *Baillieres Clin Haematol.* 1993;6:117–150.
32. Rees DC, Williams TN, Maitland K, Clegg JB, Weatherall DJ. Alpha thalassaemia is associated with increased soluble transferrin receptor levels. *Br J Haematol.* 1998;103:365–369.
33. Nathan DG, Gunn RB. Thalassemia: the consequences of unbalanced hemoglobin synthesis. *Am J Med.* 1966;41:815–830.
34. Wasi P, Na-Nakorn S, Pootrakul S. The α thalassaemias. *Clin Haematol.* 1974;3:383–410.
35. Maude GH, Higgs DR, Beckford M, et al. Alpha thalassaemia and the haematology of normal Jamaican children. *Clin Lab Haematol.* 1985;7:289–295.
36. Higgs DR, Pressley L, Clegg JB, et al. Detection of alpha thalassemia in Negro infants. *Br J Haematol.* 1980;46:39–46.
37. Kyriacou K, Kyrri A, Kalogirou E, et al. Hb Bart's levels in cord blood and alpha-thalassemia mutations in Cyprus. *Hemoglobin.* 2000;24:171–180.
38. Rugless MJ, Fisher CA, Stephens AD, Amos RJ, Mohammed T, Old JM. Hb Bart's in cord blood: an accurate indicator of alpha-thalassemia. *Hemoglobin.* 2006;30:57–62.
39. Wasi P, Pravatmuang P, Winichagoon P. Immunologic diagnosis of alpha-thalassemia traits. *Hemoglobin.* 1979;3:21–31.
40. Chui DH, Wong SC, Chung SW, Patterson M, Bhargava S, Poon MC. Embryonic zeta-globin chains in adults: a marker for alpha-thalassemia-1 haplotype due to a greater than 17.5-kb deletion. *N Engl J Med.* 1986;314:76–79.
41. Lafferty JD, Barth DS, Sheridan BL, et al. A multicenter trial of the effectiveness of zeta-globin enzyme-linked immunosorbent assay and hemoglobin H inclusion body screening for the detection of alpha^{0}-thalassemia trait. *Am J Clin Pathol.* 2008;129:309–315.
42. Galanello R, Paglietti E, Melis MA, Giagu L, Cao A. Hemoglobin inclusions in heterozygous alpha-thalassemia according to their alpha-globin genotype. *Acta Haematol.* 1984;72:34–36.
43. Gibbons RJ, Wilkie AO, Weatherall DJ, Higgs DR. A newly defined X linked mental retardation syndrome associated with alpha thalassaemia. *J Med Genet.* 1991;28:729–733.
44. Sabath DE, Cross ST, Mamiya LY. An improved method for detecting red cells with hemoglobin H inclusions that does not require glass capillary tubes. *Clin Lab Haematol.* 2003;25:87–91.
45. Lam YH, Ghosh A, Tang MH, Chan V. The risk of alpha-thalassaemia in offspring of beta-thalassaemia carriers in Hong Kong. *Prenat Diagn.* 1997;17:733–736.
46. Letsky EA, Redman CWG. Blood disorders in pregnancy. In: Weatherall DJ, Ledingham JGG, Warrell DA, eds. *Oxford Textbook of Medicine.* Vol 1. Oxford: Oxford University Press; 1987:11.31–11.35.
47. O'Donnell A, Raiko A, Clegg JB, Weatherall DJ, Allen SJ. Alpha+ -thalassaemia and pregnancy in a malaria endemic region of Papua New Guinea. *Br J Haematol.* 2006;135:235–241.
48. Diejomaoh FM, Haider MZ, Dalai H, Abdulaziz A, D'Souza TM, Adekile AD. Influence of alpha-thalassemia trait on the prevalence and severity of anemia in pregnancy among women in Kuwait. *Acta Haematol.* 2000;104:92–94.
49. White JM, Richards R, Byrne M, Buchanan T, White YS, Jelenski G. Thalassaemia trait and pregnancy. *J Clin Pathol.* 1985;38:810–817.
50. Paglietti E, Galanello R, Moi P, Pirastu M, Cao A. Molecular pathology of haemoglobin H disease in Sardinians. *Br J Haematol.* 1986;63:485–496.
51. Higgs DR, Goodbourn SE, Lamb J, Clegg JB, Weatherall DJ, Proudfoot NJ. Alpha-thalassaemia caused by a polyadenylation signal mutation. *Nature.* 1983;306:398–400.
52. Arnon S, Tamary H, Dgany O, et al. Hydrops fetalis associated with homozygosity for hemoglobin Taybe (alpha 38/39 THR deletion) in newborn triplets. *Am J Hematol.* 2004;76:263–266.
53. Charoenkwan P, Sirichotiyakul S, Chanprapaph P, et al. Anemia and hydrops in a fetus with homozygous hemoglobin constant spring. *J Pediatr Hematol Oncol.* 2006;28:827–830.
54. Lie-lnjo LE, Ganesan J, Clegg JB, Weatherall DJ. Homozygous state for Hb Constant Spring (slow-moving Hb X components). *Blood.* 1974;43:251–259.
55. Lie-lnjo LE, Ganesan J, Lopez CG. The clinical, hematological and biochemical expression of hemoglobin constant spring and its distribution. In: Schmidt RM ed. *Abnormal Hemoglobins and Thalassemia – Diagnostic Aspects.* New York: Academic Press; 1975.
56. Pongsamart S, Pootrakul S, Wasi P, Na-Nakorn S. Hemoglobin Constant Spring: hemoglobin synthesis in heterozygous and homozygous states. *Biochem Biophys Res Commun.* 1975;64:681–686.
57. Pootrakul P, Winichagoon P, Fucharoen S, Pravatmuang P, Piankijagum A, Wasi P. Homozygous haemoglobin Constant Spring: a need for revision of concept. *Hum Genet.* 1981;59:250–255.
58. Viprakasit V, Veerakul G, Sanpakit K, Pongtanakul B, Chinchang W, Tanphaichitr VS. Acute haemolytic crisis in a Thai patient with homozygous haemoglobin Constant Spring (Hb CS/CS): a case report. *Ann Trop Paediatr.* 2004;24:323–328.
59. Deny S, Wood WG, Pippard M, et al. Hematologic and biosynthetic studies in homozygous hemoglobin Constant Spring. *J Clin Invest.* 1984;73:1673–1682.
60. Fei YJ, Oner R, Bozkurt G, et al. Hb H disease caused by a homozygosity for the AATAAA–>AATAAG mutation in the polyadenylation site of the alpha 2-globin gene: hematological observations. *Acta Haematol.* 1992;88:82–85.
61. Galanello R, Aru B, Dessi C, et al. HbH disease in Sardinia: molecular, hematological and clinical aspects. *Acta Haematol.* 1992;88:1–6.
62. Kanavakis E, Papassotiriou I, Karagiorga M, et al. Phenotypic and molecular diversity of haemoglobin H disease: a Greek experience. *Br J Haematol.* 2000;111:915–923.
63. Khan SN, Butt Fl, Riazuddin S, Galanello R. Hb Sallanches [alpha104(G11)Cys->Tyr]: a rare alpha2-globin chain variant found in the homozygous state in three members of a Pakistani family. *Hemoglobin.* 2000;24:31–35.
64. Morle F, Francina A, Ducrocq R, et al. A new alpha chain variant Hb Sallanches [alpha 2 104(G11) Cys->Tyr] associated with HbH disease in one homozygous patient. *Br J Haematol.* 1995;91:608–611.
65. Oner C, Gurgey A, Oner R, et al. The molecular basis of Hb H disease in Turkey. *Hemoglobin.* 1997;21:41–51.
66. Pressley L, Higgs DR, Clegg JB, Perrine RP, Pembrey ME, Weatherall DJ. A new genetic basis for hemoglobin-H disease. *N Engl J Med.* 1980;303:1383–1388.

67. Waye JS, Walker L, Chui DH, Lafferty J, Kirby M. Homozygous Hb Sallanches [alpha104(G11)Cys->Tyr] in a Pakistani child with Hb H disease. *Hemoglobin.* 2000;24:355–357.
68. Benesch RE, Ranney HM, Benesch R, Smith GM. The chemistry of the Bohr effect. II. Some properties of hemoglobin H. *J Biol Chem.* 1961;236:2926–2929.
69. Papassotiriou I, Traeger-Synodinos J, Kanavakis E, Karagiorga M, Stamoulakatou A, Kattamis C. Erythroid marrow activity and hemoglobin H levels in hemoglobin H disease. *J Pediatr Hematol Oncol.* 1998;20:539–544.
70. Schrier SL, Rachmilewitz E, Mohandas N. Cellular and membrane properties of alpha and beta thalassemic erythrocytes are different: implication for differences in clinical manifestations. *Blood.* 1989;74:2194–2202.
71. Schrier SL, Bunyaratvej A, Khuhapinant A, et al. The unusual pathobiology of hemoglobin constant spring red blood cells. *Blood.* 1997;89:1762–1769.
72. Chen FE, Ooi C, Ha SY, et al. Genetic and clinical features of hemoglobin H disease in Chinese patients. *N Engl J Med.* 2000;343:544–550.
73. Origa R, Sollaino MC, Giagu N, et al. Clinical and molecular analysis of haemoglobin H disease in Sardinia: haematological, obstetric and cardiac aspects in patients with different genotypes. *Br J Haematol.* 2007;136:326–332.
74. Knox-Macaulay HH, Weatherall DJ, Clegg JB, Bradley J, Brown MJ. The clinical and biosynthetic characterization of -thalasasemia. *Br J Haematol.* 1972;22:497–512.
75. Pearson HA, McFarland W. Erythrokinetics in thalassemia. II. Studies in Lepore trait and hemoglobin H disease. *J Lab Clin Med.* 1962;59:147–157.
76. Rigas DA, Koler RD. Decreased erythrocyte survival in hemoglobin H disease as a result of the abnormal properties of hemoglobin H: the benefit of splenectomy. *Blood.* 1961;18:1–17.
77. Woodrow JC, Noble RL, Martindale JH. Haemoglobin H disease in an English family. *Br Med J.* 1964;1:36–38.
78. Srichaikul T, Tipayasakda J, Atichartakarn V, Jootar S, Bovornbinyanun P. Ferrokinetic and erythrokinetic studies in alpha and beta thalassemia. *Clin Lab Haematol.* 1984; 6:133–140.
79. Wongchanchailert M, Laosombat V, Maipang M. Hemoglobin H disease in children. *J Med Assoc Thai.* 1992;75:611–618.
80. Piankijagum A, Palungwachira P, Lohkoomgunpai A. Beta thalassemia, hemoglobin E and hemoglobin H disease. Clinical analysis 1964–1966. *J Med Assoc Thai.* 1978;61:50.
81. Bunn HF, Forget BG. *Hemoglobin: Molecular, Genetic and Clinical Aspects.* Philadelphia: W.B. Saunders; 1986.
82. Waye JS, Eng B, Patterson M, et al. Hemoglobin H (Hb H) disease in Canada: molecular diagnosis and review of 116 cases. *Am J Hematol.* 2001;68:11–15.
83. Fucharoen S, Winichagoon P, Pootrakul P, Piankijagum A, Wasi P. Differences between two types of Hb H disease, alpha-thalassemia 1/alpha-thalassemia 2 and alpha-thalassemia 1/Hb constant spring. *Birth Defects Orig Artic Ser.* 1987;23:309–315.
84. Galanello R, Pirastu M, Melis MA, Paglietti E, Moi P, Cao A. Phenotype-genotype correlation in haemoglobin H disease in childhood. *J Med Genet.* 1983;20:425–429.
85. Pootrakul S, Wasi P, Na-Nakorn S. Studies on haemoglobin Bart's's (Hb-gamma-4) in Thailand: the incidence and the mechanism of occurrence in cord blood. *Ann Hum Genet.* 1967;31:149–166.
86. Wasi P, Na-Nakorn S, Pootrakul S, et al. Alpha- and beta-thalassemia in Thailand. *Ann NY Acad Sci.* 1969;165:60–82.
87. Rachmilewitz EA, Harari E. Slow rate of haemichrome formation from oxidized haemoglobin Bart's ($\gamma 4$): a possible explanation for the unequal quantities of haemoglobins H ($\gamma 4$) and Bart's in alpha-thalassemia. *Br J Haematol.* 1972;22:357–364.
88. Baysal E, Kleanthous M, Bozkurt G, et al. alpha-Thalassemia in the population of Cyprus. *Br J Haematol.* 1995;89:496–499.
89. Higgs DR, Weatherall DJ. Alpha-thalassemia. *Curr Top Hematol.* 1983;4:37–97.
90. Ramot B, Sheba C, Fisher S, Ager JA, Lehmann H. Haemoglobin H disease with persistent haemoglobin "Bart's" in an Oriental Jewess and her daughter: a dual alpha-chain deficiency of human haemoglobin. *Br Med J.* 1959;2:1228–1230.
91. Chui DH, Patterson M, Dowling CE, Kazazian HH Jr, Kendall AG. Hemoglobin Bart's disease in an Italian boy. Interaction between alpha-thalassemia and hereditary persistence of fetal hemoglobin. *N Engl J Med.* 1990;323:179–182.
92. Adirojnanon P, Wasi P. Levels of haemoglobin H and proportions of red cells with inclusion bodies in the two types of haemoglobin H disease. *Br J Haematol.* 1980;46:507–509.
93. Weatherall DJ, Clegg JB. The alpha-chain-termination mutants and their relation to the alpha-thalassaemias. *Philos Trans R Soc Lond B Biol Sci.* 1975;271:411–455.
94. George E, Ferguson V, Yakas J, Kronenberg H, Trent RJ. A molecular marker associated with mild hemoglobin H disease. *Pathology.* 1989;21:27–30.
95. Kattamis C, Tzotzos S, Kanavakis E, Synodinos J, Metaxotou-Mavrommati A. Correlation of clinical phenotype to genotype in haemoglobin H disease. *Lancet.* 1988;1:442–444.
96. Wasi P. Hemoglobinopathies in Southeast Asia. In: Bowman JE, ed. *Distribution and Evolution of the Hemoglobin and Globin Loci.* New York: Elsevier; 1983:179–209.
97. Wong HB. Thalassemias in Singapore. *J Singapore Paediatr Soc.* 1984;26:1–14.
98. Lorey F, Cunningham G, Vichinsky EP, et al. Universal newborn screening for Hb H disease in California. *Genet Test.* 2001;5:93–100.
99. Au WY, Cheung WC, Hu WH, et al. Hyperbilirubinemia and cholelithiasis in Chinese patients with hemoglobin H disease. *Ann Hematol.* 2005;84:671–674.
100. Wu JH, Shih LY, Kuo TT, Lan RS. Intrathoracic extramedullary hematopoietic tumor in hemoglobin H disease. *Am J Hematol.* 1992;41:285–288.
101. Vaeusorn O, Fucharoen S, Wasi P. A study of thalassemia associated with pregnancy. *Birth Defects Orig Artic Ser.* 1988;23:295–299.
102. Tantiweerawong N, Jaovisidha A, Israngura Na Ayudhya N. Pregnancy outcome of hemoglobin H disease. *Intl J Gynecol Obstetr.* 2005;90:236–237.
103. Ong HC, White JC, Sinnathuray TA. Haemoglobin H disease and pregnancy in a Malaysian woman. *Acta Haematol.* 1977;58:229–333.
104. Lin CK, Lin JS, Jiang ML. Iron absorption is increased in hemoglobin H diseases. *Am J Hematol.* 1992;40:74–75.

105. Chim CS, Chan V, Todd D. Hemosiderosis with diabetes mellitus in untransfused Hemoglobin H disease. *Am J Hematol.* 1998;57:160–163.
106. Tso SC, Loh TT, Todd D. Iron overload in patients with haemoglobin H disease. *Scand J Haematol.* 1984;32:391–394.
107. Sonakul D, Sook-aneak M, Pacharee P. Pathology of thalassemic diseases in Thailand. *J Med Assoc Thai.* 1978;61:72.
108. Hsu HC, Lin CK, Tsay SH, et al. Iron overload in Chinese patients with hemoglobin H disease. *Am J Hematol.* 1990;34:287–290.
109. Lin CK, Peng HW, Ho CH, Yung CH. Iron overload in untransfused patients with hemoglobin H disease. *Acta Haematol.* 1990;83:137–139.
110. Ooi GC, Chen FE, Chan KN, et al. Qualitative and quantitative magnetic resonance imaging in haemoglobin H disease: screening for iron overload. *Clin Radiol.* 1999;54:98–102.
111. Thakerngpol K, Fucharoen S, Boonyaphipat P, et al. Liver injury due to iron overload in thalassemia: histopathologic and ultrastructural studies. *Biometals.* 1996;9:177–183.
112. Chan JC, Chim CS, Ooi CG, et al. Use of the oral chelator deferiprone in the treatment of iron overload in patients with Hb H disease. *Br J Haematol.* 2006;133:198–205.
113. Feder JN, Gnirke A, Thomas W, et al. A novel MHC class l-like gene is mutated in patients with hereditary haemochromatosis. *Nat Genet.* 1996;13:399–408.
114. Daneshmend TK, Peachey RD. Leg ulcers in alpha-thalassemia (haemoglobin H disease). *Br J Dermatol.* 1978; 98:233–235.
115. Cao A, Rosatelli C, Pirastu M, Galanello R. Thalassemias in Sardinia: molecular pathology, phenotype-genotype correlation, and prevention. *Am J Pediatr Hematol Oncol.* 1991;13:179–188.
116. Daneshmend TK. Ocular findings in a case of haemoglobin H disease. *Br J Ophthalmol.* 1979;63:842–844.
117. Eldor A, Rachmilewitz EA. The hypercoagulable state in thalassemia. *Blood.* 2002;99:36–43.
118. Kanavakis E, Traeger-Synodinos J, Papasotiriou I, et al. The interaction of alpha zero thalassemia with Hb Icaria: three unusual cases of haemoglobinopathy H. *Br J Haematol.* 1996;92:332–335.
119. Nathan DG, Oski FA. *Hematology of Infancy and Childhood.* 3rd ed. Philadelphia: W.B. Saunders; 1987.
120. Shojania AM, Gross S. Hemolytic anemias and folic acid deficiency in children. *Am J Dis Child.* 1964;108:53–61.
121. Kanavakis E, Tzotzos S, Liapaki A, Metaxotou-Mavromati A, Kattamis C. Frequency of alpha-thalassemia in Greece. *Am J Hematol.* 1986;22:225–232.
122. Wagner GM, Liebhaber SA, Cutting HO, Embury SH. Hematologic improvement following splenectomy for hemoglobin-H disease. *West J Med.* 1982;137:325–328.
123. Hirsh J, Dacie JV. Persistent post-splenectomy thrombocytosis and thrombo-embolism: a consequence of continuing anaemia. *Br J Haematol.* 1966;12:44–53.
124. Sonakul D, Fucharoen S. Pulmonary thromboembolism in thalassemic patients. *Southeast Asian J Trop Med Public Health.* 1992;23(Suppl 2):25–28.
125. Tso SC, Chan TK, Todd D. Venous thrombosis in haemoglobin H disease after splenectomy. *Aust NZ J Med.* 1982; 12:635–638.
126. Chapman RW, Williams G, Bydder G, Dick R, Sherlock S, Kreel L. Computed tomography for determining liver iron content in primary haemochromatosis. *Br Med J.* 1980;280:440–442.
127. Jensen PD, Jensen FT, Christensen T, Ellegaard J. Non-invasive assessment of tissue iron overload in the liver by magnetic resonance imaging. *Br J Haematol.* 1994;87:171–184.
128. Arcasoy MO, Gallagher PG. Hematologic disorders and non-immune hydrops fetalis. *Semin Perinatol.* 1995;19:502–515.
129. Holzgreve W, Curry CJ, Golbus MS, Callen PW, Filly RA, Smith JC. Investigation of nonimmune hydrops fetalis. *Am J Obstet Gynecol.* 1984;150:805–812.
130. Jauniaux E, Van Maldergem L, De Munter C, Moscoso G, Gillerot Y. Nonimmune hydrops fetalis associated with genetic abnormalities. *Obstet Gynecol.* 1990;75:568–572.
131. Nicolaides KH, Rodeck CH, Lange I, et al. Fetoscopy in the assessment of unexplained fetal hydrops. *Br J Obstet Gynaecol.* 1985;92:671–679.
132. Suwanrath-Kengpol C, Kor-anantakul O, Suntharasaj T, Leetanaporn R. Etiology and outcome of non-immune hydrops fetalis in southern Thailand. *Gynecol Obstet Invest.* 2005;59:134–137.
133. Clarke C, Whitfield AG. Deaths from rhesus haemolytic disease in England and Wales in 1977: accuracy of records and assessment of anti-D prophylaxis. *Br Med J.* 1979;1:1665–1669.
134. Machin GA. Differential diagnosis of hydrops fetalis. *Am J Med Genet.* 1981;9:341–350.
135. Ko TM, Hsieh FJ, Hsu PM, Lee TY. Molecular characterization of severe alpha-thalassemias causing hydrops fetalis in Taiwan. *Am J Med Genet.* 1991;39:317–320.
136. Liang ST, Wong VC, So WW, Ma HK, Chan V, Todd D. Homozygous alpha-thalassemia: clinical presentation, diagnosis and management. A review of 46 cases. *Br J Obstet Gynaecol.* 1985;92:680–684.
137. Lie-lnjo Luan ENG. Haemoglobin of new-born infants in Indonesia. *Nature.* 1959;183:1125–1126.
138. Tan SL, Tseng AM, Thong PW. Bart's hydrops fetalis-clinical presentation and management – an analysis of 25 cases. *Aust NZ J Obstet Gynaecol.* 1989;29:233–237.
139. Thumasathit B, Nondasuta A, Silpisornkosol S, Lousuebsakul B, Unchalipongse P, Mangkornkanok M. Hydrops fetalis associated with Bart's hemoglobin in northern Thailand. *J Pediatr.* 1968;73:132–138.
140. Lau YL, Chan LC, Chan YY, et al. Prevalence and genotypes of alpha- and beta-thalassemia carriers in Hong Kong – implications for population screening. *N Engl J Med.* 1997;336:1298–1301.
141. Tongsong T, Boonyanurak P. Placental thickness in the first half of pregnancy. *J Clin Ultrasound.* 2004;32:231–234.
142. Xu XM, Zhou YQ, Luo GX, et al. The prevalence and spectrum of alpha and beta thalassaemia in Guangdong Province: implications for the future health burden and population screening. *J Clin Pathol.* 2004;57:517–522.
143. Fischel-Ghodsian N, Vickers MA, Seip M, Winichagoon P, Higgs DR. Characterization of two deletions that remove the entire human zeta-alpha globin gene complex (--THAI and --FIL). *Br J Haematol.* 1988;70:233–238.
144. Diamond MP, Cotgrove I, Parker A. Case of intrauterine death due to alpha-thalassaemia. *Br Med J.* 1965;2:278–279.

145. Kattamis C, Metaxotou-Mavromati A, Tsiarta E, et al. Haemoglobin Bart's hydrops syndrome in Greece. *Br Med J.* 1980;281:268–270.
146. Pressley L, Higgs DR, Clegg JB, Weatherall DJ. Gene deletions in alpha thalassemia prove that the 5′ zeta locus is functional. *Proc Natl Acad Sci USA.* 1980;77:3586–3589.
147. Sharma RS, Yu V, Walters WA. Haemoglobin Bart's hydrops fetalis syndrome in an infant of Greek origin and prenatal diagnosis of alpha-thalassaemia. *Med J Aust.* 1979;2:404,:33–34.
148. Nicholls RD, Higgs DR, Clegg JB, Weatherall DJ. Alpha zero-thalassemia due to recombination between the alpha 1-globin gene and an AluI repeat. *Blood.* 1985;65:1434–1438.
149. Sophocleous T, Higgs DR, Aldridge B, et al. The molecular basis for the haemoglobin Bart's hydrops fetalis syndrome in Cyprus. *Br J Haematol.* 1981;47:153–156.
150. Galanello R, Sanna MA, Maccioni L, et al. Fetal hydrops in Sardinia: implications for genetic counselling. *Clin Genet.* 1990;38:327–331.
151. Gurgey A, Altay C, Beksac MS, Bhattacharya R, Kutlar F, Huisman TH. Hydrops fetalis due to homozygosity for alpha-thalassemia-1,-(alpha)-20.5 kb: the first observation in a Turkish family. *Acta Haematol.* 1989;81:169–171.
152. Vaeusorn O, Fucharoen S, Ruangpiroj T, et al. Fetal pathology and maternal morbidity in hemoglobin Bart's hydrops fetalis: an analysis of 65 cases. Paper presented at International Conference on Thalassemia. Bangkok, Thailand, 1985.
153. Chui DH, Waye JS. Hydrops fetalis caused by alpha-thalassemia: an emerging health care problem. *Blood.* 1998;91:2213–2222.
154. Peschle C, Mavilio F, Care A, et al. Haemoglobin switching in human embryos: asynchrony of zeta – alpha and epsilon – gamma-globin switches in primitive and definite erythropoietic lineage. *Nature.* 1985;313:235–238.
155. Horton BF, Thompson RB, Dozy AM, Nechtman CM, Nichols E, Huisman TH. Inhomogeneity of hemoglobin. VI. The minor hemoglobin components of cord blood. *Blood.* 1962;20:302–314.
156. Tuchinda S, Nagai K, Lehmann H. Oxygen dissociation curve of haemoglobin Portland. *FEBS Lett.* 1975;49:390–391.
157. Ausavarungnirun R, Winichagoon P, Fucharoen S, Epstein N, Simkins R. Detection of zeta-globin chains in the cord blood by ELISA (enzyme-linked immunosorbent assay): rapid screening for alpha-thalassemia 1 (Southeast Asian type). *Am J Hematol.* 1998;57:283–286.
158. Chui DH, Mentzer WC, Patterson M, et al. Human embryonic zeta-globin chains in fetal and newborn blood. *Blood.* 1989;74:1409–1414.
159. Kutlar F, Gonzalez-Redondo JM, Kutlar A, et al. The levels of zeta, gamma, and delta chains in patients with Hb H disease. *Hum Genet.* 1989;82:179–186.
160. Tang W, Luo HY, Albitar M, et al. Human embryonic zeta-globin chain expression in deletional alpha-thalassemias. *Blood.* 1992;80:517–522.
161. Nakayama R, Yamada D, Steinmiller V, Hsia E, Hale RW. Hydrops fetalis secondary to Bart's hemoglobinopathy. *Obstet Gynecol.* 1986;67:176–180,
162. Isarangkura P, Siripoonya P, Fucharoen S, Hathirat P. Hemoglobin Bart's disease without hydrops manifestation. *Birth Defects Orig Artic Ser.* 1987;23:333–342.
163. Beutler E, Lichtman MA, Coller BS, Kipps TJ. *Williams Hematology.* 5th ed. New York: McGraw-Hill; 1995.
164. Guy G, Coady DJ, Jansen V, Snyder J, Zinberg S. alpha-Thalassemia hydrops fetalis: clinical and ultrasonographic considerations. *Am J Obstet Gynecol.* 1985;153:500–504.
165. Abuelo DN, Forman EN, Rubin LP. Limb defects and congenital anomalies of the genitalia in an infant with homozygous alpha-thalassemia. *Am J Med Genet.* 1997;68:158–161.
166. Adam MP, Chueh J, El-Sayed YY, et al. Vascular-type disruptive defects in fetuses with homozygous alpha-thalassemia: report of two cases and review of the literature. *Prenat Diagn.* 2005;25:1088–1096.
167. Carr S, Rubin L, Dixon D, Star J, Dailey J. Intrauterine therapy for homozygous alpha-thalassemia. *Obstet Gynecol.* 1995;85:876–879.
168. Chitayat D, Silver MM, O'Brien K, et al. Limb defects in homozygous alpha-thalassemia: report of three cases. *Am J Med Genet.* 1997;68:162–167.
169. Harmon JV Jr, Osathanondh R, Holmes LB. Symmetrical terminal transverse limb defects: report of a twenty-week fetus. *Teratology.* 1995;51:237–242.
170. Lam YH, Tang MH, Sin SY, Ghosh A, Lee CP. Limb reduction defects in fetuses with homozygous alpha-thalassaemia-1. *Prenat Diagn.* 1997;17;1143–1146.
171. Fung TY, Kin LT, Kong LC, Keung LC. Homozygous alpha-thalassemia associated with hypospadias in three survivors. *Am J Med Genet.* 1999;82:225–227.
172. Ongsangkoon T, Vawesorn O, Pootakul S-N. Pathology of hemoglobin Bart's hydrops fetalis. 1. Gross autopsy findings. *J Med Assoc Thai.* 1978;61:71.
173. Thornley I, Lehmann L, Ferguson WS, Davis I, Forman EN, Guinan EC. Homozygous alpha-thalassemia treated with intrauterine transfusions and postnatal hematopoietic stem cell transplantation. *Bone Marrow Transplant.* 2003;32:341–342.
174. Chan V, Chan VW, Tang M, Lau K, Todd D, Chan TK. Molecular defects in Hb H hydrops fetalis. *Br J Haematol.* 1997;96:224–228.
175. Chan V, Chan TK, Liang ST, Ghosh A, Kan YW, Todd D. Hydrops fetalis due to an unusual form of Hb H disease. *Blood.* 1985;66:224–228.
176. Oron-Karni V, Filon D, Shifrin Y, et al. Diversity of alpha-globin mutations and clinical presentation of alpha-thalassemia in Israel. *Am J Hematol.* 2000;65:196–203.
177. McBride KL, Snow K, Kubik KS, et al. Hb Dartmouth. alpha66(E15)Leu–>Pro (alpha2) (CTG–>CCG)]: a novel alpha2-globin gene mutation associated with severe neonatal anemia when inherited in trans with Southeast Asian alpha-thalassemia-1. *Hemoglobin.* 2001;25:375–382.
178. Li DZ, Liao C, Li J, Xie XM, Huang YN, Wu QC. Hemoglobin H hydrops fetalis syndrome resulting from the association of the --SEA deletion and the a Quong Sze a mutation in a Chinese woman. *Eur J Haematol.* 2005;75:259–261.
179. Traeger-Synodinos J, Papassotiriou I, Karagiorga M, Premetis E, Kanavakis E, Stamoulakatou A. Unusual phenotypic observations associated with a rare HbH disease genotype (-Med/alphaTSaudialpha): implications for clinical management. *Br J Haematol.* 2002;119:265–267.
180. Viprakasit V, Green S, Height S, Ayyub H, Higgs DR. Hb H hydrops fetalis syndrome associated with the interaction

of two common determinants of alpha thalassaemia (-MED/(alpha) TSaudi (alpha)). *Br J Haematol.* 2002;117:759–762.

181. Henderson S, Chappie M, Rugless M, Fisher C, Kinsey S, Old J. Haemoglobin H hydrops fetalis syndrome associated with homozygosity for the alpha2-globin gene polyadenylation signal mutation AATAAA~>AATA. *Br J Haematol.* 2006;135:743–745.
182. Trent RJ, Mickleson KN, Wilkinson T, et al. Globin genes in Polynesians have many rearrangements including a recently described gamma gamma gamma gamma. *Am J Hum Genet.* 1986;39:350–360.
183. Hofstaetter C, Gonser M, Goelz R. Perinatal case report of unexpected thalassemia Hb Bart's. *Fetal Diagn Ther.* 1993;8:418–422.
184. Monaco SE, Davis M, Huang AC, et al. Alpha-thalassemia major presenting in a term neonate without hydrops. *Pediatr Dev Pathol.* 2005;8:706–709.
185. Ng PC, Fok TF, Lee CH, et al. Is homozygous alpha-thalassemia a lethal condition in the 1990s? *Acta Paediatr.* 1998;87:1197–1199.
186. Lee SY, Chow CB, Li CK, Chiu MC. Outcome of intensive care of homozygous alpha-thalassaemia without prior intra-uterine therapy. *J Paediatr Child Health.* 2007;43:546–550.
187. Bianchi DW, Beyer EC, Stark AR, Saffan D, Sachs BP, Wolfe L. Normal long-term survival with alpha-thalassemia. *J Pediatr.* 1986;108:716–718.
188. Chik KW, Shing MM, Li CK, et al. Treatment of hemoglobin Bart's hydrops with bone marrow transplantation. *J Pediatr.* 1998;132:1039–1042.
189. Jackson DN, Strauss AA, Groncy PK, Bianchi DW, Akabutu J. Outcome of neonatal survivors with homozygous a-thalassemia. *Pediatr Res.* 1990;27:266A.
190. Lam TK, Chan V, Fok TF, Li CK, Feng CS. Long-term survival of a baby with homozygous alpha-thalassemia-1. *Acta Haematol.* 1992;88:198–200.
191. Liu CA, Huang HC, Chou YY. Retrospective analysis of 17 liveborn neonates with hydrops fetalis. *Chang Gung Med J.* 2002;25:826–831.
192. Singer ST, Styles L, Bojanowski J, Quirolo K, Foote D, Vichinsky EP. Changing outcome of homozygous alpha-thalassemia: cautious optimism. *J Pediatr Hematol Oncol.* 2000;22:539–542.
193. Zhou X, Ha SY, Chan GC, et al. Successful mismatched sibling cord blood transplant in Hb Bart's disease. *Bone Marrow Transplant.* 2001;28:105–107.
194. Bizzarro MJ, Copel JA, Pearson HA, Pober B, Bhandari V. Pulmonary hypoplasia and persistent pulmonary hypertension in the newborn with homozygous alpha-thalassemia: a case report and review of the literature. *J Matern Fetal Neonatal Med.* 2003;14:411–416.
195. Dame C, Albers N, Hasan C, et al. Homozygous alpha-thalassemia and hypospadias-common aetiology or incidental association? Long-term survival of Hb Bart's hydrops syndrome leads to new aspects for counselling of alpha-thalassaemic traits. *Eur J Pediatr.* 1999;158:217–220.
196. Fung TY, Lau TK, Tarn WH, Li CK. In utero exchange transfusion in homozygous alpha-thalassaemia: a case report. *Prenat Diagn.* 1998;18:838–841.
197. Hayward A, Ambruso D, Battaglia F, et al. Microchimerism and tolerance following intrauterine transplantation and transfusion for alpha-thalassemia-1. *Fetal Diagn Ther.* 1998;13:8–14.
198. Joshi DD, Nickerson HJ, McManus MJ. Hydrops fetalis caused by homozygous alpha-thalassemia and Rh antigen alloimmunization: report of a survivor and literature review. *Clin Med Res.* 2004;2:228–232.
199. Leung WC, Oepkes D, Seaward G, Ryan G. Serial sonographic findings of four fetuses with homozygous alpha-thalassemia-1 from 21 weeks onwards. *Ultrasound Obstet Gynecol.* 2002;19:56–59.
200. Lucke T, Pfister S, Durken M. Neurodevelopmental outcome and haematological course of a long-time survivor with homozygous alpha-thalasasemia: case report and review of the literature. *Acta Paediatr.* 2005;94:1330–1333.
201. Naqvi A, Waye JS, Morrow R, Nisbet-Brown E, Olivieri NF. Normal development of an infant with homozygous a-thalassemia. *Blood.* 1997;90:132A.
202. Sohan K, Billington M, Pamphilon D, Goulden N, Kyle P. Normal growth and development following in utero diagnosis and treatment of homozygous alpha-thalassaemia. *Br J Obstet Gynaecol.* 2002;109:1308–1310.
203. Westgren M, Ringden O, Eik-Nes S, et al. Lack of evidence of permanent engraftment after in utero fetal stem cell transplantation in congenital hemoglobinopathies. *Transplantation.* 1996;61:1176–1179.
204. Petrou M, Brugiatelli M, Old J, Hurley P, Ward RH, Wong KP, et al. Alpha thalassaemia hydrops fetalis in the UK: the importance of screening pregnant women of Chinese, other South East Asian and Mediterranean extraction for alpha thalassaemia trait. *Br J Obstet Gynaecol.* 1992;99:985–989.
205. Ghosh A, Tang MH, Lam YH, Fung E, Chan V. Ultrasound measurement of placental thickness to detect pregnancies affected by homozygous alpha-thalassaemia-1. *Lancet.* 1994;344:988–989.
206. Kanokpongsakdi S, Fucharoen S, Vatanasiri C, Thonglairoam V, Winichagoon P, Manassakorn J. Ultrasonographic method for detection of haemoglobin Bart's hydrops fetalis in the second trimester of pregnancy. *Prenat Diagn.* 1990;10:809–813.
207. Saltzman DH, Frigoletto FD, Harlow BL, Barss VA, Benacerraf BR. Sonographic evaluation of hydrops fetalis. *Obstet Gynecol.* 1989;74:106–111.
208. Tongsong T, Wanapirak C, Srisomboon J, Piyamongkol W, Sirichotiyakul S. Antenatal sonographic features of 100 alpha-thalassemia hydrops fetalis fetuses. *J Clin Ultrasound.* 1996 24:73–77.
209. Ghosh A, Tang MH, Liang ST, Ma HK, Chan V, Chan TK. Ultrasound evaluation of pregnancies at risk for homozygous alpha-thalassaemia-1. *Prenat Diagn.* 1987;7:307–313.
210. Lam YH, Tang MH. Prenatal diagnosis of haemoglobin Bart's disease by cordocentesis at 12–14 weeks' gestation. *Prenat Diagn.* 1997;17:501–504.
211. Li Q, Wei J, Li D. Prenatal Ultrasonographic prediction of homozygous alpha-thalassemia disease at midpregnancy. *Int J Gynaecol Obstet.* 2007;97:156–157.
212. Liao C, Li Q, Wei J, Feng Q, Li J, Huang Y, et al. Prenatal control of Hb Bart's disease in southern China. *Hemoglobin.* 2007;31:471–475.
213. Diukman R, Golbus MS. In utero stem cell therapy. *J Reprod Med.* 1992;37:515–520.

214. Eddleman K. In utero transfusion and transplantation in α-thalassaemia. In: Migliaccio, AR ed. *Stem Cell Therapy of Inherited Disorders*. Rome; 1996.
215. Paszty C, Mohandas N, Stevens ME, Loring JF, Liebhaber SA, Brion CM, et al. Lethal alpha-thalassaemia created by gene targeting in mice and its genetic rescue. *Nat Genet.* 1995;11:33–39.
216. Paszty C. Transgenic and gene knock-out mouse models of sickle cell anemia and the thalassemias. *Curr Opin Hematol.* 1997;4:88–93.
217. Huisman THJ, Carver MFH, Efremov GD. *A Syllabus of Human Hemoglobin Variants*. Augusta, GA: The Sickle Cell Anemia Foundation; 1996.
218. Bruzdzinski CJ, Sisco KL, Ferrucci SJ, Rucknagel DL. The occurrence of the alpha G-Philadelphia-globin allele on a double-locus chromosome. *Am J Hum Genet.* 1984;36:101–109.
219. Molchanova TP, Pobedimskaya DD, Ye Z, Huisman TH. Two different mutations in codon 68 are observed in Hb G-Philadelphia heterozygotes. *Am J Hematol.* 1994;45:345–346.
220. Milner PF, Huisman TH. Studies of the proporation and synthesis of haemoblogin C Philadelphia in red cells of heterozygotes, a homozygote, and a heterozygote for both haemoglobin G and alpha thalassaemia. *Br J Haematol.* 1976;34:207–220.
221. Pardoll DM, Charache S, Hjelle BL, et al. Homozygous alpha thalassemia/Hb G Philadelphia. *Hemoglobin.* 1982;6:503–515.
222. Sancar GB, Tatsis B, Cedeno MM, Rieder RF. Proportion of hemoglobin G Philadelphia (alpha 268 Asn leads to Lys beta 2) in heterozygotes is determined by alpha-globin gene deletions. *Proc Natl Acad Sci USA.* 1980;77:6874–6878.
223. Rieder RF, Woodbury DH, Rucknagel DL. The interaction of alpha-thalassaemia and haemoglobin G Philadelphia. *Br J Haematol.* 1976;32:159–165.
224. Schwartz E, Atwater J. alpha-thalassemia in the American negro. *J Clin Invest.* 1972;51:412–418.
225. Liebhaber SA, Rappaport EF, Cash FE, Ballas SK, Schwartz E, Surrey S. Hemoglobin I mutation encoded at both alpha-globin loci on the same chromosome: concerted evolution in the human genome. *Science.* 1984;226:1449–1451.
226. Bunn HF, McDonald MJ. Electrostatic interactions in the assembly of haemoglobin. *Nature.* 1983;306:498–500.
227. Bunn HF. Subunit assembly of hemoglobin: an important determinant of hematologic phenotype. *Blood.* 1987;69:1–6.
228. Whitten WJ, Rucknagel DL. The proportion of Hb A2 is higher in sickle cell trait than in normal homozygotes. *Hemoglobin.* 1981;5:371–378.
229. Stallings M, Abraham A, Abraham EC. a-thalassemia influences the levels of fetal hemoglobin components in new born infants. *Blood.* 1983;62:75a.
230. Rombos J, Voskaridou E, Vayenas C, Boussiou M, Papadakis M, Loukopoulos D. Hemoglobin H in association with the Greek type of HPFH. Paper presented at International Congress on Thalassemia. Sardinia, 1989.
231. Giordano PC, Harteveld CL, Michiels JJ, et al. Atypical HbH disease in a Surinamese patient resulting from a combination of the -SEA and -alpha 3.7 deletions with HbC heterozygosity. *Br J Haematol.* 1997;96:801–805.
232. Thonglairuam V, Winichagoon P, Fucharoen S, Wasi P. The molecular basis of AE-Bart's disease. *Hemoglobin.* 1989;13:117–124.
233. Matthay KK, Mentzer WC Jr, Dozy AM, Kan YW, Bainton DF. Modification of hemoglobin H disease by sickle trait. *J Clin Invest.* 1979;64:1024–1032.
234. Svasti S, Yodsowon B, Sriphanich R, et al. Association of Hb Hope [beta136(H14)Gly–>Asp] and Hb H disease. *Hemoglobin.* 2001;25:429–435.
235. Vichinsky E. Hemoglobin e syndromes. *Hematology Am Soc Hematol Educ Program.* 2007:79–83.
236. Su CW, Liang S, Liang R, Wen XJ, Tang CN. Hb H disease in association with the silent beta chain variant Hb Hamilton or alpha 2 beta 2(11)(A8)Val -- lie. *Hemoglobin.* 1992;16:403–08
237. Rahbar S, Bunn HF. Association of hemoglobin H disease with Hb J-Iran (beta 77 His -- Asp): impact on subunit assembly. *Blood.* 1987;70:1790–1791.
238. Chan V, Chan TK, Tso SC, Todd D. Combination of three alpha-globin gene loci deletions and hemoglobin New York results in a severe hemoglobin H syndrome. *Am J Hematol.* 1987;24:301–306.
239. Wilkie AOM. The a thalassaemia/mental retardation syndromes: model systems for studying the genetic contribution to mental handicap. Doctor of Medicine, 1991, University of Oxford.
240. Dallman PR. The red cell. In: Dallman, PR ed. *Blood and Blood-forming Tissues.* New York: Appleton-Century-Crofts; 1977:1109–1113.
241. Dallman PR, Siimes MA. Percentile curves for hemoglobin and red cell volume in infancy and childhood. *J Pediatr.* 1979;94:26–31.
242. Lubin BH. Reference values in infancy and childhood. In: Nathan DG, OskiFA, eds. *Hematology of Infancy and Childhood.* Philadelphia: W.B. Saunders; 1987:1677–1697.
243. Llewellyn-Jones D. *Obstetrics.* London: Faber and Faber; 1969.

15

Unusual Types of α Thalassemia

Douglas R. Higgs, Veronica J. Buckle, Richard Gibbons, and David Steensma

INTRODUCTION

In this chapter we describe three relatively rare, clinically complex syndromes in which the occurrence of α thalassemia provided the clue to understanding the molecular basis of each condition. These conditions exemplify the important interplay between clinical observation and human molecular genetics. Two of these syndromes (ATR-16 [OMIM: 141750] and ATR-X [OMIM: 301040]) in which α thalassemia is associated with multiple developmental abnormalities (including mental retardation, MR) are inherited. The third condition (ATMDS [OMIM: 300448]) is an acquired disorder in which α thalassemia appears for the first time in the context of myelodysplasia.

α THALASSEMIA ASSOCIATED WITH MENTAL RETARDATION AND DEVELOPMENTAL ABNORMALITIES

The rare association of α thalassemia and mental retardation (MR) was recognized more than 25 years ago by Weatherall and colleagues.[1] It was known that α thalassemia arises when there is a defect in the synthesis of the α-globin chains of adult hemoglobin (HbA, $\alpha_2\beta_2$). When these authors encountered three mentally retarded children with α thalassemia and a variety of developmental abnormalities, their interest was stimulated by the unusual nature of the α thalassemia. The children were of northern European origin, where α thalassemia is uncommon, and although one would have expected to find clear signs of this inherited anemia in their parents, it appeared to have arisen de novo in the affected offspring. It was thought that the combination of α thalassemia with MR (ATR), and the associated developmental abnormalities represented a new syndrome and that a common genetic defect might be responsible for the diverse clinical manifestations. What emerged was the identification of two quite distinct syndromes in which α thalassemia is associated with MR.[2,3] In the first condition (ATR-16, OMIM: 141750) there are large (1–2 Mb) chromosomal rearrangements that delete many genes, including the α-globin genes from the tip of the short arm of chromosome 16 and this is an example of a contiguous gene syndrome.[4] In the second syndrome (ATR-X, OMIM 301040), a complex phenotype, including α thalassemia, results from mutations in an X-encoded factor (now called the ATRX protein), which is a putative regulator of gene expression. Mutations in this gene down regulate α globin gene expression and also perturb the expression of other as yet unidentified genes.

THE ATR-16 SYNDROME

To date we know of 40 individuals (from 32 families) who have well-characterized ATR-16 syndrome (Table 15.1a and b). Often one is alerted to this condition by observing the unusual association of α thalassemia and MR in individuals originating from outside of the areas where thalassemia commonly occurs (see Chapters 13 and 14). There are two common patterns of inheritance. In many cases neither parent has α thalassemia ($\alpha\alpha/\alpha\alpha \times \alpha\alpha/\alpha\alpha$) and the affected offspring has the phenotype of severe α thalassemia trait (genotype $--/\alpha\alpha$). Less commonly, one parent has the phenotype of mild α thalassemia trait, the other parent is nonthalassemic ($-\alpha/\alpha\alpha \times \alpha\alpha/\alpha\alpha$) and the child has HbH disease (genotype $--/-\alpha$). In addition to α thalassemia, these patients have variable degrees of facial dysmorphism (Fig. 15.1) and a wide spectrum of associated developmental abnormalities (Table 15.2a and b). In all such cases, initial molecular genetic analyses have shown that affected individuals fail to inherit the entire ζ–α globin cluster from one or other of the parents.

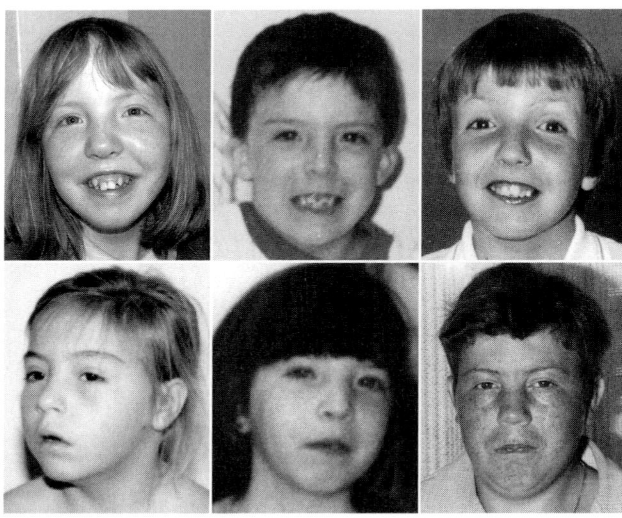

Figure 15.1. The facial appearance of patients with the ATR-16 syndrome. Common features include relative hypertelorism, a small chin and mouth, a "beaked" nose, downslanting palpebral fissures, and crowded teeth.

Table 15.1. Cytogenetic and hematological data and origin of ATR-16 mutations

Case	Sex	MR	Phenotype	Genotype	Conventional cytogenetics	Chromosomal abnormality	Parental origin	Mechanism	Reference
(a) Pure monosomy patients									
JT	F	Normal	Trait	--/αα	Normal	46.XX, del(16)(p13.3)	Maternal	De novo interstitial deletion 268 kb	[19]
OY	F	Normal	HbH	--/-α	Normal	46.XX, del(16)(p13.3)	Paternal	De novo truncation	Unpublished
AB	M	Normal	na	na	na	46.XY, del(16)(p13.3)	na	na	[16]
TY(MI)	F	Normal	Trait	--/αα	Normal	46.XX, del(16)(p13.3)	Paternal	Inherited truncation	Unpublished
TY(Mi)	M	Normal	Trait	--/αα	Normal	46.XY, del(16)(p13.3)	Unknown	Unknown truncation	Unpublished
YA	F	na	Trait	--/αα	Normal	46.XX, del(16)(p13.3)	Unknown	Unknown	Unpublished
BA	F	Normal	HbH	--/-α	Normal	46.XX, del(16)(p13.3)	Paternal	De novo truncation	[18]
GZ	M	Normal	Trait	--/αα	na	46.XY, del(16)(p13.3)	Maternal	Inherited deletion	[15]
TN (Pa)	F	Borderline	Trait	--/αα	Normal	46.XX, del(16)(p13.3)	Maternal	De novo truncation	[18]
TN (Pe)	M	Mild	Trait	--/αα	Normal	46.XY, del(16)(p13.3)	Maternal	Inherited truncation	Unpublished
TN (Al)	M	Mild	Trait	--/αα	Normal	46.XY, del(16)(p13.3)	Maternal	Inherited truncation	Unpublished
SH (Pa)	M	Moderate	Trait	--/αα	Normal	46.XY, del(16)(p13.3)	Maternal	Inherited	Unpublished
SH (Ju)	F	Normal	Trait	--/αα	Normal	46.XX, del(16)(p13.3)	Unknown	Unknown	Unpublished
DO	F	Mild	HbH	--/-α	Normal*	46.XX, del(16)(p13.3)	Maternal	Unknown	[2]
CJ	M	Mild	Trait	--/αα	Normal	46.XY, del(16)(p13.3)	Maternal	De novo interstitial deletion 1258 kb	Unpublished
MY	F	Mild	Trait	--/αα	Normal	46.XX, del(16)(p13.3)	Maternal	De novo truncation	Unpublished
PV	M	Mild	Trait	--/αα	Normal	46.XY, del(16)(p13.3)	Unknown	De novo deletion	[15]
FT	F	Mild	Trait	--/αα	Normal	46.XX, del(16)(p13.3)	Unknown	De novo deletion	[15]
BO	M	Mild	HbH	--/-α	Normal	46.XY, del(16)(p13.3)	Paternal	De novo truncation	[2,17,18]
HN	M	Mild	Trait	--/αα	Normal	46.XY, del(16)(p13.3)	Unknown	De novo deletion	[15]
LIN	F	Mild	Trait**	--/αα	Deleted	46.XX, del(16)(p13.3)	Paternal	De novo	[18,109]
IM	F	Mild	HbH	--/-αα	Normal	46.XX, del(16)(p13.3)	Unknown	Unknown	[18,110,111]
(b) Translocation patients									
JPS	M	na	Trait	--/αα	Abnormal	46,XY, -16,+der(16)t(9;16)(p13;p13.3)	na	na	A Villegas (personal communication)
MR	F	Mild	Trait	--/αα	Abnormal	46,XX, -16,+der(16)t(9;16)(p21.2;p13.3)	Paternal	De novo	[112]
BE(C)	F	Mild	HbH	--/-αα	Normal	46.XX, -16,+der(16)(qter->q24::p13.3->qter)mat	Maternal	Inversion/deletion	[113] and unpublished
BE (Ch)	F	Mild	Trait	--/αα	Normal	46,XX, -16,+der(16)(qter->q24::p13.3->qter)	Unknown	Inversion/deletion	[113] and unpublished
BE(W)	M	Mild	Trait	--/αα	Normal	46,XY, -16,+der(16)(qter->q24::p13.3->qter)	Unknown	Inversion/deletion	[113] and unpublished
SS	F	na	Trait	--/αα	Abnormal	46,XX, der(16)(qter->p13.3::p13.3->p13.13:)	Paternal	De novo duplication with deletion	Unpublished
CU	M	Mild	Trait	--/αα	Abnormal	46,XY, -16+der(16)t(9;16)(p21.2;p13.3)	Maternal	De novo	[2,112]
WA(C)	F	Borderline	Trait	--/αα	Normal	46,XX, -16,+der(16)t(16;20)(p13.3;q13.3)mat	Maternal	Derived from parental balanced translocation	Unpublished
WA (Cj)	F	Mild	Trait	--/αα	Normal	46,XX, -16,+der(16)t(16;20)(p13.3;q13.3)mat	Maternal	Derived from parental balanced translocation	Unpublished
Aa	F	Borderline	Trait	--/αα	Abnormal	46,XX, -16,+der(16)t(10;16)(q26.13;p13.3)mat	Maternal	Derived from parental balanced translocation	[2,8]
HA	M	Borderline	HbH	--/-α	Normal	46,XY, -16,+der(16)(qter->q24::p13.3->qter)	Paternal	De novo inversion/deletion	[2]
GR(M)	M	Mild	Trait	--/αα	Normal	46,XY, -16,+der(16)t(16;21)(p13.3;p13) mat	Maternal	Derived from parental balanced translocation	[18]
GR (J)	F	Mild	Trait	--/αα	Normal	46,XX, -16,+der(16)t(16;21)(p13.3;p13)mat	Maternal	Derived from parental balanced translocation	[18]
WI	M	Borderline	Trait	--/αα	Normal	46,XY, -16, +der(16)t(16;20)(p13.3;p13)	Paternal	De novo	[2]
OD	M	Moderate	HbH	--/-α	Normal	46,XY, -16, +der(16)t(1;16)(p36;p13.3)	Maternal	Derived from parental balanced translocation	[2,9]
LF	M	na	na	na	Abnormal	46,XY, -16+der(16)t(X;16)(p11.4;p13.3)mat	Maternal	Derived from parental balanced translocation	K May (personal communication)
DA	M	Mild	Trait	--/αα	Abnormal	45,XY, -15, --16 +der (16)t(15;16)(q13.1;p13.3)	Paternal	De novo	[2]
BAR	M	Mild	Trait	--/αα	Abnormal	46XY, -16, +der (16)(qter->q22::p13.3->qter)	Maternal	De novo inversion/deletion	[114]

na = data not available

* at low resolution

** Although LIN had 30% Hb Bart's at birth, neither parent appears to have an inherited form of α thalassemia that would account for the HbH chains reported in LIN.

Additional cases of ATR-16 whose deletions have not been fully characterized at the molecular level have been described in refs. 114–118.

Table 15.2. Clinical findings in patients with ATR-16 syndrome

Case	MR	Speech delay	Developmental delay	Short stature	Facial dysmorphism	Genital abnormalities	Skeletal abnormalities	Miscellaneous abnormalities
(a) Pure monosomy patients								
JT	Normal*	−	−	−	−	−	−	
OY	Normal*	−	−	−	−	−	−	
AB	Normal*	−	−	−	−	−	−	
TY(MI)	Normal*	−	−	−	−	−	−	
TY(Mi)	Normal*	−	−	−	−	−	−	
YA	na	+	+	+	+	−	−	Macroglossia Supernumery nipples, umbilical hernia and developmental delay. Fx of umbilical hernia, pyloric stenosis and omphalocele.
BA	Normal*	−	−	−	−	−	−	Poor motor skills
GZ	Normal*	−	−	−	−	−	−	Pyloric stenosis
TN (Pa)	Borderline	+	+	−	+	−	−	Less affected than sons
TN (Pe)	Mild	+	+	−	+	−	−	
TN (Al)	Mild	+	+	−	+	−	−	Left iris coloboma
SH (Pa)	Moderate	na	+	−	+	+	+	Fine motor problems, asthma, bronchitis, myopic
SH (Ju)	Normal*	−	−	−	−	−	−	Severe anxiety/depression
DO	Mild	+	+	+	+	−	−	IC, seizures,
CJ	Mild	+	+	−	+	−	−	Heart murmur, macrocephalic, no speech at age 4, slow cognitive, social, and motor development
MY	Mild	+	+	na	+	−	−	Developmental delay. Plagiocephaly. Patient and normal sister had ASD.
PV	Mild	+	+	−	+	−	+	Recurrent chest infections and asthma, epilepsy, pectus excavatum
FT	Mild	+	+	−	+	−	+	Pectus excavatum
BO	Mild	na	+	+	+	+	+	IC, P, microcephaly, clubfoot, ductus arteriosus, pneumonia
HN	Mild	+	+	−	+	−	+	Recurrent chest infections and asthma, L clubfoot, arachnoid cyst in R temporal lobe
LIN	Mild	+	+	−	+	−	na	
IM	Mild	na	+	na	+	−	+	Bilat clubfoot
(b) Translocation patients								
JPS	na							
MR	Mild	+	+	+	+	−	+	SPC
BE (C)	Mild			+	−	na	na	s
BE (Ch)	Mild			+	na	na	na	na
BE (W)	Mild			+	na	na	na	na

Table 15.2 (*continued*)

Case	MR	Speech delay	Developmental delay	Short stature	Facial dysmorphism	Genital abnormalities	Skeletal abnormalities	Miscellaneous abnormalities
SS	na	na	+	+	+	na	na	Rash, recurrent chest and ear infections, multiple developmental abnormalities
CU	Mild	+	+	−	+	−	+	SPC
WA (C)	Borderline	+	+	+	+	−	+	S, PVC, LFW, SD, NW, asthma, special school
WA (Cj)	Mild	na	na	+	+	na	na	Broadly spaced, wide-open eyes, not sloping, rash
Aa	Borderline	+	+	−	+	−	−	UG, HPN
HA	Borderline	+	+	−	+	−	+	E, clubfoot
GR (M)	Mild	+	+	−	+	−	+	Bronchitis, pneumonia, reactive airway disease, heart murmur
GR (J)	Mild	+	+	−	+	−	+	CHD
WI	Borderline	+	+	−	+	−	+	AN, IC
OD	Moderate	+	+	−	+	+	−	CAL
LF	na	na	na	na	+	+	na	T, CS, CHD, H died at 49 d
DA	Mild			−	+	+	+	SPC, HT
BAR	Mild	+	+	−	+	−	+	Bilat equinovarus

* normal phenotype, included to define critical regions.
na = data not available; U = unable to assess at time of death; CAL = cafe-au-lait patches; SPC = single palmar crease; HT = hypoplastic enamel of teeth; UG = unsteady gait; HPN = high placed nipples; IC = impaired coordination; P = ptosis; E = epilepsy; AN = accessary nipple; T = tracheobronchomalacia; CS = choanal stenosis; CHD = congenital heart disease; H = hydrocephalus; S = strabismus; PVC = paralyzed vocal cord (unilateral); LFW = left facial weakness; SD = sacral dimple; NW = neck webbing; M = myopia; TS = tuberous sclerosis; RC = renal cysts; PL = pigmented lesions (hypo & hyper). ASD = atrial septal defect; Fx = family history.

Defining the Genetic Abnormalities in Patients with ATR-16 Syndrome

In some cases, conventional cytogenetic analysis demonstrated the underlying genetic abnormality. Because the α–globin complex lies very close to the 16p telomere (16p13.3, Fig. 15.2) any chromosomal abnormality affecting this region may give rise to α thalassemia.[2] In some patients with putative ATR-16 syndrome, gross chromosomal abnormalities resulting in deletions,[2] formation of ring chromosomes,[5–7] and translocations[8] have been observed. Although such abnormalities may arise as de novo genetic events, often one parent carries a preexisting balanced translocation, which the child inherits in an unbalanced fashion (Fig. 15.3, summarizing the findings in ref. 9), resulting in monosomy for 16p and loss of the α cluster.

In many cases of ATR-16, initial high-resolution cytogenetic analysis appeared entirely normal. In some of these cases the pattern of inheritance of polymorphisms (such as variable number tandem repeats) within the α-cluster revealed the nature of the underlying molecular defect. In the example given in Fig. 15.3 the parental 16p alleles could be distinguished from each other. The mother in this family was shown to carry a balanced 1:16 translocation, which both of her children inherited in an unbalanced fashion. Her son OD (Tables 15.1 and 15.2) was monosomic for 16p, and therefore was shown to have α thalassemia (in this case HbH disease), whereas her daughter was trisomic for 16p. Both children had MR, dysmorphic facies, and a variety of associated developmental abnormalities.

Fluorescence in situ hybridization (FISH) studies have also been used to analyze ATR-16 families. In this type of study, large segments (∼40 kb) of chromosome 16 in cosmid vectors are used as probes to demonstrate the presence or absence of the corresponding sequences in the 16p telomeric region by using fluorescence microscopy.[10] By analyzing the chromosomes of both parents and the affected child it has been possible to define the extent of 16p monosomy and the mechanism by which it has arisen. In the example shown in Figure 15.4, FISH analysis demonstrated that the mother of an affected child with the ATR-16 syndrome carries a balanced 16:20 translocation, which was inherited in an unbalanced fashion (as in Fig. 15.3) by her offspring. Some chromosomal abnormalities can only be detected by FISH or molecular analyses and they are referred to as "cryptic."

Over the past 10 years other methods have also been applied systematically to the characterization of the chromosome abnormalities in these patients. M-TEL FISH[11] involves the hybridization of a panel of subtelomeric probes from each human chromosome to detect both loss of material from and additional material on the short arm

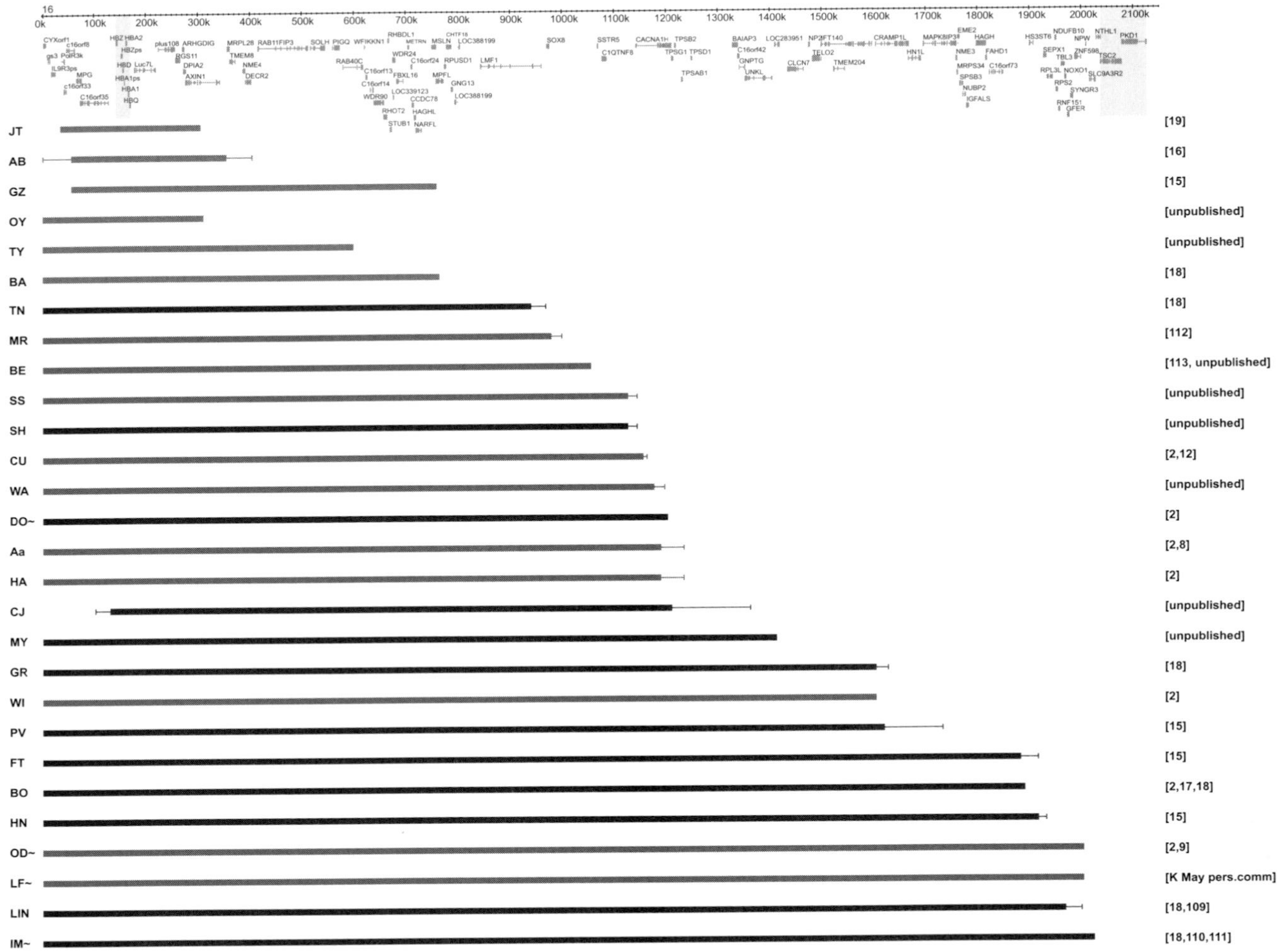

Figure 15.2. Summary of known ATR-16 deletions. The positions of the α-globin cluster and other genes within this region are indicated. Below, the extent of each deletion is shown with the patient code alongside (see Table 15.1). Deletions known to result from pure monosomy for this region are shown in either green (no abnormalities other than thalassemia) or red (ATR-16 phenotype). Chromosomal translocations (all with ATR-16 phenotypes) are shown in blue. Solid bars indicate regions known to be deleted and fine lines indicate the region of uncertainty of the breakpoints. The α genes and the genes that when mutated are associated with tuberous sclerosis and adult polycystic kidney disease are shown (shaded boxes). (See color plate 15.2.)

of chromosome 16. For example, abnormal chromosome 16 in HA (Table 15.1) was shown by this method to be not only monosomic for part of 16p13.3 but also trisomic for part of 16q24 (derived from an inversion/deletion event).

Recently there have been several technical developments that have narrowed the gap between cytogenetics and molecular analyses, enabling high-resolution analysis of the entire human genome. In the first of these types of analyses a large proportion of the genome is interrogated using microarrays consisting of DNA from bacterial artificial chromosomes spanning the genome. Using a competitive genome hybridization (CGH) approach, comparing DNA from one genome with another, it has been possible to detect large regions of monosomy in patients with ATR-16 syndrome.[12] More recently using oligo-based microarrays or bead technologies (originally made to identify single nucleotide polymorphisms) with a modified analysis it has been possible to identify deletions and duplications of greater than approximately 1 kb.[13] The resolution of this type of analysis is continuously improving. One of these approaches (using microbead technology[14]) has recently been applied to previously characterized (and new) cases of ATR-16, nicely demonstrating the large deletions from 16p13.3 and identifying any associated aneuploidy (V. Buckle et al., in preparation). Figure 15.5 shows an example of this type of analysis in a patient (BO, Tables 15.1 and 15.2) with ATR-16 syndrome due to a deletion of 1900 kb from 16p13.3.

In addition to these approaches Harteveld et al.[15] have developed a rapid and simple high-resolution approach to identify and characterize deletions of the terminal 2 Mb of 16p13.3 using the multiplex ligation–dependent probe amplification technique. An established panel of specific, synthetic oligonucleotides can now be used to detect

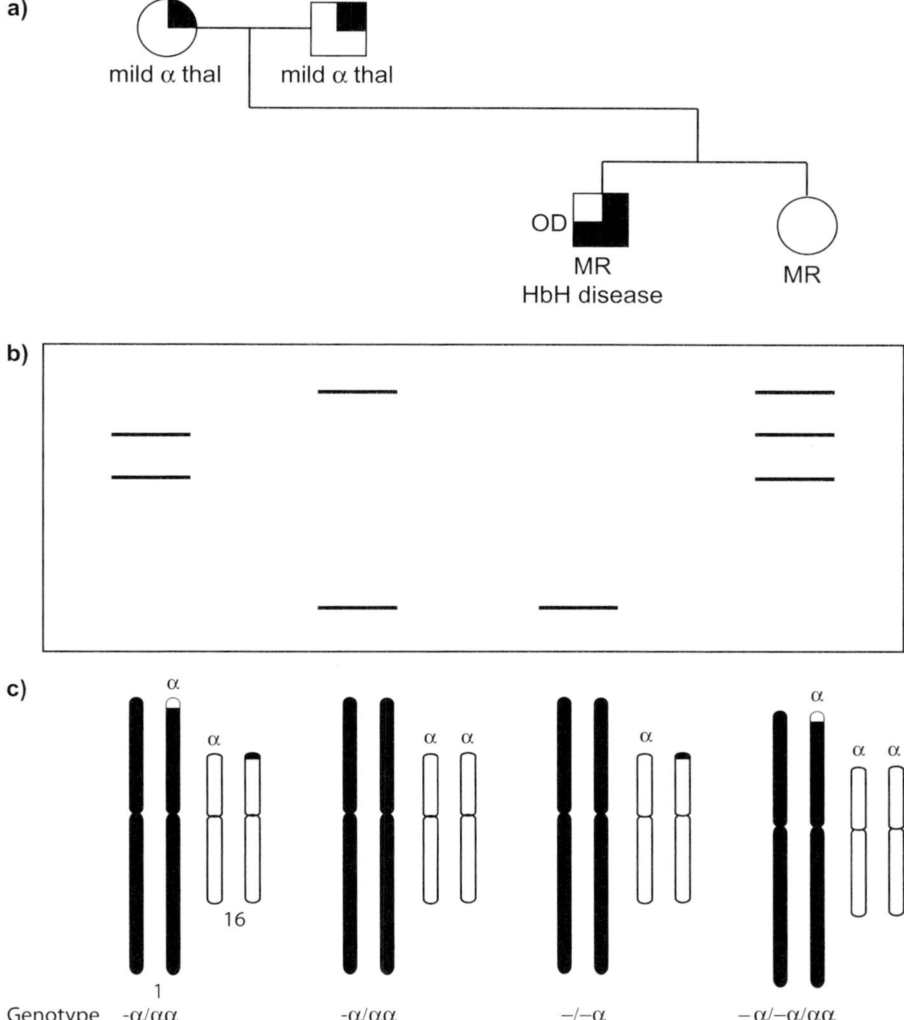

Figure 15.3. Familial subcytogenetic translocation (from ref. 9). **(a)** Pedigree indicating parents with mild α thalassemia only; son (OD) with MR and severe α-thalassemia (HbH disease) and daughter with MR. **(b)** Schematic representation of restriction fragment length polymorphism analysis using a fully informative marker closely linked to the α-globin cluster. Each track corresponds to the individual shown above. **(c)** Segregation of 1:16 translocation and α-globin complex (α) in each family member. The resulting genotype is shown. Note that both children have inherited the paternal chromosome carrying the (-α) allele; it has not been determined whether the mother's normal or translocated chromosome 16 bears her (-α) allele.

deletions in 16p13.3.[15,16] Clearly the resolution of this technique is only limited by the spacing of the appropriate oligonucleotides. An example of this type of analysis applied to a patient with ATR-16 syndrome is shown in Figure 15.5.

Using a combination of conventional cytogenetics, FISH, and molecular analysis at least three types of chromosomal rearrangements (translocation, inversion/deletion, and truncation) have now been found in ATR-16 patients (Fig. 15.2 and Table 15.1). To date, few breakpoints have been fully characterized. The telomeric truncations seen in BO, BA, and MY (Table 15.1 and Fig. 15.2) have been fully analyzed[17] (Green et al., unpublished) and it appears that these chromosomes have been broken, truncated, and "healed" by the direct addition of telomeric repeats $(TTAGGG)_n$ as described for some less extensive 16p deletions in patients with α thalassemia but no MR (e.g., TY in Fig. 13.2 and Chapter 13). In addition, another 11 ATR16 cases, shown to have pure monosomy for 16p13.3 (Fig. 15.2), are likely to fall into this same class.

Although many cases of ATR-16 have doubtless been overlooked, it is nevertheless likely that this syndrome is rare, because each case found to date has been the result of a unique and independent chromosome mutation.

How Do Chromosomal Abnormalities Give Rise to the ATR-16 Syndrome?

Because individuals with ATR-16 syndrome may have quite different degrees of chromosomal imbalance, there is considerable variation in the associated phenotypes

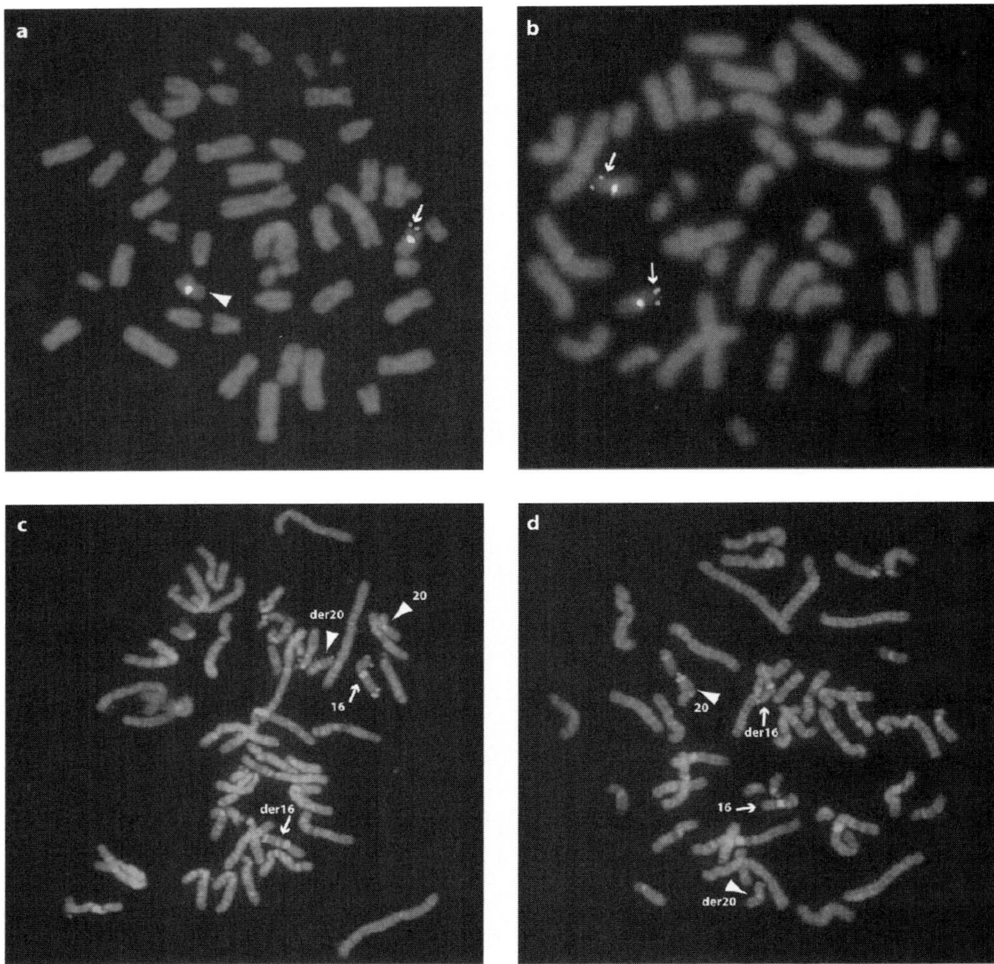

Figure 15.4. High-resolution chromosome analysis using FISH. **(a** and **b)** Examples of FISH on metaphase chromosomes of deletion patient JT. In each case chromosome 16 is identified by a chromosome 16–specific centromere probe. In **(a)** using a cosmid (cGG1) located close to the telomere, fluorescent signal was seen on the normal chromosome (arrow) but not the abnormal copy of chromosome 16 (arrowhead). **(b)** Using a second cosmid located closer to the centromere (not deleted in JT) a signal is seen on both normal and abnormal chromosomes (arrows). **(c** and **d)** FISH on metaphase chromosomes of the mother of WA showing a balanced translocation. In **(c)** and **(d)** both homologs of chromosome 16 are indicated by arrows and chromosome 20 by arrowheads. In **(c)** the subtelomeric probes for 16p and 16q were hybridized to metaphase chromosomes. Green fluorescent signal was seen on the q arm of both homologs of chromosome 16. Red fluorescent signal was seen on the p arm of the normal chromosome 16 and the q arm of the derivative chromosome 20 (der 20) but was absent from the deleted chromosome 16 (der 16). In **(d)** the subtelomeric probe for 20p (red) was seen on both homologs of chromosome 20. Fluorescent signal for 20q (green) was seen on the normal chromosome 20 and the p arm of the derivative 16 (der 16). (See color plate 15.4.)

(Table 15.2). The degree of monosomy in 16p13.3 varies from 0.3 to 2 Mb (Fig. 15.2) but many patients have additional chromosomal aneuploidy and in some cases imbalance of the non-16 material may dominate the clinical picture. For example in DA (Table 15.1) loss of material from chromosome 15 while forming the abnormal derivative t(15:16) chromosome produced the striking phenotype associated with the Prader–Willi syndrome.

Because many patients with ATR-16 have complex genomic rearrangements, to determine the role played by any gene(s), within 16p13.3, in the developmental abnormalities associated with ATR-16 syndrome, future analysis should focus on patients who have pure monosomy for 16p13.3. Clearly, patients with the common forms of α thalassemia have small deletions ($\sim$5–40 kb) from the α-globin cluster (Chapter 13) with no abnormalities other than α thalassemia. Nevertheless, rare individuals with much more extensive deletions have been identified. Surprisingly, these studies have shown that patients with deletions of up to 900 kb of 16p13.3 (including 52 genes) have α thalassemia but may be minimally affected[18] (unpublished data) or even normal[2,15–19] (unpublished data). At the other

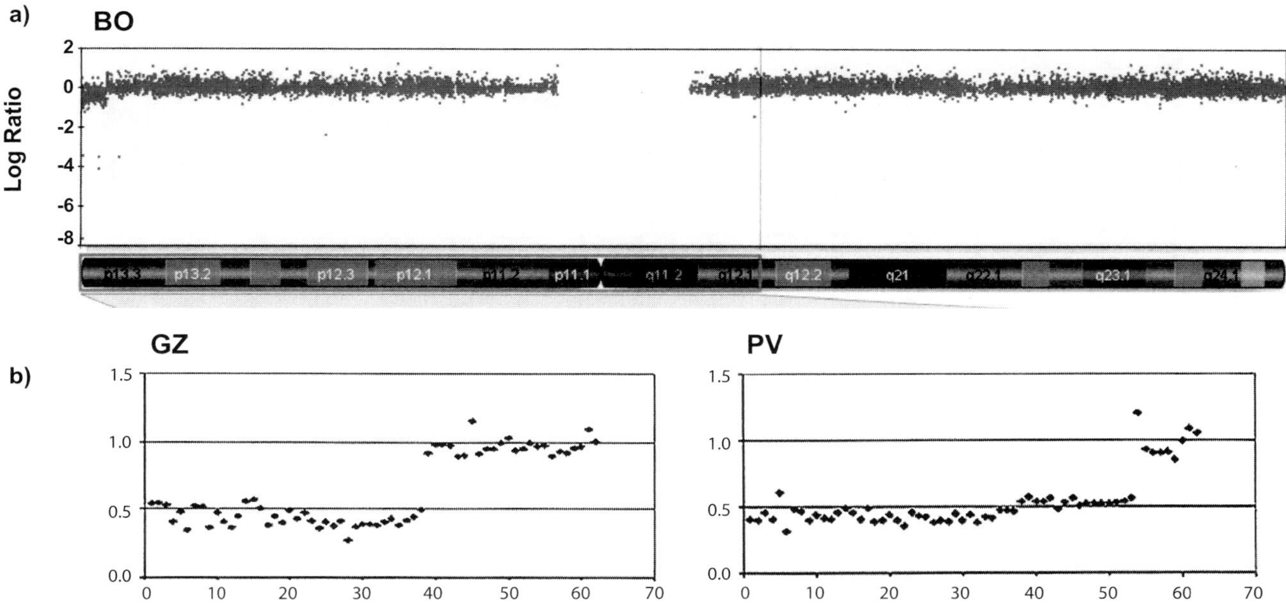

Figure 15.5. Detection of deletions. **(a)** Analysis of chromosome 16 in patient BO[18] with ATR-16 using the QuantiSNP protocol.[14] The Y-axis indicates the log ratio between normal and the test and the X-axis represents the distance along chromosome 16. **(b)** Analysis of two patients (GZ and PV[15] and Fig. 15.2) with large deletions of 16p13.3 using the multiplex ligation–dependent probe amplification protocol[15]). The Y-axis represents the ratio peak height of the test divided by the normal control and the X-axis represents the distance along chromosome 16. (See color plate 15.5.)

extreme, patients with 16p monosomy for the entire terminal region of 16p (e.g., BO, LIN, and IM) have a relatively severe phenotype with α thalassemia, MR, and dysmorphic features and skeletal abnormalities. All patients with deletions from 900 to 1700 kb have some degree of MR and shared but variable dysmorphic features (Table 15.2). In patients whose deletions extend beyond 2000 kb the clinical picture is dominated by more severe MR, tuberous sclerosis, and polycystic kidney disease.[20]

How might monosomy for 16p13.3 cause such developmental abnormalities? One possibility is that deletion of a large number of genes from one copy of chromosome 16 may unmask mutations in its homolog; the more genes that are deleted the greater the probability of this occurring. This is unlikely to be the explanation for most ATR-16 cases because it is estimated that normal individuals only carry a few harmful mutations of this type in the entire genome.[21] A further possibility is that some genes in 16p are imprinted[22] so that deletions could remove the only active copy of the gene. At present there is no evidence for imprinting of the 16p region (reviewed in ref. 23) and in the relatively few ATR-16 cases analyzed there appears to be no major clinical differences between patients with deletions of the maternally or paternally derived chromosomes (Tables 15.1 and 15.2). It therefore seems more likely that there are some genes in the 16p region that encode proteins whose effect is critically determined by the amount produced; so-called dosage-sensitive genes.[24] Examples of such genes include those encoding proteins that form heterodimers, those required at a critical level for a rate-determining step of a regulatory pathway, and tumor suppressor genes (e.g., TSC2). Removal of genes from one copy of 16p13.3 consistently reduces their levels of expression to approximately 50% of normal (Buckle et al., unpublished). If the deletion includes one or more dosage-sensitive genes this could account for the clinical effects seen in ATR-16 patients.

The region lying between 900 and 1700 kb from the 16p telomere, deleted in all patients with the characteristic features of ATR-16 syndrome, contains 16 genes and gene families of known function,[15,18] which have been implicated in a wide range of disorders with few or no features in common with ATR-16. One of these (SOX8) was considered as strong candidate because it is involved in the regulation of embryonic development and is strongly expressed in the brain.[25]A recently described Brazilian patient with a deletion that removes both the α-globin locus and SOX8 was not associated with MR or any dysmorphism however (Harteveld, personal communication, 2007). Clearly, further examples of ATR-16 due to monosomy for 16p13.3 must be characterized to identify the gene(s) responsible for the MR and other developmental abnormalities associated with this condition.

Summary of the ATR-16 Syndrome

The ATR-16 syndrome has served as an important model for improving our general understanding of the molecular basis for MR. It provided the first examples of MR due to a cryptic chromosomal translocation and truncation. Further work has shown that such telomeric rearrangements may underlie a significant proportion of unexplained MR.[26] The current challenge is to understand in detail the mechanisms by which monosomy causes developmental abnormalities; the ATR-16 syndrome provides an excellent model for addressing this issue.

THE ATR-X SYNDROME

As additional patients with α thalassemia and MR were identified throughout the 1980s, it became clear that a second group of affected individuals existed in whom no structural abnormalities in the α-globin cluster or 16p could be found. In contrast to those with ATR-16 syndrome, this group of patients was all male, presented with a much more uniform phenotype, and had a remarkably similar facial appearance.[3] That this group had a distinct and recognizable dysmorphism was underscored when additional cases were identified on the basis of their facial features alone.[27,28] Ultimately, it was shown that this unusual syndrome of α thalassemia with severe MR results from an X-linked abnormality (see later) and the condition is now referred to as the ATR-X syndrome (OMIM: 301040).

The Clinical Findings of the ATR-X Syndrome

Cases of ATR-X syndrome from over 150 families have now been characterized, and in contrast to ATR-16 a definite phenotype is emerging. The cardinal features of this condition are severe MR and developmental abnormalities associated with a characteristic facial appearance and α thalassemia. The frequency and nature of the most commonly encountered clinical features are summarized in Tables 15.3 and 15.4.

Neonates with ATR-X syndrome usually have marked hypotonia and associated feeding difficulties. Seizures have also been noted in some patients. In early childhood, all milestones are delayed. Many patients do not walk until late in childhood, and some never do so. Most have no speech, although some patients have a handful of words or signs. With some notable exceptions[29–32] most patients with ATR-X syndrome have only situational understanding and are dependent for almost all activities of daily living.

Although head circumference is usually normal at birth, postnatal microcephaly usually develops. As affected individuals age, there is often a tendency toward spasticity and seizures occur in approximately one-third of cases. Vision usually appears normal but sensorineural deafness may occur in some patients. Computed tomography or magnetic resonance brain imaging is generally unremarkable, although mild cerebral atrophy may be seen. In two cases, partial or complete agenesis of the corpus callosum was

Table 15.3. Summary of the major clinical manifestations of the ATR-X syndrome

Clinical feature	Total*	%
Profound MR	160/168	96
Characteristic face	138/147	94
Skeletal abnormalities	128/142	90
HbH inclusions	130/147	88
Neonatal hypotonia	88/105	84
Genital abnormalities	119/150	79
Microcephaly	103/134	77
Gut dysmotility	89/117	76
Short stature	73/112	65
Seizures	53/154	34
Cardiac defects	32/149	21
Renal/urinary abnormalities	23/151	15

* Total represents the number of patients for whom appropriate information is available and includes patients who do not have α-thalassemia but in whom *ATRX* mutations have been identified.

Table 15.4. Clinical manifestations of the ATR-X syndrome

Genital abnormalities	Small/soft testes, cryptorchidism, gonadal dysgenesis, inguinal hernia, micropenis, hypospadias, deficient prepuce, shawl scrotum, hypoplastic scrotum, ambiguous genitalia, female external genitalia (male pseudohermaphroditism)
Skeletal abnormalities	Delayed bone age, tapering fingers, drumstick distal phalanges, brachydactyly, clinodactyly, bifid thumb, fixed flexion deformities of joints, overriding toes, varus or valgus deformities of feet, scoliosis, kyphosis, hemivertebra, spina bifida, coxa valga, chest wall deformity
Renal/urinary abnormalities	Renal agenesis, hydronephrosis, small kidneys, vesicoureteric reflux, pelvoureteric junction obstruction, exstrophy of bladder, urethral diverticulum, urethral stricture
Cardiac defects	Atrial septal defect, ventricular septal defect, patent ductus arteriosus, tetralogy of Fallot, transposition of the great arteries, dextrocardia with situs solitus, aortic stenosis, pulmonary stenosis
Gut dysmotility	Discoordinated swallowing, eructation, gastroesophageal reflux, vomiting, gastric pseudovolvulus, hiatus hernia, hematemesis, recurrent ileus/small bowel obstruction, volvulus, intermittent diarrhea, severe constipation
Miscellaneous	Apneic episodes, cold/blue extremities, blepharitis, conjunctivitis, entropion, cleft palate, pneumonia, umbilical hernia, encephalitis, iris coloboma, optic atrophy, blindness, sensorineural deafness, prolonged periods of screaming/laughing, self injury

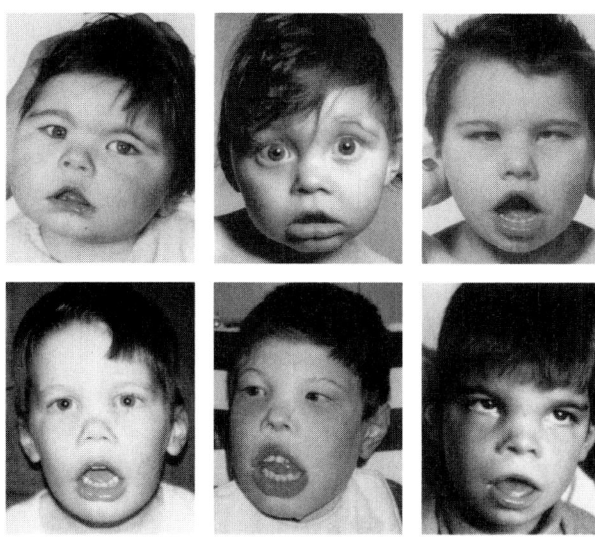

Figure 15.6. The facial appearance of patients with ATR-X syndrome as described in the text.

reported.[33] There have been autopsy reports in only three cases. The brain was small in each; in two the morphology was normal, and in one the temporal gyri on the right were indistinct, with hypoplasia of the cerebral white matter.

No systematic study of behavior has been performed in ATR-X syndrome but some recurrent themes are emerging.[34,35] Patients are usually described by their parents as content and of a happy disposition but may exhibit unprovoked emotional outbursts with sustained laughing or crying. Whereas many individuals are affectionate to their caregivers, others exhibit autistic-like behavior. They may be restless, exhibiting choreoathetoid movements and some have repetitive, stereotypic movements (pill-rolling or hand-flapping). Frequently, they put their hands into their mouths and may induce vomiting and sometimes they may engage in self-injurious behavior.

The characteristic facial appearance in ATR-X syndrome is most readily recognized in early childhood (Fig. 15.6). The frontal hair is often upswept and there is telecanthus, epicanthic folds, flat nasal bridge, midface hypoplasia, and a small triangular upturned nose with the alae nasi extending below the columella and septum. The upper lip is tented and the lower lip full and everted, giving the mouth a "carp-like" appearance. The frontal incisors are frequently widely spaced, the tongue protrudes, and there is prodigious dribbling. The ears may be simple, slightly low-set, and posteriorly rotated.

Urogenital abnormalities are seen in 80% of children. These may be very mild, for example, undescended testes or deficient prepuce; the spectrum of abnormality extends through hypospadias to micropenis to ambiguous or external female genitalia. The most severely affected children, who are clinically defined as male pseudohermaphrodites, are usually raised as females. It is of interest that these abnormalities breed true within families.[36] Renal abnormalities (hydronephrosis, renal hypoplasia or agenesis, polycystic kidney, and vesicoureteric reflux) may present with recurrent urinary tract infections.

Various relatively mild skeletal abnormalities have been noted; some of which are probably secondary to hypotonia and immobility.[37] Fixed flexion deformities, and other abnormalities, particularly of the fingers, are common. Short stature is seen in two-thirds of cases.

A wide range of gastrointestinal abnormalities have been reported in patients with this syndrome. Vomiting, regurgitation, and gastroesophageal reflux are particularly common in early childhood. An apparent reluctance to swallow has been reported by several parents and probably reflects the discoordinated swallowing that has been observed radiologically (unpublished). The tendency for aspiration is commonly implicated as a cause of death in early childhood. Excessive drooling is very common, as is frequent eructation. Constipation occurs often, and in some individuals is a major management problem. Martucciello et al.[38] demonstrated ultra-short Hirschsprung disease and colonic hypoganglionosis in two affected children. This may be a consequence of a widespread abnormality in the enteric nervous system leading to abnormal gut motility. Affected individuals may be susceptible to peptic ulceration. Esophagitis, esophageal stricture, and peptic ulcer have been observed endoscopically in single cases.

Finally, a wide range of cardiac abnormalities have also been noted including septal defects (10 cases), patent ductus arteriosus (6 cases), pulmonary stenosis (3 cases), aortic stenosis (2 cases), tetralogy of Fallot (2 cases), and single cases of transposition of the great arteries, dextrocardia with situs solitus, and aortic regurgitation.

Of the 168 patients described to date, there have been 25 deaths. The cause was established in just over half, of which there were 6 cases of pneumonia and four of aspiration of vomitus. Cases appear to be particularly vulnerable in early childhood, with 19 of the deaths occurring before the age of 5 years; this may be associated with the fact that gastroesophageal reflux and vomiting are often more severe in the early years. There are no long-term longitudinal data in this relatively newly described syndrome, but a number of affected individuals are fit and well in their 30s and 40s.

The Hematological Findings of the ATR-X Syndrome

The presence of α-thalassemia (in the form of thalassemia trait or mild HbH disease) with HbH inclusions (see Chapter 14) was one of the original diagnostic criteria for ATR-X syndrome; however, with the identification of further cases, it became clear that the hematological findings (e.g., levels of Hb, mean corpuscular volume [MCV], and mean corpuscular hemoglobin [MCH]) were different from those seen in the common types of α thalassemia. Now

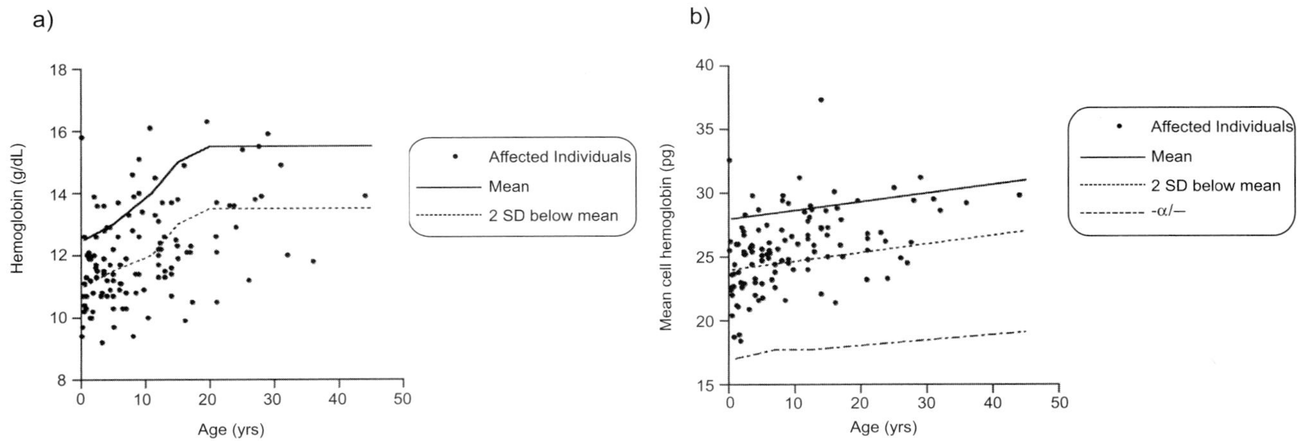

Figure 15.7. (a) Hemoglobin levels in subjects with ATR-X syndrome at various ages. Solid line indicates the mean and dashed line is 2 standard deviations below the mean.[119] For any given subject, only one result within each consecutive 5-year period is given. **(b)** MCH levels in subjects with ATR-X syndrome at various ages. Mean values for individuals with α thalassemia resulting from an -α/-- genotype are shown.

that the disease can be identified via the clinical phenotype or the ATR-X genotype, it is clear that there is considerable variation in the hematological manifestations associated with mutations of the *ATRX* gene. In fact, a number of families have been identified in which some or all of the affected members with mutations of ATRX, and the characteristic phenotype described previously, have no signs of α thalassemia.[39,40] Nevertheless, when the family history and phenotype are strongly suspect, a careful search for HbH inclusions should be made in all affected individuals and repeated if necessary as they may be very infrequent.

The hematology is often surprisingly normal considering the presence of α thalassemia (Fig. 15.7). Neither the level of hemoglobin nor the mean cell hemoglobin is as severely affected as in the classic forms of α thalassemia associated with *cis*-acting mutations in the α-globin complex (see Chapters 13 and 14), and this probably reflects the different pathophysiology of the conditions. In most cases of ATR-X, there is insufficient HbH to be detected by electrophoresis and the number of HbH inclusions is quite variable among different patients, although relatively constant over time in any affected individual.

The ATR-X Syndrome is an X-linked Condition

The five original "nondeletion" cases described by Wilkie et al.[3] were sporadic in nature, and apart from all being male, there were no immediate clues to the genetic etiology. Somatic cell hybrids composed of a mouse erythroleukemia cell line containing chromosome 16 (wherein the α-globin genes lie) derived from an affected boy produced human α-globin in a manner indistinguishable from a similar hybrid containing chromosome 16 from a normal individual. It therefore seemed likely that the defect in globin synthesis lay in *trans* to the globin cluster. This was confirmed in a family with four affected siblings in whom the condition segregated independently of the α-globin cluster.[41]

Because affected individuals were always related via the female line, this suggested that the syndrome mapped to the X chromosome and hence the condition was named the ATR-X syndrome. Subsequently linkage analysis in 16 families mapped the disease interval to Xq13.1-q21.1, confirming that the associated α thalassemia results from a *trans*-acting mutation.[42]

Early genetic studies showed that the ATR-X syndrome behaves as an X-linked recessive disorder; boys are affected almost exclusively. Furthermore, almost all female carriers have a normal appearance and intellect, although approximately one in four carriers has subtle signs of α thalassemia with very rare cells containing HbH inclusions.[42] The majority of carriers have a highly skewed pattern of X inactivation in leukocytes (derived from mesoderm), hair roots (ectoderm), and buccal cells (endoderm). In each case the disease-bearing X chromosome is preferentially inactivated. There is evidence from a recently reported mouse model of ATR-X syndrome[43] that skewed X inactivation results from selection, at key steps during development, against cells that are deficient for ATRX.[44]

Together, these findings showed that ATR-X is an X-linked disease and when the gene is mutated, among many other effects, this leads to downregulation of expression of the α-globin genes on chromosome 16.

Identification of the ATR-X Disease Gene

The isolation of cDNA fragments mapping to Xq13.1-q21.1 provided an opportunity to study candidate genes for ATR-X.[45] A number of these cDNA fragments were hybridized to DNA from a group of affected individuals. An absent

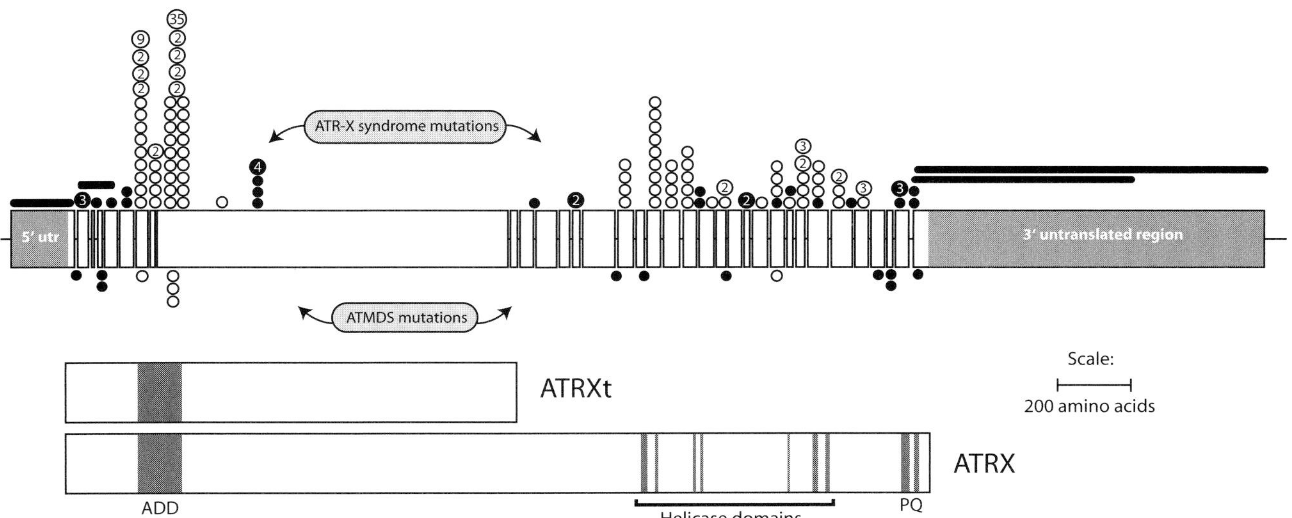

Figure 15.8. Schematic diagram of the *ATRX* gene: boxes represent the 35 exons (excluding the alternatively spliced exon 7); thin horizontal lines represent introns (not to scale). The 3′ and 5′ untranslated regions (utr) are shown flanking the open reading frame. The two protein products ATRX and ATRXt are shown as rectangles. The principal domains, the zinc finger motif (ADD), and the highly conserved helicase motif are indicated, as are the P box (P) and a glutamine-rich region (Q). In the lower part of the figure is a graphic representation of the amino acid similarity between human and mouse ATRX proteins. In the upper part of the figure is illustrated the spectrum of *ATRX* mutations described in boys with ATR-X syndrome (above the gene) and in ATMDS (below the gene). The positions of the mutations are shown by circles: filled circles represent mutations (nonsense or leading to a frameshift) that would cause protein truncation; open circles represent missense mutations and small deletions that maintain the reading frame; deletions are indicated by horizontal lines. Recurrent mutations are illustrated by larger circles, and the number of independent families is indicated.

hybridization signal was noted in one patient when an 84-bp cDNA fragment (E4) was used. E4 was shown to be part of a gene known as XH2/XNP.[46] Subsequently, a 2-kb genomic deletion was demonstrated in this individual with ATR-X syndrome. Subsequently, analysis of a segment of cDNA corresponding to XH2/XNP identified disease-causing mutations in several individuals with the clinical and hematological features of ATR-X syndrome. The X-linked gene was thus renamed as the *ATRX* gene.

Characterization of the *ATRX* Gene and Its Protein Product

We now know that the *ATRX* gene spans approximately 300 kb of genomic DNA and contains 36 exons,[47] although exon 7 may be nonfunctional. It encodes at least two alternatively spliced, 10.5-kb mRNA transcripts that differ at their 5′ ends and are predicted to give rise to slightly different proteins of 265 and 280 kD (Fig. 15.8). A further transcript of approximately 7 kb represents an isoform that retains intron 11 and truncates at this point. This gives rise to a truncated protein isoform (ATRXt) that is conserved between mouse and human.[48]

Within the N-terminal region lies a complex cysteine-rich segment (called the ADD, domain, Fig. 15.8). This comprises a PHD-like zinc finger and an additional C_2C_2 motif just upstream, which is structurally similar to the GATA-1 zinc finger.[49,50] The PHD finger is a zinc-binding domain (Cys_4-His-Cys_3), 50–80 amino acids in length and is a common feature of chromatin-related proteins and thought to mediate protein–protein interactions.[51] The structure of the ADD domain shows that it is highly related to the zinc finger domains of DNA methyltransferases.[50] Several lines of evidence suggest that this domain may bind the N-terminal tail of histone H3 and it is also possible that the upstream GATA-1-like motif in this domain may bind DNA.[52] Both of these issues are under investigation. The functional importance of the ADD segment in *ATRX* is clear. It is highly conserved throughout evolution and it contains over 50% of all mutations found in patients with ATR-X syndrome (Fig. 15.8 and see later).

The central and C-terminal regions of *ATRX* show the greatest conservation between murine and human sequences (94%).[53] The central portion of the molecule contains motifs that identify ATRX as a member of the SNF2 group of proteins. These proteins are characterized by seven highly conserved, colinear helicase motifs. Other members of the SNF2 subfamily are involved in a wide variety of cellular functions, including regulation of transcription (SNF2, MOT1, and brahma), control of the cell cycle (NPS1), DNA repair (RAD16, RAD54, and ERCC6), and mitotic chromosomal segregation (lodestar). An interaction with chromatin has been shown for SNF2 and brahma and this may be a common theme for all members of this group (reviewed by Carlson and Laurent[54]). The ATRX protein, although showing higher sequence homology to RAD54 than other members of this group, does not obviously fall into a particular functional category by virtue of homology in these flanking segments. RAD54 is a DNA repair enzyme, but there is no clinical evidence of ultraviolet sensitivity or the premature development of malignancy in the ATR-X syndrome, which might point to this being a defect in DNA repair. Furthermore, cytogenetic analysis has not demonstrated any evidence of abnormal chromosome breakage or segregation. Rather, the consistent association of ATR-X with α thalassemia suggests that the protein normally exerts its effect at one or more of the many stages involved in gene expression.

Mutations of the *ATRX* Gene and Their Associated Phenotype

In addition to ATR-X syndrome, mutations in the *ATRX* gene have now been found in many other forms of syndromal X-linked MR (reviewed in ref. 55) and it is also the disease gene associated with the occurrence of α thalassemia in myelodysplasia (discussed later).

To date, 113 different constitutional mutations have been documented in 182 independent families with ATR-X syndrome (reviewed in ref. 55). Missense mutations are clustered in two regions: the ADD domain and the helicase domain. Analysis of the mutations and their resulting phenotypes allows important conclusions to be drawn.

It seems likely that complete absence of ATRX, a true null, would be lethal because in a mouse ATRX knockout (null) model no affected embryos develop beyond approximately 8.5 dpc.[43] Therefore it was surprising to find a number of mutations, predicted to cause protein truncation, scattered throughout the gene in patients with ATR-X syndrome (Fig. 15.8). Such mutations would be expected to result in a major loss of function and yet they are clearly not lethal. In fact, their phenotypes are similar to (and in some cases milder than) those seen with other mutations. For example, one premature stop mutation (R37X) predicted to make a very small, truncated protein produced almost full-length protein.[32,56] This could result from translational initiation at a downstream codon[56] or by skipping the mutation via alternate splicing;[32] whatever the mechanism, this mutation was associated with a remarkably mild phenotype. In fact, similar phenotypic rescue has been seen for all the stop codons upstream of the catalytic domain studied to date.[55]

ATR-X syndrome is frequently caused by missense mutations (Fig. 15.8) and the levels of ATRX protein were shown to be substantially reduced in patients with such mutations involving the ADD domain.[52,57] The structure of the ADD domain casts light on how mutations might affect protein folding and stability.[50] Most mutations affect zinc-binding cysteine residues or residues in the tightly packed hydrophobic core thus reducing its stability. Of greater interest, there is a small cluster of surface mutations (e.g., R246C, G249D) that are associated with higher levels of stable protein. These mutations may interfere with protein function, possibly by disrupting an important protein–protein interaction.

Missense mutations affecting the helicase domain are located adjacent to, rather than within, the seven highly conserved motifs that characterize the SNF2 helicase/adenosine triphosphatase (ATPase) proteins. In other SNF2 proteins, mutations that fall in the motifs completely abolish activity. It is possible that the ATRX mutations alter, rather than abolish, the protein activity. Together, these findings are consistent with a view that mutations seen in patients who survive with ATR-X syndrome decrease rather than abolish ATRX activity.

Is There Any Relationship Between the Types of ATRX Mutation and the Phenotype?

Since the discovery of the *ATRX* gene, most new cases have been defined on the basis of severe MR, with the typical facial appearance associated with a mutation in the *ATRX* gene. This allows a less biased evaluation of the effect of *ATRX* mutations on the commonly associated clinical manifestations. The severity of three aspects of the phenotype (MR, genital abnormality, and α thalassemia) is quantifiable, to some degree.

The greatest variation in intellectual handicap is associated with a truncating mutation (R37X) at the N terminus of the protein.[30] As discussed previously, protein analysis by Western blotting has shown small amounts of full-length protein for each patient affected by this mutation. This may be associated with the use of an alternative, downstream translational initiation codon or alternative splicing. Nevertheless, there is no correlation between the degree of retardation and the amount of full-length protein seen in lymphoblastoid cell lines derived from these patients.

A number of other cases have been described with mild to moderate learning difficulties (reviewed in ref. 55). In a recent small study of 22 patients it was noted that cases with mutations in the ADD domain were less likely to walk than those with mutations affecting the helicase domain.[58] We have now confirmed this finding in a cohort of 83 affected individuals. Whereas 75% of cases with helicase mutations were able to walk only 25% of those with ADD mutations were able to do so (Fig. 15.9).

There are now eight different mutations associated with the most severe urogenital abnormalities.[55] In five, the protein is truncated, resulting in loss of the C-terminal domain, including a conserved element (P in Fig. 15.8) and polyglutamine tract (Q in Fig. 15.8). From the available data, it appears that, in the absence of the C-terminal domain, severe urogenital abnormalities are likely (although not inevitable as one mutation in this region was associated with cryptorchidism), suggesting that this region may play a specific role in urogenital development. Consistent with

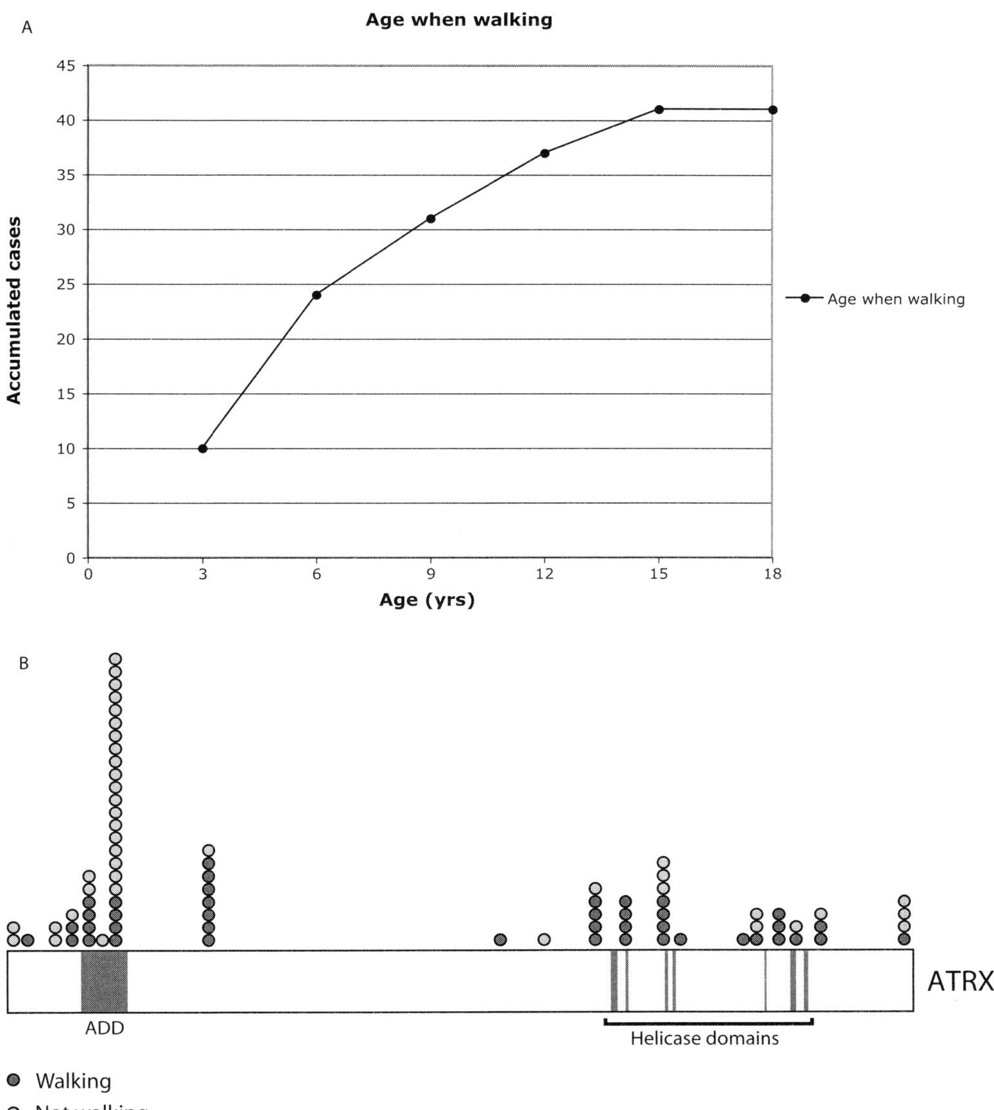

Figure 15.9. A measure of gross motor function is whether the children are able to walk and the age at which this is achieved. Forty-one affected individuals were able to walk. **(A)** Shows the age at which this was achieved. Approximately 75% of these were able to walk by the age of 9 years. None learned to walk after the age of 15 years. **(B)** This figure correlates the ability to walk with the location of the mutation. The 42 individuals who were unable to walk excluded cases who were younger than the age of 9 years at the time of assessment; the range of the ages for this group was 9–30 years. (See color plate 15.9.)

this, in families with such mutations, severe urogenital abnormalities breed true,[36,59] and a nonsense mutation (R2386X) gives rise to a similar phenotype in three unrelated families. In other regions of the protein, however, there is no obvious link between phenotype and genotype, and there is considerable variation in the degree of abnormality seen even in individuals with identical mutations.

The Relationship Between the Types of Mutation in ATRX and Thalassemia

The relationship between *ATRX* mutations and α thalassemia is unclear. Because the presence of excess β chains (HbH inclusions) was originally used to define the ATR-X syndrome, current observations are inevitably biased. Nevertheless, there is considerable variability in the degree to which α-globin synthesis is affected by these mutations, as judged by the frequency of cells with HbH inclusions. Up to 15% of patients do not have HbH inclusions[39,40,60] (Fig. 15.10), although this does not rule out downregulation of α-globin expression because inclusions may not appear until there is 30%–40% reduction in α-chain synthesis (Chapter 14).

It is interesting that patients with identical mutations may have very different, albeit stable, degrees of α thalassemia, suggesting that the effect of the ATRX protein

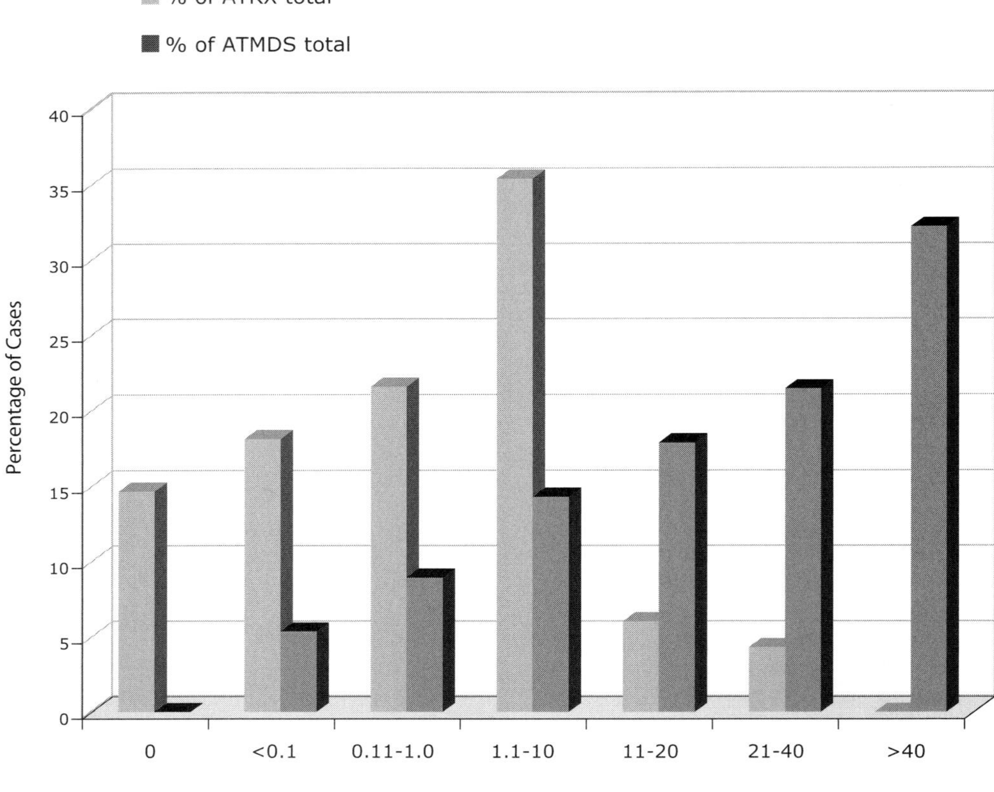

Figure 15.10. Percentage of cells with HbH inclusions in cases of ATR-X syndrome in which the presence of inclusions has been demonstrated and quantified. (See color plate 15.10.)

on α-globin expression may be modified by other genetic factors. This is most clearly illustrated by comparing the hematology of cases with identical mutations. Comparison of the 41 cases from 34 pedigrees with the common 736C>T; R246C mutation shows a wide range in the frequency of cells with HbH inclusions (0%–14%). Preliminary studies indicate that the haplotype of the α-globin locus influences the severity of the thalassemia and presumably there is a feature within this region that is variable and confers different degrees of ATRX dependency (unpublished observation).

What is the Normal Functional Role of ATRX?

In the adult, ATRX mRNA is widely expressed early in development, and continues to be widely expressed throughout development with particularly high expression in the brain, heart, and skeletal muscle.[61] Both isoforms, ATRX (280 kD) and ATRXt (200 kD), are readily detected on Western blots.[48,57] Immunocytochemical analysis and indirect immunolocalization demonstrate that both isoforms are nuclear proteins that predominantly associate with heterochromatin (in interphase and metaphase).[48,57] A significant proportion of ATRX (but not ATRXt) is also found in nuclear speckles (called promyelocytic leukemia bodies) in human cells.[62,63] One additional, striking finding in human metaphase preparations is that ATRX antibodies localize to the short arms of acrocentric chromosomes associated with the rDNA arrays.[64] Undoubtedly, a significant proportion of ATRX can be seen to be associated with heterochromatin and it is possible that the remainder of ATRX, which cannot yet be visualized, may be associated with euchromatic regions of the genome. The next questions are how is ATRX recruited to chromatin and what does it do when it gets there?

Like other members of the SNF2 family, ATRX appears to be part of a multiprotein complex. Preliminary experiments show that ATRX fractionates as a very large complex (approximately 1 Md) by Superose 6 gel filtration. These protein interactions could mediate both recruitment and contribute to ATRX function. One of the proteins with which ATRX has been shown to interact is the heterochromatin protein HP1, a structural adapter, implicated in both gene silencing and supranucleosomal chromatin structure. This interaction has been observed by the yeast two-hybrid experiments,[65] immunoprecipitation,[62] and indirect immunofluorescence,[57] and the observations are supported by genetic manipulation of the system (SuVar39H1) by which HP1 (and possibly ATRX) is recruited to heterochromatin.[66] ATRX may also be recruited to heterochromatin via other, similar interactions. For example it has been shown that in postmitotic neurons ATRX is recruited to heterochromatin via $MeCP_2$.[67]

The ADD domain of ATRX is another potential site for protein interactions that may recruit ATRX to chromatin. One component of this domain is a PHD zinc finger that, in other proteins, appears to mediate an interaction with chromatin.[51] Recent studies have shown that the PHD finger domains of at least two chromatin-associated proteins (BPTF and ING1) specifically recognize H3 histone tails (H3K4me3).[68,69] In addition, the ADD domain of Dnmt3a binds to the sequence-specific DNA-binding protein RP58.[70] A similar interaction between ATRX and other sequence-specific DNA-binding proteins may be responsible for targeting ATRX to specific loci or alternatively recruiting specific loci to repressive heterochromatin.

What role might ATRX play at chromatin? Like other members of the SNF2 family, both recombinant ATRX[71] and endogenous ATRX (isolated from cells by immunoprecipitation)[63] have been shown to have ATPase activity and weak nucleosome remodeling activity.[63] The ATRX protein (complex) exhibits an impressive ability to move (translocate) along double-stranded DNA[63] (and Mitson et al. in preparation), suggesting that ATRX may be able to move nucleosomes to facilitate access of transcription factors or DNA modifying enzymes, for example. Identifying the preferred substrate that is associated with maximal ATPase activity and the assay best suited to reveal the manner by which ATRX interacts with chromatin requires further work.

Finally a variety of other potential protein interactions with ATRX may be relevant. The strongest candidate is the protein Daxx,[63] which has been implicated in both apoptotic pathways and in the regulation of transcription. It has also been shown that the ADD domain of Dnmt3a interacts with the histone deacetylase HDAC1.[70] Interestingly, the PHD motif of Mi2b also binds HDAC1, and it is possible that this component of the ATRX-associated ADD domain may also bind HDAC. In a directed use of the yeast two-hybrid system, Cardoso et al.[72] investigated the interaction of ATRX with a variety of heterochromatin-associated proteins. An interaction was demonstrated between ATRX (475–734) and the SET domain of polycomb group protein EZH2, an enzyme that modifies chromatin. More work is required to substantiate the importance of these observations in vivo.

Functional Consequences of Mutations

Some clues to the normal role of ATRX may come from observing what happens when the gene is mutated. Perhaps the most striking observation is that mutations in ATRX are associated with changes in gene expression (hence α thalassemia) but the mechanism underlying this is currently unknown.

The effects of ATRX mutations on the chromatin structure of the rDNA arrays located at the tips of acrocentric chromosomes have been studied. Although no gross changes in DNase 1, micrococcal nuclease, or endonuclease accessibility were detected, striking differences were noted in the pattern of rDNA methylation between normal controls and patients with ATR-X syndrome.[64] In normal individuals, approximately 20% of the transcribed units were methylated, whereas in ATR-X patients, rDNA genes were substantially unmethylated. The hypomethylated regions in ATR-X individuals localized within the CpG-rich region of the rDNA repeat, which contains the transcribed 28S, 18S, and 5.8S genes and resembles a large CpG island.

Because ATRX is also associated with heterochromatin, which contains a substantial proportion of the highly repetitive DNA in mammalian genomes, these methylation studies were extended to other repetitive sequences containing CpG dinucleotides known to be epigenetically modified by methylation. In this way, two additional sequences were identified that were abnormally methylated in ATR-X patients. Y-specific repeats (DYZ2) were almost all methylated in ATR-X patients, whereas approximately 6% were unmethylated in peripheral blood of normal individuals. Subtle changes in the pattern of methylation were also observed in the TelBam3.4 family of repeats, which are mainly found in the subtelomeric regions.

Perturbations in CpG methylation have been observed with mutations in another mammalian SWI-SNF protein PASG (also known as Lsh and HELLS)[73] and its plant homolog, DDM1.[74] This raises the possibility that ATPase-dependent chromatin-remodeling activities are involved in the establishment or maintenance of DNA methylation and that different SWI/SNF proteins (e.g. ATRX and PASG) may be required for different chromatin environments. To date, no change in the pattern of methylation has been detected in the α-globin gene cluster to explain the presence of α thalassemia.

Summary of the ATR-X Syndrome

Despite considerable progress in defining the phenotype in ATR-X syndrome, describing the properties of the protein and the consequence of mutations, little is known about the function of this protein. In particular, its role in α–globin expression remains elusive. A key puzzle to be solved is how a protein that associates with heterochromatin, and is required for a normal pattern of DNA methylation at repetitive DNA, influences the expression of euchromatic genes. Further progress needs to be made to identify ATRX

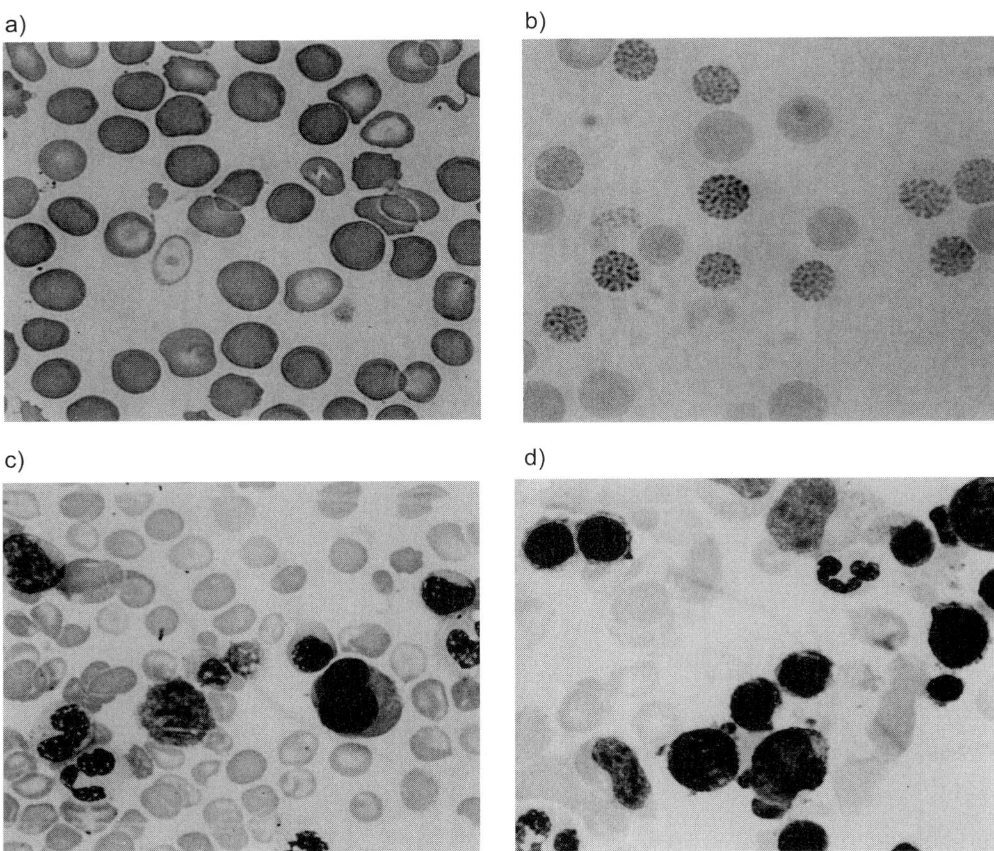

Figure 15.11. **(a)** May-Grünwald-Giemsa–stained peripheral blood smear from an elderly woman with ATMDS (original magnification, 400X). Many red cells are hypochromic, microcytic, or both, whereas others look relatively normal. As expected, the red blood cell distribution width (RDW) was elevated (19%; normal range, 11%–15%) in this patient. Iron studies were unremarkable. **(b)** Brilliant cresyl blue–stained peripheral blood smear from a 56-year-old man with ATMDS who had characteristic microcytic, hypochromic red cell indices: in this case, an MCH of 19 pg and MCV of 66 fL (original magnification, 600X). Abnormal inclusion-containing "golf ball cells" are easily distinguished from normal reticulocytes and red cells and confirm the presence of HbH (β-globin tetramers.) In this case, supravital staining was performed by incubating fresh blood for 24 hours with 1% brilliant cresyl blue in 0.9% normal saline. **(c)** and **(d)** Bone marrow samples from patients with ATMDS showing dyserythropoietic erythroblasts including binucleate cells. (See color plate 15.11.)

target genes and understand the role it plays at these loci.

AN ACQUIRED FORM OF α THALASSEMIA ASSOCIATED WITH MYELOID MALIGNANCY (ATMDS SYNDROME)

Occasionally, patients who previously exhibited normal erythropoiesis will develop an acquired form of α thalassemia, which most commonly arises within the context of hematological malignancy.[75] The first cases of this "acquired hemoglobin H (HbH) disease" were described in 1960.[76,77] Over the past half century, it has become clear that all cases of acquired α thalassemia arise in the context of an underlying clonal disorder of hematopoiesis, most commonly a form of the myelodysplastic syndromes (MDS) as defined by the latest World Health Organization hematopoietic neoplasia classification scheme.[78] Therefore, this condition is now commonly referred to as α thalassemia–myelodysplastic syndrome (ATMDS; Mendelian Inheritance in Man (OMIM) #300448).[79]]. Although other acquired hemoglobin synthetic defects such as acquired β thalassemia or perturbations in the level of HbF and HbA_2 can complicate MDS or other chronic myeloid disorders, these appear to be less common than α thalassemia, and they have not received a specific syndromic designation.[80–83]

The most dramatic and easily recognized ATMDS phenotype is that of a severe form of HbH disease, characterized by striking hypochromic microcytic anemia, numerous HbH inclusions detectable by supravital staining of peripheral blood (Fig. 15.11), and measurable amounts of HbH in the hemolysate.[84] There are also milder forms of ATMDS, in which rare HbH-containing erythrocytes can be detected on the peripheral smear. In these cases, inclusion-containing cells make up less than 1% of anucleate erythrocytes, and HbH represents such a small fraction of the total hemoglobin that it is not easily demonstrable by routine chromatographic or gel electrophoretic techniques.[85] Some of these mildly affected patients – along with others with more severe forms of ATMDS who have been recently transfused with red blood cells from healthy donors – exhibit normocytic or even macrocytic red cell indices, and thus may not be recognized by clinicians.

In the past, most mildly affected ATMDS cases were detected incidentally when a supravital stain of the peripheral blood was performed for another reason, usually to evaluate the reticulocyte count. Many clinical hematology laboratories now quantify reticulocytes by dye-based flow cytometric methods rather than by supravital staining, and thus it is likely that many ATMDS cases, especially those cases with small numbers of HbH cells, now go undetected.[86]

General Clinical Features

More than 80 well-documented patients with ATMDS have been described to date; a global ATMDS Case Registry is maintained in Oxford, and can be viewed at: http://www.imm.ox.ac.uk/groups/mrc_molhaem/home_pages/Higgs/ATMDS.xls. Case clustering among clinical groups who have developed an interest in the disorder suggests that the condition is likely to be underreported. Additionally, most described patients with ATMDS have been of European origin (88% of cases in the Registry), yet current understanding of the molecular pathology of the disease (see later) does not offer a reason for such an imbalanced geographical distribution. Instead, the global distribution of reported cases may reflect detection and reporting bias. Patients diagnosed with MDS who have microcytic red cell indices, and who originate from regions of the world where inherited forms of thalassemia are common, might reasonably be assumed to have a previously undetected inherited disorder of hemoglobin synthesis. Regardless, in all ATMDS cases for which archival data are available, there has been no evidence of a preexisting inherited form of α thalassemia.[87]

At present, other than the disease-defining red cell changes, there are no clinical features that clearly distinguish ATMDS from MDS more generally, although there is a greater male predominance than is observed in chronic myeloid disorders overall (85% of ATMDS cases have been men, whereas the male/female ratio in MDS in general is ~1.5:1).[75] The reason for this dramatic sex imbalance in ATMDS is unclear. Patients with ATMDS are diagnosed at similar ages to patients with chronic myeloid disorders who lack thalassemia (median age, 68 years), have similar marrow findings and karyotypic results, have a median survival typical for MDS overall (2–3 years), and die of the same complications – primarily death from infection and, in approximately 25% of cases, of complications of progression to acute myeloid leukemia.[75] When ATMDS progresses to acute myeloid leukemia, and the ability of hematopoietic cells to differentiate is further impaired, some patients still continue to have detectable HbH, whereas in other cases the HbH inclusions disappear entirely.

Most patients with acquired α thalassemia have MDS (>80%), but a few have chronic idiopathic myelofibrosis or another form of myeloproliferative disease, and rarely patients with acquired HbH disease present with acute myeloid leukemia without an apparent antecedent chronic myeloid disorder.[75] There was also a single case report of acquired α thalassemia in association with TdT-positive acute lymphoblastic leukemia; this case predated the modern era of molecular diagnostics and leukemia immunophenotyping.[88] No other cases of acquired thalassemia have been described in association with a lymphoproliferative disorder or plasma cell dyscrasia.

α/β Globin mRNA and Globin Chain Synthesis Ratios in Patients with ATMDS

The α- to β-globin mRNA ratio has only been studied in a few patients with ATMDS, but it was severely reduced in all these cases (range, 0.06–0.50).[89] Likewise, the reticulocyte α/β-globin chain synthesis ratio was similarly reduced in all 25 patients in whom this ratio has been analyzed (mean 0.28, range 0.05–0.67; normal 0.9–1.2). In the most severely affected individuals, α-chain synthesis is almost completely abolished (Fig. 15.12). The α/β-chain synthesis ratio may vary quite considerably during the course of the disease, and this is reflected in varying proportions of HbH-containing cells on serial supravital staining.[89] In contrast to the typical findings in ATMDS, the α/β-chain synthesis ratio was reported as elevated in a small series of MDS patients without thalassemic red cell indices.[90]

Red Cell Indices and Hematological Findings in ATMDS

Patients with ATMDS are always anemic at presentation (mean hemoglobin 8.5 g/dL), with a reduced red blood cell count (mean 4.3×10^{12}/L) and markedly hypochromic and microcytic red cell indices (average MCH 22 pg and MCV 75 fL).[75] These abnormalities are even more striking when compared with a control population of patients with MDS without thalassemia, who at presentation tend to have slightly higher than normal MCH and MCV values (average MCH 31 pg and MCV 97 fL) (Fig. 15.13). The red cell distribution width has been increased in all ATMDS patients studied.

These hematological findings are reflected in the typical peripheral blood red cell morphology (Fig. 15.11). All patients examined have had at least some hypochromic microcytic red cells, and in many cases there is marked anisopoikilocytosis. In some cases, it appears that there are at least two populations of red cells: some are quite well hemoglobinized and of relatively normal appearance, whereas others contain scant hemoglobin and are often

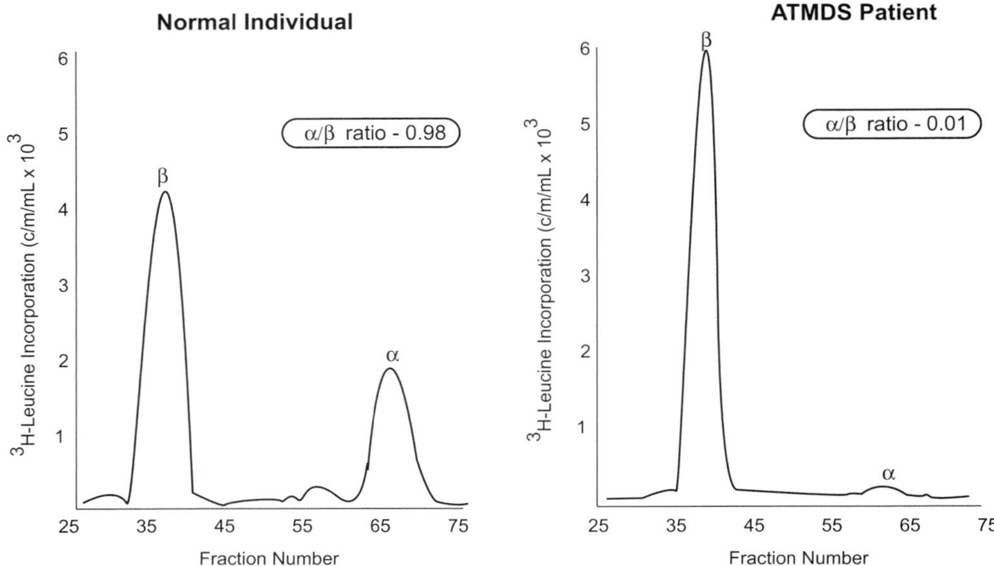

Figure 15.12. Measurement of reticulocyte α/β-globin chain synthesis ratio by radioisotope labeling and CM cellulose chromatography in a patient with ATMDS. In this case, α-globin production was markedly downregulated, and the α/β-chain synthesis ratio estimated by an area-under-the-curve method was only 0.01 (normal, 0.9–1.2). A normal chromatogram is depicted at left, for comparison. (See color plate 15.12.)

little more than "ghost cells." This picture is likely to be a consequence of mixed clonality of the bone marrow in MDS and ATMDS, with residual normal hematopoietic cells coexisting with dysplastic clones, including (in ATMDS) progenitor cells with thalassemic erythrocyte progeny that have HbH inclusions and synthesize little or no normal hemoglobin.

Hemoglobin Analysis in ATMDS

All patients with ATMDS by definition have detectable amounts of HbH in their peripheral red blood cells at some stage of the disease. In general, levels of HbH measured by column chromatography or agarose gel electrophoresis are lower than the proportion of anucleate erythrocytes that contain HbH inclusions on a supravital stained-peripheral blood smear. At the time of first detection of ATMDS, the proportion of red cells containing HbH inclusions after incubation with brilliant cresyl blue varies between less than 0.1% and 95% (median, 30%). HbH as a proportion of total hemoglobin ranges between 1% and 57% (median, 15%). Often it is not possible to obtain accurate estimations of HbH in a given ATMDS case because of prior blood transfusions. In some patients, trace amounts of Hb Bart's

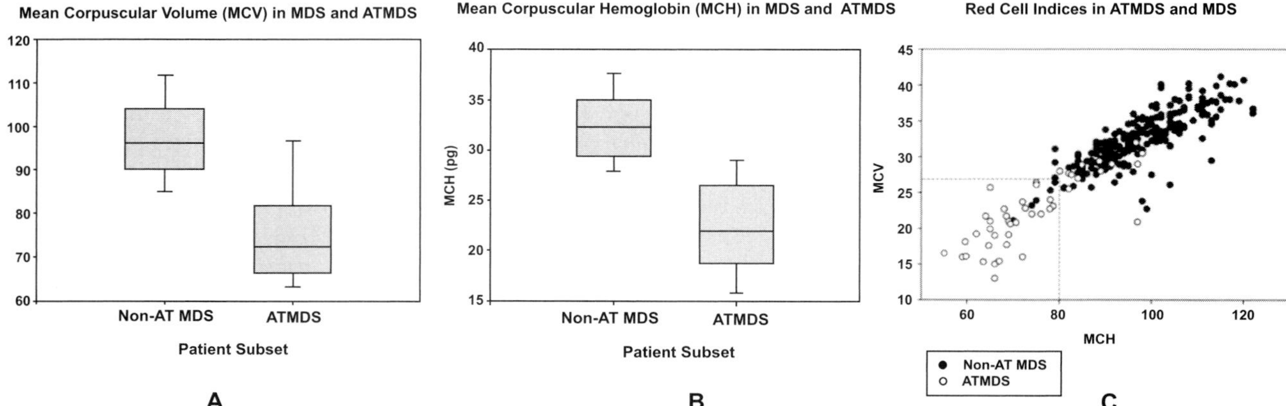

Figure 15.13. Distribution of red cell indices in patients with ATMDS compared with a more general population of patients with MDS. **(A)** MCV at the time of initial presentation in ATMDS (n = 55) vs. MDS (n = 282). Boxes enclosed 25th through 75th percentiles; middle bar denotes the median; whiskers outline the 10th through 90th percentiles. **(B)** MCH in ATMDS vs. MDS. **(C)** Scattergram of MCH vs. MCV distribution in patients with ATMDS (open circles) vs. MDS (closed circles). Dashed lines highlight limits of normal range reported in most clinical laboratories. (Reprinted from ref. 75 with permission.)

(γ globin tetramers) can be found. In the presence of these high oxygen affinity hemoglobins, the whole blood oxygen dissociation curve is shifted to the left, exacerbating the physiological consequences of anemia.[1] Levels of HbA_2 and HbF in ATMDS are variable and inconsistently abnormal.

The Molecular and Cellular Basis for ATMDS

For many years, the molecular etiology of ATMDS was mysterious, but recently, considerable progress toward a mechanistic explanation has been made.[91] It is now clear that most patients with ATMDS have an acquired, somatic point mutation or an mRNA intron–exon splicing abnormality involving *ATRX*, the X-linked gene that encodes the chromatin remodeling factor ATRX (Fig. 15.8).[92,93] This exciting finding provides a partial explanation for the ATMDS phenotype.

Although almost all of the common inherited forms of α thalassemia worldwide are due to deletions or, less commonly, point mutations involving the α-globin gene cluster and its major upstream regulatory element (HS-40), this class of mutation is not typically found in ATMDS.[94] ATMDS cases selected for initial molecular evaluation were those with less than 10% of the normal levels of α-globin mRNA and α-globin synthesis. This extreme degree of impairment of α-globin synthesis is even greater than one typically sees in patients with only a single functional α-globin gene, suggesting that all four α genes are downregulated in ATMDS. Detailed structural analysis of the α-globin genes and approximately 130 kb of their flanking regions on chromosome 16p in these cases consistently revealed no abnormalities, even in the most severely affected patients.[79] In addition, direct sequencing of the globin genes was unremarkable.

In a single reported ATMDS case, the telomeric end of chromosome 16p, including the α-globin cluster, was deleted in a clonally restricted fashion as part of a complex MDS-associated karyotype with numerous large chromosomal rearrangements.[95] This case – in which the extent of the deletion was mapped by FISH – proved exceptional, and no other ATMDS cases have been found to harbor rearrangements of chromosome 16p. Because the presence of multiple cryptic *cis*-acting mutations seemed an unlikely basis for ATMDS, investigators' attention focused next on the possibility of a *trans*-acting mutation, either involving a factor that normally controls α-globin gene expression or a novel gene that exerts a dominant negative effect.

Further support for the possibility of a *trans*-acting defect came from the generation of an interspecific hybrid between bone marrow from an ATMDS patient and adenine phosphoribosyl transferase (APRT)–deficient mouse erythroleukemia (MEL) cells.[96] (APRT is encoded on chromosome 16q24 in humans.) After selection for restored APRT activity, such hybrids retained human chromosome 16 derived from the ATMDS patient in a murine erythroid background, and the human chromosome directed normal levels of human α-globin synthesis. Although these findings would appear to exonerate chromosome 16p in ATMDS, it is also possible that the human cell that originally fused with the MEL cell could have been from an unaffected hematopoietic clone in view of the mixed clonality of MDS. Thus, even this result was not considered definitive evidence of a *trans*-acting defect.

The major clue that led directly to identification ATRX mutations as the specific *trans*-acting molecular defect underlying most ATMDS cases came from a cDNA microarray experiment, in which granulocyte RNA from a patient with severe, newly diagnosed ATMDS was compared with pooled granulocyte RNA from seven healthy donors.[92] Granulocyte RNA was chosen because it is likely to be enriched for mutant clones in chronic myeloid neoplasia, compared with other easily isolated blood cell populations that might also have been suitable for genetic analysis. Strikingly, in this pilot cDNA microarray study, *ATRX* was one of the genes with the very lowest expression in the patient with ATMDS compared with the healthy controls. Sequencing of granulocyte-derived genomic DNA from the ATMDS patient demonstrated a G>A point mutation in the canonical splice donor motif of *ATRX* intron 1, probably resulting in nonsense-mediated decay of the ATRX transcript.[92] In contrast to granulocytes, the patient's buccal cells were ATRX wild type, supporting the clonally restricted nature of the mutation. In view of the important role that ATRX mutations play in congenital ATR-X syndrome (including an association with variable degrees of α thalassemia), ATRX mutations seemed biologically plausible as the cause of α-globin downregulation in ATMDS.[97] Precisely how mutations in ATRX result in down-regulation of α-globin expression is the subject of active investigation, and our current understanding is discussed in detail elsewhere in this text.

Subsequent molecular analysis of archival material from 18 other ATMDS patients revealed ATRX mutations or pre-mRNA splicing abnormalities in almost all cases (14 of 19 total).[93] There is considerable allelic heterogeneity (Fig. 15.8). Reassuringly, when new ATMDS cases with substantial amounts of HbH have come to light, they have also consistently had point mutations involving evolutionarily conserved regions of ATRX.[98–100] This is true not only for men, who have hemizygous ATRX mutations, but also for the rare women with ATMDS, who can be demonstrated to have heterozygous mutations in ATRX.[100] Presumably, the retained wild-type ATRX allele in these women is located on the copy of the X chromosome that was inactivated during embryogenesis, and it is not expressed at a high enough level to "rescue" α-globin expression in the progeny of the ATRX-mutant clone.

Implications of ATRX Mutations in ATMDS

In general, patients with ATMDS have a more severe form of α thalassemia than boys with inherited ATR-X syndrome.

More than 30% of described ATMDS patients have had more than 50% of circulating erythrocytes containing HbH inclusions, whereas 90% of boys with ATR-X syndrome have less than 10% HbH-containing cells.[93,101] Even when an identical or similar ATRX mutation is detected in the germline in ATR-X syndrome and as a somatic change in the hematopoietic cells in ATMDS, the thalassemic phenotype is consistently more severe in ATMDS than in ATR-X. For instance, a boy with germline c.576G>S, p.L192F ATRX mutation had 0.1% HbH, whereas a man with ATMDS who had the identical mutation as an acquired phenomenon had 50% HbH. The reason for this striking difference is unclear and is suspected to be dependent on the cellular context, perhaps pointing to an interaction between ATRX mutations and a disturbed genetic or epigenetic background in MDS cells that is due to other mutations not present in boys with inherited ATR-X syndrome.

In a few patients with ATMDS, an ATRX point mutation has not been detected, despite careful investigation. Most of these patients have had less than 10% HbH, and issues related to sensitivity of the tools used for mutation detection may account for the negative results, although it remains possible that mutations in another as yet undefined *trans*-acting factor can cause an ATMDS phenocopy. Direct fluorescent dye chemistry-based DNA sequencing can only detect mutations at a level of approximately 20%–30% mutant DNA in a wild-type background, and may miss acquired mutations that are present at lower levels of clonality.[93] Other mutation screening techniques, such as denaturing high-performance liquid chromatography and denaturing-gradient gel electrophoresis, offer higher analytical sensitivity (down to ~1% mutant DNA), but these techniques also do not detect ATRX mutations in all ATMDS cases. In some ATMDS cases, only genomic DNA has been available for screening, and it is possible that some of these cases actually have an alteration in ATRX pre-mRNA splicing, as has been described in several ATMDS cases in which both DNA and RNA were accessible for analysis.[92,93,98,102]

Supravital staining of unselected MDS cases (i.e., without regard for red cell indices) demonstrates small numbers of HbH inclusion-containing cells in 8% of cases; these cells are not present in other forms of anemia not associated with a clonal myeloid disorder, and therefore are not simply a byproduct of disordered erythropoiesis.[85] It seems likely that α thalassemic clones arise fairly commonly in the marrow milieu of MDS, for unclear reasons, and that these changes alone do not give the cells that bear them any sort of competitive advantage. Additional mutations are probably required to provide a clone that happens to be thalassemic with a survival or proliferative advantage, leading ultimately to clonal dominance, and these secondary changes may account for the more dramatic ATMDS phenotypes.

Remaining Questions About ATMDS

One of the most exciting prospects for the discovery of ATRX mutations in ATMDS is that this finding may yield some new general insights into the pathobiology of MDS. Such advances would be welcome, as MDS has proven to be a rather intractable disorder, both from the standpoint of analysis of disease mechanism and from a therapeutic perspective.[103] Since the discovery of ATRX mutations in ATMDS, candidate gene analysis in MDS has focused on genes encoding known or suspected ATRX binding partners (HP1, DAXX, EZH2) or homologous SWI/SNF2 family members implicated in leukemogenesis (HELLS/LSH/SMARCA6), but these studies have thus far been unrevealing.

The reason for the sex imbalance in ATMDS remains unclear. The fact that ATRX is an X-linked factor can provide only a partial answer, as other conditions that are caused by acquired mutations in genes on the X chromosome (e.g., paroxysmal nocturnal hemoglobinuria) do not display such a striking sex distinction.

The fact that germline ATRX mutations are known to be associated with diverse alterations in DNA methylation across the genome has particular relevance in MDS, in which methylation changes are common and which some investigators have labeled an "epigenetic disease."[64,104,105] Two of the first three drug therapies approved by the United States Food and Drug Administration for the treatment of MDS – azacitidine (approved in 2004) and decitabine (approved in May 2006) – are aza-substituted cytosine nucleoside analogs that irreversibly bind to DNA methyltransferase 1 (DNMT1) and inhibit its enzymatic activity.[106–108] DNMT1 inhibition that persists through the cell cycle results in alteration in the 5′ methylation status of cytosine in CpG dinucleotides in gene promoters, with subsequent changes in gene expression. Anecdotally, one ATMDS patient treated with hypomethylating therapy experienced unusually profound and prolonged marrow aplasia, but it is uncertain whether this is merely a coincidence or is mechanistically related.[99]

Summary of ATMDS Syndrome

Over the past few years, considerable progress has been made in understanding the molecular basis for the rare syndrome of ATMDS, when α thalassemia is acquired as a "passenger" mutation (rather than a causative mutation) in MDS. We now know that the associated α thalassemia results from mutation in the X-encoded *ATRX* gene, which is also the disease gene in the inherited condition ATR-X syndrome. A remaining puzzle is why the same mutation in ATRX causes a mild form of thalassemia, whereas in ATMDS it causes severe HbH disease. It seems likely that the ATRX mutation is somehow made more severe when it interacts with one or more of the common genetic or epigenetic mutations in MDS. Understanding the mechanism underlying the severe α thalassemia in this fascinating syndrome may shed some light on the molecular basis of the common forms of MDS.

REFERENCES

1. Weatherall DJ, Higgs DR, Bunch C, et al. Hemoglobin H disease and mental retardation. A new syndrome or a remarkable coincidence? *N Engl J Med.* 1981;305:607–612.
2. Wilkie AOM, Buckle VJ, Harris PC, et al. Clinical features and molecular analysis of the α thalassaemia/mental retardation syndromes. I. Cases due to deletions involving chromosome band 16p13.3. *Am J Hum Genet.* 1990;46:1112–1126.
3. Wilkie AOM, Zeitlin HC, Lindenbaum RH, et al. Clinical features and molecular analysis of the α thalassemia/mental retardation syndromes. II. Cases without detectable abnormality of the α globin complex. *Am J Hum Genet.* 1990;46: 1127–1140.
4. Schmickel RD. Contiguous gene syndromes: a component of recognizable syndromes. *J Pediatr.* 1986;109:231–241.
5. Callen DF, Hyland VJ, Baker EG, et al. Mapping the short arm of human chromosome 16. *Genomics.* 1989;4:348–354.
6. Neidengard L, Sparkes RS. Ring chromosome 16. *Hum Genet.* 1981;59:175–177.
7. Quintana A, Sordo MT, Estevez C, Ludena MC, San Roman C. 16 Ring chromosome. *Clin Genet.* 1983;23:243.
8. Buckle VJ, Higgs DR, Wilkie AOM, Super M, Weatherall DJ. Localisation of human α globin to 16p13.3-pter. *J Med Genet.* 1988;25:847–849.
9. Lamb J, Wilkie AOM, Harris PC, et al. Detection of breakpoints in submicroscopic chromosomal translocation, illustrating an important mechanism for genetic disease. *Lancet.* 1989;ii:819–824.
10. Buckle VJ, Kearney L. New methods in cytogenetics. *Curr Opin Genet Dev.* 1994;4:374–382.
11. Brown J, Saracoglu K, Uhrig S, Speicher MR, Eils R, Kearney L. Subtelomeric chromosome rearrangements are detected using an innovative 12-color FISH assay (M-TEL). *Nat Med.* 2001;7:497–501.
12. Price TS, Regan R, Mott R, et al. SW-ARRAY:a dynamic programming solution for the identification of copy-number changes in genomic DNA using array comparative genome hybridization data. *Nucl Acids Res.* 2005;33:3455–3464.
13. Redon R, Ishikawa S, Fitch KR, et al. Global variation in copy number in the human genome. *Nature.* 2006;444:444–454.
14. Colella S, Yau C, Taylor JM, et al. QuantiSNP: an Objective Bayes Hidden-Markov Model to detect and accurately map copy number variation using SNP genotyping data. *Nucl Acids Res.* 2007;35:2013–2025.
15. Harteveld CL, Kriek M, Bijlsma EK, et al. Refinement of the genetic cause of ATR-16. *Hum Genet.* 2007;122:283–292.
16. Harteveld CL, Voskamp A, Phylipsen M, et al. Nine unknown rearrangements in 16p13.3 and 11p15.4 causing alpha- and beta-thalassaemia characterised by high resolution multiplex ligation-dependent probe amplification. *J Med Genet.* 2005;42:922–931.
17. Lamb J, Harris PC, Wilkie AOM, Wood WG, Dauwerse JG, Higgs DR. *De novo* truncation of chromosome 16p and healing with (TTAGGG)n in the α-thalassemia/mental retardation syndrome (ATR-16). *Am J Hum Genet.* 1993;52:668–676.
18. Daniels RJ, Peden JF, Lloyd C, et al. Sequence, structure and pathology of the fully annotated terminal 2 Mb of the short arm of human chromosome 16. *Hum Mol Genet.* 2001;10:339–352.
19. Horsley SW, Daniels RJ, Anguita E, et al. Monosomy for the most telomeric, gene-rich region of the short arm of human chromosome 16 causes minimal phenotypic effects. *Eur J Hum Genet.* 2001;9:217–225.
20. European Polycystic Kidney Disease Consortium. The polycystic kidney disease 1 gene encodes a 14 kb transcript and lies within a duplicated region on chromosome 16. *Cell.* 1994;77:881–894.
21. Vogel F, Motulsky AG. *Human Genetics. Problems and Approaches.* 2nd ed. Berlin: Springer-Verlag; 1986.
22. Hall JG. Genomic imprinting: review and relevance to human diseases. *Am J Hum Genet.* 1990;46:857–873.
23. Schneider AS, Bischoff FZ, McCaskill C, Coady ML, Stopfer JE, Shaffer LG. Comprehensive 4-year follow-up on a case of maternal heterodisomy for chromosome 16. *Am J Med Genet.* 1996;66:204–208.
24. Fisher E, Scambler P. Human haploinsufficiency – one for sorrow, two for joy. *Nat Genet.* 1994;7:5–7.
25. Pfeifer D, Poulat F, Holinski-Feder E, Kooy F, Scherer G. The SOX8 gene is located within 700 kb of the tip of chromosome 16p and is deleted in a patient with ATR-16 syndrome. *Genomics.* 2000;63:108–116.
26. Flint J, Wilkie AOM, Buckle VJ, Winter RM, Holland AJ, McDermid HE. The detection of subtelomeric chromosomal rearrangements in idiopathic mental retardation. *Nat Genet.* 1995;9:132–140.
27. Wilkie AOM, Pembrey ME, Gibbons RJ, et al. The non-deletion type of α thalassaemia/mental retardation: a recognisable dysmorphic syndrome with X-linked inheritance. *J Med Genet.* 1991;28:724.
28. Gibbons RJ, Wilkie AOM, Weatherall DJ, Higgs DR. A newly defined X linked mental retardation syndrome associated with α thalassaemia. *J Med Genet.* 1991;28:729–733.
29. Carpenter NJ, Qu Y, Curtis M, Patil SR. X-linked mental retardation syndrome with characteristic "coarse" facial appearance, brachydactyly, and short stature maps to proximal Xq. *Am J Med Genet.* 1999;85:230–235.
30. Guerrini R, Shanahan JL, Carrozzo R, Bonanni P, Higgs DR, Gibbons RJ. A nonsense mutation of the ATRX gene causing mild mental retardation and epilepsy. *Ann Neurol.* 2000;47:117–121.
31. Yntema HG, Poppelaars FA, Derksen E, et al. Expanding phenotype of XNP mutations: mild to moderate mental retardation. *Am J Med Genet.* 2002;110:243–247.
32. Abidi FE, Cardoso C, Lossi AM, et al. Mutation in the 5′ alternatively spliced region of the XNP/ATR-X gene causes Chudley-Lowry syndrome. *Eur J Hum Genet.* 2005;13:176–183.
33. Wada T, Gibbons RJ. ATR-X syndrome. In: Fisch GS, ed. *Genetics and Genomics of Neurobehavioral Disorders.* Totowa, NJ: Humana Press; 2003:309–334.
34. Kurosawa K, Akatsuka A, Ochiai Y, Ikeda J, Maekawa K. Self-induced vomiting in X-linked α-thalassemia/mental retardation syndrome. *Am J Med Genet.* 1996;63:505–506.

35. Wada T, Nakamura M, Matsushita Y, et al. [Three Japanese children with X-linked alpha-thalassemia/mental retardation syndrome (ATR-X)]. *No To Hattatsu.* 1998;30:283–289.
36. McPherson E, Clemens M, Gibbons RJ, Higgs DR. X-linked alpha thalassemia/mental retardation (ATR-X) syndrome. A new kindred with severe genital anomalies and mild hematologic expression. *Am J Med Genet.* 1995;55:302–306.
37. Gibbons RJ, Brueton L, Buckle VJ, et al. The clinical and hematological features of the X-linked α thalassemia/mental retardation syndrome (ATR-X). *Am J Med Genet.* 1995; 55:288–299.
38. Martucciello G, Lombardi L, Savasta S, Gibbons RJ. The gastrointestinal phenotype of ATR-X syndrome. *Am J Med Genet.* 2006;140:1172–1176.
39. Villard L, Gecz J, Mattel JF, et al. XNP mutation in a large family with Juberg-Marsidi syndrome. *Nat Genet.* 1996;12:359–360.
40. Villard L, Lacombe D, Fontes M. A point mutation in the XNP gene, associated with an ATR-X phenotype without α-thalassemia. *Eur J Hum Genet.* 1996;4:316–320.
41. Donnai D, Clayton-Smith J, Gibbons RJ, Higgs DR. The non-deletion α thalassaemia/mental retardation syndrome. Further support for X linkage. *J Med Genet.* 1991;28:742–745.
42. Gibbons RJ, Suthers GK, Wilkie AOM, Buckle VJ, Higgs DR. X-linked α thalassemia/mental retardation (ATR-X) syndrome: Localisation to Xq12-21.31 by X-inactivation and linkage analysis. *Am J Hum Genet.* 1992;51:1136–1149.
43. Garrick D, Sharpe JA, Arkell R, et al. Loss of Atrx affects trophoblast development and the pattern of X-inactivation in extraembryonic tissues. *PLoS Genet.* 2006;2:e58.
44. Muers MR, Sharpe JA, Garrick D, et al. Defining the cause of skewed X-chromosome inactivation in X-linked mental retardation by use of a mouse model. *Am J Hum Genet.* 2007;80:1138–1149.
45. Gecz J, Pollard H, Gonzalez G, et al. Cloning and expression of the murine homologue of a putative human X-linked nuclear protein gene closely linked to PGK1 in Xq13.*3. Hum Mol Genet.* 1994;3:39–44.
46. Gibbons RJ, Picketts DJ, Villard L, Higgs DR. Mutations in a putative global transcriptional regulator cause X-linked mental retardation with α-thalassemia (ATR-X syndrome). *Cell.* 1995;80:837–845.
47. Picketts DJ, Higgs DR, Bachoo S, Blake DJ, Quarrell OWJ, Gibbons RJ. *ATRX* encodes a novel member of the SNF2 family of proteins: mutations point to a common mechanism underlying the ATR-X syndrome. *Hum Mol Genet.* 1996;5:1899–1907.
48. Garrick D, Samara V, McDowell TL, et al. A conserved truncated isoform of the ATR-X syndrome protein lacking the SWI/SNF-homology domain. *Gene.* 2004;326:23–34.
49. Gibbons RJ, Bachoo S, Picketts DJ, et al. Mutations in a transcriptional regulator (hATRX) establish the functional significance of a PHD-like domain. *Nat Genet.* 1997;17:146–148.
50. Argentaro A, Yang JC, Chapman L, et al. Structural consequences of disease-causing mutations in the ATRX-DNMT3-DNMT3L (ADD) domain of the chromatin-associated protein ATRX. *Proc Natl Acad Sci USA.* 2007;104:11939–11944.
51. Bienz M. The PHD finger, a nuclear protein-interaction domain. *Trends Biochem Sci.* 2006;31:35–40.
52. Cardoso C, Lutz Y, Mignon C, et al. ATR-X mutations cause impaired nuclear location and altered DNA binding properties of the XNP/ATR-X protein. *J Med Genet.* 2000;37:746–751.
53. Picketts DJ, Tastan AO, Higgs DR, Gibbons RJ. Comparison of the human and murine ATRX gene identifies highly conserved, functionally important domains. *Mammal Genome.* 1998;9:400–403.
54. Carlson M, Laurent BC. The SNF/SWI family of global transcriptional activators. *Curr Opin Cell Biol.* 1994;6:396–402.
55. Gibbons RJ, Wada T, Fisher C, et al. Mutations in the chromatin associated protein ATRX. *Hum Mutat.* 2008:29:796–802.
56. Howard MT, Malik N, Anderson CB, Voskuil JL, Atkins JF, Gibbons RJ. Attenuation of an amino-terminal premature stop codon mutation in the ATRX gene by an alternative mode of translational initiation. *J Med Genet.* 2004;41:951–956.
57. McDowell TL, Gibbons RJ, Sutherland H, et al. Localization of a putative transcriptional regulator (ATRX) at pericentromeric heterochromatin and the short arms of acrocentric chromosomes. *Proc Natl Acad Sci USA.* 1999;96:13983–13988.
58. Badens C, Lacoste C, Philip N, et al. Mutations in PHD-like domain of the ATRX gene correlate with severe psychomotor impairment and severe urogenital abnormalities in patients with ATRX syndrome. *Clin Genet.* 2006;70:57–62.
59. Ion A, Telvi L, Chaussain JL, et al. A novel mutation in the putative DMA Helicase *XH2* is responsible for male-to-female sex reversal associated with an atypical form of the ATR-X syndrome. *Am J Hum Genet.* 1996;58:1185–1191.
60. Villard L, Toutain A, Lossi A-M, et al. Splicing mutation in the ATR-X gene can lead to a dysmorphic mental retardation phenotype without α-thalassemia. *Am J Hum Genet.* 1996;58:499–505.
61. Stayton CL, Dabovic B, Gulisano M, Gecz J, Broccoli V, Giovanazzi S et al. Cloning and characterisation of a new human Xq13 gene, encoding a putative helicase. *Hum Mol Genet.* 1994;3:1957–1964.
62. Berube NG, Smeenk CA, Picketts DJ. Cell cycle-dependent phosphorylation of the ATRX protein correlates with changes in nuclear matrix and chromatin association. *Hum Mol Genet.* 2000;9:539–547.
63. Xue Y, Gibbons R, Van Z, et al. The ATRX syndrome protein forms a chromatin-remodeling complex with Daxx and localizes in promyelocytic leukemia nuclear bodies. *Proc Natl Acad Sci USA.* 2003;100:10635–10640.
64. Gibbons RJ, McDowell TL, Raman S, et al. Mutations in ATRX, encoding a SWI/SNF-like protein, cause diverse changes in the pattern of DNA methylation. *Nat Genet.* 2000;24:368–371.
65. Le Douarin B, Nielsen AL, Gamier JM, et al. A possible involvement of TIF1 alpha and TIF1 beta in the epigenetic control of transcription by nuclear receptors. *EMBO J.* 1996;15:6701–6715.
66. Kourmpuli N, Sun YM, Van Der Sar S, Singh PB, Brown JP. Epigenetic regulation of mammalian pericentric heterochromatin in vivo by HP1. *Biochem Biophys Res Commun.* 2005;337:901–907.
67. Nan X, Hou J, Maclean A, et al. Interaction between chromatin proteins MECP2 and ATRX is disrupted by mutations that cause inherited mental retardation. *Proc Natl Acad Sci USA.* 2007;104:2709–2714.
68. Wysocka J, Swigut T, Xiao H, et al. A PHD finger of NURF couples histone H3 lysine 4 trimethylation with chromatin remodelling. *Nature.* 2006;442:86–90.
69. Pena PV, Davrazou F, Shi X, et al. Molecular mechanism of histone H3K4me3 recognition by plant homeodomain of ING2. *Nature.* 2006;442:100–103.

70. Fuks F, Burgers WA, Godin N, Kasai M, Kouzarides T. Dnmt3a binds deacetylases and is recruited by a sequence-specific represser to silence transcription. *EMBO J.* 2001;20:2536–2544.
71. Tang J, Wu S, Liu H, et al. A novel transcription regulatory complex containing death domain-associated protein and the ATR-X syndrome protein. *J Biol Chem.* 2004;279:20369–20377.
72. Cardoso C, Timsit S, Villard L, Khrestchatisky M, Fontes M, Colleaux L. Specific interaction between the *XNP/ATR-X* gene product and the SET domain of the human EZH2 protein. *Hum Mol Genet.* 1998;7:679–684.
73. Dennis K, Fan T, Geiman T, Van Q, Muegge K. Lsh, a member of the SNF2 family, is required for genome-wide methylation. *Genes Dev.* 2001;15:2940–2944.
74. Jeddeloh JA, Stokes TL, Richards EJ. Maintenance of genomic methylation requires a SWI2/SNF2-like protein [see comments]. *Nat Genet.* 1999;22:94–97.
75. Steensma DP, Gibbons RJ, Higgs DR. Acquired α thalassemia in association with myelodysplastic syndrome and other hematologic malignancies. *Blood.* 2005;105:443–452.
76. Bergren WR, Sturgeon PH. *Hemoglobin H: Some Additional Findings.* New York: Proceedings of the 7th International Congress in Hematology; 1960:488.
77. White JC, Ellis M, Coleman PN, et al. An unstable haemoglobin associated with some cases of leukaemia. *Br J Haematol.* 1960;6:171–177.
78. Harris NL, Jaffe ES, Diebold J, et al. World Health Organization classification of neoplastic diseases of the hematopoietic and lymphoid tissues: report of the Clinical Advisory Committee meeting-Airlie House, Virginia, November 1997. *J Clin Oncol.* 1999;17:3835–3849.
79. Higgs DR, Wood WG, Barton C, Weatherall DJ. Clinical features and molecular analysis of acquired hemoglobin H disease. *Am J Med.* 1983;75:181–191.
80. Bradley TB, Ranney HM. Acquired disorders of hemoglobin. *Prog Hematol.* 1973;8:77–98.
81. Dibenedetto SP, Russo Mancuso G, Di Cataldo A, Schiliro G. Non inherited hemoglobin anomalies. *Haematologica.* 1991;76:414–420.
82. Hoyle C, Kaeda J, Leslie J, Luzzatto L. Acquired beta thalassaemia trait in MDS. *Br J Haematol.* 1991;79:116–117.
83. Weinberg RS, Leibowitz D, Weinblatt ME, Kochen J, Alter BP. Juvenile chronic myelogenous leukaemia: the only example of truly fetal (not fetal-like) erythropoiesis. *Br J Haematol.* 1990;76:307–310.
84. Old J, Longley J, Wood WG, Clegg JB, Weatherall DJ. Molecular basis for acquired haemoglobin H disease. *Nature.* 1977;269:524–525.
85. Steensma DP, Porcher JC, Hanson CA, et al. Prevalence of erythrocyte haemoglobin H inclusions in unselected patients with clonal myeloid disorders. *Br J Haematol.* 2007;139:439–442.
86. Siekmeier R, Bierlich A, Jaross W. Determination of reticulocytes:three methods compared. *Clin Chem Lab Med.* 2000;38:245–249.
87. Higgs DR, Garrick D, Anguita E, et al. Understanding α-globin gene regulation: aiming to improve the management of thalassemia. *Ann NY Acad Sci.* 2005;1054:92–102.
88. Kueh YK. Acute lymphoblastic leukemia with brilliant cresyl blue erythrocytic inclusions-acquired hemoglobin H? *N Engl J Med.* 1982;307:193–194.
89. Higgs DR, Wood WG, Barton C, Weatherall DJ. Clinical features and molecular analysis of acquired HbH disease. *Am J Med.* 1983;75:181–191.
90. Peters RE, May A, Jacobs A. Increased alpha:non-alpha globin chain synthesis ratios in myelodysplastic syndromes and myeloid leukaemia. *J Clin Pathol.* 1986;39:1233–1235.
91. Higgs DR. Ham-Wasserman lecture: gene regulation in hematopoiesis: new lessons from thalassemia. *Hematology Am Soc Hematol Edu Program.* 2004:1–13.
92. Gibbons RJ, Pellagatti A, Garrick D, et al. Identification of acquired somatic mutations in the gene encoding chromatin-remodeling factor ATRX in the alpha-thalassemia myelodysplasia syndrome (ATMDS). *Nat Genet.* 2003;34:446–449.
93. Steensma DP, Higgs DR, Fisher CA, Gibbons RJ. Acquired somatic ATRX mutations in myelodysplastic syndrome associated with alpha thalassemia (ATMDS) convey a more severe hematologic phenotype than germline ATRX mutations. *Blood.* 2004;103:2019–2026.
94. Weatherall DJ, Higgs DR, Clegg JB. The molecular pathology of the alpha globin genes. *Br J Cancer.* 1988;9(Suppl):17–22.
95. Steensma DP, Viprakasit V, Hendrick A, et al. Deletion of the alpha-globin gene cluster as a cause of acquired alpha-thalassemia in myelodysplastic syndrome. *Blood.* 2004;103:1518–1520.
96. Helder J, Deisseroth A. S1 nuclease analysis of α-globin gene expression in preleukemic patients with acquired hemoglobin H disease after transfer to mouse erythroleukemia cells. *Proc Natl Acad Sci. USA.* 1987;84:2387–2390.
97. Gibbons RJ, Wada T. ATRX and X-linked α-thalassemia mental retardation syndrome. In: Epstein CJ, Erickson RP, Wynshaw-Boris A, eds. *Inborn Errors of Development.* Oxford: Oxford University Press; 2004:747–757.
98. Nelson ME, Thurmes PJ, Hoyer JD, Steensma DP. A novel 5′ ATRX mutation with splicing consequences in acquired alpha thalassemia-myelodysplastic syndrome. *Haematologica.* 2005;90:1463–1470.
99. Costa DB, Fisher CA, Miller KB, et al. A novel mutation in the last exon of ATRX in a patient with alpha-thalassemia myelodysplastic syndrome. *Eur J Haematol.* 2006;76:432–435, 53.
100. Haas PS, Schwabe M, Fisher C, et al. Two novel somatic mutations of the ATRX gene in female patients with acquired alpha thalassemia in myelodysplastic syndrome (ATMDS). *Blood.* 2006;108:A1765.
101. Gibbons RJ, Higgs DR. The Molecular-Clinical Spectrum of the ATR-X Syndrome. *Am J Med Genet.* 2000;97:204–212.
102. Steensma DP, Allen S, Gibbons RJ, Fisher CA, Higgs DR. Abstract 3606: A novel splicing mutation in the gene encoding the chromatin-associated factor *ATRX* associated with acquired hemoglobin H disease in myelodysplastic syndrome (ATMDS). *Blood.* 2004;104(11):A3606.
103. Steensma DP, Bennett JM. The myelodysplastic syndromes: diagnosis and treatment. *Mayo Clin Proc.* 2006;81:104–130.
104. Jones PA, Baylin SB. The fundamental role of epigenetic events in cancer. *Nat Rev Genet.* 2002;3:415–428.
105. Leone G, Teofili L, Voso MT, Lubbert M. DMA methylation and demethylating drugs in myelodysplastic syndromes and secondary leukemias. *Haematologica.* 2002;87:1324–1341.
106. Kantarjian H, Issa JP, Rpsenfeld CS, et al. Decitabine improves patient outcomes in myelodysplastic syndromes:

results of a phase III randomized study. *Cancer.* 2006;106: 1794–1803.

107. Silverman LR, Demakos EP, Peterson BL, et al. Randomized controlled trial of azacitidine in patients with the myelodysplastic syndrome: a study of the cancer and leukemia group B. *J Clin Oncol.* 2002;20:2429–2440.

108. Silverman LR. DMA methyltransferase inhibitors in myelodysplastic syndrome. *Best Pract Res Clin Haematol.* 2004;17:585–594.

109. Lindor NM, Valdes MG, Wick M, Thibodeau SN, Jalal S. De novo 16p deletion:ATR-16 syndrome. *Am J Med Genet.* 1997;72:451–454.

110. Fei YJ, Liu JC, Walker ELDI, Huisman THJ. A new gene deletion involving the α2-, α1-, and θ1-globin genes in a Black family with HbH disease. *Am J Hematol.* 1992;39:299–303.

111. Felice AE, Cleek MP, McKie K, McKie V, Huisman THJ. The rare α-thalassemia-1 of Blacks is a ζα-thalassemia-1 associated with deletion of all α- and ζ-globin genes. *Blood.* 1984;63:1253–1257.

112. Rack KA, Harris PC, MacCarthy AB, et al. Characterization of three de novo derivative chromosomes 16 by 'reverse chromosome painting' and molecular analysis. *Am J Hum Genet.* 1993;52:987–997.

113. Rönich P, Kleihauer E. Alpha-thalassamie mit HbH und Hb Bart's in einer deutschen Familie. *Klin Wochenschrift.* 1967;45:S1193–1200.

114. Gallego MS, Zelaya G, Feliu AS, et al. ATR-16 due to a de novo complex rearrangement of chromosome 16. *Hemoglobin.* 2005;29:141–150.

115. Gibson WT, Harvard C, Qiao Y, Somerville MJ, Lewis MES, Rajcan-Separovic E. Phenotype-genotype characterization of alpha-thalassemia mental retardation syndrome due to isolated monosomy of 16p13.3. *Am J Med Genet.* 2008;146A:225–232.

116. Kamei M, Ades LC, Eyre HJ, Callen DF, Campbell HD. *SOLH,* a human homologue of the *Drosophila melanogaster small optic lobes* gene is deleted in ATR-16 syndrome. *Appl Genom Proteom.* 2002;1:65–71.

117. Villegas A, Ropero P, Gonzalez FA, Anguita E, Espinos D. The thalassemia syndromes: molecular characterization in the Spanish population. *Hemoglobin.* 2001;25:273–283.

118. Hjelle B, Charache S, Phillips JAR. Hemoglobin H disaese and multiple congenital anomalies in a child of northern European origin. *Am J Hematol.* 1982;13:319–322.

119. Dallman PR. The red cell. In: Dallman PR, ed. *Blood and Blood-forming Tissues.* New York: Appleton-Century-Crofts; 1977:1109–1113.

SECTION FOUR

THE β THALASSEMIAS

Bernard G. Forget

Over the years, study of the thalassemia syndromes has served as a paradigm for gaining insights into the factors that can regulate or disrupt normal gene expression. The thalassemias constitute a heterogeneous group of naturally occurring, inherited mutations characterized by abnormal globin gene expression resulting in total absence or quantitative reduction of α- or β-globin chain synthesis in human erythroid cells. α Thalassemia is associated with absent or decreased production of α-chains, whereas in the β thalassemias, there is absent or decreased production of β-chains. In those cases in which some of the affected globin chain is synthesized, early studies demonstrated no evidence of an amino acid substitution. In all cases in which genetic evidence was available, the thalassemia gene appeared to be allelic with the structural gene encoding α- or β-globin. The elucidation of the nature of the various molecular lesions in thalassemia has been a fascinating process, and full of surprises. Increase in our knowledge of the molecular basis of β thalassemia has closely followed and depended on progress and technical breakthroughs in the fields of biochemistry and molecular biology. In particular, recombinant DNA and polymerase chain reaction–based technologies have contributed to a virtual explosion of new information on the precise molecular basis of most forms of thalassemia. The accrual of this knowledge has, to a great degree, paralleled the acquisition of new, detailed information on the structure, organization, and function of the normal human globin genes, as described in the preceding chapters. Historically, as new techniques have been developed for the study of protein synthesis and gene expression, they have been rapidly applied to the study of normal human hemoglobin synthesis and the abnormalities associated with abnormal globin gene expression in thalassemia. As a result, there has gradually emerged a progressively clearer and increasingly complex picture of the molecular pathology of this group of genetic disorders. One major conclusion that was drawn as this mystery unfolded was that a relatively limited number of phenotypes can result from a surprisingly large number of varied genotypes.

The chapters that follow will describe in detail the knowledge and progress that have accrued over the last 3–4 decades on the understanding of the pathophysiology, the molecular genetics, and the clinical manifestations and management of the various β thalassemia syndromes and related disorders.

There are many primary and secondary causes for the anemia observed in β thalassemia. It is easy to understand how reduced synthesis of β-globin chains of Hb A ($\alpha_2\beta_2$) will result in an overall deficit of hemoglobin accumulation in red cells and cause a hypochromic, microcytic anemia with a low mean corpuscular hemoglobin concentration in affected erythrocytes. This is true in both the heterozygous and homozygous states. In the homozygous state, however, another pathophysiological process worsens the anemia and is responsible for the major clinical manifestations in the syndrome referred to as β thalassemia major or Cooley's anemia. The continued synthesis in normal amounts of normal α-globin chains results in the accumulation, within the erythroid cells, of excessive amounts of these chains. Not finding complementary globin chains with which to bind, these chains form insoluble aggregates and precipitate within the cell, causing membrane damage and premature destruction of the red cells. The α-chain aggregates are called inclusion bodies or, perhaps improperly, Heinz bodies. In contrast to true Heinz bodies, which are made up of total precipitated hemoglobin tetramers, these inclusion bodies have been shown to consist only of α-globin chains, which do have some attached heme in the form of hemichromes. The process of inclusion body formation occurs not only in mature erythrocytes, but in particular in the erythroid precursor cells of the bone marrow. As a result, there is extensive intramedullary destruction of erythroid precursor cells, a process that is called ineffective erythropoiesis.

The severity of the clinical manifestations in β thalassemia generally correlates well with the size of the free α-chain pool and the degree of α- to non-α-globin chain imbalance. Therefore, the fortuitous coinheritance of α thalassemia together with homozygous β thalassemia reduces the degree of α- to non-α-globin chain imbalance and leads to a milder clinical course. Similarly, coinheritance of β thalassemia with conditions that are associated with increased levels of synthesis of γ-chains of HbF ($\alpha_2\gamma_2$) leads to less imbalance between α- and non-α-globin chain synthesis, resulting in decreased formation of α-chain inclusion bodies, increased effective production of red cells, and their prolonged survival in the circulation.

The clinical course in most cases of homozygous β thalassemia is severe. Although anemia is not evident at birth, severe hypochromic, microcytic, hemolytic anemia develops during the first year of life and a regular transfusion program must be undertaken to maintain an adequate circulating hemoglobin level. The clinical manifestations of homozygous β thalassemia in childhood have changed considerably over the last 3–4 decades, owing to changes in the philosophy and practice of transfusion therapy. With modern transfusion therapy, most children will develop normally, with few or no skeletal abnormalities, and will have a reasonably good quality of life. To avoid iron overload from transfusional hemosiderosis, transfusion therapy is usually coupled with a vigorous program of iron chelation, typically using parenterally administered desferrioxamine and more recently, orally effective iron-chelating agents. Although it is possible to maintain iron balance with such a management program, compliance is often difficult to achieve. Iron overload eventually develops in most patients and is the major cause of morbidity and mortality in young adults. The one therapy that is curative is bone marrow or stem cell transplantation, which is being increasingly practiced when feasible. The hope for the future is the development of even more effective oral iron-chelating agents and improved approaches to gene therapy.

Studies of the molecular basis of β thalassemia have demonstrated that the gene defects responsible for the disorder are quite heterogeneous. In contrast to α thalassemia, in which deletions in the α-globin gene cluster account for most of the mutations, the molecular defects associated with β thalassemia are usually point mutations involving only one (or a limited number of) nucleotide(s), but resulting in a major defect of β-globin gene expression either at the transcriptional or posttranscriptional level, including translation. Practically every conceivable type of defect in gene expression has been identified in one form or another of β thalassemia. Over 175 point mutations have been identified. Some deletion types of β thalassemia have also been described. In cases of β thalassemia in which β-globin gene expression is not totally absent (so-called β^+ thalassemia), the β-chain that is synthesized is usually structurally normal. There is a syndrome called dominant β thalassemia in which a highly unstable, structurally abnormal β-globin chain is synthesized, resulting in inclusion body formation in the heterozygous state. The coinheritance of HbE ($\alpha_2\beta_2$ glu26lys) with β thalassemia is very prevalent in southeast Asia and results in markedly variable and heterogeneous clinical manifestations, the basis for which is poorly understood. Finally, there are a number of β thalassemia-like disorders, called δβ thalassemia and hereditary persistence of fetal hemoglobin, that are distinguished from the more typical forms of β thalassemia by the presence of a substantial elevation of HbF in heterozygotes, as well as in homozygotes and compound heterozygotes. These disorders are usually due to deletions of different sizes involving the β-globin gene cluster, although nondeletion types of these disorders have also been identified.

The great heterogeneity of molecular lesions causing β thalassemia may appear at first glance to create insurmountable problems in putting this knowledge to practical use in the form of prenatal diagnosis and genetic counseling. The availability of rapid and accurate polymerase chain reaction–based assays for the detection of specific mutations in small samples of DNA has resulted in a number of surveys for the detection of the prevalence of different β thalassemic mutations in various population groups. The results of these surveys indicate that a given mutation is usually found only within one racial group and not another. Furthermore, a small number of different mutations, usually five or six, frequently accounts for 90% or more of the cases of β thalassemia in a given population group. Thus, it is possible to devise efficient and precise prenatal diagnosis programs using DNA-based approaches. Such programs have led to a striking decrease in the number of births of infants with homozygous β thalassemia in many countries where the disease is prevalent.

16

The Molecular Basis of β Thalassemia, δβ Thalassemia, and Hereditary Persistence of Fetal Hemoglobin

Swee Lay Thein and William G. Wood

INTRODUCTION

The β thalassemias and related disorders are characterized by a quantitative reduction in the production of β-globin chains of HbA. More than 200 β thalassemia alleles have now been characterized (http://globin.cse.psu.edu) involving mutations affecting any of the steps in the transcription of the β-globin gene, posttranscriptional processing of its pre-mRNA, or the translation of its mRNA into protein. The vast majority of simple β thalassemias are caused by point mutations within the gene or its immediate flanking sequences, although small deletions involving the β gene may also occur. If β-chain production is totally abolished by the mutation it is referred to as β^0 thalassemia, whereas reduced output of β-chains (of normal structure) produces β^+ thalassemia, with the mildest forms sometimes referred to as β^{++} or "silent" β thalassemia. These common forms of β thalassemias are inherited as haploinsufficient mendelian recessives.

Some structurally abnormal β-chain variants are also associated with quantitative deficiencies of β-globin chain production and have a phenotype of β thalassemia, in which case they are referred to as "thalassemic hemoglobinopathies," for example, HbE (β26 Glu→Lys). In others, the β-globin variants are so unstable that they undergo very rapid postsynthetic degradation giving rise to a functional deficiency. These hyperunstable β-chain variants act in a dominant negative fashion, causing a disease phenotype even when present in the heterozygous state, and hence have been referred to as "dominantly inherited β thalassemia."[1] β Thalassemia mutations that segregate independently of the β-globin cluster have been described in occasional families. In such cases, *trans*-acting regulatory factors are implicated.[2–4]

The δβ thalassemias and hereditary persistence of fetal hemoglobin (HPFH) are disorders related to the β thalassemias that also involve down-regulation of β-globin gene expression. In δβ thalassemia the δ gene is also affected and there is variable compensation from increased HbF production. These disorders result from more extensive deletions within the β-globin gene cluster, as do the deletion forms of HPFH in which HbF compensation is sufficient to minimize hematological abnormalities. Other forms of HPFH result from mutations in the promoters of the γ-globin genes that not only increase HbF production in adult life but are accompanied by reduced β-chain production.

This chapter outlines the molecular mechanisms underlying the different types of β thalassemia. The common denominator is absent or decreased synthesis of β-globin chains, resulting in the accumulation of excess α-globin chains that are responsible for the pathophysiology of the disorder. The severity of the phenotype is usually related to the degree of imbalance between α- and non-α-globin chain synthesis, and the size of the free α-chain pool. Hence severity is related to the type of β allele (β^0, β^+, β^{++}), ameliorated by an interacting α thalassemia (by reducing the α-chain excess) and any increased production of γ-chains (that decrease the excess of free a α-chains by binding to them to form HbF).

The molecular bases of β thalassemia and related conditions have provided a paradigm for our understanding of much of human genetics. Detailed references to earlier work are not provided here but readers are referred to the chapters by Forget,[2,5] Thein,[6] and Wood[7] in the first edition of this book, as well as to the comprehensive monograph by Weatherall and Clegg.[4]

The β THALASSEMIAS

Nondeletion Forms of β Thalassemia

These defects account for the majority of the β thalassemia alleles. They involve single base substitutions, small insertions or deletions within the gene or its immediate flanking sequences, and affect almost every known stage of gene expression. Allele frequency varies widely from one population to another but within any population there are usually a small number of common alleles together with many alleles that are rare for that population (see Chapter 15). They are listed in Table 16.1 according to the mechanism by which they affect gene function: transcription, RNA processing, or RNA translation. The mutations have been cataloged by Huisman et al.[8] and the updated listing is accessible electronically through the Globin Gene Server Website:[9] http://globin.cse.psu.edu. Heterozygotes have minimal anemia but hypochromic (mean corpuscular hemoglobin [MCH] 18–24 pg), microcytic (mean corpuscular volume [MCV] 65–80 fL) red blood cells. They are characterized by an increased proportion of HbA_2 (normal <3.2%, β thalassemia trait 3.5%–6.0%), and HbF levels that vary from normal (<1.0%) to slightly raised (1.0%–3.0%).

Table 16.1. Nondeletion mutants that cause β thalassemia

Mutation		Type	Distribution	References
I. Transcriptional mutations				
Promoter regulatory elements				
1)	−101 (C→T)	β^{++} (silent)	Mediterranean	4, 13
2)	−101 (C→G)	β^{++} (silent)	Ashkenazi Jew	68
3)	−92 (C→T)	β^{++} (silent)	Mediterranean	4, 13
4)	−90 (C→T)	β^{+}	Portuguese	4, 13
5)	−88 (C→T)	β^{++}	US Blacks, Asian Indians	4, 13
6)	−88 (C→A)	β^{+}	Kurds	4, 13
7)	−87 (C→G)	β^{++}	Mediterranean	4, 13
8)	−87 (C→T)	β^{++}	German, Italian	4, 13
9)	−87 (C→A)	β^{++}	US Blacks	4, 13
10)	−86 (C→G)	β^{+}	Thai, Lebanese	4, 13
11)	−86 (C→A)	β^{++}	Italian	4, 13
12)	−73 (A→T)	β^{++}	Chinese	10
13)	−32 (C→A)	β^{+}	Taiwanese	4, 13
14)	−32 (C→T)	β^{+}	Hispanic	198
15)	−31 (A→G)	β^{+}	Japanese	4, 13
16)	−31 (A→C)	β^{+}	Italian	8
17)	−30 (T→A)	β^{+}	Mediterranean, Bulgarian	4, 13
18)	−30 (T→C)	β^{+}	Chinese	4, 13
19)	−29 (A→G)	β^{+}	US Blacks, Chinese	4, 13
20)	−29 (A→C)	β^{+}	Jordanian	199
21)	−29 (G→A)	β^{+}	Turkish	200
22)	−28 (A→C)	β^{+}	Kurds	4, 13
23)	−28 (A→G)	β^{+}	Blacks, SE Asians	4, 13
24)	−27 (A→T)	β^{+}	Corsican	13
25)	−27 to −26_ (−AA)	β^{+}	African American	201
26)	−25 (G→C)	β^{+}	African American	198
5′ UTR				
27)	CAP +1 (A→C)	β^{++} (silent)	Asian Indian	4, 13
28)	CAP +8 (C→T)	β^{++} (silent)	Chinese	4, 13
29)	CAP +10 (−T)	β^{++} (silent)	Greeks	4, 13
30)	CAP +20 (C→T)***	?	Bulgarian	4, 13
31)	CAP +22 (G→A)	β^{++}	Mediterranean, Bulgarian	4, 13
32)	CAP +33 (C→G)	β^{++} (silent)	Greek Cypriot	4, 13
33)	CAP +40 to +43 (−AAAC)	β^{+}	Chinese	4, 13
34)	CAP +45 (G→C)	β^{+}	Italian	202
II. RNA processing				
Splice junction				
1)	IVS1−(−2) CD30 (**A**GG→**G**GG)	β^{0}	Sephardic Jews	4
2)	IVS1−(−2) CD30 (**A**GG→**C**GG)	β^{0}	Italian Canadian	203
3)	IVS1−(−1) CD30 (A**G**G→A**C**G) (Arg→Thr)	β^{0}	Mediterranean, US Blacks, N. African, Kurds, UAE	4, 13
4)	IVS1−(−1) CD30 (A**G**G→A**A**G)	β^{0}	Bulgaria, UAE	4, 13
5)	IVS1−1 (G→A)	β^{0}	Mediterranean	4, 13
6)	IVS1−1 (G→T)	β^{0}	Asian Indian, SE Asian, Chinese	4, 13
7)	IVS1−1 (G→C)	β^{0}	Italian Canadian, Japanese	203, 204
8)	IVS1−2 (T→G)	β^{0}	Tunisian	4, 13
9)	IVS1−2 (T→C)	β^{0}	US Blacks	4, 13
10)	IVS1−2 (T→A)	β^{0}	Algerian, Italian	4, 13
11)	IVS2−1 (G→A)	β^{0}	Mediterranean, US Blacks	4, 13
12)	IVS2−1 (G→C)	β^{0}	Iranian	4, 13
13)	IVS2−2 (T→A)	? β^{0}	Turkish	205
14)	IVS2−2 (−T)	β^{0}	Chinese	4

Mutation		Type	Distribution	References
15)	IVS1–3′ end del 17 bp	β^0	Kuwaiti	4, 13
16)	IVS1–3′ end del 25 bp	β^0	Asian Indian, UAE	4, 13
17)	IVS1–3′ end del 44 bp	β^0	Mediterranean	4, 13
18)	IVS1–3′ end duplication 22 bp	β^0	Thai	206
19)	IVS1–130 (G→C)	β^0	Italian, Japanese, UAE	4, 13
20)	IVS1–130 G→A	β^0	Egyptian	4, 13
21)	IVS1–130 (+1) CD30 (AG**G**→AG**C**) (Arg→Ser)	β^0	Middle East	4, 13
22)	IVS2–849 (A→G)	β^0	US Blacks	4, 13
23)	IVS2–849 (A→C)	β^0	US Blacks	4, 13
24)	IVS2–850 (G→C)	β^0	Yugoslavian	4, 13
25)	IVS2–850 (G→A)	β^0	N European	4, 13
26)	IVS2–850 (G→T)	β^0	Japanese	4, 13
27)	IVS2–850 (–G)	β^0	Italian	4, 13
Consensus splice sites				
28)	IVS1–5 (G→C)	β^0	Asian Indian, SE Asian, Melanesian	4, 13
29)	IVS1–5 (G→T)	β^+	Mediterranean, N European	4, 13
30)	IVS1–5 (G→A)	β^+	Mediterranean, Algerian	4, 13
31)	IVS1–6 (T→C)	β^{++}	Mediterranean	4, 13
32)	IVS1–(–3) CD29 (GG**C**→GG**T**)	β^+	Lebanese	4, 13
33)	IVS1–128 (T→G)	β^+	Saudi Arabian	4, 13
34)	IVS1–129 (A→G)		German	4, 13
35)	IVS2–5 (G→C)	β^+	Chinese	4, 13
36)	IVS2–843 (T→G)	β^+	Algerian	4, 13
37)	IVS2–844 (C→G)	β^{++} (silent)	Italian	4, 13
38)	IVS2–844 (C→A)	β^{++} (silent)	Ghanaian	207
39)	IVS2–848 (C→A)	β^+	UB Blacks, Egyptian, Iranian	4, 13
40)	IVS2–848 (C→G)	β^+	Japanese	4, 13
Cryptic splice sites in introns				
41)	IVS1–110 (G→A)	β^+	Mediterranean	4, 13
42)	IVS1–116 (T→G)	β^0	Mediterranean	4, 13
43)	IVS2–654 (C→T)	β^0/β^+	Chinese, SE Asians, Japanese	4, 13
44)	IVS2–705 (T→G)	β^+	Mediterranean	4, 13
45)	IVS2–745 (C→G)	β^+	Mediterranean	4, 13
46)	IVS2–837 (T→G)	?	Asian Indian	4, 13
Cryptic splice sites in exons				
47)	CD10 (GC**C**→GC**A**)		Asian Indian	4, 13
48)	CD19 (A**A**C→A**G**C) Hb Malay (Asn→Ser)	β^{++}	SE Asian	4, 13
49)	CD24 (GG**T**→GG**A**)	β^{++}	US Black, Japanese	4, 13
50)	CD26 (**G**AG→**A**AG) (Glu→Lys, Hb E)	β^+	SE Asian, European	4, 13
51)	CD26 (G**A**G→G**C**G) (Glu→Ala, Hb Tripoli)	β^+	Libyan	208
52)	CD27 (GCC→TCC) (Ala→Ser, Knossos)$^{++}$	β^+	Mediterranean	4, 13
3′ UTR				
RNA Cleavage – Poly A signal				
53)	AA**T**AAA→AA**C**AAA	β^{++}	US Blacks	4, 13
54)	AAT**A**AA→AAT**G**AA	β^{++}	Mediterranean	4, 13
55)	AATA**A**A→AATA**G**A	β^{++}	Malay	4, 13
56)	AATAA**A**→AATAA**G**	β^{++}	Kurd	4, 13
57)	AATAAA→AA--AA	β^+	French, US Blacks	4, 13
58)	AATAAA→A-----	β^+	Kurd, UAE	4, 13
59)	AA**T**AAA→AA**A**AAA	β^+	Tunisian	209
60)	**A**ATAAA→**C**ATAAA	β^{++} (silent)	Chinese	210
61)	**A**ATAAA→**G**ATAAA	β^+	Czechoslovakian, Mediterranean, Yugoslavian, Canadian	211
62)	**A**ATAAA→------	β^+	Nigerian	212

(continued)

Table 16.1 *(continued)*

Mutation		Type	Distribution	References
Others				
63)	Term CD +6, C→G	β^{++} (silent)	Greek	4
64)	Term CD +90, del 13 bp	β^{+}	Turkish	4
65)	Term CD +47 (C→G	β^{++}	Armenian	4
III. RNA translation				
Initiation codon				
1)	**A**TG→**G**TG	β^0	Japanese	4
2)	**A**TG→**C**TG	β^0	Northern Irish	213
3)	A**T**G→A**C**G	β^0	Yugoslavian	4
4)	A**T**G→A**G**G	β^0	Chinese	4
5)	A**T**G→A**A**G^{+++}	β^0	N European	4
6)	AT**G**→AT**C**	β^0	Japanese	4
7)	AT**G**→AT**A**	β^0	Italian, Swedish	4
8)	AT**G**→AT**T**	β^0	Iranian	4
9)	45 bp insertion (−22 to +23)	?	Maori, Polynesian	35
Nonsense codons				
1)	CD6 **G**AG→**T**AG,	β^0	Brazilian	214
2)	CD7 **G**AG→**T**AG	β^0	English	4, 13
3)	CD15 T**G**G→T**A**G	β^0	Asian Indian, Japanese	4, 13
4)	CD15 TG**G**→TG**A**	β^0	Portuguese, Japanese	4, 13
5)	CD17 **A**AG→**T**AG	β^0	Chinese, Japanese	4, 13
6)	CD22 **G**AA→**T**AA	β^0	Reunion Island	4, 13
7)	CD26 **G**AG→**T**AG	β^0	Thai	4, 13
8)	CD35 TA**C**→TA**A**	β^0	Thai	4, 13
9)	CD37 TG**G**→TG**A**	β^0	Saudi Arabian	4, 13
10)	CD39 **C**AG→**T**AG	β^0	Mediterranean	4, 13
11)	CD43 **G**AG→**T**AG	β^0	Chinese, Thai	4, 13
12)	CD59 **A**AG→**T**AG	β^0	Italian American	215
13)	CD61 **A**AG→**T**AG	β^0	Blacks	4, 13
14)	CD90 **G**AG→**T**AG	β^0	Japanese	4, 13
15)	CD112 TG**T**→TG**A**	β^0	Slovenian	4, 13
16)	CD121 **G**AA→**T**AA*	β^0	Czechoslovakian	4, 13
Frameshift				
1)	CD1 −G	β^0	Mediterranean	4, 13
2)	CD2/3/4 (−9 bp, +31 bp)	β^0	Algerian	4, 13
3)	CD2−4, 5−9, 7, 10	β^0	Algerian	4, 13
4)	CD5−CT	β^0	Mediterranean	4, 13
5)	CD6 −A	β^0	Mediterranean, US Blacks	4, 13
6)	CD8 −AA	β^0	Mediterranean	4, 13
7)	CD8/9 +G	β^0	Asian Indian, Japanese	4, 13
8)	CD9 +TA	? β^0	Tunisian	209
9)	CD9/10 +T	β^0	Greek, Arab	4, 13
10)	CD11 −T	β^0	Mexican	4, 13
11)	CD14/15 +G	β^0	Chinese	4, 13
12)	CD15 −T	β^0	Malay	4, 13
13)	CD15/16 −G	β^0	German	4, 13
14)	CD15/16 +G	β^0	Chinese	216
15)	CD16 −C	β^0	Asian Indian	4, 13
16)	CD22/23/24 −7 bp (−AAGTTGG)	β^0	Turkish	4, 13
17)	CD24 −G; +CAC	β^0	Egyptian	4, 13
18)	CD24/25 −GGT	?	No additional information	4, 13
19)	CD25/26 +T	β^0	Tunisian	4, 13
20)	CD26 +T	β^0	Japanese	4, 13
21)	CD27/28 +C	β^0	Chinese, Thai	4, 13

Mutation		Type	Distribution	References
22)	CD28 −C	β^0	Egyptian	4, 13
23)	CD28/29 −G	β^0	Japanese, Egyptian	4, 13
24)	CD31 −C	β^0	Chinese	4, 13
25)	CD35 −C	β^0	Malay	4, 13
26)	CD36/37 −T	β^0	Kurd, Iranian	4, 13
27)	CD37/38/39 del 7 bp (−GACCCAG)	β^0	Turkish	4, 13
28)	CD38/39 −C	β^0	Czechoslovakian	4, 13
29)	CD38/39 −CC	β^0	Belgian	4, 13
30)	CD40 −G	β^0	Japanese	4, 13
31)	CD40/41 +T	β^0	Chinese	4, 13
32)	CD41 −C	β^0	Thai	4, 13
33)	CD41/42 −TTCT	β^0	Chinese, SE Asian, Indian	4, 13
34)	CD42/43 +T	β^0	Japanese	4, 13
35)	CD42/43 +G	β^0	Japanese	4, 13
36)	CD44 −C	β^0	Kurdish	4, 13
37)	CD45 −T	β^0	Pakistani	4, 13
38)	CD45 +T	β^0	Turkish	217
39)	CD47 +A	β^0	Surinamese	4, 13
40)	CD47/48 +ATCT	β^0	Asian Indian	4, 13
41)	CD49 −C	β^0	Jordanian	199
42)	CD51 −C	β^0	Hungarian	4, 13
43)	CD53/54 +G	β^0	Japanese	4, 13
44)	CD54 −T	β^0	Swedish	4, 13
45)	CD55 −A	β^0	Asian Indian	218
46)	CD54/55 +A	β^0	Asian Indian	4, 13
47)	CD56−60 +14 bp	β^0	Iranian	4, 13
48)	CD57/58 +C	β^0	Asian Indian	4, 13
49)	CD59 −A	β^0	Italian	4, 13
50)	CD62/63/64 del 7 bp (−TCATGGC)	β^0	Asian Indian	219
51)	CD64 −G+++	β^0	Swiss	4, 13
52)	CD67 −TG	β^0	Filipino	4, 13
53)	CD71/72 +T	β^0	Chinese	4, 13
54)	CD71/72 +A	β^0	Chinese	4, 13
55)	CD72/73 −AGTGA, +T	β^0	British	4, 13
56)	CD74/75 −C	β^0	Turkish	4, 13
57)	CD76 GCT → --T	β^0	North African	220
58)	CD76 −C	β^0	Italian	4, 13
59)	CD82/83 −G	β^0	Czech, Azerbaijani	4, 13
60)	CD81−87 (−22 bp)	β^0	Asian Indian	221
61)	CD83−86 del 8 bp (−CACCTTTG)+++	β^0	Japanese	4
62)	CD84/85 +C	β^0	Japanese	4, 13
63)	CD84/85/86 +T	β^0	Japanese	4, 13
64)	CD88 +T	β^0	Asian Indian	4, 13
65)	CD88 −TG	β^0	Japanese	4, 13
66)	CD89/90 −GT	β^0	Japanese	4, 13
67)	CD95 +A	β^0	SE Asian	4, 13
68)	CD106/107 +G	β^0	US Blacks, Egyptian	4, 13
69)	CD109 (GTG → GT−)	?	Irish	213
70)	CD120/121 +A**	β^0	Filipino	4, 13
71)	CD130/131 +GCCT	? β^0	German	222
72)	CD142/143 (−CC)	?	French Caucasian	217

* Unlike the majority, some heterozygotes for the CD121 G→T mutation do not have an unusually severe phenotype.

** This frameshift leads to predicted truncated β variant of 138aa with an abnormal carboxy terminal. Heterozygotes do not appear to have an unusually severe phenotype.

*** Occurs *in-cis* to the IVS2-745 C→G mutation.

+ Also occurs *in-cis* to 7201-bp deletion involving δ gene.

++ Occurs *in-cis* to δ59-A.

+++ Probably de novo.

TRANSCRIPTIONAL MUTANTS

Mutations affecting transcription involve the conserved DNA sequences that form the β-globin promoter (from 100 bp upstream to the site of the initiation of transcription, including the functionally important CACCC, CCAAT, and ATAA boxes) and the stretch of 50 nucleotides in the 5′ untranslated region (UTR).

Mutations in all of the three conserved sequence motifs in the β promoter, the two CACCC, CCAAT,[10] and ATAA boxes, have been identified in different patients with β thalassemia. In general, the degree of diminished β-globin synthesis associated with mutations of the β-globin gene promoter including the latest mutation (−73 A–T) within the CCAAT box[10] is relatively minor. This finding is consistent with transcription studies of the mutant genes in tissue culture cells, which reveal only a mild-to-moderate decrease in transcriptional activity of these genes.[2]

Although these defects have been described in diverse ethnic groups, ethnic variation in phenotype has been observed. Black individuals homozygous for the −29 A→G mutation have an extremely mild disease,[11] whereas a Chinese individual homozygous for the same mutation had thalassemia major.[12] The cause of this striking difference in phenotype is not known but may be related to the different chromosomal backgrounds on which the apparently identical mutations have arisen or to the C-T polymorphism at position −158 upstream of the $^{G}\gamma$ globin gene (*Xmn*1-$^{G}\gamma$ site), which is associated with increased HbF production under conditions of erythropoietic stress. The *Xmn*1-$^{G}\gamma$ site is present in the β chromosome carrying the −29 A→G mutation in Blacks but absent in that of the Chinese.[13]

Of the mutations in this category, the C-T mutation at position −101 to the β-globin gene appears to cause an extremely mild deficit of β-globin. The allele is so mild that heterozygotes are "silent" with borderline reduced/normal red cell indices.[14,15]

An increasing number of mutations in the 5′ UTR have been characterized since the original CAP +1 A-C allele.[16] The defects include single base substitutions and minor deletions distributed along the stretch of 50 nucleotides. As in the −101 C-T mutation, heterozygotes for this class of mutations are silent; the extremely mild phenotype is exemplified in a homozygote for the +1 A-C mutation who has the hematological values of a thalassemia carrier.[16] It is not known whether the CAP mutation causes β thalassemia by decreasing β-globin gene transcription or by decreasing the efficiency of capping (posttranscriptional addition of m^7G) and mRNA translation. In vivo and in vitro studies show that the +33 C→G mutation leads to a reduction of β mRNA that is 33% of the output from a normal β gene, milder than the mutations involving the promoter elements.[17] Compound heterozygotes for these transcriptional mutations and the more severe β thalassemia alleles tend to have a milder disease.

MUTANTS AFFECTING RNA PROCESSING

Mutations of the Splice Site Junction

Intervening sequences must be precisely removed from the precursor mRNA and the coding regions spliced to produce functional mRNA. Sequences critical in the splicing process include the invariant dinucleotides GT at the 5′ (Donor) and AG at the 3′ (Acceptor) splice junctions in the introns.[5] Mutations that affect either of the invariant dinucleotides in the splice junction completely abolish normal splicing and produce the phenotype of β^0 thalassemia. These mutations can be base substitutions that change one or the other of invariant dinucleotides or short deletions that remove them. Genes bearing these mutations appear to transcribe normally and, although some alternative splicing occurs using "cryptic" donor or acceptor sites, the misspliced mRNA do not translate into functional β-globin. The misspliced mRNA species can sometimes be detected in small amounts in affected erythroid cells. They are nonfunctional because translation of the abnormally spliced or frameshifted mRNAs would usually stop prematurely due to the introduction of chain termination (nonsense) codons.[18]

Mutations of Splice Site Consensus Sequence

Flanking these invariant dinucleotides are sequences that are fairly well conserved and a consensus sequence can be recognized at the exon–intron boundaries. They encompass the last three nucleotides of the exon and the first six nucleotides of the intron for the 5′ donor site; and the last 10 nucleotides of the intron and the first nucleotide of the exon for the 3′ acceptor site. Mutations within the consensus sequences at the splice junctions reduce the efficiency of normal splicing to varying degrees and produce a β thalassemia phenotype that ranges from mild to severe. For example, mutations at IVS1 position 5, G→C, T, or A considerably reduce splicing at the mutated donor site compared with normal. The mutations appear to activate the use of three "cryptic" donor sites (sequences that mimic the consensus sequence for a splice site but are not normally used), two in exon 1 and one in IVS1, which are utilized in preference to the mutated donor site.[19] On the other hand, the substitution of C for T in the adjacent nucleotide, IVS1 position 6, only mildly affects normal RNA splicing even though it activates the same three cryptic donor sites as seen in the IVS1–5 mutants.[19] Although the IVS1–6 T-C mutation is generally associated with milder β thalassemia, studies have shown that in some cases apparently identical mutations can be severe;[20–22] and again this is presumably related to the chromosomal background on which the mutations have arisen.

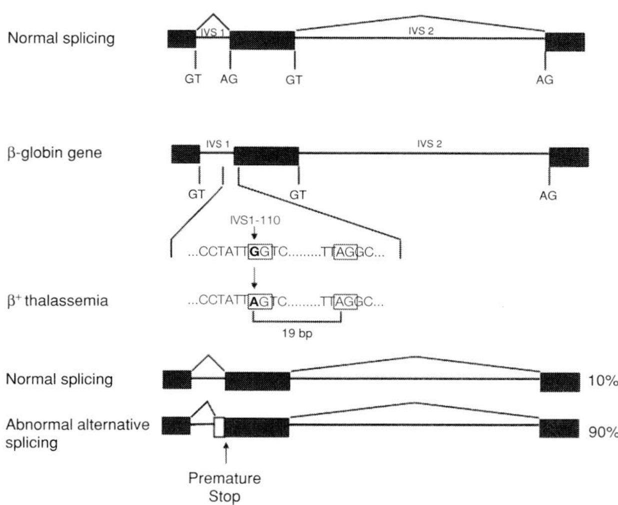

Figure 16.1. Alternative splicing of precursor β-globin mRNA resulting in β^+ thalassemia associated with the IVS1–110 G→A mutation. The G to A substitution at position 110 creates an AG dinucleotide within a potential 3′ acceptor splice site resulting in approximately 90% mRNA aberrantly spliced and 10% normally spliced.

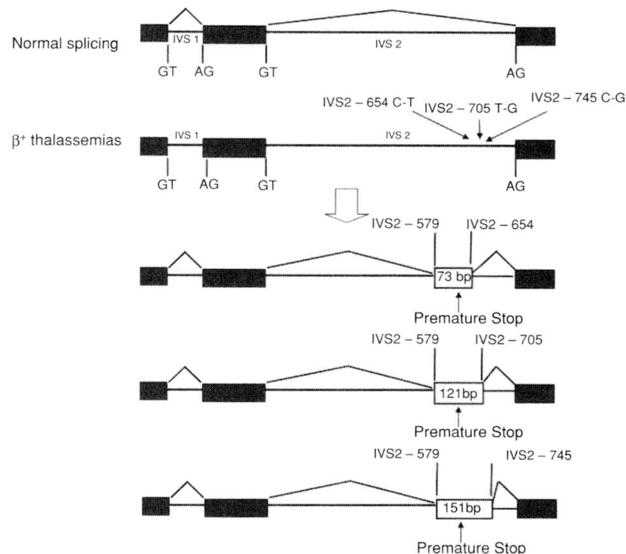

Figure 16.2. Alternative splicing of precursor β-globin mRNA due to three base substitutions; C→T at position 654, T→G at position 705, and C→G at position 745 in intron 2 of the β-globin gene. Each of these mutations creates a 5′ donor site that is preferentially spliced to the normal 3′ acceptor site, whereas the same acceptor site is activated upstream at position 579 in intron 2 and spliced to the normal donor site at the exon 2–intron 2 junction. This results in the incorporation of 73, 121, and 151 nucleotides of intron 2 into the aberrantly spliced mRNA associated with each of the different intron 2 mutations, respectively.

Mutations that Create New Alternative Splice Sites in Introns

A third category of splicing mutation is due to base substitutions in introns that generate new splicing signals, which are preferentially used instead of the normal splice sites. Five such mutations have been identified in the β-globin gene: two in IVS1 and three in IVS2 (Table 16.1).[2,13] The associated phenotype may be either β^+ or β^0 thalassemia, depending on the site and nature of the mutation.

The splicing mutation at position 110 of IVS1 was the first base substitution identified in a β thalassemia gene.[2,23,24] This mutation has subsequently been shown to be one of the most common form of β thalassemia in the Mediterranean population. The mutation is a substitution of G to A that creates an acceptor AG in a favorable consensus sequence environment, 19 bp 5′ to the normal acceptor AG of IVS1 (Fig. 16.1). In vitro expression studies have shown that this newly created alternative splice site is preferentially used in 80%–90% of the transcripts, whereas the normal splice site is used in only 10%–20% of the transcripts,[25,26] thus giving the phenotype of β^+ thalassemia (Fig. 16.1). The mutant mRNA is hardly detected in affected erythroid cells presumably because the 19-bp segment of retained intronic sequence contains an in-phase premature termination codon and thus subjected to the nonsense mediated decay surveillance mechanism (see section on dominantly inherited β thalassemia and Huang and Benz 2001[18]).

Another β thalassemia gene with a T→G substitution in position 116 of IVS1, leads to a newly created 3′ acceptor site. In this case, the normal acceptor sequence, although intact, is not used, and little or no normal β mRNA is produced resulting in a β^0 thalassemia phenotype.[27]

Three other β thalassemia genes have substitutions within IVS2 that generate new donor sites[2–4] (Fig. 16.2). They include the IVS2 position 654 C→T, 705 T→G, and 745 C→G. In each case, an upstream acceptor site at position 579 is activated such that the normal 5′ donor site at exon 2/IVS2 is spliced to the activated site at position 579 and the newly created donor site is spliced to the normal 3′ acceptor site at IVS1/exon 3. This two-stage splicing results in the retention of 73 bp of IVS2 in the misspliced β mRNA for the IVS2 654 mutation. Variable amounts of splicing from the normal donor to the normal acceptor also occurs, resulting in phenotypes that range from β^+ to β^0 thalassemia. Several individuals heterozygous for the IVS2 654 C-T mutation with an unusually severe phenotype have been described.[13] In a father and son, the ratio of aberrant β mRNA to normal β mRNA was 10-fold that in asymptomatic heterozygotes for the same mutation.[28] The unusually severe disease in these individuals is thought to result from the accumulation of the misspliced mRNA, which was predicted to translate into a highly unstable β chain variant with a dominant negative effect.

The mutation at position 745 also creates a new alternative donor splice site and is associated with a similar two-step excision of IVS2 with utilization of the newly created acceptor at position 579.[19] Some normal splicing of IVS2 occurs; therefore, this mutation results in β^+ rather than β^0 thalassemia. The β^0 versus β^+ phenotype associated with these different mutations must be related to different affinities of the enzymatic splicing complex for a given mutant splice site versus the normal splice sites.[5]

Mutations that Create Alternative Splice Sites in Exons

Four mutations have been identified in exon 1 that are associated with activation of cryptic or alternative splice sites.[2,4,13] Three of these mutations modify the cryptic splice site spanning codons 24–27 in exon 1 so that it more closely resembles the consensus splice sequence AAGGTGAGT and activates it. The reduction in normal splicing is the molecular basis for the mild β^+ thalassemic phenotype of these variants, including the β^E allele. The β^E allele is particularly prevalent in southeast Asia where it can reach up to a frequency of 75% in northeast Thailand. Its interaction with β thalassemia accounts for a large proportion of the thalassemia major in southeast Asia.[4]

Similarly, the A→G mutation in codon 19 activates another cryptic donor site spanning codons 17–19 in exon 1 resulting in a reduced level of normally spliced β mRNA that contains the codon 19 mutation encoding Hb Malay.[29]

MUTATIONS CAUSING ABNORMAL POSTTRANSCRIPTIONAL MODIFICATION

The nascent precursor globin mRNA molecule is modified at both of its ends; a methylated (m^7G) cap structure is added at the 5′ end, and a poly(A) tail is added at the 3′ end of the mRNA. One mutation of the cap site has been described,[16] although it is not known whether the principal effect of the mutation is on transcription or on the capping modification. On the other hand, a number of different β thalassemias have been associated with defective polyadenylation owing to mutations involving the consensus sequence AATAAA required for the cleavage–polyadenylation reaction. Mutations involving the polyadenylation signal include seven base substitutions at different positions of the consensus sequence, two short deletions of 2 and 5 bp each, and one deletion of the total AATAAA sequence (Table 16.1). These mutations markedly decrease the efficiency of the cleavage–polyadenylation process but do not abolish it completely. Therefore, the associated phenotype is that of β^+ thalassemia of moderate severity because approximately 10% of the mRNA is properly modified. The remainder of the transcripts extend far beyond the normal polyadenylation site and are probably cleaved and polyadenylated after the next AATAAA consensus sequences, which occur approximately 0.9–3 kb downstream.[30] Mutations affecting other sites in the 3′ UTR, a C→G substitution at nucleotide 6, and a 13-bp deletion at nucleotides 90 downstream of the termination codon, also result in β^+ thalassemia.[2,13]

MUTANTS RESULTING IN PREMATURE TERMINATION OF TRANSLATION

Approximately half the β thalassemia alleles result from the introduction of premature termination codons, either due to direct mutations creating a stop codon or to a change in the reading frame by insertion or deletion of a single to a few nucleotides. These frameshift defects cause premature termination further downstream when the next nonsense codon is reached.[5]

One of the first nonsense mutations to be characterized and extensively studied was the mutation at codon 39 (CAG–TAG). This mutation is the second most common cause of β thalassemia in the Mediterranean population and accounts for most of the cases of β thalassemia in Sardinia. An interesting feature of this and other nonsense mutations is the finding of very low levels of the mutant β-globin mRNA in affected erythroid cells. Initial studies of this phenomenon revealed that the gene was transcribed normally, but there appeared to be defective β mRNA stability in the nucleus or defective processing and/or transport of the mRNA from nucleus to cytoplasm; mRNA stability in the cytoplasm appeared to be normal.[18] It is now clear that reduced levels of the mutant β mRNA is a result of the nonsense mediated decay quality control mechanism.[31]

The frameshift and nonsense mutations that result in typical recessively inherited β^0 thalassemia all result in premature termination within exon 1 and 2 with a couple of exceptions terminating prematurely in exon 3.[13] In recent years it has become clear that the concentration of the different in-phase termination mutants in exon 1 and 2 is related to the "positional" effect on nonsense mediated decay of the mutant β mRNA (for reviews see[31–33]) that are associated with minimal steady-state levels of abnormal β mRNA.[18] In heterozygotes for such cases, no β chain is produced from the mutant allele, resulting in a typical asymptomatic phenotype. In contrast, in mutations that produce in-phase termination later in the β sequence, in exon 3, the mRNA does not undergo nonsense-mediated decay and produce normal amounts of mutant β mRNA, which presumably gets translated into variant β-chains.[34] As these cells have to deal with the excess α-chains as well as the abnormal β-chains, the proteolytic machinery is overcome and a severe phenotype results. These mutants are usually dominantly inherited, therefore, in contrast to the typical recessive inheritance of β thalassemia (see later). It is not clear how nonsense-mediated decay takes place but the mechanism could be related to coupling between transcription and translation and exerted at the nuclear membrane.[32]

MUTATIONS AFFECTING THE INITIATION CODON

Nine mutations affecting the initiation codon (ATG) have been described and all produce β^0 thalassemia (Table 16.1).

(β112 Cys→Arg,[42] which was subsequently reported in two families [Spanish and Italian] in whom affected members had evidence of mild hemolytic anemia with 2%–4% reticulocytosis[43,44]). In two patients heterozygous for Hb Terre Haute, globin-chain biosynthesis studies showed an α/non-α ratio of approximately 1.0 in bone marrow erythroblasts compared with a ratio of approximately 2.0 in peripheral blood reticulocytes. Although the variant β-globin chain was synthesized at a level almost equal to that of the normal β-globin chain, most of it was rapidly precipitated on the red cell membrane. The half-life of this globin variant was less than 10 minutes, and the abnormal hemoglobin was not detectable by standard techniques. Other examples of missense variants include Hb Chesterfield, Hb Cagliari, Hb Showa-Yakushiji, Hb Durham NC/Brescia, Hb Houston, and more recently, Hb Mont Saint Aignan.[1,6,45] In the example of Hb Chesterfield, an abnormal peak in the position expected for the β-globin chain variant but without detectable corresponding protein was demonstrated by globin-chain biosynthesis studies.[46] Hb Mont Saint Aignan [β128 (Hb) Ala→Pro], in comparison, appeared mildly unstable;[45] the abnormal β-chain could be isolated by selective isopropanol precipitation and the structure determined by protein chemistry methods.

Most of the other abnormal hemoglobins were not detected by routine hemoglobin electrophoresis. Hb Cagliari was identified postsplenectomy on isoelectrical focusing (IEF) and formed 9% of the total hemoglobin.[47] Mass spectrometry electrospray analysis estimated Hb Mont Saint Aignan to be approximately 20% of total hemoglobin.[45] Hb Indianapolis was mildly unstable; on IEF, the variant β-globin chain formed 38%–45% of the total β-globin chains.

Deletion or Insertion of Intact Codons

Deletions or insertions of entire codons allow the reading frame to remain in phase, and the remaining amino acids are normal. Both Hb Korea and Hb Gunma have 145–amino acid residues each; in Hb Gunma, the β127–128 Gln-Ala dipeptide is replaced by a proline residue due to the deletion of three bases (AGG),[48] whereas in Hb Korea, the deletion of three bases (GGT) removes one of the Val residues from codons 32–34.[49] Other β-globin chain variants have extra residues and include the insertion of Arg in codons 30–31 in a Spanish family[50] and insertion of a single proline in codons 124–126 in an Armenian patient.[51]

In all cases, no trace of abnormal hemoglobin could be detected by the standard techniques of IEF, high-performance liquid chromatography, or heat stability tests. One mechanism that could explain the lack of detection of these structural β-globin chain variants is that the affected amino acids are involved in α1β1 contacts. In the normal β-globin chain, β30 Arg (β 12), β33 Val (β 15), β34 Val (β 16), β108 Asn (γ 10), β112 Cys (γ 14), β124 Pro (H2), β125 Pro (H3), β127 Gln (H5), and β128 Ala (H6) are essential for α1β1 dimer formation.[52] Deletion or substitution of these critical amino acids would be likely to prevent the formation of αβ subunits and, effectively, lead to a functional loss of half of the β-globin chains.

The third example in this category involved a deletion of 12 nucleotides and an insertion of 6 nucleotides, leading to the substitution of the normal Val-Ala-Gly-Val by Gly-Arg in codons 134–137 and a β-globin subunit that was two amino acids shorter than normal. Affected individuals of this Portuguese family had moderately severe anemia, splenomegaly, and leg ulcers.[53]

A recent example of a hyperunstable β chain variant in this category is Hb Stara Zagnora (codons 137–139 [−6 bp]) found in a 2-year-old Bulgarian boy. Deletions of 6 bp spanning β codons 137–139 replaces Val-Ala-Asn with Asp and results in a hyperunstable variant associated with hemolysis and dyserythropoietic anemia with mild globin chain imbalance (α/β synthesis ratio 1.40), although HbA_2 levels were within normal limits.[54]

Premature Termination (Nonsense Mutation)

Probably the most common of the dominantly inherited β thalassemia alleles is a GAA→TAA termination codon at codon 121, which leads to the synthesis of a truncated β-globin chain. Although substantial amounts of mutant β-globin mRNA could be demonstrated in individuals with such mutations, showing the presence of the truncated β-globin variant has been difficult.[34] Presence of the predicted truncated variant was implicated from a large difference between the total radioactivity incorporated into newly synthesized chains and the total amount of protein in globin biosynthesis studies.[55] In another study, the truncated β-globin chain was estimated to comprise only 0.05% −0.1% of the total non-α-globin.[56] Another case of thalassemia intermedia caused by heterozygosity for the premature stop codon in β127 was recently reported in a 29-year-old French Caucasian woman.[57]

Elongated or Truncated Variants with Abnormal Carboxy Terminal Ends

In general, the elongated or truncated β-globin gene variants in this group have arisen from frameshift mutations that generated distal premature termination codons. Despite the altered charge created by the abnormal carboxy terminal end, the abnormal β-globin variants were not detected in any of the cases by hemoglobin electrophoresis or globin biosynthesis studies; however, in all cases an imbalanced synthesis of α- and β-globin chains was present.

Elongated β-globin subunits could also arise from aberrant splicing of precursor mRNA, as described in a deletion of two nucleotides affecting the IVS2 consensus donor splice site.[58] Unusually severe anemia associated with intraerythroblastic inclusions was transmitted as a single allele in five generations of this Portuguese family and the disorder was transmitted in a dominant fashion.

Since the last edition, eight additional hyperunstable β variants belonging to this category have been described (Table 16.2). Hb Jambol[54] has an unusual molecular defect caused by a complex rearrangement involving an insertion of 23 nucleotides after position 535 of βIVS2 and deletion of 310 nucleotides from position 550 of βIVS2 to the first nucleotide of β codon 108 interrupted by an insertion of 28 nucleotides at the deletion junctions. The mutation results in the replacement of Leu-Leu-Glu-Asn at codon 105–108 with nine residues (Table 16.2) and was associated with severe hemolytic anemia and mildly imbalanced globin synthesis ratio.

Pathophysiology of Dominant β Thalassemia

The common denominator of these mutations is the synthesis of the highly unstable β-chain variants. In many cases, the variants are so unstable that they can be detected only when newly synthesized, whereas in others, they are not detectable but predicted from the DNA sequence. The predicted synthesis is supported by the presence of substantial amounts of mutant β-globin gene mRNA in the peripheral blood reticulocytes, comparable in amounts to that of the other normal β-globin allele.[34,55] Indeed, the large intraerythroblastic inclusions, which are so characteristic of this form of β thalassemia, have subsequently been shown to be composed of both α- and β-globin chains.[55] In contrast, the inclusion bodies in homozygous β thalassemia consisted only of precipitated α globin.[55]

The molecular mechanisms underlying the instability include: substitution of the critical amino acids in the hydrophobic heme pocket displacing heme, leading to aggregation of the globin variant; disruption of secondary structure due to replacement of critical amino acids; substitution or deletion of amino acids involved in αβ dimer formation; and elongation of subunits by a hydrophobic tail.

Nonsense-mediated Decay

How is it that some premature termination mutations cause thalassemia intermedia whereas the majority are clinically asymptomatic in the heterozygous state? The answer appears to lie in the differential effects of these in-phase termination mutants on the accumulation of mutant mRNA.

Nonsense-mediated decay is an mRNA quality-control mechanism that degrades abnormal mRNAs that arise from mistakes in gene expression such as those caused by premature termination codons. In mammalian cells, a termination codon is recognized as premature if it is located upstream of a boundary of 50–55 nucleotides 5′ to the final exon–exon junction.[59] In the β-globin gene, this corresponds to exon 1 and the 5′ region of exon 2. Hence, in the β-globin gene, premature termination condons that terminate in exon 1 or 2 are recessively inherited, whereas those that are dominantly inherited terminate much later in the sequence of the β-globin gene, in the 3′ part of exon 2 and exon 3. Premature stop codons near the 3′ end of the gene, in exon 3 of β gene, are less likely to trigger the surveillance mechanism of nonsense-mediated decay, leading to an accumulation of the mutant β mRNA and to the synthesis of unstable β-chain variants. These in-phase termination mutations exemplify how shifting the position of a nonsense codon can alter the phenotype of recessive inheritance caused by haploinsufficiency to a dominant negative effect due to the synthesis of an abnormal and deleterious protein. Exceptions to the 50–55 nucleotide boundary rule have been reported.[60] β mRNA with nonsense mutations in codons 5, 15, and 17 within exon 1 were detected at high levels, similar to those of wild-type β-globin mRNA. It is possible that early premature termination condons within β-globin mRNA and proximity to the translation initiation codon (ATG) can override the 50–55 nucleotide boundary rule.[31]

Similarly, frameshift mutations that occur later in the sequences terminate later and tend to lead to accumulation of the mutant message and the synthesis of elongated β-globin variants. These elongated variants have abnormal carboxy-terminal ends made up of hydrophobic sequences, which cause their instability. Furthermore, these β-globin variants would not be able to form αβ dimers as most of the α1β1 contact residues would have been removed.[52] Because the heme contact site codons – mostly located in exon 2 – are retained, these elongated variants should have some tertiary structure, be less susceptible to proteolytic degradation, and presumably, form the characteristic inclusion bodies. Prominent inclusions were noted in individuals heterozygous for Hb Geneva, Hb Makabe, Hb Agnana, Hb Vercelli, and the frameshift mutation at codon 128 – the original Irish family reported by Weatherall et al. 1973.[38]

VARIANTS OF β THALASSEMIA

Normal HbA_2 β Thalassemias

The diagnostic feature of β thalassemia is the hypochromic microcytic red cells and an elevated level of HbA_2 in heterozygotes, whether β^+ or β^0. Normal HbA_2 β thalassemias (previously referred to as type 2) refers to the form in which the blood picture is typical of heterozygous β thalassemia except for the normal levels of Hb A_2,the red cell phenotype being similar to that in carriers for β thalassemia. Most cases of normal HbA_2 β thalassemia result from coinheritance of δ thalassemia (δ^0 or δ^+) in *cis* or *trans* to a β^0 or β^+ thalassemia gene.

One relatively common form of normal HbA_2 thalassemia in the Middle East and Mediterranean is that associated with Hb Knossos (β27 Ala→Ser). Like HbE, the mutation β27(GCC→TCC) activates an alternative splice site, reducing the amount of normal transcript that contains the variant. Unlike HbE, the HbA_2 level is not elevated in heterozygotes as there is a δ^0 thalassemia (Cd59-A) mutation in *cis* to the β27 Ala→Ser mutation.[61]

Another relatively common cause of normal HbA_2 β thalassemia phenotype in the Greek population is the Corfu form of δβ thalassemia, a 7.2-kb deletion that includes the 5′ part of the δ gene.[62,63] Commonly the β-globin gene in *cis* is down regulated by a G→A mutation in position 5 of the IVS1. Heterozygotes have a slight increase in HbF (1.1%–2.8%) and low to normal HbA_2 levels but homozygotes have a milder than expected phenotype of thalassemia intermedia. They have almost 100% HbF with no HbA_2 and trace levels of HbA, suggesting that the effect of the deletion is to allow increased γ chain production under the stress of anemia. Studies in primary erythroid cell cultures from heterozygotes, homozygotes and compound heterozygotes for the Corfu deletion suggest that γ mRNA accumulation and HbF expression is indirectly dependent on the total amount of viable β mRNA.[64] Reduction of β mRNA below a critical threshold, as in compound heterozygotes and homozygotes, allows full expression of HbF, and hence the unusually high HbF in such individuals. The Corfu mutation has been described as separate lesions in two different populations. The normal β gene in *cis* to the 7.2-kb deletion in an Italian individual is expressed at normal levels,[65] whereas Algerian homozygotes for the βIVS1–5 G→A mutation have a severe transfusion-dependent anemia.[66]

The phenotype of normal HbA_2 β thalassemia is also seen in heterozygotes for εγδβ thalassemia (see later).

"Silent" β Thalassemia

Heterozygotes for 'silent' β thalassemias do not have any evident hematological phenotype; the only abnormality being a mild imbalance of globin chain synthesis. These mutations have been identified in homozygotes who have a typical β thalassemia trait phenotype[16] or in the compound heterozygous state with a severe β thalassemia allele where they cause thalassemia intermedia.[14] Silent β thalassemia alleles are not common except for the C→T mutation at position −101 of the β-globin gene, which accounts for most of the milder forms of β thalassemia in the Mediterranean.[15] It has been noted that carriers for this mutation have highly variable HbA_2 levels despite similar hematological parameters and globin chain synthesis ratios.[15] Coinheritance of δ thalassemia mutations were implicated but sequence analysis of the δ globin genes in one family excluded this possibility.[67] Recently, a C→G transversion has also been reported in the same −101 position and heterozygotes have a silent phenotype.[68] Several other mutations in the 5′ and 3′ UTRs are also silent.[4]

It has been suggested that the $[TA]_x[T]_y$ sequence variation at position −530 of the β-globin gene may be responsible for some silent β thalassemia carriers and that the reduced β-globin expression may be related to increased binding of the BP1 repressor protein.[69] Population surveys and clinical studies do not show a consistent correlation between the $[TA]_x[T]_y$ variants and a β thalassemia phenotype, suggesting that it is a neutral polymorphism.[70]

β Thalassemia Trait with Unusually High HbA_2

Despite the vast heterogeneity of mutations, the increased levels of HbA_2 observed in heterozygotes for the different β thalassemia alleles in different ethnic groups are remarkably uniform, usually 3.5%–5.5% and rarely exceeding 6%.[71] Unusually high levels of HbA_2 over 6.5% seem to characterize the subgroup of β thalassemias caused by lesions that affect the regulatory elements in the β promoter. As discussed earlier, the unusually high HbA_2, often accompanied by modest increases in HbF, may be related to the removal of competition for the upstream LCR and transcription factors, allowing an increased interaction with the *cis* δ and γ genes.[72]

UNUSUAL CAUSES OF β THALASSEMIA

Insertion of a Transposable Element Causing β Thalassemia

Transposable elements may occasionally disrupt human genes and result in their inactivation. The insertion of such an element, a retrotransposon of the L1 family has been reported with the phenotype of β^+ thalassemia.[73] Despite the insertion of 6–7 kb DNA into its IVS2, the affected gene expresses full-length β-globin transcripts at a level corresponding to approximately 15% of normal β-globin mRNA.[73]

Trans-acting Mutations

Population studies have shown that approximately 1% of β thalassemias remain uncharacterized despite extensive sequence analysis, including the flanking regions of the β-globin genes.[13] Recently, it has been found that mutations in *XPD* that cause trichothiodystrophy are frequently associated with a phenotype of β thalassemia trait,[74] supported by reduced levels of β-globin synthesis and reduced β-globin mRNA. The *XPD* protein is a subunit of the general transcription factor TF11H that is involved in basal transcription and DNA repair. Some mutations in the transcription factor *GATA-1* on the X-chromosome have also been reported to cause β thalassemia in association with thrombocytopenia.[75,76] This was the first example of β thalassemia in humans caused by a mutation in the erythroid-specific transcription factor. There are several other families with β thalassemia in which no mutations have been detected and *trans*-acting regulatory factors have been implicated.[77–79]

Somatic Deletion of β-Globin Gene

This novel mechanism was recently described in three unrelated families of French[80] and Italian origins.[81] Affected individuals had moderately severe anemia with hepatosplenomegaly despite being constitutionally heterozygous for a typical β thalassemia mutation (β^0 39 C→T) with a normal α genotype. Subsequent investigations revealed a somatic deletion of chromosome 11p15, including the β-globin complex, in *trans* to the mutation in a subpopulation of erythroid cells. This results in a somatic mosaic: 10%–20% of erythroid cells were heterozygous with one normal copy of β-globin gene and the rest hemizygous, that is, without any normal β-globin gene. These unusual cases once again illustrate that the severity of anemia of β thalassemia reflects the quantitative deficiency of β-globin production. The implication for gene therapy is that expression in approximately 20% of erythroid cells may be sufficient to convert a transfusion-dependent state to transfusion independence.[3,82]

εγδβ THALASSEMIA

Clinically, the εγδβ thalassemias are characterized in newborns by anemia and hemolysis, which is self-limited, and in adults by the hematological phenotype of β thalassemia trait with normal levels of HbA_2 and HbF.[4] The severity of anemia and hemolysis may be variable (even within a family) and in some cases, blood transfusions are necessary during the neonatal period.[83,84] Only heterozygotes have been identified; homozygotes, presumably, would not survive early gestation. At the molecular level, the deletions fall into two categories: group I removes all or a greater part of the β-globin complex, including the β-globin gene; group II removes extensive upstream regions leaving the β-globin gene itself intact, despite which, its expression is silenced because of absence of the upstream β LCR. To date, a total of 18 deletions causing εγδβ thalassemia have been described – eight group II upstream deletions[13,84–86] and 10 in group I[13,83,84] that includes the β-globin gene (see Fig. 16.5). All these deletions are extremely rare and unique to the families in which they have been described. The associated phenotypes of the two groups are similar.

HEREDITARY PERSISTENCE OF FETAL HEMOGLOBIN AND δβ THALASSEMIA

HPFH[87] and δβ thalassemia are descriptive terms used for a range of disorders that are characterized by decreased or absent β-globin production and a variable compensatory increase in γ-chain synthesis. HPFH was first observed in two healthy West African individuals with only Hbs S and F[88] who produced children with HbA and with a high level of HbF. Further cases were discovered in the West Indies and the United States, and the first homozygote was found.[89] He was clinically normal and had 100% HbF, indicating a complete absence of δ and β chain production.

The first type of δβ thalassemia to be described was Hb Lepore[90] containing a fusion δβ-globin chain produced by a misaligned crossover between the δ and β genes.[91] Soon afterward a form of thalassemia with normal HbA_2 and unusually high levels of HbF was described in several different racial groups.[92,93] When the first homozygote for this condition was observed[94] with a thalassemic disorder and 100% HbF, it was clear that no δ- or β-chains were produced in this condition and hence it became known as δβ thalassemia.

Further heterogeneity in these conditions was demonstrated after it was discovered that there are two types of γ chain.[95] Although the HbF in many HPFHs and δβ thalassemias contained both $^G\gamma$ and $^A\gamma$ chains, other cases had one or the other.

Once the β-like globin genes had been cloned, these conditions were analyzed at the molecular level and it became clear that different deletions within the β-globin gene cluster underlay most cases of δβ thalassemia and many cases of HPFH. The size and positions of the deletions bore no obvious relationship to the underlying phenotypes, but these studies demonstrated that HPFH and δβ thalassemia were closely related conditions. The discovery that some HPFH conditions were not due to deletions demonstrated that there was even further heterogeneity within these disorders.

Classification

HPFH and δβ thalassemia were originally distinguished on what appeared to be clear-cut hematological and clinical grounds. Heterozygous δβ thalassemia had a similar red cell picture to β thalassemia, with hypochromic and microcytic erythrocytes, but a normal level of HbA_2 (<3.0%). In addition, there was a raised level of HbF (5%–15%) that had a heterogeneous intercellular distribution. Homozygotes or compound heterozygotes with β thalassemia had a clinical picture of thalassemia intermedia or major. In contrast, HPFH heterozygotes had essentially normal red cell indices, a normal level of HbA_2 and even higher levels of HbF (15%–30%) with a more homogeneous, pancellular distribution. HPFH homozygotes were clinically normal, albeit with reduced MCV and MCH, whereas compound heterozygotes with β thalassemia were clinically very mild. As more and more cases and different molecular types of the two conditions were described, these differences became blurred and it is now clear that there is considerable overlap in many of the parameters that were initially used to differentiate them (see later).

Many forms of HPFH and most types of δβ thalassemia are due to gene deletions and are classified as either HPFH or δβ thalassemia largely on the basis of the level of HbF in the heterozygotes and the clinical severity in homozygotes or compound heterozygotes with β thalassemia, when known. Included within the HPFH conditions is Hb Kenya, in which production of a hybrid $^A\gamma\beta$-chain is accompanied by increased $^G\gamma$-chain synthesis.

The δβ thalassemias are subdivided into those that produce both $^G\gamma$- and $^A\gamma$-chains, $^G\gamma^A\gamma(\delta\beta)^0$ thalassemia

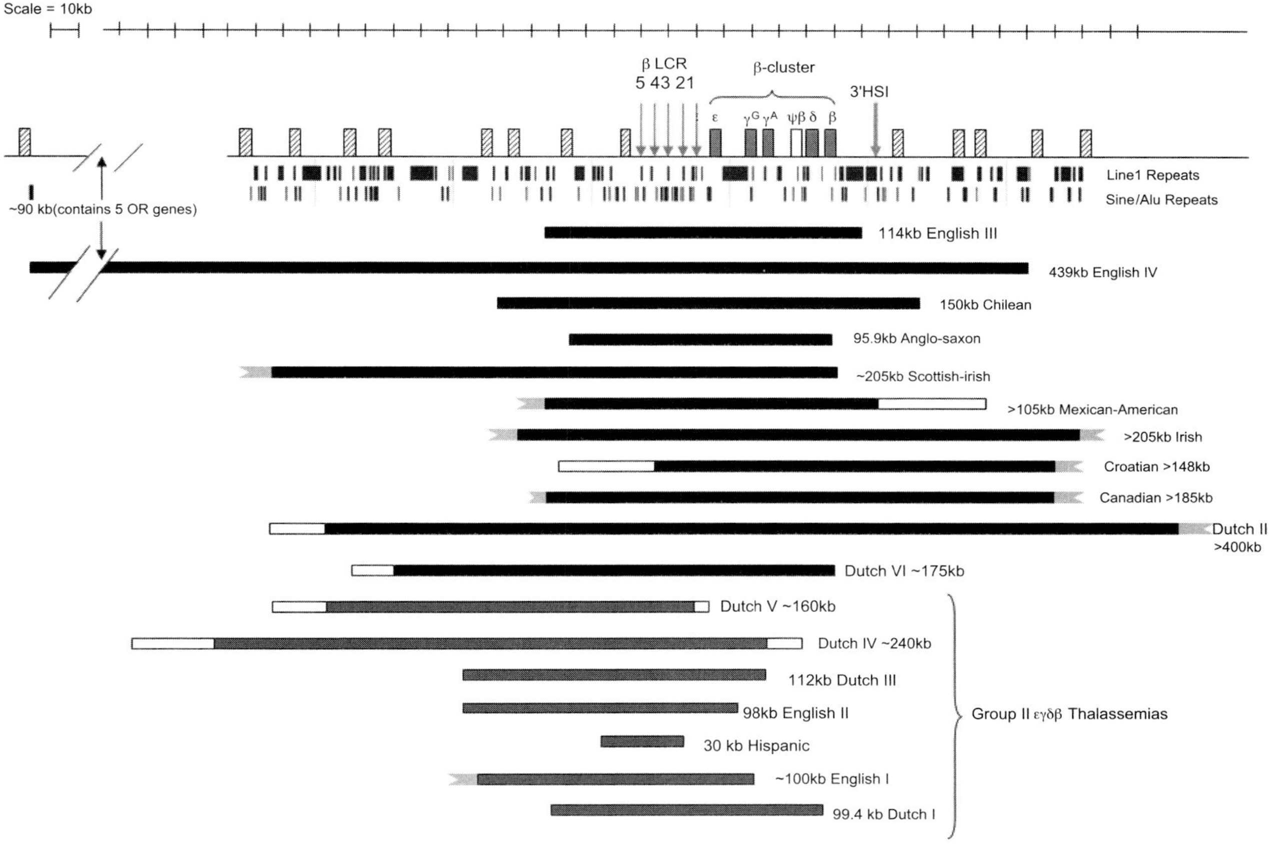

Figure 16.5. Deletions of the β-globin gene cluster causing $(\varepsilon\gamma\delta\beta)^0$ thalassemia. Top part of the figure shows the β-globin cluster and its flanking regions on chromosome 11p. The ε, $^G\gamma$, $^A\gamma$, δ, and β-globin genes are shown as gray boxes, whereas the hatched boxes represent the human olfactory receptor genes (HOR) named according to ensemble database (Ch 11:5110000–5600000). The 5′ hypersensitive sites that comprise the β LCR and the 3′ hypersensitive site (3′HS1) are shown as vertical arrows. The Line 1 and Sine/Alu repeat sequences are shown below the β-globin gene cluster as short vertical lines and boxes. The 18 deletions causing εγδβ thalassemia are shown below; the extents of the deletions are marked as complete boxes if endpoints have been determined precisely, jagged ends if undetermined, and white boxes as endpoint regions. Boxes in black are the deletions that include the β-globin gene (group I) and gray boxes represent the group II upstream deletions that leave the β-globin intact. (See color plate 16.5.)

(including Hb Lepore with a hybrid δβ-chain) and those that only contain $^G\gamma$-chains, $^G\gamma(^A\gamma\delta\beta)^0$ thalassemia. Within each of these three groups, there are several different deletions that share a similar clinical and hematological phenotype; they are usually named after the region in which they were first described.

Conditions associated with increased HbF in adult life that are not due to deletions of the β-globin cluster can also be subclassified. Those in which there is an increase of only the $^G\gamma$- or $^A\gamma$-chains are usually due to mutations in the promoters of the respective genes, resulting in a variable level of persistent HbF. Several other inherited conditions have been characterized and shown to be due to genes that increase γ gene expression but that are not linked to the β-globin complex. These include ones localized to chromosomes 2, 6, and 8 and another that appears to be X-linked. Additional genes are known to occur but have yet to be localized.

The broad classification of the deletion conditions into three groups, although useful, is rather arbitrary. When the mean levels of HbF and red cell indices are plotted out for each individual deletion it becomes apparent that there is a continuum between δβ thalassemia and the HPFHs and that not all conditions fit neatly into one of these groups.[7] For instance, the condition referred to as Indian HPFH or HPFH 3 has 20%–25% HbF in heterozygotes, consistent with an HPFH condition but it produces a relatively severe disease when inherited together with β thalassemia, a feature usually associated with δβ thalassemia. The two common types of HPFH of African origin are asymptomatic as homozygotes and appear to be mild in combination with β thalassemia. The most common Black β thalassemia alleles are themselves mild, and it is possible that if these HPFHs were coupled with a severe β thalassemia allele, a more severe clinical picture might emerge.[96] Among the $^G\gamma(^A\gamma\delta\beta)^0$ thalassemias, the Thai type has unusually high

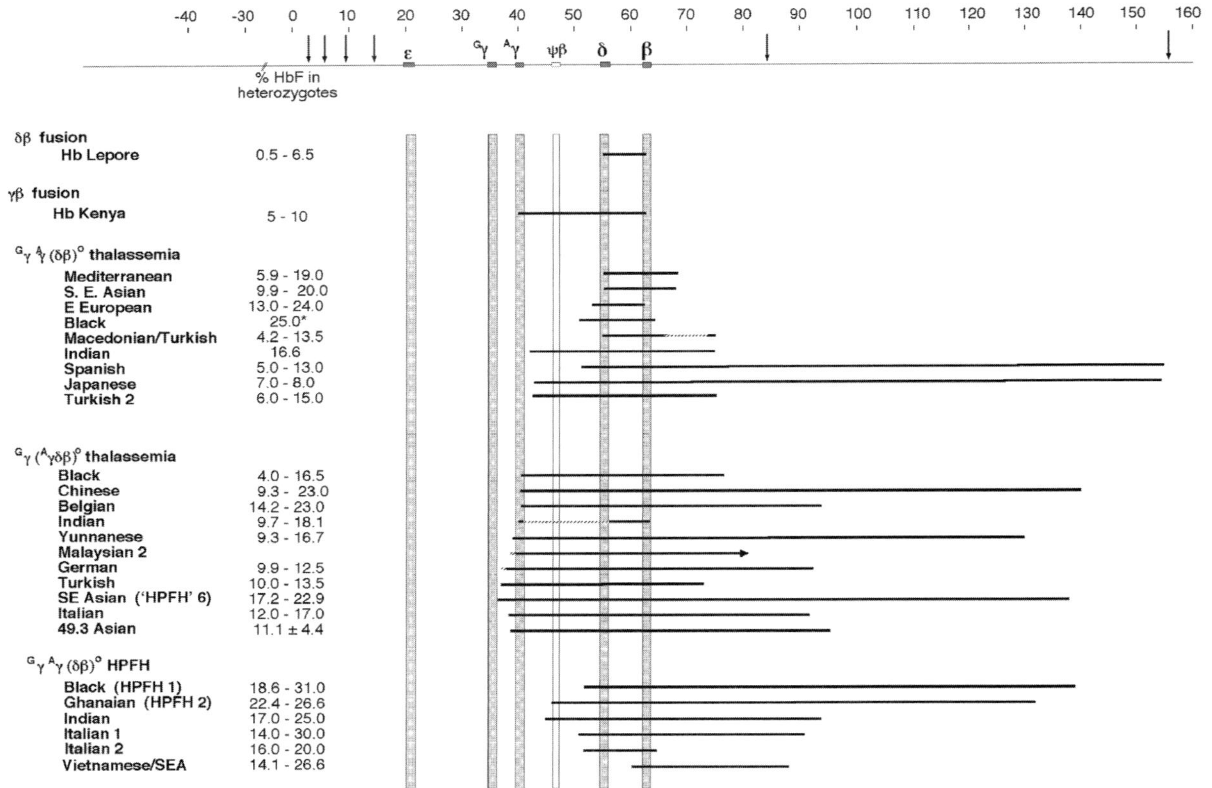

Figure 16.6. Deletions of the β-globin cluster causing HPFH, $^{G}\gamma(^{A}\gamma\delta\beta)^0$ thalassemia, and $^{G}\gamma^{A}(\gamma\delta\beta)^0$ thalassemia. Arrows in the cluster at the top of the diagram indicate DNase1 hypersensitive sites; those to the left of the ε gene define the LCR. The inverted region in the two double-deletion/inversion cases are shown as a dashed line. * This deletion has only been found in *trans* to HbS.

levels of HbF and it has been referred to as HPFH 6,[97] but from a structural point of view it clearly belongs to the $^{G}\gamma(^{A}\gamma\delta\beta)^0$ thalassemias.

Deletions that remove only the β-globin gene and hence produce a β thalassemia phenotype with a raised HbA_2 also tend to have increased HbF levels compared with nondeletion β thalassemias. The levels in some of these individuals overlap with those seen in δβ thalassemia. There are grounds, therefore, for abandoning this classification and combining all the deletion conditions into one group. Because we do not fully understand the mechanisms responsible for the increased HbF in these conditions, this might be premature and a different classification might naturally emerge with increased knowledge. In the meantime, therefore, we have retained the scheme with which most people are conversant.

DELETIONS RESULTING IN HPFH OR δβ THALASSEMIA

The structure of the β-globin gene cluster and the surrounding area is illustrated in Figures 16.5 and 16.6. The β LCR, the major regulatory region marked by erythroid-specific DNase1 hypersensitive sites, lies 5′ to the ε gene. Loss of the β LCR, which occurs in the $(\varepsilon^{G}\gamma^{A}\gamma\delta\beta)^0$ thalassemia, results in inactivation of any remaining β-globin genes. The erythroid-specific DNase1 hypersensitive sites that have been mapped around the cluster are shown by arrows on the map. Additional regulatory regions include sequences that have enhancer-like activity in transient transfection assays. These have been identified 3′ to the $^{A}\gamma$ gene, within IVS2 of the β gene, 3′ to the β gene and at three sites in the downstream region, immediately beyond the breakpoints of HPFH-1, HPFH-5, and the SE Asian $^{G}\gamma(^{A}\gamma\delta\beta)^0$ thalassemia. These are illustrated on the map with filled circles. Olfactory receptor genes have been localized in the vicinity of the cluster and the area is rich in repetitive sequences, particularly Alu and L1 repeats.

The deletions resulting in HPFH or δβ thalassemia that have been characterized to date are illustrated in Fig. 16.6 and details of characterized breakpoints are given in Table 16.3. The hematological and clinical aspects of these conditions will be dealt with in a later section. In both the $^{G}\gamma^{A}\gamma(\delta\beta)^0$ HPFHs and the $^{G}\gamma^{A}\gamma(\delta\beta)^0$ thalassemias the deletions remove both the δ and β genes and extend a variable degree 3′ to the cluster, in some cases for up to 100 kb. The $^{G}\gamma(^{A}\gamma\delta\beta)^0$ thalassemias differ in that the 5′ end of the deletion partially or totally removes the $^{A}\gamma$ gene in addition to the δ and β genes.

Table 16.3. Deletion breakpoints in δβ thalassemia and HPFH

Condition	Type	5′ Break-point	3′ Break-point	Deletion size (kb)
δβ fusion	Hb Lepore	54874–55238	62483–63572	7.398
δ thalassemia	Corfu	48841	56051	7.201
γβ fusion	Hb Kenya	39846–39869	62521–62543	22.675
$^G\gamma^A\gamma$ $(\delta\beta)^0$ HPFH	Black	51086	136004	84.918
	Ghanaian	46495	130174	83.679
	Indian	45027	94759	47.733
	Italian	50375	~91000	~40
	Sicilian	51504	64414	12.910
	SE Asian	60150	~88000	~28
$^G\gamma^A\gamma$ $(\delta\beta)^0$ thalassemia	Mediterranean	55943	69320	13.378
	SE Asian	55989	68573	12.584
	E European	53177	62301	9.124
	Black	52285	64052	11.767
	Macedonian/Turkish	54686	66151	11.465
	Macedonian/Turkish	73795	75388	1.593
	Indian	42149	74772	32.624
	Spanish	51985	~147000	~95
	Japanese	43122	156750	113.629
	Turkish	~43000	~73000	~30
$^G\gamma$ $(^A\gamma\delta\beta)^0$ thalassemia	Black	40681	76491	35.811
	Chinese	40454	119300	78.847
	Indian	40054	40887	0.834
	Indian	56174	63634	7.460
	Italian	39758	~92000	~52
	Belgian	40712	~94000	~50
	Yunnanese	39297	~127000	~88
	German	~38000	~90000	~52
	Turkish	37057	73267	36.211
	SE Asian	37242	116449	79.208
	Malay 2	~39000	~81000	~42
	49.3-kb Asian			

Breakpoints are given according to the reference sequence entry in GenBank U01317 for the β-like globin genes.

DELETION HPFHs

Six deletion forms of HPFH have been described in Africans, Mediterraneans, Indians and southeast Asians. Their size ranges from 13 to 85 kb resulting in HbF levels in heterozygotes that overlap within the range of 14%–31% (Fig. 16.6). Both δ and β genes are deleted in five cases but the δ gene remains intact in the southeast Asian form. The most common forms are the Black HPFH-1 and -2, which have large (>80 kb) deletions staggered by approximately 5 kb at the 5′ and 3′ ends. Details of the individual types and their breakpoints and original references are given in Wood.[7]

Hb Kenya. Structural analysis of the abnormal β chain in Hb Kenya showed it to be a hybrid chain in which the 5′ end was derived from γ and the 3′ end from β.[98,99] The interpretation that this resulted from crossover between the $^A\gamma$ gene and the β gene, with deletion of the sequences that lie between them was confirmed by molecular analysis.[100] The frequency of Hb Kenya is unknown but is clearly relatively rare and most cases appear to originate from East Africa.

$^G\gamma^A\gamma(\delta\beta)^0$ THALASSEMIAS

$^G\gamma^A\gamma(\delta\beta)^0$ thalassemias have a broad worldwide distribution although many of the nine characterized deletions are restricted to one or a few families. The exception to this is the Mediterranean type, which is relatively common and may comprise up to 5% of all β thalassemias in some regions. The deletions all encompass parts or all of the δ and β genes and most are of a restricted size of 10–30 kb. A Macedonian/Turkish form consists of two deletions separated by an inverted sequence, whereas a Japanese and a Turkish case are greater than 100 kb and extend beyond 3′ ends of the large HPFH 1 and 2 deletions. The HbF levels range mostly between 5% and 20% and do not distinguish the various molecular types.

Table 16.4. Hematological data (mean ± SD) on $\delta\beta$ thalassemia and deletion HPFH heterozygotes and homozygotes (defined by molecular analysis)

Condition	Hb g/dL	MCV fL	MCH pg	HbA_2%	HbF	$^G\gamma$	α/non-α synthesis	Distribution
Heterozygotes								
$^G\gamma^A\gamma\ (\delta\beta)^0$ thalassemia	12.3 ± 0.9	68.3 ± 4.7	23.6 ± 1.8	2.6 ± 0.3	10.5 ± 3.7	35–72	1.4–1.5	Heterocellular
$^G\gamma\ (^A\gamma\delta\beta)^0$ thalassemia	13.1 ± 0.6	75.1 ± 3.6	24.4 ± 1.5	2.3 ± 0.3	12.2 ± 1.5+	83–100	1.4–2.0	Heterocellular
HPFH	13.2 ± 0.6	82.6 ± 4.1	26.3 ± 1.4	2.2 ± 0.4	24.1 ± 2.7	16–71	1.1–1.5	Pancellular
Homozygotes								
$^G\gamma^A\gamma\ (\delta\beta)^0$ thalassemia	10.9 ± 0.9	78.4 ± 2.7	24.2 ± 2.4	0	100	50–61	2.3–5.2	Pancellular
$^G\gamma\ (^A\gamma\delta\beta)^0$ thalassemia	10.5 ± 1.2	71.2 ± 5.8	21.6 ± 1.6	0	100	100	3.8–4.9	Pancellular
HPFH	16.6 ± 1.1	71.9 ± 3.4	24.5 ± 1.3	0	100	54–65	1.7–2.5	Pancellular

$^\alpha$ Thalassemia not excluded in all cases; extreme outliers omitted. + not including southeast Asian form with a HbF level of 18.8 ± 2.3%.

Hb Lepore. The Lepore globin chain is a hybrid $\delta\beta$-chain produced by misaligned crossing over between the δ- and β-globin genes. Three different types have been distinguished depending on the position of the crossover: Lepore Washington/Boston, δ87-β116, Lepore Baltimore, δ50-β86, and Lepore Hollandia, δ22-β50. Lepore Washington/Boston is the most common but both it and Lepore Baltimore have been found in Mediterraneans and those of African origin. Lepore Hollandia has been found in individuals from Papua New Guinea and Bangladesh.

$^G\gamma(^A\gamma\delta\beta)^0$ THALASSEMIA

$^G\gamma\ (^A\gamma\delta\beta)^0$ thalassemias are due to deletions that include part or all of the $^A\gamma$ gene and produce HbF containing only $^G\gamma$ chains. They are also geographically widespread and mostly restricted to a few families. In size, they are more extensive than most $^G\gamma^A\gamma\ (\delta\beta)^0$ thalassemias (Fig. 14.6) and the Indian type has two deletions separated by an inverted region similar to the Macedonian/Turkish form of $^G\gamma^A\gamma\ (\delta\beta)^0$ thalassemia. The HbF levels generally are between 10% and 20% but in southeast Asian type these tend to be higher and this condition has been referred to as HPFH 6.[97,101]

Nondeletion $\delta\beta$ Thalassemia

Two Chinese families have been described with the phenotype of $\delta\beta$ thalassemia (hypochromia, microcytosis, normal HbA_2, and a raised HbF of ~22%) but with no detectable deletion.[102,103]

HEMATOLOGY RESULTS AND HEMOGLOBIN ANALYSIS

The hematology results and hemoglobin analyses on the deletion conditions are listed in Table 16.4. In these analyses, only cases for which the molecular basis has been determined have been included.

Hb Kenya. Hb Kenya carriers have near-normal hematological findings. Hemoglobin analysis reveals low-normal levels of HbA_2 (1.4%–1.8%), raised HbF levels (7%–12%), Hb Kenya, and HbA. The proportion of Hb Kenya is more variable, with levels ranging from 5% to 23% and some suggestion of bimodality, with peaks at approximately 10% and 20%. The HbF contains only $^G\gamma$-chains. On interaction with HbS, higher levels of Hb Kenya (17%–19%) are observed than in HbA/Kenya cases, whereas the HbF level (6.6%–11%) remains unchanged.[99]

$^G\gamma^A\gamma(\delta\beta)^0$ HPFH. Heterozygotes for $^G\gamma^A\gamma(\delta\beta)^0$ HPFH are characterized by normal HbA_2 levels and HbF levels of 15%–30%. There are only minor reductions in the red cell indices, which are frequently within the normal range (Table 16.4). In many of the reported cases, the presence of α thalassemia was not excluded and may explain some cases with reduced MCV and MCH.

Homozygotes have been described for both HPFH-1[89,104–106] and HPFH-2[107–111] and they are indistinguishable; their hemoglobin consists entirely of HbF (Table 16.4). They are clinically unaffected and have normal or high Hb levels (15 g/dL–18 g/dL), presumably as a result of the higher oxygen affinity of HbF. They have microcytic, hypochromic red cells, and globin chain imbalance can be demonstrated, with α/γ ratios of approximately 2.0. This shows that the output of γ chains is not sufficient to compensate fully for the lack of β-chains.

Compound heterozygotes with β thalassemia are usually clinically silent and have similar hematological indices to β thalassemia heterozygotes. Most cases were reported before characterization of the β thalassemia alleles was feasible and presumably involved mild β thalassemia mutations, as they are the most common in this racial group. HbA_2 levels are normal or slightly raised and HbF levels usually fall within the range of 60%–75%. Compound heterozygotes with the Indian type of HPFH with β thalassemia, observed in four families, were all anemic with Hb levels of 5.5 g/dL–9.0 g/dL and were classified clinically as thalassemia intermedia.

Compound heterozygotes for HPFH and HbS are generally healthy and have a mild sickling disorder. They are not usually anemic and there is little evidence of hemolysis. This is ascribed to the high level of HbF contributed by

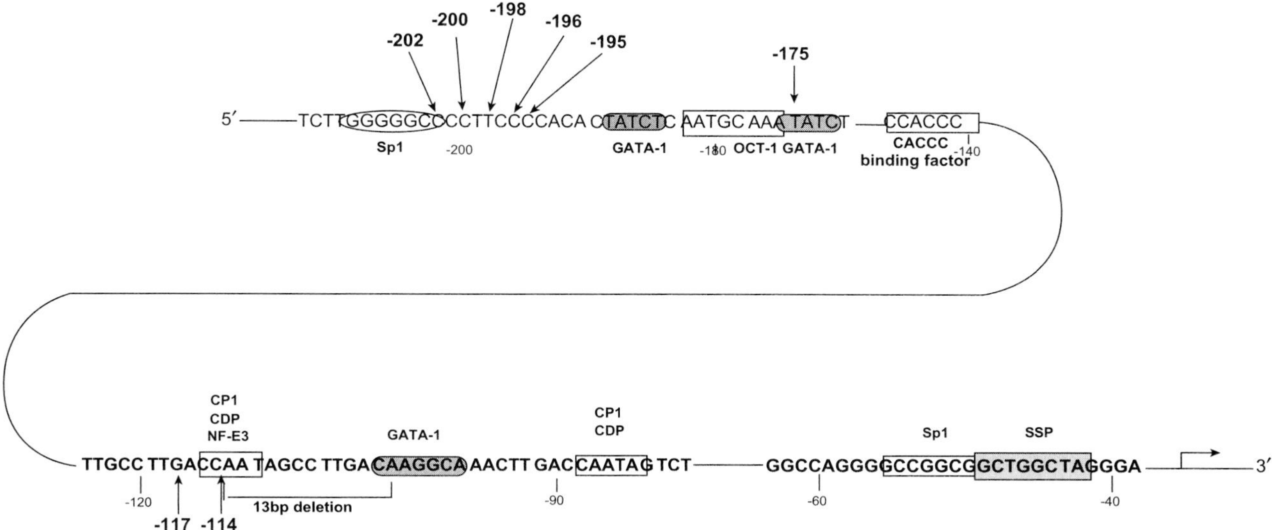

Figure 16.7. Transcription factor binding sites in the promoters of the γ-globin genes; $^A\gamma$ and $^G\gamma$ genes are identical in this region. The positions of mutations that result in nondeletion HPFH are indicated.

COMPETITION BETWEEN γ AND β GENES IN NONDELETION HPFH

Individuals with γ promoter mutations have balanced globin chain synthesis and a normal MCH (Table 16.5). When combined with a β^S or β^C gene in *trans*, the hemoglobin in the $^G\gamma$ −200 and −175 mutations and the $^A\gamma$ −175 and −114 to −102 deletion mutants has a composition of approximately 25% HbF, 25% HbA, and 50% HbS or HbC. This indicates that the combined output from the γ and β^A genes on the affected chromosome is approximately normal. The mild anemia seen in compound heterozygotes for β thalassemia and the $^A\gamma$ −196 and −117 mutations may indicate that the total γ + β chain output from the HPFH chromosome in these cases is slightly less than normal. Nevertheless, it would appear that the increased γ chain production is matched by a decrease in β chain output and that this reciprocity only occurs in *cis*. This reciprocal relationship could be explained if there was competition between these two genes for access to the β LCR. Altered binding of transcription factors to the γ gene promoter as a result of the base substitutions might well alter the balance of association with the β LCR, resulting in a more stable binding than would normally occur in adult red cells. It is known that during the normal developmental switch from γ to β gene expression, both genes are transcriptionally active in the same cell and that there is continual alternation of activation of the two genes.[171] Decreased binding of a repressor protein or increased binding of an activator to the γ gene promoter could therefore increase the gene's competitiveness. Different mutants would result in different probabilities of a productive interaction with the β LCR, hence the variability in the amount of HbF produced.

HPFH UNLINKED TO THE β-GLOBIN CLUSTER

A number of families have been reported in which an inherited increase in the level of HbF, usually demonstrated in an interaction with β thalassemia or sickle cell disease, apparently segregates independently of the β-globin gene cluster.[172–179] Genetic analysis of these cases is made difficult by the possibility that there is genetic heterogeneity and that there may be incomplete penetrance. Furthermore, the distribution of HbF levels in these families may be continuous, making phenotypic identification of normal and affected individuals difficult. Thus the pattern of inheritance is rarely clear in these families and examples of autosomal, sex-linked, dominant, codominant, or recessive patterns have all been reported.

X-linked. Analysis of HbF levels in healthy Japanese adults led to the suggestion that an X-linked gene was involved in increasing HbF levels with a frequency of 11% of males affected and 21% of females being carriers.[180] Support for the possibility of an X-linked locus affecting HbF levels came from analyses of the F reticulocytes in male and female sickle cell patients and from sibling-pair studies in the same population. Dover et al.[181] suggested that a codominant, biallelic F cell production locus (with high and low alleles) resided on the A chromosome and showed linkage to markers at Xp22.2–22.3. Furthermore, it was proposed that this locus accounts for 40% of the variability in sickle cell HbF levels, an effect of much greater magnitude than β-globin haplotype, age, sex, or α gene status, which together could only account for approximately 10% of the variability.[182]

Chromosome 6–linked. The value of a single large family in the study of unlinked HPFH has been dramatically demonstrated.[179] Starting with an Asian Indian patient homozygous for β^0 thalassemia who had an extremely mild course, with 10 g/dL–12g/dL HbF, a family study was performed that showed clear-cut evidence for an HPFH-like gene unlinked to the β-globin cluster. The family study was extended until more than 200 members were accumulated. The pattern of inheritance in this family was initially unclear and assignments of phenotypes were made difficult by not only the interacting β thalassemia but also α thalassemia. Nevertheless, by using statistical analysis to take account of the influence of α and β thalassemia, $^G\gamma$ −158 status, age, and sex, it was possible by multiple regression analysis to demonstrate the presence of a major gene affecting F cell levels in this family.[183] By using polymorphic markers covering the whole genome it proved possible to localize this gene to a small area of chromosome 6, 6q22.3-q24,[172] which was further refined to a 1.5-Mb region containing five coding genes (*AH11, MYB, ALDH8, HBS1L,* and *PDE7B*) and four noncoding RNAs.[184]

Chromosome 8–linked. Further analysis of the Asian Indian kindred showed an F cell quantitative trait locus at 8q that was conditional on the *Xmn*1-$^G\gamma$ polymorphism.[185] This linkage was confirmed in a study of twin pairs,[186] raising the possible action of an unlinked gene on 8q on the globin gene locus itself.

Chromosome 2–linked. Genome-wide association mapping of individuals with contrasting F cell values (F cell levels above 95th or below the 5th percentile points) from a panel of 5,000 individuals identified not only the β-globin locus (probably the *Xmn*1 −158 polymorphism) and chromosome 6 locus but also a quantitative trait locus influencing Fcell production on chromosome 2.[187] It mapped to a zinc-finger protein, BCL11A, previously implicated in leukemias.

The mechanism by which the chromosome 2-, 6-, 8-, or X-linked genes affect HbF levels and F cells remains unknown. It is possible that these loci code for *trans*-acting factors that bind within the β-globin gene cluster and directly affect gene transcription. It is equally plausible that there are genes that act much more indirectly, perhaps by altering the kinetics of erythropoiesis and mimicking the increased HbF seen in stress erythropoiesis.

OTHER SEQUENCE DIFFERENCES WITHIN THE β-CLUSTER AFFECTING HbF PRODUCTION

Within the β-cluster there are numerous polymorphisms affecting either single nucleotides or oligonucleotide motifs. Associations have been noted between the inheritance of some of these alleles and higher HbF levels, usually only under conditions of erythroid expansion such as in sickle cell disease or β thalassemia. The best known of these is the C→T polymorphism at position −158 of the $^G\gamma$ promoter, creating an *Xmn*1 restriction site.[188–190] Normal individuals who are homozygous for T at −158 may have a slight increase in F cells and individuals with a $^G\gamma$-$^G\gamma$ gene arrangement (as a result of a gene conversion event) in which both genes have the T at −158 have HbF levels of 2%–6%.[191] Among sickle cell disease and β thalassemia patients, those with −158 T tend to have higher HbF levels and a higher proportion of $^G\gamma$ chains. Additional differences within the cluster also influence HbF levels in these patients because even among haplotypes that contain the −158 T residue, there are haplotype-linked differences.

Other polymorphic regions within the cluster associated with variability in HbF levels in sickle cell and β thalassemia include an $(AT)_x(T)_y$ polymorphism upstream of the β-globin gene promoter,[192] substitutions upstream of the $^G\gamma$ gene and in $^G\gamma$ IVS2,[193,194] and a $(AT)_xN_{12}(AT)_y$ polymorphism within the HS2 element of the β LCR.[195–197] In none of these cases is there direct evidence from functional studies that different alleles at these sites are responsible for altering γ gene expression and the possibility remains that they are markers in linkage disequilibrium with as yet unidentified elements.

δβ THALASSEMIA AND HPFH CONCLUSIONS

The discovery that HPFH homozygotes with 100% HbF are clinically unaffected promoted the idea that reactivation of HbF production in adult life would be an effective therapeutic strategy for the severe disorders of the β-globin gene such as β thalassemia and sickle cell disease. It was hoped that an understanding of the natural mutations that cause HPFH might provide sufficient insight into the regulation of the γ and β genes to allow manipulation of the hemoglobin switching process. Although considerable progress has been made to identify the molecular basis of many of the HPFH conditions, a complete understanding of how these lead to persistent HbF still eludes us. Among the deletion conditions, the influence of the newly apposed sequences may be responsible for maintaining the γ genes in an active state in some cases but remains to be proven and other mechanisms have not been excluded.

Many of the nondeletion conditions are due to base substitutions in the promoters of the γ genes, altering the binding of transcription factors and preventing suppression of these genes in adult life. The lack of any consistent pattern to these protein binding site changes suggests that the developmental regulation of these genes is a complex multifactorial process and additional investigations are required to provide a more detailed understanding of the way these disruptions enable the mutant γ genes to compete with the β genes in adult erythroid cells.

Identifying the genes that influence adult HbF levels but are not linked to the β-globin cluster may identify other players in the process of γ- and β-globin gene regulation. Positional cloning has localized at least three such genes, but whether they have more than minor modifying roles awaits elucidation.

To date, the knowledge we have gained about the molecular basis of HPFH and δβ thalassemia mutations has considerably increased our understanding of the regulation of the globin genes. It is to be hoped that continued progress in this understanding will ultimately allow us to manipulate the expression of these genes for the benefit of patients with severe hemoglobinopathies.

REFERENCES

1. Thein SL. Is it dominantly inherited β thalassaemia or just a β-chain variant that is highly unstable? *Br J Haematol.* 1999;107:12–21.
2. Forget BG. Molecular mechanisms of beta thalassemia. In: Steinberg MH, Forget BG, Higgs DR, Nagel RL, eds. *Disorders of Hemoglobin: Genetics, Pathophysiology and Clinical Management.* Cambridge: Cambridge University Press; 2001:252–276.
3. Thein SL. Pathophysiology of beta thalassemia – a guide to molecular therapies. *Hematology (Am Soc Hematol Educ Program).* 2005:31–37.
4. Weatherall DJ, Clegg JB. *The Thalassaemia Syndromes.* 4th ed. Oxford: Blackwell Science; 2001.
5. Forget BG. Molecular genetics of the human globin genes. In: Steinberg MH, Forget BG, Higgs DR, Nagel RL, eds. *Disorders of Hemoglobin: Genetics, Pathophysiology and Clinical Management.* Cambridge: Cambridge University Press; 2001:117–130.
6. Thein SL. Structural variants with a beta-thalassemia phenotype. In: Steinberg MH, Forget BG, Higgs DR, Nagel RL, eds. *Disorders of Hemoglobin: Genetics, Pathophysiology and Clinical Management.* Cambridge: Cambridge University Press; 2001:342–355.
7. Wood WG. Hereditary persistence of fetal hemoglobin and delta beta thalassemia. In: Steinberg MH, Forget BG, Higgs DR, Nagel RL, eds. *Disorders of Hemoglobin: Genetics, Pathophysiology, and Clinical Management.* Cambridge: Cambridge University Press; 2001:356–388.
8. Huisman THJ, Carver MFH, Baysal E. *A Syllabus of Thalassemia Mutations.* Augusta, GA: The Sickle Cell Anemia Foundation; 1997.
9. Hardison R, Riemer C, Chui DH, Huisman TH, Miller W. Electronic access to sequence alignments, experimental results, and human mutations as an aid to studying globin gene regulation. *Genomics.* 1998;47(3):429–437.
10. Chen XW, Mo QH, Li Q, Zeng R, Xu XM. A novel mutation of −73(A→T) in the CCAAT box of the beta-globin gene identified in a patient with the mild beta-thalassemia intermedia. *Ann Hematol.* 2007;86(9):653–657.
11. Safaya S, Rieder RF, Dowling CE, Kazazian HHJ, Adams JG. Homozygous β-thalassemia without anemia. *Blood.* 1989;73:324–328.
12. Huang S-Z, Wong C, Antonarakis SE, Ro-Lein T, Lo WHY, Kazazian HHJ. The same TATA box β-thalassemia mutation in Chinese and U.S. blacks: another example of independent origins of mutation. *Hum Genet.* 1986;74:162–164.
13. Thein SL. Beta thalassaemia. In: Rodgers GP, ed. *Bailliere's Clinical Haematology, Sickle Cell Disease and Thalassaemia.* London: Bailliere Tindall; 1998:91–126.
14. Gonzalez-Redondo JH, Stoming TA, Kutlar A, et al. A C→T substitution at nt −101 in a conserved DNA sequence of the promoter region of the β-globin gene is associated with "silent" β-thalassemia. *Blood.* 1989;73:1705–1711.
15. Maragoudaki E, Kanavakis E, Traeger-Synodinos J, et al. Molecular, haematological and clinical studies of the −101 C→T substitution of the β-globin gene promoter in 25 β-thalassaemia intermedia patients and 45 heterozygotes. *Br J Haematol.* 1999;107:699–706.
16. Wong C, Dowling CE, Saiki RK, Higuchi RG, Erlich HA, Kazazian HHJ. Characterization of β-thalassaemia mutations using direct genomic sequencing of amplified single copy DNA. *Nature.* 1987;330:384–386.
17. Ho PJ, Rochette J, Fisher CA, et al. Moderate reduction of β-globin gene transcript by a novel mutation in the 5′ untranslated region: a study of its interaction with other genotypes in two families. *Blood.* 1996;87:1170–1178.
18. Huang S-C, Benz EJJ. Posttranscriptional factors influencing the hemoglobin content of the red cells. In: Steinberg MH, Forget BG, Higgs DR, Nagel RL, eds. *Disorders of Hemoglobin: Genetics, Pathophysiology and Clinical Management.* Cambridge: Cambridge University Press; 2001:252–276.
19. Treisman R, Orkin SH, Maniatis T. Specific transcription and RNA splicing defects in five cloned β-thalassaemia genes. *Nature.* 1983;302:591–596.
20. Camaschella C, Mazza U, Roetto A, et al. Genetic interactions in thalassemia intermedia: analysis of β-mutations, α-genotype, γ-promoters, and β-LCR hypersensitive sites 2 and 4 in Italian patients. *Am J Hematol.* 1995;48:82–87.
21. Ho PJ, Hall GW, Luo LY, Weatherall DJ, Thein SL. Beta thalassaemia intermedia: is it possible to predict phenotype from genotype? *Br J Haematol.* 1998;100:70–78.
22. Rund D, Oron-Karni V, Filon D, Goldfarb A, Rachmilewitz E, Oppenheim A. Genetic analysis of β-thalassemia intermedia in Israel: diversity of mechanisms and unpredictability of phenotype. *Am J Hematol.* 1997;54:16–22.
23. Spritz RA, Jagadeeswaran P, Choudary PV, et al. Base substitution in an intervening sequence of a β^+ thalassemic human globin gene. *Proc Natl Acad Sci USA.* 1981;78:2455–2459.
24. Westaway D, Williamson R. An intron nucleotide sequence variant in a cloned β^+-thalassemia globin gene. *Nucl Acids Res.* 1981;9:1777.
25. Busslinger M, Moschanas N, Flavell RA. β^+ thalassemia: aberrant splicing results from a single point mutation in an intron. *Cell.* 1981;27:289.
26. Fukumaki Y, Ghosh PK, Benz EJ, Jr., et al. Abnormally spliced messenger RNA in erythroid cells from patients with β^+ thalassemia and monkey cells expressing a cloned β^+-thalassemic gene. *Cell.* 1982;28:585–593.
27. Metherall JE, Collins FS, Pan J, Weissman SM, Forget BG. β^0-thalassemia caused by a base substitution that creates an alternative splice acceptor site in an intron. *EMBO J.* 1986; 5:2551–2557.
28. Ho PJ, Hall GW, Watt S, et al. Unusually severe heterozygous β-thalassemia: evidence for an interacting gene affecting globin translation. *Blood.* 1998;92:3428–3435.
29. Yang KG, Kutlar F, George E, et al. Molecular characterization of β-globin gene mutations in Malay patients with Hb E-β-thalassaemia and thalassaemia major. *Br J Haematol.* 1989;72:73–80.
30. Orkin SH, Cheng T-C, Antonarakis SE, Kazazian HH. Thalassaemia due to a mutation in the cleavage-polyadenylation signal of the human β-globin gene. *EMBO J.* 1985;4:453–456.

31. Maquat LE. Nonsense-mediated mRNA decay: splicing, translation and mRNP dynamics. *Nat Rev Mol Cell Biol.* 2004;5(2):89–99.
32. Lejeune F, Maquat LE. Mechanistic links between nonsense-mediated mRNA decay and pre-mRNA splicing in mammalian cells. *Curr Opin Cell Biol.* 2005;17(3):309–315.
33. Maquat LE. Nonsense-mediated mRNA decay. *Curr Biol.* 2002;12(6):R196–197.
34. Hall GW, Thein SL. Nonsense codon mutations in the terminal exon of the β-globin gene are not associated with a reduction in β-mRNA accumulation: a mechanism for the phenotype of dominant β-thalassemia. *Blood.* 1994;83:2031–2037.
35. Blacklock HA, Case J, Chan T, et al. Novel sequence insertion in a Maori patient with transfusion-dependent beta-thalassaemia. *Br J Haematol.* 2005;131(3):400–402.
36. Andersson BA, Wering ME, Luo HY, et al. Sickle cell disease due to compound heterozygosity for Hb S and a novel 7.7-kb beta-globin gene deletion. *Eur J Haematol.* 2007;78(1):82–85.
37. Codrington JF, Li H-W, Kutlar F, Gu L-H, Ramachandran M, Huisman THJ. Observations on the levels of Hb A2 in patients with different β thalassemia mutations and a d chain variant. *Blood.* 1990;76:1246–1249.
38. Weatherall DJ, Clegg JB, Knox-Macaulay HHM, Bunch C, Hopkins CR, Temperley IJ. A genetically determined disorder with features both of thalassaemia and congenital dyserythropoietic anaemia. *Br J Haematol.* 1973;24:681–702.
39. Stamatoyannopoulos G, Woodson R, Papayannopoulou T, Heywood D, Kurachi MS. Inclusion-body β-thalasemia trait. A form of β thalassemia producing clinical manifestations in simple heterozygotes. *N Engl J Med.* 1974;290:939–943.
40. Thein SL, Hesketh C, Taylor P, et al. Molecular basis for dominantly inherited inclusion body β thalassemia. *Proc Natl Acad Sci USA.*1990;87:3924–3928.
41. Coleman MB, Steinberg MH, Adams JG 3rd. Hemoglobin Terre Haute arginine beta 106. A posthumous correction to the original structure of hemoglobin Indianapolis. *J Biol Chem.* 1991;266(9):5798–5800.
42. Adams JG, Boxer LA, Baehner RL, Forget BG, Tsistrakis GA, Steinberg MH. Hemoglobin Indianapolis (β112(G14) arginine). An unstable β-chain variant producing the phenotype of severe β thalassemia. *J Clin Invest.* 1979;63:931–938.
43. Baiget M, Gomez Pereira C, Jue DL, Johnson MH, McGuffey JE, Moo-Penn WF. A case of hemoglobin Indianapolis [beta 112(G14) Cys→Arg] in an individual from Cordoba, Spain. *Hemoglobin.* 1986;10(5):483–494.
44. De Biasi R, Spiteri D, Caldora M, et al. Identification by fast atom bombardment mass spectrometry of Hb Indianapolis [beta 112(G14)Cys→Arg] in a family from Naples, Italy. *Hemoglobin.* 1988;12(4):323–336.
45. Wajcman H, Lahary A, Prome D, et al. Hb Mont Saint Aignan [beta128(H6)Ala→Pro]: a new unstable variant leading to chronic microcytic anemia. *Hemoglobin.* 2001;25(1):57–65.
46. Thein SL, Best S, Sharpe J, Paul B, Clark DJ, Brown MJ. Hemoglobin Chesterfield (β 28 Leu→Arg) produces the phenotype of inclusion body β thalassemia. *Blood.* 1991;77:2791–2793.
47. Podda A, Galanello R, Maccioni L, et al. Hemoglobin Cagliari (β 60 [E4] Val-Glu): a novel unstable thalassemic hemoglobinopathy. *Blood.* 1991;77:371–375.
48. Fucharoen S, Fucharoen G, Fukumaki Y, et al. Three-base deletion in exon 3 of the β-globin gene produced a novel variant (βGunma) with a thalassemia-like phenotype. *Blood.* 1990;76:1894–1896.
49. Park SS, Barnetson R, Kim SW, Weatherall DJ, Thein SL. A spontaneous deletion of β 33/34 Val in exon 2 of the β globin gene (Hb Korea) produces the phenotype of dominant β thalassaemia. *Br J Haematol.* 1991;78:581–582.
50. Arjona SN, Eloy-Garcia JM, Gu LH, Smetanina NS, Huisman THJ. The dominant β-thalassaemia in a Spanish family is due to a frameshift that introduces an extra CGG codon (arginine) at the 5′ end of the second exon. *Br J Haematol.* 1996;93:841–844.
51. Çürük MA, Molchanova TP, Postnikov YV, et al. β-thalassemia alleles and unstable hemoglobin types among Russian pediatric patients. *Am J Hematol.* 1994;46:329–332.
52. Bunn HF, Forget BG. *Hemoglobin: Molecular, Genetic and Clinical Aspects.* Philadelphia: W.B. Saunders; 1986.
53. Öner R, Öner C, Wilson JB, Tamagnini GP, Ribeiro LML, Huisman THJ. Dominant β-thalassaemia trait in a Portuguese family is caused by a deletion of (G)TGGCTGGTGT(G) and an insertion of (G)GCAG(G) in codons 134, 135, 136 and 137 of the β-globin gene. *Br J Haematol.* 1991;79:306–310.
54. Efremov GD. Dominantly inherited beta-thalassemia. *Hemoglobin.* 2007;31(2):193–207.
55. Ho PJ, Wickramasinghe SN, Rees DC, Lee MJ, Eden A, Thein SL. Erythroblastic inclusions in dominantly inherited β thalassaemias. *Blood.* 1997;89:322–328.
56. Adams JGI, Steinberg MH, Kazazian HHJ. Isolation and characterization of the translation product of a β-globin gene nonsense mutation (β121 GAA→TAA). *Br J Haematol.* 1990;75:561–567.
57. Prehu C, Pissard S, Al-Sheikh M, et al. Two French Caucasian families with dominant thalassemia-like phenotypes due to hyper unstable hemoglobin variants: Hb Sainte Seve [codon 118 (−T)] and codon 127 [CAG→>TAG (Gln→stop]). *Hemoglobin.* 2005;29(3):229–333.
58. Faustino P, Osorio-Almeida L, Romao L, et al. Dominantly transmitted beta-thalassemia arising from the production of several aberrant mRNA species and one abnormal peptide. *Blood.* 1998;91(2):685–690.
59. Nagy E, Maquat LE. A rule for termination-codon position within intron-containing genes: when nonsense affects RNA abundance. *Trends Biochem Sci.* 1998;23(6):198–199.
60. Romao L, Inacio A, Santos S, et al. Nonsense mutations in the human beta-globin gene lead to unexpected levels of cytoplasmic mRNA accumulation. *Blood.* 2000;96(8):2895–2901.
61. Olds RJ, Sura T, Jackson B, Wonke B, Hoffbrand AV, Thein SL. A novel δ^0 mutation in cis with Hb Knossos: a study of different genetic interactions in three Egyptian families. *Br J Haematol.* 1991;78:430–436.
62. Traeger-Synodinos J, Tzetis M, Kanavakis E, Metaxotou-Mavromati A, Kattamis C. The Corfu δβ thalassaemia mutation in Greece: haematological phenotype and prevalence. *Br J Haematol.* 1991;79:302–305.
63. Wainscoat JS, Thein SL, Wood WG, et al. A novel deletion in the β globin gene complex. *Ann NY Acad Sci.* 1985;445:20–27.
64. Chakalova L, Osborne CS, Dai YF, et al. The Corfu deltabeta thalassemia deletion disrupts gamma-globin gene silencing and reveals post-transcriptional regulation of HbF expression. *Blood.* 2005;105(5):2154–2160.
65. Galanello R, Melis MA, Podda A, et al. Deletion δ-thalassemia: the 7.2 kb deletion of Corfu δ-thalassemia in a non-β-thalassemia chromosome. *Blood.* 1990;75:1747–1749.
66. Lapoumeroulie C, Pagnier J, Bank A, Labie D, Kirshnamoorthy R. β-thalassemia due to a novel mutation in IVS-1

sequence donor site consensus sequence creating a restriction site. *Biochem Biophys Res Commun.* 1986;139:709–713.

67. Ristaldi MS, Casula S, Porcu S, Cao A. Normal delta globin gene sequence in carrier of the silent −101 (C→T) beta-thalassemia mutation with normal HbA2 level. *Am J Hematol.* 2001;67(1):58.
68. Moi P, Faa V, Marini MG, et al. A novel silent beta–thalassemia mutation in the distal CACCC box affects the binding and responsiveness to EKLF. *Br J Haematol.* 2004; 126(6):881–884.
69. Berg P, Mittleman M, Elion J, Labie D, Schechter AN. Increased protein binding to a −530 mutation of the human β-globin gene associated with decreased β-globin synthesis. *Am J Hematol.* 1991;36:42–47.
70. Thein SL. Genetic modifiers of beta-thalassemia. *Haematologica* 2005;90(5):649–660.
71. Nagel RL, Steinberg MH. Hemoglobins of the embryo and fetus and minor hemoglobins of adults. In: Steinberg MH, Forget BG, Higgs DR, Nagel RL, eds. *Disorders of Hemoglobin: Genetics, Pathophysiology and Clinical Management.* Cambridge: Cambridge University Press; 2001:252–276.
72. Huisman THJ. Levels of Hb A_2 in heterozygotes and homozygotes for beta-thalassemia mutations: influence of mutations in the CACCC and ATAAA motifs of the beta-globin gene promoter. *Acta Haematol.* 1997;98:187–194.
73. Kimberland ML, Divoky V, Prchal J, Schwahn U, Berger W, Kazazian HH Jr. Full-length human L1 insertions retain the capacity for high frequency retrotransposition in cultured cells. *Hum Mol Genet.* 1999;8(8):1557–1560.
74. Viprakasit V, Gibbons RJ, Broughton BC, et al. Mutations in the general transcription factor TFIIH result in β-thalassaemia in individuals with trichothiodystrophy. *Hum Mol Genet.* 2001;10(24):2797–2802.
75. Mehaffey MG, Newton AL, Gandhi MJ, Crossley M, Drachman JG. X-linked thrombocytopenia caused by a novel mutation of GATA-1. *Blood.* 2001;98(9):2681–2688.
76. Yu C, Niakan KK, Matsushita M, Stamatoyannopoulos G, Orkin SH, Raskind WH. X-linked thrombocytopenia with thalassemia from a mutation in the amino finger of GATA-1 affecting DNA binding rather than FOG-1 interaction. *Blood.* 2002;100(6):2040–2045.
77. Murru S, Loudianos G, Porcu S, et al. A β-thalassaemia phenotype not linked to the β-globin cluster in an Italian family. *Br J Haematol.* 1992;81:283–287.
78. Pacheco P, Peres MJ, Faustino P, et al. β-thalassaemia unlinked to the β-globin gene interacts with sickle-cell trait in a Portuguese family. *Br J Haematol.* 1995;91:85–89.
79. Thein SL, Wood WG, Wickramasinghe SN, Galvin MC. β-thalassemia unlinked to the β-globin gene in an English family. *Blood.* 1993;82:961–967.
80. Badens C, Mattei MG, Imbert AM, et al. A novel mechanism for thalassaemia intermedia. *Lancet.* 2002;359(9301):132–133.
81. Galanello R, Perseu L, Perra C, et al. Somatic deletion of the normal beta-globin gene leading to thalassaemia intermedia in heterozygous beta-thalassaemic patients. *Br J Haematol.* 2004;127(5):604–606.
82. Malik P, Arumugam PI. Gene therapy for {beta}-thalassemia. *Hematology Am Soc Hematol Educ Program.* 2005:45–50.
83. Game L, Bergounioux J, Close JP, Marzouka BE, Thein SL. A novel deletion causing (εγδβ)^{o} thalassaemia in a Chilean family. *Br J Haematol.* 2003;123(1):154–159.
84. Rooks H, Bergounioux J, Game L, et al. Heterogeneity of the εγδβ-thalassaemias: characterization of three novel English deletions. *Br J Haematol.* 2005;128(5):722–729.
85. Harteveld CL, Osborne CS, Peters M, et al. Novel 112 kb (epsilonGgammaAgamma) deltabeta-thalassaemia deletion in a Dutch family. *Br J Haematol.* 2003;122(5):855–858.
86. Harteveld CL, Voskamp A, Phylipsen M, et al. Nine unknown rearrangements in 16p13.3 and 11p15.4 causing alpha- and beta-thalassaemia characterised by high resolution multiplex ligation-dependent probe amplification. *J Med Genet.* 2005;42(12):922–931.
87. Jacob GF, Raper AB. Hereditary persistence of foetal haemoglobin production, and its interaction with the sickle-cell trait. *Br J Haematol.* 1958;4:138.
88. Edington GM, Lehmann H. Expression of the sickle-cell gene in Africa. *BMJ.* 1955;i:1308–1311.
89. Wheeler JT, Krevans JR. The homozygous state of persistent fetal hemoglobin and the interaction of persistent fetal hemoglobin with thalassemia. *Bull Johns Hopkins Hosp.* 1961;109:217.
90. Gerald PS, Diamond LK. The diagnosis of thalassemia trait by starch block electrophoresis of the hemoglobin. *Blood.* 1958;13:61–69.
91. Baglioni C. The fusion of two peptide chains in hemoglobin Lepore and its interpretation as a genetic deletion. *Proc Natl Acad Sci USA.* 1962;48:1880–1886.
92. Fessas P, Stamatoyannopoulos G, Karaklis A. Hereditary persistence of foetal haemoglobin and its combination with alpha and beta-thalassaemia. In: *8th Congress of the European Society of Haematology.* Vienna: Karger; 1961:302.
93. Zuelzer WW, Robinson AR, Booker CR. Reciprocal relationship of hemoglobins A2 and F in beta chain thalassemias, a key to the genetic control of hemoglobin F. *Blood.* 1961; 17:393.
94. Brancati C, Baglioni C. Homozygous β thalassaemia (β-microcythaemia). *Nature.* 1966;212:262–264.
95. Schroeder WA, Huisman THJ, Shelton JR, et al. Evidence for multiple structural genes for the γ-chain of human fetal hemoglobin. *Proc Natl Acad Sci USA.* 1968;60:537–544.
96. Fogarty WM, Vedvick TS, Itano HA. Absence of haemoglobin A in an individual simultaneously heterozygous in the genes for hereditary persistence of foetal haemoglobin and beta-thalassaemia. *Br J Haematol.* 1974;26:527.
97. Kosteas T, Palena A, Anagnou NP. Molecular cloning of the breakpoints of the hereditary persistence of fetal hemoglobin type-6 (HPFH-6) deletion and sequence analysis of the novel juxtaposed region from the 3′ end of the β-globin gene cluster. *Hum Genet.* 1997;100:441–445.
98. Huisman THJ, Wrightstone RN, Wilson JB, Schroeder WA, Kendall AG. Hemoglobin Kenya, the product of fusion of γ and β polypeptide chains. *Arch Biochem Biophys.* 1972;153:850.
99. Kendall AG, Ojwang PJ, Schroeder WA, Huisman THJ. Hemoglobin Kenya, the product of a γ-β fusion gene: studies of the family. *Am J Hum Genet.* 1973;25:548.
100. Ojwang PJ, Nakatsuji T, Gardiner MB, Reese AL, Gilman JG, Huisman THJ. Gene deletion as the molecular basis for the Kenya-$^{G}\gamma$-HPFH condition. *Hemoglobin.* 1983;7:115–123.
101. Kosteas T, Moschonas N, Anagnou NP. The molecular basis for the phenotypic differences between δβ-thalassemia and HPFH: the role of the two silencers upstream of the δ-globin gene. *Blood.* 1996;88:105a.

102. Atweh GF, Zhu X-X, Brickner HW, Dowling CH, Kazazian HH, Forget BG. The β-globin gene on the Chinese δβ-thalassemia chromosome carries a promoter mutation. *Blood.* 1987;70:1470–1474.
103. Zeng Y-T, Huang S-Z, Chen B, et al. Hereditary persistence of fetal hemoglobin or $(\delta\beta)^o$-thalassemia: three types observed in South-Chinese families. *Blood.* 1985;66:1430–1435.
104. Forget BG, Hillman DG, Lazarus H, et al. Absence of messenger RNA and gene DNA for β-globin chains in hereditary persistence of fetal hemoglobin. *Cell.* 1976;7:323–329.
105. Fritsch EF, Lawn RM, Maniatis T. Characterisation of deletions which affect the expression of fetal globin genes in man. *Nature.* 1979;279:598.
106. Orkin SH, Alter BP, Altay C, et al. Application of endonuclease mapping to the analysis and prenatal diagnosis of thalassemias caused by globin-gene deletion. *N Engl J Med.* 1978;299:166–172.
107. Acquaye CTA, Oldham JH, Konotey-Ahulu FID. Blood donor homozygous for hereditary persistence of fetal haemoglobin. *Lancet.* 1977;i:796–797.
108. Huisman TH. The first homozygote for the hereditary persistence of fetal hemoglobin observed in the southeastern United States. *Hemoglobin.* 1981;5(4):411–416.
109. Kutlar A, Gardiner MB, Headlee MG, et al. Heterogeneity in the molecular basis of three types of hereditary persistence of fetal hemoglobin and the relative synthesis of the $^G\gamma$ and $^A\gamma$ types of γ chain. *Biochem Genet.* 1984;22:21.
110. Ringelhann B, Konotey-Ahulu FID, Lehmann H, Lorkin PA. A Ghanaian adult, homozygous for hereditary persistence of foetal haemoglobin and heterozygous for elliptocytosis. *Acta Haematol.* 1970;43:100.
111. Tuan D, Murnane MJ, de Riel JK, Forget BG. Heterogeneity in the molecular basis of hereditary persistence of fetal haemoglobin. *Nature.* 1980;285:335.
112. Ferrara M, Matarese SM, Francese M, et al. Hematological and molecular analysis of beta-thalassemia and Hb Lepore in Campania, Italy. *Hemoglobin.* 2001;25(1):29–34.
113. Ribeiro ML, Cunha E, Goncalves P, et al. Hb Lepore-Baltimore (δ^{68Leu}-β^{84Thr}) and Hb Lepore-Washington-Boston (δ^{87Gin}-$\beta^{IVS\text{-}II\text{-}8}$) in Central Portugal and Spanish Alta Extremadura. *Hum Genet.* 1997;99:669–673.
114. Waye JS, Walker L, Kyriakopoulou LG, Potter MA, Eng B. Characterisation of a novel 49.3 kb $^G\gamma(^A\gamma\delta\beta)^0$-thalassaemia deletion in seven families of Asian descent. *Br J Haematol.* 2007;138(1):125–126.
115. Wood WG, Clegg JB, Weatherall DJ, et al. $^G\gamma\delta\beta$ thalassaemia and $^G\gamma$ HPFH (Hb Kenya type). Comparison of two new cases. *J Med Genet.* 1977;14:237.
116. Wood WG, Macrae IA, Darbre PD, Clegg JB, Weatherall DJ. The British type of non-deletion HPFH: characterisation of developmental changes *in vivo* and erythroid growth *in vitro*. *Br J Haematol.* 1982;50:401.
117. Henthorn PS, Smithies O, Mager DL. Molecular analysis of deletions in the human β-globin gene cluster: deletion junctions and locations of breakpoints. *Genomics.* 1990;6:226–237.
118. Huisman THJ, Schroeder WA, Efremov GD, et al. The present status of the heterogeneity of fetal hemoglobin in β-thalassemia; an attempt to unify some observations in thalassemia and related conditions. *Ann NY Acad Sci.* 1974; 232:107–124.
119. Bernards R, Flavell RA. Physical mapping of the globin gene deletion in hereditary persistence of foetal haemoglobin. *Nucl Acids Res.* 1980;8:1521.
120. Calzolari R, McMorrow T, Yannoutsos N, Langeveld A, Grosveld F. Deletion of a region that is a candidate for the difference between the deletion forms of hereditary persistence of fetal hemoglobin and δβ-thalassemia affects β- but not γ-globin gene expression. *EMBO J.* 1999;18:949–958.
121. Gribnau J, Diderich K, Pruzina S, Calzolari R, Fraser P. Intergenic transcription and developmental remodeling of chromatin subdomains in the human beta-globin locus. *Mol Cell.* 2000;5(2):377–386.
122. Gaensler KM, Zhang Z, Lin C, Yang S, Hardt K, Flebbe-Rehwaldt L. Sequences in the $^A\gamma\delta$ intergenic region are not required for stage-specific regulation of the human beta-globin gene locus. *Proc Natl Acad Sci USA.* 2003;100(6):3374–3379.
123. Townes TM, Behringer RR. Human globin locus activation region (LAR): Role in temporal control. *Trends Genet.* 1990;6:219–223.
124. Wood WG. Hb F production in adult life. In: Stamatoyannopoulos G, Nienhuis AW, eds. *Hemoglobin Switching, Part B: Cellular and Molecular Mechanisms.* New York: AR Liss; 1989:251–267.
125. Arcasoy MO, Romana M, Fabry ME, Skarpidi E, Nagel RL, Forget BG. High levels of human γ-globin gene expression in adult mice carrying a transgene of deletion-type hereditary persistence of fetal hemoglobin. *Mol Cell Biol.*1997;17:2076–2089.
126. Dillon N, Grosveld F. Human γ-globin genes silenced independently of other genes in β-globin locus. *Nature.* 1991;350:252–254.
127. Peterson KR, Li QL, Clegg CH, et al. Use of yeast artificial chromosomes (YACs) in studies of mammalian development: production of β-globin locus YAC mice carrying human globin developmental mutants. *Proc Natl Acad Sci USA.* 1995;92:5655–5659.
128. Feingold EA, Forget BG. The breakpoint of a large deletion causing hereditary persistence of fetal hemoglobin occurs within an erythroid DNA domain remote from the β-globin gene cluster. *Blood.* 1989;74:2178–2186.
129. Tuan D, Feingold E, Newman M, Weissman SM, Forget BG. Different 3′ end points of deletions causing δβ-thalassemia and hereditary persistence of fetal hemoglobin; Implications for the control of γ-globin gene expression in man. *Proc Natl Acad Sci USA.* 1983;80:6937.
130. Elder JT, Forrester WC, Thompson C, et al. Translocation of an erythroid-specific hypersensitive site in deletion-type hereditary persistence of fetal hemoglobin. *Mol Cell Biol.* 1990;10:1382–1389.
131. Forrester WC, Epner E, Driscoll MC, et al. A deletion of the human β-globin locus activation region causes a major alteration in chromatin structure and replication across the entire β-globin locus. *Genes Dev.* 1990;4:1637–1649.
132. Xiang P, Han H, Barkess G, et al. Juxtaposition of the HPFH2 enhancer is not sufficient to reactivate the gamma-globin gene in adult erythropoiesis. *Hum Mol Genet.* 2005; 14(20):3047–56.
133. Anagnou NP, Perez-Stable C, Gelinas R, et al. Sequences located 3′ to the breakpoint of the hereditary persistence of fetal hemoglobin-3 deletion exhibit enhancer activity and

can modify the developmental expression of the human fetal $^{A}\gamma$-globin gene in transgenic mice. *J Biol Chem.* 1995; 270:10256–10263.
134. Katsantoni EZ, Langeveld A, Wai AW, et al. Persistent gamma-globin expression in adult transgenic mice is mediated by HPFH-2, HPFH-3, and HPFH-6 breakpoint sequences. *Blood.* 2003;102(9):3412–3419.
135. Fessas P. The beta-chain thalassaemias. In: Lehmann H, Betke K, eds. *Haemoglobin Colloquium.* Vienna: Thieme; 1961:90.
136. Fessas P, Stamatoyannopoulos G. Hereditary persistence of fetal hemoglobin in Greece. A study and a comparison. *Blood.* 1964;24:223.
137. Huisman THJ, Schroeder WA, Stamatoyannopoulos G, et al. Nature of fetal hemoglobin in the Greek type of hereditary persistence of fetal hemoglobin with and without concurrent β-thalassemia. *J Clin Invest.* 1970;49:1035.
138. Huisman THJ, Miller A, Schroeder WA. A $^{G}\gamma$ type of the hereditary persistence of fetal hemoglobin with beta chain production in cis. *Am J Hum Genet.* 1975;27:765–777.
139. Weatherall DJ, Cartner R, Clegg JB, Wood WG, Macrae IA, MacKenzie A. A form of hereditary persistence of fetal haemoglobin characterised by uneven cellular distribution of haemoglobin F and the production of haemoglobins A and A_2 in homozygotes. *Br J Haematol.* 1975;29:205.
140. Jones RW, Old JM, Wood WG, Clegg JB, Weatherall DJ. Restriction endonuclease maps of the β-like globin gene cluster in the British and Greek forms of HPFH, and for one example of $^{G}\gamma^{+}$ HPFH. *Br J Haematol.* 1982;50:415–422.
141. Collins FS, Stoeckert CJ, Serjeant GR, Forget BG, Weissman SM. $^{G}\gamma^{+}$ hereditary persistence of fetal hemoglobin: cosmid cloning and identification of a specific mutation 5′ to the $^{G}\gamma$ gene. *Proc Natl Acad Sci USA.* 1984;81:4894–4898.
142. Collins FS, Metherall JE, Yamakawa M, Pan J, Weissman SM, Forget BG. A point mutation in the $^{A}\gamma$-globin gene promoter in Greek hereditary persistence of fetal haemoglobin. *Nature.* 1985;313:325.
143. Gelinas R, Bender M, Lotshaw C, Waber P, Kazazian HHJ, Stamatoyannopoulos G. Chinese $^{A}\gamma$ fetal hemoglobin: C to T substitution at position −196 of the $^{A}\gamma$ gene promoter. *Blood.* 1986;67:1777–1779.
144. Giglioni B, Casini C, Mantovani R, et al. A molecular study of a family with Greek hereditary persistence of fetal hemoglobin and β-thalassemia. *EMBO J.* 1984;3:2641–2645.
145. Metherall JE, Gillespie FP, Forget BG. Analyses of linked β-globin genes suggest that nondeletion forms of hereditary persistence of fetal hemoglobin are bona fide switching mutants. *Am J Hum Genet.* 1988;42:476–481.
146. Tate VE, Wood WG, Weatherall DJ. The British form of hereditary persistence of fetal haemoglobin results from a single base mutation adjacent to an S1 hypersensitive site 5′ to the $^{A}\gamma$ globin gene. *Blood.* 1986;68:1389–1393.
147. Waber PG, Bender MA, Gelinas RE, et al. Concordance of a point mutation 5′ to the $^{A}\gamma$ globin gene in $^{A}\gamma\beta^{+}$ HPFH in Greeks. *Blood.* 1986;67:551–554.
148. Berry M, Grosveld F, Dillon N. A single point mutation is the cause of the Greek form of hereditary persistence of fetal haemoglobin. *Nature.* 1992;358:499–502.
149. Starck J, Sarkar R, Romana M, et al. Developmental regulation of human γ- and β-globin genes in the absence of the locus control region. *Blood.* 1994;84:1656–1665.
150. Bacolla A, Ulrich MJ, Larson JE, Ley TJ, Wells RD. An intramolecular triplex in the human gamma-globin 5′-flanking region is altered by point mutations associated with hereditary persistence of fetal hemoglobin. *J Biol Chem.* 1995; 270(41):24556–24563.
151. Fischer K-D, Nowock J. The T→C substitution at −198 of the $^{A}\gamma$-globin gene associated with the British form of HPFH generates overlapping recognition sites for two DNA-binding proteins. *Nucl Acids Res.* 1990;18:5685–5693.
152. Fucharoen S, Shimizu K, Fukumaki Y. A novel C-T transition within the distal CCAAT motif of the $^{G}\gamma$-globin gene in the Japanese HPFH: implication of factor binding in elevated fetal globin expression. *Nucl Acids Res.* 1990;18:5245–5253.
153. Gumucio DL, Rood KL, Gray TA, Riordan MF, Sartor CI, Collins FS. Nuclear proteins that bind the human γ-globin gene promoter: alterations in binding produced by point mutations associated with hereditary persistence of fetal hemoglobin. *Mol Cell Biol.*1988;8:5310–5322.
154. Gumucio DL, Rood KL, Blanchard-McQuate KL, Gray TA, Saulino A, Collins FS. Interaction of Sp1 with the human γ globin promoter: binding and transactivation of normal and mutant promoters. *Blood.* 1991;78:1853–1863.
155. Jane SM, Gumucio DL, Ney PA, Cunningham JM, Nienhuis AW. Methylation-enhanced binding of Sp1 to the stage selector element of the human γ-globin gene promoter may regulate developmental specificity of expression. *Mol Cell Biol.* 1993;13(6):3272–3281.
156. Mantovani R, Malgaretti N, Nicolis S, Ronchi A, Giglioni B, Ottolenghi S. The effects of HPFH mutations in the human γ-globin promoter on binding of ubiquitous and erythroid specific nuclear factors. *Nucl Acids Res.* 1988;16:7783–7797.
157. Mantovani R, Superti-Furga G, Gilman J, Ottolenghi S. The deletion of the distal CCAAT box region of the A gamma-globin gene in black HPFH abolishes the binding of the erythroid specific protein NFE3 and of the CCAAT displacement protein. *Nucl Acids Res.* 1989;17(16):6681–91.
158. Martin DIK, Tsai S-F, Orkin SH. Increased γ-globin expression in a nondeletion HPFH mediated by an erythroid-specific DNA-binding factor. *Nature.* 1989;338:435–438.
159. Ronchi A, Nicolis S, Santoro C, Ottolenghi S. Increased Sp1 binding mediates erythroid-specific overexpression of a mutated (HPFH) γ-globin promoter. *Nucl Acids Res.* 1989;17: 10231–10241.
160. Superti-Furga G, Barberis A, Schaffner G, Busslinger M. The −117 mutation in Greek HPFH affects the binding of three nuclear factors to the CCAAT region of the γ-globin gene. *EMBO J.* 1988;7:3099–30107.
161. Sykes K, Kaufman R. A naturally occurring gamma globin gene mutation enhances SP1 binding activity. *Mol Cell Biol.* 1990;10:95–102.
162. Ulrich MJ, Gray WJ, Ley TJ. An intramolecular DNA triplex is disrupted by point mutations associated with hereditary persistence of fetal hemoglobin. *J Biol Chem.* 1992;267:18649–18658.
163. Gumucio DL, Lockwood WK, Weber JL, et al. The −175 T-C mutation increases promoter strength in erythroid cells: correlaion with evolutionary conservation of binding sites for two *trans*-acting factors. *Blood.* 1990;75:756–761.
164. Lanclos KD, Michael SK, Gu TC, Howard EF, Stoming TA, Huisman THJ. Transient chloramphenicol acetyltransferase

expression of the $^G\gamma$ globin gene 5′-flanking regions containing substitutions of C→T at position −158, G→A at position −161, and T→A at position −175 in K562 cells. *Biochim Biophys Acta.* 1989;1008:109–112.
165. Motum PI, Lindeman R, Harvey MP, Trent RJ. Comparative studies of nondeletional HPFH γ-globin gene promoters. *Exp Hematol.* 1993;21:852–858.
166. Nicolis S, Ronchi A, Malgaretti N, Mantovani R, Giglioni B, Ottolenghi S. Increased erythroid-specific expression of a mutated HPFH γ globin promoter requires the erythroid factor NFE-1. *Nucl Acids Res.* 1989;17:5509–5516.
167. Rixon MW, Gelinas RE. A fetal globin gene mutation in $^A\gamma$ nondeletion HPFH increases promoter strength in a non-erythroid cell. *Mol Cell Biol.* 1988;8:713–721.
168. Ulrich MJ, Ley TJ. Function of normal and mutated γ-globin gene promoters in electroporated K562 erythroleukemia cells. *Blood.* 1990;75:990–999.
169. Roberts NA, Sloane-Stanley JA, Sharpe JA, Stanworth SJ, Wood WG. Globin gene switching in transgenic mice carrying HS2-globin gene constructs. *Blood.* 1997;89:713–723.
170. Ronchi A, Berry M, Raguz S, et al. Role of the duplicated CCAAT box region in γ-globin gene regulation and hereditary persistence of fetal haemoglobin. *EMBO J.* 1996;15:143–149.
171. Wijgerde M, Grosveld F, Fraser P. Transcription complex stability and chromatin dynamics. *Nature.* 1995;377:209–213.
172. Craig JE, Rochette J, Fisher CA, et al. Haemoglobin switch: dissecting the loci controlling fetal haemoglobin production on chromosomes 11p and 6q by the regressive approach. *Nat Genet.* 1996;12:58–64.
173. Craig JE, Rochette J, Sampietro M, et al. Genetic heterogeneity in heterocellular hereditary persistence of fetal hemoglobin. *Blood.* 1997;90:428–434.
174. Giampaolo A, Mavilio F, Sposi NM, et al. Heterocellular HPFH: molecular mechanisms of abnormal γ gene expression in association with β thalassemia and linkage relationship with the β globin gene cluster. *Hum Genet.* 1984;66:151–156.
175. Gianni AM, Bregni M, Cappellini MD, et al. A gene controlling fetal hemoglobin expression in adults is not linked to the non-α globin cluster. *EMBO J.* 1983;2:921–926.
176. Martinez G, Novelletto A, Di Renzo A, Felicetti L, Colombo B. A case of hereditary persistence of fetal hemoglobin caused by a gene not linked to the β-globin cluster. *Hum Genet.* 1989;82:335–337.
177. Oppenheim A, Yaari A, Rund D, et al. Intrinsic potential for high fetal hemoglobin production in a Druz family with β-thalassemia is due to an unlinked genetic determinant. *Hum Genet.* 1990;86:175–180.
178. Seltzer WK, Abshire TC, Lane PA, Roloff JS, Githens JH. Molecular genetic studies in black families with sickle cell anemia and unusually high levels of fetal hemoglobin. *Hemoglobin.* 1992;16:363–377.
179. Thein SL, Weatherall DJ. A non-deletion hereditary persistence of fetal hemoglobin (HPFH) determinant not linked to the β-globin gene complex. In: Stamatoyannopoulos G, Nienhuis AW, eds. *Hemoglobin Switching, Part B: Cellular and Molecular Mechanisms.* New York: Alan R. Liss; 1989:97–112.
180. Miyoshi K, Kaneto Y, Kawai H, Huisman THJ. X-linked dominant control of F-cells in normal adult life. *Blood.* 1988;72:1854.
181. Dover GJ, Smith KD, Chang YC, et al. Fetal hemoglobin levels in sickle cell disease and normal individuals are partially controlled by an X-linked gene located at Xp22.2. *Blood.* 1992;80:816–824.
182. Chang YC, Smith KD, Moore RD, Serjeant GR, Dover GJ. An analysis of fetal hemoglobin variation in sickle cell disease: the relative contributions of the X-linked factor, β-globin haplotypes, α-globin gene number, gender and age. *Blood.* 1995;85:1111–1117.
183. Thein SL, Sampietro M, Rohde K, Weatherall DJ, Lathrop GM, Demenais F. Detection of a major gene for heterocellular HPFH after accounting for genetic modifiers. American Journal of *Hum Genet.* 1994;54:214–228.
184. Close J, Game L, Clark B, Bergounioux J, Gerovassili A, Thein SL. Genome annotation of a 1.5 Mb region of human chromosome 6q23 encompassing a quantitative trait locus for fetal hemoglobin expression in adults. *BMC Genomics.* 2004;5(1):33.
185. Garner CP, Tatu T, Best S, Creary L, Thein SL. Evidence of genetic interaction between the beta-globin complex and chromosome 8q in the expression of fetal hemoglobin. *Am J Hum Genet.* 2002;70(3):793–799.
186. Garner C, Menzel S, Martin C, et al. Interaction between two quantitative trait loci affects fetal haemoglobin expression. *Ann Hum Genet.* 2005;69(Pt 6):707–714.
187. Menzel S, Garner C, Gut I, et al. A QTL influencing F cell production maps to a gene encoding a zinc-finger protein on chromosome 2p15. *Nat Genet.* 2007;39(10):1197–1199.
188. Gilman JG, Huisman THJ. DNA sequence variation associated with elevated fetal $^G\gamma$ globin production. *Blood.* 1985;66:783–787.
189. Labie D, Pagnier J, Lapoumeroulie C, et al. Common haplotype dependency of high $^G\gamma$-globin gene expression and high Hb F levels in β-thalassemia and sickle cell anemia patients. *Proc Natl Acad Sci USA.* 1985;82:2111–2114.
190. Labie D, Dunda-Belkhodja O, Rouabhi F, Pagnier J, Ragusa A, Nagel RL. The −158 site 5′ to the $^G\gamma$ gene and $^G\gamma$ expression. *Blood.* 1985;66:1463–1465.
191. Gilman JG, Huisman THJ. Two independentgenetic factors in the β-globin gene cluster are associated with high $^G\gamma$-levels in the HbF of SS patients. *Blood.* 1984;64:452–457.
192. Elion J, Berg PE, Lapoumeroulie C, et al. DNA sequence variation in a negative control region 5′ to the β-globin gene correlates with the phenotypic expression of the β^S mutation. *Blood.* 1992;79:787–792.
193. Lanclos KD, Oner C, Dimovski AJ, Gu Y-C, Huisman THJ. Sequence variations in the 5′ flanking and IVS-II regions of the $^G\gamma$- and $^A\gamma$-globin genes of β^S chromosomes with five different haplotypes. *Blood.* 1991;77:2488–2496.
194. Pissard S, Beuzard Y. A potential regulatory region for the expression of fetal hemoglobin in sickle cell disease. *Blood.* 1994;84:331–338.
195. Beris P, Kitundu MN, Baysal E, et al. Black β-thalassemia homozygotes with specific sequence variations in the 5′ hypersensitive site-2 of the locus control region have high levels of fetal hemoglobin. *Am J Hematol.* 1992;41:97–101.

196. Merghoub T, Perichon B, Maier-Redesperger M, et al. Variation of fetal hemoglobin and F-cell number with the LCR-HS2 polymorphism in nonanemic individuals. *Blood.* 1996;87:2607–2609.

197. Öner C, Dimovski AJ, Altay C, et al. Sequence variations in the 5′ hypersensitive site-2 of the locus control region of β^S chromosomes are associated with different levels of fetal globin in hemoglobin S homozygotes. *Blood.* 1992;79:813–819.

198. Eng B, Walker L, Nakamura LM, et al. Three new beta-globin gene promoter mutations identified through newborn screening. *Hemoglobin.* 2007;31(2):129–134.

199. Sadiq MF, Eigel A, Horst J. Spectrum of beta-thalassemia in Jordan: identification of two novel mutations. *Am J Hematol.* 2001;68(1):16–22.

200. Akar E, Ozdemir S, Hakki Timur I, Akar N. First observation of homozygous hemoglobin hamadan (B 56 (D7) GLY-ARG) and beta thalassemia (−29 G >A)-hemoglobin Hamadan combination in a Turkish family. *Am J Hematol.* 2003;74(4):280–282.

201. Basran RK, Reiss UM, Luo HY, Ware RE, Chui DH. Beta-thalassemia intermedia due to compound heterozygosity for two beta-globin gene promoter mutations, including a novel TATA box deletion. *Pediatr Blood Cancer.* 2008;50(2):363–366.

202. De Angioletti M, Lacerra G, Sabato V, Carestia C. Beta + 45 G→C: a novel silent beta-thalassaemia mutation, the first in the Kozak sequence. *Br J Haematol.* 2004;124(2):224–231.

203. Waye JS, Walker L, Patterson M, Chui DH. Identification of two new beta-thalassemia splice mutations: IVS-I-1 (G→>C) and IVS-I (−2) (A→C). *Hemoglobin.* 2002;26(1):87–89.

204. Fujihara N, Tozuka M, Ueno I, et al. Novel beta-thalassemia trait (IVS I-1 G→C) in a Japanese family. *Am J Hematol.* 2003;72(1):64–66.

205. Basak AN. The molecular pathology of beta-thalassemia in Turkey: the Bogazici university experience. *Hemoglobin.* 2007;31(2):233–241.

206. Rojnuckarin P, Settapiboon R, Vanichsetakul P, Sueblinvong T, Sutcharitchan P. Severe β^0 thalassemia/hemoglobin E disease caused by de novo 22-base pair duplication in the paternal allele of beta globin gene. *Am J Hematol.* 2007;82(7):663–665.

207. Cross TJ, Berry PA, Akbar N, Wendon J, Thein SL, Harrison PM. Sickle liver disease–An unusual presentation in a compound heterozygote for HbS and a novel beta-thalassemia mutation. *Am J Hematol.* 2007;82(9):852–854.

208. Lacan P, Becchi M, Zanella-Cleon I, et al. Two new beta-chain variants: Hb Tripoli [beta26(B8)Glu→Ala] and Hb Tizi-Ouzou [beta29(B11)Gly→Ser]. *Hemoglobin.* 2004;28(3):205–212.

209. Jacquette A, Le Roux G, Lacombe C, Goossens M, Pissard S. Compound heterozygosity for two new mutations in the beta-globin gene [codon 9 (+TA) and polyadenylation site (AATAAA→AAAAAA)] leads to thalassemia intermedia in a Tunisian patient. *Hemoglobin.* 2004;28(3):243–248.

210. Ma SK, Lee ACW, Chan AYY, Chan LC. A novel AATAAA→CATAAA mutation at the polyadenylation site of the β-globin gene. *Br J Haematol.* 2001;115(1):231–231.

211. Waye JS, Eng B, Patterson M, Reis MD, Macdonald D, Chui DH. Novel beta-thalassemia mutation in a beta-thalassemia intermedia patient. *Hemoglobin.* 2001;25(1):103–105.

212. Lacan P, Ponceau B, Aubry M, Francina A. Mild Hb S-beta(+)-thalassemia with a deletion of five nucleotides at the polyadenylation site of the beta-globin gene. *Hemoglobin.* 2003;27(4):257–259.

213. Knott M, Ramadan KM, Savage G, et al. Novel and Mediterranean beta thalassemia mutations in the indigenous Northern Ireland population. *Blood Cells Mol Dis.* 2006;36(2):265–268.

214. Grignoli CR, Carvalho MH, Kimura EM, et al. Beta^0-thalassemia resulting from a novel mutation: beta66/u→stop codon. *Eur J Haematol.* 2000;64(2):137–138.

215. Patterson M, Walker L, Chui DH, Cohen AR, Waye JS. Identification of a new beta-thalassemia nonsense mutation [codon 59 (AAG→TAG)]. *Hemoglobin.* 2003;27(3):201–203.

216. Mo QH, Li XR, Li CF, He YL, Xu XM. A novel frameshift mutation (+G) at codons 15/16 in a beta^0 thalassaemia gene results in a significant reduction of beta globin mRNA values. *J Clin Pathol.* 2005;58(9):923–926.

217. Lacan P, Aubry M, Couprie N, Francina A. Two new beta^o-thalassemic mutations: a deletion (-CC) at codon 142 or overlapping codons 142–143, and an insertion (+T) at codon 45 or overlapping codons 44–45(45–46 of the beta-globin gene. *Hemoglobin.* 2007;31(2):159–165.

218. Nadkarni A, Sakaguchi T, Takaku H, et al. A novel beta^o-thalassemia mutation at codon 55 (−A) and a rare 17 bp deletion at codons 126–131 in the Indian population. *Hemoglobin.* 2002;26(1):41–47.

219. Shaji RV, Gerard N, Krishnamoorthy R, Srivastava A, Chandy M. A novel beta-thalassemia mutation in an Asian Indian. *Hemoglobin.* 2002;26(1):49–57.

220. Foulon K, Rochette J, Cadet E. A novel beta-thalassemic allele due to a two nucleotide deletion: beta76 (−GC). *Hemoglobin.* 2007;31(1):31–37.

221. Shaji RV, Srivastava A, Krishnamoorthy R, Chandy M. Coexistence of a novel beta-globin gene deletion (codons 81–87) with the codon 30 (G→C) mutation in an Indian patient with beta0-thalassemia. *Hemoglobin.* 2002;26(3):237–243.

222. Flatz G, Wilke K, Syagailo YV, Eigel A, Horst J. Beta-thalassemia in the German population: mediterranean, Asian and novel mutations. Mutations in brief no. 228. Online. *Hum Mutat.* 1999;13(3):258.

223. Giordano PC, Addo-Daaku A, Sander MJ, et al. The rare Hb Showa-Yakushiji [beta110(G12)Leu→Pro, CTG→CCG] in combination with an alpha gene triplication found in a Dutch patient during her first pregnancy examination. *Hemoglobin.* 2007;31(2):167–171.

224. Keser I, Kayisli OG, Yesilipek A, Ozes ON, Luleci G. Hb Antalya [codons 3–5 (Leu-Thr-Pro→Ser-Asp-Ser)]: a new unstable variant leading to chronic microcytic anemia and high Hb A2. *Hemoglobin.* 2001;25(4):369–373.

225. Hall GW, Franklin IM, Sura T, Thein SL. A novel mutation (nonsense β127) in exon 3 of the β globin gene produces a variable thalassaemia phenotype. *Br J Haematol.* 1991;79:342–344.

226. Luo HY, Tang W, Eung SH, et al. Dominantly inherited beta thalassaemia intermedia caused by a new single nucleotide deletion in exon 2 of the beta globin gene: Hb morgantown (beta91 CTG>CG). *J Clin Pathol.* 2005;58(10):1110–1112.

227. Lahr G, Brintrup J, Over S, Feurle GE, Debatin K-M, Kohne E. Codon 104(→G), a heterozygous frameshift mutation in exon 2 of HBB, resulted in a dominantly inherited

beta-phenotype with mild anemia in a German kindred, and thalassemia intermedia in the index patient. A co-inherited a gene triplication, long-term transfusion therapy, and ineffective erythropoiesis were confounding factors. *Haematologica.* 2007;92:1264–1265.

228. Waye JS, Walker L, Lafferty J, Lemire EG, Chui DH. Dominant beta-thalassemia due to a newly identified frameshift mutation in exon 3 (codon 113, GTG→Tg). *Hemoglobin.* 2002;26(1):83–86.

229. Ropero P, Villegas A, Martinez M, Ataulfo Gonzalez Fernandez F, Benavente C, Mateo M. A deletion of 11 bp (CD 131–134) in exon 3 of the beta-globin gene produces the phenotype of inclusion body beta-thalassemia. *Ann Hematol.* 2005;84(9):584–587.

230. Weinstein BI, Erramouspe B, Albuquerque DM, et al. Hb Florida: a novel elongated C-terminal beta-globin variant causing dominant beta-thalassemia phenotype. *Am J Hematol.* 2006;81(5):358–360.

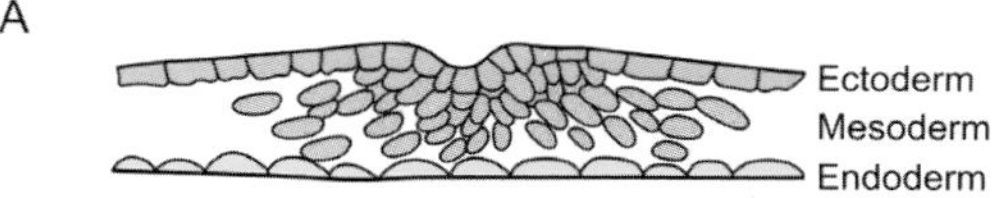

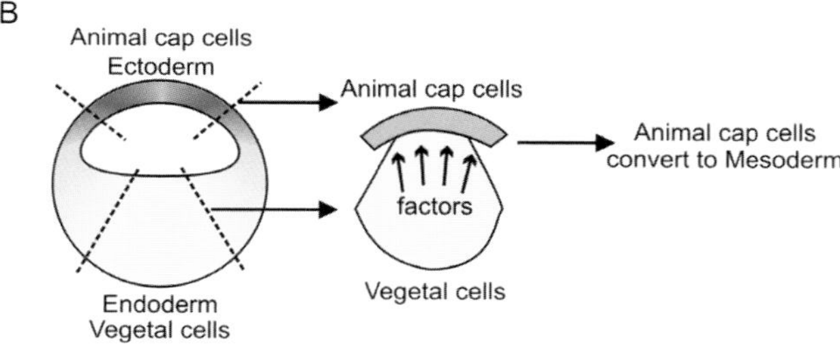

Plate 1.1. Schematic diagram of germ layer development in vertebrate embryos. **(A)** Mesoderm arises from an inductive interaction between ectoderm and endoderm. **(B)** Experimental scheme in Xenopus embryos that shows that mesodermal cells arise from the ectoderm (animal cap cells) under the inductive influence of the endodermal vegetal fragment.

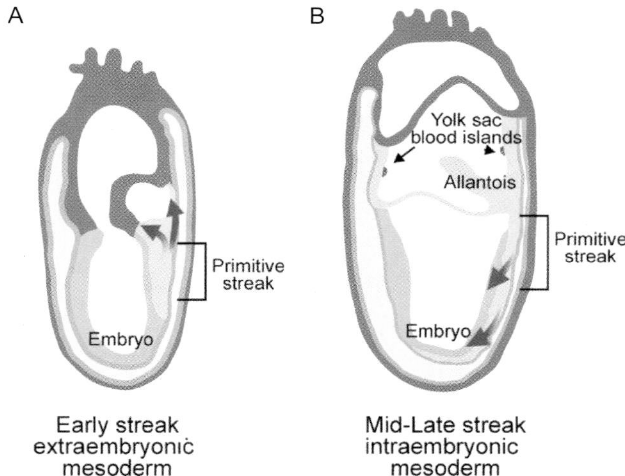

Plate 1.2. Mesodermal migration during mouse embryogenesis. **(A)** Schematic diagram of a mouse conceptus at the early primitive streak stage. Emerging from the posterior primitive streak are waves of yolk sac mesoderm (red arrows) migrating to form this extraembryonic tissues. Slightly later, this mesoderm also forms the allantois. Hemangioblasts are found in the posterior primitive streak. **(B)** Schematic diagram of a mouse conceptus at the mid–late primitive streak stage. Mesoderm emerging from the anterior primitive streak forms the paraxial and lateral mesoderm of the trunk region of the embryo (mesoderm for the prospective PAS/AGM region). At this stage the allantois is visible, as are the first primitive erythroid cells in the yolk sac blood islands. (Drawings adapted from ref. 3.)

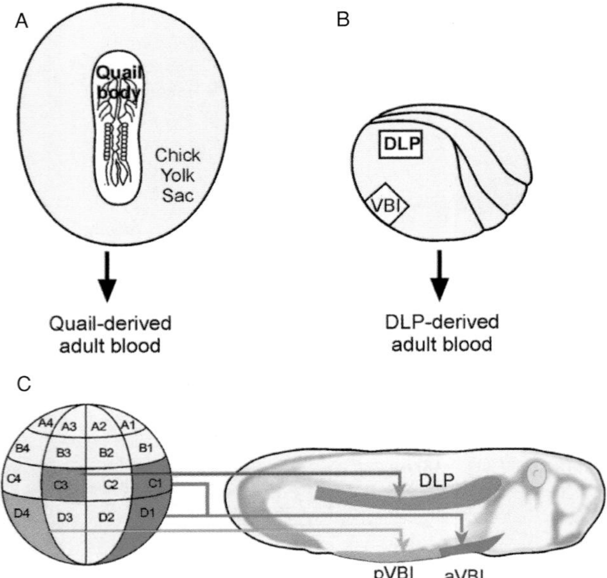

Plate 1.3. Nonmammalian vertebrate embryo–grafting experiments used for determining the origin of the adult hematopoietic system. **(A)** A schematic diagram of the avian embryo grafting strategy in which quail embryo bodies were grafted onto chick yolk sacs at the precirculation stage of development. **(B)** A schematic diagram of the amphibian embryo grafting strategy in which genetically marked dorsal lateral plate (DLP) or ventral blood island (VBI) regions were transplanted onto unmarked Xenopus or Rana embryos. **(C)** Genetic marking experiment in 32 blastomere Xenopus embryo (left). Marking of the C3 blastomere, D4 blastomere, and C1 and D1 blastomeres allowed the tracing of progeny cells to the DLP, pVBi, and aVBl, respectively, at the larval stage (right). (Drawings adapted from ref. 3.)

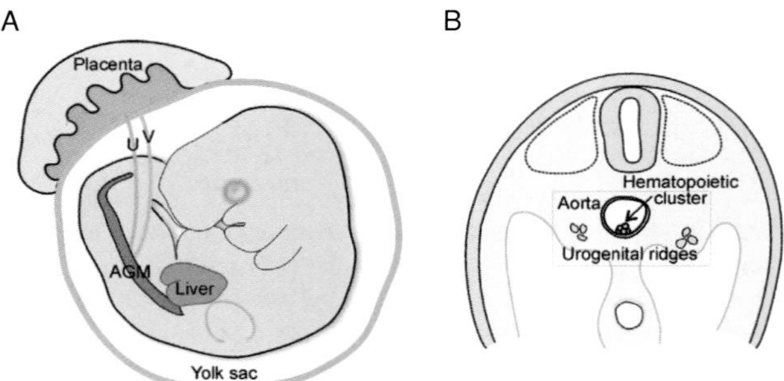

Plate 1.4. Sites of hematopoietic activity in the midgestation mouse conceptus. **(A)** A whole E10.5 mouse conceptus is shown. The placenta, AGM, yolk sac, and the vitelline (V) and umbilical (U) vessels harbor and/or generate hematopoietic cells at this time. **(B)** Transverse section through the AGM region of an E10.5 mouse embryo is shown. The dorsal aorta is located in the midline, with the neural tube on the dorsal and gut on the ventral side. The urogenital ridges laterally flank the aorta. Hematopoietic cell clusters are found in the lumen of the dorsal aorta as they emerge from the ventral hemogenic endothelium.

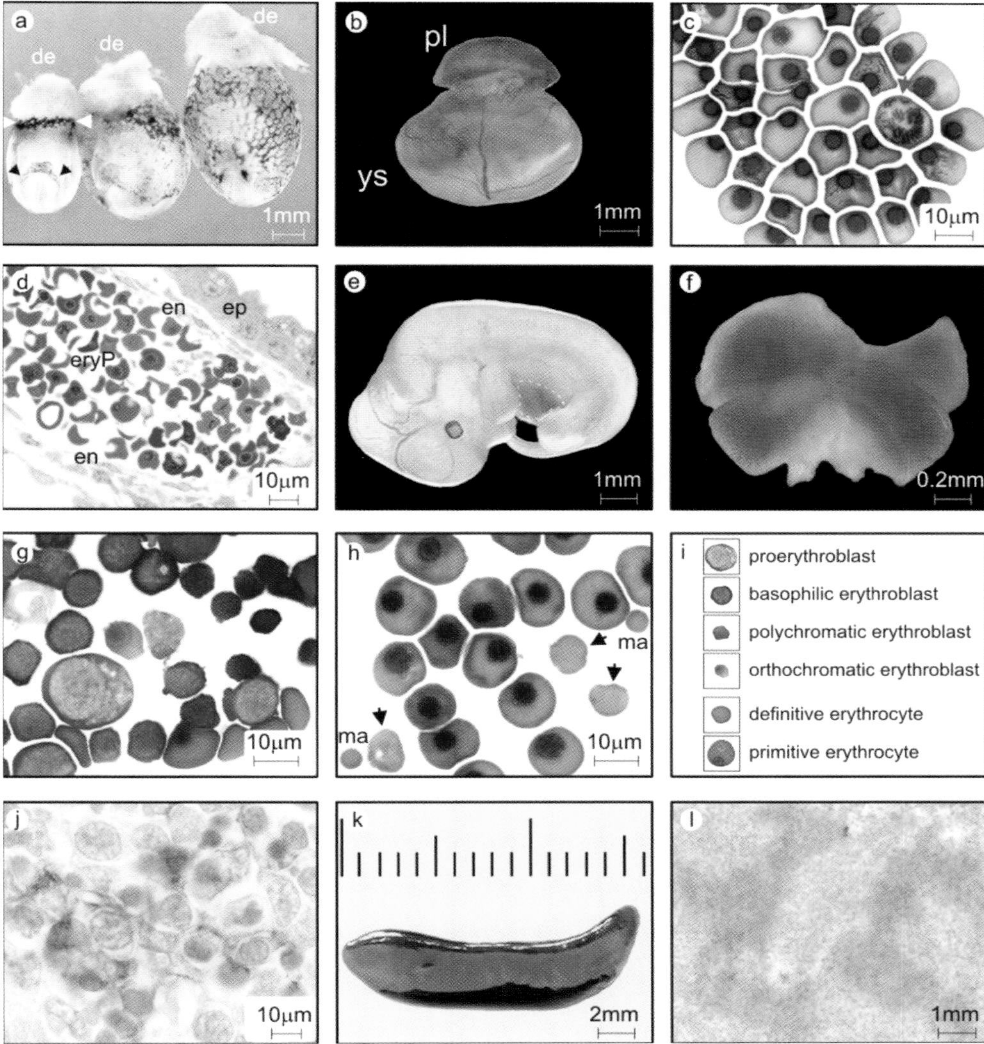

Plate 2.1. Erythropoiesis during mouse development. **(a)** E8.5 embryos, inside their yolk sacs, carrying a *LacZ* reporter gene driven by *β-globin* regulatory elements. Erythroid cells appear blue after staining for LacZ activity. White arrowheads point at the blood islands emerging as a ring at the top of the yolk sac. These are spreading through the developing vasculature, illustrated by the two embryos on the right that are progressively more advanced in development. The black arrowheads indicate the linear heart tube that already appears to contain erythroid cells before the yolk sac cells have reached the embryo. de = decidua, remaining maternal tissue. **(b)** E11.5 embryo inside its yolk sac. The blood-filled yolk sac vasculature is apparent. ys = yolk sac; pl = placenta. **(c)** Cytospin of E11.5 peripheral blood, stained with dianisidine and histological dyes.[207] Nuclei are blue, the hemoglobin-filled cytoplasm brown. Red arrow: cell in mitosis. **(d)** Section of a yolk sac vessel at E12.5, stained with toluidine/methylene blue. eryP = primitive erythrocytes; en = endothelial cells; ep = columnar epithelial cells. **(e)** E12.5 mouse embryo; the fetal liver area is indicated by a dotted line. **(f)** E12.5 fetal liver. **(g)** Cytospin of E12.5 fetal liver cells, stained as in (c). **(h)** Cytospin of E12.5 blood, stained as in (c). ma = contaminating maternal erythrocyte **(i)** key to (g) and (h). **(j)** Erythroblastic island in E13.5 fetal liver. The cytoplasmic extensions of the central macrophage (stained with the F4/80 antibody [brown]) are surrounding erythroid cells at various stages of differentiation. **(k)** Spleen of an adult mouse. **(l)** Section of adult mouse spleen stained as in (c). Red pulp, containing the erythroid cells, is stained brown; white pulp is stained blue.

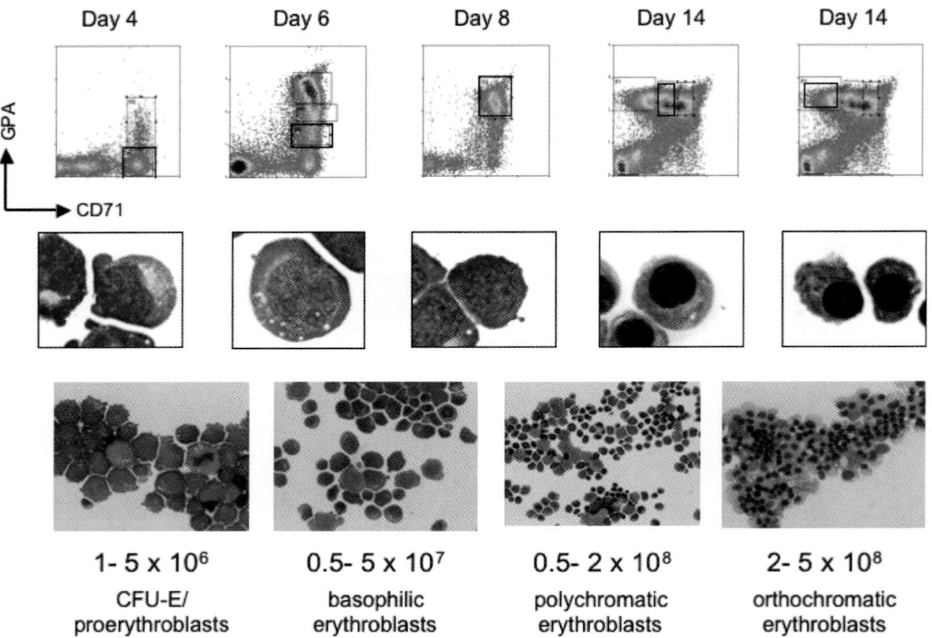

Plate 2.3. Purification of human erythroblasts. Top: FACS analysis of human erythroblasts grown in vitro by the method of Fibach et al; days refers to the time in phase 2 of culture. Middle: High-power view of cells sorted from the gate shown as a bold rectangle in the plot above. Bottom: Low-power view of the same sorted cells, together with representative cell numbers obtainable from mononuclear cells from 1 U of blood.

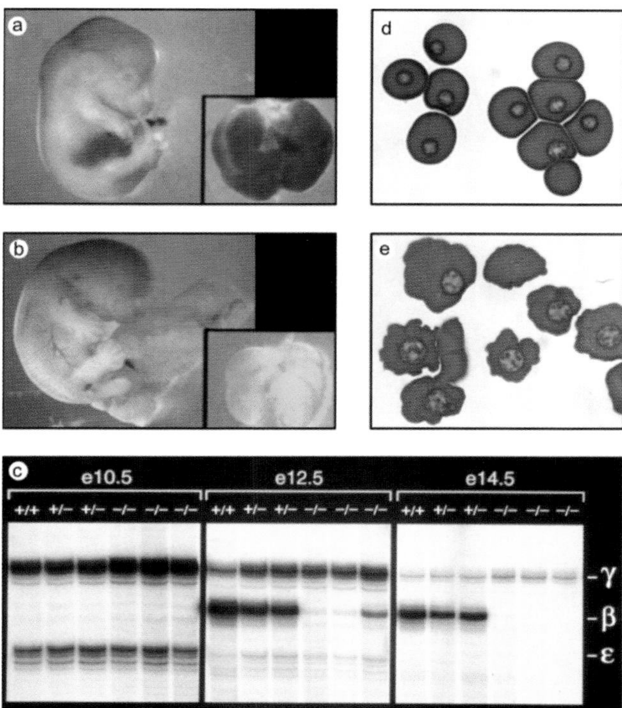

Plate 2.8. Phenotype of EKLF knockout fetuses. **(a)** E13.5 wild-type fetus. Inset: fetal liver. **(b)** E13.5 EKLF knockout fetus, displaying obvious pallor of the fetal liver (inset). **(c)** Mice carrying a human β-globin locus transgene were crossed with EKLF knockout mice. Expression analysis of the human *β-like globin* genes is shown at various gestational ages. Note that in the EKLF knockout background (−/−) the adult *β-globin* gene fails to be activated, whereas expression of the embryonic *ε-globin* and *fetal γ-globin* genes is not affected. **(d)** Cytospin of E12.5 blood from wild-type fetus, displaying primitive erythrocytes. **(e)** Cytospin of E12.5 blood from EKLF knockout fetus displaying primitive erythrocytes. Note the irregular shape of the cell membranes, compared with (d). (d) and (e) Adapted from ref. 191.

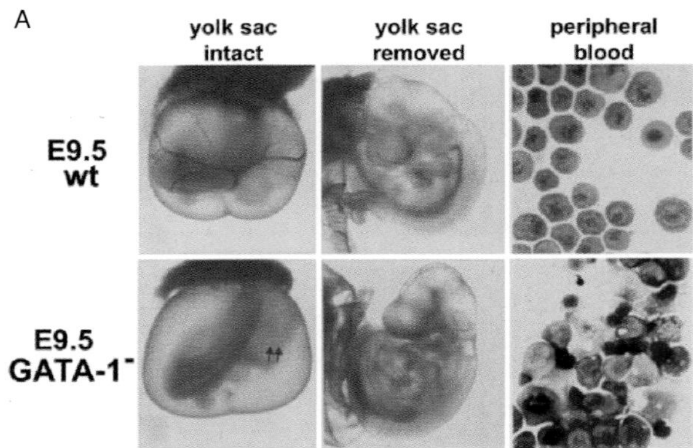

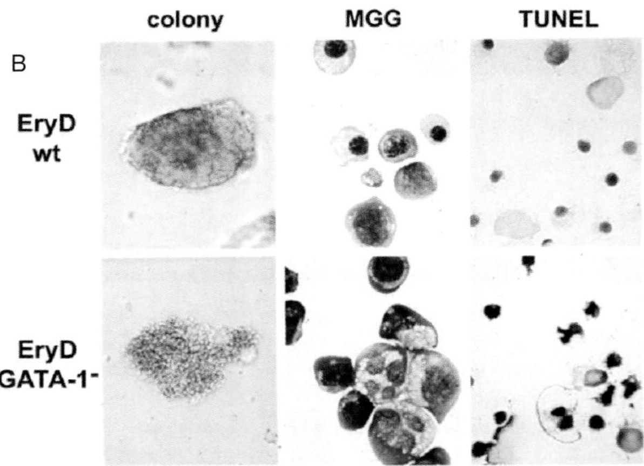

Plate 4.5. Loss of GATA-1 blocks erythroid maturation. **(A)** Impaired primitive erythropoiesis in *Gata1*-embryos. **(B)** Developmental arrest and apoptosis of cells within definitive erythroid (EryD) colonies generated by in vitro differentiation of *Gata1*-ESCs. (Modified from Weiss et al. and Fujiwara et al. Copyright 1995 and 1996, National Academy of Sciences, U.S.A. Photographs in panel A provided by Yuko Fujiwara and Stuart Orkin.)

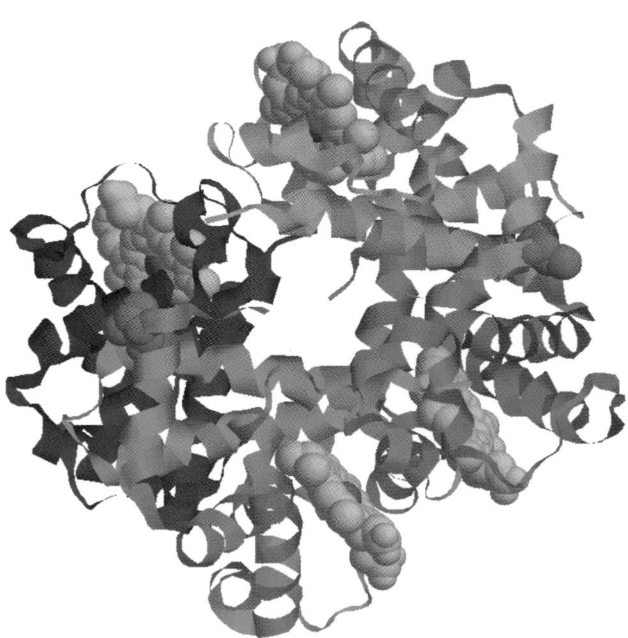

Plate 6.1. Ribbon diagram of a sickle cell hemoglobin tetramer. Each of the four subunits is shown in a different color. Four heme groups (yellow-orange) are shown with an iron (red) atom in the middle. The valine residues resulting from the single point mutation causing sickle cell disease are shown at the β6 position on each β subunit (purple). The molecule is shown looking down the axis where 2,3 bisphosphoglycerate binds. Except for the substitution of valine for glutamate, normal HbA would appear the same as the molecule shown. (The illustration was derived from the Protein Explorer (http://www.umass.edu/microbio/rasmol/) and data from the Protein Data Bank.)

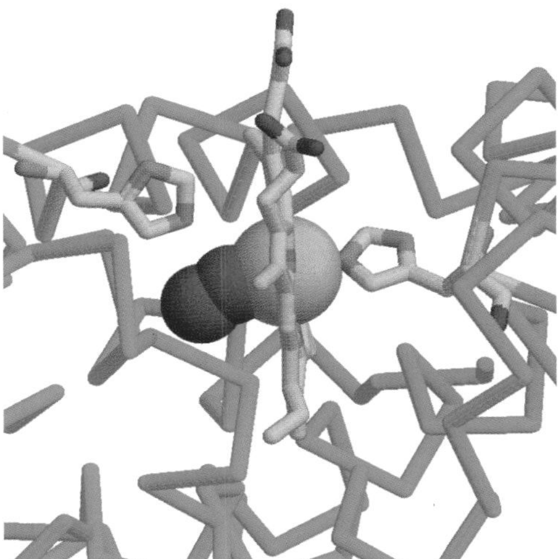

Plate 6.2. Close up of oxygen bound to the heme. Looking down the heme, the iron atom (yellow-orange) is shown bound to an oxygen molecule (red). The proximal histidine side chain is also shown bound to the iron and the distal histidine is also clearly visible on the other side of the proximal one. (The illustration was derived from the Protein Explorer (http://www.umass.edu/microbio/rasmol/) and data from the Protein Data Bank.)

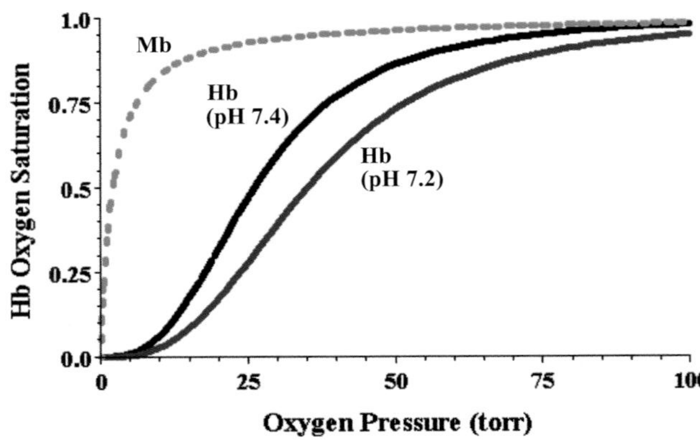

Plate 6.3. Hemoglobin and myoglobin oxygen binding curves. The myoglobin oxygen binding curve was drawn according to Equation 6.1 with P_{50} taken as 2 mm Hg. The hemoglobin oxygen binding curves were drawn using Equation 6.2 with $n = 2.8$ and P_{50} taken as 26 mm Hg at pH 7.4 and as 35 mm Hg for pH 7.2.

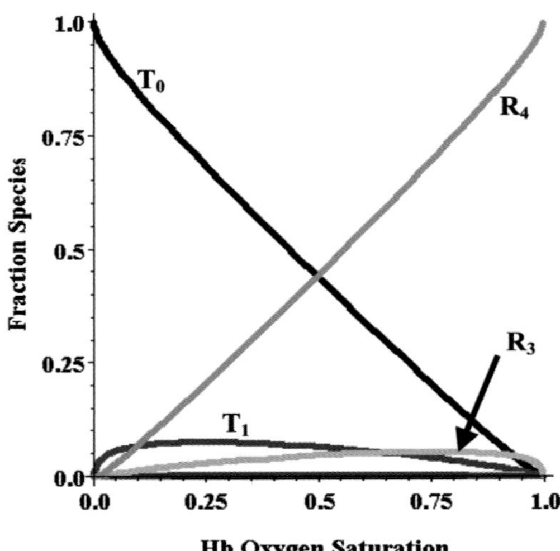

Plate 6.4. Fraction of hemoglobin states. The fraction of each state is plotted vs. hemoglobin oxygen saturation. Only the species T_0, T_1, R_3, and R_4 are present at large enough fractions to be visible. At zero oxygen saturation the hemoglobin is virtually all in the T_0 state and at 100% oxygen saturation it is all in the R_4 state. The parameters used were $L = 2 \times 10^6$, $c = 0.001$, and $K_T = 1/(75\ \text{mm Hg})$.

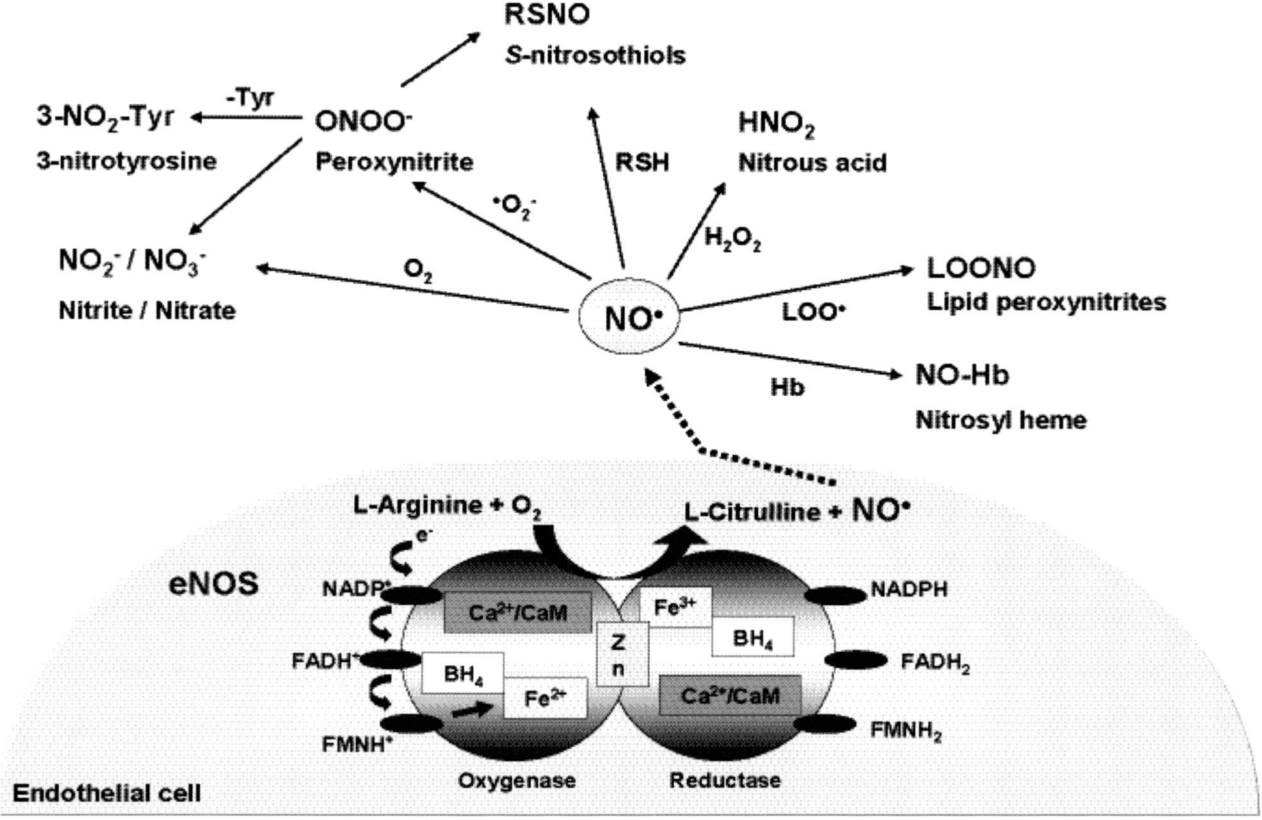

Plate 10.1. Biological source and reactions of nitric oxide. Nitric oxide ($NO^{\bullet}$) is synthesized in endothelial cells by the endothelial isoform of nitric oxide synthase (eNOS) via the five-electron oxidation reaction of L-arginine to L-citrulline. eNOS is activated by Ca^{2+}/calmodulin (Ca^{2+}/CaM) and the reaction requires molecular O_2 and NADPH as cosubstrates and flavin adenine dinucleotide ($FADH^{+}$), flavin mononucleotide ($FMNH^{+}$), and tetrahydrobiopterin (BH_4) as cofactors to facilitate electron transfer to the NOS heme moiety. Once generated, $NO^{\bullet}$ diffuses into the interstitium and the bloodstream where it reacts with molecular O_2, superoxide anion ($^{\bullet}O_2^{-}$), R-SH groups, hydrogen peroxide (H_2O_2), lipid oxides ($LOO^{\bullet}$), and hemoglobin (Hb) to generate NO species – some of which have biological activity.

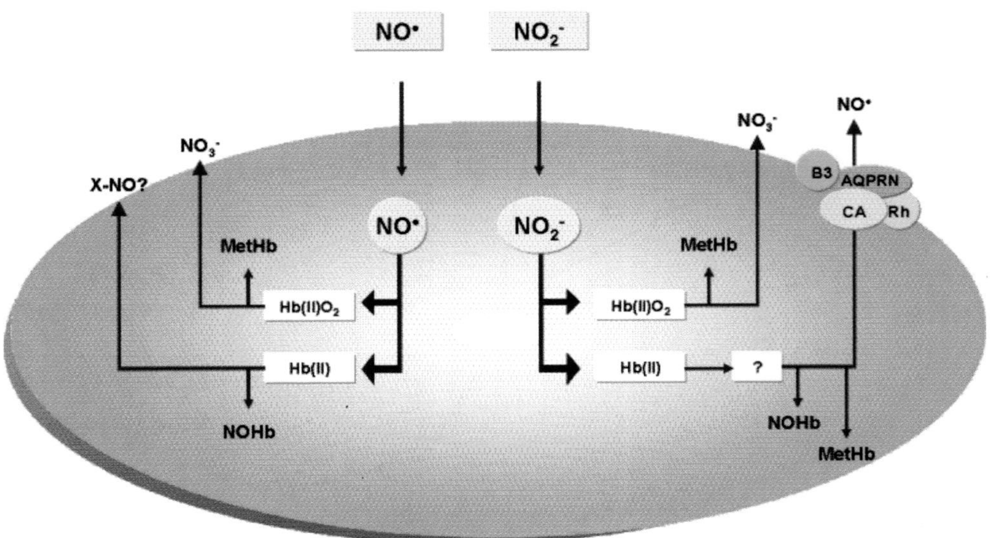

Plate 10.2. Reactions between NO and hemoglobin in erythrocytes. Nitric oxide (NO•), synthesized by the endothelium, or nitrite (NO_2^-) circulating in plasma, diffuses into the erythrocyte where it reacts with oxyhemoglobin [Hb(II)O_2] to yield methemoglobin (MetHb) and nitrate (NO_3^-), or with deoxyhemoglobin [Hb(II)] to generate nitrosylhemoglobin (NOHb) and NO adducts (X-NO). Nitrite also diffuses into the erythrocyte and reacts with deoxyhemoglobin and, via a possible intermediate species (?), produces nitrosylhemoglobin and methemoglobin. Once formed, NO• and NO• adducts are thought to exit the cell through a functional metabolon that is composed of oxy- and deoxyhemoglobin, Rh channels (Rh), aquaporin (AQPRN), band-3 complex (B3), and carbonic anhydrase (CA). These channels theoretically may transport NO• through the erythrocyte membrane.

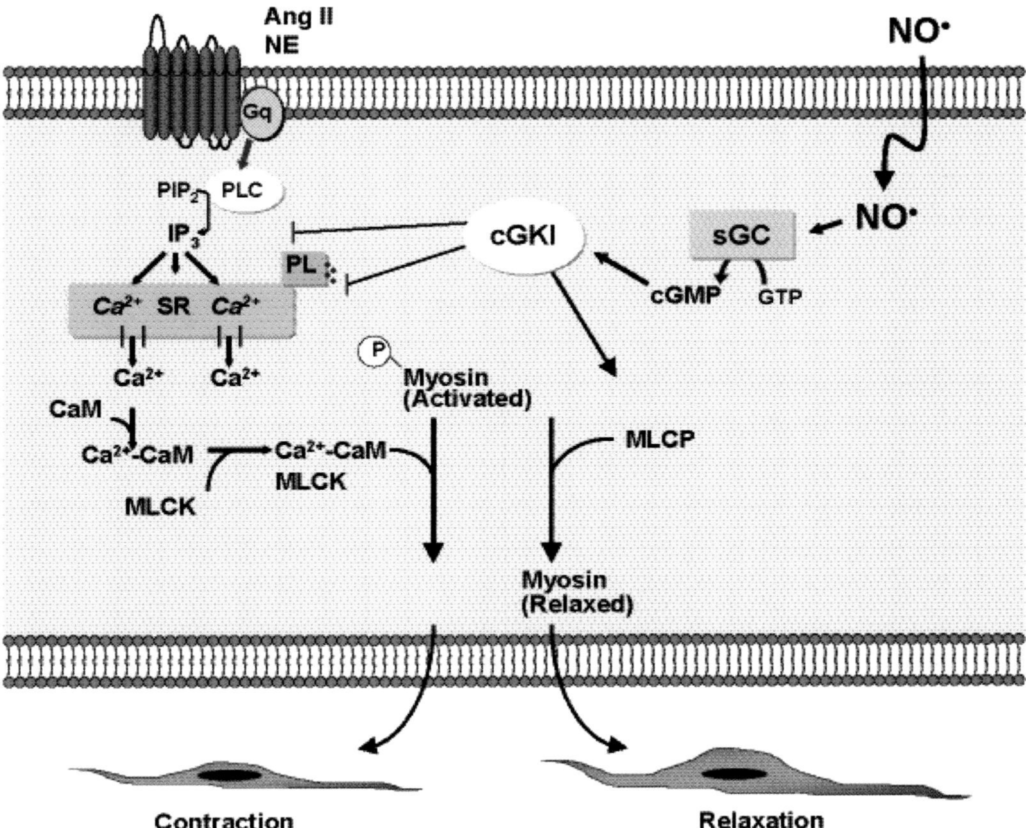

Plate 10.3. NO and vascular smooth muscle relaxation. NO•, synthesized by the endothelium, diffuses into the vascular smooth muscle cytosol and reacts with the heme iron of soluble guanylyl cyclase (sGC). This activates the enzyme, which in turn generates cGMP. As cGMP levels rise, cGMP-dependent kinase I (cGKI) is activated to inhibit inositol 1,4,5,trisphosphate (IP_3)-mediated release of Ca^{2+} from the sarcoplasmic reticulum (SR). cGKI activates phospholamban (PL), which facilitates this process by stimulating Ca^{2+} sequestration by the SR. This effect in turn also limits the ability of the Ca^{2+}-calmodulin (CaM)-myosin-light chain kinase (MLCK) complex to phosphorylate myosin and initiate contraction. cGKI also promotes vascular smooth muscle relaxation by stimulating myosin-light chain phosphatase (MLCP) to dephosphorylate myosin.

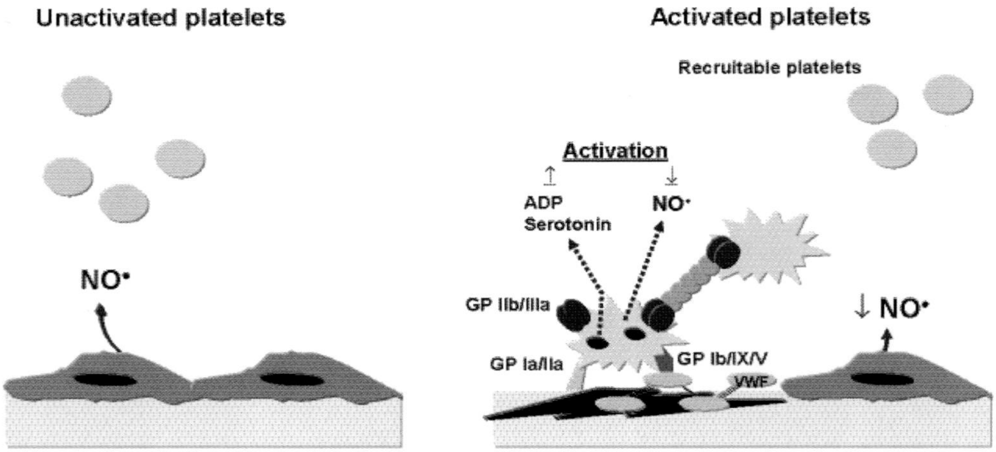

Plate 10.4. NO and platelet activation. Under basal conditions, the vascular endothelium elaborates NO• to maintain a nonthrombogenic surface. In contrast, when the endothelium is disrupted and NO• levels are decreased, platelets become activated and adhere to collagen via the cell surface receptor glycoprotein Ib/IIa (GP Ia/IIa) and glycoprotein Ib/IX/V (GP Ib/IX/V) that binds to the interstitium by von Willebrand factor (VWF). These activated platelets undergo shape change and release adenosine diphosphate (ADP) and serotonin to recruit and activate additional circulating platelets to the growing thrombus, and increase expression of the conformationally active fibrinogen receptor, glycoprotein IIb/IIIa (GP IIb/IIIa) to increase platelet aggregation and thrombus formation; the concomitant release of NO limits platelet aggregation. Platelet-derived NO limits recruitment of platelets to the growing platelet-rich hemostatic plug (or thrombus).

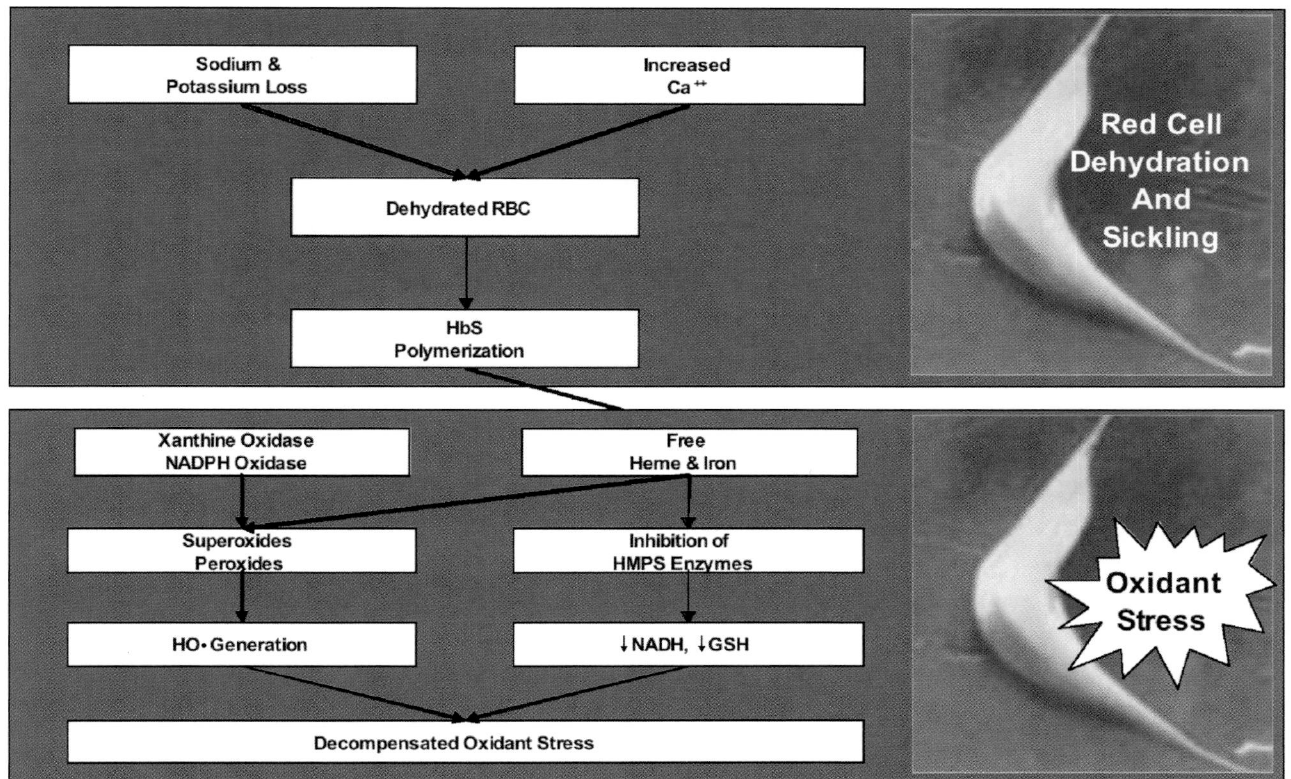

Plate 11.1. Factors leading to sickling and oxidant stress in erythrocytes in sickle cell disease. Solute loss and increased intracellular calcium promote red cell dehydration, which raises the intracellular concentration of sickle hemoglobin. This promotes polymerization of sickle hemoglobin, which is associated with generation of increased levels of oxidant species and depletion of cellular antioxidants, leading to a heightened state of oxidative stress. Each of these steps is described in the text, although the exact sequence of these events is somewhat speculative.

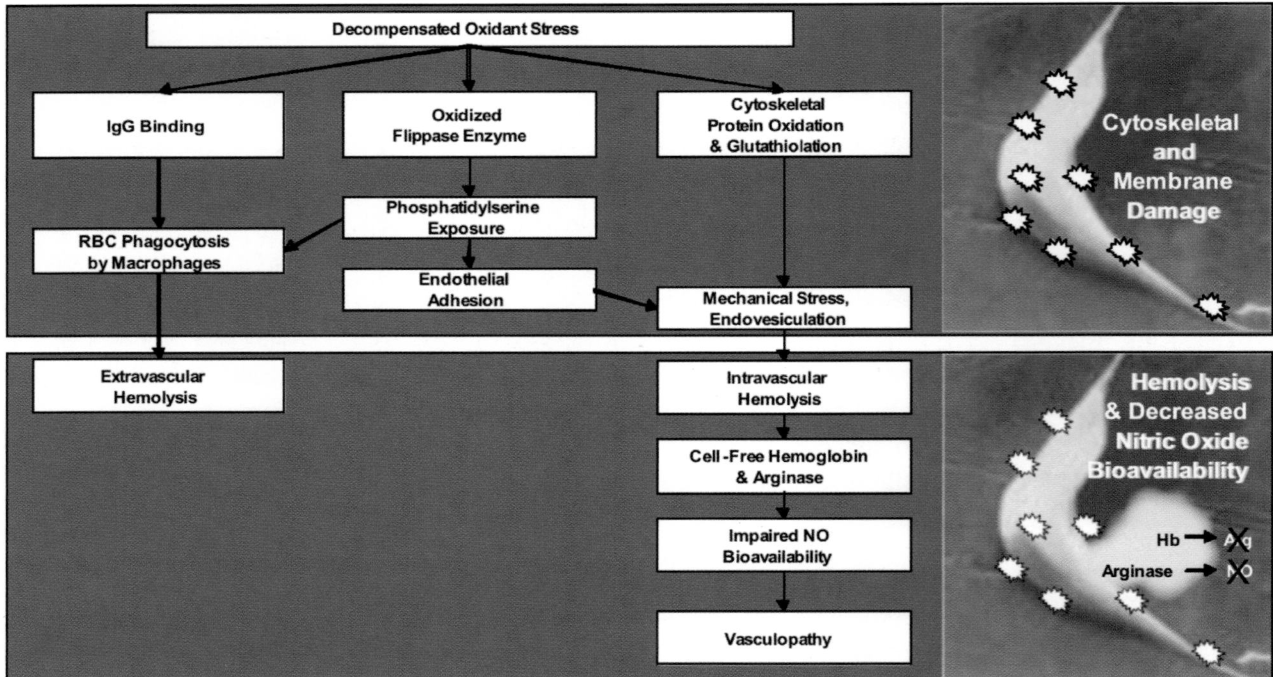

Plate 11.2. Factors promoting hemolysis in sickle cell disease. Decompensated oxidative stress in the sickle erythrocyte is associated with multiple lesions in its cytoskeleton and membrane. These lesions are responsible for binding of immunoglobulin to the membrane, promoting Fc receptor–mediated endocytosis of the damaged red cell by reticuloendothelial macrophages, considered extravascular hemolysis. Oxidative damage to the flippase enzyme is proposed to cause externalization of phosphatidylserine and phosphatidylethanolamine that also stimulate uptake of the red cell by macrophages, in addition to adhesion to endothelium. Oxidative damage and glutathiolation of the cytoskeleton can trigger endovesiculation of the membrane and release of membrane microparticles, and mechanical fragility of the damaged red cell. These latter events tend to produce intravascular hemolysis, resulting in the decompartmentalization of erythrocyte contents into plasma.

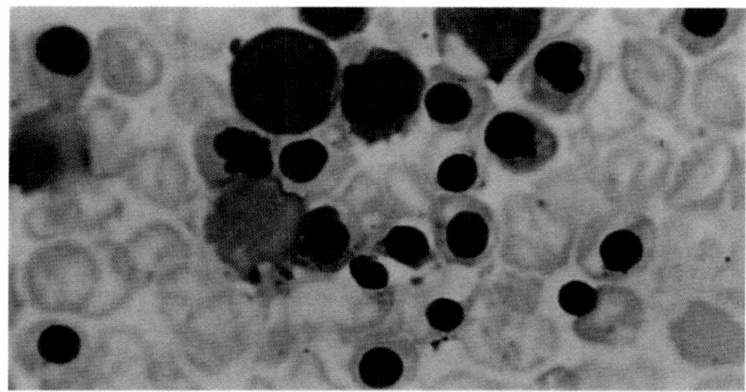

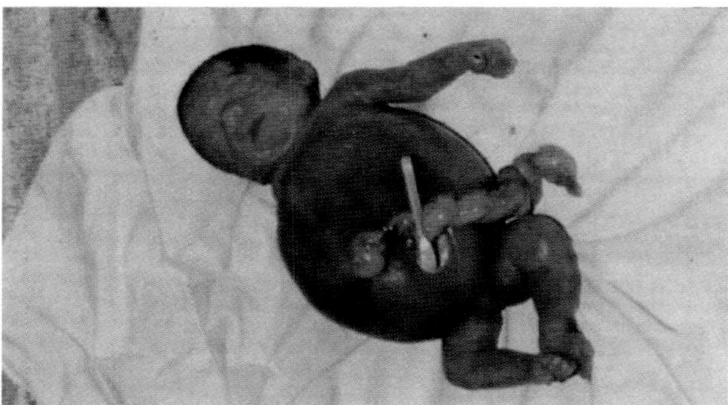

Plate 14.9. Upper the typical peripheral blood films of an infant with the Hb Bart's hydrops fetalis syndrome, showing many immature red cell precursors and hypochromic, microcytic, and anisopoikiolytic red cells. Lower the typical clinical features of a hydropic infant at birth (see text).

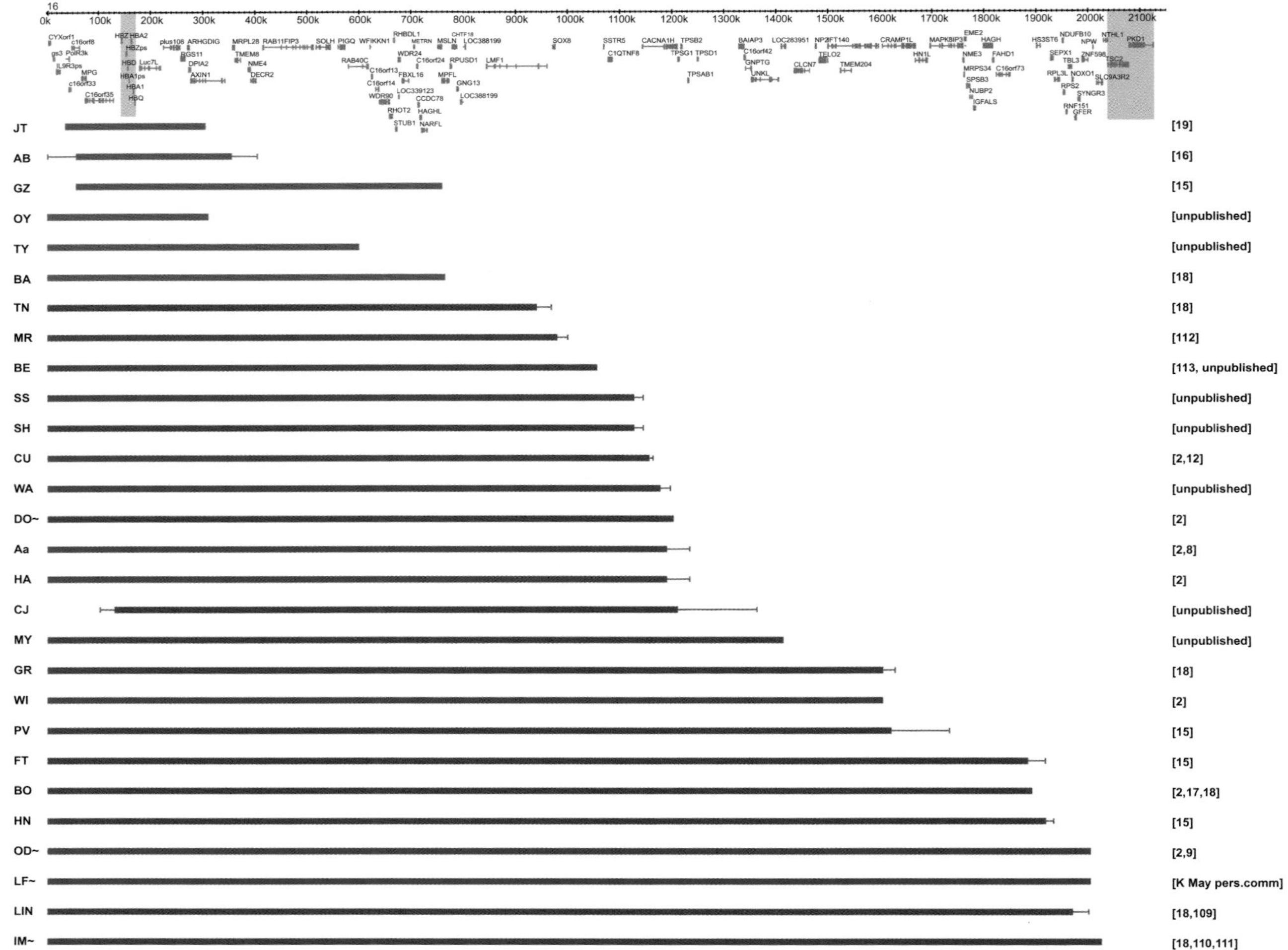

Plate 15.2. Summary of known ATR-16 deletions. The positions of the α-globin cluster and other genes within this region are indicated. Below, the extent of each deletion is shown with the patient code alongside (see Table 15.1). Deletions known to result from pure monosomy for this region are shown in either green (no abnormalities other than thalassemia) or red (ATR-16 phenotype). Chromosomal translocations (all with ATR-16 phenotypes) are shown in blue. Solid bars indicate regions known to be deleted and fine lines indicate the region of uncertainty of the breakpoints. The α genes and the genes that when mutated are associated with tuberous sclerosis and adult polycystic kidney disease are shown (shaded boxes).

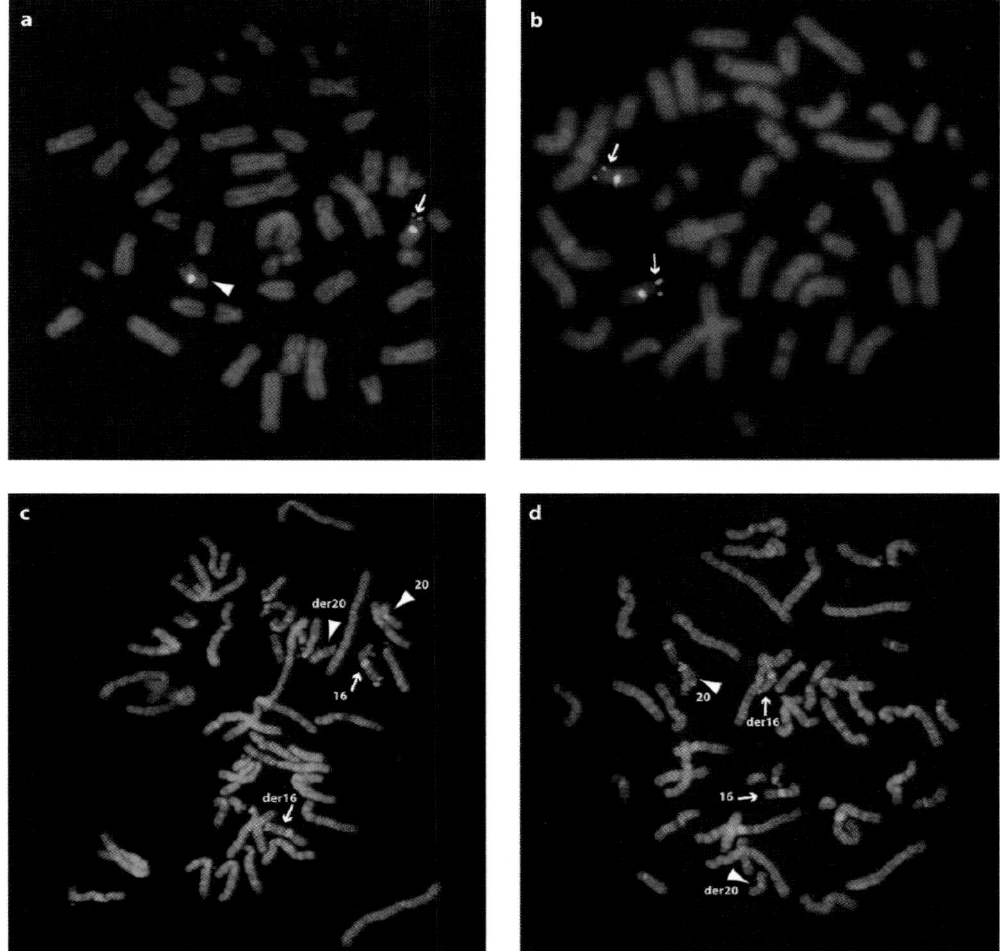

Plate 15.4. High-resolution chromosome analysis using FISH. **(a** and **b)** Examples of FISH on metaphase chromosomes of deletion patient JT. In each case chromosome 16 is identified by a chromosome 16–specific centromere probe. In **(a)** using a cosmid (cGG1) located close to the telomere, fluorescent signal was seen on the normal chromosome (arrow) but not the abnormal copy of chromosome 16 (arrowhead). **(b)** Using a second cosmid located closer to the centromere (not deleted in JT) a signal is seen on both normal and abnormal chromosomes (arrows). **(c** and **d)** FISH on metaphase chromosomes of the mother of WA showing a balanced translocation. In **(c)** and **(d)** both homologs of chromosome 16 are indicated by arrows and chromosome 20 by arrowheads. In **(c)** the subtelomeric probes for 16p and 16q were hybridized to metaphase chromosomes. Green fluorescent signal was seen on the q arm of both homologs of chromosome 16. Red fluorescent signal was seen on the p arm of the normal chromosome 16 and the q arm of the derivative chromosome 20 (der 20) but was absent from the deleted chromosome 16 (der 16). In **(d)** the subtelomeric probe for 20p (red) was seen on both homologs of chromosome 20. Fluorescent signal for 20q (green) was seen on the normal chromosome 20 and the p arm of the derivative 16 (der 16).

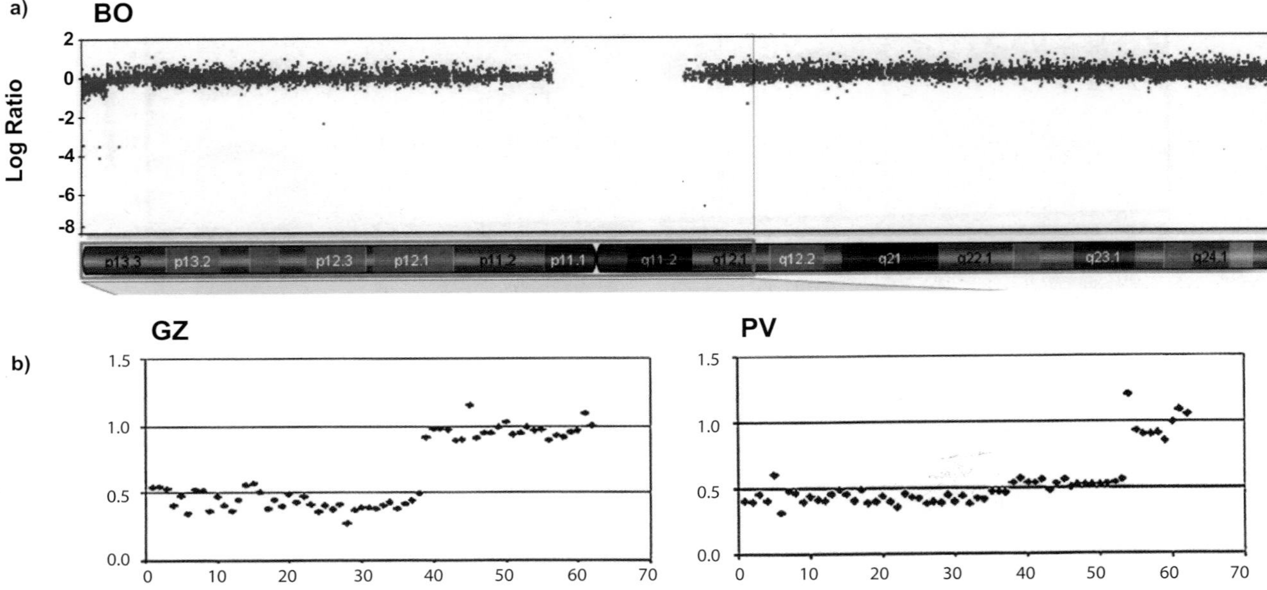

Plate 15.5. Detection of deletions. **(a)** Analysis of chromosome 16 in patient BO with ATR-16 using the QuantiSNP protocol. The Y-axis indicates the log ratio between normal and the test and the X-axis represents the distance along chromosome 16. **(b)** Analysis of two patients (GZ and PV and Fig. 15.2) with large deletions of 16p13.3 using the multiplex ligation–dependent probe amplification protocol). The Y-axis represents the ratio peak height of the test divided by the normal control and the X-axis represents the distance along chromosome 16.

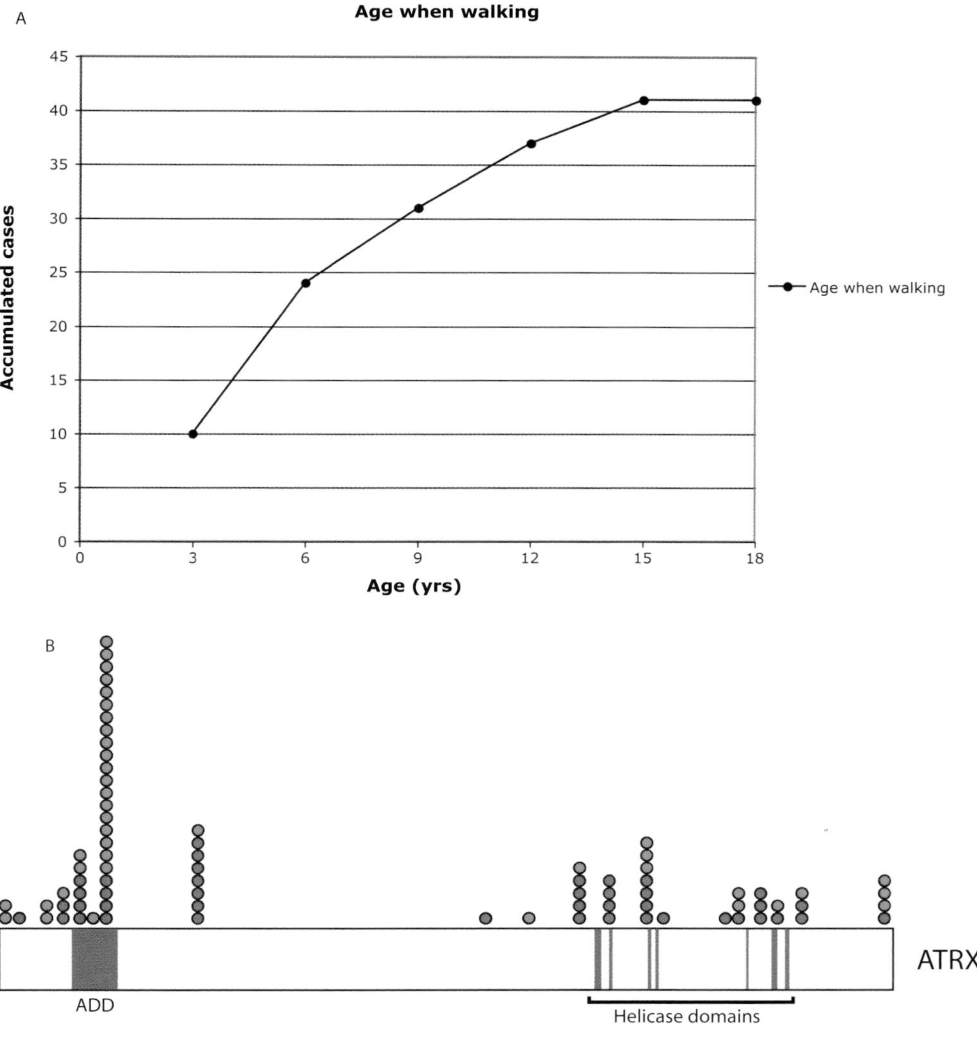

Plate 15.9. A measure of gross motor function is whether the children are able to walk and the age at which this is achieved. Forty-one affected individuals were able to walk. **(A)** Shows the age at which this was achieved. Approximately 75% of these were able to walk by the age of 9 years. None learned to walk after the age of 15 years. **(B)** This figure correlates the ability to walk with the location of the mutation. The 42 individuals who were unable to walk excluded cases who were younger than the age of 9 years at the time of assessment; the range of the ages for this group was 9–30 years.

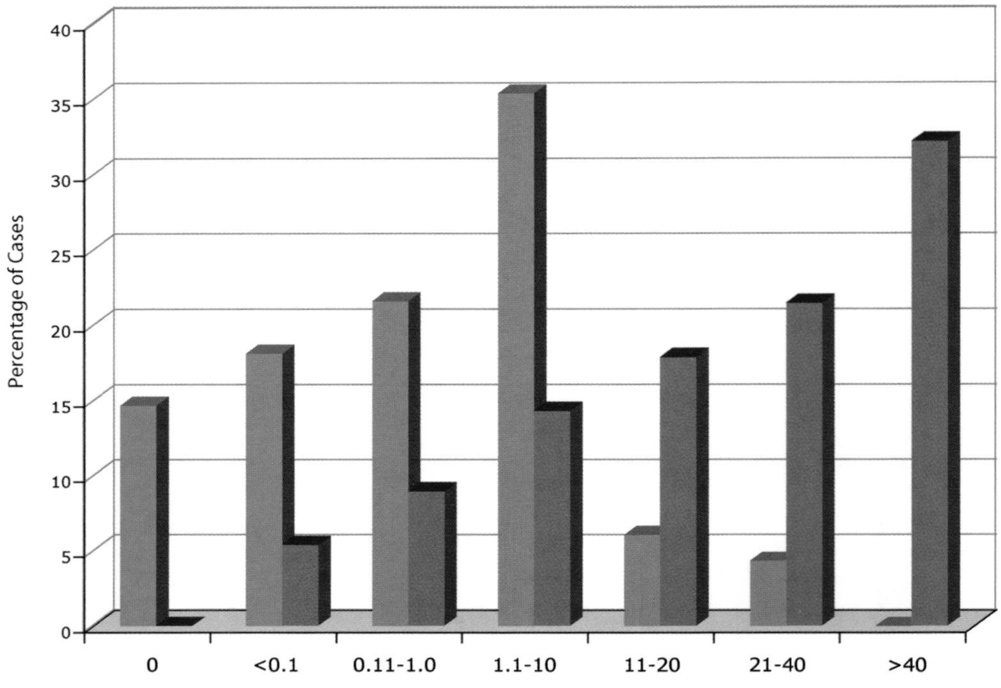

Plate 15.10. Percentage of cells with HbH inclusions in cases of ATR-X syndrome in which the presence of inclusions has been demonstrated and quantified.

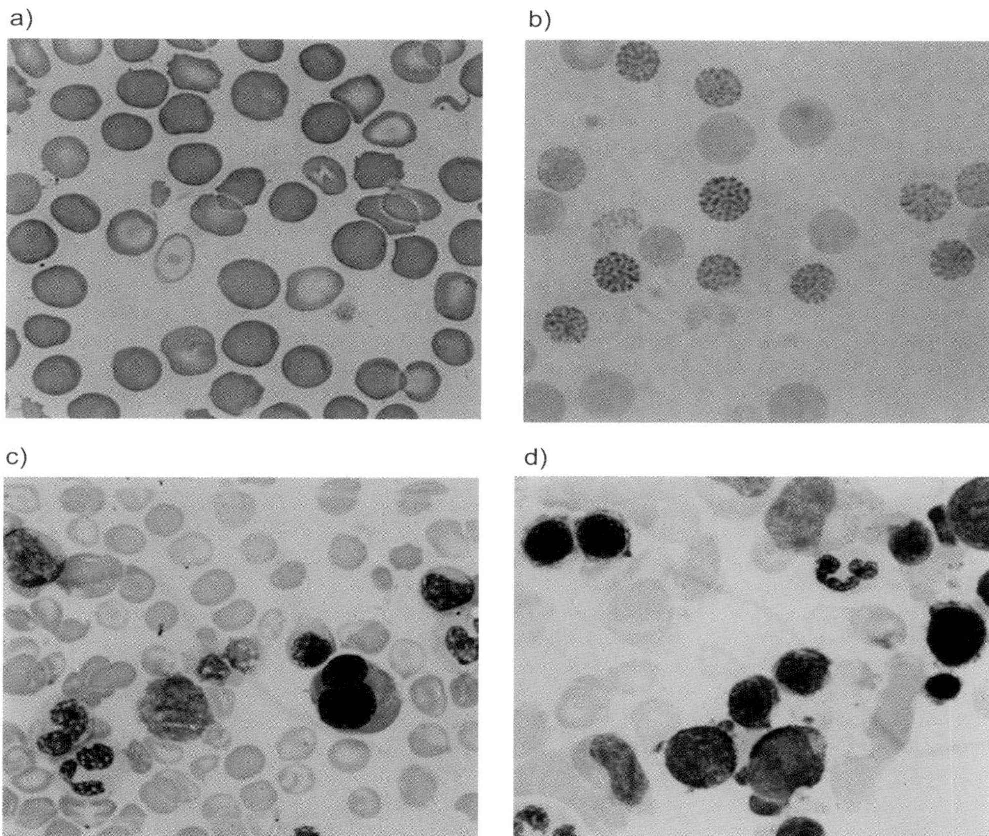

Plate 15.11. (a) May-Grünwald-Giemsa–stained peripheral blood smear from an elderly woman with ATMDS (original magnification, 400X). Many red cells are hypochromic, microcytic, or both, whereas others look relatively normal. As expected, the red blood cell distribution width (RDW) was elevated (19%; normal range, 11%–15%) in this patient. Iron studies were unremarkable. **(b)** Brilliant cresyl blue–stained peripheral blood smear from a 56-year-old man with ATMDS who had characteristic microcytic, hypochromic red cell indices: in this case, an MCH of 19 pg and MCV of 66 fL (original magnification, 600X). Abnormal inclusion-containing "golf ball cells" are easily distinguished from normal reticulocytes and red cells and confirm the presence of HbH (β-globin tetramers.) In this case, supravital staining was performed by incubating fresh blood for 24 hours with 1% brilliant cresyl blue in 0.9% normal saline. **(c)** and **(d)** Bone marrow samples from patients with ATMDS showing dyserythropoietic erythroblasts including binucleate cells.

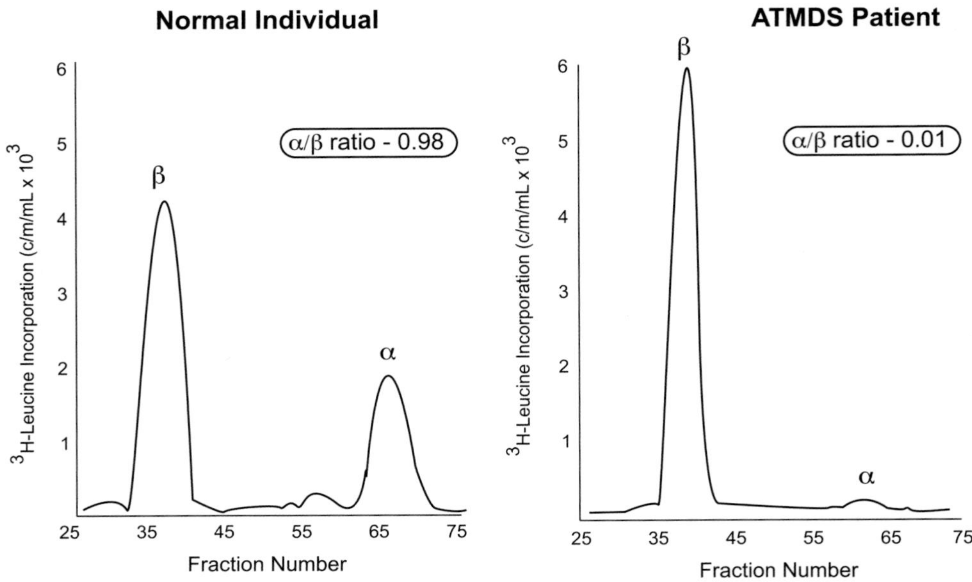

Plate 15.12. Measurement of reticulocyte α/β-globin chain synthesis ratio by radioisotope labeling and CM cellulose chromatography in a patient with ATMDS. In this case, α-globin production was markedly downregulated, and the α/β-chain synthesis ratio estimated by an area-under-the-curve method was only 0.01 (normal, 0.9–1.2). A normal chromatogram is depicted at left, for comparison.

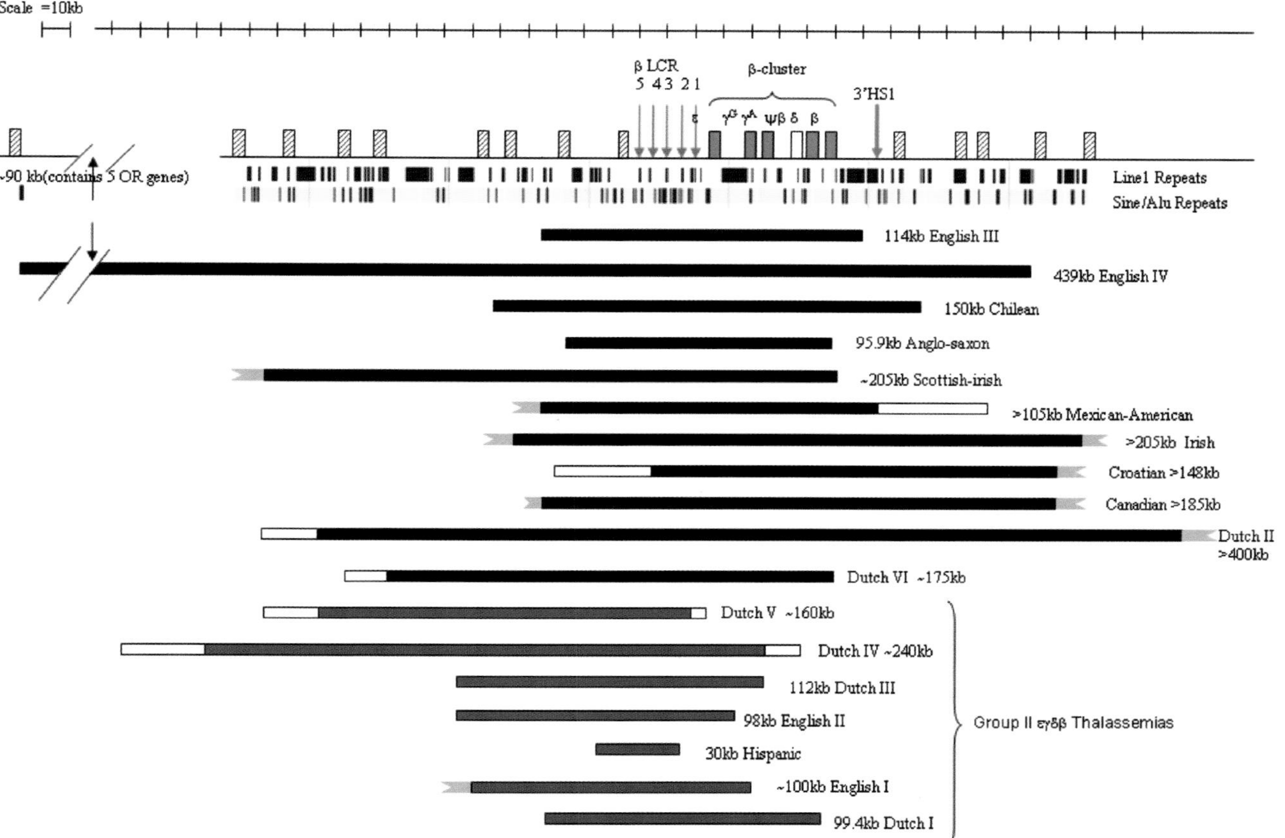

Plate 16.5. Deletions of the β-globin gene cluster causing $(\varepsilon\gamma\delta\beta)^{\circ}$ thalassemia. Top part of the figure shows the β-globin cluster and its flanking regions on chromosome 11p. The ε, ${}^{G}\gamma$, ${}^{A}\gamma$, δ, and β-globin genes are shown as gray boxes, whereas the hatched boxes represent the human olfactory receptor genes (HOR) named according to ensemble database (Ch 11:5110000–5600000). The 5′ hypersensitive sites that comprise the β LCR and the 3′ hypersensitive site (3′HS1) are shown as vertical arrows. The Line 1 and Sine/Alu repeat sequences are shown below the β-globin gene cluster as short vertical lines and boxes. The 18 deletions causing εγδβ thalassemia are shown below; the extents of the deletions are marked as complete boxes if endpoints have been determined precisely, jagged ends if undetermined, and white boxes as endpoint regions. Boxes in black are the deletions that include the β-globin gene (group I) and gray boxes represent the group II upstream deletions that leave the β-globin intact.

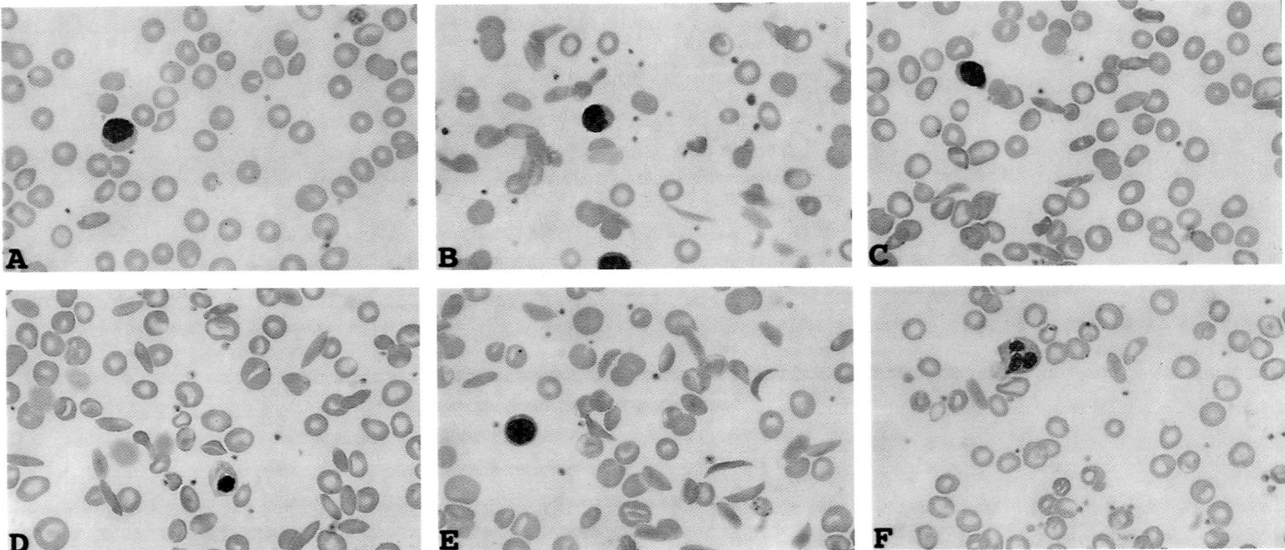

Plate 19.1. Blood films in patients with sickle cell anemia and average or low HbF levels. HbF in these patients are **A**-0.5%, **B**-1%, **C**-4%, **D**-5%, **E**-7%, and **F**-10%. Patients C and F were taking hydroxyurea. Although some of these patients have more ISCs than patients depicted in Figure 19.2 who have high HbF concentrations, note that patient A with the lowest HbF level has very few sickled cells.

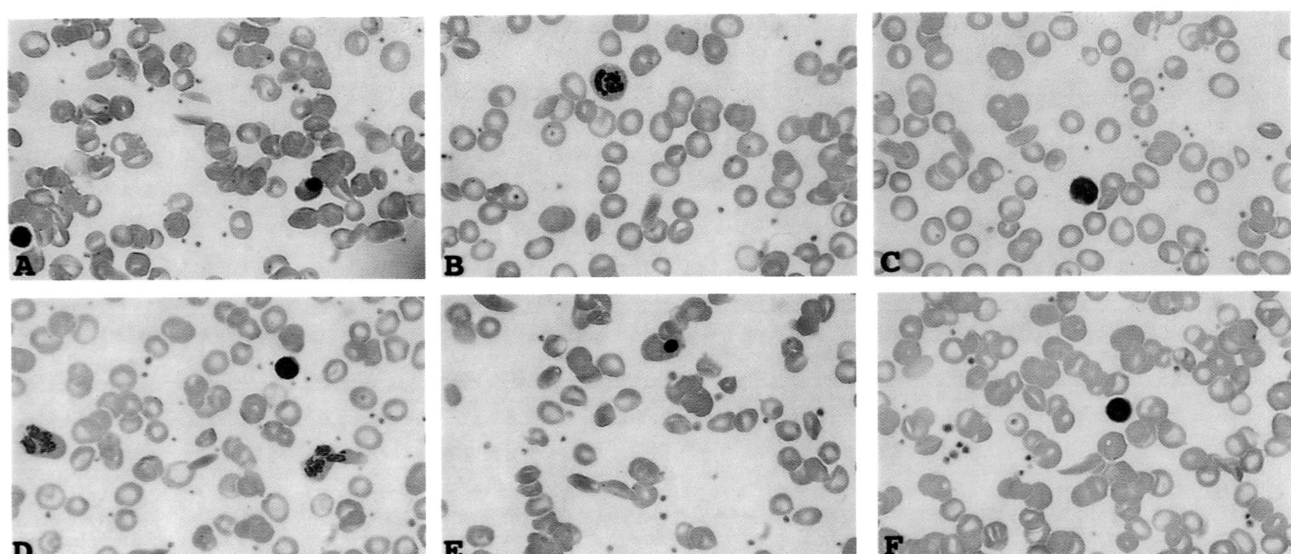

Plate 19.2. Blood films in patients with sickle cell anemia and high HbF levels. HbF in these six patients are **A**-19%, **B**-18%, **C**-19%, **D**-21%, **E**-20%, and **F**-23%. All patients were receiving hydroxyurea. All still have sickled cells in the blood and these are particularly prominent in patient A. Also note nucleated red cells in A and E.

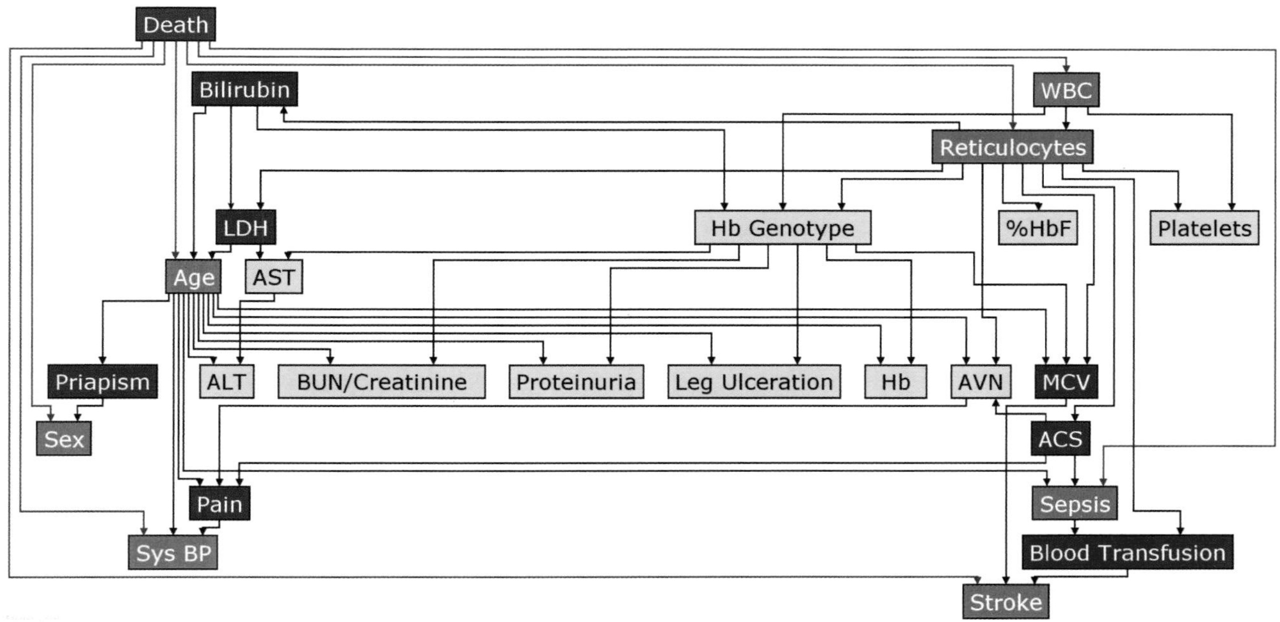

Plate 19.3. A Bayesian network model of the risk of death in sickle cell disease.[44]

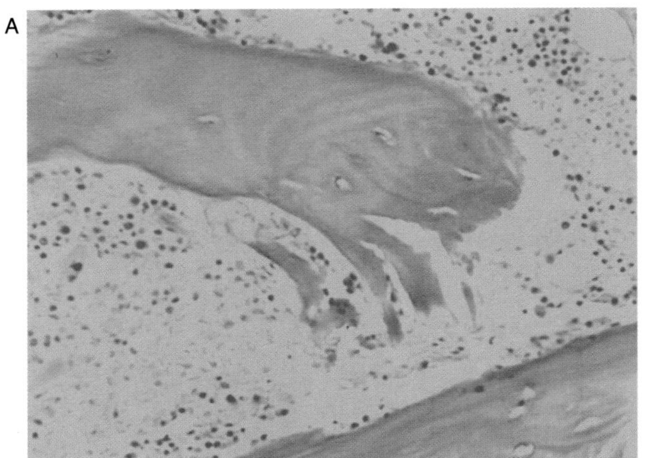

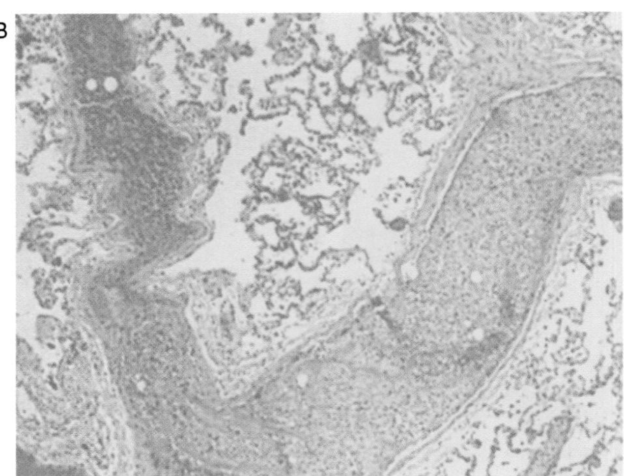

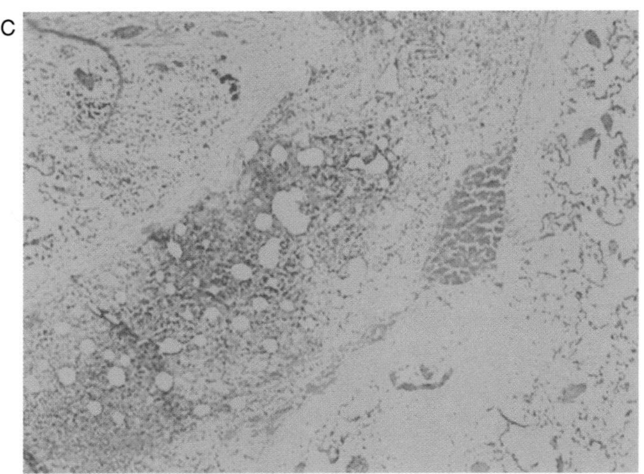

Plate 19.5. Necrotic bone marrow in the lungs of a patient with HbSC disease, who was in reasonable health, and died suddenly with severe acute chest syndrome and multiorgan failure. **(A)** Necrotic bone marrow. **(B)** Pulmonary embolus of fatty, necrotic marrow (low power). **(C)** Higher power view of necrotic marrow in a pulmonary artery.

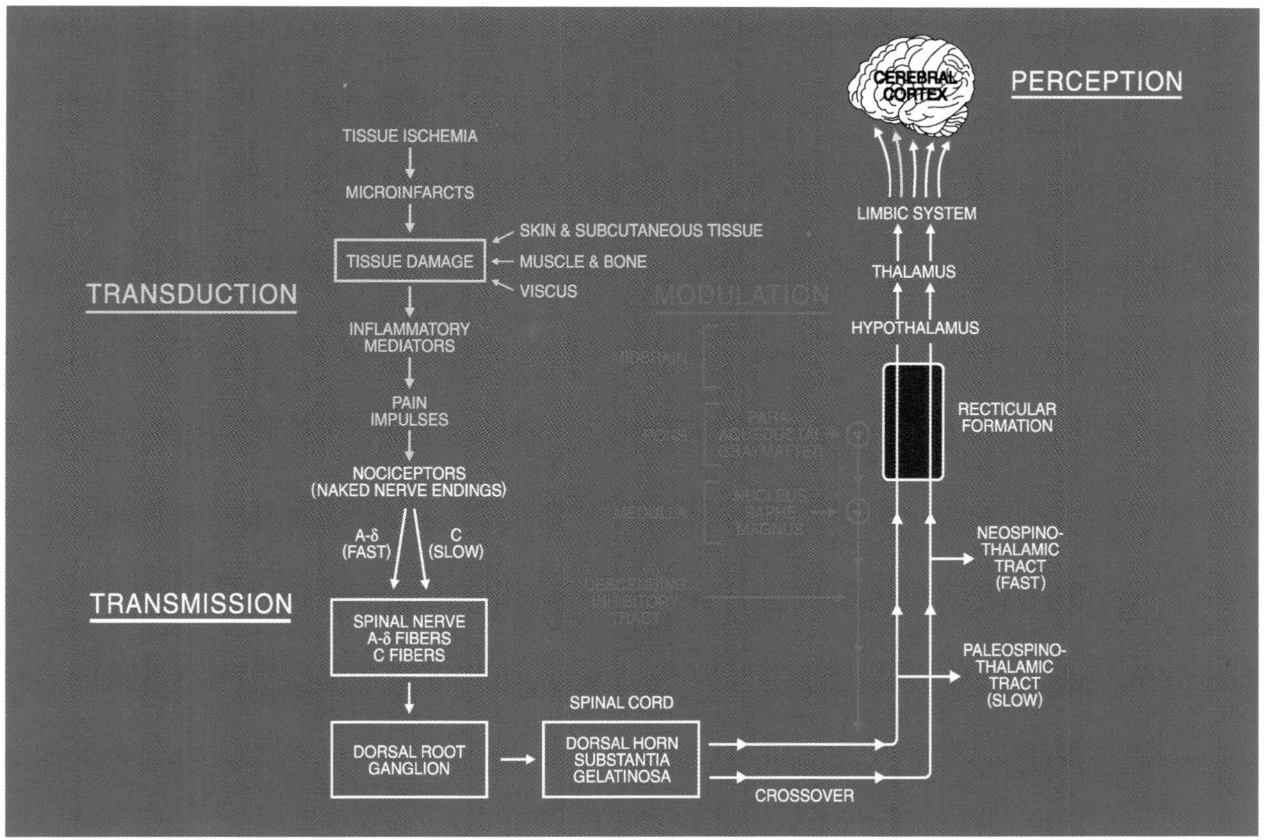

Plate 20.2. Anatomical pathways of pain in sickle cell disease. (Modified from ref. 39 with permission.)

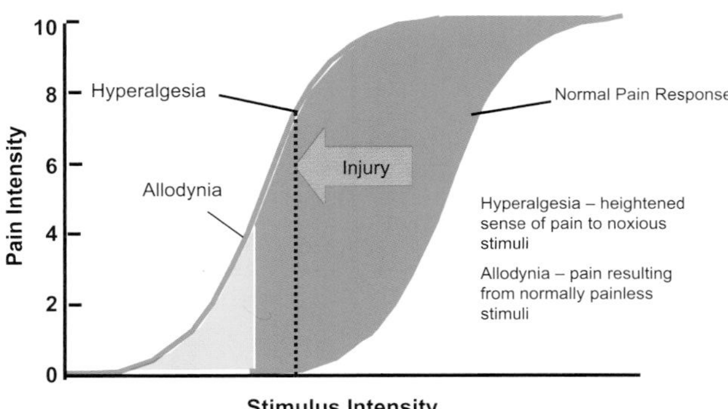

Plate 20.8. Pain hypersensitivity induced by injury. In the normal pain response, pain intensity increases as the stimulus intensity increases. Sensitization following injury causes the curve to shift to the left, resulting in hyperalgesia, in which noxious stimuli cause greater and more prolonged pain, as well as allodynia, in which pain results from normally painless stimuli. Sensitization is the manifestation of neuronal plasticity. (From ref. 139 with permission.)

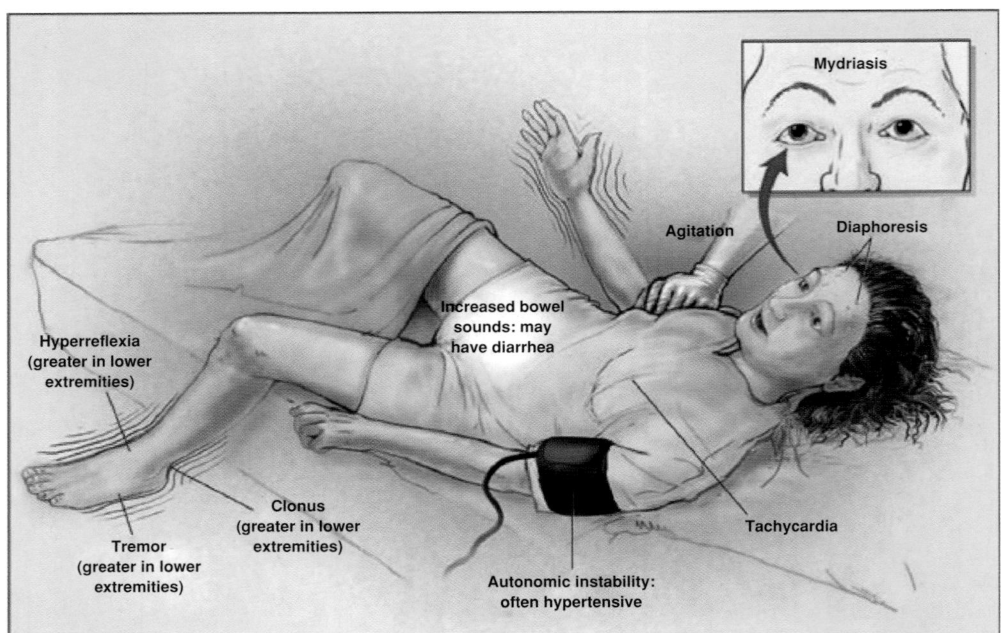

Plate 20.9. Findings in patients with moderately severe serotonin syndrome. Hyperkinetic neuromuscular findings of tremor or clonus and hyperreflexia should lead the clinician to consider the diagnosis of the serotonin syndrome. (From ref. 149 with permission.)

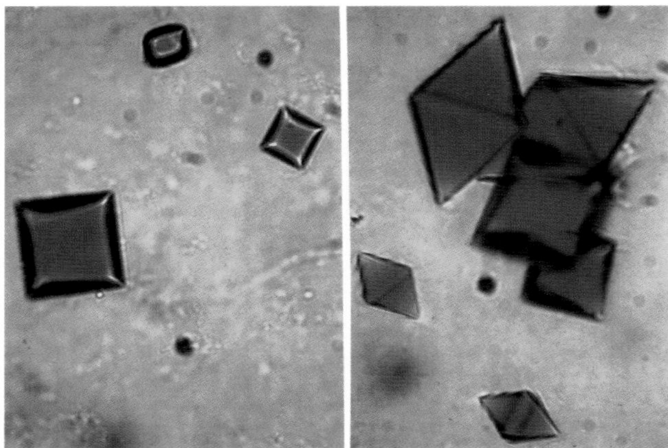

Plate 21.2. Crystal forms observed in hemolysates of patients with HbC. **(A)** Cubic crystals, generated in hemolysates of compound heterozygotes for HbC and Hb Korle-Bu. **(B)** Tetragonal crystals observed intracellularly and in hemolysates of patients homozygous for HbC, with HbSC disease and compound heterozygotes for HbC and HbA and other mutants.

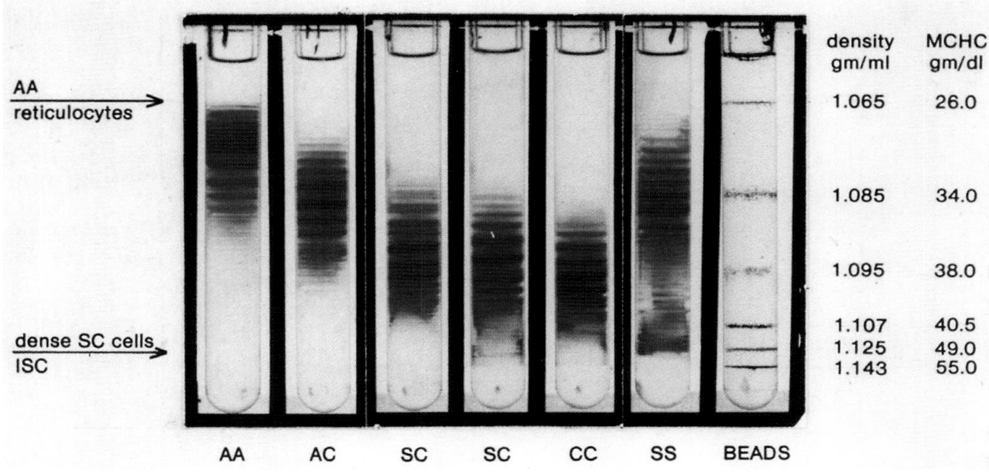

Plate 21.10. Percoll–Strachan (Larex) density separation of whole blood from normal hemolysate (AA), HbC trait (AC), and three different HbSC disease individuals and one sickle cell anemia patient. Beads: Color-coded density beads to establish the density at different levels of the gradient after centrifugation.

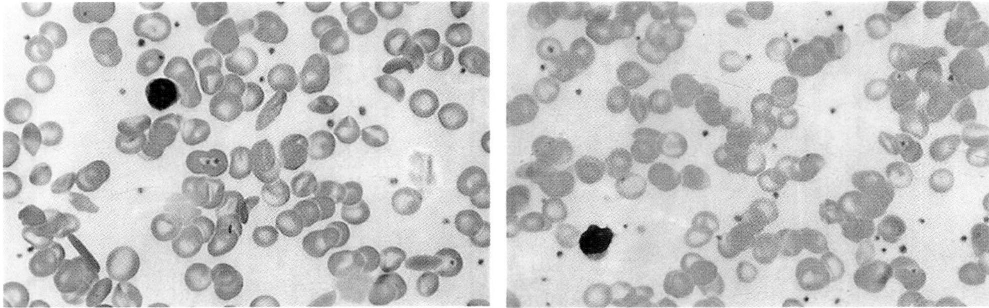

Plate 23.1. Blood films in two patients with HbS–β^0 thalassemia. In the left panel, the patient has an HbF level of 5%. Sickled cells are prominent beside microcytosis. In the right panel, with an HbF of 2%, microcytosis and hypochromia are prominent and few typical sickled cells are seen. Despite similar HbF levels, for unknown reasons, the numbers of sickled cells are quite different. This suggests the possibility of different cellular distributions of HbF or other genetic modifiers.

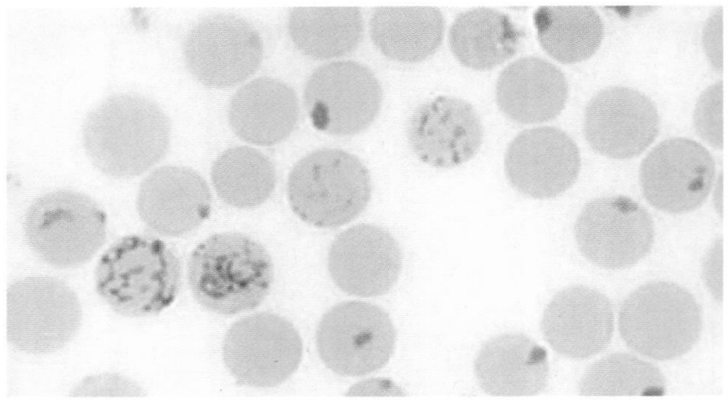

Plate 24.2. Heinz bodies. Heinz bodies are the large, single basophilic inclusions inside erythrocytes. Other red cell inclusions represent reticulocytes.

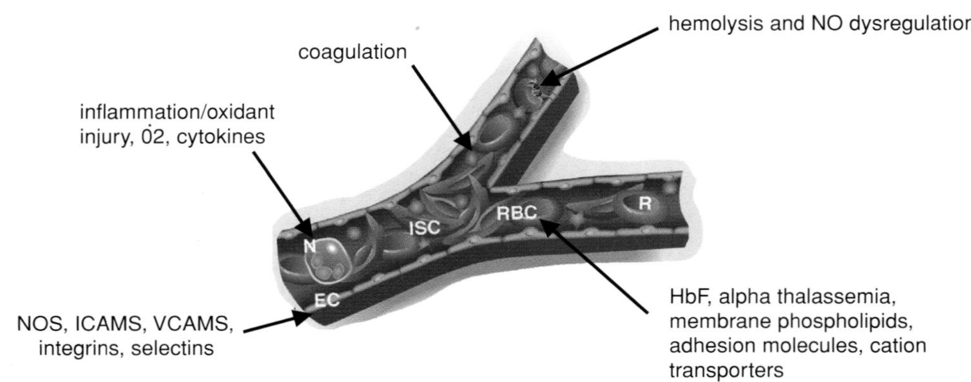

Plate 27.3. Some facets of sickle cell disease pathobiology that might be genetically modulated.

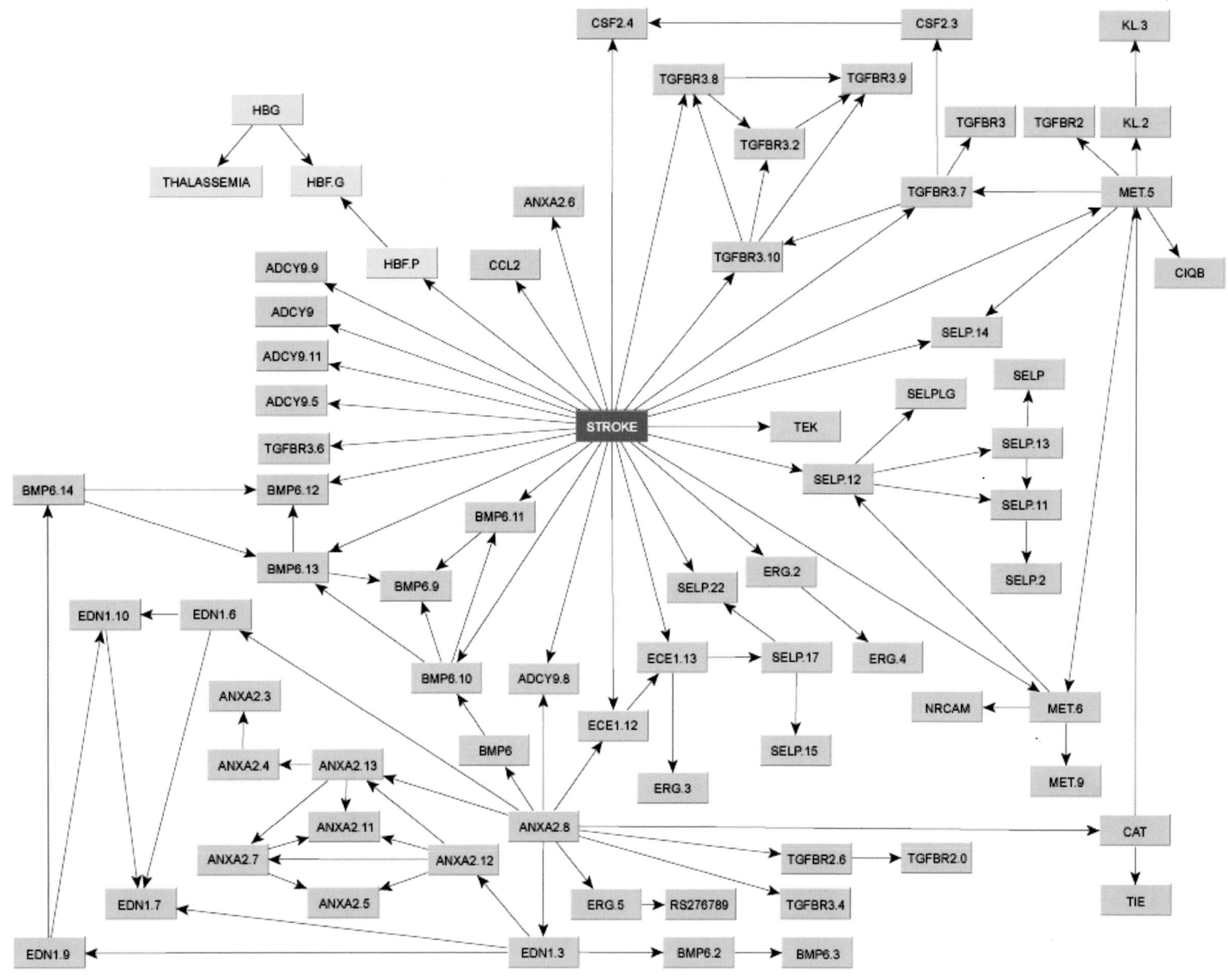

Figure 27.5. A bayesian network describing the associations of SNPs in candidate genes with the likelihood of developing nonhemorrhagic stroke in sickle cell anemia.[72]

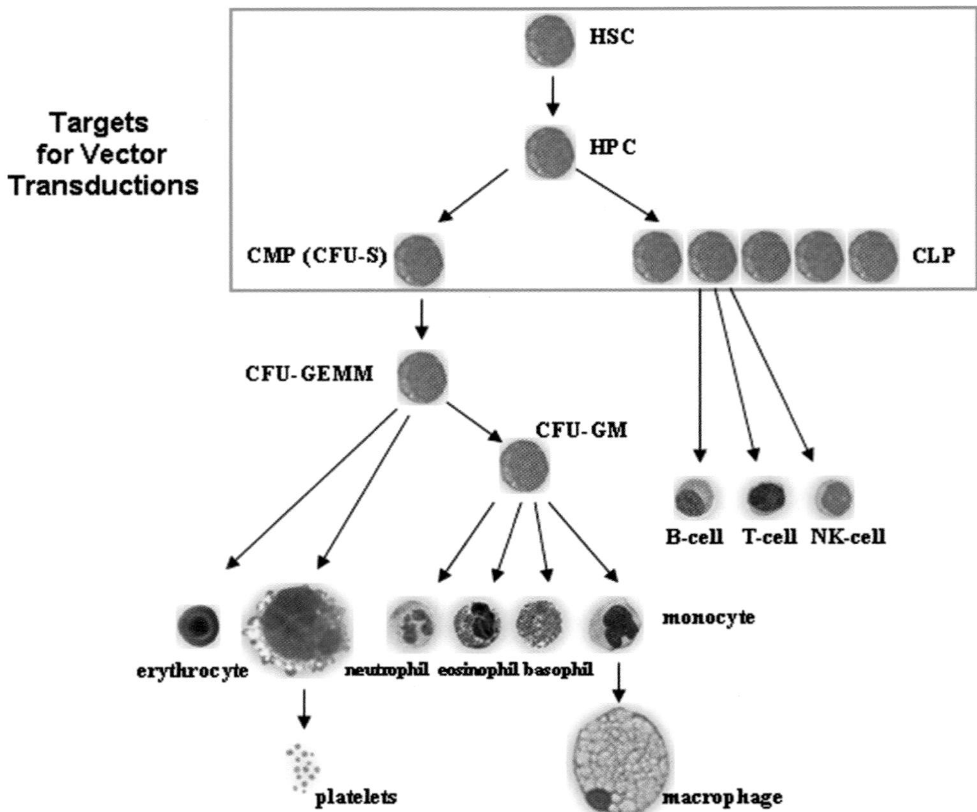

Plate 33.1. Hematopoietic cell targets for gene therapy. This figure shows the general hierarchical structure of hematopoiesis. Hematopoietic stem cells (HSCs) give rise to primitive progenitor cells (HPC), which in turn generate common myeloid progenitors (CMP) and common lymphoid progenitors (CLP). These progenitor cells then give rise to all formed elements of the blood through a number of intermediates including the granulocyte/erythrocyte/monocyte/macrophage colony forming unit (CFU-GEMM) and the granulocyte/monocyte colony forming unit (CFU-GM). The cells contained within the green outline are the desired targets for retroviral vectors because they all give rise to multiple mature cell types and because, to greater or lesser degrees, they can self-renew and lead to the persistence of genetically modified cells over time. The target cell population can differ for various diseases. For instance, for SCID, targeting of the CLP with an appropriate vector will result in long-term reconstitution of all lymphocyte subsets. In contrast, treatment of hemoglobin disorders required targeting of the most primitive HSC to have long-term persistence of stably modified erythrocytes after transplantation. The biology and frequency of the various target cell populations differs and are variable in determining the gene transfer efficiency.

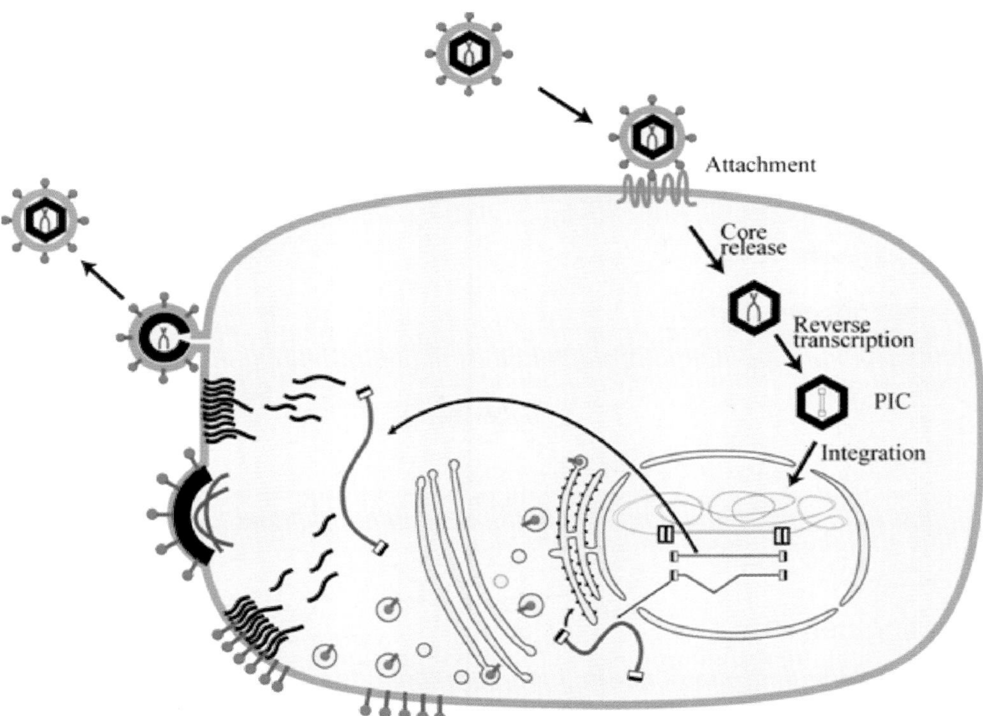

Plate 33.2. Retroviral life cycle. Entry of a retrovirus into a cell is initiated by interaction of its envelope proteins with one or more cellular membrane proteins that act as a receptor followed by internalization through membrane fusion or phagocytosis. The vector core is released and the RNA serves as a template for formation of the reverse transcription complex (RTC). The RTC includes additional viral proteins and is moved by the microtubule system from the cell periphery to the nucleus as it matures to become the preintegration complex (PIC). The PIC gains access to chromatin during mitosis, or in the case of lentiviruses, by ingress through the nuclear membrane. Following integration into host-cell DNA, the retroviral genome is expressed in RNA molecules that are transported to the cytoplasm to serve as a template for synthesis of new viral proteins and, in the case of unspliced RNA species, as a substrate for formation of new viral particles.

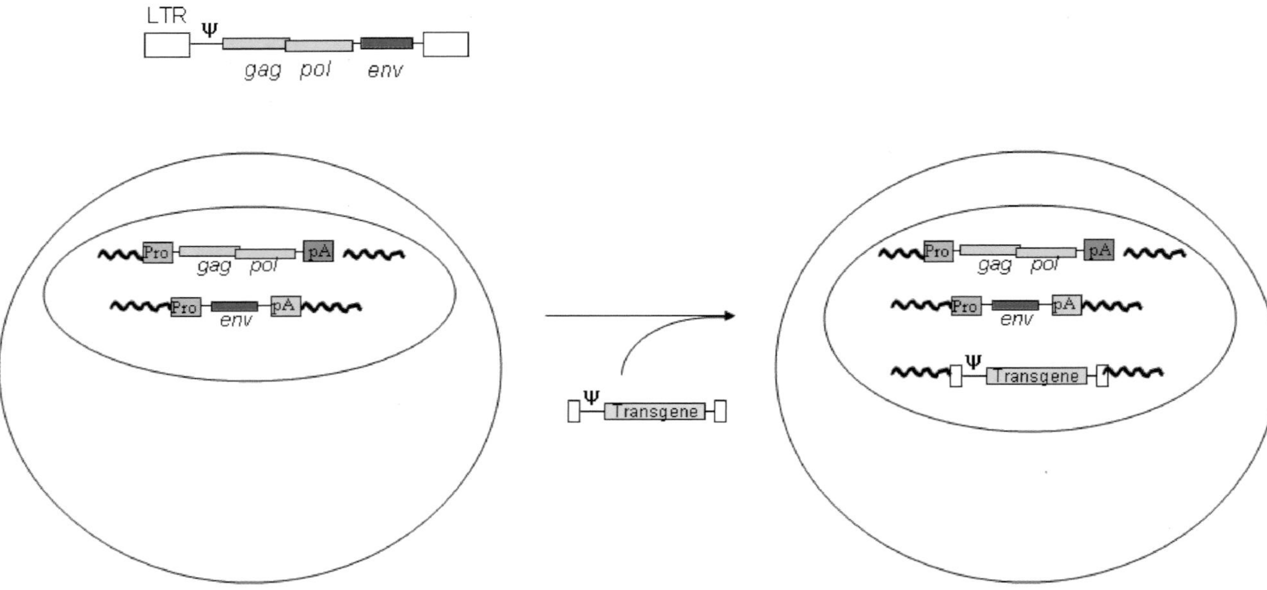

Plate 33.3. Production of retroviral vector particles. This figure illustrates the concept of the strategy used to derive retroviral vector preparations free of replication-competent virus. The diagram at the top shows the organization of a retroviral genome. Murine oncoretroviruses have coding sequences for matrix proteins (gag), reverse transcriptase, integrase and protease (pol), and envelope proteins (env). The LTR contains the viral promoter and enhancer. Immediately downstream is a sequence essential for packaging the genomic RNA (ψ). To reduce the risk of recombination and generation of replication-competent particles, these coding sequences are separated on two or more expression cassettes before transfer into a tissue culture cell line. The coding sequences for viral proteins are replaced by the coding sequences for the intended therapeutic protein in the vector. Various strategies are used for introducing the vector genome into the packaging cell that initiates production of replication-defective retroviral vector particles that can be used to introduce the therapeutic transgene into target cells. In the packaging and producer cells, the viral protein constructs are driven by exogenous promoters (Pro).

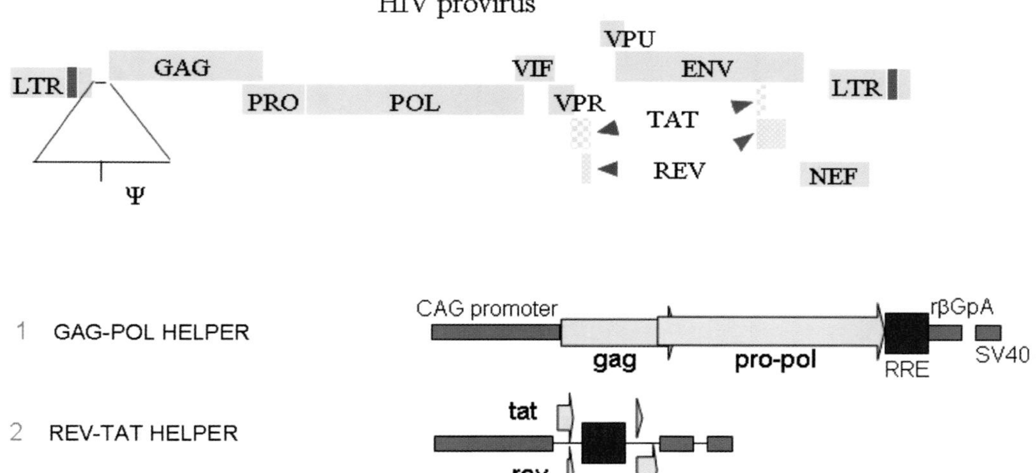

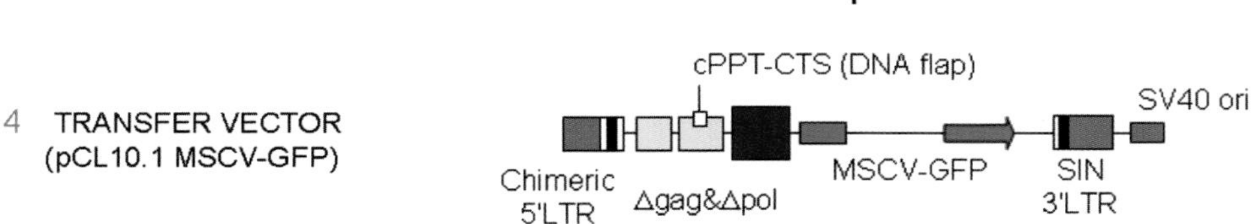

Plate 33.4. Organization of the HIV provirus and development of a packaging system for generation of vector particles free of replication competent retrovirus. The HIV-1 genome encodes 15 proteins as shown in the top row of this figure. The GAG polyprotein is processed to yield viral core proteins including MA (matrix), CA (capsid), NC (nucleocapsid), and p6. The ENV protein product is processed to yield two proteins, SU (surface) and TM (transmembrane) components of the mature envelope proteins. The POL region encodes the enzymes PR (protease), RT (reverse transcriptase), and IN (integrase). TAT and REV are regulatory proteins that facilitate transcription or nuclear to cytoplasmic transport of unspliced RNA species, respectively. The accessory proteins NEF, VIF, VPR, and VPU are viral virulence factors, which are not required for vector particle formation. Shown below in rows 1–4 are components of a system developed to generate vector particles. Each of the transcriptional units encoding viral proteins includes the powerful chimeric CMV enhance/β-actin promoter, the β-globin large intron (CAG promoter), the rabbit β-globin polyadenylation sequence (rβGpA), and the rev responsive element (RRE), which facilitate nuclear to cytoplasmic transport. The SV40 origin of replication (ORI) is included in each expression plasmid to allow its amplification in cells expressing SV40T antigen. Three separate helper plasmids are used as shown in 1–3. The transfer vector includes a portion of the gag region required for packaging and a portion of the pol region, which includes the central polypurine tract (cPPT) and the central termination sequence (CTS). These elements together constitute the DNA flap that was described as a crucial determinate for lentiviral vector nuclear import and gene transduction of primitive human hematopoietic cells. The U3 region of the 5′ LTR in the vector has been replaced with the CMV enhancer and a deletion in the U3 region of the 3′ LTR renders the vector SIN. Not shown is the fact that a portion of the U5 region of the 3′ LTR has been removed and replaced with rabbit β-globin polyadenylation site to enhance safety and improve the efficiency of vector production. Vector production occurs when a mixture of the four plasmid DNAs are transfected into human embryonic kidney (293T) cells and conditioned media is harvested over the next 3–4 days. Depending on the envelope used, the vector preparation may be concentrated by ultracentrifugation or ultrafiltration.

A. Initial MuLV vector

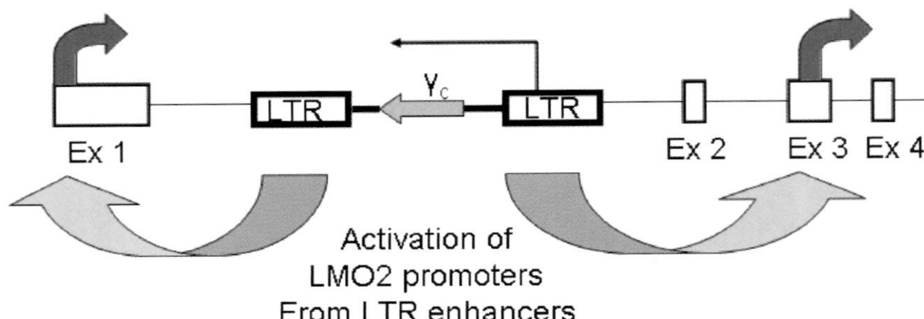

B. SIN lentivector with internal promoter and insulator

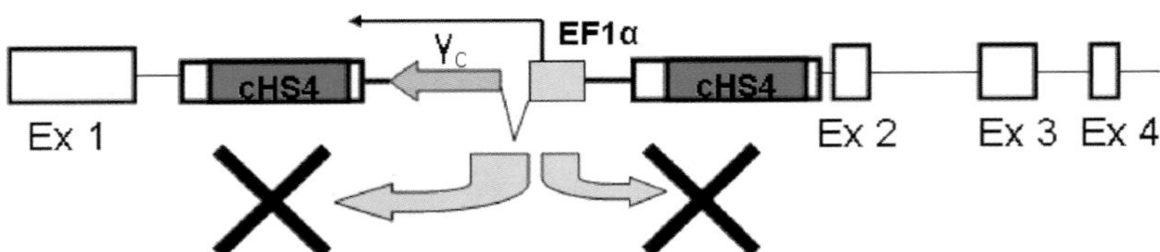

Plate 33.6. Safety design considerations for lentiviral vectors. **(A)** The upper diagram shows the safety problems associated with using γ-retroviral vectors with intact LTRs in the French X-SCID trial. In this case, the vector has integrated into the first intron of the LMO2 gene in a reverse orientation. The strong viral enhancers present in the LTRs activate both cellular LMO2 promoters as shown by the blue and red arrows. This results in oncogene expression in cells that normally would not express LMO2. **(B)** This is a safety modified lentiviral vector that has inactivating mutations in the viral LTRs creating a so-called self-inactivating or SIN design. A copy of the cHS4 chromatin insulator is present in each LTR so that any internal enhancer activity will be blocked from interacting with adjacent cellular promoters (large X). The γ_c transgene is expressed from a single cellular promoter, in the case from the EF1α gene. This promoter itself has much little enhancer activity on its own. This design has been shown to result in no significant LMO2 activation when inserted into the LMO2 locus in a human T cell line.

17

Clinical Aspects of β Thalassemia and Related Disorders

Nancy F. Olivieri and David J. Weatherall

INTRODUCTION

Clinically, either alone or through their interactions with β-globin structural hemoglobin variants, the β thalassemias are by far the most important forms of thalassemia. Their control and management will pose a major drain on health care resources in the new millennium, particularly in emerging countries in which improvements in sanitation and public health measures have dramatically reduced the number of infant deaths from malnutrition and infection, and hence in which babies with these forms of thalassemia increasingly will survive long enough to present for diagnosis and treatment.[1]

In this chapter we describe the clinical and laboratory features of the severe, transfusion-dependent forms of β thalassemia and their carrier states, and discuss what is known of the diverse family of disorders that fall between these extremes, the β thalassemia intermedias. Readers who wish to learn more about the historical development of this field are referred to the monograph of Weatherall and Clegg.[2] The public health and economic aspects of the thalassemias in the developing countries are discussed in detail by Weatherall et al.[3]

CLASSIFICATION, NOMENCLATURE, AND GENOTYPE/PHENOTYPE RELATIONSHIPS

Despite our increasing knowledge of the molecular pathology of the β thalassemias, it is still useful to retain a broad classification based on their clinical manifestations. The severe, transfusion-dependent forms are designated β thalassemia major, or Cooley anemia, and the symptomless carrier states, thalassemia minor. The term thalassemia intermedia is retained for want of anything better to describe the broad spectrum of different forms of thalassemia in which the clinical manifestations lie between these extremes.

Because of the wide variability of the hemoglobin constitution in all the severe forms of β thalassemia, it has been necessary to resort to describing the different subtypes by the more consistent findings in carriers, particularly the level of HbA_2. Most of the common forms of β thalassemia are associated with increased levels of HbA_2 in heterozygotes. There are, however, varieties in which it is in the normal range. These "normal" HbA_2 varieties of β thalassemia are further subdivided into those in which carriers have typical thalassemic morphology of their red cells, and those in which there are no hematological changes, the "silent" β thalassemias. Other forms of β thalassemia have been identified in which carriers have unusually high levels of HbF or HbA_2. Finally, there is a group characterized by a dominant rather than the usual recessive from of inheritance. A classification based on this descriptive approach to defining the different forms of β thalassemia is shown in Table 17.1.

β Thalassemia major usually results from the compound heterozygous state for two different β-globin gene mutations, or less commonly and usually in populations with a high frequency of consanguineous marriages, from the homozygous state for the same mutation. The majority of the β thalassemias are caused by mutations at the β-globin gene loci, which result in no output of β-globin chains, β^0 thalassemia, or a reduced output β^+ thalassemia. Hence compound heterozygotes may be heterozygous for both β^+ and β^0 thalassemia or for two different forms of either β^0 or β^+ thalassemia. The term β^{++} thalassemia is sometimes used to describe β thalassemia with a particularly mild reduction in β-globin chain synthesis.

Because many different mutations underlie the β thalassemias, and those that cause β^+ thalassemia vary in their overall effect on β-chain synthesis, it is not surprising that either alone or through their interactions with structural hemoglobin variants or with α thalassemia, they generate a wide variety of different clinical phenotypes. In the sections that follow the main clinical, laboratory, and diagnostic features of these different forms of β thalassemia are described.

THE SEVERE TRANSFUSION-DEPENDENT FORMS OF β THALASSEMIA: β THALASSEMIA MAJOR

The major forms of β thalassemia are defined as genetic disorders of β-globin chain synthesis in which life can only be sustained by regular blood transfusion.

The early descriptions of severe thalassemia by Cooley and others, reviewed by Weatherall and Clegg,[2] present a picture of the disease as it was and unfortunately still is seen in children who have either not been transfused at all or given inadequate transfusion. If children are adequately treated in this way many of the "typical" features of thalassemia do not appear in early childhood and most of the clinical problems that occur after the first decade are the result of iron accumulation. For this reason it is necessary to consider this disease in two settings: the inadequately

Table 17.1. The different phenotypes of β thalassemia

β thalassemia major
β^0 thalassemia
β^+ thalassemia
(β^{++} thalassemia)
β thalassemia intermedia
β thalassemia minor (trait)
With raised level of HbA_2
Low or slightly elevated level of HbF
Unusually high levels of HbF
Unusually high levels of HbA_2
Normal levels of HbA_2
β thalassemia with δ thalassemia
Mild β thalassemia
'Silent' β thalassemia
β thalassemia with α thalassemia
Symptomatic
Dominant β thalassemia
β thalassemia trait with ααα or αααα
β thalassemia with genetic determinant unlinked to β globin gene locus

treated child and the child who has been transfused from early in life.

General Clinical Features and Course

Age and Symptoms at Presentation

Because β-chain synthesis replaces γ-chain synthesis during the first months of life it might be expected that β thalassemia would become manifest at approximately that time. This is usually the case. Severe forms of β thalassemia commonly present during the first year. For example, Kattamis et al.[4] noted that the mean age at presentation was 13.1 months (±8.1 months), with a range from 2 to 36 months. In reviewing 121 patients, Modell and Berdoukas[5] found that 60% presented within the first year; the mean age at presentation was 6 months (Table 17.2). Similarly, Cao[6] found that, comparing a group of transfusion-dependent with nontransfusion-dependent β thalassemics, the mean age of presentation of the former was 8.4 ± 9.1 months whereas in the latter it was 17.4 ± 11.8 months. The mean hemoglobin level at presentation in the

Table 17.2. Age at presentation of infants with thalassemia major or intermedia

Age (y)	Thalassemia major	Thalassemia intermedia
<1	75 (62%)	4 (11%)
1–2	35 (29%)	11 (30%)
>2	11 (9%)	22 (59%)
Total	121	37

From ref. 5.

transfusion-dependent group was 8.28 g/dL compared with 9.16 ± 1.2 g/dL in the group with milder disease.

Some infants with severe β thalassemia present later than the first year. Their hemoglobin values are in the 6–9 g/dL range and it is not clear whether they are going to fall into the major or intermediate category. After observation for several months it is apparent that they are failing to thrive or not growing adequately, and it is clear that they require regular transfusion. The same reasoning applies to even older children who have been categorized as having thalassemia intermedia but in whom poor growth or the development of other complications indicate that they are transfusion dependent.

A wide variety of symptoms may alert the parents to the fact that the child has a serious illness. Frequently, infants fail to thrive and to gain weight normally and become progressively pale. Feeding problems, diarrhea, irritability, recurrent bouts of infection, progressive enlargement of the abdomen due to splenomegaly, or failure to recover from an infective episode are common presenting symptoms. Less usual presentations include the incidental finding of an enlarged spleen, a fever of unknown origin, or the mother noticing that the infant's urine stains the napkin (diaper) pink or brown.[5] At this stage the infant may look pale but otherwise there may be no abnormal signs. On the other hand, splenomegaly may already be present. Thus an accurate diagnosis depends on the hematological findings described later in this chapter, together with the demonstration of the β thalassemia trait in both parents.

If a firm diagnosis is made at this stage and the infant is started on a regular blood transfusion regimen, subsequent growth and development may be relatively normal over the next decade. If the child is not adequately transfused, however, the typical clinical picture of β thalassemia major develops over the next few years.

Diagnostic Difficulties at Presentation

When babies with β thalassemia major present with failure to thrive and anemia, whether or not splenomegaly is already present, the diagnosis is usually made from the appearance of the peripheral blood film, the finding of an unusually high level of fetal hemoglobin, and the demonstration of the carrier state in both parents. Infants often present with an acute infective episode and it is not clear the extent to which their anemia reflects infection rather than severe thalassemia. Although the blood picture can be examined first it is often necessary to transfuse them to tide them over this acute episode. All too often the infant is then assumed to be transfusion dependent, and labeled as having the major form of the illness. It is very important to stop transfusions, either immediately or after an interval to allow the child to recover fully and to observe the steady-state hemoglobin off transfusion. Only in this way is it possible to identify the milder, intermediate forms of the disease that have been exacerbated by intercurrent illness.

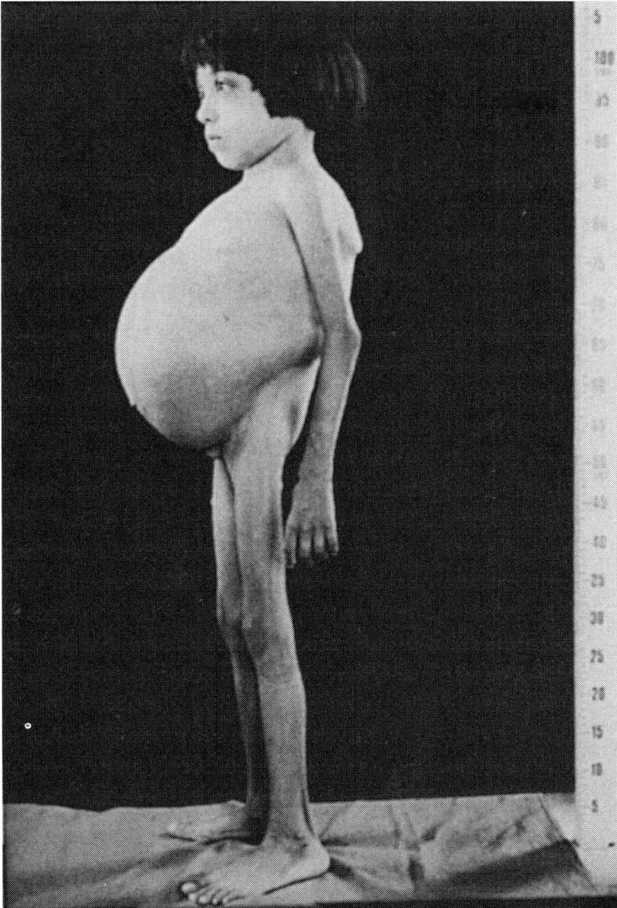

Figure 17.1. A child with β thalassemia maintained on a low-transfusion regimen. There is massive hepatosplenomegaly and marked wasting of the limbs. The peculiar stance with arching of the back is typical of this condition. (From ref. 2 with permission.)

Although the diagnosis of β thalassemia major is usually fairly straightforward we have observed a number of cases, particularly in the developing countries, in which difficulties arose. For example, the disease may present with an acute illness, and there are certain infections that can mimic β thalassemia. Malaria causes anemia and splenomegaly, and although the peripheral blood findings are quite different it may be necessary to administer antimalarial agents and carefully reexamine the child to see if the spleen has regressed, and to assess the hematological findings, before the diagnosis of β thalassemia is confirmed. Occasionally, the anemia and splenomegaly associated with leukemia may superficially resemble β thalassemia; juvenile chronic myeloid leukemia, particularly because of the associated high level of fetal hemoglobin production, may sometimes cause confusion. Severe iron deficiency can usually be diagnosed from the hematological picture together with the low serum iron and ferritin values, whereas the blood pictures associated with other congenital hemolytic anemias are sufficiently different to make them unlikely to be confused with β thalassemia. We have seen several patients with congenital dyserythropoietic anemia who were thought to have β thalassemia; although the blood pictures are quite different the associated splenomegaly and dyserythropoiesis may cause confusion.

Course Through Childhood in Inadequately Transfused Patients

The undertransfused thalassemic child may be growth retarded; some are noticeably smaller than their normal siblings, although, in general, slowing of growth is more marked as puberty approaches. There is pallor of the mucous membranes and skin, a variable degree of icterus, and the dirty gray-brown pigmentation, first noticed by Cooley in his early descriptions of the disease. These children fail to thrive and show features of a hypermetabolic state, including poor musculature, reduction in body fat, recurrent fever, poor appetite, and lethargy; the neglected child with β thalassemia, with the characteristic protuberant abdomen, poor musculoskeletal development, and spindly legs looks very much like a child with malignant disease (Fig. 17.1). There is a variable degree of hepatosplenomegaly together with skeletal changes that produce a characteristic facial appearance, with bossing of the skull (Fig. 17.2), hypertrophy of the maxilla that tends to

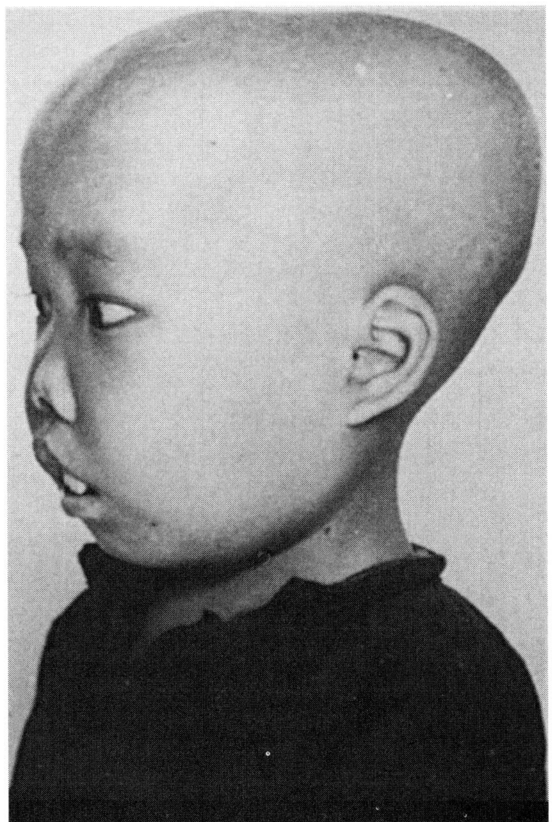

Figure 17.2 Changes in the skull in a child with thalassemia major. (From ref. 2 with permission.)

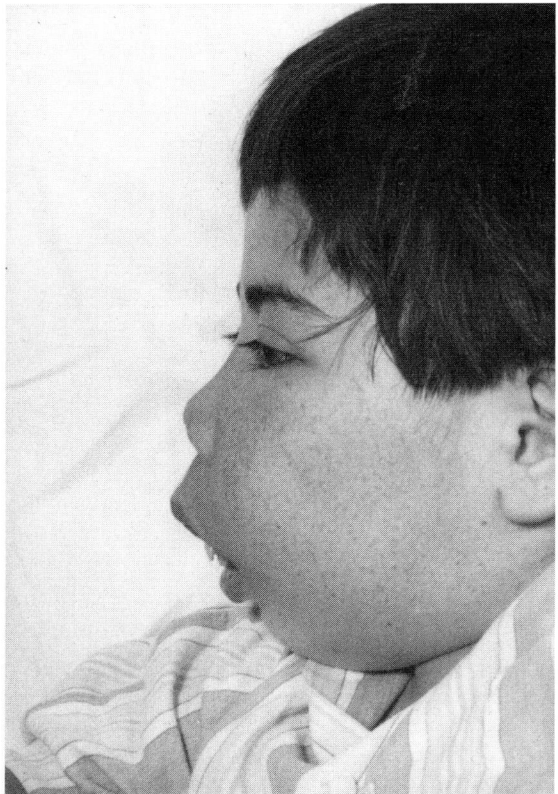

Figure 17.3. A child with thalassemia major showing typical deformities of the jaw and dentition. (From ref. 2 with permission.)

expose the upper teeth, prominent malar eminences with depression of the bridge of the nose (Fig. 17.3), puffiness of the eyelids, and a tendency to a mongoloid slant of the eyes. There may also be proximal muscle weakness and a genu valgum. Recurrent ulceration of the legs may occur at any time throughout childhood.

The skeletal changes are mirrored by characteristic radiological changes of the skull, long bones, and hands. The skull shows dilatation of the diploic space, and the subperiosteal bone grows in a series of radiating striations, giving a typical "hair on end" appearance (Fig. 17.4). There is cortical thinning of the long bones with porous rarefaction; similar changes are found in the small bones of the hands and feet (Fig. 17.5). These radiological changes, noted as early as 1930 by Voght and Diamond, have been the subject of many reviews.[7–9] Pathological fractures are also a major feature of inadequately transfused children.[10]

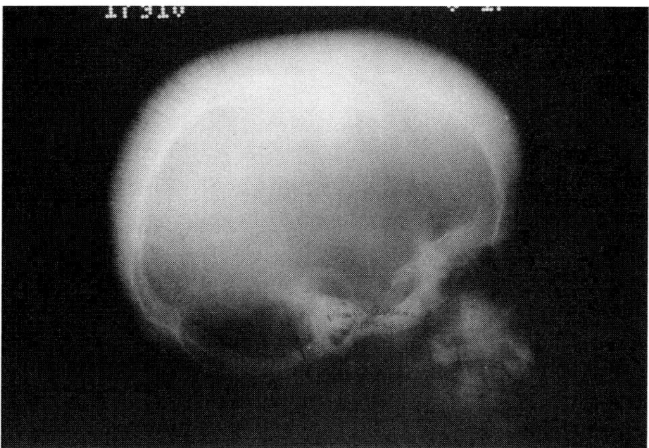

Figure 17.4. The skull in homozygous β thalassemia showing the typical "hair on end" appearance.

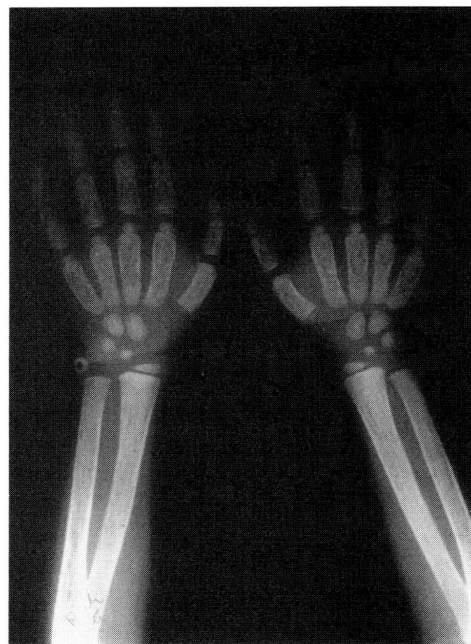

Figure 17.5. Radiological changes in the bones of the hands in thalassemia major.

The early childhood of these patients is interspersed with numerous complications. They include recurrent infections associated with worsening of the anemia, compression syndromes due to progressive bone deformity, folate deficiency, a bleeding tendency, increasing hypersplenism, gallstones, leg ulcers, and a variety of neurological conditions due to tumor masses resulting from extramedullary hematopoiesis. If they survive to puberty they often develop similar complications to children who, because they have been adequately transfused, have had a relatively trouble-free childhood.

The Well-transfused Thalassemic Child

Well-transfused thalassemic children often remain asymptomatic until early puberty. Their future course then depends on whether they have received adequate iron chelation. If not, they begin to show signs of hepatic, endocrine, and cardiac disturbances resembling those seen in adults with familial hemochromatosis. The first observable changes are often a failure or reduction of the pubertal growth spurt, sometimes associated with delayed sexual maturation. Throughout their teenage life these children suffer from a variety of complications due to different endocrine deficiencies and they nearly all develop cardiac symptoms in the latter half of the second decade.

Children who are adequately transfused and are fully compliant with respect to iron chelation may grow and develop normally, enter puberty, and become sexually mature. Even within this group, however, there is a disappointingly high frequency of growth retardation and retarded sexual maturation.

This subdivision of the course of severe β thalassemia is, of course, rather artificial; many patients are encountered who fall between one or the other group. In the sections that follow we consider the major complications of the severe β thalassemias; in many cases they are also relevant to the intermediate forms, described later in this chapter.

Complications

The frequency and severity of the complications of β thalassemia depend to a large extent on the way that patients are managed, particularly with respect to their steady-state hemoglobin level and effectiveness of chelation therapy. They can all be related to the primary defect in globin-chain synthesis (Fig. 17.6).

Hypersplenism and Plasma-Volume Expansion

All the early literature on thalassemia stresses the occurrence of progressive splenomegaly in the major form of the illness (see Weatherall and Clegg[2]). Splenectomy for the treatment of thalassemia has also been practiced from the time that the disease was first identified.

As soon as there was sufficient experience with children who had been maintained at relatively high hemoglobin levels it became apparent that marked splenomegaly and hypersplenism were being seen much less frequently.[11,12] In a series of careful measurements of the annual blood requirements of her patients, Modell demonstrated that it was possible to calculate an average annual transfusion requirement to maintain a mean hemoglobin level of approximately 10 g/dL. Patients who exceeded this figure by 50% or more almost invariably returned to their "ideal" transfusion requirements after splenectomy.[5,11,13] These observations were confirmed by others, who found that children who need more than 200–250 mL of packed cells/kg body weight/year to maintain average hemoglobins at approximately 10 g/dL have significant hypersplenism, and that splenectomy significantly reduces these requirements.[14] More recent experience suggests that hypersplenism may usually be avoided by early and regular transfusion and that many patients reaching adolescence after following a regimen of this type do not require splenectomy.[15]

Splenic enlargement may cause a variety of complications. Occasionally, there is physical discomfort simply due to the size of the spleen. The formed elements of the blood may be trapped in the splenic pool, producing anemia,

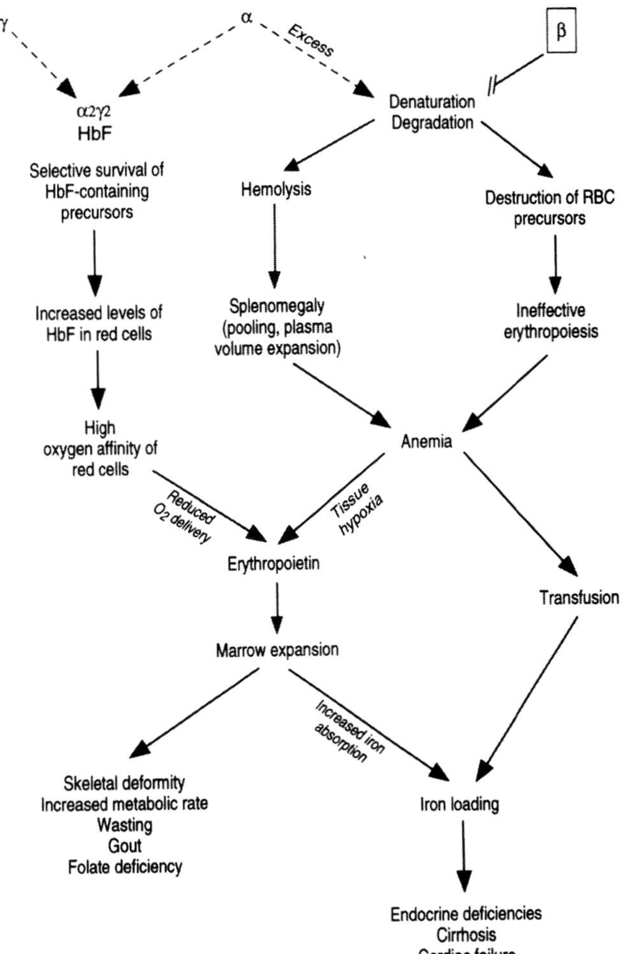

Figure 17.6. The pathophysiology of β thalassemia.

thrombocytopenia and some degree of neutropenia. The anemia of hypersplenism has a complex pathophysiology. Several early studies reported red cell mass and survival data in thalassemic children with large spleens.[16–19] There is invariably some shortening of the autologous red cell survival, trapping of a proportion of the red cells in the splenic red cell pool, and a marked expansion of the total blood volume. In the study of Blendis et al.[16] the trapped cells in the splenic pool accounted for between 9% and 40% of the total red cell mass. There is marked expansion of the plasma volume, which has the effect of worsening the anemia and, incidentally, producing a greater load on the myocardium. The reasons for the changes in plasma volume, which occur in patients with splenomegaly associated with other diseases, is not entirely clear. It is not due entirely to splenomegaly or hepatosplenomegaly; the plasma volume may remain significantly expanded after splenectomy for many months.[16] One factor that has been incriminated is expansion of the bone marrow, which may act as a vascular shunt, a mechanism that is thought to result in plasma volume expansion in a number of other settings.

Finally, it should be remembered that a very large spleen constitutes an extensive mass of ineffective hematopoietic tissue. Thus, as it enlarges, it increases the metabolic demands of the growing child while, at the same time, causing hemodilution and plasma volume expansion.

Iron Overload

Iron overload has been a recognized feature of severe forms of thalassemia since the first autopsy reports.[20] The mechanisms of iron toxicity, its tissue distribution, and the way that it causes organ failure are discussed in Chapter 29, and the methods by which the total body iron burden can be assessed are discussed later in this chapter. Here, we outline the main features of iron accumulation as a background to the description of its effects on individual organs that follow.

It was quite apparent from the results of the first iron absorption studies, and the transfusion histories of thalassemic children in the days before high transfusion regimens were instituted, that iron loading was the result of increased absorption and transfusion, however inadequate. When assessing the results of higher transfusion regimens, Modell[11] estimated that by the time children maintained asymptomatic at a relatively high hemoglobin level reached the age of 11 years they would have accumulated approximately 28 g of iron. She suggested that it was only at approximately this level of iron loading that patients begin to show signs of hepatic, cardiac, and endocrine disturbance.

Because iron overload was to become the major cause of death in thalassemia it was clearly important to attempt to derive more accurate approaches to assessing the level of iron accumulation that would render patients at risk from life-threatening complications. Letsky et al.[21] found that there was a good correlation between the serum-ferritin and liver-iron concentrations in β thalassemics maintained on high transfusion regimens. The values in most of their older patients were extremely high and well within the range seen in untreated hereditary hemochromatosis. These workers noticed that during the period over which the first 50–100 U of blood was transfused there was a steep rise in ferritin levels, after which the rate of increase was less marked. Later studies also indicated that the correlation between transfusion load and serum ferritin may not be so clear-cut.[22] Indeed, Worwood et al.[23] found that a maximum plasma ferritin concentration of approximately 5,000 μg/L probably reflects the upper physiological limit of the rate of its synthesis; higher concentrations are now thought to be caused by the release of intracellular ferritin from damaged cells. Several other factors probably determine the level of circulating ferritin, including ascorbate deficiency, infection, hepatic damage, hemolysis, and ineffective erythropoiesis.[24,25]

Unequivocal evidence that the serum ferritin level cannot be relied on as an accurate assessment of total body iron burden was reported by Olivieri et al.[26] who found that over a wide range of serum ferritin levels and hepatic iron values, there was a wide scatter and, indeed, that the 95% prediction intervals in hepatic-iron concentrations for a given plasma ferritin were so broad as to make determination of plasma ferritin a poor predictor of body iron stores.

Later work, reviewed by Olivieri and Brittenham,[15] provided more accurate information about the levels of hepatic iron at which patients are at risk of serious complications of iron overload. These studies, which extrapolate from data obtained from patients with genetic hemochromatosis, showed that patients with hepatic iron levels of approximately 80 μmol iron/g liver, wet weight, which is approximately 15 mg iron/g liver, dry weight, are at an increased risk of hepatic disease and endocrine organ damage. Patients with higher body-iron burdens are at particular risk of cardiac disease and early death. Recently, noninvasive approaches to assessing these critical liver-iron concentrations using magnetic resonance imaging have been developed[27] (see later section).

Although in the following sections we shall focus our attention on the consequence of iron loading of the heart, endocrine glands, and liver, it is likely that excess body iron has other, less dramatic pathological consequences. For example, it is responsible for the curious gray pigmentation that has been a well-recognized feature of the severe forms of thalassemia ever since they were first described. The complex relationship between iron loading and increased susceptibility to infection will be considered further later in this chapter.

Cardiac Complications

The cardiac complications of β thalassemia are the most important factors in determining the survival in both transfused and untransfused patients. Although they have been recognized for decades, many aspects of cardiac disease in β thalassemia are still poorly understood. It is clear that they are multifactorial, reflecting chronic anemia, iron overload, the consequences of pulmonary disease, myocarditis, pericarditis, and probably many other mechanisms.

Mechanisms. Many of the cardiological changes observed in undertransfused children with severe thalassemia are part of the adaptive changes to hypoxia that occur in all forms of anemia. They include enhanced left ventricular contractility, an elevated cardiac output, left ventricular hypertrophy, and ultimately, dilation, and, in cases of profound anemia, all the manifestations of congestive cardiac failure.

The advent of high transfusion regimens rescued many thalassemic children from these distressing complications in early life but, until the development of effective chelation regimens, only bought time until they died of a cardiac disease or other complications of iron loading toward the end of the second decade of life.[28] There is now good evidence

Table 17.3. Cardiac complications of β thalassemia

Cardiac failure due to severe anemia
Iron loading of the myocardium
Cardiac failure with or without arrhythmias
Right-sided failure
Recurrent pulmonary emboli
Obliterative pulmonary artery disease*
Lung disease due to iron overload
Pericarditis
Myocarditis

* Thought to be due to platelet aggregation, particularly postsplenectomy in intermediate forms of thalassemia.

that effective chelation may protect transfusion-dependent patients from developing cardiac disease. Because many patients do not adhere sufficiently strictly to their chelation programs, and because their expense precludes their use in many developing countries, cardiac disease remains a major challenge in the management of patients with severe forms of thalassemia.

It should be emphasized that the cardiological complications of thalassemia are not restricted to the effects of anemia and iron loading, although they are by far the most important factors (Table 17.3). For example, it has been recognized that, at least in some countries, patients with thalassemia major may be unusually prone to myocarditis.[29] In addition, some patients with severe forms of β thalassemia have an additional burden of right-heart strain due to chronic pulmonary hypertension.[30] It has been suggested that this too may be related to iron overload (see later section), but it may also follow recurrent, small pulmonary emboli. Unfortunately, except for data from Thailand on the frequent occurrence of this type of complication in splenectomized patients with HbE–β thalassemia,[31] there have been few studies that have pursued this possibility. Hoeper et al.[32] have suggested that there is an increased risk of pulmonary hypertension in patients who have undergone splenectomy for any cause; autopsy data showed abundant pulmonary thrombotic lesions. The relationship of these changes to persistent thrombocytosis and an increased propensity to thromboembolic disease is discussed later in this chapter.

Children with severe β thalassemia were also prone to recurrent attacks of pericarditis. Smith et al.[19,33] first reported that a benign, transient pericarditis often develops after splenectomy. This complication was later well documented by others.[34,35] Engle[28] also observed this complication but could find no causal or temporal relationship with splenectomy and suggested that these events may coincide toward the end of the first decade of life. Several workers, notably Orsini et al.,[34] examined the relationship between pericarditis and iron loading but could find no convincing evidence that the two are connected. Over recent years this complication has been seen less frequently.

Pathology. Most of the information on the pathology of the myocardium in β thalassemia comes from autopsy studies, many of which were published in the era before the introduction of iron chelation therapy. In most cases a diffuse, rust-brown staining of the myocardium was observed, together with right and left ventricular hypertrophy, dilation, and a greatly increased cardiac weight (see Engle[28]). In most of the early series, evidence of pericarditis was found.[28,36] Interestingly, an autopsy series of 19 patients with cardiac iron loading and anemia due to causes other than thalassemia did not mention pericarditis.[37]

Estimations of the iron content of the myocardium have shown gross elevations to as much as 20 times normal. They have also underlined the marked variation in cardiac iron content, in two studies, from 0.9 to 9.2 mg/iron/g of heart, dry weight, for example.[37,38] In an extensive examination of iron-loaded hearts in patients who had received transfusions for conditions other than thalassemia,[37] iron was present in myocardial fibers as well as in the connective tissue. The endocardium was reported to have an iron concentration equal to less than 50% of that in the epicardium; iron was concentrated in the left ventricular septum and free wall, with maximal concentration in the left ventricular epicardium. The preferential deposition of iron in the epicardium, only later involving the remainder of the myocardium, may explain the preservation of systolic ventricular function early in the course of the disease. Attempts to relate cardiac function to the degree of iron overload suggest that high concentrations of iron correlate reasonably well with the degree of dysfunction, although, surprisingly, in many patients iron deposition in the conduction system appears to be relatively mild, even in those who die of cardiac arrhythmias.[37,38]

Other changes that have been observed at autopsy include extensive myocardial fibre disruption and variable fibrosis.[38–40] Witzleben and Wyatt reported findings in two children aged 8 and 10 years, respectively. There was prominent right ventricular hypertrophy and pericarditis, but cardiac fibrosis was absent or minimal, despite the presence of hepatic cirrhosis. Although these studies suggested that iron deposition alone might not be enough to produce a fibrotic reaction, later work showed that iron loading is probably the major factor in generating these changes.[41] Endomyocardial biopsies have demonstrated that interstitial fibrosis correlates reasonably well with persistent electrophysiological disturbances, at least in primary hemochromatosis.[42]

Pathophysiology. It is clear from the concentrations observed in autopsy studies that the heart can accommodate less iron load than the liver, possibly because cardiac cells have a relatively small amount of storage protein and may be more sensitive to free-iron–induced oxygen radicals. There is some evidence that very low levels of myocardial iron may interfere directly with diastolic function,[43] a process that resembles the effect of hypercalcemia, and which is characterized by inadequate relaxation, spontaneous early depolarization, and subsequent failure of contractility.[44] The generation of free hydroxyl radicals may result in damage to the lysosomal membrane of cardiac cells and lead to the disruption of the sarcolemmal membrane and inhibition of the mitochondrial respiratory chain.[45–47] The effects of iron may be augmented by a number of variables, including the reduction of ferric to ferrous iron and the addition of low concentrations of ascorbic acid; conversely, the effects of iron may be inhibited by high concentrations of ascorbic acid, α-tocopherol, and desferrioxamine.[45,48] More recent studies, reviewed by Wood et al.[49] have emphasized the role of nontransferrin-bound iron (NTBI) in the pathogenesis of cardiac damage due to iron loading. In culture, NTBI uptake into myocytes is rapid and may be increased by prior exposure to iron. Both the level and duration of NTBI exposure are important components of cardiac iron uptake. Once NTBI enters the myocyte it is rapidly buffered by ferritin, hence limiting its potential for redox damage. Ferritin–iron complexes enter intracellular siderosomes, where they are stored. Because these buffering systems have a limited capacity, or may be disrupted by other factors, free-iron levels increase within the myocyte. Through the Haber–Weiss reaction, iron catalyses free-radical production, leading to widespread oxidative damage, mitochondrial dysfunction, impairment of cellular energy production and to a wide variety of alterations in cardiac gene expression. Cardiac arrhythmias may be potentiated by the direct action of ferrous iron with the ryanodine-sensitive calcium channel in the sarcoplasmic reticulum. Intracellular iron also impairs function of membrane-bound fast-sodium channels.

In inadequately transfused patients, the magnitude of the body-iron burden is the chief factor in the development of cardiac disease.[15] This appears to be true even though lung disease and myocarditis may aggravate iron-induced cardiac disease, as shown in a 5-year study of more than 1,000 thalassemic patients, of whom approximately 5% developed serious cardiac disease secondary to myocarditis with no evidence of iron overload.[29] Although the low incidence of iron-induced cardiac disease in this young and well-treated population is not surprising, it should be emphasized that infectious myocarditis may play a role in the development of cardiac disease and, conversely, that iron-promoted free radical formation may contribute to the pathogenesis of infectious myocarditis.

Clinical presentations. Considering this complex pathology it is not surprising that the clinical presentation of cardiac disease in thalassemia is extremely variable. It should be anticipated in any patient over the age of 15 years who has been inadequately transfused and chelated, who has been maintained at a high hemoglobin level with inadequate chelation, and, in particular, who has a hepatic iron concentration in excess of 15 mg/g liver dry weight[15] or an equivalent value as assessed by magnetic resonance imaging (MRI).[27]

The clinical descriptions of recent years have never bettered those of Engle,[28] who described a progressive staging for cardiac disease in irregularly transfused patients. In the first stage, observed at approximately the age of 10 years, asymptomatic but progressive cardiac enlargement was noted. This was often followed by attacks of pericarditis at a mean age of approximately 11 years, sometimes associated with large pericardial effusions. This complication was observed in nearly half the patients; no infective cause could be found. The third stage was characterized by the appearance of first-degree heart block, occasional atrial premature beats, and abnormal T waves. Finally, the typical signs of congestive cardiac failure appeared, with features of both right and left ventricular failure in parallel with serious disturbances of rhythm and conduction. The peak incidence of the final stage was between 10 and 15 years. The duration of life after the onset of failure was less than 3 months in more than half the patients, and one-third died within a month of the appearance of cardiac failure.

This general pattern of progression of cardiac disease is still observed, although, as mentioned earlier, pericarditis is seen much less frequently. Occasionally the picture may be predominantly of right heart failure.[28,50,51] As pointed out by Jessup and Manno,[52] in older, adequately chelated patients who are often asymptomatic there may be more subtle abnormalities of both systolic and diastolic function that are multifactorial in origin.

The clinical diagnosis of iron-induced cardiomyopathy is extremely difficult. The symptoms parallel that of left ventricular function, but there may be no abnormalities until the rapid onset of overt cardiac failure. Palpitations may simply be related to anemia or other cardiac abnormalities. Similarly, a poor exercise tolerance may also be related to anemia.

Detection of cardiac dysfunction. The investigation of cardiac function in thalassemia remains problematic. Conduction/rhythm abnormalities correlate poorly with conduction–tissue iron infiltration in autopsy sections of patients who have died of cardiac arrhythmias. Moreover, the subendocardial iron concentration is much less than that found in the epicardial region, so that endomyocardial biopsy may underestimate the degree of iron deposition.[53] There is no particular electrocardiographic finding indicative of iron-induced cardiac dysfunction, although serial tracings may be useful in that a significant change is often indicative of a process other than increased iron deposition. Holter monitoring has been shown to be of little value in predicting the onset of cardiac disease.[54] There is a large literature on the value of echocardiography in the diagnosis of iron loading of the myocardium. In general, systolic function, cardiac dimensions, and myocardial wall thickness are normal until there are unequivocal symptoms of cardiac failure. Measurements of resting ejection fraction by radionuclide angiography or MRI are, on the other hand, more effective approaches to identifying early systolic dysfunction.[49,58] As pointed out by Wood et al.,[49] because of the complex cardiac physiology in thalassemic patients, including the reduced afterload consequent on anemia, the expected cardiac parameters for patients who are not iron loaded remain poorly characterized.

Early approaches to the assessment of the risk of cardiac disease by imaging of tissue iron were reviewed by Olivieri and Brittenham.[15] Reasonable correlations between MRI were observed in a thalassemic mouse model,[59] and MRI changes consistent with a reduction of cardiac iron, paralleled by improvement in cardiac function, were reported in individual patients.[60] More recently the MRI-related parameters T2 and T2* have been investigated for their ability to assess iron levels in the heart.[49,61] It appears that myocardial T2 and T2* shorten in patients with thalassemia; those with normal T2* values have normal function, but the relative prevalence of myocardial dysfunction and arrhythmias increases at lower T2* values. Several uncertainties about the myocardial T2* technique have been raised and its calibration against myocardial iron levels has not yet been carried out. As pointed out by Wood et al.,[49] like many other biomarkers, abnormal T2* conveys only a relative risk; many patients with high iron burdens are asymptomatic at the time of study. The predictive value of abnormal T2*, though implied, has not yet been demonstrated. Recent studies have shown limited or no correlation between cardiac T2* values and hepatic iron levels and have suggested that cardiac dysfunction may occur in the absence of increased hepatic iron.[62,63] It is difficult to understand these findings in the light of the extensive data relating the marked reduction in cardiac disease in patients whose body iron burdens have been maintained at a low level (see later). Clearly a great deal more work is required to clarify these issues, a topic to which we will return later in this chapter.

The measurement of serum atrial natriuretic peptide levels has been reported to be of value in the identification of preclinical cardiac involvement,[64] although further experience of this approach is still required. Decreased antioxidant activity of apolipoprotein E, related to the frequency of the apolipoprotein E4 allele, has been proposed as a genetic risk for left ventricular failure in thalassemia.[65]

In a critical review of the current state of assessing cardiac function in iron-loaded patients, Jessup and Manno[52] emphasized that none of the methods that have been used to assess early myocardial impairment have been rigorously tested in a prospective manner. They suggested that the combined information obtained from the patient's transfusion record, serial serum ferritin levels, details of their adherence to a chelation regimen, and, most important, hepatic iron concentration, provides as much predictive power as any of the noninvasive tests. Although some progress has been made more recently toward improving the latter, given the complexity of the pathophysiology of cardiac disease in thalassemia more prospective studies involving these new noninvasive approaches to assessing cardiac function are still required.[49]

Changing pattern of cardiac disease. With the advent of adequate chelation therapy there was a major change in the frequency of cardiac disease.[15] Two long-term trials showed quite unequivocally that the effective use of desferrioxamine results in long-term survival and the absence of cardiological complications. In one, which used the serum ferritin as a measure of iron loading, those who maintained concentrations of less than 2,500 μg/L had an estimated cardiac-free survival of 91% after 15 years; patients in whom most of the serum ferritin concentrations exceeded this figure had an estimated cardiac disease–free survival after 15 years of less than 20%.[66] The other study assessed chelation therapy in terms of hepatic iron storage; values of 80 μmol of iron/g liver weight (15 mg iron/g liver, dry weight) were used as a cut-off point above and below which patients were classified as having received ineffective or effective chelation therapy, respectively. The probability of survival to at least 25 years was only 32% among patients above the threshold.[67] These findings have been confirmed more recently in a long-term follow-up study involving seven Italian centers.[68]

Lung Disease and Pulmonary Hypertension

Over the last three decades there has been an increasing recognition of the occurrence of chronic lung disease in β thalassemia, which may aggravate cardiac disease.

A variety of functional abnormalities have been reported, including small airway obstruction, hyperinflation, and hypoxemia, possibly as the result of several different pathological processes.[30,69–71] Other studies have described a primarily restrictive pattern of lung disease, with abnormalities consistent with obstructive airways disease.[30,72–75] Studies of total lung capacity have given inconsistent results, as have the effects of transfusion on pulmonary function.[71,75]

These abnormalities have been related to autopsy findings, which have shown massive accumulation of hemosiderin in alveolar phagocytes in the perivascular and supporting framework.[40,73] In some but not all series, fibrosis was noted in the majority of cases. In addition, sclerotic vascular lesions and thromboemboli have been observed and have been attributed to platelet thrombi.[76,77] A variety of mechanisms have been proposed to account for this pathology. They include tissue damage due to the generation of free hydroxyl radicals secondary to iron deposition, ferrugination of connective tissue resulting in reduced capillary compliance, and other less well-defined abnormalities of the alveolar capillary membrane.[78,79] Abnormal growth and development of the alveolus, secondary either to intrinsic disease or due to frequent transfusions, has also been proposed as a contributing factor.[79]

Pulmonary hypertension and right heart failure is being recognized increasingly frequently, particularly in patients with β thalassemia major who have been inadequately treated or in those with β thalassemia intermedia. Although structural changes in the lung may play a role, the pathophysiology is multifactorial and extremely complex (reviewed by Aessopos and Farmakis[80]). There is increasing evidence that pulmonary hypertension may occur in a variety of chronic hemolytic states as a result of erythrocyte release of arginase coupled with liberation of cell-free hemoglobin leading to dysregulated arginine metabolism and decreased nitric oxide availability. Vascular damage, reflected in a diffuse elastic tissue defect that resembles pseudoxanthoma elasticum, has been observed in patients with β thalassemia, especially thalassemia intermedia. The endothelial dysfunction resulting from these mechanisms may also be involved in in situ thrombus formation within the pulmonary vascular bed. These changes may be enhanced in patients with β thalassemia due to oxidative stress resulting from iron overload and the structural changes outlined earlier. In addition, as outlined in the next section, the hypercoagulable state that occurs in patients with thalassemia intermedia may lead to extensive thromboembolic disease, which leads to further right-heart strain. Finally, chronic hypoxia tends to lead to further vasoconstriction and increase in pulmonary vascular resistance. In short, the complex interaction of increased cardiac output and chronic pulmonary vascular resistance combine to produce chronic pulmonary hypertension and right heart failure.

Thromboembolic Disease

There is clear evidence that patients with β thalassemia are at increased risk of thromboembolic disease. In a 1989 study conducted in Italy that examined the causes of death in thalassemia major, it was found that thromboembolism was the primary cause in four of 159 thalassemic patients.[51] In Israel, Michaeli et al.[81] reported thromboembolic events, either recurrent arterial occlusion or, more commonly, pulmonary thromboembolism, in 4% of patients with thalassemia major. Borgna-Pignatti et al.[82] identified 32 patients with thromboembolic episodes of a total of 735 patients with β thalassemia, 683 with thalassemia major and 52 with thalassemia intermedia. The most common variety was stroke, which made up half of their cases. Other manifestations included pulmonary embolism, mesenteric or portal thrombosis, and deep venous thrombosis in either the upper or lower limbs. In an analysis of more than 8,000 patients in Italy it was found that the total number of thrombotic events was 1.65%, with a prevalence in those with thalassemia major of 0.9% and with thalassemia intermedia of 4%. There was a significant increase in the prevalence in splenectomized patients.[83]

The mechanisms that underlie the increased risk of thromboembolic disease in patients with β thalassemia are complex and multifactorial.[83,84] They include endothelial activation and vascular occlusion, as evidenced by elevated levels of endothelial adhesion proteins, vasoconstriction through a nitric oxide–mediated mechanism as outlined in the previous section, thrombocytosis, and, in particular, the procoagulant properties of the thalassemic red cells. The latter appears to be the result of an increased expression of anionic phospholipids such as phosphatidylserine. This phenomenon may be more marked in splenectomized patients or in those with thalassemia intermedia because of the higher frequency of abnormal red cells in the circulation. These damaged red cells may exhibit alterations of the phospholipid in a "flip-flop" mechanism, favoring exposure of negatively charged procoagulant phospholipids. Furthermore, other factors, both genetic and acquired, may contribute toward an increased likelihood of thromboembolic disease (reviewed by Weatherall and Clegg[2]). For example, as mentioned earlier, thalassemic patients with heart failure have a higher risk of thrombosis if they carry the apolipoprotein E4 allele.[65] It has also been observed that thalassemic patients with hepatitis C may have an increased frequency of anticardiolipin antibodies and lupus anticoagulant and that this may also be associated with an increased risk of thromboembolic events.[85]

Endocrine Dysfunction

It was recognized many years ago that the iron loading of the tissues that occurs in severe forms of β thalassemia has a particular predilection for the endocrine organs. The early literature on this topic is reviewed by Weatherall and Clegg.[2] Although these studies were conducted in very heterogeneous populations of patients it became apparent that the most common endocrine abnormalities are hypogonadotropic hypogonadism, growth hormone deficiency, and diabetes mellitus; the frequencies of hypothyroidism, hypoparathyroidism, and adrenal insufficiency seem to be much lower.

Retarded growth and development. The early literature on thalassemia major frequently emphasized defective growth and development (see Weatherall and Clegg[2]). Later studies confirmed these observations and suggested that linear growth rates and final heights are related to the hemoglobin levels that have been maintained throughout early life.[86] Growth disturbances associated with low transfusion regimens are characterized by lack of weight gain and, in particular, a reduced muscle mass, which often gives the limbs a characteristic sticklike appearance and limits exercise tolerance through weakness. Modell and Berdoukas[5] observed that undertransfused patients have a much lower level of creatinine excretion in their urine than those maintained on higher transfusion regimens. Because approximately 2% of muscle creatine is broken down to creatinine each day, and this provides the only source of urinary creatinine, these studies were compatible with the

Table 17.4. Some suggested mechanisms of defective growth in β thalassemia

Inadequate transfusion
Iron overload
Selective central hypogonadism
Defective production of insulin-like growth factor 1
Impaired growth hormone response to growth-hormone releasing hormone
Abnormal growth hormone secretion
Abnormality of growth hormone receptor
Reduced secretion of adrenal androgen
Zinc deficiency
Free-hemoglobin-induced inhibition of cartilage growth
Desferrioxamine toxicity

concept that a low-transfusion regimen is associated with a reduced muscle mass and development.

The introduction of high-transfusion regimens for thalassemic children did not entirely solve the problem of growth retardation, however. Indeed, as pointed out by Modell[11,87] one of the first indications of tissue damage due to iron overload is a failure of the normal pubertal growth spurt. This is not the whole story because even children who are well transfused and adequately chelated, and apparently who have normal sexual development, may still show some degree of growth retardation and a reduced final height.[5,88,89]

The reasons for growth retardation in well-transfused children are extremely complex, multifactorial, and not entirely understood (Table 17.4). Undoubtedly, iron accumulation due to variability in the effectiveness of chelation therapy plays a major role. Here again, several mechanisms may be involved. Delayed pubertal growth has been attributed to iron-induced selective central hypogonadism[90–93] or interference by iron with the production of insulin-like growth factor (IGF-1).[94–96] Other mechanisms that have been proposed include impaired growth hormone (GH) response to growth hormone–releasing hormone (GH-RH),[97] abnormalities in GH secretion[98] and, because GH reserves appear to be normal in many patients[99–101] a defect in its receptor, although it has not been possible to demonstrate a lesion of this kind in hepatic tissues.

Several reported studies underline the complexities of these issues. In one, nearly half of a group of patients, most of whom had received regular transfusions and chelation therapy from an early age, had evidence of reduced GH reserve and low IGF-1 levels, with a substantial proportion also demonstrating reduced levels of IGF-BP3, the predominant IGF-1 binding protein, which prolongs the serum half-life of IGF peptides, and which is GH dependent. However, the reduction in GH reserve was not shown to be correlated with short height or delay in bone age.[102]

In a similar analysis of 32 patients with thalassemia major, 14 of whom were short in stature, Roth et al.[103] investigated 13 of the group who exhibited a particularly short stature or reduced growth rate. The stimulated GH secretion in 10 was in the normal range. However, studies of their spontaneous GH secretion during the night revealed that they had markedly reduced amplitudes of their GH peaks (see next section). Low IGF-1 levels were also seen in growth-retarded patients. Stimulation tests showed a marked increase in both IGF-1 and IGF-BP3 levels, indicating intact IGF-1 generation by the liver. After priming with gonadotrophin-releasing hormone (GnRH), no change in either estradiol or testosterone levels or in LH or FSH response was observed, suggesting a severe degree of pituitary gonadotrophin insufficiency. These results indicate that low GH secretion and low levels of IGF-1 in thalassemic patients are related to severe neurosecretory dysfunction rather than liver damage. In short, it was apparent that hypogonadotrophic hypogonadism was a major factor, particularly in the growth-retarded patients who had impaired sexual development.

Evidence has also been presented for the existence of a state of partial growth hormone insensitivity due to a postreceptor defect in growth hormone action, which can be overcome with supraphysiological doses of exogenous GH.[104,105] Other factors that may play a role include a reduced level of secretion of adrenal androgen,[106,107] zinc deficiency,[108] and free-hemoglobin-induced inhibition of cartilage growth.[109] It has also been recognized that short stature, related primarily to disproportionate truncal growth and loss of sitting height, may be caused by desferrioxamine [86,110] and may reflect its damaging effect on spinal cartilage.[26,111]

It is clear, therefore, that growth retardation in thalassemia is both multifactorial and extremely common (Table 17.4). In inadequately transfused patients it seems likely that hypoxia plays a role, while in those who are well transfused but inadequately chelated, iron-mediated damage to the hypothalamic/pituitary axis is the main factor. Because of the extreme sensitivity of some of the endocrine organs to iron excess, and the fact that chelating agents such as desferrioxamine in therapeutic doses can inhibit fibroblast proliferation and collagen formation and chelate other metals, even for thalassemic children who have, by all other criteria, received ideal treatment the potential for growth retardation is still considerable.

Delayed puberty and defective function of the hypothalamic/pituitary axis. Arrest or failure of puberty occurs in approximately 50% of both male and female patients. In one large series secondary amenorrhea was documented in 23% of females and 2% of males, and arrested puberty was observed in 16% of males and 13% of females. Oligomenorrhea or irregular menstrual cycles were reported in approximately 13% of females.[112] Although a conflicting literature has accumulated regarding the overall effects of iron chelation on sexual maturation, most studies have observed an improvement, with significantly reduced serum ferritin concentrations in those who achieve a normal puberty.[112,113] However, there have been no studies of this type involving patients whose body iron loads have been assessed by hepatic biopsy.

Although in inadequately treated patients hypogonadism may be a reflection of chronic anemia, deficiency of IGF-1 secondary to liver dysfunction, cirrhosis, diabetes, and low adrenal-androgen production, there is now abundant evidence that, in those who are more adequately managed, the major mechanism involved in failure of sexual maturation is selective central hypogonadism.[91–93,114–116] Some males tend to have a low baseline testosterone level but their response to human chorionic gonadotrophin is usually normal. Although defective ovarian function has been reported in some cases,[115] patients who show retarded sexual development usually demonstrate blunted responses to GnRH rather than to FSH.

The hypothalamic/pituitary axis appears to be particularly vulnerable to the effects of iron loading. This is supported by histological studies showing selective deposition in pituitary gonadotropes [117] and the observation of loss of anterior pituitary volume in iron-loaded patients, demonstrated by MRI.[118]

Over recent years the importance of linking the function of endocrine organs to circadian cycles has been emphasized. One of the most extensively studied systems is the pulsatile secretion of LSH and FSH, which reflects the intermittent release of GnRH from the hypothalamus. In a long-term prospective study of thalassemic women with secondary amenorrhea, it was found that all of them developed gonadotrophin-pulse abnormalities together with evidence of GnRH-gonadotrophin secretory insufficiency;[114] over the 10-year period there was a progressive deterioration of hypothalamic pituitary function, and 66% of the patients became apulsatile with marked reduction in the levels of GnRH-stimulating gonadotrophin. The different approaches to the diagnosis of gonadotrophin deficiency are discussed by Chatterjee and Katz.[119]

These studies emphasize the importance of studying the hypothalamic/pituitary axis in patients with amenorrhea or other evidence of failure of sexual development. Although there were early reports of testicular and ovarian iron loading,[120] it seems likely that, with improvements in the management of β thalassemia, end-organ unresponsiveness will play a relatively small role in problems of sexual maturation and function in the future.

Thus, although there has been an increase in fertility in men and women with thalassemia over the last decade, it is disappointing that secondary amenorrhea may eventually develop in approximately one-quarter of thalassemic women. This suggests that the anterior pituitary may be particularly susceptible over time to iron-induced damage and that, unlike the heart and liver, the consequences of iron deposition may be irreversible. There are no reports in the literature describing improvement in potency, fertility, or normalization of testosterone levels and sperm counts after reduction of iron load in thalassemia major, although this may occur in primary hemochromatosis. It has been suggested that body iron burdens corresponding to a hepatic iron concentration between 9 and 30 mg/g/liver, dry weight, may be associated with a high risk of development of pituitary failure.[121] Further studies to quantitate body iron and anterior pituitary function in patients from early in life should provide more secure conclusions with respect to the threshold of risk.

Diabetes mellitus. Diabetes is relatively common in children who have been inadequately iron chelated and is also observed in those who have been well-transfused and chelated; in an extensive study of transfused and chelated patients it occurred in 4%–6% of cases.[112] It has been attributed to impaired secretion of insulin secondary to chronic pancreatic iron overload.[122–127] There have also been a number of reports of insulin-resistant diabetes,[128–131] although the mechanism is not absolutely clear. It has also been linked temporally to episodes of acute viral hepatitis.[123,132]

It appears, however, that iron-mediated damage to the pancreas is the major factor in producing diabetes in iron-loaded children; there is a good relationship between the development of diabetes and the severity and duration of iron overload.[123,133] This conclusion is strengthened by consecutive studies over a long period that have shown early and progressive loss of pancreatic β-cell mass, manifested by decreased insulin release in response to secretagogues before the development of significant insulin resistance or diabetes.[134,135] In addition, there appears to be a reduction in the frequency of diabetes in patients who have been more adequately chelated.[67]

Hypothyroidism. Mild abnormalities of thyroid function were described in some iron-loaded patients with β thalassemia by Lassman et al.[136] and Flynn et al.[137] These findings have been substantiated in later studies,[138,139] including patients who had been well managed by transfusion and iron chelation. Grundy et al.[140] described two adolescents with moderately reduced levels of plasma thyroxine and marked elevations in thyroid-stimulating hormone; both had clinical features of hypothyroidism. In the study of Jensen et al.[113] there was a strong correlation between serum ferritin concentrations and the presence of thyroid dysfunction. Although it appears that hypothyroidism is relatively uncommon in transfusion-dependent thalassemia[141] because its clinical onset is so insidious it is very important to bear this complication in mind.

Hypoparathyroidism. Defective parathyroid function has been well documented for many years[90,137,142,143] and florid, clinical hypoparathyroidism has been described in a few cases.[106,137,144,145] The symptoms and signs are all attributable to hypocalcemia and hyperphosphatemia. The early signs, which are nonspecific, include neuromuscular irritability, paresthesiae involving the face, fingers, and toes, and abdominal cramps. The full clinical picture of acute irritability, emotional ability, memory impairment, lethargy, and convulsions has been rarely reported in thalassemia. The diagnosis is easily made by the finding of hypocalcemia and hyperphosphatemia, together with a reduction in the level of plasma parathyroid hormone (PTH). In a study of 113 transfusion-dependent cases, 12.4% showed subnormal PTH levels, suggesting that subclinical hypoparathyroidism may be relatively common.[146]

Adrenal insufficiency. The limited information about functional adrenal insufficiency in thalassemic patients suggests that it is uncommon and that, although there may be measurable abnormalities of adrenal function,[125] they are rarely associated with the clinical picture of adrenal failure.[106,120,141,147] Interestingly, there seems to be some dissociation of the different adrenal hormone functions in cases in which defects have been observed. For example, Sklar et al.[107] observed low levels of adrenal androgen secretion with a normal glucocorticoid reserve. Early suggestions that part of the skin pigmentation in thalassemia might be due to the melanophore-stimulating effect of raised plasma ACTH levels were not confirmed.[90]

It is clear, therefore, that one of the relative failures of high transfusion and adequate chelation that has otherwise changed the lives of thalassemic patients has been the persistence of endocrine dysfunction, particularly involving the hypothalamic/pituitary axis. Although the reasons are not clear, it is possible that the pituitary is particularly sensitive to even mild degrees of iron overload, and that even chelation regimens that are adequate to retain the function of other organs may simply not always be good enough to protect it.

Bone Disease

The bone changes in inadequately transfused thalassemic children were described earlier in this chapter. As soon as the high transfusion regimens were instituted in the mid-1960s it became apparent that the gross skeletal deformities that had been seen earlier could be prevented.[148,149] It seems likely, therefore, that they reflect expansion of the bone marrow mass, a process that can lead to a variety of other distressing symptoms, particularly pathological fractures.[150,151] Similarly, poor dentition[152] and attacks of recurrent sinusitis due to inadequate drainage[153] are much less common.

The pathophysiology of bone disease in thalassemia is not well understood. Although it is clear that marrow expansion plays a major role in inadequately treated patients, the osteoporosis that occurs in many patients who have been reasonably well transfused, but in whom there is severe iron loading, may be related to hypogonadism.[154,155] Indeed, it is apparent that even in well-transfused patients with thalassemia major there may be a relatively high frequency of osteoporosis, at least in part due to this mechanism.[156–158]

Jensen et al.[159] investigated 82 transfusion-dependent patients of both sexes, with a mean age of 27 years. The incidence of osteoporosis was 51%. Multivariate analysis showed that hypogonadotropic-hypogonadism, sex, and diabetes were significant risk factors. There was no association between ethnic group, smoking, exercise, calcium supplementation or age at starting chelation therapy or, indeed, the serum ferritin concentration. This study also highlighted some features of osteoporosis in thalassemia that are different from those in the postmenopausal variety. In thalassemia, men are more commonly and more severely affected and their lumbar vertebrae and femoral necks are involved, whereas in women osteoporosis mainly involves the spine. This is surprising because most of the women in this study were receiving hormone replacement therapy. Many of these patients were symptomatic with varying degrees of bone pain. This study, which confirms the earlier findings of Fabri et al.,[155] Giuzio et al.,[160] and Anapliotou et al.[154] in incriminating hypogonadism as an important factor in the development of osteoporosis in thalassemia, further underlines the importance of pituitary failure, even in patients who have been treated adequately.

There has been considerable interest in the possibility that there may be subsets of individuals who are genetically susceptible to developing osteoporosis.[161] Rees et al.[162] found that there was a significant correlation between homozygosity of the SS polymorphism of vitamin D receptor and the likelihood of developing osteoporosis of the femoral neck but not the lumbar spine. Jensen et al.[159] could find no relationship between osteoporosis and polymorphisms of the gene for the estrogen receptor. Hanslip et al.[163] found a correlation between osteoporosis and a promoter polymorphism of the COLIAI gene in males but not in females. A more recent study was unable to find any correlation between osteoporosis and the candidate genes; curiously, although the study found correlations with diabetes, chronic hepatitis, and other parameters, it did not find a correlation between hypogonadism and osteoporosis in males, although the methods for assessing gonadal function were not given.[164]

It is possible that these genetic associations of osteoporosis will vary between different ethnic groups; further work is required to test this hypothesis. Although there seems little doubt that hypogonadism is a major factor underlying osteoporosis, further work is required to clarify these complex issues. Suspicions that β thalassemia minor might be a risk factor for osteoporosis have not been confirmed.[165]

Infection

The notion that thalassemic children are particularly prone to infection has been an accepted part of the thalassemia literature for many years. As symptomatic management improved this concept was questioned[166] and it was suggested that the incidence of infection in early childhood had been markedly reduced in children maintained at an adequate hemoglobin level.[11] In recent years, although there is still an awareness of the dangers of infection, particularly after splenectomy, there has been a major change in emphasis toward concerns about blood-borne infection, notably hepatitis B and C, human immunodeficiency virus (HIV), and malaria. Recent studies of the patterns of infection in thalassemia are reviewed by Vento et al.[167] and Rahav et al.[168]

Patterns of infection with changing management. In an extensive retrospective study of the patterns of infection in thalassemic children maintained at different hemoglobin levels, Modell and Berdoukas[5] concluded that the most serious infections were pneumonia, pericarditis, the sequelae of streptococcal infections, meningitis, peritonitis, and osteomyelitis. Further analysis suggested that pneumonia and septicemia were significantly associated with splenectomy and a low transfusion regimen, and that in patients who had been maintained at a satisfactory hemoglobin level these infections had almost disappeared. They also observed that other serious infections including meningitis, peritonitis, and osteomyelitis are only seen in splenectomized patients and that they have no obvious relationship to anemia. Finally, they noted that pericarditis is also unrelated to anemia and splenectomy but is very clearly related to age, occurring in childhood or later. They suggested that this might reflect a relationship between iron overload and pericarditis. Modell and Berdoukas also provided some comparative information from other countries, indicating that this overall pattern of infection is common in most thalassemic populations. These observations were in keeping with the earlier studies of the dangers of infection in splenectomized thalassemic children[169,170] and, indeed, in any child who has had the spleen removed early in life.[171,172] In this case the most important organisms are *Streptococcus pneumoniae*, *Haemophilus influenzae*, and *Neisseria meningitis*.

The widespread use of prophylactic penicillin and appropriate immunization after splenectomy has undoubtedly reduced the frequency of severe infections in splenectomized thalassemic children.

Organisms that attack iron-loaded patients. Although, as discussed earlier, there has been a great deal of controversy as to whether the frequent attacks of pericarditis in thalassemic children are related to iron loading, no organism has ever been implicated. The only pathogens that have been shown quite unequivocally to occur with an increased frequency in iron-loaded patients are those of the *Yersinia* genus, which normally have a low pathogenicity and an unusually high requirement for iron. They do not secrete siderophores but have receptors for ferrioxamine and become pathogenic in the presence of iron bound to desferrioxamine.[173] There are numerous reports of severe infections in thalassemic patients due to infections with *Yersinia* spp.[173–176] These infections are usually characterized by severe abdominal pain, diarrhea, vomiting, fever, and sore throat. They may also be associated, on occasion, with rupture of the bowel.[177]

HEPATITIS B VIRUS. It is estimated that approximately 350 million people worldwide are persistent carriers of hepatitis B virus (HBV). The virus persists in approximately 10% of infected immunocompetent adults. Approximately 25% of all patients with chronic hepatitis progress to cirrhosis, approximately 20% of whom develop hepatocellular carcinoma. During the first phase of chronicity, virus replication continues in the liver; markers of this stage include HBV DNA and a soluble antigen, hepatitis Be antigen (HBeAg). In most persons there is immune clearance of infected hepatocytes associated with seroconversion from HBeAg to anti-HBe.

Because HBV is primarily a blood-borne infection, transfusion-dependent thalassemic children are at particular risk, depending on its prevalence in their community and the effectiveness of donor screening programs. The early experience in Europe was summarized by Schanfield et al.[178] and by Modell and Berdoukas.[5] At that time, in British, Cypriot, Sardinian, and Greek populations the frequency of antibody positivity ranged from 30% to 90% with an appropriately low level of those with persistent antigen positivity. Later studies from Greece demonstrated how the application of adequate screening and vaccination programs results in a major fall in the frequency of HBV infection.[179] Although the frequency of HBV infection is now very low in countries in which screening and immunization programs have been established, HBV-related hepatitis is still seen frequently in parts of the world where these precautions are not taken. The diagnosis of chronic active hepatitis depends on the presence of abnormal liver function tests, particularly elevated transaminases, the appearances on liver biopsy, and, in the early stages, the presence of HBeAg antigens and, later, the presence of anti-HBe. In the early phase there is an HBe-positive viremia that usually becomes negative as the disease progresses.

HEPATITIS C VIRUS. Following the identification of hepatitis C virus (HCV) it soon became clear that this infection is widespread and presents a serious risk to patients with transfusion-dependent thalassemia. The prevalence of anti-HCV in patients with thalassemia major varies in different parts of the world, ranging from 11.7% in Turkish Cypriots, through 30% in Malaysians and Chinese to nearly 75% in Italians.[180–186]

An initial HCV infection is almost invariably anicteric and can only be diagnosed by screening for elevated serum transaminases; jaundice is rare. Unfortunately, only 50% of patients recover, and the remainder develop persistent viremia with hepatitis. Of these approximately one in five develops cirrhosis and run the risk of hepatocellular carcinoma. Antibodies to structural and nonstructural proteins of the virus can be detected at various times after infection. Viremia is detected by polymerase chain reaction (PCR), which can identify HCV-RNA. Patients with chronic active hepatitis are invariably HCV-RNA positive and also have IgG anti-HCV, which is also present after recovery. There is some evidence that the liver damage associated with persistent HCV infection, or response to therapy, may be modified by the presence of excess iron.[187–189]

Clearly, therefore, any patient with persistently raised serum transaminases must be screened for HCV antibody and by using PCR to identify HCV-RNA. If this test is positive it is important to proceed to a liver biopsy to identify those who have histological changes of chronic active hepatitis. The liver histology shows predominantly chronic persistent hepatitis with a low incidence of periportal, piecemeal necrosis and lobular hepatitis.

OTHER FORMS OF VIRAL HEPATITIS. Hepatitis D virus (HDV) only replicates in patients already infected with HBV. Infection is common among HBV carriers in the Mediterranean region and may occur at the same time as HBV. The clinical course is that outlined earlier for HBV infection. Hepatitis E virus (HEV) is enterically transmitted and, like HAV, although it may produce acute hepatitis is not associated with persistent infection. Evidence of infection with HEV was obtained in 2.4% of transfusion-dependent thalassemic patients in Athens[190] and in 10.7% of a similar population in Saudi Arabia.[191]

Hepatitis G virus (HGV) was discovered in 1995 (reviewed by Stransky[192]). It produces a mild form of hepatitis but there is little evidence that patients go on to develop chronic hepatitis. It can be diagnosed by the demonstration of HGV-RNA by PCR in a similar way to HCV. Its prevalence in U.S. blood donors is approximately 1.5%. In a study of 40 Italian transfusion-dependent β thalassemics, HGV-RNA was detected in 22% of cases. In patients who were also viremic for HCV the clinical manifestations of the co-infection were no different from those of patients with HVC alone. The authors concluded that although HGV is highly prevalent among Italian polytransfused individuals there is no evidence for a clinically significant role in liver disease.[193] Similar conclusions came from a study of Chung et al.[194] in Taiwan, where the prevalence of HGV-RNA positivity was 14%; again the presence of the virus did not seem to be associated with significant hepatitis. In a further follow-up of Italian patients with HGV it was concluded that in over 25% of cases the infection resolved within 6 years.[195] Similar conclusions were reported by Zemel et al.,[196] who found an incidence of HGV infection of 19.4% in a population in Tel Aviv; follow-up studies suggested that there is persistent viremia but no significant biochemical evidence of liver damage. The frequency of HGV infections in southeast Asia seems to be even higher, with reports of frequencies in transfusion-dependent thalassemic children of 32%.[197]

All these studies suggest that HGV infection, although very common, does not seem to be associated with a serious form of hepatitis or long-term liver damage. A more recent review of HGV and its strain variant, GBVC, also suggests that this is the case, although more data are required.[198]

HUMAN IMMUNODEFICIENCY VIRUSES. The HIVs HIV-1 and HIV-2 belong to the lentivirus subfamily of retroviruses. They can both give rise to the acquired immunodeficiency syndrome (AIDS). Globally, HIV-1 is responsible for the worldwide pandemic of AIDS, although HIV-2, though mainly confined to western Africa, also spread rapidly, notably in India. It is estimated that by the end of 2005 40 million people worldwide were living with HIV infection or disease, a notable rise from the 35 million in 2001, whereas sub-Saharan Africa remains the most severely affected region the virus is still spreading rapidly in parts of Asia and eastern Europe.[199]

It should be remembered that most people in the world with HIV infections are asymptomatic. Prospective studies of cohorts of infected people with known dates of seroconversion have suggested that 50% to 60% of them will develop symptoms and signs of disease within 10 years of infection. During the asymptomatic phase many individuals show abnormal laboratory tests such as low CD4 lymphocyte counts and hypergammaglobulinemia. It is beyond our scope to deal with the various symptom complexes of AIDS, which have been classified by the Centers for Disease Control and Prevention (CDC) into several subgroups (Table 17.5).

Table 17.5. Centers for Disease Control classification for HIV infection

Group I	Acute infection
Group II	Asymptomatic infection
Group III	Persistent, generalized lymphadenopathy
Group IV	Other disease
Subgroup A	Constitutional disease (1 or more of: fever for more than 1 month; weight loss >10% baseline; diarrhea for more than 1 month
Subgroup B	Neurological disease
Subgroup C	Secondary infection
	C1 As specified by CDC surveillance definition
	C2 Others
Subgroup D	Secondary cancers
Subgroup E	Other conditions

It is not surprising, therefore, that HIV infection has become a major concern for multitransfused patients with thalassemia[200] In the mid-1980s, when it was becoming apparent that HIV infection would pose a serious problem for children who had received regular blood products, a European–Mediterranean WHO Working Group on Hemoglobinopathies together with the Cooleycare Group established a program to coordinate data collection. Work from this group and others has provided valuable information about the change in prevalence of HIV infection after donor screening was established and about the course of the illness in those who were affected[201] Early prevalence figures from Italy and Greece ranged from 2.3% to 11%,[202–204] and the infection rate in transfused thalassemic patients in the United States was reported to be approximately 12%.[205] The European–Mediterranean WHO Working Group carried out a further study of 3,633 patients in 36 centers from 13 countries and found an overall frequency of HIV positivity of 1.56%. Further data collected after establishment of screening (reviewed by Girot et al.[201]) revealed a sharp fall in the number of HIV-positive patients, although there is still a very low level of transmission from HIV blood obtained from seronegative donors.[206] In the period after 1988 an analysis of nearly 3,000 patients in 13 European centers found no HIV-1-positive patients.

The same WHO Working Group started a follow-up study of 75 seropositive thalassemic patients to observe the natural history of HIV infection in thalassemic children.[207] The median follow-up period was 4 years 11 months. At the end of the study, 43 patients were CDC stage II, 23 CDC stage III, and 13 CDC stage IV, including seven patients with AIDS, of whom three had died. The rate of progression to AIDS was not associated with intercurrent infection, splenectomy, age, or sex. For the group, a cumulative AIDS incidence rate of 1.4% was observed at 3 years, and of 9% at 5 years.

The situation in other parts of the world, where screening started later, is much less encouraging. In a study of 203 children in New Dehli, Sen et al.[208] reported a frequency of 8.9% for HIV positivity. Kumar et al.[209] found a frequency of 8.9% in a transfusion clinic in Manapur, India. These data provide some indication of the magnitude of the problem that will be posed by HIV infection in thalassemic children in many parts of the world unless urgent steps are taken to institute donor screening. This problem was highlighted by Kumar and Khuranna,[210] who reported on a prospective analysis of the outcome of pregnancies in 123 women with transfusion-dependent β thalassemia, of whom 81 were HIV positive; using the CDC classification, 39 were stage CII and 42 stage AII (see Table 17.5). All 22 preterm babies of mothers with stage CII had positive viral cultures for HIV-1 within 1 week of birth; 10 of these neonates died of AIDS by 8 weeks, and the remaining 12 by 15 months of age. Of 39 CII-stage pregnancies, five infants died undelivered at 32 weeks gestation due to fulminating *Pneumocystis carinii* pneumonia.

Currently, the effectiveness of HIV control measures, including screening of blood donors, vary widely in different developing countries. The present position, together with a detailed analysis of the public health approaches to the prevention of blood-borne HIV infection, is summarized by Bertozzi et al. [199]

MALARIA. Following early hopes on the part of the WHO that malaria was being contained in many parts of the world, events of the last few years have proved just how unpredictable the control of an important infection can be. The disease has returned to many countries from which it seemed to have disappeared and, even more frighteningly, drug resistance is now widespread. Children with severe forms of thalassemia are subject to attacks of acute malaria like any other child; the protective effect of thalassemia trait against malaria, reviewed by Weatherall and Clegg,[2] is relative; no form of thalassemia protects any individual completely against the infection. Chronic malaria, as well as exacerbating the anemia of thalassemia, may also increase the degree of splenomegaly.

Thalassemic children are particularly at risk from blood-borne malaria. For example, in a study from India of the blood of children immediately after transfusion, Choudhury et al.[211] found that in 6.4% of cases there was evidence of transfusion-transmitted malaria infection. Thus it is clear that there must be a high frequency of chronic malaria in blood donors in endemic regions.

Another important question regarding malarial infection in thalassemic children relates to the effects of splenectomy on the course of the disease. This complex issue was reviewed by Looareesuwan et al.[212] Although there have been anecdotal reports suggesting that malaria may be particularly severe in those who have been splenectomized, he could not find convincing evidence that this is the case. Recent studies of patients with HbE–β thalassemia in Sri Lanka suggest that they are more prone to malarial infection than normal controls and that, furthermore, there is a highly significant increase in the serological evidence of previous infection in those who have been splenectomized.[213] These observations suggest that, at least in the case of patients with β thalassemia intermedia, there may be an increased susceptibility to malaria, part of which is related to splenectomy.

Severe *P. falciparum* malaria is not always associated with high parasitemias. Therefore, in any thalassemic child in a malarious area who presents with fever, drowsiness progressing to coma, renal failure, hemoglobinuria, hypoglycemia, or simply a rapidly worsening anemia, a diagnosis of malaria must be considered, regardless of the number of parasites in the peripheral blood. Similarly, because *P. vivax* malaria, due to persistent parasites in the liver, may cause recurrent infections, any child in a malarious area who presents with recurrent fevers and increasing enlargement of the spleen should be investigated for this condition by thin and thick blood-film studies.

Liver disease

In young adults with thalassemia major liver disease remains a common cause of morbidity. Although it has been realized for many years that iron overload, acquired through transfusion and increased gastrointestinal absorption, is a major factor in the generation of liver disease, more recently, with the increasing recognition of blood-related viral hepatitis, it has become clear that the pathogenesis of liver damage is extremely complex.

Mechanisms of liver damage. Iron produces cellular injury with progression to fibrosis and cirrhosis (Fig. 17.7). This may be mediated in several ways. It promotes free-radical mediated lipid peroxidation and mitochondrial dysfunction.[48,214–216] The deposition of hemosiderin in lysosomes may lead to fragility and subsequent rupture of their membranes. Iron-promoted catalysis of collagen synthesis or decreased collagen breakdown due to lysosomal blockade following iron overload may promote excess collagen deposition; a similar mechanism has been observed in other storage diseases.[217] Furthermore, iron overload may potentiate further iron loading; upregulation of the transport of nontransferrin-bound iron has been observed in cultured hepatocytes.[218]

As mentioned earlier, blood-borne viral infection is another major factor in the high frequency of liver disease in thalassemic patients, and iron may potentiate the effects of viral hepatitis. Agents such as alcohol may act synergistically in accelerating the development of liver damage. Clearly, therefore, hepatic pathology in patients with thalassemia is extremely complex and many questions about the mechanisms of tissue damage and its pattern of progression remain to be worked out.

Assessment of iron loading and liver damage. The methods for assessing body-iron burden in general, and the level of liver iron in particular, are discussed later in this chapter.

Early findings in inadequately treated patients. Over the last five decades, as survival has extended, severe hepatic fibrosis and siderosis have been regular findings at autopsy.[39,40,124,219] In the absence of adequate chelation therapy it is an inevitable consequence of iron overload; in most patients fibrosis develops during childhood and progresses to frank cirrhosis during the second decade.[116,217,220–222]

It appears that pathological changes in the liver occur very early during the course of the disease. In an early series of studies, the relationship between liver iron content and liver damage was examined in babies of younger than 2 years of age.[217,223–225] Hepatic fibrosis of varying degree was reported in five of these 16 babies, although the liver iron content was not reported. Importantly, screening tests were of limited clinical value and there was no biochemical evidence of hepatic damage. Consecutive histological and

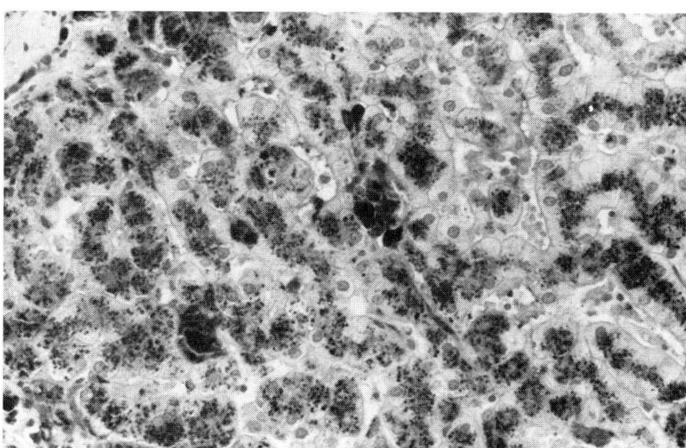

Figure 17.7. A liver biopsy obtained at autopsy from a child with thalassemia major, showing extensive iron loading (Perl's stain x510).

electron-microscopic changes in liver pathology in early childhood are reported by Iancuet al.[217]

Early studies in older children[20,40,124,219,224,226,227] suggested that fibrosis and cirrhosis were common in transfused, nonchelated children after the age of 3 years. The age and iron content at which significant fibrosis and cirrhosis are likely to develop is still unclear. The relationship between liver-iron concentration and transfusional iron overload was best expressed as an exponential, nonlinear function of the transfused iron load.[228] In these early studies the imperfect correlation between the amount of iron administered by transfusion and the development of fibrosis may be accounted for, in part, by the fact that many children were maintained on low-transfusion regimens that would not have substantially reduced gastrointestinal iron loading.

Later studies of factors influencing the rate of development of liver disease. Age, the iron content of the liver, associated hepatitis, and, possibly, splenectomy may all play roles in determining the time at which liver disease is established.

Risdon et al.[222] suggested that the severity of fibrosis is related to age in a normal linear fashion, but that even when iron accumulation is rapid, severe fibrosis may not be expected before 10 years of age. This pattern of fibrosis does not seem to have been consistent between series of transfused, poorly chelated children with thalassemia. One study reported fibrosis as early as 3 years of age, and cirrhosis as early as 8 years; by the age of 16 years, almost all children showed cirrhosis.[221] Liver biopsies obtained in 51 regularly transfused patients, aged 5–36 years (mean 18 years), showed that only six did not have some degree of fibrosis; in five, cirrhosis was fully developed.[220] Similarly, of 16 patients aged 3–17 years, all but two, both aged 3 years at the time of the biopsy, had moderate to massive fibrosis or cirrhosis; three older patients, aged 4 and 5 years, already demonstrated a severe degree of hepatic fibrosis.[116] Angelucci et al.[229] found that fibrosis was established in approximately 50% of transfused, irregularly chelated patients younger than the age of 6 years, and in 90% of similarly treated children older than the age of 5 years, an observation that has been confirmed in more recent studies of poorly chelated patients.[230]

It has been suggested that, following splenectomy, the iron content of the liver may increase and fibrosis may be accelerated.[40] Studies of the iron content of spleens in iron-loaded patients have given inconsistent results. Furthermore, Risdon et al.[222] could demonstrate no increase in fibrosis in splenectomized patients. Thus, although the question of the relationship between splenectomy and iron loading remains open, the balance of evidence is against this being an important mechanism for potentiating liver damage.

There is extensive evidence that the major factor in the development of fibrosis is the concentration of iron in the liver. Risdon et al.[222] noted an exponential relationship between iron content and fibrosis in a series of 52 liver biopsies in 19 patients studied over 13 years. The relationship between tissue iron concentration and hepatic cirrhosis was explored in children maintained on a high transfusion regimen who did, or did not, receive intramuscular desferrioxamine, and demonstrated a clear reduction in the degree of fibrosis in the former.[228] In early attempts to establish a threshold of hepatic iron associated with the development of hepatic damage, it was observed that fibrosis was only present in patients in whom the iron levels exceeded 7.6 mg/g dry weight.[40] Later, De Virgillis et al.[231] reported chronic persistent hepatitis, or chronic active hepatitis with periportal lesions, but only in patients with liver-iron concentrations exceeding 10 mg/g dry weight. Aldouri et al.[220] found a mean hepatic-iron concentration of approximately 12.5 mg/g dry weight, in patients with moderate or severe fibrosis, although fibrosis was observed in the presence of lower concentration of hepatic iron.

As mentioned earlier, the first clear evidence that fibrosis can be arrested by iron-chelating therapy was obtained by Barry et al.[228] This effect was observed at a dose that would now be considered inadequate, and at a liver-iron concentration in excess of 20 mg/g dry weight, a level that was subsequently shown to be associated with a heightened risk of cardiac disease and early death.[232] Arrest of fibrosis was observed in several other small studies.[116,220]

In the absence of prospective clinical trials to evaluate life-long therapy for the prevention of tissue damage in thalassemia, guidance about the risk of hepatic fibrosis has had to be derived from the clinical experience with hereditary hemochromatosis.[15] Minor iron loading develops in approximately a quarter of heterozygotes for this condition, although their body iron stores do not seem to increase beyond two–fourtimes the upper limit of normal, that is, up to approximately 7 mg/g dry weight. In contrast, homozygotes who have iron burdens exceeding 7 mg/g dry weight have a definite increased risk of hepatic fibrosis.

It is clear, however, that the toxic manifestations of iron overload do not depend entirely on the amount of excess iron in the liver. They are also modified by the rate of iron accumulation, the duration of exposure to increased iron, the partition of the iron load between relatively harmless sites in macrophages and more hazardous deposits in parenchymal cells, ascorbate status, which may help to determine this partition effect, the extent of internal redistribution of iron between macrophages and parenchymal sites, and noniron-related factors, particularly viral hepatitis. In early studies of patients with hepatitis C liver damage associated with persistent infection, or response to therapy, was considerably modified by the presence of excess iron,[187–189] although this was not observed in a more recent series.[233] Early experience with the oral chelating agent deferiprone suggested that it may result in progression of hepatic fibrosis.[234] In a small retrospective study it was observed that cirrhotic changes appeared to reverse after marrow transplantation.[235]

Assessment of liver function. Given the extremely complex and multifactorial nature of liver disease in β thalassemia, assessment of liver function and determining the reasons for abnormalities of liver function tests may be extremely difficult. As mentioned earlier, there may be significant liver damage due to iron excess without any changes in standard liver function tests. Most patients with β thalassemia, unless their bone marrow is suppressed by transfusion, have elevated serum bilirubin levels, reflecting both ineffective erythropoiesis and a shortened red cell survival. The level of bilirubin is extremely variable and, as mentioned later in this chapter, it is becoming apparent that some patients who remain deeply jaundiced may have an additional genetic defect in bilirubin conjugation. Hepatocellular damage is reflected by a rise in the activity of serum aspartate aminotransferase and alanine aminotransferase (ALT). Because these enzymes are not specific for the liver, elevated levels must be assessed with caution. Because gallstones occur quite frequently in patients with β thalassemia, particularly of the intermediate variety, a typical picture of obstructive jaundice may occur, with raised levels of serum alkaline phosphatase, 5′ nucleotidase, and γ-glutamyl-transferase.

In assessing patients with suspected liver disease an estimation of the size of the liver may be helpful. A moderate degree of hepatomegaly is quite common in patients who have been maintained at a relatively low hemoglobin level. A large, tender liver should raise the suspicion of an underlying hepatitis or, in grossly iron-loaded patients, cardiac failure. An elevation of the liver enzymes should always be investigated, particularly if the level is rising with time. It is essential to screen for the different forms of hepatitis, as discussed earlier. A liver biopsy should be performed and, when possible, the liver-iron level estimated chemically. The liver should be examined histologically with appropriate stains to demonstrate iron, collagen, and, where applicable, hepatitis antigen.

Exocrine Pancreas

As well as diabetes, described earlier in this chapter, there is increasing evidence that iron may also cause damage to the exocrine pancreas.[236] In a combined ultrasonographic and pancreatic enzyme determination study, the frequency of exocrine pancreatic damage was assessed in 39 consecutive patients with β thalassemia and iron overload. Most of them had markedly increased echogenicity of the pancreas, with decreased size of the gland, as compared with controls. These changes showed a significant correlation with age and the duration of transfusion. Serum concentrations of trypsin and lipase were significantly lower in patients than controls. The lowest values were found in older patients with a longer duration of transfusion therapy, who also had the most marked sonographic changes. Although the functional significance of these findings is not clear, it is possible that in cases of extreme damage to the exocrine pancreas malabsorption may occur.

Folic Acid and Vitamin B_{12} Deficiency

The early literature on thalassemia offered clear evidence that in inadequately treated patients folate deficiency is relatively common.[237–239] These findings were confirmed in studies conducted in Thailand.[240] Chanarin[241] pointed out that the bone marrow may not show features that are absolutely typical of a megaloblastic anemia in patients with thalassemia and coexistent folate deficiency. In several of the early reports it was noted that severe bone pain may follow the administration of folic acid to folate-deficient patients. Folate deficiency is seen less commonly in well-transfused patients although it is still an important problem in those with the intermediate forms of thalassemia.

Vitamin B_{12} levels are usually normal or elevated.[242]

Other Vitamin and Trace Metal Deficiencies

A variety of deficiencies of vitamins and trace metals have been reported in all forms of β thalassemia.

Ascorbic acid. Early studies suggested that leukocyte ascorbic acid concentrations are significantly reduced in patients with severe forms of β thalassemia.[87,243] Subsequent work confirmed that low ascorbic acid levels are found in iron-loaded thalassemic patients.[244–246] It seems likely that ascorbic acid, because of its role as a biological reducing agent, may well be utilized in combating some of the complex free-radical damage that is mediated by excess iron in the tissues. Its role in this process, and how this may differ at varying tissue concentrations of ascorbate, is reviewed by Gutteridge and Halliwell.[215] Although clinical scurvy must be unusual in iron-loaded patients,[245] ascorbate deficiency is of great importance in determining the response to chelating agents such as desferrioxamine. Although the mechanism is uncertain, it seems likely that this effect is mediated by expansion of the chelatable iron pool to which desferrioxamine has access.[246–248]

Vitamin E deficiency. It has long been established that severe β thalassemics may be vitamin E depleted.[87,249] Hyman and her colleagues found that baseline serum DL-α-tochophoral levels and vitamin E stores were low, and that serial biopsies of skin, liver, thyroid and testes showed increased deposits of lipofuscin, which are associated with vitamin E deficiency. These findings were corroborated by Rachmilewitz,[250] who suggested that, because of the continual process of peroxidation of thalassemic red cell membranes, low serum vitamin E levels reflect its consumption as an antioxidant rather than a primary defect in vitamin E absorption or metabolism. The antioxidant properties of vitamin E are discussed by Gutteridge and Halliwell.[215] In their studies of the effects of vitamin E supplementation, Rachmilewitz et al.[251] showed that it was possible to produce a fourfold increase in both serum and red cell vitamin E levels, that the serum vitamin E level dropped rapidly after discontinuation of therapy, that there was a reduction in oxidant stress in red cells due to reduced peroxidative damage, and that in three of seven patients treated there was a significant increase in red cell survival. These findings, although they confirmed the function of vitamin E as an antioxidant in thalassemic red cells, did not define its role, if any, in the treatment of β thalassemia.

Trace metal deficiencies. There have been conflicting reports about the levels of certain trace metals in the blood of thalassemic patients, and even less is known about their significance. Erlandson et al.[252] found increased serum copper and decreased magnesium levels. Prasad et al.[253] also reported increased serum copper levels and Hyman et al.[254] confirmed that at least some patients have decreased serum magnesium levels. The significance of these observations is not clear although Hyman et al. suggested that markedly reduced magnesium levels might have a deleterious effect on cardiac function.

Prasad et al.[253] reported a reduction in serum zinc levels. Again the mechanism is not clear although it appears to be a general feature of hemolytic states, including sickle cell anemia. Low levels of serum zinc were also found in a study in Thailand by Silprasert et al.[255] Incidentally, this study also confirmed the earlier findings of elevated levels of serum copper, although there was no correlation between copper and zinc levels. These authors point out that, at least in experimental animals with zinc and vitamin A deficiency, there is lack of response to vitamin A that can be corrected by zinc supplementation. Zinc deficiency has also been incriminated in growth retardation, although this has not been documented in thalassemia.

Overall, we know very little about the significance of these changes in the levels of trace elements. Because many chelating agents remove metals other than iron, and even desferrioxamine is not entirely specific for iron, trace metal deficiency may also be exacerbated by treatment.

Gallstones

Gallstone formation is common in undertransfused β thalassemic patients and in thalassemia intermedia.[256]

Secondary Gout

Because of the rapid turnover of red cells in their bone marrow, many patients with β thalassemia who are maintained on a low transfusion regimen are hyperuricemic. Secondary gout has been well documented[257] and gouty arthropathy has been reported.[258]

Neuromuscular Abnormalities

Neuromuscular complications of thalassemia are not common. Logothetis et al.[259] summarized their studies on 138 consecutive patients with thalassemia major who had been maintained on only a moderate transfusion regimen. They noted that walking was delayed beyond 18 months in approximately one-third of the patients, whereas speech and intellectual development appeared to proceed normally. Twenty-six of their patients developed a curious myopathic syndrome with proximal weakness, mostly in the lower extremities, and a myopathic electromyographic pattern. This complication was associated with severe skeletal stigmata, suggesting that it occurred in inadequately transfused patients. It does not seem to be a feature of adequately transfused thalassemic children.

In the series of Logothetis et al. 27 patients had histories of episodes suggesting cerebral ischemia, with focal neurological episodes. Similar episodes were described by Sinniah et al.[260] Neurosensory deafness has been noted by McIntosh,[106] who described improvement in hearing after commencement of regular blood transfusion and, in the same article, noted that deafness was relatively common in inadequately transfused young thalassemics. This complication was also reported by Hazell and Modell.[153] There is no doubt that severe cranial deformities resulting from massive expansion of the bone marrow can result in symptoms of this kind, or involvement of the optic nerve, but these complications are only seen in patients who have been maintained at extremely low hemoglobin levels.

The increased incidence in thrombotic strokes, particularly in patients with thalassemia intermedia and in those who have been splenectomized, was discussed earlier in this section. It is becoming clear however that there is also an elevated risk for subclinical infarction, or silent stroke, in patients with thalassemia intermedia or β thalassemia major. For example, Manfre et al.[261] found evidence of silent infarcts in 37.5% of individuals with thalassemia intermedia compared with 52% in those with HbS–β thalassemia. Those with thalassemia showed milder atrophy and a greater number of single lesions than those with HbS–β thalassemia. These findings were confirmed in a more recent study.[262] It seems likely that these lesions reflect the hypercoagulable state as defined earlier in this chapter. Their neurocognitive significance is considered below.

We discuss the various neurological syndromes that can follow compression by hematopoietic cell tumor masses when we describe the complications of thalassemia intermedia. There are several neurological and sensory complications of desferrioxamine therapy; these are also discussed later.

Intelligence and Behavioral Patterns

Logothetis et al.[263] evaluated the status of 138 consecutive cases of thalassemia major in Greece. Intelligence testing revealed no difference from normal children of the same age and social group. A trend to lower IQ scores was found in those subjected to less vigorous transfusion regimens. Abnormalities of behavior and character were noted in 96 cases and abnormal emotional responses, mainly depression and anxiety, were observed in 67 of the children. In summarizing their experience these workers concluded that their findings were similar to those in any group of children with chronic disease.

More recent studies have used the modern techniques of psychology and psychiatry to assess the behavioral and emotional problems of young children with thalassemia. For example, Tsiantis[264] assessed a group of Greek children by using the methods that were pioneered by Rutter and colleagues[265] for studying the reliability and validity of psychiatric assessment of children. Using these strict criteria it was found that approximately 40% of the thalassemic children, compared with approximately 30% of a control group of chronically sick children, had an emotional or behavioral disorder that would be classified as requiring some kind of psychiatric help. Problems relating to denial and displacement, which are considered to be maladaptive mechanisms, were particularly common. In a further study of group interactions with the parents of thalassemic children a number of factors were defined that may have contributed to the children's problems: death anxiety; denial; overprotective behavior; and, surprisingly, excessive pressure on the sick child to achieve.

Because of growing concerns about these problems the WHO undertook a large multicenter study in 1985 to evaluate the psychosocial aspects of thalassemia and sickle cell anemia. As an approach to data collection they produced an extremely complex questionnaire. To make this more useful for studying thalassemic populations a simpler and more practical program was developed by Ratnip (quoted by Klein et al.[266]). In particular, this attempts to define major psychosocial burdens, but also tries to put them into perspective as seen through the very different eyes of patients and parents. A pilot study carried out on the Toronto thalassemic population using this questionnaire showed just how dangerous it is to generalize about psychosocial problems based on studies in any one group of patients or their relatives. For example, it found that the clinical and psychosocial burdens were not correlated between parents and their children, parents' perception of their child's psychological burden correlated well although the child was young but not when they reached adulthood, the burden experienced by children was affected by that felt by their parents and vice versa, and although the overall psychosocial burden was similarly perceived by children and their parents, the value placed on individual aspects may differ considerably among family members.

The neurocognitive implications of the silent infarcts, which have been demonstrated frequently in patients with different forms of β thalassemia are discussed by Armstrong.[267] He points out that most of the current studies of neurocognitive function in children with hemoglobin disorders have been restricted to the sickle cell syndromes. Their chronic anemia has been associated with a decline in neurocognitive function, even in the absence of structural changes on MRI. Currently, it is unclear to what extent the presence of silent infarcts are associated changes in neurocognitive function. He emphasizes the importance of carrying out well-controlled studies of this type on children with different forms of thalassemia, particularly with the increasingly good prognosis for patients with these conditions.

Pregnancy

Until the era of adequate transfusion and chelation, pregnancy was not observed in patients with severe forms of β thalassemia. Many patients are now passing through a relatively normal puberty and most centers that look after large numbers of thalassemic patients have had some experience of managing pregnancy in those who are on regular transfusion and chelation therapy.

Several series of successful pregnancies in transfusion-dependent β thalassemic patients have been reported. They have included both spontaneous pregnancies, twin pregnancies, and pregnancies following in vitro fertilization.[268,269] Presumably because pregnancy would only be likely to occur in women who had been adequately chelated, and therefore in whom it is unlikely that there would be serious hepatic, cardiac, or endocrine complications, most of these pregnancies seem to have gone to term and there have been no major problems. Deaths due to cardiac failure have occurred and it is essential that pregnancy be avoided in women with evidence of cardiac iron loading. The patients have maintained their usual hemoglobin levels by regular transfusion. There are limited data on the outcome of pregnancies in which desferrioxamine has been administered in the first trimester.[270] It is currently suggested that, if indicated, it is restricted to later than 16 weeks gestation until one week before delivery. It should be avoided during breastfeeding. Because of lack of data, the use of oral chelators (see later section and Chapter 29) should be avoided during pregnancy.

Autopsy Findings

With one notable exception the recent literature of the thalassemia field has, like that of the rest of medicine, completely neglected the value of the autopsy. The exception is the beautifully illustrated atlas produced by Sonakul.[271]

There are, however, many excellent descriptions of the morbid anatomy of thalassemia in its earlier literature.[20,124,272–274] Perhaps the most valuable information to come from these reports is the distribution of iron among the different organs. Extensive data, together with the weight of iron per organ, were summarized by Modell and Matthews.[274] Most of the findings at autopsy reflect the various pathologies that have been described in different sections of this chapter. The most striking finding in all these reports is the widespread deposition of iron with varying degrees of organ fibrosis. As might be expected the organs most affected include the liver, spleen, endocrine glands, pancreas, heart, and kidneys. The degree of fibrosis varies widely, and is most marked in the liver and least noticeable in the thyroid gland. The spleen is enlarged and congested with thickened reticulum. It may contain Gaucher-like cells similar to those seen in the marrow. Detailed studies of the myocardium and conductive tissues are reported by Buja and Roberts[37] and Modell and Matthews[274] (see earlier section). As shown most elegantly in the atlas of Sonakul,[271] there may be extensive extramedullary hematopoiesis. This work is also notable for the illustrations of obliterative changes in the small vessels of the lungs seen in some Thai patients with HbE thalassemia and pulmonary hypertension.

Hematological Findings

Peripheral Blood and Marrow

There is always a severe degree of anemia that is typically hypochromic and microcytic with a low mean cell hemoglobin (MCH) and mean cell volume (MCV). Presumably because of the marked changes in the shape and size of the red cells, red cell indices derived from electronic cell counters do not always reflect the degree of hemoglobinization of the red cells as judged from an inspection of the peripheral blood film. They show marked anisocytosis and poikilocytosis, with many misshapen microcytes, occasional macrocytes, and variable numbers of target cells. Erythroblasts are always present and may reach extremely high levels after splenectomy (Fig. 17.8). The appearances of the red cells are different in splenectomized patients. In particular, large hypochromic cells are found together with small piscine forms that are little more than fragments of

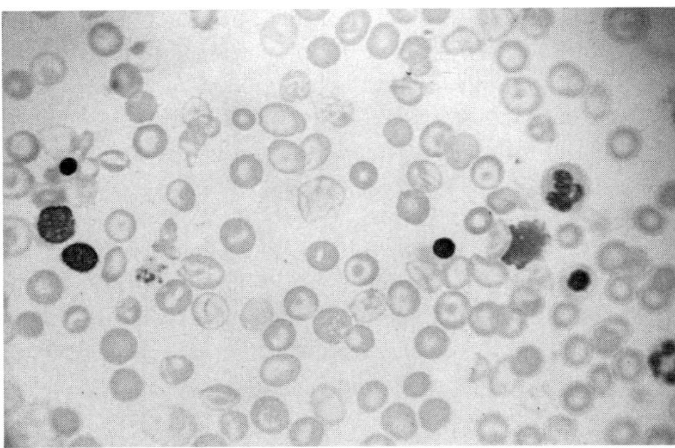

Figure 17.8 The blood smear of a patient with thalassemia major showing the typical morphological changes (Wright's stain, x438).

stroma. Ragged inclusion bodies can be seen in the cytoplasm of both nucleated and nonnucleated red cells after incubation with methyl violet. Their ultrastructural characteristics have been described in several studies.[275–278] The absolute reticulocyte count is rarely high although it tends to increase after splenectomy. The total white cell count and differential is usually normal but may also increase after splenectomy. A reduction in white cell count, particularly if there is a shift to the right with hyperlobulation of the neutrophils, is indicative of folate deficiency. Severe neutropenia may occur occasionally as part of the picture of hypersplenism. The platelet count is usually normal or slightly elevated, particularly after splenectomy; thrombocytopenia usually reflects hypersplenism or folate deficiency.

The bone marrow shows marked erythroid hyperplasia with a reversal of the myeloid/erythroid ratio. Iron staining reveals an abundance in the reticuloendothelial elements and also in the red cell precursors. On incubation of the marrow with methyl violet it is always possible to demonstrate inclusion bodies in the erythroblasts.[279] Their identification as precipitated α chains, kinetics of precipitation, distribution in red cell precursors at different stages of maturation, and ultrastructure, together with the pathophysiological consequences of α-chain precipitation, are reviewed in detail by Weatherall and Clegg[2] (see Chapters 9 and 11).

The cytoplasm of thalassemic erythroblasts contains an accumulation of glycogen, most marked in the G1 phase of early polychromatic erythroblasts.[280] It has been suggested that this reflects the storage of unused energy in cells that are blocked in this phase of the cell cycle. The marrow also shows intense phagocytic activity, with the presence of large foamy cells resembling Gaucher cells.[281]

Red Cell Survival and Metabolism

Red cell survival is reduced, with published figures ranging from 7 to 22 days. Several studies have shown that there are two populations of red cells, one that is rapidly destroyed and another with a longer survival.[282–284] The short-lived population appears to be low in HbF and to contain predominantly small amounts of HbA or α-chain precipitates.[285] Although external scanning suggests that some red cell destruction occurs in the spleen, the main effect of increasing splenomegaly is to trap a large number of red cells with consequent hypervolemia and hemodilution.[16,286]

There are several distinctive metabolic abnormalities of the red cells; the mechanisms and relationship to red cell membrane damage by excess α chains are discussed elsewhere in Chapter 9. The red cell osmotic fragility is markedly decreased. The metabolic changes reflect the marked heterogeneity of the different red cell populations in the peripheral blood. After centrifugation, cells from the "younger," upper layers contain more inclusion bodies, have a lower hemoglobin content, and show a remarkable increase in the rate of flux of potassium, with higher rates of glycolysis and lactate formation and low and unstable levels of adenosine triphosphate (ATP).[275,287,288] These changes are less marked in the "older," HbF-rich population, underlining the protective effect of increased γ-chain synthesis on both red cell metabolism and survival. Changes in other red cell enzymes and porphyrins are reviewed by Weatherall and Clegg.[2]

Iron Metabolism

As discussed earlier, iron loading is a constant feature of transfusion-dependent β thalassemia. Although the majority of the iron load is derived from blood transfusion, there may, in certain circumstances, be increased gastrointestinal absorption. As will be described later in this chapter, this is certainly the case in the intermediate forms of β thalassemia.

Iron Absorption

The inconsistent results of some iron absorption studies almost certainly relate to the transfusional status of the patients at the time of study. Heinrich et al.[289] found that inorganic-iron absorption was markedly increased 64–300 days after transfusion, whereas it fell into the normal range if performed 3–17 days after transfusion. Presumably, therefore, the level of iron absorption is related to the degree of ineffective erythropoiesis and erythroid hyperplasia; if this is reduced by transfusion iron absorption is also reduced.

Serum Iron

Serum iron is elevated in children with severe β thalassemia, and in older patients the iron-binding capacity is fully saturated. The serum of such patients contains 2–7 μmol/L of nonspecifically bound iron that is dialyzable and can be bound by transferrin from normal sera.[290]

Serum Ferritin

The measurement of plasma or serum ferritin is the most commonly used estimate of body iron stores in thalassemia. As discussed earlier, it has serious limitations, particularly in severely iron-loaded patients. The wide fluctuations that may occur at high ferritin levels may reflect a variety of mechanisms that alter the concentration independently of body iron load. These include ascorbate deficiency, acute and chronic infection, liver damage, hemolysis, and ineffective erythropoiesis. The 95 prediction intervals for hepatic iron concentration, related to the serum ferritin, are so broad that it is not possible to use the serum ferritin levels as a reliable predictor of body stores[15] (see earlier section).

Hepatic Iron Concentration

Until recently the hepatic iron concentration has been the most effective guide to assessing body iron stores, and the likelihood of tissue damage. The main disadvantage of this approach is, of course, that it is invasive; there is also the possibility of sampling error, particularly in livers that are involved by increased fibrosis of frank cirrhosis. There is now increasing evidence that adequately calibrated MRI techniques can enable safe and accurate non-invasive measurement and imaging of liver iron concentrations. The technique is based on the measurement and imaging of proton transverse relaxation times (R_2) in the liver. This approach has been reviewed recently by St. Pierre et al.,[27] who provide a comparison of the sensitivity of MRI data with different values of hepatic iron concentration. The only other approach that provides data equivalent to the latter is magnetic susceptometry using a super-conducting quantum interference device.[15]

Ferrokinetics and Erythrokinetics

Ferrokinetic and erythrokinetic studies in severe β thalassemia show a marked degree of ineffective erythropoiesis.[291,292] On the one hand there is evidence of increased red cell production as judged by bone marrow hyperplasia, plasma iron turnover, and fecal urobilinogen production, although effective red cell production as assessed by the hemoglobin level, absolute reticulocyte count, and iron incorporation is not increased, indicating an extreme degree of intramedullary destruction of red cells.

Hemoglobin Constitution

The red cells in all the severe forms of β thalassemia contain increased amounts of HbF. Homozygous β^0 thalassemics have only Hbs F and A_2; HbA is absent. The level of HbF in β^+ thalassemia homozygotes or compound heterozygotes is variable but is always elevated above normal after the first few months of life. Hemoglobin-A_2 levels are variable and of no diagnostic value. The only other abnormal finding is the presence of free α chains, which can sometimes be demonstrated using appropriate electrophoretic techniques.

Hemoglobin F

The complex and still ill-understood mechanisms for the production of HbF in β thalassemia are reviewed in detail by Weatherall and Clegg.[2] In short, it seems to reflect marked erythroid expansion, which may favor γ-chain synthesis in the postnatal period, together with selective survival of red cell precursors and mature red cells that have relatively higher levels of γ-chain production. This latter mechanism reflects the extreme heterogeneity of the level of γ-chain synthesis between different red cell precursors after birth; those that produce relatively more γ-chains, and hence in which the degree of globin-chain balance is less, come under intensive selection in the marrow and blood. By these routes alone, together with the major expansion of the total red cell precursor mass, it is possible to account for between 2 and 4 g/dL HbF without the necessity of invoking other mechanisms. This hypothesis received some experimental verification when it was observed that in patients with HbE–β thalassemia who were regularly transfused at a hemoglobin level of approximately 10 g/dL, and hence in whom there was limited erythroid expansion and endogenous erythropoiesis, there was virtually no synthesis of HbF; only HbE production could be identified. Yet the steady state HbF in untransfused patients with this condition, and hence with expanded marrows and anemia, is in the 30%–40% range.[293]

Despite some reports to the contrary, it is clear that from studies of the hemoglobin constitution of young patients with β^0 or β^+ thalassemia major before their first transfusion, that the predominant form of hemoglobin produced in all the severe forms of β thalassemia is HbF. The ${}^G\gamma/{}^A\gamma$ ratios of HbF in severe thalassemia has been reported by Schroeder and Huisman[294] and Huisman et al.[295] There was a broad scatter with a mean of approximately 3:2, regardless of the findings in the parents.

Hemoglobin A_2

The difficulties in interpreting HbA_2 levels in severe forms of β thalassemia are similar in many ways to those in interpreting the level of HbF. In a series of pretransfusion patients described by Kattamis et al.,[4] the HbA_2 level in 54 homozygotes, of whom 11 were of the β^+ variety, was 3.0 with a range from 0.8% to 5.5%. Several differential centrifugation studies have shown that the absolute level of HbA_2 in the HbF-rich population is much lower than that in cells that contain predominantly HbA (reviewed by Weatherall and Clegg[2]). Thus, it is clear that the distribution of HbA_2 is uneven and that the level that is measured in the peripheral blood is an average of cells with widely differing amounts; it is of no diagnostic value.

In Vitro Hemoglobin Synthesis

In vitro globin-chain synthesis studies have provided a clear picture of hemoglobin production in the severe forms of β thalassemia.[296–300] In nonthalassemic reticulocytes α- and β-chain synthesis is almost synchronous and there is only a small pool of free α chains. In reticulocytes or marrow cells from patients with severe β thalassemia there is always marked globin-chain imbalance, with published α/β + γ production ratio ranging from 1.5 to 30. Imbalanced globin-chain synthesis leads to substantial number of free α chains in the cells, which can be demonstrated by both gel filtration and DEAE cellulose chromatography.[299,300] The α chains in this pool exist both as monomers and dimers, and either combine with newly made β and γ chains to produce Hbs A and F, respectively, are destroyed by proteolysis, or form hemichromes and become associated with the red cell membrane.

The problems and pitfalls with this approach to measuring globin-chain production in β thalassemia have been reviewed in detail.[2] It should be remembered that the excess of α chains that are produced in β thalassemia are unstable and hence in order to obtain an estimate of the absolute amount of globin chain produced in radioactive labeling experiments it is necessary to carry out a time course experiment and extrapolate to zero time. Furthermore, many of the early discrepancies that were reported in α/β+γ-chain production ratios between the peripheral blood and bone marrow were the result of artifacts caused by the contamination of globin chains with nonglobin radioactive proteins produced in the bone marrow.

In short, because of the rapid destruction and turnover of excess α chains, particularly in the bone marrow, and the heterogeneity of cell populations with respect to γ-chain synthesis, the measurement of globin-chain synthesis in the marrow and blood at a single time point does not give information about the absolute rates of synthesis of individual chains. Nevertheless, it provides a reasonable indication of the overall severity of the defect in β-globin production. Provided that the various pitfalls associated with the measurements of total counts or specific activities, as outlined in detail by Weatherall and Clegg,[2] are taken into consideration, this approach can be used for diagnostic purposes, or to monitor the effects of different forms of therapy designed to augment γ-chain synthesis, or other modalities, to a reasonable degree of accuracy.

β THALASSEMIA INTERMEDIA

It has been apparent since the earliest descriptions of thalassemia that there are forms characterized by moderate anemia, jaundice, and splenomegaly that, although not as severe as the transfusion-dependent varieties, are clearly worse than the carrier states. In the extensive Italian literature on this subject these conditions have been variously described as La Malattia-di-Rietti-Greppi-Micheli (reviewed by Bannerman[301] and Weatherall[302]), the anemic form of the Mediterranean hematological disorder,[303] microcitica costituzionale,[304] and thalassemia intermedia.[305] Over recent years it has been apparent that this clinical picture can result from the interaction of many different thalassemia alleles, either one with another or with those for structural hemoglobin variants. Hence, the term is simply a descriptive title for a particular clinical disorder and has no clear-cut genetic meaning. Because we are still not at a stage at which we can always describe precisely the genetic interactions that can produce this clinical picture, it seems useful to retain it.

Thalassemia intermedia has been the subject of a number of articles and reviews that focus either on the molecular pathology and pathophysiology in general,[2,306,307] the molecular basis in certain populations,[308–314] or the clinical features.[2,315–317]

How is β Thalassemia Intermedia Defined?

There is no adequate definition of β thalassemia intermedia. As discussed later in this chapter, the hematological findings in heterozygous β thalassemia are remarkably uniform, and are characterized by a mild degree of anemia; splenomegaly is extremely unusual. Hence, any thalassemic patient with a hemoglobin level persistently below 9–10 g/dL, particularly if there is associated splenomegaly, falls into the intermediate class of β thalassemias. It is at the more severe end of the spectrum that the difficulty in definition arises. Some children survive early life with hemoglobin levels in the 5–6 g/dL range. Although they are often classified as having thalassemia intermedia, particularly if they present relatively late, many do not thrive or develop normally, and may grow up with gross skeletal deformities. It is now believed that these children should be transfused to avoid these distressing complications. Whether they should be classified as having severe thalassemia intermedia or thalassemia major is, therefore, a question of semantics that is of little importance.

Some children with β thalassemia have hemoglobin values between 6 and 9 g/dL. They grow and develop reasonably well, and reach adult life, and it is also useful to retain the term thalassemia intermedia for this type of patient. It should be remembered that they may become transfusion dependent if complications such as hypersplenism develop, or if the disorder is complicated by other factors such as folate deficiency or intercurrent infection. Clearly, the term thalassemia intermedia can cover a broad and shifting clinical spectrum, from almost complete health to a condition characterized by severe growth retardation and skeletal deformity that requires transfusion therapy; it is a diagnosis that can be made only after a considerable period of observation and that often requires revision.

Table 17.6. Thalassemia intermedia

1. Mild deficit in β-globin chain production
   - Homozygous mild β^+ thalassemia
   - Compound heterozygosity for severe β^0 or β^+ and mild β^+ thalassemia
   - Interactions of β^0 with 'silent' β thalassemia
   - Homozygosity for 'silent' β thalassemia
2. Reduced globin chain imbalance due to coinheritance of α and β thalassemia
   - Homozygous or compound heterozygous β^0 or β^+ thalassemia with 2 or 3 α gene deletions
   - Homozygous or compound heterozygous severe β^0 or β^+ thalassemia with nondeletion α2 gene mutation
   - Homozygous or compound heterozygous severe β^+ thalassemia with 1 or 2 α gene deletions
3. Severe β thalassemia with increased capacity for γ-chain synthesis
   - Homozygous or compound heterozygous β^0 or β^+ thalassemia with heterocellular HPFH
   - Homozygous or compound heterozygous β^0 or β^+ thalassemia with particular β-globin RFLP haplotype
   - Mechanism unknown
4. Deletion forms of δβ thalassemia and HPFH
   - Homozygous $(\delta\beta)^0$ or $(^A\gamma\delta\beta)^0$ thalassemia
   - Compound heterozygosity for β^0 or β^+ and $(\delta\beta)^0$ or $(^A\gamma\delta\beta)^0$ thalassemia
   - Homozygosity for Hb Lepore (some cases)
   - Compound heterozygosity for Hb Lepore and β^0 or β^+ thalassemia (some forms)
   - Compound heterozygosity for $(\delta\beta)^0$, $^G\gamma\beta^+$ or $^A\gamma\beta^+$ HPFH and β^0 or β^+ thalassemia
   - Compound heterozygosity for $(\delta\beta)^0$ thalassemia and $(\delta\beta)^0$ HPFH
5. Compound heterozygosity for β or δβ thalassemia and β-chain structural variants
   - Hb S, C, E/β or δβ thalassemia
   - Many other rare interactions
6. Other β thalassemia alleles or interactions
   - Dominant β thalassemia
   - β thalassemia trait associated with ααα or αααα globin gene duplications
   - Highly unstable β-globin chain variants

Genetic Interactions that Result in the Phenotype of β Thalassemia Intermedia

The main interactions that are known to modify the phenotype of β thalassemia are summarized in Table 17.6 and Figure 17.9. Other conditions that produce the clinical picture of thalassemia intermedia, the interactions of the β thalassemias with structural hemoglobin variants, the δβ thalassemias and their interactions, and so on, are considered elsewhere in this book. It is still difficult to predict phenotypes from genotypes with certainty; some guidelines are summarized in the following sections.

Interactions of "Silent" or "Mild" β

Thalassemia Alleles. It is customary to divide the mild β thalassemia alleles, which can interact with one another or with more severe alleles to produce thalassemia intermedia, into the "silent" and "mild" β^+ thalassemias. Although useful in practice, this is a somewhat artificial classification. Although many of the so-called silent alleles show no hematological changes in individual cases, if large numbers are studied it is apparent that some of them have slightly reduced MCV or MCH values, and slightly elevated HbA_2 or α/β-globin chain synthesis ratios. There is so much overlap with normal values, however, that for practical purposes it is reasonable to classify these extremely mild alleles as "silent," not in the least because they would not be identified by standard screening techniques to detect β thalassemia carriers. We shall return to this question later in this chapter. It is now apparent that interactions of both silent and mild β thalassemia alleles may be responsible for some forms of β thalassemia intermedia.

Several of the "silent" β thalassemia alleles, when coinherited with more severe β thalassemia alleles, have been shown to produce the picture of β thalassemia intermedia. For example, the β-101 C→T allele has been observed in the compound heterozygous state with a variety of different β thalassemia alleles, including codon 39 (C→T), IVS-1-110 (G→A), IVS-1-1 (G→A), IVS-2-745 (C→G), codon 44 (–C–C), and others.[312,318–320] All these interactions result in mild

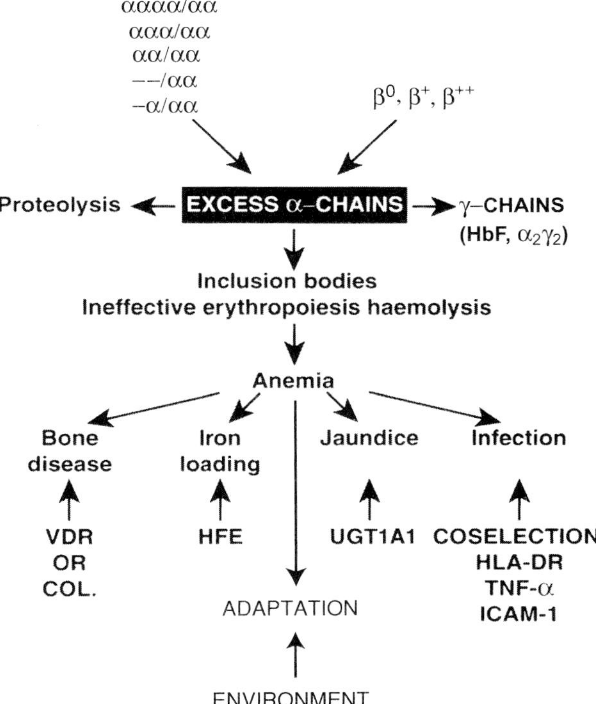

Figure 17.9. Some of the factors that modify the phenotype of β thalassemia. They include variable output from the β-globin genes, different forms of α thalassemia, variation in the level of fetal hemoglobin production, and a variety of secondary genetic modifiers. VDR, vitamin D receptor; OR, estrogen receptor; COL, collagen genes; HFE, primary hemochromatosis gene; UGT1A1, glucuronosyl transferase. Coselection indicates a number of genetic polymorphisms that are, like the thalassemias, modified by malaria resistance.

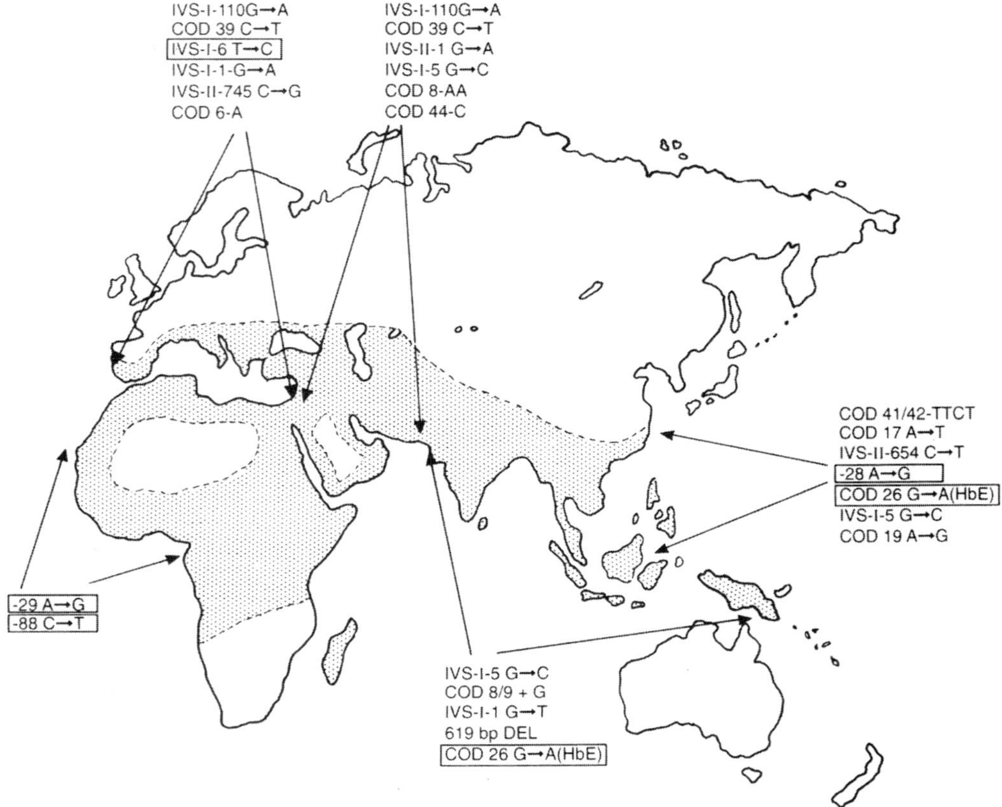

Figure 17.10. The world distribution of the thalassemia alleles. The common mild alleles are shown in boxes. In these populations, many of the intermediate forms of β thalassemia result from the different interactions of these milder alleles. (From ref. 2 with permission.)

forms of β thalassemia with steady-state hemoglobin values in the 9–12 g/dL range, a marked reduction in the MCV and MCH, elevated HbA_2 levels of 4.5–6.0, and HbF values ranging from 10% to 45%. They are a very common cause of β thalassemia intermedia in Mediterranean populations.

Other silent β thalassemia alleles that interact with more severe alleles to produce β thalassemia intermedia include β CAP+1 (A→C),[321] β 5′ UTR+10 (–T),[322] β CAP+33 (C→G),[323] and IVS-2-844 (C→G).[324]

These silent mutations produce the clinical picture of β thalassemia trait in their homozygous state. In families in which they interact with severe alleles to produce β thalassemia intermedia it is usual to find one parent with typical β thalassemia trait, although the other shows no hematological abnormality.

Interactions of Mild β Thalassemia Alleles

There are many mild β thalassemia alleles. For most of them there are very few published data about their hematological characteristics or about the results of their interactions with more severe β thalassemia alleles (Fig. 17.10).

The β-88 (C→T) allele is relatively common among Africans and African-Americans.[325,326] Its heterozygous phenotype is typical of β thalassemia trait. The homozygous condition is characterized by a relatively mild form of β thalassemia intermedia, with hemoglobin values in the 9–12 g/dL range, HbA_2 values in the 4%–8% range, and surprisingly high levels of HbF, in the range 40%–72%. In the compound heterozygous state with the other common promoter allele in this racial group, β-29 (A→G), the phenotype is also an extremely mild form of β thalassemia intermedia.

The β-87 (C→G) allele has been observed in Mediterranean populations, particularly in Italy and Turkey. The homozygous state is characterized by a mild form of β thalassemia intermedia.[327,328] This mutation has been observed in the compound heterozygous state with several β thalassemia alleles including codon 39 (C→T),[329] IVS-1-110 (G→A).[314] The best characterized of these interactions are with the codon 39 nonsense mutation; these patients have thalassemia intermedia with steady-state hemoglobin levels of approximately 10 g/dL and fetal hemoglobin values in the 30%–80% range.

There have been a few reports of individuals homozygous for the β-31 (A→G) and β-30 (T→A) alleles.[330,331] These conditions have not been observed in their compound heterozygous state with other β thalassemia alleles; their homozygous states are characterized by extremely mild forms of β thalassemia intermedia.

The β-29 (A→G) mutation is probably the most common form of β thalassemia in African populations. The homozygous state is characterized by a mild form of β thalassemia intermedia and there have been no reported transfusion-dependent cases.[325,332] Steady-state hemoglobin values range between 10 and 12 g/dL and HbF values between 50% and 70%. In the compound heterozygous state with the β codon 24 (T→A) allele, the clinical picture is again a mild form of β thalassemia intermedia, with hemoglobin values in the 9–13 g/dL range and HbF levels in the 25%–70% range.

In view of the mildness of the promoter mutations it is surprising that the β-29 (A→G) allele, observed in a Chinese family, is described as having a severe, transfusion-dependent phenotype.[333] Although it has been suggested that the different phenotype to that observed in Black populations with the same mutation may reflect the fact that, in the latter, it is on a chromosome carrying the Xmn-1 $^{G}\gamma$ polymorphism, although this is not the case in the Chinese patient, it is not clear whether this difference alone is sufficient to explain the wide difference between the phenotypes in different populations.

Mutations in β codons 19, 26, and 27, in addition to reducing β-globin output, are also associated with the production of the structural hemoglobin variants, Hbs Malay, E, and Knossos, respectively. The homozygous states for Hb Malay and Knossos are characterized by mild forms of thalassemia intermedia, with hemoglobin values in the 9–12 g/dL range and moderately elevated levels of HbF. Because of its common occurrence in the Mediterranean region, Hb Knossos has been found in the compound heterozygous state with several severe β thalassemia alleles.[314,334,335] All these interactions are associated with the clinical picture of a mild to moderate form of β thalassemia intermedia. In the case of compound heterozygosity for Hb Knossos and the IVS-1-110 G→A allele, the disorder has been severe enough to require occasional blood transfusions, and splenectomy. The clinical phenotypes of the many HbE interactions are described in Chapter 18.

The β IVS-1-6 (T→C) splice mutation, sometimes called the Portuguese β thalassemia variant, is widespread among the Mediterranean population. Unlike the other mild forms of β thalassemia, the homozygous state for this condition is not always associated with a mild phenotype.[312,314,336–339] In the first descriptions of this condition, and in the extensive study of Efremov et al.,[336] it was found that homozygotes had a relatively mild form of thalassemia intermedia; none had required regular transfusion. On the other hand, in a later report from Israel, Rund and her colleagues describe a much more variable clinical phenotype. At one extreme nine patients had baseline hemoglobin levels of 10–11 g/dL, none had been splenectomized, and transfusions had either been rare or never required. At the other extreme, however, there were nine patients with baseline hemoglobin levels of 6–7 g/dL who were transfused either infrequently or regularly, even though they had undergone splenectomy. This latter group also had growth retardation, pronounced bone changes and thalassemic bone changes, absent puberty, and evidence of iron overload. The reasons for this remarkable clinical heterogeneity are not clear. Because this mutation is so common there have been numerous opportunities for studying its interaction with other β thalassemia alleles, particularly the more severe forms that are common in the Mediterranean population. The most extensive data relate to interactions with the IVS-1-110 G→A and codon 39 C→T alleles. Overall, it appears that the interactions with β^0 thalassemia alleles are more severe and result in a picture at the most severe end of the spectrum of β thalassemia intermedia. On the other hand, those with β^+ mutations are more varied in their phenotype, some of them being described as moderately severe, others mild; many of the latter cases may have, in addition, one or more α thalassemia alleles.[314]

Finally, there are several different mutations that involve the poly-A addition site of the β-globin gene. From the limited number of interactions that have been described it seems likely that these are fairly mild alleles. A homozygote for the AATAAA→AACAAA allele, first described by Orkin et al.,[340] has been encountered (Dr. J. Old, personal communication). This patient has never required transfusion and has a mild form of β thalassemia intermedia with moderate splenomegaly and no skeletal deformities. His steady-state hemoglobin level is approximately 7–8 g/dL, with HbF and HbA_2 values of 13.3% and 9.2%, respectively. Other interactions of this family of β thalassemia alleles are summarized by Weatherall and Clegg.[2]

Interactions between α and β Thalassemia

The extensive literature on the ameliorating effect of the co-inheritance of α thalassemia on the different forms of β thalassemia has been reviewed.[2] The concept that defective α-chain synthesis might reduce the severity of β thalassemia by lessening the degree of globin-chain excess was suggested both by biosynthetic studies[341] and by direct gene analysis.[342] It was later confirmed by larger population studies.[310,313,343–346] From these investigations it was possible to determine, at least in outline, how different α and β thalassemia alleles can interact to produce forms of β thalassemia intermedia of varying severity. It appears that, overall, there is a reasonable correlation between the homozygous states for β^0 or β^+ thalassemia, together with the homozygous state for α^+ thalassemia, and a mild phenotype. On the other hand, the loss of a single α-globin gene seems to have minimal phenotypic effect on homozygosity for β^0 thalassemia, except for a slightly later presentation, and an unpredictable effect on compound heterozygosity for β^+ or β^0 thalassemia or homozygosity for β^+ thalassemia. Reports of the occurrence of homozygous β thalassemia in association with a genotype of HbH disease in the same individual suggests that this rare interaction produces the clinical picture of a severe form of β thalassemia intermedia.[347,348]

Unusually High Levels of HbF Production in Generating β Thalassemia Intermedia

It has long been realized that variation in the ability to produce HbF in the postnatal period must be a major factor in the generation of the phenotype of β thalassemia intermedia. Although many threads of evidence have pointed in this direction, some of the most convincing were early reports of individuals apparently homozygous for β^0 thalassemia who ran relatively mild clinical courses.[318,349–352] In the families of some of these patients a determinant for heterocellular hereditary persistence of fetal hemoglobin (HPFH) appeared to be segregating. Detailed studies of the HbF of parents and relatives, however, sometimes did not show any evidence for a second determinant of this type.[352] Later studies, relating HbF production to particular restriction fragment length polymorphism (RFLP) haplotypes in the β-globin gene cluster, together with detailed family studies, suggest that some of the determinants that are associated with an unusually high level of HbF production in β thalassemia lie within the β-globin gene cluster, whereas others segregate quite independently. Although this work has gone some way to explaining the heterogeneity of HbF production in β thalassemia, in many cases the reasons for unusually high levels of HbF are not clear (see Chapter 16).

Determinants for Increased HbF Production within the β-Globin Gene Cluster

A variety of studies have suggested that the β-globin gene RFLP haplotypes associated with the Xmn-1 $^G\gamma$ polymorphism associated with a C→T change at position-158 in the $^G\gamma$-globin gene are associated with an increased propensity for HbF production in β thalassemia.[310,353,354] In both African-Asian and Italian populations this has been the only change found in a number of patients homozygous for β^0 thalassemia whose clinical course has been that of a moderate to severe form of β thalassemia intermedia. This conclusion was strengthened in later comparisons of the β-globin gene RFLP haplotypes of patients with thalassemia major and intermedia.[309,314]

A word of caution is necessary, however. In all these studies there has been a wide spectrum of phenotypes associated with homozygosity for the $^G\gamma$ polymorphism. Overall, homozygotes for β^0 of β^+ thalassemia who are also homozygous for this polymorphism have a milder disease, manifested by a late presentation and the picture of a moderately severe form of β thalassemia intermedia. This is not always the case, however, and some of them subsequently become transfusion dependent in later life or even have severe disease from early in childhood. In the study of Ho et al.[314] there was a wide variation in the phenotypic severity, even among those who fell into the β thalassemia intermedia category. It is also apparent that certain β thalassemia mutations are, themselves, associated with an increased propensity for fetal hemoglobin production. Although this relates particularly to promoter mutations it is also observed in the rare deletional forms of β thalassemia that remove the 5′ end of the β-globin gene (reviewed by Thein[355]).

Determinants for Increased HbF Production Not Encoding in the β-Globin Gene Complex

Several families have been reported in which there is very good evidence that homozygotes or compound heterozygotes for β thalassemia produce unusually high levels of HbF and have the phenotype of β thalassemia intermedia, due to the coinheritance of a gene for heterocellular HPFH.[356,357] In both the families described in these reports subsequent studies showed that the genetic determinant for heterocellular HPFH did not segregate in the β-globin gene cluster.[357,358] Later studies indicated that the determinant in the large family described by Thein and Weatherall showed strong linkage to chromosome 6, whereas that in the family originally described by Cappellini et al. does not. Further families have been reported by Ho et al;[314] again it is clear that heterocellular HPFH is an important factor in the generation of β^0 thalassemia intermedia. It appears, therefore, that there are a number of determinants for a form of heterocellular HPFH that can modify the β thalassemic phenotype; one is on chromosome 6, but this form of heterocellular HPFH is quite heterogeneous and other varieties exist that are encoded on other chromosomes (see Chapter 16). The role of the locus on the X chromosome, which seems to be involved in setting the level of F cells in adults[359] in determining the level of HbF in β thalassemia is still not clear.

Heterozygous β Thalassemia with an Unusually Severe Phenotype

There are two mechanisms whereby heterozygous β thalassemia can be associated with the phenotype of β thalassemia intermedia. First, there are cases in which β thalassemia is complicated by the inheritance of chromosomes carrying more than the usual number of α-globin genes, ααα or αααα. Second, there are particular β-globin gene mutations that, because of the unusual properties of their products, give rise to severe phenotypes in heterozygotes. The latter are usually referred to as the dominant β thalassemias.

The extensive literature on the ααα and αααα interactions is summarized in detail by Weatherall and Clegg[2] and by Premawardhena et al.[360] It is clear that the inheritance of triplicated or quadruplicated α-globin gene arrangements, either in homozygous or heterozygous states, can, together with the heterozygosity for β^0 or β^+ thalassemia, produce a wide spectrum of phenotypes ranging from extremely mild to quite severe forms of β thalassemia intermedia.[314,315,319,360–364]

Families with dominantly inherited forms of β thalassemia were first described by Weatherall et al.[365] and Stamatoyannopoilos et al.[366] Their relationship to exon 3 mutations is described elsewhere in this book. This condition is characterized by a form of thalassemia intermedia of varying severity together with typical thalassemic changes in the blood and bone marrow. The most striking feature is the presence of inclusion bodies in the marrow and, after splenectomy, in the peripheral blood. It seems likely, although it has not been firmly established, that these consist of excess α chains and quite possibly the unstable β chain products.

There is one remarkable characteristic of the forms of β thalassemia intermedia associated with heterozygosity for β thalassemia. In all these conditions there are unusually low levels of HbF for the β thalassemia intermedia phenotype. This observation was emphasized in the recent description of the homozygous state for the quadruplicated α-globin genes associated with heterozygous β thalassemia. The phenotype was a moderately severe form of β thalassemia intermedia yet the fetal hemoglobin level was only 4.6%.[360] The degree of globin chain imbalance in this patient was similar to that in other forms of β thalassemia intermedia associated with extremely high levels of HbF. In reviewing the literature on both varieties of β thalassemia intermedia associated with β thalassemia trait it was clear that a low level of HbF in these conditions is nearly always found. Whether this reflects a requirement for defective β-globin synthesis in both *cis* and *trans* for the production of high levels of HbF, or some more subtle effect whereby red cell precursors that contain relatively mild HbF do not come under selection in these conditions is not clear. But there is no question that the low level of HbF is characteristic of all of them.

Summary

Considering the remarkable heterogeneity of the various interactions that can produce the clinical phenotype of β thalassemia intermedia, it is not surprising that this condition has a remarkably variable clinical course. Although hitherto ignored, it should be remembered that other factors including adaptation to anemia may play an important role in this diversity. For example, patients with HbE–β thalassemia, the most common form of thalassemia intermedia globally, are able to grow and develop normally at hemoglobin levels which would be associated with a much more severe phenotype in other genetic forms of thalassemia intermedia. Recent studies suggest that this relates to the level of HbF and hence the oxygen affinity of the red cells of patients with these different conditions; the relatively low levels of HbF in HbE–β thalassemia compared with other forms of thalassemia intermedia allow much better adaptation to anemia (unpublished observations), and the action of environmental factors, notably malaria, may have a profound effect on phenotypes of these intermediate forms of thalassemia in many of the developing countries. It is also apparent that much remains to be learnt about the genetic factors that are involved in HbF production in these conditions. Given these factors, it is not surprising that it is difficult to predict the clinical course for any particular form of thalassemia intermedia, even when the genetic basis is apparently well established.

Clinical Features

One of the hallmarks of β thalassemia intermedia is its late presentation compared with transfusion-dependent forms of the disease.[4–6] Although there is considerable individual variation, overall it is usual for transfusion-dependent patients to come to medical attention in the first year of life, whereas those with thalassemia intermedia tend to present during the second year or later. There are few good published data on the hemoglobin levels over the first few years of life. Although some children maintain a steady-state hemoglobin value that seems to vary little, others do not. Although it has been suggested that a fall in hemoglobin over the first few years may reflect increasing hypersplenism[5] it is not clear whether this is always the case. From our own experience many children with intermediate forms of β thalassemia do not reach a steady-state hemoglobin level for several years, and it is very important not to draw conclusions about their likely prognosis without a long period of observation.

The clinical manifestations are extremely variable. In some cases the disorder presents early in life with relatively severe anemia, while in others it may not appear until later due to a complication such as hypersplenism. Many patients have been found to have this condition on routine clinical examination. Growth and development may be normal or there may be a similar pattern of retardation as occurs in undertreated transfusion-dependent β thalassemia. The most common symptoms are those of anemia and mild jaundice. There is always some degree of splenomegaly. Bone changes are variable and range from none at all to the severe skeletal deformities characteristic of transfusion-dependent β thalassemia. Some infants, who have presented relatively late with hemoglobin values in the 7 g/dL range, are clearly destined for transfusion from the beginning. When observed over a few months there is failure to thrive, listlessness, proneness to infection, and a poor appetite. Sequential studies over even a short period make it clear that these infants are not developing normally and that they should be considered to have thalassemia major, and treated accordingly. The course for infants who, despite their relatively low hemoglobin levels, are fully active and thriving, is usually one of chronic well-compensated anemia that may be exacerbated during periods of infection or folate deficiency or with increasing hypersplenism.

Complications

Hypersplenism

Increasing splenomegaly leading to hypersplenism is a relatively common feature of β thalassemia intermedia. In most of the larger series cited earlier, a significant proportion of the patients had undergone splenectomy for worsening of their anemia, thrombocytopenia, or neutropenia.

Iron Loading

There is increasing evidence that although the rate of iron loading is much slower than in transfusion-dependent β thalassemia, patients with β thalassemia intermedia do iron load and this may become of clinical importance in adult life. Bannerman et al.[367] described a 41-year-old Sicilian patient with β thalassemia intermedia who had gross iron loading with associated cardiac failure, diabetes mellitus, and hypopituitarism. On the other hand, Erlandson et al.[368] did not consider that iron loading was a major problem in this disorder. In a later study Pippard et al.[317] examined the rate of iron loading in 15 patients with this condition. There was a highly significant increase in plasma ferritin levels with age and the majority of patients older than 20 years had totally saturated iron-binding capacities. Liver biopsies of three of the older patients showed excessive iron deposition associated with portal cirrhosis in each case. Iron absorption studies, described in a later section, showed that the rate of iron loading from the gastrointestinal tract was approximately three–four times normal.

Later studies confirmed these observations. Cossu et al.[369] reported an increasing serum ferritin level with age and increased urinary iron excretion in response to desferrioxamine. Fiorelli et al.,[370] in attempting to explain some of the variability in the degree of iron loading among 38 adult patients with β thalassemia intermedia, described significant differences between patients who had undergone splenectomy compared with those with intact spleens; the iron burden was considerably greater in the former. This may simply reflect the greater severity and hence more marked marrow expansion and higher rate of iron absorption of these children. Although these data are limited, there seems little doubt that iron loading is an important feature of β thalassemia intermedia. It can undoubtedly lead to liver damage and cirrhosis and to other complications of iron excess. It is not clear how often it causes cardiac damage; as discussed later, there are very few data relating to the cardiac status of older adult patients with this condition.

Endocrine Function

The fact that in many of the larger series of patients with β thalassemia intermedia cited earlier there was a history of a normal puberty and menarche, even though the latter was sometimes delayed, suggests that overall endocrine function is often maintained up to and beyond puberty. From such limited data as there are it appears that by the time these patients reach the third or fourth decades there is a significant incidence of diabetes mellitus, and other endocrine deficiencies. Of the 15 patients reported by Pippard et al.[317] one was frankly diabetic and three showed a reduced first-stage insulin response associated with a high-normal fasting plasma glucose concentration during standard glucose tolerance tests, findings that suggest impairment of pancreatic β-cell function. Similar results were obtained in three of 11 patients studied by De Sanctis et al.[132] In the series reported by Pippard et al.[317] all had normal thyroid-stimulating hormone reponses to thyroid-releasing hormone, and a normal fasting prolactin concentration, but two had a reduced luteinizing hormone response to luteininzing hormone–releasing hormone. Plasma cortisol response to synacthen was normal in four of five patients tested. McIntosh[106] described a woman with multiple endocrine deficiencies; replacement therapy was followed by a normal pregnancy.

Cardiac Function

Because of the slower rate of iron loading in β thalassemia intermedia than in transfusion-dependent forms of the disease it would be expected that, if cardiac complications occur at all, they would only be manifest in adult life. Although there have been single case reports of cardiac failure associated with iron loading in this disorder,[367,371] there is very little information about the dangers of iron loading of the myocardium in this condition.

In the series of patients reported by Pippard et al.,[317] a high proportion complained of exertional dyspnea, palpitations, or both. The electrocardiogram showed only minor abnormalities in a few cases; there were inverted T waves over the right ventricular leads in one, and evidence of left-ventricular hypertrophy in four of the older patients. Holter monitoring over a 24-hour period revealed marked abnormalities in eight of the nine patients studied. These included periods of bradycardia and tachycardia, and supraventricular extrasystoles. This was in marked contrast to the absence of rhythm abnormalities in nine cases of well-transfused patients with β thalassemia major, including five older than the age of 14 years. Echocardiography showed that four of the older patients with thalassemia intermedia had enlarged diastolic dimensions. Both the ejection fractions and fractional shortening, however, were normal in all eight cases studied. Fiorelli et al.[316] described the cardiac status of 18 patients with thalassemia intermedia in Italy. All had cardiomegaly and systolic flow murmurs compatible with the degree of anemia. Their electrocardiograms showed some modifications of the QRS complexes compatible with ventricular hypertrophy. No consistent abnormalities of rhythm or conduction were observed. In five of the patients, echocardiography showed enlarged diastolic dimensions and some rather nonspecific functional alterations. Most of these changes could be ascribed to moderate to severe anemia and none were characteristic of iron loading of the myocardium.

Olivieri et al.[372] reported detailed studies on a 29-year-old Italian man who, although he had not received transfusions after the age of 5 years, nevertheless presented with hepatomegaly, abnormal liver function tests, an elevated serum ferritin level, and marked iron loading of the liver as judged by biopsy and quantitative MRI. Before treatment the left ventricular ejection fraction was 60% at rest, with no increase at peak exercise, and there was mild right ventricular dilation and abnormalities in diastolic function. These changes did not alter after intensive chelation therapy, except that there was some improvement in the atrial contribution. Although these are relatively mild changes the fact that they altered after treatment suggests that there may have been some functional cardiac anomalies secondary to iron loading.

Clearly, it will be important to try to follow larger series of adult patients with β thalassemia intermedia with consecutive studies of cardiac function; currently there is no way of knowing what proportion of older patients with this condition are at risk from cardiac disease.

Over recent years there has been considerable interest in the syndrome of pulmonary hypertension and right heart failure in patients with HbE–β thalassemia, particularly those who have undergone a splenectomy (see Chapter 18). This complication has also been reported in β thalassemia intermedia.[373] In seven patients who presented with congestive cardiac failure and pulmonary hypertension after splenectomy, there was dilation of the main pulmonary artery with cardiac enlargement, signs of right ventricular hypertrophy, and a dilated right ventricle, but good left ventricular function as judged by echocardiography. Right heart catheterization showed markedly raised pulmonary pressure with increased pulmonary vascular resistance. Whether this picture results from platelet aggregation in the pulmonary circulation, as suggested in the case of HbE–β thalassemia, remains to be determined.

Gallstones

Probably as a result of both ineffective erythropoiesis and hemolysis there is a high frequency of pigment stones.[316,368,374]

Folic Acid Deficiency

There are many well-documented cases of folate deficiency occurring in patients with β thalassemia intermedia.[5,367,368] The degree of anemia may be profound and patients may present in cardiac failure.

Skeletal Deformities and Bone and Joint Disease

As mentioned earlier, some patients with β thalassemia intermedia develop severe skeletal deformities, similar in every way to those seen in the undertreated transfusion-dependent forms of the disease. Pathological fractures are also a major feature, particularly in older patients. There is also a particularly distressing complication involving the bones and joints that has been called "thalassemic osteoarthropathy."[375] This takes the form of a curious periarticular disease characterized by dull aching pains in the ankles, exacerbated by weight bearing and relieved by rest. Radiological changes include widening of the medullary spaces, thin cortices with coarse trabeculation, and evidence of microfractures in the region of the joints. Histological analysis confirmed the presence of the latter and, in addition, showed osteomalacia and increased osteoblastic surface areas with iron deposition in the calcification front and cement lines. We have observed this complication in a number of adult patients with β thalassemia intermedia, at least one of whom required an arthrodesis of the ankle joint for relief of intractable pain. Acetabular protrusion has also been reported in patients with severe bone involvement.

Extramedullary Erythropoiesis

The generation of tumor masses composed of extramedullary erythropoietic tissue is a frequent complication.[368,376,377] The most common site is in the paraspinal region. Alam et al.[378] give a valuable summary of the radiological characteristics of these lesions. Although they do not usually cause symptoms there have been well-documented case reports of spinal cord compression,[379,380] cauda equina lesions,[381] and hemorrhage causing a massive hemothorax.[382]

Although these masses are usually identified by conventional radiography,[378] the diagnosis can be confirmed, particularly if they are in an unusual site, by both computed tomography (CT) and MRI analysis.[383] They produce a low-intensity signal similar to that of adjacent marrow of the thoracic spine and are surrounded by a characteristically high-intense rim attributed to a layer of fat surrounding the masses.

Total body CT analyses of adults with β thalassemia intermedia suggest that some degree of extramedullary erythropoiesis is probably quite common; it was detected in 65% of patients by Sergiacomi et al.[384] It seems likely that at least some of these lesions may undergo fatty transformation with time, particularly if the hemoglobin level is raised by splenectomy.[385]

Infection

Although it is suspected that patients at the severe end of the spectrum of β thalassemia intermedia have increased susceptibility to infection, there are very few supporting data. Such that there are suggest that the pattern of infection is similar to that outlined for transfusion-dependent β thalassemia earlier in this chapter. As is the case in thalassemia major, severe *Yersinia* infection associated with iron chelation, and aplastic or hypoplastic episodes due to parvovirus infection have been recorded.[386] There is increasing evidence that those patients who require occasional transfusion are prone to contract hepatitis B and C.[387] Although there have been attempts at defining specific abnormalities of neutrophil function or of the immune system, as in the case of the more severe forms of β thalassemia there have been no consistent findings. The problem of infection in thalassemia intermedia is discussed in more detail by Weatherall and Clegg.[2]

Hyperuricemia and Gout

Although in several reported series patients with β thalassemia had elevated uric acid levels, secondary gout seems to be uncommon.[375]

Leg Ulcers

This is a relatively common complication of β thalassemia intermedia.[5,315,316] The cause is unknown; the possible relationship to the rheological properties of the red cells is discussed by Gimmon et al.[388]

Pregnancy

Because many patients with thalassemia intermedia pass through a normal puberty, pregnancy is not uncommon.[389,390] In most of these reports it is stressed that these patients may become quite profoundly anemic during pregnancy, but if they are maintained at a relatively normal hemoglobin level there seems to be no increased rate of fetal loss.

Thromboembolic Disease

The "hypercoagulable state" associated with platelet activation, which correlates with abnormal red cell phospholipid exposure, is reviewed by Ruf et al.[391] In fact, much of the experimental work that underlies this concept was performed on the blood of patients with β thalassemia intermedia. In a review of thromboembolic complications of β thalassemia from Italy Borgna-Pignatti et al.[82] discussed earlier in this chapter, five of the 32 affected patients had thalassemia intermedia. There have been occasional reports of severe thromboembolic disease following splenectomy, but in the series described by Skarsgard et al.[392] several nonthalassemic patients presented with the same complication. From these limited data it is not possible to assess the overall risk of thrombotic disease, nor is it clear whether it is related to the occurrence of recurrent priapism following splenectomy in patients with this type of thalassemia.[393]

Hematological Findings

There is a variable degree of anemia, with hemoglobin values in the 5–10 g/dL range. The red cell indices are typically

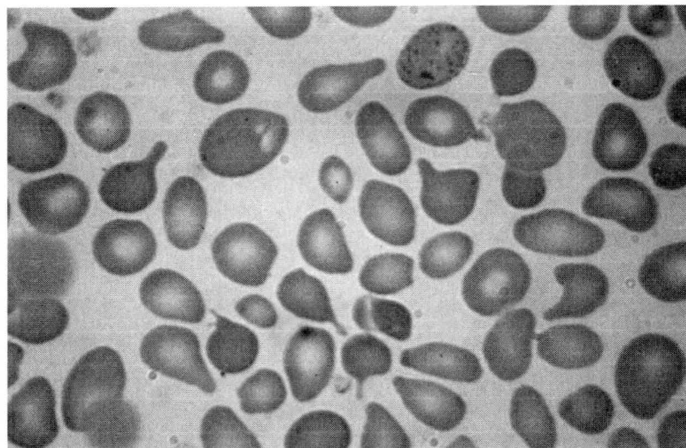

Figure 17.11. A peripheral blood smear from the propositus from the first family to be reported with dominantly inherited β thalassemia.[365] Hypochromia is not a major feature but there is a remarkable degree of poikilocytosis and heavy basophilic stippling.

thalassemic and the peripheral blood findings are indistinguishable from those of the more severe forms of β thalassemia. In some of the dominantly inherited forms of β thalassemia, hypochromia is less marked, and poikilocytosis is the main feature (Fig. 17.11). Except when there is hypersplenism the white cell and platelet counts are usually normal. The reticulocyte count is elevated and, following splenectomy, on staining with methyl violet nucleated red cells show ragged inclusions similar to those observed in thalassemia major. The bone marrow shows marked erythroid hyperplasia and, again, many of the red cell precursors contain inclusion bodies.

Red Cell Survival, Ferrokinetics, and Erythrokinetics

Red cell survival studies have shown a moderate reduction in survival times, with $^{Cr}51$ T1/2 values ranging from 10 to 16 days.[368,394]

Iron-absorption studies have shown an increase in the rate of iron accumulation.[289,317,395–397] In the studies of Pippard et al. the patients were in positive balance of between 2.6 and 8.6 mg iron per day. Cavill et al.[398] found that the marrow turnover was approximately six times normal but that most of this increase in activity was ineffective. Similar results were reported by Najean et al.[399] The serum-transferrin-receptor level has been used to assess the degree of erythroid expansion. In a study by Dore et al.[400] of untransfused patients with a steady-state hemoglobin level of 9.6 g/dL the mean basal transferrin receptor level was 30.3 compared with 12.8 in a series of age-matched healthy controls.

There have been several studies of serum erythropoietin (Epo) levels in β thalassemia intermedia.[401,402] Although overall elevated levels were found, and there was evidence of a reciprocal relationship with the hemoglobin level, in one study there appeared to be inappropriately low Epo levels for the degree of anemia. Because of the increased oxygen affinity of red cells with high levels of HbF, erythropoietin levels may be particularly high in patients with HbF levels in excess of 50%.[403] More extensive data on Epo response in HbE–β thalassemia are discussed in Chapter 18.

Hemoglobin Constitution

Considering the extraordinarily diverse genotypes that underlie the phenotype of β thalassemia intermedia, it is not surprising that it is characterized by a wide range of different hemoglobin constitutions, particularly with respect to the levels of HbF. In the intermediate forms of the β^0 thalassemias the hemoglobin consists entirely of HbF, with HbA_2 values in the low-normal range. There is a wide range of HbF levels in the β^+ thalassemia intermedias and it is possible only to make some broad generalizations about how these relate to the underlying genotypes.

In the β^+ thalassemia intermedias that reflect the homozygous state for mild β^+ thalassemia mutations the level of HbF tends to be low compared with those that result from the interaction of two severe alleles. This is exemplified in the homozygous state for the common Mediterranean mutation, IVS-1-6 (T→C), in which the fetal hemoglobin level tends to be in the region of 20% of the total, although even here there is considerable scatter.[404] The exception to this rule is the homozygous or compound heterozygous states for promoter mutations of the β-globin gene. In this case there tends to be an unexpectedly high level of fetal hemoglobin, usually in excess of 50% of the total.[325] In both these conditions homozygotes have, as a rule, increased levels of HbA_2.

In interactions between homozygous or compound heterozygous states for β^+ or β^0 thalassemia and the heterozygous states for α^+ or α^0 thalassemia, the hemoglobin pattern does not seem to alter from that found with the β thalassemia mutations alone. In the interactions between these forms of β thalassemia and the genotype of HbH disease there is quite a different pattern. In this case, although the amounts of Hbs A and F do not differ significantly from those seen with β^+ or β^0 thalassemia alone, there is an unusually high level of HbA_2 and traces of Hb Bart's can be demonstrated.[347,348] The unusually low levels of HbF in the forms of thalassemia intermedia associated with β thalassemia trait were discussed earlier in this chapter.

Hemoglobin Synthesis

Early studies that provided data on α/non-α-globin-chain synthesis ratios in patients with β thalassemia intermedia showed that, overall, the degree of imbalance of globin-chain synthesis was less than that observed in the more severe forms of β thalassemia.[394,405] Although there have been sporadic reports none have related the degree of globin-chain imbalance to the underlying molecular pathology in sufficient numbers to be able to offer any firm conclusions about the degree of globin-chain imbalance associated with the different combinations of mutations that underlie the intermediate forms of β thalassemia.

THE HETEROZYGOUS FORMS OF β THALASSEMIA

The heterozygous states for the different forms of β thalassemia are summarized in Table 17.1. The most common varieties are associated with an elevated level of HbA_2 and normal or slightly elevated levels of HbF. There is another group that is characterized by normal levels of HbA_2. This is subdivided into Type 1, in which there are no hematological changes; this corresponds to the "silent" β thalassemias. In Type 2, the hematological changes are indistinguishable from the β thalassemia trait with elevated levels of HbA_2. There are other rare groups characterized by unusually high levels of Hbs A_2 or F, or by a much more severe course.

The Common Forms of Heterozygous β Thalassemia

The heterozygous states for most forms of β thalassemia are characterized by mild anemia, characteristic changes in the MCV and MCH, an elevated level of HbA_2, and normal or only slightly elevated levels of HbF.

Clinical Features

Patients heterozygous for β thalassemia are believed to be symptom-free; the condition is diagnosed as part of a family study, as an incidental finding during an intercurrent illness, or as part of a population survey. Recently, however, a population study that compared the symptoms and quality of life of adult patients with thalassemia trait with age-matched controls found that the former had a highly significant increase in symptoms attributable to mild anemia and, possibly, increased rates of infection.[406] Occasionally, and particularly during pregnancy, the mild anemia may bring a carrier to the notice of the physician.

There are no characteristic clinical findings, and palpable splenomegaly is most unusual.

Hematological Findings

The larger reported series, when adequately analyzed by sex and age, have shown that although there is a considerable scatter in hemoglobin levels, most heterozygous β thalassemics have a significant degree of anemia compared with controls drawn from the same population.[351,407,408] The red cell indices are a valuable diagnostic feature. There is a relatively high red cell count but the cells are small and poorly hemoglobinized and the MCH and MCV are markedly reduced. On the other hand, the MCHC is usually in the normal range or only moderately reduced. There may be a slightly elevated reticulocyte count. The red cells show characteristic morphological changes; there is microcytosis and hypochromia with variation in the size and shape. The presence of target cells, much stressed by early workers, is very variable and although some are usually found their absence is of little diagnostic value. Basophilic stippling is a frequent finding, particularly in patients with more severe β thalassemia alleles.

Completely normal hematological findings in heterozygous β thalassemia are very unusual. They are usually found in individuals with β thalassemia trait who have coinherited one or other forms of α thalassemia. These interactions, and their implications for screening programs, are discussed by Weatherall and Clegg.[2]

The bone marrow shows a variable degree of erythroid hyperplasia, in which polychromatic and pyknotic normoblasts predominate. The cytoplasm of the red cell precursors is often ragged and shows basophilic stippling. Iron is usually plentiful and is distributed normally between the reticuloendothelial elements and the red cell precursors. On incubation of the marrow with methyl violet, a few of the red cell precursors show small inclusions, similar to those seen in abundance in homozygous individuals.[409]

Red Cell Survival, Iron Metabolism, and Ferrokinetics

The ^{51}Cr T1/2 of the red cells have given mean values just below the normal range in several reported series.[292,410–412] Serum iron and ferritin estimations have shown that, although there is considerable variability, the mean values are little different from normal.[351,412–416]). Iron loading, as evidenced by increased serum iron or ferritin levels, or iron deposition in the tissues, is unusual. In the series described by Knox-Macaulay et al.,[351] five females and four males had iron-binding saturations of 50% or more; one 68-year-old woman, who had received oral iron intermittently for 15 years due to a mistaken diagnosis of iron-deficiency anemia, had a totally saturated iron-binding capacity and clinical evidence of iron overload. There have been other reports of iron loading in heterozygous β thalassemics.[417,418] In addition to these isolated case reports, Fargion et al.[419] described a group of Italian males with very high serum ferritin levels. Whether some of these patients were also carrying genes for hereditary hemochromatosis is not known.

The rate of iron absorption is either normal or slightly elevated [367,420] Iron is rapidly removed from the plasma, the rate of plasma iron turnover is increased, but it appears in red cells relatively slowly. In an extensive series of ferrokinetic studies, Pippard and Wainscoat[412] found that the overall efficiency of erythropoiesis is significantly reduced, with a mean of 76 ± 17 standard deviations of normal. Serum erythropoietin levels are slightly elevated, more so in females than males, but there appears to be no correlation with the hemoglobin level.[421]

These findings suggest that there is a mild degree of ineffective erythropoiesis in β thalassemia carriers and that the anemia is predominantly due to intramedullary destruction of red cell precursors rather than hemolysis.

Complications

Most patients heterozygous for β thalassemia go through life without any manifestations that can be ascribed to the disease. The only complication of any importance is worsening of the anemia during pregnancy.

Pregnancy. Although it is clear that the hemoglobin level falls to a greater degree during pregnancy than in normal women, the resulting anemia is usually mild; most of the reports of more severe forms of anemia in pregnancy probably reflect the added complications of either iron or folic acid deficiency.[351,422,423]

In normal women there is an increase in both plasma volume and red cell mass that commences at the end of the first trimester. Schuman et al.[424] found that pregnant thalassemic women are unable to increase their red cell mass to the same degree as normal women; there is no difference between them in the degree of expansion of the plasma volume. On average, the decrease in the hemoglobin level between the first and second trimester is comparable with that of normal women, in the range of 7%–10%. In the large series of White et al.[423] and Landman[422] there were minimal changes in the red cell indices during pregnancy. From these studies it is clear that any pregnant β thalassemia carrier with a hemoglobin value of less than 8–9 g/dL should be investigated for other causes for anemia. Because of the unreliability of serum iron and iron-binding capacity estimations in pregnancy, it is helpful to assess the patient's iron status by the serum ferritin level.

Folic acid deficiency. Folic acid deficiency has been reported in heterozygous β thalassemia in nonpregnant persons, but this must be extremely rare.[425,426]

Failure of diagnosis. In populations in which β thalassemia is not common the trait may be misdiagnosed as iron-deficiency anemia or attract a number of other diagnostic labels. This can lead to a variety of unnecessary investigations, considerable anxiety, and inappropriate treatment with iron.

Life Expectancy

In one extensive study aimed at defining the lifespan of individuals heterozygous for β thalassemia, no significant differences were found between β thalassemia heterozygotes and normals.[427] Surprisingly, in a prospective study of 4,401 subjects in Ferrara over a 7-year period of observation by the same group, it was concluded that male β thalassemia heterozygotes show a significant degree of protection against myocardial infarction.[428] At first sight these observations seem contradictory although it is possible that the relatively small effect on cardiac disease was masked in the life expectancy survey. A more recent study in Greece also has found a significant degree of protection against cardiac disease, and suggests that the lipoprotein and blood rheology profiles may be the underlying cause of the protective effect.[429]

Hemoglobin Constitution

The cardinal finding in the common forms of heterozygous β thalassemia is an elevated level of HbA_2. In most of the larger series the HbA_2 levels ranged from 3.5% to 7% with a mean of approximately 5% (reviewed by Weatherall and Clegg[2]). By relating the percentage of HbA_2 to the MCH it is clear that this reflects an absolute increase in δ-chain production. Studies of patients with β thalassemia trait who are also heterozygous for δ-chain variants have shown that the increased output is both cis and trans to the β thalassemia gene.[430–433] The level of HbA_2 may be reduced in association with coexistent iron deficiency, but although it has been reported that it may fall into the normal range and is restored to its elevated level after iron therapy,[415,434] this must be unusual. What usually happens is that the level falls but it remains elevated in the β thalassemia trait range.[435]

In most large series the HbF level is elevated in approximately 50% of cases, in the range 1%–2%.[436] The distribution of HbF within the red cells, as judged either by acid elution or fluorescent antibody techniques, is heterogeneous.

In all the larger reported series of HbF levels a few individuals fall outside the distribution of normal to 2%–3%, and have values ranging between 4% and 15%. Knox-Macaulay et al.[351] showed that at least some of them have, in addition, determinants for heterocellular HPFH. In one family it was possible to demonstrate independent segregation of β thalassemia and HPFH genes. Similar families have been reported by Mazza et al.[408] Wood et al.,[437] and Thein and Weatherall.[357] It seems likely, therefore, that the majority of β thalassemia heterozygotes with unusually high levels of HbF carry one or more genes for heterocellular HPFH.

There is no evidence that acquired factors alter the level of HbF to any significant degree; the only one that has been adequately documented is pregnancy, during which the normal rise in HbF that occurs at midterm is mirrored in heterozygous β thalassemias by an increase at approximately the same time. It returns to its basal level some time toward the end of pregnancy.[438] The level of HbF is not modified by coexistent iron deficiency.[415]

Red Cell Metabolism

One of the characteristic changes of the red cells in β thalassemia heterozygotes is their decreased osmotic fragility, which in contrast to normal red cells, becomes even more marked after sterile incubation for 24 hours.[439] These altered osmotic properties have formed the basis for several population screening tests.

There have been a variety of studies of membrane function.[440–443] Using radioactive tracers it has been shown that there is an increased flux of K^+, an effect that is accentuated when the cells are incubated for 24 hours at 37°C. This increased permeability to K^+ appears to occur in cells of all ages, although it may be slightly more marked in younger cells. ATP levels are normal or slightly reduced, but on sterile incubation the red cells lose ATP more rapidly than normal; this can be reversed by glucose. It appears that heterozygous β thalassemic red cells can compensate for their increased cation loss by upregulating the transport-regulated component of glycolysis, and hence can maintain normal ATP levels, but when they are stressed by in vitro incubation this mechanism breaks down.

In some of the studies cited previously similar membrane function abnormalities were found in other hypochromic anemias such as iron deficiency. It is likely, therefore, that these abnormalities reflect an underhemoglobinized red cell as well as globin-chain imbalance. In favor of this concept is the observation that similar changes have been described in cells of α/β thalassemics in which there is minimal globin-chain imbalance.[444]

These observations suggest a possible mechanism for the further increase in osmotic resistance on sterile incubation of β thalassemic red cells. With successive loss of K^+ and water, and cellular dehydration, there must be a decrease in red cell volume and hence in osmotic activity. If glucose is added to the incubation this probably provides adequate energy for ATP regeneration and hence for maintaining the Na^+-K^+ pump to counteract excessive loss of K^+ and water from the cells. Further evidence that this is the case is derived from the observation that the increased osmotic resistance can be demonstrated, even in the presence of glucose, by inhibition of the Na^+-K^+ pumps by ouabain or ethacrynic acid.[442]

Globin-Chain Synthesis

In vitro hemoglobin synthesis studies indicate that α/β-globin-chain production ratios range from approximately 1.5–2.5, both in the bone marrow and in peripheral blood. Reports of more balanced globin-chain synthesis in the bone marrow[410,445,446] were later found to be based on artifacts produced by the presence of radioactively labeled nonglobin proteins that cochromatograph with β-globin chains.[447,448] Hence the measurement of globin-chain synthesis, particularly if peripheral blood reticulocytes are used, provides a valuable confirmatory test for heterozygosity for β thalassemia in cases in which the diagnosis is uncertain.

Developmental Changes in Hematological Findings and Hemoglobin Constitution

The changes in the red cells of infants heterozygous for β thalassemia over the first few months of life are of considerable importance with respect to the diagnosis of the condition over this period. Because of the alterations that occur both in the red cell indices and in the hemoglobin pattern of normal infants over the first year, studies that set out to describe these changes in β thalassemia heterozygotes must be carefully controlled with a population of normal infants at exactly the same stage of development. Data of this kind have been reported by Galanello et al.[449] and Wood et al.[450] Galanello et al.[451] have produced useful percentile curves for the red cell indices in β thalassemia heterozygotes in infancy and childhood. Further information on these changes is reported by Metaxatou-Mavromati et al.[452]

From these studies it is apparent that the hemoglobin values and red cell indices of heterozygous β thalassemic newborns do not differ significantly from normal. By the age of 3 months, however, clear differences emerge, which become highly significant by 6 months and remain so during the rest of development. It appears, therefore, that carrier screening by MCV or MCH determination is feasible from approximately 3 months onward. Similarly, there is clear distinction in HbA_2 values by 3 months. In all these studies it was observed that the rate of decline of HbF is retarded in β thalassemia heterozygotes and does not reach its adult level until well into childhood.

Phenotypic Characteristics in Relationship to Different Molecular Forms of β Thalassemia

Limited data have been published that relate the hematological findings and HbA_2 and F levels to particular mutations in β thalassemia heterozygotes.[325,453–455] Although there is some overlap, it is evident that the common, mild β thalassemia mutations, IVS-1-6 T→C, β-29 A→G, β-87 C→G, and β-88 T→G, for example, have slightly higher hemoglobin levels and, more important, higher MCH and MCV values than the more severe β^0 or β^+ thalassemia alleles. Other mild alleles for which sufficient data are available, including the forms of β thalassemia associated with Hbs E, Malay, and Knossos, are also associated with MCH and MCV values that are either normal or only slightly reduced. Indeed, the pattern that is emerging is of a continuous spectrum of hematological findings, ranging from the typical characteristics of β thalassemia trait associated with severe β^0 or β^+ thalassemia alleles, through milder changes associated with less severe alleles, to complete normality in the "silent" alleles. There are insufficient data to make it possible to be dogmatic about what is a "typical" set of red cell indices for a particular allele.

The HbA_2 levels in relationship to underlying mutations were reviewed by Huisman.[456] Overall, and although there is considerable overlap, several groups can be defined. Carriers of β^0 or severe β^+ thalassemia alleles have HbA_2 levels between 4.5% and 5.5%, whereas those with mild β^+ alleles have values between 3.6% and 4.2%. There are exceptions, however. Carriers of β-globin gene promoter mutations tend to have relatively high levels of HbA_2, even though these are mild β thalassemia alleles. The highest HbA_2 values in heterozygotes appear to be associated with deletional forms of β thalassemia (see later section and Chapter 16).

The relationship between the underlying mutation and HbF levels in β thalassemia heterozygotes has been reviewed by Kutlar et al.[457] These analyses are complicated by the presence or absence of the C→T polymorphism at $-158^G\gamma$, which is known to modify both the $^G\gamma/^A\gamma$ ratio of the HbF and, probably, its level under conditions of erythropoietic stress. It appears that β thalassemia heterozygotes with certain mutations, notably –88 (C→T), –29 (A→G), and IVS-1-1 (C→A), appear to have relatively higher levels of HbF that are independent of the C→T polymorphism at $-158^G\gamma$. Carriers of mutations such as IVS-1-6 (T→C), IVS-1-110 (G→A), codon 24 (T→A), codon 39 (C→T), and codons 41–42 (-TCTT) tend to fall into two groups, that is, with high $^G\gamma$ and low $^G\gamma$ varieties of HbF; neither is associated with high HbF values.

Association with Other Genetic Disorders

Because the heterozygous state for β thalassemia is so common, it is not surprising that it has been found in association with a variety of other genetic disorders.

In many populations glucose-6-phosphate dehydrogenase (G6PD) deficiency and β thalassemia are found at high frequencies and hence they are not infrequently encountered together in the same individual. This interaction was analyzed in Sardinia by Piomelli and Siniscalco.[458] The mean hemoglobin levels in hemizygous G6PD-deficient males was 14.1 g/dL, thalassemic males 13.6 g/dL, and males with both conditions 12.5 g/dL. The red cell indices in the thalassemic males were not altered by coexistent G6PD deficiency. In a later study Sanna et al.[459] found no interaction between the two traits.

Another common occurrence is the co-inheritance of the genetic determinant for Gilbert syndrome.[193,460] There is a polymorphic variation in the promoter of the bilirubin UDP-glucuronosyl transferase gene (UGT1A1); the particular motif is a $A(TA)_n$ TAA. Some individuals with Gilbert syndrome have an additional TA, that is, the arrangement $A(TA)_7TAA$ rather than the more usual $A(TA)_6TAA$. It has been found that the expanded variety of promoter polymorphism is found commonly in heterozygous β thalassemics with unusually high bilirubin levels. Interestingly, homozygosity for the $(TA)_7$ motif is not always associated with an elevated bilirubin in otherwise normal persons and hence it is likely that the increased production of bilirubin as a result of the ineffective erythropoiesis in β thalassemia heterozygotes is sufficient to cause unusually high blood levels.

Several families have been reported in which the genes for hereditary elliptocytosis (HE) and β thalassemia were segregating.[461–463] In these cases there did not seem to be any summation of the effects of the two disorders, although in the family reported by Perillie and Chernoff[464] there may have been some interaction. Similarly, there have been reports of the interaction of β thalassemia trait and hereditary spherocytosis (HS.[465–468] Although it has been reported to cause relatively severe hemolysis it is difficult to determine whether this is a true summation effect; HS is very variable in its expression even within members of the same family. Similarly, in the few reported instances of the coinheritance of β thalassemia and pyruvate kinase deficiency, the red cell enzyme deficiency has not had any deleterious effect on the phenotype of β thalassemia trait [469,470]

Variant Forms of Heterozygous β Thalassemia

The more unusual forms of heterozygous β thalassemia are summarized in Table 17.1. The most common and most important are the normal HbA_2-β thalassemias.

Normal HbA_2–β Thalassemia

Based on the hematological findings it has been useful to divide the normal HbA_2–β thalassemias into Type 1, in which there are minimal red cell abnormalities and in which the thalassemia allele is clinically "silent," and Type 2, in which the hematological changes are indistinguishable from those of heterozygous β thalassemia with an elevated level of HbA_2.[471]

"Silent" β Thalassemia *(Normal HbA_2–β thalassemia type 1).* As described by Schwartz[472] and discussed earlier in this chapter, the importance of the "silent" β thalassemias is that they can interact with more severe β thalassemia alleles to produce β thalassemia intermedia. Their molecular basis is described in Chapter 16 and the clinical consequences of their interaction with different β thalassemia alleles are summarized earlier in this chapter. There are no significant hematological abnormalities but on globin-chain synthesis analysis there is mild imbalance, with α/β-chain production ratios in the 1.2–1.3/1 range.

Normal HbA_2–β thalassemia type 2. This condition is heterogeneous. One of the most common causes is the compound heterozygous inheritance of both δ and β thalassemia.[473] A variety of different forms of δ^0 or δ^+ thalassemia mutations have been found, either in cis or trans to β thalassemia mutations, and in some cases β haplotypes containing β and δ thalassemia genes in *cis* have been disseminated throughout populations. For example, in the mild form of β thalassemia, Hb Knossos, carriers have minimal hematological changes and low levels of HbA_2. This phenotype results from a mild β^+ thalassemia mutation (β27 G→T) together with a deletion of an A in codon 59 of the δ gene in *cis*, which completely inactivates it.[335] The same δ^0 59 (-A) mutation has been found in *cis* to the β^0 39 and β^+ IVS-1-110 mutations in Mediterranean populations[474] and δ+27 (G→T) has been reported in both *cis* and *trans* to the β^+ IVS-2-745 mutation.[475,476] Although on average, the HbA_2 levels fall into the normal range, there is considerable scatter and in some cases values in the 3–3.7 range are observed.

Although the diagnosis of coexistent β and δ thalassemia is best made by analysis of the respective globin genes, some clues can be obtained from family studies. Where the two mutations exist in *cis*, the condition will be transmitted both vertically and laterally. On the other hand, if the two thalassemia mutations are in trans they will separate and individuals with both high HbA_2– and normal HbA_2–β thalassemia may be found in different generations.

When considering the differential diagnosis of normal HbA_2–β thalassemia, and if different forms of δ thalassemia have been excluded, it is important to remember that there are certain unusual phenocopies of this condition. For example, some forms of εγδβ thalassemia, which involve long deletions of the β-globin gene complex, are characterized by a picture that is indistinguishable from normal HbA_2–β thalassemia in heterozygotes. Similarly, the Corfu form of δβ thalassemia, in which a 7.2-kb deletion involves the δ gene but leaves the β gene intact is also associated with this phenotype. This is because the β gene in *cis* to this deletion carries an additional β thalassemia mutation.

Heterozygous β Thalassemia with Unusually High Levels of HbA_2 or HbF

There is a rare group of β thalassemias in which levels of HbA_2 in excess of 5%–6% are observed. They all seem to result from deletions of the β-globin gene, which remove its 5′ promoter region, including sequences from −125 to +78 relative to the CAP site; in each case the promoter boxes are lost (reviewed by Thein[355]). The HbA_2 levels associated with these β thalassemias may be as high as 8%–9% (see Chapter 16).

These deletion forms of β thalassemia are also associated with unusually high HbF levels in heterozygotes. The first variety to be described, which became known as the Dutch form of β thalassemia,[477] was found in a large kindred with 13 heterozygotes; their HbF levels ranged from 5.1% to 14.4% with a mean value of 8.3%. Similar values have been reported in heterozygotes for several other deletional forms of β thalassemia.

Isolated Elevated HbA_2 Levels: Heterozygous β Thalassemia with α Thalassemia and Related Conditions

Occasionally, during population screening or family studies, individuals are encountered who have elevated HbA_2 levels in the absence of the usual hematological findings of heterozygous β thalassemia. Because the coinheritance of α^+ or α^0 thalassemia with β thalassemia may result in normalization of the red cell indices and balanced globin-chain synthesis, leaving a raised HbA_2 as the sole abnormality, it seems likely that many of the reported cases of isolated HbA_2 elevation reflect these interactions.[478,479]

Several families have been described in which there were otherwise normal individuals with raised HbA_2 levels in whom detailed analyses of the α-, β-, and δ-globin genes showed no abnormalities.[480]

Heterozygous β Thalassemia with an Unusually Severe Clinical Course

There are two main mechanisms whereby heterozygous thalassemia may run a more severe course. First, there is the coinheritance of a chromosome containing additional α-globin genes, either ααα or αααα. The forms of β thalassemia intermedia associated with these genotypes were discussed earlier in this chapter. Second, there are the dominant β thalassemias, which result from mutations that give rise to products that are able to form inclusion bodies in the red cell precursors.[365,366] These conditions, which give rise to a wide spectrum of forms of β thalassemia intermedia of varying clinical severity, together with the underlying molecular mechanism, are described in Chapter 16.

β Thalassemia Unlinked to the β-Globin Gene Complex

Several families have been reported in which a form of β thalassemia trait appears to segregate independently from the β-globin gene complex.[481–484] Although subsequent analyses have shown some problems of interpretation in one of these families there seems little doubt from the study of Thein et al. that there is a form of phenotypically characteristic heterozygous β thalassemia that segregates independently of the β-globin genes. It seems likely that this reflects the action of a mutant *trans*-acting factor that is involved with β-globin gene regulation. The red cell indices, HbA_2 levels, and globin-chain synthesis findings are indistinguishable from the forms of β thalassemia trait associated with mutations in the β-globin genes.

Other β Thalassemias of Unknown Cause

Most laboratories that have sequenced large numbers of β-globin genes during their studies of families with the phenotype of β thalassemia have amassed varying numbers of cases in which no abnormality has been found. For example, Kazazian[485] reported that this was the case in nine of the 100 alleles that his laboratory had sequenced in detail. Because in many cases it has not been possible to conduct the kind of genetic studies required, it is quite possible that at least some of these undefined disorders reflect the type of unlinked forms of β thalassemia described previously.

The Problem of Borderline Red Cell Indices or HbA_2 Levels

In heterozygotes for very mild β thalassemia alleles, or those for severe alleles who have coinherited α thalassemia, the red cell indices may be almost normal. The usual levels of the MCH and MCV below which further study is advised, less than 27 pg and 80 fl, respectively, may miss these conditions in screening programs.

In clinical practice it is also not infrequent to encounter individuals with HbA_2 levels that appear to be very marginally raised, that is, in the 3%–3.5% range. These cases pose considerable diagnostic and counseling difficulties. What action should be taken? Probably the first thing to do is to repeat the estimation, but if similar values are obtained again, the finding cannot be ignored.

Galanello et al.[486] have analyzed 125 individuals with HbA_2 values in this range. In 37 cases they were able to detect an underlying molecular defect in the β-, δ-, or α-globin genes. Twenty-three were carriers of mild β-thalassemia alleles, 16 were compound heterozygotes for δ and β thalassemia, two had triplicated α-globin genes, and two had single α-globin gene deletions. The finding of this relatively high percentage of abnormalities, and the fact that many of them can interact with β thalassemia to produce severe phenotypes, suggests that in any screening program, particularly when an individual who has a borderline HbA_2 is planning to have a child with a partner with typical β thalassemia trait, it is important to investigate the cause for the marginally elevated HbA_2 level.

AVOIDANCE AND POPULATION CONTROL

Because of the changing demography of disease in many countries the thalassemias will be a major health problem in the new millennium.[1,2,487] As populations become richer, and standards of nutrition and public health improve, there is a fall in childhood mortality. Hence, an increasing number of babies with genetic diseases such as thalassemia will survive the early months of life and present for treatment. It is essential, therefore, that some form of program for the population control of these diseases is initiated.

It is beyond the scope of this chapter to deal with the complex ethical, economic, and organizational problems of establishing screening programs for the thalassemias. They must be backed up by adequate facilities for counseling and each individual society has to decide whether it wishes to try to reduce the frequency of births of children with serious forms of thalassemia by counseling and marital advice or by establishing a program of prenatal diagnosis. These complex issues are discussed in detail by Weatherall and Clegg[2] and Weatherall et al.[3] and the extensive experience gained from the successful population programs that have been carried out over the last 20 years in the Mediterranean island populations are reviewed by Cao et al.[488] The methods that are currently established for prenatal diagnosis of β thalassemia are described in Chapter 28 and Weatherall and Clegg.[2]

MANAGEMENT

Advances in the management of thalassemia major have greatly improved the prognosis for patients over recent years. Although bone marrow transplantation, for those with appropriate donors and in countries in which the facilities exist, now offers the possibility of curing the condition, the mainstays of treatment are still adequate transfusion, backed up with iron chelation therapy and the judicious use of splenectomy. Some of these topics are dealt with in detail in other chapters. Here we simply outline the principles of management. The broader population, social, and psychological aspects are reviewed elsewhere.[2]

It is very important before embarking on any form of treatment to establish the particular variety of β thalassemia and to obtain a full blood group genotype of the patient. It is also essential to assess the patient carefully over the first few months after the diagnosis is established and not to embark on a transfusion regimen too hastily. Many patients with intermediate forms of β thalassemia, who may not need regular transfusion, embark on a life of unnecessary treatment of this kind, particularly if they present with an unusually low hemoglobin level during a period of intercurrent infection. The important indications for transfusion are not the steady-state hemoglobin level, but the child's well-being, particularly with respect to activity, growth, development, and the early appearance of skeletal changes.

Transfusion and Splenectomy

Transfusion Regimens. Long-term transfusion programs form the cornerstone of treatment for most patients with thalassemia major[149] (see Chapter 29). Avoidance or reduction of the frequency of transfusions in an effort to ameliorate iron loading does not prevent this complication; when erythropoietic activity is increased more than fivefold, as it may be in severe thalassemia, the amount of iron absorbed surpasses iron loss, resulting in an increase in body iron.[489] The goals of transfusion, therefore, include not only correction of the anemia but also suppression of erythropoiesis and inhibition of increased gastrointestinal absorption of iron. Both "hypertransfusion" and "supertransfusion" regimens, in which pretransfusion hemoglobins are maintained above 10 and 12 g/dL, respectively, prevent most complications of anemia and ineffective erythropoiesis[490] but are associated with substantial iron loading. The maintenance of pretransfusion hemoglobin concentrations that did not exceed 9.5 g/dL were found to reduce transfusion requirements and body iron loading, as estimated by serum ferritin concentrations; in parallel, marrow activity did not increase more than threefold over normal, and a lower incidence of endocrine and cardiac complications was observed.[491]

Type of Red Cell Concentrates

Most centers still use washed or filtered red cells. Early clinical experience of the use of neocytes, young red blood cells separated from older cells by density centrifugation,[492] suggested that a modest extension of the transfusion interval could be achieved.[493] Later studies, which used a simpler method of preparation,[494] confirmed these findings.[495] A more recent report observed that the reduction in total annual transfusional iron load during neocyte transfusions varied widely: from less than 10% to greater than 25%[496] The cost–benefit relationship of neocyte transfusions is unclear; the benefits of reduced iron administration are offset by an up to fivefold increase in preparation expenses over those of standard concentrates.[497]

Further details of the practical aspects of transfusion therapy are discussed in Chapter 29 and by Weatherall and Clegg.[2]

Splenectomy

In the past, it was quite common to observe an increase in transfusion requirements at approximately the age of 10 years. In many cases it was apparent that this reflected the effects of hypersplenism (see Modell and Berdoukas[5]). More recent experience, however, suggests that many patients who have received adequate transfusion therapy from an early age do not show this phenomenon and hence splenectomy is now required less often.[15] Splenectomy has been recommended when transfusion requirements exceed 250 mL[498] or 200 mL packed cells/kg body weight.[14] Concerns that it may be associated with acceleration of iron loading in other organs[499,500] are not supported by one study that reported that the spleen is not a significant repository of transfused iron.[501] Because of the risk of infection, splenectomy should be delayed until the age of 5 years. Splenic embolization[502] and partial splenectomy[503,504] have been used to preserve splenic function, but an early response has often been followed by recurrence of hypersplenism, and these approaches are not generally recommended.

At least 6 weeks before splenectomy, patients should be vaccinated with pneumococcal, *Haemophilus influenzae* type B and meningococcal vaccines, and after surgery, daily prophylactic penicillin should be administered, at least during childhood and probably indefinitely. Erythromycin may be substituted for those who are allergic to penicillin. Antimalarials should be given to those traveling to countries in which malaria is endemic and to those who live in these regions.

Iron Chelation

Background. In the absence of iron chelating therapy, transfusional iron overload is progressive and ultimately fatal.[15] For many years, cardiac iron loading has been the leading cause of death in transfusion-dependent thalassemia patients and it is still observed at the present time. The beneficial effects of iron chelation therapy with the agent desferrioxamine mesylate on survival and the prevention of cardiac disease are reviewed earlier in this chapter. In short, two extensive studies reported the influence of effective long-term use of desferrioxamine mesylate on the prevention of cardiac disease,[66,232] findings that were later confirmed by a multicenter study in Italy.[68] As well as providing clear evidence of the efficacy of desferrioxamine in compliant patients these studies also provided evidence about the level of body iron that should be maintained to maintain transfusion-dependent thalassemic patients in good health.[15]

Assessment and Maintenance of Body Iron Levels

Methods for the assessment of body iron levels were discussed earlier in this chapter and are also summarized in Chapter 29. Data that have accumulated over the past 10 years permit a quantitative approach to the management of iron overload and provide guidelines for the control of body iron burden in chelated patients. Chelating therapy should not be aimed at maintenance of a normal body iron (~0.2–1.6 mg iron/g liver dry weight), as this greatly increases the probability of desferrioxamine toxicity.[505] By contrast, maintenance of hepatic iron concentrations exceeding 15 mg iron/g liver dry weight is associated with a greatly increased risk of cardiac disease and early death.[232] Slightly lower iron burdens (between ~7 and 15 mg iron/g liver dry weight) are associated with an increased risk of other complications of iron overload, including hepatic fibrosis, in homozygotes for hereditary hemochromatosis.[506,507]

It has been proposed therefore that a conservative goal for chelating therapy is the maintenance of hepatic storage iron concentrations of approximately 3–7 mg iron/g liver dry weight[15] in the range found in asymptomatic heterozygotes for hereditary hemochromatosis.[508] If measurement of hepatic iron by liver biopsy or MRI is not feasible, the serum ferritin provides an alternative but less reliable means of determining whether the body iron is within an optimal range. A serum ferritin level of 2,500 μg/L, maintained over a period of more than 10 years, may reflect a threshold of increased risk of cardiac disease and early death.[66] Recent studies using MRI approaches to the assessment of myocardial iron levels (reviewed by Pennell[61]) have suggested that there may not be a clear cut relationship between hepatic iron or serum ferritin levels and cardiac iron. The current status of these new approaches to the assessment of cardiac iron was discussed earlier in this chapter and is considered in more detail in Chapter 29. Until more is known about the clinical efficacy of this new technology, particularly from prospective studies, and given the overwhelming evidence for the prolonged survival of patients who are compliant to chelation therapy, it is essential that monitoring of transfusion-dependent patients continues to be carried out by assessment of body iron burden by hepatic MRI or direct iron measurements.

The initiation of desferrioxamine therapy. The adverse effects associated with desferrioxamine, and the balance between its effectiveness and toxicity, are reviewed by Olivieri and Brittenham.[15] It has been recommended that initiation of desferrioxamine should be guided by the concentration of hepatic iron, obtained by liver biopsy under ultrasound guidance, after approximately 1 year of regular transfusions. If a liver biopsy is not possible at the start of therapy, subcutaneous infusions of desferrioxamine, not exceeding 25–35 mg/kg/day, should be initiated after approximately 1 year of regular transfusions. Titration of hepatic iron, as above, should avert the potential toxic effects of desferrioxamine.[505] If the hepatic iron concentration is not regularly assessed, a "toxicity" index, defined as the mean daily dose of desferrioxamine (mg/kg) divided by the serum ferritin concentration (g/L) should be calculated for each patient every 6 months and should not exceed 0.025.[505] Doses of desferrioxamine should not usually exceed 50 mg/kg/day, and all patients should undergo regular examination for ophthalmological or auditory complications and abnormalities of growth (see Chapter 29).

Alternatives to subcutaneous infusions. Regimens of continuous ambulatory intravenous desferrioxamine infused through implantable subcutaneous ports, in which the infusion site cannot be manipulated by the patient, overcome the disadvantages of drug preparation and self-administration, eliminate the irritation associated with subcutaneous infusions, and improve compliance.[60] Because this system requires that the site be changed weekly by medical personnel at a clinic visit, it is not popular with many patients. Those unwilling to visit the clinic frequently, and those for whom standard pumps are unwieldy, may benefit from systems in which the desired concentrations of continuous subcutaneous or intravenous desferrioxamine can be infused using a lightweight, disposable, silent balloon infuser (Baxter) that produces continuous pressure without a battery or other mechanical device.[509,510]

Desferrioxamine "allergy". Reactions to desferrioxamine include acute inflammation, itching, and edema at the site of infusion, increasing in severity, to wheezing, tachypnea, tachycardia, hypotension, and coma. Although these reactions suggest an allergic mechanism, evidence supporting an immunological basis for this is lacking; direct, IgE-independent activation of dermal mast cells by desferrioxamine has been demonstrated.[511] These severe reactions may be effectively managed using rapid intravenous desensitization similar to protocols recommended for penicillin-allergic individuals,[512–514] followed by long-term, continuous, subcutaneous or intravenous infusion.

Rescue of patients with severe iron loading and organ damage. There is limited evidence that it is possible to improve both liver and cardiac function in patients who are heavily iron loaded and in whom there is evidence of defective organ function. These patients are best managed by the administration of desferrioxamine intravenously through implantable venous ports, although scrupulous attention has to be paid to the care of access sites. Because of the dangers of high-dose desferrioxamine administration it is recommended that the drug is given by continuous infusion at a dose of up to 50 mg/kg/day. Further details of this topic are reviewed by Davis and Porter[515] and Weatherall and Clegg.[2]

Orally active iron chelators. The expense and inconvenience of desferrioxamine, and problems with compliance, have led to a search for orally active iron chelators. The pharmacology and clinical experience with these agents is discussed in detail in Chapter 29. Here we summarize only particular issues of their use in patients with severe forms of thalassemia.

The most extensive experience has been obtained with deferiprone (L1). Although support for a long-term open label study and randomized trial of deferiprone and desferrioxamine was terminated prematurely by the corporate sponsor, follow-up of hepatic storage iron concentrations in both cohorts indicated that in approximately one-third of the deferiprone-treated patients the hepatic iron stabilized at, or increased concentrations that would have placed patients at risk for cardiac disease. Despite the fact that compliance was better in the deferiprone-treated group,[26,516,517] these findings, and subsequent studies[518] suggested that long-term therapy with deferiprone might not provide adequate control of body iron in a significant proportion of patients with thalassemia major.[519] The administration of deferiprone is also associated with a number of side effects including neutropenia, gastrointestinal upset, and painful arthritis; importantly, the latter seems to vary in frequency between different racial groups and has been reported as occurring in between 30% and 50% of patients on the Indian subcontinent, although in many cases the arthritis is transient in some there has been both clinical and radiological evidence of destructive joint disease.[520] The reasons why a proportion of patients do not maintain iron balance while receiving deferiprone, and why there are differences in the frequency of complications in different ethnic backgrounds remain unexplained (see Chapter 29).

Recent uncontrolled retrospective studies, or short-term prospective studies, have suggested that deferiprone might be more effective in reducing the level of cardiac iron loading than desferrioxamine.[521,522] Until the results of longer-term prospective controlled studies are available, the potential role for deferiprone, alone or combined with desferrioxamine in the management of cardiac iron loading, remains unclear.[523]

The more recently developed oral tridentate chelator, Deferasirox (ICL670, Exjade) has also shown promise in early clinical trials[524,525] (see Chapter 29). So far the effects on maintaining iron balance look promising and the side effects have been restricted to abdominal discomfort, rashes, and a mild increase in the creatinine level.

Clearly the current position regarding the place for the use of oral chelating agents compared with the well-proven gold standard of desferrioxamine remains uncertain. It is absolutely vital that new agents are subjected to long-term prospective controlled studies; the natural history of iron loading and its associated toxicity renders short-term observational studies completely inadequate. This is of particular importance with respect to the problem of thalassemia in developing countries in which the cost of any therapeutic agents is in competition with drugs required for the major communicable diseases. In these populations it is particularly difficult to monitor patients regularly for potential side effects and until the true place of these agents has been determined by adequate studies their widespread use in the developing world should be monitored with extreme caution.

Other novel oral chelating agents that are being developed are considered in Chapter 29.

Blood-Borne Infections

As discussed earlier, liver disease due to transfusion-transmitted viruses, hepatitis B, C, HIV, and malaria are now a major cause of morbidity and mortality in patients with β thalassemia. HBV infection is still the most important worldwide, while HCV is a major problem in Europe, North America, and Japan. Since the introduction of HIV donor screening, the risk of acquisition of HIV by transfusion has been greatly reduced in Europe and the United States. In patients becoming HIV seropositive the risk of progression to AIDS appears to be approximately 9% at 5 years. It is beyond our scope to discuss the treatment of HIV infections. Here we will focus on the management of HCV, because this is an important and increasing problem in patients with β thalassemia. The prevention and management of blood-borne malaria has been reviewed recently.[526]

Hepatitis C. Iron overload and infection with HCV are cofactors in the evolution of chronic liver disease, a common cause of death after age 15 years in thalassemia major.[51]

When recombinant α-interferon was the only effective therapy for chronic infection with HCV,[527] a study of the long-term efficacy of α-interferon in patients with thalassemia major[528] reported a complete response, defined as both sustained normalization of serum ALT and clearance of HCV-RNA from serum, in 40% of patients over a mean follow-up period of 3 years. The rate of relapse was much lower in thalassemic (18%) than in nonthalassemic individuals (50%). This suggested that in most patients with thalassemia, α-interferon should not be stopped after 3–6 months, but should be continued at least until the serum ALT level declines to normal. This and other studies[187,529] also highlighted the importance of compliance with desferrioxamine during α-interferon therapy. When it was found that responses to α-interferon were improved by its coadministration with ribavirin,[530,531] concerns were raised about the effect that the hemolytic complications of ribavirin administration might have on the anemia of thalassemic patients. Recent studies suggest that, although transfusion requirements may increase, it is possible to treat successfully thalassemic patients with interferon in combination with ribavirin although the results of more extensive trials are required to confirm the efficacy and safety of this type of regimen.[532]

Other infections. Although in the past infectious complications were a major problem in thalassemic children, this seems to be less common in those who are maintained on an adequate transfusion and chelation regimen. The one important exception is infections with the *Yersinia* genus of bacteria. The pathophysiology and clinical features were described in a previous section. Treatment with desferrioxamine should be stopped, stool cultures examined for *Yersinia* spp, and appropriate antibiotic treatment started, either an aminoglycoside or cotrimoxazole. The management of other infections in patients with thalassemia is reviewed by Vento et al.[167]

Bone and Endocrine Disease

The mechanisms of the reduction in bone density in β thalassemia were discussed earlier. It is recommended that bone densitometry, using dual-energy x-ray absorptiometry or in vivo neutron activation, is included in the evaluation of thalassemia patients to guide treatment.[533] Appropriate hormonal replacement therapy in hypogonadal patients, exercise programs, and the administration of elemental calcium and vitamin D may be of benefit. The value of bisphosphonates, calcitonin,[534] and fluoride remains to be determined.

Other endocrine disorders are discussed in detail earlier in this chapter. They should be managed by appropriate replacement therapy.

Bone Marrow Transplantation

Bone marrow transplantation is now an important option for transfusion-dependent patients with β thalassemia who have appropriate donors. This topic is discussed in full in Chapter 32.

Thalassemia Intermedia

Patients who are growing and developing adequately without transfusion, and who fall into the β thalassemia intermedia category, should be maintained on folate supplementation and have regular assessment of their iron status, with appropriate chelation therapy if there is evidence of iron loading. In the face of a falling hemoglobin level and progressive splenomegaly, splenectomy may be indicated, although the results are unpredictable. Symptomatic extramedullary hematopoietic masses have been treated successfully with various combinations of hypertransfusion, x-ray therapy and the administration of hydroxyurea.[2,535]

Other issues relating to the management of the complications of thalassemia intermedia are discussed in detail by Weatherall and Clegg.[2]

Experimental Therapies

As well as work directed toward the development of new chelating agents (Chapter 28) the major areas of research toward improvements in the management of the thalassemias include attempts to increase the level of fetal hemoglobin production (Chapter 30), the development of noninvasive approaches for prenatal diagnosis (Chapter 32) and the application of somatic gene therapy (Chapter 33). Other approaches at the molecular level, including the use of RNA interference technology, homologous recombination and therapeutic cloning, antisense messenger RNA and others, have been reviewed recently.[536]

Global Health Issues

Although the β thalassemias and different interactions are of increasing importance in richer countries, their major public health impact is in the poorer countries of the Middle East, the Indian subcontinent, and south and east Asia. It is beyond the scope of this Chapter to discuss the economic aspects of the control and management of the thalassemias, particularly in the developing countries. These issues, together with some recommendations for the future control of these conditions in the developing world have been summarized recently.[3]

It should be remembered that any form of treatment and particularly pharmacological approaches, are in direct competition with the costs of managing the major killers in the developing countries, notably AIDS, malaria, and tuberculosis. Hence, in assessing therapy for thalassemia in these countries, the "better than nothing" approach to drug therapy is simply not possible; treatment has to be of genuine proven value if it is to compete with some of the costs of the major killers in these countries.

Because research into more effective management or cure of the thalassemias is still at an early stage, and even if some of it comes to fruition it is likely to be extremely expensive, the more conservative approaches to the prevention and management of the β thalassemias outlined in this chapter are likely to be the major approach that is possible in many countries of the world for the foreseeable future. Given the heavy pressures on healthcare provision in the developing world it is absolutely critical that the richer countries take every opportunity to fully confirm the efficacy of any new forms of investigation or treatment, even if they appear to be cost-effective, before they are introduced into the developing countries.

FORMS OF THALASSEMIA RELATED TO β THALASSEMIA

There are several forms of thalassemia or thalassemia-like disorders that are related to the β thalassemias. They include the δβ, εγδβ and δ thalassemias and hereditary persistence of fetal hemoglobin (HPFH). The molecular basis and hemoglobin constitution of these conditions are described in detail in Chapter 16 and original references to their clinical manifestations are given in detail in Weatherall and Clegg.[2] Here, their major clinical manifestations are summarized briefly.

The δβ Thalassemias

The δβ thalassemias are subdivided into the $(\delta\beta)^+$, $(\delta\beta)^0$, and $(^A\gamma\delta\beta)^0$ thalassemias. There is considerable clinical variation associated with these different conditions and their various interactions with structural hemoglobin variants.

$(\delta\beta)^+$ Thalassemia

These disorders are also known as the hemoglobin Lepore thalassemias because they are associated with the production of δβ fusion variants. Over 20 individuals have been reported as being homozygous for different molecular forms of Hb Lepore. Despite the fact that they synthesize no normal β or δ chains these patients have a remarkably diverse series of clinical phenotypes, ranging from conditions that are very similar to the homozygous state for β^0 thalassemia to relatively mild forms of β thalassemia intermedia.[2] Many of the reports of these patients did not include studies to search for ameliorating factors such as the coexistence of α thalassemia or heterocellular HPFH and where these factors had been looked for, and excluded, the phenotype has usually been similar to the homozygous state for β^0 thalassemia.[537]

The heterozygous states for the Hb Lepore thalassemias are symptomless and the hematological changes are similar to those of heterozygous β thalassemia except that the level of HbF is significantly higher. There is an extensive literature on the interaction of this condition with the β and $(\delta\beta)^0$ thalassemias.[2] These conditions also show remarkable clinical diversity which, in the case of the β thalassemia interactions, seems to depend mainly on whether they are between β^0 or β^+ thalassemias; in the former case the phenotype is of severe β thalassemia major, whereas in the latter the phenotype is in the more severe spectrum of β thalassemia intermedia.[538] Compound heterozygosity for hemoglobin Lepore and $(\delta\beta)^0$ thalassemia also produces the phenotype of thalassemia intermedia. The hemoglobin Lepore thalassemias have also been found in compound heterozygotes for Hbs S, C, and E. Here again, the clinical phenotypes have been extremely variable but, overall, resemble those of Hbs S, C or E–β thalassemia (see Chapters 18, 19, and 21). Except when coinherited with other hemoglobin variants or β thalassemia, the anti-Lepore hemoglobins are not associated with any clinical abnormalities. The rare interactions between the anti-Lepore hemoglobins and β thalassemia have been associated with very mild forms of β thalassemia intermedia.

$(\delta\beta)^0$ and $(^A\gamma\delta\beta)^0$ Thalassemia

The homozygous states for these conditions, that are associated with 100% HbF production, usually result in the phenotype of a variable form of β thalassemia intermedia with hemoglobin values in the 7–9 g/dL range. Compound heterozygotes for these conditions and β thalassemia are also characterized by β thalassemia intermedia of widely varying severity; those with $(^A\gamma\delta\beta)^0$ thalassemia seem to be at the more severe end of the spectrum of this phenotype.

The $(\delta\beta)^0$ thalassemias have been observed in the compound heterozygous state with a variety of hemoglobin variants, including Hbs S, C, and E. The combination with HbS produces a relatively mild sickling disorder and in some cases there has been no history of sickle cell crises. Again, however, there is considerable heterogeneity and at least one family has been reported in which children with sickle cell $(^A\gamma\delta\beta)^0$ had a condition which was similar to sickle cell disease.[539] From the limited amount of data it appears that HbC–$(\delta\beta)^0$ thalassemia is a milder condition than HbC disease or HbC–β^0 thalassemia. Similar, HbE–$(\delta\beta)^0$ thalassemia is characterized by a very mild phenotype, which is significantly less severe than HbE–β thalassemia.

Finally, the phenocopies of δβ thalassemia that arise from the acquisition of two different mutations in the β-globin gene cluster that involve the γ gene promoters, the β genes or the δ genes, Sardinian δβ thalassemia and Corfu δβ thalassemia for example,[540,541] behave clinically in the same way as the other forms of δβ thalassemia.

δ Thalassemia

Although the δ thalassemias are clinically and hematologically silent, they may cause problems for genetic counseling. They may occur in *cis* or *trans* to a β thalassemia mutation, and produce the hematological phenotype of normal Hb A_2–β thalassemia trait. Although the gene frequencies have not been determined it appears that δ thalassemia may occur in *trans* with a variety of different β thalassemia mutations in the Mediterranean population.[542]

$(\varepsilon\gamma\delta\beta)^0$ Thalassemia

This rare condition is characterized by a complete absence of output from the β globin gene cluster and therefore, in the homozygous state, would not be compatible with survival. Although this disorder results from two distinct forms of molecular pathology (see Chapter 16), the clinical features in heterozygotes are similar although remarkably variable even within the same family. In newborn babies there is a moderate degree of anemia, with hemoglobin values in the 7–10 g/dL range. As these patients get older the anemia becomes less severe and in adult life the disorder behaves like the heterozygous state for normal Hb A_2–β thalassemia trait. But the clinical variability after birth is quite remarkable. In some patients there is pallor, jaundice and splenomegaly whereas others, in the same family, may go through completely uneventful postnatal periods. The reasons for this clinical diversity have not been determined.[2,543]

Hereditary Persistence of Fetal Hemoglobin

A classification together with the molecular pathology of these conditions is described in Chapter 16. Overall, they fall into two main groups depending on whether they result from deletions or point mutations. They are further classified into whether the distribution of HbF in the red cells is pancellular or heterocellular. Their clinical importance is related mainly to their interaction and modifying effect on other β-globin disorders.

$(\delta\beta)^0$ Hereditary Persistence of Fetal Hemoglobin

These conditions have been observed in the homozygous state and in the heterozygous state, either alone or in combination with other disorders of β globin.

There have been a number of detailed descriptions of the homozygous state for $(\delta\beta)^0$ thalassemia including the underlying pathophysiological mechanisms.[2,544] These individuals have no clinical disability or abnormal physical signs. The characteristic hematological finding is a moderately elevated red cell count, probably reflecting a low P_{50} due to the very high level of HbF. The hemoglobin levels are normal or slightly elevated and the red cell indices show moderately reduced MCV and MCH values. These findings, with biosynthetic studies showing a mild defect in non-α-chain synthesis, indicate that HbF production is not quite sufficient to compensate for an absence of β-chain production and hence the phenotype of β thalassemia trait. Heterozygotes, apart from an increased level of HbF and a slightly reduced MCV, show no hematological abnormalities. They have significantly reduced HbA_2 levels.

There are extensive data on the clinical and hematological changes in compound heterozygotes for $(\delta\beta)^0$ HPFH and HbS. These individuals are not anemic and have very few episodes suggestive of sickle cell crises, although occasional mild bone or joint pains have been reported. Splenomegaly has not been a regular feature of this condition in the US, although it has been observed in approximately 40% of cases in West Africa. There have been occasional reports of aseptic necrosis of the femoral heads. Clearly, the uniform distribution of approximately 25% HbF in the red cells of these patients protects them from most of the deleterious effects of the sickle cell gene. Compound heterozygotes for $(\delta\beta)^0$ HPFH and HbC are usually symptomless and show normal or slightly reduced hemoglobin levels with minimal reticulocytosis. A small proportion of patients show mild splenomegaly. Compound heterozygotes with HbE also have an extremely mild phenotype with no anemia or other hematological changes. Compound heterozygotes with β thalassemia are also very mildly affected, if at all. Their hemoglobin levels are similar to those of heterozygous β thalassemia, as are the red cell indices, and splenomegaly is extremely rare. There have been occasional exceptions however. For example in one well-documented family that described the interaction of the Indian form of $(\delta\beta)^0$ HPFH, or HPFH 3, the three affected children had a relatively severe form of thalassemia intermedia with hemoglobin values in the 5–9 g/dL range.[545] Presumably these cases reflect the inability of the level of HbF to compensate for defective β-globin production.

Nondeletional HPFH

As described in Chapter 16 these heterogeneous conditions are divided into those in which there is a mutation in either the $^G\gamma$- or $^A\gamma$-gene promoters, and a group of conditions that are characterized by persistently low levels of HbF that is heterogeneously distributed among the red cells. As a group, they have very little clinical implication except for their interactions with other β-globin gene abnormalities.

$^G\gamma\beta^+$ HPFH results from a number of different mutations at the $^G\gamma$ locus. It has only been observed in the homozygous form in Tunisian $^G\gamma\beta^+$ HPFH. These individuals have approximately 50% HbF but are clinically and hematologically completely normal. Many different varieties have been found in the heterozygous state but in no case has there been any hematological abnormalities. Similarly, in the compound heterozygous state with HbS or β^0 thalassemia there have been no clinical or hematological changes; in the latter interaction the patient had a hemoglobin level of 13.1 g/dL and red cell indices typical of β thalassemia trait, although the HbF level was 64%.

The $^A\gamma\beta^+$ forms of HPFH, also heterogeneous at the molecular level, have also been observed in the homozygous and heterozygous states, either alone or in combination with β thalassemia or structural hemoglobin variants. The homozygous state was identified in the Greek form. These individuals showed no clinical abnormalities and were not anemic although at least in one case there was a slightly reduced MCV and MCH. The HbF value was approximately 24% which is twice that found in heterozygotes for this particular mutation. There are no clinical or hematological abnormalities in the heterozygotes. In compound heterozygotes with β thalassemia there appears to be no clinical disability although there is usually pallor, icterus and splenomegaly. There is mild anemia with hemoglobin values in the 9–11 g/dL range and the red cells show typical thalassemic red cell indices. Fetal hemoglobin levels range from 25%–45%. Similarly, in homozygotes for the British form of $^{A}\gamma\beta^{+}$ HPFH both homozygotes and heterozygotes show no clinical or hematological abnormality. The compound heterozygous states for Black $^{A}\gamma\beta^{+}$ HPFH together with HbS or HbC are also associated with no significant clinical or hematological changes.

Heterocellular HPFH

Heterocellular HPFH is undoubtedly a heterogeneous condition in which there are relatively low levels of persistent HbF production distributed in a heterogeneous fashion among the red cells. Although genetic linkage studies have shown that this condition is quite heterogeneous at the molecular level, none of the genes involved have been identified with certainty. Heterozygotes have approximately 5%–10% HbF heterogeneously distributed among their red cells with no associated clinical or hematological abnormalities. It is clear, however, that the coinheritance of this condition with β thalassemia or the sickle cell genes can modify the phenotypes of their associated diseases quite considerably by increasing the output of HbF.[2] They are usually ascertained when one or other heterozygous parent of a patient with these disorders has an unusually high level of HbF; an extended family study may demonstrate other normal individuals with an elevated HbF. It is important, therefore, to carefully measure the level of HbF in heterozygous members of families in which there are patients with either β thalassemia intermedia or sickle cell anemia with unusually mild features.

The Diagnostic Value of the Cellular Distribution of Hemoglobin F in δβ Thalassemia and HPFH

In $(\delta\beta)^{0}$, $^{G}\gamma\beta^{+}$ and $^{A}\gamma\beta^{+}$ HPFH HbF is uniformly distributed among the red cells. There is one exception. In the British form of $^{A}\gamma\beta^{+}$ HPFH HbF is quite heterogeneously distributed, both in homozygotes and heterozygotes.[2] In all these conditions the red cell indices are normal.

In the δβ thalassemias and heterocellular HPFH the HbF is heterogeneously distributed. They can be distinguished by the higher levels of HbF (greater than 10% in heterozygotes) and reduced MCH and MCV in δβ thalassemia. In heterocellular HPFH the HbF level rarely exceeds 5% and the red cell indices are normal.

REFERENCES

1. Weatherall DJ, Clegg JB. Inherited haemoglobin disorders: an increasing global health problem. *Bull WHO.* 2001;79:704–712.
2. Weatherall DJ, Clegg JB. *The Thalassaemia Syndromes.* 4th ed. Oxford: Blackwell Science; 2001.
3. Weatherall DJ, Akinyanju O, Fucharoen S, Olivieri NF, Musgrove P. Inherited disorders of hemoglobin. In: Jamison DT, Breman JG, Measham AR, et al, eds. *Disease Control Priorities in Developing Countries.* New York, Washington: Oxford University Press and the World Bank; 2006:663–680.
4. Kattamis C, Ladis V, Metaxatou-Mavromati A. Hemoglobins F and A2 in Greek patients with homozygous β and β/δβ thalassemia. In: Schmidt RM, ed. *Abnormal Haemoglobins and Thalassaemia: Diagnostic Aspects.* New York: Academic Press; 1975:209–228.
5. Modell CB, Berdoukas VA. *The Clinical Approach to Thalassaemia.* New York: Grune and Stratton; 1984.
6. Cao A. Diagnosis of β-thalassemia intermedia at presentation. *Birth Defects: Origin Artic Series.* 1988;23:219–226.
7. Baker DH. Roentgen manifestations of Cooley's anemia. *Ann NY Acad Sci.* 1964;119:641–661.
8. Cammisa M, Sabella G. Clinico-radiological considerations on the pathogenesis of bone changes in thalassemia major. *Nunt Radiol.* 1967;33:77–101.
9. Middlemis JH, Raper AB. Skeletal changes in the haemogobinopathies. *J Bone Joint Surg.* 1966;48:693.
10. Michelson J, Cohen A. Incidence and treatment of fractures in thalassemia. *J Orthop Trauma.* 1988;2:29–32.
11. Modell CB. Management of thalassaemia major. *Br Med Bull.* 1976;32:270–276.
12. O'Brien RT, Pearson HA, Spencer RP. Transfusion-induced decrease in spleen size in thalassemia major: documentation by radioisotope scan. *J Pediatr.* 1972;81:105–107.
13. Modell CB. Total management in thalassaemia major. *Arch Dis Child.* 1977;52:489–500.
14. Cohen A, Gayer E, Mizanin J. Long-term effect of splenectomy on transfusion requirements in thalassemia major. *Am J Hematol.* 1989;30:254–256.
15. Olivieri NF, Brittenham GM. Iron-chelating therapy and the treatment of thalassemia. *Blood.* 1997;89:739–761.
16. Blendis LM, Modell CB, Bowdler AJ, Williams R. Some effects of splenectomy in thalassaemia major. *Br J Haematol.* 1974;28:77–87.
17. Lichtman HC, Watson RJ, Feldman F, Ginsberg V, Robinson J. Studies on thalassemia. I. An extracorpuscular defect in thalassemia major. II. The effects of splenectomy in thalassemia major with an associated acquired hemolytic anemia. *J Clin Invest.* 1953;32:1229–1235.
18. Reemsta K, Elliot RH. Splenectomy in Mediterranean anemia: an evaluation of long-term results. *Ann Surg.* 1956;144:999–1007.
19. Smith CH, Schulman I, Ando RE, Stern G. Studies in Mediterranean (Cooley's) anemia. I. Clinical and hematologic aspects of splenectomy with special reference to fetal hemoglobin synthesis. *Blood.* 1955;10:582–599.
20. Whipple GH, Bradford WL. Mediterranean disease-thalassemia (erythroblastic anemia of Cooley); associated pigment abnormnalities simulating hemochromatosis. *J Pediatr.* 1936;9:279–311.
21. Letsky EA, Miller F, Worwood M, Flynn DM. Serum ferritin in children with thalassaemia regularly transfused. *J Clin Pathol.* 1974;27:652–655.
22. Pippard MJ, Callender ST, Weatherall DJ. Intensive iron-chelation therapy with desferrioxamine in iron loading patients. *Clin Sci Mol Med.* 1978;54:99–106.
23. Worwood M, Cragg SJ, McLaren C, Ricketts C, Economidou J. Binding of serum ferritin to concanavalia A: patients with

homozygous β thalassaemia and transfusional iron overload. *Br J Haematol.* 1980;46:409–416.

24. Baynes R, Bezwoda W, Bothwell T, Khan Q, Mansoor N. The non-immune inflammatory response: serial changes in plasma iron, iron-binding capacity, lactoferrin, ferritin and C-reactive protein. *Scand J Clin Lab Invest.* 1986;46:695–704.
25. Roeser HP, Halliday JW, Sizemore DEA. Serum ferritin in ascorbic acid deficiency. *Br J Haematol.* 1980;45:457–466.
26. Olivieri NF, Brittenham GM, Matsui D, et al. Iron-chelation therapy with oral deferiprone in patients with thalassemia major. *N Engl J Med.* 1995;332:918–922.
27. St Pierre TG, Clark PR, Chua-Anusorn W. Measurement and mapping of liver iron concentrations using magnetic resonance imaging. *Ann NY Acad Sci.* 2005;1054:379–385.
28. Engle MA. Cardiac involvement in Cooley's anemia. *Ann NY Acad Sci.* 1964;119:694–702.
29. Kremastinos DT, Tiniakos G, Theodorakis GN, Katritsis DG, Toutouzas PK. Myocarditis in beta-thalassemia major. A cause of heart failure. *Circulation.* 1996;91:66–71.
30. Grisaru D, Rachmilewitz EA, Mosseri M, et al. Cardiopulmonary assessment in beta-thalassemia major. *Chest.* 1990;98:1138–1142.
31. Wasi P, Fucharoen S, Younghchaiyud P, Sonakul D. Hypoxemia in thalassemia. *Birth Defects: Origin Artic Series.* 1982;18:213–217.
32. Hoeper MM, Niedermeyer J, Hoffmeyer F, Flemming P, Fabel H. Pulmonary hypertension after splenectomy. *Ann Intern Med.* 1999;130:506–509.
33. Smith CH, Erlandson ME, Stern G, Scholman I. The role of splenectomy in the management of thalassemia. *Blood.* 1960;15:197–211.
34. Orsini A, Louchet E, Raybaud C, Brusquet Y, Perrimond H. Les pericardites de la maladie de Cooley. *Pediatrie.* 1970;15:831–842.
35. Wasi P. Adverse effects of splenectomy. *J Med Assoc Thailand.* 1972;55:1.
36. Arnett EN, Nienhuis AW, Henry WL, Ferrans VJ, Redwood DR, Roberts WC. Massive myocardial hemosiderosis: a structure-function conference at the National Heart and Lung Institute. *Am Heart J.* 1975;90:777–787.
37. Buja LM, Roberts WC. Iron in the heart: etiology and clinical significance. *Am J Med.* 1971;51:209–221.
38. Schellhammer PF, Engle MA, Hagstrom JWC. Histochemical studies of the myocardium and conduction system in acquired iron-storage disease. *Circulation.* 1967;35:631–637.
39. Howell J, Wyatt JP. Development of pigmentary cirrhosis in Cooley's anaemia. *Arch Pathol.* 1953;55:423–431.
40. Witzleben CL, Wyatt JP. The effect of long-survival on the pathology of thalassaemia major. *J Pathol Bacteriol.* 1961;82:1–12.
41. Lombardo T, Tamburino C, Bartoloni G, et al. Cardiac iron overload in thalassemic patients: an endomyocardial biopsy study. *Ann Hematol.* 1995;71:135–141.
42. Short EM, Winkle RA, Billingham ME. Myocardial involvement in idiopathic hemochromatosis. Morphologic and clinical improvement following venisection. *Am J Med.* 1981;70:1275–1279.
43. Spirito P, Lupi G, Melevendi C, Vecchio C. Restrictive diastolic abnormalities identified by Doppler echocardiography in patients with thalassemia major. *Circulation.* 1990;82:88–94.
44. Liu P, Olivieri N. Iron overload cardiomyopathies: new insights into an old disease. *Cardiovasc Drugs Ther.* 1994;8:101–110.
45. Hershko C, Konijn AM, Link G. Iron chelators for thalassaemia. *Br J Haematol.* 1998;101:399–406.
46. Link G, Pinson A, Hershko C. The ability of orally effective iron chelators dimethyl- and diethyl-hydroxypyrid-4-one and of deferoxamine to restore sarcolemmal thiolic enzyme activity in iron-loaded heart cells. *Blood.* 1994;83:2692–2697.
47. Link G, Tirosh R, Pinson A, Hershko C. Role of iron in the potentiation of anthracycline toxicity: identification of heart cell mitochondria as the site of iron-anthracycline interaction. *J Lab Clin Med.* 1996;127:272–278.
48. Hershko C, Link G, Cabantchik I. Pathophysiology of iron overload. *Ann NY Acad Sci.* 1998;850:191–201.
49. Wood JC, Enriquez C, Ghugre N, et al. Physiology and pathophysiology of iron cardiomyopathy in thalassemia. *Ann NY Acad Sci.* 2005;1054:386–395.
50. Ehlers KH, Levin AR, Markenson AL, et al. Longitudinal study of cardiac function in thalassemia major. *Ann NY Acad Sci.* 1980;344:397–404.
51. Zurlo MF, De Stefano P, Borgna-Pignatti C, et al. Survival and causes of death in thalassaemia major. *Lancet.* 1989;ii:27–30.
52. Jessup M, Manno CS. Diagnosis and management of iron-induced heart disease in Cooley's anemia. *Ann NY Acad Sci.* 1998;850:242–250.
53. Fitchett DH, Coltart DJ, Littler WA, et al. Cardiac involvement in secondary haemochromatosis: a catheter biopsy study and analysis of myocardium. *Cardiovas Res.* 1980;14:719–724.
54. Qureshi N, Avasarala K, Foote D, Vichinsky EP. Utility of Holter electrocardiogram in iron-overloaded hemoglobinopathies. *Ann NY Acad Sci.* 2005;1054:476–480.
55. Bahl VK, Malhotra OP, Kumar D, et al. Noninvasive assessment of systolic and diastolic left ventricular function in patients with chronic severe anemia: a combined M-mode, two-dimensional, and Doppler echocardiographic study. *Am Heart J.* 1992;124:1516–1523.
56. Henry WL, Nienhuis AW, Wiener M, Miller DR, Canale VC, Piomelli S. Echocardiographic abnormalities in patients with transfusion-dependent anemia and secondary myocardial iron deposition. *Am J Med.* 1978;64:547–555.
57. Lattanzi F, Bellotti P, Picano E, et al. Quantitative ultrasonic analysis of myocardium in patients with thalassemia major and iron overload. *Circulation.* 1993;87:748–754.
58. Davis BA, O'Sullivan C, Jarritt PH, Porter JB. Value of sequential monitoring of left ventricular ejection fraction in the management of thalassemia major. *Blood.* 2004;104(1):263–269.
59. Liu P, Henkelman M, Joshi J, et al. Quantitation of cardiac and tissue iron by nuclear magnetic resonance in a novel murine thalassemia-cardiac iron overload model. *Can J Cardiol.* 1996;12:155–164.
60. Olivieri NF, Berriman AM, Davis SA, Tyler BJ, Ingram J, Francombe WH. Continuous intravenous administration of deferoxamine in adults with severe iron overload. *Am J Hematol.* 1992;41:61–63.

61. Pennell DJ. T2* magnetic resonance and myocardial iron in thalassemia. *Ann NY Acad Sci.* 2005;1054:373–378.
62. Anderson LJ, Holden S, Davis B, et al. Cardiovascular T2-star (T2*) magnetic resonance for the early diagnosis of myocardial iron overload. *Eur Heart J.* 2001;22(23):2171–2179.
63. Westwood MA, Anderson LJ, Tanner MA, Pennell DJ. The relationship between myocardial iron deposition and left ventricular dysfunction in thalassemia using cardiovascular magnetic resonance. *J Cardiovasc Magn Reson.* 2005;7:46–47.
64. Derchi G, Bellone P, Forni GL, et al. Cardiac involvement in thalassaemia major: altered atrial natriuretic peptide levels in asymptomatic patients. *Eur Heart J.* 1992;13:1368–1372.
65. Economou-Petersen E, Aessopos A, Kladi A, et al. Apolipoprotein E epsilon4 allele as a genetic risk factor for left ventricular failure in homozygous beta-thalassemia. *Blood.* 1998;92:3455–3459.
66. Olivieri NF, Nathan DG, MacMillan JH, et al. Survival of medically treated patients with homozygous β thalassemia. *N Engl J Med.* 1994;331:574–578.
67. Brittenham GM. Disorders of iron metabolism: deficiency and overload. In: Hoffman R, Benz EJ, Shattil SJ, Furie B, Cohen HJ, Silberstein LE, eds. *Hematology: Basic Principles and Practice.* New York: Churchill Livingstone; 1994:492–523.
68. Borgna-Pignatti C, Rugolotto S, De Stefano P, et al. Survival and complications in patients with thalassemia major treated with transfusion and deferoxamine. *Haematologica.* 2004;89(10):1187–1193.
69. Hoyt RW, Scarpa N, Wilmott RW, Cohen A, Schwartz E. Pulmonary function abnormalities in homozygous β-thalassemia. *J Pediatr.* 1986;109:452–455.
70. Keens TG, O'Neal MH, Ortega JA, Hyman CB, Platzker ACG. Pulmonary function abnormalities in thalassemia patients on a hypertransfusion program. *Pediatrics.* 1980;65:1013–1017.
71. Santamaria F, Villa MP, Werner B, Cutrera R, Barreto M, Ronchetti R. The effect of transfusion on pulmonary function in patients with thalassemia major. *Pediatr Pulmonol.* 1994;18:139–143.
72. Bacalo A, Kivity S, Heno N, Greif J, Topilsky M. Blood transfusion and lung function in children with thalassemia major. *Chest.* 1992;101:362–370.
73. Cooper DM, Mansell AL, Weiner MA, et al. Low lung capacity and hypoxemia in children with thalassemia. *Am Rev Respir Dis.* 1980;121:639–646.
74. Factor JM, Pottipati SR, Rappaport I, Rosner IK, Lesser ML, Giardini PJ. Pulmonary function abnormalities in thalassemia major and the role of iron overload. *Am J Respir Crit Care Med.* 1994;149:1570–1574.
75. Grant GP, Graziano Jh, Seaman C, Mansell AL. Cardiorespiratory response to exercise in patients with thalassemia major. *Am Rev Respir Dis.* 1987;136:92–97.
76. Sonakul D, Pacharee P, Thakerngpol K. Pathologic findings in 76 autopsy cases of thalassemia. *Birth Defects: Origin Artic Series.* 1988;23:157–176.
77. Sonakul D, Suwananagool P, Sirivaidyapong P, Fucharoen S. Distribution of pulmonary thromboembolic lesions in thalassemic patients. *Birth Defects: Origin Artic Series.* 1988; 23:375–384.
78. Koren A, Garty I, Antonelli D, Katzuni E. Right ventricular cardiac dysfunction in β-thalassemia major. *Am J Dis Child.* 1987;141:93–96.
79. Tai DYH, Wang YT, Lou J, Wang WY, Mak Kh, Cheng HK. Lungs in thalassaemia major parients receiving regular transfusion. *Eur Respir.* 1996;9:1389–1394.
80. Aessopos A, Farmakis D. Pulmonary hypertension in beta-thalassemia. *Ann NY Acad Sci.* 2005;1054:342–349.
81. Michaeli J, Mittelman M, Grisaru D, Rachmilewitz EA. Thromboembolic complications in beta thalassemiua major. *Acta Haematol.* 1992;87:71–74.
82. Borgna-Pignatti C, Carneli V, Caruso V, et al. Thromboembolic events in beta thalassemia major: an Italian multicenter study. *Acta Haematol.* 1998;99:76–79.
83. Cappellini MD, Grespi E, Cassinerio E, Bignamini D, Fiorelli G. Coagulation and splenectomy: an overview. *Ann NY Acad Sci.* 2005;1054:317–324.
84. Barker JE, Wandersee NJ. Thrombosis in heritable hemolytic disorders. *Curr Opin Hematol.* 1999;6:71–75.
85. Giordano P, Galli M, Del Vecchio GC, et al. Lupus anticoagulant, anticardiolipin antibodies and hepatitis C virus infection in thalassaemia. *Br J Haematol.* 1998;102:903–906.
86. De Sanctis V, Katz M, Vullo C, Bagni B, Ughi M, Wonke B. Effect of different treatment regimes on linear growth and final height in β-thalassaemia major. *Clin Endocrinol.* 1994;40:791–798.
87. Modell CB, Beck J. Long-term desferrioxamine therapy in thalassemia. *Ann NY Acad Sci.* 1974;232:201–210.
88. Borgna-Pignatti C, de Stafano P, Zonta L, et al. Growth and sexual maturation in thalassemia major. *J Pediatr.* 1985;106:150–155.
89. Kattamis C, iakopoulou T, Kattamis A. Growth and development in children with thalassaemia major. *Acta Paediatr Scand.* 1990;366:111.
90. Costin G, Kogut MD, Hyman CB, Ortega JA. Endocrine abnormalities in thalassemia major. *Am J Dis Child.* 1979;133:497–502.
91. Kletsky OA, Costin G, Marrs RP, Bernstein G, March CM, Mishell DR. Gonadotrophin insufficiency in patients with thalassemia major. *J Clin Endocrinol Metab.* 1979;48:901–905.
92. Landau H, Matoth I, Landau-Cordova Z, Goldfarb A, Rachmilewitz EA, Glaser B. Cross-sectional and longitudinal study of the pituitary-thyroid axis in patients with thalassaemia major. *Clin Endocrinol.* 1993;38:55–61.
93. Wang C, Tso SC, Todd D. Hypogonadotropic hypogonadism in severe beta-thelassemia: effect of chelation and pulsatile gonadotrophin-releasing hormone therapy. *J Clin Endocrinol Metab.* 1989;68:511–516.
94. Herington AC, Werthe GA, Matthews RN, Burger HG. Studies on the possible mechanism for deficiency of nonsuppressible insulin-like activity in thalassemia major. *J Clin Endocrinol Metab.* 1981;52:393–398.
95. Saenger P, Schwartz E, Markenson AL, et al. Depressed serum somatomedin activity in beta-thalassemia. *J Pediatr.* 1980;96:214–218.
96. Werther GA, Matthews RN, Burger HG, Herington AC. Lack of response of nonsuppressible insulin-like activity to short term administration of human growth hormone in thalassemia major. *J Clin Endocrinol Metab.* 1981;53:806–809.

97. Pintor C, Cella SG, Manso P, et al. Impaired growth hormone (GH) response to GH-releasing hormone in thalassemia major. *J Clin Endocrinol Metab.* 1986;62:263–267.
98. Shehadeh N, Hazani A, Rudolf MCJ, Benderly A, Hochberg Z. Neurosecretory dysfunction of growth hormone secretion in thalassaemia major. *Acta Paediatr Scand.* 1990;79:790–795.
99. Leger J, Girot R, Crosnier H, Postel-Vinay MC, Rappaport R. Normal growth hormone (GH) response to GH-releasing hormone in children with thalassemia major before puberty: a possible age-related effect. *J Clin Endocrinol Metab.* 1989;69:453–456.
100. Masala A, Meloni T, Gallisai D, et al. Endocrine functioning in multitransfused prepubertal patients with homozygous beta-thalassemia. *J Clin Endocrinol Metab.* 1984;58:667–670.
101. Tolis G, Politis C, Kontopoulou I, et al. Pituitary somatotropic and corticotropic function in patients with β-thalassaemia on iron chelation therapy. *Birth Defects.* 1988;23:449–452.
102. Cavallo L, Gurrado R, Gallo F, Zacchino C, de Mattia D, Tato L. Growth deficiency in polytransfused beta-thalassaemia patients is not growth hormone dependent. *Clin Endocrinol.* 1997;46:701–706.
103. Roth C, Pekrun A, Bartz M, et al. Short stature and failure of pubertal development in thalassaemia major: evidence for hypothalamic neurosecretory dysfunction of growth hormone secretion and defective pituitary gonadotropin secretion. *Eur J Pediatr.* 1997;156:777–783.
104. Low LC, Kwan EYW, Lim YJ, Lee ACW, Tam CF, Lam KSL. Growth hormone treatment of short Chinese children with β-thalassaemia major without growth hormone deficiency. *Clin Endocrinol.* 1995;42:359–363.
105. Scacchi M, Damesi L, De Martin M, et al. Treatment with biosynthetic growth hormone of short thalassaemic patients with impaired growth hormone secretion. *Clin Endocrinol.* 1991;35:335–339.
106. McIntosh N. Endocrinopathy in thalassaemia major. *Arch Dis Child.* 1976;51:195–201.
107. Sklar CA, Lew LQ, Yoon DJ, David R. Adrenal function in thalassemia major following long-term treatment with multiple transfusions and chelation therapy. Evidence for dissociation of cortisol and adrenal androgen secretion. *Am J Dis Child.* 1987;141:327–330.
108. Arcasoy A, Cavdar A, Cin S, et al. Effects of zinc supplementation on linear growth in beta thalassemia (a new approach). *Am J Hematol.* 1987;24:127–136.
109. Vassilopoulou-Sellin R, Oyedeji CO, Foster PL, Thompson MM, Saman NA. Haemoglobin as a direct inhibitor of cartilage growth *in vitro. Horm Metab Res.* 1989;21:11.
110. Rodda CP, Reid ED, Johnson S, Doery J, Matthews R, Bowden DK. Short stature in homozygous β-thalassaemia is due to disproportionate truncal shortening. *Clin Endocrinol.* 1995;42:587–592.
111. Hatori M, Sparkman J, Teixeira CC, et al. Effects of deferoxamine on chondrocyte alkaline phosphatase activity: pro-oxidant role of deferoxamine in thalassemia. *Calif Tissue Intl.* 1995;57:229–236.
112. Italian working Group on Endocrine Complications in Non-endocrine Diseases. Multicentre study on prevalence of endocrine complications in thalassaemia major. *Clin Endocrinol.* 1995;42:581–586.
113. Jensen CE, Tuck SM, Old J, et al. Incidence of endocrine complications and clinical disease severity related to genotype analysis and iron overload in patients with β-thalassaemia. *Eur J Haematol.* 1997;59:76–81.
114. Chatterjee R, Katz M, Cox TF, Porter JB. A prospective study of the hypothalmic-pituitary axis in thalassaemic patients who developed secondary amenorrhoea. *Clin Endocrinol.* 1993;39:287–296.
115. De Sanctis V, Vullo C, Katz M, Wonke B, Tanas R, Bagni B. Gonadal function in patients with beta thalassaemia major. *J Clin Pathol.* 1988;41:133–137.
116. Maurer HS, Lloyd-Still JD, Ingrisano C, Gonzalez-Crussi F, Honig CR. A prospective evaluation of iron chelation therapy in children with severe β-thalassemia: a six-year study. *Am J Dis Child.* 1988;142:287–292.
117. Bergeron C, Kovacs K. Pituitary siderosis. A histologic, immunocytologic, and ultrastructural study. *Am J Pathol.* 1978;93:295–309.
118. Chatterjee R, Katz M, Oatridge A, Bydder GM, Porter JB. Selective loss of anterior pituitary volume with severe pituitary-gonadal insufficiency in poorly compliant male thalassemic patients with pubertal arrest. *Ann NY Acad Sci.* 1998;850:479–482.
119. Chatterjee R, Katz M. Evaluation of gonadotrophin insufficiency in thalassemic boys with pubertal failure: spontaneous versus provocative test. *J Pediatr Endocrinol Metab.* 2001;14(3):301–312.
120. Canale VC, Steinherz P, New M, Erlandson M. Endocrine function in thalassemia major. *Ann NY Acad Sci.* 1974; 232:333–345.
121. Berkovitch M, Bistritzer T, Milone SD, Perlman K, Kucharczyk W, Olivieri NF. Iron deposition in the anterior pituitary in homozygous beta-thalassemia: MRI evaluation and correlation with gonadal function. *J Pediatr Endocrinol Metab.* 2000;13(2):179–184.
122. Costin G, Kogut MD, Hyman C, Ortega JA. Carbohydrate metabolism and pancreatic islet-cell function in thalassemia major. *Diabetes.* 1977;26:230–240.
123. De Sanctis V, Zurlo MG, Senesi E, Boffa C, Cavallo L, Di Gregorio F. Insulin dependent diabetes in thalassaemia. *Arch Dis Child.* 1988;63:58–62.
124. Ellis JT, Schulman I, Smith CH. Generalized siderosis with fibrosis of liver and pancreas in Cooley's (Mediterranean) anemia; with observations on the pathogenesis of the siderosis and fibrosis. *Am J Pathol.* 1954;30:287–309.
125. Lassman MN, Genel M, Wise JK, Hendler R, Felig P. Carbohydrate homeostasis and pancreatic islet cell function in thalassemia. *Blood.* 1974;80:65–69.
126. Saudek CD, Hemm RM, Peterson CM. Abnormal glucose tolerance in beta-thalassemia major. *Metabolism.* 1977;26:43–52.
127. Zuppinger K, Molinari B, Hirt A, et al. Increased risk of diabetes mellitus in beta-thalassaemia major. *Hel Paediat Acta.* 1979;4:197–207.
128. Cavello-Perin P, Pacini B, Cerutti F, et al. Insulin resistance and hyperinsulinemia in homozygous β-thalassemia. *Metabolism.* 1995;44:281–286.
129. Dandona P, Hussain MAM, Varghese Z, Politis D, Flynn DM, Hoffbrand AV. Insulin resistance and iron overload. *Ann Clin Biochem.* 1983;20:77–79.

130. Dmochowski K, Finegood DT, Francombe WH, Tyler B, Zinman B. Factors determining glucose tolerance in patients with thalassemia major. *J Clin Endocrinol Metab.* 1993; 77:478–483.
131. Merkel PA, Simonson DC, Amiel SA, et al. Insulin resistance and hyperinsulinemia in patients with thalassemia major treated by hypertransfusion. *N Engl J Med.* 1988;318:809–814.
132. De Sanctis V, D'Ascola G, Wonke B. The development of diabetes mellitus and chronic liver disease in long term chelated β-thalassaemic patients. *Postgrad Med J.* 1986;62:831–836.
133. Olivieri NF, Ramachandran S, Tyler B, Bril V, Moffatt K, Daneman D. Diabetes mellitus in older patients with thalassemia major: relationship to severity of iron overload and presence of microvascular complications. *Blood.* 1990;76:72a.
134. Karahanyan E, Stoyaniva A, Moumdzhiev I, Ivanov I. Secondary diabetes in children with thalassaemia major (homozygous thalassemia). *Folia Med Plovdiv.* 1994;35:29–34.
135. Soliman AT, el-Banna N, Al Salmi I, Asfour M. Insulin and glucagon responses to provocation with glucose and arginine in prepubertal children with thalassemia major before and after long-term blood transfusion. *J Trop Pediatr.* 1996;42:291–296.
136. Lassman MN, O'Brien RT, Pearson HA, et al. Endocrine evaluation in thalassemia major. *Ann NY Acad Sci.* 1974;232:226.
137. Flynn DM, Fairney A, Jackson D, Clayton BE. Hormonal changes in thalassemia major. *Arch Dis Child.* 1976;51:828–836.
138. Magro S, Puzzonia P, Consarino C, et al. Hypothyroidism in patients with thalassemia syndromes. *Acta Haematol.* 1990;84:72–76.
139. Sabato A, De Sanctis V, Atti G, Capra L, Bagni L, Vullo C. Primary hypothyroidism and the low T3 syndrome in thalassemia major. *Arch Dis Child.* 1983;58:120–127.
140. Grundy RG, Woods RA, Savage MO, Evans JPM. Relationship of endocrinopathy to iron chelation status in young patients with thalassaemia major. *Arch Dis. Child.* 1994;71:128–132.
141. Vullo C, De Sanctis V, Katz M, et al. Endocrine abnormalities in thalassemia. *Ann NY Acad Sci.* 1990;612:293–310.
142. De Sanctis V, Vullo C, Bagni B, Chiccoli L. Hypoparathyroidism in β-thalassemia major. Clinical and laboratory observations in 24 patients. *Acta Haematol.* 1992;88:105–108.
143. Gertner JM, Broadus AE, Anast CS, Grey M, Pearson H, Genel M. Impaired patathyroid response to induced hypocalcemia in thalassemia major. *J Pediatr.* 1979;95:210–213.
144. Gabrielle O. Hypoparathyroidism associated with thalassemia. *Southern Med J.* 1971;64:115–116.
145. Oberklaid F, Seshadri R. Hypoparathyroidism and other endocrine dysfunction complicating thalassaemia major. *Med J Aust.* 1975;1:304–306.
146. Pratico G, Di Gregorio F, Caltabiano L, Palano GM, Caruso-Nicoletti M. Calcium phosphate metabolism in thalassemia. *Pediatr Med Chir.* 1998;20:265–268.
147. Kuo B, Zaino E, Roginsky MS. Endocrine function in thalassemia. *J Clin Endocrinol Metab.* 1968;28:805–808.
148. Johnston FE, Roseman JM. The effects of more frequent transfusions upon bone loss in thalassemia major. *Pediatr Res.* 1967;1:479–483.
149. Piomelli S, Danoff SJ, Becker MH, Lipera MJ, Travis SF. Prevention of bone malformations and cardiomegaly in Cooley's anemia by early hypertransfusion regimen. *Ann NY Acad Sci.* 1969;165:427.
150. Herrick RT, Davis GL. Thalassemia major and non-union of pathologic fractures. *J LA State Med Sci.* 1975;127:341–347.
151. Wolman IJ. Transfusion therapy in Cooley's anemia: growth and health as related to long-range hemoglobin levels, a progress report. *Ann NY Acad Sci.* 1964;119:736–747.
152. Tas I, Smith P, Cohen T. Metric and morphologic characteristics of the dentition in beta thalassaemia major in man. *Arch Oral Biol.* 1976;21:583–586.
153. Hazell JW, Modell CB. E.N.T. complications in thalassaemia major. *J Laryngol Otol.* 1976;90:877–881.
154. Anapliotou ML, Kastanias IT, Psara P, Evangelou EA, Liparaki M, Dimitriou P. The contribution of hypogonadism to the development of osteoporosis in thalassaemia major: new therapeutic approaches. *Clin Endocrinol.* 1995;42:279–287.
155. Fabbri G, Petraglia F, Segre A, et al. Reduced spinal bone density in young women with amenorrhoea. *Eur J Obstet Gynecol Reprod Biol.* 1991;41:117–122.
156. Giardina PJ, Schneider R, Lesser M, et al. Abnormal bone metabolism in thalassemia. In: Ando S, Brancati C, eds. *Endocrine Disorders in Thalassemia.* Berlin: Springer; 1995:38–46.
157. Vichinsky EP. The morbidity of bone disease in thalassemia. *Ann NY Acad Sci.* 1998;850:344–348.
158. Wonke B. Annotation: Bone disease in β-thalassaemia major. *Br J Haematol.* 1998;103:897–901.
159. Jensen CE, Tuck SM, Agnew JE, et al. High prevalence of low bone mass in thalassaemia major. *Br J Haematol.* 1998;103:911–915.
160. Giuzio E, Bria M, Bisconte MG, et al. Osteoporosis in patients affected with thalassemia. Our experience. *Chir Organ Mov.* 1991;76:369–374.
161. Eisman JA. Vitamin D receptor gene variants: implications for therapy. *Curr Opin Genet Dev.* 1996;6:361–365.
162. Rees DC, Basran RK, Hum B, Peto TEA, Weatherall DJ, Olivieri NF. Genetic influences on bone disease in thalassemia. *Blood.* 1998;92, Suppl 1:532a.
163. Hanslip JI, Prescott E, Lalloz M, Layton M, Wonke B. The role of the Sp1 polymorphism in the development of osteoporosis in patients with thalassaemia major. *Br J Haematol.* 1998;101:26.
164. Origa R, Fiumana E, Gamberini MR, et al. Osteoporosis in beta-thalassemia: Clinical and genetic aspects. *Ann NY Acad Sci.* 2005;1054:451–456.
165. Kalef-Exra J, Challa A, Chaliasos N, et al. Bone minerals in beta-thalassemia minor. *Bone.* 1995;16:651–655.
166. Valassi-Adam H, Nassika E, Kattamis C, Matsaniotis N. Immunoglobulin levels in children with homozygous beta-thalassemia. *Acta Paediatr Scand.* 1976;65:23–27.
167. Vento S, Cainelli F, Cesario F. Infections and thalassaemia. *Lancet Infect Dis.* 2006;6(4):226–233.
168. Rahav G, Volach V, Shapiro M, Rund D, Rachmilewitz EA, Goldfarb A. Severe infections in thalassaemic patients: prevalence and predisposing factors. *Br J Haematol.* 2006;133(6):667–674.
169. Smith CH, Erlandson ME, Stern G, Hilgartner MW. Postsplenectomy infection in Cooley's anemia. An appraisal of the problem in this and other blood disorders, with consideration of prophylaxis. *N Engl J Med.* 1962;266:737–743.

170. Smith CH, Erlandson ME, Stern G, Hilgartner H. Post-splenectomy infection in Cooley's anemia. *Ann NY Acad Sci.* 1964;119:748–757.
171. Eraklis AJ, Kevy SV, Diamond LK, Gross RE. Hazard of overwhelming infection after splenectomy in childhood. *N Engl J Med.* 1967;276:1225–1229.
172. Erikson WD, Burgert EO, Lynn HB. The hazard of infection following splenectomy in children. *Am J Dis Child.* 1968;116:1–12.
173. Green NS. Yersinia infections in patients with homozygous beta-thalassemia associated with iron overload and its treatment. *Pediatr Hematol Oncol.* 1992;9:247–254.
174. Gallant T, Freedman MH, Vellend H, Francombe WH. Yersinia sepsis in patients with iron overload treated with deferoxamine [letter]. *N Engl J Med.* 1986;314:1643.
175. Kelly DA, Price E, Jani B, Wright V, Rossiter M, Walker-Smith JA. Yersinia entercolitis in iron overload. *J Pediatr Gastroenterol Nutr.* 1987;6:643–645.
176. Robins-Browne RM, Prpic JK. Effects of iron and desferrioxamine in infections with *Yersinia enterocolitica. Infect Immunol.* 1985;47:774–779.
177. Mazzoleni G, de Sa D, Gately J, Riddell RH. Yersinia entercolotica infection with ileal perforation associated with iron overload and deferoxamine therapy. *Dig Dis Sci.* 1991;36:1154–1160.
178. Schanfield MS, Scalise G, Economidou I, Modell CB, Bate C, Zuckerman AJ. Immunogenetic factors in thalassemia and hepatitis B infection. A multicentre study. *Dev Biol Stand.* 1975;30:257–269.
179. Politis C. Complications of blood transfusion in thalassemia. In: Buckner CD, Gale RP, Lucarelli G, eds. *Advances and Controversies in Thalassemia Therapy: Bone Marrow Transplantation and Other Approaches.* New York: Alan R. Liss; 1989:67–76.
180. Bozkurt G, Dikengil T, Alimoglu O, et al. Hepatitis C among Turkish Cypriot thalassemic patients. In: Fifth International Conference on Thalassemias and Hemaglobinopathies; 1993; Nicosia, Cyprus; 1993:176.
181. Cancado RD, Guerra LGM, Rosenfeld MOJA, et al. Prevalence of hepatitis C virus antibody in beta thalassemic patients. In: Fifth International Conference on Thalassemia and Hemoglobinopathies; 1993; Nicosia, Cyprus; 1993: 176.
182. Cao A, Galanello Renzo M, Rosatelli MC, Argiolu F, De Virgilis S. Clinical experience of management of thalassemia: the Sardinian experience. *Semin Hematol.* 1996;33:66–75.
183. Kaur P, Kaur B. Thalassemia in Penang. In: First Asian Congress on Thalassemia; 1995; Penang, Malaysia; 1995:70–72.
184. Lau YL, Chow CB, Lee AC, et al. Hepatitis C virus antibody in multiply transfused Chinese with thalassaemia. *Bone Marrow Transplant.* 1993;12:26–28.
185. Wonke B, Hoffbrand VA, Brown D, Dusheiko G. Antibody to hepatitis C virus in multiply transfused patients with thalassaemia major. *J Clin Pathol.* 1990;43:638–640.
186. Wonke B, Hoffbrand AV, Bouloux P, Jensen C, Telfer P. New approaches to the management of hepatitis and endocrine disorders in Cooley's anemia. *Ann NY Acad Sci.* 1998;850:232–241.
187. Clemente MG, Congia M, Lai ME, et al. Effect of iron overload on the response to recombinant interferon-alfa treatment in transfusion-dependent patients with thalassemia major and chronic hepatitis C. *J Pediatr.* 1994;125:123–128.
188. Olynyk JK, Bacon BR. Hepatitis C. Recent advances in understanding and management. *Postgrad Med J.* 1995;98:79–81.
189. Rubin RB, Barton AL, Banner BF, Bonkovsky HL. Iron and chronic viral hepatitis: emerging evidence for an important interaction. *Dig Dis.* 1995;13:223–238.
190. Psichogiou M, Tzala E, Boletis J, et al. Hepatitis E virus infection in individuals at high risk of transmission of non-A, non-B hepatitis and sexually transmitted diseases. *Scand J Infect Dis.* 1996;28:443–445.
191. al-Fawaz I, al-Rasheed S, al-Mugeiren M, al-Salloum A, al-Sohaibani M, Ramia S. Hepatitis E virus infection in patients from Saudi Arabia with sickle cell anaemia and β-thalassemia major: possible transmission by blood transfusion. *J Virol Hepatol.* 1996;3:203–205.
192. Stransky J. The discovery of hepatitis G virus. *Cas Lek Cesk.* 1996;135:99–101.
193. Sampietro M, Lupica L, Perrero L, et al. The expression of uridine diphosphate glucuronosyltransferase gene is a major determinant of bilirubin level in heterozygous β-thalassaemia and in glucose-6-phosphate dehydrogenase deficiency. *Br J Haematol.* 1997;99:437–439.
194. Chung JL, Kao JH, Kong MS, Yang CP, Hung IJ, Lin TY. Hepatitis C and G virus infections in polytransfused children. *Eur J Pediatr.* 1997;156:546–549.
195. Prati D, Zanella A, Bosoni P, et al. The incidence and natural course of transfusion-associated GB virus C/hepatitis G virus infection in a cohort of thalassemic patients. The Cooleycare Cooperative Group. *Blood.* 1998;91:774–777.
196. Zemel R, Dickman R, Tamary H, Bukh J, Zaizov R, Tur-Kaspa R. Viremia, genetic heterogeneity, and immunity to hepatitis G/GB-C virus in multiply transfused patients with thalassemia. *Transfusion.* 1998;38:301–306.
197. Poovorawan Y, Theamboonlers A, Chongsrisawat V, Jantaradsamee P. Prevalence of infection with hepatitis G virus among various groups in Thailand. *Ann Trop Med Parasitol.* 1998;92:89–95.
198. Luban NL. Transfusion safety: Where are we today? *Ann NY Acad Sci.* 2005;1054:325–341.
199. Bertozzi S, Padian NS, Wegbreit J, et al. HIV/AIDS Prevention and Treatment. In: Jamison DT, Breman JG, Measham AR, et al., eds. *Disease Control Priorities in Developing Countries.* New York, Washington: Oxford University Press and the World Bank; 2006:331–370.
200. Manconi PE, Dessi C, Sanna G, et al. Human immunodeficiency virus infection in multi-transfused patients with thalassaemia major. *Eur J Pediatr.* 1998;147:304–307.
201. Girot R, Lefrère JJ, Schettini F, Kattamis C, Ladis V. HIV infection and AIDS in thalassemia. In: Rebulla P, Fessas P, eds. *Thalassemia 1990 5th Annual Meeting of the COOLEYCARE Group, 1991.* Athens: Centro trasfusionale Ospedale Naggiore Policlinico Dio Milano Editore; 1991:69–73.
202. De Martino M, Quarta G, Melpignano A, et al. Antibodies to HTLV III and the lymphadenopathy syndrome in multi-transfused beta-thalassemia patients. *Vox Sang.* 1985;41:230–233.

203. Politis C, Roumeliotou A, Germenis A, Papaevangelou G. Risk of acquired immune deficiency syndrome in multi-transfused patients with thalassemia major. *Plasma Ther Transfus Technol.* 1986;7:41–43.
204. Zanella A, Mozzi F, Ferroni P, Sirchia G. Anti-HTLV III screening in multi-transfused thalassaemia patients. *Vox Sang.* 1986;50:192.
205. Robert-Guroff M, Giardina PJ, Robey WG, et al. HTLV III neutralizing antibody development in transfusion-dependent seropositive patients with β-thalassemia. *J Immunol.* 1987;138:3731–3736.
206. Jullien AM, Courouce AM, Richard D, Favre M, Lefrere JJ, Habibi B. Transmission of HIV blood from seronegative donors. *Lancet.* 1988;2:1248–1249.
207. Costagliola DG, Girot R, Rebulla P, Lefrère J-J. Incidence of AIDS in HIV-1 infected thalassaemia patients. *Br J Haematol.* 1992;81:109–112.
208. Sen S, Mishra NM, Giri T, et al. Acquired immunodeficiency syndrome (AIDS) in multitransfused children with thalassemia. *Indian Pediatr.* 1993;30:455–460.
209. Kumar RM, Uduman S, Hamo IM, Morrison J, Khaurana AK. Incidence and clinical manifestations of HIV-1 infection in multitransfused thalassaemia Indian children. *Trop Geogr Med.* 1994;46:163–166.
210. Kumar RM, Khuranna A. Pregnancy outcome in women with beta-thalassemia major and HIV infection. *Eur J Obstet Gynecol Reprod Biol.* 1998;77:163–169.
211. Choudhury NV, Dubey ML, Jolly JG, Kalra A, Mahajan RC, Gangury NK. Post-transfusion malaria in thalassaemia patients. *Blut.* 1990;61:314–316.
212. Looareesuwan S, Suntharasamai P, Webster HK, Ho M. Malaria in splenectomized patients: report of four cases and review. *Clin Infect Dis.* 1993;16:361–366.
213. Olivieri NF, Muraca GM, O'Donnell A, Premawardhena A, Fisher C, Weatherall DJ. Studies in haemoglobin E beta-thalassaemia. *Br J Haematol.* 2008;141:388–397.
214. Grinberg LN, Rachmilewitz EA. Oxidative stress in β-thalassemic red blood cells and potential use of antioxidants. In: Beuzard Y, Lubin B, Rosa J, eds. *Sickle Cell Disease and Thalassaemia: New Trends in Therapy.* Colloque INSERN/John Libby Eurotext Ltd.; 1995:519–524.
215. Gutteridge JMC, Halliwell B. Iron toxicity and oxygen radicals. *Clin Haematol.* 1989;2:195–256.
216. Tsukamoto H, Horne W, Kimimura S, et al. Experimental liver cirrhosis induced by alcohol and iron. *J Clin Invest.* 1995;96:620–630.
217. Iancu TC, Neustein HB, Landing BH. The liver in thalassaemia major: ultrastructural observations. In: *Iron Metabolism Ciba Symposium No 51.* Amsterdam: Excerpta Medica; 1977:293–316.
218. Parkes JG, Randell EW, Olivieri NF, Templeton DM. Modulation by iron loading and chelation of the uptake of non-transferrin-bound iron by human liver cells. *Biochim Biophys Acta.* 1995;1243:373–380.
219. Frumin AM, Waldman S, Morris P. Exogenous hemochromatosis in Mediterranean anemia. *Pediatrics.* 1952;9:290–294.
220. Aldouri MA, Wonke B, Hoffbrand AV, et al. Iron state and hepatic disease in patients with thalassaemia major treated with long term subcutaneous desferrioxamine. *J Clin Pathol.* 1987;40:1352–1359.
221. Jean G, Terzoli S, Mauri R, et al. Cirrhosis associated with multiple transfusions in thalassemia. *Arch Dis Child.* 1984;59:67–70.
222. Risdon AR, Barry M, Fynn DM. Transfusional iron overload: the relationship between tissue iron concentration and hepatic fibrosis in thalassaemia. *J Pathol.* 1975;116:83–95.
223. Koch LA, Shapiro B. Erythroblastic anemia; review of cases reported showing roentgenographic changes in bones and 5 additional cases. *Am J Dis Child.* 1932;44:318–335.
224. Panizon F, Vullo C. Sulla envoluzione della siderosi e fibrosi epatica nella malattia di Cooley. Studio bioptico su 20 casi. *Acta Paediatr Lat.* 1952;10:71.
225. Wollstein M, Kreidel KV. Familial hemolytic anemia of childhood – von Jaksch. *Am J Dis Child.* 1930;39:115–130.
226. Baty JM, Blackfan KD, Diamond LK. Blood studies in infancts and in children. I. Erythroblastic anemia; a clinical and pathologic study. *Am J Dis Child.* 1932;43:667–704.
227. Cooley TB, Witwer ER, Lee P. Anemia in children with splenomegaly and peculiar changes in bones; report of cases. *Am J Dis Child.* 1927;34:347.
228. Barry M, Flynn DN, Letsky EA, Risdon RA. Long-term chelation therapy in thalassaemia major: effect on liver iron concentration, liver histology and clinical progress. *Br Med J.* 1974;i:16–20.
229. Angelucci E, Baronciani D, Lucarelli G, et al. Liver iron loverload and liver fibrosis in thalassemia. *Bone Marrow Transplant.* 1993;1:29–31.
230. Thakerngpol K, Fucharoen S, Boonyaphipat P, et al. Liver injury due to iron overload in thalassemia: histopathologic and ultrastructural studies. *Biometals.* 1996;9:177–183.
231. De Virgillis S, Sanna G, Carnacchia G, et al. Serum ferritin, liver iron stores and liver histology in children with thalassaemia. *Arch Dis Child.* 1980;55:43–45.
232. Brittenham GM, Griffith PM, Nienhuis AW, et al. Efficacy of deferoxamine in preventing complications of iron overload in patients with thalassemia major. *N Engl J Med.* 1994;331:567–573.
233. Sievert W, Pianko S, Warner S, et al. Hepatic iron overload does not prevent a sustained virological response to interferon-alpha therapy: a long term follow-up study in hepatitis C-infected patients with beta thalassemia major. *Am J Gastroenterol.* 2002;97(4):982–987.
234. Olivieri NF, Brittenham GM, McLaren CE, et al. Long-term safety and effectiveness of iron chelation therapy with deferiprone for thalasemia major. *N Engl J Med.* 1998;339:417–423.
235. Muretto P, Angelucci E, Lucarelli G. Reversibility of cirrhosis in patients cured of thalassemia by bone marrow transplantation. *Ann Intern Med.* 2002;136(9):667–672.
236. Gullo L, Corcioni E, Brancati C, Bria M, Pezzelli R, Sprovieri G. Morphologic and functional evaluation of the exocrine pancreas in beta-thalassemia. *Pancreas.* 1993;8:176–180.
237. Jandl JH, Greenberg MS. Bone marrow failure due to relative nutritional deficiency in Cooley's hemolytic anemia. *N Engl J Med.* 1959;266:461–468.
238. Luhby AL, Cooperman JM. Folic acid deficiency in thalassaemia major. *Lancet.* 1961;ii:490–491.
239. Luhby AL, Cooperman JM, Feldman R, Ceraolo J, Herrero J, Marley JF. Folic acid deficiency as a limiting factor in the anemias of thalassemia major. *Blood.* 1961;18:786.

240. Vatanavicharn S, Anuvatanakulchai M, Na-Nakorn S, Wasi P. Serum erythrocyte folate levels in thalassaemia patients in Thailand. *Scand J Haematol.* 1979;22:241–245.
241. Chanarin I. *The Megaloblastic Anaemias.* 2nd ed. Oxford: Blackwell Scientific Publications; 1980.
242. Luhby AL, Cooperman JM, Lopez R, Giorgio AJ. Vitamin B12 metabolism in thalassemia major. *Ann NY Acad Sci.* 1969;165:443–460.
243. Wapnick AA, Lynch SR, Charlton RW, Seftel HC, Bothwell TH. The effect of ascorbic acid deficiency on desferrioxamine-induced iron excretion. *Br J Haematol.* 1969;17:563–568.
244. Chapman RWG, Hussein MAM, Gorman A, et al. Effect of ascorbic acid deficiency on serum ferritin concentrations in patients with β-thalassaemia major and iron overload. *J Clin Pathol.* 1982;35:487–491.
245. Cohen A, Cohen IJ, Schwartz E. Scurvy and altered iron stores in thalassemia major. *N Engl J Med.* 1981;304:158–160.
246. O'Brien RT. Ascorbic acid enhancement of desferrioxamine induced urinary iron excretion in thalassemia major. *Ann NY Acad Sci.* 1974;232:221–225.
247. Bridges KR, Hoffman KE. The effects of ascorbic acid on the intracellular metabolism of iron and ferritin. *J Biol Chem.* 1986;261:14273–14277.
248. Nienhuis AW. Vitamin C and iron. *N Engl J Med.* 1981;304:170–171.
249. Hyman CB, Landing B, Alfin-Slater R, Kozak L, Weitzman J, Ortega JA. D1-alpha-tocopherol, iron and lipofuscin in thalassemia. *Ann NY Acad Sci.* 1974;232:211.
250. Rachmilewitz EA. The role of intracellular hemoglobin precipitation, low MCHC and iron overload on red blood cell membrane peroxidation in thalassemia. In: Bergsma D, Cerami A, Peterson CM, Graziano JH, eds. Birth Defects: Original Article Series. New York: Liss; 1976:123–128.
251. Rachmilewitz EA, Shifter A, Kahane I. Vitamin E deficiency in β-thalassemia major: changes in hematological and biochemical parameters after a therapeutic trial with α-tocopherol. *Am J Clin Nutr.* 1979;32:1850–1858.
252. Erlandson ME, Golubow J, Smith CH. Bivalent cations in homozygous thalassemia. *J Pediatr.* 1965;66:637–648.
253. Prasad AS, Diwany M, Gabr M, Sandstead HH, Mokhtar N, El Hefny A. Biochemical studies in thalassemia. *Ann Intern Med.* 1965;62:87–96.
254. Hyman CB, Ortega JA, Costin G, Takahashi M. The clinical significance of magnesium depletion in thalassaemia. *Ann NY Acad Sci.* 1980;344:436.
255. Silprasert A, Laokuldilok T, Kulapongs P. Zinc deficiency in β-thalassemic children. *Birth Defects: Origin Artic Series.* 1998;23:473–476.
256. Dewey KW, Grossman H, Canale VC. Cholelithiasis in thalassemia major. *Radiology.* 1970;96:385–388.
257. Fessas P, Loukopoulos D. The β thalassaemias. *Clin Haematol.* 1974;3:411–435.
258. Paik CH, Alavi L, Dunea G, Weiner L. Thalassemia and gouty arthritis. *JAMA.* 1970;213:296–297.
259. Logothetis J, Constantoulakis M, Economidou J, et al. Thalassemia major (homozygous beta-thalassemia): a survey of 138 cases with emphasis on neurological and muscular aspects. *Neurology.* 1972;22:294–304.
260. Sinniah D, Vegnaendra V, Kammaruddin A. Neurological complications of beta-thalassaemia major. *Arch Dis Child.* 1977;52:977–979.
261. Manfre L, Giarratano E, Maggio A, Banco A, Vaccaro G, Lagalla R. MR imaging of the brain: findings in asymptomatic patients with thalassemia intermedia and sickle cell-thalassemia disease. *AJR Am J Roentgenol.* 1999;173(6):1477–1480.
262. Matarugcheep P, Chanyawattjwongs M, Srisubat K. Clinical silent cerebral infarct (SCI) in patients with thalassemia diseases assessed by magnetic resonsance imaging (MRI). In: *The Eighth Cooley's Anemia Symposium*; 2005; Lake Buena Vista, FL; 2005. Poster presentation.
263. Logothetis J, Haritos-Fatouros M, Constantoulakis M, Economidou J, Augoustaki P, Loewensen RB. Intelligence and behavioural patterns in patients with Cooley's anemia (homozygous beta-thalassemia); a study based on 138 consecutive cases. *Pediatrics.* 1971;48:740.
264. Tsiantis J. Family reactions and relationships in thalassemia. *Ann NY Acad Sci.* 1990;612:451–461.
265. Rutter M, Graham P. The reliability and validity of psychiatric assessment of the child: Interview with the child. *Br J Psychiatry.* 1968;114:581–592.
266. Klein, N., Sen A, Rusby J, Ratip S, Modell B, Olivieri NF. The psychosicial burden of Cooley's anemia in affected children and their parents. *Ann NY Acad Sci.* 1998;850:512–513.
267. Armstrong FD. Thalassemia and learning: neurocognitive functioning in children. *Ann NY Acad Sci.* 2005;1054:283–289.
268. Seracchioli R, Porcu E, Colombi C, et al. Transfusion-dependent homozygous β-thalassaemia major: successful twin pregnancy following in vitro fertilization and tubal embryo transfer. *Hum Reprod.* 1994;9:1964–1965.
269. Tampakoudis P, Tsatalas C, Mamopoulos M, et al. Transfusion-dependent homozygous β-thalassaemia major: successful pregnancy in five cases. *Eur J Obstet Gynecol Reprod Biol.* 1997;74:127–131.
270. Singer ST, Vichinsky EP. Deferoxamine treatment during pregnancy: is it harmful? *Am J Hematol.* 1999;60:24–26.
271. Sonakul D. *Pathology of Thalassaemic Diseases.* Thailand: Amarin Printing Group; 1989.
272. Astaldi G, Tolentino P, Sacchetti G. La talassemia (Morbo di Cooley e forme affini). In: *Biblioteca Haematologica.* Pavia: Tipografia del libro; 1951.
273. Fink HE. Transfusion hemochromatosis in Cooley's anemia. *Ann NY Acad Sci.* 1964;119:680–685.
274. Modell CB, Matthews R. Thalassemia in Britain and Australia. In: Bergsma D, Cerami A, Peterson CH, Graziano JH, eds. *Birth Defects: Original Article Series.* New York: Liss; 1976:13–29.
275. Nathan DG, Gunn RB. Thalassemia: the consequences of unbalanced hemoglobin synthesis. *Am J Med.* 1966;41:815–830.
276. Polliack A, Rachmilewitz EA. Ultrastructural studies in β-thalassaemia major. *Br J Haematol.* 1973;24:319–326.
277. Rifkind RA. Heinz body anemia: an ultrastructural study. II. Red cell sequestration and destruction. *Blood.* 1965;26:433–448.
278. Zaino EC, Rossi MB. Ultrastructure of the erythrocytes in β-thalassemia. *Ann NY Acad Sci.* 1974;232:238–260.
279. Fessas P. Inclusions of hemoglobin in erythroblasts and erythrocytes of thalassemia. *Blood.* 1963;21:21–32.
280. Yataganas X, Gahrton G, Fessas P, Kesse-Elias M, Thorell B. Proliferative activity and glycogen accumulation of erythroblasts in β-thalassaemia. *Br J Haematol.* 1973;24:651–659.

281. Zaino EC, Rossi MB, Pham TD, Azar HA. Gaucher's cells in thalassemia. *Blood.* 1971;38:457–462.
282. Bailey IS, Prankerd TAJ. Studies in thalassaemia. *Br J Haematol.* 1958;4:150–155.
283. Hillcoat BL, Waters AH. The survival of 51Cr labelled autotransfused red cells in a patient with thalassaemia. *Aust Med J.* 1962;11:55–58.
284. Kaplan E, Zuelzer WW. Erythrocyte survival studies in childhood. II. Studies in Mediterranean anemia. *J Lab Clin Med.* 1950;36:517–523.
285. Gabuzda TG, Nathan DG, Gardner FH. The turnover of hemoglobins A, F and A2 in the peripheral blood of three patients with thalassemia. *J Clin Invest.* 1963;42:1678–1688.
286. Prankerd TAJ. The spleen and anaemia. *Br Med J.* 1963;ii:517–524.
287. Loukopoulos D, Fessas P. The distribution of hemoglobin types in thalassemic erythrocytes. *J Clin Invest.* 1965;44:231.
288. Nathan DG, Stossel TB, Gunn RB, Zarkowsky HS, Laforet MT. Influence of hemoglobin precipitation on erythrocyte metabolism in alpha and beta thalassemia. *J Clin Invest.* 1969;48:33–41.
289. Heinrich HC, Gabbe EE, Oppitz KH, et al. Absorption of inorganic and food iron in children with heterozygous and homozygous beta-thalassemia. *Z Kinderheilkd.* 1973;115:1–22.
290. Hershko C, Graham G, Bates CW, Rachmilewitz ES. Nonspecific serum iron in thalassaemia: an abnormal serum iron fraction of potential toxicity. *Br J Haematol.* 1978;40:255–263.
291. Finch CA, Deubelbeiss K, Cook JD, et al. Ferrokinetics in man. *Medicine (Baltimore).* 1970;49:17–53.
292. Malamos B, Belcher EH, Gyftaki E, Binopoulos D. Simultaneous studies with Fe59 and Cr51 in congenital haemolytic anaemias. *Nucl Med (Stuttg).* 1961;2:1–20.
293. Rees DC, Porter JB, Clegg JB, Weatherall DJ. Why are hemoglobin F levels increased in Hb E/β thalassemia? *Blood.* 1999;94:3199–3204.
294. Schroeder WA, Huisman THJ. Nonallelic structural genes and hemoglobin synthesis. In: *XIIth International Congress of Hematology Plenary Sessions,* Lehmanns Munich; 1970:26.
295. Huisman THJ, Schroeder WA, Efremov GD, et al. The present status of the heterogeneity of fetal hemoglobin in β-thalassemia; an attempt to unify some observations in thalassemia and related conditions. *Ann NY Acad Sci.* 1974; 232:107–124.
296. Weatherall DJ, Clegg JB, Naughton MA. Globin synthesis in thalassaemia: an *in vitro* study. *Nature.* 1965;208:1061–1065.
297. Bank A, Marks PA. Excess a chain synthesis relative to β chain synthesis in thalassaemia major and minor. *Nature.* 1966;212:1198–1200.
298. Bargellesi A, Pontremoli S, Conconi F. Absence of beta globin synthesis and excess alpha globin synthesis in homozygous β thalassemia. *Eur J Biochem.* 1967;1:73–79.
299. Modell CB, Latter A, Steadman JH, Huehns ER. Haemoglobin synthesis in β-thalassaemia. *Br J Haematol.* 1969;17:485–501.
300. Weatherall DJ, Clegg JB, Na-Nakorn S, Wasi P. The pattern of disordered haemoglobin synthesis in homozygous and heterozygous β-thalassaemia. *Br J Haematol.* 1969;16:251–267.
301. Bannerman RM. *Thalassemia. A Survey of Some Aspects.* New York: Grune and Stratton; 1961.
302. Weatherall DJ. Toward an understanding of the molecular biology of some common inherited anemias: the story of thalassemia. In: Wintrobe MM, ed. *Blood, Pure and Eloquent.* New York: McGraw–Hill; 1980:373–414.
303. Chini V, Valeri CM. Mediterranean hemopathic syndromes. *Blood.* 1949;4:989–1013.
304. Bianco I, Montalenti G, Silvestroni E, Siniscalco M. Further data on genetics of microcythemia or thalassaemia minor and Cooley's disease or thalassaemia major. *Ann Eugen.* 1952;16:299–314.
305. Sturgeon P, Itano HA, Bergren WR. Genetic and biochemical studies of 'intermediate' types of Cooley's anaemia. *Br J Haematol.* 1955;1:264–277.
306. Cao A, Gasperini D, Podda A, Galanello R. Molecular pathology of thalassemia intermedia. *Eur J Int Med.* 1990;1:227–236.
307. Wainscoat JS, Thein SL, Weatherall DJ. Thalassaemia intermedia. *Blood Rev.* 1987;1:273–279.
308. Antonarakis SE, Kang J, Lam VMS, Tam JWO, Li AMC. Molecular characterization of β-globin gene mutations in patients with β-thalassemia intermedia in South China. *Br J Haematol.* 1988;70:357–361.
309. Camaschella C, Mazza U, Roetto A, et al. Genetic interactions in thalassemia intermedia: analysis of β-mutations, α-genotype, γ promoters, and β-LCR hypersensitive sites 2 and 4 in Italian patients. *Am J Hematol.* 1995;48:82–87.
310. Galanello R, Dessi E, Melis MA, et al. Molecular analysis of β^0-thalassemia intermedia in Sardinia. *Blood.* 1989;74:823–827.
311. Kanavakis E, Traeger-Synodinos J, Tzetis M, Metataxatou-Mavromati A, Ladis V, Kattamis C. Molecular characterization of homozygous (high Hb A_2) β-thalassemia intermedia in Greece. *Pediatr Hematol Oncol.* 1995;12:37–45.
312. Rund D, Oron-Karni V, Filon D, Goldfarb A, Rachmilewitz E, Oppenheim A. Genetic analysis of β-thalassemia intermedia in Israel: diversity of mechanisms and unpredictability of phenotype. *Am J Hematol.* 1997;54:16–22.
313. Thein SL, Hesketh C, Wallace RB, Weatherall DJ. The molecular basis of thalassaemia major and thalassaemia intermedia in Asian Indians: application to prenatal diagnosis. *Br J Haematol.* 1988;70:225–231.
314. Ho PJ, Hall GW, Luo LY, Weatherall DJ, Thein SL. Beta thalassaemia intermedia: is it possible to predict phenotype from genotype? *Br J Haematol.* 1998;100:70–78.
315. Camaschella C, Cappellini MD. Thalassemia intermedia. *Haematologica.* 1995;80:58–68.
316. Fiorelli G, Sampietro M, Romano M, Albano M, Cappellini MD. Clinical features of thalassemia intermedia in Italy. *Birth Defects: Origin Artic Series.* 1988;23:287–295.
317. Pippard MJ, Rajagopalan B, Callender ST, Weatherall DJ. Iron loading, chronic anaemia, and erythroid hyperplasia as determinants of the clinical features of β-thalassaemia intermedia. In: Weatherall DJ, Fiorelli G, Gorini S, eds. *Advances in Red Blood Cell Biology.* New York: Raven Press; 1982:103–113.
318. Bianco I, Cappabianca MP, Foglietta E, et al. Silent thalassemias: genotypes and phenotypes. *Haematologica.* 1997;82:269–280.
319. Bianco I, Lerone M, Foglietta E, et al. Phenotypes of individuals with a β thal classical allele associated either with a β thal silent allele or with a globin gene triplicate. *Haematologica.* 1997;82:513–525.

320. Ristaldi MS, Pirastu M, Murru S, et al. A spontaneous mutation produced a novel elongated β^0 globin chain structural variant (Hb Agnana) with a thalassemia-like phenotype. *Blood.* 1990;75:1378–1380.
321. Wong C, Dowling CE, Saiki RK, Higuchi RG, Erlich HA, Kazazian HHJ. Characterization of β-thalassaemia mutations using direct genomic sequencing of amplified single copy DNA. *Nature.* 1987;330:384–386.
322. Athanassiadou A, Papachatzopoulou A, Zoumbos N, Maniatis G, Gibbs R. A novel b-thalassaemia mutation in the 5′ untranslated region of the β-globin gene. *Br J Haematol.* 1994;88:307–310.
323. Ho PJ, Rochette J, Fisher CA, et al. Moderate reduction of β-globin gene transcript by a novel mutation in the 5′ untranslated region: a study of its interaction with other genotypes in two families. *Blood.* 1996;87:1170–1178.
324. Murru S, Loudianos G, Deiana M, et al. Molecular characterization of β-thalassemia intermedia in patients of Italian descent and identification of three novel β-thalassemia mutations. *Blood.* 1991;77:1342–1347.
325. Gonzalez-Redondo JH, Stoming TA, Lanclos KD, et al. Clinical and genetic heterogeneity in Black patients with homozygous β-thalassemia from the Southeastern United States. *Blood.* 1988;72:1007–1014.
326. Orkin SH, Antonarakis SE, Kazazian HHJ. Base substitution at position –88 in a β-thalassemic globin gene. Further evidence for the role of distal promoter element ACACCC. *J Biol Chem.* 1984;259:8679–8681.
327. Camaschella C, Alfarano A, Gottardi E, Serra A, Revello D, Saglio G. The homozygous state for the -87 C→G β^+ thalassaemia. *Br J Haematol.* 1990;75:132–133.
328. Diaz-Chico JC, Yang KG, Stoming TA, et al. Mild and severe b-thalassemia among homozygotes from Turkey: identification of the types by hybridization of amplified DNA with synthetic probes. *Blood.* 1988;71:248–251.
329. Rosatelli C, Oggiano L, Leoni GB, et al. Thalassemia intermedia resulting from a mild beta-thalassemia mutation. *Blood.* 1989;73:601–605.
330. Fattoum S, Guemira F, Öner C, et al. β-thalassemia, Hb S-β-thalassemia and sickle cell anemia among Tunisians. *Hemoglobin.* 1991;15:11–21.
331. Takihara Y, Nakamura T, Yamada H, Takagi Y, Fukumaki Y. A novel mutation in the TATA box in a Japanese patient with β^+-thalassemia. *Blood.* 1986;67:547–550.
332. Safaya S, Rieder RF, Dowling CE, Kazazian HHJ, Adams JG. Homozygous β-thalassemia without anemia. *Blood.* 1989;73:324–328.
333. Huang S-Z, Wong C, Antonarakis SE, Ro-Lein T, Lo WHY, Kazazian HHJ. The same TATA box β-thalassemia mutation in Chinese and U.S. blacks: another example of independent origins of mutation. *Hum Genet.* 1986;74:162–164.
334. Galacteros F, Delanoe-Garin J, Monplaisir N, et al. Two new cases of heterozygosity for hemoglobin Knossos $\alpha_2\beta_2$ Ala→Ser detected in the French West Indies and Algeria. *Hemoglobin.* 1984;8:215–228.
335. Olds RJ, Sura T, Jackson B, Wonke B, Hoffbrand AV, Thein SL. A novel δ^0 mutation in cis with Hb Knossos: a study of different genetic interactions in three Egyptian families. *Br J Haematol.* 1991;78:430–436.
336. Efremov D, Dimovsky A, Baysal E, et al. Possible factors influencing the haemoglobin and fetal haemoglobin levels in patients with β-thalassaemia due to a homozygosity for the IVS-1-6 (T-C) mutation. *Br J Haematol.* 1994;86:824–830.
337. Öner R, Altay C, Aksoy M, et al. β-thalassemia in Turkey. *Hemoglobin.* 1990;14(1):1–13.
338. Scerri CA, Abela W, Galdies R, Pizzuto M, Grech JL, Felice AE. The β^+ IVS, I-NT no. 6 (T→C) thalassaemia in heterozygotes with an associated Hb Valletta or Hb S heterozygosity in homozygotes from Malta. *Br J Haematol.* 1993;83:669–671.
339. Tamagnini GP, Lopes MC, Castanheira ME, Wainscoat JS, Wood WG. b+ thalassaemia – Portuguese type: clinical, haematological and molecular studies of a newly defined form of β thalassaemia. *Br J Haematol.* 1983;54:189–200.
340. Orkin SH, Cheng T-C, Antonarakis SE, Kazazian HH. Thalassaemia due to a mutation in the cleavage-polyadenylation signal of the human β-globin gene. *EMBO J.* 1985;4:453–456.
341. Kan YW, Nathan DG. Mild thalassemia: the result of interactions of alpha and beta thalassemia genes. *J Clin Invest.* 1970;49:635–642.
342. Weatherall DJ, Pressley L, Wood WG, Higgs DR, Clegg JB. The molecular basis for mild forms of homozygous β thalassaemia. *Lancet.* 1981;i:527–529.
343. Furbetta M, Tuveri T, Rosatacelli C, et al. Molecular mechanism accounting for milder types of thalassemia major. *J Pediatr.* 1983;103:35–39.
344. Wainscoat JS, Kanavakis E, Wood WG, et al. Thalassaemia intermedia in Cyprus: the interaction of alpha and beta thalassaemia. *Br J Haematol.* 1983;53:411–416.
345. Galanello R, Dessi E, Melis MA, et al. Molecular analysis of β^0-thalassemia intermedia in Sardinia. *Blood.* 1989;74:823–827.
346. Winichagoon P, Fucharoen S, Weatherall DJ, Wasi P. Concomitant inheritance of α-thalassemia in β^0-thalassemia/Hb E. *Am J Hematol.* 1985;20:217–222.
347. Furbetta M, Galanello R, Ximenes A, et al. Interaction of alpha and beta thalassaemia genes in two Sardinian families. *Br J Haematol.* 1979;41:203–210.
348. Loukopoulos D, Loutradi A, Fessas P. A unique thalassaemia syndrome: homozygous α-thalassaemia$^+$ homozygous β-thalassaemia. *Br J Haematol.* 1978;39:377–389.
349. Cividalli G, Kerem H, Execkiel E, Rachmilewitz EA. β^+-thalassemia intermedia. *Blood.* 1978;52:345.
350. Godet J, VErdier G, Nigon V, et al. β^0-thalassemia from Algeria: genetic and molecular characterization. *Blood.* 1977; 50:463.
351. Knox-Macaulay HHM, Weatherall DJ, Clegg JB, Pembrey ME. Thalassaemia in the British. *Br Med J.* 1973;iii:150–155.
352. Weatherall DJ, Clegg JB, Wood WG, et al. The clinical and molecular heterogeneity of the thalassaemia syndromes. *Ann NY Acad Sci.* 1980;344:83–100.
353. Labie D, Pagnier J, Lapoumeroulie C, et al. Common haplotype dependency of high $^G\gamma$-globin gene expression and high Hb F levels in β-thalassemia and sickle cell anemia patients. *Proc Natl Acad Sci USA.* 1985;82:2111–2114.
354. Thein SL, Sampietro M, Old JM, et al. Association of thalassaemia intermedia with a beta-globin gene haplotype. *Br J Haematol.* 1987;65:370–373.
355. Thein SL. β-Thalassaemia. In: Higgs DR, Weatherall DJ, eds. *Baillière's Clinical Haematology International Practice and Research: The Haemoglobinopathies.* London: Baillière Tindall; 1993:151–176.

356. Cappellini MD, Fiorelli G, Bernini LF. Interaction between homozygous β^0 thalassaemia and the Swiss type of hereditary persistence of fetal haemoglobin. *Br J Haematol.* 1981;48:561–572.
357. Thein SL, Weatherall DJ. A non-deletion hereditary persistence of fetal hemoglobin (HPFH) determinant not linked to the β-globin gene complex. In: Stamatoyannopoulos G, Nienhuis AW, eds. *Hemoglobin Switching, Part B: Cellular and Molecular Mechanisms.* New York: Alan R. Liss; 1989:97–112.
358. Gianni AM, Bregni M, Cappellini MD, et al. A gene controlling fetal hemoglobin expression in adults is not linked to the non-α globin cluster. *EMBO J.* 1983;2:921–926.
359. Dover GJ, Smith KD, Chang YC, et al. Fetal hemoglobin levels in sickle cell disease and normal individuals are partially controlled by an X-linked gene located at Xp22.2. *Blood.* 1992;80:816–824.
360. Premawardhena A, Fisher CA, Olivieri NF, et al. A novel molecular basis for β thalassemia intermedia poses new questions about its pathophysiology. *Blood.* 2005;106:3251–3255.
361. Galanello R, Ruggeri R, Paglietti E, Addis M, Melis MA, Cao A. A family with segregating triplicated alpha globin loci and beta thalassemia. *Blood.* 1983;62:1035–1040.
362. Sampietro M, Cazzola M, Cappellini MD, Fiorelli G. The triplicated alpha-gene locus and heterozygous beta thalassaemia: a case of thalassaemia intermedia. *Br J Haematol.* 1983;55:709–710.
363. Thein SL, Al-Hakim I, Hoffbrand AV. Thalassaemia intermedia: a new molecular basis. *Br J Haematol.* 1984;56:333–337.
364. Traeger-Synodinos J, Kanavakis E, Vrettou C, et al. The triplicated α-globin gene locus in β-thalassaemia heterozygotes: clinical, haematological, biosynthetic and molecular studies. *Br J Haematol.* 1996;95:467–471.
365. Weatherall DJ, Clegg JB, Knox-Macaulay HHM, Bunch C, Hopkins CR, Temperley IJ. A genetically determined disorder with features both of thalassaemia and congenital dyserythropoietic anaemia. *Br J Haematol.* 1973;24:681–702.
366. Stamatoyannopoulos G, Woodson R, Papayannopoulou T, Heywood D, Kurachi MS. Inclusion-body b-thalasemia trait. A form of β thalassemia producing clinical manifestations in simple heterozygotes. *N Engl J Med.* 1974;290:939–943.
367. Bannerman RM, Keusch G, Kreimer-Birnbaum M, Vance VK, Vaughan S. Thalassemia intermedia, with iron overload, cardiac failure, diabetes mellitus, hypopituitarism and porphyrinuria. *Am J Med.* 1967;42:476–486.
368. Erlandson ME, Brilliant R, Smith CH. Comparison of sixty-six patients with thalassemia major and thirteen patients with thalassemia intermedia: including evaluations of growth, development, maturation and prognosis. *Ann NY Acad Sci.* 1964;119:727–735.
369. Cossu P, Toccafondi C, Vardeu F, et al. Iron overload and desferrioxamine chelation therapy in beta-thalassemia intermedia. *Eur J Pediatr.* 1981;137:267–271.
370. Fiorelli G, Fargion S, Piperno A, Battafarano N, Cappellini MD. Iron metabolism in thalassemia intermedia. *Haematologica.* 1990;75:89–95.
371. Mancuso L, Iacona MA, Marchi S, Rigano P, Geraci E. Severe cardiomyopathy in a woman with intermediate beta-thalassemia. Regression of cardiac failure with desferrioxamine. *G Ital Cardiol.* 1985;15:916–920.
372. Olivieri NF, Koren G, Matsui D, et al. Reduction of tissue iron stores and normalization of serum ferritin during treatment with the oral iron chelator L1 in thalassemia intermedia. *Blood.* 1992;79:2741–2748.
373. Aessopos A, Stamatelos G, Skoumas V, Vassilopoulos G, Mantzourani M, Loukopoulos D. Pulmonary hypertension and right heart failure in patients with b-thalassemia intermedia. *Chest.* 1995;107:50–53.
374. Goldfarb A, Grisaru D, Gimmon Z, Okon E, Lebensart P, Rachmilewitz EA. High incidence of cholelithiasis in older patients with homozygous β-thalassemia. *Acta Haematol.* 1990;83:120–122.
375. Gratwick GM, Bullough PG, Bohne WHO, Markenson AL, Peterson CM. Thalassemia osteoarthropathy. *Ann Intern Med.* 1978;88:494–501.
376. Ben-Bassat I, Hertz M, Selzer G, Ramot B. Extramedullary hematopoiesis with multiple tumor-simulating mediastinal masses in a patient with β-thalassemia intermedia. *Israel J Med Sci.* 1977;13:1206–1210.
377. Yu YC, Kao EL, Chou SH, Lin TJ, Chien CH. Intrathoracic extremedullary hematopoiesis simulating posterior mediastinal mass – report of a case in a patient with beta-thalassemia intermedia. *Kao Hsiung I Hsueh Ko Hsueh Tsa Chih.* 1991;7:43–48.
378. Alam R, Padmanabhan K, Rao H. Paravertebral mass in a patient with thalassemia intermedia. *Chest.* 1997;112:265–267.
379. Cardia E, Toscano S, La Rosa G, Zaccone C, d'Avella D, Tomasello F. Spinal cord compression in homozygous β-thalassemia intermedia. *Pediatr Neurosurg.* 1994;20:186–189.
380. David CV, Balusubramaniam P. Paraplegia with thalassemia. *Aust NZ J Med.* 1983;53:283–284.
381. Mancuso P, Zingale A, Basile L, Chiaramonte I, Tropea R. Cauda equina compression syndrome in a patient affected by thalassemia intermedia: complete regression with blood transfusion therapy. *Childs Nerv Syst.* 1993;9:440–441.
382. Smith PR, Manjoney DL, Teitcher JB, Choi KN, Braverman AS. Massive hemothorax due to intrathoracic extramedullary hematopoiesis in a patient with thalassemia intermedia. *Chest.* 1988;94:658–660.
383. Papavasiliou C, Gouliamos A, Vlahos L, Trakadas S, Kalovidouris A, Pouliades G. CT and MRI of symptomatic spinal involvement by extramedullary haemopoiesis. *Clin Radiol.* 1990;42:91–92.
384. Sergiacomi G, Palma E, Cianciulli P, Forte L, Papa G, Simonetti G. Correlazioni clinico-radiologiche nella talassemia intermedia. *Radiol Med Torino.* 1993;85:570–573.
385. Martin J, Palacio A, Petit J, Martin C. Fatty transformation of thoracic extramedullary hematopoiesis following splenectomy: CT features. *J Comput Assist Tomogr.* 1990;14:477–478.
386. Brownell AI, McSwiggan DA, Cubitt WD, Anderson MJ. Aplastic and hypoplastic episodes in sickle cell disease and thalassaemia. *J Clin Pathol.* 1986;39:121–124.
387. Mela QS, Cacace E, Ruggerio V, Frigerio R, Pitzus F, Carcassi U. Virus infection in β-thalssemia intermedia. *Birth Defects: Origin Artic Series.* 1988;23:557–564.
388. Gimmon Z, Wexler MR, Rachmilewitz EA. Pathogenesis of juvenile leg ulcers in β-thalassaemia major and intermedia. *Plast Reconstruct Surg.* 1982;69:320–323.

389. Afifi AM. High transfusion regime in the management of reproductive wastage and maternal complications of pregnancy in thalassaemia major. *Acta Haematol.* 1974;52:331–335.

390. Walker EH, Whelton MJ, Beaven GH. Successful pregnancy in a patient with thalassaemia major. *J Obstet Gynaecol Br Commonw.* 1969;76:549–553.

391. Ruf A, Pick M, Deutsch V, et al. In vivo platelet activation correlates with red cell anionic phospholipid exposure in patients with β-thalassaemia major. *Br J Haematol.* 1997;98:51–56.

392. Skarsgard E, Doski J, Jaksic T, et al. Thrombosis of the portal venous system after splenectomy for pediatric hematologic disease. *J Pediatr Surg.* 1993;28:1109–1112.

393. Dore F, Bonfigli S, Pardini S, Pirozzi F, Longinotti M. Priapism in thalassemia intermedia. *Haematologica.* 1991;76:523.

394. Gallo E, Massaro P, Miniero R, David D, Tarella C. The importance of the genetic picture and globin synthesis in determining the clinical and haematological features of thalassaemia intermedia. *Br J Haematol.* 1979;41:211–221.

395. De Alarcon PA, Donovan ME, Forbes GB, Landau SA, Stockman JA. Iron absorption in the thalassemia syndromes and its inhibition by tea. *N Engl J Med.* 1979;300:5–8.

396. Pippard MJ, Warner GT, Callender ST, Weatherall DJ. Iron absorption and loading in β-thalassaemia intermedia. *Lancet.* 1979;ii:819–821.

397. Pippard MJ, Weatherall DJ. Iron absorption in non-transfused iron loading anaemias: prediction of risk for iron loading, and response to iron chelation treatment, in β thalassaemia and congenital sideroblastic anaemias. *Haematologica.* 1984;17:17–24.

398. Cavill I, Ricketts C, Jacobs A, Letsky E. Erythropoiesis and the effect of transfusion in homozygous beta-thalassemia. *N Engl J Med.* 1978;298:776–778.

399. Najean Y, Deschryver F, Henni T, Girot R. Red cell kinetics in thalassaemia intermedia: its use for a prospective prognosis. *Br J Haematol.* 1985;59:533–539.

400. Dore F, Bonfigli S, Gaviano E, Pardini S, Longinotti M. Serum transferrin receptor levels in patients with thalassemia intermedia during rHuEPO administration. *Haematologica.* 1996;81:37–39.

401. Camaschella C, Gonella S, Calabrese R, et al. Serum erythropoietin and circulating transferrin receptor in thalassemia intermedia patients with heterogeneous genotypes. *Haematologica.* 1996;81:397–403.

402. Dore F, Bonfigli S, Gaviano E, et al. Serum erythropoietin levels in thalassemia intermedia. *Ann Hematol.* 1993;67:183–186.

403. Galanello R, Barella S, Turco MP, et al. Serum erythropoietin and erythropoiesis in high- and low-fetal hemoglobin β-thalassemia intermedias patients. *Blood.* 1994;83:561–565.

404. Efremov DG, Efremov GD, Zisovski N, et al. Variation in clinical severity among patients with Hb Lepore-Boston-β-thalassaemia is related to the type of b-thalassaemia. *Br J Haematol.* 1988;68:351–355.

405. Bianco I, Graziani B, Carboni C. Genetic patterns in thalassemia intermedia (constitutional microcytic anemia). Familial, hematologic and biosynthetic studies. *Hum Hered.* 1977;27:257.

406. Premawardena A, Arambepola M, Katugaha N, Weatherall DJ. Is the β thalassaemia trait of clinical importance. *Br J Haematol.* 2008:141:407–410.

407. Castaldi G, Zavagli G, Ambroso G, Dallapiccolas B, Trotta F. Anaemia in beta-thalassaemia carriers. *Br Med J.* 1974;i:518.

408. Mazza U, Saglio G, Cappio FC, Camaschella C, Neretto G, Gallo E. Clinical and haematological data in 254 cases of beta-thalassaemia trait in Italy. *Br J Haematol.* 1976;33:91–99.

409. Yataganas X, Fessas P. The pattern of hemoglobin precipitation in thalassemia and its significance. *Ann NY Acad Sci.* 1969;165:270–287.

410. Gallo E, Pich PG, Ricco G, Saglio G, Camaschella C, Mazza U. The relationship between anemia, fecal stercobilinogen, erythrocyte survival and globin synthesis in heterozygotes for β-thalassemia. *Blood.* 1975;46:692–698.

411. Pearson HA, McFarland W, King ER. Erythrokinetic studies in thalassemia trait. *J Lab Clin Med.* 1960;56:866–873.

412. Pippard MJ, Wainscoat JS. Erythrokinetics and iron status in heterozygous β thalassaemia, and the effect of interaction with α thalassaemia. *Br J Haematol.* 1987;66:123–127.

413. Galanello R, Turco MP, Barella S, et al. Iron stores and iron deficiency anemia in children heterozygous for β-thalassemia. *Haematologica.* 1990;75:319–322.

414. Huisman THJ, Gravely ME, Sox R. A note on the inheritance of the hereditary persistence of fetal haemoglobin and the delta chain variant HbA2. *J Med Genet.* 1976;13:62.

415. Kattamis C, Lagos P, Metaxatou-Mavromati A, Matsaniotis N. Serum iron and unsaturated iron-binding capacity in the β-thalassaemia trait: their relation to the levels of haemoglobins A, A_2 and F. *J Med Genet.* 1972;9:154–159.

416. Pootrakul P, Wasi P, Na-Nakorn S. Haematological data in 312 cases of β thalassaemia trait in Thailand. *Br J Haematol.* 1973;24:703–712.

417. Bowdler AJ, Huehns ER. Thalassaemia major complicated by excessive iron storage. *Br J Haematol.* 1963;9:13–24.

418. Tolot F, Bocquet B, Baron M. Hemochromatosis and pigmentary cirrhosis in minor thalassemia in adults. *J Med Lyon.* 1970;51:655–660.

419. Fargion S, Piperno A, Panaiotopoulos N, Taddei MT, Fiorelli G. Iron overload in subjects with β-thalassaemia trait: role of idiopathic haemochromatosis gene. *Br J Haematol.* 1985;61:487–490.

420. Crosby WH, Conrad ME. Iron imbalance in thalassaemia minor. A preliminary report. *Ann NY Acad Sci.* 1964;119:616.

421. Vedovato M, Salvatorelli G, Taddei-Masieri M, Vullo C. Epo serum levels in heterozygous β-thalassemia. *Haematologia-Budap.* 1993;25:19–24.

422. Landman H. *Haemoglobinopathies and Pregnancy.* Groningen: Van Denderen Printing; 1988.

423. White JM, Richards R, Byrne M, Buchanan T, White YS, Jelenski G. Thalassaemia trait and pregnancy. *J Clin Pathol.* 1985;38:810–817.

424. Schuman JE, Tanser CL, Peloquin R, de Leeuw NKM. The erythropoietic response to pregnancy in β thalassaemia minor. *Br J Haematol.* 1973;25:249–260.

425. Chanarin I, Dacie JV, Mollin DL. Folic-acid deficiency in haemolytic anaemia. *Br J Haematol.* 1959;5:245–256.

426. Silva AE, Varella-Garcia M. Plasma folate and vitamin B12 levels in β-thalassemia heterozygotes. *Braz J Med Biol Res.* 1989;22:1225–1226.

427. Gallerani M, Cicognani I, Ballardini P, et al. Average life expectancy of heterozygous β thalassemia subjects. *Haematologica.* 1990;75:224–227.
428. Gallerani M, Scapoli C, Cicognani I, et al. Thalassaemia trait and myocardial infarction: low infarction incidence in male subjects confirmed. *J Intern Med.* 1991;230:109–111.
429. Tassiopoulos S, Deftereos S, Konstantopoulos K, et al. Does heterozygous beta-thalassemia confer a protection against coronary artery disease? *Ann NY Acad Sci.* 2005;1054:467–470.
430. Ceppellini R. Discussion. Biochemistry of human genetics. In: Wolstenholme GEW, O'Connor CM, eds. *Ciba Foundation Symposium.* Boston: Little, Brown; 1959:133–134.
431. Huisman THJ, Punt K, Schaad JDG. Thalassemia minor associated with hemoglobin B2 heterozygosity. *Blood.* 1961;17:747.
432. Weatherall DJ, Clegg JB, Milner PF, Marsh GW, Bolton FG, Serjeant GR. Linkage relationships between β- and δ-structural loci and African forms of thalassaemia. *J Med Genet.* 1976;13:20–26.
433. Codrington JF, Li H-W, Kutlar F, Gu L-H, Ramachandran M, Huisman THJ. Observations on the levels of Hb A_2 in patients with different β thalassemia mutations and a δ chain variant. *Blood.* 1990;76:1246–1249.
434. Wasi P, Disthasongchan P, Na-Nakorn S. The effect of iron deficiency on the levels of hemoglobins A_2 and E. *J Lab Clin Med.* 1968;71:85–91.
435. Steinberg MH. Case report: effects of iron deficiency and the −88 C→T mutation on Hb A_2 levels in β-thalassemia. *Am J Med Sci.* 1993;305:312–313.
436. Beaven GH, Ellis MJ, White JC. Studies in human foetal haemoglobin. III. The hereditary haemoglobinopathies and thalassaemia. *Br J Haematol.* 1961;7:169–186.
437. Wood WG, Weatherall DJ, Clegg JB. Interaction of heterocellular hereditary persistence of foetal haemoglobin with β thalassaemia and sickle cell anaemia. *Nature.* 1976;264:247–249.
438. Popat N, Wood WG, Weatherall DJ, Turnbull AC. The pattern of maternal F-cell production during pregnancy. *Lancet.* 1977;ii:377–379.
439. Selwyn JG, Dacie JV. Autohemolysis and other changes resulting from the incubation in vitro of red cells from patients with congenital hemolytic anemia. *Blood.* 1954;9(5):414–438.
440. Chapman SJ, Allison JV, Grimes AJ. Abnormal cation movements in human hypochromic red cells incubates *in vitro.* *Scand J Haematol.* 1973;10:225–231.
441. Gunn RB, Silvers ND, Rosse WF. Potassium permeability in β-thalassemia minor red blood cells. *J Clin Invest.* 1972;51:1043–1050.
442. Knox-Macaulay HHM, Weatherall DJ. Studies of red-cell membrane function in heterozygous β thalassaemia and other hypochromic anaemias. *Br J Haematol.* 1974;28:277–297.
443. Vettore L, Falezza GC, Cetto GL, de Matteis MC. Cation content and membrane deformability of heterozygous beta-thalassemia red blood cells. *Br J Haematol.* 1974;27:429–437.
444. Knox-Macaulay HHM, Weatherall DJ, Clegg JB, Bradley J, Brown MJ. Clinical and biosynthetic characterization of αβ-thalassaemia. *Br J Haematol.* 1972;22:497–512.
445. Kan YW, Nathan DG, Lodish HF. Equal synthesis of α and β globin chains in erythroid precursors in heterozygous β thalassemia. *J Clin Invest.* 1972;51:1906–1909.
446. Schwartz E. Heterozygous beta thalassemia: balanced globin synthesis in bone marrow cells. *Science.* 1970;167:1513–1514.
447. Chalevelakis G, Clegg JB, Weatherall DJ. Imbalanced globin chain synthesis in heterozygous β-thalassemia bone marrow. *Proc Natl Acad Sci USA.* 1975;72:3853–3857.
448. Chalevelakis G, Clegg JB, Weatherall DJ. Globin synthesis in normal human bone marrow. *Br J Haematol.* 1976;34:535–557.
449. Galanello R, Melis MA, Ruggeri R, Cao A. Prospective study of red blood cell indices, hemoglobin A_2 and hemoglobin F in infants heterozygous for b-thalassemia. *J Pediatr.* 1981;99:105–108.
450. Wood WG, Weatherall DJ, Hart GH, Bennett M, Marsh GW. Hematologic changes and hemoglobin analysis in β thalassemia heterozygotes during the first year of life. *Pediatr Res.* 1982;16:286–289.
451. Galanello R, Lilliu F, Bertolino F, Cao A. Percentile curves for red cell indices of β^0-thalassaemia heterozygotes in infancy and childhood. *J Pediatr.* 1991;150:413–415.
452. Metaxatou-Mavromati AD, Antonopoulou HK, Laskari SS, Tsiarta HK, Ladis VA, Kattamis CA. Developmental changes in hemoglobin F levels during the first two years of life in normal and heterozygous β-thalassemia infants. *Pediatrics.* 1982;69:734–738.
453. Rosatelli C, Leoni GB, Tuveri T, et al. Heterozygous β-thalassemia: relationship between the hematological phenotype and the type of β-thalassemia mutation. *Am J Hematol.* 1992;39:1–4.
454. Rund D, Filon D, Dowling C, Kazazian HHJ, Rachmilewitz EA, Oppenheim A. Molecular studies of β-thalassemia in Israel. Mutational analysis and expression studies. *Ann NY Acad Sci.* 1990;612:98–105.
455. Stefanis L, Kanavakis E, Traeger-Synodinos J, Tzetis M, Metaxotou-Mavromati A, Kattamis C. I: Hematologic phenotype of the mutations IVS1-n6 (T→C), IVS1-n110 (G→A), and CD39 (C→T) in carriers of beta-thalassemia in Greece. *Pediatr Hematol Oncol.* 1994;11:509–517.
456. Huisman THJ. Levels of Hb A_2 in heterozygotes and homozygotes for beta-thalassemia mutations: influence of mutations in the CACCC and ATAAA motifs of the beta-globin gene promoter. *Acta Haematol.* 1997;98:187–194.
457. Kutlar A, Kutlar F, Gu L-G, Mayson SM, Huisman TH. Fetal hemoglobin in normal adults and β-thalassemia heterozygotes. *Hum Genet.* 1990;85:106–110.
458. Piomelli S, Siniscalco M. The haematological effects of glucose-6-phosphate dehydrogenase deficiency and thalassaemia trait: interaction between the two genes at the phenotype level. *Br J Haematol.* 1969;16:537–549.
459. Sanna G, Frau F, Melis MA, Galanello R, de Virgiliis S, Cao A. Interaction between glucose-6-phosphate dehydrogenase deficiency and thalassaemia genes at phenotype level. *Br J Haematol.* 1980;44:555–561.
460. Galanello R, Perseu L, Melis MA, et al. Hyperbilirubinaemia in heterozygous β-thalassaemia is related to co-inherited Gilbert's syndrome. *Br J Haematol.* 1997;99:433–436.
461. Frick P. Congenital elliptocytosis. Elliptocytosis and thalassemia in the same family. *Schweiz Med Wschr.* 1970;100:1009–1012.

462. Pavri RS, Baxi AJ, Grover S, Parande RA. Study of glycolytic intermediates in hereditary elliptocytosis with thalassemia. *J Postgrad Med.* 1977;23:189–192.
463. Ros G, Seynhaeve V, Fiasse L. Beta$^+$-thalassaemia, haemoglobin A and hereditary elliptocytosis in a Zairian family. Ischaemic costal necroses in a child with sickle-cell beta$^+$ thalassaemia. *Acta Haematol.* 1976;56:241–252.
464. Perillie PE, Chernoff AI. Heterozygous beta-thalassemia in association with hereditary elliptocytosis. *Blood.* 1965;25:494–501.
465. Aksoy M, Eredem S. Combination of hereditary elliptocytosis and heterozygous beta-thalassaemia: a family study. *J Med Genet.* 1968;5:298–301.
466. Cohen F, Zuelzer WW, Neel JV, Robinson AR. Multiple inherited erythrocyte abnormalities in an American Negro family: hereditary spherocytosis, sickling and thalassemia. *Blood.* 1959;14:816–827.
467. Cunningham TA, Vella F. Combination of spherocytosis and a variant of beta thalassaemia ('isolated raised Hb A2'). *J Med Genet.* 1967;4:109.
468. Swarup-Mitra S, Ghosh SK, Chatterjea JB. Haemolytic anaemia due to interaction of genes for spherocytosis and beta-thalassaemia. *Indian J Med Res.* 1969;57.
469. Baughan MA, Paglia DE, Schneider AS, Valentine WN. An unusual haematological syndrome with pyruvate-kinase deficiency and thalassaemia minor in the kindreds. *Acta Haematol.* 1968;39:345–358.
470. Zoratto E, Norelli MT, Lumare A. Hemolytic anemia caused by association of a double anomaly beta-thalassemia and deficiency of G6PD. *Minerva Pediatr.* 1969;21:605–610.
471. Kattamis C, Metaxatou-Mavromati A, Wood WG, Nash JR, Weatherall DJ. The heterogeneity of normal Hb A_2-β thalassaemia in Greece. *Br J Haematol.* 1979;42:109–123.
472. Schwartz E. The silent carrier of beta thalassaemia. *N Engl J Med.* 1969;281:1327–1333.
473. Silvestroni E, Bianco I, Graziani B, Carboni C. Heterozygous β-thalassaemia with normal haemoglobin pattern. *Acta Haematol.* 1978;59:332–340.
474. Tzetis M, Traeger-Synodinos J, Kanavakis E, Metaxotou-Mavromati A, Kattamis C. The molecular basis of normal Hb A_2 (type 2) β-thalassemia in Greece. *Hematol Pathol.* 1994;8:25–34.
475. Loudianos G, Cao A, Ristaldi MS, et al. Molecular basis of $\delta\beta$-thalassemia with normal fetal hemoglobin. *Blood.* 1990;75:526–528.
476. Trifillis P, Ioannou P, Schwartz E, Surrey S. Identification of four novel δ-globin gene mutations in Greek Cypriots using polymerase chain reaction and automated fluorescence-based DNA sequence analysis. *Blood.* 1991;78:3298–3305.
477. Schokker RC, Went LN, Bok J. A new genetic variant of beta-thalassaemia. *Nature.* 1966;209:44–46.
478. Kanavakis E, Wainscoat JS, Wood WG, et al. The interaction of α thalassaemia with heterozygous β thalassaemia. *Br J Haematol.* 1982;52:465–473.
479. Melis MA, Pirastu M, Galanello R, Furbetta M, Tuveri T, Cao A. Phenotypic effect of heterozygous α and β^0-thalassemia interaction. *Blood.* 1983;62:226–229.
480. Gasperini D, Cao A, Paderi L, et al. Normal individuals with high Hb A_2 levels. *Br J Haematol.* 1993;84:166–168.
481. Murru S, Loudianos G, Porcu S, et al. A β-thalassaemia phenotype not linked to the β-globin cluster in an Italian family. *Br J Haematol.* 1992;81:283–287.
482. Schwartz E, Cohen A, Surrey S. Overview of the β thalassemias: genetic and clinical aspects. *Hemoglobin.* 1988;12:551–564.
483. Semenza GL, Delgrosso K, Poncz M, Mallidi P, Schwartz E, Surrey S. The silent carrier allele: β thalassemia without a mutation in the β-globin gene or its immediate flanking regions. *Cell.* 1984;39:123–128.
484. Thein SL, Wood WG, Wickramasinghe SN, Galvin MC. β-thalassemia unlinked to the β-globin gene in an English family. *Blood.* 1993;82:961–967.
485. Kazazian HH. The thalassemia syndromes: molecular basis and prenatal diagnosis in 1990. *Semin Hematol.* 1990;27:209–228.
486. Galanello R, Barella S, Ideo A, et al. Genotype of subjects with borderline hemoglobin A_2 levels: Implication for β-thalassemia carrier screening. *Am J Hematol.* 1994;46:79–81.
487. Weatherall DJ, Clegg JB. Thalassemia – a global public health problem. *Nat Med.* 1996;2(8):847–849.
488. Cao A, Galanello R, Rosatelli MC. Prenatal diagnosis and screening of the haemoglobinopathies. *Clin Haematol.* 1998;11:215–238.
489. Pootrakul P, Kitcharoen K, Yansukon P, et al. The effect of erythroid hyperplasia on iron balance. *Blood.* 1988;71:1124–1129.
490. Fosburg MT, Nathan DG. Treatment of Cooley's anemia. *Blood.* 1990;76:435–444.
491. Cazzola M, Borgna-Pignatti C, Locatelli F, Ponchio L, Beguin Y, De-Stefano P. A moderate transfusion regimen may reduce iron loading in β-thalassemia major without producing excessive expansion of erythropoiesis. *Transfusion.* 1997;37:135–140.
492. Piomelli S, Seaman C, Reibman J, Tyrun A, Graziano J, Tabachnik N. Separation of younger red cells with improved survival *in vivo*: an approach to chronic transfusion therapy. *Proc Natl Acad Sci USA.* 1978;75:3474–3478.
493. Cohen AR, Schmidt JM, Martin MB, Barnsley W, Schwartz E. Clinical trial of young red cell transfusions. *J Pediatr.* 1984;104:865–868.
494. Simon TL, Sohmer P, Nelson EF. Extended survival of neocytes produced by a new system. *Transfusion.* 1989;29:221–225.
495. Kevy SV, Jacobson MS, Fosburg M, et al. A new approach to neocyte transfusion: preliminary report. *J Clin Apher.* 1988;4:194–197.
496. Spanos T, Ladis V, Palamidou F, et al. The impact of neocyte transfusion in the management of thalasssaemia. *Vox Sang.* 1996;70:217–223.
497. Collins AF, Dias GC, Haddad S, et al. Evaluation of a new neocyte transfusion preparation vs. washed cell transfusion in patients with homozygous beta thalassemia. *Transfusion.* 1994;34:517–520.
498. Graziano JH, Piomelli S, Hilgartner M, et al. Chelation therapy in beta-thalassemia major. III. The role of splenectomy in achieving iron balance. *J Pediatr.* 1981;99:695–699.
499. Okon E, Levij IS, Rachmilewitz EA. Splenectomy, iron overload and liver cirrhosis in beta-thalassemia major. *Acta Haematol.* 1976;56:142–150.

500. Pootrakul P, Rugkiatsakul R, Wasi P. Increased tranbsferrin iron saturation in splenectomized thalassaemia patients. *Br J Haematol.* 1980;46:143–145.
501. Borgna-Pignatti C, de Stefano P, Bongo IG, Avato F, Cazzola M. Spleen iron content is low in thalassemia. *Am J Pediatr Hematol Oncol.* 1984;6:340–343.
502. Politis C, Spigos DG, Georgiopoulou P, et al. Partial splenic embolisation for hypersplenism of thalassaemia major: five year follow-up. *Br Med J.* 1987;294:665–667.
503. de Montalembert M, Gitor R, Revillon Y, et al. Partial splenectomy in homozygous β thalassemia. *Arch Dis Child.* 1990;65:304–307.
504. Kheradpir MH, Albouyeh M. Partial splenectomy in the treatment of thalassaemia major. *Kinderchirurgie.* 1985;40:195–198.
505. Porter J, Huehns ER. The toxic effects of desferrioxamine. *Clin Haematol.* 1989;2:459–474.
506. Loreal O, Deugnier Y, Moirand R, et al. Liver fibrosis in genetic hemochromatosis. Respective roles of iron and non-iron related factors in 127 homozygous patients. *J Hepatol.* 1992;16:122–127.
507. Niederau C, Fischer R, Purschel A, Stremmel W, Haussinger D, Strohmeyer G. Long-term survival in patients with hereditary hemochromatosis. *Gastroenterology.* 1996;110:1304–1307.
508. Cartwright GE, Edwards CQ, Kravitz K, et al. Hereditary hemochromatosis: phenotypic expression of the disease. *N Engl J Med.* 1979;301:175–179.
509. Araujo A, Kosaryan M, MacDowell A, et al. A novel delivery system for continuous desferrioxamine infusion in transfusional iron overload. *Br J Haematol.* 1996;93:835–837.
510. Lombardo T, Frontini V, Ferro G, Sergi P, Guidice A, Lombardo G. Laboratory evaluation of a new delivery system to improve patient compliance with chelation therapy. *Clin Lab Haematol.* 1996;18:13–17.
511. Shalit M, Tedeschi A, Miadonna A, Levi-Shaffer A. Desferal (desferrioxamine) – A novel activator of connective tissue-type mast cells. *J Allergy Clin Immunol.* 1991;6:854–860.
512. Bousquet J, Navarro M, Robert G, Aye P, Michel FB. Rapid desensitization for desferrioxamine anaphylactoid reactions. *Lancet.* 1983;ii:859–860.
513. Lombardo T, Ferro G, Frontini V, Percolla S. High-dose intravenous desferrioxamine (DFO) delivery in four thalassemic patients allergic to subcutaneous DFO administration. *Am J Hematol.* 1996;51:90–92.
514. Miller KB, Rosenwasser LJ, Bessette JA, Beer DJ, Rocklin RE. Rapid desensitisation for desferrioxamine anaphylactic reaction. *Lancet.* 1981;i:1059.
515. Davis BA, Porter JB. Long-term outcome of continuous 24-hour deferoxamine infusion via indwelling intravenous catheters in high-risk beta-thalassemia. *Blood.* 2000; 95(4):1229–1236.
516. Olivieri NF. Long-term follow-up of body iron in patients with thalassemia major during therapy with the orally active iron chelator deferiprone (L1). *Blood.* 1996;88:310a.
517. Olivieri NF. Randomized trial of deferiprone (L1) and deferoxamine (DFO) in thalssemia major. *Blood.* 1996;88:651a.
518. Hoffbrand AV, al-Refaie F, Davis B, et al. Long-term trial of deferiprone in 51 transfusion-dependent iron overloaded patients. *Blood.* 1998;91:295–300.
519. Hoffbrand AV, Cohen A, Hershko C. Role of deferiprone in chelation therapy for transfusional iron overload. *Blood.* 2003;102(1):17–24.
520. Choudhry VP, Pati HP, Saxena A, Malaviya AN. Deferiprone, efficacy and safety. *Indian J Pediatr.* 2004;71(3):213–216.
521. Borgna-Pignatti C, Cappellini MD, De Stefano P, et al. Cardiac morbidity and mortality in deferoxamine- or deferiprone-treated patients with thalassemia major. *Blood.* 2006;107(9):3733–3737.
522. Pennell DJ, Berdoukas V, Karagiorga M, et al. Randomized controlled trial of deferiprone or deferoxamine in beta-thalassemia major patients with asymptomatic myocardial siderosis. *Blood.* 2006;107(9):3738–3744.
523. Neufeld EJ. Oral chelators deferasirox and deferiprone for transfusional iron overload in thalassemia major: new data, new questions. *Blood.* 2006;107(9):3436–3441.
524. Nisbet-Brown E, Olivieri NF, Giardina PJ, et al. Effectiveness and safety of ICL670 in iron-loaded patients with thalassaemia: a randomised, double-blind, placebo-controlled, dose-escalation trial. *Lancet.* 2003;361(9369):1597–1602.
525. Piga A, Galanello R, Cappellini MD, et al. Phase II study of ICL670, an oral chelator, in adult thalassaemia patients with transfusional iron overload: efficacy, safety, pharmaco kinetics (PK) and pharmacodynamics (PD) after 18 months of therapy. *Blood.* 2003;102:121a (Abstract 412).
526. Weatherall D, Kwiatkowski D, Roberts D. Hematologic manifestations of systemic disaeses in children of the developing world. In: Orkin SH, Ginsburg D, Nathan DG, Look AT, Fisher DE, Lux SE, eds. *Nathan and Oski's Hematology of Infancy and Childhood.* 7th ed. Elsevier; 2008:in press.
527. Tin F, Magrin S, Crax A, Pagliaro L. Interferon for non-A, non-B chronic hepatitis: a meta-analysis of randomized clinical trials. *J Hepatol.* 1991;13:192–199.
528. Di Marco V, Lo Iacono O, Almasio P, et al. Long-term efficacy of α-Interferon in β-thalassemics with chronic hepatitis C. *Blood.* 1997;90:2207–2212.
529. Donohue SM, Wonke B, Hoffbrand AV, et al. Alpha interferon in the treatment of chronic hepatitis C infection in thalassaemia major. *Br J Haematol.* 1993;83:491–497.
530. Preston H, Wright TL. Interferon therapy for hepatitis C. *Lancet.* 1996;348:973–974.
531. Sherlock S. Antiviral therapy for chronic hepatitis C viral infection. *J Hepatol.* 1995;23:3–7.
532. Butensky E, Pakbaz Z, Foote D, Walters MC, Vichinsky EP, Harmatz P. Treatment of hepatitis C virus infection in thalassemia. *Ann NY Acad Sci.* 2005;1054:290–299.
533. Orvieto R, Leichter I, Rachmilewitz EA, Margulies JY. Bone density, mineral content, and cortical index in patients with thalassemia major and the correlation to their bone fractures, blood transfusions, and treatment with desferrioxamine. *Calcif Tissue Int.* 1992;50:397–399.
534. Catanan D, Akar N, Arcasoy A. Effects of calcitonin therapy on osteoporosis in patients with thalassemia. *Acta Haematol.* 1995;93:20–24.
535. Saxon BR, Rees D, Olivieri NF. Regression of extramedullary haemopoiesis and augmentation of fetal haemoglobin concentration during hydroxyurea therapy in β thalassaemia. *Br J Haematol.* 1998;101:416–419.

536. Quek L, Thein SL. Molecular therapies in beta-thalassaemia. *Br J Haematol.* 2007;136(3):353–365.
537. Olivieri NF, Rees DC, Ginder GD, et al. Treatment of thalassaemia major with phenylbutyrate and hydroxyurea. *Lancet.* 1997;350:491–492.
538. Efremov DG, Efremov GD, Zisovski N, et al. Variation in clinical severity among patients with Hb Lepore-Boston-β-thalassaemia is related to the type of β-thalassaemia. *Br J Haematol.* 1988;68:351–355.
539. Henthorn PS, Smithies O, Nakatsuji T, et al. $(^{A}\gamma\delta\beta)^0$-Thalassaemia in Blacks is due to a deletion of 34 kbp of DNA. *Br J Haematol.* 1985;59:343–356.
540. Cao A, Melis MA, Galanello R, et al. δβ(F)-thalassaemia in Sardinia. *J Med Genet.* 1982;19:184–192.
541. Traeger-Synodinos J, Tzetis M, Kanavakis E, Metaxotou-Mavromati A, Kattamis C. The Corfu δβ thalassaemia mutation in Greece: haematological phenotype and prevalence. *Br J Haematol.* 1991;79:302–305.
542. Tzetis M, Traeger-Synodinos J, Kanavakis E, Metaxotou-Mavromati A, Kattamis C. The molecular basis of normal Hb A_2 (type 2) β-thalassemia in Greece. *Hematol Pathol.* 1994;8:25–34.
543. Trent RJ, Williams BG, Kearney A, Wilkinson T, Harris PC. Molecular and hematologic characterization of Scottish-Irish type $(\varepsilon\gamma\delta\beta)^0$ thalassemia. *Blood.* 1990;76:2132–2138.
544. Charache S, Clegg JB, Weatherall DJ. The Negro variety of hereditary persistence of fetal haemoglobin is a mild form of thalassaemia. *Br J Haematol.* 1976;34:527.
545. Wainscoat JS, Old JM, Wood WG, Trent RJ, Weatherall DJ. Characterization of an Indian $(\delta\beta)^0$ thalassaemia. *Br J Haematol.* 1984;58:353–360.

18

Hemoglobin E Disorders

Suthat Fucharoen and David J. Weatherall

INTRODUCTION

Hemoglobin E (HbE) is the most common abnormal hemoglobin in Southeast Asians, especially among the Khmer, Laotians, and Mon/Khmer speaking people, the Zhuang in Guangxi, People's Republic of China, and in India, Bangladesh, and Sri Lanka. The occurrence of HbE is most concentrated at the border of Thailand, Laos, and Cambodia, an area dubbed the HbE triangle.[1–4] The gene frequency of HbE is between 0.05 and 0.10, reaching 0.5 in certain parts of Cambodia and the northeast of Thailand. It is estimated that 30 million Southeast Asians are heterozygous for HbE and 1 million are homozygous. The maintenance of so high a gene frequency indicates that the HbE variant somehow improves fitness. Correlation of HbE frequency with the incidence of malaria has been noted, suggesting the action of a balanced polymorphism.[5] Studies of malaria and HbE are detailed in Chapter 26.

CLASSIFICATION OF HbE DISORDERS

In 1954, HbE became the fourth abnormal hemoglobin to be identified by electrophoresis,[6] and a substitution of lysine for glutamic acid at position 26 of the β-globin chain was found in 1961.[7] Many different syndromes are observed when HbE is variously combined with different α and β thalassemias and with other abnormal hemoglobins (Fig. 18.1). They can be classified into asymptomatic and symptomatic forms (Table 18.1).

Asymptomatic Forms

HbE Heterozygotes. HbE heterozygotes are clinically normal with minimal changes in blood counts and erythrocyte indices. Red cell morphology is similar to that in thalassemia minor with normocytic or slightly microcytic red cells (mean corpuscular volume [MCV] 84 ± 5 fL). A few target cells may be present in the blood smear. Osmotic fragility curves may be within normal limits or moderately shifted to the right, indicating slightly decreased osmotic fragility. Hemoglobin electrophoresis reveals both HbA and HbE. Quantifying the amount of HbE is crucial for the diagnosis of various HbE syndromes that occur from the interaction of HbE with other genetic hemoglobin abnormalities and nongenetic factors (Table 18.2). HbE constitutes 25%–30% of the hemolysate in HbE trait and with double heterozygosity for HbE and α^+ thalassemia ($-\alpha/\alpha\alpha$). HbE–α^+ thalassemia trait cannot be differentiated from simple HbE trait by hematological screening. The amount of HbE is reduced by coexistent α thalassemia. Lower levels of HbE suggest concomitant inheritance of the α^0 thalassemia ($--/\alpha\alpha$) gene.[8,9] In double heterozygotes for α^0 thalassemia and HbE, the amount of HbE ranges between 19% and 21%. A marked decrease of HbE to 13%–15% is observed in individuals who are double heterozygotes for HbH disease and HbE and have the HbAE Bart's disease syndrome.[10–12] Interactions between HbE and various α thalassemia genes are illustrated in Figure 18.2. HbE levels of 30% or above suggest the interaction of HbE with β thalassemia.[13–16] HbE heterozygotes who have iron deficiency anemia may have lowered amounts of HbE and further reduced MCV and mean corpuscular hemoglobin (MCH) values, depending on the degree of anemia.[17] The changes in the hematological parameters and amount of HbE in compound heterozygotes of HbE with other abnormal hemoglobins are summarized later in this chapter.

Homozygous HbE. Homozygotes for HbE usually have normal hemoglobin levels but some may be mildly anemic; clinical symptoms are rare. Most patients are not jaundiced and the liver and spleen are usually not enlarged. Reticulocyte counts are consistently normal, and nucleated red cells are not seen in the blood. Bone marrow examination shows a normal cellular pattern or minimal erythrocytic hyperplasia. Bone changes are not present. Osmotic fragility studies show a marked increase in the resistance of erythrocytes to hypotonic saline, indicating decreased osmotic fragility. In addition to a slightly reduced hemoglobin level and microcytic, poorly hemoglobinized red cells[18–20] (Table 18.2), the most unique finding is the red cell morphology, with 20%–80% target red cells (Fig. 18.3). Hemoglobin analysis reveals approximately 85%–95% HbE with the remainder HbF. There is defective β^E-globin chain synthesis in all HbE homozygotes with an average α/non-α biosynthesis ratio of 2, equivalent to the ratio found in β^+ thalassemia heterozygotes.[18–21] Defective β^E-chain synthesis is due to decreased β^E mRNA production, a result of abnormal RNA splicing caused by the HbE mutation[22–24] (see Chapter 16).

Symptomatic Forms

HbE–β Thalassemia. Generally, HbE–β thalassemia disease is a thalassemia syndrome of intermediate severity, although the clinical spectrum can be very heterogeneous.[14,16] Two types of HbE–β thalassemia disease have

Table 18.1. Summary of the common HbE syndromes in Thailand

Phenotype	Genotype	Anemia	Distinguishing features
Asymptomatic			
HbE heterozygote	β^A/β^E	No	Hbs E (25–30%) + A
HbE $-\alpha^+$ thalassemia heterozygote	β^A/B^E $-\alpha/\alpha\alpha$	No	Hbs E (25–30%) + A
HbE $-\alpha^0$ thalassemia heterozygote	β^A/B^E $--/\alpha\alpha$	No	Hbs E (19–21%) + A
HbE homozygote	β^E/β^E	No	only HbE
HbE homozygote $-\alpha^+$ or α^0 thalassemia heterozygote	β^E/β^E $-\alpha/\alpha\alpha$ or $--/\alpha\alpha$	No	only HbE
HbE/Hb C	β^E/β^C	No	HbE (32%) + Hb C(56%)
Symptomatic			
HbE homozygote-Hb CS homozygote	β^E/β^E $-\alpha^{CS}\alpha/\alpha^{CS}\alpha$	Mild	Hbs E $(\alpha_2\beta_2{}^E) + \alpha_2{}^{CS}\beta_2{}^E$
β^0 Thalassemia/HbE	β^o/β^E	Moderate–severe	Hbs E + F
$\beta+$ Thalassemia/HbE	$\beta+/\beta^E$	Mild	Hbs E + F + A
EA Bart's			
- HbH disease with HbE heterozygote	$-\alpha/--$ β^A/β^E	Moderate	Hbs E + A + Bart's
- HbH-CS disease with HbE heterozygote	$\alpha^{CS}\alpha/--$ β^A/β^E	Moderate	Hbs CS + E + A + Bart's
EF Bart's			
- HbH disease with HbE homozygote	$-\alpha/--$ β^E/β^E	Moderate–severe	Hbs E + F + Bart's
- Hb H-CS disease with HbE homozygote	$\alpha^{CS}\alpha/--$ β^E/β^E	Moderate–severe	Hbs CS + E + F + Bart's
- HbH disease with β thal/HbE disease	$-\alpha/--$ β^o/β^E	Moderate–severe	Hbs E + F + Bart's
- HbH-CS disease with β thal/HbE disease	$\alpha^{CS}\alpha/--$ β^o/β^E	Moderate–severe	Hbs CS + E + F + Bart's

CS = Hb Constant Spring.

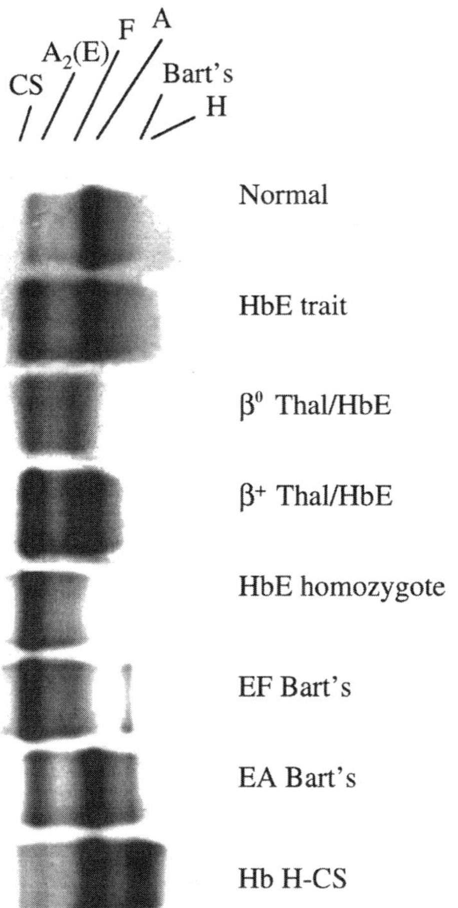

Figure 18.1. Hemoglobin types of various HbE syndromes performed by electrophoresis in an alkaline pH buffer.

been described that depend on the presence or absence of HbA. In HbE–β^0 thalassemia, β^A-globin chains are not present. This genotype results in HbE–β^0 thalassemia disease characterized by HbE and HbF without detectable HbA (Fig. 18.1). HbE constitutes between 40% and 60% of the hemolysate with the remainder HbF (Table 18.2). Clinically, HbE–β^0 thalassemia and homozygous HbE are quite different; the latter is asymptomatic and the level of HbF much lower. In exceptionally rare cases the amount of HbE in HbE–β^0 thalassemia and homozygous HbE may overlap, requiring family studies and further investigation to define the genotype. In HbE–β^+ thalassemia, some HbA is detected in addition to HbE and HbF. Different β^+-thalassemia genes result in a variable severity of disease because of different levels of HbA.[25]

HbAE Bart's Diseases. Because α chains appear to have a lower affinity for β^E chains than β^A chains, HbE heterozygotes who inherit different forms of α thalassemia, and in whom α chain synthesis is decreased, tend to have relatively lower levels of HbE than in unaffected HbE heterozygotes. This particular thalassemia syndrome is characterized by the presence of HbA, HbE, and Hb Bart's and results from the interaction of the genotype of HbH disease with heterozygous HbE.[10–12] Two common subtypes of HbAE Bart's disease have been observed: α^+ thalassemia/α^0 thalassemia $-\beta^A/\beta^E$ and α^0 thalassemia/Hb Constant Spring – β^A/β^E. The latter disorder has a more severe clinical syndrome than the former type of HbAE Bart's disease. Usually the HbE level ranges from 13% to 15% (Table 18.2). Small amounts of Hb Bart's are always present in this genotype and intraerythrocytic inclusion bodies (HbH inclusions) can be demonstrated in approximately 5% of the

Table 18.2. Hematological data in various Hb EHbE syndromes

	Hb (g/dL)	MCV (fL)	MCH (pg)	MCHC (g/dL)	RDW (%)	Osmotic fragility	DCIP	Alkaline denaturation test (%)	Hb typing
Normal	M15.9 ± 0.9 F12.5 ± 2.0	87 ± 6	31 ± 1.1	33 ± 0.9	13.1 ± 0.8	N	–	0.5 ± 0.2	A_2 (2.5 ± 0.2) + A
HbE trait	12.8 ± 1.5	84 ± 5	30 ± 2.4	33 ± 1.8	14.1 ± 0.6	N or D	+	0.9 ± 0.7	E (29.4 ± 2.3%) + A
HbE trait $-\alpha/\alpha\alpha$	13.1 ± 1.4	88 ± 4	ND	ND	ND	N or D	+		E (28.5 ± 1.5%) + A
HbE trait $--/\alpha\alpha$	12.5 ± 1.4	77 ± 5	23 ± 1.1	32 ± 1.6	ND	D	+	0.9 ± 0.4	E (20.7 ± 1.2%) + A
Homozygous HbE	11.4 ± 1.8	70 ± 4	22 ± 1.9	33 ± 1.7	15.6	D	+	1.8 ± 1.4	EE (E87.7 ± 5.9%)
β^o thal/HbE	7.8 ± 2.6	67 ± 6	19 ± 3.6	28 ± 4.8	26.5 ± 5.6	D	+	42 ± 11.5	E (58±11.5%) + F
EA Bart's disease $-\alpha/--\ \beta^A/\beta^E$ or $\alpha^{CS}\alpha/--\ \beta^A/\beta^E$	9.1 ± 1.1	60 ± 3	17 ± 2	31 ± 4	ND	D	+	2.0 ± 0.7	E (13.0 ± 2.1%) + A + Bart (2.2 ± 1.8%)
EF Bart's disease $-\alpha/--\ \beta^E/\beta^E$ or $\alpha^{CS}/--\ \beta^E/\beta^E$	8.0 ± 0.9	67 ± 4	19 ± 2	29 ± 2	ND	D	+	2.3 ± 1.4	CS (1.1 ± 0.4%) + E (13.9 ± 1.8%) + A + Bart's (3.9 ± 1.5%)
	8.0 ± 1.3	63 ± 6	18 ± 2	29 ± 2	ND	D	+	5.8 ± 3.7	E (80%) + F + Bart's (5%) or CS (1.9 ± 0.9%) + E (86.4 ± 8%) + F + Bart's (3.7 ± 1.9%)

ND = not determined; N = normal; D = decreased.

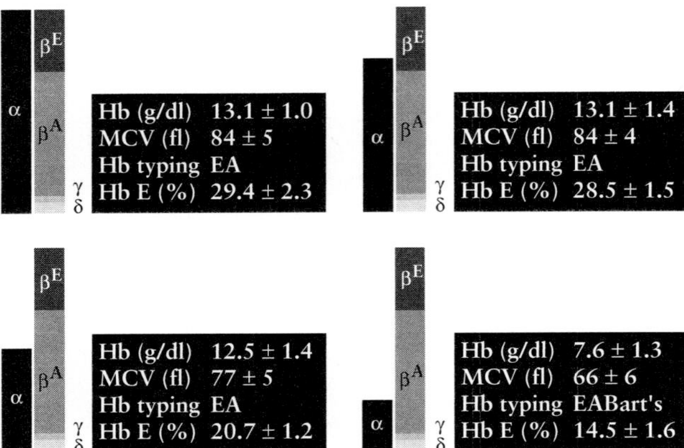

Figure 18.2. HbE heterozygote versus α thalassemia. Interaction of different α thalassemia genes and HbE heterozygote leads to changes in the hematologic parameters.

erythrocytes, indicating the presence of small amounts of HbH (β_4); this amount is insufficient to be resolved by electrophoresis.

HbEF Bart's Disease. HbEF Bart's disease is characterized by HbE, HbF, and Hb Bart's.[10] HbE constitutes 80% and HbF 10% of the hemolysate, with the remainder Hb Bart's. The presence of Hb Bart's indicates that there is excess γ-globin chain; however, no inclusion bodies or HbH are present, probably because the abnormal β^E-globin chains do not form tetramers. Four genotypes of HbEF Bart's disease can be found. These result from the interaction between the genotype for HbH disease, either α^0 thalassemia/α^+ thalassemia or α^0 thalassemia/Hb Constant Spring, with either homozygous HbE or HbE–β thalassemia.[26] Hb Constant Spring and small amounts of HbA may be observed in patients with the α^0 thalassemia/Hb Constant Spring and HbE–β^+ thalassemia genotype. To differentiate among these genotypes, family studies and further investigation by DNA analysis are required.

Homozygous HbE–Homozygous Hb Constant Spring Syndrome. It is difficult to identify the existence of the α thalassemia gene in homozygous HbE without DNA analysis. Individuals have been encountered who were homozygous for HbE and homozygous for Hb Constant Spring. They had thalassemia intermedia with a mild degree of anemia, jaundice, and splenomegaly. Their MCV ranged from 75 to 80 fL, and their MCH was between 23 and 25 pg (Table 18.2). Compared with homozygous HbE alone there were minimal red cell changes. This may be due to the interaction of α thalassemia with the β thalassemia–like reduced globin synthesis typical of HbE.

HEMOGLOBIN E–β THALASSEMIA

Because of the extremely high gene frequency for HbE and the widespread occurrence of β thalassemia, in many Asian countries HbE–β thalassemia is the most common form of severe thalassemia in the population. For example, in parts of India, Bangladesh, Myanmar, Thailand, and Indonesia it is the most common severe form of β thalassemia. In these countries it is causing an increasingly serious burden on healthcare resources and, because of its extraordinary phenotypic diversity, presents particular management problems.[16,25]

Pathophysiology

Individuals homozygous for HbE are usually clinically normal but compound heterozygotes with HbE–β thalassemia may have thalassemia major.[14] The abnormal β^E gene results in reduced amounts of β^E-mRNA and β^E-globin chains, leading to a mild β^+ thalassemia phenotype.[21,23] This occurs because the G→A mutation in codon 26 (Glu→Lys) of the β^E-globin gene activates a cryptic splice site at codon 25, leading to alternative mRNA splicing with reduced β^E-globin chain production[22] (see Chapter 16). A reduction in β^E-chain synthesis results in α/β synthesis ratios from 1.2 to 2.1 in HbE heterozygotes. In addition to the reduction of β^E-globin chains, the tertiary conformation of the HbE molecule is also affected. This is because the inhibitory effect of the β-26 substitution on the α1β1 contact may lead to the exposure of certain sulfhydryl groups and precipitation under conditions of oxidative stress.[27] The phenotypic implications of the inherent instability of HbE are not clear and require further investigation. Finally, the low percentage of HbE may also be partly attributed to the defective assembly of α_2 $\beta^E{}_2$ tetramers[28] (see Chapter 4).

The pathophysiology of HbE–β thalassemia therefore reflects both the reduced output of HbE together with the added globin-chain imbalance consequent on the coinheritance of β thalassemia. Hence the pathophysiology of this condition has many features in common with that of the intermediate forms of β thalassemia (see Chapter 17). As well as the deleterious effects of excess α globin chain production the inherent instability of HbE, as described previously, undoubtedly contributes to the overall damage to erythroid precursors and red cells. On the other hand, patients with this condition appear to be able to adapt more effectively to their anemia than those with other forms of β thalassemia intermedia at similar hemoglobin levels. This may reflect the relatively lower levels of HbF that are produced in HbE–β thalassemia and hence the lower oxygen affinity of the red cells.[16] Recent studies have also suggested that developmental changes in erythropoietin response to severe anemia in this condition may have important pathophysiological implications. It was found that hemoglobin levels and age are independent variables and that, for a given hemoglobin level, the erythropoietin response decreases with increasing age. Hence the hematopoietic drive, with resultant erythroid expansion, is greater in very young children with this condition, possibly explaining some of the phenotypic instability during early life.[29]

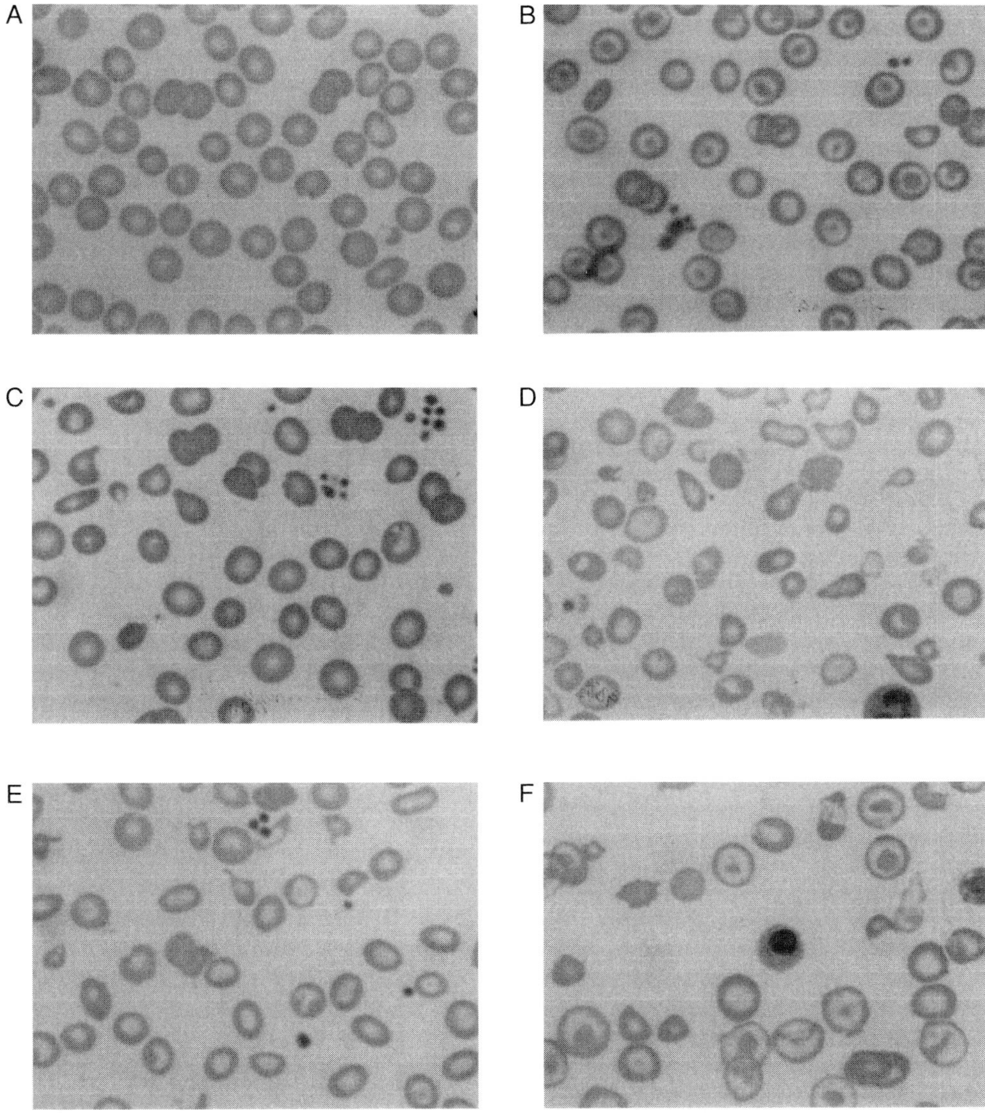

Figure 18.3. Morphology of red cells with Wright's staining in various HbE syndromes. **(A)** HbE heterozygote; **(B)** HbE homozygote; **(C)** HbE–α thalassemia-1; **(D)** HbE–β thalassemia; **(E)** AE Bart's disease; **(F)** EF Bart's disease.

Genotype–Phenotype Interaction

Definition of Severity. Despite seemingly identical genotypes, compound heterozygotes for β thalassemia and HbE have remarkably variable phenotypes. Notable are variations in anemia, growth, development, hepatosplenomegaly, and transfusion requirements (Fig. 18.4). A novel scoring system based on six independent parameters – hemoglobin level, age at disease presentation, age at receiving first blood transfusion, requirement for transfusion, spleen size, growth and development – was able to separate patients into three distinctive severity categories: mild, moderate and severe courses. The scoring system consisting of six clinical criteria scored as 0, 0.5, 1 or 2, according to clinical presentation. HbE–β thalassemia patients with total scores ranging from 0 to 3.5, 4 to 7, and 7.5 to 10 are grouped as mild, moderate, and severe cases, respectively. The severe patients are very anemic and are usually transfusion dependent; some may have marked growth retardation and skeletal deformities, whereas the mild cases have mild anemia and usually have normal growth and development.[30] A spectrum of severity with hemoglobin levels from 2.5 to 13.5 g/dL, in the steady state, was found in 803 patients with HbE–β^0 thalassemia.[14] Because β^0 thalassemia is associated with an absence of β-globin chain synthesis, the causes of phenotype heterogeneity in these patients is likely to be a result of factors other than reduced β-globin chain synthesis.

As suggested by recent studies in Sri Lanka, the application of a clearly defined scoring system for severity

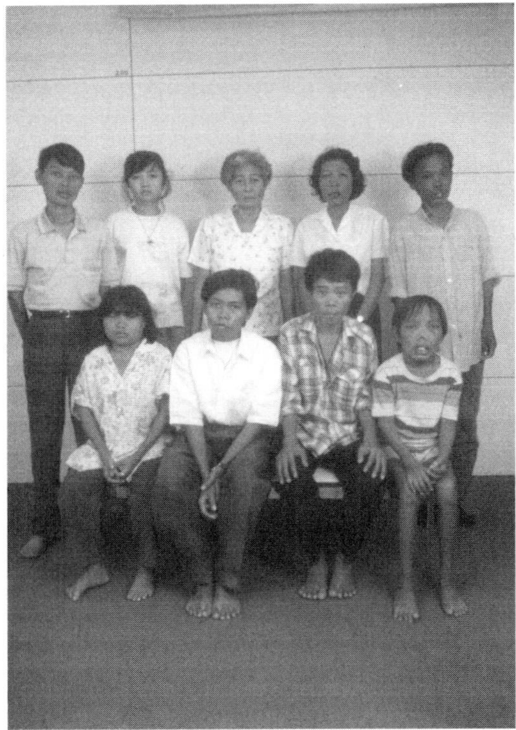

Figure 18.4. A group of β-thalassemia patients with variation of anemia and clinical phenotypes.

combined with a long period of observation and genetic analysis[31] may help us to understand the factors that determine the severity of anemia in HbE–β^0 thalassemia. Analysis of concordance and discordance of hemoglobin levels in 216 sibling pairs from 98 families showed a remarkable skew toward the lower values with a mode at 0–0.5 g/dL.[32] Concordance of hemoglobin levels between sibling pairs greatly exceeded discordance, indicating that severity of anemia in these patients is determined by polygenic factors, rather than a single gene effect. The factors that influence the severity of anemia are discussed later.

β Thalassemia Mutations. Although β^0 thalassemia is caused by many mutations, all result in absence of β-globin chain production by the abnormal gene (see Chapter 16). β^0 Thalassemia is usually more severe than β^+ thalassemia, in which a wide range of β-globin chain production is observed. Some β^+ thalassemia mutations may produce only very small amounts of β-globin chains and have a phenotype similar to that of β^0 thalassemia (e.g., C→T in IVS-II-654) (see Chapter 16). Alternatively, interaction between HbE and mild β^+ thalassemia, such as A→G at position –28 or A→G in codon 19 of the β-globin gene usually results in a mild thalassemic phenotype. Table 18.3 shows the hematological data and hemoglobin analysis, in the steady state, in mild HbE–β^+ thalassemia compared with homozygous HbE and severe types of HbE–β^+ thalassemia.[25] In mild HbE–β^+ thalassemia, HbE formed approximately 60% of total hemoglobin and HbF levels were approximately 3%–10%, which is the same effect produced by the mutation in codon 19 (Hb Malay, β19(B1) Asn→Ser). HbF is minimally increased in the absence of severe hemolytic stress. In a few cases, the hemoglobin phenotype was "HbE + HbA" with 60% HbE. In contrast, in the two types of severe HbE–β^+ thalassemia shown in Table 18.3 with mutations at IVS-II-654 and IVS-I-5, the mutations lead to severe hemolytic stress with HbF increased to a similar degree as in HbE–β^0 thalassemia. Therefore, these severe HbE–β^+ thalassemias are similar to HbE–β^0 thalassemia. Compound heterozygotes for β^+ and β^0 thalassemia genes also show variable severity similar to HbE–β^0 thalassemia (see Chapter 16). We can conclude that 1) patients with mild β^+ thalassemia and HbE have mild disease; and 2) patients with severe β^+ or β^0 thalassemia alleles and HbE have moderate to severe disease. These observations suggest that additional factors may be involved in determining disease severity.

Coinheritance of α Thalassemia. Concomitant inheritance of α thalassemia or Hb Constant Spring may be responsible for mildness of anemia in β or HbE–β thalassemia.[31, 33–35] HbE–β^0 thalassemia patients who have coinherited α^+ thalassemia have hemoglobin levels of 7.4 g/dL or above, whereas those without detectable α thalassemia have hemoglobin levels higher or lower than 7.4 g/dL. Coinheritance of α^0 thalassemia with HbE–β^0 thalassemia may lead to so mild a condition that the individuals do not have a clinical abnormality that requires medical attention.[33] This effect is more evident in the

Table 18.3. Hb levels and Hb analysis in two types of mild HbE-β^+ thalassemia, severe HbE-β^+ thalassemia and homozygous HbE

		Mild HbE–β^+ thalassemia		Severe HbE–β^+ thalassemia	
	Homozygous HbE	−28/HbE	Codon 19/HbE	IVS-II-654/HbE	IVS-I-5/HbE
No.	39	16	7	13	5
Hb type	EE	EFA	EF + Malay	EF	EF
Hb (g/dL)	11.4 ± 1.2	9.5 ± 1.5	9.2 ± 2.8	6.6 ± 0.9	7.9 ± 1.0
HbE (%)	95.2 ± 2.1	57.1 ± 5.9	58.2 ± 3.4	57.5 ± 11.6	52.2 ± 8.0
HbF (%)	4.8 ± 2.1	10.1 ± 5.6	3.4 ± 1.1	39.2 ± 13.7	47.7 ± 8.0

Table 18.4. Genetic determinants for the severity difference in 80 patients with HbE–β thalassemia disease

		Type of mutation		α-Genotype				Xmn I $^{G}\gamma$-gene			
Phenotype	No.	β+ Thal/HbE	β° Thal/HbE	αα/αα	--/αα	-α/αα	$\alpha^{CS}\alpha/\alpha\alpha$	+/+	+/−	−/−	ND*
Mild	27	4	23	15	0	8	4	1	22	2	2
Moderate	42	0	42	40	0	0	2	1	32	6	3
Severe	11	0	11	11	0	0	0	0	8	3	0

Thal = thalassemia.

HbE–β^0 thalassemia or β^+ thalassemia/β^0 thalassemia and minimal in β^0 thalassemia/β^0 thalassemia compound heterozygotes.

Association with Increased HbF. Coinheritance of determinants that increase HbF expression can ameliorate the severity of β thalassemia. Inheritance of a β thalassemia chromosome with the *Xmn*-1 cleavage site at position –158 5′ to the $^{G}\gamma$-globin gene is associated with increased HbF and milder anemia.[34] Two copies of this allele are necessary to produce a significant clinical effect. Hemoglobin levels of patients with an *Xmn*-$1^{+/+}$ genotype were greater than 8.5 g/dL, whereas those of patients with the *Xmn*-$1^{-/-}$ genotype were less than 7 g/dL. Increased expression of the $^{G}\gamma$-globin gene was also detected in the *Xmn*-$1^{+/+}$ patients. This increase of γ-globin gene activity helps to reduce the overall globin-chain imbalance and thus ameliorates the anemia. A similar effect, however, is not seen in individuals heterozygous for the *Xmn*-l site polymorphism. Patients with a single copy of the *Xmn*-l-positive allele have a variable clinical course and a wide range of hemoglobin levels and HbF production.

The association between the *Xmn*-$1^{+/+}$ genotype and a highly significant increase in the absolute level of HbF and a milder phenotype has also been observed in patients with HbE–β thalassemia in Sri Lanka.[31] In this study, it was clear that there must be other genetic determinants in the population that are responsible for an elevation of HbF, although so far these have not been identified.

Table 18.4 shows the effect of the type of β-thalassemia mutation, α thalassemia, and the *Xmn*l restriction site in determining severity in 80 Thai HbE–β thalassemia patients. The presence of a mild β thalassemia mutation, α thalassemia, and homozygosity for the *Xmn*l restriction site was associated with a mild phenotype in 17 of 27 (63%) patients. Although two cases were *Xmn*l negative, one had HbE–β^+ thalassemia and the other had the Hb Constant Spring gene. These findings suggest that the three factors can account for the mildness of the disease in 21% of cases. In severe cases, none had coinherited α thalassemia or an Hb Constant Spring gene and 3 of 11 cases (27%) were also *Xmn*l negative. Six of 42 patients with moderate severity also lacked an *Xmn*l restriction site.

Amount of Alternative Spliced β^E-Globin mRNA. An underproduction of β-globin chains from the β^E-globin gene strongly suggests that alternative RNA splicing is of physiological significance. The percentage of alternative spliced β^E globin mRNA was determined by the reverse transcriptase polymerase chain reaction technique in 14 patients with the same β thalassemia mutation.[36] Variation in clinical phenotype and degree of anemia were present. Preliminary results showed abnormally spliced β^E globin mRNA in patients with severe symptoms and low hemoglobin levels between 2.9% and 6.1%, whereas those with higher hemoglobin levels had values from 1.6% to 2.6%. The majority of patients with the *Xmn*l-negative genotype had more severe anemia and a higher percentage of abnormally spliced β^E globin mRNA. This indicated that the amount of alternatively spliced β^E globin mRNA was a more predominant factor in determining severity of anemia than the pattern of *Xmn*l polymorphism or the level of HbF. If confirmed, β-globin mutations resulting in abnormal pre-mRNA processing should result in variable degrees of gene expression and greater severity of anemia. Further investigation is needed to clarify this point.

Pyrimidine 5′ Nucleotidase Deficiency. In one Bangladeshi family, an individual homozygous for both HbE and pyrimidine 5′ nucleotidase deficiency was found. The patient had a severe hemolytic anemia in contrast with HbE homozygotes. Globin–chain synthesis experiments showed that the mechanism underlying the interaction between these two genotypes was a marked decrease in the stability of HbE in pyrimidine 5′ nucleotidase–deficient red blood cells. In these cells, free α-globin chains but not β^E-globin chains accumulated on the membrane. It was hypothesized that the marked instability of HbE in the enzyme-deficient cells resulted from oxidant damage to mildly unstable HbE.[37] Clearly this interaction also has the potential to modify the phenotype of HbE–β thalassemia.

Severe jaundice. In Sri Lanka, and probably in other regions of the Indian subcontinent, patients with HbE–β thalassemia are encountered quite commonly who have severe and persistent jaundice in the absence of definable liver disease. It turns out that this is due to the homozygous inheritance of the $TA_{(7)}$ allele of the promoter of the glucuronyltransferase 1 gene, a polymorphism that is particularly common in this population.[38] These patients have a highly significant increase in the incidence of gallstones. Homozygosity for the $TA_{(7)}$ allele occurs in 10%–25% of some populations of Africa and the Indian subcontinent but at a much lower frequency in Southeast Asia.[39]

Conclusion. The genotypic factors that can be used to predict a mild phenotype in HbE–β thalassemia are mild β^+ thalassemia mutations, the coinheritance of α thalassemia, and the homozygosity for *Xmn*-I restriction site 5′ to the $^G\gamma$ globin gene. The *Xmn*-I-$^G\gamma$ site may not consistently predict the phenotype of HbE–β thalassemia. It is also clear that the complications of the disease, severe jaundice for example, may be affected by genetic modifiers.

Clinical Manifestations

HbE–β thalassemia is an important cause of childhood chronic disease in Southeast Asia. In contrast to thalassemia patients in developed countries, and for economic reasons, most Southeast Asian patients do not undergo transfusion or the transfusion is suboptimal, and iron chelation is uncommon. Patients show remarkable variability in the clinical expression of HbE–β thalassemia, ranging from a mild form of thalassemia intermedia to transfusion-dependent conditions clinically indistinguishable from homozygous β^0 thalassemia (Fig. 18.4). Approximately half of the patients have the thalassemia intermedia and half have the thalassemia major phenotype. In 803 HbE–β thalassemia patients, hemoglobin levels ranged from 3 to 13 g/dL and averaged 7.7 g/dL in the steady state.[14] As discussed earlier this remarkable variability in severity reflects the heterogeneity of β thalassemia mutations present with HbE and other modulating factors. A similar degree of phenotypic heterogeneity is also well characterized in patients living in Sri Lanka[31,40] and in immigrants, mainly from Bangladesh, living in the United Kingdom.[16,41]

At birth, infants with severe HbE–β thalassemia are asymptomatic because HbF levels are high. As HbF production wanes and is replaced by HbE at 6–12 months of age, anemia with splenomegaly develops. In the more severe phenotypes, almost without exception signs of impaired health are noted during the first decade of life. Clinical data in 378 patients with HbE–β thalassemia in Thailand are shown in Table 18.5. The initial complaints varied from patient to patient, and several symptoms usually appeared simultaneously. Most common was the development of a mass in the left upper quadrant and pallor. With time and without transfusions, anemia, jaundice, hepatosplenomegaly, retardation of physical development, and thalassemic facies evolve. Absence of secondary sexual development is common and chronic leg ulcers are sometimes observed. These clinical manifestations are secondary to decreased oxygen delivery to tissues, ineffective erythropoiesis and iron overload, and resemble those of untreated β thalassemia major (see Chapter 17).

The milder, nontransfusion-dependent phenotypes of HbE–β thalassemia also show considerable heterogeneity. Some patients grow and develop normally with only modest splenomegaly, despite having hemoglobin levels that are only 2–3 g/dL higher than those with more severe disease. Yet some of these patients pass through a normal puberty with good growth and sexual development, whereas others who have been asymptomatic through early childhood have delayed puberty with or without defective growth. Detailed studies in a group of children with HbE–β thalassemia in Sri Lanka, performed over 10 years,

Table 18.5. Clinical data in 378 patients with HbE–β thalassemia disease

	No.	Percent
Age onset (y)		
0–9	299	79.10
10–19	49	12.96
20–29	23	6.09
30–39	7	1.85
Growth development		
Normal	94	24.87
Retardation	284	75.13
Mongoloid facies		
Absent	65	17.20
Slight	159	42.06
Obvious	154	40.74
Hepatomegaly		
Absent	41	10.85
<5 cm	247	65.34
5–8 cm	66	17.46
>8 cm	24	6.35
Splenomegaly		
Absent	9	2.38
<5 cm	132	34.92
5–8 cm	62	16.40
>8 cm	75	19.84
First menstruation (y)		
10–14	15	8.72
15–19	86	50.00
20–24	10	5.81
None	54	31.40
No record	7	4.07
Splenectomy (y)	134	35.45
0–9	52	38.81
10–19	63	47.01
20–29	12	8.96
>30	7	5.22
Blood transfusion (U)	231	61.11
<5	115	49.78
5–9	47	20.35
10–14	22	9.52
15–19	11	4.76
>20	12	5.19
Unknown	24	10.39

have emphasized the instability of the phenotype during early development.[31,40,42]

Complications

Expanded Erythropoiesis. Erythrpoiesis is massively increased to 10–15 times normal because anemia stimulates erythropoietin production. Extensive erythropoiesis can be found in the liver, spleen, and bone and in extramedullary sites. Erythropoietic masses in the spinal canal can cause spinal cord compression and paraplegia, and when they occur intracranially convulsions may result.[43–45] Massive erythropoiesis leads to fragility and distortion of the bones and decreases bone density because of osteoporosis and osteomalacia, as observed in irregularly transfused thalassemia major patients.[46] Bone marrow expansion also increases blood volume, leading to high-output cardiac failure.

Iron Overload. Iron overload occurs without exception.[47] Excessive iron accumulates because of blood transfusions and enhanced gastrointestinal absorption.[48] The skin is darkened and iron deposition occurs in the bone marrow, liver, spleen, heart, pancreas, and elsewhere.[49–51] Arrhythmias are not as frequently encountered as in thalassemia major and although liver fibrosis from iron overload is common, ascites and other signs of cirrhosis are very rare. Diabetes mellitus secondary to iron deposition in the pancreas frequently develops in untreated adult patients if they live long enough.[52] We have observed a terminal wasting stage in some patients who lived into their third and fourth decades. These patients developed more skin pigmentation, poor appetite, weight loss, and increasing anemia, and eventually died. This is believed to result from organ failure caused by uncontrolled tissue oxidation from chronic, severe iron overload. As iron overload is a constant complication of thalassemia and iron is a strong oxidant, reduced levels of antioxidants such as vitamins C and E are common in these patients.[53]

Heart Disease. Half of the patients with HbE–β thalassemia in Thailand die of heart failure. This is associated with failure of other organs, delayed growth and sexual maturation, hepatomegaly, and endocrinopathies. Organ failure results from iron deposition in the heart and other tissues.[49–52] Myocardial iron deposition is mostly slight, occurring primarily as small granules in perinuclear areas, with later accumulation throughout the fibers, predominantly subepicardial, occasionally subendocardial.[54] The small amount of iron deposited in the heart is in marked contrast to enormous iron deposition in the liver and pancreas. Other causes of death are anemia, infection, constrictive pericarditis, and pulmonary artery occlusion. Cardiomegaly is proportional to the severity of anemia and systolic murmurs are frequently present.[55–57]

Chronic pericarditis following upper respiratory tract infection is frequently encountered, more so in splenectomized patients. A pericardial rub may be detected, often transiently. Intractable pericardial effusion may follow, causing cardiac tamponade and failure, and requires aspiration. In a very few cases chronic constrictive pericarditis develops, requiring surgical intervention. Histological examination of the pericardium shows nonspecific pericarditis.[54] Viral infection has been suspected as the cause of this pericarditis but has not been proven.

Infections. Prospective studies showed increased susceptibility to viral, bacterial, and fungal infection that may be causes of death in severe HbE–β thalassemia.[58–61] In splenectomized patients, septicemia can be very acute and overwhelming, leading to death in a short period. Gram-negative and Gram-positive bacteria are frequent causes of septicemia. Fungal infection with *Pythium* can lead to arterial occlusion and gangrene of the legs.[60,61] Investigators have not yet pinpointed the mechanisms that cause increased susceptibility to infections but iron overload and severe anemia may be involved.

Recent studies have suggested that patients with HbE–β thalassemia may be more prone to infection by both *Plasmodium falciparum* and *Plasmodium vivax* malaria and that those who have undergone splenectomy may be even more susceptible. The clinical significance of these findings remain to be determined.[62]

Jaundice and Gallstones. Stones are found in approximately 50% of patients.[63] As discussed earlier, they occur most frequently in a genetic subset of individuals with very high bilirubin levels in some populations.[38,39] For the detection of biliary calculi, ultrasonography is more sensitive than oral cholecystography and plain abdominal films. Cholecystitis and ascending cholangitis may occur with abdominal pain, fever, and increasing jaundice.[64] Antibiotics alone are usually not effective and cholecystectomy is necessary.

Hypertension, Convulsions, and Cerebral Hemorrhage. After multiple blood transfusions some patients in Thailand developed hypertension, convulsions, and cerebral hemorrhage after transfusion of 2 U or more of blood and many of them died.[65] This complication may develop as late as 2 weeks after multiple transfusions, suggesting that blood volume overload is not the cause of hypertension. Monitoring blood pressure during and after blood transfusions with prompt antihypertensive intervention has reduced deaths from this complication. This complication has not been reported in other populations.

Hypoxemia. A great majority of splenectomized HbE–β^0 thalassemia patients in Thailand develop hypoxemia with low arterial pO_2.[66] Platelet counts in splenectomized thalassemia patients are double that of nonsplenectomized patients; young and larger platelets are also observed in the absence of the spleen. Platelet microaggregates have been detected in the circulation of these splenectomized patients.[67] One hypothesis for the pathogenesis of hypoxemia in HbE–β^0 thalassemia is that platelets increase in number, are younger and more active after splenectomy, and aggregate in the circulation and in the pulmonary vasculature. Substances released during platelet aggregation may cause constriction of the terminal bronchioles leading to decreased oxygenation and hypoxemia. A canine model showed that induction of platelet aggregation in the circulation reproduced the hypoxemia observed in splenectomized thalassemia patients.

Administration of aspirin to inhibit platelet aggregation reduces the degree of hypoxemia in the majority of cases,[68] suggesting that these agents should be routinely given to splenectomized patients with HbE–β thalassemia.

Interestingly, the combination of pulmonary hypertension and consequent hypoxemia has not been observed so frequently in other populations, suggesting that other factors may be involved in the Thai population.

Thromboembolism. Autopsy findings in a large number of patients with HbE–β thalassemia revealed striking pulmonary artery occlusion. Serial sections of the lungs revealed in some patients as many as 24 lesions/cm^2, the distribution of which indicated an embolism.[69,70] Thromboembolism in HbE–β thalassemia seems to involve platelets, a reactive thalassemic red cell surface, coagulation factors, and abnormal endothelium, but this problem is still under study.

Autoimmune Hemolytic Anemia. Some patients develop autoimmune hemolytic anemia with worsening anemia and a positive Coombs' test.[71] The condition is responsive to corticosteroids. Studies of HbE thalassemia patients with this condition showed that their red cell surface is an active site of complex immune reactions that are likely to be associated with many pathophysiological phenomena.[72]

Treatment

Because HbE–β thalassemia has such a variable phenotype and patients with this disorder, probably because they have relatively lower levels of HbF and reflecting the oxygen affinity of HbE, are able to adapt to anemia better than patients with other forms of β thalassemia intermedia, it is vital to observe young children with this condition after presentation for a reasonable period before deciding on the best approach to management. It is important to remember that they may present with a particularly low hemoglobin level consequent to a recent infection and it is particularly important therefore not to establish them on a regular transfusion until their steady-state hemoglobin level and level of growth and degree of splenomegaly has been assessed. Particularly in areas where malaria is endemic it is important to exclude chronic *P. vivax* infection as a possible cause of rapidly progressive splenomegaly.

The hemoglobin level alone should not be the major factor in initiating transfusion. Rather, the broader picture should be taken into account with particular attention to growth failure, lack of activity, and the earlier appearance of skeletal change. If it is clear that the patient will require regular transfusion the regimen to be followed, including chelation, is similar to that for the management of β thalassemia major (see Chapter 17). Those who do not require transfusion should be maintained on folic acid supplements and advised about the early treatment of infective episodes. Although some patients with increasing splenomegaly and evidence of hypersplenism may benefit from splenectomy, this should be avoided when possible because of the particularly high risk of infection.

Patients who do not require regular transfusion have serum ferritin estimations at least twice per year. Increased iron levels should be controlled by intermittent courses of chelating agents to maintain safe ferritin levels (see Chapter 17).

Hydroxyurea therapy may increase HbF levels,[73] although recent studies in other populations have shown that this effect is not great, even when combined with erythropoietin.[74] For those who present early with severe disease bone marrow transplantation remains an important option[75,76] (see Chapters 31 and 32).

Rapidly expanding extramedullary hemopoietic masses, particularly involving the brain or spinal cord, require urgent treatment by blood transfusion, hydroxyurea, or possibly, radiotherapy. Limited experience in those with profound jaundice due to genetic inability to conjugate bilirubin suggest that at least in some cases very low doses of phenobarbitone may be helpful.

Conclusions

HbE-β thalassemia is a major public health problem in Southeast Asia and in other Asian countries. Although some progress has been made toward a better understanding of its pathophysiology and clinical management a great deal remains to be learned. Recent work has made it absolutely clear that there must be other genetic modifiers to be discovered that are responsible for the variable phenotype. A better approach to predicting the phenotype is urgently required, particularly if prenatal diagnosis is to be widely used for the control of this condition and, even more so, if experimental forms of gene therapy become available in the future.

Because it may be some time before there are more definitive forms of treatment it is important to utilize the information that we already have more effectively. For example, in malarious areas it will be very important to conduct trials of malaria prophylaxis with particular respect to the phenotype of patients with this condition early in life. Because recent evidence suggests that the erythropoietin response to anemia tends to decline with age, the possibility of transient periods of transfusion during maximum erythroid expansion should be seriously considered.[29] Because genetic evidence indicates that the phenotype in this condition may be improved quite dramatically with only a modest increase in steady-state hemoglobin level,

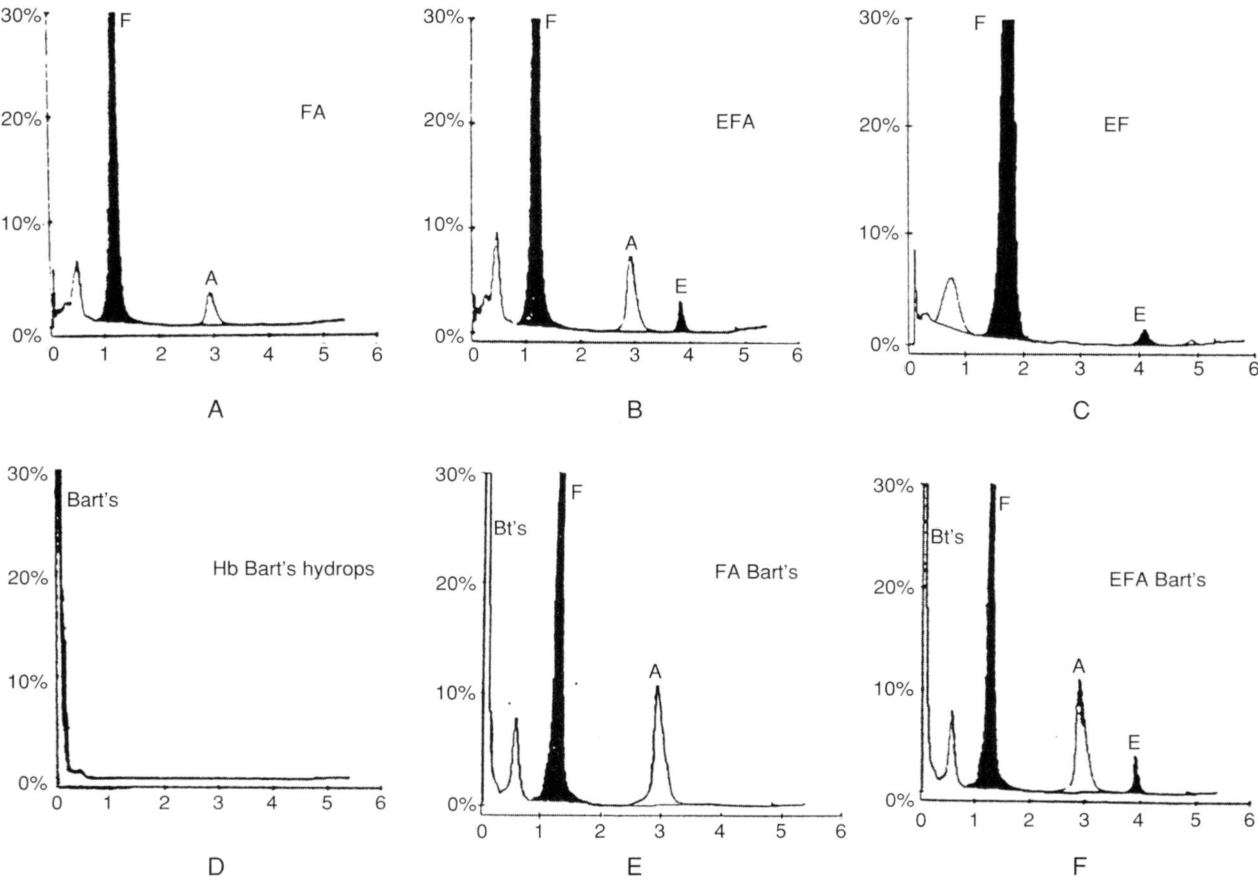

Figure 18.5. Chromatograms of newborns with HbE syndromes detected by automated HPLC. **(A)** Healthy newborn; **(B)** newborn with HbE trait; **(C)** newborn with HbE–β thalassemia; **(D)** newborn with Hb Bart's hydrops fetalis; **(E)** newborn with HbH disease; **(F)** newborn with HbAE Bart's disease.

more efforts should be directed at trying to raise the HbF level in these patients.

NEONATAL AND PRENATAL DIAGNOSIS

The amount of HbA_2 in normal newborns is lower than in adults and usually is not visualized by hemoglobin electrophoresis. Pootrakul et al.[77] observed a "slow" hemoglobin component at the position of HbA_2 that proved to be HbE. The mean HbE level, quantitated by cellulose-acetate electrophoresis, was 3.7%. An automatic high-performance liquid chromatography (HPLC) system (Variant™, Bio-Rad) was used to study various HbE disorders in cord blood (Fig. 18.5). HbE concentrations in homozygous HbE ranged between 3.9% and 14.9%. In HbE heterozygotes, HbE was between 2.1% and 10.3% with a mean of 4.5% (Table 18.6).[78] These data suggest that newborns with homozygous HbE have a tendency to have higher concentration of HbE than those with heterozygous HbE, but some overlap occurs. Furthermore, both homozygous HbE and HbE–β^0 thalassemia patients had similar chromatograms composed of HbE and HbF with similar amounts of HbE. DNA analysis is necessary to differentiate between these two syndromes.

Diagnosis of HbE syndromes can also be performed prenatally by cordocentesis at the gestational ages of 16–24 weeks.[79] The chromatograms obtained from cordocentesis using the automatic HPLC system were similar to those of the cord blood specimens. In the HbE heterozygote, 0.8%–1.5% of HbE was detected in addition to HbA. HbA was not present in fetuses homozygous for HbE or with HbE–β^0 thalassemia (Table 18.7). These two conditions were distinguished only by DNA analysis. Prenatal diagnosis of Hb–β thalassemia is now performed, if requested, by chorion-villus sampling and DNA analysis.

LABORATORY DIAGNOSIS IN ADULTS

The diagnosis of HbE is based on the electrophoretic or chromatographic separation of hemoglobins from peripheral blood. In alkaline buffer (pH 8.6), HbE migrates like HbA_2 on cellulose-acetate membranes but can be distinguished from HbA_2 by its higher concentration, more than 10% of the total hemoglobin. HbE also migrates like HbA_2 on HPLC columns.[78] Variable concentrations of HbE may reflect the genotypes of HbE disorders. In general, as

Table 18.6. Hematologic data and hemoglobin analysis in cord blood samples

Condition	No.	Hb g/dL	MCV fL	MCH pg	MCHC g/dL	Hb type	% Hemoglobin (HPLC)				Genotype
							A_2 (E)	F	A	Barts	
Normal	326	15.4 ± 1.7	105 ± 6.2	35 ± 2.2	33 ± 1.0	FA	0.6 ± 0.4	74.1 ± 6.4	17.8 ± 6.3	0.7 ± 0.4	$\alpha\alpha/\alpha\alpha\text{-}\beta^A/\beta^A$
EA Bart's disease	1	13.0	72	22	30	EFA Bart's	3.6	80.6	12.2	27.9	$\text{--}/\text{-}\alpha\text{-}\beta^A/\beta^E$
EF Bart's disease	1	11.2	70	21	30	EF Bart's	30.1	64.4	0.9	17.5	$\text{--}/\text{-}\alpha\text{-}\beta^E/\beta^E$
β thal/HbE disease	1	13.1	99	33	34	EF	2.0	93.0	0.1	1.0	$\alpha\alpha/\alpha\alpha\text{-}\beta^{thal}/\beta^E$
HbE homozygote	9	14.5 ± 2.1	103 ± 6.7	34 ± 2.5	33 ± 1.2	EF	8.0 ± 3.6	81.4 ± 4.5	0.6 ± 0.6	0	$\alpha\alpha/\alpha\alpha\text{-}\beta^E/\beta^E$
HbE trait	114	15.4 ± 1.6	104 ± 7.5	35 ± 6.6	33 ± 1.0	EFA	4.5 ± 1.5	76.7 ± 4.8	10.1 ± 3.5	0.7 ± 0.4	$\alpha\alpha/\alpha\alpha\text{-}\beta^A/\beta^E$
EE-α^+ thal trait	1	13.8	96	31	33	EF Bart's	11.6	76.1	0.4	1.9	$\text{-}\alpha/\alpha\alpha\text{-}\beta^E/\beta^E$
EE-α^0 thal trait	1	13.5	82	27	33	EF Bart's	7.6	81.3	0.3	8.8	$\text{--}/\alpha\alpha\text{-}\beta^E/\beta^E$
HbE trait α^0 thal trait	5	14.0 ± 1.3	89 ± 4.8	28 ± 1.5	32 ± 0.5	EFA Bart's	5.1 ± 1.1	72.8 ± 4.4	15.6 ± 3.6	8.6 ± 1.7	$\text{--}/\alpha\alpha\text{-}\beta^A/\beta^E$
HbE trait α^+ thal/Hb CS	1	15.0	106	32	30	EFA Bart's	3.0	66.0	22.1	9.3	$\text{-}\alpha/\alpha^{CS}\alpha\text{-}\beta^A/\beta^E$
HbE trait	3	13.2	78	25	32	EFA Bart's	5.6	72.0	15.9	3.7	$\text{-}\alpha/\text{-}\alpha\text{-}\beta^A/\beta^E$
Homozygous α^+ thal		14.3	91	28	31	EFA Bart's	4.2	79.3	12.3	5.3	$\text{-}\alpha/\text{-}\alpha\text{-}\beta^A/\beta^E$
		14.9	98	31	31	EFA Bart's	2.2	88.2	4.9	2.8	$\text{-}\alpha/\text{-}\alpha\text{-}\beta^A/\beta^E$

Table 18.7. The amounts of Hbs A_2 (E), F, and a from a normal fetus and fetuses with thalassemias and HbE

			Hb Analysis (%)			
Phenotype	No.	Hb Type	A_2/E	F	A	Bart's
Normal	1	FA	0	94.0	5.8	–
β Thal trait	6	FA	0	94.8–96.3	4.0–5.2	–
β Thal/HbE	7	EF	1.0–1.7	89.4–98.6	0	–
Homozygous HbE	2	EF	3.0, 2.1	96.8, 97.3	0	–
HbE trait	4	EFA	0.8–1.4	94.0–97.2	2.0–2.8	–
Hb Bart's hydrops	10	Bart's	0	0	0	@100%

mentioned previously, HbE is 25%–30% of the hemolysate from heterozygotes and lower amounts of HbE are found with coinheritance of α thalassemia (Table 18.2) or with coexistence of iron-deficiency anemia. Lower proportions of HbE in heterozygotes indicate a concomitant inheritance of the more pronounced defects of α-globin chain synthesis as in HbAE Bart's disease.[10–12] In contrast, the amount of HbE is higher in HbE–β thalassemia and HbE levels of 85%–95% of total hemoglobin are found with homozygous HbE. Compound heterozygotes with HbE and HbC also appear to have very high HbE levels because HbC ($\alpha_2\beta^{6Glu\rightarrow Lys}{}_2$) coelectrophoreses with HbE ($\alpha_2\beta^{6Glu\rightarrow Lys}{}_2$) in the standard alkaline buffer. These two variants can be distinguished by agar gel electrophoresis at acid pH, or by reverse phase HPLC, and by the presence of approximately 45% HbC in the heterozygous state.[80]

The blue dye dichlorophenolindophenol can be used as a screening test for HbE, which has a weakened $\alpha_1\beta_1$ contact and precipitates on incubation with the dye at 37° C.[27] Homozygous HbE produces heavy sediments at the bottom of the tube whereas heterozygous HbE, HbH disease, and HbE–β thalassemia produce a cloudy or evenly distributed particulate appearance.

INTERACTIONS OF HEMOGLOBIN E WITH OTHER β-GLOBIN CHAIN VARIANTS

As well as the common interactions of hemoglobin E with the α and β thalassemias described in this chapter there have been occasional reports of interactions between HbE and other β-chain structural hemoglobin variants (Table 18.8). Although most of these interactions result in a

Table 18.8. Hemoglobin analysis of HbE/other β variants

Hb variants	α-Genotype	Hb (g/dL)	MCV (fL)	HbE (%)	Hb variant (%)	HbF (%)	References
Hb Pyrgos	ND	9.5	76.5	26.5	71.2	ND	[82–84]
	$-\alpha^{3.7}/\alpha\alpha$	12.4	86	25.5	63.6	5.1	
	$\alpha^{CS}\alpha/\alpha\alpha$	14.1	72.6	22.8	77.2	ND	
	$--/\alpha\alpha$ $-\alpha^{3.7}/\alpha\alpha$	11.1	68.4	19.4	73.9	2.2	
Hb D-Punjab	αα/αα	14.1	77.2	29.7	73.3	<2	[85,86]
	ND	12	84	33.5	59	0.9	
Hb Hope	ND	10.5	63	40	60	ND	[87,88]
	αα/αα	10.5	78.3	32.3	60.9	1.0	
Hb New York	ND	14.6	ND	33.2	60	1.6	[89]
Hb J-Bangkok	ND	12.3	79.7	32.3	67.7	ND	[82,86]
	ND	12.8, 15.5	95, 84	31.9, 30.4	68.9, 69.6	ND, 0.76	
Hb Dhonburi	ND	12.1	77	38.9	55	4.5	[81,86]
Hb Tak	ND	14.3	77.4	24.1	58.8	2.8	[86,90]
	ND	17.8	80	35.2	62.2	ND	
Hb C	ND	14	ND	37	50	ND	[86,91–93]
	ND	9.5, 10.1	61, 59.5	35.2, 36.9	55.9, 53.6	2.1, 3.1	
	ND	11.8	59	40.6	56	1.9	
	αα/αα	11.3 (11.0–12.0)	81.7(74.1–88.0)	35.6(32.0–39.7)	56.4(53.7–57.5)	ND	
Hb S	ND	12.7	71	34.6	64.2	1.3	[93–95]
	ND	14.6	ND	32	60	ND	
	ND	12.9	74	36	60	4	
Hb Korle-Bu	$-\alpha^{3.7}/\alpha\alpha$	9.5, 12.2	77.5, 73.2	21.8, 22.4	71.1, 69.3	3.2, 2.6	[96]
Hb T-Cambodia	ND	10.1	64	57.3	39.3	3.4	[97]
Hb Lepore-Hollandia	αα/αα	10.2, 8.9	62.5, 61.3	51.7, 50.6	9.0, 11.0	39.3, 38.4	[98–100]
	-α/αα	10.1	58.5	59.4	20.3	20.3	
	ND	8.3, 6	60.3, 54.1	64, 75	10, 8	26, 17	
	ND	10.1	64.7	67.6	ND	27.8	
Hb Lepore-Washington-Boston	ND	11.4	70	53	12.7	34.3	[101]
Hb Malay	αα/αα	7.6, 8.5, 8.5	61.5, 53.4, 63	59.9, 64.1, 48.8	27.1, 30.3, 20.9	12.1, 3.6, 24.4	[86,102]
	ND	8.7	60.1	53.6	34.6	11.8	

ND = indicates no available data.

relatively mild clinical phenotype, because of their rarity they may cause difficulties in both diagnosis and for genetic counseling, particularly if prenatal diagnosis is being considered.

The interaction of HbE with HbS, HbSE disease, has been accounted occasionally in India and Sri Lanka and in other populations. The clinical features of this rare condition are discussed in Chapter 23.

The interactions between HbE and Hb Malay are of particular interest. Hb Malay occurs not uncommonly in Malaysia and Thailand and, like HbE, results from a mutation (β codon 19 AC-AGC; β19 Asn-Ser) that creates an alternative splice site, in this case between codons 17 and 18 (see Chapter 16). Hence it is synthesized at a slightly reduced rate and has a phenotype of the mild form of β thalassemia. From the limited amount of published data it appears that this interaction is associated with a relatively mild phenotype similar to that described earlier for the milder forms of HbE β thalassemia (see Weatherall and Clegg[16] and Table 18.8). Similarly, although the number of reported cases is too small to make any dogmatic statements, as shown in Table 18.8 interactions of HbE with unstable hemoglobin variants, Hb Dhonburi for example,[81] also seem to have been associated with mild phenotypes, and the same seems to apply to the few reported interactions with different forms of Hb Lepore.

ACKNOWLEDGMENTS

This work was supported by the Prajadhipok Rambhai Barni Foundation and the National Center for Genetic Engineering and Biotechnology (BIOTEC), Thailand and The Wellcome Trust, UK. S.F is a senior research scholar of The Thailand Research Fund.

REFERENCES

1. Na-Nakorn S, Minnich mV, Chernoff AI, Quagqui-Puag S, Chavalekviraj K. Studies on hemoglobin E II. The incidence of hemoglobin E in Thailand. *J Lab Clin Med.* 1956;47:490–498.
2. Flatz G. Hemoglobin E in Southeast Asia. In: *Felicitation Volumes of Southeast-Asian Studies.* Bangkok: Siam Society; 1965;1:96–106.
3. Flatz G. Hemoglobin E: Distribution and population dynamics. *Humangenetik.* 1967;3:189–234.
4. Wasi P. Geographic distribution of hemoglobin variants in Southeast Asia. In: Winter WP, ed. *Hemoglobin Variants in Human Populations.* Vol 2. Florida: CRC Press; 1986;111–127.
5. Kwiatkowski DP. How malaria has affected the human genome and what human genetics can teach us about malaria. *Am J Hum Genet.* 2005;77:171–192.
6. Itano HA, Bergren WR, Sturgeon P. Identification of a fourth abnormal human hemoglobin. *J Am Chem Soc.* 1954;76:2278.
7. Hunt JA, Ingram VM. Abnormal human haemoglobins. VI. The chemical difference between haemoglobins A and E. *Biochim Biophys Acta.* 1961;49:520–536.
8. Wasi P, Na-Nakorn S, Pootrakul S, Sookanek M, Disthasongcham P, Pornpatkul M et al. Alpha- and beta-thalassemia in Thailand. *Ann NY Acad Sci.* 1969;165:60–82.
9. Fucharoen S, Winichagoon P, Thonglairuam V. Beta-thalassemia associated with alpha-thalassemia in Thailand. *Hemoglobin.* 1988;12:581–592.
10. Wasi P, Sookanek M, Pootrakul S, Na-Nakorn S, Suingdumrong A. Haemoglobin E and alpha-Thalassaemia. *Br Med J.* 1967;4:29–32.
11. Fucharoen S, Winichagoon P, Prayoonwiwat W, Pootrakul P, Piankijagum A, Wasi P. Clinical and hematologic manifestations of AE Bart's disease. *Birth Defects Orig Artic Series.* 1987;23:327–332.
12. Thonglairuam V, Winichagoon P, Fucharoen S, Wasi P. The molecular basis of AE-Bart's disease. *Hemoglobin.* 1989; 13:117–24.
13. Chernoff AI, Minnich V, Na-Nakorn S, Tuchinda S, Kashamsant C, Chernoff RR. Studies on hemoglobin E: I. The clinical, hematologic, and genetic characteristics of the hemoglobin E syndromes. *J Lab Clin Med.* 1956;47:455–89, 90–98.
14. Fucharoen S, Winichagoon P, Pootrakul P, Piankijagum A, Wasi P. Variable severity of Southeast Asian beta^0 thalassemia/Hb E disease. *Birth Defects Orig Artic Series.* 1987; 23:241–248.
15. Minnich V, Na-Nakorn S, Chongchareonsuk S, Kochaseni S. Mediterranean anemia: a study of 32 cases in Thailand. *Blood.* 1954;9:1–23.
16. Weatherall DJ, Clegg JB. *The Thalassaemia Syndromes.* 4th ed. Oxford: Blackwell Science; 2001.
17. Wasi P, Disthasongchan P, Na-Nakorn S. The effect of iron deficiency on the levels of hemoglobins A2 and E. *J Lab Clin Med.* 1968;71:85–91.
18. Fairbanks VF, Oliveros R, Brandabur JH, Willis RR, Fiester RF. Homozygous hemoglobin E mimics beta-thalassemia minor without anemia or hemolysis: hematologic, functional, and biosynthetic studies of first North American cases. *Am J Hematol.* 1980;8:109–121.
19. Na-Nakorn S, Minnich V. Studies on hemoglobin E. III. Homozygous hemoglobin E and variants of thalassemia and hemoglobin E; a family study. *Blood.* 1957;12:529–538.
20. Pootrakul S, Assawamunkong S, Na-Nakorn S. Beta$^+$-Thalassemia trait: hematologic and hemoglobin synthesis studies. *Hemoglobin.* 1976;1:75–83.
21. Traeger J, Wood WG, Clegg JB, Weatherall DJ, Wasi P. Defective synthesis of Hb E is due to reduced levels of beta^E mRNA. *Nature.* 1980;288:497–499.
22. Orkin SH, Kazazian HH, Antonarakis SE, Ostrer H, Goff SC, Sexton JP. Abnormal RNA processing due to the exon mutation of beta^E-globin gene. *Nature.* 1982;300:768–769.
23. Traeger J, Winichagoon P, Wood WG. Instability of beta^E-messenger RNA during erythroid cell maturation in hemoglobin E homozygotes. *J Clin Invest.* 1982;69:1050–1053.
24. Wasi P, Winichagoon P, Baramee T, Fucharoean S. Globin chain synthesis is heterozygous and homozygous hemoglobin E. *Hemoglobin.* 1982;6:75–78.
25. Fucharoen S, Winichagoon P. Hemoglobinopathies in Southeast Asia: molecular biology and clinical medicine. *Hemoglobin.* 1997;21:299–319.
26. Fucharoen S, Winichagoon P, Thonglairuam V, Wasi P. EF Bart's disease: interaction of the abnormal alpha- and beta-globin genes. *Eur J Haematol.* 1988;40:75–78.

27. Frischer H, Bowman J. Hemoglobin E, an oxidatively unstable mutation. *J Lab Clin Med.* 1975;85:531–539.
28. Huisman TH. Hb E and alpha-thalassemia; variability in the assembly of beta E chain containing tetramers. *Hemoglobin.* 1997;21:227–236.
29. O'Donnell A, Premawardhena A, Arambepola M, Allen SJ, Peto TE, Fisher CA et al. Age-related changes in adaptation to severe anemia in childhood in developing countries. *Proc Natl Acad Sci USA.* 2007;104:9440–9444.
30. Sripichai O, Makarasara W, Munkongdee T, et al. A scoring system for the classification of beta-thalassemia/Hb E disease severity. *Am J Hematol.* 2008;83:482–484.
31. Premawardhena A, Fisher CA, Olivieri NF, et al. Haemoglobin E beta thalassaemia in Sri Lanka. *Lancet.* 2005;366:1467–1470.
32. Fucharoen S, Winichagoon P, Pootrakul P, Wasi P. Determination for different severity of anemia in thalassemia: concordance and discordance among sib pairs. *Am J Med Genet.* 1984;19:39–44.
33. Winichagoon P, Fucharoen S, Weatherall DJ, Wasi P. Concomitant inheritance of alpha-thalassemia in beta^0-thalassemia/Hb E. *Am J Hematol.* 1985;20:217–222.
34. Winichagoon P, Fucharoen S, Thonglairoam V, Wasi P. Different severity of homozygous beta-thalassemia among siblings. *Hum Genet.* 1987;76:296–297.
35. Winichagoon P, Thonglairoam V, Fucharoen S, Wilairat P, Fukimaki Y, Wasi P. Severity differences in beta-thalassaemia haemoglobin E syndromes: implication of genetic factors. *Br J Haematol.* 1993;83:633–639.
36. Winichagoon P, Fucharoen S, Wilairat P, Chihara K, Fukumaki Y. Role of alternatively spliced beta E-globin mRNA on clinical severity of beta-thalassemia/hemoglobin E disease. *Southeast Asian J Trop Med Public Health.* 1995;26 Suppl **1**:241–245.
37. Rees DC, Duley J, Simmonds HA, et al. Interaction of hemoglobin E and pyrimidine 5′ nucleotidase deficiency. *Blood.* 1996;88:2761–2767.
38. Premawardhena A, Fisher CA, Fathiu F, et al. Genetic determinants of jaundice and gallstones in haemoglobin E beta thalassaemia. *Lancet.* 2001;357:1945–1946.
39. Premawardhena A, Fisher CA, Liu YT, et al. The global distribution of length polymorphisms of the promoters of the glucuronosyltransferase 1 gene (UGT1A1): hematologic and evolutionary implications. *Blood Cells Mol Dis.* 2003;31:98–101.
40. Premawardhena A, De Silver S, Arambepola M, et al. Hemoglobin E-beta-thalassemia: progress report from the International Study Group. *Ann NY Acad Sci.* 2005;1054:33–39.
41. Rees DC, Styles J, Vichinsky EP, Clegg JB, Weatherall DJ. The hemoglobin E syndromes. *Ann NY Acad Sci.* 1998;850:334–343.
42. De Silva S, Fisher CA, Premawardhena A, et al. Thalassaemia in Sri Lanka: implications for the future health burden of Asian populations. *Lancet.* 2000;355:786–791.
43. Fucharoen S, Tunthanavatana C, Sonakul D, Wasi P. Intracranial extramedullary hematopoiesis in beta-thalassemia/hemoglobin E disease. *Am J Hematol.* 1981;10:75–78.
44. Fucharoen S, Suthipongchai S, Poungvarin N, Ladpli S, Sonakul D, Wasi P. Intracranial extramedullary hematopoiesis inducing epilepsy in a patient with beta-thalassemia/hemoglobin E. *Arch Intern Med.* 1985;145:739–742.
45. Issaragrisil S, Piankigagum A, Wasi P. Spinal cord compression in thalassemia. Report of 12 cases and recommendations for treatment. *Arch Intern Med.* 1981;141:1033–1036.
46. Pootrakul P, Hungsprenges S, Fucharoen S, et al. Relation between erythropoiesis and bone metabolism in thalassemia. *N Engl J Med.* 1981;304:1470–1473.
47. Pootrakul P, Vougsmasa V, Laongpanich P, Wasi P. Serum ferritin levels in thalassemias and the effect of splenectomy. *Acta Haematol.* 1981;66:244–250.
48. Vatanavicharn S, Anuwatanakulchai M, Tuntawiroon M, Suwanik R, Wasi P. Iron absorption in patients with beta-thalassaemia/haemoglobin E disease and the effect of splenectomy. *Acta Haematol.* 1983;69:414–416.
49. Sonakul D, Pacharee P, Thakerngpol K. Pathologic findings in 76 autopsy cases of thalassemia. *Birth Defects Orig Artic Series.* 1988;23:157–176.
50. Thakerngpol K, Sonakul D, Fucharoen S, Vathanopas V, Stitnimankarn T. Histochemical study of liver tissue from thalassemic patients. *Birth Defects Orig Artic Series.* 1988;23:193–198.
51. Tran KC, Webb DJ, Pootrakul P. Beta-thalassaemia/haemoglobin E tissue ferritins: II: A comparison of heart and pancreas ferritins with those of liver and spleen. *Biol-Met.* 1990;3:227–231.
52. Vannasaeng S, Ploybutr S, Visutkul P, Tandhanand S, Suwanik R, Wasi P. Endocrine function in thalassaemia. *Clin Endocrinol.* 1981;14:165–173.
53. Vatanavicharn S, Yenchitsomanus P, Siddhikol C. Vitamin E in beta-thalassaemia and alpha-thalassaemia (HbH) diseases. *Acta Haematol.* 1985;73:183.
54. Sonakul D, Pacharee P, Wasi P, Fucharoen S. Cardiac pathology in 47 patients with beta thalassaemia/haemoglobin E. *Southeast Asian J Trop Med Public Health.* 1984;15:554–563.
55. Yipintsoi T, Haraphongse M, Wasi P, Na-Nakorn S. Cardiological examinations in hemoglobin E and thalassemia diseases. *J Med Assoc Thailand.* 1968;51:131–141.
56. Sudhas Na Ayuthya P, Pongpanich B, Damrongwatna T, Isarangkura P, Hathirat P, Pintadit P. Cardiac study in thalassemic children. *Birth Defects Orig Artic Series.* 1987;23:351–354.
57. Jootar P, Fucharoen S. Cardiac involvement in beta-thalassemia/hemoglobin E disease: clinical and hemodynamic findings. *Southeast Asian J Trop Med Public Health.* 1990;21:269–273.
58. Aswapokee N, Aswapokee P, Fucharoen S, Wasi P. A study of infective episodes in patients with beta-thalassemia/Hb E disease in Thailand. *Birth Defects Orig Artic Series.* 1988;23:513–520.
59. Aswapokee P, Aswapokee N, Fucharoen S, Sukroongreung S, Wasi P. Severe infection in thalassemia: a prospective study. *Birth Defects Orig Artic Series.* 1988;23:521–526.
60. Sathapatayavongs B, Leelachaikul P, Prachaktam R, et al. Human pythiosis associated with thalassemia hemoglobinopathy syndrome. *J Infect Dis.* 1989;159:274–280.
61. Wanachiwanawin W, Thianprasit M, Fucharoen S, et al. Fatal arteritis due to Pythium insidiosum infection in patients with thalassaemia. *Trans R Soc Trop Med Hyg.* 1993;87:296–298.
62. Weatherall D. 2009: Manuscript in preparation.

63. Chandcharoensin-Wilde C, Chairoongruang S, Jitnuson P, Fucharoen S, Vathanopas V. Gallstones in thalassemia. *Birth Defects Orig Artic Series.* 1988;23:263–267.
64. Vathanopas V, Fucharoen S, Chandrcharoensin-Wilde C, Sukroongreung S, Nilakul C. Cholecystectomy in thalassemia. *Birth Defects Orig Artic Series.* 1988;23:269–273.
65. Wasi P, Na-Nakorn S, Pootrakul P, Sonakul D, Piankijagum A, Pacharee P. A syndrome of hypertension, convulsions, and cerebral haemorrhage in thalassaemic patients after multiple blood transfusions. *Lancet.* 1978;ii:602–604.
66. Wasi P, Fucharoen S, Younghchaiyud P, Sonakul D. Hypoxemia in thalassemia. *Birth Defects Orig Artic Series.* 1982;18:213–217.
67. Winichagoon P, Fucharoen S, Wasi P. Increased circulating platelet aggregates in thalassaemia. *Southeast Asian J Trop Med Public Health.* 1981;12:556–560.
68. Fucharoen S, Youngchaiyud P, Wasi P. Hypoxaemia and the effect of aspirin in thalassaemia. *Southeast Asian J Trop Med Public Health.* 1981;12:90–93.
69. Sonakul D, Pacharee P, Laohapand T, Fucharoen S, Wasi P. Pulmonary artery obstruction in thalassaemia. *Southeast Asian J Trop Med Public Health.* 1980;11:516–523.
70. Sonakul D, Suwananagool P, Sirivaidyapong P, Fucharoen S. Distribution of pulmonary thromboembolic lesions in thalassemic patients. *Birth Defects Orig Artic Series.* 1988;23:375–384.
71. Kruatrachue M, Sirisinha S, Pacharee P, Chandarayingyong D, Wasi P. An association between thalassaemia and autoimmune haemolytic anaemia (AIHA). *Scand J Haematol.* 1980;25:259–263.
72. Malasit P, Mahasorn W, Mongkolsapaya J, Singhathong B, Fucharoen S, Wasi P, et al. Presence of immunoglobulin, C3 and cytolytic C5b-9 complement components on the surface of erythrocytes from patients with beta-thalassaemia/Hb E disease. *Br J Haematol.* 1997;96:507–513.
73. Fucharoen S, Siritanaratkul N, Winichagoon P, et al. Hydroxyurea increases hemoglobin F levels and improves the effectiveness of erythropoiesis in beta-thalassemia/hemoglobin E disease. *Blood.* 1996;87:887–892.
74. Singer ST, Kuypers FA, Olivieri NF, et al. Fetal haemoglobin augmentation in E/beta(0) thalassaemia: clinical and haematological outcome. *Br J Haematol.* 2005;131:378–388.
75. Issaragrisil S. Bone marrow transplantation in Thailand. *Bone Marrow Transplant.* 1994;13:721–723.
76. Issaragrisil S, Visuthisakchai S, Suvatte V, et al. Brief report: transplantation of cord-blood stem cells into a patient with severe thalassemia. *N Engl J Med.* 1995;332:367–369.
77. Pootrakul S, Muang-sup V, Fucharoen S, Wasi P. Cord blood study on beta-thalassemia and hemoglobin E. *Am J Med Genet.* 1988;29:49–57.
78. Fucharoen S, Winichagoon P, Wisedpanichkij R, Sae-Ngow B, Sriphanich R, Oncoung W et al. Prenatal and postnatal diagnoses of thalassemias and hemoglobinopathies by HPLC. *Clin Chem.* 1998;44:740–748.
79. Fucharoen S, Winichagoon P, Siritanaratkul N, Chowthaworn J, Pootrakul P. Alpha- and beta-thalassemia in Thailand. *Ann NY Acad Sci.* 1998;850:412–414.
80. Siriboon W, Srisomsap C, Winichagoon P, Fucharoen S, Svasti J. Identification of Hb C [beta 6(A3)Glu-->Lys] in a Thai male. *Hemoglobin.* 1993;17:419–425.
81. Viprakasit V, Chinchang W. Two independent origins of Hb Dhonburi (Neapolis) [beta 126 (H4) Val-->Gly]: an electrophoretically silent hemoglobin variant. *Clin Chim Acta.* 2007;376:179–183.
82. Fucharoen S, Singsanan S, Sanchaisuriya K, Fucharoen G. Molecular and haematological characterization of compound Hb E/Hb Pyrgos and Hb E/Hb J-Bangkok in Thai patients. *Clin Lab Haematol.* 2005;27:184–189.
83. Jetsrisuparb A, Sanchaisuriya K, Fucharoen G, Fucharoen S, Wiangnon S, Komwilaisak P. Triple heterozygosity of a hemoglobin variant: hemoglobin Pyrgos with other hemoglobinopathies. *Int J Hematol.* 2002;75:35–39.
84. Sawangareetrakul P, Svasti S, Yodsowon B, et al. Double heterozygosity for Hb Pyrgos [beta83(EF7)Gly-->Asp] and Hb E [beta26(B8)Glu-->Lys] found in association with alpha-thalassemia. *Hemoglobin.* 2002;26:191–196.
85. Fucharoen S, Changtrakun Y, Surapot S, Fucharoen G, Sanchaisuriya K. Molecular characterization of Hb D-Punjab [beta121(GH4)Glu-->Gln] in Thailand. *Hemoglobin.* 2002; 26:261–269.
86. Svasti S, Winichagoon P, Svasti J, Fucharoen S. 2008: in press.
87. Chunpanich S, Fucharoen S, Sanchaisuriya K, Fucharoen G, Kam-itsara K. Molecular and hematological characterization of hemoglobin Hope/hemoglobin E and hemoglobin Hope/alpha-thalassemia 2 in Thai patients. *Lab Hematol.* 2004;10:215–220.
88. Pillers DA, Jones M, Head C, Jones RT. Hb Hope [beta 136(H14) Gly---Asp] and HbE [beta 26(B8)Glu----Lys]: compound heterozygosity in a Thai Mien family. *Hemoglobin.* 1992;16: 81–84.
89. Pootrakul S, Wasi S, NaNakorn S, Dixon GH. Double heterozygosity for hemoglobin E and hemoglobin New York in a Thai family. *J Med Assoc Thai.* 1971;54:688–697.
90. Hoyer JD, Wick MJ, Thibodeau SN, Viker KA, Conner R, Fairbanks VF. Hb Tak confirmed by DNA analysis: not expressed as thalassemia in a Hb Tak/HbE compound heterozygote. *Hemoglobin.* 1998;22:45–52.
91. Fucharoen S, Fucharoen G, Sanchaisuriya K, Surapot S. Compound heterozygote states for Hb C/Hb Malay and Hb C/Hb E in pregnancy: a molecular and hematological analysis. *Blood Cells Mol Dis.* 2005;35:196–200.
92. Sanchaisuriya K, Fucharoen G, Sae-ung N, Siriratmanawong N, Surapot S, Fucharoen S. Molecular characterization of hemoglobin C in Thailand. *Am J Hematol.* 2001;67:189–193.
93. Schroeder WA, Powars D, Reynolds RD, Fisher JI. Hb-E in combination with Hb-S and Hb-C in a black family. *Hemoglobin.* 1977;1:287–289.
94. Altay C, Niazi GA, Huisman TH. The combination of Hb S and Hb E in a black female. *Hemoglobin.* 1976;1:100–102.
95. Gupta R, Jarvis M, Yardumian A. Compound heterozygosity for haemoglobin S and haemoglobin E. *Br J Haematol.* 2000;108:463.
96. Changtrakun Y, Fucharoen S, Ayukarn K, Siriratmanawong N, Fucharoen G, Sanchaisuriya K. Compound heterozygosity for Hb Korle-Bu (beta(73); Asp-Asn) and HbE (beta(26); Glu-Lys) with a 3.7-kb deletional alpha-thalassemia in Thai patients. *Ann Hematol.* 2002;81:389–393.
97. Hutt PJ, Fairbanks VF, Thibodeau SN, et al. Hb T-Cambodia, a beta chain variant with the mutations of Hb E and

Hb D-Punjab, confirmed by DNA analysis. *Hemoglobin*. 1997;21:205–218.

98. Waye JS, Eng B, Patterson M, et al. Hb E/Hb Lepore-Hollandia in a family from Bangladesh. *Am J Hematol*. 1994;47:262–265.

99. Edison ES, Shaji RV, Srivastava A, Chandy M. Compound heterozygosity for HbE and Hb Lepore-Hollandia in India; first report and potential diagnostic pitfalls. *Hemoglobin*. 2005;29:221–224.

100. Viprakasit V, Pung-Amritt P, Suwanthon L, Clark K, Tanphaichtr VS. Complex interactions of deltabeta hybrid haemoglobin (Hb Lepore-Hollandia) Hb E (beta(26G-->A)) and alpha+ thalassaemia in a Thai family. *Eur J Haematol*. 2002;68:107–111.

101. Boontrakoonpoontawee P, Svasti J, Fucharoen S, Winichagoon P. Identification of Hb Lepore-Washington-Boston in association with Hb E [beta 26(B8)Glu----Lys] in a Thai female. *Hemoglobin*. 1987;11:309–316.

102. Fucharoen S, Sanchaisuriya K, Fucharoen G, Surapot S. Molecular characterization of thalassemia intermedia with homozygous Hb Malay and Hb Malay/HbE in Thai patients. *Haematologica*. 2001;86:657–658.

SECTION FIVE

SICKLE CELL DISEASE

Martin H. Steinberg

PATHOPHYSIOLOGY

A β-hemoglobin gene mutation results in the synthesis of the sickle β-globin chain. Sickle hemoglobin (HbS) polymerizes when deoxygenated, and polymer-associated injury to the sickle erythrocyte is the proximate cause of sickle cell disease. The principal pathophysiological features of this disease are shown in the figure and can be grouped as vasoocclusive/blood viscosity related and hemolysis/vasculopathy related. This complex pathophysiology involves diverse molecular and cellular defects that include abnormal erythrocyte volume regulation, impaired nitric oxide bioavailability, reperfusion injury and inflammation, altered hemostasis, defects of intercellular interactions, endothelial cell damage, leukocyte and platelet activation, and in all probability, other perturbations of normal physiology.

DIAGNOSIS

Sickle cell disease is a constellation of similar but not identical disorders, all of which have at least 50% HbS in the blood. The phenotype of sickle cell disease is caused by several common and some less common genotypes; homozygotes for the HbS gene are said to have sickle cell anemia; common compound heterozygous forms of disease include HbSC disease and HbS-β thalassemia. The cornerstone of the clinical laboratory diagnosis is the detection and quantification of HbS. Depending on the context of the diagnostic situation, direct detection of the HbS and other globin gene mutations can be warranted. Sickle cell trait is clinically benign and not considered a form of sickle cell disease.

CLINICAL FEATURES

The complications of sickle cell disease can occur acutely, producing dramatic clinical findings, or they can be chronic, disabling, and cause premature death. For example, pulmonary hypertension is usually silent but is associated with a grave prognosis. The clinical features of sickle cell disease are heterogeneous. Fetal hemoglobin, α thalassemia, and compound heterozygosity for other variant hemoglobins such as HbC or β thalassemia are well-known determinants of the phenotype.

Acute painful episodes are the most common clinical events. Most often they begin with little warning. In some patients it is difficult to distinguish among new episodes of acute pain, chronic pain with acute exacerbations, therapy-induced pain, and pain made worse by major psychosocial issues. Insufficient doses of opioid analgesics, given at infrequent intervals, is the most common deficiency in pain treatment.

The acute chest syndrome, with fever, chest pain, cough, hypoxia, and lung infiltrates affects more than half of all sickle cell anemia patients. It is most common but least severe in young children, in whom it is often secondary to infection. In adults, pain often precedes this event, and mortality is higher than in children. Fat embolism from necrotic bone marrow is a common cause of the most severe acute chest events. Sometimes, fat embolization is accompanied by dramatic falls in the hemoglobin and platelet levels, marked leukocytosis, and multiorgan failure. Recognizing acute chest syndrome is critical because aggressive treatment with oxygen, blood transfusions, bronchodilators, and antimicrobials can be lifesaving.

Strokes occur in approximately 10% of children with sickle cell anemia and are more rare in other genotypes.

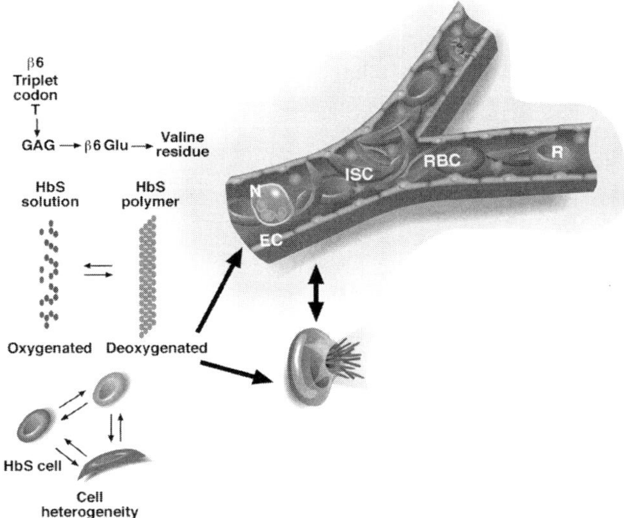

Pathophysiology of sickle cell disease. The nucleotide and amino acid substitution of HbS leads to the replacement of a glutamic acid residue by a valine residue. On deoxygenation, HbS polymer forms, causing cell sickling and damage to the erythrocyte membrane. Some cells adhere to the endothelium and cause vasoocclusion. Other cells are destroyed within the circulation, releasing hemoglobin and arginase and depleting bioavailable nitric oxide (Chapters 10 and 11).

Prophylactic blood transfusion can prevent a stroke in high-risk individuals. A current focus is how better to predict who will have clinically significant cerebrovascular disease and how this might best be managed. Survival decreases and the risk of stroke increases as blood pressure increases, even though it is within the "normal" range.

Osteonecrosis, seen in approximately half of all patients, most often affects the heads of the femur and humerus. In some individuals, it culminates in a severely painful or a useless joint that requires surgery.

Pulmonary hypertension affects approximately a third of adults with sickle cell anemia. Although usually mild, when defined in terms of pulmonary artery systolic pressure, its presence portends a poor prognosis as at least a quarter of patients die within 2 years of its detection.

Other severe complications are leg ulcers, priapism, nephropathy with renal failure and severe anemia with advancing age, and sickle retinopathy, especially in HbSC disease and liver disease. Infections are common and major causes of death in children and adults.

Treatment. Treatment for sickle cell disease is evolving and many clinical trials of new agents are in progress. With the exceptions of transfusions to prevent stroke, hydroxyurea for prevention of painful episodes, and prophylactic penicillin for prevention of pneumococcal disease in children, controlled clinical trials have not established the superiority of any treatment modality. Nevertheless, much can be done to promote better health of the individual, including good nutrition and avoidance of extremes of temperature and dehydration, genetic counseling for couples at risk for having affected children, and neonatal screening to identify infants with sickle cell disease and directing their parents toward comprehensive care programs that provide recommended immunizations and prophylactic penicillin.

The following five chapters discuss in detail the topics outlined previously.

19

Clinical and Pathophysiological Aspects of Sickle Cell Anemia

Martin H. Steinberg, Kwaku Ohene-Frempong, and Matthew M. Heeney

INTRODUCTION

Many authors have recounted the history of sickle cell disease in Africa and its first recognition in the United States[1–3] Sickle-shaped red cells were first described in 1910 in the blood of a sick, anemic student from Grenada.[4,5] Sickle hemoglobin (HbS) was identified in 1949 and the mechanism of inheritance of sickle cell anemia was established afterward.[6–8] A single amino acid difference was found to distinguish the sickle β-globin chain from the normal one.[9] The breadth of clinical and laboratory manifestations of sickle cell disease and its multitudinous complications still challenge the pediatrician, internist, general surgeon, obstetrician, orthopedist, ophthalmologist, psychiatrist, and subspecialists in each of these disciplines.

The features of sickle cell anemia change as life advances. Life's first decade, with declining fetal hemoglobin (HbF) levels, is typified by a risk of severe life-threatening infection, dactylitis, acute chest syndrome, splenic sequestration, and stroke; pain is often the torment of adolescence. If the worst of childhood and adolescent problems are survived or escaped, young adulthood can be a time of relative clinical quiescence, but sickle vasculopathy is likely to progress despite producing few symptoms. Chronic organ damage leading to pulmonary hypertension, deteriorating pulmonary function, renal failure, and late affects of previous cerebrovascular disease, including neurocognitive impairment, become paramount as years advance. Sickle cell anemia is noted for its clinical heterogeneity (Chapter 27). Any patient can have nearly all known disease complications; some have almost none, but die with a sudden acute problem. Some skip one or more phases of the disease but suffer intensely from others.

For convenience, when discussing the most common clinical events of sickle cell anemia, we have grouped these by the age group in which a complication is most likely to occur, although nearly every complication can occur at any age. As in other chapters, because of space constraints, many early references are omitted to allow inclusion of new material. Most of these citations can be found in the first edition of this book.[10]

PREVALENCE OF DISEASE AND LABORATORY DIAGNOSIS

Prevalence

Outside Africa, the prevalence of HbS depends primarily on gene flow from Africa to the Middle East, Asia, Europe, and the New World, modulated by genetic admixture with indigenous populations. Variations in the prevalence of HbS from within a country or geographic region are due to the presence of malaria, population isolates, altitude, and miscegenation. Although HbS is widely distributed in Caucasian populations, this is usually not the result of selection, but of ancient wars and migration, the slave trade, and generations of genetic admixture. In India, Greece, Turkey, Italy, and elsewhere in the Old World, HbS, excluding recent migrants from Africa or the Caribbean, is found mainly in Caucasians. In the United States, the prevalence of HbS in Caucasians varies according to the population examined, but it is usually less than 0.1% and is invariably found with African or Arab–Indian β-globin gene cluster haplotypes (Chapter 27). Table 22.1 in Chapter 22 shows the prevalence of the HbS gene in some African locations and throughout the world.

In African Americans, the incidence of sickle cell anemia at birth was estimated to be approximately 1 in 600 and the incidence of all genotypes of sickle cell disease approached 1 in 300.[11] These estimates and the distribution of disease in the United States have surely changed because of new immigrants from the Caribbean region, Central and South America, the Middle East, Africa, and India. In Paris, 1 in 900 newborns has sickle cell disease and in Salvador, Bahia, Brazil, approximately 1 in 500 newborns is affected. Although the treatment of complications of sickle cell disease differs little among its genotypes, knowing the genotype is critical for genetic counseling.

Diagnosis

Imprecision defining sickle hemoglobinopathies has permeated the medical literature. Sickle cell disease is a phenotype, expressed in patients with different genotypes. We use the following definitions:

- Sickle cell disease – at least half the hemoglobin is HbS and patients have distinguishing clinical and hematological features
- Sickle cell trait (HbAS; Chapter 22) is clinically benign and blood counts are normal, so it is not a form of sickle cell disease
- Individuals homozygous for the HbS gene (*HBB*, glu6val) are said to have sickle cell anemia

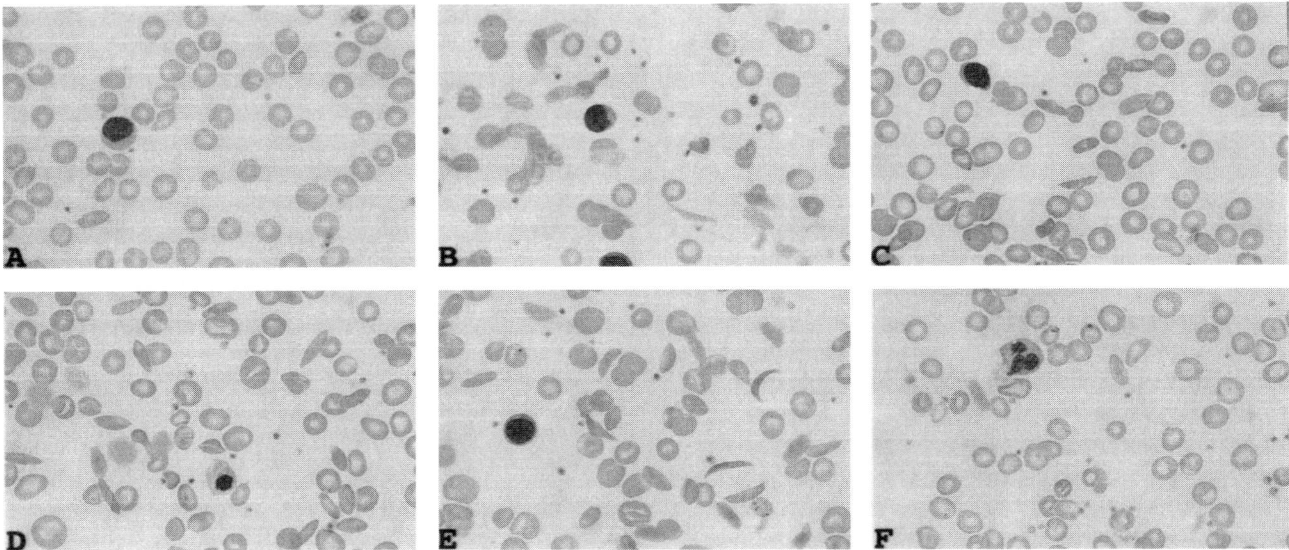

Figure 19.1. Blood films in patients with sickle cell anemia and average or low HbF levels. HbF in these patients are **A**-0.5%, **B**-1%, **C**-4%, **D**-5%, **E**-7%, and **F**-10%. Patients C and F were taking hydroxyurea. Although some of these patients have more ISCs than patients depicted in Figure 19.2 who have high HbF concentrations, note that patient A with the lowest HbF level has very few sickled cells. See color plates.

- Compound heterozygous forms of sickle cell disease include HbSC disease (*HBB* glu6val, glu6lys), HbS-β thalassemia (*HBB* glu6val and a β thalassemia mutation), and less common types (Chapters 21 and 23).

Diagnosing sickle cell disease is not difficult but determining the correct genotype can be problematic if family studies and access to molecular diagnostic methods are not available. Examining the blood of parents or siblings of affected patients is the least costly way of establishing the genotype and can be done with simple combinations of blood counts and quantitative studies of hemoglobin fractions.

Blood Counts and Erythrocyte Indices

In sickle cell anemia, the erythrocytes are normocytic or macrocytic, depending on the reticulocyte count and the presence or absence of confounding conditions such as iron or folic acid deficiency and coincident α thalassemia (Chapter 23). Microcytosis in a suspected case of sickle cell anemia can be seen very early in life before erythropoiesis has fully matured, when iron deficiency has developed or when α thalassemia is present. HbS–β^0 thalassemia, a phenocopy of sickle cell anemia but with microcytosis, and sickle cell anemia–α thalassemia are addressed in Chapter 23. These two conditions are very alike hematologically and clinically and their distinction from each other is difficult lacking genetic testing or family studies. In an individual, they cannot be separated using hemoglobin analysis or blood counts alone. Typical blood counts and erythrocyte indices in these genotypes are shown in Table 23.2 of Chapter 23.

Blood Films

Sickled cells are nearly always seen in sickle cell anemia and HbS–β^0 thalassemia but are less common in other genotypes. Typical blood films from patients with sickle cell anemia with high, average, and low HbF concentrations are shown in Figures 19.1 and 19.2. Some patients have many irreversibly sickled cells (ISCs), nucleated red cells, Howell–Jolly bodies, and polychromatophilic cells, whereas others have far fewer. In adults, ISCs remain relatively constant over time, although their percentage increases early in a painful episode (Chapter 20).[12]

Detecting HbS and Measuring Hemoglobin Fractions

From neonatal life through early adult life, there is a slow but continual fall in HbF, whereas HbA_2 levels increase until ages 1–2 years. With few exceptions, the hemoglobin fractions present at age 1 year are sufficiently stable to be relied on for diagnosis. In untreated sickle cell anemia, HbS nearly always forms more than 80% of the hemolysate, except in infancy when the γ- to β-globin gene switch is incomplete. HbS can be detected by isoelectric focusing, hemoglobin electrophoresis, or high-performance liquid chromatography (HPLC). Hemoglobin fractions are best measured by HPLC or capillary electrophoresis. Sickling hemoglobins can be detected chemically because they are insoluble and precipitate in high-molarity phosphate buffer when

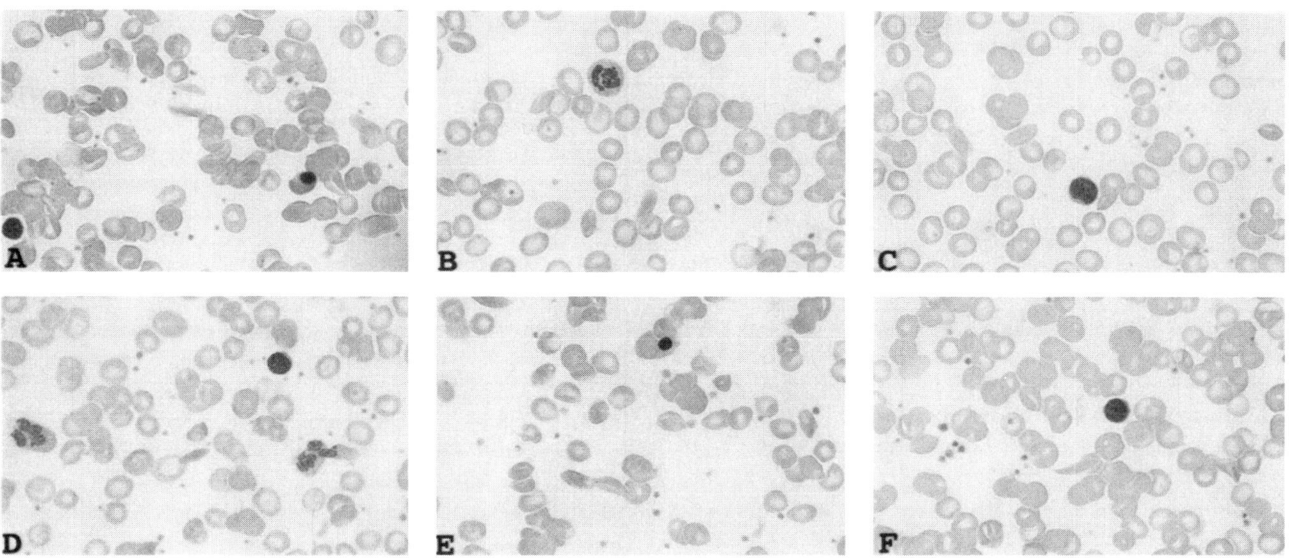

Figure 19.2. Blood films in patients with sickle cell anemia and high HbF levels. HbF in these six patients are **A**-19%, **B**-18%, **C**-19%, **D**-21%, **E**-20%, and **F**-23%. All patients were receiving hydroxyurea. All still have sickled cells in the blood and these are particularly prominent in patient A. Also note nucleated red cells in A and E. (See color plate 19.2.)

reduced with sodium dithionite, but these sickle solubility tests should not be used as the sole means of detecting HbS or other sickling variants because their results are not quantifiable and they cannot reliably distinguish among genotypes of sickle cell disease and HbAS. DNA-based methods of detecting the HbS mutation are now widely available and are definitive (Chapter 28).

PATHOPHYSIOLOGY

Major features of the pathophysiology of sickle cell disease such as HbS polymer, erythrocyte membrane abnormalities, sickle vasculopathy, and hemolytic anemia are discussed in Chapters 6, 8, 9, 10, and 11. Sickle vasoocclusion and hemolytic anemia are the two major features of disease pathophysiology. Reappraisals of the contributions of hemolysis and sickle vasoocclusion to the phenotypes of the disease and novel insights into the role of nitric oxide (NO) in sickle vasculopathy have led to new pathophysiological insights (Chapters 10 and 11).

A New View of Sickle Cell Pathophysiology: Hemolysis and Viscosity–Vasoocclusive Phenotypes (for a more detailed discussion, see Chapter 11)

Hemolysis, long discounted as a critical measure of sickle cell disease severity when compared with sickle vasoocclusion, might be the proximate cause of some severe disease complications and a major predictor of mortality. Hemolytic anemia is most severe in patients with sickle cell anemia, less severe in individuals with sickle cell anemia and concurrent α thalassemia, and least severe in patients with HbSC disease and HbS–β^+ thalassemia. Even within a single genotype, the hemoglobin concentration is variable because of different rates of hemolysis.[13–17]

Intravascular heme reduces NO bioavailability. NO binds soluble guanylate cyclase, which converts guanosine triphosphate to cyclic guanosine monophosphate (cGMP), relaxing vascular smooth muscle and causing vasodilation. A state of reduced endothelial NO bioavailability in sickle cell disease impairs downstream homeostatic vascular functions of NO, such as inhibition of platelet activation and aggregation and transcriptional repression of the cell adhesion molecules, vascular cell adhesion molecule (VCAM)-1, intercellular adhesion molecule (ICAM)-1, P-selectin, and E-selectin. Hemoglobin, heme, and heme iron catalyze the production of oxygen radicals, further limiting NO bioavailability and activating endothelium. Lysed erythrocytes also liberate arginase that destroys L-arginine, the substrate for the NO synthases. Reactive oxygen species, generated at high rates in patients with sickle cell anemia, also consume NO. The normal balance of vasoconstriction to vasodilation is therefore skewed toward vasoconstriction, endothelial activation, and proliferation. Both hemolysis and splenectomy are associated with red cell membrane damage, phosphatidylserine exposure at the red cell membrane surface, activation of tissue factor, and thrombosis. Chronic anemia and tissue ischemia might also contribute to a proliferative vasculopathy via activation of hypoxia inducible factor (HIF)-1α–dependent factors such as inducible nitric oxide synthase (iNOS), erythropoietin, and vascular endothelial growth factor (VEGF).[18]

Clinical studies suggest a close association of hemolysis with the subphenotypes of pulmonary hypertension, priapism, leg ulceration, and perhaps ischemic stroke.[19–26] Individuals with the highest rates of hemolysis also had a greater risk of death.[27] The frequency of painful episodes has also been associated with mortality.[28] Perhaps this association is mediated by increased hemolysis during painful episodes with a rise in pulmonary artery systolic pressure.[29] Hemolysis-related complications occur less often in patients with HbSC disease and sickle cell anemia–α thalassemia. HbF appears to have a lesser effect in modulating these phenotypes compared with the viscosity–vasoocclusive phenotypes of painful episodes, acute chest syndrome, and osteonecrosis.

Hemolysis might also be linked to vasoocclusive disease via the adhesive properties of the sickle reticulocyte. Sickle reticulocytes, whose numbers reflect in part the bone marrow response to hemolysis, adhere to endothelium and to leukocytes and are the most adherent of the heterogeneous population of sickle erythrocytes. Sickle erythrocyte adherence varies according to the hemoglobin genotype being most manifest in sickle cell anemia. Even among patients with this genotype, adherence varies approximately 20-fold. Because most of the endothelial cell adhesion molecules that bind sickle reticulocytes are normally suppressed by NO, decreased NO bioavailability might also contribute to sickle erythrocyte adherence.

Distinct from the hemolysis-related phenotypes are ones associated with increased blood viscosity and vasoocclusion, such as osteonecrosis, acute chest syndrome and painful episodes. Adversely affected by α thalassemia, their prevalence is directly associated with hemoglobin concentration; high HbF levels have a protective effect.

Hemolytic anemia–induced phenotypes are likely to be improved by transfusion, by agents that increase NO bioavailability and drugs that reduce intravascular hemolysis, but helped to a lesser extent by drugs that induce HbF expression.[30,31] Drugs that induce the production of HbF appear to reduce the incidence of painful episodes and acute chest syndrome.[32,33]

Hemolytic and viscosity–vasoocclusive phenotypes must have substantial areas of overlap and HbF is likely to play a role in all disease complications. Nevertheless, this dichotomization of pathophysiology helps place subphenotypes of sickle cell disease into a new context with implications for therapeutics, for example, by devising drug combinations that target multiple limbs of the pathophysiological tree.[18] One can envision combining a drug or drugs that induce HbF expression with agents that reduce sickle erythrocyte density, adhesive interactions of sickle cells, and the inflammatory response.[34]

Chronic activation of the hemostatic system has also been considered part of the pathobiology of sickle cell disease and might be the consequence of the exposure of aminophospholipids in the sickle erythrocyte, endothelial dysfunction with thrombin generation, and platelet activation, among other factors.[35,36] Platelet activation was correlated with the severity of pulmonary hypertension and also with reticulocyte count but not with lactate dehydrogenase (LDH). When exposed to cell-free hemoglobin, basal- and agonist-stimulated platelet activation was increased. In patients, sildenafil reduced platelet activation. These findings suggested a possible interaction among hemolysis, decreased NO bioavailability, and pathological platelet activation that might contribute to thrombosis and pulmonary hypertension.[37]

CLINICAL FEATURES OF SICKLE CELL ANEMIA

In the following discussion of the clinical features of sickle cell anemia complications are grouped by the age at which each is paramount. Painful episodes and their management are discussed separately in Chapter 20. Two large observational studies, one in Jamaica and the other in the United States, have provided much of our most reliable information on the clinical course and complications of sickle cell disease in developed countries. The Cooperative Study of Sickle Cell Disease (CSSCD) followed nearly 4,000 patients, including a newborn cohort of 694 patients, over a span of 20 years.[38–40] In Jamaica, a newborn cohort of more than 300 individuals and their matched controls, have been followed even longer.[41] Both studies have substantial patient numbers, longitudinal data collection, and biological sample repositories that can be used for genetic studies and measurement of newly developed disease markers. The inclusion of newborn cohorts in these studies eliminated the bias of studying only patients seeking medical care. Nevertheless, these studies are now decades old and their databases do not include complications of disease that were more recently recognized and do not report current methods of clinical and laboratory testing. Newly ascertained patient databases with their associated biological samples are needed.

Few controlled clinical trials of the treatment of the complications of sickle cell anemia are published and progress in this area has been slow. There were a number of questions posed in the first edition of this book: How should acute chest syndrome be managed? Is exchange transfusion superior to simple transfusion? Can preoperative transfusion sometimes be avoided? Do angiotensin-converting enzyme inhibitors delay sickle nephropathy? How is priapism best managed? How aggressively should blood pressure be lowered to decrease the chance of stroke? These questions have yet to be answered.

We will summarize recent information about the complications of sickle cell disease and provide explicit recommendations for treatment based on controlled clinical trials, in the few instances where they are available. In most cases, however, lacking the results of such studies, we will recommend management strategies based on experience with similar problems in other diseases, data from observational studies, expert opinion, and our understanding of the pathophysiology of sickle cell disease.

Assessing the Severity of Sickle Cell Disease

Knowing the elements of disease that put patients at risk for selected complications, overall disease severity and death

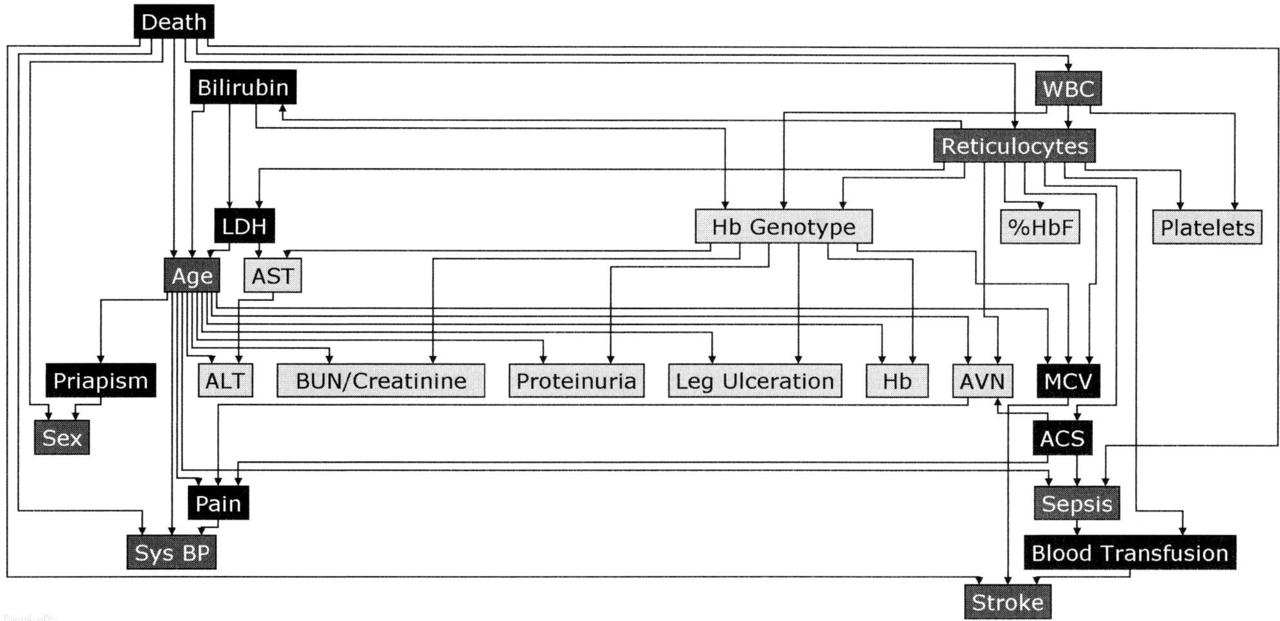

Figure 19.3. A Bayesian network model of the risk of death in sickle cell disease.[44] (See color plate 19.3.)

would have great value for patient counseling, planning therapy, and the development of novel treatments. A study was done of 392 infants with sickle cell anemia or HbS–β^0 thalassemia from the CSSCD. Nine years of clinical and laboratory data were available for analysis and an additional 115 infants were used for validation. Severe outcomes were defined as death, stroke, two or more painful episodes per year for 3 consecutive years, and one or more acute chest events per year for 3 years. Seventeen percent of the newborn cohort was identified as severe. A severe endpoint was achieved at a mean age of 5.6 ± 3.8 years. Hemoglobin levels of less than 8 g/dL, leukocyte counts more than 20,000/mm^2, an episode of dactylitis in patients aged younger than 1 year, and an elevated percentage of "pocked" red blood cells by age 1 year were significant predictors of adverse outcomes and combined identified 10.5% of the cohort, with a 0.35–0.71 probability of a severe outcome by age 10 years. Application of the severity model to the validation cohort yielded 100% positive predictive value and an 88% negative predictive value.[42] Unfortunately, in another study of children, this result could not be replicated.[43] In 168 children followed for up to 7.1 years, no relationship existed between these early clinical predictors and later adverse outcomes, with the possible exception of leukocyte count. At this moment, clinical and laboratory features seem unreliable means of making prognoses in young children.

Using Bayesian network modeling and data from 3,380 sickle cell disease patients of all ages and multiple genotypes, a severity score was constructed that estimated the risk of death within 5 years.[44] The predictive value of this score was validated in two independent patient groups: 140 adults and children in whom severity was assessed by expert clinicians and 210 adults in whom severity was also assessed by the echocardiographic diagnosis of pulmonary hypertension and death. A network of 24 variables described complex associations among complications of sickle cell disease and its laboratory variables (Fig. 19.3). In addition to known risk factors, the severity of hemolytic anemia and clinical events associated with hemolytic anemia were major contributors to risk for death. By capturing multiple effects that could be synergistic or antagonistic, according to the overall clinical presentation, the model could be used to compute a personalized measure of disease severity. A model calculator can be used to assess the clinical severity of patients with sickle cell disease, given any clinical profile (www.bu.edu/sicklecell/downloads/Projects).

This analysis suggested that the intensity of hemolytic anemia, estimated by LDH, reticulocyte count, and aspartate aminotransferase (AST), is an important contributor to death. Systolic hypertension, associated with pulmonary hypertension in patients with sickle cell disease, is an important predictor of mortality and might reflect the decrease in NO bioavailability that characterizes hemolytic anemia. Polymorphisms in key genes that modulate the pathobiology of disease that might underlie severity and the propensity to develop subphenotypes of disease are discussed in Chapter 27.

THE NEONATE

At birth and for the first few months of life, children with sickle cell disease usually do not have typical vasoocclusive complications. This is likely to be due to the persistence of very high HbF levels. The CSSCD reviewed birth outcome

Table 19.1. Incidence of major clinical events in children with sickle cell anemia in the first decade

Age (y)	Hand–foot syndrome	Painful event	Acute chest	CVA	Acute anemia: Spleen	Acute anemia: Other	Bacteremia
< 0.5	14.6	2.9	6.8	0.0	1.0	2.9	1.9
0.5–1	31.3	9.5	16.4	0.0	5.5	5.0	9.9
1	20.0	24.0	26.8	0.3	6.2	1.7	6.5
2	11.0	38.3	26.3	1.3	5.3	3.3	8.7
3	3.5	42.4	34.2	0.4	2.0	5.9	4.7
4	2.0	49.6	25.5	1.5	1.5	3.9	2.0
5	0.0	40.8	22.5	0.7	1.4	2.0	0.0
6	0.0	39.2	28.9	2.1	1.0	8.3	4.1
7	0.0	41.6	20.8	1.5	0.0	3.0	1.5
8–10	0.0	37.9	15.2	0.0	0.0	1.9	0.0

Incidence rates per 100 person-years from 427 children with sickle cell anemia observed in the Cooperative Study of Sickle Cell Disease, from October 1978 to October 1988.[38]

and neonatal clinical course of 480 infants with sickle cell disease. Rates of preterm birth (aged <37 weeks), low birth weight (<2500 g) and small for gestational age were 9%, 10%, and 8%, respectively, and similar to those in all African Americans. These figures were similar among the different genotypes of sickle cell disease. Fifty-nine percent of newborns with sickle cell disease with a low birth weight were born at term compared with 41% of all African Americans with low birth weight, a significant difference.[45]

Although the onset of clinical manifestations of vasoocclusive disease can be delayed, laboratory evidence of the presence of hemolytic disease is present early. Neonatal hyperbilirubinemia has been reported at a higher rate in newborns with sickle cell disease. The prevalence of anemia in newborns with sickle cell disease in the United States is unknown because hemoglobin levels are not measured routinely on full-term, well-appearing newborns. The Jamaican cohort study reported that compared with controls, neonates with sickle cell anemia had a lower than normal hemoglobin concentration as early as age 2 weeks. In a longitudinal study on the hematological changes in children with sickle cell disease followed from birth to age 5 years, the CSSCD reported that anemia and reticulocytosis were apparent by age 10 weeks in patients with sickle cell anemia.[46] There are no physical features in a newborn with sickle cell disease that would raise the clinician's suspicion of this diagnosis. That is why screening programs are the most effective way to identify patients prior to the onset of clinical complications and at present, such programs are in place in all states (http://genes-r-us.uthscsa.edu/nbsdisorders.pdf) and in may sites in countries with a high incidence of disease.

INFANTS

The CSSCD collected data prospectively on clinical complications of disease in 694 babies.[38] Table 19.1 shows the frequency of the most common complications and their prevalence or incidence at different ages in children with sickle cell anemia up to age 10 years. With the exception of acute chest syndrome, which occurred more frequently in boys than in girls (29.1 vs. 20.1 per 100 person-years), and painful events, which had a higher incidence in girls (35.7 vs. 28.9), there were no sex differences in the occurrence of most of these complications. Constant or episodic scleral icterus and the pattern of recurrent pain in limbs and abdomen often become established in the first year of life. Splenomegaly, another manifestation of sickle cell disease in children, is present in a few infants with sickle cell anemia aged younger than 6 months. The spectrum of complications was the same in children with HbSC disease but complications occurred at lower rates and at later ages. It is evident that even at the ages when HbF levels are expected to be high, some children with sickle cell disease face increased risk for vasoocclusive complications. The high incidence of pneumococcal bacteremia in infancy is explainable by the documentation of early splenic dysfunction (discussed later).

In children not detected through newborn screening, it is difficult for unsuspecting physicians to determine the existence of sickle cell disease on the basis of physical examination alone. The earliest physical sign of the disease is often dactylitis ("hand–foot syndrome"), manifested as painful swollen hands and feet. In sickle cell anemia, anemia is present early, with a mean hemoglobin level of 9.3 g/dL at age 3 months, and remains at the same level until after age 18 months, when it falls below 9.0 g/dL. Over the same period, the mean HbF level drops from 40.4% to 17.1%.[46] It is unclear why this large fall in HbF concentration has so little effect on the degree of anemia, but it could be related to the rise (5.4%–10.4%) in mean reticulocyte count over the same period.

FIRST 10 YEARS

In the first decade of life, the most common sickle cell disease–related clinical events are painful episodes and acute chest syndrome. Pain, presumed to be caused by vasoocclusive ischemia, often starts as the hand–foot syndrome, when the feet and hands become swollen and tender because of inflammation of the metacarpal and/or metatarsal periosteum. When accompanied by fever and persistent localized tenderness and erythema, osteomyelitis should be ruled out. Beyond infancy, the pattern of recurrent pain, typical of sickle cell disease, usually becomes established. The management and pathophysiology of sickle cell disease–related pain is discussed in Chapter 20.

The Spleen in Early Childhood

The spleen undergoes immense changes in function and size in the early life of children with severe forms of sickle cell disease. In sickle cell anemia and HbS–β^0 thalassemia, splenic dysfunction begins in infancy. This has been demonstrated in a series of studies first using technetium-99m sulfur-colloid liver-spleen scans, and later by the presence of increased circulating "pocked" or "pitted" red cells as measures of splenic function. Splenic dysfunction is the primary cause of the increased incidence of and mortality from bacterial infection in young children with sickle cell disease. Splenomegaly is a common feature of sickle cell disease in early life. The onset of splenomegaly and the prevalence of splenomegaly at different ages are different among the major genotypes and among different sickle cell disease populations around the world. In the United States, splenomegaly is seen in children with sickle cell anemia who are aged 1–5 years, but it is rare in older children. Splenomegaly persists longer in patients with HbS–β^0 thalassemia and in patients with HbSC disease in whom it is present over a wider age range. In Jamaica, early splenomegaly was found to be associated with increased susceptibility to infection and low HbF concentrations. Greek patients with sickle cell anemia had persistent splenomegaly at a higher rate than did Jamaicans.

When 43 children with sickle cell disease had splenic function measured before and during treatment with hydroxyurea for a median duration of 2.6 years, six patients (14%) completely recovered splenic function and two (5%) had preserved splenic function, suggesting that hydroxyurea might help preserve or recover splenic function.[47]

Persistent gross splenomegaly, related to endemic malaria, is common in patients with sickle cell disease residing in Africa. The frequency of splenomegaly was higher in a group of Nigerian children with sickle cell anemia compared with age-matched patients from the United States. Nigerian children with persistent gross splenomegaly had more frequent episodes of acute anemia, a complication commonly associated with acute attacks of malaria. Persistent massive splenomegaly is often associated with a hematological picture of hypersplenism with lower hemoglobin levels, platelet, and leukocyte counts than expected for age and hemoglobin genotype.

Growth and Development: Nutrition

Growth, Development, and Energy Expenditure. Delayed growth and sexual development become major issues of concern to the adolescent. Growth delay starts in early childhood but becomes more apparent during adolescence when the growth spurt of normal children separates them from patients with sickle cell disease. Children and adolescents with sickle cell disease have impaired growth compared with controls.[48–51] The growth deficit tends to be greater in weight than in height, and is more severe in patients with sickle cell anemia and HbS–β^0 thalassemia compared with HbSC disease and HbS–β^+ thalassemia. Bone age is often less than chronological age in both boys and girls. In a more recent study of 148 children, 38% fell below the 5th percentile in one or more measures such as height, weight, or body mass index.[52]

In parallel with delayed growth in weight and height, adolescents with sickle cell disease are delayed in sexual maturation. There was a 1–2 year delay in attaining Tanner stages 2–5 in both males and females with sickle cell anemia, and menarche was delayed by 2–3 years. Puberty was delayed 1–2 years, and median age at menarche was 13.2 years.[52] Fortunately, sexual maturation is eventually achieved and the height, but not the weight, gap is closed by adulthood in most patients. Nevertheless, size and rate of sexual development are constant measures of comparison among adolescents and those who are delayed often face severe emotional consequences.

To see if reduced height and weight were associated with abnormalities of the growth hormone (GH)/insulin-like growth factor–I (IGF-I)/IGF-binding protein-3 (IGFBP-3) axis, 21 children with sickle cell disease were examined. Nearly half had a defective GH response to both clonidine and glucagon and they had slower linear growth velocity, lower circulating IGF-I and IGFBP-3, and either partial or complete empty sellae by computed tomography (CT) scanning. A single injection of GH produced a smaller increase in circulating IGF-I in children with or without defective GH secretion when compared with age-matched children with idiopathic short stature and children with isolated GH deficiency, suggesting partial GH resistance in the sickle cell disease group. Defective GH secretion, decreased IGF-I synthesis, and partial resistance to GH in these short children suggest that treatment with IGF-I may be superior to GH therapy.[53] Five patients treated for more than 3 years with GH had improvement in their height.[54]

Delayed growth and skeletal and sexual maturation in sickle cell disease could be a result of energy deficiency and chronic malnutrition. Children and adults with sickle cell disease had increased resting energy expenditure.[55–59] Resting metabolic rate in patients with sickle cell anemia was 19% higher than that in control subjects, and this difference was not accounted for by differences in lean body mass. Increased energy expenditure could lead to a marginal nutritional state that contributes to abnormal growth.

When basal rates of whole body protein, glucose, lipid metabolism, and resting energy expenditure were measured, resting energy expenditure was 15% greater in the patients than controls. Whole body protein breakdown and protein synthesis were 32% and 38% greater, respectively, in patients, but whole body amino acid oxidation, glucose, and lipid metabolism were similar to controls. Isotope infusions studies and indirect calorimetry reflected hypermetabolism, and suggested that hemolysis and increased cardiac workload might contribute to this.[60] Additional energy required for the greater rates of whole body protein breakdown and synthesis contributed significantly to the observed increase in resting energy expenditure, suggesting that dietary energy and protein requirements are increased in sickle cell disease. Supplemental oral glutamine decreased resting energy expenditure and might improve growth.[61]

Voluntary energy intake in sickle cell anemia appears to be similar to that of control subjects with a normal hemoglobin genotype despite their higher resting metabolic rate. This observation suggests a suboptimal nutritional state. Patients might therefore conserve energy by reducing their physical activities. This hypothesis was tested by comparing resting metabolic rate, total daily energy expenditure, and physical activity level in postpubertal boys with sickle cell disease and in normal matched controls. Resting metabolic rate of patients exceeded that of the controls, but total energy expenditure was greater in controls. Control subjects had nearly 50% more physical activity than patients, suggesting that reducing physical activity is a compensatory mechanism for energy deficiency in sickle cell disease.[57]

Nearly all studies of energy expenditure in sickle cell disease are flawed by the difficulty of choosing appropriate controls, making their interpretation difficult. Although matching for age and sex is fine as far as it goes, controls for hemolysis or anemia are not included. Therefore, results of these studies are not specific for sickle cell disease, but compare patients with hemolytic anemia with hematologically normal controls. Ideally, to ensure that results reflect the pathophysiology of sickle cell anemia and not hemolytic anemia in general, controls should include individuals with other chronic hemolytic anemias.

Nutrition

Dietary intake of multiple vitamins and minerals, calcium, and fiber was low, and declined steeply during 3 years of observation.[62] Poor dietary intake might be contributed to by frequent hospitalizations for pain.[63] A long-standing and still unanswered question centers about the contribution, if any, of nutritional deficits to the pathophysiology of disease. In developed countries nutritional deficiencies do not seem to be a major factor in the course of the disease in most patients. No evidence exists that the many vasoocclusive complications of sickle cell disease or its hemolytic anemia are, except in extreme circumstances, affected by a patients' nutritional status or that nutritional supplementation, with the exception of the rare case of megaloblastic arrest of erythropoiesis due to folic acid deficiency, can change the course of disease.

Zinc deficiency has been found in some patients with sickle cell anemia and treatment with supplemental zinc has been claimed to reverse the sexual immaturity of some patients, promote the healing of leg ulcers, reduce infections, and have some effect on the sickling process. The relationship between zinc deficiency and delayed growth and sexual development in children with sickle cell disease has been confirmed.[64]

Several lines of evidence indicate that tissue zinc deficiency is present in some patients with sickle cell anemia but there are some inconsistencies in the data. Among most experienced practitioners, supplemental zinc has not been widely used. Whether or not zinc deficiency plays an important role in the pathophysiology of well-nourished patients with sickle cell anemia is doubtful, but this has not been the subject of many controlled trials. One trial of 130 patients compared the effects of zinc with a placebo in the reduction of painful episodes. After 18 months of observation, approximately half as many episodes occurred in the zinc-treated group compared with the placebo-treated patients.[65] As zinc deficiency adversely affects helper T cells and cell-mediated immunity, the role of supplemental zinc for preventing infection was studied in 32 patients with sickle cell disease, aged 19–49 years.[66] Twenty-one zinc-deficient patients were divided in two groups: 11 subjects were observed for 1 year, following which they received, for 3 years, 50–75 mg of elemental zinc daily, as oral zinc acetate; and 10 patients were observed for 1 year, following which they received placebo for 1 year and then switched to zinc supplementation for 2 years. A third group of 11 patients were zinc sufficient and not treated. Zinc supplementation increased lymphocyte and granulocyte zinc, and increased in interleukin-2 production. Documented bacteriologically positive infections, hospitalizations, and number of vasoocclusive pain episodes were significantly decreased.

Vitamin A status, estimated by a reduced serum retinol level, was less than normal in 66% of children with sickle cell anemia. This was associated with increased hospitalizations, poor growth, and lower hemoglobin concentration.[67] Among 65 children with sickle cell anemia, aged 5–18 years, 65% had reduced levels of vitamin D (25 OHD), and this was associated with season of the year and dietary intake.[68] Bone metabolism in sickle cell disease is discussed later.

Because of the relationship between plasma homocysteine concentration and folate status, plasma homocysteine concentrations were measured in 120 children with sickle cell anemia who had never received supplemental folic acid.[69] Plasma homocysteine levels in sickle cell anemia patients and controls were similar. In 34 children, simultaneous serum folate, red cell folate, and total homocysteine concentrations were measured and their serum folate and red cell folate concentrations were normal. There was no correlation of plasma homocysteine concentration with various clinical or laboratory measures or with red cell folate concentration. These children, who likely had good nutritional status, had normal folate stores in the absence of supplemental folic acid, making daily folic acid supplementation in well-nourished patients unlikely to be necessary.

Stroke, Neurological, and Neurocognitive Manifestations

Pathophysiology

One of the best examples of the vasculopathy of sickle cell disease is the extensive cerebrovascular damage that often leads to stroke and subtle neuropsychological dysfunction. Many recent reviews have discussed the pathophysiology and management of sickle cerebrovascular disease.[70–73]

Most cases of sickle cell stroke are due to stenosis and/or occlusion of major vessels of the Circle of Willis, the internal carotid arteries, and less frequently, the vessels of the vertebrobasilar system. These large arteries show fragmentation and duplication of the internal elastic lamina with extensive intimal hyperplasia encroaching on the vascular lumen. Some vessels also show aneurysmal formation. Strokes are caused by in situ occlusion or embolism from thrombi formed at the point of vascular damage or formed at areas of turbulent blood flow. Stenosis of the major vessels results in increased blood flow velocity, which can be measured with transcranial Doppler (TCD) ultrasonography.[74,75]

Gene expression profiling in blood outgrowth endothelial cells has been used to understand the biological systems that might mediate stroke in sickle cell disease.[76] In endothelial cells grown from the blood of 11 patients with sickle cell anemia at risk for stroke because of Circle of Willis disease, compared with nine patients not at risk for stroke, genes mediating inflammation were differentially expressed.

Hemorrhagic stroke is thought to be caused often by rupture of aneurysms formed in the vessels of the Circle of Willis or the fragile vessels of moyamoya disease that results from stenotic lesions of the major intracranial vessels. Angiographic studies following hemorrhagic stroke have shown the presence of multiple aneurysms, although not all cases of hemorrhage were associated with aneurysm. Bleeding is commonly subarachnoid but can be intraventricular or parenchymal.

Epidemiology

Strokes in sickle cell disease are classified into three clinical types: infarctive, hemorrhagic, and transient ischemic attacks. Although all types are seen in all age groups, infarctive strokes were generally believed to be more common in children.

The overall prevalence of stroke and incidence of a first stroke in patients with sickle cell anemia in the United States are, respectively, 4.96% and 0.61 per 100 person-years as reported in the CSSCD.[22] In HbSC disease, the rate and prevalence are 0.84% and 0.15 per 100 person-years; in HbS–β^+ thalassemia and HbS–β^0 thalassemia, these figures are 1.29% and 0.09 and 2.43% and 0.08, respectively.

Stroke is rare in infants with sickle cell disease; however beyond age 1 year, stroke incidence in sickle cell anemia patients is relatively uniform at approximately 0.5 per events per 100 patient-years until age 40 years, except for peaks of 1.02 events per 100 person-years in patients aged 2–5 years and 0.8 in patients aged 6–9 years. In 39 children with sickle cell anemia between ages 7 and 48 months without a history of clinical stroke – three had a history of seizures – who were examined with magnetic resonance imaging (MRI) and magnetic resonance angiography (MRA), the overall prevalence of abnormalities in these "asymptomatic" children was 11%. One patient had a silent infarct observed on MRI and a stenotic lesion on MRA; three other patients had stenotic lesions on MRA. Patients with a history of seizures all had lesions consistent with infarcts on MRI. Of the patients who had psychometric testing, 1 of 18 was developmentally delayed. One of 3 patients with a history of seizures had mild developmental delay.[77] Therefore, very young children with sickle cell anemia without a history of clinical stroke can have infarction in the brain and/or stenosis of major cerebral arteries, similar to those reported in older children. The high incidence in the first decade and the absence of a direct correlation between the incidence of stroke and advancing age, suggest that cerebrovascular disease is not likely to be simply the result of cumulative damage caused by sickle cells and abnormal blood flow. Rather, those children experiencing stroke in the first decade might have an additional risk factor, genetic or acquired, which predisposes them to early stroke (Chapter 27). The risk of stroke persists throughout life for sickle cell disease patients. In sickle cell anemia, the risk of having a first stroke is 11% by age 20 years, 15% by age 30 years, and 24% by age 45 years. The absence of an antecedent or concurrent medical event associated with an initial stroke is a major risk factor for subsequent stroke in patients on a regular transfusion program.[78] Approximately 60% of patients with moyamoya and an incident stroke will have at least one recurrent cerebrovascular event despite transfusion, an incidence approximately twice that of individuals without moyamoya.[79]

The only reliable data to compare with the rates of stroke in the United States is from the Jamaican cohort study. In this study, 5.5% of 310 children with sickle cell anemia had a stroke by age 14 years.[80] This rate seems lower than that of children in the United States where approximately 8% of those with sickle cell anemia would have had a stroke by this age.

Stroke in adults can be infarctive or hemorrhagic. In the CSSCD, the incidence of stroke in patients aged 20 years or older was 0.59 per 100 person-years. Of the 27 first strokes occurring in adults, 52% were hemorrhagic, 30% were infarctive, 11% were transient ischemic attacks, and two were unclassified. The risk of hemorrhagic stroke was highest in patients aged 20–29 years, at 0.44 per 100 patient-years. In contrast, only 5 of 52 first strokes in sickle cell anemia patients younger than 20 years were hemorrhagic. Hemorrhagic stroke has a reported mortality rates of 24%–65%. In 15 children, aged approximately 10 years, compared with 29 control subjects, an increased risk of hemorrhagic stroke was associated with a history of hypertension, recent transfusion, and treatment with corticosteroids and possibly nonsteroidal antiinflammatory drugs.[81]

Stroke is associated with a high mortality rate. In the CSSCD, 10% of patients with stroke died within 2 weeks following the incident event. All patients who died had sickle cell anemia; almost all had a hemorrhagic stroke that was associated with a mortality rate of 26%. No deaths occurred soon after infarctive stroke. In the Jamaican cohort, in which stroke is not managed routinely with blood transfusion, 6 of 15 children with presumed infarctive stroke died, two immediately after the initial stroke and four after a recurrent stroke; one of two patients with a hemorrhagic stroke died.

Several factors were identified with increased risk for stroke. In decreasing order of risk, prior transient ischemic attack, level of anemia at steady state, rate of acute chest syndrome, acute chest syndrome 2 weeks prior to the stroke event, and elevated systolic blood pressure were associated with infarctive stroke. In 95 patients aged 1–23 years, without a previous stroke, and followed for a median of 6 years, 19 patients had central nervous system (CNS) events. Mean overnight oxygen saturation and TCD velocity were independently associated with risk.[82] Risk factors for hemorrhagic stroke were anemia and elevated leukocyte count at steady state. In the CSSCD study, no association was found between stroke and the frequency of painful episodes, priapism, or transfusion therapy within 2 weeks before the stroke event. Increased level of HbF has been reported in two smaller series to be protective of stroke, an association not noted in the CSSCD.[80,83] Scant data exist on the association of stroke in sickle cell disease with either inherited or acquired thrombophilia.[84]

High homocysteine levels have been associated with stroke in one study, whereas another correlated homocysteine levels with acquired folic acid deficiency.[85,86] Correction of the folic acid deficiency led to lower levels of homocysteine. Systolic hypertension is another risk factor for stroke.[87]

Coincident α thalassemia is associated with protection from stroke, perhaps because these patients have less hemolysis and a higher hemoglobin concentration (Chapter 23). Only 20% of pediatric patients with sickle cell anemia who had a stroke had α thalassemia, whereas 35% of individuals without a history of stroke had α thalassemia. The incidence of infarctive strokes in sickle cell anemia with coincident α thalassemia was reduced by more than 50%, and none of 48 patients with homozygous α thalassemia-two had a stroke. Nevertheless, in the Jamaican study, α thalassemia was not a deterrent for stroke.[80] α Thalassemia was associated with reduced TCD flow rate and hemolysis, estimated by serum LDH, is an independent risk factor for cerebral vasculopathy.[27,88] Serum LDH correlated with TCD flow velocity in children with sickle cell anemia, supporting the notion that hemolytic anemia was a determinant of cerebrovascular disease.[89]

Diagnosis

Stroke can be diagnosed by clinical presentation or history. The most common presenting symptoms of infarctive stroke are hemiparesis, aphasia, dysphagia, seizure, and monoparesis. The diagnosis is often confirmed or defined further with brain imaging studies that are also performed to exclude hemorrhage, which could require surgical intervention. Hemorrhagic stroke often presents as severe headache with vomiting and depressed consciousness. MRI or CT scanning is able to demonstrate parenchymal infarct or hemorrhage, although changes in CT can lag behind the event by several days (Fig. 19.4). Cerebrovascular lesions can also be delineated using MRA. Traditional angiography involving catheterization and injection of radiographic dyes is used less frequently, although this method might still be a more sensitive and specific than MRA.

Positron emission tomography (PET) added to MRI can improve the detection of cerebral vasculopathy and PET excels at assessing the functional metabolic state by permitting glucose utilization and microvascular blood flow to be measured. Forty-nine children with sickle cell anemia were studied using PET and MRI, 19 who had clinically overt stroke, 20 who had life-threatening hypoxic episodes or "soft" neurological signs, and 10 who were normal based on neurological history and examination. Sixty-one percent of all patients had abnormal MRI findings, 73% had abnormal PET findings, and 90% showed abnormalities on either the MRI or the PET or both. Eighty-nine percent of patients with overt stroke had an abnormal MRI, 89% had abnormal PET, and all had either abnormal MRI or PET or both. In the 20 subjects with "soft" neurological signs, half had abnormal MRI, 65% had abnormal PET, and 85% had abnormal MRI and/or PET. Sixty percent of the 10 neurologically normal subjects had abnormal PET. Eighty-three percent of patients without an overt stroke had imaging abnormalities based on either MRI or PET or both, suggesting silent ischemia. These imaging abnormalities were associated with lower than average full-scale intelligence quotient whether there was an overt stroke or silent ischemia. Chronic red blood cell transfusion in four patients improved metabolic and perfusion status on repeated PET scans. Using both PET and MRI identified a much greater proportion of children with sickle cell anemia who had neuroimaging abnormalities, even in the absence of a history of overt neurological events. In addition, the PET lesions were more extensive and bihemispheric.[90] These data suggest that PET can be useful a tool to evaluate metabolic improvement after therapeutic interventions.

Six patients with sickle cell disease and a history of stroke, aged 10–28 years, had PET scans using ^{18}F-fluorodeoxyglucose as a tracer. MRI demonstrated that two patients had only small vessel disease and four had both large and small vessel disease. In two of four subjects with large vessel disease, PET showed a corresponding

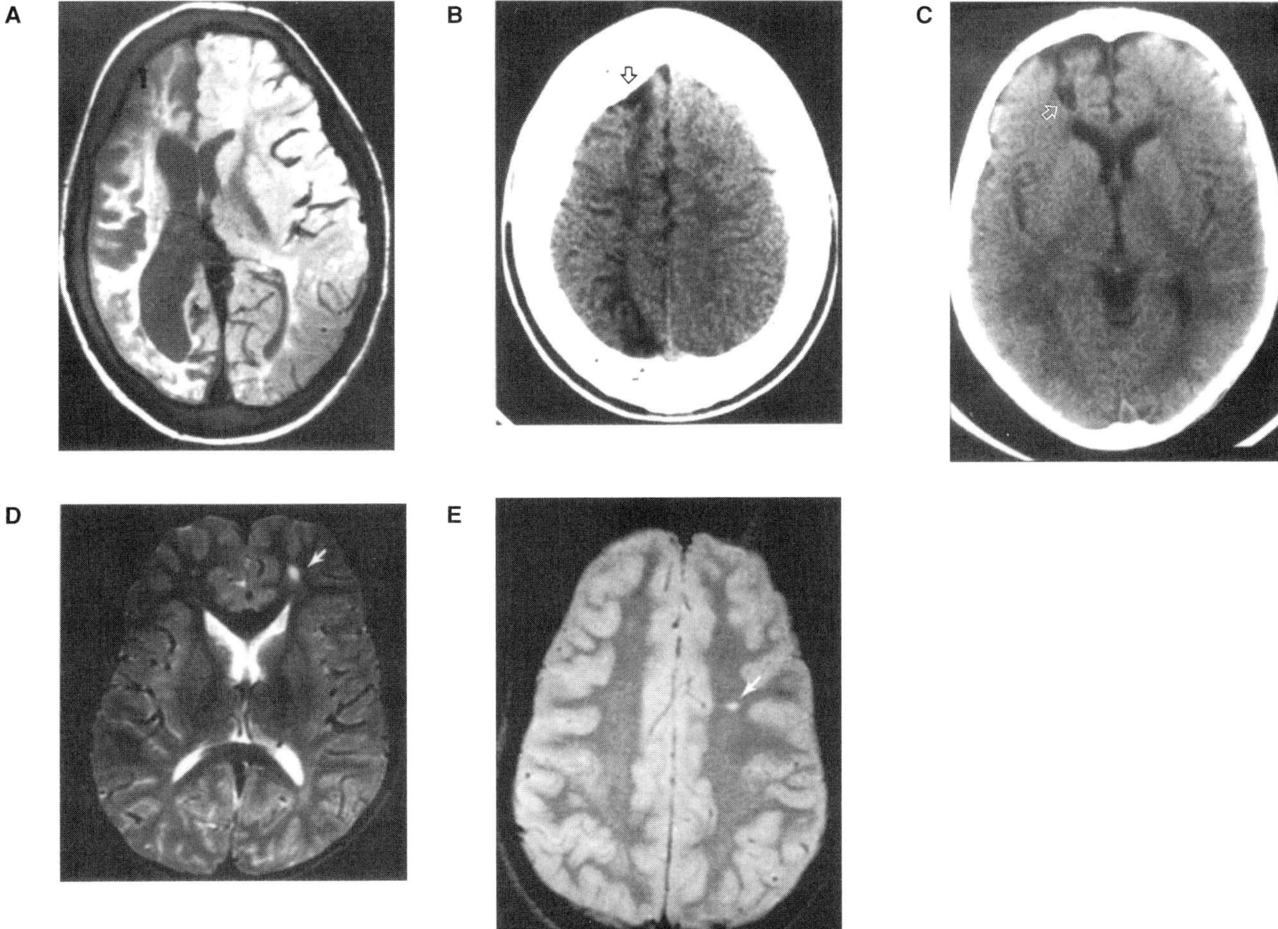

Figure 19.4. MRI and CT scans of cerebral infarction in sickle cell anemia. CT and MRI patterns of cerebrovascular disease. The left side of the photo represents the right side of the brain. **(A)** Tl-weighted MRI from a 12-year-old girl who suffered a right internal carotid artery occlusion 1 year before this study. There is severe loss of cortical and subcortical brain and massive dilation of the ventricular system. The anterior cerebral (ACA) and middle cerebral artery (MCA) territories are involved. This is an example of a major vessel occlusion pattern. **(B)** CT showing a linear area (open arrow) of infarction defining the border zone between the MCA and ACA territories. This 10-year-old boy developed mild left hemiparesis. Angiography showed an occluded right internal carotid artery (ICA) with extensive collateral flow from the vertebrobasilar system. **(C)** CT demonstrating another "border zone" infarction with a wedge-shaped area of infarction extending from the cortical surface to near the frontal pole of the lateral ventricle on the right (open arrow). This 14-year-old boy had a stroke at age 10 years. When studied at age 14 years after 4 years of chronic transfusion he had bilateral border zone infarcts (only right side shown), but both carotid systems were patent on angiography. These lesions are typically seen in cases with large artery, usually the ICA, stenosis or occlusion. In this case the absence of carotid lesions could indicate another mechanism, perhaps repeated bouts of severe anemia or resolution of lesions after years of transfusion. **(D)** T2-weighted MRI showing what is also considered by some to be a border zone lesion. The area of high signal near the frontal pole of the left lateral ventricle (white arrow) is an abnormal area of ischemia in the border zone between the deep and superficial vessels. This area is often abnormal on MRI in sickle cell disease when the CT is normal, and the patient may have little if any deficit. This 10-year-old boy was neurologically asymptomatic but had this MRI because of abnormal TCD studies. **(E)** Tl-weighted MRI from a 13-year-old girl who was neurologically asymptomatic except for headaches. The white arrow shows what has been called an "unidentified bright object." Similar lesions have been noted in asymptomatic elderly patients with vascular risk factors. Although not yet proven by pathological studies, it is likely that these small lesions, usually appearing in the subcortical white matter, are areas of small infarction caused by microvascular occlusion. Their presence does not imply concomitant large artery stenosis, and the risk of subsequent clinical stroke associated with these lesions is unknown. The patient whose MRI is shown in this panel remained asymptomatic without evidence of stroke 6 years after this study was performed.[74]

metabolic abnormality and also identified an area of hypometabolism extending beyond the anatomical lesion revealed by MRI. PET did not demonstrate an abnormality corresponding with small vessel disease. Detailed neuropsychological testing demonstrated cognitive dysfunction in all cases.[91] For some patients, PET might add sensitivity in detecting impaired metabolism in the area surrounding a major vessel infarct.

The magnitude of initial brain damage, degree of cerebrovascular disease, age at first stroke, type of stroke, and management determine the long-term outcome of stroke. Children with infarctive stroke often recover motor deficits, but recovery might depend on their age at the time of the first stroke. In one report, only one-third of children younger than 5 years, compared with two-thirds of those older than 5 years, recovered from motor deficits after initial stroke.[92]

In addition to motor deficits, cognitive abnormalities occur in sickle cell disease patients with cerebrovascular disease and stroke. Abnormal neuropsychometric studies are common both in the short-term and long-term periods after stroke. Brain MRI and neuropsychological evaluations were conducted to determine whether neuroradiographic evidence of infarct in children with sickle cell disease aged 6–12 years would result in impairment in cognitive and academic functioning. In 194 children, 135 of whom had sickle cell anemia, MRIs were categorized according to the presence of T2-weighted, high-intensity images suggestive of infarct and were further categorized on the basis of a clinical history of stroke. An abnormal MRI but no clinical history of cerebrovascular accident was classified as a silent infarct. Neuropsychological evaluations included assessment of both global intellectual functioning and specific academic and neuropsychological functions. Nearly 18% of all patients and 22% of patients with sickle cell anemia had MRI abnormalities. A clinical history of stroke was found only in children with sickle cell anemia (4.6%). Children with a history of stroke performed significantly more poorly than children with silent infarcts or no MRI abnormality on most neuropsychological evaluation measures, and individuals with silent infarction performed significantly more poorly than children with no MRI abnormality on tests of arithmetic, vocabulary, and visual motor speed and coordination.[93,94] Neurocognitive abnormalities in neurologically intact adults are discussed later.

It might be useful to obtain a thorough family history of stroke and other thrombotic events and to include evaluation for thrombophilia in laboratory assessment of sickle cell disease patients, particularly those with silent infarcts and stroke. Patients with hemorrhage should also be evaluated for coagulopathy.

Treatment recommendations. Initial management of infarctive stroke should include stabilization of the patient, judicious intravenous hydration, and transfusion (Chapter 29).[95] The goal of initial transfusion is to improve oxygenation and reduce the risk of further vasoocclusive and hypoxic damage. Exchange transfusion is preferable to simple transfusion because it allows a rapid decrease in the percentage of sickle cells. In a retrospective analysis, children receiving simple transfusion as an initial treatment had a fivefold greater relative risk of a second stroke during follow-up than those receiving exchange transfusion.[96]

Patients with persistent neurological deficits should be started on rehabilitation therapy as soon as possible. Long-term care centers and chronic transfusion therapy should be used to reduce the chance of recurrent stroke and management of iron overload. In untransfused patients the risk of recurrent stroke is as high as 70%, whereas it is approximately 10% in those maintained at HbS levels of less than 30% by chronic transfusion therapy.[97] In patients who remain stable neurologically, the HbS level can be allowed to rise to approximately 50% after several years at a level of 30% or less, with no added risk of a recurrent stroke.[78,98] This reduces the transfusion requirement and the rate of iron accumulation.

The duration of chronic transfusion is undetermined. In children, strokes have recurred when transfusion therapy was discontinued after 1–2 years or after 5–12 years. It is unknown whether continued chronic transfusion therapy will reduce the risk of hemorrhagic stroke later in life.

Iron overload in sickle cell disease patients receiving chronic transfusion occurs at rates similar to those in transfusion-dependent thalassemia. Iron chelation therapy, when adhered to, is equally effective in reducing iron stores (Chapter 29). Partial exchange transfusion reduces the rate of iron accumulation. This method of chronic transfusion is applicable to young children, as long as they have good venous access required for the procedure, and has eliminated iron overload in many patients receiving chronic transfusions.[99]

Although chronic transfusion therapy is effective in decreasing the rate of recurrent infarctive stroke in children, this has not been proven to be an effective measure in patients who have their first stroke in adulthood. Moreover, transfusion therapy is often stopped when children make the transition from the pediatric to the adult clinic. Hemorrhagic stroke might be a late sequela of infarctive stroke, suggesting that progressive vascular damage could eventually lead to rupture of abnormal vessels. Such bleeding has occurred even in patients maintained on chronic transfusion therapy. Encephaloduroarteriosynangiosis, to establish anastomoses between external and internal carotid arteries, has been used in patients with moyamoya and recurrent cerebrovascular events with a good outcome in a small series of patients.[100]

Management of hemorrhagic stroke includes careful hydration, nimodipine to reduce vasospasm, surgical evacuation of blood, and ligation of accessible aneurysms. Long-tem management of hemorrhagic stroke is unclear. The risk of recurrence is unknown, and the value of chronic transfusion in preventing recurrence is unproven. A high fatality rate within 2 weeks of a hemorrhagic stroke illustrates the need for ways to prevent this complication. Routine evaluation for aneurysms is not standard practice, although surgical intervention is usually successful in the treatment of those with aneurysm.

In 35 children with sickle cell anemia and stroke, transfusions were discontinued, hydroxyurea initiated, and phlebotomy was used to reduce iron stores. Initially, patients discontinued transfusions before hydroxyurea therapy was started, but later patients overlapped transfusions with hydroxyurea until the full dose was achieved. After 3–104 months of treatment, the stroke recurrence rate was 5.7 events per 100 patient-years, but children receiving overlapping hydroxyurea therapy had 3.6 events per 100 patient-years. With more than 6 months of phlebotomy, serum ferritin decreased from a median of 2,722 to 298 ng/mL and liver biopsy showed normal histology and iron stores.[101]

Stroke prevention. It is now possible to prevent the first occurrence of stroke in most children with sickle cell anemia. TCD ultrasonography, which measures blood flow velocity through intracranial vessels, was shown to be capable of selecting children with a high risk of stroke based on blood flow velocity in the major intracranial arteries.[102] Blood flow velocity is higher than normal in stenotic vessels. In a study of children with sickle cell anemia and no history of stroke, when blood flow velocity of 170 cm/second or higher in a middle cerebral artery was defined as abnormal, 6 of 23 patients with abnormal TCD ultrasonography had a stroke compared with only 1 of 167 with normal TCD ultrasonography. In a subsequent multicenter controlled study, 130 children with sickle cell anemia and internal carotid artery or middle cerebral artery blood flow velocity of 200 cm/second or higher were randomized to chronic transfusion therapy or standard care. After 1–26 months of observation, 11 of the patients on standard care had a stroke compared with only one in the transfusion group, a risk reduction of 92%.[103,104]

On the basis of these studies, patients with sickle cell anemia and HbS–β^0 thalassemia are screened – sometimes biannually, depending on their blood velocity value – for cerebrovascular blood flow by TCD ultrasonography, and individuals at high risk of stroke are chronically transfused. Nevertheless, most high-risk patients will not have a stroke during a given year and this must be weighed in the decision to transfuse. Additional prognostic variables that could help gauge the risk of stroke are being sought. In one study, a Bayesian network was able to predict, based on clinical variables and polymorphisms in candidate genes, the likelihood of developing a stroke (Chapter 27).[105]

The question of how long these transfusions should be continued was partially answered in a follow-up study.[106] When children at high risk of stroke were transfused for 30 months or longer, and their TCD flow rates became normal, they were randomly assigned to continue or discontinue transfusion. Children with severe stenotic lesions on MRA were excluded. The study was stopped after only 79 of the planned 100 patients were randomized as high-risk TCD flow rate developed in the 14 of the 41 children in the transfusion-halted group and two had a stroke within 2.1 to 10.1 months of their last transfusion. Neither high-risk TCD flow rate nor stroke occurred in the 38 children randomized to continue transfusions. It was concluded that discontinuation of transfusion for the prevention of stroke in children with sickle cell disease results in a high rate of reversion to abnormal blood flow velocities and stroke. Interestingly, the serum LDH level increased in patients randomized to stop transfusions, suggesting that increased intravascular hemolysis and decreased NO bioavailability might play a role in stroke recurrence. It was suggested that stem cell transplantation might be one approach to recurrent stroke prevention.

Hydroxyurea can reduce TCD flow rates, sometimes to normal values, raising the possibility that it could be useful in some instances for primary stroke prevention.[107–109] In the largest of these studies that included 37 children, HbF increased from 10.3% ± 6.6% to 22.7% ± 7.9% and the maximum transcranial velocity fell from 173 ± 22 to 129 ± 20 after 1 year at maximum tolerated dose.[107] The use of hydroxyurea to prevent recurrent stroke (ClinicalTrials.gov NCT0012298) is now the subject of a randomized clinical trial. Until these results are reported, prophylactic transfusion remains the standard unless there is no possibility of successfully transfusing the patient.

Silent infarction. MRI studies have identified brain infarcts in 18%–20% of patients who have had not had a clinical stroke. These "silent" infarcts are usually located in the deep white matter in the junctional areas ("border zones") between the tributaries of the anterior and middle cerebral and the posterior and middle cerebral arteries. Patients with complete strokes usually have infarcts in the cortical regions. In an analysis of risk factors for silent infarct among the infant cohort of the CSSCD who underwent MRI studies after age 5.9 years, 18% had a silent infarct. History of seizure, lower rates of painful episodes, and lower hemoglobin level were associated with silent infarcts, as were increased leukocyte count, elevated "pocked" red cell count, and the numbers of patients with a Senegal β-globin gene haplotype.[110] Silent infarcts are associated with increased neuropsychometric abnormalities. Infants with silent infarcts on MRI performed significantly more poorly than children with no MRI abnormality on tests of arithmetic, vocabulary, and visual motor speed and coordination.[111] Children with a history of stroke scored lower than those with silent infarcts or no MRI abnormality on most neuropsychological evaluation measures.

Although clinicians suspect that "silent" infarcts are associated with increased risk of clinical stroke, this has not been proven conclusively. A broadened definition of stroke that included significant changes in neuropsychometric studies in association with infarcts or vascular changes on brain imaging studies would identify a large number of children with sickle cell disease who might require therapy to prevent further brain damage and overt (motor) stroke. The management of children with sickle cell anemia should include annual TCD ultrasonography, starting at age 2 years, to identify those with high risk of stroke for consideration of preventive chronic transfusion therapy. Annual MRI studies might also identify those with "silent" infarcts and cerebrovascular damage.

Neuropathy. Peripheral neuropathies have been described but are not common. Most often they seem to result from adjoining bone disease and nerve entrapment, as when the mental nerve becomes entrapped in the mandibular canal due to bone infarction and in spinal radiculopathy, when bone infarction compresses a nerve root. Less often a mononeuropathy can occur.[112] One conjecture is that the richly anastomosing arteriolar and capillary network supplying peripheral nerves and the large diameter of these vessels helps preclude vasoocclusive damage. Some reports suggest that children with sickle cell anemia who become lead intoxicated are prone to peripheral neuropathy.[113]

Sensorineural hearing loss, particularly in the high-frequency 2,000–8,000-Hz range, has been encountered in up to 22% of patients with sickle cell disease.[114,115] Sometimes this has been observed in the course of a painful episode with resolution thereafter. Although the cause of this defect is uncertain it has been ascribed to vasoocclusive damage to inner and outer hair cells and the stria vascularis. Some patients also have transitory vertigo from apparent labyrinthitis. Although it is not possible to dissociate infectious causes from a vasoocclusive etiology, the latter remains a possibility.

Acute Anemic Episodes

Except for acute and usually small changes during vasoocclusive events – sometimes with severe acute chest syndrome, the packed cell volume (PCV) can fall dramatically – steady-state hemoglobin levels remain more or less constant over time unless erythropoiesis is depressed. Acute anemic episodes describe the episodic lowering of hemoglobin levels below the usual steady-state level in patients with sickle cell disease. The two common causes of acute anemia occurring in sickle cell disease, splenic sequestration and the B19 parvovirus–associated acute aplastic crisis, occur mainly in children. Other acute anemic events are seen in all age groups.

Acute Splenic Sequestration

Because it is initially enlarged, the spleen in sickle cell anemia becomes dysfunctional as early as the first 6 months of life and then begins a slow process of involution that in over 90% of patients outside of Africa culminates in a total loss of functional splenic tissue in late childhood. HbF levels determine, at least partially, the rate of splenic atrophy so that individuals with the highest levels of HbF maintain splenic function longer than those with lower levels. Some individuals with unusually high HbF levels continually have an enlarged functional spleen and these patients become susceptible to complications of splenomegaly in sickle cell anemia such as sequestration crisis, splenic infarction, intrasplenic hemorrhage, rupture, and abscess. Acute splenic sequestration, the sudden trapping of red cells in the sinuses of an enlarging spleen accompanied by severe anemia, mild thrombocytopenia, and hypovolemia has been defined by the CSSCD as a decrease of the hemoglobin or PCV of at least 20% from baseline, accompanied by an increase in palpable spleen size of at least 2 cm from baseline. Acute splenic sequestration often occurs in association with a febrile upper respiratory illness but its pathophysiology is not clearly understood. Sickle cells trapped for any duration of time in a hypoxic environment might be expected to hemolyze. It might therefore be inaccurate to describe acute splenic sequestration as trapping of sickled cells as it is neither acute nor followed by increased hemolysis and plasma is sequestered along with cells. Moreover, the "trapped" red cells are easily released into the general circulation as the acute anemia and hypovolemia are corrected when the spleen shrinks following therapeutic blood transfusion. It is more likely that blood continues to flow into the sinuses of the spleen but leaves at a much slower rate. A phenomenon causing expansion and subsequent shrinkage of the sinus vascular space within the spleen is a more likely mechanism. This could be due to hypoxic injury to the splenic microvasculature. Splenic sequestration is not always severe, and mild forms with less than 2 cm enlargement of the spleen and less than a 2-g/dL drop in hemoglobin level probably predominate. Rapid enlargement of the liver can also be associated with blood pooling and acute anemia, albeit much less often than splenic sequestration. Management of both conditions are similar (see later).

Acute splenic sequestration can occur in patients younger than 6 months. Cases of acute splenic sequestration in a 5-week-old and 2-month-old with sickle cell anemia have been reported. Although rare, acute splenic sequestration can occur in adults with sickle cell anemia and HbSC disease. Sometimes this occurs in adult patients with typical sickle cell anemia with low HbF levels and without any suggestion of having coincident α thalassemia.[116] The incidence of acute splenic sequestration in children with sickle cell anemia was 1.0 per 100 person-years by age 6 months, 6.2 by 1 year, 5.3 by 2 years, 2.0 by 3 years, and 1.0 by 6 years.[38] Acute splenic sequestration is less common in young children with HbSC disease and its peak incidence of 2.9 per 100 person-years by age 4 years is not reached as early as it is in patients with sickle cell anemia. Acute splenic sequestration in HbSC disease might occur over a broader age range and is seen in adults and children. α Thalassemia, by its effects on the rheology of sickle erythrocytes, might help preserve splenic function into adulthood and increase the incidence of acute splenic sequestration episodes in children and adults with sickle cell anemia (Chapter 23).[16] Among French and Guadeloupean children with sickle cell disease, the incidence of splenic sequestration was approximately 13% and 29%, respectively.[117,118]

Among the CSSCD cohort of newborns, 43 of 694 patients experienced 62 episodes of acute splenic sequestration over a 10-year observation period. Many patients develop episodes of subacute sequestration with the spleen frequently showing enlargement and reduction in size associated with mild changes in hemoglobin level. In a few patients, there is a chronic hypersplenism with lower hemoglobin level, platelet, and leukocyte counts than usual. Sixteen of the 43 children experiencing acute splenic sequestration underwent splenectomy. Those who had splenectomy were aged 0.3–4.1 years (median 1.6 years) at the time of the initial acute splenic sequestration event and were splenectomized at a median age of 2.6 years (range 0.8–5.3 years). None of the splenectomized sickle cell anemia patients developed postsplenectomy invasive bacterial infection during follow-up. Early splenectomy has been performed in the management of acute splenic sequestration without apparent increased risk of postsplenectomy bacterial infection.[119] The concern that splenectomy could pose additional risk for bacterial infection in young children with sickle cell disease has led some centers to the use of partial splenectomy, although the protective value of this procedure is uncertain as overwhelming septicemia has followed partial splenectomy.

Treatment recommendations. Acute splenic sequestration is a potentially life threatening and should be managed with urgency. Deaths often result from hypovolemic shock and not from anemia. Immediate management of acute splenic sequestration should be directed toward correction of hypovolemia with volume expanders. In an autopsy-based study, approximately 7% of deaths were due to splenic sequestration.[120] Transfusion of red cells can follow restoration of blood volume and blood pressure but this should be performed with caution because an acutely enlarged spleen has a tendency to release sequestered blood, and hemoglobin levels a few hours after transfusion tend to be higher than expected from the amount of red cells transfused. Red cells should be given in small portions and allowed to equilibrate to avoid hypervolemia. One guide to transfusion for splenic sequestration is that when the observed hemoglobin level is less than 5 g/dL, the initial volume of transfused red cells should be the equal in milliliters/kilograms to the observed hemoglobin level. For example, a child with hemoglobin concentration of 3 g/dL would then receive as an initial transfusion, 3 mL/kg of packed red cells. Subsequent transfusion amounts, if clinically indicated, should be estimated based on the hemoglobin level after equilibration of the initial transfusion. The use of diuretics might be advisable in those in whom hypervolemia is imminent or present.

Long-term management for individuals with recurrent acute splenic sequestration or severe hypersplenism includes parental retraining in the palpation of the spleen – this is a part of the initial training of parents of all infants with sickle cell disease – limited-term chronic transfusion therapy, or splenectomy. In facing the issue of splenectomy following one or more episodes of acute splenic sequestration, the ease of accessibility of the child to a competent medical facility in the event of an acute event and the functional state of the spleen must be considered. In situations where it is deemed unlikely that the child can reach a competent medical facility in time, splenectomy should be performed after the first episode of acute splenic sequestration. Where medical access is not a problem, the function of the spleen can be assessed through technetium-99m sulfur colloid scan or pocked red cell counts. If the spleen is judged functional, it might be prudent to delay splenectomy through chronic transfusion therapy until the child is 3 years or older. Partial splenectomy could be an alternative solution.

In regions of the world where sickle cell anemia is accompanied by high HbF levels, such as the eastern province of Saudi Arabia, the features of splenic sequestration are different. The age of onset is later and chronic splenomegaly is often present. In 44 sickle cell disease patients who had a splenectomy, more than half had high HbF levels and hypersplenism and most had some type of sequestration crisis, which could be minor. The spleen showed histological features of fibrocongestive splenomegaly.[121] Among 134 patients with sickle cell anemia who had splenectomy, recurrent acute splenic sequestration crisis was the most common indication, followed by hypersplenism. The mean HbF level was 20.5%.[122]

Aplastic Crisis and B19 Parvovirus Infection

Beyond malaria endemic areas, the most common cause of acute anemia in children with sickle cell disease is the so-called "aplastic crisis." This is defined as a transient erythroid aplasia or hypoplasia and is usually associated with parvovirus B19 infection, an agent that preferentially attacks erythroid precursors – the P antigen of erythrocytes is its receptor – so that the bone marrow has few primitive red cells and reticulocytes might be absent. Recovery occurs in 1–2 weeks. Not every patient with evidence of B19 parvovirus infection becomes acutely anemic and the reason for this is not known. Patients who have been infected with this virus appear to develop life-long immunity due to the presence of neutralizing antibodies. Transient cessation of red cell production in the marrow, coupled with the continued rapid destruction of sickle erythrocytes in the periphery, results in a rapidly developing severe anemia. The incidence of transient erythroid aplasia has not been determined in many sickle cell disease populations. In the 64 acute anemic episodes not due to acute splenic sequestration that occurred in 33 children aged 10 years and younger, the CSSCD did not report the specific incidence of erythroid aplasia. The largest reported series of transient erythroid aplasia comes from the Jamaican cohort study. All 91 episodes of "aplastic crisis" occurring in 308 sickle cell anemia patients were associated with parvovirus B19 and the rate of parvovirus B19 infection was the same in both the patients and their normal age-matched controls. An additional 23 sickle cell anemia patients with parvovirus B19 infection showed mild or no hematological changes. In one United States institution, parvovirus accounted for only 70% of the episodes of "aplastic crisis." Other viruses and bacteria have been associated with transient erythroid aplasia.

The clinical course of transient erythroid aplasia is usually insidious and is often discovered during evaluation of febrile children. Older children can report headache or that they are easily tired. The diagnostic hallmark of transient erythroid aplasia is reticulocytopenia (often <2%) associated with either a minimal or a clinically significant fall in hemoglobin concentration from its usual level. Usually erythropoiesis alone is affected, but concomitant neutropenia and thrombocytopenia have also been reported. Because of its relatively gradual development – in contrast, acute splenic sequestration develops rapidly – transient erythroid aplasia is often well tolerated. Hemoglobin levels of less than 4 g/dL can be seen in patients whose only complaint might be fever. In patients without evidence of previous parvovirus B19 infection and who do not have increased IgG for parvovirus B19, it is important to document whether parvovirus B19 is responsible for any episode of reticulocytopenia by obtaining antiparvovirus B19 IgM and IgG levels. Aside from searching for possible bacterial causes of the febrile illness, it is generally not useful clinically to test for other viral infections in establishing etiology of erythroid aplasia. B19 parvovirus is often asymptomatic and more than 70% of patients aged 17–21 years have IgG antibodies but less than 30% of individuals had a history of acute anemic episodes.[123] Parvovirus B19 is also associated with acute splenic sequestration, acute chest syndrome, stroke, nephrotic syndrome, encephalopathy, and myocarditis.[124–126]

The prevalence and incidence rates of B19 parvovirus infection were determined in 633 patients with sickle cell disease. Thirty percent were B19 IgG positive at intake into the study. On annual testing the incidence rate was 11.3 per 100 patient-years. In 68 patients who developed transient red cell aplasia, pain was present in 61.8%, acute splenic sequestration in 19.1%, and acute chest syndrome in 11.8%.[127] Virtually identical findings were reported from Jamaica.[128]

Acute anemia with reticulocytopenia can also accompany oxygen treatment in sickle cell disease[129,130] and bone marrow necrosis.

Treatment recommendations. The management of transient erythroid aplasia starts with awareness of whether the patient has had prior infection with parvovirus B19. Routine screening of children with sickle cell disease for parvovirus B19 IgG helps to identify patients who remain at risk and in whom parvovirus B19 infection should be considered whenever they are evaluated for a febrile illness. Patients at risk or whose parvovirus B19 status is unknown should be isolated from pregnant women until the reticulocyte count is determined because this virus might have untoward affects on the fetus of susceptible women. In the future, when a vaccine is available, patients without B19 parvovirus immunity should be recipients. Unlike normal children, children with sickle cell disease are instructed to seek medical attention for all febrile illnesses. This increases the chances of those with parvovirus B19 being exposed to medical staff. A cluster of parvovirus B19 infections in nurses traced to two sickle cell disease patients hospitalized for transient erythroid aplasia has been reported.

During the earliest phases of acute illness, antiparvovirus IgM and IgG levels can be negative. It is advisable to repeat these tests 1 week or so later for evidence of recent parvovirus B19 reflected by an increase of IgM antibody. The main therapeutic decision considered in erythroid aplasia is whether or not transfusion of red cells is required. Patients with a 25% or more drop in their hemoglobin level from baseline with reticulocyte counts that are falling or are absent and those who are symptomatic from severe anemia should be transfused early to shorten the period of the acute anemia. In a series of 80 children with strokes at the Children's Hospital of Philadelphia at least four had a stroke during a period of severe anemia due to erythroid aplasia. Transfusion should be performed cautiously similar to that described for splenic sequestration to avoid hypervolemia and complications due to a sharp rise in blood viscosity. Typically, a patient with transient erythroid aplasia begins to show nucleated red cells and reticulocytes within a week of the severe reticulocytopenia. In untransfused patients, the reticulocyte counts can rise to dramatic levels during recovery.

Hyperhemolysis

Hemolysis in sickle cell disease is discussed in detail in Chapter 11. An increase in the rate of hemolysis, in conjunction with specific clinical complications of sickle cell disease, has been called hyperhemolysis and is a third potential cause of acute anemia in sickle cell disease. Nevertheless, most experts, in the absence of malaria, have had difficulty documenting a convincing case of acute hyperhemolysis. Hyperhemolysis should be typified by an acute reduction in hemoglobin level associated with higher than usual reticulocyte counts and perhaps an unaccountable and sudden increase in LDH. In some reported cases of hyperhemolysis, the patient might have been examined during the recovery phase of an acute erythroid aplastic episode and the reticulocytosis was not reflective of increased red cell production due to hemolysis. Other cases could be a result of extensive bone marrow necrosis, although in this instance, reticulocytopenia should be present. Acute chest syndrome is often associated with a 0.5–1 g/dL drop in steady-state hemoglobin level. Also, during hospitalization for acute painful events, the hemoglobin concentration usually falls modestly. These observations are likely to be the result of a combination of events such as blood loss due to phlebotomy, acute bone marrow suppression due to associated inflammation, and small increases in hemolysis.

There is little evidence to implicate G6PD deficiency in accelerated hemolysis and acute anemia. Although reported, the lack of a sex difference in the incidence of acute anemic events argues against such an association.

Autoimmune hemolytic anemia is found in some patients with sickle cell disease who have been transfused and can be responsible for the fall in hemoglobin concentration from baseline (Chapter 29).

Perhaps the most clinically significant cause of acute hemolysis in sickle cell disease occurs in the context of malaria infection. Acute hemolytic anemia due to malaria is the leading cause of death in children with sickle cell disease living in malaria-endemic areas of Africa.

Bacterial infection can transiently reduce erythropoiesis and worsen the usual anemia of sickle cell disease. Rarely, in developed countries, when severe anemia develops, megaloblastic arrest of erythropoiesis is present. This is usually due to marginal nutrition that causes folic acid deficiency.

Erythropoietin in Sickle Cell Disease

Serum erythropoietin levels in sickle cell anemia have been measured and are inappropriately low for the level of hemoglobin.[131] This might be explained by the right-shifted blood hemoglobin–oxygen dissociation curve in sickle cell anemia that enhances the delivery of oxygen to tissues, and the observation that red cell precursor mass appears to be an independent determinant of erythropoietin levels. An expanded erythroid marrow of sickle cell anemia would offset the reduction in peripheral red cell mass, reducing erythropoietin concentrations.[132] Erythropoietin has been used successfully to treat the severe anemia that often develops as sickle nephropathy progresses. In this case, care must be taken to avoid untoward increases in PCV so that increased blood viscosity from sickle erythrocytes does not lead to an increased incidence of vasoocclusive events.

In a review of 39 patients with sickle cell disease treated with erythropoietin or darbepoietin the median dose range was more than 200 U/kg. It was suggested that this treatment might allow more aggressive dosing of hydroxyurea in the setting of mild renal insufficiency.[133]

Treatment recommendations. Increased hemolysis in a patient with sickle cell disease should be investigated to exclude autoimmune hemolysis that is found accompanying alloimmunization in heavily transfused patients. In these patients, because of the presence of antibodies that are usually panagglutinins, finding blood compatible for transfusion is difficult. Corticosteroids can be used effectively, as in other types of autoimmune hemolytic anemia.

Judicious use of blood transfusion is warranted when anemia is severe. Hemolysis related to malaria infection must be corrected as the infection is treated. It is generally recommended that children with sickle cell disease living in malaria-endemic areas should be protected from malaria. It is unclear whether this protection should be in the form of antimalarial prophylaxis or patient/family education on how to respond to febrile illness. The widespread selection of chloroquine-resistant *P. falciparum* in Africa and elsewhere makes that drug unsuitable for routine prophylaxis. It is also unclear whether sulfadoxine-pyrimethamine preparations recommended for malaria prophylaxis during pregnancy are suitable for long-term use in patients with sickle cell disease.

Infection

Epidemiology

Infection is the major cause of mortality and morbidity in children in the first years of life, when the most common offending agent is *Streptococcus pneumoniae*. The spectrum of infection changes with age, where Gram-negative organisms acquired via the urinary, respiratory, and gastrointestinal tract become more common and indwelling venous access devices are a common locus of infection.

Prior to the institution of universal newborn screening for sickle cell disease, pneumococcal vaccination, and penicillin prophylaxis therapy, *S. pneumoniae* bacteremia was the leading cause of death in patients aged younger than 2 years in the United States. Patients with sickle cell disease lose splenic reticuloendothelial function in early life. This was demonstrated by technetium-99m sulfur colloid liver-spleen scans, which showed absence of splenic uptake in young sickle cell anemia patients even when their spleen was enlarged, an entity termed functional hyposplenism. The dysfunction of the spleen appears to be unrelated to its size fluctuation in the early years; gradual enlargement occurs until ages 3–4 years, followed by gradual regression into a contracted fibrotic, but possibly revivable organ. Splenic dysfunction is also inferred from the appearance in circulation of red cells containing Howell–Jolly bodies – remnants of nuclear chromatin, normally "culled" from red cells by the spleen – and by the rise in "pocked," more correctly, pitted, red cells in circulation. The rate of splenic regression is related to the natural reduction in HbF levels that occurs during postnatal development. Ten Saudi Arabs, aged 4–26 years, with sickle cell anemia and mean HbF of 20% were found to have splenic abscesses. Tender, enlarged spleen, abdominal pain, and fever were common presenting features. Six patients had evidence of infection with *Salmonella* sp.

Hyposplenic patients are susceptible to infection with encapsulated bacteria such as *S. pneumoniae* and *Haemophilus influenzae*. There is also evidence of abnormal granulocyte function in sickle cell anemia. Circulating neutrophils appear to be activated in the "steady state" as they have increased activity of phospholipase A_2.[134] Although these cells might contribute to the initiation of vasoocclusion, they also respond poorly to priming by cytokines and have approximately half the nicotinamide adenine dinucleotide phosphate (NADPH) oxidase response as control cells. An impaired response would affect killing of microorganisms requiring high levels of oxidant radicals for their death, such as *S. pneumoniae* and *H. influenzae*. Sepsis, pneumonia, meningitis, and otitis are the most frequent infections and they can progress with devastating rapidity.

The immune defect in sickle cell disease appears to be specific for certain organisms; primary among these is *S. pneumoniae*. Early studies had demonstrated a defect in opsonization of *S. pneumoniae* antecedent to phagocytosis. This opsonic defect was initially thought to reside in the alternate pathway of complement activation, but later it was shown that the opsonic defect was due to a lack of specific antibodies against pneumococci, perhaps due to early loss of splenic antibody production function. This opsonic defect is not generalized to all microorganisms.

The relatively high risk of overwhelming pneumococcal infection in patients with sickle cell disease and the associated high rate of mortality have been well documented. The incidence of bacteremia in sickle cell disease varies with age and the genotype of the disease. Overall, the rate of bacteremia seems to have declined in the United States since the early reports of children with sickle cell disease having bacteremia at 300–600 times the rate of normal children. Factors accounting for the declining rate of bacteremia include the institution of penicillin prophylaxis and the use of conjugate pneumococcal and *H. influenzae* type b vaccination. In its cohort of 427 infants with sickle cell anemia followed from 1978–1988, the CSSCD reported that bacteremia occurred in babies younger than 6 months. The peak incidence of bacteremia, 9.9 events per 100 person-years, occurred in babies aged 6–12 months, declining to less than 5 per 100 person-years after age 3 years. The second 6 months of life also saw the highest incidence of bacteremia in children with HbSC disease. The CSSCD had reported an incidence of bacteremia of 7.98 per 100 person-years for children younger than 3 years with sickle cell anemia; this declined to 2.54 in those aged 3–5 years. *S. pneumoniae* was responsible for 67% of the cases of bacteremia in those younger than 6 years but only 19% of cases in individuals older than 6 years. Twenty-four percent of children younger than 3 years with sickle cell anemia who had pneumococcal bacteremia died. In 75% of the patients who died of sepsis, death occurred within 24 hours after hospitalization.

Recent changes in management of febrile illness in young children with sickle cell disease have reduced the rate of mortality. In the CSSCD infant cohort of 427 children with sickle cell anemia, there were 62 cases of *S. pneumoniae* bacteremia with a 14.5% mortality rate, after 1,781.4 person-years of observation.

With increasing age, the cause of bacterial infection in sickle cell disease changes from the pneumococcus to Gram-negative organisms such as *Escherichia coli*, *Klebsiella* and *Salmonella* species.[135,136] Acquisition of natural antibodies, subclinical infection, and in recent years, protection offered by conjugated pneumococcal vaccination might account for the decline in relative risk of pneumococcal infection despite the permanent loss of splenic function. Until the widespread use of *H. influenza* type b vaccination, this organism was the second leading cause of sepsis and meningitis in children with sickle cell disease. As the rate of *H. influenzae* infection has declined in the general childhood population so has it declined in children with sickle cell disease, although it remains higher than that in the general population.

In addition to bacterial sepsis and meningitis, patients with sickle cell disease have increased risk of osteomyelitis. In the United States, *Salmonella* sp. are the most common cause of osteomyelitis followed by *Staphylococcus aureus*.[137] In recent literature from other parts of the world, *Salmonella* sp. are reported also as the most frequent causes of osteomyelitis in sickle cell disease patients. Other Gram-negative organisms such as *Klebsiella* and staphylococcal species are the leading causes of osteomyelitis in some regions.

Eighteen African American patients with sickle cell disease with human immunodeficiency virus (HIV)-1 infection were reported, 11 who had quantitative studies of viral load and were under treatment or follow-up. Although data are scanty, it might be that these HIV-1–infected sickle cell anemia individuals have a lower viral load and higher CD4 cell counts than HIV-1–infected control patients and include more asymptomatic long-term non-progressors than controls. It was hypothesized that asplenia removes an important site for viral replication and accounts for a more indolent disease when HIV-1 and sickle cell anemia coexist.[138]

Prevention

Invasive pneumococcal infection was the nemesis of children with sickle cell anemia, a major contributor to morbidity and the leading cause of death in children, adolescents and young adults prior to the initiation of penicillin prophylaxis.[139] More than 20 years ago, in a randomized, controlled clinical trial, Gaston and colleagues[140] showed that when children with sickle cell disease received penicillin prophylactically, they had an 84% reduction in pneumococcal infection. The results of this landmark study lead to a rapid medical response that improved the care of children with sickle cell disease. Prevention of mortality from pneumococcal infection is the basis for the establishment of newborn screening for sickle cell disease as these infections can occur shortly after birth. Since 2006, all states now universally screen for sickle cell disease so that affected infants can be identified and given prophylactic penicillin. When identified, infants at risk, when possible, are followed in special Pediatric programs, and in addition to being given prophylactic penicillin, a polysaccharide pneumococcal vaccine was administered, most commonly at age 2–5 years.[140] Parents should be taught to understand the importance of the appearance of fever and the need for rapid treatment should pneumococcal infection "breakthrough" the antibiotic-vaccination barrier. This approach was believed to reduce the high mortality rate of pneumococcal infection.

Nevertheless, infections continued to occur because of vaccine ineffectiveness and the lack of compliance with prophylaxis. A recent study examined the incidence of invasive pneumococcal disease before and after the introduction of the 7-valent pneumococcal conjugate vaccine.[141] The results were remarkable: an average 92% decline in infection in children younger than 5 years when the post–conjugate vaccine era was compared with the pre–conjugate vaccine era. A similar effect was not seen in older children. Only a small number of individuals developed pneumococcal disease, the surveillance had a limited geographical distribution, and all drug recipients were Medicaid enrollees, so that replication of these results is warranted.

Penicillin remains highly efficacious prophylaxis for most strains of *S. pneumoniae*. What makes this treatment a less effective approach to disease prevention is that compliance with treatment is suboptimal. Penicillin should be given twice daily and the solution used for the youngest children remains stable for only 2 weeks. In one study, only 25%–30% of Medicaid program enrollees were likely to receive prophylactic penicillin for at least 270 days per year, and this failure to achieve maximal prophylaxis seemed likely to be generalizable, at least to the Medicaid population.[141] Perhaps the financial difficulties encountered by state Medicaid programs accounted for this poor record of prophylaxis.

Although a polysaccharide pneumococcal vaccine was first introduced in the late 1940s and a 23-valent vaccine was available by 1986, the babies with sickle cell disease, who are at highest risk for infection, often have a poor antibody response. The risk of infection in children younger than 3 years might also not be reduced. The loss of splenic function in older children retards their response to this vaccine. In contrast, the conjugate pneumococcal vaccine is given in the first months of life when the risk infection in sickle cell disease begins and this immunization is associated with a superior antibody response.[142]

How long penicillin prophylaxis should be continued is unclear. A follow-up study to the prophylactic penicillin trial whose purpose was to determine the efficacy of penicillin prophylaxis in children older than 5 years with sickle cell anemia failed to show any significant difference between the penicillin and placebo groups.[143]

These results do not apply to children with a history of severe pneumococcal infection or splenectomy as they were excluded from the study. Some clinicians might conclude that penicillin prophylaxis is unnecessary for patients older than 5 years. Splenic dysfunction remains present however, and older children and adults have died of overwhelming pneumococcal infection. The decision to discontinue penicillin prophylaxis for any child should be carefully considered, taking into account parental understanding of and the ability to respond appropriately to signs of infection and the prior history of pneumococcal infection.

With effective vaccines to prevent infection with *S. pneumoniae*, the question of whether or not prophylactic penicillin is needed arises. Widespread penicillin use is not risk free. Penicillin-resistant strains of *S. pneumoniae* are increasing in number and approximately 4% of isolates in sickle cell disease have some measure of resistance; most patients taking prophylaxis harbor some resistant strains. The susceptibility of these organisms to penicillin might be declining and prophylaxis is less effective in carriers of intermediate resistance and resistant serotypes. In North America, the 7-valent conjugate vaccine protects against more than 70% of the serotypes isolated from patients in the pre–conjugate vaccine era; however, two-thirds of the serotypes not included in the vaccine were susceptible to penicillin and the use of this vaccine appeared to decrease the number of antibiotic-resistant invasive pneumococcal infections.[144] To increase vaccine efficacy a 13-valent vaccine is being developed. Although patterns of penicillin resistance and vaccine susceptibility are likely to continue to change and to differ throughout the world, until a conjugate vaccine with greater coverage is available, antibiotic prophylaxis could still be useful.[145]

Is a conjugate vaccine useful in other parts of the world where sickle cell disease is more common than in North America and where the spectrum of pneumococcal disease might be different? In developing countries, a vaccine that is affordable, deliverable, and covers the spectrum of infectious strains of the pneumococcus could have a major impact on the public's heath. Although only 32% of infected patients in an urban hospital and 23% of pneumococcus carriers from rural villages in The Gambia had serotypes represented in the vaccine, in both studies approximately twice as many individuals had serotypes related to those in the vaccine.[146,147] Despite some concerns, because of the benefits of vaccination in the general population, experts have suggested that vaccination should start now if the obstacles to vaccine delivery can be overcome.[148] Sickle cell disease patients will be special beneficiaries of this policy. Another caveat to consider is that *S. pneumoniae* can switch capsular serotypes by conjugation and adapt to the presence of vaccine pressure. This is one mechanism by which virulent nonvaccine serotypes could arise in the face of vaccine pressure.[144]

Treatment. Young children with sickle cell disease who have a febrile illness are managed as if they have pneumococcal sepsis until proven otherwise. This practice mandates that all children with sickle cell disease with significant fever or who simply look or act ill need medical evaluation and prompt antibiotic therapy. Their evaluation should consist at minimum of a physical examination, complete blood count, reticulocyte count (to exclude erythroid aplasia), and a blood culture. Lumbar puncture should be performed if meningitis is suspected based on the examination or cannot be ruled out because of the young age of the patient. Immediately after the specimens for culture are obtained, broad-spectrum antibiotics should be administered intravenously. A chest x-ray is advisable in children younger than 3 years because physical signs of acute chest syndrome can be less obvious in young children, and because the presence of acute chest syndrome would alter the course of therapy.

Children younger than 6 years with fever, or who appeared ill were hospitalized and treated with intravenous antibiotics until bacterial cultures were negative. The standard practice has shifted to outpatient management of febrile children with sickle cell disease who are not ill appearing. Children are given ceftriaxone, a long-acting cephalosporin with excellent antipneumococcal sensitivity, watched for a few hours to ensure their continued well-being, and discharged home for outpatient follow-up. In some institutions, infants are excluded from outpatient management of febrile illness, and in others, children are given oral antibiotics for a few days following the intravenous ceftriaxone. This practice change has succeeded largely because in the era of penicillin prophylaxis, pneumococcal vaccination, and comprehensive care, the incidence of pneumococcal sepsis, bacteremia, and meningitis has become very low at major clinical centers. With good follow-up, outpatients whose cultures grow pathogenic bacteria are returned for further evaluation and appropriate treatment. An unusual fatal hemolytic reaction to ceftriaxone in a child with sickle cell disease has been reported. This underscores the need for close follow-up of those managed as outpatients after receiving ceftriaxone.

The standardized incidence rates for second and third infections in patients with sickle cell anemia were 4.8 and 15.8 times greater, respectively, than the rate of infection in the sickle cell anemia population at large. This implied that the susceptibility to infection is characteristic of a subgroup of patients and that sick patients with prior bacteremia should be assessed early and aggressively for further infection. A possible genetic basis for bacteremia is discussed in Chapter 27.

Acute Chest Syndrome

Epidemiology

Characterized by fever, chest pain, cough, and lung infiltrates, this sometimes lethal complication affects more than half of all sickle cell disease patients and is the second most common reason for hospitalization. Acute chest syndrome was defined in the CSSCD as, "the new appearance of an infiltrate on chest radiograph or, in the presence of pulmonary symptoms and negative chest radiograph, abnormalities on an isotopic scan of the lungs." This broad definition attempted to unify a condition characterized by chest pain, varying degrees of respiratory distress, fever, cough, and leukocytosis. In many instances, particularly in young children, the new pulmonary infiltrate is discovered incidentally as part of the evaluation of fever. Acute chest syndrome has its highest incidence in the more severe forms of sickle cell disease, but also occurs and can be lethal in HbSC disease and HbS–β^+ thalassemia.

In 3,751 patients who were observed for a total of 19,867 person-years, 1,085 (29.2%) had at least one episode of acute chest syndrome. Of these individuals, 56% had only one episode, whereas 6% had five or more episodes.[149] Acute chest syndrome occurred more often in sickle cell anemia (12.8/100 person-years) and HbS–β^0 thalassemia (9.4/100 person-years) than in HbSC disease (5.2/100 person-years) and HbS–β^+ thalassemia (3.9/100 person-years). Risk factors for acute chest syndrome in sickle cell anemia patients were low age, low HbF level, high total hemoglobin level, and high steady-state leukocyte count. Children aged 2–4 years with sickle cell anemia had the highest incidence of acute chest syndrome (25.3/100 person-years) The direct relationship between hemoglobin concentration level and acute chest syndrome is unexplained, but it is thought to be related to the higher blood viscosity associated with a high PCV. The role of asthma is discussed later.

Pathophysiology

The etiology of acute chest syndrome is usually not defined, and in most instances is likely to be multifactorial. Its pathogenesis is summarized in Table 19.2. Pulmonary infarction, pulmonary infection with all types of microorganisms, atelectasis secondary to rib infarction and involuntary splinting, pulmonary embolism, necrotic bone marrow emboli, and in situ thrombosis all might eventuate in acute chest syndrome. Lungs are particularly vulnerable to vasoocclusive damage in sickle cell disease. Deoxygenated sickle cells that manage to escape trapping in the peripheral microcirculation are returned to the lungs where they are

Table 19.2. Pathogenesis of the acute chest syndrome

Mechanism	Evidence
Bone infarction with atelectasis and regional hypoxia	Bone infarctions cause pain with hypoventilation, atelectasis, and subsequent hypoxia
	Incentive spirometry reduces radiographic atelectasis in patients with sickle cell anemia and vasoocclusive crisis
Fat emboli	Bone marrow embolization found in many patients
	Lipid-laden alveolar macrophages are recovered from bronchopulmonary lavage fluids in acute chest episodes
	Secretory phospholipase A_2 levels elevated and may liberate free fatty acids and promote inflammation
Infection	Seasonal predilection, pathogenic microorganisms recovered from lung and blood
Thromboembolic disease	Microvascular in situ thrombosis
	Increased adherence of erythrocytes to endothelial cells
	Pulmonary hypoxia results in entrapment of sickle erythrocytes
	Pulmonary emboli documented
Vascular injury and inflammation	Endothelin-1 levels elevated during acute chest syndrome
	Elevated levels of inflammatory mediators
	Clinical progression to acute respiratory distress syndrome

Adapted from ref. 161.

reoxygenated. It is conceivable that those cells that become fully sickled by the time they reach the lungs and before they are reoxygenated would be trapped in pulmonary precapillary arterioles, particularly in atelectatic areas, before reoxygenation and unsickling. Large and small branches of pulmonary arteries probably undergo damage similar to that seen in cerebral arteries in sickle cell disease, leading to stenosis and occlusion of the vessels and diminished blood flow and infarction in some areas of the lung. Cumulative microinfarction of the lung might lead to progressive pulmonary dysfunction and chronic lung disease with advancing age (see later). Shunting of deoxygenated and partially oxygenated red cells from the alveolar microcirculation is likely to deposit into the peripheral circulation cells that might readily sickle on further deoxygenation. Partially oxygenated sickle cells have been described in the circulation of patients with sickle cell disease.

Isolation of microorganisms in pulmonary secretions or from the blood during the course of acute chest syndrome does not necessarily establish that they are etiologically related to acute chest syndrome, and their presence might represent superinfection in damaged pulmonary tissue. It is believed that acute chest syndrome can be triggered by lung infection. Unsurprisingly, a wide variety or organisms have been associated with acute chest syndrome, and the recovery of an offending agent is greatly increased by bronchopulmonary lavage. Such agents include, *S. pneumoniae, H. influenzae, Mycoplasma pneumoniae, and Chlamydia pneumoniae.*[150] Recent data indicate that approximately 5% of acute chest syndrome episodes are associated with recent B19 parvovirus infection. In most cases of acute chest syndrome, an aggressive search for all possible causes of infections is not done. Therefore, many of the published studies on the frequency infection in acute chest syndrome underreport the possibility of such a causative linkage. A pathogen isolated from blood at the time of acute chest syndrome is often assumed to be its causative agent. Bacteremia was present in only 3.5% of the 1,772 episodes of acute chest syndrome reported by the CSSCD. The most frequent organism was *S. pneumoniae*, followed by *H. influenza*, a pathogen much less common now as a cause of serious infection in the United States than in the CSSCD report. Children were more likely to have infection-associated acute chest syndrome than were adults. In children younger than 2 years, 14% of the episodes of acute chest syndrome were associated with bacteremia and *S. pneumoniae* was the pathogen in 78% of cases. In contrast, only 1.8% of patients older than 10 years had bacteremia, and *S. pneumoniae* accounted for only 25% of the positive cultures.

Acute chest syndrome is a frequent postoperative complication of sickle cell disease. It is presumed that this is an extension of the common atelectasis that tends to follow prolonged anesthesia. The likelihood, however, that pulmonary infarction initiated by sickled red cells returning to the lungs after slow flow through anesthetized tissue cannot be discounted.

Clinical Course

The course of acute chest syndrome is variable. Fever, cough, and chest pain are the most common presenting symptoms. Children younger than 5 years presented more frequently with fever and cough, whereas older children and adults tended to also have shortness of breath, wheezing, productive cough, chest pain, and chills. Pain and fever are the most frequent acute events associated with acute chest syndrome. Thirty percent of the patients with acute chest syndrome had pain, but adults tended to have pain prior to acute chest syndrome more often than did children. Rib infarction was a common precipitating factor of acute chest syndrome. Incentive spirometry was able to reduce the incidence of acute chest syndrome following rib infarction.

Fat embolism from necrotic bone marrow is a common cause of the most severe acute chest events during which hemoglobin and platelet levels fall and the leukocyte count increases.[151] Fat embolism, with its poor prognosis, can be identified by finding lipid within pulmonary macrophages

A
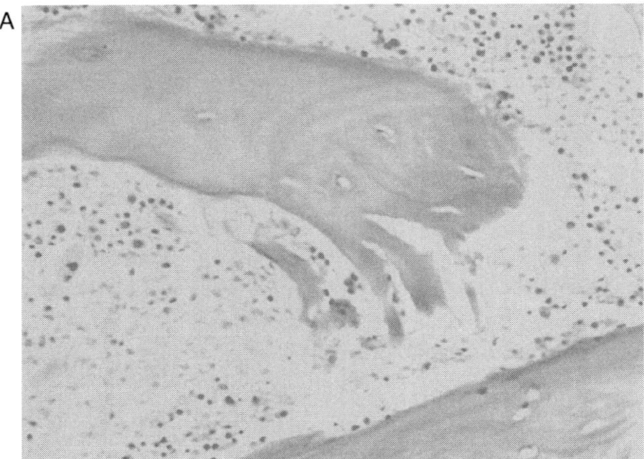

B
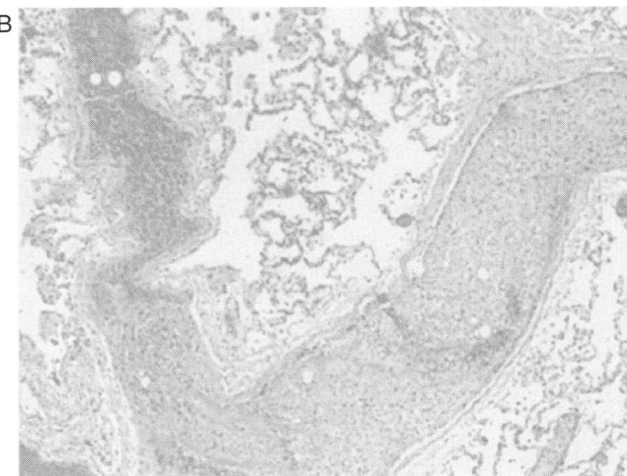

C
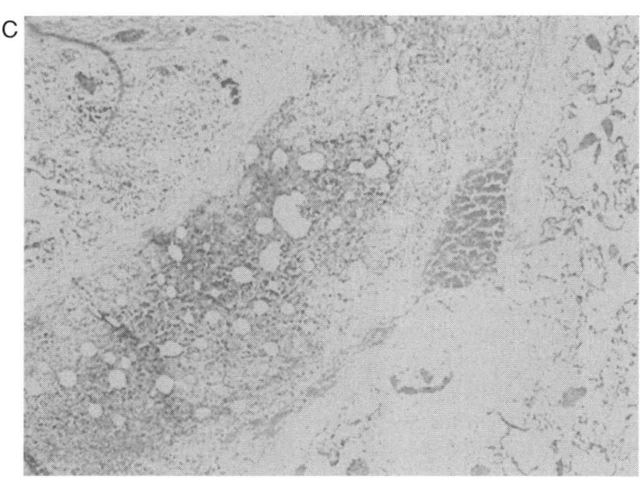

Figure 19.5. Necrotic bone marrow in the lungs of a patient with HbSC disease, who was in reasonable health, and died suddenly with severe acute chest syndrome and multiorgan failure. **(A)** Necrotic bone marrow. **(B)** Pulmonary embolus of fatty, necrotic marrow (low power). **(C)** Higher power view of necrotic marrow in a pulmonary artery. (See color plate 19.5.)

obtained by bronchopulmonary lavage; however, this test is rarely done. Fat-laden necrotic bone marrow has been found on autopsy of sickle cell disease patients dying from severe acute chest syndrome (Fig. 19.5). The detection of fat in the circulation and in pulmonary macrophages can also help make this diagnosis. Sometimes, bone marrow fat embolization causes an adult respiratory distress–like syndrome, in which maintaining adequate oxygenation is difficult and multiorgan failure develops. This is characterized by central nervous system disease including lethargy progressing to coma, renal failure, hepatic failure, rhabdomyolysis, severe anemia, thrombocytopenia, and marked leukocytosis. Fat emboli, in addition to being prominent in the pulmonary vasculature, can be seen in the brain and other organs. In the full-blown multiorgan failure syndrome, which might develop over the course of hours, death might at times be inevitable despite the rapid institution of treatment.

Although it is generally believed that repeated episodes of acute chest syndrome lead to restrictive and obstructive lung disease, to date, no longitudinal studies have confirmed this supposition. A history of acute chest syndrome was associated with lower transcutaneous oxygen saturation in one study. A similar finding was made when children older than 5 years were compared with younger children. Acute chest syndrome is often recurrent and a few patients have repeated severe episodes. Such patients and those with chronic hypoxia after surviving severe acute chest syndrome or adult respiratory distress syndrome might benefit from chronic transfusion therapy.

Prevention

Prevention of acute chest syndrome should be among the goals of managing sickle cell disease patients in pain, particularly when they are bedridden. The use of incentive spirometry in all patients should be strongly encouraged.[152] Routine assessment of oxygen saturation by using pulse oximetry at steady state should be part of general care of sickle cell disease patients. A drop of 3% or more from baseline level at presentation with acute illness was predictive of acute chest syndrome.[153]

Elevated levels of phospholipase A_2 have been found in sickle cell disease patients in association with acute chest syndrome. Free fatty acids released from embolized fat by phospholipase A_2 were suspected of causing further damage to lung tissue. It was hypothesized that elevated levels of serum phospholipase A_2 might predict the occurrence of acute chest syndrome. In a pilot study, when patients were hospitalized with an acute painful episode, but without evidence of acute chest syndrome, they were randomized to receive either a simple blood transfusion or standard care. Five of eight patients who received standard care developed acute chest syndrome compared with none of the seven patients who were transfused. These promising results have lead to the planning of a larger clinical trial of the ability of serum phospholipase A_2 levels to predict development of acute chest syndrome and of transfusion to thwart its occurrence.[154–159]

Hydroxyurea (see Chapter 30) reduced the frequency of acute chest syndrome in adults with sickle cell anemia but it is unclear whether hydroxyurea alone will prevent recurrent acute chest syndrome.

Management

Severe acute chest syndrome is a medical emergency, as progression to hypoxia and circulatory collapse with multiorgan failure requiring intensive care can rapidly develop. Vigilance and a high index of suspicion that this can occur should dictate the management of most cases of acute chest syndrome, especially when on presentation, pain is severe, hypoxia present, the hemoglobin concentration is lower than the baseline level, the leukocyte count is elevated beyond that customary for a painful event, and the platelet count is depressed from its baseline. Repeating a previously normal chest x-ray, especially if chest pain is present, and continuous, or very frequent measurement of blood oxygenation by pulse oximetry will permit the early detection of hypoxia that might signal the need for transfusion.

Successful management of severe acute chest syndrome depends to a large degree on the experience of the intensive care unit in managing such patients. Close coordination of intensive care among internists, pulmonologists, hematologists, infectious disease experts, nursing, and respiratory therapists is necessary for achievement of a successful outcome. Response to treatment was evaluated in 671 episodes of the acute chest syndrome in 538 patients.[150] Treatment included phenotypically matched blood transfusions, bronchodilators, and bronchoscopy. Thirteen percent of patients required mechanical ventilation; 3% died and 81% recovered. As in prior studies, adults older than 20 years were more severely affected than younger patients. Transfusions improved oxygenation with a 1% rate of alloimmunization. Twenty percent of the patients treated with bronchodilators improved. Eighteen patients died, and the most common causes of death were pulmonary emboli and infectious bronchopneumonia, with infection contributing to 56% of the deaths. Regardless of its etiology, management of acute chest syndrome includes intravenous broad-spectrum antibiotics, careful hydration, aggressive respiratory therapy with bronchodilators, incentive spirometry, and maintenance of tissue oxygenation. Antibiotics are usually given although documented bacterial infection is found in less than 10% of cases. The choice of antimicrobial can be predicated on the algorithm for community-acquired pneumonia; however, some patients with sickle cell disease are frequent hospital visitors and this might modify the choice of a drug. It has become customary to add erythromycin or another agent to cover mycoplasma or chlamydiae infection. Oxygen therapy should be given when the patient is hypoxic or tachypneic with signs of respiratory distress. Hydration should be used carefully to avoid pulmonary edema and should not exceed maintenance and replacement of losses. In the context of pain management with opioid analgesics, care should be taken to balance the analgesic need and the danger of respiratory suppression.

Simple or exchange transfusion to reduce the percentage of HbS containing cells and increase the baseline hemoglobin concentration level is useful in hypoxic patients. The timing of transfusion is unclear as is whether exchange transfusion is superior to simple transfusion. Although some experts prefer the former, a controlled study of the merits of any form of transfusion for acute chest syndrome has not been conducted. It is the impression of clinicians that patients with infarctive acute chest syndrome, as opposed to infectious acute chest syndrome, if this distinction can be made, have a more rapid recovery in response to blood transfusion, suggesting that early transfusion might prevent progression to severe acute chest syndrome. This also has not been tested in a controlled study. In patients with moderate to severe acute chest syndrome, the goals of transfusion should be to maintain a hemoglobin concentration of 10 g/dL and HbS level of less than 30%, levels similar to those used in the management of stroke. Blood less than 5 days old is preferable because banked blood has low 2,3 bisphosphoglycerate levels and a high affinity for oxygen. Transfusing old blood into a hypoxic sickle cell disease patient could worsen the condition of the patient in the immediate posttransfusion period as transfused cells have a higher oxygen affinity than normal until the 24 hours that it takes to restore 2,3, bisphosphoglycerate levels passes.

Recent studies suggest that NO could be involved in the pathogenesis of acute chest syndrome and that inhaled NO could be a useful treatment (summarized in ref. 162). It must be emphasized that despite apparent responses to 80 ppm inhaled NO for 15 minutes in acute chest syndrome, with increases in pO_2 and reductions in pulmonary artery pressure, there have been no careful clinical trials of this treatment and this treatment has not yet improved mortality in adult respiratory distress syndrome.

ADOLESCENCE

Adolescents with sickle cell disease face both the physical limitations associated with this disease and the psychological impact of a serious chronic disease. Although sickle cell disease in older children and adolescents is not fundamentally different, there are a few problems that are more or less common during adolescence. In the second decade of life patients with sickle cell anemia have a lower incidence of bacteremia, dactylitis, acute splenic sequestration, acute chest syndrome, stroke, and mortality, but higher incidence of cholelithiasis and cholecystectomy and severe pain episodes.

Psychosocial Issues

Although adolescence can be a period of relative stability medically, it is not so psychologically. In fact, much of medical literature dealing with adolescents with sickle cell disease concentrates on psychosocial issues. The management of adolescents with sickle cell disease has been reviewed.[163] Some of the major issues in adolescents with sickle cell disease include, growth and development, management of pain, the psychological impact of, and psychosocial adjustment to a chronic disease and their transition to adult care.

Psychosocial problems reported in adolescents with sickle cell disease include low social adjustment, depression, anxiety, acting out behavior, and negative body image. These are not unexpected outcomes from a chronic disease, which is associated with severe pain, physical limitations, and an unpredictable course. Adolescent boys are more vulnerable to psychosocial problems than are girls and demonstrate more difficulties coping with sickle cell disease. Older boys were more likely to be socially withdrawn and were more depressed than younger boys and girls. Family competence was associated with fewer internalizing and externalizing behaviors by the adolescent. Difficulties with medical staff often begin in adolescence and frequently revolve around issues of pain management and inpatient stay. Unpredictable painful episodes can hamper the adolescent's development of a sense of control.[163]

Psychosocial difficulties of adolescents with sickle cell disease often go unaddressed by pediatric staff who feel unqualified to handle such issues. Those unresolved difficulties become magnified when adolescents are transferred to adult care. Independent of parents, transferred patients might fail to comply with recommended medical therapy and follow-up. There is growing interest in ensuring that the transition from pediatric to adult care proceed successfully for adolescents with sickle cell disease. Programs caring for adolescents with sickle cell disease need to be aware of these psychosocial issues and adopt measures to ensure optimal physical and psychological wellness for their patients. A series of guidelines on psychosocial issues are recommended for professionals taking care of adolescents and others with sickle cell disease.[164,165]

YOUNG ADULTS

Pregnancy and Contraception

The obstetrical and gynecological issues of sickle cell disease, including recommendations for management, have been reviewed. Pregnancy in sickle cell disease is not contraindicated. Complications of pregnancy are most prevalent in sickle cell anemia and HbS–β^0 thalassemia and less common in HbSC disease and HbS–β^+ thalassemia.[166] Routine sterilization or interruption of pregnancy in women with sickle cell anemia is not medically indicated. Women with sickle cell disease appeared to be as fertile as controls, although they had a delay in menarche and for their first pregnancy. In the Jamaican study, the number of infants born to patients with sickle cell disease was less at all ages compared with controls, perhaps reflecting lesser fertility after a first pregnancy.

The Placenta

The placenta in sickle cell anemia weighs less than that of age-matched controls and shows villous sclerosis, intervillous fibrin deposits, and infarction.[167] Umbilical veins have irregularly elongated and round cells suggesting hypoxia and proliferation of the smooth muscle cells, absence of an inner elastic lamina in the tunica media, and varying thickness of the basement membrane.[168] These changes are possibly related to hypoxia-induced cytokines in the placenta and umbilical vein.[169,170]

Hazards of Pregnancy

A low birth rate may be explained in part by the anemia and vasculopathy of sickle cell disease and perhaps poor access to health care. One hundred twenty-seven deliveries in women with sickle cell anemia and HbSC disease that occurred between 1980 and 1999 were compared with a control group of 129 deliveries in African American women with normal hemoglobin. Compared with controls, deliveries among women with sickle cell disease were at increased risk for intrauterine growth restriction, antepartum hospital admission, and postpartum infection. They were also more likely to be complicated by low birth weight, prematurity, and preterm labor or premature rupture of membranes. Perinatal deaths were similar and there were no maternal deaths.[171]

The hazards of pregnancy in sickle cell anemia are many, especially for the fetus. Older medical literature suggested that pregnancy in sickle cell anemia was not worth the risk and that therapeutic abortion and early sterilization was desirable. Modern medical management of pregnancy generally achieves good results but the rate of obstetrical complications is still higher than in normals. Among more than 9,300 African American women delivering at a single maternity center, the combined prenatal and perinatal losses in women with sickle cell anemia were 20% compared with 10% in women with HbAS or normal hemoglobin.[172] Four percent of women with sickle cell anemia had pyelonephritis (0.3% in controls); pregnancy-induced hypertension was found in 20% (9.6% in controls); caesarian sections were performed in 44% of patients (22% in controls); gestational ages were approximately 1 week less than in controls; and birth weight was 2,700 g (3,010 g in controls). Patients with sickle cell anemia have approximately twice the normal rate of multiple pregnancy, placenta previa, abruptio placentae, preterm delivery, fetal distress, and caesarean sections and a fivefold increased occurrence of toxemia.[172] Twenty-one percent of infants born to mothers with sickle cell anemia were small for gestational age when compared with the general population; the incidence in mothers with HbSC disease and HbS–β thalassemia is unknown but presumed to be less. Small-for-gestational-age fetuses are likely a result of placental insufficiency and patients with preeclampsia and acute anemic events are especially prone to this complication.[173] In a cohort individuals with sickle cell anemia residing in Jamaica and their matched normal controls who were followed from birth, patients had later menarche and age of first pregnancy by several years. Thirty-seven percent of patients had spontaneous abortions compared with 10% of controls and babies of subjects had a lower gestational age and lower birth weight. In this study, the death rate was 2.1%.[175]

Given access to modern obstetrical care, maternal mortality has been reported to range from less than 0.5% to 2.1%.[173–177] In pregnancy, the B19 parvovirus may cause fetal loss and hydrops fetalis. In the general population, parvovirus-infected patients have a 10% risk of fetal loss before 20 weeks gestation, falling to 1% afterward. The incidence and risk in pregnant sickle cell disease patients are unknown and the role of intrauterine blood transfusion and intravenous immunoglobulin has not been studied.[178,179]

Sickle cell patients have an increased risk of developing preeclampsia after 20 weeks of gestation when hypertension coexists with edema and proteinuria. The pathophysiology of preeclampsia lies in utero-placental insufficiency, which activates endothelial cells with release of oxygen free radials, endothelial reactive substances, and consumption of NO and prostacyclins. As noted in Chapters 10 and 11, sickle vasculopathy is associated with similar abnormalities.

Treatment recommendations. Pregnant patients should be seen by their obstetrician at least twice monthly and their labor closely supervised with frequent fetal monitoring. Antenatal care is best provided by an obstetrician familiar with sickle cell disease patients in conjunction with an experienced hematologist. Prenatal visits serve to collect background data, establish the hemoglobin phenotype, and catalog the existing complications of the disease. Other than HbF level, maternal steady-state hematology has little influence on fetal outcome. Pertinent data include previous pregnancies and their outcomes, previous complications during pregnancy with emphasis on spontaneous abortions, preeclampsia, low-birth weight infants, and complications from sickle cell disease such as acute chest syndrome, stroke, cardiac disease, pulmonary hypertension, and history of blood transfusions. Some patients with frequent vasoocclusive complications, renal failure, pulmonary hypertension, prior spontaneous abortions, and frequent blood transfusion warrant even more intense observation.

As a group, patients with sickle cell anemia have relative hypertension as their blood pressure is higher than expected when compared with a control group with similar levels of anemia. This is associated with an increased risk of stroke. Even "normal" blood pressure might be "abnormal," so this should be carefully followed. Similarly, significant renal damage can be present with normal serum creatinine levels because of the very high glomerular filtration rates in young patients with sickle cell anemia (see later). Prognostically, women with the highest levels of HbF had a lower rate of fetal perinatal death.[179]

A medication profile with particular attention to hydroxyurea use should be documented. Although patients have become pregnant or fathered children while taking hydroxyurea or having taken hydroxyurea in the past, this drug is a teratogen in animals and should not be used if pregnancy is planned. Pregnancy has been reported in at less than two dozen individuals receiving hydroxyurea, usually for myeloproliferative disorders, but sometimes in sickle cell anemia.[33] In this very small experience there have been no adverse outcomes. Developmental defects have not been reported in pregnant patients who took hydroxyurea for other diseases. Contraception should be practiced by both women and men receiving hydroxyurea and the uncertain outcome of unplanned pregnancy discussed frankly. If pregnancy occurs while taking hydroxyurea there is little information on which to base a decision for continuation or termination of the pregnancy. So far, congenital defects have not been described in pregnancies followed to term and developmental defects have not been reported in infants of mothers who took hydroxyurea for other diseases. This is no cause for complacency and careful studies of this issue have not yet been reported.

Antenatal testing should include, hemoglobin fraction quantification by HPLC to establish the hemoglobin phenotype and HbF level. HPLC is also used to measure HbA and HbS concentration after transfusion. In addition to blood counts and serum chemistries, other laboratory tests should include hepatitis A, B, C, and HIV testing, electrolytes, urinalysis, urine culture, rubella antibody titer, and serum ferritin. All patients should have their red cell phenotype recorded and alloantibodies identified so that if the need arises for blood transfusion, phenotypically matched blood can be used. When antenatal diagnosis is contemplated, the parental genotypes must be determined by DNA-based methods.

Folic acid should be taken at a dose of 1 mg/day. The decision to place a patient with sickle cell disease on iron supplementation during pregnancy depends on their iron status. For patients who are already iron overloaded, there is no indication for supplemental iron. When iron stores are low or marginal, especially in patients transfused infrequently, routine iron supplementation is advisable.

Blood transfusion during pregnancy continues to be debated and the practice of transfusion varies according to locale and individual practice customs. A common, but questioned, practice is to place all patients on a transfusion regimen. The benefits of this practice have not been proven.[180–183] Transfusions are warranted preoperatively for caesarian section, during some episodes of acute chest syndrome, during acute neurologic events and with severe anemia. Lacking a history of complicated pregnancies, prior miscarriage and frequent difficult to manage vasoocclusive events, most pregnancies can be successfully managed without regular transfusions. Multiple birth pregnancies appear to benefit from transfusion.[183,184]

The mode of delivery of the patient with sickle cell disease depends on the clinical/obstetric indications, such as fetal distress and abruptio placentae and nonobstetrical emergencies. Prior to surgery, preoperative transfusion should be used to reduce the level of HbS to less than 30% of total hemoglobin (Chapter 29). When the PCV is less than 25%, simple transfusion can be used because hyperviscosity is minimal if PCV remains below 30%. If the baseline PCV is more than 25%, exchange transfusion is preferable.

The treatment of preeclampsia and eclampsia is beyond the scope of this chapter but should include a low threshold for exchange blood transfusion and if preeclampsia progresses, careful thought should be given to delivery.

If pregnancy must be terminated, some have advised against using hypertonic saline because of the theoretical possibility of it inducing a vasoocclusive episode. Little information on the choice of method for abortion is available.

During the puerperium, the main concerns are pain control, adequate hydration, and the prevention of pulmonary complications, such as acute chest syndrome that might be favored by immobility and hypoventilation. Patients should be provided with an incentive spirometer to help lung expansion and prevent atelectasis.[173,175,176]

Any approved form of contraception is acceptable in sickle cell anemia. The dangers and the consequences of unwanted pregnancies outweigh the very small risks of contraceptive devices or drugs and the complications of these methods do not seem to exceed those in the normal population.[185]

In summary, obstetricians should establish strong lines of communication with hematologists so that care can be coordinated. In the primigravida, careful observation and intervention with transfusions only if complications such as toxemia, severe anemia, or worsening symptoms of sickle cell disease ensue is a reasonable plan. In multigravida, the experience of prior pregnancies helps guide the clinician. Uncomplicated previous pregnancies might be managed like those in primigravidae. Individuals who have lost previous pregnancies might benefit from the early use of transfusions aimed at keeping the hemoglobin level above 9 g/dL.

Surgery and Anesthesia

Surgery and anesthesia in sickle cell disease are safe, but not complication free. Precautions must be observed and the major issue is the use of preoperative blood transfusion.[152] Anesthesia in sickle cell disease has been comprehensively reviewed; the principles of best preoperative and intraoperative anesthetics should be followed.[188,189]

In an analysis of more than 700 surgical procedures in sickle cell anemia, mortality was approximately 1% with no deaths in children.[190] In this report, transfused patients undergoing moderate-risk surgery had fewer postoperative acute chest syndromes and painful episodes. Low-risk surgeries did not have any acute chest syndromes even if patients were untransfused. Nearly 90% of patients were transfused preoperatively but this was not a clinical trial of perioperative management or the effects of preoperative transfusion. Even complicated surgery including heart, liver, and renal transplantation can be accomplished.

Although common sense suggests that tourniquets be avoided and arterial cross-clamping eschewed, most reports do not indicate problems with these procedures.[191,192]

The major issue in preoperative management is the question of blood transfusion. Whether or not preoperative blood transfusion forestalled intraoperative or postoperative complications has been partially answered by a clinical trial that compared simple transfusion to a hemoglobin level of approximately 10 g/dL before surgery under general anesthesia to exchange transfusion that reduced HbS levels to 30% or less.[193] Both regimens were effective in preventing postoperative complications but simple transfusion exposed patients to half as much blood and these individuals had fewer transfusion-related complications. Regardless of the type of transfusion regimen, complications, often minor, were seen in approximately a third of surgeries and acute chest syndrome, a major problem occurred in 10%. When acute chest syndrome occurs after cholecystectomy or splenectomy it has a preference for basal lung regions and for the lung on the side of surgery.[194] In one retrospective analysis, laparoscopic cholecystectomy did not decrease the incidence of acute chest syndrome when compared with an open approach; however, preoperative transfusion was not uniformly used.[195]

What remains unclear is the complication rate of surgery without routine transfusion. The need to resolve this issue was suggested by a prospective survey of preoperative transfusion practice in the United Kingdom where 43%, 39%, and 23% of patients, respectively, received no transfusion, simple transfusion, or exchange transfusion preoperatively. All groups had similar postoperative complication rates and sickle cell–related complication rates of 12%, 8%, and 0%, respectively. Undergoing moderate high-risk procedures was a predictor of postoperative complications.[197] In another study, 28 children with sickle cell disease had a total of 38 minor surgical procedures and no preoperative transfusions were given in 34 cases. Only minor postoperative complications occurred and the absence of postoperative acute chest syndrome suggested that minor or low-risk elective surgical procedures in children might not routinely require preoperative transfusion.[198] The authors of both studies concluded that the lack of clear benefit of transfusion confirmed the need for a randomized controlled trial of transfusion versus no transfusion.

After tonsillectomy and myringotomy, more than a third of patients had postoperative complications regardless of the method of transfusion, and a history of pulmonary disease was predictive of these complications.[199] These results were confirmed in 41 children who underwent transfusion to a hemoglobin level of 10 g/dL and underwent tonsillectomy. Postoperative complications including hypoxia, fever, and acute chest syndrome were noted in 22% of patients and the majority of patients were managed with less than 24 hours of hospitalization.[200]

Treatment recommendations. Lacking a randomized direct comparison of preoperative transfusion compared with no transfusion in sickle cell anemia, a reasonable approach would be to recommend simple transfusion to a hemoglobin level of 10 g/dL in all patients with sickle cell disease undergoing intraabdominal and thoracic surgery, tonsillectomy, and other procedures while receiving a general anesthetic with moderate or high risk. Incentive spirometry might help prevent acute chest syndrome. Minor elective procedures in children might be performed without preoperative transfusions.[201]

Venous Access Devices

Indiscriminate use of intravenous fluid therapy and blood transfusion early in life often culminates in difficulty finding venous access in teenagers and adults requiring implantable intravenous access devices. Infusion ports and central venous catheters are associated with a 5–10 times higher risk of complications in sickle cell anemia than when they are used in other diseases.[202] The risks include thrombosis, at times involving large veins and causing superior vena cava syndrome, and sepsis. Some reports found serious complications associated with more than half of the devices implanted. Infections have been estimated to occur at a rate of 1.5/1,000 catheter days depending on the indication for catheter placement.[203] In one analysis, 41% of bacteremias in adults were associated with venous access devices.[204] Another study suggested that more than 80% of bacteremias in adults were related to indwelling catheters.[205] Approximately 60% of infections were due to coagulase-positive or coagulase-negative staphylococci. Fungemia is usually associated with indwelling catheters and *Candida albicans* is the usual organism. Some experts recommend using low doses of warfarin, 2 mg daily, to retard thrombosis of implantable ports and catheters.

Treatment recommendations. Preservation of veins by using oral hydration when possible early in life and meticulous care of short-term intravenous lines should delay the destruction of veins that leads to indwelling line placement. After a line is placed, special attention should be devoted to its care. Most often, successful treatment of catheter-associated bacteremia requires that the device be removed.

Osteonecrosis

Epidemiology

Painful, often disabling, and frequently requiring surgical treatment, the age-adjusted incidence rate of osteonecrosis in sickle cell anemia is 2.5 per 100-patient years for both hip and shoulder joints.[206,207] About three-quarters of individuals with shoulder disease also have hip involvement. By age 35 years, half of all individuals with sickle cell anemia have evidence of hip and shoulder osteonecrosis and in childhood, sickle cell disease is the most common cause of this lesion. Among 1,056 patients with sickle cell anemia, 21% had osteonecrosis and the median age at diagnosis was 32 years.[208] In 64 adults with 92 symptomatic hips who were followed for a mean duration of 17 years, nearly 90% of hips collapsed within 5 years of diagnosis. The average time between the diagnosis and collapse was 42 months for stage I hips and 30 months for stage II hips.[209]

One hundred twenty-one patients with sickle cell disease and asymptomatic osteonecrosis of the femoral head contralateral to a hip with symptomatic osteonecrosis were identified by MRI and followed with annual hip x-rays for a mean duration of follow-up of 14 years. At the initial evaluation, 56 asymptomatic hips were classified as stage 0, 42 as stage I, and 23 as stage II. At the most recent follow-up, pain had developed in 110 previously asymptomatic hips and collapse had occurred in 93. Symptoms always preceded collapse. Of the 56 hips that were classified as stage 0 at the time of the initial evaluation, 47 had symptomatic osteonecrosis and 34 had collapse. Of the 42 asymptomatic stage I hips, 40 became symptomatic within 3 years and 36 had collapse of the femoral head. Of 23 asymptomatic stage II hips, all became symptomatic within 2 years and all collapsed; the mean interval between the onset of pain and collapse was 11 months. At final follow-up, 91 hips had intractable pain and required surgery. These prospectively collected data strongly suggest that osteonecrosis in sickle cell disease follows an inexorable path that ends with joint failure.[210]

Table 19.3. A modified Ficat system of grading osteonecrosis of the femoral head[211, 212]

	Imaging results	Clinical
Stage 0	MRI normal (marrow necrosis may be present histologically)	Normal
Stage I	Normal radiograph and CT; abnormal MRI with necrosis (marrow and bone necrosis)	Usually painless
Stage II	Sclerosis and lytic areas on x-ray; CT and MRI abnormal with necrosis and reactive interface	Pain not always present
Stage III	Femoral head flattening and crescent sign on x-ray; MRI, crescent sign	Pain present, especially with weight bearing, relieved with rest
Stage IV	Femoral head collapse; joint space narrowing; osteoarthritis	Pain at rest, joint stiffness and weakness; secondary arthritis

Pathogenesis

A complete understanding of the pathogenesis of osteonecrosis in sickle cell anemia is lacking but it might begin with microinfarction of the trabeculae of cancellous bone. Pressure within the marrow of the femoral head is increased when osteonecrosis is recognized clinically or by MRI, but whether or not this is a cause or a result of osteonecrosis is unclear. It has been reported in nonsickle cell disease–related osteonecrosis, that asymptomatic "normal" hips contralateral to involved hips can have increased pressure and it has been claimed that it is these, rather than "normal" hips with normal pressure, which will ultimately develop clinical disease. Patients with higher PCV and with sickle cell anemia–α thalassemia have a higher prevalence of osteonecrosis.[206,207] In studies of osteonecrosis in patients who did not have sickle cell disease, there has been some association of this lesion with low levels of protein S and protein C and hypofibrinolysis and the strong impression that coagulation plays some role in the genesis of this lesion.[211] The genetic modulation of sickle cell osteonecrosis is discussed in Chapter 27.

Clinical Aspects

Osteonecrosis of the hip, because of pain and loss of joint function, can dominate the clinical manifestation of sickle cell anemia. Presenting with pain in and about the affected joint, at times with spasm of the surrounding musculature, hip disease can also present acutely and mimic septic arthritis or synovitis.

More often, the onset of osteonecrosis is insidious. Hip necrosis is often bilateral although both hips need not develop disease simultaneously or progress symmetrically. Activity-limiting symptoms do not often accompany shoulder disease that is asymptomatic in 80% of patients when discovered.

Osteonecrosis can be detected very early in its evolution by MRI and only more advanced disease is radiographically visible (Table 19.3). MRI can be used to quantify the extent of damage to the femoral head. Hip disease can be scored by the system of Ficat, a simplification of an earlier categorization, that classifies by x-ray and MRI the progressive features of this disorder (Fig. 19.6 and Table 19.3).[212] The crescent sign, present in stage III disease, represents an intracapital fracture that begins at the interface of the necrotic lesion and subchondral bone and extends through the area of bone necrosis. Fibrous metaplasia beneath this fracture prevents revascularization and repair, making this lesion irreversible. Many other more or less complicated classification systems have been proposed, some including objective measurements of femoral head involvement and joint destruction. These more elaborate systems might be useful when evaluating and comparing new methods of treatment.[213]

Treatment recommendations. Because symptoms of hip disease often are present in children and can progress rapidly to disability, management poses a dilemma that must balance the relief of pain and avoidance of loss of joint function with the knowledge that total joint replacement is not yet a permanent "cure" and reoperation, especially of the hip, is likely to be required.

Until now, conservative treatment with bed rest and wheelchair, crutches to reduce the load on weight-bearing joints, nonsteroidal antiinflammatory drugs, and physical therapy have been the sole means of managing early disease. Pain relief is problematic, relying on joint protection, rest, heat, hydrotherapy, relaxation techniques, and analgesics. Milder analgesics are often ineffective. If not guarded against, prolonged bed rest can cause flexion contractures. Physical therapy is directed to stretching and strengthening hip adductors and other hip muscles, releasing muscle spasm, training in the proper uses of crutches, quadriceps strengthening, improving upper body strength, and posture retraining. Whether any conservative treatment delays the progression of sickle osteonecrosis is unclear, but the bulk of the evidence suggests that it does not.[214,215] As pain becomes intolerable and joint function is lost, as a final resort, joint replacement is done. Transfusions have not proved useful for pain relief or halting disease progression.[216]

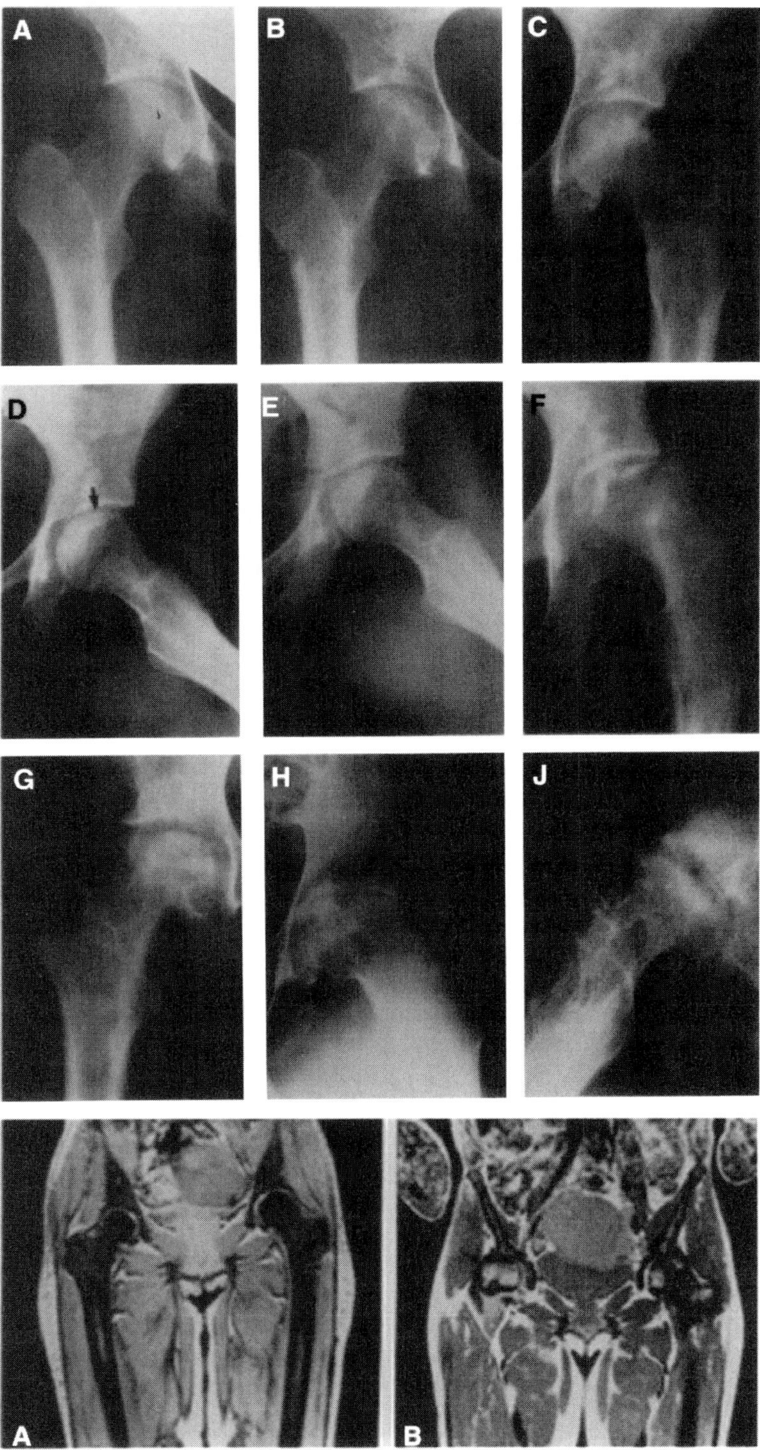

Figure 19.6. Osteonecrosis of the hip in sickle cell disease. **(A)** Subpanels **A** through **C**, the progression of osteonecrosis in a 19-year-old woman with sickle cell anemia is shown. Although the hip was painful, the x-ray was initially normal **(A)** but MRI showed osteonecrosis. Core decompression was done (note track) **(B)**. In **(C)** the joint space is normal but there is sclerosis. In another patient, a crescent sign appears in a painful hip **(D)**. Five weeks later, there is collapse of this segment **(E)**. After an additional 15 months there is extensive joint destruction and total hip replacement was done. (**G**, **H**, and **J**) Show in three different patients with sickle cell disease advanced degenerative changes. **(B)** MRI of the hips in a 30-year-old woman with sickle cell anemia. In subpanel **A**, the femoral heads are normal. After 1 year changes of osteonecrosis are evident **(B)**. (From Embury et al. Sickle Cell Disease: Basic Principles and Clinical Practice, NY, Lippincott-Raven 1994, with permission.)

Pain in osteonecrosis tends to be chronic, and, if possible, narcotic analgesics should be limited. Nevertheless, other analgesics often fail to provide the same measure of comfort as in degenerative joint disease. As destruction progresses, pain becomes severe and joint function is lost, the effected joint needs replacement.

Total hip arthroplasty can be very successful, but using older prostheses, by 4 to 5 years after surgery, approximately one-third have failed and pain can remain a major problem. Cementless components have been tried, and the results of their use are said to be encouraging, but their ultimate value in sickle cell disease is still unknown.[217,218] Postoperative complications of total hip arthroplasty, including infection, fracture, and acute chest syndrome, with persistent pain are very common. Among different series, the need for revision ranged from 30% to 50%, infection occurred in 8%–30%, and failure occurred approximately 40% of cases followed for approximately 5–8 years.[211] It seems prudent to delay this type surgery until symptoms interfere with the activities of daily living.

The inexorable progress of this complication once pain and radiographic abnormalities have appeared has prompted a search for treatment that could stabilize disease progression and relieve its pain. Core decompression is one approach to arresting the progression of osteonecrosis of the hip. Its possible value was discovered serendipitously during measurements of bone marrow pressure and femoral head biopsies when pain decreased after removal of a bone core, and controversy has dogged its application. In this method, a core of bone is removed from the femoral neck, stopping well short of the subchondral plate. This procedure has been studied most intensively in osteonecrosis from causes other than sickle cell anemia and the results, if variable, have been encouraging. An analysis of more than 1,000 hips from 24 different studies, with a 30-month follow-up, showed a clinical and radiographic success rate of 64%.[219] Eighty-five percent of stage I patients had a good result. In comparison, only 23% of patients who did not undergo surgery had a successful outcome. Reports that formed the basis for this synthesis were largely uncontrolled retrospective studies. Treatment of sickle cell osteonecrosis by core decompression decreased pain, restored function, and promoted healing in some patients, but the results of a randomized prospective study were disappointing and did not suggest an advantage for core decompression compared with physical therapy alone.[220] In this prospective multicenter study, the safety of hip core decompression was evaluated and the results of decompression and physical therapy were compared with those of physical therapy. Forty-six patients with stage I, II, or III osteonecrosis of the femoral head were randomized and 38 completed the study. After a mean of 3 years, the hip survival rate was 82% in the group treated with decompression and physical therapy and 86% in the group treated with physical therapy alone. In a review of 312 total hip arthroplasties in sickle cell disease, the mean age of the patients was 32 years. With a minimum follow-up of 5 years, 10 hips were revised for infection and 21 cups and 17 stems required revision for aseptic loosening at a mean of 14 years. Although the medical complication rate was 27% and orthopedic complications were 13%, the results were generally considered successful, given the severity of the problem.[221]

Rotational osteotomy has been considered when pain is severe and normal activities impossible. Although some good results have been seen in sickle cell anemia, adverse outcomes also occur and there are few or no data to recommend when this procedure is indicated or to judge its effectiveness. Expert orthopedic advice should be sought.

Occasionally shoulder disease becomes severely painful and joint destruction can require total shoulder arthroplasty. There is no published experience with core decompression of the humeral head in osteonecrosis associated with sickle cell anemia, but in uncontrolled studies it has been used with good results in steroid- or alcohol-induced disease.

Other Disorders of Bone and Joints

Joint symptoms in addition to hand–foot syndrome and osteonecrosis are commonly encountered but are usually minor compared with other complications of sickle cell anemia. Joint effusions can be monoarticular or polyarticular, noninflammatory or inflammatory and contain sickled cells. Noninflammatory effusions of the knee can be managed successfully by rest and nonsteroidal antiinflammatory drugs. Acute hematogenous osteomyelitis causes acute pain and swelling and can involve periarticular bone, extend into the joint space, and cause effusion. MRI is a more sensitive diagnostic method than technetium or gallium scanning. Because of increased production of uric acid and impaired renal function, approximately one quarter of patients have elevated uric acid levels and some will have attacks of acute gouty arthritis. Lupus erythematosus is very common in African American women and the coincidence of lupus and its articular manifestations with sickle cell anemia is not rare. Backaches may often be ascribed to osteoporosis from expanded hematopoiesis, sometime with vertebral collapse, and can be treated with physical therapy and mild analgesics. Myofascial inflammation has also been found and is associated with localized edema, severe pain, inflammatory tissue changes, and myonecrosis.[222,223]

Orbital complications are uncommon in sickle cell disease. In one patient with fever, headache, orbital swelling, and optic nerve dysfunction, CT displayed bilateral superior subperiosteal cystic masses that during surgical exploration were found to be bilateral liquefied hematomas.[115] A review of the literature showed 16 young patients with sickle cell disease with rapidly developing findings ranging from frontal headache, fever, and eyelid edema to bilateral complete orbital compression syndrome. Sixty percent had orbital hemorrhage on CT and 80% of 12 patients tested were had orbital bone marrow infarction. Recovery was complete in 94% of cases, 74% of whom were treated conservatively and 11% had a recurrence. These unusual events are likely to arise from vasoocclusive disease in the marrow space surrounding the orbits.

Overgrowth of the maxilla and mandible can lead to facial deformity with separation and anterior angulation of the incisors called sickle gnathopathy. Rare in developed countries, it has been more characteristic of the disease in Africa and the deformities can be of a severity to necessitate surgical correction. Diploic spaces of the skull are also widened giving, at times, a "hair-on-end" radiographic picture, but these changes are not as prominent as described in patients with poorly treated β thalassemia.

Bone Marrow Necrosis

Bone marrow infarction may be associated with painful episodes. Humerus, tibia, and femur were the most common sites of bone marrow infarction when symptomatic sickle cell disease patients were studied by bone marrow scintigraphy.[224] Thirty-four percent of infarcts eventually healed.

An unusual but serious disease complication is diffuse bone marrow necrosis without signs of acute chest syndrome. Diffuse bone marrow necrosis is suspected clinically by an acute, and unusually severe painful episode; patients have fever, leukocytosis, worsening anemia and a rapidly rising LDH.[225] Bone marrow necrosis has been associated with infection with the B19 parvovirus. In many respects, diffuse marrow necrosis resembles the acute chest syndrome caused by embolization of necrotic bone marrow but chest involvement and the development of multiorgan failure are not present. Bone marrow MRI and scintigraphy can suggest the presence of regional or diffuse marrow necrosis but are not needed for the diagnosis of severe, diffuse marrow necrosis.[226] Patients have been treated with transfusion and recovery seems to be the rule.

Endocrinopathies

Sex Hormones

In 10 sickle cell anemia patients with a mean age of 17.5 years who had delayed menarche, luteinizing hormone (LH), follicle-stimulating hormone (FSH), and prolactin levels were reduced compared with normal and

HbAS controls.[227] It was concluded that these patients with delayed menarche had a hypothalamopituitary axis dysfunction.

Thirty-two men with sickle cell anemia, mean age 26.5 years, had reduced testosterone and dihydrotestosterone levels and increased LH and FSH levels consistent with primary gonadal failure. Zinc levels were decreased in hair and erythrocytes, and their erythrocyte zinc content correlated with serum testosterone. These patients had abnormal secondary sexual characteristics and eunuchoid skeletal proportions.[228] Male and female sickle cell disease patients, aged 4–50 years, had gonadal hypofunction with low LH, FSH, cortisol, and testosterone levels compared with age- and sex-matched normal controls.

Semen analysis in 25 patients with sickle cell anemia showed significantly reduced ejaculate volume, sperm motility, and sperm density compared with controls. A significant increase was also observed in the percentage of spermatids and in abnormal spermatozoa with amorphous and tapered heads in the patients' semen. These abnormalities could result from testicular dysfunction and abnormalities in the accessory sex organs, such as the seminal vesicles and prostate. To assess the role of the gonads and anterior pituitary gland in the production of poor-quality semen of males with sickle cell anemia, FSH, LH, prolactin, and serum testosterone were assayed radioimmunologically in 33 men with sickle cell disease and in 29 age-matched normal controls. Individuals with sickle cell disease had significantly lower mean serum testosterone, higher mean FSH, and higher prolactin levels than controls. Higher gonadotrophins associated with lower testosterone suggested an intact hypothalamic–pituitary axis and a primary testicular defect.[229] Testicular failure might also result from repeated infarction.[230]

Hypogonadism in sickle cell anemia could also have a hypothalamic origin.[231] In two 19-year-old men with sickle cell anemia and hypogonadism, hypothalamic dysfunction responded to oral clomiphene therapy. Partial hypothalamic hypogonadism was shown by low levels of testosterone, low to low-normal levels of LH and FSH, and a nearly normal rise in gonadotropin levels in response to exogenous gonadotropin-releasing hormone. Treatment with oral clomiphene raised LH, FSH, and testosterone levels to normal, inducing puberty in both patients.

Parathyroid and Bone Mineral Metabolism

In a cross-sectional study of 32 adults (mean age 34 years) with sickle cell disease, nearly 74% had low bone mineral density at one or more anatomical sites.[232] In 52 patients with HbS–β thalassemia 32% had osteopenia/osteoporosis and 57% had osteosclerosis. Bone resorption was diminished in patients with osteosclerosis and increased in those with osteopenia/osteoporosis. The sRANKL/osteoprotegerin ratio was elevated in the osteosclerotic group. Osteoporosis patients had mild renal impairment and their bone mineral density correlated with osteoprotegerin and bone resorption markers. Osteosclerosis patients had multiple infarctions in the studied bones that led to reduced osteoclast activity and increased bone mineral density.[233]

In children with frequent hospitalizations, growth delay, or need for chronic red cell transfusions, bone density was assessed at the lumbar spine and proximal femur. Calcium intake was inadequate in 60%, and serum (25(OH)D (25-hydroxyvitamin D) [25 OHD] level was less than 50 nmol in 74%. Median Z-scores for lumbar spine (-2.3) and proximal femur (-1.7) were markedly reduced, and 64% of patients had low bone density.[234] In another study of children, 65% of subjects had low vitamin D levels and all were vitamin D deficient in the spring.[68] In contrast, in the tropics, vitamin D levels were normal.[235] Bone mineral density is reduced 6%–20% in most patients with sickle cell anemia.[236] Generalized osteoporosis is commonly present, especially in the spine where vertebrae display a typical "fish mouth" appearance.

Limited studies of parathyroid function in sickle cell disease have been reported. Concentrations of serum calcium, parathyroid hormone (PTH), 25 OHD, and 1,25 dihydroxyvitamin D (1,25(OH)2D) were determined in 99 Saudi sickle cell disease patients and in 104 healthy controls. Serum calcium and 25 OHD were significantly lower in the patients and 14% and 12% had serum calcium and 25 OHD concentrations, respectively, below normal. Thirty-one percent had PTH above normal. These results suggested that sickle cell disease patients have a tendency toward hypocalcemia associated with high PTH levels, implying impaired intestinal absorption of calcium and vitamin D.[237] In 18 children with a median age of 8 years with sickle cell anemia living in the tropical island of Curacao, serum calcium concentration was slightly lower than in controls but no individual was hypocalcemic. In contrast to the studies in Saudis, there were no differences in serum concentrations of phosphate, total protein, albumin, PTH, 25 OHD, and 1,25(OH)2D in patients and controls.

In 14 adults with sickle cell disease 25 OHD and bone mineral density at the femoral neck, lumbar spine, and distal third of the ulna plus radius, along with markers of bone resorption and bone formation was measured before and after 12 months of vitamin D_2 and calcium carbonate treatment. Pretreatment, all patients were vitamin D–deficient, had low bone mineral density at the lumbar spine, femoral neck and the distal radius and ulna, and had elevated collagen type I (CTx) and osteocalcin levels. After treatment, all patients corrected their 25 OHD level with a significant increase in bone mineral density at the lumbar spine and the femoral neck. CTx, osteocalcin and PTH(i) levels were unchanged. These results suggest that treatment of adult sickle cell disease with vitamin D and calcium can restore 25 OHD levels to normal and improve bone mineral density, but markers of bone resorption remained unchanged.[238] These results suggest that early detection and treatment of sickle cell bone disease might prevent its progression and continued bone resorption.

Miscellaneous

Basal and stimulated cortisol levels and the increment of cortisol at 30, 50, and 120 minutes after adrenocorticotropic hormone infusion were similar in patients with sickle cell anemia and controls, suggesting normal adrenal function.[239]

Studies of thyroid function in sickle cell disease have been normal and have also shown mild primary thyroid failure, occasionally associated with iron overload.[240–242]

Some clinicians believe that diabetes is underrepresented among patients with sickle cell disease but cases of this association have been reported. Advanced glycation end-products (AGEs) have been implicated in the oxidant-induced vascular pathology of diabetes and other diseases and were measured in normoglycemic patients with sickle cell anemia and controls.[243] Plasma AGE levels and the rate of erythrocyte AGE accumulation were significantly higher in patients compared with controls. Oxidized glutathione (GSSG) was lower and the GSH/GSSG ratio was higher when a vasoocclusive episode was present, suggesting that this ratio might be an objective indicator or a risk factor for an acute event.

Patients with sickle cell disease who are iron overloaded due to transfusion are less likely to develop endocrinopathies than chronically transfused patients with thalassemia. Fifty-six percent of thalassemia patients had more than one endocrinopathy compared with only 13% of sickle cell disease patients. An endocrinopathy was approximately 10 times more likely in thalassemia and this was related to the duration of chronic transfusion.[244]

Pulmonary Hypertension and Pulmonary Function (also see Chapter 11)

Epidemiology and Diagnosis

Pulmonary hypertension in sickle cell disease has been recognized since at least 1982,[245] and recent studies have suggested that it is present in approximately one-third of adults with sickle cell anemia and lesser numbers of patients with HbSC disease and HbS–β^+ thalassemia.[246] As an increasing number of studies are reported, it is becoming clear that this problem begins in childhood.[247] Although symptoms other than dyspnea on exertion might be lacking, pulmonary hypertension, defined as the presence of a tricuspid regurgitant jet (TRJ) velocity of 2.5 m/second or higher on echocardiographic measurement is associated with a 20%–50% risk of death over a 2-year follow-up period, regardless of whether a patient has sickle cell anemia or HbSC disease.[19,246,248–254] Autopsy studies suggest that 75% of patients have some evidence of pulmonary hypertension, although the typical plexiform arterial lesions are not often seen.[255] Pulmonary hypertension is rarely a result of pulmonary artery obstruction.[256] The high mortality rate may reflect the severity of the underlying sickle vasculopathy, and death might not always be a direct result of pulmonary hypertension.

Pulmonary hypertension might be less common in children and adolescents.[257,258] When 32 children with sickle cell anemia were compared with age-matched controls, their right ventricular free-wall mass index continued to rise gradually throughout childhood and a TRJ velocity of more than 2.5 m/second was found in 16% of patients older than 9 years.[259] In 224 children with sickle cell disease, 44 had echocardiographic measurement of TRJ velocity and 26.2% were found to have pulmonary hypertension. This was associated with anemia, reticulocytosis, and cerebral vasculopathy.[260] In 38 of 43 patients with varied genotypes of sickle cell disease, in whom the TRJ velocity was measurable and whose mean age was 14 years, the TRJ velocity was 2.5 m/second or greater in 34% and was associated with markers of hemolysis.[261] In another study by this same group, TRJ velocity was correlated with LDH, hemoglobin concentration, reticulocyte count, and AST.[262] A study of 228 children with a mean age of 12 years revealed that the TRJ velocity was significantly higher than in age-matched controls and was independently associated with systolic blood pressure and LDH concentration, but not with vasoocclusive events.[263]

In sickle cell pulmonary hypertension, pulmonary artery pressure and pulmonary vascular resistance is only moderately elevated, whereas the cardiac output and pulmonary capillary wedge pressures are high. Echocardiography is an excellent and simple screening test for pulmonary hypertension and some studies have shown an excellent correlation between the TRJ velocity and pulmonary arterial systolic pressure measured directly during right heart catheterization. During echocardiography, it is important to search diligently for and measure the TRJ velocity as this allows calculation of pulmonary artery systolic pressure. The definitive diagnosis of pulmonary hypertension can only be made by right heart catheterization and this should be done before beginning specific treatment.

As the symptoms of idiopathic pulmonary hypertension can be lacking or overlap with symptoms of anemia and findings on physical examination are few or present only with advanced disease, the diagnosis of pulmonary hypertension can be difficult and relies on screening (Chapter 11).

In contrast to pulmonary arterial hypertension in other diseases, pulmonary hypertension in sickle cell disease is mild to moderate, with pulmonary artery systolic pressures in the range of 30–40 mm Hg, and often increased pulmonary capillary wedge pressure, suggesting that in some patients diastolic dysfunction contributes to pulmonary hypertension. It has been recommended that an exercise echocardiogram with assessment of pulmonary pressures be used to evaluate patients with significant exertional dyspnea and a normal resting TRJ velocity. Patients with sickle cell disease, in contrast to most individuals with pulmonary hypertension, have moderate to severe levels of anemia and this might make any degree of pulmonary hypertension poorly tolerated. This might account for the morbidity and mortality of otherwise 'mild' pulmonary hypertension. The 6-minute walk distance correlates with functional status, peak oxygen consumption, and with survival in patients with pulmonary arterial hypertension.[264]

When 26 patients were studied by echocardiography before and during a vasoocclusive episode, TRJ velocity increased during the event, and this was associated with decreases in hemoglobin concentration and increases in LDH and plasma hemoglobin levels. In 21 additional subjects with pulmonary hypertension, mean pulmonary artery pressures and pulmonary vascular resistance increased during exercise performed during cardiac catheterization. These results suggested that acute elevations in pulmonary pressures during painful episodes or exercise might contribute to morbidity and mortality and that screening studies should be conducted at a time remote from an acute sickle cell vasoocclusive event.[29] The sudden, unexplained death that sometimes accompanies the acute painful episode might be explained by this rise in pulmonary artery pressure in an anemic patient with many comorbidities. TRJ velocity also can increase during acute chest syndrome, and a level of more than 3 m/second was associated with mortality.[265]

N-terminal pro-brain natriuretic peptide (NT-proBNP), released from ventricles under stress, is a biomarker of idiopathic pulmonary arterial hypertension. NT-proBNP levels were measured in 230 sickle cell disease patients screened for pulmonary hypertension and in an independent sample of 121 patients, and a threshold level predictive of high pulmonary artery pressure and mortality was identified. NT-proBNP levels were higher in patients with sickle cell pulmonary hypertension and correlated directly with TRJ velocity. A level of 160 pg/mL or greater had a 78% positive predictive value for the diagnosis of pulmonary hypertension and was an independent predictor of mortality. In the independent sample, 30% of patients had an NT-proBNP level of 160 pg/mL or greater that was associated with mortality. These data suggest that in sickle cell anemia, a NT-proBNP level of 160 pg/mL or higher was a predictor of mortality that was associated with hemolytic anemia and pulmonary hypertension.[266]

Pathogenesis and Clinical Aspects

The pathogenesis of pulmonary hypertension is likely to be multifactorial and related in part to reduced NO bioavailability (Chapters 10 and 11). Also, endothelial cell adhesion molecules mediate binding of inflammatory cells to vascular endothelium and their levels are modulated by NO and increase with endothelial dysfunction and vascular injury. In sickle cell disease, levels of adhesion molecules are related to measures of NO bioavailability. In 160 sickle cell disease patients, increased soluble adhesion molecule expression correlated with severity of pulmonary hypertension, and soluble VCAM-1, ICAM-1, and E-selectin were associated with the risk of mortality.[267] Individuals with sickle cell pulmonary hypertension had higher levels of soluble VCAM activation, thrombin–antithrombin complexes, prothrombin fragment F1+2, D-dimer, and interleukins 6, 8, and 10 compared with patients without hypertension.[268]

Patients with pulmonary hypertension were more likely to have had priapism, iron overload, reduced oxygen saturation, increased creatinine, and a reduced arginine:ornithine ratio compared with controls.[19,254] The history of acute chest syndrome, osteonecrosis, and emergency department visits were not different in cases and controls, whereas leg ulcers, history of stroke, systolic hypertension, and HbF showed disparate associations.[19,250,269] All these studies compared less than 200 cases and controls, and this might account for the difference in the distribution of clinical events and laboratory measurements.

Erythrocyte glutathione depletion is linked to hemolysis and oxidative stress. Glutamine preserves intracellular NADPH levels, which is required for glutathione recycling. Glutathione and glutamine were significantly lower in plasma and erythrocytes of sickle cell disease patients than in controls and were independently associated with pulmonary hypertension and hemolysis.[270]

Pulmonary hypertension[19] is likely to be modulated by the effects of genes that control NO and oxidant radical metabolism, cell–cell interaction, vasculogenesis, and vasoreactivity. For example, mutations in bone morphogenetic protein receptor–2 (*BMPR2*) and other genes have been associated with both familial and sporadic pulmonary hypertension.[271–273] The genetic basis of pulmonary hypertension in sickle cell disease is poorly understood but polymorphisms in genes of the TGFβ/BMP pathway might be involved (Chapter 27).

Pulmonary Function

Dyspnea is a frequent complaint in patients with sickle cell disease. Studies of lung function to date in this population have often involved less than 50 patients and yielded a spectrum of abnormalities including restrictive lung disease, abnormal diffusion capacity for carbon monoxide (D_LCO), obstructive disease, and hypoxemia.[264,274–276]

Using maximal respiratory flow-volume curves, body plethysmography and the response to bronchodilators, a normal pattern of pulmonary function was detected in 57%, obstructive disease in 35%, and restrictive lung disease in 8% of pediatric age group patients with sickle cell anemia. Almost 80% of patients with obstructive disease and 70% with restrictive disease responded to bronchodilators. Lung function was not associated with painful episodes, acute chest syndrome, or asthma.[277]

Spirometry, lung volumes and D_LCO were studied in 310 adults with sickle cell anemia to determine the pattern of pulmonary dysfunction and their association with other systemic complications of sickle cell disease.[278] Normal pulmonary function tests were present in only 10% of patients. Adult sickle cell anemia was characterized by decreased total lung capacities and D_LCO, and the most common abnormalities were restrictive physiology in 36%, low lung volume in 34% and an isolated low D_LCO in 13% of patients. Decreased D_LCO was associated with thrombocytosis, increased ALT, and renal dysfunction. Based on these studies, pulmonary function was abnormal in 90% of adults with sickle cell anemia. In contrast, preliminary studies in children suggest that D_LCO is not reduced and that obstructive and restrictive disease is associated with TRJ velocity.[279]

Asthma

Asthma and bronchial hyperactivity were more than twice as common in patients with sickle cell disease than in controls.[280] In 74 children evaluated for a painful episode, 36 were diagnosed with asthma. Among children with pain and asthma, the odds ratio of having antecedent or concurrent respiratory symptoms was 4.9 when compared with children with pain and without asthma, suggesting that asthma is a risk factor for painful episodes within 96 hours of an attack.[281] Asthma was also associated with a near doubling of the incidence of acute chest syndrome,[280–283] a twofold increase in mortality[284] and has also been associated with stroke in children with sickle cell disease.[285] Segregation analysis performed in 104 families ascertained through sickle cell anemia probands with asthma found that 19.7% of the parents and 31.8% of siblings of affected probands reported a history of asthma, suggesting that asthma is a comorbid condition.[286] Careful management of asthma might reduce the rates of pain and acute chest syndrome, but no controlled trials of the efficacy of bronchodilators during acute chest syndrome have been reported.

Treatment recommendations. Although the clinical significance of pulmonary hypertension in sickle cell disease is being defined and refined, exactly how this problem should be managed remains unclear (Chapter 11). A standard of treatment based on controlled clinical trials is not available. It is also not clear when and if treatment should be started or how often patients should be screened by echocardiography. Some believe that adults should be screened yearly, whereas in younger individuals screening intervals can be longer. Presently, it appears that few asymptomatic patients are being treated. If treatment appears needed because of symptoms, first, the use of transfusions and hydroxyurea should be optimized even though the HbF levels achieved with hydroxyurea treatment do not appear to protect against the development of this complication (Fig. 19.7).[19] Other complications of sickle cell disease such as iron overload, HIV infection, hypoxemia, especially nocturnal hypoxia, relative systemic hypertension and thromboembolic disease, should be effectively managed before turning to therapies directed more specifically to pulmonary hypertension.[264] Based on the value of anticoagulation in idiopathic pulmonary arterial hypertension, anticoagulation with warfarin might be considered if a specific contraindication does not exist.

Prostanoids such as epoprostenol, treprostinil, iloprost, and beraprost and endothelin-1 (ET-1) antagonists such as bosentan and sitaxsentan and possibly phosphodiasterase-5 (PDE5) inhibitors such as sildenafil are used in other types of pulmonary arterial hypertension, but studies in sickle cell disease are just starting.

The main toxicity of ET-1 receptor antagonists is hepatocellular injury, which could limit their use in sickle cell disease with its high incidence of liver disease of various types. The fall in hemoglobin concentration associated with these agents might lead to symptomatic anemia.

Because of the relationship of reduced NO bioavailability to the development of pulmonary hypertension, the use of PDE5 inhibitors has been explored. The safety and efficacy of sildenafil in 12 patients with sickle cell disease and pulmonary hypertension, NYHA/WHO classes I–III, were studied. Sildenafil, given for 6 ± 1 months, decreased the estimated pulmonary artery systolic pressure and increased the 6-minute walk distance. Three men were studied and none had priapism; however, two received chronic exchange transfusions and one had erectile dysfunction.[287]

Oral arginine, the substrate for NOS, was associated with a 15% reduction in pulmonary artery systolic pressure when given for 5 days to 10 patients.[31]

In summary, adults with sickle cell disease should have yearly screening for pulmonary hypertension by echocardiography. Symptomatic individuals should have elevated TRJ velocity values confirmed by right heart catheterization. If symptoms are judged to be a result of pulmonary hypertension, therapy for sickle cell disease and its complications should be optimized and reevaluated (Fig. 19.7). Presently, the choice of treatment specifically for the pulmonary hypertension should be made with consultation with a pulmonologist with experience managing this condition, as evidence-based approaches to this treatment in sickle cell disease are not yet available.

Leg Ulcers

Epidemiology

On entry into the CSSCD, approximately 5% of patients with sickle cell anemia older than 10 years had leg ulcers. Less than 1% of individuals with HbS–β^0 thalassemia had an ulcer and no ulcers were seen in HbSC disease or HbS–β^+ thalassemia, although they have been reported in these genotypes. When incidence rates were examined according to the genotype of sickle cell disease, individuals aged 20 years and older with sickle cell anemia had a rate of nearly 20 per 100 patient-years, whereas in sickle cell anemia–α

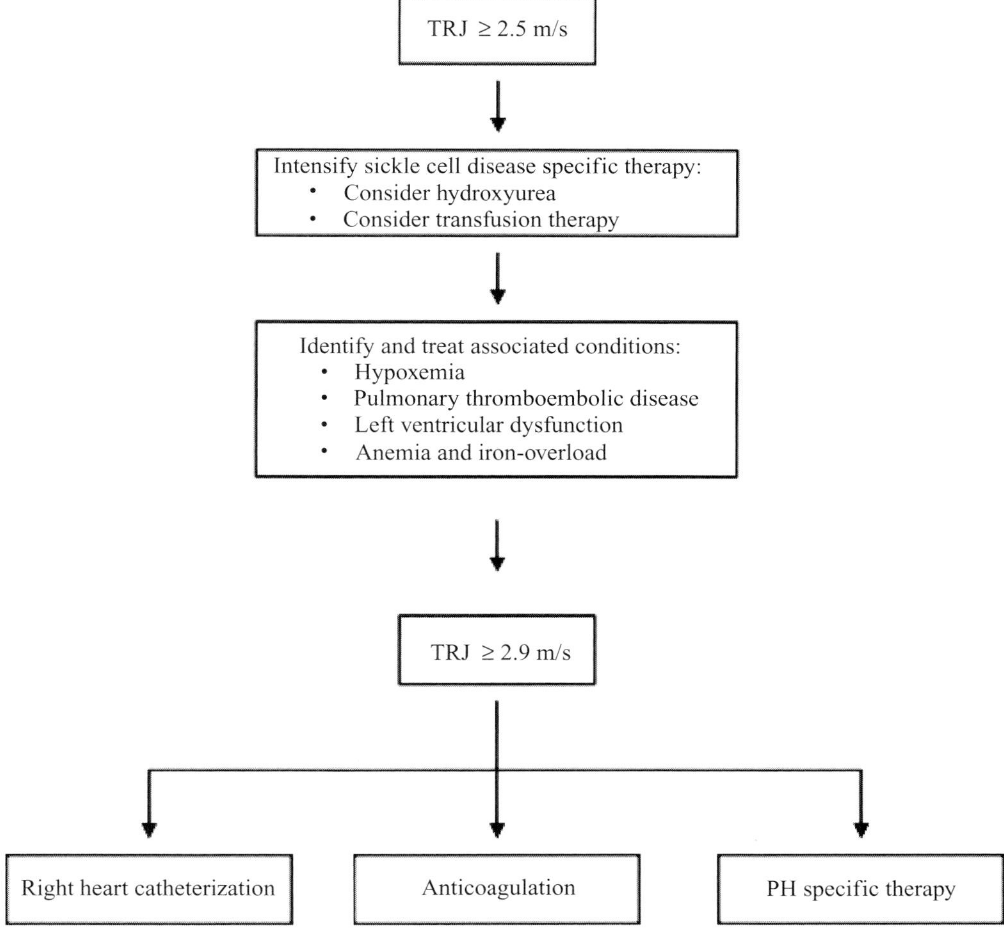

Figure 19.7. Approach to management of pulmonary hypertension.[264]

thalassemia the rate was approximately 10 per 100 patient-years. In total, approximately a quarter of patients had a history of leg ulcer or developed a leg ulcer during an observation period, which was variable but no more than 8 years. Leg ulcers were uncommon in children – none of 1,700 children younger than 10 years had an ulcer – and begin to make their appearance during the early teen years when activities that are most apt to cause trauma to the lower legs become commonplace.[288] Beyond age 20 years, the incidence of ulcers increased sharply. Males were more likely to have ulcers than females whether or not they also had α thalassemia. In Los Angeles, 14% of patients had leg ulcers with a median age at diagnosis of 30 years.[208] In Jamaica, more than 40% of patients and in Africa, between 1.5% and 13.5% of sickle cell disease patients were reported to have leg ulcers.[289]

Leg ulcers are a complication of hydroxyurea treatment in myeloproliferative disorders and new leg ulcers have appeared after institution of hydroxyurea in sickle cell anemia. In the controlled clinical trial of hydroxyurea in sickle cell anemia, the patients randomized to treatment did not have an increase in leg ulcers, but the number of patients was relatively small and the observation period, short.[32,290–293]

Pathophysiology

The cause of leg ulcers in sickle cell disease and in other types of chronic hemolytic anemia is unknown.[10,294,295] Chronic venous ulcers have been associated with thrombophilia, perhaps because of the relationship between thrombophilia and venous thrombosis.[296] Whether or not venous pressure abnormalities contribute to the development of sickle cell leg ulcers is inconclusive.[289,297–299]

Hemolysis, with its associated reduction in NO bioavailability is likely to be a major contributor to the development of leg ulcers.[18] Among the patients enrolled in the CSSCD, 387 patients with sickle cell anemia had a confirmed history of leg ulcers or had leg ulcers at the time of examination,[21] and they were compared with 928 patients without a leg ulcer. Leg ulcer patients had more severe hemolytic anemia than did controls, as shown by their higher reticulocyte counts, LDH, bilirubin, and AST. Cases also had higher leukocyte counts than controls. Leg ulcer

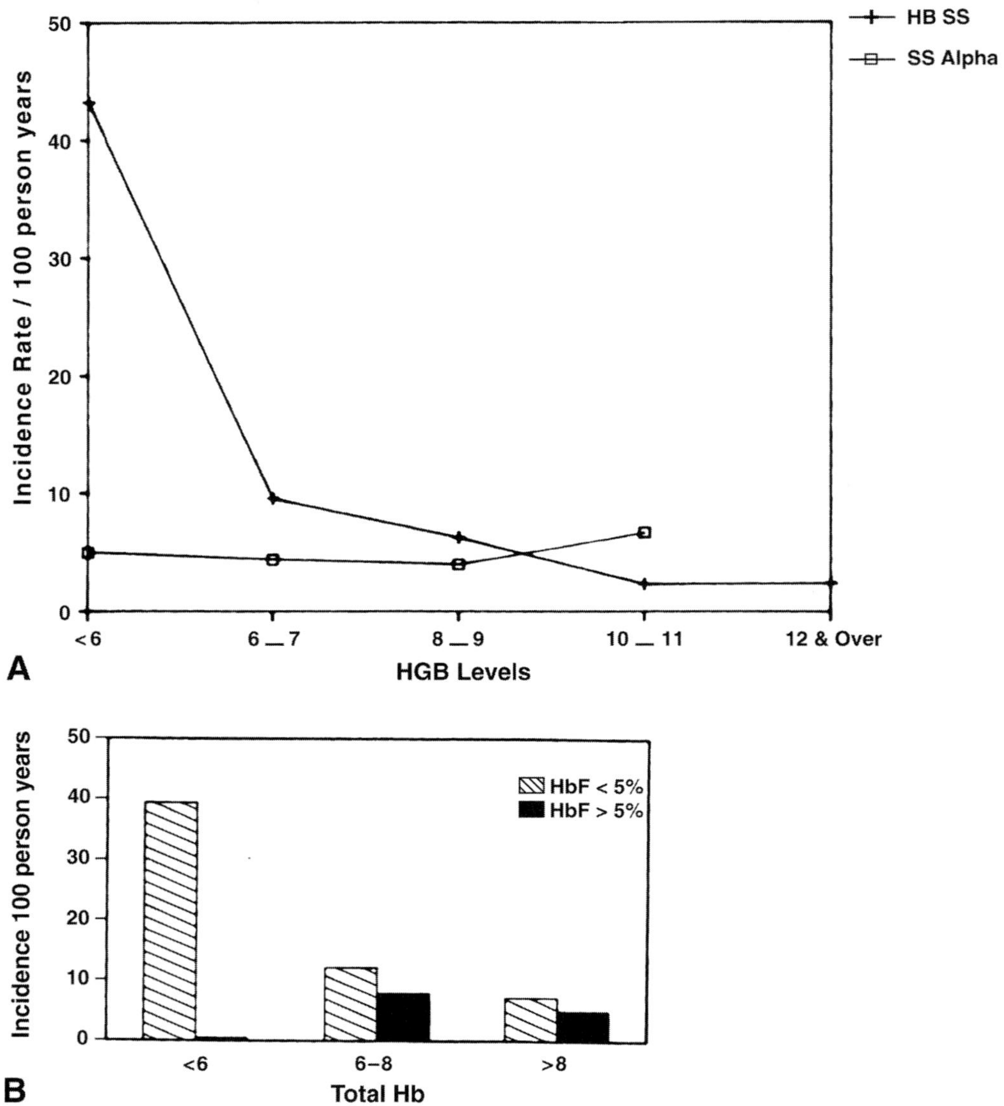

Figure 19.8. Incidence of leg ulcers per 100 patient-years in patients with sickle cell anemia without α thalassemia according to total hemoglobin concentration and HbF level.[288]

patients had lower total hemoglobin and HbF levels and ulcers were more common in males. Individuals with sickle cell anemia–homozygous α thalassemia-2 had an incidence of ulcers less than half that of individuals with sickle cell anemia–heterozygous α thalassemia-2.[288]

Among other elements likely to contribute to the development of leg ulcers in sickle cell anemia are tropical climate, circulatory dynamics, the "exposed" environment of the leg and erythrocyte and vascular injury triggered by the polymerization of HbS and local infection. Both anaerobes and aerobes can be cultured from the base of ulcers more than half of the time.[300,301] It is likely that the ulcer flora varies from clinic to clinic and by region to region. Their role in the development or enlargement of ulcers is unknown. The development of leg ulcers might also be modulated by polymorphic variants of certain genes (Chapter 27).[21]

The higher incidence of leg ulcers in sickle cell anemia compared with thalassemia and other types of hemolytic anemia might be a result of the special characteristics of the sickle erythrocyte (Fig. 19.8).

Clinical Features

Most small and superficial ulcers usually appear on the lower leg and about the medial malleolus[302] and heal spontaneously with rest and careful local hygiene. At times leg ulcers are deep, huge and circumferential, exceedingly painful, disabling, and defy all simple and many complex therapeutic measures.

The first appearance of a leg ulcer usually signifies the high likelihood of their recurrence over a period of many years. Sometimes an ulcer will appear, disappear with treatment or spontaneously, and never recur. More often, they

Table 19.4. Treatment of leg ulcers in sickle cell disease

Débridement
Wet to dry saline dressings
Hydrocolloid dressings
Surgical
Prevent local edema
Support hose PRN
Bed rest and leg elevation PRN
Local treatments
Unna boots (zinc oxide impregnated)
Hydrocolloid dressings
Topical antibiotic PRN
Skin grafting as final alternative
Systemic treatments
Transfusions
Systemic antibiotic PRN
Oral zinc sulfate
Bed rest

All patients should be treated with combinations of local treatments. Systemic treatment has not been proven effective. Adapted from ref. 295.

recur after healing but sometimes only after many years. Leg ulcers can occur on the dorsum of the foot and the anterior or posterior aspects of the leg and be bilateral or unilateral. It has been said that skin ulceration can occur on the arms and other locations but if they have the same cause as the typical sickle cell leg ulcer, they must be quite rare. Ulcers often are first found following trauma to the leg that can seem trivial or appear to be the sequelae of an insect bite.

Treatment recommendations. As expected, there are no trials comparing therapies and only a few controlled trials of any type of ulcer treatment. Perhaps nowhere in the annals of treatment of sickle cell anemia have more untested remedies been applied than in the therapy of leg ulceration (Table 19.4). In the CSSCD, recurrence of ulcers was unaffected by treatment that included transfusions, the Unna gel dressing, zinc, skin grafts, and topical medications of different types, including antibiotics. There are reports touting the use of erythropoietin, antithrombin III, propionyl-L-carnitine, perilesional injection of colony-stimulating factors such as GM-CSF, arginine butyrate, pentoxifylline, DuoDERM, Solcoseryl, isoxsuprine, zinc sulfate, ozone, oxygen, topical opioids, honey, various gels, human skin equivalent, and hyperbaric oxygen.[10] All patients, especially those who have had leg ulcers, should be urged to protect their legs with support hose, avoid activities that cause swelling, such as prolonged standing, and use local lubricants that might help prevent excessive skin dryness and cracking. Control of local inflammation and infection ensuring a clean granulating surface for reepithelialization remains the mainstay of treatment. Wet to dry dressings applied several times a day provide debridement. Occasionally surgical debridement is needed to cleanse the ulcer base. Although cultures of the ulcer base are most often positive, topical antibiotics do not uniformly help healing, and systemic and antimicrobials are usually not indicated. When erythema of the ulcer borders and a purulent exudate are present that do not rapidly resolve after débridement, topical neomycin-bacitracin-polymyxin ointment and systemic antibiotics, chosen on the basis of culture, can be considered.[303] A preliminary report suggested that some chronic ulcers resistant to treatment and accompanied by antibodies to staphylolysin and antinuclease antibodies healed after treatment with flucloxacillin, but this has not been followed by any confirmatory data. Dressing the ulcer with an Unna boot protects the involved area and is a reasonable method of conservative management. Zinc sulfate, 220 mg orally three times daily has also been recommended.

Even small ulcers can be excruciatingly painful and require large amounts of narcotic analgesics for relief. Some patients get good analgesia from narcotic-containing skin patches. When healing occurs, the pain usually disappears.

When healing fails after a trial of conservative treatment that should last 6–8 weeks, difficult choices for more radical treatment must be faced. Prolonged bed rest might be helpful but is usually impractical. Controlled studies of transfusion have not been reported, but reducing HbS level to less than 30% by periodic transfusion can be considered. Surgery is a last resort because the recurrence rate and chance of graft failure are high. Different procedures have been used including free flaps, myocutaneous flaps, and simple skin grafts. The type of grafting used depends on the size of the ulcer and surgeon's experience.

Priapism

Priapus, the mythological god of procreation who is associated with debauchery, is personified by an enlarged tumescent phallus. Priapism is a prolonged, undesirable, painful erection, often occurring without sexual stimulation. Rather than provoking sexual profligacy, priapism can terminate in impotence. Regardless of the initial stimulus for priapism, the normal process of detumescence fails, and this is almost always a result of impaired venous outflow.

Pathophysiology

Vascular communication between the paired corpora cavernosa and the single corpus spongiosum does not exist. Draining the corporal sinusoids are emissary veins that enter progressively larger vessels forming the internal pudendal vein. Sinusoids of the glans drain directly into deep dorsal veins, allowing, when medically indicated, therapeutic shunts to be created that permit blood to flow from the corpora cavernosa to the corpus spongiosum (Fig. 19.9).

Normal erection is initiated by psychogenic, tactile, and neural stimuli, mediated partly by reduced α-adrenergic activity. Relaxed arterial vessels enhance blood delivery to the corporal bodies. Venous outflow is restricted as draining veins are compressed against the surrounding fascia

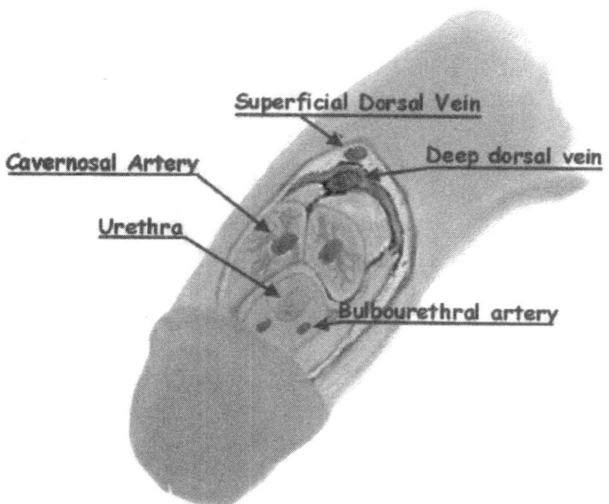

Figure 19.9. Anatomy of the penis. Fed by anastomosing branches of the internal pudendal artery, the erectile apparatus consists of two longitudinal cylinders of sinusoidal tissue: the paired corpora cavernosa with their associated arteries. Ventral to the corpora cavernosa is the corpus spongiosum, pierced by the urethra and terminating in the glans penis. A bulbourethral artery feeds the corpus spongiosum. The corporal bodies – except the glans – are encased in fibrous fascial tunics, the tunica albuginea. There is no vascular communication between the corpora cavernosa and the corpus spongiosum. Draining the corporal sinusoids are emissary veins that enter progressively larger vessels to form the internal pudendal vein. Sinusoids of the glans drain directly into the deep dorsal veins.

by distended sinusoids. As the circumference of the penis is limited by the fascial wrapping of the corpora, when sinusoids become engorged, elongation is paramount. Detumescence reverses this process as α-adrenergic activity increases, feeding arterioles constrict and venous return is reestablished.

Typically, priapism in sickle cell anemia is said to be bicorporeal – only the corpora cavernosa are affected – and is "low flow" – venous outflow is obstructed rather than arterial flow increased. In children, priapism is often associated with normal vascular flow, perhaps accounting for their better prognosis. Tricorporeal priapism has been described in sickle cell anemia and rarely a "high-flow" state, in the absence of penile vascular injury, is present.[303,304] With bicorporeal priapism, the glans remains soft and urination is normal. A tense glans and impaired urination signals involvement of the spongiosa that usually implies infarctive damage to the corpora cavernosa.

An alternative construct of priapism in sickle cell anemia holds that prepubertal patients have bicorporal priapism with high blood flow. Priapic episodes in this population usually last less than 48 hours, tend not to recur, and potency is preserved. In contrast, priapism in adults is usually tricorporal, low flow, recurrent, and long-lasting, and impotence results in over half of these cases, regardless of treatment.[304] These patients have been said to have a higher incidence of stroke, lung disease, renal failure, leg ulcers, and premature death than individuals without priapism.

Priapism is a hemolysis-related complication of sickle cell disease (Chapter 11).[18,20] Penile NO, originating from both neurons and endothelium, modulates penile vascular and smooth muscle relaxation.[305] Low-flow priapism may be the result of venous outflow occlusion because of reduced NO availability.[306,307] Priapic activity and pronounced erectile responses to stimulation are seen in transgenic mice in which both neuronal *(nos1)* and endothelial *(nos3)* NO synthase genes are knocked out and in sickle transgenic mice expressing HbS and lacking any murine hemoglobin.[308] This was thought to be a consequence of dysregulated activity of downstream signaling in the phosphodiesterase type 5 *(pde5a)* pathway. Depleted NO may cause *pde5a* down-regulation, less enzyme available for hydrolysis of cGMP, a reduction in its effector protein kinase G, and supersensitization to local cGMP from other sources. NO deficiency secondary to intravascular hemolysis might down-regulate *PDE5A* and its downstream effectors so that non–NO-mediated uninhibited increases in cGMP result in uncontrolled erection. Sildenafil and similar PDE5A inhibitors might paradoxically alleviate or prevent priapism in these states and pilot studies suggest that sildenafil might be useful in sickle cell priapism.[30] How sickle erythrocytes, neutrophils, and platelets contribute to this pathophysiology is unknown.

In preliminary studies, erythrocytes from patients with priapism had increased adhesion to thrombospondin compared with controls.[309]

The likelihood of developing priapism might be influenced by the presence of polymorphisms in genes associated with NO metabolism and cell adhesion (see Chapter 27).

Epidemiology and Clinical Features

Where sickle cell anemia is common, it is a leading cause of priapism. Less is known about the incidence of priapism in other genotypes of sickle cell disease. Most cases of priapism in sickle cell disease are seen in individuals with sickle cell anemia; in sickle cell anemia–α thalassemia the incidence of priapism decreases; and in HbSC disease the incidence is even lower.[20,304] This is likely to be a result of the less hemolysis in these genotypes and perhaps the greater likelihood of maintaining splenic function.

The incidence of priapism is highly dependent on the assiduousness of questioning. Many different age groups have been studied, most retrospectively: observation periods vary greatly, definitions may be vague, and self-reporting can be poor. In one study of children and adolescents, the actuarial probability of experiencing priapism by age 20 years was 89% ± 9%.[310] The mean age at the initial episode was 12 years, the mean number of episodes per patient was 15.7, and the mean duration of an episode was 125 minutes. Episodes typically occurred around 4:00 AM, and 75% of the patients surveyed had at least one episode starting during sleep or upon awakening from sleep. Other studies of different populations suggested a lower incidence.[312–316] In another study the mean age of onset was 19 years but priapism was reported in children as young as 5 years.[317]

Recurrent attacks of priapism can last for several hours with tolerable discomfort, and they can be self-limited. These episodes have been termed stuttering priapism and they usually have a nocturnal onset. Erectile function is mostly preserved between these attacks, which can recur over a period of years and number in the dozens. Major episodes of priapism often, but not always, follow a history of stuttering attacks, last for days, and can be excruciatingly painful. They often destroy sexual function by causing irreversible corporal damage. Prolonged or recurrent episodes of priapism cause edema of the vascular septa of the corpora cavernosa leading to fibrosis, destruction of the normal distensible sinusoidal anatomy, and culminate in impotence.[313] In children, impotence seems to be a less common result of priapism, the incidence of which varies directly with age.[318,319] One attack of priapism presages multiple episodes. This may be an indication that sufficient vascular damage is present to alter normal erectile function. It seems reasonable to suspect that subclinical vascular damage precedes overt priapism and to some extent determines the end result of priapic episodes.

A rare complication of priapism is megalophallus. In a well-studied case, in which penile enlargement followed a prolonged severe priapic event, the proximal two-thirds of the penis had a circumference of nearly 20 cm. Using Doppler measurements, penile blood flow was high and MRI showed deoxyHbS in the corpora cavernosa. At least in this instance, corporal fibrosis did not seem to be present and erectile function was preserved. It was hypothesized that sudden loss of elasticity of the tunica albuginea allowed painless penile expansion.[320]

Diagnosis

History and physical examination establish this diagnosis. Six patients, five with a history of priapism, were studied by nocturnal tumescence testing with polysomnography and penile MRI. Nocturnal erections and detumescence times were prolonged and corporal anatomy varied from normal to intracorporeal fibrosis.[321] These studies correlated well with clinical examinations and history, suggesting to the authors that their routine use was not warranted.

Penile scans using technetium-99m can distinguish between low and high blood flow states and which corporal bodies are affected. They may not be helpful in predicting the clinical course of the event. Intracorporeal pressure and blood gases can be monitored. Doppler flow studies and MRI can also provide information on blood flow and which of the corporal bodies are involved. There is little information on how any of these tests can be used to direct therapy or establish a prognosis.

Treatment recommendations. The Cochrane Database Reviews concluded that there is no evidence for the benefits or risks of the different treatments for both stuttering and fulminant sickle cell priapism.[322] Clinicians must decide when "conservative" treatment with analgesics, hydration, and perhaps transfusions should be stopped and operative intervention initiated. Small retrospective case studies comprise the only information available to assist in this decision.[318] Retrospectively, when the adverse outcome of impotence has occurred after a severe bout of priapism, it is easy to assume that earlier operative intervention would have preserved erectile function. It is possible that the natural history of priapism is unaffected by any presently used treatment, conservative or surgical, and that the ultimate loss of potency is governed by the interplay of intracorporeal and systemic factors.

Most "authorities" believe that 24–48 hours is the maximum time that should elapse before treatment of priapism should be converted from "conservative" to operative intervention. There are several difficulties with this pronouncement. No scale is available to gauge the severity of the priapic episode or account for the preceding history of priapism. Conceivably, extreme turgidity with excruciating pain should be managed differently from lesser degrees of penile engorgement. Most episodes of priapism are preceded by a history of other episodes; these can be similar, more severe, or less severe, and have resolved with erectile function preserved. How should this history be incorporated into the treatment plan? It would be invaluable to know how hydration, sedation, and simple or exchange transfusions, compare with aspiration and irrigation and with surgical shunts. One small study found automated exchange transfusions to be ineffective.[323] Whether or not transfusions are helpful, especially if a major episode has occurred, is not known, and a recent review found no benefit of this treatment.[324] If surgery is superior, what type of operation is best? Although priapism is a common complication, the experience of any single urologist or hematologist is limited and their favorite treatment is likely to be biased by their own limited observations. Because of this uncertainty, the many published schema for managing priapism, including our own, cannot be taken as a "standard of care" dictating rigid adherence, but are general guidelines only.

Pain should be relieved with narcotic analgesics and adequate fluids provided. If the episode differs from prior episodes of stuttering priapism according to the patient history and physician experience, aspiration and irrigation should be done within a 12-hour window from the onset of erection. In a prospective study in children, aspiration of blood from the corpora cavernosa and irrigation with a dilute epinephrine solution while the patient received local anesthetic was used to relieve priapism if hydration and analgesics failed to produce detumescence or if priapism had lasted more than 4 hours. Fifteen patients with sickle cell anemia were treated 39 times and detumescence occurred 95% of the time without serious side effects. All patients whose priapism resolved had self-reported normal erectile function at a median of 40 months after the last procedure.[325] Self-limited attacks of stuttering priapism often resolve after masturbation, cold showers, or exercise.

Invasive treatment for priapism in sickle cell anemia is designed to evacuate stagnant blood within the corpora cavernosa and to prevent immediate recurrence of corporal expansion. The simplest surgical procedure is aspiration of the corporal bodies with irrigation; however, when a major episode of priapism has been present for 24–48 hours aspiration of blood is usually difficult. Creation of shunts between the glans penis and the distal corpora cavernosa with a Tru-cut biopsy needle is an alternate approach favored by most urologists if corporal irrigation fails. This procedure, popularized by Winter and bearing his name, allows blood from the distended corpora cavernosa to drain into the uninvolved corpus spongiosa. If there is tricorporal involvement, this shunt is unlikely to be effective. An operative intervention to create larger shunts between the corpora cavernosa and corpus spongiosum can be considered if detumescence is not achieved with the Winter shunt.

α-Adrenergic activity maintains the vessels feeding the corporal bodies in a constricted state when the penis is flaccid. This suggested that oral and intracavernous administration of α-adrenergic agonists, with or without drainage, may help reverse priapism.[326–328] Etilefrine, an α-adrenergic agonist, and other α-adrenergic agents were used in patients with sickle cell anemia and stuttering or acute priapism.[329,330] When Etilefrine was used orally in stuttering episodes, recurrence was claimed to be prevented, and acute, more severe episodes were reversed after intracavernous injection. These observations do not warrant a general recommendation for using these agents because there are some dangers associated with α-adrenergic agonists, and the reports available do not substitute for well-controlled trials. Vasodilators and even β-adrenergic agents have also been used but there are no good studies of their efficacy.

In perhaps the sole double-blind, placebo-controlled trial of treatment for priapism, stilbestrol was found to reduce attacks of stuttering priapism.[312] Eleven patients with a history of two attacks of priapism weekly were enrolled and after a 2-week baseline were randomized to receive either 5 mg of stilbestrol daily or a placebo. Two individuals stopped having attacks during the baseline period. Five placebo-treated patients continued their attacks and when they switched to active drug ceased having priapism. Four patients randomized to receive active drug stopped their attacks in 1–3 days. A maintenance dose of 2.5–5 mg every few days or weekly was usually effective. Stilbestrol can cause gynecomastia, prevent desired erections, and have other undesirable consequences. This was a short-term study of a small and very select group of patients. The general usefulness of this treatment and its ability to stop major episodes of priapism is unknown.

Low doses of the androgen antagonist, bicalutamide, have been successful in preventing recurrent priapism but very few cases have been reported, and this form of treatment might also have troubling consequences.[331]

In five patients with stuttering priapism who were started on hydroxyurea, four had a reduction in the number and severity of episodes and in two patients the episodes stopped.[332] Two patients had HbF levels of approximately 20%. The absence of an association of HbF levels with priapism raise some skepticism about this approach, although the NO donor properties of hydroxyurea might, in conjunction with an exuberant HbF increase, be useful.

Seven patients with priapism were given sildenafil and tadalafil and followed for 2 years. A retrospective analysis suggested that treatment was successful in alleviating or resolving priapism recurrences in six of the seven patients, and erectile function was unchanged in six patients and improved in one patient at last follow-up. All the patients tolerated the treatment well. The investigators concluded that a rigorously implemented controlled clinical trial was necessary to confirm the utility of this treatment.[30,333] It seems unlikely that when the anatomy of the erectile apparatus is permanently damaged, treatment with sildenafil will be effective for regaining lost erectile function.

When impotence results from priapism, implantable penile prostheses have been used with success, although they might be difficult to insert in fibrotic corporal bodies and might be associated with more complications than when used in cases of idiopathic priapism.[334]

Digestive Diseases

Biliary tract disease and parenchymal liver disease are the most prevalent and serious complications of sickle cell anemia that affect the digestive system. Abdominal pain is a frequent complaint of patients with sickle cell disease. Whether pain results from cholelithiasis or cholecystitis, has its roots in intraabdominal vasoocclusive disease, or is related to intraabdominal pathology unrelated to sickle cell anemia, it is often a difficult to resolve. Some causes of abdominal pain in sickle cell anemia are shown in Table 19.5. In one series, over half of the episodes of abdominal pain were thought to be due to vasoocclusive episodes, approximately a quarter were due to gall bladder disease or appendicitis, 13% had a renal origin, and some were due to pneumonia and gynecological disease.[188]

There is little reliable information on other abnormalities of the digestive system. Documented episodes of bowel ischemia are rare. Pancreatitis has been reported but appears to be uncommon. Controversy surrounds the incidence of peptic ulcer disease in sickle cell anemia, and whether or not these individuals have reduced acid secretion.[313]

Sickle Cell Liver Disease

Hepatomegaly is found in 80%–100% of patients. Liver disease is often a mélange of diverse pathologies that might

Table 19.5. Potential causes of abdominal pain in sickle cell anemia

Enlarged mesenteric and retroperitoneal nodes
Bone and spinal abnormalities
marrow hyperplasia
bone infarction
ribs
spine
femoral head
osteoporosis and vertebral collapse
Nerve root compression
Hepatobiliary disease
hepatitis
acute hepatic enlargement
sequestration
intrahepatic cholestasis
cholelithiasis
Spleen
hemorrhage
infarction
sequestration
abscess
Mesenteric ischemia
Pneumonia
Renal
obstructive uropathy
stone
clot
papillary necrosis
cystitis

Modified from ref. 188.

be contributed to by intra- and extrahepatic cholestasis, viral hepatitis, cirrhosis, hypoxia and infarction, erythrocyte sequestration, iron overload, and drug reactions. Often it is difficult to differentiate among these causes in an individual and more than one cause of liver disease is often present. In common with liver disease in the general population, treatment options are limited.

Abnormal "liver" tests are often present but might not always reflect hepatocellular disease or even be related to the hemoglobinopathy.[335] Unconjugated hyperbilirubinemia is an expression of hemolytic anemia. Bilirubin levels vary considerably and this is likely a reflection of liver disease, hemolysis, and genetic differences in bilirubin metabolism. Increased levels of alkaline phosphatase, especially in children and adolescents, could be from growing or injured bones. Protein C and protein S levels are lower in sickle cell anemia when compared with controls, an observation that was accounted for by hepatic dysfunction rather than consumptive coagulopathy.[336]

Hepatic drug metabolism is variously affected with some drugs, such as morphine, having increased clearance, others, such as lidocaine, having decreased clearance, and still others, such as meperidine, being unaffected. These differences could exist because of genetic differences and the different routes of drug metabolism, for example glucuronidation or deethylation.[337] Insufficient information is available on which to base changes in drug dosing.

An occasional otherwise well patient will have an isolated elevation of unconjugated bilirubin beyond the usual values seen in sickle cell anemia,[13] with normal liver tests and no indication of hepatic disease. Perhaps some of these individuals have Gilbert syndrome, now known to be associated with polymorphisms of the UDP-glucuronyltransferase (*UDPGT1*) gene promoter (see Chapter 27).

Results of liver biopsy are highly dependent on the clinical events that prompted biopsy. Hemosiderosis is often present, a result of chronic transfusions and parenchymal liver disease. Chronic hepatitis and cirrhosis might suggest transfusion-transmitted diseases.[338] When biopsy was performed during cholecystectomy, sinusoidal dilation and perisinusoidal fibrosis were the pervasive lesions.[339] Kupffer cells often contain phagocytized erythrocytes.

As expected in patients who have often received multiple blood transfusions, viral hepatitis is common. Bilirubin levels may be much higher than found in viral hepatitis uncomplicated by the hemolysis and other liver-related complications of disease.[340] Viral hepatitis B was often present in transfused patients before it was possible to screen blood for its presence.

In 141 patients with sickle cell disease, hepatitis B core antibodies were positive in 14% and hepatitis C viral antibody titers were positive in 16.5%. Hepatitis C positivity was related to transfusion.[341] These observations are unlikely to be representative of the world's population as transmission of hepatitis C by transfusions is dependent on the incidence of this disease in the population of blood donors. Worldwide, hepatitis C viral antibodies are present in 2%–20% of transfused patients. When serum ALT levels were persistently elevated, 90% of these patients were hepatitis C viral antibody positive. Hepatitis E infection has been noted, and as new blood borne viral hepatitides appear, undoubtedly they will be found among transfused patients. Autoimmune hepatitis diagnosed by biopsy and responsive to immunosuppressive therapy has been described.

Sickle hepatopathy, hepatic crisis, and the right upper quadrant syndrome of sickle cell disease have been variously defined. Syndromes of "benign" intrahepatic cholestasis and acute hepatic sequestration – akin to the splenic sequestration syndrome – have been described. Nevertheless, it is difficult from descriptions in the literature to differentiate among these entities, probably because their causes include viral hepatitis and vasoocclusive disease compounded by hemolysis and cholestasis. A syndrome of increasing hepatomegaly, extreme hyperbilirubinemia with levels approaching 100 mg/dL, has been recognized. In this syndrome there are only modest increases in transaminase levels, high alkaline phosphatase and γ-glutamyltransferase levels, right upper quadrant pain, increasing anemia, fever, coagulation abnormalities, and differing degrees of hepatic failure.

When sickle hepatopathy was defined by a total serum bilirubin concentration of more than 13 mg/dL in the absence of acute hemolysis, viral hepatitis, extrahepatic obstruction, or hepatic sequestration, 44 patients were categorized based on whether hepatic dysfunction at presentation was mild or severe. Mild patients were younger with lower maximum bilirubin levels than severe patients (36.2 mg/dL vs. 76.8 mg/dL) and had a 4% mortality compared with a 64% mortality. Two of nine patients who received exchange transfusion died compared with 12 of 13 who did not receive exchange transfusion.[342]

About 11% of deaths in one analysis were attributable to cirrhosis.[251] Liver disease can also be present in HbSC disease and HbS–β^+ thalassemia.

Treatment recommendations. There are no data on the value of interferon for chronic active hepatitis C in sickle cell anemia. Its use should be based on the experience in other diseases. Individuals with the severe right upper quadrant syndrome can reasonably be offered exchange transfusions, although there is not proof of their efficacy. Unless it is unequivocally clear that extrahepatic obstruction is present, surgery should be avoided. The management of iron overload is discussed in Chapter 29.

Gallstones

Hyperbilirubinemia is associated with a high prevalence of gallstones. In Jamaica, 31% of sickle cell anemia and 11% of HbSC disease patients aged 17–24 years who participated in the cohort study had gallstones, but specific symptoms necessitating cholecystectomy occurred in only 2% of sickle cell anemia cases.[343] Gallstones were found in approximately 16% of Kuwaiti children with sickle cell anemia, aged 10.8 ± 5.5 years.[344] Individuals with stones had a lower hemoglobin level and were less likely to have α thalassemia. Although α thalassemia might reduce the development of cholelithiasis by reducing hemolysis, the genotype of the *UGT1A* gene seems of greater importance (Chapter 27).[345]

Patients with sickle cell anemia had a lower frequency of the common *UGT1A* promoter polymorphism $(TA)_6$ and a higher frequency of the $(TA)_7$ allele.[346] Children with the $(TA)_6$ allele had a lower serum bilirubin (2.4 ± 0.8 mg/dL) and had less than half the rate of cholecystectomy than those with the $(TA)_7$ allele who had higher bilirubin levels (5.8 ± 3.1 mg/dL). This polymorphisms is also related to the age of onset of cholelithiasis.[347] In children taking hydroxyurea the hydroxyurea-related decreases in serum bilirubin levels were dependent on the *UGT1A* genotype with individuals with the wild-type promoter genotype having lower levels.[348]

Pigmented gallstones in sickle cell disease can be either radiopaque or radiolucent. Ultrasonography is the preferred means of their detection. Open cholecystectomy accounted for 20% of all operations in 717 patients with sickle cell anemia with only one death.[191] In a study of the effects of preoperative transfusion in sickle cell anemia, 211 open cholecystectomies and 153 laparoscopic cholecystectomies were performed.[349] Nineteen percent of these patients had intraoperative, 11% transfusion related, and 10% postoperative complications, for a total complication rate of 39%. Untransfused patients had the highest rate of postoperative acute chest syndrome and painful episodes. When common duct stones were suspected on the basis of a dilated duct, high alkaline phosphatase levels, and bilirubin that exceeded baseline by 5 mg/dL, endoscopic retrograde cholangiopancreatography, sphincterotomy, and stone extraction followed by laparoscopic cholecystectomy was an effective approach.[350]

Treatment recommendations. Unequivocal episodes of acute cholecystitis are not common and typical obstructive jaundice is equally infrequent. When stones are asymptomatic or symptoms and laboratory findings are equivocal, it is probably best not to do elective cholecystectomy. Laparoscopic cholecystectomy patients were hospitalized for a shorter time period but had a similar rate of complications as those who underwent open cholecystectomy.

Neurocognitive Dysfunction in Adults

Although neurocognitive abnormalities are well known to be present in children with cerebrovascular disease, few studies have been done in adults. To study this problem, adults with sickle cell anemia or HbS–β^0 thalassemia who were neurologically normal and did not have a history of stroke or an abnormal MRI examination were given a standard group of neuropsychological tests and underwent MRI.[351]

Forty percent of young adult patients had abnormal scans. Abnormalities included frontal and parietal atrophy, lacunae and white matter lesions, and reduced intracranial and hippocampal volumes. Mean IQ scores were below average with more than twice as many patients scoring less than 85 on the Wechsler Adult Intelligence and Memory Scales compared with 16% of controls. Approximately 40% of patients had IQ scores 1 standard deviation or more below the normative population mean. Memory, reading, and math performance were also decreased. Hemoglobin concentration was positively associated with IQ, and IQ tended to be associated with hippocampal volume.

Although preliminary, these findings suggest that even neurologically normal adults can be neurocognitively impaired. They could explain some of the unusual behaviors seen in some adults and attributed to "poor adjustment" and other nonorganic psychological problems. A pilot trial is being conducted to see if transfusion can improve neurocognitive function. Perhaps more important is the realization that central nervous system disease, like disease of other organs, can be "silent" but progressive and

Table 19.6. Laboratory values and clinical events in septuagenarians with sickle cell anemia

Age (y)	Sex	Hb	MCV	Retic	WBC	PLT	HbF	HAPLO	α genes	Cr	ALT	Bili
75	M	5.6	80	13	6.4	249	4.0	BEN/Atyp	3	1.5	23	3.3
71	M	7.8	86	7	6.8	170	5.3	BEN/BEN	3	1.3	27	2.4
71	F	7.5	95	14	10.7	433	2.8	BEN/CAR	4	1.5	22	1.7
76	M	5.5	96	7	7.6	162	0.2	–	4	4.2	25	2.9
80	M	8.8	84	1.9	11.4	340	5.0	–	–	–	24	0.7
73	M	5.5	91	5	11.4	272	–	–	–	1.5	7	4.7

Age (y)	Pain	CHF	Leg ulcer	Acute chest	ON	CVA	Retina	TX
75	0	Y	Y	N	N	N	N	Y
71	10	Y	Y	Y	Y	Y	N	N
71	3	N	Y	N	Y	N	N	N
76	0	Y	Y	N	N	N	N	Y
80	<1	Y	N	N	N	N	N	–
73	0	Y	N	N	Y	N	N	Y

Hb, hemoglobin level in g/dL; MCV, mean corpuscular volume (fL); Retic, reticulocyte count (percent); WBC, leukocyte count (10^6/L); PLT, platelet count (10^9/L); HbF, fetal hemoglobin (percent); HAPLO, β-globin gene cluster haplotype [BEN-Benin; CAR Central African Republic; Atyp-atypical]; α genes, α-globin genotype; Cr, creatinine (mg/dL); ALT, alanine aminotransferase (units); Pain, average numbers of pain crises yearly, CHF, congestive heart failure (Y, yes; N, no); Leg ulcer, presence or history of leg ulcers; ON, osteonecrosis, CVA, history of cerebrovascular accidents; Retina, sickle retinopathy; TX, regular transfusions.[353]

that early treatment with drugs such as hydroxyurea might prevent or retard its development.

OLDER ADULTS

Sickle cell anemia, first considered a disease of childhood, is now found in the elderly. Most clinics have seen individuals in their sixth and seventh decades and some individuals have survived into the ninth decade. Increasing numbers of older adults with sickle cell anemia are probably a result of higher standards of supportive care. In follow-up of the Jamaican sickle cell study patients, it was noted that of the 102 patients who had survived their 60th birthday, 40 were known to be alive and were aged 60.2–85.6 years and females predominated.[352]

Older adults with sickle cell anemia have their own array of complications.[353,354] Laboratory and clinical features of a small group of septuagenarians with sickle cell anemia are shown in Table 19.6. In such a small number of cases, generalizations are difficult, but several features of these patients deserve comment. Although their lifespan was near normal, they were not unaffected; most of their serious complications became apparent in later life. Although their HbF levels, the best predictor of morbidity and mortality, were lower than average, Jamaican "survivors" had HbF levels approximately 5% higher than expected. HbF constantly falls with aging in sickle cell anemia and there is very little information on HbF in patients aged 60–80 years.[354] Leukocyte counts, also associated with morbidity and mortality in sickle cell anemia, were lower than average. As both leukocyte counts and HbF fall with age in sickle cell anemia the levels observed may be an effect, not a cause, of longevity. With aging, hemoglobin levels fall and renal function declines.[352] One other septuagenarian with sickle cell anemia had a PCV of 18, HbF of 6.4%, and a leukocyte count of 10.3×10^6/L.[354]

We do not understand why some patients with sickle cell anemia survive their peers by decades. These unusual patients can be examples of the possibility of a long life and should alert physicians that this diagnosis need not be excluded by age alone. Old age in sickle cell anemia does not imply that these are the "golden years." Decades of vascular injury – much of which is subclinical – begins to result in chronic organ damage and failure. The lung, heart, bones, and kidneys are primarily affected.

Eye Disease

Sickle retinopathy is discussed in detail in Chapter 21 and the treatment of hyphema in HbAS is discussed in Chapter 22. Present in approximately one to two thirds of adults with HbSC disease, depending on their ages, proliferative sickle retinopathy is far less common in sickle cell anemia. As hydroxyurea treatment makes sickle cell anemia erythrocytes more like HbSC disease cells, the prevalence of proliferative retinopathy could begin to increase in young sickle cell anemia patients treated with this drug.

In distinction to proliferative retinopathy, central retinal artery occlusion is a rare cause of sudden blindness and is more common in sickle cell anemia than HbSC disease.[355] Approximately half of the reported cases were in association with a vasoocclusive episode and 7 of 17 cases were bilateral. Most patients had partial recovery of vision, although any relationship of recovery to transfusion, which is usually used for treatment, is unclear.

Some patients with sickle cell anemia have abnormal dark adaptation.[356] This defect is related to tissue zinc deficiency, a consequence of hyperzincuria and improves with zinc replacement. Any clinical consequences of this laboratory observation have not been reported.

Conjunctival vessels in sickle cell anemia are damaged by vasoocclusion and develop corkscrew- and comma-shaped forms, show dropped out segments, and can become obliterated causing avascular regions of the bulbar conjunctiva. These abnormalities have been considered pathognomonic of sickle cell disease, and their presence is inversely correlated with HbF level and directly related to the numbers of ISCs.[357] Conjunctival abnormalities are less often present in HbSC disease and HbS–β^+ thalassemia.

Cardiovascular Complications

Cardiac abnormalities may be present in children with sickle cell anemia. When 23 patients aged 7–17 years underwent exercise myocardial scintigraphy, myocardial perfusion was abnormal in 61%; some patients had irreversible abnormalities and others had cardiac failure, angina, or ventricular tachycardia.[358] Children with a median age of 10.1 years had larger left ventricular and atrial volumes than controls and some had left ventricular hypertrophy and stiffness.[359] Perhaps such changes antedate cardiac disease in adults.

Physical work capacity is reduced by approximately half in adults, and 60%–70% in children with sickle cell anemia, and is related to the severity of the anemia. Cardiac examinations in adults are rarely normal; the heart is usually enlarged and the precordium hyperactive, systolic murmurs are found in most patients, and premature contractions are often present.[360] Cardiomegaly and heart murmurs often raise the question of whether congestive heart failure is present, but contractility is usually normal and overt congestive heart failure is uncommon, especially in children.[361] Preliminary studies of transfused and nontransfused patients with sickle cell disease suggest that left ventricular dysfunction is relatively uncommon compared with transfused patients with β thalassemia. When heart failure is present, it often can be related to secondary causes such as fluid overload.

Hypertension can cause ventricular hypertrophy and heart failure. Cardiac output is increased at rest in individuals with sickle cell anemia and rises further with exercise. Electrocardiograms often have nonspecific abnormalities and can show sign of ventricular hypertrophy. Cardiac index is increased approximately twice normal at rest and increases further during exercise. Cardiac index was not related to hemoglobin level or oxygen content suggesting increased tissue extraction of oxygen. This was postulated to be due to the increased capillary diffusing surface.

Cardiac abnormalities in almost 200 patients aged 13 years and older with sickle cell anemia were studied echocardiographically by investigators of the CSSCD.[361] Compared with normal controls, patients had increased left and right ventricular and left atrial chamber dimensions, increased interventricular septal thickness, and normal contractility. These dimensions, except for those of the right ventricle, were inversely related to the hemoglobin level and indicated cardiac dilation. Cardiac dilation was also dependent on age. Pericardial effusions were present in 10% of patients. When homozygous α thalassemia-2 was present, left ventricular dimensions were more normal but wall thickness was increased.[362] This difference was postulated to be a result of the higher hemoglobin levels caused by α thalassemia. Nevertheless, the response to exercise was not improved.

Diastolic dysfunction was found in 18% of 141 patients with different genotypes of sickle cell disease. A combination of diastolic dysfunction and pulmonary hypertension was present in 11% but diastolic dysfunction explained only 10%–20% of the variability in TRJ velocity. Diastolic dysfunction independently contributes to prospective mortality.[363] Most patients had no evidence of impaired right or left ventricular systolic function.

Chest pain, a common entity in sickle cell anemia, often leads to patients being told they have had a "heart attack." In fact, obvious myocardial infarction is unusual, but has been reported. Paradoxically, coronary artery occlusion is not common, suggesting that small vessel disease is responsible for the cardiac damage.[364] Gross and microscopic findings consistent with acute (three patients) and healed (four patients) myocardial infarction were found in seven (9.7%) of 72 consecutive hearts from patients with sickle cell disease studied at autopsy. Gross obstructive and atherosclerotic lesions were absent in all seven patients, whereas microthrombi were present in the arterioles of infarcted tissue in two. Chest pain occurred clinically in six of the seven patients and electrocardiographic findings typical of infarction were found in two. One patient died suddenly. These findings suggest that ischemic heart disease can be present in patients with sickle cell disease and should not be categorically excluded in patients with chest pain.[365]

Sudden unexpected and unexplained death is common in adults with sickle cell anemia. In postmortem examinations of the cardiac conduction system and coronary chemoreceptors from the hearts of two black males who died suddenly there were abundant foci of old and recent degeneration in the sinus node, atrioventricular node, and His bundle, and also the coronary chemoreceptor.[366] Many capillaries and small arteries were packed with sickled erythrocytes, among which small groups of aggregated platelets were also present. Focal fibromuscular dysplasia caused moderate to severe narrowing of many small coronary arteries, including those supplying the conduction system and chemoreceptor. These abnormalities suggest that electrical instability might be one component of the lethal terminal events in some individuals. Cardiovascular autonomic function tests were performed in 24 patients with sickle cell anemia and 38 healthy white controls. Fifty-eight percent had cardiovascular autonomic dysfunction based on abnormal values for at least two cardiovascular autonomic function tests, whereas 41.7% had preserved autonomic function.[367]

Treatment recommendations. Overt congestive heart failure in sickle cell anemia is not common and when present should be treated with the usual methods. When "rehydrating" patients during treatment of acute vasoocclusive events, care should be taken so that excessive fluids do not lead to iatrogenic congestive failure. Severely anemic patients with symptoms of congestive heart failure or angina pectoris might be helped by cautiously increasing their hemoglobin concentration by transfusion or erythropoietin treatment.

Renal Disease

Renal complications are a common cause of morbidity and mortality in sickle cell disease and the incidence of renal failure increases as overall patient survival increases. Early elements of sickle cell renal disease include increased renal plasma flow, glomerular hyperfiltration, increased proximal tubular function and hematuria. Subsequently, reduced concentrating ability, focal segmental glomerulosclerosis with proteinuria, papillary necrosis, impaired urine acidification and potassium secretion and reduced glomerular filtration can develop.[368–375]

Epidemiology

In the United States, between 1992 and 1996, there were 345 reported new cases of end-stage renal disease in sickle cell anemia (U.S. Renal Data System 1997 Annual Report, NIDDK, NIH). In one study, patients with a Bantu β-globin gene cluster haplotype were most likely to develop renal failure.[376,377] This study was a prospective, 25-year longitudinal demographic and clinical cohort study of 725 patients with sickle cell anemia and 209 patients with HbSC disease. Approximately 4% of sickle cell anemia and 2.4% of HbSC disease patients developed renal failure, with median ages of onset of 23 and 50 years, respectively. Sixty percent of patients older than 40 years had proteinuria and 30% had renal insufficiency. Nephrotic syndrome was found in 40% of patients with creatinine levels above 1 mg/dL for children and 1.5 mg/dL for adults. In the Jamaican cohort study, subjects with sickle cell disease, aged 18–23 years had lower blood pressure and normal or increase glomerular filtration rate and renal plasma flow compared with controls. Twenty-six percent of patients had microalbuminuria, and this correlated positively with glomerular filtration rate and blood pressure.[375] Approximately 20% of children aged 3–20 years had microalbuminuria.[378]

Survival time for patients with sickle cell anemia after the diagnosis of sickle renal failure was 4 years even when on dialysis, and the median age at the time of death was 27 years. Case-control analysis showed that ineffective erythropoiesis with increasingly severe anemia, hypertension, proteinuria, the nephrotic syndrome, and microscopic hematuria were significant preazotemic predictors of chronic renal failure. Perhaps the lower levels of HbF associated with the Bantu haplotype was responsible for more rapid organ failure.

α Thalassemia might prevent or retard sickle glomerulopathy. In 76 adults with sickle cell anemia, albumin excretion of more than 300 mg/g creatinine was found in 13% of patients with heterozygous or homozygous α thalassemia-2 compared with 40% of patients with a normal α-globin gene haplotype.[379] Renal failure is a risk factor for early death with survival reduced by nearly half compared with patients having normal renal function.[207,250,377]

Pathophysiology

Two major abnormalities characterize the renal lesions associated with sickle cell disease. The first, and least important, is medullary disease that is found in most individuals with sickle cell anemia and even in carriers of HbAS (Chapter 22). Acidosis, hypoxia, and hyperosmolarity, conditions that favor HbS polymerization, typify the conditions in the renal medulla. Even HbAS cells deform in this environment, leading to hyposthenuria and occasionally hematuria. In sickle cell anemia, the vasa recta may be severely damaged or lost entirely. Isosthenuria, distal renal tubular acidosis, and impaired potassium excretion are signs of medullary dysfunction. Clinically, the loss of concentrating ability is not important unless access to fluid is restricted. Systemic acidosis is not a clinical problem despite the acidification defect. Hyperkalemia can accompany renal failure and the use of angiotensin-converting enzyme (ACE) inhibitors and might be worsened by type IV renal tubular acidosis. Hematuria and papillary necrosis are also seen. The former is almost always benign as it is in HbAS. Proximal renal tubular function is supranormal and creatinine secretion and phosphate reabsorption are increased. This is of no clinical significance but can lead to overestimation of glomerular filtration rate.

The major renal abnormality of sickle cell disease is a glomerulopathy, characterized by glomerular hypertrophy, hypercellularity, mesangial proliferation, and segmental glomerulosclerosis.[380,381] Why glomerular hypertrophy occurs is unclear, but might be related to increased renal plasma flow, hypoxia, increased prostaglandin production, and dilation of afferent glomerular arterioles. Arteriolar dilation could produce glomerular hypertension, which is ultimately responsible for loss of filtration. Glomerular permeability is increased before renal insufficiency develops and decreases with chronic renal failure.[382] When macroalbuminuria occurs, glomerulopathy is present, and the

Table 19.7. Renal abnormalities in sickle cell disease

Distal Nephron
Impaired urine-concentrating ability
Impaired urine acidification–incomplete renal tubular acidosis
Impaired K^+ excretion
Medullary carcinoma
Hematuria
Papillary necrosis
Proximal Tubule
Increased phosphate reabsorption
Increased β_2-microglobulin reabsorption
Increased uric acid secretion
Increased creatinine secretion
Hemodynamic Changes
Increased glomerular filtration rate
Increased renal plasma flow
Glomerular Abnormalities
Proteinuria
Nephrotic syndrome with focal glomerular sclerosis
Chronic renal failure; decreased filtration fraction

glomerular filtration ability is reduced to approximately 40%, even in patients with a preserved glomerular filtration rate.[369] Glomerular hypertrophy and hyperfiltration lead to increased secretion of creatinine and explain the very low creatinine levels of children and adolescents with sickle cell anemia and their increased creatinine clearance. A "normal" creatinine level in teenagers and young adults with sickle cell anemia is "abnormal" and is evidence for sickle nephropathy.[375]

Acute reversible deterioration of renal function due to tubular necrosis, occasionally severe and requiring dialysis, sometimes develops in hospitalized patients. It is often associated with volume contraction, anemia, and infection, but most patients recover with time. Renal cortical necrosis can also occur and here, recovery is less likely. Renal abnormalities in sickle cell anemia are shown in Table 19.7.

Diagnosis

Albuminuria is a sensitive marker of glomerular damage in sickle cell disease and precedes the development of overt renal insufficiency. In 300 patients with sickle cell disease, including 184 with sickle cell anemia, albumin excretion rates and renal function were measured. Micro- and macroalbuminuria occurred in 68% and macroalbuminuria in 26% of adults with sickle cell anemia, whereas in other disease genotypes, micro- and macroalbuminuria occurred in 32% and macroalbuminuria in 10%. In one study, development of albuminuria was age dependent and correlated with serum creatinine, but not with blood pressure.[383] In a cross-sectional study, albuminuria was associated with blood pressure.[375]

Yearly screening, by measuring the albumin/creatinine ratio in a random urine specimen, might help identify patients for treatment with ACE inhibitors or ACE receptor antagonists should controlled clinical trials shown that they can retard the progression of disease. Other proposed markers for renal failure and injury are urinary kallikrein,[384] cystatin-C and N-acetyl-beta-D-glucosaminidase,[232] the ^{51}Cr EDTA measurement of glomerular filtration rate,[385] and endothelin-1.[386]

Transgenic sickle mice also have glomerular hyperfiltration and hyposthenuria, excrete increased amounts of stable NO metabolites, and have raised levels of glomerular iNOS.[387]

Treatment recommendations. Nonsteroidal antiinflammatory drugs that inhibit the production of prostaglandins can reduce glomerular filtration rate in sickle cell anemia and might best be avoided in older individuals with signs of incipient renal failure. Dialysis and renal transplantation are used in end-stage sickle cell nephropathy with outcomes less favorable than in other types of renal failure.[388] If drugs such as hydroxyurea that increase HbF concentration can be used successfully in young children, presumably the glomerulopathy of sickle cell disease can be forestalled or prevented. Medullary disease precedes glomerular damage so that drug therapy will need to be started earlier in life to prevent this type of damage; however, these lesions are not as critical as glomerulopathy.

Concordant with the rise in creatinine, PCV begins to fall and, not infrequently, symptoms of severe anemia and congestive heart failure appear and dominate the clinical picture. In sickle cell anemia, erythropoietin levels are lower than predicted and the judicious use of erythropoietin can return hemoglobin to the prerenal failure baseline.[389] If this approach is chosen, care should be taken not to increase the PCV beyond the level present prior to the onset of renal disease because this might have the potential of promoting vasoocclusive episodes. Larger than customary doses of erythropoietin might be needed.

Hemodialysis can be an effective in end-stage renal failure in sickle cell disease. Renal transplantation has also been advocated. In the most comprehensive examination of the results of renal transplantation in sickle cell disease, the incidence of acute rejection, mean serum creatinine after surgery, and 1-year graft survival in 82 patients with end-stage sickle cell nephropathy who underwent renal transplantation after an average dialysis period of 41 months was similar to age-matched African American controls. The 3-year cadaveric graft survival of 61% was poorer than that of controls (86%). Patient survival at 1 and 3 years posttransplantation was also worse in the sickle cell disease. Compared with patients treated with dialysis and wait-listed for transplantation, there was a trend toward improved survival.[390] This report, in which the results differ from earlier smaller studies which concluded that renal transplantation in sickle cell anemia had poor

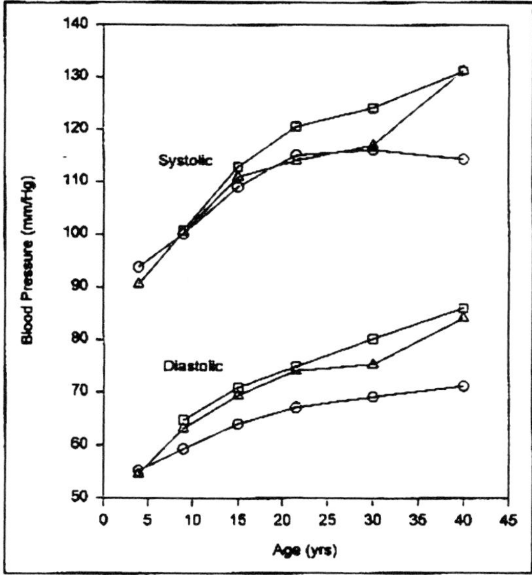

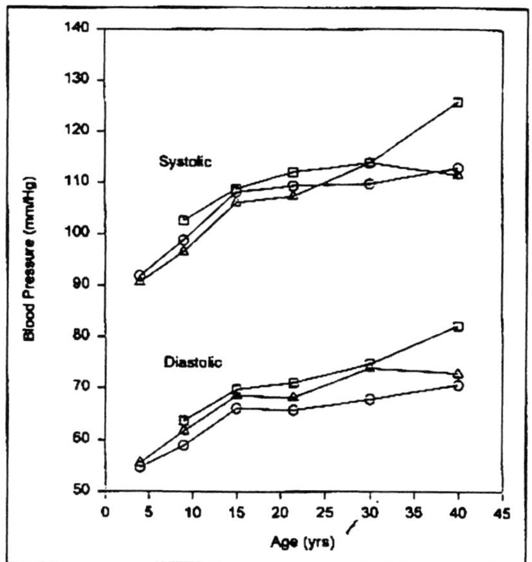

Figure 19.10. Systolic and diastolic blood pressure in male (left panel) and female (right panel) patients with sickle cell anemia (○) and HbSC disease (ˉ) and in African American participants in the NHANES II study (□). In most age categories, both men and women with sickle cell anemia had lower systolic and diastolic blood pressure than NHANES II controls and individuals with HbSC disease.[87]

results, suggests that the outcome of renal transplantation in sickle cell anemia can be at least as good as dialysis and should be seriously considered for individuals with end-stage renal failure.

ACE inhibitors and receptor antagonists that can decrease glomerular pressure by dilating the efferent arterioles can reduce the proteinuria of sickle cell anemia and are being studied as treatment for sickle nephropathy.[378,380,391,392] In a randomized double-blind study of 22 patients, after 6 months treatment, 25 mg/day of captopril caused a 37% reduction in microalbuminuria compared with a 17% increase in placebo-treated patients. A small but significant reduction in diastolic blood pressure was seen in captopril-treated patients. At present, no controlled clinical trial has examined the efficacy of these drugs in sickle nephropathy.

In a pilot trial, effects of angiotensin blockade with losartan were studied in 15 patients with biopsy-proven sickle cell glomerulopathy and macroalbuminuria. Losartan, at a dose of 50–100 mg given for 4–8 weeks, reduced proteinuria in all individuals by an average 40% and did not reduce glomerular filtration rate or blood pressure; hyperkalemia, requiring diuretics or weekly oral kayexalate, occurred in three patients.[393]

Blood Pressure and Hypertension

Patients with anemia have lower than expected blood pressure and individuals with sickle cell anemia are no exception. This could be due to renal sodium wasting; however, its cause is not known for certain.[87] Compared with individuals with β thalassemia who had similar hemoglobin concentrations, the blood pressure of patients with sickle cell anemia was higher than expected, suggesting the possibility that they had "relative" hypertension.[304] In this study of 89 patients, there was an association between higher blood pressures and stroke. Figure 19.10 shows blood pressure as a function of age in more than 2,500 African Americans with sickle cell anemia and 800 with HbSC disease.[87] Compared with controls, individuals with sickle cell anemia had significantly lower systolic and diastolic blood pressures. Survival decreased and the risk of stroke increased as blood pressure rose (Fig. 19.11), even though the blood pressure at which these risks increased was below the level defining early hypertension in the normal population. This suggests that "relative" hypertension was pathogenetically important. "Relative" hypertension in sickle cell anemia might reflect impaired NO bioactivity due to intravascular hemolysis. Higher systemic blood pressure is associated with sickle cell pulmonary hypertension and renal dysfunction.[19,268] Systolic blood pressure was also a component of a network model predicting survival.[44]

Treatment recommendations. Although blood pressure is a major contributor to mortality, there are no trials in patients with sickle cell anemia that can guide the decision of when to begin antihypertensive treatment, what agents are most effective, what the blood pressure goals of treatment should be, and if blood pressure reduction can reduce the incidence of stroke or prolong life. A reasonable approach, based on experience in the general hypertensive population in which the risk of stroke begins well below

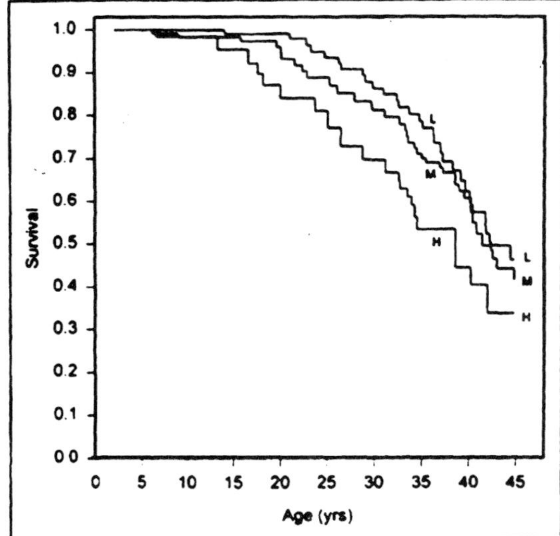

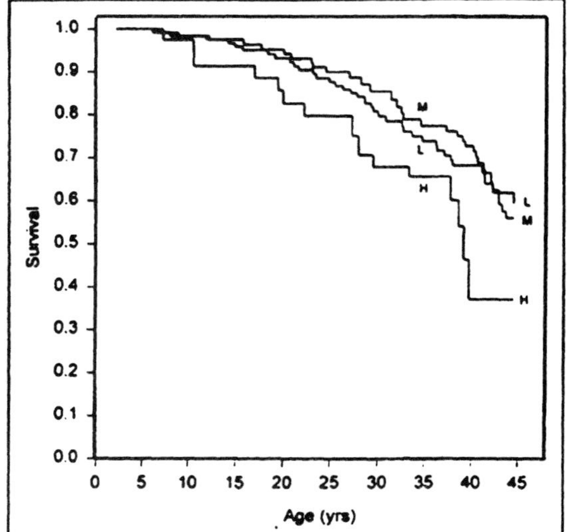

Figure 19.11. Survival of male (left panel) and female (right panel) patients with sickle cell anemia classified according to their diastolic blood pressures. High diastolic press (H) is the 90th percentile or above, medium diastolic blood pressure (M) in the 50th through 89th percentile, and low (L) diastolic pressure, below the 50th percentile. Mortality is increased for men ($p = 0.007$) and women whose diastolic blood pressure is above the 90th percentile but only the result in males is significant. Blood pressure in the 90th percentile of these sickle cell anemia patients overlaps with "normal" blood pressure.[87]

the "normal" blood pressure, is to make a careful evaluation of the patient and consider beginning antihypertensive treatment when systolic blood pressure is greater than 120/80 mm Hg or when there is evidence of target organ damage that includes heart disease, nephropathy, and peripheral vascular disease. Theoretically, diuretics, by causing hemoconcentration, might predispose to vasoocclusion. In practice, it is not clear if this occurs, and their use is not contraindicated. β-Adrenergic receptor blocking agents can also be used. Renin-dependent hypertension can result from focal area of renal ischemia. Severe blood pressure increases in sickle cell anemia should be evaluated thoroughly to exclude this and other forms of secondary hypertension.

Mortality

In the United States, median ages of death for males and females are were 42 and 48 years, respectively, when reported in 1994. These data do not reflect many children who now survive because of prophylactic penicillin and other treatment innovations.[371] In Jamaica, where over 3,000 patients with sickle cell anemia were followed, Kaplan–Meier survival curves estimated a life expectancy of 58 years for men and 66 years for women, a reduction of 14 and 10 years, respectively, compared with all Jamaicans.[394]

In a study of 232 deaths in more than 1,000 patients, the leading primary causes of death were chronic lung disease (including pulmonary hypertension) in 20%, renal disease in 14%, cerebrovascular disease in 10%, sepsis in 8%, and acute chest syndrome in 5%.[207] Left ventricular diastolic dysfunction and pulmonary hypertension are independent risk factors for mortality. Diastolic dysfunction alone is associated with a risk ratio of 3.5, whereas combined with increased TRJ velocity the risk ratio increases to 12%.[363]

In the CSCCD, acute chest syndrome was the leading specific cause of death in the patients aged 20 years or older.[371] There were 32 deaths in 1,741 acute chest syndrome events in 949 patients for an overall death rate of 1.8%.[395] Fourteen of the deaths were in patients younger than 20 years for a death rate of 1.1%, whereas the death rate in adults was 4.3%. Patients with sickle cell anemia and HbSC disease had similar rates of death from acute chest syndrome (1.9% and 1.6%). Pulmonary embolism, with or without fat embolism, pneumococcal sepsis, extremity pain episode, and respiratory failure within 48 hours of admission were all common in those who died. Preliminary studies suggest that prolongation of the QTc interval is common in sickle cell disease, associated with death, and that QTc prolongation is related to elevated serum ferritin levels.[396]

For comparison, in a study of 306 autopsies of sickle cell disease patients, the most common cause of death was infection (33%–48%) associated with respiratory tract syndromes in 72.6% and gastroenteritis in 13.7%. Other causes of death included stroke (9.8%), therapy-related complications (7.0%), splenic sequestration (6.6%), pulmonary thromboembolism (4.9%), renal failure (4.1%), pulmonary hypertension (2.9%), hepatic failure (0.8%), hemolysis/red cell aplasia (0.4%), and left ventricular failure (0.4%). Consistent with clinical observations, approximately 40% of deaths were sudden and unexpected and usually associated with acute events.[120] The discrepancy among these results is likely to result from the respective difficulties of assigning causes of death by autopsy and by clinical impressions and the very selective nature of the autopsy-based sample.

Bayesian network modeling, discussed previously, identified laboratory markers of the severity of hemolytic anemia and its associated clinical events as contributing risk factors for mortality.[44]

GENERAL MEASURES OF TREATMENT

Most general measures to preserve good health have been discussed earlier. Sickle cell disease is a chronic disorder, and attention should be paid to good nutrition, immunizations, and avoidance of extremes of temperature and activity. Work should be encouraged, but for most individuals it is best to avoid overly strenuous occupations.

Oxygen

Oxygen is considered by many to be a mainstay of treatment; however, there have been few studies of the value of oxygen in normoxic patients with sickle cell anemia. Inhaled oxygen did reduce the numbers of reversible sickled cells but not ISCs, when given to children with acute painful episodes and had no effects on the intensity and duration of pain.[397] When hypoxia or oxygen desaturation accompanies surgery, acute chest syndrome, or occurs nocturnally,[398] oxygen treatment can reverse the abnormality. There is no evidence that high concentrations of inhaled oxygen can curtail or prevent deoxyHbS polymerization. Moreover, inhaled oxygen can have adverse effects in sickle cell anemia as discussed previously. Although hyperbaric oxygen has been used for treatment of pain, ocular disease, and leg ulceration, controlled studies of its effectiveness have not been conducted.

CONCLUSIONS

Until cures of disease by stem cell transplantation or gene therapy become feasible and widely applicable, drug treatment will remain of paramount importance. Using a single agent to prevent or reverse disease pathophysiology seems an unlikely prospect. This suggests that combinations of agents that increase HbF and decrease hemolysis might be more effective than any single agent. Trials of combined treatments might include one or more HbF-inducing agents. To this could be added agents that target facets of pathophysiology other than HbS polymerization. One can imagine clinical trials that combine agents that increase NO bioavailability, reduce intercellular interactions, reduce hemolytic anemia, and are antiinflammatory, used along with one or more HbF-inducing drug. The pathophysiology of disease argues that treatment should be started as early as safely possible to avoid chronic irreversible organ damage.[34]

Current treatments for the complications of sickle cell anemia are rarely guided by the results of controlled clinical trials. Better understanding of the use of mainstay treatments, such as transfusion and opioids, coupled with the advent of new treatments have likely improved and prolonged life. Discussed elsewhere in this volume are blood transfusion (Chapter 29), hydroxyurea (Chapter 30), stem cell transplantation (Chapter 32), and various experimental therapies (Chapter 31), including gene therapy (Chapter 33).

REFERENCES

1. Ranney HM. Historical Milestones. In: Embury SH, Hebbel RP, Mohandas N, Steinberg MH, eds. *Sickle Cell Disease: Basic Principles and Clinical Practice.* 1st ed. New York: Lippincott-Raven; 1994:1–5.
2. Pauling L. Foreword. In: Embury SH, Hebbel RP, Mohandas N, Steinberg MH, eds. *Sickle Cell Disease: Basic Principles and Clinical Practice.* 1st ed. New York: Lippincott-Raven; 1994: xvii–xix.
3. Conley CL. Sickle-cell anemia-the first molecular disease. In: Wintrobe M, ed. *Blood, Pure and Eloquent.* 1st ed. New York: McGraw-Hill; 1980:319–371.
4. Herrick JB. Peculiar elongated and sickle-shaped red blood corpuscles in a case of severe anemia. *Arch Intern Med.* 1910;6:517–521.
5. Savitt TL, Goldberg MF. Herrick's 1910 case report of sickle cell anemia: the rest of the story. *JAMA.* 1989;261:266–271.
6. Pauling L, Itano H, Singer SJ, Wells IC. Sickle cell anemia: a molecular disease. *Science.* 1949;110:543–548.
7. Beet EA. The genetics of sickle cell trait in a Bantu tribe. *Ann Eugen.* 1949;14:279–284.
8. Neel JV. The inheritance of the sickling phenomenon with particular reference to sickle cell disease. *Blood.* 1951;6:389–412.
9. Ingram VM. A specific chemical difference between the globins of normal human and sickle-cell anaemia haemoglobin. *Nature.* 1956;178:792–794.
10. Frempong KO, Steinberg MH. Clinical aspects of sickle cell anemia in adults and children. In: Steinberg MH, Forget BG, Higgs DR, Nagel RL, eds. *Disorders of Hemoglobin: Genetics, Pathophysiology, and Clinical Management.* 1st ed. Cambridge: Cambridge University Press; 2001:611–710.
11. Motulsky AG. Frequency of sickling disorders in US blacks. *N Engl J Med.* 1973;288:31–33.
12. Ballas SK, Smith ED. Red blood cell changes during the evolution of the sickle cell painful crisis. *Blood.* 1992;79:2154–2163.
13. West MS, Wethers D, Smith J, Steinberg MH, Coop Study of Sickle Cell Disease. Laboratory profile of sickle cell disease: a cross-sectional analysis. *J Clin Epidemiol.* 1992;45:893–909.
14. Hayes RJ, Beckford M, Grandison Y, Mason K, Serjeant BE, Serjeant GR. The haematology of steady state homozygous sickle cell disease: frequency distributions variation with age and sex, longitudinal observations. *Br J Haematol.* 1985;59:369–382.
15. Kato GJ, McGowan V, Machado RF, et al. Lactate dehydrogenase as a biomarker of hemolysis-associated nitric oxide resistance, priapism, leg ulceration, pulmonary

hypertension, and death in patients with sickle cell disease. *Blood.* 2006;107(6):2279–2285.

16. De Ceulaer K, Serjeant GR. Acute splenic sequestration in Jamaican adults with homozygous sickle cell disease: a role of alpha thalassaemia. *Br J Haematol.* 1991;77:563–564.
17. Reiter CD, Wang X, Tanus-Santos JE, et al. Cell-free hemoglobin limits nitric oxide bioavailability in sickle-cell disease. *Nat Med.* 2002;8(12):1383–1389.
18. Kato GJ, Gladwin MT, Steinberg MH. Deconstructing sickle cell disease: Reappraisal of the role of hemolysis in the development of clinical subphenotypes. *Blood.* Rev 2007;21:37–47.
19. Gladwin MT, Sachdev V, Jison ML, et al. Pulmonary hypertension as a risk factor for death in patients with sickle cell disease. *N Engl J Med.* 2004;350(9):886–895.
20. Nolan VG, Wyszynski DF, Farrer LA, Steinberg MH. Hemolysis-associated priapism in sickle cell disease. *Blood.* 2005;106(9):3264–3267.
21. Nolan VG, Adewoye A, Baldwin C, et al. Sickle cell leg ulcers: associations with haemolysis and SNPs in Klotho, TEK and genes of the TGF-beta/BMP pathway. *Br J Haematol.* 2006;133(5):570–578.
22. Ohene-Frempong K, Weiner SJ, Sleeper LA, et al. Cerebrovascular accidents in sickle cell disease: rates and risk factors. *Blood.* 1998;91(1):288–294.
23. Adams RJ, Kutlar A, McKie V, et al. Alpha thalassemia and stroke risk in sickle cell anemia. *Am J Hematol.* 1994;45(4): 279–282.
24. Hsu LL, Miller ST, Wright E, et al. Alpha Thalassemia is associated with decreased risk of abnormal TCD ultrasonography in children with sickle cell anemia. *J Pediatr Hematol Oncol.* 2003;25(8):622–628.
25. Lezcano NE, Odo N, Kutlar A, Brambilla D, Adams RJ. Regular transfusion lowers plasma free hemoglobin in children with sickle-cell disease at risk for stroke. *Stroke.* 2006;37(6):1424–1426.
26. Kato GJ, Hsieh M, Machado R, et al. Cerebrovascular disease associated with sickle cell pulmonary hypertension. *Am J Hematol.* 2006;81(7):503–510.
27. Taylor JG, Nolan VG, Kato GJ, Gladwin MT, Steinberg MH. The hyperhemolysis phenotype in sickle cell anemia: increased risk of leg ulcers, priapism, pulmonary hypertension and death with decreased risk of vasoocclusive events. *Blood.* 2006;108:236a.
28. Platt OS, Thorington BD, Brambilla DJ, et al. Pain in sickle cell disease-rates and risk factors. *N Engl J Med.* 1991;325:11–16.
29. Machado RF, Kyle MA, Martyr S, et al. Severity of pulmonary hypertension during vaso-occlusive pain crisis and exercise in patients with sickle cell disease. *Br J Haematol.* 2007;136(2):319–325.
30. Burnett AL, Bivalacqua TJ, Champion HC, Musicki B. Long-term oral phosphodiesterase 5 inhibitor therapy alleviates recurrent priapism. *Urology.* 2006;67(5):1043–1048.
31. Morris CR, Morris SM Jr, Hagar W, et al. Arginine therapy: a new treatment for pulmonary hypertension in sickle cell disease? *Am J Respir Crit Care Med.* 2003;168(1):63–69.
32. Charache S, Terrin ML, Moore RD, et al. Effect of hydroxyurea on the frequency of painful crises in sickle cell anemia. *N Engl J Med.* 1995;332:1317–1322.
33. Steinberg MH, Barton F, Castro O, et al. Effect of hydroxyurea on mortality and morbidity in adult sickle cell anemia: risks and benefits up to 9 years of treatment. *JAMA.* 2003;289(13):1645–1651.
34. Steinberg MH. Clinical trials in sickle cell disease: adopting the combination chemotherapy paradigm. *Am J Hematol.* 2008;83(1):1–3.
35. Stuart MJ, Setty BN. Hemostatic alterations in sickle cell disease: relationships to disease pathophysiology. *Pediatr Pathol Mol Med.* 2001;20(1):27–46.
36. Setty BN, Rao AK, Stuart MJ. Thrombophilia in sickle cell disease: the red cell connection. *Blood.* 2001;98(12):3228–3233.
37. Villagra J, Shiva S, Hunter LA, Machado RF, Gladwin MT, Kato GJ. Platelet activation in patients with sickle disease, hemolysis-associated pulmonary hypertension, and nitric oxide scavenging by cell-free hemoglobin. *Blood.* 2007; 110(6):2166–2172.
38. Gill FM, Sleeper LA, Weiner SJ, et al. Clinical events in the first decade in a cohort of infants with sickle cell disease. *Blood.* 1995;86:776–783.
39. Gaston M, Smith J, Gallagher D, et al. Recruitment in the Cooperative Study of Sickle Cell Disease (CSSCD). *Control Clin Trials.* 1987;8:131S–140S.
40. Gaston M, Rosse WF. The cooperative study of sickle cell disease: review of study design and objectives. *Am J Pediatr Hematol Oncol.* 1982;4:197–201.
41. Bainbridge R, Higgs DR, Maude GH, Serjeant GR. Clinical presentation of homozygous sickle cell disease. *J Pediatr.* 1985;106:881–885.
42. Miller ST, Sleeper LA, Pegelow CH, et al. Prediction of adverse outcomes in children with sickle cell disease. *N Engl J Med.* 2000;342(2):83–89.
43. Quinn CT, Lee NJ, Shull EP, Ahmad N, Rogers ZR, Buchanan GR. Prediction of adverse outcomes in children with sickle cell anemia: a study of the Dallas Newborn Cohort. *Blood.* 2008;111(2):544–548.
44. Sebastiani P, Nolan VG, Baldwin CT, et al. Predicting severity of sickle cell disease. *Blood.* 2007;110:2727–2735.
45. Brown AK, Sleeper LA, Pegelow CH, et al. The influence of infant and maternal sickle cell disease on birth outcome and neonatal course. *Am J Dis Child.* 1994;148:1156–1162.
46. Brown AK, Sleeper LA, Miller ST, Pegelow CH, Gill FM, Waclawiw MA. Reference values and hematologic changes from birth to 5 years in patients with sickle cell disease. *Am J Dis Child.* 1994;148:796–804.
47. Hankins JS, Helton KJ, McCarville MB, Li CS, Wang WC, Ware RE. Preservation of spleen and brain function in children with sickle cell anemia treated with hydroxyurea. *Pediatr Blood Cancer.* 2007;50:293–297.
48. Platt OS, Rosenstock W, Espeland M. Influence of S hemoglobinopathies on growth and development. *N Engl J Med.* 1984;311:7–12.
49. Singhal A, Thomas P, Cook R, Wierenga K, Serjeant G. Delayed adolescent growth in homozygous sickle cell disease. *Arch Dis Child.* 1994;71:404–408.
50. Caruso-Nicoletti M, Mancuso M, Spadaro G, Samperi P, Consalvo C, Schiliro G. Growth and development in white patients with sickle cell diseases. *Am J Pediatr Hematol Oncol.* 1992;14(4):285–288.
51. Modebe O, Ifenu SA. Growth retardation in homozygous sickle cell disease: role of calorie intake and possible gender-related differences. *Am J Hematol.* 1993;44(3):149–154.

52. Zemel BS, Kawchak DA, Ohene-Frempong K, Schall JI, Stallings VA. Effects of delayed pubertal development, nutritional status, and disease severity on longitudinal patterns of growth failure in children with sickle cell disease. *Pediatr Res.* 2007;61(5 Pt 1):607–613.
53. Soliman AT, El Banna N, AlSalmi I, De Silva V, Craig A, Asfour M. Growth hormone secretion and circulating insulin-like growth factor-I (IGF-I) and IGF binding protein-3 concentrations in children with sickle cell disease. *Metabolism.* 1997;46(11):1241–1245.
54. Nunlee-Bland G, Rana SR, Houston-Yu PE, Odonkor W. Growth hormone deficiency in patients with sickle cell disease and growth failure. *J Pediatr Endocrinol Metab.* 2004;17(4):601–606.
55. Badaloo A, Jackson AA, Jahoor F. Whole body protein turnover and resting metabolic rate in homozygous sickle cell disease. *Clin Sci (Lond).* 1989;77(1):93–97.
56. Singhal A, Davies P, Sahota A, Thomas PW, Serjeant GR. Resting metabolic rate in homozygous sickle cell disease. *Am J Clin Nutr.* 1993;57:32–34.
57. Singhal A, Davies P, Wierenga KJ, Thomas P, Serjeant G. Is there an energy deficiency in homozygous sickle cell disease? *Am J Clin Nutr.* 1997;66(2):386–390.
58. Kopp-Hoolihan LE, van L, Mentzer WC, Heyman MB. Elevated resting energy expenditure in adolescents with sickle cell anemia. *J Am Diet Assoc.* 1999;99(2):195–199.
59. Borel MJ, Buchowski MS, Turner EA, Peeler BB, Goldstein RE, Flakoll PJ. Alterations in basal nutrient metabolism increase resting energy expenditure in sickle cell disease. *Am J Physiol Endocrinol Metab.* 1998;274(2):E357–E364.
60. Salman EK, Haymond MW, Bayne E, et al. Protein and energy metabolism in prepubertal children with sickle cell anemia. *Pediatr Res.* 1996;40:34–40.
61. Williams R, Olivi S, Li CS, et al. Oral glutamine supplementation decreases resting energy expenditure in children and adolescents with sickle cell anemia. *J Pediatr Hematol Oncol.* 2004;26(10):619–625.
62. Kawchak DA, Schall JI, Zemel BS, Ohene-Frempong K, Stallings VA. Adequacy of dietary intake declines with age in children with sickle cell disease. *J Am Diet Assoc.* 2007;107(5): 843–848.
63. Jacob E, Miaskowski C, Savedra M, Beyer JE, Treadwell M, Styles L. Changes in sleep, food intake, and activity levels during acute painful episodes in children with sickle cell disease. *J Pediatr Nurs.* 2006;21(1):23–34.
64. Leonard MB, Zemel BS, Kawchak DA, Ohene-Frempong K, Stallings VA. Plasma zinc status, growth, and maturation in children with sickle cell disease. *J Pediatr.* 1998;132(3 Pt 1): 467–471.
65. Gupta VL, Chaubey BS. Efficacy of zinc therapy in prevention of crisis in sickle cell anemia: a double blind randomized controlled clinical trial. *J Assoc Physicians India.* 1995;43:467–469.
66. Prasad AS, Beck FWJ, Kaplan J, et al. Effect of zinc supplementation on incidence of infections and hospital admissions in sickle cell disease (SCD). *Am J Hematol.* 1999;61(3):194–202.
67. Schall JI, Zemel BS, Kawchak DA, Ohene-Frempong K, Stallings VA. Vitamin A status, hospitalizations, and other outcomes in young children with sickle cell disease. *J Pediatr.* 2004;145(1):99–106.
68. Buison AM, Kawchak DA, Schall J, Ohene-Frempong K, Stallings VA, Zemel BS. Low vitamin D status in children with sickle cell disease. *J Pediatr.* 2004;145(5):622–627.
69. Rodriguez-Cortes HM, Griener JC, Hyland K, et al. Plasma homocysteine levels and folate status in children with sickle cell anemia. *J Pediatr Hematol Oncol.* 1999;21(3):219–223.
70. Wang WC. The pathophysiology, prevention, and treatment of stroke in sickle cell disease. *Curr Opin Hematol.* 2007;14(3):191–197.
71. Wang WC. Central nervous system complications of sickle cell disease in children: an overview. *Child Neuropsychol.* 2007;13(2):103–119.
72. Platt OS. Prevention and management of stroke in sickle cell anemia. *Hematology Am Soc Hematol Educ Program.* 2006;54–57.
73. DeBaun MR, Derdeyn CP, McKinstry RC, III. Etiology of strokes in children with sickle cell anemia. *Ment Retard Dev Disabil Res Rev.* 2006;12(3):192–199.
74. Adams R, McKie V, Nichols F, et al. The use of transcranial ultrasonography to predict stroke in sickle cell disease. *N Engl J Med.* 1992;326:605–610.
75. Adams RJ. Neurologic complications. In: Embury SH, Hebbel RP, Mohandas N, Steinberg MH, eds. *Sickle Cell Disease: Basic Principles and Clinical Practice.* 1 ed. New York: Raven Press; 1994:599–621.
76. Milbauer LC, Wei P, Enenstein J, et al. Genetic endothelial systems biology of sickle stroke risk. *Blood.* 2008:111:3872–3879.
77. Wang WC, Langston JW, Steen RG, et al. Abnormalities of the central nervous system in very young children with sickle cell anemia. *J Pediatr.* 1998;132(6):994–998.
78. Scothorn DJ, Price C, Schwartz D, et al. Risk of recurrent stroke in children with sickle cell disease receiving blood transfusion therapy for at least five years after initial stroke. *J Pediatr.* 2002;140(3):348–354.
79. Dobson SR, Holden KR, Nietert PJ, et al. Moyamoya syndrome in childhood sickle cell disease: a predictive factor for recurrent cerebrovascular events. *Blood.* 2002;99(9):3144–3150.
80. Balkaran B, Char G, Morris JS, Thomas PW, Serjeant BE, Serjeant GR. Stroke in a cohort of patients with homozygous sickle cell disease. *J Pediatr.* 1992;120:360–366.
81. Strouse JJ, Hulbert ML, DeBaun MR, Jordan LC, Casella JF. Primary hemorrhagic stroke in children with sickle cell disease is associated with recent transfusion and use of corticosteroids. *Pediatrics.* 2006;118(5):1916–1924.
82. Kirkham FJ, Hewes DKM, Prengler M, Wade A, Lane R, Evans JPM. Nocturnal hypoxaemia and central-nervous-system events in sickle-cell disease. *Lancet.* 2001;357(9269):1656–1659.
83. Powars D, Wilson B, Imbus C, et al. The natural history of stroke in sickle cell disease. *Am J Med.* 1978;65:461–470.
84. Francis RB, Jr., Hebbel RP. *Hemostasis.* In: Embury SH, Hebbel RP, Mohandas N, Steinberg MH, eds. *Sickle Cell Disease: Basic Principles and Clinical Practice.* 1st ed. New York: Lippincott-Raven; 1994:299–310.
85. Houston PE, Rana S, Sekhsaria S, Perlin E, Kim KS, Castro OL. Homocysteine in sickle cell disease: relationship to stroke. *Am J Med.* 1997;103(3):192–196.

86. Van Der Dijs FPL, Schnog JJB, Brouwer DAJ, et al. Elevated homocysteine levels indicate suboptimal folate status in pediatric sickle cell patients. *Am J Hematol.* 1998;59(3):192–198.
87. Pegelow CH, Colangelo L, Steinberg M, et al. Natural history of blood pressure in sickle cell disease: risks for stroke and death associated with relative hypertension in sickle cell anemia. *Am J Med.* 1997;102:171–177.
88. Bernaudin F, Verlhac S, Coic L, et al. High LDH level, G6PD deficiency and absence of alpha-thalassemia are significant independent risk factors of abnormally high cerebral velocities in patients with sickle cell anemia. *Blood.* 2008;112: 4314–4317.
89. O'Driscoll S, Height SE, Dick MC, Rees DC. Serum lactate dehydrogenase activity as a biomarker in children with sickle cell disease. *Br J Haematol.* 2008:140(2):206–209.
90. Powars DR, Conti PS, Wong WY, et al. Cerebral vasculopathy in sickle cell anemia: diagnostic contribution of positron emission tomography. *Blood.* 1999;93(1):71–79.
91. Reed W, Jagust W, Al Mateen M, Vichinsky E. Role of positron emission tomography in determining the extent of CNS ischemia in patients with sickle cell disease. *Am J Hematol.* 1999;60(4):268–272.
92. Ohene-Frempong K. Stroke in sickle cell disease: demographic, clinical, and therapeutic considerations. *Semin Hematol.* 1991;28(3):213–219.
93. Berkelhammer LD, Williamson AL, Sanford SD, et al. Neurocognitive sequelae of pediatric sickle cell disease: a review of the literature. *Child Neuropsychol.* 2007;13(2):120–131.
94. Tarazi RA, Grant ML, Ely E, Barakat LP. Neuropsychological functioning in preschool-age children with sickle cell disease: the role of illness-related and psychosocial factors. *Child Neuropsychol.* 2007;13(2):155–172.
95. Switzer JA, Hess DC, Nichols FT, Adams RJ. Pathophysiology and treatment of stroke in sickle-cell disease: present and future. *Lancet Neurol.* 2006;5(6):501–512.
96. Hulbert ML, Scothorn DJ, Panepinto JA, et al. Exchange blood transfusion compared with simple transfusion for first overt stroke is associated with a lower risk of subsequent stroke: a retrospective cohort study of 137 children with sickle cell anemia. *J Pediatr.* 2006;149(5):710–712.
97. Pegelow CH, Adams RJ, McKie V, et al. Risk of recurrent stroke in patients with sickle cell disease treated with erythrocyte transfusions. *J Pediatr.* 1995;126:896–899.
98. Cohen AR, Martin MB, Silber JH, Kim HC, Ohene-Frempong K, Schwartz E. A modified transfusion program for prevention of stroke in sickle cell disease. *Blood.* 1992;79:1657–1661.
99. Singer ST, Quirolo K, Nishi K, Hackney-Stephens E, Evans C, Vichinsky EP. Erythrocytapheresis for chronically transfused children with sickle cell disease: an effective method for maintaining a low hemoglobin S level and reducing iron overload. *J Clin Apher.* 1999;14(3):122–125.
100. Fryer RH, Anderson RC, Chiriboga CA, Feldstein NA. Sickle cell anemia with moyamoya disease: outcomes after EDAS procedure. *Pediatr Neurol.* 2003;29(2):124–130.
101. Ware RE, Zimmerman SA, Sylvestre PB, et al. Prevention of secondary stroke and resolution of transfusional iron overload in children with sickle cell anemia using hydroxyurea and phlebotomy. *J Pediatr.* 2004;145(3):346–352.
102. Adams RJ. Stroke prevention and treatment in sickle cell disease. *Arch Neurol.* 2001;58(4):565–568.
103. Adams RJ, McKie VC, Brambilla D, et al. Stroke prevention trial in sickle cell anemia. *Control Clin Trials.* 1998;19(1):110–129.
104. Adams RJ, McKie VC, Hsu L, et al. Prevention of a first stroke by transfusions in children with sickle cell anemia and abnormal results on transcranial Doppler ultrasonography [see comments]. *N Engl J Med.* 1998;339(1):5–11.
105. Sebastiani P, Ramoni MF, Nolan V, Baldwin CT, Steinberg MH. Genetic dissection and prognostic modeling of overt stroke in sickle cell anemia. *Nat Genet.* 2005;37(4):435–440.
106. Adams RJ, Brambilla D. Discontinuing prophylactic transfusions used to prevent stroke in sickle cell disease. *N Engl J Med.* 2005;353(26):2769–2778.
107. Zimmerman SA, Schultz WH, Burgett S, Mortier NA, Ware RE. Hydroxyurea therapy lowers transcranial Doppler flow velocities in children with sickle cell anemia. *Blood.* 2007;110:1043–1047.
108. Gulbis B, Haberman D, Dufour D, et al. Hydroxyurea for sickle cell disease in children and for prevention of cerebrovascular events: the Belgian experience. *Blood.* 2005;105(7): 2685–2690.
109. Kratovil T, Bulas D, Driscoll MC, Speller-Brown B, McCarter R, Minniti CP. Hydroxyurea therapy lowers TCD velocities in children with sickle cell disease. *Pediatr Blood Cancer.* 2006;47(7):894–900.
110. Kinney TR, Sleeper LA, Wang WC, et al. Silent cerebral infarcts in sickle cell anemia: a risk factor analysis. *Pediatrics.* 1999;103(3):640–645.
111. Armstrong FD, Thompson RJ Jr, Wang W, et al. Cognitive functioning and brain magnetic resonance imaging in children with sickle cell disease. *Pediatrics.* 1996;97:864–870.
112. Shields RW Jr, Harris JW, Clark M. Mononeuropathy in sickle cell anemia: anatomical and pathophysiological basis for its rarity. *Muscle Nerve.* 1991;14:370–374.
113. Imbus CE, Warner J, Smith E, Pegelow CH, Allen JP, Powars DR. Peripheral neuropathy in lead-intoxicated sickle cell patients. *Muscle Nerve.* 1978;1:168–171.
114. Donegan JO, Lobel JS, Gluckman JL. Otolaryngologic manifestations of sickle cell disease. *J Otolaryngol.* 1982;3:141–144.
115. Curran EL, Fleming JC, Rice K, Wang WC. Orbital compression syndrome in sickle cell disease. *Ophthalmology.* 1997;104(10):1610–1615.
116. Koduri PR. Acute splenic sequestration crisis in adults with sickle cell anemia. *Am J Hematol.* 2007;82(2):174–175.
117. Neonato MG, Guilloud-Bataille M, Beauvais P, et al. Acute clinical events in 299 homozygous sickle cell patients living in France. French Study Group on Sickle Cell Disease. *Eur J Haematol.* 2000;65(3):155–164.
118. Tarer V, Etienne-Julan M, Diara JP, et al. Sickle cell anemia in Guadeloupean children: pattern and prevalence of acute clinical events. *Eur J Haematol.* 2006;76(3):193–199.
119. Wright JG, Hambleton IR, Thomas PW, Duncan ND, Venugopal S, Serjeant GR. Postsplenectomy course in homozygous sickle cell disease. *J Pediatr.* 1999;134(3):304–309.
120. Manci EA, Culberson DE, Yang YM, et al. Causes of death in sickle cell disease: an autopsy study. *Br J Haematol.* 2003;123(2):359–365.

121. Chopra R, Al-Mulhim AR, Al-Baharani AT. Fibrocongestive splenomegaly in sickle cell disease: a distinct clinicopathological entity in the Eastern province of Saudi Arabia. *Am J Hematol.* 2005;79(3):180–186.
122. Al-Salem AH. Indications and complications of splenectomy for children with sickle cell disease. *J Pediatr Surg.* 2006;41(11):1909–1915.
123. Zimmerman SA, Davis JS, Schultz WH, Ware RE. Subclinical parvovirus B19 infection in children with sickle cell anemia. *J Pediatr Hematol Oncol.* 2003;25(5):387–389.
124. Krishnamurti L, Lanford L, Munoz R. Life threatening parvovirus B19 and herpes simplex virus associated acute myocardial dysfunction in a child with homozygous sickle cell disease. *Pediatr Blood Cancer.* 2007;49:1019–1021.
125. Bakhshi S, Sarnaik SA, Becker C, Shurney WW, Nigro M, Savasan S. Acute encephalopathy with parvovirus B19 infection in sickle cell disease. *Arch Dis Child.* 2002;87(6):541–542.
126. Wierenga KJ, Serjeant BE, Serjeant GR. Cerebrovascular complications and parvovirus infection in homozygous sickle cell disease. *J Pediatr.* 2001;139(3):438–442.
127. Smith-Whitley K, Zhao H, Hodinka RL, et al. Epidemiology of human parvovirus B19 in children with sickle cell disease. *Blood.* 2004;103(2):422–427.
128. Serjeant BE, Hambleton IR, Kerr S, Kilty CG, Serjeant GR. Haematological response to parvovirus B19 infection in homozygous sickle-cell disease. *Lancet.* 2001;358(9295):1779–1780.
129. Lane PK, Embury SH, Toy PT. Oxygen-induced marrow red cell hypoplasia leading to transfusion in sickle painful crisis. *Am J Hematol.* 1988;27:67–68.
130. Embury SH, Garcia JF, Mohandas N, Pennathur-Das R, Clark MR. Effects of oxygen inhalation on endogenous erythropoietin kinetics erythropoiesis and properties of blood cells in sickle cell anemia. *N Engl J Med.* 1984;311:291–295.
131. Sherwood JB, Goldwasser E, Chilcote R, Carmichael LD, Nagel RL. Sickle cell anemia patients have low erythropoietin levels for their degree of anemia. *Blood.* 1986;67:46–49.
132. Cazzola M, Guarnone R, Cerani P, Centenara E, Rovati A, Beguin Y. Red blood cell precursor mass as an independent determinant of serum erythropoietin level. *Blood.* 1998;91:2139–2145.
133. Little JA, McGowan VR, Kato GJ, et al. Combination erythropoietin-hydroxyurea therapy in sickle cell disease: experience from the National Institutes of Health and a literature review. *Haematologica.* 2006;91(8):1076–1083.
134. Mollapour E, Porter JB, Kaczmarski R, Linch DC, Roberts PJ. Raised neutrophil phospholipase A2 activity and defective priming of NADPH oxidase and phospholipase A2 in sickle cell disease. *Blood.* 1998;91(9):3423–3429.
135. Wright J, Thomas P, Serjeant GR. Septicemia caused by Salmonella infection: An overlooked complication of sickle cell disease. *J Pediatr.* 1997;130:394–399.
136. Magnus SA, Hambleton IR, Moosdeen F, Serjeant GR. Recurrent infections in homozygous sickle cell disease. *Arch Dis Child.* 1999;80(6):537–541.
137. Overturf GD. Infections and immunizations of children with sickle cell disease. *Adv Pediatr Infect Dis.* 1999;14:191–218.
138. Bagasra O, Steiner RM, Ballas SK, et al. Viral burden and disease progression in HIV-1-infected patients with sickle cell anemia. *Am J Hematol.* 1998;59(3):199–207.
139. Leikin SL, Gallagher D, Kinney TR, Sloane D, Klug P, Rida W. Mortality in children and adolescents with sickle cell disease. *Pediatrics.* 1989;84:500–508.
140. Gaston MH, Verter J, Woods G, et al. Prophylaxsis with oral penicillin in children with sickle cell anemia. *N Engl J Med.* 1986;314:1593–1599.
141. Halasa NB, Shankar SM, Talbot TR, et al. Incidence of invasive pneumococcal disease among individuals with sickle cell disease before and after the introduction of the pneumococcal conjugate vaccine. *Clin Infect Dis.* 2007;44(11):1428–1433.
142. Davies EG, Riddington C, Lottenberg R, Dower N. Pneumococcal vaccines for sickle cell disease. *Cochrane Database Syst Rev.* 2004;(1):CD003885.
143. Falletta JM, Woods GM, Verter JI, et al. Discontinuing penicillin prophylaxis in children with sickle cell anemia. *J Pediatr.* 1995;127:685–690.
144. Kyaw MH, Lynfield R, Schaffner W, et al. Effect of introduction of the pneumococcal conjugate vaccine on drug-resistant Streptococcus pneumoniae. *N Engl J Med.* 2006; 354(14):1455–1463.
145. Adamkiewicz TV, Sarnaik S, Buchanan GR, et al. Invasive pneumococcal infections in children with sickle cell disease in the era of penicillin prophylaxis, antibiotic resistance, and 23-valent pneumococcal polysaccharide vaccination. *J Pediatr.* 2003;143(4):438–444.
146. Hill PC, Onyeama CO, Ikumapayi UN, et al. Bacteraemia in patients admitted to an urban hospital in West Africa. *BMC Infect Dis.* 2007;7:2.
147. Hill PC, Akisanya A, Sankareh K, et al. Nasopharyngeal carriage of Streptococcus pneumoniae in Gambian villagers. *Clin Infect Dis.* 2006;43(6):673–679.
148. Levine OS, O'Brien KL, Knoll M, et al. Pneumococcal vaccination in developing countries. *Lancet.* 2006;367(9526):1880–1882.
149. Castro O, Brambilla DJ, Thorington B, et al. The acute chest syndrome in sickle cell disease: Incidence and risk factors. *Blood.* 1994;84:643–649.
150. Vichinsky EP, Neumayr LD, Earles AN, et al. Causes and outcomes of the acute chest syndrome in sickle cell disease. *N Engl J Med.* 2000;342(25):1855–1865.
151. Vichinsky E, Williams R, Das M, et al. Pulmonary fat embolism: a distinct cause of severe acute chest syndrome in sickle cell anemia. *Blood.* 1994;83:3107–3112.
152. Bellet PS, Kalinyak KA, Shukla R, Gelfand MJ, Rucknagel DL. Incentive spirometry to prevent acute pulmonary complications in sickle cell diseases. *N Engl J Med.* 1995;333:699–703.
153. Rackoff WR, Kunkel N, Silber JH, Asakura T, Ohene-Frempong K. Pulse oximetry and factors associated with hemoglobin oxygen desaturation in children with sickle cell disease. *Blood.* 1993;81:3422–3427.
154. Styles LA, Schalkwijk CG, Aarsman AJ, Vichinsky EP, Lubin BH, Kuypers FA. Phospholipase A2 levels in acute chest syndrome of sickle cell disease. *Blood.* 1996;87:2573–2578.
155. Styles LA, Aarsman AJ, Vichinsky EP, Kuypers FA. Secretory phospholipase A2 predicts impending acute chest syndrome in sickle cell disease. *Blood.* 2000;96(9):3276–3278.
156. Miller ST, Wright E, Abboud M, et al. Impact of chronic transfusion on incidence of pain and acute chest syndrome during the Stroke Prevention Trial (STOP) in sickle–cell anemia. *J Pediatr.* 2001;139(6):785–789.

157. Styles LA, Abboud M, Larkin S, Lo M, Kuypers FA. Transfusion prevents acute chest syndrome predicted by elevated secretory phospholipase A2. *Br J Haematol.* 2007;136(2):343–344.
158. Kuypers FA, Styles LA. The role of secretory phospholipase A2 in acute chest syndrome. *Cell Mol Biol.* 2004;50(1):87–94.
159. Naprawa JT, Bonsu BK, Goodman DG, Ranalli MA. Serum biomarkers for identifying acute chest syndrome among patients who have sickle cell disease and present to the emergency department. *Pediatrics.* 2005;116(3):e420–e425.
160. Dworkis DA, Nolan VG, McMahon L, Klings ES, Steinberg MH. Predicting acute chest syndrome in sickle cell disease patients hospitalized for acute vasoocclusive events. *Blood.* 2007.
161. Gladwin MT, Schechter AN, Shelhamer JH, Ognibene FP. The acute chest syndrome in sickle cell disease – Possible role of nitric oxide in its pathophysiology and treatment. *Am J Respir Crit Care Med.* 1999;159(5):1368–1376.
162. Kinney TR, Ware RE. The adolescent with sickle cell anemia. *Hematol Oncol Clin North Am.* 1996;10:1255–1264.
163. Kell RS, Kliewer W, Erickson MT, Ohene-Frempong K. Psychological adjustment of adolescents with sickle cell disease: relations with demographic, medical, and family competence variables. *J Pediatr Psychol.* 1998;23(5):301–312.
164. Treadwell MJ, Gil KM. *Psychosocial Aspects.* In: Embury SH, Hebbel RP, Mohandas N, Steinberg MH, eds. *Sickle Cell Disease: Basic Principles and Clinical Practice.* New York: Lippincott-Raven; 1994:517–530.
165. Adewoye AH, Steinberg MH. Hemoglobinopathies in pregnancy. In: Bick RL, Frenkel EP, Baker WF, Sarode R, eds. *Hematological Complications in Obstetrics, Pregnancy and Gynecology.* Cambridge: Cambridge University Press; 2006: 442–468.
166. Serjeant GR, Hambleton I, Thame M. Fecundity and pregnancy outcome in a cohort with sickle cell-haemoglobin C disease followed from birth. *Br J Obstet Gynaecol.* 2005;112(9):1308–1314.
167. Anyaegbunam A, Mikhail M, Axioitis C, Morel MI, Merkatz IR. Placental histology and placental/fetal weight ratios in pregnant women with sickle cell disease: relationship to pregnancy outcome. *J Assoc Acad Minor Phys.* 1994;5(3):123–125.
168. Decastel M, Leborgne-Samuel Y, Alexandre L, Merault G, Berchel C. Morphological features of the human umbilical vein in normal, sickle cell trait, and sickle cell disease pregnancies. *Hum Pathol.* 1999;30(1):13–20.
169. Granger JP, Alexander BT, Llinas MT, Bennett WA, Khalil RA. Pathophysiology of preeclampsia: linking placental ischemia/hypoxia with microvascular dysfunction. *Microcirculation.* 2002;9(3):147–160.
170. Sun PM, Wilburn W, Raynor BD, Jamieson D. Sickle cell disease in pregnancy: twenty years of experience at Grady Memorial Hospital, Atlanta, Georgia. *Am J Obstet Gynecol.* 2001;184(6):1127–1130.
171. Williams-Murphy M, Thorneycroft I, Little F, Hoff C. Pregnancy outcome in women with sickle-cell disease in Mobile Alabama. *J Invest Med.* 1999;47:123A.
172. Koshy M, Burd L. Obstetric and Gynecologic Issues. In: Embury SH, Hebbel RP, Mohandas N, Steinberg MH, eds. *Sickle Cell Disease: Basic Principles and Clinical Practice.* 1st ed. New York: Lippincott-Raven; 1994:689–702.
173. Smith JA, Espeland M, Bellevue R, Bonds D, Brown AK, Koshy M. Pregnancy in sickle cell disease: Experience of the cooperative study of sickle cell disease. *Obstet Gynecol.* 1996;87:199–204.
174. Serjeant GR, Loy LL, Crowther M, Hambleton IR, Thame M. Outcome of pregnancy in homozygous sickle cell disease. *Obstet Gynecol.* 2004;103(6):1278–1285.
175. Howard RJ, Tuck SM, Pearson TC. Pregnancy in sickle cell disease in the UK: results of a multicentre survey of the effect of prophylactic blood transfusion on maternal and fetal outcome. *Br J Obstet Gynaecol.* 1995;102:947–951.
176. Powars DR, Sandhu M, Nilland-Weiss J, Johnson C, Bruce S, Manning PR. Pregnancy in sickle cell disease. *Obstet Gynecol.* 1986;67:217–228.
177. Fairley CK, Smoleniec JS, Caul OE, Miller E. Observational study of effect of intrauterine transfusions on outcome of fetal hydrops after parvovirus B19 infection. *Lancet.* 1995;346(8986):1335–1337.
178. Selbing A, Josefsson A, Dahle LO, Lindgren R. Parvovirus B19 infection during pregnancy treated with high-dose intravenous gammaglobulin. *Lancet.* 1995;345(8950):660–661.
179. Morris JS, Dunn DT, Poddar D, Serjeant GR. Haematological risk factors for pregnancy outcome in Jamaican women with homozygous sickle cell disease. *Br J Obstet Gynaecol.* 1994;101(9):770–773.
180. Koshy M, Burd L, Wallace D, Moawad A, Baron J. Prophylactic red-cell transfusions in pregnant patients with sickle cell disease. A randomized cooperative study. *N Engl J Med.* 1988;319:1447–1452.
181. El-Shafei AM, Kaur Dhaliwal J, Kaur Sandhu A, Rashid Al-Sharqi M. Indications for blood transfusion in pregnancy in sickle cell disease. *Aust NZ J Obstet Gynaecol.* 1995;35:405–408.
182. Mahomed K. Prophylactic versus selective blood transfusion for sickle cell anaemia during pregnancy. *Cochrane Database Syst Rev.* 2000;CD000040.
183. Koshy M, Burd L. Mangement of pregnancy in sickle cell syndromes. *Hematol Oncol Clin North Am.* 1991;5:585–596.
184. ACOG practice bulletin. *No.* 73: Use of hormonal contraception in women with coexisting medical conditions. *Obstet Gynecol.* 2006;107(6):1453–1472.
185. Halvorson DJ, McKie V, McKie K, Ashmore PE, Porubsky ES. Sickle cell disease and tonsillectomy – Preoperative management and postoperative complications. *Arch Otolaryngol Head Neck Surg.* 1997;123(7):689–692.
186. Scott-Conner CEH, Brunson CD. The pathophysiology of the sickle hemoglobinopathies and implications for perioperative management. *Am J Surg.* 1994;168:268–274.
187. Scott-Conner CEH, Brunson CD. Surgery and Anesthesia. In: Embury SH, Hebbel RP, Mohandas N, Steinberg MH, eds. *Sickle Cell Disease: Basic Principles and Clinical Practice.* 1st ed. New York: Lippincott-Raven; 1994:809–827.
188. Firth PG. Anaesthesia for peculiar cellsa century of sickle cell disease. *Br J Anaesth.* 2005;95(3):287–299.
189. Firth PG, Head CA. Sickle cell disease and anesthesia. *Anesthesiology.* 2004;101(3):766–785.
190. Koshy M, Weiner SJ, Miller ST, et al. Surgery and anesthesia in sickle cell disease. *Blood.* 1995;86:3676–3684.
191. Stein RE, Urbaniak J. Use of the tourniquet during surgery in patients with sickle cell hemoglobinpathies. *Clin Orthop.* 1980;151:231–233.
192. Vipond AJ, Caldicott LD. Major vascular surgery in a patient with sickle cell disease. *Anaesthesia.* 1998;53(12):1204–1206.

193. Vichinsky EP, Haberkern CM, Neumayr L, et al. A comparison of conservative and aggressive transfusion regimens in the perioperative management of sickle cell disease. *N Engl J Med.* 1995;333:206–213.
194. Crawford MW, Speakman M, Carver ED, Kim PC. Acute chest syndrome shows a predilection for basal lung regions on the side of upper abdominal surgery. *Can J Anaesth.* 2004;51(7):707–711.
195. Wales PW, Carver E, Crawford MW, Kim PCW. Acute chest syndrome after abdominal surgery in children with sickle cell disease: is a laparoscopic approach better? *J Pediatr Surg.* 2001;36(5):718–721.
196. Buck J, Casbard A, Llewelyn C, Johnson T, Davies S, Williamson L. Preoperative transfusion in sickle cell disease: a survey of practice in England. *Eur J Haematol.* 2005; 75(1):14–21.
197. Fu T, Corrigan NJ, Quinn CT, Rogers ZR, Buchanan GR. Minor elective surgical procedures using general anesthesia in children with sickle cell anemia without pre-operative blood transfusion. *Pediatr Blood Cancer.* 2005;45(1):43–47.
198. Waldron P, Pegelow C, Neumayr L, et al. Tonsillectomy, adenoidectomy, and myringotomy in sickle cell disease: perioperative morbidity. Preoperative Transfusion in Sickle Cell Disease Study Group. *J Pediatr Hematol Oncol.* 1999;21(2): 129–135.
199. Duke RL, Scott JP, Panepinto JA, Flanary VA. Perioperative management of sickle cell disease children undergoing adenotonsillectomy. *Otolaryngol Head Neck Surg.* 2006;134(3):370–373.
200. Griffin TC, Buchanan GR. Elective surgery in children with sickle cell disease without preoperative blood transfusion. *J Pediatr Surg.* 1993;28:681–685.
201. Jeng M, Feusner J, Vichinksy EP. Risk factors for central venous catheter infections in sickle cell disease. 23rd Annual Meeting of the National Sickle Cell Disease Program. 1999;106.
202. Wagner SC, Eschelman DJ, Gonsalves CF, Bonn J, Sullivan KL. Infectious complications of implantable venous access devices in patients with sickle cell disease. *J Vasc Interv Radiol.* 2004;15(4):375–378.
203. Zarrouk V, Habib A, Zahar JR, et al. *Blood.* stream infection in adults with sickle cell disease: association with venous catheters, Staphylococcus aureus, and bone-joint infections. *Medicine (Baltimore).* 2006;85(1):43–48.
204. Chulamokha L, Scholand SJ, Riggio JM, Ballas SK, Horn D, DeSimone JA. Bloodstream infections in hospitalized adults with sickle cell disease: a retrospective analysis. *Am J Hematol.* 2006;81(10):723–728.
205. Milner PF, Kraus AP, Sebes JI, et al. Sickle cell disease as a cause of osteonecrosis of the femoral head. *N Engl J Med.* 1991;325:1476–1481.
206. Milner PF, Kraus AP, Sebes JI, et al. Osteonecrosis of the humeral head in sickle cell disease. *Clin Orthop.* 1993;289: 136–143.
207. Powars DR, Chan LS, Hiti A, Ramicone E, Johnson C. Outcome of sickle cell anemia: a 4-decade observational study of 1056 patients. *Medicine (Baltimore).* 2005;84(6):363–376.
208. Hernigou P, Bachir D, Galacteros F. The natural history of symptomatic osteonecrosis in adults with sickle-cell disease. *J Bone Joint Surg Am.* 2003;85(3):500–504.
209. Hernigou P, Habib A, Bachir D, Galacteros F. The natural history of asymptomatic osteonecrosis of the femoral head in adults with sickle cell disease. *J Bone Joint Surg Am.* 2006;88(12):2565–2572.
210. Osteonecrosis-etiology, diagnosis, and treatment. American Orthopaedic Association;1997.
211. Ficat R. Idiopathic bone necrosis of the femoral head. *Soc Bone Joint Surg.* 1985;67:3–9.
212. Aguilar CM, Neumayr LD, Eggleston BE, et al. Clinical evaluation of avascular necrosis in patients with sickle cell disease: Children's Hospital Oakland Hip Evaluation Scale – a modification of the Harris Hip Score. *Arch Phys Med Rehabil.* 2005;86(7):1369–1375.
213. Mankin H. Nontraumatic necrosis of bone (osteonecrosis). *N Engl J Med.* 1992;326:1473–1479.
214. Washington E, Root L. Conservative treatment of sickle cell avascular necrosis of the femoral head. *J Pediatr Orthop.* 1985; 5:192–194.
215. Dunsmore K, Ware R, Frush D, Kinney T. Short-term transfusion therapy for avascular necrosis of the hips in children with sickle cell disease. *Int J Pediatr Hematol Oncol.* 1995;2:79–83.
216. Hickman JM, Lachiewicz PF. Results and complications of total hip arthroplasties in patients with sickle-cell hemoglobinopathies – Role of cementless components. *J Arthroplasty.* 1997;12:420–425.
217. Jeong GK, Ruchelsman DE, Jazrawi LM, Jaffe WL. Total hip arthroplasty in sickle cell hemoglobinopathies. *J Am Acad Orthop Surg.* 2005;13(3):208–217.
218. Mont MA, Carbone JJ, Fairbank AC. Core decompression versus non-operative management for osteonecrosis of the hip. *Clin Orthop Rel Res.* 1996;324:169–178.
219. Neumayr LD, Aguilar C, Earles AN, et al. Physical therapy alone compared with core decompression and physical therapy for femoral head osteonecrosis in sickle cell disease. Results of a multicenter study at a mean of three years after treatment. *J Bone Joint Surg Am.* 2006;88(12):2573–2582.
220. Hernigou P, Zilber S, Filippini P, Mathieu G, Poignard A, Galacteros F. Total THA in adult osteonecrosis related to sickle cell disease. *Clin Orthop Rel Res.* 2008;466(2):300–308.
221. Dorwart BB, Gabuzda T. Symmetric myositis and faciitis: a complication of sickle cell anemia during vasoocclusion. *J Rheumatol.* 1985;12:590–595.
222. Malekgoudarzi B, Feffer S. Myonecrosis in sickle cell anemia. *N Engl J Med.* 1999;340(6):483.
223. Kim SK, Miller JH. Natural history and distribution of bone and bone marrow infarction in sickle hemoglobinopathies. *J Nucl Med.* 2002;43(7):896–900.
224. Ataga KI, Orringer EP. Bone marrow necrosis in sickle cell disease: A description of three cases and a review of the literature. *Am J Med Sci.* 2000;320(5):342–347.
225. Mankad VN, Williams JP, Harpen MD, et al. Magnetic resonance imaging of bone marrow in sickle cell disease: clinical, hematologic, and pathologic correlations. *Blood.* 1990;75(1):274–283.
226. Abbiyesuku FM, Osotimehin BO. Anterior pituitary gland assessment in sickle cell anaemia patients with delayed menarche. *Afr J Med Med Sci.* 1999;28(1–2):65–69.
227. Abbasi AA, Prasad AS, Ortega J, Congco E, Oberleas D. Gonadal function abnormalities in sickle cell anemia: studies in male patients. *Ann Intern Med.* 1976;85:601–605.

228. Osegbe DN, Akinyanju OO. Testicular dysfunction in men with sickle cell disease. *Postgrad Med J.* 1987;63(736):95–98.
229. Li M, Fogarty J, Whitney KD, Stone P. Repeated testicular infarction in a patient with sickle cell disease: a possible mechanism for testicular failure. *Urology.* 2003;62(3):551.
230. Landefeld CS, Schambelan M, Kaplan SL, Embury SH. Clomiphene-responsive hypogonadism in sickle cell anemia. *Ann Intern Med.* 1983;99(4):480–483.
231. Miller RG, Segal JB, Ashar BH, et al. High prevalence and correlates of low bone mineral density in young adults with sickle cell disease. *Am J Hematol.* 2006;81(4):236–241.
232. Voskaridou E, Stoupa E, Antoniadou L, et al. Osteoporosis and osteosclerosis in sickle cell/beta-thalassemia: the role of the RANKL/osteoprotegerin axis. *Haematologica.* 2006;91(6):813–816.
233. Lal A, Fung EB, Pakbaz Z, Hackney-Stephens E, Vichinsky EP. Bone mineral density in children with sickle cell anemia. *Pediatr Blood Cancer.* 2006;47(7):901–906.
234. Van Der Dijs FP, Van Der Klis FR, Muskiet FD, Muskiet FA. Serum calcium and vitamin D status of patients with sickle cell disease in Curacao. *Ann Clin Biochem.* 1997;34(Pt 2):170–172.
235. Almeida A, Roberts I. Bone involvement in sickle cell disease. *Br J Haematol.* 2005;129(4):482–490.
236. Mohammed S, Addae S, Suleiman S, et al. Serum calcium, parathyroid hormone, and vitamin D status in children and young adults with sickle cell disease. *Ann Clin Biochem* 1993;30(Pt 1):45–51.
237. Adewoye AH, Chen TC, Ma Q, et al. Sickle cell bone disease: Response to vitamin D and calcium. *Am J Hematol.* 2008;83(4):271–274.
238. Saad STO, Costa FF. Glucose-6-phosphate dehydrogenase deficiency and sickle cell disease in Brazil. *Hum Hered.* 1992;42:125–128.
239. Phillips G Jr, Becker B, Keller VA, Hartman J. Hypothyroidism in adults with sickle cell anemia. *Am J Med.* 1992; 92:567–570.
240. Parshad O, Stevens MC, Hudson C, et al. Abnormal thyroid hormone and thyrotropin levels in homozygous sickle cell disease. *Clin Lab Haematol.* 1989;11(4):309–315.
241. el-Hazmi MA, Bahakim HM, Al-Fawaz I. Endocrine functions in sickle cell anaemia patients. *J Trop Pediatr.* 1991;38(6):307–313.
242. Somjee SS, Warrier RP, Thomson JL, Ory-Ascani J, Hempe JM. Advanced glycation end-products in sickle cell anaemia. *Br J Haematol.* 2005;128(1):112–118.
243. Fung EB, Harmatz PR, Lee PD, et al. Increased prevalence of iron-overload associated endocrinopathy in thalassaemia versus sickle-cell disease. *Br J Haematol.* 2006;135(4):574–582.
244. Collins FS, Orringer EP. Pulmonary hypertension and cor pulmonale in the sickle hemoglobinopathies. *Am J Med.* 1982;73(6):814–821.
245. Taylor JG, Ackah D, Cobb C, et al. Mutations and polymorphisms in hemoglobin genes and the risk of pulmonary hypertension and death in sickle cell disease. *Am J Hematol.* 2008;83:6–14.
246. Kato GJ, Onyekwere OC, Gladwin MT. Pulmonary hypertension in sickle cell disease: relevance to children. *Pediatr Hematol Oncol.* 2007;24(3):159–170.
247. Castro O, Hoque M, Brown BD. Pulmonary hypertension in sickle cell disease: cardiac catheterization results and survival. *Blood.* 2003;101(4):1257–1261.
248. Castro O, Gladwin MT. Pulmonary hypertension in sickle cell disease: mechanisms, diagnosis, and management. *Hematol Oncol Clin North Am.* 2005;19(5):881–896.
249. Ataga KI, Moore CG, Jones S, et al. Pulmonary hypertension in patients with sickle cell disease: a longitudinal study. *Br J Haematol.* 2006;134(1):109–115.
250. Darbari DS, Kple-Faget P, Kwagyan J, Rana S, Gordeuk VR, Castro O. Circumstances of death in adult sickle cell disease patients. *Am J Hematol.* 2006; 80(11):858–863.
251. Sutton LL, Castro O, Cross DJ, Spencer JE, Lewis JF. Pulmonary hypertension in sickle cell disease. *Am J Cardiol.* 1994;74:626–628.
252. Ataga KI, Sood N, De GG, et al. Pulmonary hypertension in sickle cell disease. *Am J Med.* 2004;117(9):665–669.
253. De Castro LM, Jonassaint JC, Graham FL, Ashley-Koch A, Telen MJ. Pulmonary hypertension associated with sickle cell disease: clinical and laboratory endpoints and disease outcomes. *Am J Hematol.* 2008;83(1):19–25.
254. Haque AK, Gokhale S, Rampy BA, Adegboyega P, Duarte A, Saldana MJ. Pulmonary hypertension in sickle cell hemoglobinopathy: a clinicopathologic study of 20 cases. *Hum Pathol.* 2002;33(10):1037–1043.
255. van Beers EJ, van Eck-Smit BL, Mac Gillavry MR, et al. Large and medium sized pulmonary artery obstruction does not play a role of primary importance in the, etiology of sickle cell disease associated pulmonary hypertension. *Chest.* 2008;ePub.
256. Suell MN, Bezold LI, Okcu MF, Mahoney DH, Jr., Shardonofsky F, Mueller BU. Increased pulmonary artery pressures among adolescents with sickle cell disease. *J Pediatr Hematol Oncol.* 2005;27(12):654–658.
257. Joyce K, Sable C, Martin B, Minniti CP. Pulmonary artery hypertension in children with sickle cell disease: Is chronic transfusion protective? *Blood.* 2006;108:356a.
258. Qureshi N, Joyce JJ, Qi N, Chang RK. Right ventricular abnormalities in sickle cell anemia: evidence of a progressive increase in pulmonary vascular resistance. *J Pediatr.* 2006;149(1):23–27.
259. Ambrusko SJ, Gunawardena S, Sakara A, et al. Elevation of tricuspid regurgitant jet velocity, a marker for pulmonary hypertension in children with sickle cell disease. *Pediatr Blood Cancer.* 2006;47(7):907–913.
260. Liem RI, Willingham NM, Young LT, Thompson AA. Tricuspid regurgitant jet velocity is significantly associated with hemolysis in the evaluation of pulmonary hypertension in children and young adults with sickle cell disease. *Blood.* 2006;108:356a.
261. Liem RI, Young LT, Thompson AA. Tricuspid regurgitant jet velocity is associated with hemolysis in children and young adults with sickle cell disease evaluated for pulmonary hypertension. *Haematologica.* 2007;92:1549–1552.
262. Campbell AD, Minniti C, Sable C, et al. Prospective evaluation of the prevalence of elevated tricuspid regurgitant jet velocity and associated clinical and echocardiographic factors in children and adolescents with sickle cell disease. *Blood.* 2007;110:993a.
263. Machado RF, Gladwin MT. Chronic sickle cell lung disease: new insights into the diagnosis, pathogenesis and treatment

of pulmonary hypertension. *Br J Haematol.* 2005;129(4):449–464.

264. Mekontso Dessap A, Leon R, Habib A, et al. Pulmonary Hypertension and Cor Pulmonale during Severe Acute Chest Syndrome in Sickle Cell Disease. *Am J Respir Crit Care Med.* 2008;177(6):646–653.
265. Machado RF, Anthi A, Steinberg MH, et al. N-terminal pro-brain natriuretic peptide levels and risk of death in sickle cell disease. *JAMA.* 2006;296(3):310–318.
266. Kato GJ, Martyr S, Blackwelder WC, et al. Levels of soluble endothelium-derived adhesion molecules in patients with sickle cell disease are associated with pulmonary hypertension, organ dysfunction, and mortality. *Br J Haematol.* 2005;130(6):943–953.
267. Ataga KI, Moore CG, Hillery CA, et al. Coagulation activation and inflammation in sickle cell disease-associated pulmonary hypertension. *Haematologica.* 2008;93(1):20–26.
268. Gordeuk VR, Sachdev V, Taylor JG, Gladwin MT, Kato G, Castro OL. Relative systemic hypertension in patients with sickle cell disease is associated with risk of pulmonary hypertension and renal insufficiency. *Am J Hematol.* 2008;83(1):15–18.
269. Morris CR, Suh JH, Hagar W, et al. Erythrocyte glutamine depletion, altered redox environment, and pulmonary hypertension in sickle cell disease. *Blood.* 2008;111(1):402–410.
270. Ameshima S, Golpon H, Cool CD, et al. Peroxisome proliferator-activated receptor gamma (PPARgamma) expression is decreased in pulmonary hypertension and affects endothelial cell growth. *Circ Res.* 2003;92(10):1162–1169.
271. Nichols WC, Koller DL, Slovis B, et al. Localization of the gene for familial primary pulmonary hypertension to chromosome 2q31–32. *Nat Genet.* 1997;15(3):277–280.
272. Machado RD, Pauciulo MW, Thomson JR, et al. BMPR2 haploinsufficiency as the inherited molecular mechanism for primary pulmonary hypertension. *Am J Hum Genet.* 2001;68(1):92–102.
273. Santoli F, Zerah F, Vasile N, Bachir D, Galacteros F, Atlan G. Pulmonary function in sickle cell disease with or without acute chest syndrome. *Eur Respir J.* 1998;12(5):1124–1129.
274. Powars D, Weidman JA, Odom-Maryon T, Niland JC, Johnson C. Sickle cell chronic lung disease: prior morbidity and the risk of pulmonary failure. *Medicine (Baltimore).* 1988;67(1):66–76.
275. Akgul F, Yalcin F, Babayigit C, Seyfeli E, Seydaliyeva T, Gali E. Right ventricular and pulmonary function in sickle cell disease patients with pulmonary hypertension. *Pediatr Cardiol.* 2006;27(4):440–446.
276. Zar HA, Wu WW. The inability to detect expired carbon dioxide after endotracheal intubation as a result of one-way valve obstruction of the endotracheal tube. *Anesth Analg.* 2001;93(4):971–972, table.
277. Klings ES, Wyszynski DF, Nolan VG, Steinberg MH. Abnormal pulmonary function in adults with sickle cell anemia. *Am J Respir Crit Care Med.* 2006;173:1264–1269.
278. Arteta M, Campbell AD, Minniti C, et al. Pulmonary function tests and their correlation with tricuspid regurgitant jet velocity in pediatric sickle cell disease patients. *Blood.* 2007;110:670a.
279. Knight-Madden JM, Forrester TS, Lewis NA, Greenough A. Asthma in children with sickle cell disease and its association with acute chest syndrome. *Thorax.* 2005;60(3):206–210.
280. Glassberg J, Spivey JF, Strunk R, Boslaugh S, DeBaun MR. Painful episodes in children with sickle cell disease and asthma are temporally associated with respiratory symptoms. *J Pediatr Hematol Oncol.* 2006;28(8):481–485.
281. Boyd JH, Macklin EA, Strunk RC, DeBaun MR. Asthma is associated with acute chest syndrome and pain in children with sickle cell anemia. *Blood.* 2006;108:2923–2927.
282. Boyd JH, Moinuddin A, Strunk RC, DeBaun MR. Asthma and acute chest in sickle-cell disease. *Pediatr Pulmonol.* 2004;38(3):229–232.
283. Boyd JH, Macklin EA, Strunk RC, DeBaun MR. Asthma is associated with increased mortality in individuals with sickle cell anemia. *Haematologica.* 2007;92(8):1115–1118.
284. Nordness ME, Lynn J, Zacharisen MC, Scott PJ, Kelly KJ. Asthma is a risk factor for acute chest syndrome and cerebral vascular accidents in children with sickle cell disease. *Clin Mol Allergy.* 2005;3(1):2.
285. Phillips KL, An P, Boyd JH, et al. Major gene effect and additive familial pattern of inheritance of asthma exist among families of probands with sickle cell anemia and asthma. *Am J Hum Biol.* 2007;ePub.
286. Machado RF, Martyr S, Kato GJ, et al. Sildenafil therapy in patients with sickle cell disease and pulmonary hypertension. *Br J Haematol.* 2005;130(3):445–453.
287. Koshy M, Entsuah R, Koranda A, et al. Leg ulcers in patients with sickle cell disease [see comments]. *Blood.* 1989;74:1403–1408.
288. Clare A, FitzHenley M, Harris J, Hambleton I, Serjeant GR. Chronic leg ulceration in homozygous sickle cell disease: the role of venous incompetence. *Br J Haematol.* 2002; 119(2):567–571.
289. Best PJ, Daoud MS, Pittelkow MR, Petitt RM. Hydroxyurea-induced leg ulceration in 14 patients. *Ann Intern Med.* 1998;128(1):29–32.
290. Weinlich G, Schuler G, Greil R, Kofler H, Fritsch P. Leg ulcers associated with long-term hydroxyurea therapy. *J Am Acad Dermatol.* 1998;39(2 Pt 2):372–374.
291. Ravandi-Kashani F, Cortes J, Cohen P, et al. Cutaneous ulcers associated with hydroxyurea (HU) therapy in myeloproliferative disorders. *Blood.* 1998;92:248b.
292. Chaine B, Neonato MG, Girot R, Aractingi S. Cutaneous adverse reactions to hydroxyurea in patients with sickle cell disease. *Arch Dermatol.* 2001;137(4):467–470.
293. Giraldi S, Abbage KT, Marinoni LP, et al. Leg ulcer in hereditary spherocytosis. *Pediatr Dermatol.* 2003;20(5):427–428.
294. Eckman JR. Leg ulcers in sickle cell disease. *Hematol Oncol Clin North Am.* 1996;10:1333–1344.
295. Mackenzie RK, Ludlam CA, Ruckley CV, Allan PL, Burns P, Bradbury AW. The prevalence of thrombophilia in patients with chronic venous leg ulceration. *J Vasc Surg.* 2002;35(4):718–722.
296. Billett HH, Patel Y, Rivers SP. Venous insufficiency is not the cause of leg ulcers in sickle cell disease. *Am J Hematol.* 1991;37:133–134.
297. Chalchal H, Rodino W, Hussain S, et al. Impaired venous hemodynamics in a minority of patients with chronic leg ulcers due to sickle cell anemia. *Vasa.* 2001;30(4):277–279.
298. Mohan JS, Vigilance JE, Marshall JM, Hambleton IR, Reid HL, Serjeant GR. Abnormal venous function in patients with homozygous sickle cell (SS) disease and chronic leg ulcers. *Clin Sci (Lond).* 2000;98(6):667–672.

299. Ademiluyi SA, Rotimi VO, Coker AO, Banjo TO, Akinyanju O. The anaerobic and aerobic bacterial flora of leg ulcers in patients with sickle-cell disease. *J Infect.* 1988;17:115–120.
300. MacFarlane DE, Baum KF, Serjeant GR. Bacteriology of sickle cell leg ulcers. *Trans R Soc Trop Med Hyg.* 1986;80:553–556.
301. Sawhney H, Weedon J, Gillette P, Solomon W, Braverman A. Predilection of hemolytic anemia-associated leg ulcers for the medial malleolus. *Vasa.* 2002;31(3):191–193.
302. Baum KF, MacFarlane DE, Maude GH, Serjeant GR. Topical antibiotics in chronic sickle cell leg ulcers. *Trans R Soc Trop Med Hyg.* 1987;81:847–849.
303. Ramos CE, Park JS, Ritchey ML, Benson GS. High flow priapism associated with sickle cell disease. *J Urol.* 1995; 153:1619–1621.
304. Sharpsteen JR Jr, Powars D, Johnson C, Rogers ZR, Williams WD, Posch RJ. Multisystem damage associated with tricorporal priapism in sickle cell disease. *Am J Med.* 1993;94:289–295.
305. Burnett AL. Role of nitric oxide in the physiology of erection. *Biol Reprod.* 1995;52(3):485–489.
306. Burnett AL. Neurophysiology of erectile function: androgenic effects. *J Androl.* 2003;24(6 Suppl):S2–S5.
307. Burnett AL. Pathophysiology of priapism: dysregulatory erection physiology thesis. *J Urol.* 2003;170(1):26–34.
308. Champion HC, Bivalacqua TJ, Takimoto E, Kass DA, Burnett AL. Phosphodiesterase-5A dysregulation in penile erectile tissue is a mechanism of priapism. *Proc Natl Acad Sci USA.* 2005;102(5):1661–1666.
309. Brandow AM, Rennie KM, Scott JP, Hillery CA, Panepinto JA. Increased red blood cell adhesion is associated with priapism in sickle cell disease. *Blood.* 2006;108:363a.
310. Mantadakis E, Cavender JD, Rogers ZR, Ewalt DH, Buchanan GR. Prevalence of priapism in children and adolescents with sickle cell anemia. *J Pediatr Hematol Oncol.* 1999;21(6):518–522.
311. Fowler JE, Jr., Koshy M, Strub M, Chinn SK. Priapism associated with the sickle cell hemoglobinopathies: Prevalence, natural history and sequelae. *J Urol.* 1991;145:65–68.
312. Serjeant GR. *Sickle Cell Disease.* 2nd ed. Oxford: Oxford Medical Publications; 1992.
313. Serjeant GR, De Ceulaer K, Maude GH. Stilboestrol and stuttering priapism in homozygous sickle cell disease. *Lancet.* 1985;2:1274–1276.
314. Adeyoju AB, Olujohungbe AB, Morris J, et al. Priapism in sickle-cell disease; incidence, risk factors and complications – an international multicentre study. *Br J Urol. Int.* 2002;90(9):898–902.
315. Hakim LS, Hashmat AI, Macchia RJ. Priapism. In: Embury SH, Hebbel RP, Mohandas N, Steinberg MH, eds. *Sickle Cell Disease: Basic Principles and Clinical Practice.* 1st ed. New York: Lippincott-Raven; 1994:633–643.
316. Miller ST, Rao SP, Dunn EK, Glassberg KI. Priapism in children with sickle cell disease. *J Urol.* 1995;154:844–847.
317. Chakrabarty A, Upadhyay J, Dhabuwala CB, Sarnaik S, Perlmutter AD, Connor JP. Priapism associated with sickle cell hemoglobinopathy in children: Long-term effects on potency. *J Urol.* 1996;155:1419–1423.
318. Tarry WF, Duckett JW Jr, Snyder HMI. Urological complications of sickle cell disease in a pediatric population. *J Urol.* 1987;138:592–594.
319. Kassim AA, Umans H, Nagel RL, Fabry ME. Megalophallus as a sequela of priapism in sickle cell anemia: use of blood oxygen level-dependent magnetic resonance imaging. *Urology.* 2000;56(3):509.
320. Burnett AL, Allen RP, Tempany CM, Dover GJ, Brendler CB. Evaluation of erectile function in men with sickle cell disease. *Urology.* 1995;45:657–663.
321. Chinegwundoh F, Anie KA. Treatments for priapism in boys and men with sickle cell disease. *Cochrane Database Syst Rev.* 2004;(4):CD004198.
322. McCarthy LJ, Vattuone J, Weidner J, et al. Do automated red cell exchanges relieve priapism in patients with sickle cell anemia? *Ther Apher.* 2000;4(3):256–258.
323. Merritt AL, Haiman C, Henderson SO. Myth: blood transfusion is effective for sickle cell anemia-associated priapism. *CJEM.* 2006;8(2):119–122.
324. Mantadakis E, Ewalt DH, Cavender JD, Rogers ZR, Buchanan GR. Outpatient penile aspiration and epinephrine irrigation for young patients with sickle cell anemia and prolonged priapism. *Blood.* 2000;95(1):78–82.
325. Virag R, Bachir D, Lee K, Galacteros F. Preventive treatment of priapism in sickle cell disease with oral and self-administered intracavernous injection of etilefrine. *Urology.* 1996;47:777–781.
326. Virag R, Bachir D, Floresco J, Galacteros F, Dufour B. Ambulatory treatment and prevention of priapism using alpha-agonists. Apropos of 172 cases. *Chirurgie.* 1997;121:648–652.
327. Bachir D, Virag R, Lee K, et al. Prevention and treatment of erectile disorders in sickle cell disease [in French]. *Rev Med Interne.* 1997;18(Supp 1):46S–51S.
328. Okpala I, Westerdale N, Jegede T, Cheung B. Etilefrine for the prevention of priapism in adult sickle cell disease. *Br J Haematol.* 2002;118(3):918–921.
329. Gbadoe AD, Atakouma Y, Kusiaku K, Assimadi JK. Management of sickle cell priapism with etilefrine. *Arch Dis Child.* 2001;85(1):52–53.
330. Dahm P, Rao DS, Donatucci CF. Antiandrogens in the treatment of priapism. *Urology.* 2002;59(1):138.
331. Saad ST, Lajolo C, Gilli S, et al. Follow-up of sickle cell disease patients with priapism treated by hydroxyurea. *Am J Hematol.* 2004;77(1):45–49.
332. Burnett AL, Bivalacqua TJ, Champion HC, Musicki B. Feasibility of the use of phosphodiesterase type 5 inhibitors in a pharmacologic prevention program for recurrent priapism. *J Sex Med.* 2006;3(6):1077–1084.
333. Monga M, Broderick GA, Hellstrom WJG. Priapism in sickle cell disease: the case for early implantation of the penile prosthesis. *Eur Urol.* 1996;30:54–59.
334. Johnson CS, Omata M, Tong MJ, Simmons JF Jr, Weiner J, Tatter D. Liver involvement in sickle cell disease. *Medicine.* 1985;69:833–837.
335. Wright JG, Cooper P, Malia RG, et al. Activated protein C resistance in homozygous sickle cell disease. *Br J Haematol.* 1997;96:854–856.
336. Gremse DA, Fillingim E, Hoff CJ, Wells DJ, Boerth RC. Hepatic function as assessed by lidocaine metabolism in sickle cell disease. *J Pediatr.* 1998;132(6):989–993.
337. Comer GM, Ozick LA, Sachdev RK, et al. Transfusion-related chronic liver disease in sickle cell anemia. *Am J Gastroenterol.* 1991;86:1232–1234.
338. Charlotte F, Bachir D, Nénert M, et al. Vascular lesions of the liver in sickle cell disease: a clinicopathological study in 26 living patients. *Arch Pathol Lab Med.* 1995;119:46–52.

339. Achord JL. Gastroenterologic and hepatobiliary manifestations. In: Embury SH, Hebbel RP, Mohandas N, Steinberg MH, eds. *Sickle Cell Disease: Basic Principles and Clinical Practice*. 1st ed. New York: Lippincott-Raven; 1994:663–672.
340. Richard S, Billett HH. Liver function tests in sickle cell disease. *Clin Lab Haematol.* 2002;24(1):21–27.
341. Ahn H, Li CS, Wang W. Sickle cell hepatopathy: clinical presentation, treatment, and outcome in pediatric and adult patients. *Pediatr Blood Cancer.* 2005;45(2):184–190.
342. Walker TM, Hambleton IR, Serjeant GR. Gallstones in sickle cell disease: observations from The Jamaican Cohort study. *J Pediatr.* 2000;136(1):80–85.
343. Haider MZ, Ashebu S, Aduh P, Adekile AD. Influence of a-thalassemia on cholelithiasis in SS patients with elevated Hb F. *Acta Haematol.* 1998;100(3):147–150.
344. Chaar V, Keclard L, Etienne-Julan M, et al. UGT1A1 polymorphism outweighs the modest effect of deletional (−3.7 kb) alpha-thalassemia on cholelithogenesis in sickle cell anemia. *Am J Hematol.* 2006;81(5):377–379.
345. Passon RG, Howard TA, Zimmerman SA, Schultz WH, Ware RE. Influence of bilirubin uridine diphosphate-glucuronosyltransferase 1A promoter polymorphisms on serum bilirubin levels and cholelithiasis in children with sickle cell anemia. *J Pediatr Hematol Oncol.* 2001;23(7):448–451.
346. Chaar V, Keclard L, Diara JP, et al. Association of UGT1A1 polymorphism with prevalence and age at onset of cholelithiasis in sickle cell anemia. *Haematologica.* 2005;90(2):188–199.
347. Heeney MM, Howard TA, Zimmerman SA, Ware RE. UGT1A promoter polymorphisms influence bilirubin response to hydroxyurea therapy in sickle cell anemia. *J Lab Clin Med.* 2003;141(4):279–282.
348. Haberkern CM, Neumayr LD, Orringer EP, et al. Cholecystectomy in sickle cell anemia patients: perioperative outcome of 364 cases from the national preoperative transfusion study. *Blood.* 1997;89:1533–1542.
349. Al-Salem AH, Nourallah H. Sequential endoscopic/laparoscopic management of cholelithiasis and choledocholithiasis in children who have sickle cell disease. *J Pediatr Surg.* 1997;32(10):1432–1435.
350. Vichinksy E, Gold J, Rule R, et al. Neuropsychological (NP) dysfunction and neuroimaging abnormalities in neurologically intact adult patients with sickle cell disease (SCD). *Blood.* 2007;110:132a.
351. Serjeant GR, Higgs DR, Hambleton IR. Elderly survivors with homozygous sickle cell disease. *N Engl J Med.* 2007; 356(6):642–643.
352. Steinberg MH, Ballas SK, Brunson CY, Bookchin R. Sickle cell anemia in septuagenarians. *Blood.* 1995;86:3997–3998.
353. Rucknagel DL, Hanash SH, Sing CF, Winter WP, Whitten CF, Prasad AS. Age and sex effects on hemoglobin F in sickle cell anemia. In: Stammatoyannopoulos JA, Nienhius AW, eds. *Cellular and Molecular Regulation of Hemoglobin Switching.* New York: Grune and Stratton; 1979:107–118.
354. Shurafa MS, Prasad AS, Rucknagel DL, Kan YW. Long survival in sickle cell anemia. *Am J Hematol.* 1982;12:357–365.
355. Liem RI, Calamaras DM, Chhabra MS, Files B, Minniti CP, Thompson AA. Sudden onset blindness in sickle cell disease due to retinal artery occlusion. *Pediatr Blood Cancer.* 2007;50(3):624–627.
356. Warth JA, Prasad AS, Zwas F, Franke U. Abnormal dark adaptation in sickle cell anemia. *J Lab Clin Med.* 1981;98:189–194.
357. Serjeant GR, Serjeant BE, Condon PI. The conjunctival sign in sickle cell anemia. A relationship with irreversibly sickled cells. *JAMA.* 1972;219:1428–1431.
358. Acar P, Maunoury C, de MM, Dulac Y. Abnormalities of myocardial perfusion in sickle cell disease in childhood: a study of myocardial scintigraphy. *Arch Mal Coeur Vaiss.* 2003;96(5):507–510.
359. Zilberman MV, Du W, Das S, Sarnaik SA. Evaluation of left ventricular diastolic function in pediatric sickle cell disease patients. *Am J Hematol.* 2007;82(6):433–438.
360. Leight L, Snider TH, Clifford GO, Hellems HK. Hemodynamic studies in sickle cell anemia. *Circulation.* 1954;10:653–662.
361. Covitz W, Espeland M, Gallagher D, Hellenbrand W, Leff S, Talner N. The heart in sickle cell anemia – The cooperative study of sickle cell disease (CSSCD). *Chest.* 1995;108:1214–1219.
362. Braden DS, Covitz W, Milner PF. Cardiovascular function during rest and exercise in patients with sickle-cellanemia and coexisting alpha thalassemia-2. *Am J Hematol.* 1996;52:96–102.
363. Sachdev V, Machado RF, Shizukuda Y, et al. Diastolic dysfunction is an independent risk factor for death in patients with sickle cell disease. *J Am Coll Cardiol.* 2007;49(4):472–479.
364. Covitz W. Cardiac Disease. In: Embury SH, Hebbel RP, Mohandas N, Steinberg MH, eds. *Sickle Cell Disease: Basic Principles and Clinical Practice.* 1st ed. New York: Lippincott-Raven; 1994:725–734.
365. Martin CR, Johnson CS, Cobb C, Tatter D, Haywood LJ. Myocardial infarction in sickle cell disease. *J Natl Med Assoc.* 1996;88(7):428–432.
366. James TN, Riddick L, Massing GK. Sickle cells and sudden death: morphologic abnormalities of the cardiac conduction system. *J Lab Clin Med.* 1994;124:507–520.
367. Romero Mestre JC, Hernandez A, Agramonte O, Hernandez P. Cardiovascular autonomic dysfunction in sickle cell anemia: a possible risk factor for sudden death? *Clin Auton Res.* 1997;7(3):121–125.
368. Ataga KI, Orringer EP. Renal abnormalities in sickle cell disease. *Am J Hematol.* 2000;63(4):205–211.
369. Guasch A, Cua M, Mitch WE. Early detection and the course of glomerular injury in patients with sickle cell anemia. *Kidney Int.* 1996;49:786–791.
370. Pham PT, Pham PC, Wilkinson AH, Lew SQ. Renal abnormalities in sickle cell disease. *Kidney Int.* 2000;57(1):1–8.
371. Platt OS, Brambilla DJ, Rosse WF, et al. Mortality in sickle cell disease. Life expectancy and risk factors for early death. *N Engl J Med.* 1994;330(23):1639–1644.
372. Schmitt F, Martinez F, Brillet G, et al. Early glomerular dysfunction in patients with sickle cell anemia. *Am J Kidney Dis.* 1998;32(2):208–214.
373. Wong WY, Elliott-Mills D, Powars D. Renal failure in sickle cell anemia. *Hematol Oncol Clin North Am.* 1996;10:1321–1331.
374. Scheinman JI. Sickle cell disease and the kidney. *Semin Nephrol.* 2003;23(1):66–76.
375. Thompson J, Reid M, Hambleton I, Serjeant GR. Albuminuria and renal function in homozygous sickle cell disease: observations from a cohort study. *Arch Intern Med.* 2007;167(7):701–708.

376. Powers JS, Krantz SB, Collins JC, et al. Erythropoietin response to anemia as a function of age. *J Am Geriatr Soc.* 1991;39:30–32.
377. Powars DR, Elliott Mills DD, Chan L. Chronic renal failure in sickle cell disease: Risk factors, clinical course, and mortality. *Ann Intern Med.* 1991;115:614–620.
378. McKie KT, Hanevold CD, Hernandez C, Waller JL, Ortiz L, McKie KM. Prevalence, prevention, and treatment of microalbuminuria and proteinuria in children with sickle cell disease. *J Pediatr Hematol Oncol.* 2007;29(3):140–144.
379. Guasch A, Zayas CF, Eckman JR, Muralidharan K, Zhang W, Elsas LJ. Evidence that microdeletions in the a globin gene protect against the development of sickle cell glomerulopathy in humans. *J Am Soc Nephrol.* 1999;10(5):1014–1019.
380. Falk RJ, Scheinman J, Phillips G, Orringer E, Johnson A, Jennette JC. Prevalence and pathologic features of sickle cell nephropathy and response to inhibition of angiotensin-converting enzyme. *N Engl J Med.* 1992;326:910–915.
381. Falk RJ, Jennette JC. Renal disease. In: Embury SH, Hebbel RP, Mohandas N, Steinberg MH, eds. *Sickle Cell Disease: Basic Principles and Clinical Practice.* 1st ed. New York: Raven-Lippincott; 1994:673–680.
382. Guasch A, Cua M, You W, Mitch WE. Sickle cell anemia causes a distinct pattern of glomerular dysfunction. *Kidney Int.* 1997;51:826–833.
383. Guasch A, Navarrete J, Nass K, Zayas CF. Glomerular involvement in adults with sickle cell hemoglobinopathies: prevalence and clinical correlates of progressive renal failure. *J Am Soc Nephrol.* 2006;17(8):2228–2235.
384. Bergmann S, Zheng D, Barredo J, Abboud MR, Jaffa AA. Renal kallikrein: a risk marker for nephropathy in children with sickle cell disease. *J Pediatr Hematol Oncol.* 2006;28(3):147–153.
385. Barros FB, Lima CS, Santos AO, et al. 51Cr-EDTA measurements of the glomerular filtration rate in patients with sickle cell anaemia and minor renal damage. *Nucl Med Commun.* 2006;27(12):959–962.
386. Tharaux PL, Hagege I, Placier S, et al. Urinary endothelin-1 as a marker of renal damage in sickle cell disease. *Nephrol Dial Transplant.* 2005;20(11):2408–2413.
387. Bank N, Aynedjian HS, Qiu JH, et al. Renal nitric oxide synthases in transgenic sickle cell mice. *Kidney Int.* 1996;50:184–189.
388. Montgomery R, Zibari G, Hill GS, Ratner LE. Renal transplantation in patients with sickle cell nephropathy. *Transplantation.* 1994;58:618–620.
389. Steinberg MH. Erythropoietin in anemia of renal failure in sickle cell disease. *N Engl J Med.* 1991;324:1369–1370.
390. Ojo AO, Govaerts TC, Schmouder RL, et al. Renal transplantation in end-stage sickle cell nephropathy. *Transplantation.* 1999;67(2):291–295.
391. Aoki RY, Saad STO. Enalapril reduces the albuminuria of patients with sickle cell disease. *Am J Med.* 1995;98:432–435.
392. Foucan L, Bourhis V, Bangou J, Mérault L, Etienne-Julan M, Salmi RL. A randomized trial of captopril for microalbuminuria in normotensive adults with sickle cell anemia. *Am J Med.* 1998;104(4):339–342.
393. Rabala A, Guasch A. Effects of angiotensin blockade with losartan on glomerular function in patients with sickle cell glomerulopathy. *J Am Soc Nephrol.* 2002;13:265A.
394. Wierenga KJ, Hambleton IR, Lewis NA. Survival estimates for patients with homozygous sickle-cell disease in Jamaica: a clinic-based population study. *Lancet.* 2001;357(9257):680–683.
395. Vichinsky EP, Styles LA, Colangelo LH, et al. Acute chest syndrome in sickle cell disease: clinical presentation and course. *Blood.* 1997;89:1787–1792.
396. Upadhya B, Ntim W, Dworkin J, et al. Prolongation of QTc intervals and risk of sudden death among patients with sickle cell diseases. *Blood.* 2007;110:667a.
397. Zipursky A, Robieux IC, Brown EJ, et al. Oxygen therapy in sickle cell disease. *Am J Pediatr Hematol Oncol.* 1992; 14(3):222–228.
398. Hargrave DR, Wade A, Evans JP, Hewes DK, Kirkham FJ. Nocturnal oxygen saturation and painful sickle cell crises in children. *Blood.* 2003;101(3):846–848.

20

Sickle Cell Pain: Biology, Etiology, and Treatment

Samir K. Ballas and James R. Eckman

INTRODUCTION

Definition of Acute Pain Episodes

Pain is an unpleasant sensory and emotional experience. Acute pain episodes in sickle cell disease are mildly to excruciatingly unpleasant sensory and emotional experiences that occur episodically and unpredictably in one or many parts of the body, lasting from hours to weeks for which there is no other pathological explanation. Episodes of acute pain are the most common and distressing manifestations of sickle cell disease for the affected individual and their families. Their onset is early in life and unpredictable recurrences cause life-long suffering; they are disruptive to social and psychological functioning; they result in frequent utilization of healthcare resources, and they are a predictor of reduced survival.[1–4]

Pain can occur anywhere, be localized to one or a few areas, be migratory, or be generalized. Back, chest, extremities, and joints are most often involved. Swelling and tenderness over affected areas and low-grade fever are common.[5–7] The pain episode occurs in phases[8–10] with an average length of approximately 10 days in adults.[11]

The pathophysiology of painful episodes is poorly understood despite years of investigation. Observations during acute painful events suggest they result from diffuse ischemia of bones and muscles caused by disruption of blood flow in small and large blood vessels.[12–14] The pathogenesis of the disruption of blood flow is complex and not well understood and is likely to be related to sickle cell–related vasoocclusion and vasculopathy, whose proximate cause is polymerization of deoxygenated sickle hemoglobin (HbS).[15–17] Factors that contribute to vasoocclusion include blood viscosity, entrapment of irreversibly sickled cells (ISCs), adhesion of sickle erythrocytes to vascular endothelium and other cells, changes in vascular tone from nitric oxide (NO) consumption, activation of coagulation, inflammation, and vascular remodeling.[17–22] The onset of sickle pain episodes simultaneously in many different parts of the body suggests that circulating factors such as inflammatory cytokines, free hemoglobin, and activated coagulation proteins could be of cardinal importance.

Pain is reported as intense and unremitting. One patient characterized his pain as, "like all of the bones in my body breaking at once." Another reported, "the pain of childbirth was nowhere near as severe." The life-long occurrence, intensity, unpredictable nature, and its duration make sickle pain unique, which causes psychological and social problems for patients.

As patients age, and if their acute pain is not appropriately treated, they can develop chronic pain syndromes that make coping more difficult. Repeated bone infarctions, spinal changes, and avascular necrosis of the hips and shoulders can cause severe unremitting pain that becomes a challenge for the patient and healthcare provider. Inadequate treatment and also overtreatment can lead to severe disability and chronic suffering.[23]

ACUTE PAIN EPISODES

Pathophysiology of Pain

Vasoocclusion, which can involve the micro- and macrovasculature, is a key pathophysiological event that explains many of the clinical manifestations of sickle cell disease and is the presumed prerequisite for the development of acute pain.[18,19,24–30] Tissue damage due to vasoocclusion initiates a series of complex biochemical, neurological, and electrochemical events, collectively referred to as nociception, that culminate in the perception of acute pain. Acute pain can become chronic.[31,32] Vasoocclusion is also responsible for creating a state of chronic vascular inflammation.[33,34] Psychological, social, cultural, and spiritual factors often interact with vasoocclusion to produce the unique nature of sickle cell pain.

Cellular and Molecular Mechanisms of Pain

Nociception involves four major pathophysiological processes that seem to occur in tandem to explain the pain experience (Table 20.1, Fig. 20.1). They are transduction, transmission, modulation, and perception (Fig. 20.2).[31,32,35–38]

Transduction

Transduction is the process through which noxious inflammatory mediators (collectively referred to as inflammatory soup) activate nociceptors (naked nerve endings) by converting chemical, mechanical, or thermal energy to an electrochemical impulse in the primary afferent nerve fibers. The "soup" contains prostaglandins, histamine, bradykinin, H^+, K^+, cytokines, serotonin, substance P, calcitonin gene–related peptide (CGRP), leukotrienes, and

Table 20.1. Pathophysiology of sickle cell pain

- Vasoocclusion
  - Tissue Damage
    - Nociception
      - Transduction
        - Transmission
          - Modulation
            - Perception

These pathophysiological events seem to occur in tandem.

more (Fig. 20.3).[39] These inflammatory mediators sensitize or activate nociceptors in the primary afferent nerve fibers. The relative abundance of these mediators might explain some clinical findings. Interleukin-1 is an endogenous pyrogen and also activates the cyclooxygenase gene, which leads to synthesis of prostaglandins E_2 and I_2. Bradykinin, potassium, and hydrogen ions, and serotonin activate nociceptive afferent nerve fibers and evoke a pain response.[40,41] Prostaglandins, leukotrienes, nerve growth factor, and bradykinin also sensitize peripheral nerve endings and facilitate the transmission of painful stimuli that reach the cerebral cortex via the spinal cord and the thalamus. Moreover, activated nociceptors release stored substance P in peripheral nerves and in the spinal cord, which facilitates the transmission of painful stimuli. Bradykinin and substance P also cause vasodilation with extravasation of fluids that can lead to local swelling and tenderness.[41] Prostaglandins increase the effective renal blood flow and effective renal plasma flow in children and young adults (Chapter 19).[42]

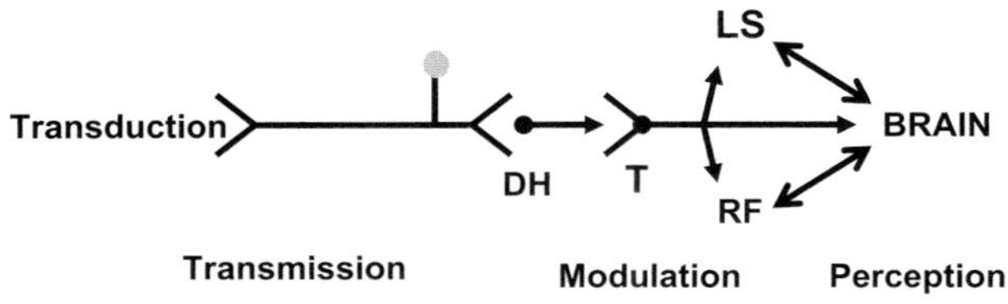

Figure 20.1. Molecular mechanisms of pain. DH, dorsal horn; T, thalamus; LS, limbic system; RF, reticular formation.

The conversion of chemical, mechanical, or thermal energy into electrochemical impulses occurs by depolarization of the neuronal membrane (Fig. 20.4). Depolarization occurs by simple diffusion of Na^+ and K^+ into and out of the axon fiber, thus decreasing the normal action potential or the threshold for electrical excitability to propagate the painful stimulus.[43] Many drugs such as anesthetics, anticonvulsants, opioids, and benzodiazepines exert their effect by causing hyperpolarization of the cell membrane. Hyperpolarization can be achieved by decreasing

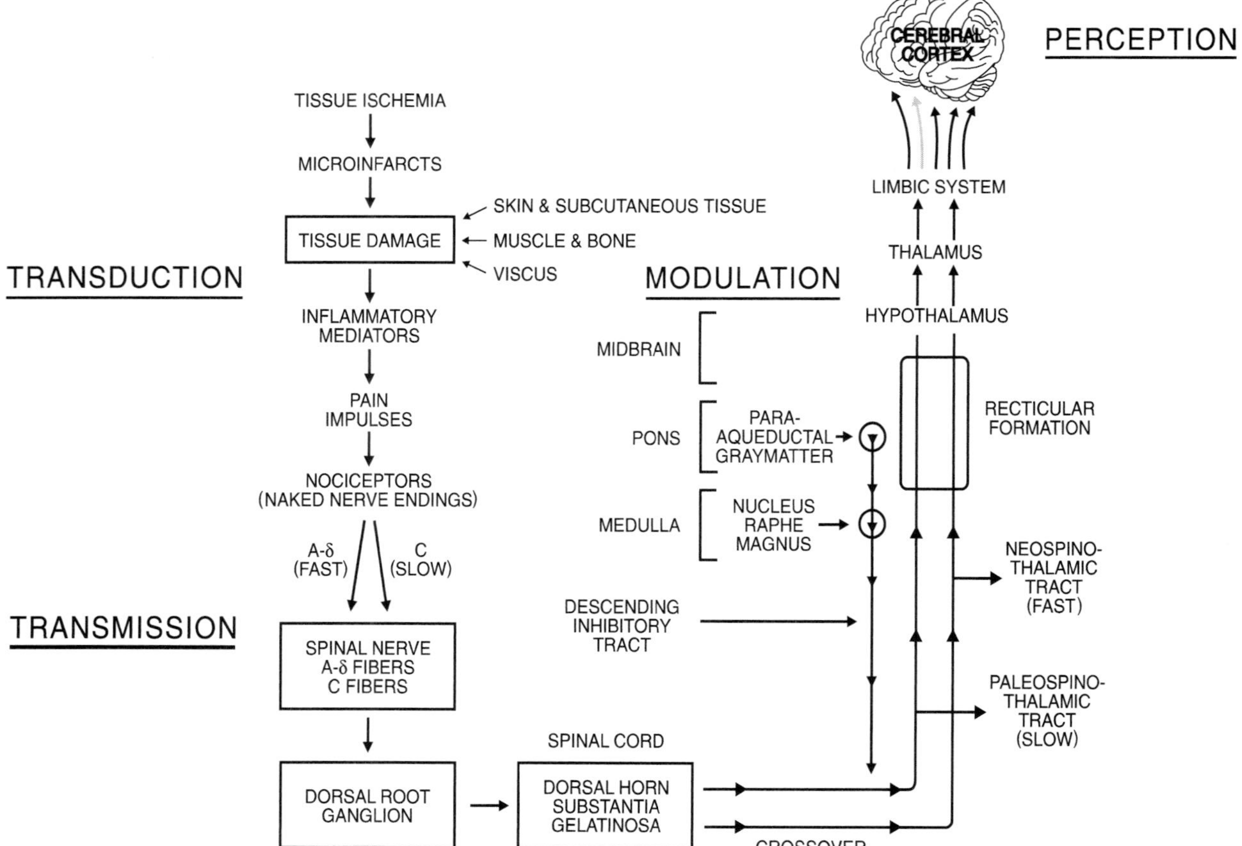

Figure 20.2. Anatomical pathways of pain in sickle cell disease. (Modified from ref. 39 with permission.) (See color plate 20.2.)

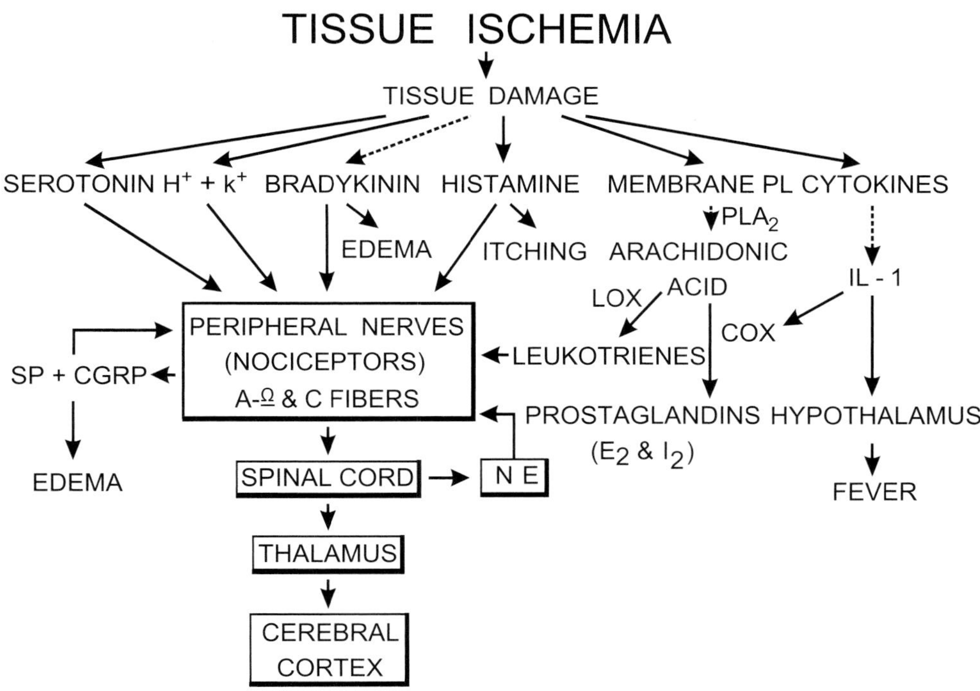

Figure 20.3. Pain pathways. Tissue damage results in the release of numerous inflammatory mediators that initiate the production of noxious stimuli. These activate peripheral nerves that in turn transmit painful stimuli to the central nervous system. (Modified from ref. 40 with permission.)

the entry of Na^+ into the cell (anesthetics and anticonvulsants), enhancing the exit of K^+ from cells (opioids), enhancing the entry of Cl^- into cells (benzodiazepines), or by other mechanisms.[40] Sudden discontinuation of medications that cause hyperpolarization might result in rebound depolarization, increased pain intensity, seizures, or status epilepticus.

Transmission

Transmission is a process by which electrical impulses carrying coded information about noxious stimuli are relayed to and through the central nervous system to brain regions where pain sensation is perceived. The neural pathways established in transmission include primary afferent nociceptor nerves, the dorsal root ganglion, dorsal horn cells of the spinal cord, spinothalamic tracts, the thalamus, and the thalamocortical projections to the somatosensory cortex. These sites also have connections with other areas of the nervous system including but not limited to the sympathetic system, microglia, the limbic system, the hypothalamus, and reticular formation (Figs. 20.1 and 20.2).[44]

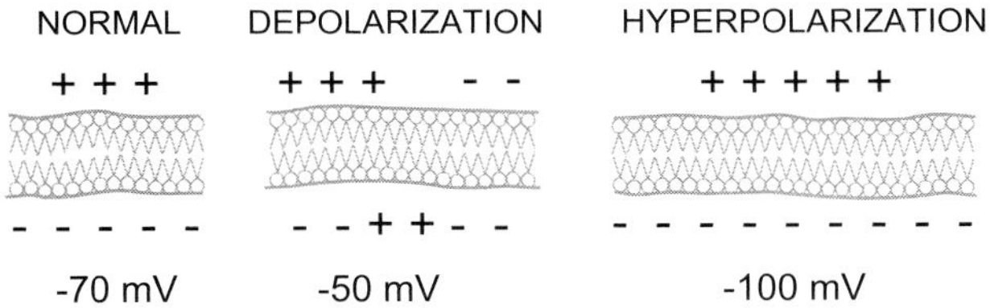

Figure 20.4. Action potential across axonal membrane during depolarization and hyperpolarization compared with normal.

Primary afferent nociceptors (PANS) are involved in both transduction and transmission. Several somatic PANS are located in skin, subcutaneous tissue, muscles, and joints. These subtypes are defined by their microscopic appearance, conduction, velocity, and pattern of response to chemical, thermal, and mechanical stimuli. Visceral PANS are found in the gastrointestinal tract, cardiopulmonary system, and genitourinary tract; they are activated by irritation, torsion, traction, and distention, particularly in conjunction with inflammation. Impulses generated by visceral nociceptors are conducted via splanchnic nerve fibers.

Impulses generated by activation of nociceptors are conducted by specific fibers within peripheral nerves. Table 20.2 summarizes the characteristics of these nerve fibers, which are classified into types A, B, and C according to size and conduction velocity of noxious stimuli.[31,43] The Aδ and C fibers are most important in transmitting the painful stimuli of acute sickle cell pain. Aδ fibers are thin myelinated fibers, approximately 50% of which respond to noxious mechanical, thermal, or chemical stimuli. They elicit sharp, localized pain. In contrast, C fibers, conducting at less than 2 m/s, are unmyelinated, respond to mechanical, thermal, and chemical stimuli, and elicit dull, diffuse pain sensations.

Central pain mechanisms involve the dorsal horn of the spinal cord, ascending spinothalamic tracts, and the cerebral cortex. The dorsal horn region of the spinal cord receives pain stimuli from the Aδ and C fibers of the spinal

Table 20.2. Characteristics of primary afferent nociceptors

Type	Stimulus	Conduction velocity (m/s)	Diameter (μm)	Sensation
Aβ	Mechanical, motor, pressure, proprioception	30–70	5–15	Sharp pain, allodynia
Aδ	Mechanical, thermal, nociception	5–30	1.4	Sharp, localized pain
C	Mechanical, thermal, chemical	0.2–1.5	0.5–1.5	Dull, diffuse pain

From ref. 44 with permission.

and cranial nerves via the dorsal root ganglion (Fig. 20.2). Afferent fibers that enter the spinal cord laterally in the dorsal root bifurcate, ascend, and descend in the Lissauer tract, and synapse in the dorsal horn with a complex structure consisting of six laminae, with lamina I the most dorsal. Each lamina corresponds to some of the horn's anatomical and functional characteristics. Cells in laminae I, II, and V respond preferentially to noxious stimuli. Laminae II and III constitute the substantia gelatinosa, where nociceptive and nonnociceptive input into the spinal cord are integrated.[45,46]

Primary afferent nociceptors form synaptic connections with neurons in laminae I, II, and V in the dorsal horn. Some of these dorsal horn neurons cross over to form the contralateral spinothalamic tract that sends connections to the brainstem, hypothalamus, and thalamus. Some thalamic relay neurons connect to limbic forebrain structures associated with the emotional aspect of pain (Fig. 20.2). In addition to the spinothalamic tract, other afferent systems such as the spinoreticular and spinomesencephalic tracts provide ascending pathways for noxious stimuli.

Important events occur along the route of transmission of the painful stimulus from the afferent nerve fibers to the somatosensory cortex. These events affect the final outcome of the pain experience due to tissue damage. Some of these events are[44]

- At the level of the dorsal horn, painful stimuli may be enhanced or suppressed by several receptors. Most important among these is the N-methyl-D-aspartate (NMDA) receptors that facilitate the transmission of painful stimuli once activated.
- Excitatory amino acids are the major neurotransmitters and their receptors are located in the presynaptic terminals of primary afferents, on dorsal root ganglion cells, and at postsynaptic sites in the dorsal horn. Table 20.3 lists the major endogenous neurotransmitters and their effect on pain transmission. The most important and best-studied excitatory amino acid is glutamate, which facilitates the transmission of the painful stimulus.

Table 20.3. Major endogenous neurotransmitters and their effect on pain transmission

Neurotransmitter	Effect of pain transmission
Substance P	Excitation
L-Glutamate	Excitation
Somatostatin	Excitation
Norepinephrine	Inhibition (central) Excitation (peripheral?)
Serotonin	Inhibition (central)
Opioid peptides	
Enkephalin	Inhibition
β-Endorphin	Inhibition
Dynorphin	Inhibition

From ref. 44 with permission.

- The primary afferents are unique neurons in that their cell bodies are located in the dorsal root ganglion. The majority of primary root afferent axons project from the dorsal root ganglion to the spinal cord mostly through the dorsal root. Substance P and CGRP, which are synthesized in the dorsal root ganglion, are thus transmitted either to the spinal cord or antidromically to the periphery at the site of injury. This antidromic transmission mediates neuroinflammation characterized by pain, redness, and swelling due to the presence of substance P and CGRP. A patient with sickle cell disease who develops sudden onset of pain and swelling of a joint most likely has nociceptive inflammation due to tissue damage and edema due mostly to bradykinin. Sudden onset of pain, followed by swelling 1 or 2 days later, represents neuroinflammation where the swelling and redness is most likely due to the antidromic accumulation of substance P and CGRP. Careful history can differentiate the two types that could affect management (Table 20.4). Definite differentiation, however, requires the measurement of the mediators in tissue fluids at the affected sites.
- Activated by the primary nerve afferents, the dorsal root ganglion forms fibers that in turn activate adjacent mechanoreceptor neurons located in the intermediolateral column of the spinal cord. These activated neurons stimulate their respective sympathetic ganglia to release norepinephrine that is transmitted antidromically to the periphery via postganglionic fibers. Norepinephrine, in the setting of tissue injury, causes more spastic tissue

Table 20.4. Types of inflammation associated with acute pain

- Nociceptive inflammation
  - Release of peripheral proinflammatory metabolites
  - Acute onset of pain and swelling
- Neuroinflammation
  - Antidromic release of cytokines, substance P, and calcitonin gene–related peptide (CGRP)
  - Delayed onset of swelling and redness
  - Neuropathic pain

ischemia thus creating a vicious circle of pain (Fig. 20.3). This is the coupling of the somatosensory system (tissue damage) and the sympathetic system (neuroinflammatory response) that makes sickle cell pain unique.

- Repetitive transmission of the painful stimuli activates the dorsal root ganglion that in turn activates the astrocytes and the microglia in the spinal cord. Once activated, microglia and astrocytes upregulate the immune system to secrete proinflammatory cytokines such as tumor necrosis factor–α, interleukin-6, NO, excitatory amino acids, prostaglandins, and adenosine triphosphate that influence the induction and maintenance of pain, especially its neuropathic component. It is this novel immune-mediated pathway that seems responsible for opioid-induced hyperalgesia (see later).
- The hippocampus is the most important organelle of the limbic system.[47] As the site of memory, the memory of a previous pain experience might affect the characteristics of subsequent painful events. A relationship between memory and pain is suggested by the observation that patients with chronic pain who developed sudden onset of amnesia had pain relief without medication.[48]

Modulation

Modulation is the process by which transmission of nociceptive stimuli are modified. The mechanisms involved can enhance or inhibit their transmission (Table 20.3).[44] Pain modulation occurs at the level of the dorsal horn of the spinal cord. Proposed neural mechanisms include segmental sensory inputs and the descending inhibitory tract.

The supraspinal descending neural systems have considerable modulating influence on dorsal horn pain transmission neurons.[49,50] One such pathway begins in the periaqueductal gray matter (Fig. 20.2) of the midbrain and descends to the nucleus raphe magnus. From here, long fibers descend via the dorsolateral funiculus to terminate in laminae I, II, and V of the dorsal horn, where they modulate afferent nociceptive impulses.[39] Both electrical stimulation and opiate microinjection of the periaqueductal gray matter result in analgesia; both these forms of analgesia are abolished by naloxone. Neurotransmitters of the inhibitory descending pathway include norepinephrine and serotonin.

Perception

Perception is the final outcome of the interactions of transduction, transmission, and modulation with the unique environment, genetic makeup, and the psychosocial status of the individual to perceive mild, moderate, or severe pain.

EPIDEMIOLOGY OF PAIN IN SICKLE CELL DISEASE

Acute Pain Episodes

Acute pain punctuates the clinical course of most patients with sickle cell disease. These episodes include, among others, acute painful episodes, dactylitis, acute splenic sequestration, splenic infarcts or subcapsular hemorrhage, avascular necrosis of joints, bone infarcts, acute chest syndrome, priapism, hepatic crises, and leg ulcers (Chapter 19).[24,25,44] The acute sickle cell painful episode, however, is the hallmark of sickle cell disease, the number one cause of treatment in the Emergency Department (ED) and of hospitalization.[51]

The frequency of acute pain episodes varies within and among individuals from rare occurrences during a lifetime to many times a month.[7] Approximately 30% of patients have rare or no pain episodes, 50% have occasional episodes, and 20% have weekly or monthly episodes requiring medical attention.[52] The frequency of pain episodes increases late in the second decade of life and decreases in frequency after the fourth decade, for reasons that are not understood.[1,7] More than three episodes a year is associated with a reduced life expectancy.[1] A small number of patients account for the majority of patients requiring healthcare for acute pain episodes.[1] Among the predisposing factors, there are at least three elements that seem to predict the frequency and severity of the acute sickle cell painful episode. They include genetic, cellular, and environmental factors.

Genetic factors include fetal hemoglobin (HbF) level, the coinheritance of α or β thalassemia, the coinheritance of other hemoglobin variants such as HbC, the nature of the β-like globin gene cluster haplotype, and sex. Unknown genetic factors are also likely to be important. As a rule, the higher the level of HbF, the milder is the disease and the less frequent are the painful episodes.[30,53,54] The coinheritance of β^+ thalassemia, HbC, and hyperhemolysis decreases the frequency of episodes. The Senegalese β-gene haplotype seems to be associated with fewer episodes than the Benin or the CAR haplotypes, most likely because of the higher HbF level in these patients (Chapter 27).[55] Females are admitted less frequently to the hospital than males, but they have longer hospital stays.[51,56]

Cellular factors associated with decreased erythrocyte deformability and increased numbers of dense cells in the steady state have a salutary effect, most likely because these are associated with more severe anemia and, hence, relatively decreased whole blood viscosity.[57,58] Conversely, patients with sickle cell anemia and relatively high hemoglobin levels are more likely to experience more frequent episodes than those patients with lower hemoglobin levels.[59,59a]

Nocturnal hypoxia, sleep apnea, and nutritional factors such as vitamin A deficiency are environmental factors amenable to preventative therapy.[60,61]

Patients often relate onset of pain to emotional stress, changes in weather, exposure to cold, dehydration, infection, fatigue, and overexertion. Major reported factors that seem to precipitate vasoocclusive events include dehydration; physical, traumatic, physiological, psychosocial, or emotional stress; infection; acidosis; sleep apnea; climate; and pregnancy.[23,44] Nevertheless, most painful episodes are not preceded by an obvious precipitating factor. Daily mood and stress predict painful events, utilization of healthcare facilities, and work activity in adults.[62]

Anecdotally, many patients report that sudden changes in temperature seem to precipitate acute painful episodes. Several studies have found an increased incidence of pain episodes during cold and rainy weather.[63–65] Others have disputed this association, although these studies were underpowered because of sample size.[66–69] The effect of high wind and low humidity is likely to be related to skin cooling. More recent studies suggest that windy dry weather and increased air pollution might precipitate pain episodes.[70,71,71a] Patients' suggestion that swimming or exposure to cold water is a precipitant was directly supported in one study.[72]

Frequent or Chronic Pain

Studies using pain diaries in children, adolescents, and adults show that much of the pain experience in sickle cell disease does not come to the attention of the health professionals as acute pain episodes because it is managed successfully at home.[3,73–78] A recent study in 232 adults characterized pain over 6 months. Pain was reported on 54.5% of analyzed patient days; pain without healthcare utilization was present on 12.7% of days; pain resulting in healthcare utilization occurred on only 3.5% of analyzed days.[78] Only 14.2% of patients reported pain on less than 5% of days and 29.3% reported pain on more than 95% of days.[78] This suggests that the majority of patients have frequent pain and that previous studies based on ED visits and hospitalizations have greatly underestimated the frequency and severity of pain in adults with sickle cell disease. These findings have importance in defining the epidemiology of pain in sickle cell disease, managing pain, and in designing outcome studies in which impact on pain frequency and severity is important.

Phases of the Acute Painful Episode

The concept that the painful episode evolves in phases was introduced by Ballas and Smith[9] and Akinola et al.[79] who, in prospective longitudinal studies of adults, independently described the presence of two phases of the uncomplicated painful episode. Akinola et al. studied 20 patients over 16 months, and Ballas and Smith studied 117 painful events affecting 36 patients with sickle cell anemia over 6 years. Both studies indicated the presence of two phases. The initial phase was associated with increasing pain, decreased red cell deformability, increases in the number of dense cells, red cell distribution width ([RDW], see Chapter 28), hemoglobin distribution width (HDW), reticulocyte count, leukocyte count, and a decrease in the number of platelets. The second phase was characterized by established pain of maximum severity and gradual reversal of the abnormalities of the first phase. Later, Ballas[80] revised the description of the painful episode and redefined its evolution into four

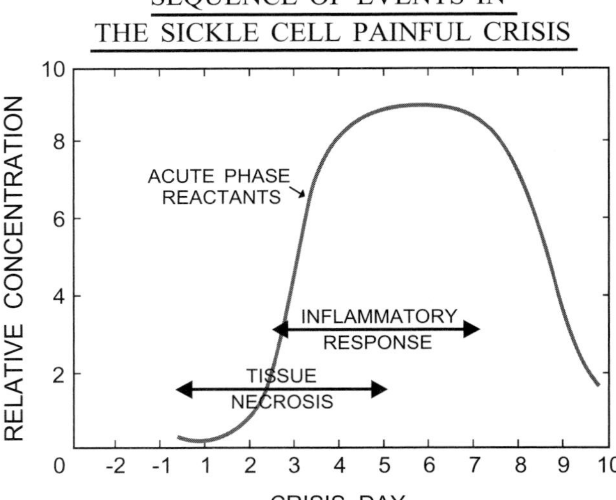

Figure 20.5. In situ sickling initiates a vicious circle of ischemic tissue damage and subsequent inflammatory response.

phases by including observations by several other investigators. The characteristics of these phases are described and illustrated in Figure 20.5 and are termed, prodromal, initial, established, and resolving. Subsequent studies in children found that the painful episodes also evolved in phases, although the phases were named differently.[10,81]

The evolution of the uncomplicated painful episode allows the observer to determine the presence of objective signs. This requires careful baseline observations when the individual is well and serial laboratory studies during the episode. The presence of phases permits the provider to monitor the progress of the event and manage it rationally, thus avoiding the conflicts that often arise between patients and providers about the authenticity of pain. Several parameters change at variable points in the progression of a painful episode.

Outcomes of the Painful Episode

Objective Signs

Severe painful events are usually associated with fever up to 101°F (38.3°C) and sometimes more. Fever develops after the onset of pain and gradually declines as the pain severity decreases.[5,25,57] Up to 21% of the painful episodes that required hospitalization were accompanied by fever of at least 100°F (37.8°C) in the absence of infection whereas another nearly 15% of the events were associated with swelling, tenderness, or vomiting.[57] Passage of dark urine is common and could reflect increased urinary porphyrin excretion.[82] Painful episodes can also be associated with joint effusion.[25,83,84] Aspirates are usually sterile and are thought to result from nociceptive or neuroinflammation, as described previously. Joint effusions can be mild and unilateral or severe and migratory.[85,86] These signs of the painful episode reflect the accumulation of inflammatory mediators such as bradykinin and substance P that are known to cause local pain, vasodilation, extravasations of fluids, and edema.[87] Other clinical signs include tenderness or pressure over affected sites, usually over bone.[88–90] Acute urinary retention and muscle swelling and tenderness due to myonecrosis can also occur.[89–91]

Erythrocyte Changes

Red blood cell changes during the acute sickle cell painful episode have centered on hemoglobin levels, the percentages of ISCs and dense cells, RDW, HDW, and red cell deformability. Erythrocyte changes are biphasic. Early in the event the number of dense cells, RDW, and HDW increase, whereas red cell deformability and hemoglobin concentration level decrease. Three to 5 days into the episode, there is reversal in these parameters to levels higher than those in the steady state. Serial examination of the peripheral smear also reflects these changes. Early in the episode there is abundance of ISCs that disappear almost completely when the episode resolves.

Hyperhemolysis

The decrease in hemoglobin level with concomitant increase in reticulocyte count seems to be most probably due to transient hyperhemolysis that occurs in some patients during uncomplicated painful episode. This has been confirmed in selected patients by finding decreased red cell survival during the evolution of the painful episode.[92]

Changes in Leukocytes

The white blood cell count increases during painful episodes to levels higher than those of the steady state.[93] This occurs in the absence of overt infection and might be secondary to the inflammatory response to ischemic tissue damage. If an infectious process complicates the painful episode, the leukocyte count will increase further and be associated with an increase in the percentage of band cells. One study reported no significant change in leukocyte count from steady state to painful episode, but a decrease from days 1–3 to 6–9 of hospitalization.[94] Others found that the white blood cell count was elevated on day 1 of the episode, reached a peak on days 3–5, and then decreased toward steady state values after the day 6.[79]

Changes in Platelets

Patients with sickle cell anemia usually have increased platelet counts in the steady state, with a mean value of $320 \times 10^3/\mu L$.[95–97] Some studies reported that platelet counts did not change during painful episodes irrespective of the presence or absence of infection.[94,95,98] The lifespan of autologous platelets in adult patients is one-third of normal. Platelet counts decrease during an acute pain episode,

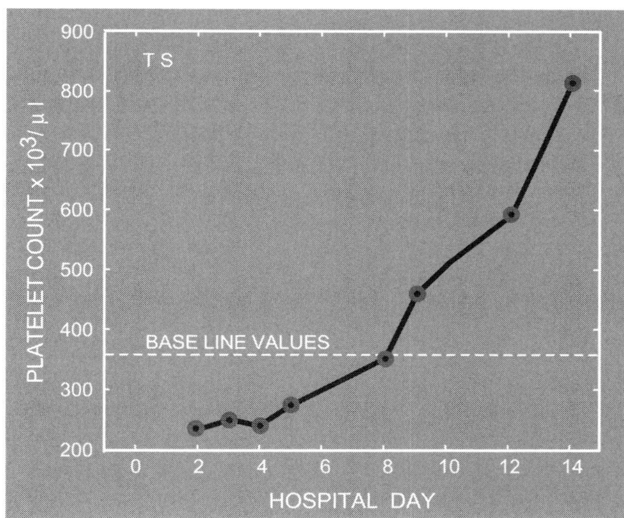

Figure 20.6. Typical changes in the platelet count during an acute sickle cell painful episode.

rebound to levels above those of the steady state during the second week following the onset of pain, and platelet aggregation, normal during the acute episode, increases during the period of rebound thrombocytosis (Fig. 20.6).[96,99–101]

Blunted Pain Relief

In some patients, a blunted response to analgesic therapy with failure to achieve adequate pain relief occurs after the fourth–sixth hospital day.[51,102,103] Although these patients had significant decrease in intensity of pain from the first day of hospitalization to the fourth–sixth day, they continued to have severe pain with an intensity score of more than 6/10 at discharge (Fig. 20.7). These patients were the most likely to be readmitted within a few days to 1 week after discharge. The reasons for this blunting in pain relief are unknown. Possible causes include inadequate pain management, increase in the level of acute phase reactants that bind to opioids and make them unavailable for pain relief, the development of tolerance to opioids, hyperalgesia, or changes at the opioid receptor sites.

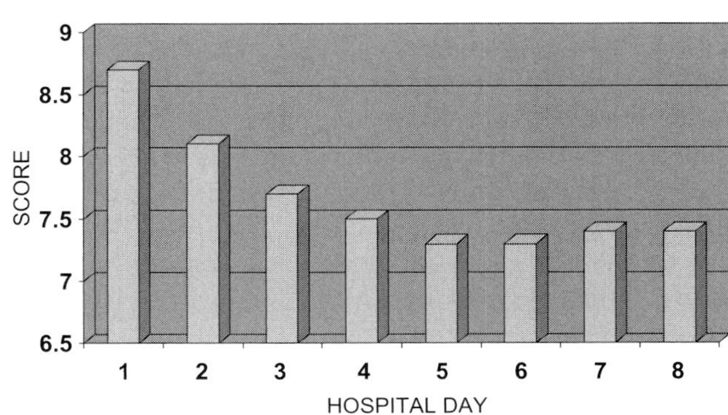

Figure 20.7. Pain intensity scores during hospitalization for acute painful episodes in 1998–2002. (Adopted from ref. 51 with permission.)

Hypercoagulability

As the acute episode resolves, markers of hypercoagulability can be seen. These include, increased serum fibrinogen, increased orosomucoid, thrombocytosis, increased sedimentation rate, and increased plasma viscosity.[80] Together these suggest a hypercoagulable state that could promote further vasoocclusion.[104]

Relapsing Pain Episodes and Hospital Readmission

Approximately 16% of patients with sickle cell disease are readmitted to the hospital with a painful episode within 1 week and approximately 50% within 1 month of discharge.[9,51] Other studies reported an average time between admissions of 10.7 days, with 50% readmissions within 8 days, and 77% within 21 days after discharge.[105]

Possible reasons for rapid hospital readmission include premature discharge, opioid withdrawal, a new acute painful episode, and maladaptive behavior. Withdrawal syndrome can precipitate a new acute painful episode and might be iatrogenic in nature. Providers who are unfamiliar with the patients or the disease often feel uncomfortable writing prescriptions for outpatient opioids. Consequently, patients might go home with no prescription or with one for insufficient medication. The dose taken at home would then be much smaller than the dose taken in the hospital. This sudden decrease in opioid dose precipitates withdrawal syndrome in some patients. Another reason for readmission is the occurrence of a genuinely new acute painful episode that could be due to the hypercoagulable state generated by a previous resolving episode or a change in the distribution of circulating sickle erythrocytes. Patient outcomes after hospital discharge can be improved if their postdischarge care is with physicians who treated them in the hospital rather than with other physicians.[106] Adverse events occurred in approximately 20% of patients in the peridischarge period with adverse drug events and medical errors occurring most frequently during the first 2 weeks of discharge.[107] Although not specific to patients with sickle cell disease, the postdischarge period is one of vulnerability that could conceivably contribute to early readmission.

Maladaptive behavior could potentially be a cause of readmission. This seems to be the exception rather than the rule and seems to apply to approximately 3% of readmitted patients.[51] Morbidity and mortality rates seem to be higher in patients with frequent painful episodes that require hospital admission and readmission.

These data suggest that special attention must be paid to the resolving phase of the painful episode. Providers using aggressive pain therapy during hospitalization should exclude the possibility of tolerance, consider opioid rotation, and design discharge instructions that avoid causing withdrawal. The establishment of a clinic to evaluate patients within a few days after discharge to ensure compliance with discharge instructions is recommended.

PHARMACOLOGICAL MANAGEMENT OF SICKLE CELL PAIN

Complementary and Alternative Medications

Rational and effective management of sickle cell pain relies on thorough assessment and individualization of therapy coupled with the use of nonpharmacological and pharmacological approaches.

Pharmacological management of sickle cell pain entails the use of three major classes of compounds: nonopioids, opioids, and adjuvants (Tables 20.5–20.7). Some patients use complementary and alternative supplements on their own, based on hearsay, advertisements, or the media. Such medications are available over the counter or at health food outlets and include antioxidants, vitamins, herbal products, magnesium, garlic extract, glucosamine, and others. Patients should be advised to use these products only after discussion and approval by their care providers to avoid possible deleterious interactions with approved opioids and nonopioids.

Niprisan, a phytomedicine, in a phase 2B study of 82 patients with sickle cell disease, was effective in reducing episodes of painful episodes associated with severe pain over a 6-month period, without serious side effects.[108] It did not affect the risk of severe complications or the level of anemia. A phase 3 multicenter trial of this agent has not been reported. In a study of 19 hospitalized children with sickle cell disease given intravenous magnesium sulfate, the duration of hospital stay was reduced compared with historical controls.[109] It was not clear if the response to magnesium sulfate was dose dependent, and a randomized, controlled study is needed to confirm these promising findings.

Clinical Pharmacology of Analgesics: General Features

A major difference between opioids and nonsteroidal anti-inflammatory drugs (NSAIDs) is that the latter have a ceiling effect. This is a dose above which there is no additive analgesic effect. NSAIDs are associated with serious systemic side effects such as gastritis, nephropathy, and hemostatic defects.

Opioid analgesics have fewer systemic side effects than NSAIDs, but their use in sickle cell disease is associated with many misconceptions and phobias. They are the most-often used class of drug for severe sickle cell pain. Opioid agonists can be given orally, subcutaneously, intramuscularly, intravenously, transdermally, and transmucosally, and the methods of parenteral administration include continuous intravenous drip, patient-controlled analgesia (PCA) pump, or intermittent injections. Other routes of administration such as nebulization, iontophoresis, topical, epidural, or implantable intrathecal drug delivery systems are rarely, if ever, used in sickle cell disease. Meperidine, morphine, hydromorphone, and fentanyl are the major opioid analgesics used in the treatment of severe pain in the ED and the hospital. Oxycodone with codeine is most

Table 20.5. Dosing equivalents and starting doses for nonopioid analgesics*

Drug	Usual dose for adults and children >50 kg	Usual dose for children and adults <50 kg body weight	Comments
Acetaminophen	650–1000 mg q 4 h	10–15 mg/kg q 4 h 15–20 mg/kg q 4 h rectal	Liquid available, not antiinflammatory, use with caution in liver disease
NSAIDs			Use with caution with renal or heart failure
Aspirin	650–1000 mg q 4 h	10–15 mg/kg q 4 h 15–20 mg/kg q 4 h rectal	Not safe in febrile children, inhibits platelet function
Ibuprofen	400–600 mg q 6–8 h	10 mg/kg q 6–8 h	
Naproxen	500 mg initial then 250 mg q 6–8 h	10–20 mg/kg/d in divided doses q 8–12 h	Available as a liquid
Naproxen sodium	550 mg initial then 275 mg q 6–8 h	10–20 mg/kg/d in divided doses q 8–12 h	
Choline magnesium trisalicylate	1000–1500 mg q 12 h		Minimal platelet inhibition, liquid available
Diclofenac potassium	50 mg q 8 h		Maximum 200 mg first day then 150 mg/d
Diflunisal	1000 mg initial then 500 mg q 12 h		
Etodolac	200–400 mg q 6–8 h		
Flurbiprofen	50–100 mg q 8–12 h		Maximum 300 mg/d
Fenoprofen	200 mg q 4–6 h		
Ketoprofen	25–50 mg q 6–8 h		Maximum 75 mg/d
Ketorolac tromethamine	10 mg PO q 6–8 h		Not to exceed 5 d
Magnesium salsalate	650 mg q 4 h		
Meclofenamate sodium	50 mg q 4–6 h		Maximum 400 mg/d
Mefenamic acid	250 mg q 6 h		Maximum 7 d
Piroxicam	20 mg q 24 h		
Salsalate	500 mg q 6 h		
Sulindac	200 mg q 12 h		
Ketorolac tromethamine parenteral	30–60 mg initial then 15–30 mg q 6–8 h	0.5 mg/kg IM/IV q 6 h up to 72 h; 1.0 mg/kg IM/IV q 6 h 24–48 h	Maximum daily 120 mg Not to exceed 5 d

Modified from Acute pain management panel. Acute Pain Management: Operative or Medical Procedures and Trauma. Clinical Practice Guideline. AHCPR No. 92-0032. Rockville, MD Agency for Health Care Policy and Research. United State Department of Health and Human Services, 1992.

* Black box warning for heart disease and gastrointestinal bleeding. Contraindicated with congestive heart failure or renal insufficiency. Consult package insert for other Contraindications, Drug Interactions, and Adverse Reactions.

often used to treat painful episodes of mild or moderate severity at home.[110] Opioids such as extended-release (ER) oxycodone and ER morphine, or long-acting opioids such as methadone and levorphanol are useful in the management of chronic pain at home in combination with short-acting opioids for breakthrough pain.

The concurrent administration of adjuvant medications with the primary opioid analgesics can enhance their analgesic potential and obviate or ameliorate opioid side effects. Anticonvulsants can be useful especially if the pain has a neuropathic component. Adjuvant drugs commonly used in the management of sickle cell pain are listed in Table 20.7. These agents have their own set of side effects and hence, their use should be carefully monitored. Some of the side effects overlap with those of sickle cell disease. For example, some antidepressants like trazodone are associated with priapism and might best be avoided.

The choice of an opioid, its dose, and route of administration should be individualized based on history and experience. No single opioid constitutes a panacea for all patients. Any opioid might be the treatment of choice in a patient. A general trend is to avoid the use of meperidine, to administer opioids orally for mild pain and intravenously or subcutaneously for severe pain, and avoid the intramuscular route if possible.

The use of meperidine is controversial.[111–113] Meperidine is associated with seizures in 1%–12% of patients with sickle cell disease.[114] A retrospective study of hospitalized children reported a very low rate of seizures in sickle cell disease patients receiving meperidine, which was comparable with that observed in patients receiving morphine.[115] In a subset of adult patients with sickle cell disease, meperidine is the only opioid that gives relief without serious side effects.

Table 20.6. Dosing equivalents and starting doses for opioid analgesics in opioid naïve patients*

		Approximate equianalgesic dose		Appropriate starting dose adults >50 kg body weight		Appropriate starting dose children & adults <50 kg body weight†		
Opioid agonist	Active agent	Oral	Parenteral	Oral	Parenteral	Oral	Parenteral	Comments
Morphine	M6G and M3G	30 mg regular 60 mg single dose	10 mg	IR 30 mg q 3–4 h SR 90 mg q 12 h	10 mg q 3–4 h	0.3 mg/kg q 3–4 h	0.3 mg/kg q 3–4 h	Available for rectal administration
Codeine	Morphine	130 mg	75 mg	60 mg q 3–4 h	60 mg q 2 h	1 mg/kg q 3–4 h	Not used	
Hydrocodone	Hydromorphone	30 mg	Not available	10 mg q 3–4 h	Not available	0.2 mg/kg q 3–4 h	Not available	
Oxycodone	Oxymorphone	30 mg	Not available	10 q 3–4 h	Not available	0.2 mg/kg q 3–4 h	Not available	
Meperidine	Normeperidine	300 mg	100 mg	Not recommended	100 mg q 3 h	Not recommended	0.75 mg/kg q 2–3 h	
Hydromorphone	Same	7.5 mg	1.5 mg	6 mg q 3–4 h	1.5 mg q 3–4 h	0.06 mg/kg q 3–4 h	0.015 mg/kg q 3–4 h	Available for rectal administration
Methadone	Same	20 mg	10 mg	20 mg q 6–8 h	10 mg q 6–8 h	0.2 mg/kg q 6–8 h	0.1 mg/kg q 6–8 h	May accumulate with repeated dosing
Levorphanol	Same	4 mg	2mg	4 mg q 6–8 h	2 mg q 6–8 h	0.04 mg/kg q 6–8 h	0.02 mg/kg q 6–8 h	
Oxymorphone	Same	Not available	1 mg	Not available	1 mg q 3–4 h	Not available	Not recommended	Available for rectal administration
Fentanyl	Same	Transdermal fentanyl dosing does not convert to equianalgesic single-dose morphine equivalents. Dosing should be based on package insert. Doses > 25 μg/h should not be used in opioid naïve patients.						
Agonist/ antagonists		Oral equianalgesic	Parenteral equianalgesic	Oral adults >50 kg	Parenteral adults >50 kg	Oral child or adult <50 kg	Parenteral child or adult <50 kg[1]	
Nalbuphine	Same	Not available	10 mg	Not available	10 mg q 3–4 h	Not available	0.1 mg/kg q 3–4 h	Maximum 20 mg q 3 h and 160 mg in 24 h
Buprenorphine	Same	Not available	0.3–0.4 mg	Not available	0.6 mg then 0.3 mg g 6–8 h	Not available	0.004 mg/kg q 6–8 h in children >2 y	Maximum 0.6 mg q 6 h
Butorphanol	Same	Not available	2 mg	Not available	2 mg q 3–4 h	Not available	Not recommended	
Pentazocine	Same	150 mg	60 mg	50 mg q 4–6 h	Not recommended	Not recommended	Not recommended	Maximum 360 mg in 24 h

Modified from acute pain management panel. Acute Pain Management: Operative or Medical Procedures and Trauma. Clinical Practice Guideline. AHCPR No. 92-0032. Rockville, MD Agency for Health Care Policy and Research. United State Department of Health and Human Services, 1992.

* Doses do not apply for patients with hepatic disease, renal insufficiency, or diseases that alter drug metabolism or kinetics. Sickle cell disease may affect drug metabolism and kinetics; however, pharmacokinetic data specific to this population are not available in the literature. Consult package insert for other contraindications, drug interactions, and adverse reactions.

† Recommendations on use and dosing for infants younger than 6 months of age cannot be made.

Table 20.7. Adjuvant drugs useful in treating sickle cell pain

• Antihistamines	• Antidepressants
• Antiemetics	• Anticonvulsants
• Laxatives	• Benzodiazepines
• α2-Adrenergic agonists (Clonidine)	• Other miscellaneous agents
• Phenothiazines	

The use of implantable intravenous access devices in patients with sickle cell disease seems to be associated with a higher rate of infection than in other diseases.[116] Decisions to rotate opioids should follow equianalgesic dosing equivalents, taking into consideration the comparative absorption, availability, and half-life of the opioid. Thus, the dose of oral methadone to replace the dose of ER morphine will be one-sixth the dose of morphine because methadone absorption is twice that of morphine and its half-life is three times longer than that of morphine. Moreover, the dose of methadone will take five half-lives to stabilize orally. Many recommend starting the new opioid analgesic at half the equivalent dose and then titrating to control the pain.[117] If the comparative absorption and half-lives are not known, it is advisable to do gradual conversion from one opioid to another.

Basic Pharmacology of Opioids: Pharmacokinetic and Pharmacodynamics

To manage sickle pain effectively with opioid analgesics, it is essential to know their pharmacokinetics and pharmacodynamics, including their side effects and complications. Pharmacokinetics refers to "what the body does to the drug," including absorption, distribution, binding to tissues, metabolism, and excretion. Pharmacodynamics, on the other hand, refers to "what the drug does to the body" in terms of the mechanism by which the drug produces therapeutic effects.[37,38,44,118,119] An important step in the pharmacokinetics of opioids is their conversion into metabolites that could be active or inactive (Table 20.6).[37,38,44,118,119]

Prodrugs are not active by themselves but have active metabolites. Codeine is a prodrug without an analgesic effect by itself, but its metabolite, morphine, is the active analgesic. The conversion into an active metabolite depends on the presence of the required enzyme and its polymorphic variants. Approximately 5%–10% of the general population lack the enzyme *CYP2D6* and hence, will not achieve pain relief by using codeine alone. Moreover, the enzyme is polymorphic, and some variants are more efficient in the conversion into active metabolite than others. The same principles apply to the conversion of hydrocodone into hydromorphone and oxycodone into oxymorphone. Morphine is unique in that it is an active drug itself, and its metabolites, morphine-6-gluconide (M6G) and morphine-3-glucuronide (M3G) are also active (Table 20.6).

Opioid agonists produce their effect by binding to μ receptors.[37,38,118–123] The L isomers of opioids exert analgesic activity. The binding affinity, or strength with which a drug binds to its receptors, varies considerably among opioids, with fentanyl, for example, having a higher binding affinity than morphine. The binding affinity of opioids seems to correlate well with their analgesic potency. Bound opioids activate their receptors and initiate a series of biochemical events, including activation of G-proteins, inhibition of adenylate cyclase activity, and extrusion of K^+ that results in hyperpolarization of cell membranes, resulting in delay or prevention of the transmission of painful stimuli. Moreover, receptors are also polymorphic and some variants are more efficient in mediating the analgesic effect of opioids than others. Thus, the response to opioids depends not only on the type of opioid used, but also on the number and activity of the opioid receptors. An opioid that has poor affinity and that binds to one or two receptors, for example, is unlikely to produce effective analgesia in certain patients even if the dose is high. On the other hand, an opioid with moderate- or high-binding affinity that binds to several efficient receptors would provide effective analgesia even if used in small doses. This provides a possible explanation for the immense variability in patients' response to opioids.

Characteristics of Selected Opioids

Morphine

Morphine[37,38,44,118] is a strong μ-opioid agonist. It is a naturally occurring alkaloid derived from the opium poppy; it is hydrophilic and thus is rapidly distributed to tissues and organs. It can be administered by any route and is available in immediate-, controlled-, and sustained-release formulations. Morphine is metabolized by conjugation with glucuronic acid by the enzyme uridine diphosphate–glucuronosyl transferase 2B7(*UGT2B7*) into M6G and M3G.[124] The former is four times more potent and has a longer half-life than its parent drug, explaining why sometimes repeated administration of morphine results in severe sedation. Moreover, functional allelic variants of *UGT2B7* might alter the conversion of morphine to M6G and M3G. The G allele of this enzyme (*UTG2B7* promoter variant -840G-A) is associated with reduced glucuronidation of morphine.[125] Both morphine and M6G are associated with toxicity in patients with renal failure. Morphine is highly histaminergic and is often associated with pruritus that can be severe. Other reported adverse effects of morphine in sickle cell disease include increased risk of acute chest syndrome,[126,127] acceleration of renal injury,[128] and retinopathy in transgenic sickle mice. Morphine accelerates sarcoma-induced bone pain, bone loss, and spontaneous fracture in a murine model of bone cancer.[129] Morphine, hydromorphone, and fentanyl seem to heal ischemic wounds in rats.[130]

Codeine

Codeine,[37,38,44,118] like morphine, is a naturally occurring alkaloid. It is a weak μ agonist. In the liver, approximately 10% of the dose is converted to morphine via *CYP2D6* that

Table 20.8. Commonly prescribed drugs with potential for QT interval prolongation

• Methadone	• Sumatriptan
• Erythromycin	• Venlafaxine
• Clarithromycin	• Fluoxetine
• Levofloxacin	• Indapamide
• Amitriptyline	• Sertraline
• Imipramine	• Tamoxifen
• Doxepin	• Salmeterol
• Risperidone	

is part of the cytochrome P-450 system. In addition to its absence in 10% of the population, *CYP2D6* can be duplicated in some patients. In these individuals, approximately 20% of the dose of codeine is converted to morphine with better pain relief. Codeine is available in the market as schedule II (codeine), schedule III (codeine with nonopioids like acetaminophen) and schedule V (codeine in antitussive formulations).

Methadone

Methadone,[37,38,44,118] the least expensive opioid, is a potent synthetic opioid agonist. Its formulation is a racemic mixture of L and D isomers both of which are NMDA antagonists. Only the L-isomer is a μ agonist. Methadone also mildly inhibits the reuptake of serotonin and norepinephrine and suppresses heroin and other opioid craving for 24 hours. It has a half-life of at least 36 hours, but short duration of analgesia of 4–6 hours. This difference might predispose to drug accumulation following the initiation of therapy or dose escalation.

Methadone is associated with cardiotoxicity due to prolongation of the QTc interval with arrhythmia that can be fatal. It is associated with death more than any other opioid. Other medications, such as antibiotics and antidepressants (Table 20.8), contribute to its cardiotoxic effect, and their use with methadone should be avoided or monitored carefully. Nevertheless, methadone is an excellent analgesic that is useful in treating chronic pain, provided the prescriber knows its pharmacology and has experience in its use. Careful monitoring of patients coupled with initiation of a low dose followed by gradual stepwise dose escalation or reduction decreases the risk of toxicity from its accumulation. Monitoring should include performing periodic electrocardiograms. Oral and parenteral preparations of methadone are available; subcutaneous injections cause local skin toxicity and are not recommended.

Oxycodone

Oxycodone[37,38,44,118] is a semisynthetic μ opioid derivative of morphine and has a similar profile. It is available for oral but not parenteral administration. It is metabolized in the liver into noroxycodone and oxymorphone. Like codeine, oxycodone is usually admixed with nonopioid analgesics in commercial preparation for the management of mild to moderate pain. Dose escalation is limited in the combination form because of a potential toxicity from the acetaminophen or aspirin component. It is also available as a short-acting single entity and doses can be increased to achieve pain relief. A controlled-release formulation (OxyContin) is also available but has strong abuse potential.

Hydromorphone

This semisynthetic μ agonist morphine congener is five–seven times more potent than morphine.[37,38,44,118] It is more soluble and is available in a concentrated dosage form of 10 mg/mL and has been widely used by subcutaneous infusion in PCA pumps. The bioavailability of hydromorphone by continuous subcutaneous infusion is approximately 80% of the intravenous route. An ER form of hydromorphone (Palladone) was initially approved by the Food and Drug Administration and later withdrawn from the market because of fatality associated with the use of alcohol that dissolves the formulation and releases the hydromorphone as a short-acting formulation. Nevertheless the ER formulation is available outside the United States. Hydromorphone is not contraindicated in renal failure.

Oxymorphone

Oxymorphone[37,38,44,118] is a lipophilic semisynthetic μ agonist congener of morphine. When administered parenterally it is approximately 10 times more potent than morphine. It is available in rectal formulation, which is approximately one-tenth as potent as intramuscular administration. It has a half-life of 1.2–2 hours and is less likely to produce histamine release than morphine. Its major disadvantage is its high cost. Recent oral preparations of oxymorphone include immediate-release (Opana) and extended-release (Opana ER) formulations.

Meperidine

This semisynthetic μ agonist opioid is a member of the phenylpiperidine series of μ opioid agonists.[37,38,44,111–113,118] More lipophilic than morphine, it produces euphoria, and has fast onset of action after parenteral administration. Problems with meperidine center around one of its major metabolites normeperidine. Approximately 90% of a dose of meperidine undergoes N-demethylation in the liver to produce normeperidine, which has a half-life four–five times that of meperidine (18 vs. 3.5 hours) and is twice as potent a convulsant and half as potent an analgesic as its parent compound. Accumulation of normeperidine after repetitive dosing of meperidine can result in central nervous system excitability characterized by subtle mood changes, anxiety, tremor, multifocal myoclonus, and seizures. The effects of meperidine and normeperidine on seizure induction are more pronounced in the presence of renal failure. Oral meperidine has only 15%–25% of the analgesic effectiveness but produces just as much normeperidine. Oral meperidine should not be used for control of sickle pain, and prolonged high-dose therapy should be avoided if possible. Naloxone does not reverse meperidine-induced seizures and to the contrary might precipitate seizures by blocking the depressant action of meperidine and facilitating the manifestation of the convulsant activity of normeperidine. Unlike other opioids, meperidine is anticholinergic and hence, is associated with tachycardia and does not cause constriction of the pupils.

Fentanyl

This synthetic μ agonist congener of meperidine is a member of the phenylpiperidine series (Table 20.6).[37,38,44,118] Fentanyl is extremely lipophilic and is approximately 100 times more potent than morphine as an analgesic. It is available in parenteral (Sublimaze), transdermal (Duragesic), oral transmucosal (Actiq), and buccal (Fentora) formulations.

Characteristics of Selected Nonopioid Analgesics

Tramadol (Ultram)

Tramadol[37,38,44,118] is a synthetic centrally acting analgesic, not chemically related to opiates, which acts as a weak agonist at opioid receptors with preferential affinity for the μ receptor. Moreover, it inhibits neuronal uptake of both serotonin and norepinephrine and stimulates the release of serotonin. Thus, functionally, it has properties of an opioid and an antidepressant. It seems to be as effective as acetaminophen with 30 mg codeine with the added advantage of tricyclic antidepressant-like effect. Tramadol can be used by the oral or parenteral route and it is available in slow-release form. Only the oral form is approved for marketing in the United States. Major adverse effects include seizures, abuse potential, respiratory depression, and serotonin syndrome.

Ketorolac Tromethamine (Toradol)

Ketorolac tromethamine[37,38,44,118,131] is a member of the pyrrole acetic acid group of NSAIDs. It was introduced into the United States as a short-acting parenteral analgesic and is also available in an oral formulation. Ketorolac possesses many desirable features as an adjunctive or alternative medication to opioids. After intramuscular injection, analgesia is perceptible at approximately 10 minutes, similar to opioids and the duration of analgesia is approximately 6 hours. Similar to other NSAIDs, ketorolac is highly bound to plasma proteins and is metabolized to inactive products, which are excreted in the urine. Clearance is significantly reduced in patients aged 65 years or older and in patients with renal disease.

Ketorolac has analgesic potency similar to opioids. It should be given every 6 hours to maintain a steady-state plasma level. A loading dose of 30 or 60 mg intramuscularly or intravenously should be followed by 30 mg intramuscularly or intravenously every 6 hours for 3–5 days. In patients weighing less than 60 kg or aged 65 years or older or with reduced renal function, a loading dose of 30 mg intramuscularly should be followed by 15 mg intramuscularly every 6 hours. No dosage adjustment is indicated in patients with chronic cirrhosis. The coadministration of ketorolac with opioids exerts an additional analgesic effect and decreases the amount of opioids consumed for the treatment of acute sickle cell painful episodes.[132] Unlike opioids, ketorolac does not produce respiratory depression, reduction of gastrointestinal motility, psychomotor effects, or addiction. As with other NSAIDs, heart failure, gastrointestinal, hematological, and nephrotoxic side effects are possible.

Opioid Antagonists

Traditionally, the use of opioid antagonists has been primarily limited to counteract the depressive effects of opioid agonists. Recently, however, there have been reports showing that small doses of antagonists in combination with agonists appear to enhance the analgesic effect and prevent or delay tolerance to opioid agonists.[133] Moreover, new formulations in development include the use of naltrexone in combination with oxycodone or morphine to deter abuse; this is reminiscent of the use of disulfiram (Antabuse) with alcohol.

Adverse Effects and Complications of Opioids

Adverse effects of opioid analgesics include pruritus, hives, nausea, vomiting, constipation, and respiratory depression. All opioids can induce seizures – meperidine is the most frequent inducer – if used in high doses over a long period of time. The mechanism of seizure induction by other opioids is different from that by meperidine and seems to be related to their excitatory effects. The incidence of seizure due to morphine has been reported to be 1.2%.[134] Metabolites of morphine can accumulate to toxic levels in the presence of renal failure.

The serious complications of opioids that are often misunderstood and confused with each other are collectively referred to as aberrant behavior and include addiction, physical dependence, withdrawal, tolerance, and pseudoaddiction. Their definitions according to the American Academy of Pain Medicine, American Pain Society, and American Academy of Addiction Medicine consensus document are[135]

- Tolerance, a state of adaptation in which exposure to a drug induces changes that result in a diminution of one or more of the drug's effects over time.
- Physical dependence, a state of adaptation manifested by a drug class–specific withdrawal syndrome that can

be produced by abrupt cessation, rapid dose reduction, decreasing blood level of the drug, and/or administration of an antagonist. Signs and symptoms include tremor, shakiness, anxiety, depression, lacrimation, rhinorrhea, fatigue, irritability, and diarrhea.

- Addiction, a primary, chronic, neurobiological disease, with genetic, psychosocial, and environmental factors influencing its development and manifestations. It is characterized by behaviors that include one or more of the following: impaired control over drug use, compulsive use, continued use despite harm, and craving.
- Pseudoaddiction, the seeking of additional medication, secondary to undertreatment of pain. When the pain is treated properly, all inappropriate behavior ceases.
- Aberrant drug-taking behaviors less predictive of addiction include aggressive demand for more drug, drug hoarding (e.g., obtaining drug from more than one source), unsanctioned dose escalation, unapproved use of drug.
- Aberrant drug-taking behaviors more predictive of addiction, like selling prescription drugs, forging prescriptions, stealing drugs, frequent prescription "loss," injecting oral/topical formulations, concurrent abuse of illicit drugs.

Complications of opioids are best understood by knowing their mechanisms. Theses include the histaminergic, excitatory (hyperalgesia), dopaminergic, and proserotonergic effects.

Histaminergic Effects

Histamine is a neurotransmitter in the brain and an autocoid stored in the granules of mast cells and basophils that accumulate at sites of injury or potential injury. Opioids in general and morphine in particular, release both neuronal and nonneuronal histamine. Released histamine causes vasodilation, bronchoconstriction, smooth muscle activation, pruritus, and hives. It is for this reason that antihistamines are usually given as adjuvants to opioids in treating sickle cell pain. The antihistamines most commonly used include hydroxyzine (Vistaril) and diphenhydramine (Benadryl). The former is a piperazine antihistamine and the latter is an H1 receptor antagonist.

Opioid-induced Hyperalgesia

Paradoxically, the chronic administration of opioid analgesics to treat pain can contribute to or cause pain, a condition referred to as secondary hyperalgesia.[136,137] This has been described most often with morphine administration, but could occur with other opioids such as hydromorphone and methadone. The pathophysiology of this is not well understood. In the case of morphine, it seems to be due to an excitatory pathway initiated by the M3G metabolite. Morphine has a major inhibitory effect that controls pain and a minor excitatory effect that initiates tolerance

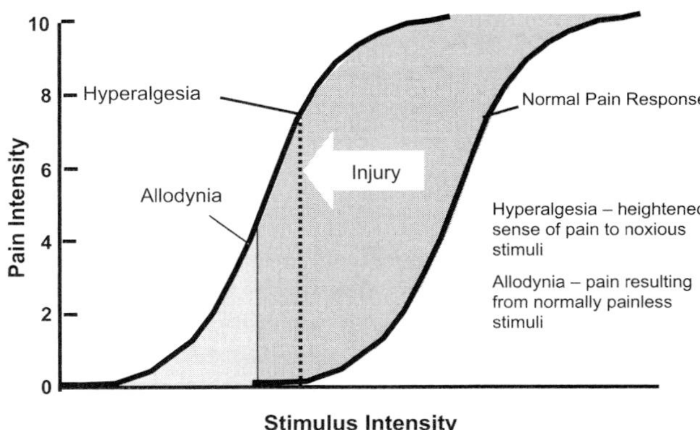

Figure 20.8. Pain hypersensitivity induced by injury. In the normal pain response, pain intensity increases as the stimulus intensity increases. Sensitization following injury causes the curve to shift to the left, resulting in hyperalgesia, in which noxious stimuli cause greater and more prolonged pain, as well as allodynia, in which pain results from normally painless stimuli. Sensitization is the manifestation of neuronal plasticity. (From ref. 139 with permission.) (See color plate 20.8.)

and hyperalgesia. With chronic use, the excitatory pathway is magnified and its effect becomes dominant. Moreover persistent nociceptive input into the central nervous system induces sensitization of the dorsal horn and other neuronal sites.[136,137] This central sensitization, in turn, produces pain hypersensitivity by shifting the response curves to the left, relative to the normal nonsensitized situation (Fig. 20.8).[138,139] Consequently, ambient stimuli that normally do not cause pain induce severe pain in the centrally sensitized patient. This sensitivity to ambient stimuli is referred to as allodynia. Chronic pain can alter brain function. Using functional magnetic resonance imaging during simple visual attention tasks in back pain patients and controls, chronic pain had a widespread impact on overall brain function that might underlie its cognitive and behavioral impairment.[140]

The molecular/cellular mechanism of hyperalgesia is poorly understood. One possible mechanism is secondary to activation of the NMDA receptor normally blocked by Mg^{++}. With persistent nociceptive input from the periphery, postsynaptic sodium channels become saturated. As a result, the Mg^{++} block from the NMDA receptor is removed allowing the entry of Ca^{++} into excitatory neurons. Ca^{++} initiates a cascade of intracellular enzymatic reactions that maintain the excitability of nociceptive neurons. Protein kinase C is activated and deactivates opioid receptors, resulting in receptor desensitization and reduced analgesia.[141–144] Another possible mechanism pertains to the activation of microglia and astrocytes to secrete proinflammatory cytokines that influence the induction and maintenance of pain.[145–147]

The pain caused by drug-induced hyperalgesia usually involves the same sites involved by the pain due to vasoocclusion, but its quality can be different. It is more neuropathic than nociceptive in nature and is usually superficial, not deep, and burning, tingling, and lancinating.

Dopaminergic Effects

All opioids have a dopaminergic effect that affects the reward/pleasure circuitry of the brain.[37,38] This circuitry includes the ventral tegmental area, nucleus accumbens, and the prefrontal cortex. The fundamental reward neurotransmitter in the brain is dopamine. This circuitry subserves natural rewards of all kinds, such as food, sex, listening to music, or watching a favorite movie. Opioids derive their abuse potential from acting on the reward/pleasure circuitry in the brain by increasing the level of dopamine, which in turn enhances the desire to achieve reward/pleasure. Depending on the environment and the genetic potential of individual patients, this dopaminergic effect of opioids can sometimes lead to addiction. Addiction is a disease by itself and should be treated as such. Recent reports suggest that topiramate is effective in the treatment of drug dependence.[148] Strategies to prevent or decrease the abuse potential of prescribed opioids include measures to uncouple the circuitry that links the dual effect of analgesia and reward.

Proserotonergic Effects

The serotonin syndrome is a clinical triad of altered mental states, autonomic dysfunction, and neuromuscular abnormalities.[149] It is not an idiopathic drug reaction but the result of excess use of central and peripheral nervous system serotonergic drugs. Table 20.9 lists some of the drugs associated with the serotonin syndrome. Signs and symptoms range from tremors and diarrhea in mild cases to delirium, neuromuscular rigidity, and hyperthermia in life-threatening cases (Fig. 20.9). The classic example of this syndrome is with the use of meperidine and monoamine oxide inhibitors.[149] Modulation of the painful stimuli includes the release of serotonin in the central nervous system to inhibit pain transmission.

Table 20.9. Drugs associated with the serotonin syndrome

- Antidepressants including selective serotonin reuptake inhibitors (SSRIs)
- Monoamine oxidase inhibitors (MAOIs)
- Anticonvulsants
- Analgesics
- Antiemetic agents
- Cough and cold remedies
- Antimigraine drugs

It is not unusual for hospitalized sickle cell disease patients to receive multiple proserotonergic medications, including an antidepressant, an opioid, an antiemetic, an anticonvulsant, and an antibiotic. The net result of such combinations can increase the level of serotonin. The signs and symptoms of the serotonin syndrome overlap with those of withdrawal, but careful history-taking can help in their differentiation.

MANAGEMENT OF ACUTE SICKLE CELL PAIN

Reviews of sickle pain management can serve as resources in guiding the treatment.[150–152] Evidenced-based reviews of the literature on management of acute pain episodes are scanty.[153]

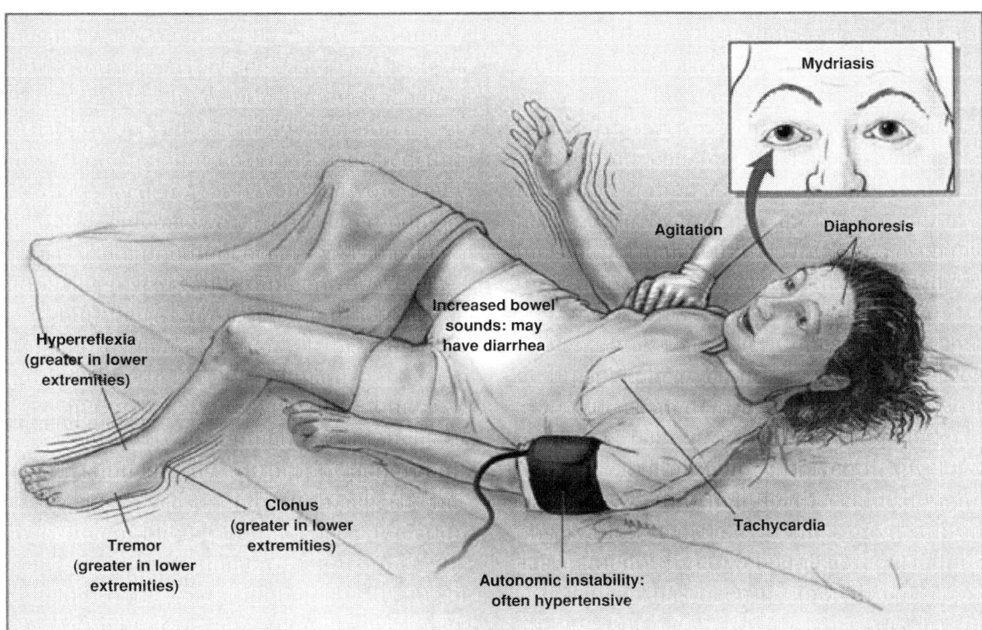

Figure 20.9. Findings in patients with moderately severe serotonin syndrome. Hyperkinetic neuromuscular findings of tremor or clonus and hyperreflexia should lead the clinician to consider the diagnosis of the serotonin syndrome. (From ref. 149 with permission.) (See color plate 20.9.)

Outpatient Pain Episode Treatment

Emerging data that suggest that individuals with sickle cell disease and their families manage the majority of pain successfully in the home.[73,78,154,155] This suggests that significant improvements in pain management and reductions in healthcare utilization could occur if individuals and their families are taught appropriate and effective methods for managing daily pain. To accomplish this, individual home management plans should be developed that include prevention, early nonpharmacological, and appropriate graded pharmacological interventions. Management plans should also incorporate guidelines for immediately seeking medical care.

Many patients have a premonition signaling the imminent onset of a pain episode. They should increase water intake, get more rest, and use behavioral and cognitive interventions to try to avoid the onset of a pain episode. Physical interventions such as taking a warm bath or shower, heating pad or blanket, and resting might prevent progression. Approaches should be individualized and patients and their families should be coached to identify successful techniques.

When these interventions fail, the World Health Organization (WHO) pain ladder approach to cancer pain is an effective approach to home management.[156] This starts with nonopioid analgesics such as acetaminophen, aspirin, and NSAIDs (Table 20.5).[157] These should be given by the clock in an appropriate dosing schedule based on the drug's half-life. Education should include discussion of the maximum doses that are safe and the ceiling effects of NSAIDs. Pain that is not controlled by these medications should be treated by the addition of oral opioid analgesics of appropriate potency.[157] Early in life, and in patients with infrequent pain, less potent oral analgesics such as codeine, hydrocodone, and tramadol (using fixed dosing based on biological half-life) should be added to the initial drugs. If the pain is not relieved, then a strong opioid such as morphine, oxycodone, hydromorphone, or methadone could be considered as a substitute for the less potent opioid. This will require that a limited supply of these analgesics be available to the individual in the home.

If the pain is not typical of the usual pain episode, fever is more that 101°F, signs of infection are present, or if the pain does not improve within 24–48 hours, immediate medical attention should be sought. It is also very important that the individuals and their caretakers understand that the pharmacological approach to the pain be graded based on the type and severity of the pain. For example, headaches and menstrual pain will often respond better to acetaminophen or NSAIDS than to opioid analgesics.

Outpatient Pain Treatment in Medical Facilities

The majority of pain episodes in the United States that require medical intervention are treated in EDs.[158] There are a limited number of day hospitals, clinics, and one 24-hour center that provide extended outpatient care for individuals with sickle pain episodes.[159–162] Guidelines have been published that provide a review of approaches to sickle cell pain management by health professionals.[23,151,163,164] Recent publications document the effectiveness of the systematic approach to outpatient management of sickle pain.[160,165,166]

Successful management of acute sickle pain is facilitated by a knowledgeable healthcare team that has a positive therapeutic relationship with the patient. Treatment should be initiated as rapidly as is possible. Significant delays occur in the initiation of care in the ED so every effort must be made to give these patients high priority for assessment and treatment.[167] Emergency treatment of sickle pain occurs in four stages; 1) assessment; 2) initiation of therapy; 3) evaluation of effectiveness; and 4) adjustment of therapy based on response. After these stages are completed, the patient is evaluated for the effectiveness of response and whether further treatment can be managed at home or in the hospital if more prolonged therapy is needed.

Initial assessment requires a history of the present episode, review of past approaches and responses to treatment, and the therapies that the individual has used prior to arriving at the hospital. It is very important to screen for precipitating complications and pain from other causes or other complications of sickle cell disease.[163] Allergies, adverse reactions to past treatment, and treatment approaches that have worked in the past should be identified. A physical evaluation should focus on exclusion of infection and other acute medical problems such as cholecystitis, acute chest syndrome, pregnancy, and so forth. Laboratory screening should include a complete blood count, reticulocyte count, platelet count, chemistry panel that includes creatinine and liver tests, and a urinalysis.[168]

The approach to initial therapy must be individualized. Acute pain intensity can be measured and recorded using a number of age-appropriate instruments that have been well validated.[151] The Attia behavioral pain scale is available for infants; the Childrens' Hospital Eastern Ontario Pain Scale for children aged 1–3 years; The Ocher, Poker-chip Tool, and Wong-Baker Faces for children; and Word Graphic Rating Scale, Numerical Pain Score-Intensity Scale, and the Visual Analog Scale for older children, adolescents, and adults.[151] Consistent use of one of these scales will allow rapid assessment and recording of pain and assessment of efficacy of treatment by frequent reassessments of the pain score by using the same instrument. The goals for therapy should also be determined based on the patient's desire for pain relief and acceptance of side effects.

The WHO analgesic ladder should also be used in acute pain management in the healthcare setting. All patients who do not have contraindications should be treated with oral or intravenous NSAIDs (Table 20.5). These should be given at analgesic doses on a fixed interval based on their half-life and not escalated because of ceiling effects. Moderate pain that has not been treated with oral opioid

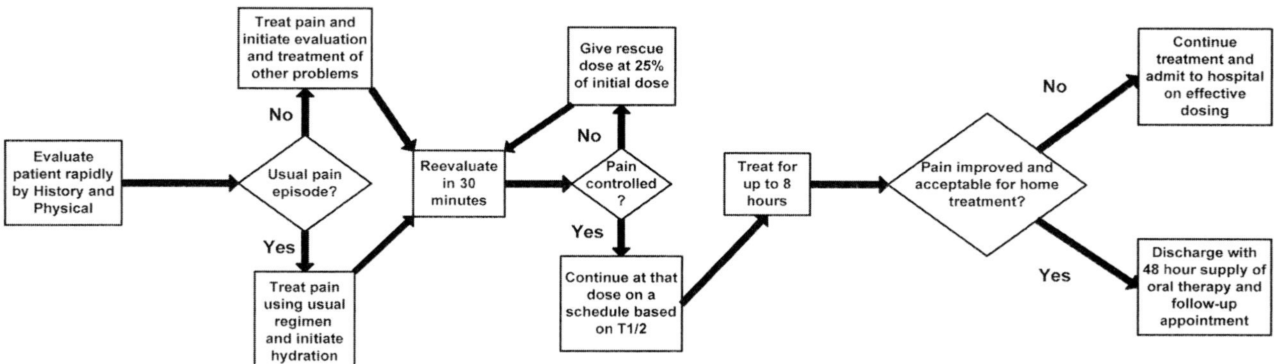

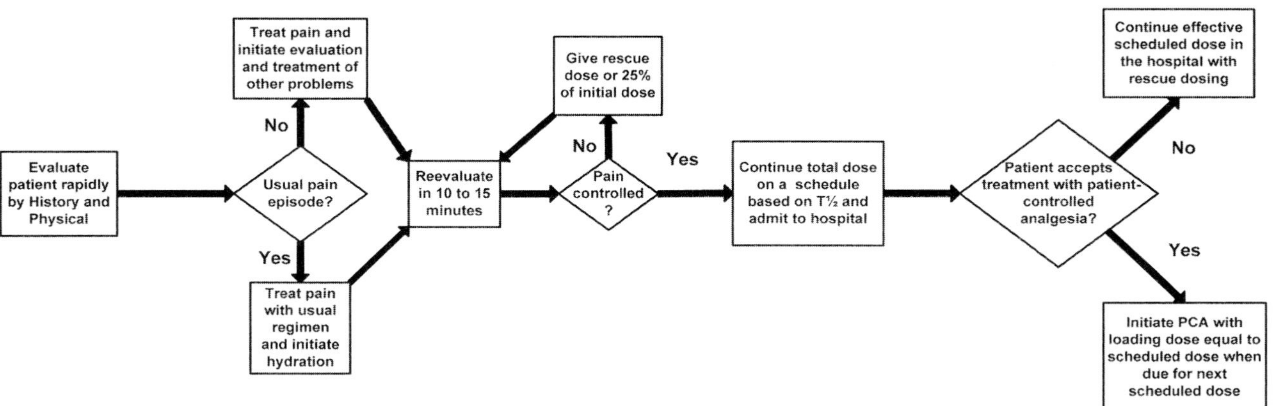

Figure 20.10. Outpatient approach to the treatment of pain in the 24 hours a day 7-day-a-week Georgia Comprehensive Sickle Cell Center at Grady. Patient's initial history-taking includes determining previous pain medication utilization and results of therapy. Patients with pain episodes and other complications such as fever, pneumonia, urinary infection, or significant changes in laboratory parameters are usually admitted without 8 hours of outpatient treatment. **(A)** Management of a patient who is known, to the Center and is presenting with a typical pain of usual intensity. **(B)** Management of a patient who is new to the Center or a known patient who presents with an unusually severe pain episode.

medications prior to presentation might respond to oral therapy.[166] More severe pain should generally be treated with intravenous, intramuscular, or subcutaneous opioid analgesics (Table 20.6). The medication should be administered using a dose based on the patient's previous response to therapy and the response reassessed in 15–30 minutes. If adequate relief is obtained, the medication can be administered using a fixed dosing interval based on the effective half-life of the medication (Fig. 20.10).

If the patient's history of opioid use is unclear or there is inadequate response to the initial dose of opioid, the drug should be administered in small doses every 15–30 minutes until an adequate response is obtained and then this amount can be given on a fixed schedule based on the effective half-life. Duration of treatment before discharge or admission to inpatient care depends on the individual's response to therapy and the ability to provide extended care in the outpatient setting. Extended care observation units allow effect treatment, and individuals may avoid hospital admission.[159–162] The decision to admit the patient to the hospital should be based on the patient's assessment of their ability to manage their pain at home and the presence of complications such as changes in baseline laboratory values, signs of infections, or other medical problems. Discharge medications should provide sufficient analgesic medications to treat the pain for 48–72 hours, and the patient should be instructed to return if pain cannot be adequately managed at home because of intensity or duration. Patients treated in EDs should be referred to their primary care provider for follow-up and provision of outpatient analgesics (Fig. 20.10). More detailed outpatient management protocols are available in monographs, on the Internet, and in books.[44,151,169]

Inpatient Pain Episode Treatment

Individuals requiring inpatient care should be treated with regimens that were effective in the outpatient setting or the treatment should be escalated if pain control was inadequate. Patients should be treated with an around-the-clock fixed-dose schedule with rescue doses of 25%–50% of the fixed dose for breakthrough pain.[23,151] Continuous intravenous dosing and long-acting oral preparations should be used instead of fixed dosing with short-acting preparations, especially if the patient reports awakening in pain.[170,171] If frequent rescue doses are required, the dose of the continuously administered analgesic can be increased.[151] If patients report that the pain is not adequately relieved by the fixed dose, it should be increased, and if the duration of pain control is inadequate, the interval of administration should be decreased.

Acute chest syndrome often develops several days after admission for an acute painful episode (Chapter 19). It should always be expected if there are increases in leukocyte count, fall in hemoglobin concentration, cough, chest pain, or fever.

Use of PCA

PCA has been used effectively in children and adults with sickle cell pain episodes[170,172–178] even though controlled studies have not validated its effectiveness compared with other treatment approaches.[153] Two studies suggest that PCA alone or PCA plus a low-dose infusion of morphine might be superior to continuous infusion or high-dose continuous infusion with rescue dosing.[175,176] Morphine PCA provides the only published experiences, although some centers use meperidine, hydromorphone, or other opioids for PCA.

Loading doses of morphine up to 0.05–15 mg/kg can be given based on severity of pain and initial response to therapy. Demand doses of 0.018–0.04 mg/kg with a 5–15-minute lockout are the usual range for sickle cell disease patients. Continuous infusion doses, if necessary, can be given at night or around the clock. The usual dose ranges are between 0.01 and 0.04 mg/kg/hour. One-hour or 4-hour limits, if required by the PCA pump, should be calculated so that the patient can get treatment for the entire period. That is, the limits should be based on the sum of the maximum demand dose plus the continuous infusion dose. Standard orders should provide for proximity to nursing station, frequent measurement of vital signs and O_2 saturation, naloxone at the bedside, and a resuscitation bag in proximity. Other narcotics and sedatives should be stopped. Orders should require that PCA should immediately be stopped and the physician notified for over sedation, respiratory rate of less than 12 per minute, or loss of intravenous access. PCA use and pain relief should be reevaluated frequently and at least every 24 hours. Once the pain episode is improving, the infusion should be tapered and the amount of the demand dose reduced. If a basilar infusion of morphine greater than 1 mg/hour is required to prevent adequately pain recurrence, oral sustained-release morphine in a dose equivalent to the infusion can be substituted for the infusion to prevent rebound pain as the infusion is stopped. Oral analgesic medications are started and the PCA discontinued when the patient's pain can be managed with oral analgesia alone.

Adjuvant Drugs

Adjuvant therapies are also very important to maximize pain management and to treat complications of therapy (Table 20.7). Morphine and all related analgesics can cause pruritus that can be controlled with antihistamines. Nausea is also common and best managed with antiemetics. Pain and opioid administration both cause in decrease in intestinal smooth muscle motility and constipation. All patients without diarrhea should be started on stool softeners and laxatives while being treated with opioids. Although it is not appropriate to substitute sedatives for appropriate analgesic drugs, most patients admitted for pain episodes have significant anxiety and might benefit form careful administration of appropriate anxiolytics. Patients also benefit from nonpharmacological interventions such as heat, cognitive and behavioral therapy, and distraction. Patients learn what works best for them over time and healthcare providers must understand that watching television, walking, playing games, doing puzzles, and other interventions are positive approaches to therapy and not indications that the patient is not in pain. The patient's assessment of their status is generally the best guide to when hospital discharge is appropriate.

CHRONIC PAIN IN SICKLE CELL DISEASE

Pain in sickle cell disease has some unique characteristics that must be appreciated for optimal management. Sickle cell pain is a lifelong experience with pain episodes beginning in early life and recurring with unpredictable frequency throughout life, resulting in physical, psychological, social, and economic impact on an individual's life experience. It results in frequent interactions with healthcare providers that can be positive or might result in negative experiences because of health professionals' attitudes and actions toward patients in pain. The negative attitudes and actions of some health professionals toward individuals with sickle cell disease have been documented.[179–184]

Another unique aspect of sickle cell pain is that early in life the pain is episodic with defined periods of pain and painfree intervals. As patients age, chronic pain becomes common. Adults have frequent pain that is not characterized as an acute pain episode and does not prompt seeking healthcare.[78] This change in pain character has important implications for pain management and requires reeducation of the individual with sickle cell disease and the families. Previous goals of being pain free are unrealistic and efforts need to be redirected at minimizing pain, maximizing functioning, optimizing positive pain coping strategies, and minimizing negative coping styles. Nonpharmacological interventions become much more important in the successful management of chronic pain.

The many sources of chronic pain have been discussed.[151] Neuropathic pain can result from frequently recurring acute pain, nerve entrapment syndromes, neuronal

Table 20.10. Nonpharmacological interventions for chronic pain in sickle cell disease

Physical measures	Psychological interventions	Behavioral interventions
Heat	Relaxation imagery	Relaxation therapy
Immobilization	Distraction	Breathing exercises
Graded exercise	Cognitive reframing	Behavioral modification
Massage	Peer support groups	Occupational therapy
Physical therapy	Psychotherapy	Biofeedback
TENS	Hypnosis	Self-hypnosis
Acupuncture	Pastoral counseling	
Acupressure	Patient education	
	Caregiver education	

ischemic damage, consequences of undertreated chronic pain, and complications of therapy.[23,44,151,185] Patients with HbSC disease and HbS–β^+ thalassemia have fewer acute pain episodes when they are younger but might have chronic pain from bone disease as they age. Each of these sources of chronic pain needs a systematic approach to management and specific therapy directed at the underlying cause.

Management of chronic pain is challenging for those affected and their care providers. Assessment includes defining the etiology of the pain, determining the pain intensity and impact on functioning and quality of life, and successful and unsuccessful coping strategies. This requires a detailed history-taking, thorough physical evaluation, assessment of psychological functioning, social functioning and support systems, and vocational activities. A detailed care plan is developed that includes pharmacological, physical, psychological, behavioral, social, and occupational pain management strategies (Table 20.10). A therapeutic agreement is developed with the individual, their caregivers, and families that clearly articulates the goals of treatment, limitations of therapy, the responsibilities of the patient, and those of the healthcare team.[186,187] The care plan is implemented with periodic review and refinement based on response to therapy. Assessing of use of medications, coping strategies, and therapeutic response can be facilitated by daily pain diaries.[3,73,75,76,188,189] Because of the complexity of chronic pain management, a multidisciplinary team that includes physicians, nurses, pharmacologists, psychologists, social workers, physical therapists, and occupation therapists is useful.[52,151,187]

The most common form of chronic pain experienced by individuals with sickle cell disease is bone pain.[190] Bone infarction often occurs during severe acute pain episodes and can last weeks to months. Avascular necrosis of the femur and humerus is also a common cause of pain.[191,192] Marrow expansion in the vertebral bodies leads to osteopenia, protrusion of the intervertebral discs, stepwise depression, and occasional compression fractures, which can contribute to the frequent occurrence of acute and chronic back pain.[190,193–195]

Management of chronic bone pain is challenging. NSAIDs and acetaminophen should be used as initial therapy if they are not contraindicated. Pain from avascular necrosis might respond well to physical therapy and could require changes in employment if prolonged standing and heavy lifting are required.[196] Avascular necrosis can require surgical intervention, which can significantly improve the pain (Chapter 19).[197–199]

Leg ulcers can cause severe chronic pain that requires opioids (Chapter 19).[200–203] Pain associated with dressing changes and debridement procedures may benefit from saturation of the area with topical anesthetics.

Neuropathic pain can be present in sickle cell disease and is underrecognized. Characteristics such as burning, lancinating, shooting, tingling, and associated numbness should suggest the presence of a neuropathic component. Specific neuropathies can cause chronic neuropathic pain.[23,204–206] Neuropathic pain responds poorly to opioid analgesics and is generally managed with topical analgesics, anticonvulsant medications, tricyclic antidepressants, and new approaches.[207–210]

Some patients develop intractable pain, without other signs or symptoms of disease pathology.[203] Acute exacerbations of pain can occur, but patients report pain on the majority of days that is severe enough to require treatment. The cause of intractable chronic pain is unknown. Central sensitization from recurrent and perhaps undertreated pain leads to allodynia and hyperalgesia.[185] Because of the frequency of chronic pain in a number of unrelated diseases, it has been suggested that persistent pain is a disease entity that might require removal of the painful stimulus and addressing the psychological and social contributors to, and the consequences of, the pain.[211] Genetic and acquired differences in pain perception might predispose some individuals to developing chronic pain because of increased baseline pain sensitivity and reduced pain inhibitory processing.[212]

Managing the individual with chronic pain is challenging. The availability of a multidisciplinary team is essential and models exist in primary care settings.[52,187] The goals of therapy are to minimize pain and negative pain–related behavior and to maximize positive behavior and quality of life. A formal care plan that is understood and followed by the patient and all members of the care team to minimize miscommunication and negative interactions is imperative. The goals of the plan and details of implementation should be negotiated with the patient, their caregivers, and family and form the basis of a therapeutic agreement.[186] Nonpharmacological approaches including psychological, behavioral and physical strategies are the primary initial methods of pain management. Pharmacological treatment should be based on the WHO analgesic ladder for cancer pain starting with acetaminophen and long-acting NSAIDs. Weaker short-acting opioid analgesics can be added for breakthrough pain. The regular use of stronger opioid analgesics in noncancer pain is still controversial, but will often be required in individuals with sickle cell disease and severe, intractable pain. Adjunct medications including antihistamines, antiemetic drugs, stool softeners, laxatives, antidepressants, and anticonvulsive medications can be added to control side effects of opioid analgesics and for specific pain syndromes and complications such as depression.

Chronic Opioids

The use of chronic opioid analgesics in sickle cell disease is problematic. Because patients median lifespan is probably in the fifth or sixth decade, pain management strategies must be continued for many years. Regular use of opioid analgesics induces physiological tolerance that reduces their efficacy and therapeutic index. Treatment of acute pain episodes can become increasing difficult if a patient has high levels of tolerance. Interruption of regular opioid use can lead to abstinence syndromes characterized by pain, often in the sites of sickle cell pain, tachycardia and increased blood pressure, piloerection, anxiety, dysphoria, irritability, insomnia, rhinorrhea, lacrimation, myalgia, nausea, vomiting, diarrhea, and other neuroendocrine responses.[213] Many patients interpret these as acute pain episodes and seek further treatment leading to continuously increasing utilization of opioid analgesics and increasing difficulty managing pain.

Chronic use of opioid analgesics in individuals with intractable nonmalignant pain was studied in 38 patients without a history of drug abuse and showed that maintenance therapy can be effective, humane, and safe.[214] Other studies have questioned the benefits of such therapy, citing its lack of efficacy in improving pain and increasing function with acceptable side effects and risks. Only a small subset of patients with chronic pain might benefit from such therapy. These include patients with ongoing nociception and moderate to severe refractory pain or neuropathic pain. The more common chronic pain patient with pain and disability out of proportion to the physical stimulus is unlikely to benefit, and that benefit should be judged on reduction in pain with stable doses of opioid analgesics, improved quality of life, and improvement in social and psychological function.[215] An excellent review outlines a realistic approach to treatment of chronic pain with opioid analgesics. This stresses development of a formal treatment plan with goals and objectives specified, use of moderate doses of medications, frequent assessment documenting improvement in pain and functioning, and avoidance of high-dose treatment over prolonged periods.[216] Accumulating evidence suggests that a conscious, structured approach in a selected subset of patients suffering chronic pain with objective evaluation of outcome in terms of pain control, quality of life, and functioning is the best treatment approach. [216–219] Little evidence is available to guide selection of sickle cell disease patients for chronic opioid treatment.

Once the decision is made to initiate chronic opiate therapy, it is generally recommended that such therapy be based on a well documented evaluation and treatment plan and that it be closely monitored.[220] Reviews have documented the limitations of monitoring of chronic opioid therapy.[221] A model policy for using controlled substances for the treatment of pain outlines recommended guidelines for the physician.[222] Many have suggested that an opioid contract for the management of chronic pain be developed and used in all individuals receiving chronic opioid treatment.[223] The elements of these agreements and model consent forms and sample agreements have been published.[223–225] These agreements stress opioids are part of a comprehensive pain treatment program, indicate the methods by which adherence and improvement will be evaluated, document the healthcare providers' responsibility to improve the patient's pain, indicate the purpose is to improve communication and reduce misunderstanding, state behaviors that will result in modification of the agreement and their specific consequences, and have a positive and cooperative tone.[223,226] Little evidence is available to determine the utility of these agreements to improve adherence to therapy and improve outcome. Some have raised concerns about their utility and purposes; however, they are recommended and widely used in chronic pain clinics.[226,227]

SPECIFIC MANAGEMENT ISSUES

Many important issues develop during the treatment of pain in all patients. They include pseudoaddiction, opioid-induced hyperalgesia, addiction, and managing the "difficult" patient. Although not unique to sickle cell disease, they might be more prevalent because of the lifelong nature of pain in this disorder.

Pseudoaddiction

Pseudoaddiction occurs in two forms. The first is the induction of pain medication–seeking behavior by undertreatment. This is easily treated by increasing the amount or frequency of the analgesic therapy, and the behavior disappears when the pain is adequately controlled. The second form is the occurrence of repeated episodes of abstinence syndrome when opioid analgesics have been discontinued abruptly after prolonged therapy induces physical dependency. This is common in sickle cell disease after prolonged therapy for an unusually severe pain episode or other major complication that results in the need for prolonged, high-dose opioid treatment. When the medication is stopped or the dose significantly decreased, the patient will experience the onset of pain approximately 48–72 hours later requiring repeated ED visits or hospitalizations. This pattern persists until the problem is recognized and treated by administration of long-acting opioid analgesics and slowly tapering the total daily dose with reductions every

2 or 3 days. Prevention requires recognizing this potential in individuals requiring prolonged inpatient treatment and discharging them on a tapering schedule when high-dose opioid therapy is required for more than 5–7 days.[151]

Opioid-induced Hyperalgesia

Opioid-induced hyperalgesia is likely much more frequent than previously thought and occurs in sickle cell disease patients receiving high-dose opioid analgesics for prolonged periods.[228] This syndrome was first recognized in individuals receiving methadone maintenance[229] but is now recognized to occur in many pain settings. Animal models exist documenting the physiological basis for the syndrome.[230–234]

Improvement in pain, quality of life, and psychosocial functioning can be achieved by recognizing the syndrome, stabilizing opioid dose with long-acting preparations, and decreasing the doses of opioid slowly over time. Diagnosis is based on lack of lasting benefit from increases in doses, rapidly developing tolerance, changes in pain pattern with increasing pain as doses are escalated, hyperalgesia, and allodynia.[228] Treatment includes decreasing doses, use of NMDA antagonists such as ketamine and dextromethorphan, α 2-agonists such as clonidine, cyclooxygenase inhibitors, and rotation of opioids.[117] Prevention includes avoidance of prolonged treatment with high-dose opioid analgesics.[233]

Addiction

The American Pain Society defines addiction as, "a pattern of compulsive drug-use behaviors characterized by continued craving for an opioid and a need to use the opioid for effects other than pain relief."[151] The *Diagnostic and Statistical Manual of Mental Disorders-IV* stresses tolerance, withdrawal, longer use than intended, repeated desire or unsuccessful attempts to cut down, spending a great deal of time obtaining substances, negative impact on social, occupational, or recreational activities, and continued use despite knowledge of psychological and physical harm.[235] Addiction is a problem distinct from sickle cell pain and is not a consequence of pain treatment. Recent research suggests that addiction results from genetic, environmental, and social vulnerabilities that when coupled with drug effects lead to changes in brain circuitry causing the addictive phenomenon.[236] Addiction does not appear to be more common in sickle cell disease than other chronic pain states.[151] Recognition of individuals who have this problem is important because the addiction needs specific and likely lifelong treatment.[237]

The "Difficult" Patient

The "difficult" patient is not unique to sickle cell disease. Studies show that 15% of patient interactions are viewed as difficult by physicians in primary care.[238] These are better characterized as difficult patient–provider interactions that arise because of patient characteristics, physician characteristics, and situational issues.[238–241] Some characteristics of sickle cell disease patients directly related to their disease can make them more likely to be perceived as difficult. These include many bothersome physical symptoms and their severity, worry about the seriousness of their illness, and mood and anxiety disorders.[238] Physician characteristics that were more commonly associated with frustration with patients include: age younger than 40 years, work hours more than 55 hour/week, subspecialty practice, and more symptoms of depression, stress, and anxiety. These characteristics may or may not be more common in the physicians caring for sickle cell disease patients.[241] The results of these interactions for the patient include poorer functional status, more unmet expectations, less satisfaction with care, and higher use of health services.[238] This sounds like the description of the "frequent flier" who is the sickle cell patient most likely to be viewed as problematic by the healthcare community.

A recent authoritative review of pain management in sickle cell disease included an excellent discussion of specific methods of approaching the sickle cell patient who is viewed as difficult. Useful approaches have defined a successful physician–patient encounter including collaboration in problem solving, direct proactive communication, appropriate use of power, showing empathy, avoiding being drawn into conflict, and being aware of one's stress, fatigue, and beliefs with limit setting.[238–240,242–245]

SUMMARY

Pain is one of the most frequent and distressing clinical problems facing individuals with sickle cell disease. Its treatment presents major challenges to healthcare providers. Pain episodes are unpredictable and severe. As the individual with sickle cell disease gets older, chronic pain becomes more common and presents new management challenges. Recent studies in adults show that acute and chronic pain is more prevalent than once appreciated because most pain is managed successfully at home and without interaction with the healthcare system.

Despite significant advances in the understanding of mechanisms of pain, new insights into complications of pain, and new information on management, the treatment of acute and chronic pain in sickle cell disease is unsatisfactory. Many healthcare providers have inadequate training in pain management. High levels of frustration for patients, their families, and their healthcare providers are common because the pain is recurrent and difficult to manage adequately. Much of the patient's frustration relates to the healthcare providers failure to believe the severity or even the presence of pain. Although there are consistent laboratory changes during a pain episode, these are only apparent after careful retrospective analysis and comparisons with baseline values and those obtained well after the pain episode has resolved. No reliable way of determining the presence or severity of the pain is available except for the patient's report and studies document that the pain is underappreciated by healthcare providers.[183] Barriers to treatment of pain in general[246] and sickle cell disease specifically have been enumerated.[179,182,247,248] These might be becoming more of a problem for both patients and providers because of the significant push to minimize utilization of inpatient services and limit outpatient visits.

A major advance in prevention of sickle pain episodes is the introduction of hydroxyurea therapy. Treatment with hydroxyurea significantly reduces the incidence of pain episodes in adults and children with sickle cell anemia and HbS–β^0 thalassemia (Chapter 30).[249] Unfortunately, there is presently no treatment that directly focuses on the immediate cause of the acute painful episode.

Chronic pain is emerging as a major problem for the older patients with sickle cell disease. Approaches to management of chronic pain are unsatisfactory. Better understanding of the effects and side effects of opioid analgesics requires reevaluation of their use in all patients with chronic nonmalignant pain.[216] NSAIDs, physical, psychological, and behavioral approaches need to be the basis for therapy in chronic pain, and multidisciplinary healthcare teams are required.

Finally, recent reviews document a lack of clinical research in sickle pain management, thus sufficient data are lacking to recommend evidence-based approaches to either acute or chronic pain.[153,250–252] New research is needed to refine pharmacological and nonpharmacological approaches to acute and chronic pain in sickle cell disease and to translate the elegant understanding of the disease pathophysiology into effective strategies to abort and prevent acute pain and nervous system adaptation that leads to chronic pain syndromes.

REFERENCES

1. Platt OS, Thorington BD, Brambilla DJ, et al. Pain in sickle cell disease. Rates and risk factors. *N Engl J Med.* 1991;325: 11–16.
2. Treadwell M, Gil KM. Psychosocial aspects. In: Embury S, Hebbel R, Mohandas N, Steinberg M, eds. *Sickle Cell Disease: Basic Principles and Clinical Practice.* New York: Raven Press, Ltd.; 1994:517–529.
3. Shapiro BS, Dinges DF, Orne EC, et al. Home management of sickle cell-related pain in children and adolescents: natural history and impact on school attendance. *Pain.* 1995;61:139–144.
4. Walco GA, Dampier CD. Pain in children and adolescents with sickle cell disease: a descriptive study. *J Pediatr Psychol.* 1990;15:643–658.
5. Diggs LW. Sickle cell crisis. *Am J Clin Pathol.* 1965;44:1–19.
6. Konotey-Ahulu FI. The sickle cell diseases. Clinical manifestations including the "sickle crisis." *Arch Intern Med.* 1974;133:611–619.
7. Serjeant GR, Ceulaer CD, Lethbridge R, Morris J, Singhal A, Thomas PW. The painful crisis of homozygous sickle cell disease: clinical features. *Br J Haematol.* 1994;87:586–591.
8. Akinola NO, Stevens SM, Franklin IM, Nash GB, Stuart J. Subclinical ischaemic episodes during the steady state of sickle cell anaemia. *J Clin Pathol.* 1992;45:902–906.
9. Ballas SK, Smith ED. Red blood cell changes during the evolution of the sickle cell painful crisis. *Blood.* 1992;79:2154–2163.
10. Beyer JE, Simmons LE, Woods GM, Woods PM. A chronology of pain and comfort in children with sickle cell disease. *Arch Pediatr Adolesc Med.* 1999;153:913–920.
11. Davies SC. The hospital management of patients with sickle cell disease. *Haematologica.* 1990;75 Suppl 5:96–106.
12. Feldman F, Zwass A, Staron RB, Haramati N. MRI of soft tissue abnormalities: a primary cause of sickle cell crisis. *Skeletal Radiol.* 1993;22:501–506.
13. Mankad VN, Williams JP, Harpen MD, et al. Magnetic resonance imaging of bone marrow in sickle cell disease: clinical, hematologic, and pathologic correlations. *Blood.* 1990;75:274–283.
14. Mankad VN, Yang YM, Williams JP, Brogdon BG. Magnetic resonance imaging of bone marrow in sickle cell patients. *Am J Pediatr Hematol Oncol.* 1988;10:344–347.
15. Bunn HF. Pathogenesis and treatment of sickle cell disease. *N Engl J Med.* 1997;337:762–769.
16. Steinberg MH. Management of sickle cell disease. *N Engl J Med.* 1999;340:1021–1030.
17. Embury SH, Hebbel RP, Steinberg MH, Mohandas N. Pathogenesis of vasoocclusion. In: Embury SH, Hebbel RP, Mohandas N, Steinberg MH, eds. *Sickle Cell Disease: Basic Principles and Clinical Practice.* New York: Raven Press, Ltd.; 1994:311–326.
18. Ballas SK, Mohandas N. Sickle red cell microrheology and sickle blood rheology. *Microcirculation.* 2004;11:209–225.
19. Chiang EY, Frenette PS. Sickle cell vasoocclusion. *Hematol Oncol Clin North Am.* 2005;19:771–784.
20. Frenette PS. Sickle cell vasoocclusion: heterotypic, multicellular aggregations driven by leukocyte adhesion. *Microcirculation.* 2004;11:167–177.
21. Frenette PS, Atweh GF. Sickle cell disease: old discoveries, new concepts, and future promise. *J Clin Invest.* 2007;117: 850–858.
22. Hebbel RP, Osarogiagbon R, Kaul D. The endothelial biology of sickle cell disease: inflammation and a chronic vasculopathy. *Microcirculation.* 2004;11:129–151.
23. Benjamin LJ. Nature and treatment of the acute painful episode in sickle cell disease. In: Steinberg MH, Forget BG, Higgs DR, Nagel RL, eds. *Disorders of Hemoglobin: Genetics, Pathophysiology, and Clinical Management.* New York: Cambridge University Press; 2001:671–710.
24. Embury S, Hebbel R, Mohandas N, Steinberg M. Sickle cell disease. *Basic Principles and Clinical Picture.* New York: Raven Press, Ltd.; 1994.
25. Serjeant GR. *Sickle Cell Disease.* 3rd ed. New York: Oxford University Press; 2001.
26. Boros L, Thomas C, Weiner WJ. Large cerebral vessel disease in sickle cell anaemia. *J Neurol Neurosurg Psychiatry.* 1976;39:1236–1239.
27. Powars D, Wilson B, Imbus C, Pegelow C, Allen J. The natural history of stroke in sickle cell disease. *Am J Med.* 1978;65:461–471.

28. Powars DR. Sickle cell anemia and major organ failure. *Hemoglobin.* 1990;14:573–598.
29. Hebbel RP. Beyond hemoglobin polymerization: the red blood cell membrane and sickle disease pathophysiology. *Blood.* 1991;77:214–237.
30. Francis RB, Jr., Johnson CS. Vascular occlusion in sickle cell disease: current concepts and unanswered questions. *Blood.* 1991;77:1405–1414.
31. Fields HL. *Pain.* New York: McGraw-Hill; 1987.
32. Katz N, Ferrante FM. Nociception. In: Ferrante FM, Vade-Boncoeur TR, eds. *Post Operative Pain Management.* New York: Churchill Livingstone; 1993:17–67.
33. Kaul DK. Hypoxia/reoxygenation causes inflammatory response in transgenic sickle mice but not in normal mice. *J Clin Invest.* 2000;106:411–420.
34. Platt OS. Sickle cell anemia as an inflammatory disease. *J Clin Invest.* 2000;106:337–338.
35. Cousins MJ, John J. Bonica distinguished lecture. Acute pain and the injury response: immediate and prolonged effects. *Reg Anesth.* 1989;14:162–179.
36. Cousins MJ. Acute post operative pain. In: Wall PD, Melzack R, eds. *Textbook of Pain.* New York: Churchill Livingstone; 1994:357–385.
37. McMahon SB, Koltzeninburg M, eds. In: *Wall and Melzack's Textbook of Pain.* 5th ed. New York: Churchill Livingstone; 2006.
38. Loeser JD, Butler SH, Chapman CR, Turk DC, eds. *Bonica's Management of Pain.* 3rd ed. Philadelphia: Lippincott Williams & Wilkins; 2001.
39. Ballas SK. The neurobiology and treatment of pain in sickle cell disease. In: Embury SH, Hebbel RP, Mohandas N, Steinberg MH, eds. *Sickle Cell Disease: Scientific Principles and Clinical Practice.* New York: Raven Press; 1994:745–772.
40. Ballas SK. Sickle cell disease. In: Rakel RE, ed. *Conn's Current Therapy.* Philadelphia: WB Saunders; 1995:318–327.
41. Meyer RA, Ringkamp M, Campbell JN, Raja SN. Peripheral mechanisms of cutaneous nociception. In: McMahon SB, Koltzeninburg M, eds. *Wall and Melzack's Textbook of Pain.* 5th ed. New York: Churchill Livingston; 2006:16.
42. Dunn MJ, Hood VL. Prostaglandins and the kidney. *Am J Physiol.* 1977;233:169–184.
43. Dyck PJ, ed. *Peripheral Neuropathy.* Philadelphia: Saunders; 1975.
44. Ballas SK. Sickle cell pain. *Progress in Pain Research and Management.* Seattle: IASP Press; 1998.
45. Melzack R. Pain questionnaire: major properties and scoring. *Pain.* 1975;1:277–299.
46. Wall PD, Melzack R, eds. *Textbook of Pain.* 3rd ed. New York: Churchill Livingstone; 1994.
47. Anderson P, Morris R, Amaral D, et al. *The Hippocampus Book.* New York: Oxford University Press; 2007.
48. Choi DS, Choi DY, Whittington RA, Nedeljkovic SS. Sudden amnesia resulting in pain relief: the relationship between memory and pain. *Pain.* 2007;132:206–210.
49. Basbaum AI. The generation and control of pain. In: Rosenberg RN, Grossman RG, Schochet Jr SS, Heinz ER, Willis WD, eds. *The Clinical Neurosciences, Neurobiology.* New York: Churchill Livingstone; 1983:V301–V24.
50. Basbaum AI, Fields HL. Endogenous pain control systems: brainstem spinal pathways and endorphin circuitry. *Annu Rev Neurosci.* 1984;7:309–338.
51. Ballas SK, Lusardi M. Hospital readmission for adult acute sickle cell painful episodes: frequency, etiology, and prognostic significance. *Am J Hematol.* 2005;79:17–25.
52. Vichinsky EP, Johnson R, Lubin BH. Multidisciplinary approach to pain management in sickle cell disease. *Am J Pediatr Hematol Oncol.* 1982;4:328–333.
53. Bonds DR. Three decades of innovation in the management of sickle cell disease: the road to understanding the sickle cell disease clinical phenotype. *Blood Rev.* 2005;19:99–110.
54. Steinberg MH. Predicting clinical severity in sickle cell anaemia. *Br J Haematol.* 2005;129:465–481.
55. Powars DR. Sickle cell anemia: beta s-gene-cluster haplotypes as prognostic indicators of vital organ failure. *Semin Hematol.* 1991;28:202–208.
56. Udezue E, Girshab AM. Differences between males and females in adult sickle cell pain crisis in eastern Saudi Arabia. *Ann Saudi Med.* 2004;24:179–182.
57. Ballas SK, Larner J, Smith ED, Surrey S, Schwartz E, Rappaport EF. Rheologic predictors of the severity of the painful sickle cell crisis. *Blood.* 1988;72:1216–1223.
58. Lande WM, Andrews DL, Clark MR, et al. The incidence of painful crisis in homozygous sickle cell disease: correlation with red cell deformability. *Blood.* 1988;72:2056–2059.
59. Baum KF, Dunn DT, Maude GH, Serjeant GR. The painful crisis of homozygous sickle cell disease. A study of the risk factors. *Arch Intern Med.* 1987;147:1231–1234.
59a. Taylor JG IV, Nolan VG, Mendelsohn L, Kato GJ, Gladwi, MT, Steinberg MH. Chronic hyper-hemolysis in sickle cell anemia: association of vascular complications and mortality with less frequent vasoocclusive pain PLoS One. 2008; 3(5)e 2095.
60. Hargrave DR, Wade A, Evans JP, Hewes DK, Kirkham FJ. Nocturnal oxygen saturation and painful sickle cell crises in children. *Blood.* 2003;101:846–848.
61. Schall JI, Zemel BS, Kawchak DA, Ohene-Frempong K, Stallings VA. Vitamin A status, hospitalizations, and other outcomes in young children with sickle cell disease. *J Pediatr.* 2004;145:99–106.
62. Gil KM, Carson JW, Porter LS, Scipio C, Bediako SM, Orringer E. Daily mood and stress predict pain, health care use, and work activity in African American adults with sickle-cell disease. *Health Psychol.* 2004;23:267–274.
63. Amjad H, Bannerman RM, Judisch JM. Letter: Sickling pain and season. *Br Med J.* 1974;2:54.
64. Ibrahim AS. Relationship between meteorological changes and occurrence of painful sickle cell crises in Kuwait. *Trans R Soc Trop Med Hyg.* 1980;74:159–161.
65. Redwood AM, Williams EM, Desal P, Serjeant GR. Climate and painful crisis of sickle-cell disease in Jamaica. *Br Med J.* 1976;1:66–68.
66. Kehinde MO, Marsh JC, Marsh GW. Sickle cell disease in North London. *Br J Haematol.* 1987;66:543–547.
67. Seeler RA. Non-seasonality of sickle-cell crisis. *Lancet.* 1973;2:743.
68. Slovis CM, Talley JD, Pitts RB. Non relationship of climatologic factors and painful sickle cell anemia crisis. *J Chronic Dis.* 1986;39:121–126.
69. Smith WR, Coyne P, Smith VS, Mercier B. Temperature changes, temperature extremes, and their relationship to emergency department visits and hospitalizations for sickle cell crisis. *Pain Manage Nurs.* 2003;4:106–111.

70. Jones S, Duncan ER, Thomas N, et al. Windy weather and low humidity are associated with an increased number of hospital admissions for acute pain and sickle cell disease in an urban environment with a maritime temperate climate. *Br J Haematol.* 2005;131:530–533.
71. Yallop D, Duncan ER, Norris E, et al. The associations between air quality and the number of hospital admissions for acute pain and sickle-cell disease in an urban environment. *Br J Haematol.* 2007;136:844–848.
71a. Nolan VG, Zhang Y, Lash T, Sebastiani P, Steinberg MH. Association of wind speed and the occurrence of sickle cell acute painful episodes: results of a case-crossover study. *Br J Haematol.* 2008; 143(3) 433–438.
72. Resar LM, Oski FA. Cold water exposure and vaso-occlusive crises in sickle cell anemia. *J Pediatr.* 1991;118:407–409.
73. Dampier C, Ely E, Brodecki D, O'Neal P. Home management of pain in sickle cell disease: a daily diary study in children and adolescents. *J Pediatr Hematol Oncol.* 2002;24:643–647.
74. Anie KA, Steptoe A, Bevan DH. Sickle cell disease: pain, coping and quality of life in a study of adults in the UK. *Br J Health Psychol.* 2002;7:331–344.
75. Fuggle P, Shand PA, Gill LJ, Davies SC. Pain, quality of life, and coping in sickle cell disease. *Arch Dis Child.* 1996;75:199–203.
76. Porter LS, Gil KM, Sedway JA, Ready J, Workman E, Thompson RJ, Jr. Pain and stress in sickle cell disease: an analysis of daily pain records. *Int J Behav Med.* 1998;5:185–203.
77. Westerman MP, Bailey K, Freels S, Schlegel R, Williamson P. Assessment of painful episode frequency in sickle-cell disease. *Am J Hematol.* 1997;54:183–188.
78. Smith WR, Penberthy LT, Bovbjerg VE, et al. Daily assessment of pain in adults with sickle cell disease. *Ann Intern Med.* 2008;148:94–101.
79. Akinola NO, Stevens SM, Franklin IM, Nash GB, Stuart J. Rheological changes in the prodromal and established phases of sickle cell vaso-occlusive crisis. *Br J Haematol.* 1992;81:598–602.
80. Ballas SK. The sickle cell painful crisis in adults: phases and objective signs. *Hemoglobin.* 1995;19:323–333.
81. Jacob E, Beyer JE, Miaskowski C, Savedra M, Treadwell M, Styles L. Are there phases to the vaso-occlusive painful episode in sickle cell disease? *J Pain Symptom Manage.* 2005; 29:392–400.
82. Neuman HN, Diggs LW, Schlenker FS, et al. Increased urinary porphyrin excretion in sickle cell crises. *Proc Soc Exp Biol Med.* 1966;123:1–4.
83. Schumaker HR. Rheumatological manifestation of sickle disease and other haemoglobinopathies. *Clin Rheum Dis.* 1975;1:37–52.
84. Schumacher HR, Andrews R, McLaughlin G. Arthropathy in sickle-cell disease. *Ann Intern Med.* 1973;78:203–211.
85. Brugsch HG, Gill D. Polyarthritis in sickle cell anemia. *N Engl J Med.* 1944;231:291–292.
86. Espinoza LR, Spilberg I, Osterland CK. Joint manifestations of sickle cell disease. *Medicine (Baltimore).* 1974;53:295–305.
87. Miller RL, Webster ME, Melmon KL. Interaction of leukocytes and endotoxin with the plasmin and kinin systems. *Eur J Pharmacol.* 1975;33:53–60.
88. Dorwart BB, Gabuzda TG. Symmetric myositis and fasciitis: a complication of sickle cell anemia during vasoocclusion. *J Rheumatol.* 1985;12:590–595.
89. Valeriano-Marcet J, Kerr LD. Myonecrosis and myofibrosis as complications of sickle cell anemia. *Ann Intern Med.* 1991;115:99–101.
90. Schumacher HR, Jr., Murray WM, Dalinka MK. Acute muscle injury complicating sickle cell crisis. *Semin Arthritis Rheum.* 1990;19:243–7.
91. Walker BK, Brownstein PK, Burka ER, Ballas SK. Urinary retention in sickle cell syndromes. *Urology.* 1980;16:33–35.
92. Ballas SK, Marcolina MJ. Hyperhemolysis during the evolution of uncomplicated acute painful episodes in patients with sickle cell anemia. *Transfusion.* 2006;46:105–110.
93. Buchanan GR, Glader BE. Leukocyte counts in children with sickle cell disease. Comparative values in the steady state, vaso-occlusive crisis, and bacterial infection. *Am J Dis Child.* 1978;132:396–398.
94. Billett HH, Nagel RL, Fabry ME. Evolution of laboratory parameters during sickle cell painful crisis: evidence compatible with dense red cell sequestration without thrombosis. *Am J Med Sci.* 1988;296:293–298.
95. Green D, Kwaan HRG. Impaired fibrinolysis in sickle cell disease. Relation to crisis and infection. *Thromb Diath Haemorrh.* 1970;24:10–16.
96. Haut MJ, Cowan DH, Harris JW. Platelet function and survival in sickle cell disease. *J Lab Clin Med.* 1973;82:44–53.
97. Kenny MW, George AJ, Stuart J. Platelet hyperactivity in sickle-cell disease: a consequence of hyposplenism. *J Clin Pathol.* 1980;33:622–625.
98. Billett HH, Fabry ME, Nagel RL. Hemoglobin distribution width: a rapid assessment of dense red cells in the steady state and during painful crisis in sickle cell anemia. *J Lab Clin Med.* 1988;112:339–344.
99. Van Der Sar A. The sudden rise in platelets and reticulocytes in sickle cell crises. *Trop Geogr Med.* 1970;22:30–40.
100. Gordon PA, Breeze GR, Mann JR, Stuart J. Coagulation fibrinolysis in sickle-cell disease. *J Clin Pathol.* 1974;27:485–489.
101. Alkjaersig N, Fletcher A, Joist H, Chaplin H, Jr. Hemostatic alterations accompanying sickle cell pain crises. *J Lab Clin Med.* 1976;88:440–449.
102. Jacob E, Miaskowski C, Savedra M, Beyer JE, Treadwell M, Styles L. Changes in intensity, location, and quality of vaso-occlusive pain in children with sickle cell disease. *Pain.* 2003;102:187–193.
103. Jacob E, Mueller BU. Pain experience of children with sickle cell disease who had prolonged hospitalizations for acute painful episodes. *Pain Med.* 2008;9:13–21.
104. Tomer A, Harker LA, Kasey S, Eckman JR. Thrombogenesis in sickle cell disease. *J Lab Clin Med.* 2001;137:398–407.
105. Frei-Jones MJ, DeBaun MR. Hospital readmission within 30 days: a new benchmark for quality care among children with sickle cell disease. *Blood.* 2007;11:3403a.
106. van Walraven C, Mamdani M, Fang J, Austin PC. Continuity of care and patient outcomes after hospital discharge. *J Gen Intern Med.* 2004;19:624–31.
107. Forster AJ, Murff HJ, Peterson JF, Gandhi TK, Bates DW. The incidence and severity of adverse events affecting patients after discharge from the hospital. *Ann Intern Med.* 2003;138:161–167.
108. Cordeiro NJ, Oniyangi O. Phytomedicines (medicines derived from plants) for sickle cell disease. *Cochrane Database Syst Rev.* 2004:CD004448.

109. Brousseau DC, Scott JP, Hillery CA, Panepinto JA. The effect of magnesium on length of stay for pediatric sickle cell pain crisis. *Acad Emerg Med.* 2004;11:968–972.
110. Benjamin LJ, Dampier CD, Jacox A, et al. Guideline for the Management of Acute and Chronic Pain in Sickle Cell Disease. In: *American Pain Society Clinical Practice Guidelines Series No 1.* Glenview, IL: American Pain Society; 1999.
111. Morgan MT. Use of meperidine as the analgesic of choice in treating pain from acute painful sickle cell crisis. *Ann Emerg Med.* 2008;51:202–203.
112. Howland MA, Goldfrank LR. Why meperidine should not make a comeback in treating patients with sickle cell disease. *Ann Emerg Med.* 2008;51:203–205.
113. Ballas SK. Meperidine for acute sickle cell pain in the emergency department: revisited controversy. *Ann Emerg Med.* 2008;51:217.
114. Tobin DL, Holroyd KA, Reynolds RV, Wigal JK. The hierarchical factor structure of the coping strategies inventory. *Cognitive Ther Res.* 1989;13:343–361.
115. Zsebik G, O'Riordan MA, Berman B, Villela A. Low risk of meperidine-induced seizures in children with sickle cell disease [abstract]. *Pediatr Blood Cancer.* 2007;48:612.
116. Chulamokha L, Scholand SJ, Riggio JM, Ballas SK, Horn D, DeSimone JA. Bloodstream infections in hospitalized adults with sickle cell disease: a retrospective analysis. *Am J Hematol.* 2006;81:723–728.
117. Koppert W. Opioid-induced hyperalgesia – Pathophysiology and clinical relevance. *Acute Pain.* 2007;9:21–34.
118. Klepstad P, Dale O, Skorpen F, Borchgrevink PC, Kaasa S. Genetic variability and clinical efficacy of morphine. *Acta Anaesthesiol Scand.* 2005;49:902–908.
119. Graham AW, Schultz TK, Mayo-Smith MF, Ries RK. *Principles of Addiction Medicine.* 3rd ed. Chevy Chase, MD: American Society of Addiction Medicine; 2003.
120. Uhl GR, Sora I, Wang Z. The mu opiate receptor as a candidate gene for pain: polymorphisms, variations in expression, nociception, and opiate responses. *Proc Natl Acad Sci USA.* 1999;96:7752–7755.
121. Compton P, Geschwind DH, Alarcon M. Association between human mu-opioid receptor gene polymorphism, pain tolerance, and opioid addiction. *Am J Med Genet B Neuropsychiatr Genet.* 2003;121:76–82.
122. Klepstad P, Rakvag TT, Kaasa S, et al. The 118 A > G polymorphism in the human mu-opioid receptor gene may increase morphine requirements in patients with pain caused by malignant disease. *Acta Anaesthesiol Scand.* 2004;48:1232–1239.
123. Mehta S, Kutlar F, Bailey L, et al. Mu opioid receptor 1 (MOR 1) polymorphisms among patients with sickle cell disease. Oral presentation. In: *27th Annual Meeting of the National Sickle Cell Disease Program.* Los Angeles, CA; April 18–21, 2004.
124. Darbari DS, Minniti CP, Rana S, Van Den Anker J. Pharmacogenetics of morphine: potential implications in sickle cell disease. *Am J Hematol.* 2008;83:233–236.
125. Darbari DS, van Schaik RH, Capparelli EV, Rana S, McCarter R, Van Den Anker J. UGT2B7 promoter variant -840G>A contributes to the variability in hepatic clearance of morphine in patients with sickle cell disease. *Am J Hematol.* 2008;83:200–202.
126. Kopecky EA, Jacobson S, Joshi P, Koren G. Systemic exposure to morphine and the risk of acute chest syndrome in sickle cell disease. *Clin Pharmacol Ther.* 2004;75:140–146.
127. Buchanan ID, Woodward M, Reed GW. Opioid selection during sickle cell pain crisis and its impact on the development of acute chest syndrome. *Pediatr Blood Cancer.* 2005;45:716–724.
128. Weber ML, Hebbel RP, Gupta K. Morphine induces kidney injury in transgenic sickle cell mice. *Blood.* 2005;106: 884a–5a.
129. King T, Vardanyan A, Majuta L, et al. Morphine treatment accelerates sarcoma-induced bone pain, bone loss, and spontaneous fracture in a murine model of bone cancer. *Pain.* 2007;132:154–168.
130. Poonawala T, Levay-Young BK, Hebbel RP, Gupta K. Opioids heal ischemic wounds in the rat. *Wound Repair Regen.* 2005;13:165–174.
131. Ferrante MF. Nonsteroidal anti-inflammatory drugs. In: Ferrante MF, Vade Bancoeur TR, eds. *Post Operative Pain Management.* New York: Churchill Livingstone; 1993a:133–143.
132. Perlin E, Finke H, Castro O, et al. Enhancement of pain control with ketorolac tromethamine in patients with sickle cell vaso-occlusive crisis. *Am J Hematol.* 1994;46:43–47.
133. Crain SM, Shen KF. Ultra-low concentrations of naloxone selectively antagonize excitatory effects of morphine on sensory neurons, thereby increasing its antinociceptive potency and attenuating tolerance/dependence during chronic cotreatment. *Proc Natl Acad Sci USA.* 1995;92:10540–10544.
134. Winkelmuller M, Winkelmuller W. Long-term effects of continuous intrathecal opioid treatment in chronic pain of nonmalignant etiology. *J Neurosurg.* 1996;85:458–467.
135. Definitions Related to the Use of Opioids for the Treatment of Pain. American Academy of Pain Medicine American Pain Society American Academy of Addiction Medicine 2001. Available at http://www.ama-assn.org/ama1/pub/upload/mm/455/opioiddefinitions.pdf. Accessed March 31, 2008.
136. Benjamin LJ, Payne R. Pain in sickle cell disease: a multidimensional construct. In: Pace B, ed. *Renaissance of Sickle Cell Disease Research in the Genomic Era.* London: Imperial College Press; 2007:99–118.
137. Mercadante S, Ferrera P, Villari P, Arcuri E. Hyperalgesia: an emerging iatrogenic syndrome. *J Pain Symptom Manage.* 2003;26:769–775.
138. Woolf CJ, Salter MW. Neuronal plasticity: increasing the gain in pain. *Science.* 2000;288:1765–1769.
139. Gottschalk A, Smith DS. New concepts in acute pain therapy: preemptive analgesia. *Am Fam Physician.* 2001;63:1979–1984.
140. Baliki MN, Geha PY, Apkarian AV, Chialvo DR. Beyond feeling: chronic pain hurts the brain, disrupting the default-mode network dynamics. *J Neurosci.* 2008;28:1398–1403.
141. Song I, Huganir RL. Regulation of AMPA receptors during synaptic plasticity. *Trends Neurosci.* 2002;25:578–588.
142. Carroll RC, Beattie EC, von Zastrow M, Malenka RC. Role of AMPA receptor endocytosis in synaptic plasticity. *Nat Rev Neurosci.* 2001;2:315–324.
143. Perez-Otano I, Ehlers MD. Homeostatic plasticity and NMDA receptor trafficking. *Trends Neurosci.* 2005;28:229–238.

144. Morishita W, Marie H, Malenka RC. Distinct triggering and expression mechanisms underlie LTD of AMPA and NMDA synaptic responses. *Nat Neurosci.* 2005;8:1043–1050.
145. Marchand F, Perretti M, McMahon SB. Role of the immune system in chronic pain. *Nat Rev Neurosci.* 2005;6:521–532.
146. Nakajima K, Kohsaka S. Microglia: activation and their significance in the central nervous system. *J Biochem.* 2001;130:169–175.
147. Deleo JA, Sorkin L, Watkins L, eds. *Immune and Glial Regulation of Pain.* Seattle: IASP Press; 2007.
148. Katz JL, Higgins ST. The validity of the reinstatement model of craving and relapse to drug use. *Psychopharmacology.* 2003;168:21–30.
149. Boyer EW, Shannon MT. The serotonin syndrome. *N Engl J Med.* 2005;352:1112–1120.
150. NIH. The Management of Sickle Cell Disease. National Heart, Lung and Blood Institute, No. 02-2117. 4th ed. Washington DC: National Institutes of Health; 2002.
151. Benjamin LJ, Dampier CD, Jacox A, et al. *Guideline for the Management of Acute and Chronic Pain in Sickle-Cell Disease.* Glenview, IL: American Pain Society; 1999.
152. Sickle Cell Education Center. Georgia Comprehensive Sickle Cell Center, 2006. Available at www.scinfo.org. Accessed March 3, 2008.
153. Dunlop RJ, Bennett KC. Pain management for sickle cell disease. *Cochrane Database Syst Rev.* 2006:CD003350.
154. Gil KM, Carson JW, Sedway JA, Porter LS, Schaeffer JJ, Orringer E. Follow-up of coping skills training in adults with sickle cell disease: analysis of daily pain and coping practice diaries. *Health Psychol.* 2000;19:85–90.
155. Gil KM, Thompson RJ Jr, Keith BR, Tota-Faucette M, Noll S, Kinney TR. Sickle cell disease pain in children and adolescents: change in pain frequency and coping strategies over time. *J Pediatr Psychol.* 1993;18:621–637.
156. WHO Pain Ladder. World Health Organization, 2008. Available at http://www.who.int/cancer/palliative/painladder/en/. Accessed March 8, 2008.
157. Jacox A, Carr DB, Payne R. New clinical-practice guidelines for the management of pain in patients with cancer. *N Engl J Med.* 1994;330:651–655.
158. Epstein K, Yuen E, Riggio JM, Ballas SK, Moleski SM. Utilization of the office, hospital and emergency department for adult sickle cell patients: a five-year study. *J Natl Med Assoc.* 2006;98:1109–1113.
159. Adewoye AH, Nolan V, McMahon L, Ma Q, Steinberg MH. Effectiveness of a dedicated day hospital for management of acute sickle cell pain. *Haematologica.* 2007;92:854–855.
160. Benjamin LJ, Swinson GI, Nagel RL. Sickle cell anemia day hospital: an approach for the management of uncomplicated painful crises. *Blood.* 2000;95:1130–1136.
161. The Georgia Comprehensive Sickle Cell Center at Grady Health System in Atlanta, Georgia: Center Description and Services. 2006. Available at http://www.scinfo.org/.
162. Wright J, Bareford D, Wright C, et al. Day case management of sickle pain: 3 years experience in a UK sickle cell unit. *Br J Haematol.* 2004;126:878–80.
163. Beyer J, Platt A, Kinney T. *Assessment of Pain in Adults and Children with Sickle Cell Disease.* Mt. Desert, ME: New England Regional Genetics Group; 1994.
164. Shapiro B, Schechter NL, Ohene-Frempong K. *The Genetic Resource, Sickle Cell Related Pain: Assessment and Management.* Mt. Desert, ME: New England Regional Genetics Group; 1994.
165. Frei-Jones MJ, Baxter AL, Rogers ZR, Buchanan GR. Vaso-occlusive episodes in older children with sickle cell disease: emergency department management and pain assessment. *J Pediatr.* 2008;152:281–285.
166. Ballas SK. Current issues in sickle cell pain and its management. *Hematology Am Soc Hematol Educ Program.* 2007; 110: 97–105.
167. Tanabe P, Myers R, Zosel A, et al. Emergency department management of acute pain episodes in sickle cell disease. *Acad Emerg Med.* 2007;14:419–425.
168. Pain Episodes. Georgia Comprehensive Sickle Cell Center, 2006. Accessed at http://www.scinfo.org/painepi.htm.
169. The Georgia Comprehensive Sickle Cell Center at Grady Health System in Atlanta, Georgia 2006. (Accessed 2008)
170. Payne R. Pain management is sickle cell disease: rationale and techniques. *Ann NY Acad Sci.* 1989;565:189–206.
171. Platt A, Eckman JR, Beasley J, Miller G. Treating sickle cell pain: an update from the Georgia comprehensive sickle cell center. *J Emerg Nurs.* 2002;28:297–303.
172. Gonzalez ER, Bahal N, Hansen LA, et al. Intermittent injection vs patient-controlled analgesia for sickle cell crisis pain. Comparison in patients in the emergency department. *Arch Intern Med.* 1991;151:1373–1378.
173. Holbrook CT. Patient-controlled analgesia pain management for children with sickle cell disease. *J Assoc Acad Minor Phys.* 1990;1:93–96.
174. Melzer-Lange MD, Walsh-Kelly CM, Lea G, Hillery CA, Scott JP. Patient-controlled analgesia for sickle cell pain crisis in a pediatric emergency department. *Pediatr Emerg Care.* 2004;20:2–4.
175. Trentadue NO, Kachoyeanos MK, Lea G. A comparison of two regimens of patient-controlled analgesia for children with sickle cell disease. *J Pediatr Nurs.* 1998;13:15–9.
176. van Beers EJ, van Tuijn CF, Nieuwkerk PT, Friederich PW, Vranken JH, Biemond BJ. Patient-controlled analgesia versus continuous infusion of morphine during vaso-occlusive crisis in sickle cell disease, a randomized controlled trial. *Am J Hematol.* 2007;82:955–60.
177. Schechter NL, Berrien FB, Katz SM. PCA for adolescents in sickle-cell crisis. *Am J Nurs.* 1988;88:719, 21–2.
178. Schechter NL, Berrien FB, Katz SM. The use of patient-controlled analgesia in adolescents with sickle cell pain crisis: a preliminary report. *J Pain Symptom Manage.* 1988;3:109–113.
179. Ballas SK. Ethical issues in the management of sickle cell pain. *Am J Hematol.* 2001;68:127–132.
180. Elander J, Lusher J, Bevan D, Telfer P, Burton B. Understanding the causes of problematic pain management in sickle cell disease: evidence that pseudoaddiction plays a more important role than genuine analgesic dependence. *J Pain Symptom Manage.* 2004;27:156–169.
181. Elander J, Marczewska M, Amos R, Thomas A, Tangayi S. Factors affecting hospital staff judgments about sickle cell disease pain. *J Behav Med.* 2006;29:203–214.
182. Elander J, Midence K. A review of evidence about factors affecting quality of pain management in sickle cell disease. *Clin J Pain.* 1996;12:180–193.

183. Armstrong FD, Pegelow CH, Gonzalez JC, Martinez A. Impact of children's sickle cell history on nurse and physician ratings of pain and medication decisions. *J Pediatr Psychol.* 1992;17:651–164.
184. Todd KH, Green C, Bonham VL, Jr., Haywood C, Jr., Ivy E. Sickle cell disease related pain: crisis and conflict. *J Pain* 2006;7:453–458.
185. Ballas SK. Current issues in sickle cell pain and its management. *Hematology Am Soc Hematol Educ Program.* 2007;2007:97–105.
186. Quill TE. Partnerships in patient care: a contractual approach. *Ann Intern Med.* 1983;98:228–234.
187. Donovan MI, Evers K, Jacobs P, Mandleblatt S. When there is no benchmark: designing a primary care-based chronic pain management program from the scientific basis up. *J Pain Symptom Manage.* 1999;18:38–48.
188. Gil KM, Carson JW, Porter LS, et al. Daily stress and mood and their association with pain, health-care use, and school activity in adolescents with sickle cell disease. *J Pediatr Psychol.* 2003;28:363–373.
189. Smith WR, Bovbjerg VE, Penberthy LT, et al. Understanding pain and improving management of sickle cell disease: the PiSCES study. *J Natl Med Assoc.* 2005;97:183–93.
190. Ennis JT, Serjeant GR, Middlemiss H. Homozygous sickle cell disease in Jamaica. *Br J Radiol.* 1973;46:943–950.
191. Milner PF, Kraus AP, Sebes JI, et al. Sickle cell disease as a cause of osteonecrosis of the femoral head. *N Engl J Med.* 1991;325:1476–1481.
192. Milner PF, Kraus AP, Sebes JI, et al. Osteonecrosis of the humeral head in sickle cell disease. *Clin Orthop Rel Res.* 1993:136–143.
193. Riggs W Jr, Rockett JF. Roentgen chest findings in childhood sickle cell anemia. A new vertebral body finding. *Am J Roentgenol Radium Ther Nucl Med.* 1968;104:838–845.
194. Diggs LW. Bone and joint lesions in sickle-cell disease. *Clin Orthop Rel Res.* 1967;52:119–143.
195. Diggs LW, ed. *Anatomic Lesions in Sickle Cell Anemia.* St. Louis: C.V. Mosby Co; 1973.
196. Neumayr LD, Aguilar C, Earles AN, et al. Physical therapy alone compared with core decompression and physical therapy for femoral head osteonecrosis in sickle cell disease. Results of a multicenter study at a mean of three years after treatment. *J Bone Joint Surg Am.* 2006;88:2573–2582.
197. Hernigou P, Habibi A, Bachir D, Galacteros F. The natural history of asymptomatic osteonecrosis of the femoral head in adults with sickle cell disease. *J Bone Joint Surg Am.* 2006;88:2565–2572.
198. Bishop AR, Roberson JR, Eckman JR, Fleming LL. Total hip arthroplasty in patients who have sickle-cell hemoglobinopathy. *J Bone Joint Surg Am.* 1988;70:853–855.
199. Hernigou P, Zilber S, Filippini P, Mathieu G, Poignard A, Galacteros F. Total THA in adult osteonecrosis related to sickle cell disease. *Clin Orthop Rel Res.* 2008;466:300–308.
200. Koshy M, Entsuah R, Koranda A, et al. Leg ulcers in patients with sickle cell disease. *Blood.* 1989;74:1403–1408.
201. Serjeant GR. Leg ulceration in sickle cell anemia. *Arch Intern Med.* 1974;133:690–694.
202. Eckman JR. Leg ulcers in sickle cell disease. *Hematol Oncol Clin North Am.* 1996;10:1333–1344.
203. Ballas SK. Pain management of sickle cell disease. *Hematol Oncol Clin North Am.* 2005;19:785–802.
204. Adams RJ. Neurologic complications. In: Embury SH, Hebbel RP, Mohondas N, Steinberg MH, eds. *Sickle Cell Disease: Basic Principles and Clinical Practice.* 1st ed. New York: Raven Press; 1994:599–621.
205. Konotey-Ahulu FI. Mental-nerve neuropathy: a complication of sickle-cell crisis. *Lancet.* 1972;2:388.
206. Asher SW. Multiple cranial neuropathies, trigeminal neuralgia, and vascular headaches in sickle cell disease, a possible common mechanism. *Neurology.* 1980;30:210–211.
207. Sommer C. Painful neuropathies. *Curr Opin Neurol.* 2003;16: 623–628.
208. Woolf CJ, Mannion RJ. Neuropathic pain: aetiology, symptoms, mechanisms, and management. *Lancet.* 1999;353: 1959–1964.
209. Harden RN. Chronic neuropathic pain. Mechanisms, diagnosis, and treatment. *Neurologist.* 2005;11:111–122.
210. Irving GA. Contemporary assessment and management of neuropathic pain. *Neurology.* 2005;64:S21–27.
211. Siddall PJ, Cousins MJ. Persistent pain as a disease entity: implications for clinical management. *Anesth Analg.* 2004;99: 510–520.
212. Edwards RR. Individual differences in endogenous pain modulation as a risk factor for chronic pain. *Neurology.* 2005;65: 437–443.
213. Krantz MJ, Mehler PS. Treating opioid dependence. Growing implications for primary care. *Arch Intern Med.* 2004;164: 277–288.
214. Portenoy RK, Foley KM. Chronic use of opioid analgesics in non-malignant pain: report of 38 cases. *Pain.* 1986;25:171–186.
215. Schofferman J. Long-term use of opioid analgesics for the treatment of chronic pain of nonmalignant origin. *J Pain Symptom Manage.* 1993;8:279–288.
216. Ballantyne JC, Mao J. Opioid therapy for chronic pain. *N Engl J Med.* 2003;349:1943–1953.
217. Ballantyne JC. Opioids for chronic pain: taking stock. *Pain.* 2006;125:3–4.
218. Kalso E, Edwards JE, Moore RA, McQuay HJ. Opioids in chronic non-cancer pain: systematic review of efficacy and safety. *Pain.* 2004;112:372–380.
219. Eriksen J, Sjogren P, Bruera E, Ekholm O, Rasmussen NK. Critical issues on opioids in chronic non-cancer pain: an epidemiological study. *Pain.* 2006;125:172–179.
220. Medicine AAoP, Society AP. The use of opioids for the treatment of chronic pain: a consensus statement. *Clin J Pain.* 1997;13:6–8.
221. Fishman SM, Wilsey B, Yang J, Reisfield GM, Bandman TB, Borsook D. Adherence monitoring and drug surveillance in chronic opioid therapy. *J Pain Symptom Manage.* 2000;20:293–307.
222. States Federation of Medical Boards, Model policy for the use of controlled substances for the treatment of pain. Available at: http://www.fsmb.org/pdf/2004_grpol_Controlled_Substances.pdf. 2004.
223. Fishman SM, Bandman TB, Edwards A, Borsook D. The opioid contract in the management of chronic pain. *J Pain Symptom Manage.* 1999;18:27–37.
224. Consent for chronic opioid therapy. American Academy of Pain Medicine, 2001. Available at: http://www.painmed.org/pdf/opioid_consent_form.pdf.

225. Long-term Controlled Substances Therapy for Chronic Pain. *Sample Agreement.* 1997 Available at: http://www.painmed.org/pdf/controlled_substances_sample_agrmt.pdf.
226. Arnold RM, Han PK, Seltzer D. Opioid contracts in chronic nonmalignant pain management: objectives and uncertainties. *Am J Med.* 2006;119:292–296.
227. Hariharan J, Lamb GC, Neuner JM. Long-term opioid contract use for chronic pain management in primary care practice. A five year experience. *J Gen Intern Med.* 2007;22:485–490.
228. Zylicz Z, Twycross R. Opioid-induced hyperalgesia may be more frequent than previously thought. *J Clin Oncol.* 2008;26:1564.
229. Doverty M, White JM, Somogyi AA, Bochner F, Ali R, Ling W. Hyperalgesic responses in methadone maintenance patients. *Pain.* 2001;90:91–96.
230. White JM. Pleasure into pain: the consequences of long-term opioid use. *Addict Behav.* 2004;29:1311–1324.
231. Angst MS, Clark JD. Opioid-induced hyperalgesia: a qualitative systematic review. *Anesthesiology.* 2006;104:570–587.
232. Chang G, Chen L, Mao J. Opioid tolerance and hyperalgesia. *Med Clin North Am.* 2007;91:199–211.
233. Mao J. Opioid-induced abnormal pain sensitivity: implications in clinical opioid therapy. *Pain.* 2002;100:213–217.
234. Mao J. Opioid-induced abnormal pain sensitivity. *Curr Pain Headache Rep.* 2006;10:67–70.
235. American Psychiatric Association. *Diagnostic and Statistical Manual of Mental Disorders, Revised.* 4th ed. Washington, DC: American Psychiatric Association; 1994.
236. Kalivas PW, O'Brien C. Drug addiction as a pathology of staged neuroplasticity. *Neuropsychopharmacology.* 2008;33:166–180.
237. O'Brien CP. Research advances in the understanding and treatment of addiction. *Am J Addict.* 2003;12 Suppl 2:S36–47.
238. Jackson JL, Kroenke K. Difficult patient encounters in the ambulatory clinic: clinical predictors and outcomes. *Arch Intern Med.* 1999;159:1069–1075.
239. Adams J, Murray R, 3rd. The general approach to the difficult patient. *Emerg Med Clin North Am.* 1998;16:689–700.
240. Hull SK, Broquet K. How to manage difficult patient encounters. *Fam Pract Manage.* 2007;14:30–34.
241. Krebs EE, Garrett JM, Konrad TR. The difficult doctor? Characteristics of physicians who report frustration with patients: an analysis of survey data. *BMC Health Serv Res.* 2006;6:128.
242. Koekkoek B, van Meijel B, Hutschemaekers G. "Difficult patients" in mental health care: a review. *Psychiatr Serv.* 2006;57:795–802.
243. Haas LJ, Leiser JP, Magill MK, Sanyer ON. Management of the difficult patient. *Am Fam Physician.* 2005;72:2063–2068.
244. Tandeter H. Making peace with your "difficult patient." *Patient Educ Couns.* 2006;62:3–4.
245. Elder N, Ricer R, Tobias B. How respected family physicians manage difficult patient encounters. *J Am Board Fam Med.* 2006;19:533–541.
246. Marks RM, Sachar EJ. Undertreatment of medical inpatients with narcotic analgesics. *Ann Intern Med.* 1973;78:173–181.
247. Marlowe KF, Chicella MF. Treatment of sickle cell pain. *Pharmacotherapy.* 2002;22:484–491.
248. Sutton M, Atweh GF, Cashman TD, Davis WT. Resolving conflicts: misconceptions and myths in the care of the patient with sickle cell disease. *Mt Sinai J Med.* 1999;66:282–285.
249. Platt OS. Hydroxyurea for the treatment of sickle cell anemia. *N Engl J Med.* 2008;358:1362–1369.
250. Eccleston C, Yorke L, Morley S, Williams AC, Mastroyannopoulou K. Psychological therapies for the management of chronic and recurrent pain in children and adolescents. *Cochrane Database Syst Rev.* 2003:CD003968.
251. Anie KA, Green J. Psychological therapies for sickle cell disease and pain. *Cochrane Database Syst Rev.* 2002:CD001916.
252. Ballas SK. Sickle cell disease: current clinical management. *Semin Hematol.* 2001;38:307–314.

21

Hemoglobin SC Disease and Hemoglobin C Disorders

Martin H. Steinberg and Ronald L. Nagel

INTRODUCTION

HbC (*HBB* glu6lys), along with HbS (*HBB* glu6val) and HbE (*HBB* glu26lys), is one of the three most common hemoglobin variants in humankind. Its positive charge that allows it to bind the erythrocyte membrane, and perhaps other unique features of this variant, lead to loss of cell K^+ and water, thereby increasing erythrocyte density. HbC disease, defined as homozygosity for the HbC gene, causes mild hemolytic anemia; simple heterozygosity for HbC (HbC trait, HbAC) is innocuous. In HbSC disease, in which the erythrocyte concentration of HbS and HbC is nearly equal, the dehydrated, dense erythrocyte accentuates the deleterious properties of HbS by producing a milieu favoring HbS polymerization. HbSC disease causes vasoocclusive disease and hemolytic anemia, albeit on average both less severe than found in sickle cell anemia (homozygosity for HbS). Like sickle cell anemia, the hematological and clinical features of HbSC disease are heterogeneous, but all of the complications that make sickle cell anemia notorious can be present; some even appear more often in HbSC disease.

HbC and HbC Disease

Origins, Selection, and Distribution of HbC

HbC, the second hemoglobin variant discovered, was described in 1950, and the first homozygous case was reported in 1953. The β^C-globin gene contains a GAG→AAG transition and codes for lysine instead of glutamic acid. Shortly after its description in African Americans, HbC was found to be common in Africa.

Origins. The HbC mutation originated on a β^A-globin gene in West Africa and by means similar to the dispersion of the HbS gene (Chapter 27) spread throughout the world. The β^C-globin gene migrated northward through ancient trans-Saharan trade routes. Predicated on the identity of their haplotypes, HbC in sub-Saharan Africa and North Africa, appears to have had the same origin as in Burkina Faso. Strong gene flow, influenced by the selective pressure of *Plasmodium falciparum* malaria, has distributed HbC throughout central West Africa and toward North Africa, particularly Morocco.

Absence of a Hpa I restriction site 3′ to the HbC gene made it doubtful that HbC arose from mutations in a HbS gene.[1] HbC, which is found in Africa in a restricted distribution, reaches its highest frequency in central West Africa and its gene frequency decreases concentrically outward from there.[2,3] Interestingly, HbC is found in Africa almost exclusively in areas where HbS exists. Although the possibility of a second origin of the HbC gene in Africa has been raised by the presence of a 3′ β-globin gene Hpa I site in several patients, this site is in the middle of an extensive L1 repeat where a high probability of rearrangement exists.

Recombination is expected to reduce the effect of selection on the extent of linkage disequilibrium. It was estimated that the HbC mutation originated less than 5,000 years ago, but despite strong selection and this recent origin, crossing-over or gene conversion present in the "hotspot" 5′ to the β-globin gene locus in more than a third of the HbC chromosomes sampled led to rapid decay in linkage disequilibrium upstream of the HbC allele mitigating the effects of positive selection.

Two instances of independent origin of the β^C have been found in Thailand and in Oman.[4] In both, a strong case for independent origin is made by the presence of the mutation in a different chromosomal framework.

Haplotypes of the HbC Gene. Haplotypes of β^C-globin gene–bearing chromosomes are shown in Figure 21.1A. Three major haplotypes of the β^C-globin gene, termed CI, CII, and CIII are found. Several minor unusual haplotypes have also been described (Fig. 21.1B). Of 90 β^C-globin gene chromosomes, 70% were CI, 20% CII, and 10% had other haplotypes that were either CIII or compatible with recombination events. Heterogeneity of haplotypes associated with the β^C gene is likely to result from crossovers in the 5′ portion of the β-globin gene cluster, an event that is common and results in atypical haplotypes of the β^S gene. In Africa, most β^C chromosomes from Burkina Faso and Benin had the C I haplotype.

HbC and Malaria

HbC provides some protection from malaria.[5] In a case-control study in Burkina Faso, HbC was associated with a 29% reduction in risk of clinical malaria in carriers and a 93% reduction in HbC disease.[6] It was also associated with reduced parasitemia and protection from malarial attacks.[7] Among children with severe malaria, asymptomatic parasitemia and no malaria studied in Ghana, HbC trait did not prevent infection with *P. falciparum* but reduced the odds of developing severe malaria and anemia, albeit to a lesser extent than sickle cell trait (HbAS). The multiplication rate

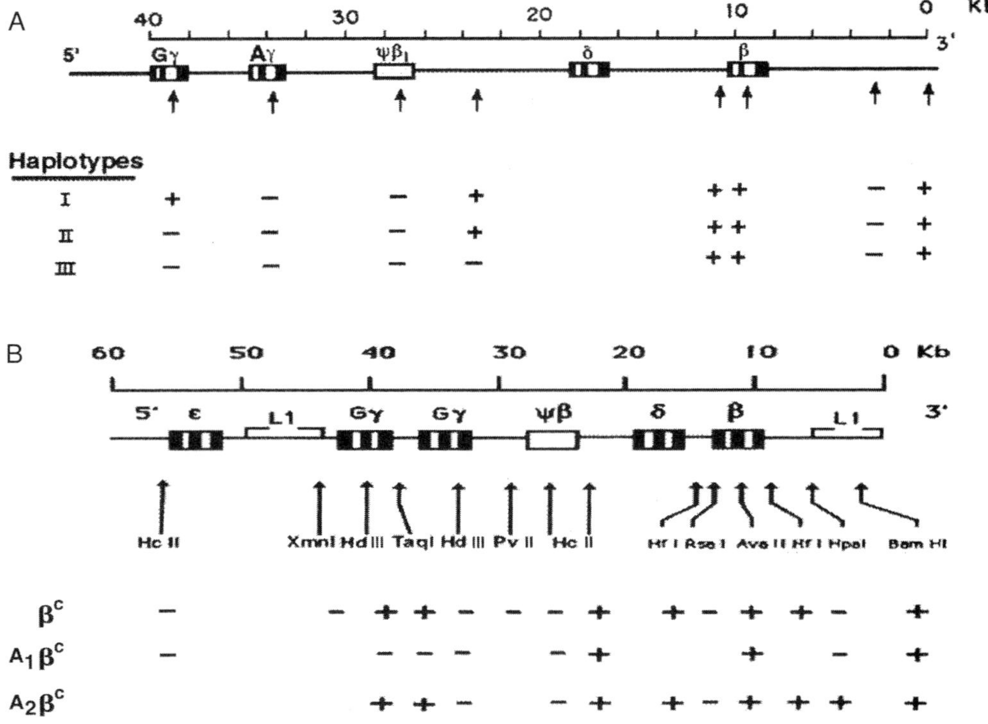

Figure 21.1. β-Globin gene cluster haplotypes associated with the β^C-globin gene. Above each section are depicted the β-like globin genes with approximate size markers in kilobases. **(A)** Haplotypes of β^C-globin gene–bearing chromosomes were determined using eight restriction fragment length polymorphisms (RFLPs). Shown are the "typical" haplotypes CI, CII, and CIII. Arrows indicate, from left to right, the polymorphic restriction sites, *Hind* III (2 sites), *Hinc* II (2 sites), *Hinf* I, *Ava* II, *Hpa* I, and *Bam* HI. **(A)** (+) indicates cleavage and a (−), lack of cleavage by the designated enzyme. **(B)** Two atypical haplotypes associated with the β^C-globin gene (A_1 β^C and A_2 β^C). These haplotypes were determined using additional RFLPs as shown.[107,108]

of *P. falciparum* in HbC disease erythrocytes is lower than in normal cells with a high proportion of ring forms and with trophozoites disintegrating. Also, knobs present on the surface of infected cells are fewer and morphologically aberrant when compared with those on normal cells.[8] These data support natural selection acting on the HbC gene because of the relative resistance it confers against severe malaria but not resistance to acquiring an infection.[9,10]

PATHOPHYSIOLOGY OF HbC DISORDERS

Biochemical Features of HbC

HbC was first detected because of its slow migration compared with HbA and HbS during cellulose acetate electrophoresis at pH 8.6, a difference caused by the net increase of two units of positive charge per molecule. Newer techniques of hemoglobin separation now allow high-performance liquid chromatography (HPLC) separation of variants with similar positive charges such as HbE and HbO-Arab (*HBB* glu121lys) and also the normal HbA_2, from HbC (Chapters 7, 23, and 28).

Carboxy HbC has decreased solubility in phosphate buffers, whereas deoxy HbC has nearly the same solubility as deoxy HbA. In concentrated phosphate buffers, deoxy HbC had even higher solubility than HbA. Oxygen affinity of HbC "stripped" of 2,3-BPG was normal.

HbC Crystallization. When concentrated solutions of purified hemoglobins are incubated in high-molarity

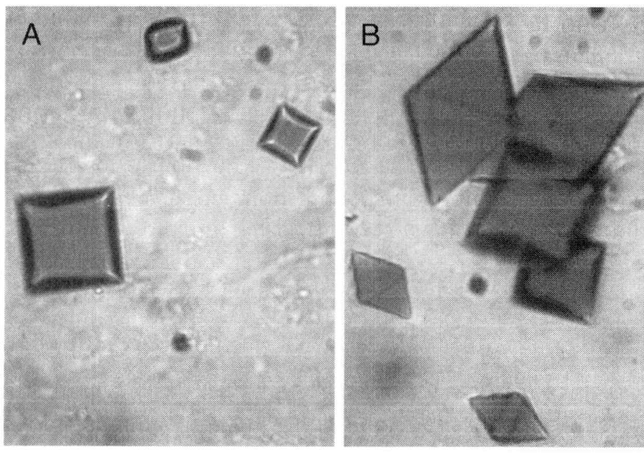

Figure 21.2. Crystal forms observed in hemolysates of patients with HbC. **(A)** Cubic crystals, generated in hemolysates of compound heterozygotes for HbC and Hb Korle-Bu. **(B)** Tetragonal crystals observed intracellularly and in hemolysates of patients homozygous for HbC, with HbSC disease and compound heterozygotes for HbC and HbA and other mutants. (See color plate 21.2.)

phosphate buffer, hemoglobin crystals usually form (Fig. 21.2). In these crystals, hemoglobin can be liganded either as cyanmet, oxy, or CO hemoglobin. HbC crystals form within 25 minutes in a 100% HbC solution and HbF appears to inhibit crystallization.[11] In HbC disease erythrocytes, cells with crystals isolated from density gradients had very low HbF concentrations.[12] In the dense cell fraction, F cells did not contain HbC crystals.

HbA_2 inhibited HbC crystallization to a greater extent than HbF. The critical residue involved is at position 87 in the δ- and γ-globin chains where a gln replaces thr. This is the same residue that might account for the inhibition of HbS polymerization by HbF and HbA_2.[11] An examination of the interactions of HbC with Hb Lepore-Boston, which inhibits HbC crystallization to a lesser extent than HbF and HbA_2, suggests that a reduction in inhibition could arise from the slight difference in hemoglobin conformation due to the shift of oxygen equilibrium observed in Hb Lepore.[11,13] Other amino acids located between positions 88 and 146 could add to the inhibitory effect of both the γ -and the δ-globin chains on HbC crystallization.

Other mutant hemoglobins that are present with HbC can affect its in vitro crystallization. Compound heterozygotes having HbC-HbN-Baltimore (*HBB* lys95glu) and HbC-Hb Riyadh (*HBB* lys120asn) suggest that β120 and β95 are additional contact sites in the crystal. Hb Riyadh inhibited the in vitro crystallization of HbC explaining the lack of overt pathology, with the exception of microcytosis, in a compound heterozygous infant. In contrast, HbN-Baltimore accelerated the crystallization of HbC and contributed to abnormal red cell morphology, suggesting that the crystal is sustained by hydrophobic interactions.[14]

Hb Korle-Bu (*HBB* asp73asn) accelerates HbC crystallization.[15] Compound heterozygotes for Hb Korle-Bu and HbC have mild microcytic hemolytic anemia and in vitro acceleration of crystal formation, where precrystal hemoglobin structures convert rapidly into cubic-like crystals as opposed to the typical tetragonal crystal structure. In vitro crystallization studies led to the conclusion that β87 and β73 are contact sites of the oxyhemoglobin crystal.[13]

Hemoglobin $\alpha_2^{G\text{-Philadelphia}}\beta_2^{C}$ has an increased rate of crystal nucleation compared with HbC, implying that position α68, the mutation site of HbG-Philadelphia, is a contact site in the crystal of HbC.[16]

Mixtures of HbA and HbC crystallize with a different morphology than the classic HbC crystal habit, raising the question of the hemoglobin composition of crystals generated in mixtures of HbC with HbF or HbA_2. As the HbA concentration of the mixture increases, more tetragonal crystals are formed as opposed to typical orthorhombic crystals. HbA alone does not form crystals under these conditions, making it likely that hybrid tetramers ($\alpha_2\beta^C\beta^A$) are incorporated into these crystals. It also suggests strongly that these two hemoglobins cocrystallize. HbS also cocrystalizes with HbC.

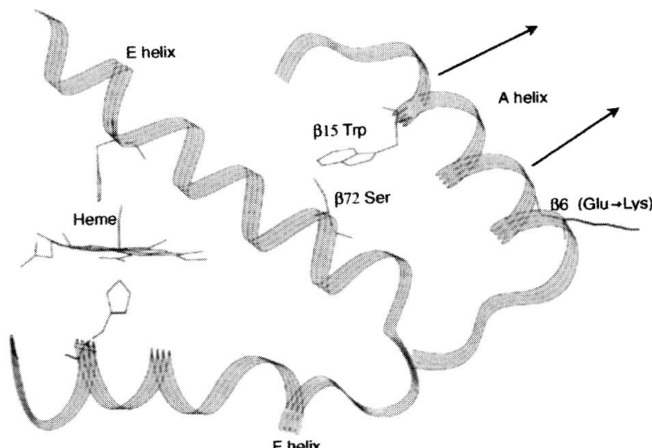

Figure 21.3. View of the F, E, and A helix in the β chains of hemoglobin. Also depicted are the heme, the β15 trp - β72 ser bond and the β6 Lys (the mutation of HbC). The arrows depict the likely movement of the A helix away from the E helix, which is compatible with conformational changes in the central cavity of the tetramer.[13]

A weakening of trpβ15–serβ72 bond most likely leads to a displacement of the A helix away from the E helix.[13] The central cavity (between the two β-globin chains of HbC, is altered compared with HbA[17] (Fig. 21.3).

HbC crystals do not grow by the alignment of the preformed strand but by the attachment of single molecules to suitable sites on the surface. These sites are located along the edges of new layers generated by two-dimensional nucleation. During growth, the steps propagate with random velocities, with the mean being an increasing function of the crystallization driving force.[18] Static and dynamic light scattering characterization of the interactions between the R-state (CO) of HbC, HbA, and HbS molecules in low-ionic-strength solutions showed that the interactions are dominated by the specific binding of solutions' ions to the proteins. Crystals of HbC nucleate and grow by the attachment of native molecules from the solution and concurrent amorphous phases. Spherulites and microfibers are not building blocks for the crystal. HbC crystallization is possible because of the huge entropy gain stemming from the release of up to 10 water molecules per protein intermolecular contact–hydrophobic interaction, suggesting that the higher crystallization propensity of R-state HbC is attributable to increased hydrophobicity.[18] Deoxy HbC formed aggregates and twisted macroribbon forms similar to those seen in the oxy liganded state. In contrast to oxy HbC, deoxy HbC favored the formation of a greater morphological variety of aggregates including polymeric unbranched fibers in radial arrays with dense centers, with infrequent crystal formation in close spatial relation to both the radial arrays and macroribbons. These results suggest that the glu6lys substitution evokes a crystallization process dependent on ligand state conformation. Oxy HbC is thermodynamically driven to a limited number of aggregation pathways with a high propensity to form the tetragonal crystal structure. In contrast, deoxy HbC energetically equally favors multiple pathways

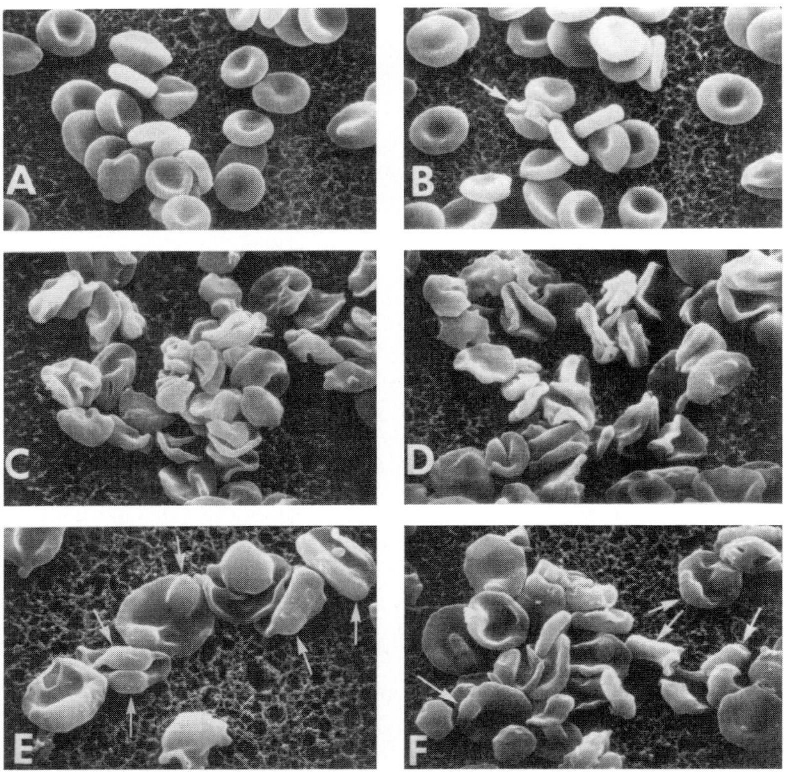

Figure 21.4. Scanning microscopy of HbC disease fractions. **(A** and **B)** Whole blood, in **B** a folded cell. **(C** and **D)** Middle density red cell fraction, notice the abundance of folded cells. **(E** and **F)** The highest density red cell fraction, arrows point to crystal containing red cells.

of aggregation, not all of which might culminate in crystal formation.[19]

Intracellular Crystals in HbC Disease. HbC crystalizes in its oxy configuration and crystals probably exist in vivo. Nevertheless, they are unlikely to play an important role in the pathophysiology of this disorder because deoxygenation will induce melting before or as they enter the microcirculation.

Observations of crystals in vivo were first made under circumstances in which crystal formation could have been induced by cell processing. When blood from splenectomized HbC disease patients was examined by continuous density gradients, a new, very dense band of cells containing crystals 1 μm or more in size were observed. This cell fraction was absent from most HbC disease individuals with intact spleens but present in smaller amounts in some HbC disease patients older than 55 years. Scanning electron microscopy of HbC cells isolated from density gradients and freeze-fracture preparations show intracellular crystals (Figs. 21.4 and 21.5). Circulating crystals can be detected in unperturbed wet preparations from individuals with HbC disease but are rare in unsplenectomized cases.[20]

HbC crystals in the red cells of a splenectomized HbC disease patient were found to be in the oxy state and melted after deoxygenation (Fig. 21.6).[12] When cells from venous and arterial blood were fixed and counted, a small but significant difference in the mean percentage of crystal-containing cells in the arterial circulation versus the venous

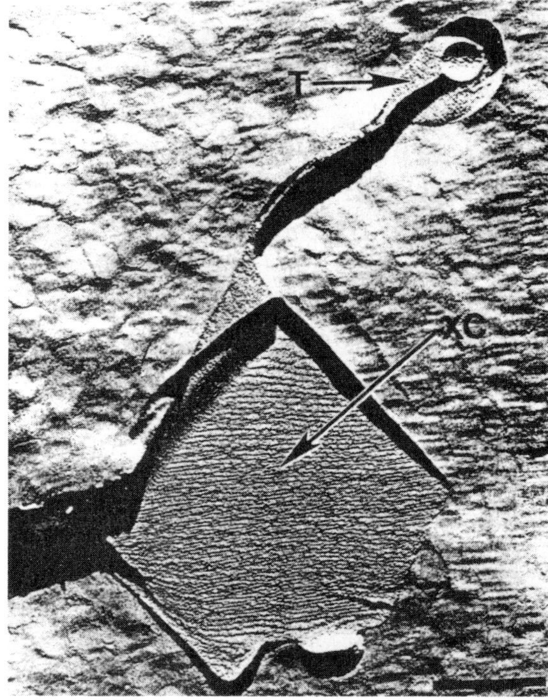

Figure 21.5. Freeze fracture of an HbC disease cell from a splenectomized patient containing a highly ordered crystal (XC) and tail portion (T) that correspond to the membrane of the cell devoid of hemoglobin. This is a negative print (light areas have accumulation of platinum) of a predominantly cross-fractured cell.

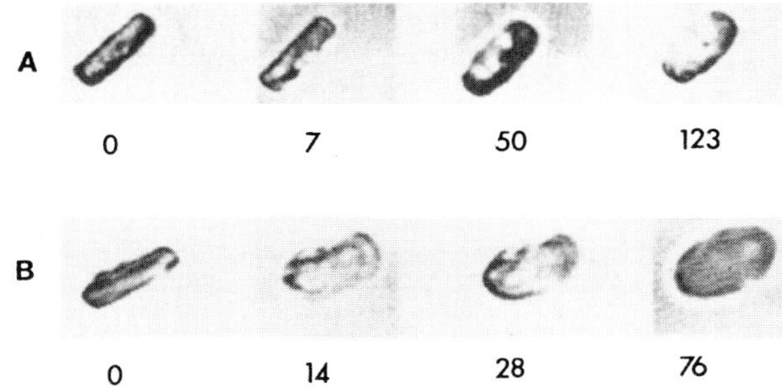

Figure 21.6. Melting of oxy HbC crystal intracellularly by deoxygenation. Time sequence (in seconds) recording of oxy HbC intracellular melting after the addition of isotonic dithionite solution for deoxygenation. Demonstration that the crystal habit of the intracellular crystal is indeed oxy, which is incompatible with the deoxy conformer of HbC.

circulation was present. HbC crystals were not observed either in vitro or in vivo in HbC trait.

PROPERTIES OF THE HbC ERYTHROCYTE

Morphology

HbC disease erythrocytes are noted for their bizarre morphology. In wet preparations, microcytic and hyperchromic cells are present, whereas in dried stained blood films, target cells, microspherocytes, and cells with crystalline inclusions are found. Target cells, a diagnostically useful artifact, are presumably the consequence of the greater surface/volume ratio of HbC disease cells, which is in turn the consequence of their reduced water content.

Ion Transport and Cation Content

Erythrocytes that contain HbC have a characteristic volume-stimulated K^+ leak. Consequently, intracellular cation and water content of HbC disease cells are strikingly reduced, whereas the cation content of HbC trait and HbSC disease cells is less prominently depleted (Chapter 9).[21,22] When the cation and water content of HbC disease cells were increased by making the membrane permeable to cations and returning the cells to an isotonic medium, they returned to their original volume by gaining K^+, a behavior that was not observed in control cells. Volume-stimulated K^+ efflux was neither inhibited by ouabain and butamide nor blocked by inhibitors of Ca^{2+}-activated K^+ permeability. A volume-regulated decrease in cell water in HbC disease cells stands in sharp contrast to the usual description of the human red cell as a passive, slightly imperfect osmometer and probably explained the reduced response of HbC disease cells to changes in the extracellular osmotic pressure. From these observations, it was concluded that HbC disease cells have a potassium transport mechanism that is either absent from, or inactive in, normal cells, and raised the possibility that the presence of the abnormal hemoglobin was responsible for the activity of this transporter. Volume-stimulated K^+ efflux occurred when osmolarity and pH were both reduced, an effect that was chloride–dependent, N-ethylmaleimde stimulated, and similar to previously reported K^+Cl^- transporters.[23–25] Transporters of this sort are present in normal and sickle reticulocytes under oxygenated conditions and decrease in activity with cell aging.[26] Although red cell lifespan is shortened to approximately 40 days in HbC disease, this is more than three times the lifespan of sickle cell anemia erythrocytes, suggesting that factors beyond a high proportion of young cells contribute to the high activity of the K^+Cl^- transporter in HbC disease. Total cellular calcium was elevated in HbC disease cells as it was in sickle cell anemia and was sequestered in endocytic vesicles.

K:Cl cotransport is a powerful volume regulator in young erythrocytes. The delay time for activation of K^+ efflux in sickle cell anemia cells was sixfold shorter than for HbC disease cells and 5.1-fold shorter than for normal cells. HbC cells were first swollen to activate the K:Cl cotransport and then shrunk by reestablishing normal osmolarity. The delay time for K^+ efflux was eightfold longer than sickle cell anemia cells. When K:Cl cotransport was activated by acidification, similar differences in the delay times for activation and deactivation were observed. Moreover, the delay time for activation increased markedly with cell density, but the delay time for deactivation was approximately equal in all density fractions. These studies suggest that K:Cl cotransport is very active in young HbC disease cells but has a longer delay time for deactivation by cell shrinkage than in sickle cell anemia or normal red cells. This suggests that transient activation of K:Cl cotransport in HbC disease reticulocytes, followed by a slow deactivation, can gradually decrease hydration and increase mean corpuscular hemoglobin concentration (MCHC). It implies that K:Cl cotransport regulation by phosphorylation/dephosphorylation might be altered either by a direct effect of HbC and/or by HbC-dependent alteration of enzymes controlling the phosphorylated state. Many of the same abnormalities in K:Cl cotransport can be found in HbC transgenic mice.[27–30]

Oxygen Affinity

P_{50} of HbC disease cells was increased to 29.5 mm Hg (normal, 26.5 mm Hg). The 2,3-BPG content of HbC disease cells was equal to that of normal cells, whereas the difference between the intracellular and extracellular pH was increased for HbC disease cells. Decreased oxygen affinity of HbC disease cells was attributed primarily to reduced intracellular pH, but the "normal" 2,3-BPG content failed to take into account the diminished intracellular water content. When this is considered, the effective 2,3-BPG content is considerably higher than normal and should further decrease oxygen affinity. Decreased oxygen affinity could modulate the anemia of HbC disease by increasing oxygen delivery to tissues.

Osmotic Response and Cell Density

High MCHC and low intracellular water content are characteristics of HbC cells, and the cells in HbC trait and HbC disease are denser than normal. Average MCHC in HbC disease, HbSC disease, HbC trait, and HbA cells were 38, 37, 34, and 33 g/dL, respectively. The youngest and lightest cells differ from the oldest and most dense cells by only 3–4 g/dL. In contrast, cells of sickle cell anemia have a very wide density distribution. HbC disease, HbSC disease, and HbC trait reticulocytes are denser than normal reticulocytes. Either these cells are denser than normal when they first enter the circulation or their density changes within 24 hours while they are still recognizable as reticulocytes. Reduced osmotic fragility in HbC disease is consistent with an increased surface to volume ratio.

Binding of HbC to Red Cell Membrane

HbC, like HbS, interacts more strongly with the erythrocyte membrane than HbA. This interaction has been studied using changes in the fluorescence intensity of the membrane-imbedded fluorescent probe, whose fluorescence is quenched when it is approached by hemoglobin. At pH 6.8, the affinity of HbC for the erythrocyte membrane was approximately five times greater than that of HbA. Deoxy HbA and HbC were less strongly bound than the oxy form. When the NaCl concentration was increased, HbC was approximately 90% dissociated from the membrane.

At higher hemoglobin concentrations, HbC binding was stronger, and higher salt concentrations were required to displace the hemoglobin from the membrane. The cytoplasmic portion of band 3 was implicated as the binding site for both HbA and HbC. HbO-Arab is more strongly bound than HbS and is even more tightly membrane bound than HbC, suggesting that both electrostatic charge and the protein conformation in the vicinity of the charged groups play roles in membrane binding. Membrane binding of abnormal hemoglobins could affect membrane proteins involved in anion or cation movement and play a role in altering red cell density.

Rheological Properties of HbC Disease Erythrocyte

HbC disease cells were less filterable than normal cells. Although the optimum filterability of normal cells occurred at 300 mOsm, HbC disease cells were maximally filterable at 200 mOsm, an observation consistent with increased density. By measuring cellular elongation in response to a fluid shear stress, cellular deformability was examined as a function of buffer osmolarity. HbC disease cells were poorly deformable in isotonic media but deformability improved when osmolarity was reduced to 100–200 mOsm.

HbC disease cells caused a 10%–20% increase in peripheral resistance when studied in a rat mesoappendix model. This minimal change is compatible with the benign clinical course of HbC disease and also suggests that the adverse affects density could be offset by their microcytosis.

HbC Disease, HbC Trait, HbC–β Thalassemia, and HbC–α Thalassemia

HbC trait is found in 2% of African Americans.[31] In parts of West Africa, the prevalence of the HbC gene can reach 0.125.[3,32] Among African Americans, the prevalence of HbC disease is 1 in 6,000. Vasoocclusive episodes are not a feature of HbC trait or HbC disease. Although poorly deformable, HbC cells are rheologically competent. Any oxy HbC crystals formed will tend to melt when cells become lodged in the microcirculation.

Laboratory Features and Diagnosis

Both HbC trait and HbC disease are characterized by target cells and other abnormal erythrocytes. Individuals with HbC trait are not anemic, have normal mean corpuscular volume (MCV) and normal red cell lifespan. MCHCs were approximately 2 g/dL higher than normal cells and 1 g/dL more than HbAS cells.[33] HbC trait erythrocytes contain approximately 40% HbC and 2%–3% HbA_2. In HbC disease, HbC is the predominant hemoglobin with normal amounts of HbA_2 and HbF. Many of the older commonly used methods of hemoglobin separation did not resolve HbC from HbA_2 and positively charged variants like HbE and HbO-Arab.

α Thalassemia can be present in individuals with HbC trait or in homozygotes with HbC disease. Trimodality in the percentage of HbC in carriers of HbC trait first suggested the presence of α thalassemia as a modulator of HbC concentration. HbC plus HbA_2 concentration was 44%, 38%, and 32% in HbC trait carriers presumed to have four, three, and two α-globin genes, respectively. In other cases in which the carrier was presumed to have heterozygous α^+ thalassemia, MCV was reduced and HbC and HbA_2 together were approximately 33%; however, the ascertainment of α thalassemia did not rely on DNA analysis. A case of HbC trait–HbH disease, caused by compound heterozygosity for the -$\alpha^{3.7}$ and SEA deletions (Chapter 13), had splenomegaly, mild anemia, MCV of 59 fl, and 24% HbC.[34] HbC disease–α thalassemia has been described with a phenotype similar to HbC disease, but again, α-globin gene mapping was not done.

In HbC trait–α thalassemia, the concentration of HbC is reduced similarly to HbS levels in HbAS–α thalassemia and this reduction depends on the number of deleted α-globin genes (Chapter 23). mRNA isolated from individuals with simple HbC trait and HbC trait with either homozygous α thalassemia-2 or HbH disease, supported balanced expression of β^C and β^S globin favoring a post translational mechanism for the modulation of HbC concentration.[35] Compared with the wealth of information on the effects of the interaction of α thalassemia and HbAS, there are few available data on the hematological and clinical aspects HbC trait or HbC disease with α thalassemia. Because both HbC trait and the -$\alpha^{3.7}$ type of α thalassemia are clinically innocuous there is no reason to believe that their concordance should be any different.

HbC crystals, very prominent target cells, and anemia are present in HbC disease. Mild hemolytic anemia is customary: the packed cell volume (PCV) is usually 32%–34% and hemoglobin concentration between 9 and 12 g/dL, with a moderate reticulocytosis of between 5% and 10%. Characteristically, the MCV is between 55 and 65 fL. Using DF ^{32}P(di-isopropylfluoropropyl phosphate)-labeled red cells, a mean red cell lifespan of 38.5 and 35.1 days was found in two individuals with a ^{51}Cr red cell survival of 19 days.

Hemolysis is unlikely to be the sole mechanism generating anemia in HbC disease. A reduced oxygen affinity of HbC cells, could account for a portion of the reduction in PCV as these red cells would more readily unload oxygen in the tissues. In turn, erythropoietin production would be stimulated at a lower hemoglobin level than normal. Anemia might therefor appear to be uncompensated because of the decreased oxygen affinity of HbC disease red cells. Dyserythropoietic features, including nuclear disorganization and altered chromatin staining, have been found in erythroblasts of HbC disease but not sickle cell anemia. These findings suggest that ineffective erythropoiesis could account for some of the anemia in this disorder although why this should be is unclear. In children with HbC disease, hemoglobin levels and reticulocyte counts were similar to those in adults and the MCV was between 60 and 80 fL.[36]

HbC–β^+ thalassemia and β^0 thalassemia have been described, and like HbS-β thalassemia, the phenotype is determined by the β thalassemia mutation. In individuals of African descent, because of the prominence of the "mild" promoter mutations in this population, HbC-β^+ thalassemia has hematological features of β thalassemia trait with microcytosis and either no anemia or very mild anemia. HbC levels are 20%–30% and similar to HbS levels in most black patients with HbS–β^+ thalassemia. Like HbS–β^+ thalassemia in Mediterranean populations, β^+ thalassemia mutations that considerably reduce gene expression produce a more severe phenotype approaching that of HbC–β^0 thalassemia.

HbC–β^0 thalassemia can be difficult to distinguish from HbC disease because HbA is absent and HbA_2 is not always easily measured when HbC is present (Table 21.1). DNA analysis or family studies are required when it is important to make the distinction between HbC disease and HbC–β^0 thalassemia. Further complicating the separation of these disorders is the possibility of α thalassemia coincidental with HbC disease, which is likely to cause a phenotype similar to HbC–β^0 thalassemia. HbC trait has been described with gene deletion hereditary persistence of HbF, Hb Lepore, and with $\delta\beta$ thalassemia. All are mild conditions resembling HbC–β^+ thalassemia because of the presence of HbF and Hb Lepore.

Table 21.1. Hematological findings in HbC disease and HbC–β^0 thalassemia*

Genotype	Hemoglobin (g/dL)/PCV	MCV (fL)	HbF (%)	Reticulocytes (%)	Spleen
HbC Disease	10–15/30–45	60–90	2–4	2–7	↑↑
Hb C–β^0 Thalassemia	8–12/25–35	55–70	3–10	5–20	↑↑↑

* These data are a composite of many cases reported in the literature.

Clinical Features and Treatment of HbC Trait and HbC Disease

HbC trait is not associated with clinical disease. Hematuria and isosthenuria, the best-characterized clinical abnormalities of HbAS, are not associated with HbC trait.

Individuals with HbC disease have hematological and clinical evidence of their hemoglobinopathy but appear to have a normal lifespan and few signs or symptoms besides splenomegaly that are attributable to their disease. They do not have vasoocclusive events typical of sickle cell disease.

Splenomegaly has been reported in most adult patients with HbC disease and is usually asymptomatic. In the past, splenectomy was frequently recommended with the hope of correcting the anemia; current practice avoids splenectomy in all but very selected cases. Splenectomy is usually followed by a slight increase in PCV and by increased numbers of circulating cells containing HbC crystals. Children might have a lower prevalence of splenomegaly.[36] Spontaneous rupture of the spleen has been described in HbC disease. Increased density of the HbC-containing erythrocytes does not impair renal concentrating ability.

Treatment Recommendations

As HbC disease is clinically asymptomatic and hematologically benign, no special treatment is needed. Iron should be avoided because it will not, in the absence of iron lack, repair anemia or microcytosis. Hemolysis is very mild, so a reasonably nutritious diet should provide sufficient folic acid, and supplementation is unnecessary. No information exists about hemolysis related pulmonary hypertension in HbC disease.

Parvovirus B19 can transiently interrupt erythropoiesis but because hemolysis is mild, the sequelae of this infection should not be as serious as when it occurs in sickle cell anemia and might not reach the threshold of clinical detection.

Patients sometimes have aches and pains and it is not clear if these can be linked to HbC disease. There is no evidence that HbC disease is accompanied by a reduction in longevity in the Western World, although this might not be true in the harsh environmental conditions of the African Sahel.

HbSC Disease

In HbSC disease the erythrocytes contain nearly equal concentrations of HbC and HbS and each hemoglobin component exerts its own special pathological effects that synergistically cause the well-delineated features of HbSC disease. HbSC disease is the neglected stepchild of sickle hemoglobinopathies. Its unique pathophysiology suggests that it could be amenable to treatments that might prevent dense cell formation, yet until very recently, therapeutic trials in HbSC disease have not been done and most often, in clinical trials, its treatment has been lumped with treatment for sickle cell anemia. This might have the dual unfortunate effect of confounding the interpretation of trials for sickle cell anemia and retarding the development of novel treatments for HbSC disease.

Cellular Determinants of Pathophysiology and Severity

HbAS and HbSC disease erythrocytes both have far lower concentrations of HbS than cells of sickle cell anemia. Nevertheless, the expectation that because of low HbS concentrations polymerization-induced defects will be attenuated or absent is realized only in HbAS. The reasons why HbAS and HbSC disease differ, which elucidate the pathophysiology of HbSC disease, are discussed in the following sections.

HbC Crystals in HbSC Disease. Crystals are the most striking and distinctive feature in circulating red cells of HbSC disease, especially when patients have a normal complement of α-globin genes (Figs. 21.7 and 21.8). HbS accelerates the crystallization of HbC in vivo and in vitro.[37] HbC crystals are observed in Wright and vital dye–stained smears and in "wet" blood preparations (Fig. 21.7).

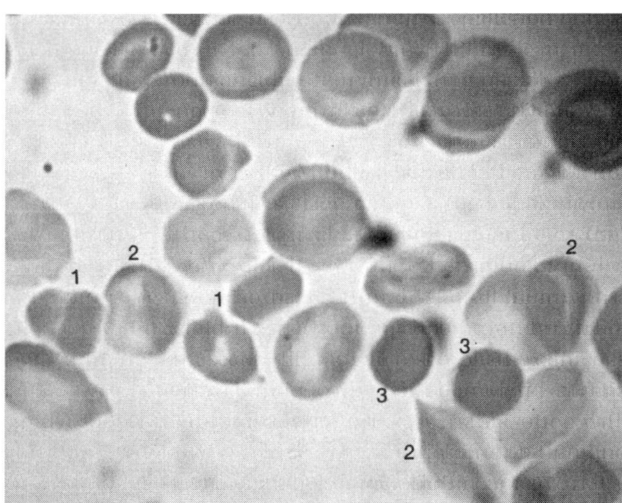

Figure 21.7. Erythrocytes in HbSC disease. These cells are characterized by sharp edges, increased red color (particularly in a reticulocyte stained smear), and often by having all the hemoglobin of the cells recruited into the crystal, leaving a ghost of the red cell without cytosolic dissolved hemoglobin. 1 = crystal containing red cell; 2 = "billiard ball" cells; 3 = folded cells. (Lawrence et al., *Blood* 1991;78: 2104–2112.)

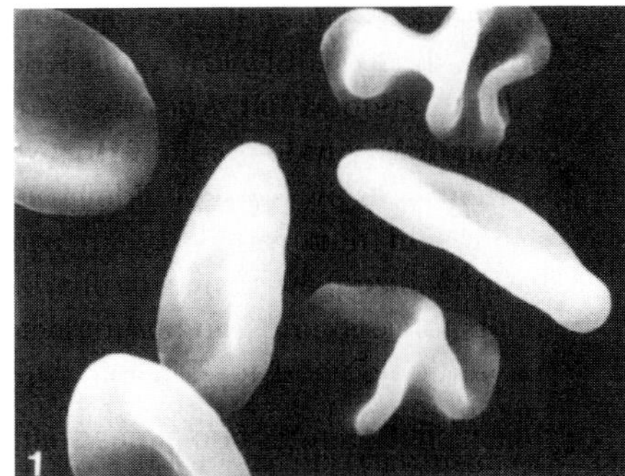

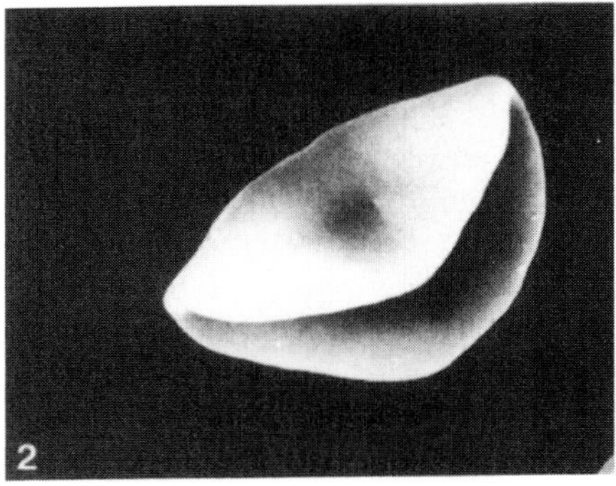

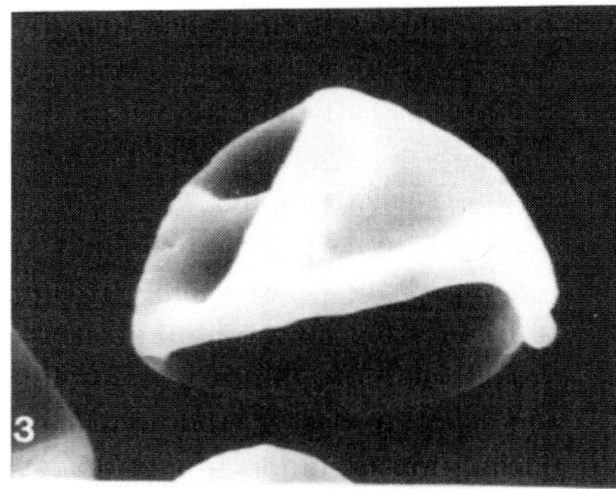

Figure 21.8. Several types of red cells found in the blood of HbSC disease patients illustrated by scanning electron microscopy: Folded red cells (Top panel), "pita bread" red cells (middle panel), and highly folded red cell (lower panel) from whole blood of a HbSC disease patient.

When α thalassemia is present with HbSC disease, typical crystals are absent in some patients. All HbSC disease patients' red cells exhibit heavily stained conglomerations of hemoglobin that appear marginated with rounded edges in distinction to the straight edged crystals. Both crystals and hemoglobin conglomerations are found in the densest fraction of HbSC disease and represent hemoglobin aggregation distinct from HbS polymer. Regardless of the α-globin gene haplotype, the blood of HbSC disease patients has additional abnormally shaped cells that are strikingly apparent upon scanning electron microcopy (Fig. 21.8). These bizarre shapes are the product of an increased surface/volume ratio. Crystals, pitted by a normal spleen might

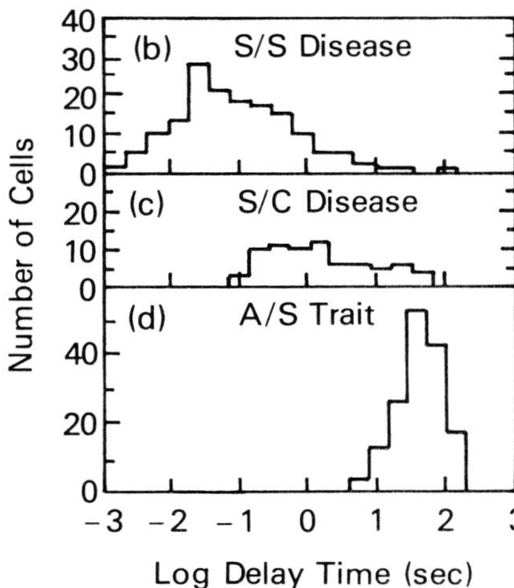

Figure 21.9. This graph depicts individual red cell delay times of polymerization in HbSC disease compared with sickle cell anemias and HbAS. Notice that many HbSC cells behave as sickle trait cells, as far as delay times, but that also some of the cells behave as the slowest sickle cell anemia cells. In effect, delay time of HbSC cells is intermediate between sickle cell anemia and sickle cell trait cells, with overlapping.[109]

remain in the cell in the presence of an enlarged, infarcted and perhaps abnormally functioning spleen.

Ratio of HbS to HbC. The ratio of HbS/HbC is approximately 50:50 compared with the 40:60 ratio of HbS/HbA in HbAS. Charge-related differences in αβ dimer assembly account for the lower proportion of HbS in HbAS and HbC in HbC trait. Although HbC has an additional positive charge compared with HbS, both these abnormal variants can compete similarly for α-globin chains equalizing the HbS/HbC ratio.

Just as HbF is unequally distributed among all cells, there is some evidence that HbC is unequally apportioned among red cells. Using single-cell electrophoresis, the distribution of HbS in HbAS and HbC in HbC trait was found to vary among cells but whether HbS concentration differs among cells in HbSC disease is unknown.

HbSC disease is associated with hemolytic anemia and vasoocclusive complications, whereas HbAS is not, a difference that might be attributed to the higher concentration of HbS in HbSC disease. Although the effects of HbA and HbC on HbS polymerization are equivalent, increasing the HbS from 40% to 50% increased the rate of polymerization nearly 15-fold. The duration of the delay time before sickling occurs could play a role in the pathophysiology of HbSC disease. A long delay might allow a cell to move through hypoxic microvasculature before rigidity and rheological incompetence ensue, whereas a shorter delay time could increase a cell's propensity to induce vasoocclusion (Fig. 21.9).

Cell Density, Cation Content, and Density-related Properties. Cation content of HbSC disease red cells is intermediate between normal and HbC disease cells. Oxygenated HbSC disease cells exhibit a volume-stimulated K^+ efflux similar to that observed in sickle cell anemia and HbC disease. HbSC disease cells also exhibit a diminished change in cell volume in response to variation of the osmolarity of the suspending medium, which is likely to be due to volume, regulated K^+ efflux. Volume-regulated K^+ efflux should impact adversely the pathophysiology of disease because any increase of MCHC will aggravate HbS polymerization.

The intracellular HbS concentration in HbSC disease is raised to a level where polymerization occurs under physiological conditions. This contrasts with HbAS cells in which polymerization occurs only at high osmolarity and low pH, such as in the renal medulla. Reducing the MCHC in HbSC disease to normal levels of 33 g/dL by osmotically swelling resulted in normalization of many of their polymerization-dependent abnormal properties.[38] Among the beneficial effects of cell rehydration were increased hemoglobin oxygen affinity, reduction of viscosity of deoxygenated erythrocyte suspensions, fall in the rate of sickling, and reduction in the deoxygenation-induced K^+ leak. At an osmolality of 240 mOsm, where the density distribution of HbSC disease cells most nearly matched normal cells, the cells were found to be biconcave disks. These observations suggest that restoring the density of HbSC cells toward normal might be an efficacious treatment.

Analogous to sickle cell anemia, when α thalassemia coexists with HbSC disease fewer dense cells are present. During the course of vasoocclusive crisis in HbSC disease, dense cells decrease just as in sickle cell anemia, suggesting their sequestration.[39,40]

HbSC disease cells exhibit pathological properties characteristic of both sickle cell anemia and HbC disease cells, and this feature helps explain the greater than anticipated severity of HbSC disease. A morphological analysis of density-separated HbSC disease cells indicated that they became progressively more aberrant in shape as their density increased. The densest fraction of the gradient contained cells with the most abnormal shapes, which were particularly noticeable for their gross pitting and membrane invaginations. HbSC disease cells destined to become extremely dense are likely also to produce crystals as a byproduct of their progressive MCHC increase as the concentration of hemoglobin within crystals is approximately 68 g/dL. Irreversibly sickled cells are rare in HbSC disease and are found in the densest cell fractions (Fig. 21.10).

α Thalassemia is associated with a decrease in the dense cell fraction. In contrast with sickle cell anemia, the highest percentage of reticulocytes is found within a fraction of dense cells, although the youngest, or stress reticulocytes, are predominant in the least dense fraction. This suggests that in HbSC disease reticulocytes exit the marrow as low-density cells and become dense within 24 hours, sinking to the next to densest fraction of cells in the blood.

Reticulocytes are almost absent from the dense cell fractions that contains the largest proportion of crystal containing cells. Hyperdense reticulocytes migrate to lower

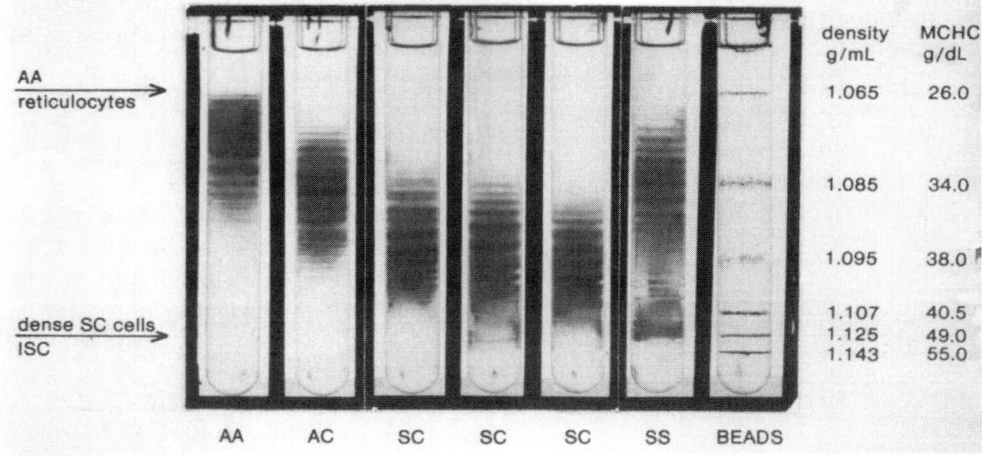

Figure 21.10. Percoll–Strachan (Larex) density separation of whole blood from normal hemolysate (AA), HbC trait (AC), and three different HbSC disease individuals and one sickle cell anemia patient. Beads: Color-coded density beads to establish the density at different levels of the gradient after centrifugation. See color plates.

densities if Cl^- is removed from the media, in concordance with a K:Cl cotransport-mediated phenomena. It seems likely that K:Cl cotransport is responsible for the presence of HbSC disease reticulocytes of unusually high densities.

β-Globin Gene Cluster Haplotypes in HbSC Disease

A Benin haplotype β^S chromosome was present in 56%, Bantu in 25%, Senegal in 6%, and other haplotypes in 12% of HbSC disease cases.[41] No hematological differences among these patients were present.[42] Hematological features of individuals with HbSC disease who had Benin or Bantu β^S chromosomes were similar whether they had a C I or C II haplotype. Most likely, the effect of β-globin gene haplotype on the hematological and clinical features of sickle cell anemia is via haplotype-linked elements that affect the levels of HbF. HbF levels in HbSC disease are lower than in sickle cell anemia, probably because there is less hemolysis and bone marrow expansion in HbSC disease. Another speculative consideration is that the β^C chromosome might not contain the critical genetic elements or polymorphisms that are present in sickle cell anemia and necessary for increased transcription of the γ-globin genes (Chapter 27).

CLINICAL FEATURES OF HbSC DISEASE

In northern Ghana, Burkina Faso, and western Nigeria, approximately a quarter of the population might have HbSC disease. Centuries of population movements have spread the HbS and HbC genes throughout the world, broadening greatly the distribution of the sickle hemoglobinopathies. HbSC disease has an incidence of approximately 1:833 live births in African Americans.[31]

All complications that are found in patients with sickle cell anemia have occurred in individuals with HbSC disease. Nevertheless, most, but not all, of these complications are less frequent and appear at a later age in the course of HbSC disease compared with sickle cell anemia. Hemolysis is less intense so that hemolysis-related complications like leg ulcer, priapism, stroke, pulmonary hypertension, aplastic episodes, and cholelithiasis are less frequent or severe. Disease complications due to blood viscosity, such as osteonecrosis of bone can be as common as in sickle cell anemia; proliferative sickle retinopathy is much more prevalent in HbSC disease than in sickle cell anemia; the mortality of acute chest syndrome might be increased.[43] Painful episodes occur at approximately half the frequency as in sickle cell anemia. The lifespan of HbSC disease patients is shortened when compared with control populations, but is longer than in sickle cell anemia.

Specific treatments that will prevent complications of this disease are not yet available. In the following sections, the clinical aspects of HbSC disease that differ most from those of sickle cell anemia are discussed. For details of treatment and many complications, which differ little among the genotype of sickle cell disease, the reader should consult Chapters 19, 20, and 29–33.

Hematology and Laboratory Findings

HPLC now provides rapid quantitative analysis of hemoglobin fractions and can distinguish HbS, HbC, and many of the variants with which they might be confused (Chapter 28). Blood films can suggest the diagnosis of HbSC disease. Except in the presence of sickle cell–related renal failure or with coincidental medical conditions that can reduce the PCV, patients with HbSC disease do not usually have overt symptoms of anemia. At any age, PCV in HbSC disease is higher than in sickle cell anemia.[44] Median values by age and sex for PCV, MCV, platelet count, and bilirubin are shown in Figure 21.11. PCV rises from 31 to 32 in

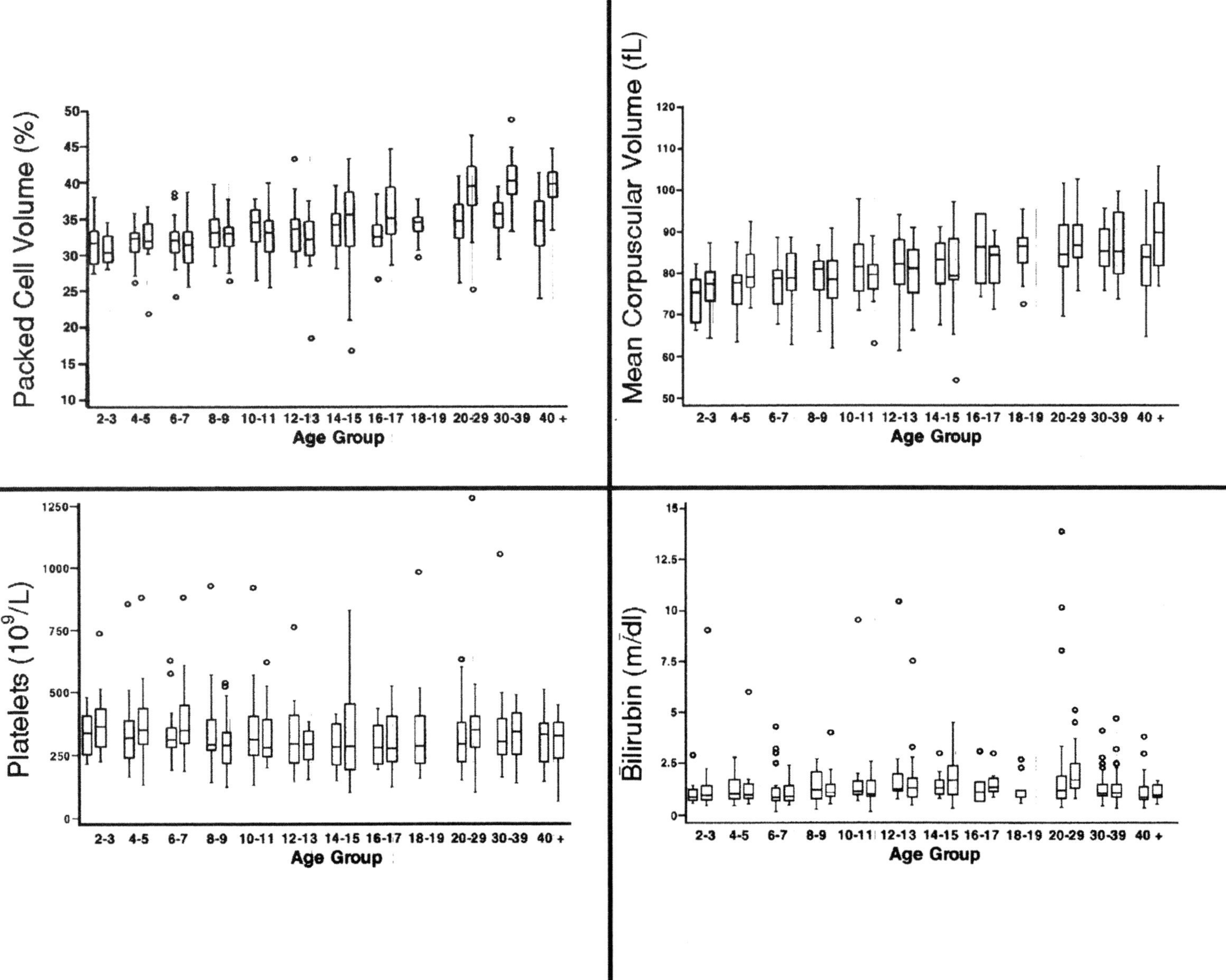

Figure 21.11. PCV, MCV, platelet count, and bilirubin levels in a cross-sectional study of patients with HbSC disease ages 2 years to older than 40 years. PCV, MCV, and reticulocyte counts were available for 586 patients and bilirubin for 467 patients. Box plots show the mean and 25th (bottom of box) and 75th percentile (top of box) of the data.[44]

children aged 2–5 years to approximately 37 in males older than 20 years, a level approximately five points higher than in females with HbSC disease. Many adult men, but fewer adult women, have a normal PCV.[44–46] Individuals with high PCV might be at greatest risk for complications such as proliferative retinopathy and osteonecrosis of the femoral head. Leukocyte counts in HbSC disease are normal or only very slightly elevated. Perhaps this is a result of more persistent splenomegaly, reduced hemolysis, and less proliferative activity of the bone marrow. Platelet counts are also lower in HbSC disease than in sickle cell anemia, perhaps for similar reasons. Some individuals with HbSC disease have mild thrombocytopenia, and this can often be related to an enlarged spleen.

Leukocytosis, thrombocytosis, and reticulocytosis have been linked to the severity of vasoocclusive disease in sickle cell anemia. Mature sickle cells circulate in the company of leukocytes, platelets, and "stress" reticulocytes that display adhesive ligands that facilitate erythrocyte–endothelial interactions. High granulocyte counts are a risk for mortality in sickle cell anemia. Perhaps some of the milder features of HbSC disease are accounted for by the lower numbers of activated neutrophils and platelets.

Bilirubin is usually normal and lactic dehydrogenase (LDH) levels are lower, reflecting mild hemolytic anemia compared with sickle cell anemia. Chromium-51 survival in HbSC disease was 13–26 days and DF ^{32}P mean lifespan was 29 days. Reticulocytes in HbSC disease ranged from less than 1%–7% supporting the lower hemolytic rate. As in sickle cell anemia, red cell volume was only modestly reduced, whereas plasma volume was more substantially elevated. Red cell survival, plasma volume, and PCV were unrelated to splenomegaly or splenic function.

Although hemolysis is only modest, compensation is incomplete. Mild anemia in HbSC disease cannot be entirely accounted for by the rate of red cell destruction because this does not exceed the potential of normal marrow to replace lost cells. In HbSC disease, the PCV and red cell mass average approximately 80%–85% of normal. As hypothesized for sickle cell anemia, it might be that increased P_{50} and enhanced tissue extraction of oxygen blunts erythropoiesis in HbSC disease. Although hemoglobin-oxygen affinity of hemoglobin isolated from HbSC disease red cells is normal, the whole blood P_{50} is increased to 32 mm Hg. Serum erythropoietin levels are higher than normal, but lower than found in sickle cell anemia.[47] These levels might be inappropriately low for the level of anemia and could also be due to subclinical renal disease or an inappropriate marrow erythroid response.

HbSC disease patients usually have HbF levels less than 2% but occasionally the HbF in adults is near 10%. HbF is unlikely to have a major affect on the hematology or clinical features of HbSC disease because of its low level in the majority of patients. In contrast to sickle cell anemia, individuals with HbSC and HbC disease, regardless of haplotype, have similar $^{G}\gamma$-globin chain levels despite different degrees of erythropoietic stress.

α Thalassemia, a known modulator of sickle cell anemia (Chapter 27), has a minor effect on the hematology of HbSC disease. Although coincident α thalassemia reduces the MCV by approximately 5 fl, there is little change in the hemoglobin concentration or HbF level.[48]

Growth and Development

Growth in HbSC disease is delayed, but less so than in sickle cell anemia. With access to reasonable nutrition, Tanner stages of adult sexual development are achieved at 14–16 and 16–18 years of age in young women and boys, respectively, 1–2 years earlier than in children with sickle cell anemia.[49] In some studies, HbSC disease does not appear to affect height, weight, and bone age.[50] A study of 298 children with sickle cell anemia and 157 children with HbSC disease revealed that after age 5 years, HbSC disease children had normal growth.

Mortality

A 1989 report indicated that 95% of patient's with HbSC disease in the United States survived to age 20 years.[51] These individuals were participants in the Cooperative Study of Sickle Cell Disease (CSSCD) (Chapter 19) and many attended comprehensive sickle cell centers, making it possible that they had more regular and skilled care than the general population of HbSC disease. Mortality in this series was greatest in children aged between 1 and 3 years, and was most often a result of pneumococcal sepsis. Another study, reported in 1990, in which 231 individuals with HbSC disease were compared with 785 sickle cell anemia patients, showed an age-specific death rate (per 100 person-years) up to age 30 years of less than one in HbSC disease compared with two–three in sickle cell anemia. Beyond this age, mortality in all patients increased. Nevertheless, the rate in HbSC disease was less than half that of sickle cell anemia.[52] In the largest study of mortality from the United States, the median survival in HbSC disease was 60 years for men and 68 years for women (Fig. 21.12).[53] Jamaican children with HbSC disease, diagnosed by cord blood screening, and so unlikely to represent a biased sample, had a 95% chance of surviving to age 2 years.

Two hundred eighty-four patients with HbSC disease, more than 80% of whom entered the study as children, were followed over a span of 40 years for nearly 3,000 person-years.[48] The median age of death in this study was 37 years and was unaffected by sex. Approximately 10% of patients died, and 60% of these entered the study prior to 1970. No single cause of death predominated. In another study of adults, the median age was 50 years.[54]

It has been theorized that since these reports, the mortality of sickle cell anemia has fallen in developed countries

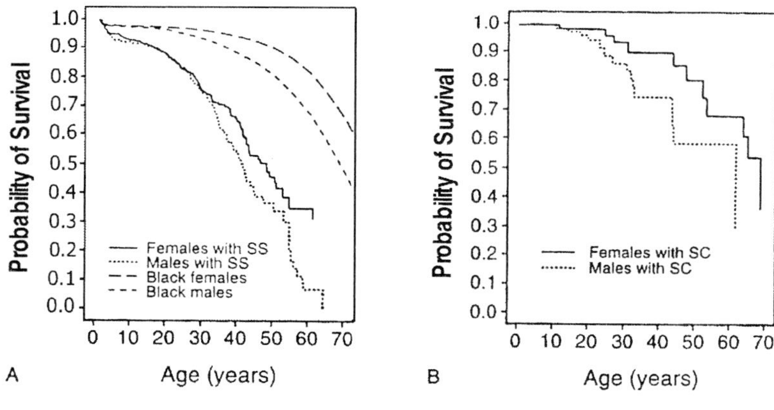

Figure 21.12. Survival curves comparing patients with HbSC disease (**A**) and sickle cell anemia (**B**).[110]

because of the widespread use of prophylactic penicillin, better supportive care for events such as acute chest syndrome and perhaps hydroxyurea. Penicillin prophylaxis is not uniformly used in HbSC disease and studies of hydroxyurea as a treatment for HbSC disease are just starting, so their effects on mortality are not known.

There are few data on risk factors for early death in HbSC disease. Median age of onset for irreversible organ failure like stroke, renal failure, and chronic lung disease, that might contribute to early mortality in HbSC disease is 10–35 years later than in sickle cell anemia.[52] Even in large series of patients, relatively small numbers of deaths occur in HbSC disease, making it difficult to assess the relationship of HbF, leukocyte count, and prior vasoocclusive episodes such as pain and acute chest syndrome to mortality. It is clear that HbSC disease has a pattern of survival that is different from sickle cell anemia. Increased mortality of HbSC disease is apparent only after age 20 years. Overall prognosis of HbSC disease is, therefore, better than that of sickle cell anemia.

CLINICAL EVENTS

Patients with HbSC disease can have all of the problems of sickle cell anemia but usually have a milder clinical course. A survey of 90 Jamaican patients with HbSC disease showed pathology similar to sickle cell anemia, but with generally reduced severity, except for retinal vascular disease. These findings might be a result of reduced hemolysis and higher hemoglobin levels in HbSC disease. In a pediatric cohort, 50% of HbSC patients were found to develop symptoms by age 5 years but 22% remained free of symptoms at age 10 years.[55] Approximately 40% of patients were found to have some chronic organ complication with a mean age of onset of approximately 30 years.[48]

Many individuals with HbSC disease are active in quite strenuous occupations. Some never have the occasion to seek medical attention for the unique events of sickle cell disease and have their diagnosis established incidental to another medical condition. Rarely, the presenting attribute of HbSC disease is calamitous, such as life-threatening acute chest syndrome, multiorgan failure, sepsis, or splenic sequestration. Therefore, although sometimes mild and needing little obvious medical supervision, HbSC disease should not be neglected. Patients with HbSC disease should be detected by neonatal screening so that they and their families can be enrolled in programs providing education about the potential complications of this disorder and the needed level of continued monitoring.

Sickle Retinopathy

Proliferative sickle retinopathy is perhaps the most typical vasoocclusive complication of HbSC disease (Fig. 21.13). More common in this genotype, where it is found in approximately a third of patients, than in sickle cell anemia where only 3% are affected, the pathology of this entity has been delineated in detail.[56,57]

Pathophysiology of Sickle Retinopathy. The primary site of vasoocclusion in sickle retinopathy was located at the precapillary level.[58] Hairpin loops, a neovascular formation that appeared to result from recanalization of occluded vessels and autoinfarcted preretinal neovascular formations are present. Small pigmented lesions consisting of retinal pigment epithelial cells ensheathing channels that resembled autoinfarcted vessels were also seen.

Macular blood flow velocity was compared in 18 patients with sickle cell disease and 45 normal controls and the relation between macular blood flow velocity and red blood cell density was examined.[59] Leukocyte velocity in the macular capillaries was negatively associated with a greater range of red cell density, suggesting that sickle red cell density heterogeneity might slow macular capillary blood flow.

The distribution and relative levels of components in the fibrinolytic system and growth factors in retina and choroid showed increased plasminogen activator inhibitor-1 immunoreactivity in retinal vessels compared with controls, whereas tissue plasminogen activator localization and immunoreactivity were similar.[60] Immunoreactive fibrin was often observed within the lumen of retinal and choroidal vessels and in choroidal neovascularization. Blood vessels containing fibrin generally exhibited elevated plasminogen activator inhibitor-1 immunoreactivity. Von Willebrand factor and basic fibroblast growth factor immunoreactivity were elevated in choriocapillaris and the walls of some retinal vessels. Transforming growth factor–β1 (TGF-β) immunoreactivity was significantly lower in

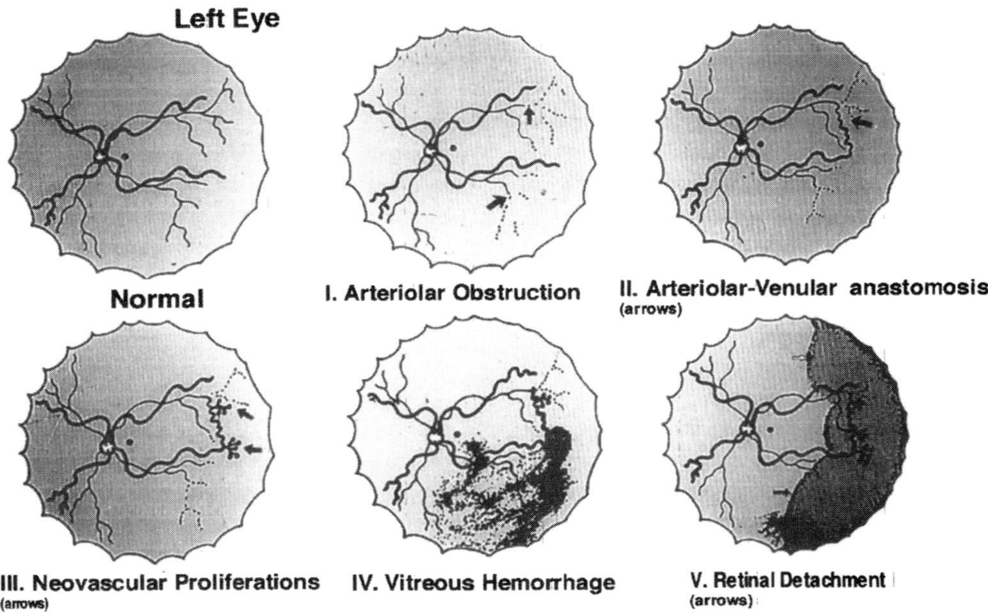

Figure 21.13. Stages of proliferative sickle retinopathy.

sickle cell choriocapillaris than in controls. In chorioretinal-pigmented lesions of an HbSC disease patient, basic fibroblast growth factor, TGF-β1, 2, 3 immunoreactivity was present within migrating retinal pigment epithelial cells. These data suggested that fibrin deposition within retinal and choroidal vessels of sickle cell disease subjects could occur due to elevated plasminogen activator inhibitor–1 activity. Vasoocclusion of choroidal vessels might influence the expression of growth factors in choriocapillaris endothelium, which could stimulate formation of choroidal neovascularization. Fibrosis and gliosis in and near chorioretinal-pigmented lesions, could be stimulated by migrating retinal pigment epithelial cell production of basic fibroblast growth factor and TGF-β.

Pigment epithelium-derived factor (PEDF) is an inhibitor of angiogenesis and a neurotrophic factor in the mammalian eye, and its level is related to retinal neovascularization Using tissue from normal eyes and subjects with sickle cell retinopathy, PEDF was mainly localized to the vitreous condensed at the internal limiting membrane, RPE-Bruch membrane-choriocapillaris complex and choroidal stroma in normal eyes. In sickle retinopathy, the ratio of PEDF/vascular endothelial growth factor (VEGF) was increased in the nonperfused area of the nonproliferative sickle cell retina and in eyes with proliferative sickle cell retinopathy. Elevated PEDF and VEGF immunostaining was present in viable vessels of sea fan neovascular formations and in feeder vessels of sea fans. Only PEDF was present in nonviable sea fans, suggesting that this might play an important role in inhibiting angiogenesis and inducing the regression of sea fans.[61]

Neovascularization is a common consequence of retina vasoocclusion. Morphometric analysis in postmortem ocular tissue from subjects with sickle hemoglobinopathies[62] showed numerous active and autoinfarcted lesions, representing virtually all stages in preretinal neovascularization. They ranged from single small loops extending from arteries and veins along the retinal surface to the typical complex, elevated sea fan formations. Sea fans developed at hairpin loops and at arteriovenous crossings. There was an average of 5.6 connections between sea fans and retinal vessels; of these, 45% were arteriolar, 52.5% were venular, and 2.6% involved capillaries. Autoinfarction appeared to occur initially within the sea fan capillaries. Preretinal neovascularization in sickle cell retinopathy might arise from both the arterial and venous sides of the retinal vasculature and assume a variety of morphological configurations. Multiple feeding arterioles and draining venules are common, and autoinfarction appears to occur initially at the preretinal capillary level rather than at feeding arterioles.

Plasma angiopoietin-1 and angiopoietin-2, soluble Tie-2, VEGF, soluble Flt-1, and von Willebrand factor were measured in patients with HbSC disease or sickle cell anemia who had proliferative and nonproliferative sickle retinopathy. In eight patients who received panretinal laser photocoagulation, plasma was obtained before and 6 months after treatment. Angiopoietin-1 and -2, VEGF, and von Willebrand factor were raised in all sickle cell patient groups compared with controls and only minor changes in were seen after treatment.[63] Angiopoietin-2, erythropoietin, VEGF, and soluble Tie-2 and VCAM were elevated suggesting a proangiogenic state. With painful crisis, only VCAM increased.[47]

Vasoocclusion in the retina has also been studied in transgenic sickle mice and in a rat animal model.[64] Retinal vascular occlusions resulted in nonperfused areas of retina and arteriovenous anastomoses. Intra- and extraretinal neovascularization was observed adjacent to nonperfused areas. Retinal pigmented lesions were formed by the migration of retinal pigment epithelial cells into sensory retina, often ensheathing choroidal neovascularization. Bilateral chorioretinopathy was present in 30% of animals older than 15 months. These ocular histopathological changes mimicked many aspects of human proliferative sickle cell retinopathy and permitted the detection of choroid abnormalities not previously characterized. Forty-two percent of $\alpha^H\beta^S[\beta^{MDD}]$ (Chapter 12) mice without any proliferative retinopathy had retinal blood vessels containing red cell plugs visualized by endogenous peroxidase activity and lacked luminal horseradish peroxidase (HRP)–reaction product.[65] In sections from whole eyes of the same animals, foci of photoreceptor degeneration were associated with areas of choriocapillaris nonperfusion. In areas with normal photoreceptors, the choriocapillaris appeared perfused and HRP-reaction product was present.

In animals with proliferative chorioretinopathy, some neovascular formations lacked luminal HRP-reaction product, suggesting autoinfarction. Nonperfused retinal and choroidal vessels were observed in mice without retinal and choroidal neovascularization, whereas, all mice with neovascularization had nonperfused areas. Small foci of HRP loss were associated with areas of nonperfused choriocapillaris. These results suggest that sickle cell–mediated retinal vasoocclusion is an initial event in the chorioretinopathy and outer retinal atrophy.

Density separated, labeled HbSC and sickle cell anemia erythrocytes infused into rats were retained in capillaries. Dense cell retention was inversely dependent on pO_2.[66] Trapping, not adhesion, appeared to be responsible for retention of sickle cells in the normal retinal vasculature because of preferential retention of dense cells with a lower adherence propensity. Paradoxically, given the prevalence of retinopathy in HbSC disease, there was low retention of HbSC cells. Fractionated sickle erythrocytes were infused into rats that were either hypoxic or were given TNFα. Sickle erythrocytes were also preincubated with a peptide that inhibits binding of VLA-4 and α4β7 integrins to their ligands. Hypoxia caused retention of dense but not reticulocyte-rich sickle cells. TNFα significantly increased retention of all types of sickle cells, and this was inhibited by VLA-4 inhibition or by monoclonal antibodies against fibronectin, a ligand for VLA-4. Similar inhibition of retention was seen in retinal vessels when a VLA-4 inhibitor was used.[67]

These studies suggested that the mechanisms for retention of sickle cells in retina and choroid appeared identical and was the result of hypoxia-mediated retention of dense red cells and adherence of sickle reticulocytes after cytokine stimulation. TNFα-stimulated retention of sickle cells in choroid appeared to be mediated by VLA-4, presumably on the surface of some reticulocytes.[68]

The expression of the adhesion molecules ICAM-1, VCAM-1, and P-selectin, and the distribution and number of polymorphonuclear leukocytes were investigated in sickle cell retinopathy and compared with the normal retina. In cryopreserved postmortem ocular tissue from subjects with sickle cell disease and one control subject, increased ICAM-1, VCAM-1, and P-selectin immunoreactivities were observed in sickle cell subjects and the highest ICAM and P-selectin immunoreactivity was associated with intraretinal vessels adjacent to the preretinal neovascular formation in subjects with proliferative sickle retinopathy. VCAM-1 immunoreactivity was highest in intraretinal vessels adjacent to the newly forming sea fans. Old sea fans had the highest levels of VCAM-1. The increase in adhesion molecule immunoreactivity was paralleled by an increase in intraretinal neutrophils that increased with progression of the disease. These data suggest that adhesion molecule mediated leukocyte adhesion might play a role in sickle cell retinopathy.[69]

Table 21.2. Age-related prevalence of proliferative sickle retinopathy in HbSC disease

Age (y)	No. of patients	Percent with retinopathy
0–9	47	0
10–14	77	6
15–19	117	14
20–24	81	27
25–29	67	60
30–39	88	57
>40	56	70
Total	533	32

Using a noninvasive method to assess the velocity, adherence, and arterial/venous transit time of normal and sickle erythrocytes in retinal and choroidal vessels, labeled red cells can be observed in the retina of pigmented rats and on the choroid of albino rats. Normal density sickle cells were transiently retained in retinal vessels. Sickle red cells were retained in larger numbers, in some cases for extended periods of time, suggesting that the choroid–capillaris vasoocclusion can play an important role in sickle retinopathy.[70]

Prevalence. Age-adjusted prevalence of proliferative retinopathy in 533 patients with HbSC disease is shown in Table 21.2. The distinctive "black sea fan," "black sunburst" and salmon patches typify this disorder and characterize the hemorrhagic, infarctive, proliferative, and resolving lesions of sickle retinopathy. Conjoint effects of a higher PCV, increased cell density, and greater blood viscosity in HbSC disease could account for the higher prevalence of retinopathy in HbSC disease than in sickle cell anemia; it is also possible that the lower HbF levels of HbSC disease play a role.

Paradoxically, the high prevalence of proliferative retinopathy in HbSC disease might be an expression of the relative benignity of this genotype. A classification of the peripheral retinal vascular changes in sickle cell disease, based on the appearance of the peripheral retinal vasculature has been proposed in which vessels are either "normal" (Type I) or abnormal (Type IIa or IIb) based on qualitative changes such as irregular vascular margins, capillary stumps, hyper- or hypofluorescence, and capillary bed thinning.[71] This classification is based on the observation that proliferative retinopathy develops in response to progressive closure of the vessels of the peripheral retina, and, the recession centripetally, of the margin of retinal perfusion.[72,73] Abnormal peripheral retinal vasculature is present in approximately 80% of adults with HbSC disease.[74] By age 17 years, the prevalence of abnormal vascular borders is approximately 60%.[71] More than 260 patients with sickle cell anemia and 154 with HbSC disease were studied with serial fluorescein angiography and retinal photography, beginning at ages 6–12 years. In the teenage years, each year there is a 6% conversion from a normal to abnormal vascular border. The occurrence of sickle proliferative retinopathy was always associated with an abnormal vascular border.

In sickle cell anemia, peripheral retinal vessels are occluded early in the course of disease so that further retinal vascular damage and proliferative lesions cannot develop. The enhanced circulatory competence of the HbSC disease cell could preserve this retinal circulation, permitting the later development of proliferative lesions. If this is true, as hydroxyurea treatment (Chapter 30) makes sickle cell anemia cells more like HbSC disease cells and improves their circulatory competence, the prevalence of proliferative retinopathy could begin to increase in young sickle cell anemia patients treated with this drug.

Diagnosis. Sickle retinopathy is recognizable by its different stages, which include nonproliferative lesions and three stages of proliferative lesions including neovascularization, vitreous hemorrhage, and retinal detachment. Whether or not there is an orderly progression from less to more serious stages that precede retinal detachment and blindness or whether catastrophic changes can arise directly from early stages of proliferative retinopathy is not well characterized. Characteristically, following vasoocclusion in the peripheral vessels of the retina – the nonproliferative stages of retinopathy – neovascular malformations called black sea fans grow from the retinal surface into the vitreous. These fragile new vessels can leak blood into the vitreous, at times in amounts sufficient to reduce vision. Organization of vitreal hemorrhages exerts traction on the inelastic retina, causing tears and allowing vitreal fluid to enter the subretinal space. Retinal detachment, a potential consequence of subretinal fluid invasion, can produce blindness. Of 14 patients with HbSC disease who were selected for study because they had nonproliferative lesions or peripheral retinal arteriolar occlusion or arteriovenous anastomoses, 21% developed new sea fans with an average interval of 18 months (range 8–36 months). Based on these rather small numbers of patients, the authors estimated that approximately 14% of young adults with HbSC disease develop neovascularization each year.[75] Complicating the evaluation of retinopathy in HbSC disease is the propensity for spontaneous regression of proliferative lesions due to autoinfarction.[76] These authors caution, however, that withholding treatment in the hopes of a spontaneous regression is dangerous because the incidence of spontaneous vitreal hemorrhage increased from 28% to 44% in patients observed for 6–77 months.[77]

Table 21.3. Prevalence of ocular lesions in HbSC disease

Ocular lesion	Percent
Nonproliferative	
Salmon patch	17
Iridescent spot	28
Black sunburst	62
Proliferative	
Stage III-Neovascularization	45
Stage IV-Vitreous hemorrhage	21
Stage V-Retinal detachment	10

Progression. Patients picked randomly from a clinic population, were enrolled and followed with annual or semiannual detailed ophthalmological examinations.[78] Initially, 11 patients had stage III retinopathy and their average duration of follow-up was 7 months. Twelve patients had normal findings or stage I or II disease (Table 21.3). The natural history of proliferative retinopathy in HbSC disease compared with sickle cell anemia in patients who presented with stage III disease is shown in Table 21.4. Forty-eight percent had proliferative disease on initial examination and 74% developed stages III–V disease at final examination; there was little change over time in the prevalence of nonproliferative retinopathy in either HbSC disease or sickle cell anemia patients.

In studies from Jamaica, 115 patients with HbSC disease were followed sequentially.[79] Efforts were made to ensure that this was a random sample of HbSC disease patients. Proliferative retinopathy was present in 24% of patients at the initial examination, arose de novo during the study in 18%, and was present at the final examination in 40%. The mean age of patients showing progression was 27.7 years. Of 43 individuals, 58 new lesions were found in 18 patients

Table 21.4. Natural history of proliferative retinopathy in sickle cell disease

	Sickle cell anemia	HbSC disease
No. of eyes	17	19
Duration of observation (mo)	69	77
Stable disease (%)	59	26
Regression (%)	18	42
Progression (%)	35	58
Vitreous hemorrhage (%)	6	37
Retinal detachment (%)	6	6

Table 21.5. Evolution of proliferative retinopathy in HbSC disease according to patient age

Age (y)	Eyes (no.)	Progression (%)	Regression (%)	Stable (%)
10–19	10	40	30	30
20–29	47	60	17	23
30–39	56	43	27	30
>40	24	29	4	67

younger than 25 years, and the highest risk period was between ages 20 and 24 years. Two thirds of patients with de novo proliferative lesions were aged 15–29 years. Approximately one-third to half of patients had autoinfarction during the course of the study. From ages 10 to 39 years, approximately 7% of individuals in each 5-year age bracket developed proliferative retinopathy per 100 patient-years of observation.[80] In follow-up, progressive disease was most frequent between ages 20 and 39 years, and visual loss occurred in only 9% of patients followed for a mean of 4.5 years.[81] (Table 21.5)

A longitudinal study spanning 20 years was performed in 307 children with sickle cell anemia and 166 children with HbSC disease detected by newborn screening. Participants had annual ophthalmological studies with angiography and angioscopy. Proliferative retinopathy developed in 14 patients with sickle cell anemia and 45 with HbSC disease, unilaterally in 36 patients and bilaterally in 23. The incidence increased with age in both genotypes, with crude annual incidence rates of 0.5 cases per 100 sickle cell anemia and 2.5 cases per 100 HbSC disease patients. By the age of 24–26 years, proliferative retinopathy had occurred in 43% of the subjects with HbSC disease compared with 14% of those with sickle cell anemia. Patients with HbSC disease and unilateral disease had a 17% probability of regression and a 13% probability of progressing to bilateral disease. Those with bilateral had half the chance of regression as those individuals with unilateral disease. Visual loss occurred in only 1 of 82 affected eyes and one required detachment surgery with recovery of normal visual acuity.[82]

In one study, 30% of patients with HbSC disease had retinopathy with a median age of onset of 28 years.[48] Data suggested that the CI β^C haplotype and Benin β^S-globin gene haplotype carriers with the CI β^C haplotype had a delayed onset of retinopathy. The numbers of cases were small and a physiological explanation for these observations was not forthcoming. Similarly, coincident α thalassemia appeared to decrease the incidence of retinopathy, but less than 30 cases were examined.

Treatment Recommendations

Management of sickle proliferative retinopathy is imperfect. Incipient proliferative disease has been treated with focal or panretinal section photocoagulation to forestall advancing pathology and impaired vision. Some of the earliest comparative trials were inconclusive and questioned the role of photocoagulation, but different techniques of treatment and new technologies now make these results difficult to interpret.[83] There are presently no data that conclusively show that prophylactic photocoagulation significantly changes the natural history of retinopathy.[78] In a randomized trial of argon laser scatter photocoagulation, 99 eyes were treated and 75 eyes served as controls, with an average follow-up of approximately 45 months.[84] There was complete or partial regression of sea fans in 81% of treated eyes and spontaneous regression in 46% of control eyes. New sea fans developed in 34% of treated compared with 41% of control eyes. Using the criteria of visual loss, five control eyes and three treated eyes lost vision during follow-up, an insignificant difference similar to that seen in an observational study. Also, the incidence of retinal detachment was not reduced.

Some data suggest that proliferative retinopathy is most prevalent in individuals with higher hemoglobin levels. Phlebotomy to reduce the hemoglobin concentration to 9–10 g/dL has been advocated as a measure to prevent retinopathy or slow its advancement without evidence of the efficacy of this approach.

In summary, proliferative retinopathy occurs often in patients with HbSC disease aged between 15 and 30 years, is progressive, can culminate in visual loss, and does not have a definitive treatment that can eliminate its most severe endpoints. Consultation with ophthalmologists experienced in managing this complication is vital.

Painful Episodes

In a given year, more than half of 806 patients with HbSC disease did not have a painful episode, one-third had a single episode of pain and less than 10% had three or more pain episodes.[85] This rate was approximately 0.4 episodes per patient-year, less than half the rate in sickle cell anemia. Forty percent of Jamaican patients with HbSC disease had at least one pain episode needing hospitalization; 17% never reported a pain crisis. Approximately 60% of HbSC disease patients in Los Angeles reported at least one pain episode.[48]

Acute Chest Syndrome

Acute chest syndrome, with its high morbidity and appreciable mortality, is seen in approximately 30% of patients with HbSC disease.[48] Although this incidence is only 50%–75% that of sickle cell anemia, progression to chronic lung disease is only 0.1 that of sickle cell anemia and the median age of onset is almost one decade later.[52,86] The incidence per 100 patient-years in patients of all ages is 5.2. Typical of this condition, the incidence in children age 5 years or younger is twice that of older individuals. Only steady-state leukocyte count was a risk factor for acute chest syndrome in HbSC disease. When compared with

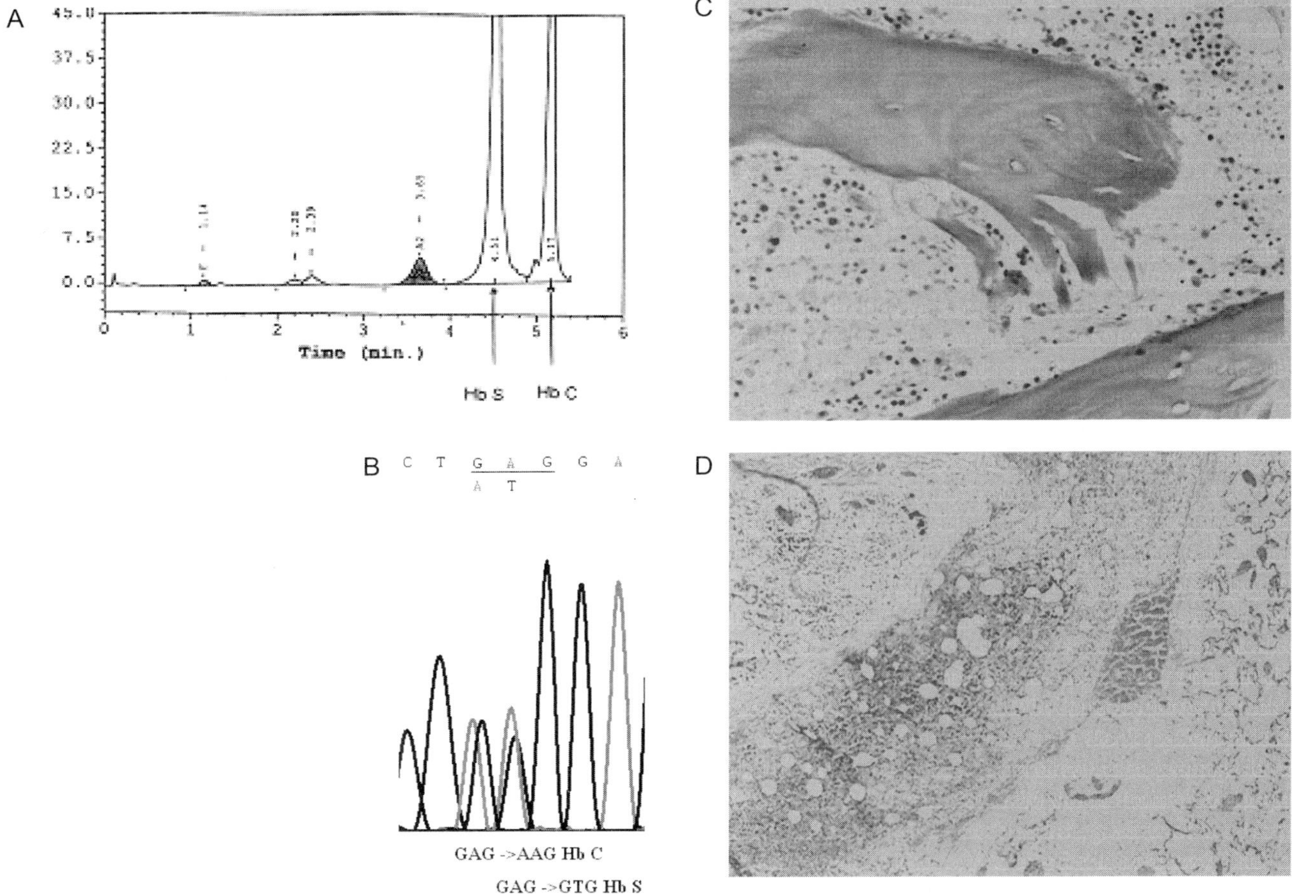

Figure 21.14. A 52-year-old man with HbSC disease and known osteonecrosis and sickle retinopathy who was never hospitalized for painful episodes; he developed severe pain in his extremities and chest and shortness of breath. The hemoglobin level was approximately 10 g/dL and white blood cell count of 25,000/mL^3. The pain soon became unbearable; he became severely hypoxic and comatose and the hemoglobin concentration and platelet count plummeted. Oxygenation was impossible to maintain and despite rapid use of blood transfusions and supportive care he died within hours of presentation with multiorgan failure. **(A)** HPLC separation of HbS and HbC. **(B)** Portion of a DNA sequencing reaction showing compound heterozygosity for HbS and HbC in *HBB* codon 6. **(C)** Bone marrow showing necrotic marrow. **(D)** Lung showing bone marrow emboli in pulmonary arteries.

sickle cell anemia, there were no differences in duration of hospitalization or death rate, but sickle cell anemia patients were more likely to present with severe pain.[87] Nevertheless, severe acute chest syndrome events due to embolization of necrotic bone marrow can occur and can terminate in multiorgan failure and death (Fig. 21.14).

Pulmonary Hypertension

The first reports of pulmonary hypertension in sickle cell disease considered HbSC disease and sickle cell anemia as a group.[88,89] More recently, in an analysis of 43 HbSC patients screened by echocardiography for pulmonary hypertension, the mean age of affected individuals was 52 years. Within this group, anemia, but not markers of hemolysis such as LDH was associated with the pulmonary hypertension phenotype. As with sickle cell anemia, pulmonary hypertension was associated with a higher risk of death.[90]

Spleen

Splenic function is often preserved in HbSC disease, whereas it is rarely preserved in adults with sickle cell anemia. A positive result of retained splenic function is the reduced incidence of infection with encapsulated bacteria. A negative result is the chance for splenic sequestration crises and splenic infarction to occur in adults.

Pocked or "pitted" red cells are found in increased numbers when splenic function declines and is lost, and can be used as a measure of functional asplenia. When pitted red cell counts were used to evaluate splenic reticuloendothelial function in HbSC disease, there were 4.9 ± 9.1% pitted cells in this disorder compared with 11.8 ± 7.0% in sickle cell anemia; however pitted cells might not always reflect splenic function. Pitted cells increased with age in sickle cell anemia but did not in HbSC disease suggesting they had stabilized splenic function.

Six percent of children with HbSC disease had splenic complications that included acute sequestration crisis, painful infarction, and hemorrhage.[91] Similar events can occur in adults with HbSC disease but are rare in adult sickle cell anemia. Slightly over one half of all adults with HbSC disease had splenomegaly, 36% were asplenic, and 12% had normal spleens when evaluated by spleen scanning. When "pit" counts were related to spleen scans, no patient with HbSC disease younger than age 4 years had functional asplenia, although this abnormality was present in 22% of individuals aged 4–12 years and 45% of individuals older than 12 years.[92]

Coexistent hereditary spherocytosis and HbSC disease were deemed responsible for multiple episodes of splenic sequestration crises in one interesting case report. It was hypothesized that the increased density and reduced deformability of red cells with membrane damage from both hereditary spherocytosis and HbSC disease caused increased splenic trapping and sickling.

Infection

The relative risk of bacteremia is less for HbSC disease patients than for sickle cell anemia patients when correction is made for the total nonhospitalized population at risk, but is much larger than that for the normal population. Gram-negative bacteremia, the systemic infection most commonly found in HbSC disease patients, was less life threatening than the pyogenic bacteremia most commonly found in sickle cell anemia. In children age 4 years and younger, normal "pit" counts suggested that prophylactic penicillin need not be given.[92] Two adolescents with functional asplenia were reported to die of pneumococcal sepsis. Fatal pneumococcal sepsis has been described in children age 5 years and younger who were not receiving penicillin but their state of splenic function was unknown.[93]

Treatment Recommendations

Some authorities question the use of prophylactic penicillin in HbSC disease.[94] A reasonable approach in children who are most susceptible to pneumococcal infection might be to assess splenic function by "pit" counts, the presence of Howell–Jolly bodies or radionuclide scanning. If splenic function is normal, prophylaxis might be withheld; however, as discussed, the evaluation of splenic function is imperfect. Also, a large spleen does not always equate with a normally functional spleen. Pneumococcal vaccines should be given and as in sickle cell anemia, parents instructed to seek immediate medical attention for febrile illnesses.

Osteonecrosis

The incidence of osteonecrosis in HbSC disease is only slightly lower than in sickle cell anemia with an age-adjusted incidence rate of 1.9/100 patient-years for the hip joints and 1.7/100 patient years for shoulders. Shoulder disease was uncommon in patients younger than age 25 years. Osteonecrosis of the femoral heads was almost as prevalent in HbSC disease as in sickle cell anemia but developed later in life.[46,52,95] The estimated age at diagnosis in HbSC disease varied from 36 to 40 years versus 36 years for sickle cell anemia.[48,95] In one study, coincident α thalassemia delayed the age of onset by approximately 15 years.[48]

Leg Ulcers

Compared with sickle cell anemia, leg ulcers are infrequent in HbSC disease and found in only approximately 3% of cases.[48,96] As in the case of priapism, this could be a result of improved nitric oxide (NO) bioavailability because of reduced hemolysis in HbSC disease compared with sickle cell anemia.

Genitourinary

The pathophysiology of renal lesions in HbSC disease is similar to that in HbAS and sickle cell anemia. Hematuria is often present and appears to be more frequent than in HbAS.[2] In HbSC disease, renal concentrating ability is lost at a time intermediate between the loss in sickle cell anemia and HbAS. Maximum concentrating ability in patients with HbSC diseases, mean age 30 years, was 537 mOsm and appeared to decline with age. The two youngest patients, aged 6 and 8 years, had maximally concentrated urines of 640 and 698 mOsms, approximately 60% of normal. In eight children with HbSC disease, mean age 11 years, none had an overnight urine concentration greater than 545 mOsm (normal, 800–1000 mOsm). Seven of eight increased their urine concentration after receiving 1-desamino-8d-arginine vasopressin, although not to normal.[97]

Renal function deteriorates with age but chronic renal failure is half as common as in sickle cell anemia (2%–3%) and its median age of onset is 25 years later.[44,48] In one study, 73% of 27 patients had papillary necrosis based on calyceal blunting by intravenous pyelography, but renal function was normal so the clinical significance of this observation is unclear.[98] Among 25 deaths in 284 HbSC disease patients, three were due to renal failure.[48]

Priapism has been estimated to occur in between 3% and 10% of patients with HbSC disease, a rate far lower than in sickle cell anemia.[48,99] Among other possible explanations, the reduced hemolysis in HbSC disease compared with sickle cell anemia with better NO bioavailability might explain this observation.[99]

Cerebrovascular Disease

Two percent to 3% of HbSC disease patients had a stroke, and 3 deaths due to stroke were noted among 248 patients.[48,52] This incidence was three–four times less than in sickle cell anemia. In the CSSCD, 0.8% of individuals with HbSC disease compared with 4% of patients with sickle cell anemia had suffered a stroke at study entry.[100]

Pregnancy

Perinatal mortality in HbSC disease has been reported to vary from 28%–nil in the absence of transfusions and from 0 to 9% when transfusions were given.[101] In a heterogeneous collection of patient series with widely different numbers of cases, more recent reports generally had lower mortality. Pregnancy-related complications are higher than in normal controls and not dissimilar to those with sickle cell anemia. The rate of caesarian sections is similar.[102] Stress or pregnancy might result in disease symptoms, and the pregnant HbSC disease patient can be as severely affected as the sickle cell anemia patient. In 95 pregnancies in 43 patients with HbSC disease followed from birth, menarche was marginally delayed compared with controls, but the age at first pregnancy was similar. The prevalence of pregnancy-induced hypertension, preeclampsia, antepartum or postpartum hemorrhage did not differ from controls. Sickle-related complications were similar to those in patients with sickle cell anemia with marginally fewer miscarriages, more live deliveries, and higher birthweight.[103]

Pregnancy and recommendations for its management are discussed in detail in Chapter 19.

HbSC/Hb-G Philadelphia

This genotype has a special phenotype because the hybrid molecule, $\alpha_2^{\text{G-Philadelphia}}\beta_2^{C}$ increases the rate of crystal nucleation compared with native HbC, and HbS enhances this effect in a pathogenetically relevant manner.[16] Heterozygotes for the β^S, β^C, and the $\alpha^{\text{G-Philadelphia}}$ genes have abundant circulating intraerythrocytic crystals and increased numbers of folded red cells with a mild clinical course. This phenotype seems to be the result of increased crystallization and decreased polymerization caused by the effects of the $\alpha^{\text{G-Philadelphia}}$ globin chain on the β^C and β^S gene products. Some of the intraerythrocytic crystals in this syndrome, unlike the typical crystal of HbSC disease, are unusually long and thin and resemble sugar cane (Fig. 21.15). A mild clinical course associated with increased crystallization implies that in HbSC disease polymerization of HbS is pathogenically more important than the crystallization induced by β^C chains.

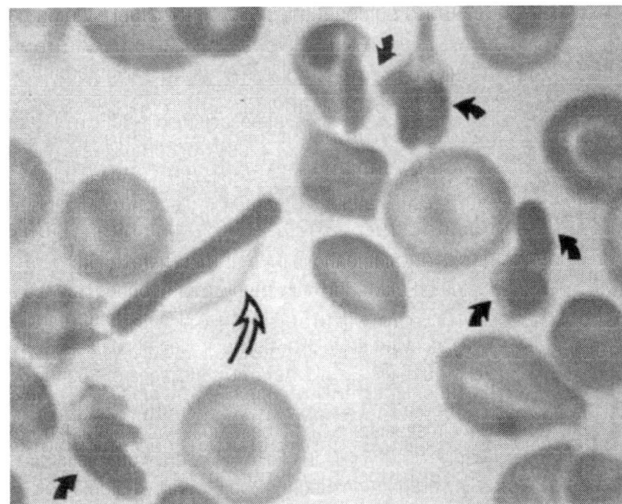

Figure 21.15. Blood smear directly from finger stick blood from a patient with $SC^{\alpha\text{G Philadelphia}}$ disease. Open arrow, depicts a "sugar cane" crystal, a shape not observed in HbC disease or HbSC disease blood. The black arrows depict red cells with more classic forms of HbC-dependent crystals.[16]

TREATMENT OF HbSC DISEASE

No currently available treatment is unique for HbSC disease. The special pathophysiological features of HbSC disease might in the future allow a direct attack on some basic disease mechanisms such as K:Cl cotransport (Chapter 9 and 31), but these approaches are still under study. Hydroxyurea can effect changes in the HbSC disease erythrocyte that might be independent of any change in HbF. Early trials of hydroxyurea in HbSC disease are discussed in Chapter 30.

Transfusions are used in HbSC disease for the same indications as in sickle cell anemia. A study was performed on preoperative transfusion in HbSC disease.[104] Eighteen percent of all patients had some postoperative complications. Postoperative events were compared between patients who received preoperative transfusions and those who were untransfused. In patients undergoing intraabdominal surgery, more than a third of untransfused patients had postoperative acute chest syndrome or painful episodes. Although this study was not randomized and both simple and exchange transfusions were used, based on these observations and the larger study of preoperative transfusion in sickle cell anemia,[105] preoperative transfusion should be considered in patients with HbSC disease who face procedures with moderate surgical risk.

Because some patients with HbSC disease have PCVs that approach normal, in emergent situations such as severe acute chest syndrome or stroke, or when preparing a patient for surgery, exchange transfusions might be the most prudent approach to treatment so as not to unduly raise the PCV and increase blood viscosity.

Because of the higher PCV, phlebotomy has been considered one approach to treating HbSC disease. In one patient, the PCV rose following splenectomy and the rate of acute painful episodes increased. Following a phlebotomy program to lower the PCV to presplenectomy values and induce iron deficiency, the symptoms regressed.[106] A controlled trial of this approach has not been reported.

SUMMARY

Positively charged HbC induces cellular changes in HbC trait, HbC disease, and HbSC disease that are a result of cellular dehydration. Although biologically interesting and producing characteristic hematological features in the erythrocyte, only trivial clinical abnormalities are associated with HbC trait and HbC disease. This is not so when HbC is present with HbS. HbSC disease is a clinically important illness with all of the complications of sickle cell anemia, albeit at a reduced rate. An effective treatment would be a major medical advance and clinical trials of agents that can reduce cell density and increase HbF concentration have started.

REFERENCES

1. Kan YW, Dozy AM. Evolution of the hemoglobin S and C genes in world populations. *Science.* 1980;209:388–391.
2. Dacie J. *The Haemolytic Anaemias.* 3 ed. Edinburgh: Churchill Livingstone; 1988.
3. Labie D, Richin C, Pagnier J, Gentilini M, Nagel RL. Hemoglobins S and C in Upper Volta. *Hum Genet.* 1984;65: 300–302.
4. Daar S, Hussain HM, Gravell D, Nagel RL, Krishnamoorthy R. Genetic epidemiology of HbS and HbC in Oman: multicentric origin for the β^S gene. *Am J Hematol.* 2000; 39–46.
5. Agarwal A, Guindo A, Cissoko Y, et al. Hemoglobin C associated with protection from severe malaria in the Dogon of Mali, a West African population with a low prevalence of hemoglobin S. *Blood.* 2000;96(7):2358–2363.
6. Modiano D, Luoni G, Sirima BS, et al. Haemoglobin C protects against clinical Plasmodium falciparum malaria. *Nature.* 2001;414(6861):305–308.
7. Rihet P, Flori L, Tall F, Traore AS, Fumoux F. Hemoglobin C is associated with reduced Plasmodium falciparum parasitemia and low risk of mild malaria attack. *Hum Mol Genet.* 2004;13(1):1–6.
8. Fairhurst RM, Fujioka H, Hayton K, Collins KF, Wellems TE. Aberrant development of Plasmodium falciparum in hemoglobin CC red cells: implications for the malaria protective effect of the homozygous state. *Blood.* 2003;101(8):3309–3315.
9. Mockenhaupt FP, Ehrhardt S, Cramer JP, et al. Hemoglobin C and resistance to severe malaria in Ghanaian children. *J Infect Dis.* 2004;190(5):1006–1009.
10. Mockenhaupt FP, Ehrhardt S, Burkhardt J, et al. Manifestation and outcome of severe malaria in children in northern Ghana. *Am J Trop Med Hyg.* 2004;71(2):167–172.
11. Hirsch RE, Lin MJ, Nagel RL. The inhibition of hemoglobin C crystallization by hemoglobin F. *J Biol Chem.* 1988;263:5936–5939.
12. Hirsch RE, Raventos-Suarez C, Olson JA, Nagel RL. Ligand state of intraerythrocytic circulating Hb C crystals in homozygous CC patients. *Blood.* 1985;66:775–777.
13. Hirsch RE, Lin MJ, Vidugirus GVA, Huang SC, Friedman JM, Nagel RL. Conformational changes in oxyhemoglobin C (Glu $\beta6\rightarrow$lys) detected by spectroscopic probing. *J Biol Chem.* 1996;271:372–375.
14. Hirsch RE, Witkowska HE, Shafer F, et al. HbC compound heterozygotes [HbC/Hb Riyadh and HbC/Hb N- Baltimore] with opposing effects upon HbC crystallization. *Br J Haematol.* 1997;97:259–265.
15. Nagel RL, Lin MJ, Witkowska HE, Fabry ME, Bestak M, Hirsch RE. Compound heterozygosity for hemoglobin C and Korle-Bu: Moderate microcytic hemolytic anemia and acceleration of crystal formation. *Blood.* 1993;82:1907–1912.
16. Lawrence C, Hirsch RE, Fataliev NA, Patel S, Fabry ME, Nagel RL. Molecular interactions between Hb α-G Philadelphia, HbC, and HbS: Phenotypic implications for SC α-G Philadelphia disease. *Blood.* 1997;90(7):2819–2825.
17. Hirsch RE, Juszczak LJ, Fataliev NA, Friedman JM, Nagel RL. Solution-active structural alterations in liganded hemoglobins C (β6 Glu $\rightarrow$ Lys) and S (β6 Glu $\rightarrow$ Val). *J Biol Chem.* 1999;274(20):13777–13782.
18. Feeling-Taylor AR, Yau ST, Petsev DN, Nagel RL, Hirsch RE, Vekilov PG. Crystallization mechanisms of hemoglobin C in the R state. *Biophys J.* 2004;87(4):2621–2629.
19. Hirsch RE, Samuel RE, Fataliev NA, et al. Differential pathways in oxy and deoxy HbC aggregation/crystallization. *Proteins.* 2001;42(1):99–107.
20. Jensen WN, Schoefield RA, Agner R. Clinical and necropsy findings in hemoglobin C disease. *Blood.* 1998;12:74–83.
21. Brugnara C, Kopin AS, Bunn HF, Tosteson DC. Regulation of cation content and cell volume in hemoglobin erythrocytes from patients with homozygous hemoglobin C disease. *J Clin Invest.* 1985;75:1608–1617.
22. Brugnara C, Kopin AS, Bunn HF, Tosteson DC. Electrolyte composition and equilibrium in hemoglobin CC red blood cells. *Trans Assoc Am Physicians.* 1984;97:104–112.
23. Canessa M, Splavins A, Nagel RL. Volume-dependent and NEM-stimulated K+Cl- transport is elevated in oxygenated SS SC and CC human cells. *FEBS Lett.* 1986;200:197–202.
24. Lauf PK, Theg BE. A chloride dependent K+ flux induced by N-ethlymaleimide in genetically low K+ sheep and goat erythrocytes. *Biochem Biophys Res Commun.* 1980;92:1422–1428.
25. Dunham PB, Ellory JC. Passive potassium transport in low potassium sheep red cells: dependence upon cell volume and chloride. *J Physiol.* 1981;318:511–530.
26. Canessa M, Fabry ME, Blumenfeld N, Nagel R. A volume-stimulated Cl-dependent K+ efflux is highly expressed in young human red cells containing normal hemoglobin or Hb S. *J Membr Biol.* 1987;97:97–105.
27. Romero-Garcia C, Navarro JL, Lam H, et al. Hb A2-Manzanares or $\alpha_2\delta_2$ 121 (GH4) Glu-Val, an unstable δ chain variant observed in a Spanish family. *Hemoglobin.* 1983;7: 435–442.

28. Fabry ME, Romero JR, Suzuka SM, et al. Hemoglobin C in transgenic mice: Effect of HbC expression from founders to full mouse globin knockouts. *Blood Cells Mol Dis.* 2000;26(4):331–347.
29. Romero JR, Suzuka SM, Nagel RL, Fabry ME. Expression of HbC and HbS, but not HbA, results in activation of K-Cl cotransport activity in transgenic mouse red cells. *Blood.* 2004;103(6):2384–2390.
30. Romero JR, Suzuka SM, Romero-Gonzalez GV, Nagel RL, Fabry ME. K:Cl cotransport activity is inhibited by HCO_3 in knockout mouse red cells expressing human hemoglobin C. *Blood Cells Mol Dis.* 2001;27(1):69–70.
31. Motulsky AG. Frequency of sickling disorders in US blacks. *N Engl J Med.* 1973;288:31–33.
32. Lehmann H, Huntsman RG. *Man's Haemoglobins.* 2nd ed. Amsterdam: North Holland; 1974.
33. Hinchliffe RF, Norcliffe D, Farrar LM, Lilleyman JS. Mean cell haemoglobin concentration in subjects with haemoglobin C, D, E and S traits. *Clin Lab Haematol.* 1996;18:245–248.
34. Giordano PC, Harteveld CL, Michiels JJ, et al. Atypical HbH disease in a Surinamese patient resulting from a combination of the -SEA and -α3.7 deletions with HbC heterozygosity. *Br J Haematol.* 1997;96:801–805.
35. Liebhaber SA, Cash FE, Cornfield DB. Evidence for posttranslational control of Hb C synthesis in an individual with Hb C trait and α-thalassemia. *Blood.* 1988;71:502–504.
36. Olson JF, Ware RE, Schultz WH, Kinney TR. Hemoglobin C disease in infancy and childhood. *J Pediatr.* 1994;125:745–747.
37. Lin MJ, Nagel RL, Hirsch RE. The acceleration of hemoglobin C crystallization by hemoglobin S. *Blood.* 1989;74:1823–1825.
38. Fabry ME, Kaul DK, Raventos-Suarez C, Chang H, Nagel RL. SC cells have an abnormally high intracellular hemoglobin concentration: Pathophysiological consequences. *J Clin Invest.* 1982;70:1315–1319.
39. Fabry ME, Benjamin L, Lawrence C, Nagel RL. An objective sign of painful crisis in sickle cell anemia. *Blood.* 1983;64:559–563.
40. Ballas SK, Smith ED. Red blood cell changes during the evolution of the sickle cell painful crisis. *Blood.* 1992;79:2154–2163.
41. Steinberg MH, Nagel RL, Lawrence C, et al. β-globin gene haplotype in Hb SC disease. *Am J Hematol.* 1996;52:189–191.
42. Talacki CA, Rappaport E, Schwartz E, Surrey S, Ballas SK. Beta-globin gene cluster haplotype in Hb C heterozygotes. *Hemoglobin.* 1990;14:229–240.
43. Embury SH, Hebbel RP, Mohandas N, Steinberg MH. *Sickle Cell Disease: Basic Principles and Clinical Practice.* 1st ed. New York: Raven Press; 1994.
44. West MS, Wethers D, Smith J, Steinberg MH, Coop Study of Sickle Cell Disease. Laboratory profile of sickle cell disease: a cross-sectional analysis. *J Clin Epidemiol.* 1992;45:893–909.
45. Bannerman RM, Serjeant B, Seakins M, England JM, Serjeant GR. Determinants of haemoglobin level in sickle cell-haemoglobin C disease. *Br J Haematol.* 1979;43:49–56.
46. Serjeant GR, Ashcroft MT, Serjeant BE. The clinical features of haemoglobin SC disease in Jamaica. *Br J Haematol.* 1973;24:491–501.
47. Duits AJ, Rodriguez T, Schnog JJ. Serum levels of angiogenic factors indicate a pro-angiogenic state in adults with sickle cell disease. *Br J Haematol.* 2006;134(1):116–119.
48. Powars DR, Hiti A, Ramicone E, Johnson C, Chan L. Outcome in hemoglobin SC disease: a four-decade observational study of clinical, hematologic, and genetic factors. *Am J Hematol.* 2002;70(3):206–215.
49. Platt OS, Rosenstock W, Espeland M. Influence of S hemoglobinopathies on growth and development. *N Engl J Med.* 1984;311:7–12.
50. Stevens MCG, Maude GH, Cupidore L, Jackson H, Hayes RJ, Serjeant GR. Prepubertal growth and skeletal maturation in children with sickle cell disease. *J Pediatr.* 1986;78:124–132.
51. Leikin SL, Gallagher D, Kinney TR, Sloane D, Klug P, Rida W. Mortality in children and adolescents with sickle cell disease. *Pediatrics.* 1989;84:500–508.
52. Powars D, Chan LS, Schroeder WA. The variable expression of sickle cell disease is genetically determined. *Semin Hematol.* 1990;27:360–376.
53. Platt OS, Brambilla DJ, Rosse WF, et al. Mortality in sickle cell disease: Life expectancy and risk factors for early death. *N Engl J Med.* 1994;330:1639–1644.
54. Koduri PR, Agbemadzo B, Nathan S. Hemoglobin S-C disease revisited: clinical study of 106 adults. *Am J Hematol.* 2001;68(4):298–300.
55. Bainbridge R, Higgs DR, Maude GH, Serjeant GR. Clinical presentation of homozygous sickle cell disease. *J Pediatr.* 1985;106:881–885.
56. Welch RB, Goldberg MF. Sickle-cell hemoglobin and its relation to fundus abnormality. *Arch Ophthalmol.* 1966;75:353–362.
57. Lutty GA, Goldberg MF. Ophthalmologic complications. In: Embury SH, Hebbel RP, Mohandas N, Steinberg MH, eds. *Sickle Cell Disease: Basic Principles and Clinical Practice.* 1st ed. New York: Raven; 1994:703–724.
58. McLeod DS, Goldberg MF, Lutty GA. Dual-perspective analysis of vascular formations in sickle cell retinopathy. *Arch Ophthalmol.* 1993;111:1234–1245.
59. Roy MS, Gascon P, Giuliani D. Macular blood flow velocity in sickle cell disease: Relation to red cell density. *Br J Ophthalmol.* 1995;79:742–745.
60. Lutty GA, Merges C, Crone S, McLeod DS. Immunohistochemical insights into sickle cell retinopathy. *Curr Eye Res.* 1994;13:125–138.
61. Kim SY, Mocanu C, McLeod DS et al. Expression of pigment epithelium-derived factor (PEDF) and vascular endothelial growth factor (VEGF) in sickle cell retina and choroid. *Exp Eye Res.* 2003;77(4):433–445.
62. McLeod DS, Merges C, Fukushima A, Goldberg MF, Lutty GA. Histopathologic features of neovascularization in sickle cell retinopathy. *Am J Ophthalmol.* 1997;124(4):455–472.
63. Mohan JS, Lip PL, Blann AD, Bareford D, Lip GY. The angiopoietin/Tie-2 system in proliferative sickle retinopathy: relation to vascular endothelial growth factor, its soluble receptor Flt-1 and von Willebrand factor, and to the effects of laser treatment. *Br J Ophthalmol.* 2005;89(7):815–819.
64. Lutty GA, McLeod DS, Pachnis A, Costantini F, Fabry ME, Nagel RL. Retinal and choroidal neovascularization in a transgenic mouse model of sickle cell disease. *Am J Pathol.* 1994;145:490–497.
65. Lutty GA, Merges C, McLeod DS, et al. Nonperfusion of retina and choroid in transgenic mouse models of sickle cell disease. *Curr Eye Res.* 1998;17(4):438–444.

66. Lutty GA, Phelan A, McLeod DS, Fabry ME, Nagel RL. A rat model for sickle cell-mediated vaso-occlusion in retina. *Microvasc Res.* 1996;52:270–280.
67. Lutty GA, Taomoto M, Cao J, et al. Inhibition of TNF-alpha-induced sickle RBC retention in retina by a VLA-4 antagonist. *Invest Ophthalmol Vis Sci.* 2001;42(6):1349–1355.
68. Lutty GA, Otsuji T, Taomoto M, et al. Mechanisms for sickle red blood cell retention in choroid. *Curr Eye Res.* 2002;25(3):163–171.
69. Kunz MM, McLeod DS, Merges C, Cao J, Lutty GA. Neutrophils and leucocyte adhesion molecules in sickle cell retinopathy. *Br J Ophthalmol.* 2002;86(6):684–690.
70. Wajer SD, Taomoto M, McLeod DS et al. Velocity measurements of normal and sickle red blood cells in the rat retinal and choroidal vasculatures. *Microvasc Res.* 2000;60(3):281–293.
71. Penman AD, Talbot JF, Chuang EL, Thomas P, Serjeant GR, Bird AC. New classification of peripheral retinal vascular changes in sickle cell disease. *Br J Ophthalmol.* 1994;78:681–689.
72. Talbot JF, Bird AC, Serjeant GR, Hayes RJ. Sickle cell retinopathy in young children in Jamaica. *Br J Ophthalmol.* 1982;66:149–154.
73. Talbot JF, Bird AC, Maude GH, Acheson RW, Moriarity BJ, Serjeant GR. Sickle cell retinopathy in Jamaican children: further observations in a cohort study. *Br J Ophthalmol.* 1996;72:727–732.
74. Kent D, Arya R, Aclimandos WA, Bellingham AJ, Bird AC. Screening for ophthalmic manifestations of sickle cell disease in the United Kingdom. *Eye.* 1994;8:618–622.
75. Raichand M, Goldberg MF, Nagpal KC, Goldbaum MH, Asdourian GK. Evolution of neovascularization in sickle cell retinopathy: a prospective flourescein angiographic study. *Arch Ophthalmol.* 1977;95:1543–1552.
76. Nagpal KC, Patrianakos D, Asdourian GK, Goldberg MF, Rabb M, Jampol L. Spontaneous regression (autoinfarction) of proliferative sickle retinopathy. *Am J Ophthalmol.* 1975;80:885–892.
77. Goldberg MF. Natural history of untreated proliferative sickle retinopathy. *Arch Ophthalmol.* 1971;85:428–437.
78. Clarkson JG. The ocular manifestations of sickle-cell disease: a prevalence and natural history study. *Trans Am Ophthalmol Soc.* 1992;90:481–504.
79. Condon PI, Serjeant GR. Behavior of untreated proliferative sickle retinopathy. *Br J Ophthalmol.* 1980;64:404–411.
80. Fox PD, Dunn DT, Morris JS, Serjeant GR. Risk factors for proliferative sickle retinopathy. *Br J Ophthalmol.* 1990;74:172–176.
81. Fox PD, Vessey SJR, Forshaw ML, Serjeant GR. Influence of genotype on the natural history of untreated proliferative sickle retinopathy – an angiographic study. *Br J Ophthalmol.* 1991;75:229–231.
82. Downes SM, Hambleton IR, Chuang EL, Lois N, Serjeant GR, Bird AC. Incidence and natural history of proliferative sickle cell retinopathy: observations from a cohort study. *Ophthalmology.* 2005;112(11):1869–1875.
83. Condon PI, Serjeant GR. Photocoagulation in proliferative sickle retinopathy: results of a 5-year study. *Br J Ophthalmol.* 1980;64:832–840.
84. Farber MD, Jampol LM, Fox P, et al. A randomized clinical trial of scatter photocoagulation of proliferative sickle retinopathy. *Arch Ophthalmol.* 1991;109:363–367.
85. Platt OS, Thorington BD, Brambilla DJ, et al. Pain in sickle cell disease – rates and risk factors. *N Engl J Med.* 1991;325:11–16.
86. Castro O, Brambilla DJ, Thorington B, et al. The acute chest syndrome in sickle cell disease: incidence and risk factors. *Blood.* 1994;84:643–649.
87. Vichinsky EP, Styles LA, Colangelo LH, et al. Acute chest syndrome in sickle cell disease: clinical presentation and course. *Blood.* 1997;89:1787–1792.
88. Gladwin MT, Sachdev V, Jison ML, et al. Pulmonary hypertension as a risk factor for death in patients with sickle cell disease. *N Engl J Med.* 2004;350(9):886–895.
89. Ataga KI, Moore CG, Jones S, et al. Pulmonary hypertension in patients with sickle cell disease: a longitudinal study. *Br J Haematol.* 2006;134(1):109–115.
90. Taylor JG, Ackah D, Cobb C, et al. Mutations and polymorphisms in hemoglobin genes and the risk of pulmonary hypertension and death in sickle cell disease. *Am J Hematol.* 2008;83:6–14.
91. Aquino VM, Norvell JM, Buchanan GR. Acute splenic complications in children with sickle cell hemoglobin C disease. *J Pediatr.* 1997;130:961–965.
92. Lane PA, Rogers ZR, Woods GM, et al. Fatal pneumococcal septicemia in hemoglobin SC disease. *J Pediatr.* 1994; 124:859–862.
93. Lane PA, O'Connell JL, Lear JL, et al. Functional asplenia in hemoglobin SC disease. *Blood.* 1995;85(8):2238–2244.
94. Rogers ZR, Buchanan GR. Bacteremia in children with sickle hemoglobin C disease and sickle beta^{+}-thalassemia: is prophylactic penicillin necessary? *J Pediatr.* 1995;127:348–354.
95. Milner PF, Kraus AP, Sebes JI, et al. Sickle cell disease as a cause of osteonecrosis of the femoral head. *N Engl J Med.* 1991;325:1476–1481.
96. Nolan VG, Adewoye A, Baldwin C, et al. Sickle cell leg ulcers: associations with haemolysis and SNPs in Klotho, TEK and genes of the TGF-beta/BMP pathway. *Br J Haematol.* 2006;133(5):570–578.
97. Iyer R, Baliga R, Nagel RL, et al. Maximum urine concentrating ability in children with Hb SC disease: effects of hydroxyurea. *Am J Hematol.* 2000;64(1):47–52.
98. Ballas SK, Lewis CN, Noone AM, Krasnow SH, Kamarulzaman E, Burka ER. Clinical hematological and biochemical features of Hb SC disease. *Am J Hematol.* 1982;13:37–51.
99. Nolan VG, Wyszynski DF, Farrer LA, Steinberg MH. Hemolysis-associated priapism in sickle cell disease. *Blood.* 2005;106(9):3264–3267.
100. Ohene-Frempong K, Weiner SJ, Sleeper LA, et al. Cerebrovascular accidents in sickle cell disease: Rates and risk factors. *Blood.* 1998;91(1):288–294.
101. Koshy M, Burd L. Obstetric and Gynecologic Issues. In: Embury SH, Hebbel RP, Mohandas N, Steinberg MH, eds. *Sickle Cell Disease: Basic Principles and Clinical Practice.* 1st ed. New York: Lippincott-Raven; 1994:689–702.
102. Koshy M, Burd L, Wallace D, Moawad A, Baron J. Prophylactic red-cell transfusions in pregnant patients with sickle cell disease. A randomized cooperative study. *N Engl J Med.* 1988;319:1447–1452.
103. Serjeant GR, Hambleton I, Thame M. Fecundity and pregnancy outcome in a cohort with sickle cell-haemoglobin C disease followed from birth. *Br J Obstet Gynaecol.* 2005; 112(9):1308–1314.

104. Neumayr L, Koshy M, Haberkern C, et al. Surgery in patients with hemoglobin SC disease. *Am J Hematol.* 1998;57(2):101–108.
105. Vichinsky EP, Haberkern CM, Neumayr L, et al. A comparison of conservative and aggressive transfusion regimens in the perioperative management of sickle cell disease. *N Engl J Med.* 1995;333:206–213.
106. Markham MJ, Lottenberg R, Zumberg M. Role of phlebotomy in the management of hemoglobin SC disease: case report and review of the literature. *Am J Hematol.* 2003;73(2):121–125.
107. Boehm CD, Dowling CE, Antonarakis SE, Honig GR, Kazazian HH. Evidence supporting a single origin of the β(C)-globin gene in blacks. *Am J Hum Genet.* 1985;37:771–777.
108. Trabuchet G, Elion J, Dunda O, et al. Nucleotide sequence evidence of the unicentric origin of the β^C mutation in Africa. *Hum Genet.* 1991;87:597–601.
109. Eaton WA, Hofrichter J. Sickle cell hemoglobin polymerization. *Adv Protein Chem.* 1990;40:63–280.
110. Platt OS, Brambilla DJ, Rosse WF, et al. Mortality in sickle cell disease. Life expectancy and risk factors for early death. *N Engl J Med.* 1994;330(23):1639–1644.

22

Sickle Cell Trait

Martin H. Steinberg

INTRODUCTION

Parents of children with sickle cell anemia seldom have the same disease as their offspring. In 1927, 17 years after the first clinical description of sickle cell anemia, it was discovered that almost 10% of African Americans had erythrocytes that sickled when deoxygenated. With the subsequent identification of HbS, and the observation that patients with sickle cell anemia had predominantly HbS in their hemolysates, whereas their parents' had both HbS and HbA, the genetics of sickle hemoglobinopathies was characterized and sickle cell trait (HbAS) was defined.

Almost 40 years ago, reports of sudden death in military recruits with HbAS triggered a push for mandatory screening for HbAS, denial of military service for some carriers, and insurance coverage cancellation for others. An astounding list of complications of HbAS appeared in the literature. The interpretation of these reports often disregarded the distinction between statistically significant associations and coincidence, and almost all lacked any control comparisons. This chapter reviews what is known, what is presumed, and what is erroneous about the pathogenicity, clinical features, and management of HbAS.

PATHOGENESIS

HbAS is usually implies simple heterozygosity for the HbS gene (*HBB* glu6val). Less than half the hemoglobin in the HbAS erythrocyte is HbS; the remainder is mainly HbA. The probability that the mixed hybrid tetramer, $\alpha_2\beta^S\beta^A$, will enter the polymer phase is only half that of the HbS tetramer, $\alpha_2\beta^S{}_2$ (Fig. 22.1A).[1] HbS polymer concentrations sufficient to injure the red cell are prerequisite for the expression of the phenotype of sickle cell disease; in HbAS, high concentrations of HbA preclude clinically significant HbS polymer formation at the oxygen saturation and physiological conditions present in most tissues (Fig. 22.1B). HbS polymer appears in HbAS cells only when oxygen saturation falls below 60%. Even when HbAS blood is completely deoxygenated, the polymer fraction is only 40% of total hemoglobin. HbAS should therefore be clinically benign, and, despite the multitudinous reports of innumerable complications associated with HbAS, very few are confirmed by careful epidemiological studies.

Diagnosis

Indications for detecting HbAS in at risk populations are limited and include genetic counseling, population surveys, evaluating hematuria, planning treatment of hyphema, pregnancy, and perhaps before complicated thoracic surgery.

Detecting HbAS requires the quantification HbS and HbA in a hemolysate. This is best accomplished by high-performance liquid chromatography (HPLC) (see Chapter 28), in which the presence and ratio of HbS to HbA are accurately determined. Isoelectric focusing does not provide quantitative data. DNA-based methods definitively detect the presence of both HbS and HbA genes but are usually unnecessary if all one desires to establish is the presence of HbAS. HbAS cannot be diagnosed by medical history, clinical examination, or routine laboratory testing. Neither hematological indices nor peripheral blood film reviews are useful for diagnosis because both are normal in HbAS. With rare exception, the sickle solubility test has no role as a primary screening test or as the sole means of detecting HbS. This test indicates only the presence of HbS and cannot reliably distinguish between HbAS, sickle cell anemia, and HbS–β^+ thalassemia. Table 22.1 shows the prevalence of HbAS in some locations in African and throughout the world.

Fetal hemoglobin (HbF) levels are usually normal in HbAS. Carriers of HbAS in whom the HbS gene is on a Senegal or Arab–Indian β-globin gene haplotype chromosome (Chapter 27) can have higher HbF levels than other individuals, but they remain within the normal range.[2] HbF and F cells (erythrocytes containing HbF) can be increased in individuals with both HbAS and coincident hereditary persistence of fetal hemoglobin (HPFH) due to point mutations in the γ-globin gene promoters (Chapters 16 and 17).

HbS Concentration in HbAS

Effects of α Thalassemia

The proportion of hemoglobins in the erythrocyte depends on the transcriptional rate of each globin gene, the stability of the mRNA and hemoglobin produced, and the posttranslational assembly and stability of the αβ dimer and hemoglobin tetramer.

αβ Dimers rapidly associate into tetramers, and oxyhemoglobin tetramers dissociate into dimers. Hybrid tetramers ($\alpha_2\beta^S\beta^A$) occur in HbAS. Normally, a slight excess of positively charged α chains are always available to bind

Table 22.1. Prevalence of HbAS in world populations

Region/country		Prevalence (%)
Africa	North Africa	1.3–6.3
	West Africa	13.2–24.4
	Central Africa	5.1–24.5
	East Africa	2–38
	Southern Africa	0.8–20
Middle East, Central Asia, & India	India	20 (in affected tribal populations)
	Transcaucasia	0.5–1
	Turkey	13 (Eti-Turks)
	Iran	
	Saudi Arabia	1–60
Europe	Greece	0–32 (mean =11 in the north)
	Italy (Sicily)	2–4
	Portugal	
United States	United States	8–9 (African Americans)
	Amerindians	rare
South America	Brazil	4–8
Caribbean		7–14 (excluding Puerto Rico)
Central America		1–20 (dependent on racial origin of population examined)

Data from Africa are summarized from the work of many investigators and adapted from ref. 24.

non-α chains. Therefore, the steady-state accumulation of hemoglobin tetramers in the erythrocyte depends predominantly on expression of the non-α-globin genes. Hemoglobin dimers are assembled by the electrostatic attraction of α- and non-α-globin chains.[3] β^S-Globin chains are more positively charged than β^A chains, and therefore, bind α chains less avidly, accounting for HbS levels in heterozygotes (and levels of other positively charged hemoglobin variants also) being less than the 50% expected based on gene dosage alone.

HbAS carriers with four α-globin genes usually have 40% ± 4% HbS. The percentage of HbS can be altered by an α-globin gene mutant, a β-globin gene variant *trans* to the HbS gene (or very rarely in *cis*), β thalassemia, iron deficiency anemia, and possibly lead poisoning and megaloblastic anemia.

HbS concentration in HbAS is trimodally distributed, with peaks at 30%, 35%, and 40%.[4] This distribution, with few exceptions, is determined by the number of α-globin genes. Mild forms of α thalassemia are extraordinarily common where HbS is prevalent (Chapters 13 and 14). Individuals with HbAS who have α thalassemia exhibit HbA/HbS ratios less than 40%. The ratio of α/β globin biosynthesis in three families with a proband with HbAS–α thalassemia is shown in Figure 22.2. As α thalassemia reduces the pool of available α-globin chains, β^A- and β^S-globin chains must compete for those available and β^A chains dimerize twice as effectively with α chains as do β^S chains. When α gene triplication or quadruplication increases the number of α-globin chains, the HbS level increases beyond 40% due to the augmented pool of available α-globin.[5] These relationships are shown in Table 22.2. Individuals with the -$\alpha^{4.2}$ deletion have lower HbS levels than those with the more common -$\alpha^{3.7}$ deletion because of the greater α-globin chain deficit associated with the former type of α thalassemia (Chapter 13). Homozygotes for the -$\alpha^{4.2}$ with HbAS deletion have approximately 20% HbS.

Rare individuals with HbAS have only a single α-globin gene, or HbH disease.[6,7] They have HbS levels of approximately 20%, mild anemia, and marked microcytosis,

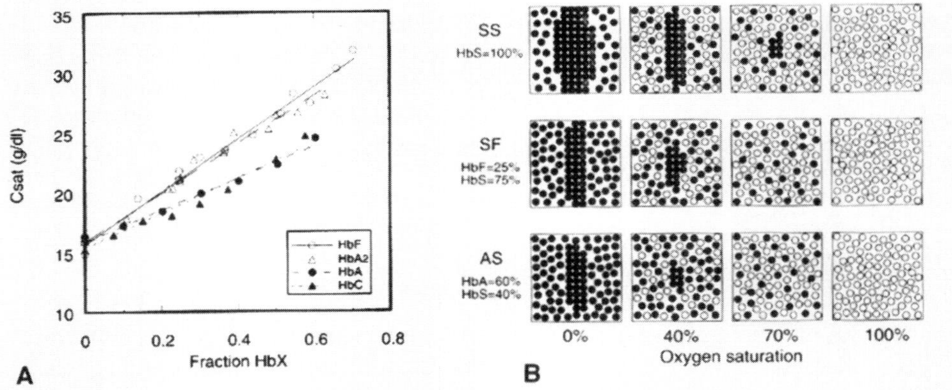

Figure 22.1. (A) Solubility of deoxygenated hemoglobin mixtures. Other hemoglobins prevent HbS polymerization by increasing HbS solubility (Csat). The percentage of increase in solubility reflects the likelihood of the other hemoglobin type being included in the deoxy HbS polymer. Neither the γ-globin chain of HbF nor the δ-globin chain of HbA_2 is incorporated into the polymer phase, so HbF and HbA_2 inhibit polymerization more than do HbA and HbC. From ref. 71, with permission. **(B)** Effects of HbA and HbF on HbS polymerization. Closed circles indicate fully deoxygenated hemoglobin and open circles indicate fully oxygenated hemoglobin. Polymer is indicated by stacked closed circles. (From ref. 71, with permission.)

Table 22.2. Hematology and percentage of HbS in HbAS with α thalassemia or β thalassemia

α-Globin genotype	Hemoglobin (g/dL)	MCV (fL)	α/β* biosynthesis	HbS§ (%)
ααα/αα	N	N	–	45
αα/αα	N	N	1	40
-α/ααα	N	N	–	40
-α/αα	N–low N	75–85	0.85	35
--α /αα codon 62 GTG>TG##	12	73	–	28
--/αα¶	?	?	?	?
-α/-α	N–low N	70–75	0.75	30
--/-α	7–10 g/dL	50–60	0.50	20–25
HbAS with β+ Thalassemia in Trans or in Cis				
β+ Thalassemia Cis	12–13	65	1.50	10
β+ Thalassemia in Trans (see Chapter 23)				

Modified from ref. 4. N signifies normal levels. * Ratio of radioactivity incorporated into α-globin chains vs. β-globin chains during incubation of reticulocytes with radioisotopes. The normal α/β ratio is 1 ± 0.15. Lower ratios suggest the presence of α thalassemia and higher ratios, β thalassemia. ## This single case is associated with a novel frameshift mutation.[116] ¶ This genotype has not been reported with HbAS. § Remainder of hemoglobin predominantly HbA.

Most values represent means from several studies. Although approximately 50 patients with HbAS and the αα/αα genotype, 40 with the -α/αα genotype, and 20 with the -α/-α have been studied, far fewer with the other genotypes have been examined, so the data presented should be interpreted with caution. HbS with β+ thalassemia assumes a normal α-globin genotype.

but no detectable HbH. It might be that in the presence of only a single normal β-globin gene, the high affinity of α-globin chains for the limited β^A-globin chains and the instability of a β^S teramer preclude HbH (β_4) formation. Heterozygotes for HbC (*HBB* glu6lys) and HbE (*HBB* glu26lys) have similar reductions in the level of the variant hemoglobin when α thalassemia coexists (Chapters 18 and 21).

Occasionally, α thalassemia is caused by a point mutation in either the α_1 or α_2 gene (*HBA1, HBA2*) (Chapter 13). When these mutations are present in individuals with HbAS, the level of HbS is likely to be dependent on the suppression of α-globin synthesis and the particular α-globin gene that is affected, but few data are available.

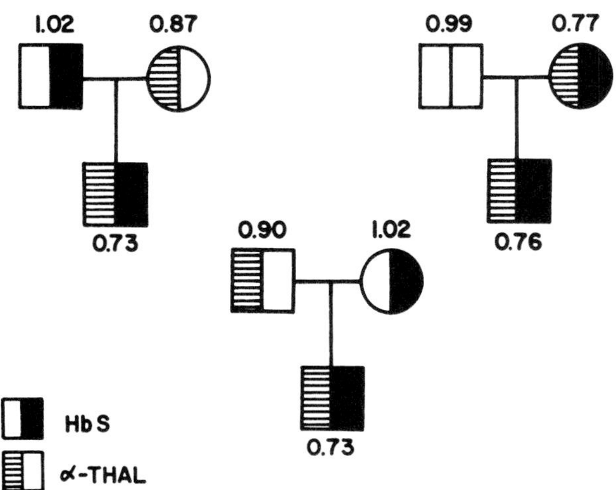

Figure 22.2. $\alpha/\beta^A + \beta^S$ biosynthesis in three families in which there was a proband with HbAS–α thalassemia. Shown beneath each individual is the $\alpha/\beta^A + \beta^S$ biosynthesis ratio. The normal ratio is 0.85–1.25.

Iron deficiency selectively inhibits the translation of α-globin mRNA and can produce an acquired form of α thalassemia. Depending on its severity, iron deficiency can mimic HbAS–α thalassemia by depressing HbS levels and causing microcytic erythrocytes. In vitro and perhaps in vivo, lead can do the same.

Effects of Variant Hemoglobins, β Thalassemia and HPFH

α-Globin variants. HbG Philadelphia (*HBA2* or *HBA1* asn68lys), an α-globin chain variant is the most common hemoglobin variant found with HbAS (Chapter 24). This mutation is usually on a chromosome with a $-\alpha^{3.7}$ deletion. Compound heterozygotes with HbAS and HbG-Philadelphia are not anemic and have no hemolysis but might have mild microcytosis. HbG-Philadelphia can be separated from normal hemoglobins by HPLC. When HbAS or HbC trait appears with HbG-Philadelphia, the HPLC and electrophoretic patterns can be confusing as normal α-globin chains and α^G-globin chains combine with non-α-globin chains to form hybrid and normal hemoglobin tetramers. These species can be resolved by HPLC that in contrast to electrophoresis can separate HbS from HbG. Other α-globin chain variants can be found with HbAS, and like the example of HbG-Philadelphia, their initial resolution could be puzzling, but, like HbG-Philadelphia with HbAS, they are clinically insignificant. Some of these variants include Hb Memphis (glu23gln), Hb Montgomery (leu48arg) Hb Mexico (gln54glu), Hb Stanleyville-II (pro77arg), Hb Nigeria (ser8cys), HbG-Georgia (pro95leu), and Hb Hopkins-II (his112asp). (The Globin Gene Server http://globin.cse.psu.edu/ provides up-to-date information on hemoglobin variants and thalassemias.)

β-Globin Variants. HbS can coexist as a compound heterozygote with many other β-globin chain variants, including HbD Ibadan (*HBB* thr87lys), HbD Iran (*HBB* glu22gln), HbG San Jose (*HBB* glu7gly), Hb Osu-Christianbourg (*HBB* asp52asn), HbE, HbG Galveston (*HBB* glu43ala), Hb Korle-Bu (*HBB* asp73asn; also known as HbG-Accra), and Hb Richmond (*HBB* asn102lys). The resulting phenotypes depend on the pathogenicity of the β-globin variant but usually resemble uncomplicated HbAS (Chapter 23). HbC-Harlem (*HBB* glu6val; asp73asn) migrates like HbC at alkaline pH, is present at a concentration of approximately 40% of the hemolysate, and gives a positive test for sickling (Chapter 23). It can be separated from HbC at acidic pH. HbC-Harlem heterozygotes do not have abnormal hematology or symptoms.

β Thalassemia, HPFH, Fusion Hemoglobins. Compound heterozygotes with β^+ thalassemia and HbS synthesize more HbS than HbA because of the reduced expression of the β thalassemia gene. Rarely, a β thalassemia mutation can be *cis* to the β^S-globin gene. A C→T mutation at position -88 5′ to the β-globin gene was found in a HbS gene on a Benin haplotype chromosome.[8] Affected patients had a normal α-globin genotype with α:β synthesis consistent with β thalassemia trait. They were mildly anemic with microcytosis, high HbA_2 concentration, and HbS levels of 10%–11%. This HbS level is much lower than those found in HbAS with HbH disease (Table 22.2).

Point mutations that produce HPFH can be found *cis* and *trans* to the HbS gene. They are not associated with a clinical phenotype but can produce confusing HPLC and electrophoretic findings. Depending on the mutation causing HPFH, there can be minor increases in HbF of approximately 5% or major increases that exceed 20% of the total hemoglobin. Individuals with HbAS who inherit the -202 C→T mutation 5′ to the $^A\gamma$ globin gene have 2%–4% HbF and more than 90% $^A\gamma$ chains.[9] Mutations associated with these conditions are shown in Table 22.3. The compound heterozygous conditions of HbS-deletion HPFH and HbS–δβ thalassemia are discussed in Chapter 23.

Hb Lepore (Chapters 16 and 17) is the product of a poorly expressed fusion gene with δ- and β-globin chain components. Hb Lepore migrates like HbS on electrophoresis at alkaline pH and like HbA at acidic pH but is separable from HbA and HbS by HPLC. Heterozygotes have approximately 10% Hb Lepore and the phenotype of β thalassemia trait. Hb Lepore heterozygotes should not be confused with HbAS or the very rare cases of HbAS–HbH disease or β thalassemia *cis* to HbAS. The anti-Lepore variants HbP Nilotic (HbP Congo) and Hb Lincoln Park exhibit the same electrophoretic behavior as HbS and form approximately 20% of the hemolysate. Unlike Hb Lepore, they do not cause a thalassemia phenotype. Hb Parchman, only reported once,

Table 22.3. Nongene deletion hereditary persistence of HbF and HbAS[24]

Mutation	HbF	HbA	HbS	$^G\gamma$ (%)
-202 C→G 5′ $^G\gamma$	20	30	50	100
-202 C→T 5′ $^A\gamma$	2–4	60	40	10
-175 T→C 5′ $^G\gamma$	30	30	40	
-175 T→C 5′ ^{A}	40	20	40	85
-158 C→T 5′ $^G\gamma$ in *cis*				

migrates electrophoretically like HbS but forms less than 2% of the hemolysate.

HbAS has been described with the γβ fusion hemoglobin, Hb Kenya (Chapters 16 and 23). Carriers are not anemic but could have mild microcytosis. The hemolysate contains approximately 20% Hb Kenya and 60%–70% HbS; the remainder is HbA_2 and HbF.

SYMPTOMATIC "HbAS"

With some exceptions, carriers of HbAS do not have the clinical features of sickle cell disease. Nevertheless, sometimes, what appears at first to be HbAS is accompanied by disease symptoms. In addition to the rare conditions discussed, it is formally possible that genetic polymorphisms in the many genes that could affect the phenotype of sickle cell anemia might lead to symptoms in HbAS, but, to date, such associations have not been studied.

Variant Hemoglobins

HbS-Antilles (*HBB* glu6val; val23Ile) migrates like HbS, giving the electrophoretic appearance of HbAS. In contrast to HbAS, HbS-Antilles is associated with sickle cell disease in the heterozygote. Its presence should be considered in patients with HbAS who have hemolytic anemia and vasoocclusive disease (Chapter 23). Heterozygotes have 40%–50% HbS-Antilles, and sickling tests are positive. Erythrocyte damage and symptoms are seen in heterozygotes because the additional val23Ile mutation in HbS-Antilles allows this variant to polymerize even when it forms only half of the hemoglobin.

A baby girl presented with symptomatic sickle cell disease despite a prior diagnosis of HbAS. One β-globin gene contained the HbS mutation and an additional *HBB* leu68phe mutation. This variant, Hb Jamaica Plain, had severely reduced oxygen affinity, suggesting destabilization of the oxy conformation at ambient partial pressures of oxygen.[10]

Pyruvate Kinase Deficiency

A unique cause of symptomatic HbAS was found with the coexistence of erythrocyte pyruvate kinase deficiency in a carrier of the HbS gene. This patient, a 42-year-old Guinean woman, had an HbS level of 44%, packed cell volume of 25, reticulocytes of $203 \times 10^9/L$, cholelithiasis, and a 35-year history of hospitalizations approximately five times yearly for painful episodes.[11] Erythrocyte density profiles resembled that seen in HbSC disease. The P_{50} was 41.5 mm Hg (normal ~25). Severe pyruvate kinase deficiency was present.

High 2,3-BPG levels, a consequence of the metabolic block caused by pyruvate kinase deficiency, increased P_{50} and decreased hemoglobin oxygen affinity allowing HbS polymerization. Intraerythrocytic HbS polymer was inferred by hysteresis – different P_{50} values during deoxygenation and reoxygenation – of the hemoglobin–oxygen dissociation curves. HbS polymerization under physiological conditions evidently increased cell density, caused hemolytic anemia, and provoked vasoocclusive episodes. Although it would be useful to know in greater detail the clinical features of the vasoocclusive disease in this patient, this case seems to be an exceptional example of a truly symptomatic individual with HbAS. It suggests that metabolic abnormalities can influence the phenotype of HbAS and, by extension, sickle cell disease.

Hereditary Spherocytosis

Rarely, HbAS and hereditary spherocytosis coexist.[12,13] The dominant phenotype is that of hereditary spherocytosis.[14] Patients with this combination have been reported to developed acute splenic sequestration crises and the post-splenectomy specimens showed erythrostasis and sickling. Perhaps these unusual events – sequestration crises are not a feature of HbAS – were the result of the splenomegaly of hereditary spherocytosis and the high mean corpuscular Hb concentration of HbS-containing hereditary spherocytosis erythrocytes.

HEMOGLOBIN VARIANTS MASQUERADING AS HbAS

Many variants of the β- and α-globin chain will migrate like HbS under the conditions of alkaline electrophoresis. Most, but not all, of these variants can be resolved by more sensitive analytical methods such as HPLC, and in principle, all can be distinguished by DNA analysis. None, except the rare variants like HbS Antilles, and Hb Jamaica Plain, with the HbS mutation and other mutations in the same β-globin gene, will polymerize. HbG Makassar (*HBB* glu6ala) cannot be separated from HbS by HPLC, isoelectric focusing, hemoglobin electrophoresis, or globin chain electrophoresis. It is present at a level of approximately 45% and has no pathological consequences.

CLINICAL FEATURES

Does HbAS interfere with any physical activities? Is it a risk factor for increased morbidity and mortality? Again, with some exceptions, there is little evidence for the pathogenicity of HbAS under conditions of ordinary living.

Hematology

Table 22.2 presents hematological data compiled from various studies of people with HbAS and either normal α-globin genotype or with α thalassemia or β^+ thalassemia. In some studies, the packed cell volume in HbAS was slightly reduced but still normal; in others, it did not differ from the packed cell volume in controls.[15,16] The disparity might have been due to differences in methodology and the examination of diverse populations with different age ranges. Differences from normal are very small and are unlikely to be clinically significant.

Hemolysis is absent in uncomplicated HbAS in which the reticulocyte count and studies of red cell survival were usually normal. The popular Variant II™ HPLC method of hemoglobin variant detection used in the United States is associated with increases in HbA_2 when HbS is present because of the coelution of glycosylated HbS.[17] A modification of this method, the Variant II HbA_2/HbA_{1c}, improves the reliability of HbA_2 measurement in the presence of HbS.[18] Gene deletion α thalassemia is associated with very small differences in HbA_2 levels that vary according to the numbers of α-globin genes.[17]

Mortality, Rhabdomyolysis, and Sudden Death

In diverse cross-sectional, longitudinal, hospital and community-based studies of thousands of subjects with HbAS, carriers did not have excess risk of mortality.[19–23] Evidence that Africans with HbAS have increased mortality rates is also lacking, but adequate data are not available.[24]

Exercise-related sudden death, or near death, in previously healthy, young athletes is always a tragic event. When an athlete dies and has HbAS, a causal relationship is often assumed, and the case reported in the medical literature and lay press. What is lacking, and needed to interpret the clinical significance of these reports and the concerns they engender, is a careful epidemiological study of exertional rhabdomyolysis, associated and not associated with sudden death, in the universe of athletes (90% of deaths in athletes are due to unsuspected cardiovascular disease). Although studies of military recruits showed that death after exertional heat illness and rhabdomyolysis was increased in carriers of HbAS, their incidence of exertional heat illness was not.

Reports of sudden death or life-threatening episodes during exercise in HbAS abound and have been extensively reviewed.[25] Most deaths were attributed to exertional heat illness, with rhabdomyolysis and idiopathic sudden death accounting for equal numbers of cases. Case reports and small clusters of unexpected sudden death in people with HbAS in special situations – military recruits undergoing basic training and athletes engaging in physically stressful sports – raised the possibility that under extremely rigorous conditions, HbAS could be associated with a higher risk of sudden death.[25]

Over a span of 5 years, during which 2.1 million recruits underwent basic training in the U.S. Armed Forces, the risk of sudden unexplained death in black recruits with HbAS compared with those without the trait was 27.6.[26] Compared with all recruits – blacks without HbAS, and whites – the relative risk was 40. Other HbAS mortality studies suffer from design flaws, principally low power due to small sample size. The risk increased progressively with increasing age from a death rate of 12 per 100,000 at ages 17–18 years to 136 per 100,000 at ages 31–34 years. Perhaps the increasing prevalence of isosthenuria with age in HbAS and the accompanying possibility of dehydration when access to fluids was limited might account for this observation. It was not possible to tell if the fractional percentage of HbS was associated with sudden death. Coincident α thalassemia in individuals with HbAS might be associated with better-preserved urine-concentrating ability.[27] Using percentage of HbS as a surrogate for α thalassemia, studies suggested that α thalassemia was underrepresented in individuals with sudden death.[25,28]

In summary, HbAS is not a risk factor for a higher mortality rate in the general population, and restraint during the rigors of conditioning should eliminate any hazard in special groups.

Treatment Recommendations

A prudent course for all exercising individuals includes gradual conditioning, liberal fluid intake, and avoidance of overexertion under all conditions, especially when temperature and humidity are high. When that strategy was adopted by the U.S. military in recruit conditioning and training, the death rate in the HbAS was said to fall to that of the recruit population overall. Unfortunately, the abandonment of this policy was associated with a return to an increased number of deaths in carriers of HbAS.

Thromboembolism

Individuals with HbAS might have increased coagulation system activity and a higher prevalence of prothrombotic mutations, but most studies reporting such association are small, poorly controlled, and inconclusive.[29,30] In one study, individuals with HbAS had increased levels of d-dimers, thrombin–antithrombin complexes, and prothrombin fragment 1.2 compared with controls.[31] The differences between HbAS and controls were small and might be attributable to a few cases with very high values. This study only included 23 individuals with HbAS, nearly half of whom appeared to be atypical with mild anemia and with a hemoglobin concentration of less than 12 g/dL.

In contrast to individuals of African descent in whom the factor V Leiden mutation is rare, in Iranians who have an HbS gene this prothrombotic mutation appears to be common.[32]

Two careful studies suggest that middle aged African Americans with HbAS have an increased risk of thromboembolic disease. In a study of 65,000 hospitalized veterans, 2.2% of individuals with HbAS had pulmonary embolism compared with 1.5% of controls, a statistically significant, albeit small, difference.[19] This study examined men nearly exclusively, and, the currently used sensitive methods to diagnose pulmonary embolism were not available. A recent case-control study examined 515 hospitalized African Americans with either deep venous thrombosis or pulmonary embolism and compared them with 555 outpatient controls. The prevalence of the HbS allele was 0.070 for cases and 0.032 for controls. The odds of a case having HbAS were approximately twice that of a control, indicating that the risk of venous thromboembolism is increased approximately twofold among individuals with HbAS. The odds ratio for pulmonary embolism was 3.9. The proportion of cases of pulmonary embolism attributable to HbAS was approximately 7%. The prevalence of sickle cell disease was also increased among cases compared with controls, but in most of these cases there was an underlying reason for thromboembolism.[33]

Treatment Recommendations

These studies show that African Americans with HbAS have an increased risk of venous thromboembolic disease. Although it was implied that African Americans should know if they carry HbAS, given its benignity, it is difficult to see how screening the adult population for HbAS would alter the management of thromboembolic disease. The importance of knowing if a patient with thromboembolic disease has HbAS is also unclear as the treatment implications of such knowledge seem nil.

Pregnancy and Contraception

It was thought that fertility was increased in women and perhaps in men with HbAS; however, this supposition is not supported by more recent studies.[34–37]

According to many reports, pregnancy complications are more frequent in HbAS. Some studies suggest that the risks for bacteriuria, pyelonephritis, and urinary tract infection might be increased as much as twofold. In a well-designed prospective study of 162 pregnancies with HbAS and 1,422 controls, the preeclampsia rate in HbAS was doubled, endometritis occurred more frequently, and gestational age and birth weight were reduced in infants.[38] In contrast, a retrospective study, in which HbAS was ascertained by solubility testing, showed no difference in the prevalence of preeclampsia in HbAS and controls.[39] A recent retrospective study using data collected from 1991 to 2006 showed that among 36,897 pregnancies, perinatal mortality and preeclampsia were not increased in HbAS.[40]

In a recent retrospective cohort study, asymptomatic bacteriuria, acute cystitis, and pyelonephritis had a similar prevalence in HbAS (n = 455) and matched pregnant control patients (n = 448). Although HbAS carriers had significantly higher rates of pyelonephritis, many affected patients had risk factors such as previous pyelonephritis or noncompliance with therapy.[41]

In a retrospective case-control study, 180 pregnant women with HbAS were compared with controls. Women with HbAS had significantly shorter average duration of pregnancy (233 ± 45 days vs. 255 ± 34 days), lower birth weight infants (2,114 ± 1,093 g vs. 2,672 ± 942 g), and a higher rate of fetal death (9.7% vs. 3.5%). Acute ascending amniotic infection and meconium histiocytosis were noted more frequently.[42] The authors speculate that placental infarction led to intrauterine hypoxia. Patients in this study might not represent the African American population overall. They had a high prevalence of comorbid conditions such as hypertension, diabetes, and obesity and the fetal loss rate in the population from which cases and controls were drawn was approximately twice the national average. Also, it was not clear that comorbidities and hematological findings, such as the prevalence of α thalassemia, were similar in HbAS and control pregnancies. In contrast, a retrospective study of more than 5,000 pregnancies showed that HbAS was associated with lower risk of preterm delivery at less than 32 weeks and increased odds of multiple gestations.[43]

The effect of maternal age on pregnancy outcomes is controversial. Some studies showed a reduced birth weight of infants born to older mothers but others did not. Pregnancy outcomes did not seem to be affected by age. Although some studies reported increased complications of many types, including prematurity and premature rupture of membranes, they often lacked appropriate controls. In Nigerian women, pregnancy outcomes were similar in HbAS and controls and HbAS women had fewer attacks of malaria.[44] Iron supplementation to pregnant African women with HbAS is of little benefit, perhaps because of an increased risk of malaria, but those results are inconclusive.

Mothers with HbAS were more likely to have HbAS children than those with only HbA.[45–47] This maternal segregation distortion could be another means of maintaining a high prevalence of HbAS.

Treatment Recommendations

Despite some uncertainties, the available data suggest that HbAS might be associated with increased risks of certain complications of pregnancy, mainly urinary tract infections, low birth weight, and possibly increased fetal loss. These observations suggest that screening for HbAS in at risk pregnancies might be useful if affected individuals are provided a higher level of antenatal care.

The scanty literature available does not suggest that any means of contraception is more hazardous in HbAS than in the general population but definitive studies have yet to be reported.

Growth and Development

Many investigators have questioned whether HbAS influences growth and development, and although some have found differences in physical and intellectual development, the best evidence suggests that children with HbAS and matched controls are similar. HbAS is not associated with an increased chance of sudden infant death syndrome.[48]

Exercise Capacity

Whether or not athletes with HbAS are at special risk of sudden death and should be treated differently from their peers is a subject of continued debate and the expression of strong opinions without the addition of new definitive studies.[49–54] It is questionable whether HbAS affects the physiological responses to exercise or impairs exercise tolerance and performance. Forty-eight people with HbAS, aged 4–21 years, underwent progressive ergometer stress testing at their voluntary maximal performance and the results were compared with 184 controls. Equivocal ischemic changes on electrocardiographic exmination were seen in four individuals with HbAS. The maximum workload and heart rate were lower in the HbAS subjects, but there were no complications of the exercise program.[55] One study comparing the response to incremental exercise in people with HbAS and controls revealed no differences in cardiovascular function but did reveal lower blood lactate concentrations in HbAS.[56] When anaerobic exercise and exercise metabolism after force-velocity tests were compared in sedentary adults with HbAS and closely matched controls, there were no differences between the groups.[57] Under laboratory conditions, when eight HbAS and eight normal individuals were subjected to an incremental exercise test, maximal oxygen uptake and ventilatory thresholds were similar, and no difference in whole blood, plasma, or red blood cell lactate concentrations were found, suggesting that lactate production and clearance is quite similar during exercise. Lactate uptake by HbAS erythrocytes is more rapid during exercise.[58] At supramaximal exercise, an increase in red cell rigidity was seen in HbAS, but it is not known if this has any clinical significance.[59,60]

Concurrent α thalassemia does not effect the oxygen response to exercise in HbAS.[61] Before and after basic training, a group of HbAS and control subjects had similar responses to exercise testing.[62,63]

In some circumstances and among some African tribes, hypoxia at high altitudes appeared to affect performance in vigorous exercise and cause changes in the splenic circulation.[64] In other studies at simulated altitude and moderate hypoxic environment, the cardiopulmonary and gas exchange responses of persons with HbAS during brief episodes of exhaustive exercise were comparable to those of controls.[65] Acute stressful exercise at an altitude of 1,270 m and a simulated altitude of 2,300 m were not associated with differences in cardiopulmonary and gas exchange between subjects with HbAS and controls. Vigorous arm exercise was associated with sickled cells in effluent venous blood, and the frequency of such cells increased fourfold at simulated altitudes of 4,000 m.[66] Performance was unimpaired, and sickled cells were not detected in arterial blood and hemolysis was not detectable. Ventilatory responses to three episodes of heavy exercise was similar in HbAS and controls.[49]

When athletes with HbAS, with and without coincident α thalassemia, were exercised on a bicycle ergometer and levels of soluble intercellular adhesion molecule–1 and vascular cell adhesion molecule–1 were measured, the HbAS group had higher vascular cell adhesion molecule–1 basal concentrations, and incremental exercise resulted in a significant increase in all subjects. Levels remained elevated in the HbAS group during recovery, and individuals with HbAS–α thalassemia had a more rapid return to baseline.[67]

Many other studies show minimal or no adverse effects of HbAS during exercise.[58,68,69] After prolonged intense exercise, prothrombin time, antithrombin III activity, and plasma fibrinogen were similar in individuals with HbAS and controls.[70] Black athletes with HbAS are well represented in elite competitive sports. The percentage of African semimarathon runners with HbAS was similar to that of the general population.[63]

Treatment Recommendations

Based on the total body of work on exercise ability and capacity, there is no reason to restrict exercise of any type in persons with HbAS. All individuals engaged in strenuous exercise, trained or untrained, should be properly conditioned, clothed, have unrestricted access to fluids, appropriate rest periods, moderation of the exercise routine when harsh atmospheric conditions like excessive heat and humidity are present, and rapid treatment should symptoms develop. Any restraints applied to carriers of HbAS need not differ from those used to forestall ill effects of exercise in the general population.

Flying and Scuba Diving

There are many reports of splenic infarction during flight in unpressurized aircraft at altitudes of 3,000–5,000 m. In the early reports, the diagnosis of HbAS was often made by tests that today would be considered inadequate, and some cases reported could have been instances of HbSC disease or HbS–β^+ thalassemia rather than HbAS. Commercial aircraft are pressurized to 2,500 m and splenic infarct – and any other complication of HbS polymerization – is unlikely to occur under that condition. As of 1996, the US Department of Defense stopped preinduction testing for HbAS and as of 2003 HbAS carriers were not restricted from flight or undersea duty.

Scuba diving, in which divers breathe compressed air, provides an environment with increased pO_2 and poses no known risk to carriers of HbAS.

Genitourinary System

Hyposthenuria. The kidney medulla is one of the few sites where under physiological conditions, HbAS erythrocytes are placed in jeopardy. Low pO_2, low pH, and high solute concentration provide a milieu where sickling of even the HbAS erythrocyte can occur.[71] Damage to the countercurrent urine-concentrating mechanism and the vasculature of the renal medulla leads to a defect in urine-concentrating ability and hyposthenuria in most adults with HbAS and hematuria in some individuals. These abnormalities might result from microvascular injury in the vasa recta of the renal medulla. A defect in urine acidification, which in sickle cell anemia is related to the severity of the concentration defect, is not seen in HbAS.

The polymerization tendency of HbS might determine the extent of the urine-concentrating defect in HbAS.[27] To test this hypothesis, urinary-concentrating ability was examined following overnight water deprivation and intranasal arginine vasopressin in HbAS subjects separated into two groups – one with a normal α-globin gene complement and one with either heterozygous or homozygous -$\alpha^{3.7}$ gene deletion α thalassemia. The ability to concentrate urine was most impaired in subjects with normal α-globin genotype and least impaired in subjects with homozygous α thalassemia. Urine osmolality was 882 ± 37 mOsm/kg H_2O in α thalassemia homozygotes and 672 ± 38 mOsm/kg H_2O in the heterozygotes. In all subjects, urinary osmolality correlated linearly and inversely with percentage of HbS. A similar correlation was found between urine-concentrating ability and HbS polymerization tendency at 0.4 oxygen saturation (Fig. 22.3), suggesting that HbS polymer, a function of percentage of HbS, is responsible for the urine-concentrating defect of HbAS.

Hematuria. Hematuria occurs episodically in approximately 5% of people with HbAS. Some studies suggest that hematuria is most common at higher HbS levels. Bleeding is more frequent from the left kidney, perhaps because of the anatomy of venous system, and men are affected four times as often as women. Although von Willebrand syndrome has been reported in HbAS, no association has been established between any coagulation abnormality and HbAS hematuria.

Papillary necrosis can cause hematuria, sometimes with renal colic. This might be more frequent in HbAS and is perhaps another consequence of sickling in the renal medulla.[72,73] Autosomal dominant polycystic kidney disease might be more prevalent and progress to renal failure more rapidly in individuals with HbAS.[74]

Medullary Carcinoma. Renal medullary carcinoma, a rare and aggressive tumor, has a unique association with HbAS.[75–82] In a retrospective analysis spanning 20 years, 33 black patients, aged 11–40 years, who presented with hematuria and pain had renal medullary carcinoma. Nine patients had proven HbAS, and one had HbSC disease, but all tumor specimens contained sickled cells. The tumors were lobulated with satellite cortical nodules and widespread metastases. Histologically, the tumors had a reticular, yolk sac–like or glandular cystic appearance, with a desmoplastic stroma, hemorrhage, necrosis, neutrophil infiltration, and lymphocyte sheathing (Fig. 22.4). Characteristic findings of renal medullary carcinoma on computed tomography and magnetic resonance imaging include an infiltrative renal mass with associated retroperitoneal adenopathy and caliectasis.[83] Chemotherapy was uniformly unsuccessful, and survival after diagnosis was approximately 4 months.[67]

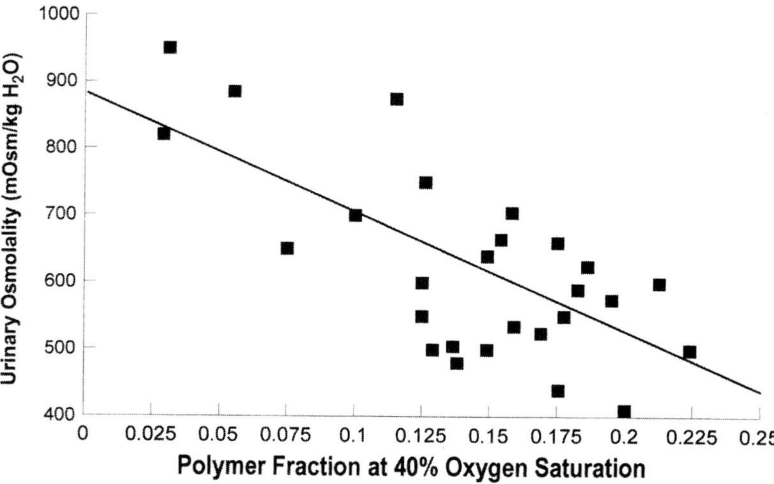

Figure 22.3. Relationship between maximum urine-concentrating ability and polymer fraction at 40% oxygen saturation in individuals with HbAS and 4, 3, and 2 α-globin genes. (From ref. 27 with permission.)

The diagnosis of HbAS for 23 of the patients was based only on histological findings because diagnostic tests documenting HbAS were not available. If HbAS was present in all 33 patients, the conclusion that the condition predisposes to this rare tumor seems inescapable. It has been hypothesized that the medullary cancers could originate in terminal collecting ducts, where epithelial cell proliferation has been noted in HbAS. Perhaps rapid cell proliferation and oxygen radicals produced by cell sickling, coupled with preexisting mutations in genes controlling cell growth, predispose to carcinogenesis. In three cases, the *ABL* gene was amplified.[81] Gene expression studies suggested that the tumor signature resembled that of urothelial tumors rather than renal cell carcinoma.

Genitourinary Lesions Probably Not Caused by HbAS. Other renal or genitourinary system disorders, such as nephrotic syndrome, pyelonephritis, hypotonic bladder, hypertension, renal failure, renal cortical infarction, renal vein thrombosis, and testicular infarction undoubtedly occur in some carriers of HbAS, but there is no evidence of their being caused by HbAS. Priapism, a serious complication of sickle cell anemia, is not associated with HbAS. Renal allograft survival in HbAS is equivalent to that in the general population.

Treatment Recommendations

No treatment can reliably stop hematuria in people with HbAS and radical treatments, such as nephrectomy, should be avoided.[84] Induced hypotonicity, alkalinization, and epsilon amino caproic acid, an antifibrinolytic agent, have all been used to control severe hematuria but controlled trials have never been reported. Epsilon amino caproic acid can be dangerous in some situations by inducing clot formation and causing obstructive uropathy.

Although often recurrent and sometimes producing anemia, hematuria is usually benign and self-limited. Nevertheless, hematuria could arise from more ominous causes than a damaged renal medulla. Renal and bladder cancer – especially medullary cancer in young patients – stones, glomerulonephritis, and infection should be excluded during the evaluation of hematuria.

SPLEEN

Young black men with HbAS who resided at altitudes up to 1,600 m for many years had normal splenic function as assessed by radionuclide scanning and by the number of

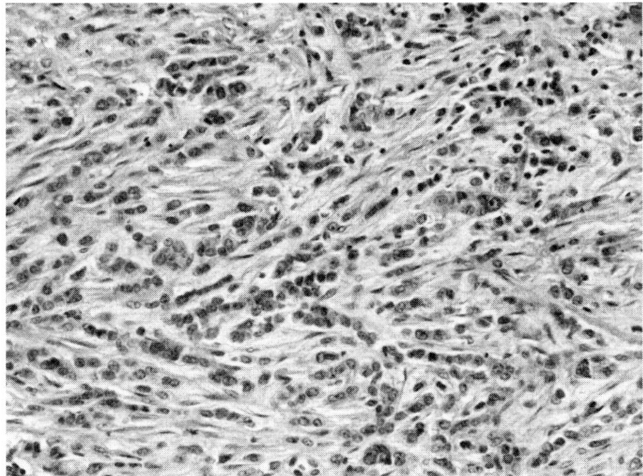

Figure 22.4. Renal medullary carcinoma showing epithelioid cells and spindle cells in a background of fibrosis and small lymphocytes (× 400). Kindly provided by R.S. Figenshau.[79]

red cells with "pits."[85] Splenic infarction can occur in individuals with HbAS when they encounter hypobaric conditions.

Splenic infarcts in African Americans with HbAS are rare, or rarely reported. Splenic infarction was not mentioned in a report of African runners with HbAS who competed at altitudes of up to 4,100 m. Especially interesting are reports of splenic infarction in Caucasians with HbAS.[86,87] Caucasian men might be overrepresented in reports of altitude-induced splenic syndrome and splenic infarcts at sea level. Twenty of 29 reported cases of splenic syndrome were in Caucasian men.[88] Most, but not all, episodes occurred shortly after ascent to approximately 3,000 m. These curious observations have led to much speculation.[28] A reasonable supposition is that an African HbS gene within the Caucasian gene pool became isolated from accompanying genes that in Africa evolved along with the HbS gene and modulated its effects. The hypothesized modulating genes could affect the mean corpuscular HbS concentration, which might differ between black and nonblack HbAS carriers. Inconclusive evidence suggests that Caucasian carriers with splenic infarction have a higher HbS concentration than black carriers and that a high mean cell HbS concentration increases the risk of intrasplenic sickling and organ damage. One Caucasian splenic infarction patient had an HbS level of 46.5% and had five α-globin genes (Table 22.1). In a report in which both father and son had a splenic infarct, the HbS levels were 41% and 45.6%. In another study, however, HbS levels in a small series of nonblack carriers differed little from those in most black carriers of HbAS. If HbS levels are truly higher in Caucasian carriers, it might be a consequence of the absence of α thalassemia and the reduced cation exchange and lower cation content in Caucasians erythrocytes, a deficit most marked in men (splenic infarction is rarely reported in women), or, differences in other "protective" genes associated with the HbS gene in black patients.

Treatment Recommendations

Fear of splenic damage should not dissuade carriers of HbAS from activities at altitude. Physicians should be aware, however, that in this setting, splenic infarction should be considered as a cause of left upper quadrant pain in any racial and ethnic group. Fortunately, most often splenic infarction is a self-limited process and needs no special treatment.

EYE

In nonhemoglobinopathic individuals, hyphema, or hemorrhage into the anterior chamber, usually clears uneventfully with topical medical therapy. Among individuals with traumatic hyphema, carriers of HbAS might be overrepresented.[89] The naturally low pO_2 in the anterior chamber causes erythrocyte sickling in HbAS and impedes cellular outflow through the trabecular meshwork and Schlemm canal, raising intraocular pressure. High pressure in the anterior chamber can reduce vascular perfusion pressure elsewhere in the eye, injuring the optic nerve and retina and causing hemorrhage and impairing vision.[90] Anterior segment hypoxia and acidosis set in place the vicious circle of erythrostasis typical of sickle cell disease. Secondary open-angle glaucoma can result from poorly treated hyphema.

Many ocular abnormalities, including internuclear ophthalmoplegia, transient monocular blindness, vitreous hemorrhage, and optic atrophy have been described in HbAS, but any association with HbAS is likely to be fortuitous.[91–93] Chronic open-angle glaucoma is no more common in HbAS than in age- and sex-matched controls.

Although proliferative retinopathy, akin to the type known to occur in sickle cell disease has been described in HbAS, in all cases, a known cause of proliferative retinopathy such as diabetes, was present, perhaps predisposing to the development of retinal lesions. Uncomplicated HbAS is not associated with sickle retinopathy.[94]

Treatment Recommendations

Black patients and others at risk of carrying the HbS gene who present with hyphema should be screened for HbAS without delay. A sickle solubility test will do, because it is important at this point to find out only whether HbS is present. Management of hyphema in HbAS is beyond the scope of this chapter; it should be supervised by an ophthalmologist who understands the special problems that can arise when the hyphema and HbAS coexist. Intraocular pressure can be controlled medically in perhaps two thirds of the cases. Anterior chamber hypertension of greater than 24 mm Hg for consecutive 24-hour periods and repeated but transient increases above 30 mm Hg should be reduced by paracentesis, which can be repeated if necessary. Normal pressure during the first 24 hours of observation suggests, but does not establish, that medical treatment will suffice.[95]

BONES AND JOINTS

Reports of osteonecrosis in HbAS make an unconvincing case for their association. Bone infarction has also been described with HbAS, also with no evidence of association beyond coincidence.[96]

NERVOUS SYSTEM

Children with HbAS had greater arterial tortuosity on magnetic resonance imaging and magnetic resonance angiography compared with controls, and this was related to the percentage of HbS.[97] The authors speculated that this was a sign of mild vasculopathy; however, the clinical implications of this observation are unknown. Cerebral infarcts have been reported in HbAS.[98] Most of the reports are of one or two cases so that given the ubiquity of both HbAS and stroke, a causal relationship cannot be established. In a retrospective study in Guadeloupe, in 295 patients hospitalized for stroke, HbAS appeared to be more prevalent in individuals with hemorrhagic stroke and less prevalent in individuals with infarctive stroke.[99] The truth of the assertion that HbAS is a risk factor for stroke cannot yet be established.[98]

SURGERY AND ANESTHESIA

Untold numbers of patients with HbAS have safely undergone anesthesia and surgery. In a matched-pair analysis of patients with HbAS and control subjects, the frequency of anesthetic, surgical, and postoperative complications was similar; however, most patients were young, and few intraabdominal and thoracic procedures were included.

Use of a tourniquet in orthopaedic procedures appears safe in HbAS (and in sickle cell anemia).

Treatment Recommendations

Most evidence suggests that anesthetic risk is not increased by HbAS, and the choice of anesthesia need not be limited.[100,101] Thus, there is no rationale for routine preoperative screening for HbAS.[102]

With open heart surgery or complicated intrathoracic surgeries, in which hypoxia might be intrinsic to the procedure, preoperative transfusion was recommended.[100,101] Screening for HbAS might be prudent under those circumstances, but there are no well-controlled studies on the preoperative management of intrathoracic surgery in HbAS.

MALARIA

The selection pressure from *Plasmodium falciparum* malaria is expressed primarily in children, and where malaria is endemic, HbAS children have reduced mortality.[103,104] HbAS retards the development of cerebral malaria in children aged younger than 5 years, and it reduces their death rate.[105] Although the clinical features, haptoglobin levels, parasite counts, and most laboratory measurements are similar in children with and without HbAS, trait carriers are transfused more often. It is estimated that HbAS is almost 90% protective for severe *P. falciparum* malaria with lesser protection against mild disease.[106]

When homozygous α thalassemia and HbAS coexist, the protection against *P. falciparum* malaria afforded by each trait individually was lost, an example of negative epistasis.[107] It was suggested that this might be explained by the reduction in HbS concentration caused by α thalassemia or effects on the erythrocyte membrane altering merozoite invasion.

Children with HbAS have an imbalanced distribution of immunoglobulin G2 (IgG2) antibodies to merozoite surface protein 2 (MSP2) and a higher frequency of infection with multiple *P. falciparum* strains. In Gabonese children with HbAS, Fc gamma receptor IIa (CD32) polymorphism and the rate of in vitro invasion of red blood cells from subjects with HbAS and controls with multiple *P. falciparum* strains were investigated. Lower levels of IgG2 subclass antibodies to MSP2 peptides were independently associated with the Fc gamma receptor IIa-R131 allele and with HbAS, suggesting that IgG3 antibody responses to MSP2 epitopes could be exacerbated by lower IgG2 levels. Longer persistence of ring forms in HbAS might reflect slower multiplication, longer circulation, and enhanced phagocytosis of these nonpathogenic forms and could contribute to the protection against malaria.[108] Some aspects of malaria and hemoglobinopathies are discussed in Chapter 26.

OTHER CONDITIONS

The grab bag of other diseases reported in individuals with HbAS has been reviewed and new "associations" continue to appear.[109] Early reports of impaired pulmonary function in HbAS have been refuted by more carefully controlled studies of diffusing capacity for CO and spirometry at simulated altitudes up to 7,500 m and pulmonary function at rest and after exhaustive exercise in men with HbAS who had been living above 1,600 m for many years. Reports of sickle cell disease–like "crises," complicated migraine with occlusion of branches of the middle cerebral artery, venous thrombosis, and retroperitoneal fibrosis could not be linked etiologically to HbAS.

Leg ulcers have been associated with HbAS in Jamaica. Of 250 patients with chromic leg ulcers, 20% had HbAS, whereas 11% of the general population carried the HbS gene. There are no data to support an increase in leg ulceration in HbAS carriers in temperate climates.

Erythrocyte glucose-6-phosphate dehydrogenase (G6PD) deficiency is common in many populations in which HbAS is found. Hemizygotes with the common African type of G6PD deficiency rarely encounter clinical difficulties. In a study of more than 65,000 hospitalized African-American men, nearly 1% had both HbAS and G6PD deficiency. Morbidity from pneumonia and mean age of death were similar for the group with HbAS alone and the group with both HbAS and G6PD deficiency.

TRANSFUSION OF HbAS BLOOD

Minor changes distinguish HbAS from normal blood under storage conditions, but transfused HbAS erythrocytes are equivalent to normal cells in safety, effectiveness, and survival. Cryopreserved red cells from individuals with HbAS could hemolyze when deglycerolized but a special deglycerolization protocol can prevent this; thus, when cryopreservation of rare blood types is undertaken, knowing if the donor has HbAS is useful.

Table 22.4. Recommendations for counseling and management of HbAS

Counseling permits informed family planning
Antenatal diagnosis for sickle cell disease is available
Occupational choice should be unrestricted
Flying in commercial aircraft is safe
Unexplained pain should not be ascribed to HbAS
Hematuria is usually benign and self-limited but should be carefully evaluated
Hyposthenuria is present in most adults with HbAS
When strenuous exercise is undertaken, fluid intake should match expected losses
Surgical intervention might be needed in hyphema
Pregnancy can have complications such as urinary tract infection
Surgery is safe
Morbidity from most associated diseases is not increased
Duration and quality of life are normal
Clinically significant anemia is not a complication
Microcytosis in HbAS is usually a sign of α thalassemia but should be evaluated.

Blood from donors with HbAS cannot be consistently leukodepleted with any available filter but cell sickling upstream of the filters was not observed.[110–112] This might be due to the low pO_2 and pH of stored blood and HbS polymerization.[113,114] Universal leukodepletion has become the standard in the United States, France, and Canada. Because HbAS carriers are a large fraction of donors in many locales, the loss of their units could seriously reduce blood supplies. Studies have suggested that storage of HbAS whole blood in large-capacity oxygen-permeable bags increases oxygen tension and allows more effective leukoreduction.[114] Units from HbAS donors should be avoided when transfusing large amounts of blood into anemic hypoxic neonates.

SCREENING AND COUNSELING

Screening for HbAS has limited indications and in most cases should be reserved for individuals likely to carry the HbS gene. The U.S. Armed Forces do not screen before induction but might conduct screening afterward. Although the screening of individuals assigned to flight duty might be prudent to detect asymptomatic individuals with sickle cell disease such as HbS–β^+ thalassemia and HbSC disease, screening the general population for HbAS serves no purpose.

Before screening prospective parents, they should be educated about sickle cell disease and HbAS and receive nondirective counseling. Antenatal diagnosis for sickle cell disease is possible in instances in which a pregnancy is at risk for an affected fetus (Chapter 28).

A byproduct of neonatal screening for sickle cell disease is the identification of babies with HbAS. The value of finding HbAS in newborns is questionable; nevertheless, notifying the parents is reasonable so they can be informed about the implications of the condition and offered further family testing.[115]

Table 22.4 summarizes an approach for counseling and management of individuals with HbAS.

REFERENCES

1. Poillon WN, Kim BC, Rodgers GP, Noguchi CT, Schechter AN. Sparing effect of hemoglobin F and hemoglobin A2 on the polymerization of hemoglobin S at physiologic ligand saturations. *Proc Natl Acad Sci USA.* 1993;90:5039–5043.
2. Kulozik AE, Thein SL, Kar BC, Wainscoat JS, Serjeant GR, Weatherall DJ. Raised Hb F levels in sickle cell disease are caused by a determinant linked to the b globin gene cluster. In: Stamatoyannopoulos G, Nienhius AW, eds. *Developmental Control of Globin Gene Expression.* New York: Alan R. Liss; 1996:427–439.
3. Bunn HF. Subunit assembly of hemoglobin: an important determinant of hematologic phenotype. *Blood.* 1987;69:1–6.
4. Steinberg MH, Embury SH. Alpha-thalassemia in blacks: genetic and clinical aspects and interactions with the sickle hemoglobin gene. *Blood.* 1986;68:985–990.
5. Higgs DR, Clegg JB, Weatherall DJ, Serjeant BE, Serjeant GR. Interaction of the a globin gene haplotype and sickle haemoglobin. *Br J Haematol.* 1984;57:671–678.
6. Felice AE, Cleek MP, McKie K, McKie V, Huisman TH. The rare alpha-thalassemia-1 of blacks is a zeta alpha-thalassemia-1 associated with deletion of all alpha- and zeta-globin genes. *Blood.* 1984;63:1253–1257.
7. Steinberg MH, Coleman MB, Adams JG, Hartmann RC, Saba H, Anagnou NP. A new gene deletion in the a-like globin gene cluster as the molecular basis for the rare a-thalassemia-1(--/a) in blacks: HbH disease in sickle cell trait. *Blood.* 1986;67:469–473.
8. Baklouti F, Ouzana R, Gonnet C, Lapillonne A, Delaunay J, Godet J. β^+ Thalassemia in *cis* of a sickle gene: occurrence of a promoter mutation on a β^S chromosome. *Blood.* 1989;74:1818–1822.
9. Gilman JG, Mishima N, Wen XJ, Kutlar F, Huisman THJ. Upstream promoter mutation associated with a modest elevation of fetal hemoglobin expression in human adults. *Blood.* 1988;72:78–81.
10. Geva A, Clark JJ, Zhang Y, Popowicz A, Manning JM, Neufeld EJ. Hemoglobin Jamaica plain – a sickling hemoglobin with reduced oxygen affinity. *N Engl J Med.* 2004;351(15):1532–1538.
11. Cohen-Solal M, Préhu C, Wajcman H, et al. A new sickle cell disease phenotype associating Hb S trait, severe pyruvate kinase deficiency (PK Conakry), and an a2 globin gene variant (Hb Conakry). *Br J Haematol.* 1998;103(4):950–956.
12. Ustun C, Kutlar F, Holley L, Seigler M, Burgess R, Kutlar A. Interaction of sickle cell trait with hereditary spherocytosis: splenic infarcts and sequestration. *Acta Haematol.* 2003;109(1):46–49.
13. Dulman RY, Buchanan GR, Ginsburg H, et al. Splenic infarction due to concomitant hereditary spherocytosis and sickle cell trait. *J Pediatr Surg.* 2007;42(12):2129–2131.
14. Yang Y-M, Donnell C, Wilborn W, et al. Splenic sequestration associated with sickle cell trait and hereditary spherocytosis. *Am J Hematol.* 1992;40:110–116.

15. Castro O, Scott RB. Red blood cell counts and indices in sickle cell trait in a black American population. *Hemoglobin.* 1985;9:65–67.
16. Rana SR, Sekhsaria S, Castro OL. Hemoglobin S and C traits: Contributing causes for decreased mean hematocrit in African-American children. *Pediatrics.* 1993;91:800–802.
17. Head CE, Conroy M, Jarvis M, Phelan L, Bain BJ. Some observations on the measurement of haemoglobin A2 and S percentages by high performance liquid chromatography in the presence and absence of alpha thalassaemia. *J Clin Pathol.* 2004;57(3):276–280.
18. Lafferty JD, McFarlane AG, DH KC. Evaluation of a dual hemoglobin A(2)/A(1c) quantitation kit on the Bio-Rad variant II automated hemoglobin analyzer. *Arch Pathol Lab Med.* 2002;126(12):1494–1500.
19. Heller P, Best WR, Nelson RB, Becktel J. Clinical implications of sickle-cell trait and glucose-6-phosphate dehydrogenase deficiency in hospitalized black male patients. *N Engl J Med.* 1979;300:1001–1005.
20. Petrakis NL, Wiesenfeld SL, Sams BJ, Collen MF, Cutler JL, Siegelaub AB. Prevalence of sickle-cell trait and glucose-6-phosphate dehydrogenase deficiency. *N Engl J Med.* 1970; 282:767–770.
21. Ashcroft MT, Desai P. Mortality and morbidity in Jamaican adults with sickle-cell trait and with normal haemoglobin followed up for twelve years. *Lancet.* 1976;2:748–786.
22. Stark AD, Janerich DT, Jereb SK. The incidence and causes of death in a follow-up study of individuals with haemoglobin AS and AA. *Int J Epidemiol.* 1980;9:325–328.
23. Castro O, Rana SR, Bang KM, Scott RB. Age and prevalence of sickle -cell trait in alarge ambulatory population. *Genet Epidemiol.* 1987;4:307–311.
24. Ohene-Frempong K, Nkrumah FK. Sickle cell disease in Africa. In: Embury SH, Hebbel RP, Mohandas N, eds. *Sickle Cell Disease: Basic Principles and Clinical Practice.* 1st ed. New York: Raven Press; 1994:423–435.
25. Kark JA, Ward FT. Exercise and hemoglobin S. *Semin Hematol.* 1994;31:181–225.
26. Kark JA, Posey DM, Schumacher HR Jr, Ruehle CJ. Sickle-cell trait as a risk factor for sudden death in physical training. *N Engl J Med.* 1987;317:781–787.
27. Gupta AK, Kirchner KA, Nicholson R, et al. Effects of a-thalassemia and sickle polymerization tendency on the urine-concentrating defect of individuals with sickle cell trait. *J Clin Invest.* 1991;88:1963–1968.
28. http:\\sickle.bwh.harvard.edu\sickle_trait.html. *Kark JA. Sickle Cell Trait.* 2007.
29. Moreira NF, Lourenco DM, Noguti MA, et al. The clinical impact of MTHFR polymorphism on the vascular complications of sickle cell disease. *Braz J Med Biol Res.* 2006;39(10): 1291–1295.
30. Isma'eel H, Arnaout MS, Shamseddeen W, et al. Screening for inherited thrombophilia might be warranted among Eastern Mediterranean sickle-beta-0 thalassemia patients. *J Thromb Thrombolysis.* 2006;22(2):121–123.
31. Westerman MP, Green D, Gilman-Sachs A, et al. Coagulation changes in individuals with sickle cell trait. *Am J Hematol.* 2002;69(2):89–94.
32. Rahimi Z, Vaisi-Raygani A, Nagel RL, Muniz A. Thrombophilic mutations among Southern Iranian patients with sickle cell disease: high prevalence of factor V Leiden. *J Thromb Thrombolysis.* 2008;25(3):288–292.
33. Austin H, Key NS, Benson JM, et al. Sickle cell trait and the risk of venous thromboembolism among blacks. *Blood.* 2007;110(3):908–912.
34. Modebe O, Ezeh UO. Effect of age on testicular function in adult males with sickle cell anemia. *Fertil Steril.* 1995;63:907–912.
35. Ezeh UO, Modebe O. Is there increased fertility in adult males with the sickle cell trait. *Hum Biol.* 1996;68:555–562.
36. Fleming AF. Maternal segregation distortion in sickle-cell trait. *Lancet.* 1996;347:1634–1635.
37. Madrigal L. Hemoglobin genotype, fertility, and the malaria hypothesis. *Hum Biol.* 1989;61:311–325.
38. Larrabee KD, Monga M. Women with sickle cell trait are at increased risk for preeclampsia. *Am J Obstet Gynecol.* 1997;177(2):425–428.
39. Stamilio DM, Sehdev HM, Macones GA. Pregnant women with the sickle cell trait are not at increased risk for developing preeclampsia. *Am J Perinatol.* 2003;20(1):41–48.
40. Tita AT, Biggio JR, Chapman V, Neely C, Rouse DJ. Perinatal and maternal outcomes in women with sickle or hemoglobin C trait. *Obstet Gynecol.* 2007;110(5):1113–1119.
41. Thurman AR, Steed LL, Hulsey T, Soper DE. Bacteriuria in pregnant women with sickle cell trait. *Am J Obstet Gynecol.* 2006;194(5):1366–1370.
42. Taylor MY, Wyatt-Ashmead J, Gray J, Bofill JA, Martin R, Morrison JC. Pregnancy loss after first-trimester viability in women with sickle cell trait: time for a reappraisal? *Am J Obstet Gynecol.* 2006;194(6):1604–1608.
43. Bryant AS, Cheng YW, Lyell DJ, Laros RK, Caughey AB. Presence of the sickle cell trait and preterm delivery in African-American women. *Obstet Gynecol.* 2007;109(4):870–874.
44. Adeyemi AB, Adediran IA, Kuti O, Owolabi AT, Durosimi MA. Outcome of pregnancy in a population of Nigerian women with sickle cell trait. *J Obstet Gynaecol.* 2006;26(2):133–137.
45. Silva ID, Ramalho AS. Maternal segregation distortion in sickle-cell and b- thalassaemia traits. *Lancet.* 1996;347:691–692.
46. Silva ID, Ramalho AS. Evidence of maternal segregation distortion in the sickle cell and bthalassaemia traits. *J Med Genet.* 1996;33:525.
47. Duchovni-Silva I, Ramalho AS. Maternal effect: an additional mechanism maintaining balanced polymorphisms of haemoglobinopathies? *Ann Hum Genet.* 2003;67(Pt 6):538–542.
48. Gozal D, Lorey FW, Chandler D, et al. Incidence of sudden infant death syndrome in infants with sickle cell trait. *J Pediatr.* 1994;124:211–214.
49. Marlin L, Connes P, ntoine-Jonville S, et al. Cardiorespiratory responses during three repeated incremental exercise tests in sickle cell trait carriers. *Eur J Appl Physiol.* 2008;102(2):181–187.
50. Connes P, Hardy-Dessources MD, Hue O. Last Word on Point:Counterpoint "Sickle cell trait should/should not be considered asymptomatic and as a benign condition during physical activity." *J Appl Physiol.* 2007;103(6):2144.
51. Tripette J, Hardy-Dessources MD, Sara F, et al. Does repeated and heavy exercise impair blood rheology in carriers of sickle cell trait? *Clin J Sport Med.* 2007;17(6):465–470.

52. Connes P, Caillaud C, Py G, Mercier J, Hue O, Brun JF. Maximal exercise and lactate do not change red blood cell aggregation in well trained athletes. *Clin Hemorheol Microcirc.* 2007;36(4):319–326.
53. Le Gallais D, Lonsdorfer J, Bogui P, Fattoum S. Last Word on Point:Counterpoint "Sickle cell trait should/should not be considered asymptomatic and as a benign condition during physical activity." *J Appl Physiol.* 2007;103(6):2143.
54. Baskurt OK, Meiselman HJ, Bergeron MF. Sickle cell trait should be considered asymptomatic and as a benign condition during physical activity. *J Appl Physiol.* 2007;103(6):2142.
55. Alpert BS, Flood NL, Strong WB, Blair JR, Walpert JB, Levy AL. Responses to exercise in children with sickle cell trait. *Am J Dis Child.* 1982;136:1002–1004.
56. Bile A, Le Gallais D, Mercier B, et al. Blood lactate concentrations during incremental exercise in subjects with sickle cell trait. *Med Sci Sports Exerc.* 1998;30(5):649–654.
57. Bile A, Le Gallais D, Mercier B, Martinez P, Ahmaidi S, Prefaut C. anaerobic exercise components during the force-velocity test in sickle cell trait. *Int J Sports Med.* 1996;17:254–258.
58. Fagnete S, Philippe C, Olivier H, Mona MH, Maryse EJ, Marie-Dominique HD. Faster lactate transport across red blood cell membrane in sickle cell trait carriers. *J Appl Physiol.* 2006;100(2):427–432.
59. Sara F, Hardy-Dessources MD, Marlin L, Connes P, Hue O. Lactate distribution in the blood compartments of sickle cell trait carriers during incremental exercise and recovery. *Int J Sports Med.* 2006;27(6):436–443.
60. Connes P, Sara F, Hardy-Dessources MD, et al. Effects of short supramaximal exercise on hemorheology in sickle cell trait carriers. *Eur J Appl Physiol.* 2006;97(2):143–150.
61. Connes P, Monchanin G, Perrey S, et al. Oxygen uptake kinetics during heavy submaximal exercise: effect of sickle cell trait with or without alpha-thalassemia. *Int J Sports Med.* 2006;27(7):517–525.
62. Weisman IM, Zeballos RJ, Johnson BD. Cardiopulmonary and gas exchange responses to acute strenuous exercise at 1,270 meters in sickle cell trait. *Am J Med.* 1988;84:377–383.
63. Le Gallais D, Prefaut C, Mercier J, Bile A, Bogui P, Lonsdorfer J. Sickle cell trait as a limiting factor for high-level performance in a semi-marathon. *Int J Sports Med.* 1994;15:399–402.
64. Thiriet P, Le Hesraan JY, Wouassi D, Bitanga E, Gozal D, Louis FJ. sickle cell trait performance in a prolonged race at high altitude. *Med Sci Sports Exerc.* 1994;26:914–918.
65. Weisman IM, Zeballos RJ, Johnson BD. Effect of moderate inspiratory hypoxia on exercise performance in sickle cell trait. *Am J Med.* 1988;84:1033–1040.
66. Martin TW, Weisman IM, Zeballos RJ, Stephson SR. Exercise and hypoxia increase sickling in venous blood from an exercising limb in individuals with sickle cell trait. *Am J Med.* 1989;87:48–56.
67. Monchanin G, Serpero LD, Connes P, et al. Effects of progressive and maximal exercise on plasma levels of adhesion molecules in athletes with sickle cell trait with or without {alpha}-thalassemia. *J Appl Physiol.* 2007;102(1):169–173.
68. Samb A, Kane MO, Ba A, et al. Physical performance and thermoregulatory study of subjects with sickle cell trait during a sub-maximal exercise. *Dakar Med.* 2005;50(2):46–51.
69. Moheeb H, Wali YA, El-Sayed MS. Physical fitness indices and anthropometrics profiles in schoolchildren with sickle cell trait/disease. *Am J Hematol.* 2007;82(2):91–97.
70. Connes P, Tripette J, Chalabi T, et al. Effects of strenuous exercise on blood coagulation activity in sickle cell trait carriers. *Clin Hemorheol Microcirc.* 2008;38(1):13–21.
71. Embury SH, Hebbel RP, Mohandas N, Steinberg MH. *Sickle Cell Disease: Basic Principles and Clinical Practice.* 1 ed. New York: Raven Press; 1994.
72. Zadeii G, Lohr JW. Renal papillary necrosis in a patient with sickle cell trait. *Am J Soc Nephrol.* 1997;8:1034–1039.
73. Lang EK, Macchia RJ, Thomas R, et al. Multiphasic helical CT diagnosis of early medullary and papillary necrosis. *J Endourol.* 2004;18(1):49–56.
74. Kimberling WJ, Yium JJ, Johnson AM, Gabow PA, Martinez-Maldonado M. Genetic studies in a black family with autosomal dominant polycystic kidney disease and sickle-cell trait. *Nephron.* 1996;72(4):595–598.
75. Adsay NV, DeRoux SJ, Sakr W, Grignon D. Cancer as a marker of genetic medical disease – An unusual case of medullary carcinoma of the kidney. *Am J Surg Pathol.* 1998;22(2):260–264.
76. Coogan CL, McKiel CF Jr, Flanagan MJ, Bormes TP, Matkov TG. Renal medullary carcinoma in patients with sickle cell trait. *Urology.* 1998;51(6):1049–1050.
77. Davidson AJ, Choyke PL, Hartman DS, Davis CJ Jr. Renal medullary carcinoma associated with sickle cell trait; radiologic findings. *Radiology.* 1995;195:83–85.
78. Davis CJ, Jr., Mostofi FK, Sesterhenn IA. Renal medullary carcinoma: The seventh sickle cell nephropathy. *Am J Surg Pathol.* 1995;19:1–11.
79. Figenshau RS, Basler JW, Ritter JH, Siegel CL, Simon JA, Dierks SM. Renal medullary carcinoma. *J Urol.* 1998; 159(3 Pt 1):711–713.
80. Friedrichs P, Lassen P, Canby E, Graham C. Renal medullary carcinoma and sickle cell trait. *J Urol.* 1997;157:1349.
81. Simpson L, He X, Pins M, et al. Renal medullary carcinoma and ABL gene amplification. *J Urol.* 2005;173(6):1883–1888.
82. Hakimi AA, Koi PT, Milhoua PM, et al. Renal medullary carcinoma: the Bronx experience. *Urology.* 2007;70(5):878–882.
83. Blitman NM, Berkenblit RG, Rozenblit AM, Levin TL. Renal medullary carcinoma: CT and MRI features. *AJR Am J Roentgenol.* 2005;185(1):268–272.
84. Yang XJ, Sugimura J, Tretiakova MS, et al. Gene expression profiling of renal medullary carcinoma: potential clinical relevance. *Cancer.* 2004;100(5):976–985.
85. Nuss R, Feyerabend AJ, Lear JL, Lane PA. Splenic function in persons with sickle cell trait at moderately high altitude. *Am J Hematol.* 1991;37:130–132.
86. Gitschier J, Thompson CB. Non-altitude related splenic infarction in a patient with sickle cell trait. *Am J Med.* 1989;87:697–698.
87. Lane PA, Githens JH. Splenic syndrome at mountain altitudes in sickle cell trait. it's occurence in nonblack persons. *JAMA.* 1985;253:2251–2254.
88. Harkness DR. Sickle cell trait revisited. *Am J Med.* 1989;87: 30N–34N.
89. Lai JC, Fekrat S, Barron Y, Goldberg MF. Traumatic hyphema in children: risk factors for complications. *Arch Ophthalmol.* 2001;119(1):64–70.
90. Nasrullah A, Kerr NC. Sickle cell trait as a risk factor for secondary hemorrhage in children with traumatic hyphema. *Am J Ophthalmol.* 1997;123(6):783–790.

91. Sear DA. The morbidity of sickle cell trait: a review of the literature. *Am J Med.* 1978;64:1021–1036.
92. Leavitt JA, Butrus SI. Internuclear ophthalmoplegia in sickle cell trait. *J Neuroophthalmol.* 1994;14:49–51.
93. Finelli PF. Sickle cell trait and transient monocular blindness. *Am J Ophthalmol.* 1976;81:850–851.
94. Nia J, Lam WC, Kleinman DM, Kirby M, Liu ES, Eng KT. Retinopathy in sickle cell trait: does it exist? *Can J Ophthalmol.* 2003;38(1):46–51.
95. Liebmann JM. Management of sickle cell disease and hyphema. *J Glaucoma.* 1996;5:271–275.
96. Lally EV, Buckley WM, Claster S. Diaphyseal bone infarctions in a patient with sickle cell trait. *J Rheumatol.* 1983;10:813–816.
97. Steen RG, Hankins GM, Xiong X, et al. Prospective brain imaging evaluation of children with sickle cell trait: initial observations. *Radiology.* 2003;228(1):208–215.
98. Golomb MR. Sickle cell trait is a risk factor for early stroke. *Arch Neurol.* 2005;62(11):1778–1779.
99. Lannuzel A, Salmon V, Mevel G, Malpote E, Rabier R, Caparros-Lefebvre D. [Epidemiology of stroke in Guadeloupe and role of sickle cell trait]. *Rev Neurol (Paris).* 1999; 155(5):351–356.
100. Scott-Conner CEH, Brunson CD. The pathophysiology of the sickle hemoglobinopathies and implications for perioperative management. *Am J Surg.* 1994;168:268–274.
101. Scott-Conner CEH, Brunson CD. Surgery and anesthesia. In: Embury SH, Hebbel RP, Mohandas N, Steinberg MH, eds. *Sickle Cell Disease: Basic Principles and Clinical Practice.* 1st ed. New York: Lippincott-Raven; 1994:809–827.
102. Crawford MW, Galton S, Abdelhaleem M. Preoperative screening for sickle cell disease in children: clinical implications. *Can J Anaesth.* 2005;52(10):1058–1063.
103. Hendrickse RG, Hasan AH, Olumide LO, Akinkunmi A. Malaria in early childhood: an investigation of five hundred seriously ill children in whom a "clinical" diagnosis of malaria was made on admission to the children's emergency room at University College Hospital, Ibadan. *Ann Trop Med Parasitol.* 1971;65:1–20.
104. Aidoo M, Terlouw DJ, Kolczak MS, et al. Protective effects of the sickle cell gene against malaria morbidity and mortality. *Lancet.* 2002;359(9314):1311–1312.
105. Olumese PE, Adeyemo AA, Ademowo OG, Gbadegesin RA, Sodeinde O, Walker O. the clinical manifestations of cerebral malaria among Nigerian children with the sickle cell trait. *Ann Trop Paediatr.* 1997;17:141–145.
106. Williams TN, Mwangi TW, Wambua S, et al. Sickle cell trait and the risk of Plasmodium falciparum malaria and other childhood diseases. *J Infect Dis.* 2005;192(1):178–186.
107. Williams TN, Mwangi TW, Wambua S, et al. Negative epistasis between the malaria-protective effects of alpha(+)-thalassemia and the sickle cell trait. *Nat Genet.* 2005; 37(11):1253–1257.
108. Ntoumi F, Flori L, Mayengue PI, et al. Influence of carriage of hemoglobin AS and the Fc gamma receptor IIa-R131 allele on levels of immunoglobulin G2 antibodies to Plasmodium falciparum merozoite antigens in Gabonese children. *J Infect Dis.* 2005;192(11):1975–1980.
109. Steinberg MH. Sickle cell trait. In: Steinberg MH, Forget BG, Higgs DR, Nagel RL, eds. *Disorders of Hemoglobin: Genetics, Pathophysiology, and Clinical Management.* 1st ed. Cambridge: Cambridge University Press; 2001:811–830.
110. Bodensteiner D. White cell reduction in blood from donors with sickle cell trait. *Transfusion.* 1994;34(1):84.
111. Leukocyte depletion of whole blood and red cells from donors with hemoglobin sickle cell trait. *Transfusion.* 1999; 39(Suppl 108S).
112. Schuetz AN, Hillyer KL, Roback JD, Hillyer CD. Leukoreduction filtration of blood with sickle cell trait. *Transfus Med Rev.* 2004;18(3):168–176.
113. Stroncek DF, Rainer T, Sharon V, et al. Sickle Hb polymerization in RBC components from donors with sickle cell trait prevents effective WBC reduction by filtration. *Transfusion.* 2002;42(11):1466–1472.
114. Stroncek DF, Byrne KM, Noguchi CT, Schechter AN, Leitman SF. Increasing hemoglobin oxygen saturation levels in sickle trait donor whole blood prevents hemoglobin S polymerization and allows effective white blood cell reduction by filtration. *Transfusion.* 2004;44(9):1293–1299.
115. Newborn screening for sickle cell disease and other hemoglobinopathies. *JAMA.* 1987;258:1205–1209.
116. Luo H-Y, Yulong M, Adewoye AH, et al. Two new a thalassemia frame-shift mutations. *Hemoglobin.* 2007;31:135.

23

Other Sickle Hemoglobinopathies

Martin H. Steinberg

INTRODUCTION

The Genotypic Complexity of Sickle Cell Disease

The sickle hemoglobin gene (*HBB* glu6val) and β thalassemia alleles are often geographically coincident. Consequently, compound heterozygotes with HbS–β thalassemia are commonplace. The incidence of this genotype is dependent on the populations' ratio of carriers of an HbS gene to carriers of β thalassemia. In the United States, and in Africa where the HbS predominates, sickle cell anemia (homozygous for *HBB* glu6val) is the prevailing genotype of sickle cell disease. Wherever β thalassemia is more frequent than sickle cell trait (HbAS) – Greece, Italy, and other Mediterranean countries are examples – HbS–β thalassemia predominates. Some β thalassemia variants, such as δβ thalassemia and Hb Lepore and gene deletion hereditary persistence of fetal hemoglobin (HPFH), can interact with HbS producing different interesting phenotypes. α Thalassemia is present in 30% of African Americans with sickle cell anemia and might be even more common in some populations from the Middle East and Indian subcontinent. Individuals with sickle cell anemia–α thalassemia have distinctive hematological and clinical features. Compound heterozygotes of HbS with other mutant α- or β-globin genes are also present in any population with a high prevalence of HbS. Depending on the other globin gene mutation, these conditions can resemble the clinically benign HbAS or have a phenotype with hemolytic anemia and vasoocclusive complications. Rare variants, often with intriguing phenotypes, have both the sickle mutation and an additional mutation in the same β-globin gene.

This chapter will examine the molecular, diagnostic, laboratory, and clinical aspects of compound heterozygous genotypes of sickle cell disease, excluding HbSC disease, which is discussed in Chapter 21. Unless there are special features associated with a genotype discussed in this chapter, its clinical aspects will be covered in chapters on sickle cell anemia (Chapter 19) and HbSC disease (Chapter 21) and in other chapters in which management is discussed (Chapters 20, section VIII, Chapters 29–33).

Whatever the hemoglobin genotype responsible for a sickle hemoglobinopathy, the treatment of its complications is nearly always the same. The critical clinical issue is to establish the correct genotypic diagnosis before counseling and when discussing prognosis.

HbS–β Thalassemia and HbS–β Thalassemia-like Conditions

β Thalassemia is classified as β^0 thalassemia or β^+ thalassemia (Chapter 16). In the former, the thalassemia-causing mutation totally abolishes expression of the affected gene; in the latter, there is a reduction in β-globin gene expression that depends on the thalassemia mutation. Lacking recent blood transfusion, HbA is not present in HbS–β^0 thalassemia; the hemolysate contains only HbS, fetal hemoglobin (HbF), and 4%–6% HbA_2. Therefore, the phenotype of HbS–β^0 thalassemia mimics that seen in sickle cell anemia and is equally variegated.

In HbS–β^+ thalassemia, HbA levels range from less than 5%–45% of the hemolysate. Given the primacy of the HbS concentration in determining the phenotype of the resulting disease, individuals with only traces of HbA have a disease resembling sickle cell anemia or HbS–β^0 thalassemia; most patients with HbA levels of 20% or more have a phenotype milder than that of HbSC disease or sickle cell anemia.

Because of the confounding influences of genetic modifiers like γ-globin gene expression, α thalassemia, and other more obscure modulators of sickle cell disease (Chapter 27), rigid genotype–phenotype correlations are difficult to establish in all instances of HbS–β thalassemia. Among the different genotypes of HbS–β^+ thalassemia, higher levels of HbA are usually associated with a milder phenotype and in all types of HbS–β thalassemia, as in sickle cell anemia, higher HbF concentrations temper the disease.

Pathophysiology

β Thalassemia Mutations in HbS–β Thalassemia

The pathophysiology of the sickle–β thalassemias is similar to the pathophysiology of sickle cell anemia (Chapters 8–11) with the major determinant of severity being the magnitude of the reduction in β^A-globin chain production caused by the thalassemia mutation. Different β thalassemia–causing mutations have been described in association with HbS and many of these are shown in Table 23.1. The β thalassemia mutations extant in each population determine the phenotypes of HbS–β thalassemia present. HbS–β thalassemia has a different clinical spectrum in different racial and ethnic groups because β thalassemia mutations vary among populations. HbS–β thalassemia is most common in selected Italian and Greek populations, in Turks,

Table 23.1. β Thalassemia mutations in HbS–β thalassemia

Mutation	PCV/Hemoglobin	HbA	HbF	MCV	Phenotype
β^+ Thalassemia*					
-90 C-T	11/33	?	5	75	? Mild
-92 C→T§	14.5/	45	1.4	83	Asymptomatic
-88 C→T	10/31	18	15	65–70	Mild
-88 C→T in *cis* to HbS§	12/35	90	3	70	Very mild New thal mutation on HbS gene
-29 A→G	11/32	20	11¶	65–70	Mild
CD24 T-A					Mild
IVS-1 -1 G→C	7.3–11.4/	0	3–9	61–72	Severe Hb Monroe
IVS-1 5 G→C	9/	<5	12	72	Severe Indian, 1 black
IVS-1 5 G→T§	8/24	~5	5–12	57	? Severe
IVS-1 5 G→A§	6/20	<5	5	68	Severe
IVS-1§ 6 T→C		35			
IVS-1, 110 G→A	9/	9–11	7	72	Severe
IVS-2 745 C→G		5			Severe
IVS-2 848 C-A§	10/33	17	3	74	
Poly A site AAT→AAC§	10/32	18	2	70	
Poly A site -5 nt AATAA---A	11/	19	3	58	Mild
β^0 Thalassemia					
CD 2/3/4 (-9,+31 bp)§	9/	–	8.5	70–80	
CD 6 -A§					
CD 15 TGG→TGA§	–	–	–	–	Vasoocclusion
CD 25/26 GGT.GAG→GGT.T.GAG§	8/	–	14	74	Severe, Tunisians
CD37 TGG-TAG	9/	–	22	75	
CD 39 C→T					
CD 44 -C§					
CD 106/007 +G§					
IVS-1 1 G-C (Hb Monroe)		–			Expressed as severe β thalassemia
IVS-1 2 T→C	7/		6	58	Severe
IVS-2 1 G→A					
IVS-2 849 A→G§					
IVS-2 849 A→C	10/28		8–35	79	
Frameshift 106/107§ (+G)					
1393 bp	11/32	–	11–19	73	Mild/severe
-532 bp§§			30		An infant when described
-468§	10		23	74	'Mild'
7733 bp	10/		15	70	'Mild'

* In many instances, few patients or only a single patient was studied so that the values reported may not necessarily be representative of the genotype.
§ Indicates those examples of HbS–β thalassemia in which information is scanty and only one or two cases are reported. Also, patient ages could differ among groups, confounding the interpretation of hemoglobin level, MCV, HbF, and HbA_2. Sometimes, no hematological values are available. Data reported were assembled from the following references and are summarized in http://globin.cse.psu.edu.[58,82–92]
¶ Mean age of patients was approximately 10 years.
§§ One individual, age 9 months, was studied. HbA_2 was 6%.

Iranians, and other Middle Eastern nationalities, in tribal groups of the Indian subcontinent and in blacks of African descent. "Mild" β-globin gene promoter mutations are prevalent in blacks, accounting for the preponderance of milder forms of HbS–β^+ thalassemia in this racial group.

As with sickle cell disease caused by other genotypes, the pathophysiology of the HbS–β thalassemias is ultimately linked to HbS polymerization and modulated by coincident genetic factors, such as the ability to make large amounts of HbF and by the cellular concentration of HbS. Two interrelated elements modulate the polymerization tendency of HbS in HbS–β thalassemia. They are mean corpuscular HbS concentration and the concentration of HbA. In both HbS–β^0 thalassemia and HbS–β^+ thalassemia, reduced β-globin chain accumulation reduces mean corpuscular hemoglobin (MCH) and mean corpuscular volume (MCV). In HbS–β^+ thalassemia, HbA concentration is the major determinant of mean corpuscular HbS concentration. HbA dilutes HbS and, depending on its concentration, variably inhibits polymerization-induced cellular damage. HbA is

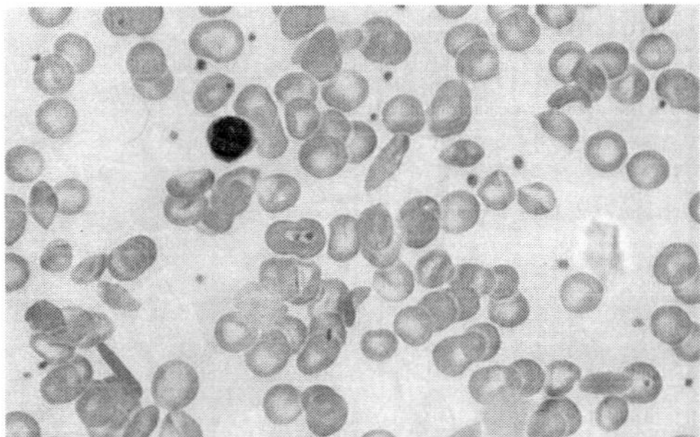
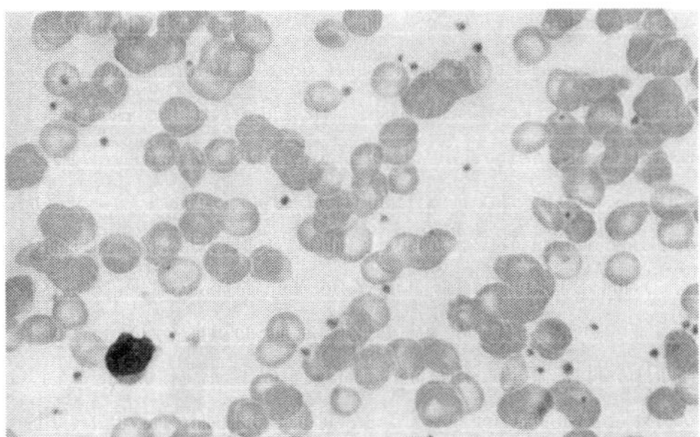

Figure 23.1. Blood films in two patients with HbS–β^0 thalassemia. In the left panel, the patient has an HbF level of 5%. Sickled cells are prominent beside microcytosis. In the right panel, with an HbF of 2%, microcytosis and hypochromia are prominent and few typical sickled cells are seen. Despite similar HbF levels, for unknown reasons, the numbers of sickled cells are quite different. This suggests the possibility of different cellular distributions of HbF or other genetic modifiers. See color plates.

only a "dilutent" and does not have the enhanced benefit of HbF, which is not incorporated into the polymer phase of HbS (Chapters 6, 7).

In HbS–β^0 thalassemia, compared with sickle cell anemia, the effects of thalassemia on sickle erythrocytes – microcytosis, hypochromia, sometimes high levels of HbF – improve the circulatory competence of these cells, marginally reduce hemolysis, and cause a small increase in total hemoglobin concentration. This suggests that as with sickle cell anemia-α thalassemia (see later) a reduction in hemolysis and improved anemia might lead to fewer of the disease complications attributable to intravascular hemolysis, although perhaps increasing the viscosity-vasoocclusive events of sickle cell disease.[1] Nevertheless, despite a few reports, comprehensive data are not yet available in HbS–β thalassemia.[2] Hemolysis-related complications have been described in HbS–β thalassemia. Reduced nitric oxide bioavailability, oxidant stress, and endothelial dysfunction are key contributors to the proliferative vasculopathy of sickle cell disease and its complications (Chapter 11). Similar to what has been found in sickle cell anemia,[3–6] in patients with HbS–β thalassemia, and normal left ventricular function, a complex vasculopathy with endothelial dysfunction, increased arterial stiffness, and a global effect on cardiovascular function was present.[7]

Table 23.2. Laboratory differentiation of sickle cell anemia, sickle cell anemia–α thalassemia and HbS–β^0 thalassemia*

Diagnosis	Hemoglobin (g/dL)	MCV (fL)	HbA_2 (%)	HbF§ (%)	α/β@
Sickle cell anemia	7–8	85–95	2.5–3.5	5	0.95
Sickle cell anemia–α thalassemia¶	8–10	70–85	3.5–4.5	5	0.75
HbS–β^0 thalassemia	8–10	65–75	4–6	8	1.50

* The laboratory values reflect ranges found in individuals aged 15 years and older.[93,94]
¶ α Thalassemia includes both heterozygotes and homozygotes for the -$\alpha^{3.7}$ deletion.
§ Average level.
@ Ratio of radioactive leucine incorporated into newly synthesized α- and β-globin chains.[9]

Diagnosis

Hematological Evaluation of HbS–β^0 Thalassemia

Microcytosis and hypochromia, noticed on blood films but best determined using automated blood cell counters, and elevated concentrations of HbA_2 are often the first clues to diagnosis of HbS–β thalassemia. Nevertheless, alone they are insufficient for diagnosis. HbS–β^0 thalassemia resembles, in many respects, sickle cell anemia, and in some cases of HbS–β^0 thalassemia the MCV is near normal and the HbA_2 is only elevated marginally. Compounding the possibilities for diagnostic confusion is that sickle cell anemia–α thalassemia is a nearly exact phenocopy of HbS–β^0 thalassemia. Iron deficiency also causes microcytosis in sickle cell anemia, but here, the level of HbA_2 is normal or low. Hematological studies, including the determination of MCV and MCH, quantification of HbS, HbA_2, HbF, and when present, HbA levels, form the cornerstone of diagnosis. Blood films from two patients with HbS–β^0 thalassemia are shown in Figure 23.1. Family studies and the demonstration by DNA analysis of heterozygosity for the sickle β-globin gene and the presence of a β-thalassemia mutation are important confirmatory analyses and are critical when antenatal diagnosis and genetic counseling are at issue.

Some hematological distinctions among these three phenocopies are shown in Table 23.2 and comparative pedigrees are displayed in Figure 23.2. Most cases of HbS–β thalassemia are accompanied by reduced MCV and MCH and increased concentration of HbA_2. Depending on the reticulocyte count, the HbF level, and the nature of the particular β thalassemia mutation, the MCV could be normal or in the lower range of normality. HbA_2 levels are low in early childhood and cannot be relied on for diagnostic discrimination at this stage of life. When the HbF level is very high, HbA_2 levels are often reduced, further compromising the utility of

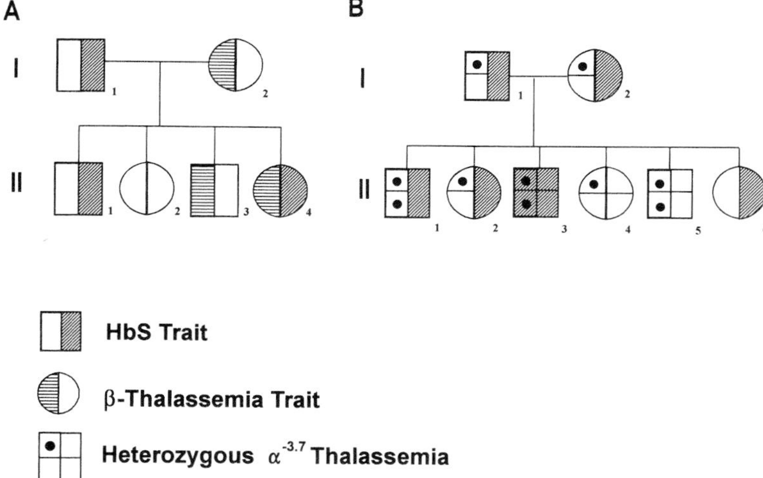

Figure 23.2. Pedigrees of families with HbS–β thalassemia **(A)** and sickle cell anemia with α thalassemia **(B)**. II 4 in family A and II 3 in family B have nearly identical hematological findings with microcytic erythrocytes and increased HbA_2 levels. Nevertheless, A II 4 has HbS–β thalassemia and B II 3 has sickle cell anemia with homozygous α thalassemia-2. The latter individual has inherited an HbS gene from each parent and an α thalassemia gene from each parent. As shown in the pedigree, because the β-globin genes and α-globin genes are on different chromosomes they are inherited independently and individuals can have HbAS (or sickle cell anemia) without α thalassemia or with one or two α thalassemia genes. The HbS and β thalassemia genes are allelic.

this measurement. Although high HbA_2 levels are typical of heterozygous β thalassemia, the increase is in part dependent on the reduction of β-globin chain synthesis. HbA_2 is also high when α thalassemia is present with sickle cell anemia. This increase is proportional to the reduction in α-globin chain synthesis and is a result of the differential affinities of non-α-globin chains for the limited numbers of α-globin chains. HbA_2 levels and MCV in sickle cell anemia, HbS-β^0 thalassemia, and sickle cell anemia–α thalassemia are shown in Figure 23.3. Although HbA_2 levels are highest in HbS-β^0 thalassemia, lowest in sickle cell anemia, and intermediate in sickle cell anemia–α thalassemia, in an individual, they have little discriminatory value and diagnostic utility. HbF levels span a very wide range in all three genotype, rendering them diagnostically useless.

Hematological Evaluation of HbS–β^+ Thalassemia

Family studies, hematological evaluation, and measuring the percentage of HbA, HbS, and HbA_2 by high-performance liquid chromatography (HPLC) are usually sufficient for establishing the presence of HbS–β^+ thalassemia. When a sickle solubility test is the sole means of diagnosis – it should never be! – or when protein-based methods, such as hemoglobin electrophoresis or HPLC, are uncritically interpreted, HbS–β^+ thalassemia might be confused with HbAS or even go unsuspected.

In HbS–β^+ thalassemia, the presence of HbA simplifies the diagnosis. Yet, the rare case with very high HbA levels – the highest level reported is 45% – might be confused with HbAS and in instances in which HbA is quite low – the lowest levels are less than 5% – its presence can be overlooked. Representative hematological findings in the different genotypes of HbS–β^+ thalassemia are presented in Table 23.1. During newborn screening for sickle cell disease, small amounts of HbA might be undetected, leading to a false diagnosis of sickle cell anemia and emphasizing the need for confirmatory testing after the initial screening.[8]

Individuals with HbS–β^+thalassemia and very low levels of HbA are often mistakenly diagnosed as having HbS–β^0 thalassemia. Four β^+ thalassemia mutations, all producing a severe phenotype, have been described at IVS-1 position 5, and two of these have been associated with severe HbS–β^+ thalassemia, masquerading as HbS–β^0 thalassemia (Table 23.1).[9] IVS-1 position 5 is part of the consensus sequence for the donor splice site of exon 1. When mutated, splicing efficiency is greatly reduced and only a small amount of mRNA is correctly spliced.

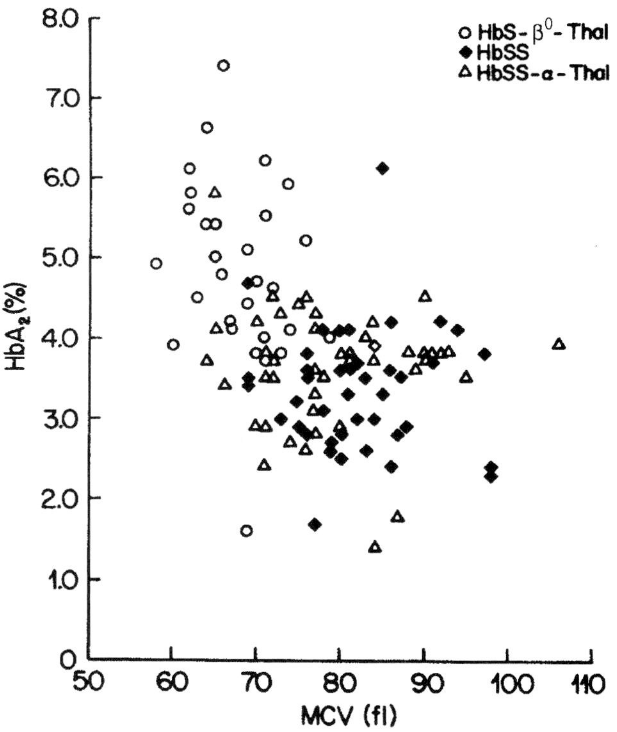

Figure 23.3. HbA_2 levels and MCV in HbS–β^0 thalassemia, sickle cell anemia–α thalassemia, and sickle cell anemia. Considerable overlap among these genotypes makes it difficult to rely on HbA_2 for diagnostic purposes in an individual case. Most reported methods of HbA_2 analysis by HPLC result in higher levels of HbA_2 when HbS is present. The data reported here are not based on HPLC.

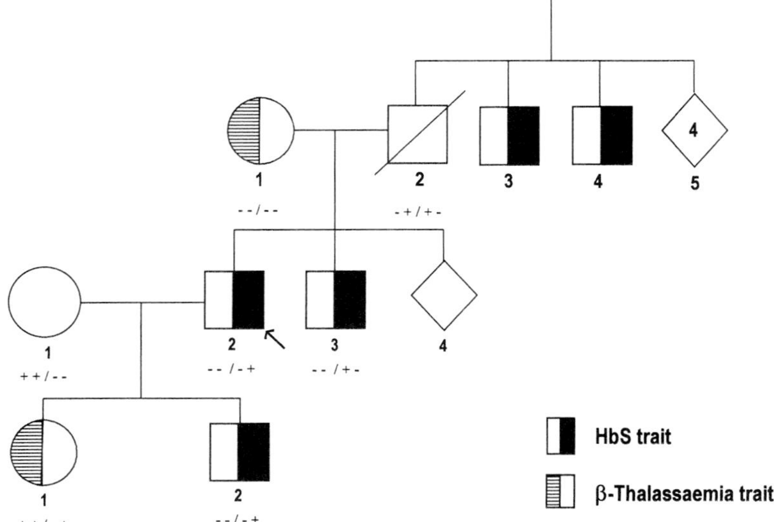

Figure 23.4. Inheritance of sickle cell trait and β thalassemia unlinked to the β-globin gene cluster. The two Hinc II/ψ β restriction length polymorphisms are shown with +/-.[12]

Molecular Evaluation

In any instance when antenatal diagnosis is contemplated or family counseling is needed, DNA-based molecular analysis is required (Chapter 28). The most confusing diagnostic problem is the differentiation of HbS–β^0 thalassemia from sickle cell anemia–α thalassemia. Microcytosis and the elevated HbA_2 level in sickle cell anemia–α thalassemia cause great confusion with HbS–β^0 thalassemia. Differentiating between these genotypes is critical during genetic counseling because hematological, HPLC or electrophoretical studies, and, for the case of sickle cell anemia–α thalassemia, family studies, cannot distinguish among these conditions.

In HbS–β^0 thalassemia, DNA analysis will show that the patient is heterozygous for the HbS gene and that the other β-globin gene contains a β thalassemia mutation. In sickle cell anemia–α thalassemia, patients are homozygous for the HbS gene and have an α thalassemia mutation, most often a deletion of one or more α-globin genes (Chapter 13).

Hb Monroe (*HBB* IVS-1 position -1, G-C), initially described in a Tunisian patient and called Hb Kairouan, has been described in several families as a compound heterozygote with HbS. IVS-1 position -1 is between the A and G of β-globin gene codon 30 (AGG), which normally codes for arginine; in Hb Monroe it is converted to a threonine codon (ACG). The mutation has dual effects: it impairs the use of the normal 5′ splice site by 98%, and the threonine residue causes hemoglobin instability. In HbS–Hb Monroe disease, Hb Monroe is not detectable by isoelectric focusing, and only in some patients is 0.6%–1.6% Hb Monroe found by HPLC.[10] Patients with HbS–Hb Monroe appear to have all the clinical and hematological features of HbS–β^0 thalassemia.

Two Moroccan adults with HbAS were found to have the -88 C-T β^+ thalassemia mutation in *cis* to the sickle mutation. Both had a normal α-globin gene haplotype. A reticulocyte count of approximately 3%, mild anemia, and microcytosis (Table 23.1), without iron deficiency suggested the presence of mild hemolysis. HbA_2 levels were 6%–7%, HbF approximately 3% and HbS, 10%–11%. In one individual, the α/β globin biosynthesis ratio was 1.35 and the ratio of $\beta^S/\beta^A+\beta^S$ was 0.17.[11] Further studies of cloned DNA in the patient's family confirmed that the thalassemia mutation was in the same gene as the HbS mutation. Analysis of polymorphisms 5′ to the β^S gene revealed a Benin haplotype chromosome, strongly suggesting that the thalassemia mutation arose anew on the HbS chromosome rather than from a recombination between a β thalassemia and an HbS chromosome. It was not clear why HbS levels were as low as they were because analysis showed a reduction of β-globin mRNA similar to that found in simple heterozygotes for the -88 C-T mutation. The authors speculated that the reduction in HbS was caused by a posttranslational event and that even without α thalassemia, the β^S chains competed less well than the β^A chains for α-globin chains.

Two Portuguese patients with HbAS had a β thalassemia determinant that was not linked to the β-globin gene (Fig. 23.4).[12] Extensive analysis of the β-globin gene DNA failed to find a thalassemia-causing mutation. Carriers had very mild microcytic anemia and increased HbA_2 levels; in vitro translation of mRNA showed an α/β ratio of 1.6. Examples of *trans*-acting β thalassemia mutations are rare.[13]

Clinical Features

Although it is possible to generalize about genotype–phenotype relationships in HbS–β thalassemia, as with sickle cell anemia, genotype–phenotype association correlations are often difficult to establish because of the many genetic and environmental modulators that impact this disease (Chapter 27).

HbS–β^0 Thalassemia

HbS–β^0 thalassemia (and HbS–β^+ thalassemia with very low levels of HbA), with some exceptions, has a pathophysiology and panoply of clinical complications very similar to sickle cell anemia. In HbS–β^0 thalassemia, the average packed cell volume (PCV) and hemoglobin concentration are higher than in sickle cell anemia, a likely result of the reduction in mean cell HbS concentration and improved red cell survival. Based on current understanding of the role of hemolysis as a risk factor for death and some complications of disease,[1,14] it might be expected that the mild reduction of hemolysis in HbS–β^0 thalassemia compared with sickle cell anemia would be beneficial in some areas. That supposition has not yet been confirmed by clinical studies. Conversely, one might expect that disease complications associated with blood viscosity might be more prevalent. In one study of HbS–β^0 thalassemia, osteonecrosis was more common than in sickle cell anemia.[15] Bacteremia occurred half as often in HbS–β^0 thalassemia as in sickle cell anemia.

An exception to the nearly uniform severe phenotype of HbS–β^0 thalassemia is the rare patient with very high HbF and HbA_2 levels. This has been associated with several small deletions that affect the 5′ portion of the β-globin gene, and, perhaps because of competition of the transcriptional apparatus for gene promoters, is typified by very high HbA_2 and HbF levels (Chapter 16). Both HbA_2 and HbF inhibit the polymerization of HbS. In families with HbS–β^0 thalassemia caused by a −1.4-kb 5′ β-globin gene deletion, the combined total of HbF and HbA_2 was more than 20% of the total hemoglobin. This was associated with a milder than expected phenotype; nevertheless, other observations suggested that all individuals with this genotype might not be similarly affected. One young child with HbS–β^0 thalassemia caused by a 532-bp deletion in the 5′ part of the β-globin gene had 29% HbF and 6% HbA_2; however, this patient's age precluded an assessment of the phenotype.

HbS–β^+ Thalassemia

The clinical features of HbS–β^+ thalassemia depend on the β thalassemia mutation and the deficit of β^A-globin chains (Table 23.1). Rare cases of HbS–β^+ thalassemia are asymptomatic, and some are quite severe; however, for the most part the phenotype of HbS–β^+ thalassemia lies between these extremes.

In one HbS–β^+ thalassemia study, the median PCV was 32 in all patients younger than age 10 years. Males aged 10–19 years and those aged 20 years and older had PCVs of 36 and 40, respectively, approximately four–six points higher than age-matched females. In all patients, the MCV was 70–72 fL compared with approximately 90 fl in sickle cell anemia. Leukocyte and platelet counts were also reduced compared with sickle cell anemia patients.[16] These data were from African American patients in whom the preponderance of β^+ thalassemia mutations is "mild" (Table 23.1 and Chapter 16).

The Cooperative Study of Sickle Cell Disease in the United States examined clinical differences among the common sickle hemoglobinopathies. Approximately 3% of patients with HbS–β^+ thalassemia died during 6–8 years of observation compared with 8% of patients with sickle cell anemia, 4% with HbS–β^0 thalassemia, and 3% with HbSC disease.[17] Patients with HbS–β^+ thalassemia had pain rates approximately half those observed in HbS–β^0 thalassemia and sickle cell anemia and similar to those of patients with HbSC disease.[18] Osteonecrosis of the femoral head rarely appeared in children with HbS–β^+ thalassemia and was less frequent in adults with this genotype (5.8%) than in sickle cell anemia (10.2%). Bacteremia was approximately half as frequent in HbS–β^+ thalassemia as in sickle cell anemia and similar to its incidence in HbSC disease. At any age, the incidence of acute chest syndrome in HbS–β^+ thalassemia was less than in sickle cell anemia or HbS–β^0 thalassemia, which did not differ, and it was similar to that in HbSC disease.[19] Strokes occur in all genotypes of HbS–β thalassemia but less often than in sickle cell anemia.[20] As in patients with sickle cell anemia, individuals with HbS–β thalassemia without overt stroke can have abnormal transcranial Doppler flow velocity and silent cerebral infarction, although in one small study patients' cognitive function seemed unimpaired.[21]

HbS–β^+ thalassemia patients with more than 20% HbA usually have milder clinical disease than those with sickle cell anemia and HbSC disease, and some patients can be asymptomatic with the diagnosis established incidental to other medical problems. Now and then, the presence of HbS is not recognized at all because the patient seems normal hematologically. Sometimes, the mildness of this genotype leads it to be confused with HbAS. Nevertheless, microcytosis and reticulocytosis are virtually always present in HbS–β^+ thalassemia, whereas reticulocytosis is not a feature of HbAS. Failing to recognize mild HbS–β^+ thalassemia can be a serious omission when surgery is planned or pneumonia-like disorders are treated because individuals with this genotype can encounter severe and devastating problems.[22] Some observations suggest that the mortality rate of acute chest syndrome is higher in HbS–β^+ thalassemia than in sickle cell anemia.[23–25]

Splenic enlargement is more likely to persist into the adult years in HbS–β thalassemia; in some studies it is present in more than half the affected patients. As a result, adults can have splenic sequestration episodes. An enlarging spleen in adults can also lead to hypersplenism with falling blood counts and splenic infarction.

In Greek patients with HbS–β thalassemia, detailed studies of renal function showed multiple abnormalities that were similar in all respects to those found in sickle cell anemia. Similarly, polymorphisms of the *UGT1A1* gene (Chapter 27) modulated serum bilirubin concentration.[26]

HbS–β Thalassemia with α Thalassemia

Although some reports suggest a milder phenotype in HbS–β thalassemia with α thalassemia,[27] when more than a few cases are available for analysis, any influence of coexistent α thalassemia on the phenotype of HbS–β^0 thalassemia or β^+ thalassemia is difficult to detect. The numbers of observations are still too small to provide firm conclusions. Not all reports used gene mapping to detect α thalassemia. When the coincidence of these disorders was based on the less reliable use of hematological, electrophoretical,

Table 23.3. HbS with hereditary persistence of HbF and δβ thalassemia (http://globin .cse.psu.edu)

Mutation	Hb/PCV	HbF	$^G\gamma$ (%)	MCV	Phenotype
Nongene-deletion HPFH					
-202 C→G 5′ $^G\gamma$		20	100		In sickle cell trait, HbA ~30%
-202 C→T 5′ $^A\gamma$	11/30	2.5	32	88	In sickle cell anemia
-175 T→C 5′ $^G\gamma$		30	100		In sickle cell trait, HbS ~40%, HbA ~28%
-175 T→C 5′ $^A\gamma$,5′ $^G\gamma$ 158 C→T in *cis*	14/42	40	35	85	In sickle cell trait, HbS ~40%, HbA ~17%
13-bp deletion -114 to -102		31	14		HbA 20%
-158 C→T 5′ $^G\gamma$					See discussion of Senegal haplotype in sickle cell anemia (Chapter 27)
Gene-deletion HPFH					
HPFH-1, ~106 kb	Normal	25	51	70–80	None
HPFH-2, ~105 kb	Normal	25	32		None
δβ Thalassemia					
~12 kb	11/34	25		85	Very mild
~36 kb	9–13/29–45	19–22	90–98	75–91	

and globin biosynthesis studies, there were no clinical or hematological differences compared with patients with HbS–β^0 thalassemia, except for the presence of balanced globin biosynthesis ratios. No clinical and hematological differences were observed when heterozygous or homozygous α thalassemia-2 was ascertained by α-globin gene mapping.

HbS–Hereditary Persistence of Fetal Hemoglobin and δβ Thalassemia

Pathophysiology

HPFH connotes the continued expression of HbF into adult life (Chapters 16 and 17). These conditions are, like all genetic abnormalities of globin, genetically and hematologically heterogeneous. They can be divided into two classes: HPFH caused by extensive deletions within the β-like globin gene complex and HPFH caused by point mutations within the promoters of the γ-globin genes. The δβ thalassemias, also caused by large gene deletions, are closely related to gene deletion HPFH. Compound heterozygotes with HbS-deletion HPFH and δβ thalassemia can be found in populations of African and Mediterranean ancestry, and some mutations described in HbS–HPFH and δβ thalassemia are shown in Table 23.3. Nongene-deletion HPFH in sickle cell anemia is difficult to recognize when lacking family studies with enumeration of F cells and determination of the HPFH mutation, so there is no reliable description of its phenotype. Therefore, we will consider mainly the HbS-deletion HPFH and δβ thalassemia syndromes. Nongene-deletion HPFH is more commonly suspected when it is present with HbAS or exists without an abnormal hemoglobin or β thalassemia.

A pancellular distribution of HbF in HbS-deletion HPFH retards HbS polymerization to the extent that hemolytic and vasoocclusive diseases are absent or very minimal. Although HbS–δβ thalassemia and HbS-deletion HPFH can have similar total HbF levels, in the former condition all cells are not equally endowed with HbF so that mild hemolytic anemia is present.

Diagnosis

In blacks, the prevalence of HbS-deletion HPFH is approximately 0.0001.[28] HbF levels are 20%–30%, and nearly equal concentrations of HbF are present in all erythrocytes leading to the designation, pancellular HPFH. Anemia and reticulocytosis are absent or mild, irreversibly sickled cells are absent, target cells are present, and HbA_2 levels are low or normal because the HPFH chromosome lacks the δ-globin gene. Thirteen unselected patients with HbS–HPFH, diagnosed because the proband had a parent with heterozygous HPFH, but not by molecular analysis, were compared with patients with sickle cell anemia and HbS–β^0 thalassemia. In all groups, patients were aged between 9 and 12 years, and all individuals had HbF levels of more than 20%. Their hematological findings are summarized in Table 23.4. Differentiating among these genotypes was possible based on the hematological findings, although the patients with sickle cell anemia and HbS–β^0 thalassemia were selected for this comparison by their high HbF levels. When HbS-gene deletion HPFH is compared with unselected cases of sickle cell anemia and HbS–β^0 thalassemia that have more ordinary HbF levels, the differentiation among these genotypes is even more dramatic.

Hb Kenya is caused by a γβ fusion gene, the product of nonhomologous crossing over between the γ- and β-globin

Table 23.4. Comparisons of HbS Gene–deletion HPFH, sickle cell anemia with high HbF, and HbS–β thalassemia

	HbS-HPFH	Sickle cell anemia	HbS–β thalassemia
Hemoglobin (g/dL)	13.4	10.2	10.9
HbF (%)	29.2	21.6	24.2
HbA_2 (%)	2.0	2.0	3.7
MCV (fL)	78.4	89.2	75
Reticulocytes (%)	1.9	7.3	3.6

Adapted from ref. 28; values given are means.

genes (Chapter 16). In compound heterozygotes with HbS, there was approximately 18% Hb Kenya, evenly distributed among the red cell population and HbF averaged approximately 8%. Hb Kenya acted as a deletion HPFH determinant, and vasoocclusive symptoms were not reported. Red cell morphology was normal, and anemia was absent or minimal.[29]

In HbS–δβ thalassemia, the HbF level is 15%–25%. Its cellular distribution is not uniform as it is in HbS-deletion HPFH, but instead HbF is unevenly spread among red cells, or, is heterocellular. Anemia is mild with the hemoglobin level averaging 10–12 g/dL, reticulocytes are approximately 2%, and the MCV is low normal. HbA_2 levels are normal or low because of the deleted δ-globin gene.

Some individuals with sickle cell anemia have very high HbF levels and seem not to have deletion HPFH, δβ thalassemia, or a Senegal haplotype chromosome (Chapter 27). Few of these patients have been carefully studied, but it is likely that some will have a nondeletion HPFH mutation. In a patient with sickle cell anemia who was heterozygous for the Benin and the "MOR" haplotype and lacked the −158 C–T polymorphism, HbF was 24%–29%. The presence of a C–T mutation at −202 5′ to the $^{A}\gamma$ globin gene was suspected to cause this marked increase in HbF. Individuals with HbAS who also inherited this mutation had 2%–4% HbF and more than 90% $^{A}\gamma$ chains.

In some cases of sickle cell anemia with unusually high HbF levels, the increase in HbF might not be linked to the β-globin gene-like cluster. Other instances could be associated with already identified or still obscure *cis*-acting elements linked to the β-globin gene that might modulate γ-globin gene expression or with *trans*-acting elements that modulate HbF expression (Chapter 27).

Clinical Aspects

HbS-deletion HPFH is not associated with hemolytic anemia or acute vasoocclusive disease, although osteonecrosis has been described. The phenotype of HbS–δβ thalassemia also seems mild. Vasoocclusive problems can occur but less often than in sickle cell anemia or HbS–β thalassemia. Splenomegaly is common.

HbS–Hb Lepore

Hb Lepore, the name given to a small group of hemoglobin variants that result from unequal crossing over between δ- and β-globin genes (Chapter 16), is characterized by the deletion of both these genes from the chromosome and their replacement by a poorly expressed, δβ hybrid, or, Hb Lepore gene. HbS–Lepore was first described in Greece but has since been found in many other geographical areas. Hb Lepore moves electrophoretically like HbS but is easily separated from HbS, HbA, and HbF, but not HbA_2, by HPLC. In heterozygotes, it accounts for approximately 10% of the total hemoglobin causing, in essence, a $\delta\beta^+$ thalassemia with levels of Hb Lepore equivalent to the levels of HbA in the IVS-1, 110 G-A HbS–β^+ thalassemia.

Compound heterozygosity for HbS and Hb Lepore is an uncommon condition, most often described in Mediterranean populations, and best diagnosed by family studies that document heterozygous Hb Lepore in a parent or sibling. Failure to note the presence of Hb Lepore by protein-based hemoglobin diagnostic studies can result in the confusion of this genotype with sickle cell anemia or HbS–β^0 thalassemia, but HPLC can now simplify this distinction, and DNA analysis can authenticate the presence of the Hb Lepore gene.[30] Because compound heterozygotes with HbS–Hb Lepore have only a single β-globin gene, amplification of the β-globin gene and allele-specific hybridization or restriction endonuclease cleavage can falsely suggest homozygosity for the HbS gene when in actuality, the patient is hemizygous at the β^6 codon.

Unsurprisingly, reported patients with HbS–Lepore have heterogeneous phenotypes. Compared with sickle cell anemia and HbS–β^0 thalassemia, there is less anemia, and a reduction in MCV, HbA_2, and reticulocyte counts. Symptoms can vary and splenomegaly is common. Only a few clinical studies of HbS–Lepore disease have been conducted, making it difficult to define completely its clinical spectrum. On average, the hemoglobin level is 11–13 g/dL, HbS and Hb Lepore comprise 70%–80%, and HbF makes up 10%–20% of total hemoglobin.

Residues δ22 (ala) and δ87 (gly) inhibit polymerization of HbS (Chapter 6). When HbA_2 and HbF levels are high, their combination might cause a mild phenotype. Hb Lepore Boston, the type most often reported with HbS, contains the δ87 glycine residue whereas Hb Lepore Hollandia contains δ22 alanine. It is possible that the presence of Hb Lepore not only reduces the concentration of HbA but also inhibits polymerization, accounting for the milder than expected phenotype.

Treatment Recommendations

With few exceptions, individuals with HbS–β thalassemia-like disorders should be managed like those with sickle cell anemia. Although serious pneumococcal infection is less common in HbS–β^+ thalassemia with high levels of HbA

Table 23.5. Sickling hemoglobins with two amino acid substitutions in the β-globin chain

Hb name	Amino acid substitution	Variant with same mutation	*HBB* mutation	Phenotype
S-Antilles	val23Ile	HbS (---)	GTT→ATT	Migrates ~HbS. Heterozygote affected; compound heterozygote with HbS or HbC severely affected
C-Ziguinchor	pro58arg	HbS (Dhofar)	CCT→CGT	Migrates ~HbC on electrophoresis. 30%–40% in the heterozygote. Normal hematology, target cells
C-Ndjamena	trp37gly	Hb Howick	TGG-GGG	Migrates like HbC on isoelectric focusing; faster than HbS on HPLC; phenotype appears severe
Jamaica Plain	leu68phe	New mutation (Rockford/ Loves Park)	CTC-TTC	Migrates like HbS on isoelectric focusing, not separable from HbS by HPLC. Moderate to severe disease in simple heterozygote
C-Harlem	asp73asn	HbS (Korle-Bu)	GAT→AAT	Migrates like HbS at alkaline pH and like HbC at acidic pH. Compound heterozygote with HbS, ~sickle cell anemia, Heterozygote ~40%, normal hematology
S-Providence	asn82asp	HbS (Providence)	AAG→AAT or AAC	Migrates like HbA. Hematology normal
S-Cameroon	glu90lys	HbS (Agenogi)	GAG-AAG	HbAS; 38% HbS-Cameroon
S-Oman	glu121lys	HbS (O-Arab)	GAA→AAA	Migrates ~HbC. Heterozygote has ~15% HbS-Oman
S-South End	lys132asn	HbS (Yamagata)	GAG-GTG	Migrates like HbA on HPLC. Severe sickle cell disease when present with HbS
S-Travis	ala142val	HbS (---)	GCC→GTC	Migrates between HbS and HbF at alkaline pH and between HbA and HbS at acidic pH. Unstable, ~15% in heterozygote. Hematology normal

Shown are the non-HbS mutation and amino acid substitution. All cases have the *HBB* glu6val HbS mutation (http://globin.cse.psu.edu[9]). The mutations have been proven by gene analysis in only a few instances.

and might be no more common than in the general population, it does occur.[31] Little consensus exists on the use of prophylactic penicillin to prevent pneumococcal sepsis in HbS–β$^+$ thalassemia or other "mild" compound heterozygous forms of sickle cell disease.[31–33] A decision to use prophylactic penicillin in HbS–β thalassemia can be based on an approach similar to that for HbSC disease and is discussed in Chapters 19 and 21. In essence, this decision is predicated on an evaluation of splenic function, which if normal, argues for withholding prophylaxis. Pneumococcal vaccinations should be given and parents instructed to seek immediate medical attention for febrile illnesses.

Patients with HbS–β thalassemia and like disorders have a higher prevalence of proliferative retinopathy than do individuals with sickle cell anemia. They should be monitored like patients with HbSC disease (Chapter 21).

Continued and sometimes advancing splenomegaly predisposes affected individuals to splenic infarction, splenic sequestration episodes, and hypersplenism. These complications raise the issue of splenectomy and its timing during the evolution of the disease. Delaying splenectomy until the first recurrence of an episode of splenic sequestration seems reasonable. Hypersplenism or subacute splenic sequestration can be associated with worsening anemia and the need for transfusion. This might then dictate the need for splenectomy. Splenic infarcts can be painful, recurrent, and associated with intrasplenic hemorrhage. They may, depending on the severity of symptoms, also require splenectomy.

When general anesthesia is planned, based on observations in HbSC disease and in sickle cell anemia, using preoperative transfusion in patients with HbS–β$^+$ thalassemia who face procedures with moderate surgical risk, such as abdominal surgery, appears prudent.[34,35] Preoperative transfusions are likely to reduce the incidence of serious complications such as the acute chest syndrome.

SICKLING HEMOGLOBINS WITH TWO SUBSTITUTIONS IN THE β-GLOBIN GENE

Nine variant hemoglobins have been described with both the *HBB* glu6val mutation and an additional amino acid substitution in the same β-globin chain (Table 23.5). Some of these variants were likely to have arisen from crossing-over between a chromosome with the HbS mutation and a chromosome containing the other mutation. Hb Korle-Bu (*HBB* asp73asn*)* and HbO-Arab (*HBB* glu121lys) are sufficiently common to suggest that crossing-over between these genes and HbS genes account for the origin of HbC-Harlem (*HBB* glu6val; asp73asn) and S-Oman (*HBB* glu6val; glu121lys), respectively. For Hb Jamaica Plain (*HBB* glu6val; leu68phe), analysis of parental alleles suggested a new mutation on the proband's HbS gene.[36] In six instances (Table 23.5), the hemoglobin variant with the second mutation was characterized before the description of the HbS variant.

HbS-Antilles

HbS-Antilles (*HBB* glu6val; val23ile) was found in a black family from Martinique. Twenty-four heterozygotes with 40%–50% HbS-Antilles had hemolytic anemia with hemoglobin levels of 11 g/dL, reticulocytes of 4.5%, and MCV of 90 fL. Irreversibly sickled cells were present in the blood film. Heterozygotes for HbS-Antilles had recurrent painful episodes and splenomegaly. Three compound heterozygotes with HbS died with severe anemia and one child with HbS-Antilles/HbC had severe disease.

Like the erythrocytes of HbS homozygotes, HbS-Antilles red cells had reduced oxygen affinity but solutions of HbS-Antilles also had a low P_{50}. This variant had a C_{sat} – a measure of hemoglobin solubility – of 11.9 g/dL compared with 18.4 g/dL for HbS and 24.1 g/dL for an equal mixture of HbS and HbA. HbS-Antilles erythrocytes sickled at physiological pO_2. Ten percent to 20% of HbS-Antilles erythrocytes had increased density. The percentage of HbS-Antilles cells that sickled at pO_2 between 0 and 70 mm Hg was identical to HbSC disease erythrocytes. At a pO_2 between 40 and 90 mm Hg, the polymer fraction in HbS-Antilles cells was calculated to be similar to that present in erythrocytes of sickle cell anemia. These findings show that this variant polymerized more readily than HbS at any pO_2. HbS-Antilles polymerizes even when it comprises only half of the cellular hemoglobin, accounting for cellular damage and the symptoms of sickle cell disease in heterozygotes (Chapter 22) and the very severe phenotype in compound heterozygotes with HbS or HbC.

HbS-Oman

This variant, containing the HbS and HbO-Arab mutation, migrates more slowly than HbC when electrophoresed at alkaline pH because of an additional positive charge; β121 lys appears to stabilize the sickle polymer. C_{sat} was 11 g/dL, nearly identical to that of HbS-Antilles and lower than that of HbS. In all cases described to date, HbS-Oman has been associated with either heterozygous or homozygous α thalassemia-2 (Fig. 23.5). Homozygotes for this variant have not been described but are predicted to have very severe disease, resembling homozygotes with HbS-Antilles and perhaps made even worse by the presence of α thalassemia. Two different phenotypes appear to exist.[37] Patients with HbS-Oman–heterozygous α thalassemia-2 had more than 20% of the variant hemoglobin, low hemoglobin levels, MCV approximately 73 fL, splenomegaly, and vasoocclusive episodes including acute chest syndrome. Their sickle cells had a peculiar morphology described as "yarn/knitting needle" believed to be a consequence of one or two domains of HbS-Oman polymerization. Individuals with

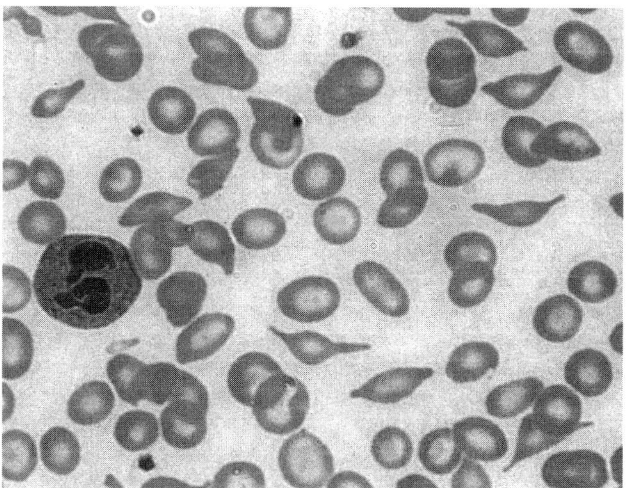

Figure 23.5. Erythrocytes in different genotypes of HbS-Oman disease. The peculiar shape of the irreversibly sickled cells has been called "yarn/knitting needle" and it presumed due to the polymerization of HbS-Oman in one or two domains.[37]

HbS-Oman–homozygous α thalassemia-2 had approximately 14% variant hemoglobin and further reduction of MCV. They were asymptomatic but had microcytosis. Interaction of this highly charged variant with the membrane, a general feature of hemoglobins with high positive charges like HbC and HbA_2, promotes dense cell formation and polymerization even at the relative low concentrations of HbS-Oman found in heterozygous HbS-Oman–heterozygous α thalassemia-2.

HbS-HbC Harlem

A compound heterozygote with HbS and HbS-HbC-Harlem had 50% HbS, 43% HbC-Harlem, and 7% HbF. Hematological findings were similar to those in sickle cell anemia, with vasoocclusive episodes and osteonecrosis of the hips requiring surgery. Heterozygous HbC-Harlem emulates HbAS. Equal mixtures of HbC-Harlem and HbS had gelling properties identical to 100% HbS, predicting that compound heterozygotes would resemble sickle cell anemia. Compound heterozygotes for HbAS and Hb Korle-Bu, however, do not differ from individuals with HbAS trait alone, indicating that in that variant, the β73 asp-asn substitution does not promote HbS polymerization.

Hb Jamaica Plain

An infant who was thought to have HbAS developed symptoms of sickle cell disease with hypoxia. The blood contained 27% of a variant hemoglobin that behaved like HbS. Genetic studies showed that the *HBB* leu68phe mutation occurred on the paternal HbS gene. Hb Jamaica Plain had reduced O_2 affinity, which was thought to account for its polymerization in the heterozygous carrier and the symptoms of sickle cell disease.[36]

HbS-South End

Another interesting variant is HbS-South End (*HBB* glu6val; lys132asn), described only in a compound heterozygote with HbS.[38] Severe sickle cell disease was present in the adult carrier of HbS-HbS-South End who, because HbS-South End comigrated with HbA on electrophoresis, was initially diagnosed as having HbS–β^+ thalassemia. It was presumed, but not proven experimentally, that the *HBB* lys132asn mutation in the HbS gene caused reduced oxygen affinity as it did when found as the simple heterozygote in Hb Yamagata.[39,40]

COMPOUND HETEROZYGOTES OF HbS WITH β-GLOBIN CHAIN VARIANTS

Examples Without a Clinical Phenotype

Many β-globin chain variants have been described as compound heterozygotes with HbS. In most examples, only one or a few cases have been reported and gauging the true extent of any hematological or clinical abnormalities is difficult because confounding genetic and acquired abnormalities are not always excluded. Most of these compound heterozygous combinations are not associated with any clinical disease, and if there are hematological abnormalities present, they are minor. Only when the site and type of amino acid substitution permits participation in the polymerization of HbS or the variant is unstable or is synthesized in vastly reduced amounts, as with Hb Monroe, is a clinically apparent phenotype apt to be present. Approximately one third of the β-globin chain variants found with HbS as compound heterozygotes do not separate from HbS by the alkaline electrophoresis as reported in the initial descriptions so the individuals who have these hemoglobins can be mistaken for patients with sickle cell anemia and counseled erroneously or treated incorrectly. More current methods of hemoglobin separation and family studies can usually resolve any confusion that might arise. Some compound heterozygotes with HbS that do not have a clinically significant phenotype are listed in Table 23.6.

Examples with a Clinical Phenotype

Some examples of compound heterozygosity for HbS and other β-globin gene variants associated with hematological or clinical findings are described only once or twice. Their associated phenotype is likely to be incompletely characterized. Often enough, the phenotype is ostensibly the result of the abnormal properties of the variant associated with HbS, usually instability, rather than due to the polymerization of HbS so that, strictly speaking, these examples might not be a type of sickle cell disease (Table 23.7).

HbO-Arab. HbO-Arab is a relatively common variant in blacks and individuals of Arabic descent and in both populations it has been associated with HbS. Together, the two variants can cause severe sickle cell disease. Because HbO-Arab migrates with HbC when electrophoresed at alkaline pH, HbS-O-Arab disease was confused often with HbSC disease. HPLC can separate HbC from HbO-Arab. Patients with unusually severe "HbSC disease" should be carefully evaluated for the presence of HbO-Arab. The β121 residue, also affected in HbD-Los Angeles, is a contact point in the HbS polymer, and substitutions at this residue increase the nucleation rate for polymer formation.

Thirty-nine patients with HbS-O-Arab have been reported, making an assessment of the clinical phenotype possible.[41] Individuals with HbS-O-Arab disease have hematological and clinical findings indistinguishable from patients with sickle cell anemia. In 13 African Americans with HbS-O-Arab disease, aged 3–63 years, mean hemoglobin concentration was 8.7 g/dL, reticulocytes 5.8%, and HbF 6.7%. Blood films showed target and sickled cells. Acute chest syndrome, stroke, leg ulcers, and painful episodes along with all of the other complications of sickle cell disease occurred in all patients. Four patients died: Two children died of pneumococcal sepsis, a teenager died of acute chest syndrome, and an adult from multiorgan failure.

HbD-Los Angeles (Punjab). Compound heterozygosity of HbD-Los Angeles (*HBB* glu121gln) with HbS, first described in Caucasians, produces hematological and clinical manifestations similar to those of sickle cell anemia. The β121 glutamine residue facilitates polymerization of HbS. This mutant, widespread throughout the world, is most common in Caucasians of Northern India. It is a typical HbD when evaluated by the older method of electrophoresis, but it can be separated from HbS and HbA by HPLC.

HbS-Oman and HbS-O-Arab, where the β 121 substitution is in *cis* or in *trans*, respectively, to the HbS mutation and where both conditions are associated with vasoocclusive disease, illustrate the clinical importance of mutations that stabilize the HbS polymer. In contrast, the *HBB* 73 residue, altered in Hb Korle-Bu, does not affect polymerization. Heterozygotes for HbC-Harlem, where the β 73 mutant is in *cis* to the sickle mutation, resemble HbAS. Only the HbS-HbC-Harlem compound heterozygote has sickle cell disease, and this is because of homozygosity for the HbS mutation and not the β 73 mutation in trans.

Hb Quebec-Chori. Hb Quebec-Chori (*HBB* thr87ile) migrated like HbA on alkaline electrophoresis and by isoelectric focusing, allowing the compound heterozygous state with HbS to be confused with HbAS. Reverse-phase HPLC and electrospray ionization mass spectroscopy separated this variant β-globin chain from β^A. Mixtures of Hb Quebec-Chori with HbS had the same delay time of

Table 23.6. Compound heterozygotes of HbS with β-globin chain variants lacking a clinical phenotype

Name	*HBB* Mutation	Properties
Hb Deer Lodge	his2arg	Migrates like HbS on alkaline electrophoresis. Compound heterozygotes appear like "sickle cell anemia"
HbG-San Jose	glu7gly	Migrates between HbF and HbS
Hb Saki	leu14arg	Migrates like HbA
HbJ-Baltimore	gly16asp	Separable by HPLC
Hb Sinai-Baltimore	val18gly	Migrates ∼HbA
HbD-Iran	glu22gln	Separable from HbA, ∼ to HbA_2 on HPLC
Hb Knossos	ala27ser	Migrates like HbA. A "thalassemic" variant. 40% in compound heterozygote with HbS
Hb Muscat	leu32val	Migrates like HbA. 48% in compound heterozygote with HbS
Hb Athens-Georgia	arg40lys	50% 'HbA' on HPLC
HbG Galveston	glu43ala	Migrates like HbS at alkaline pH, like HbA at acidic pH. Possibly mistaken for sickle cell anemia
Hb Maputo	asp47tyr	Migrates like HbS at alkaline pH, like HbA at acidic pH
Hb Osu-Christiansborg	asp52asn	Separable from HbA, ∼ to HbA_2 on HPLC. Possibly mistaken for sickle cell anemia on electrophoresis.
Hb Ocho Rios	asp52ala	Migrates like HbS at alkaline pH
Hb Korle-Bu	asp73asn	Common variant
Hb Mobile	asp73val	Can be confused electrophoretically with HbS
Hb Pyrgos	gly83asp	Migrates faster than HbA
HbD-Ibadan	thr87lys	Migrates like HbS at alkaline pH, like HbA at acidic pH
Hb Caribbean	leu91arg	Migrates between HbS and HbA
HbN-Baltimore	lys95glu	Separable by HPLC, common in blacks
Hb New Mexico	pro100arg	Migrates like HbS at alkaline pH, between HbS and HbC at acidic pH. High oxygen affinity variant with mild erythrocytosis. 54% with HbS
Hb Richmond	asn102lys	Migrates as 2 bands between HbS and HbA
HbP-Galveston	his117arg	Separable on HPLC
Hb Iowa	gly119ala	Migrates ∼HbF at alkaline pH. In neonate, electrophoresis was confused with HbSF pattern and sickle cell anemia was considered
Hb Hofu	val126glu	Migrates faster than HbA. 23% with HbS, mild anemia. This might be due to α thalassemia. No symptoms despite HbS of ∼70%
Hb Sesirade	ala129val	Unstable, 45% variant; Hb12.7
Hb K-Cameroon	ala129?	Amino acid substitution unclear, ?asp, ?glu
Hb Camden	gln131glu	Migrates faster than HbA at alkaline pH, near HbF at acidic pH
Hb K-Woolwich	lys132gln	Separable by HPLC
Hb McKees Rock	tyr145term	Migrates like HbA. High O_2 affinity variant
Hb Rainier	7tyr145cys	Migrates like HbA. High O_2 affinity variant

Many of these rare variants have not been examined by modern methods of HPLC so that their separation for other hemoglobins is reported only for electrophoresis or isoelectric focusing (http://globin.cse.psu.edu).

polymerization as pure HbS. A bulky hydrophobic isoleucine residue substituted at β87 might strengthen the hydrophobic environment in the acceptor pocket for β6 val, stabilize a lateral contact between HbS polymer strands, and accelerate polymerization. Other work has shown the importance of this site in polymer formation. Participation of this variant with HbS in the polymerization process caused vasoocclusive symptoms and the hematological phenotype of sickle cell disease in the compound heterozygote with HbS. Associated with a nonfunctional enlarged spleen, vasoocclusive episodes, mild anemia, reticulocytosis, sickled cells in the blood, HbS-Hb Quebec-Chori mimics sickle cell anemia and not HbAS. This rare condition, described in the literature twice, provides a cautionary note on the evaluation of clinically symptomatic instances of HbAS (Chapter 22). In one case, hydroxyurea treatment was associated with an increase of HbF.[42]

HbI-Toulouse. HbI-Toulouse (*HBB* lys66glu) was described in a boy with HbAS, splenomegaly, a hemoglobin level of 10.5 g/dL, reticulocytes of 7%, and MCV of 110 fL.

Table 23.7. Compound heterozygotes of HbS with β-globin chain variants with a clinical phenotype

Name	*HBB* Mutation	Phenotype
Hb Monroe	IVS-1–1 G→C; arg→thr	Severe HbS–β^0 thalassemia
HbO-Tibesti	val11ile; glu121lys	Severe, like HbS-O-Arab
HbE	glu26lys	Mild sickle cell disease
Hb Volga	ala27asp	Unstable, hemolytic anemia; Hb Volga elutes ~HbA on HPLC ~19%
Hb Lufkin	gly29asp	Migrates faster than HbA. Mildly unstable. ~45% in compound heterozygote with HbS. Mild hemolysis
Hb I-Toulouse	lys66glu	Migrates faster than HbS
Hb Quebec-Chori	thr87Ile	Causes sickle cell disease. 60% of hemolysate
Hb San Diego	val109met	Difficult to separate from HbA. High oxygen affinity variant with erythrocytosis
Hb Showa-Yakushiji	leu110pro	Unstable variant expressed as a β^0 thalassemia allele. 60% HbS, 36% HbF, Hb 10.7. MCV 63 fL
HbD-Los Angeles (Punjab)	glu121gln	Detectable by HPLC. Fourth most common Hb variant
HbO-Arab	glu121lys	Detectable using HPLC
Hb Shelby	gln131lys	Migrates like HbF at alkaline pH and between HbS and HbC at acidic pH. Mild instability, anemia, microcytosis, ~10 variant
Hb North Shore	val134glu	"Thalassemic" variant causing HbS–β^+ thalassemia-like phenotype
Hb Hope	gly136asp	Separable by HPLC

(http://globin.cse.psu.edu)[95]

Similar findings were present in a simple heterozygote for this variant, suggesting that it was the characteristics of this unstable hemoglobin rather than HbS responsible for the phenotype.

Hb San Diego. Hb San Diego (*HBB* val109met) is a high oxygen affinity variant described in diverse ethnic backgrounds and often results from a new mutation. It has been postulated that the ethnic diversity of this variant is a result of the mutation occurring at a CpG "hot spot" where deamination of methylcytosine leads to a C-T transition. In a compound heterozygote with HbS, approximately 70% of the hemolysate was Hb San Diego. Mild erythrocytosis with a hemoglobin of 18.8 g/dL and PCV 58 was caused by the high oxygen affinity variant and not by sickle cell disease.

Hb Shelby. Hb Shelby (*HBB* gln131lys), a mildly unstable variant, is associated with hemolytic anemia when present with HbS.[43] It appears to interact similarly with HbS and HbA. At age 4 years, the proband with HbS-Hb Shelby had a hemoglobin level of 9.8 g/dL, 14% reticulocytes, and MCV of 70 fL. Hb Shelby formed 43% of the hemolysate. Splenomegaly or vasoocclusive symptoms were absent. It is not clear why anemia was present in this compound heterozygote. Based on studies of simple heterozygotes for Hb Shelby, the phenotype of this combination most likely is due to Hb Shelby and not HbS polymerization.

Hb Hope. Hb Hope (*HBB* gly136asp) is mildly unstable and has reduced oxygen affinity. When present with HbS, it is associated with mild hemolytic anemia with a hemoglobin concentration of approximately 10 g/dL but normal reticulocyte counts and no symptoms of vasoocclusive disease.[44] In compound heterozygotes, approximately 50%–58% of the hemolysate was Hb Hope.[51] Cr red cell survival was reduced approximately 30%, and Heinz bodies were present in half the red cells. Hb Hope did not appear to affect HbS polymerization because the minimum gelling concentrations of mixtures of Hb Hope with HbS and HbA with HbS were similar. Lack of reticulocytosis was thought to result from the low oxygen affinity of Hb Hope. Again, the phenotype of this combination does not appear to be due to HbS polymerization.

Hb North Shore. Hb North Shore (*HBB* val134glu) is associated with the phenotype of mild β thalassemia. A patient with HbAS and Hb North Shore had mild hemolytic anemia, MCV of 71 fl, HbA_2 of 4.9%, and an α/β synthesis ratio of 3. These findings suggested that HbS polymerization did not contribute to the phenotype that was likely to be a reflection of the 'thalassemic' properties of this variant.[45]

Others. Severe sickle cell disease was associated with compound heterozygosity for HbS and two β-globin variants: HbC-Ndjamena (*HBB* glu6lys; trp37gly) and HbO-Tibesti (*HBB* val11ile; glu121lys) (Chapter 24, Table 24.8). The former contains the HbC mutation and the latter, the HbO Arab mutation, so it is not surprising that a clinically significant phenotype is found with these combinations.

HbSE Disease

HbSE disease was first reported from southern Turkey and has since been reported in the Middle East, India and Pakistan, Southeast Asia, North America, and the Caribbean.[46]

Table 23.8. Effects of α thalassemia in sickle cell anemia

Cellular
Reduced HbS polymer
Decreased cation exchange
Decreased erythrocyte density
Increased erythrocyte deformability
Prolonged erythrocyte lifespan
Clinical
Clinical events
Increased osteonecrosis
Increased splenic sequestration
Possible increased painful episodes
Increased incidence of acute chest syndrome
Fewer leg ulcers
Reduced incidence of pulmonary hypertension
Reduced incidence of priapism
Normalized transcranial Doppler flow studies
Fewer cerebrovascular accidents
Laboratory
Reduced hemolysis and increased PCV
Reduced lactate dehydrogenase, aspartate transaminase
Reduced reticulocytes

In Oman, HbSE disease was found in 0.05% of more than 600 children, a prevalence second only to sickle cell anemia, which was present in 0.2%.[47] Worldwide, HbS and HbE are the two most common variant hemoglobins, and with population migrations and intermarriages, increasingly more patients with HbSE disease will be encountered.

Hematological Findings and Diagnosis. In 26 patients with HbSE disease the hemoglobin level was either normal or mildly decreased with a mean of 11.2 +/− 1.8 g/dL in 24 individuals including children.[46] Hemoglobin levels as high as 14.6 g/dL in a 22-year-old African American man and 14.3 g/dL in a 31-year-old Turkish man were observed. Their MCV was slightly below the normal range. Data on variables that might affect the wide range of MCV, including the α-globin genotype, the degree of reticulocytosis, possible coexistent iron deficiency, or other chronic diseases were not always available. In 18 patients, reticulocyte counts varied from 0.5% to 4.3%. HbS accounted for 62.8% +/− 7.4%, and Hb E accounted for 33.3% +/− 3.6% of the hemolysate in 22 patients. HbF level varied from undetectable to 5.2%. Similarly heterogeneous hematological findings are seen in Hb S–β^+-thalassemia although in this genotype, the severity of the β^+-thalassemia mutation is the major determinant of the hematological and clinical phenotype.

The clinical laboratory diagnosis of HbSE can be problematic. HbE cannot be distinguished from some variant hemoglobins, such as HbC, by some still commonly used clinical laboratory electrophoretical techniques, but it is separable by HPLC, and DNA-based diagnostics are definitive. The level of HbS in the hemolysate is comparable to the level present in many patients with HbS–β^+ thalassemia.

Clinical Features. Although generally thought to be benign, HbSE disease can be symptomatic. Review of the literature showed that nine patients, aged 18 years and younger, were generally well; nevertheless, among 17 patients aged 20 years and older, nine presented with symptoms and findings usually ascribed to sickle cell disease.[46] Some patients had mild anemia, reticulocytosis, and hyperbilirubinemia, indicative of hemolysis. Other reported events in patients with HbSE disease included painful episodes, avascular necrosis of the hip and shoulder, acute chest syndrome, sickle cell retinopathy, bone marrow necrosis, hematuria, splenic infarction, splenic sequestration, splenomegaly, and cholelithiasis. Two patients developed acute chest syndrome, one following parvovirus B19 infection, accompanied by markedly elevated lactate dehydrogenase and hyperbilirubinemia. These sickling-related complications appeared mostly in adults who were aged 20 years or older. As asymptomatic patients with HbSE are less likely to be reported, these results are not necessarily representative of all patients with this genotype. In 12 cases of HbSE disease from six families reported from Oman, seven were aged younger than 20 years.[47] Only three individuals had symptoms of sickle cell disease.

Although patients with HbSE disease might have a relatively mild clinical course, they can develop all of the complications of sickle cell disease. Concomitant α thalassemia exerts significant effect on the clinical manifestations of patients with sickle cell anemia, and α thalassemia is likely to be present in some patients with HbSE disease. Hemoglobin subunit assembly is facilitated by electrostatic attraction between the positively charged α-globin chains and the negatively charged β-globin chains, predicting that with limiting amounts of available α-globin chains, the assembly of $\alpha\beta^S$ dimers is favored over the assembly of $\alpha\beta^E$-dimers. Consequently, the proportion of HbS might increase further, potentially causing more clinical complications. So far, none of the published reports on HbSE disease recorded the patients' α-globin genotype. Other genetic modifiers might also dictate whether patients with HbSE disease will develop sickling-related complications.

In summary, the previously held assumption that HbSE disease is a clinically benign disorder might not be entirely true. Perhaps half of patients older than 20 years have significant sickling-related complications, including the potentially serious acute chest syndrome. Although this high proportion of symptomatic adult patients with HbSE disease is possibly due to reporting bias, it underscores the importance of proper recognition and follow-up of patients with HbSE disease and the need to provide appropriate treatment when they develop sickling-related symptoms and complications.

Treatment Recommendations

Firm recommendations are hampered by the lack of knowledge of the natural history of HbSE disease. During the newborn period, patients should be vaccinated against pneumococcal and *Haemophilus influenzae* infections. The currently available and limited data show that children with HbSE disease are clinically well. Therefore, the need for penicillin prophylaxis and folic acid supplement is uncertain, and the same approach as recommended for HbSC disease might be applied. HbE is an oxidatively unstable hemoglobin and is more reactive than HbS in drug-induced oxidation. The coinheritance with pyrimidine 5′ nucleotidase deficiency or exposure to elevated temperature of 39°C–41°C in vitro have been reported to exacerbate HbE instability and hemolysis. If possible, avoiding prescribing oxidant drugs or compounds to these patients is advisable.

For surgery under general anesthesia, appropriate precautions have to be taken during the pre-, intra-, and postoperative period to guard against the development of sickling-related complications, especially acute chest syndrome. Preoperative exchange transfusions to reduce HbS concentration to less than 30% seems prudent. Simple transfusions in patients with hemoglobin levels near normal could be associated with an untoward rise in PCV and blood viscosity, suggesting that exchange transfusions might be preferable.

Hydroxyurea, used to treat sickle cell anemia has been used successfully in patients with HbS–β^+ thalassemia. When serious and/or repeated sickling-related complications occur in HbSE disease, a trial of hydroxyurea might be indicated.

SICKLE CELL ANEMIA–α THALASSEMIA

Early accounts of sickle cell anemia–α thalassemia were limited by the inability to definitively detect the common gene deletion α thalassemia. Because of this and the small number of patients studied, these reports could not accurately define the effect of α thalassemia on the phenotype of sickle cell anemia. DNA-based diagnosis of α thalassemia and its application to the study of large groups of patients have permitted the definition of the phenotype of sickle cell anemia–α thalassemia.[48–51] As the role of hemolysis as a major determinant of some subphenotypes of sickle cell anemia has emerged, the effects of α thalassemia as a genetic modulator of sickle cell disease have come into sharper focus (Chapter 27).

Among African Americans and other individuals of African descent with sickle cell anemia, 30%–40% are heterozygous and 2%–3% are homozygous for the common -$\alpha^{3.7}$ kb–deletion type of α thalassemia.[51] This genotype is also prevalent in Saudi Arabia and India. Some instances of sickle cell anemia with microcytosis without evidence of β thalassemia or gene-deletion α thalassemia could reflect the presence of nondeletion types of α thalassemia. Although uncommon in blacks, these mutations are not rare on the Arabian peninsula, the Middle East, and in North Africa and can be found with sickle cell anemia (Chapter 13) Infrequently, the $\alpha^{4.2}$-kb deletion and HbH disease have been found in individuals with the HbS gene.

Sickle cell anemia has also been described with triplicated α-globin loci. Few cases have been reported, and although they do not seem to differ from sickle cell anemia with a normal α-globin gene haplotype, it is not yet possible to know if the phenotype of the disease is affected.[52]

An extensive literature on the interaction of α thalassemia with sickle cell anemia is available and the following seems clearly established: α Thalassemia affects the cellular abnormalities, hematological values, and clinical features of sickle cell anemia; the extent of this effect is dependent on the α-globin gene haplotype; in a single patient the changes produced by α thalassemia can be subtle and difficult to detect; and differences among groups of patients are clear and clinically relevant.

Cellular Effects

α Thalassemia has multiple effects on the sickle erythrocyte that culminate in its improved cellular survival (Table 23.8). Reduced cellular hemoglobin content, a primary consequence of α thalassemia, is calculated to diminish the polymerization potential of HbS and the cascade of cellular damage that emanates from this phenomenon. Smaller sickle cells could also have rheological advantages that increase their survival. In sickle cell anemia–α thalassemia, the numbers of dense cells are reduced and fewer irreversibly sickled cells – cells that are least deformable and shortest lived – are present. The oxygen affinity of sickle cells, intrinsically low because of HbS polymer, might be increased in sickle cell anemia–α thalassemia by the improvement in cellular hydration and reduction in mean cell HbS concentration. Higher oxygen affinity should reduce the fraction of deoxy HbS, further retarding polymerization.

α Thalassemia reduces the density and increases the deformability of oxygenated sickle erythrocytes. When sickle cells of equal density were isolated from individuals with four, three, and two α-globin genes, they were equally deformable, showing that the improved deformability associated with α thalassemia was due to the presence of fewer dense cells. Improved deformability is probably related also to reduced cytoplasmic viscosity caused by a lower mean cell HbS concentration and the advantages of an increased cell surface:volume ratio. As PCV is the prime determinant of blood viscosity, the rheological benefit of enhanced deformability of the individual cell is lost when the PCV in sickle cell anemia–α thalassemia cell is increased due to improved cell survival. Whole blood viscosity in sickle cell anemia–homozygous α thalassemia-2 at a standard PCV of 45 was lower than viscosity of sickle cell anemia blood at the same PCV. When these groups were compared at the patient's original PCV, viscosity was higher in sickle cell anemia–α thalassemia.[53] An additional

Table 23.9. Effects of α-globin haplotype on the hematological features of sickle cell anemia

Genotype	Number	Hemoglobin (g/dL)	Reticulocytes (%)	MCV (fL)	HbF (%)	HbA_2 (%)
$\alpha\alpha/\alpha\alpha$	299	8.1	11.4	92	6.2	2.9
$-\alpha/\alpha\alpha$	152	8.6	9.0	83	5.7	3.3
$-\alpha/-\alpha$	66	9.2	6.7	72	5.1	3.8

The values reported are averages of studies that used gene mapping to ascertain the α-globin genotype. The series differed in the mean ages of the patients studied. One series combined the $-\alpha/\alpha\alpha$ and $-\alpha/-\alpha$ genotype together for hemoglobin, MCV, and HbF levels; only nine $-\alpha/-\alpha$ patients were in this series, and in this table these data were analyzed with the $-\alpha/\alpha\alpha$ genotype. The HbF differences are not significant; however, the patients were not segregated by β haplotype. In patients with α thalassemia and the Senegal haplotype, HbF levels are higher than in the other groups. The other differences are statistically significant.

benefit anticipated from increased cell surface: volume ratio is protection against deoxygenation-induced K^+ efflux induced by polymerization-provoked membrane distortion (Chapter 9). α Thalassemia protects against deoxygenation-induced cation leak and the rapid dehydration of reticulocytes that generates irreversibly sickled cells.[54] Effects of α thalassemia on red cell surface area to volume relationships might explain the lack of effect of α thalassemia on the severity of anemia in young children when persistent splenic function in childhood might condition sickle erythrocytes by removing excessive membrane.[55]

Hematological Effects

Hematological manifestations of sickle cell anemia–α thalassemia are a direct consequence of the cellular changes and are summarized in Table 23.9. Patients of African descent with sickle cell anemia–α thalassemia had increased levels of HbA_2, microcytosis, reduced reticulocyte counts, and higher hemoglobin levels. Patients homozygous for the $-\alpha^{3.7}$-kb deletion had more pronounced changes than heterozygotes for this haplotype. It was suggested that the lower mean corpuscular HbS concentration associated with α thalassemia resulted in retarded HbS polymerization, which reduced red cell injury. Higher hemoglobin levels and reduced reticulocyte counts suggested that hemolysis was likely to be reduced and studies of red cell survival in sickle cell anemia–α thalassemia confirmed this notion.[56]

HbA_2 levels are elevated in sickle cell anemia–α thalassemia, an effect that confounds its distinction from HbS–β^0 thalassemia. It is likely that δ-globin chains compete more effectively than β^S chains for the limited numbers of α-globin chains that are present in α thalassemia, favoring the assembly of HbA_2 over HbS.

Sickle cell anemia–α thalassemia was first thought to be associated with increased HbF levels, but subsequent studies have failed to confirm this observation, which was likely to have been the result of the examination of few patients. Hypothetically, γ-globin chains might compete more favorably than β^S chains for the reduced number of α chains available in sickle cell anemia–α thalassemia and increase HbF levels. Several large studies of sickle cell anemia–α thalassemia found little influence of α thalassemia on HbF concentration in sickle cell anemia, and other investigators found that α thalassemia reduced HbF in sickle cell anemia. It was hypothesized that the presence of both α thalassemia and HbF allowed some sickle erythrocytes to survive longer, masking the usual F cell enrichment characteristic of sickle cell anemia and reducing the total HbF level. When patients were stratified based on the β-globin gene haplotype, no effect of α thalassemia on HbF was observed.[57,58] HbF levels are unaltered by α thalassemia in children with sickle cell anemia and the Arab–India haplotype.[59]

Clinical Effects

α Thalassemia–related reduction in mean cell hemoglobin concentration lowers the polymerization tendency of HbS, forestalls erythrocyte injury, and leads to the production of smaller, less dense, more deformable cells. These cells have an increased survival and anemia is therefore improved. This reduction in hemolysis decreases the incidence of disease complications that are a consequence of the hemolysis-induced vasculopathy, but appears to increase the complications that are more dependent on blood viscosity (Chapters 11 and 19).

In one study, patients with sickle cell anemia–α thalassemia did not have an increased risk of pulmonary hypertension.[2] Priapism is more common in individuals with sickle cell anemia than in those with sickle cell anemia–α thalassemia or HbSC disease.[60,61] Age-adjusted comparisons showed that sickle cell anemia–α thalassemia and HbSC disease were more frequent among control patients than in patients with leg ulcers.[62] Coexistent α thalassemia protects patients with sickle cell anemia from stroke and is also associated with reduced cerebral blood flow.[63,64] The 'no stroke' group also had HbF levels twice as high as the stroke group but, even when controlling for the effects of HbF, α thalassemia was associated with a lower risk of stroke. Likewise, the prevalence of α thalassemia was significantly higher in children with normal transcranial Doppler flow rates than in patients with high flow velocity.[65] Chronic transfusions, by reducing plasma hemoglobin and other markers of hemolysis, might affect the risk of stroke by retarding hemolysis.[66] In several studies of stroke in sickle cell disease, stroke was associated with lower hemoglobin concentration.[20] None of 48 patients with homozygous α thalassemia-2 had a stroke. Although patients with silent cerebral infarct were more anemic than controls, there was

Table 23.10. Association of α-globin gene variants with HbS

Variant	*HBA* mutation*	Phenotype
Hb Memphis	glu23gln	Migrates like HbS at both alkaline and acidic pH
Hb Montgomery	leu48arg	Migrates between HbS and HbA at alkaline pH
Hb Mexico	gln54glu	With sickle cell trait, ~20% Hb Mexico and 50% hybrid hemoglobin
Hb G-Philadelphia	asn68lys	Migrates like HbS at alkaline pH and HbA at acidic pH. Usually, when found with HbS, mutation is linked to -$\alpha^{3.7}$ chromosome
Hb Stanleyville-II	α_2 asn78lys	Separable by HPLC or electrophoresis. Migrates like HbC at alkaline pH and HbA at acid pH and therefore, might be confused with HbSC disease
Hb Nigeria	ser81cys	Migrates faster than HbA and hybrid with β^S migrates faster than HbS at alkaline pH
HbG-Georgia	pro95leu	Migrates ~HbS at alkaline pH
Hb Hopkins-II	his112sp	Migrates ~HbA
Hb Oleander	α_2 glu116gln	20%–30% HbS; 9%–14% Hb Oleander and HbS hybrid (Also found with -$\alpha^{3.7}$ chromosome)
Hb Chicago	leu136met	Not separated by electrophoresis

* It is usually not known which of the two α-globin genes contain the mutation. (http://globin.cse.psu.edu; Chui DHK, personal communication).

no association of α thalassemia, reticulocyte count, aspartate transaminase, or bilirubin with this phenotype.[67]

Bayesian network modeling was used to estimate severity in patients with sickle cell anemia, sickle cell anemia–α thalassemia, and HbSC disease. A disease severity score ranking patients from least severe (0) to most severe (1), defining severity as risk of death within 5 years, was constructed. Subjects with sickle cell anemia were at greatest risk compared with subjects with sickle cell anemia–α thalassemia.[14]

Blood flow is optimal at the PCV found in most patients with sickle cell anemia. Presumably, as the PCV rises, viscosity-associated reductions in flow in some vascular beds promote sickle vasoocclusion. In sickle cell disease, the intrinsically abnormal properties of dense and poorly deformable sickle erythrocytes vastly increase blood viscosity at any given PCV. The common complications of acute painful episodes, acute chest syndrome, and avascular necrosis of bone might be particularly dependent on blood viscosity, and their incidence is increased by the presence of α thalassemia.[64] For example, osteonecrosis of the humeral and femoral heads had an incidence of 4.5–4.9 cases per 100 patient-years in sickle cell anemia–α thalassemia when compared with 2.4 cases for sickle cell anemia without α thalassemia.[15,68]

Cardiovascular function was examined in patients with sickle cell anemia who were homozygous for the common α thalassemia-2 deletion.[69] These individuals had increased left ventricular wall thickness with higher heart rates and blood pressure during exercise compared with patients with sickle cell anemia. The abnormalities noted in sickle cell anemia–α thalassemia suggested that the lower hemoglobin level in sickle cell anemia protects cardiac function. The inheritance of α thalassemia was associated with a 13% prevalence of macroalbuminuria compared with 40% in patients without α thalassemia.[70]

Reduced hemolysis in sickle cell anemia–α thalassemia predicts that cholelithiasis should be less common in this genotype, but any effect is outweighed by the genotype of the *UGT1A1* promoter.

α Thalassemia might increase the incidence of acute splenic sequestration episodes in children and adults with sickle cell anemia. Improved rheology of sickle erythrocytes in the presence of α thalassemia could preserve splenic function,[71] setting the stage for acute sequestration episodes at a later age than expected. A positive aspect of α thalassemia-related preserved splenic function, at least in individuals with the Arab–Indian haplotype and high HbF levels, is a reduction in bacterial infection.[59,72]

α Thalassemia was initially thought to increase survival in sickle cell anemia.[73,74] Other studies do not confirm this observation, and, in some studies, α thalassemia was a risk for increased morbidity and mortality.[48,75–78] α Thalassemia and markers of hemolysis were important elements of the modeling of near-term death.[14] Perhaps differences in the analytical approaches in these studies account for the variability of the results.

HbS with α-Globin Chain Variants

Separate inheritance of β- and α-globin genes permits a dizzying array of combinations of sickle cell disease and HbAS with α-globin gene variants and α thalassemia. In this section, the interactions of sickle cell anemia with α-globin gene variants are considered (Table 23.10). When variants of the α-globin gene are present, hybrid tetramers

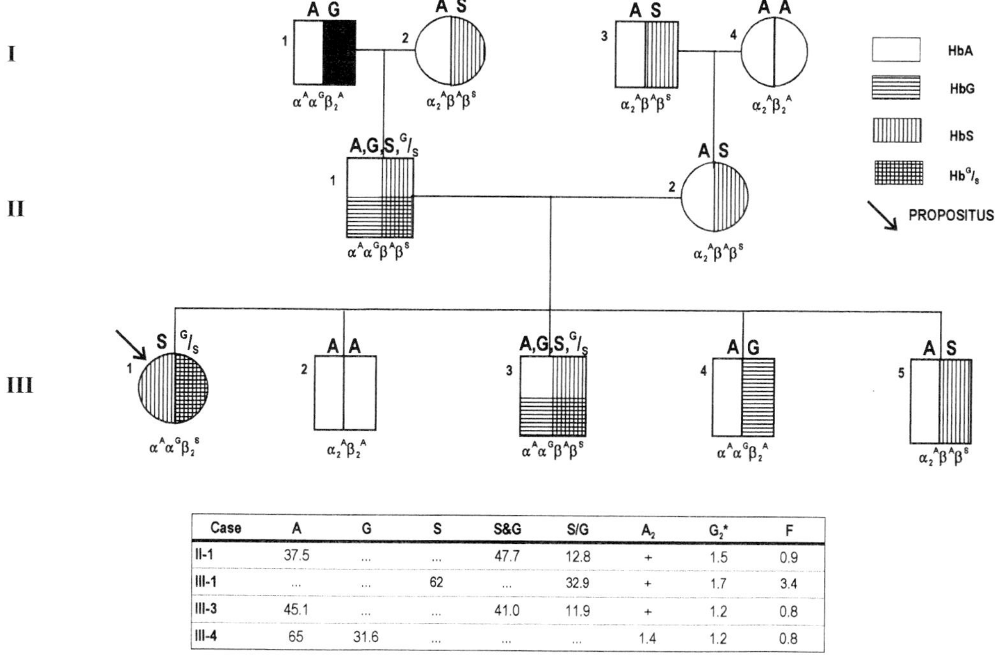

Case	A	G	S	S&G	S/G	A_2	G_2*	F
II-1	37.5	...	...	47.7	12.8	+	1.5	0.9
III-1	...	...	62	...	32.9	+	1.7	3.4
III-3	45.1	...	...	41.0	11.9	+	1.2	0.8
III-4	65	31.6	...	...	...	1.4	1.2	0.8

Figure 23.6. Pedigree of an extended family in which HbG-Philadelphia is present with sickle cell trait and sickle cell anemia. Below the pedigree, the percentage of different hemoglobin fractions is shown. (Redrawn from ref. 96.)

containing variant α-globin chains and normal α-globin chains are present. In the presence of β-globin chain mutants such as HbS and HbC additional hybrid tetramers form that can display unique electrophoretical or HPLC patterns. This often provides a clue or the diagnosis of disorders in which both α- and β-globin chain variants are present.

Many examples of the coincidence of HbG-Philadelphia (*HBA* asn68lys) and sickle cell anemia or HbAS have been described. In Figure 23.6, a pedigree and the hemoglobin fractions found in a family in which HbG-Philadelphia was present with sickle cell anemia and HbAS is shown. Figure 23.7 shows separation by HPLC of HbG-Philadelphia from HbS and HPLC separations of other variant hemoglobin from HbS. In sickle cell anemia, diagnostic confusion can occur because the hybrid molecule, $\alpha^A\alpha^G\beta_2{}^S$ might be confused with HbC if electrophoresis alkaline pH is the sole diagnostic method. Clinically and hematologically, sickle cell anemia–HbG-Philadelphia resembles sickle cell anemia and not HbSC disease. HbG-Philadelphia has been described in patients with HbSC disease in whom it was associated with a mild phenotype, perhaps because of the antipolymerization effect of the *HBA* asn68lys mutation.[79]

Sickle cell anemia has also been described with the α-globin gene variants Hb Montgomery (*HBA* leu48arg) and Hb Chicago (*HBA* leu136met).[80] An example of isoelectric focusing of these variants is shown in Figure 23.8.

Hb Memphis (*HBA* glu23gln) was described as migrating with HbS when electrophoresed at both alkaline and acidic pH. In older adults with sickle cell anemia, red cell survival was 11 days but vasoocclusive episodes were absent. The hemoglobin level was 9.5 g/dL, reticulocytes 5%–24%, MCV 88 fL, and HbF 6% and sickled cells were present in the blood. Curiously, in neither the proband nor three children in the family of the proband who had HbAS and Hb Memphis was there evidence of hybrid molecules that are typical of other α-globin gene variants. These observations anteceded the era of DNA-based diagnosis.

Hb Stanleyville-II (*HBA* pro77arg) was described in a boy from Zaïre with findings that were typical of sickle cell anemia, with 70% HbS and 30% Hb Stanleyville-II. A brother with sickle cell anemia had a more severe disease. Individuals with HbAS and Hb Stanleyville-II were well and had the expected distribution of HbA, Hb Stanleyville-II, and hybrid molecules. It was proposed that the mutation to arginine stabilized HbS fiber formation.

A report of a 3-year-old patient with sickle cell anemia and Hb Hopkins-II (*HBA* his112asp), a variant with high oxygen affinity, revealed mild anemia and reticulocytosis, no sickled cells in the blood, reduced MCV, and normal splenic function.

Mild sickle cell anemia was reported in a 34-year-old patient homozygous for the HbS gene and heterozygous for Hb Matsue-Oki (*HBA1* asp75asn).[81] This α_2-globin gene variant affects a contact site between deoxy HbS polymer strands. $\alpha^{\text{Matsue-Oki}}{}_2\beta^S{}_2$ tetramers formed 28% of the hemolysate and migrated on cellulose acetate electrophoresis like HbC. Hb Matsue-Oki migrates like HbS, and heterozygotes have between 12% and 24% of this variant. Although no clinical information was provided in the

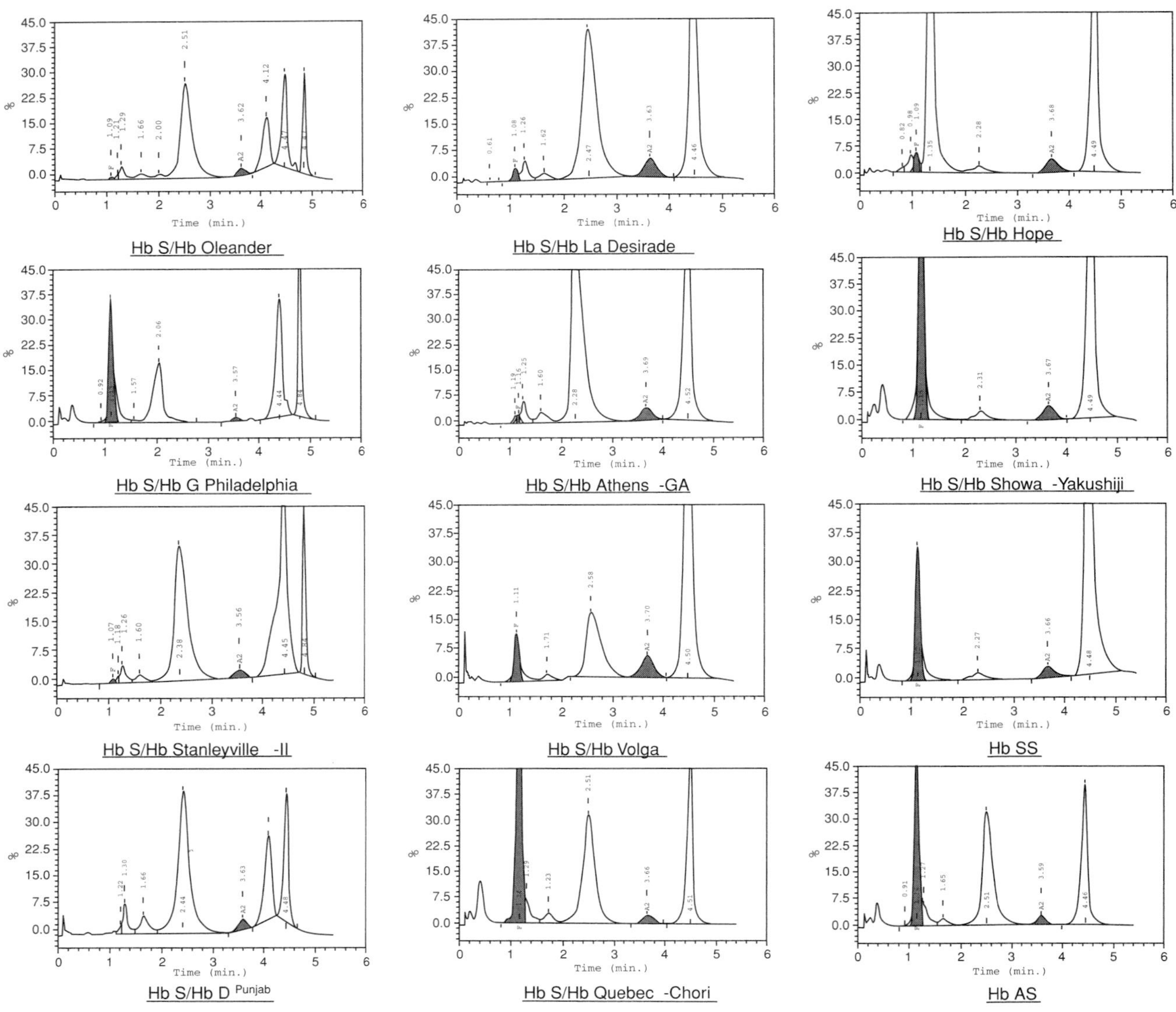

Figure 23.7. HPLC separation of variant hemoglobin found with HbS. Representative HPLC tracings of some common and rare hemoglobin variants associated with HbS. All hemoglobins were verified by DNA sequencing. For comparison, tracings from an HbS homozygote and carrier of HbAS are shown. Retention times obtained with the Beckman Variant II system are shown in or above the peaks. Note that the retention of some variants such as Hb Quebec-CHORI (*HBB* thr87ile) and Hb Volga (*HBB* ala27asp) cannot be resolved from HbA. α-Globin variants such as Hb Oleander (*HBA* glu116gln) and Hb G Philadelphia have peaks representing hybrid tetramers. Hb Showa-Yakushiji (*HBB* leu110pro) is hyperunstable and no protein can be recovered, therefore, HPLC is identical to sickle cell anemia.

initial report of this compound heterozygote, it was implied that the phenotype was milder than that of HbSC disease, with which it might be confused.

HbS with Other Globin Variants

Variants of the γ-globin chains and the δ-globin chain are also found with homozygosity and heterozygosity for the HbS gene. Although they might cause diagnostic confusion, they are not associated with hematological or clinical sequelae. γ-Globin gene variants are usually detected in infants in whom they can form up to 30% of the total hemoglobin and similar proportions of the HbF fraction. As γ-globin gene expression diminishes, these variants are reduced to a minor fraction of the small amount of remaining HbF and are usually undetectable.

HbA_2', (*HBD* gly16arg) is found in approximately 1% of individuals of African descent and is the most common δ-globin gene variant. Migrating more slowly than HbA_2 on electrophoresis at alkaline pH, it is often found in sickle cell anemia and HbAS (Chapter 22).

Individuals with HbAS have been described with the βδ-globin gene crossover variant Hb P-Nilotic (Congo) (β through residue 22, δ from residue 50). Pedigrees, in which

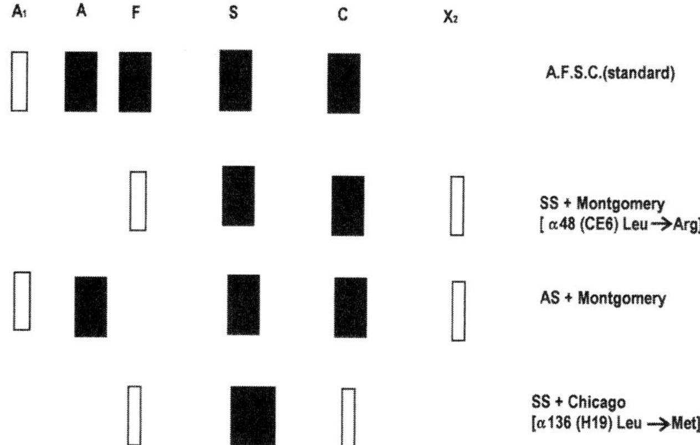

Figure 23.8. Isoelectric focusing of hemolysates from sickle cell trait and sickle cell anemia with Hb Montgomery and sickle cell anemia with Hb Chicago. These α-globin gene variants display confusing patterns by hemoglobin electrophoresis and isoelectric focusing. Redrawn from ref. 80.

the affected but hematologically normal individual had HbS, HbA, and HbP-Nilotic, confirm that the chromosome with the fusion gene contained a normal β-globin gene. In the compound heterozygote with HbS, there was 40% HbS, 35% HbA, 22% HbP-Nilotic, and 2.3% HbA_2.[29]

CONCLUSION

HbS can be present with different forms of α or β thalassemia and dozens of abnormal hemoglobins. Phenotypes associated with these genetic combinations can be pernicious or benign, and the management of clinically significant phenotypes should follow the guidelines proposed for sickle cell anemia or HbSC disease. The correct delineation of the genotype is clinically important for genetic counseling.

REFERENCES

1. Kato GJ, Gladwin MT, Steinberg MH. Deconstructing sickle cell disease: Reappraisal of the role of hemolysis in the development of clinical subphenotypes. *Blood Rev.* 2007;21:37–47.
2. Taylor JG, Ackah D, Cobb C, et al. Mutations and polymorphisms in hemoglobin genes and the risk of pulmonary hypertension and death in sickle cell disease. *Am J Hematol.* 2008;83:6–14.
3. Eberhardt RT, McMahon L, Duffy SJ, et al. Sickle cell anemia is associated with reduced nitric oxide bioactivity in peripheral conduit and resistance vessels. *Am J Hematol.* 2003;74(2):104–111.
4. Cannon RO, III, Schechter AN, Panza JA, et al. Effects of inhaled nitric oxide on regional blood flow are consistent with intravascular nitric oxide delivery. *J Clin Invest.* 2001;108(2):279–287.
5. Nath KA, Katusic ZS, Gladwin MT. The perfusion paradox and vascular instability in sickle cell disease. *Microcirculation.* 2004;11:179–194.
6. Belhassen L, Pelle G, Sediame S, et al. Endothelial dysfunction in patients with sickle cell disease is related to selective impairment of shear stress-mediated vasodilation. *Blood.* 2001;97(6):1584–1589.
7. Aessopos A, Farmakis D, Tsironi M, et al. Endothelial function and arterial stiffness in sickle-thalassemia patients. *Atherosclerosis.* 2006;92(2):427–432.
8. Strickland DK, Ware RE, Kinney TR. Pitfalls in newborn hemoglobinopathy screening: Failure to detect β^+-thalassemia. *J Pediatr.* 1995;127:304–308.
9. Huisman THJ, Carver MFH, Baysal E. *A Syllabus of Thalassemia Mutations.* 1st ed. Augusta, GA: The Sickle Cell Anemia Foundation; 1997.
10. Sweeting I, Serjeant BE, Serjeant GR, Kulozik AE, Vetter B. Hb S-Hb Monroe: a sickle cell β-thalassemia syndrome. *Hemoglobin.* 1998;22(2):153–156.
11. Baklouti F, Francina A, Dorleac E, et al. Association in cis of β^+-thalassemia and hemoglobin S. *Am J Hematol.* 1987;26:237–245.
12. Pacheco P, Peres MJ, Faustino P, et al. β-thalassaemia unlinked to the β-globin gene interacts with sickle-cell trait in a Portuguese family. *Br J Haematol.* 1995;91:85–89.
13. Viprakasit V, Gibbons RJ, Broughton BC, et al. Mutations in the general transcription factor TFIIH result in β-thalassaemia in individuals with trichothiodystrophy. *Hum Mol Genet.* 2001;10(24):2797–2802.
14. Sebastiani P, Nolan VG, Baldwin CT, et al. Predicting severity of sickle cell disease. *Blood.* 2007;110:2727–2735.
15. Milner PF, Kraus AP, Sebes JI, et al. Sickle cell disease as a cause of osteonecrosis of the femoral head. *N Engl J Med.* 1991;325:1476–1481.
16. West MS, Wethers D, Smith J, Steinberg MH, Cooperative Study of Sickle Cell Disease. Laboratory profile of sickle cell disease: A cross-sectional analysis. *J Clin Epidemiol.* 1992;45:893–909.
17. Platt OS, Brambilla DJ, Rosse WF, et al. Mortality in sickle cell disease. Life expectancy and risk factors for early death. *N Engl J Med.* 1994;330(23):1639–1644.
18. Platt OS, Thorington BD, Brambilla DJ, et al. Pain in sickle cell disease-rates and risk factors. *N Engl J Med.* 1991;325:11–16.
19. Castro O, Brambilla DJ, Thorington B, et al. The acute chest syndrome in sickle cell disease: Incidence and risk factors. *Blood.* 1994;84:643–649.
20. Ohene-Frempong K, Weiner SJ, Sleeper LA, et al. Cerebrovascular accidents in sickle cell disease: Rates and risk factors. *Blood.* 1998;91(1):288–294.
21. Zafeiriou DI, Prengler M, Gombakis N, et al. Central nervous system abnormalities in asymptomatic young patients with Sbeta-thalassemia. *Ann Neurol.* 2004;55(6):835–839.
22. Kolquist KA, Vnencak-Jones CL, Swift L, Page DL, Johnson JE, Denson MR. Fatal fat embolism syndrome in a child with undiagnosed hemoglobin S/β^+ thalassemia: a complication of acute parvovirus B19 infection. *Pediatr Pathol Lab Med.* 1996;16:71–82.
23. Desselle BC, O'Brien T, Bugnitz M, Beaty O, Wilimas JA, Helton K. Fatal fat embolism in a patient with sickle-β^+ thalassemia. *Pediatr Hematol Oncol.* 1995;12:159–162.
24. Johnson K, Stastny JF, Rucknagel DL. Fat embolism syndrome associated with asthma and sickle cell-β^+-thalassemia. *Am J Hematol.* 1994;46:354–357.
25. Zaidi Y, Sivakumaran M, Graham C, Hutchinson RM. Fatal bone marrow embolism in a patient with sickle cell β^+ thalassaemia. *J Clin Pathol.* 1996;49:774–775.

26. Kalotychou V, Antonatou K, Tzanetea R, Terpos E, Loukopoulos D, Rombos Y. Analysis of the A(TA)(n)TAA configuration in the promoter region of the UGT1 A1 gene in Greek patients with thalassemia intermedia and sickle cell disease. *Blood Cells Mol Dis.* 2003;31(1):38–42.
27. Kerkhoffs JL, Harteveld CL, Wijermans P, et al. Very mild pathology in a case of Hb S/β^0-thalassemia in combination with a homozygosity for the alpha-thalassemia 3.7 kb deletion. *Hemoglobin.* 2000;24(3):259–263.
28. Murray N, Serjeant BE, Serjeant GR. Sickle cell-hereditary persistence of fetal haemoglobin and its differentiation from other sickle cell syndromes. *Br J Haematol.* 1988;69:89–92.
29. Huisman THJ. Compound heterozygosity for Hb S and the hybrid Hb S Lepore, P- Nilotic, and Kenya: comparison of hematological end hemoglobin composition data. *Hemoglobin.* 1997;21:249–257.
30. Goncalves I, Henriques A, Raimundo A, et al. Fetal hemoglobin elevation in Hb Lepore heterozygotes and its correlation with beta globin cluster linked determinants. *Am J Hematol.* 2002;69(2):95–102.
31. Rogers ZR, Buchanan GR. Risk of infection in children with hemoglobin S-beta-thalassemia. *J Pediatr.* 1995;127:672.
32. Rogers ZR, Buchanan GR. Bacteremia in children with sickle hemoglobin C disease and sickle beta(+)-thalassemia: is prophylactic penicillin necessary? *J Pediatr.* 1995;127:348–354.
33. Buchanan GR. Infection. In: Embury SH, Hebbel RP, Mohandas N, Steinberg ME, eds. *Sickle Cell Disease: Basic Principles and Clinical Practice.* 1st ed. New York: Lippincott-Raven; 1994:567–587.
34. Vichinsky EP, Haberkern CM, Neumayr L, et al. A comparison of conservative and aggressive transfusion regimens in the perioperative management of sickle cell disease. *N Engl J Med.* 1995;333:206–213.
35. Neumayr L, Koshy M, Haberkern C, et al. Surgery in patients with hemoglobin SC disease. *Am J Hematol.* 1998;57(2):101–108.
36. Geva A, Clark JJ, Zhang Y, Popowicz A, Manning JM, Neufeld EJ. Hemoglobin Jamaica Plain–a sickling hemoglobin with reduced oxygen affinity. *N Engl J Med.* 2004;351(15):1532–1538.
37. Nagel RL, Daar S, Romero JR, et al. Hb S-Oman heterozygote: a new dominant sickle syndrome. *Blood.* 1998;92:4375–4382.
38. Luo HY, Adewoye AH, Eung SH, et al. A novel sickle hemoglobin: hemoglobin S-South End. *J Pediatr Hematol Oncol.* 2004;26(11):773–776.
39. Han JY, Wee JH, Kim JM, Kim JY, Kim IH, Rodgers GP. A new observation of Hb Yamagata with a different nucleotide substitution: beta 132 AAA-->AAT. *Hemoglobin.* 1996;20(2):165–168.
40. Harano T, Harano K, Ueda S, Imai K, Marubashi S. Hb Yamagata [beta 132(H10)Lys---Asn]: a new abnormal hemoglobin in a Japanese family. *Hemoglobin.* 1990;14(2):207–211.
41. Zimmerman SA, O'Branski EE, Rosse WF, Ware RE. Hemoglobin S/O_{ARAB}: Thirteen new cases and review of the literature. *Am J Hematol.* 1999;60(4):279–284.
42. Tubman VN, Bennett CM, Luo HY, Chui DH, Heeney MM. Sickle cell disease caused by Hb S/Quebec-CHORI: treatment with hydroxyurea and response. *Pediatr Blood Cancer.* 2007;49(2):207–210.
43. Adachi K, Surrey S, Tamary H, et al. Hb Shelby [β131(H9) Gln-->Lys] in association with Hb S [β6(A3)Glu-->Val]: characterization, stability, and effects on Hb S polymerization. *Hemoglobin.* 1993;17:329–343.
44. Ingle J, Adewoye A, Dewan R, et al. Hb Hope [β136 (H14)Gly-->Asp (GGT-->GAT)]: interactions with Hb S [β6(A3)Glu-->Val (GAG-->GTG)], other variant hemoglobins and thalassemia. *Hemoglobin.* 2004;28(4):277–285.
45. Smith CM, Hedlund B, Cich JA, et al. Hemoglobin North Shore: a variant hemoglobin associated with the phenotype of beta-thalassemia. *Blood.* 1983;61:378–383.
46. Masiello D, Heeney M, Adewoye AH, Eung SH, Steinberg MH, Chui DHK. HbSE disease; a concise review. *Am J Hematol.* 2007;82:643–649.
47. Knox-Macaulay HH, Ahmed MM, Gravell D, Al-Kindi S, Ganesh A. Sickle cell-haemoglobin E (HbSE) compound heterozygosity: a clinical and haematological study. *Int J Lab Hematol.* 2007;29(4):292–301.
48. Higgs DR, Aldridge BE, Lamb J, et al. The interaction of alpha-thalassemia and homozygous sickle-cell disease. *N Engl J Med.* 1982;306:1441–1446.
49. Embury SH, Dozy AM, Miller J, et al. Concurrent sickle-cell anemia and alpha-thalassemia: effect on severity of anemia. *N Engl J Med.* 1982;306:270–274.
50. Embury SH. The interaction of alpha-thalassemia with sickle cell anemia. *Hemoglobin.* 1988;12:509–517.
51. Steinberg MH, Embury SH. Alpha-thalassemia in blacks: genetic and clinical aspects and interactions with the sickle hemoglobin gene. *Blood.* 1986;68:985–990.
52. Higgs DR, Clegg JB, Weatherall DJ, Serjeant BE, Serjeant GR. Interaction of the ααα globin gene haplotype and sickle haemoglobin. *Br J Haematol.* 1984;57:671–678.
53. Serjeant BE, Mason KP, Kenny MW, et al. Effect of alpha thalassaemia on the rheology of homozygous sickle cell disease. *Br J Haematol.* 1983;55:479–486.
54. Embury SH, Backer K, Glader BE. Monovalent cation changes in sickle erythrocytes: a direct reflection of α-globin gene number. *J Lab Clin Med.* 1985;106:75–79.
55. Stevens MC, Maude GH, Beckford M, et al. Alpha thalassemia and the hematology of homozygous sickle cell disease in childhood. *Blood.* 1986;67:411–414.
56. De Ceulaer K, Higgs DR, Weatherall DJ, Hayes RJ, Serjeant BE, Serjeant GR. alpha-Thalassemia reduces the hemolytic rate in homozygous sickle-cell diseas. *N Engl J Med.* 1983;309:189–190.
57. Steinberg MH, Hsu H, Nagel RL, et al. Gender and haplotype effects upon hematological manifestations of adult sickle cell anemia. *Am J Hematol.* 1995;48(3):175–181.
58. Steinberg MH, Lu Z-H, Barton FB, et al. Fetal hemoglobin in sickle cell anemia: Determinants of response to hydroxyurea. *Blood.* 1997;89:1078–1088.
59. Adekile AD, Haider MZ. Morbidity, βs haplotype and α-globin gene patterns among sickle cell anemia patients in Kuwait. *Acta Haematol.* 1996;96:150–154.
60. Nolan VG, Wyszynski DF, Farrer LA, Steinberg MH. Hemolysis-associated priapism in sickle cell disease. *Blood.* 2005;106(9):3264–3267.
61. Kato GJ, McGowan V, Machado RF, et al. Lactate dehydrogenase as a biomarker of hemolysis-associated nitric oxide

resistance, priapism, leg ulceration, pulmonary hypertension, and death in patients with sickle cell disease. *Blood.* 2006;107(6):2279–2285.

62. Nolan VG, Adewoye A, Baldwin C, et al. Sickle cell leg ulcers: associations with haemolysis and SNPs in Klotho, TEK and genes of the TGF-β/BMP pathway. *Br J Haematol.* 2006;133(5):570–578.
63. Adams RJ, Kutlar A, McKie V, et al. Alpha thalassemia and stroke risk in sickle cell anemia. *Am J Hematol.* 1994;45(4): 279–282.
64. Neonato MG, Guilloud-Bataille M, Beauvais P, et al. Acute clinical events in 299 homozygous sickle cell patients living in France. French Study Group on Sickle Cell Disease. *Eur J Haematol.* 2000;65(3):155–164.
65. Hsu LL, Miller ST, Wright E, et al. Alpha thalassemia is associated with decreased risk of abnormal transcranial Doppler ultrasonography in children with sickle cell anemia. *J Pediatr Hematol Oncol.* 2003;25(8):622–628.
66. Lezcano NE, Odo N, Kutlar A, Brambilla D, Adams RJ. Regular transfusion lowers plasma free hemoglobin in children with sickle-cell disease at risk for stroke. *Stroke.* 2006;37(6):1424–1426.
67. Kinney TR, Sleeper LA, Wang WC, et al. Silent cerebral infarcts in sickle cell anemia: a risk factor analysis. *Pediatrics.* 1999;103(3):640–645.
68. Milner PF, Kraus AP, Sebes JI, et al. Osteonecrosis of the humeral head in sickle cell disease. *Clin Orthop.* 1993;289: 136–143.
69. Braden DS, Covitz W, Milner PF. Cardiovascular function during rest and exercise in patients with sickle-cell anemia and coexisting alpha thalassemia-2. *Am J Hematol.* 1996;52:96–102.
70. Guasch A, Zayas CF, Eckman JR, Muralidharan K, Zhang W, Elsas LJ. Evidence that microdeletions in the alpha globin gene protect against the development of sickle cell glomerulopathy in humans. *J Am Soc Nephrol.* 1999;10(5):1014–1019.
71. Wali YA, Al Lamki Z, Hussein SS, et al. Splenic function in Omani children with sickle cell disease: correlation with severity index, hemoglobin phenotype, iron status, and alpha-thalassemia trait. *Pediatr Hematol Oncol.* 2002;19(7):491–500.
72. Adekile AD, Tuli M, Haider MZ, Al-Zaabi K, Mohannadi S, Owunwanne A. Influence of α-thalassemia trait on spleen function in sickle cell anemia patients with high HbF. *Am J Hematol.* 1996;53:1–5.
73. Mears JG, Lachman HM, Labie D, Nagel RL. Alpha thalassemia is related to prolonged survival in sickle cell anemia. *Blood.* 1983;62:286.
74. Martinez G, Muniz A, Svarch E, Espinosa E, Nagel RL. Age dependence of the gene frequency of α-thalassemia in sickle cell anemia in Cuba. *Blood.* 1996;88:1898–1899.
75. Keclard L, Romana M, Lavocat E, Saint-Martin C, Berchel C, Merault G. Sickle cell disorder, β-globin gene cluster haplotypes and α-thalassemia in neonates and adults from Guadeloupe. *Am J Hematol.* 1997;55(1):24–27.
76. Keclard L, Ollendorf V, Berchel C, Loret H, Merault G. beta S haplotypes, α-globin gene status, and hematological data of sickle cell disease patients in Guadeloupe (F.W.I.). *Hemoglobin.* 1996;20(1):63–74.
77. Powars DR, Chan L, Schroeder WA. Beta S-gene-cluster haplotypes in sickle cell anemia: clinical implications. *Am J Pediatr Hematol Oncol.* 1990;12(3):367–374.
78. Thomas PW, Higgs DR, Serjeant GR. Benign clinical course in homozygous sickle cell disease: a search for predictors. *J Clin Epidemiol.* 1997;50:121–126.
79. Lawrence C, Hirsch RE, Fataliev NA, Patel S, Fabry ME, Nagel RL. Molecular interactions between Hb α-G Philadelphia, HbC, and HbS: phenotypic implications for SC α-G Philadelphia disease. *Blood.* 1997;90(7):2819–2825.
80. Gu L-H, Wilson JB, Molchanova TP, McKie KM, McKie VC, Huisman THJ. Three sickle cell anemia patients each with a different α chain variant. Diagnostic complications. *Hemoglobin.* 1993;17:295–301.
81. Witkowska E, Asakura T, Tang D, et al. Compound heterozygote for Hb S and Hb Matsue-Oki α75(EF4)Asp->Asn presents with a mild sickle cell disease phenotype. *Blood.* 1998;92; 525a.
82. Altay C, Öner C, Öner R, et al. Genotype-phenotype analysis in HbS-beta-thalassemia. *Hum Hered.* 1997;47:161–164.
83. Divoky V, Baysal E, Schiliro G, Dibenedetto SP, Huisman THJ. A mild type of Hb S-β^+-thalassemia [-92(C-->T)] in a Sicilian family. *Am J Hematol.* 1993;42:225–226.
84. Gonzalez-Redondo JM, Stoming TA, Lanclos KD, et al. Clinical and genetic heterogeneity in black patients with homozygous β-thalassemia from the southeastern United States. *Blood.* 1988;72:1007–1014.
85. Gonzalez-Redondo JM, Kutlar F, Stoming TA, De Pablos JM, Kilinc Y, Huisman THJ. Hb S(C)β^+-thalassaemia: different mutations are associated with different levels of normal Hb A. *Br J Haematol.* 1988;70:85–89.
86. Gonzalez-Redondo JM, Kutlar A, Kutlar F, et al. Molecular characterization of Hb S(C) β-thalassemia in American blacks. *Am J Hematol.* 1991;38:9–14.
87. Huisman TH. Combinations of β chain abnormal hemoglobins with each other or with β-thalassemia determinants with known mutations: influence on phenotype. *Clin Chem.* 1997;43(10):1850–1856.
88. Padanilam BJ, Felice AE, Huisman THJ. Partial deletion of the 5′ β-globin gene region causes β^0-thalassemia in members of an American black family. *Blood.* 1984;64:941–944.
89. Waye JS, Chui DHK, Eng B, et al. Hb S/β^0-thalassemia due to the ~1.4-kb deletion is associated with a relatively mild phenotype. *Am J Hematol.* 1991;38:108–112.
90. Patterson M, Walker L, Eng B, Waye JS. High Hb A_2 β-thalassemia due to a 468 bp deletion in a patient with Hb S/β-thalassemia. *Hemoglobin.* 2005;29(4):293–295.
91. Lacan P, Ponceau B, Aubry M, Francina A. Mild Hb S-β^+-thalassemia with a deletion of five nucleotides at the polyadenylation site of the β-globin gene. *Hemoglobin.* 2003;27(4):257–259.
92. Andersson BA, Wering ME, Luo HY, et al. Sickle cell disease due to compound heterozygosity for Hb S and a novel 7.7-kb β-globin gene deletion. *Eur J Haematol* 2007;78(1):82–85.
93. Steinberg MH, Rosenstock W, Coleman MB, et al. Effects of thalassemia and microcytosis upon the hematological

and vaso-occlusive severity of sickle cell anemia. *Blood.* 1984;63:1353–1360.

94. Serjeant GR, Asfcroft MT, Serjeant BE, Milner PF. The clinical features of sickle-cell β thalassaemia in Jamaica. *Br J Haematol.* 1973;24:1930–30.

95. Luo HY, Heeney M, Wang WC, et al. Hemoglobinopathies mimicking Hb S/beta-thalassemia: Hb S/S with α-thalassemia and Hb S/Volga. *Am J Hematol.* 2006;81(5):361–365.

96. Charache S, Zinkham WH, Dickerman JD, Brimhall B, Dover GJ. Hemoglobin SC, SS/GPhiladelphia and SO_{Arab} disease: diagnostic importance of an integrative analysis of clinical, hematologic and electrophoretic findings. *Am J Med.* 1977;62:439–446.

SECTION SIX

OTHER CLINICALLY IMPORTANT DISORDERS OF HEMOGLOBIN

Martin H. Steinberg

Three chapters discuss rare inherited hemoglobinopathies including unstable hemoglobins, hemoglobins with altered oxygen affinity, hemoglobins easily oxidized, and a miscellaneous group of hemoglobin variants with interesting biological properties, some of which are clinically important. Acquired disorders of hemoglobin can arise from heme iron oxidation due to inherited abnormalities of hemoglobin-reducing enzymes or because of exposure to exogenous oxidizing agents.

Rare hemoglobinopathies have taught us much about the structure-stability-function relationships of hemoglobin. Hemoglobin mutants have provided the most comprehensive list of mutations of any system in human biology, creating a map for understanding mutation in other genetic loci. Globin gene mutations – these include nearly every class of mutation so far described – provided an early catalog of the possible mechanisms of genetic disease.

An accounting of globin gene mutations in early 2008 listed 1,326 unique mutations (http://globin.cse.psu.edu/). Here, we discuss some rare hemoglobin mutations. As comparatively few globin residues are critical for maintaining the structural integrity and functional utility of the molecule, most hemoglobin mutations are not associated with hematological or clinical abnormalities and so escape detection. Some mutations, although not medically important, illustrate interesting biological and anthropological principles.

Abnormal hemoglobins with high or low oxygen affinity, variants that have their heme iron oxidized to the ferric form causing methemoglobinemia (HbM), or hemoglobin variants that are unstable are abnormalities seen rarely by the general physician and infrequently encountered in the practice of hematology. High oxygen affinity hemoglobin variants cause erythrocytosis; low oxygen affinity variants can be accompanied by cyanosis and anemia; HbM variants present with cyanosis. Patients with unstable hemoglobins can have hemolytic anemia that might worsen during infection and when certain drugs are given. Because these uncommon variants are unusual causes of erythrocytosis, cyanosis, and hemolytic anemia, their presence is often unsuspected. When present, their identification can prevent hazardous diagnostic tests, forestall potentially dangerous treatments, permit reassurance of the patients, and allow family counseling.

In evaluating these disorders, tests for hemoglobin instability are useful and measurement of the hemoglobin–oxygen dissociation curve is vital when a hemoglobin variant is suspected of causing erythrocytosis or cyanosis. Methemoglobins are suspected by observing an abnormal brown coloration of the blood and spectrophotometric recording of the visible spectrum of the hemolysate. Mutation detection by DNA analysis is the only way of definitively diagnosing rare hemoglobin variants.

24

Unstable Hemoglobins, Hemoglobins with Altered Oxygen Affinity, Hemoglobin M, and Other Variants of Clinical and Biological Interest

Martin H. Steinberg and Ronald L. Nagel

INTRODUCTION

Mutations of hemoglobin can be polymorphic (>1% of a population), like HbS, HbE, HbC, and the thalassemias, or rare. Our first edition listed 750 unique hemoglobin variants; this number is now more than 1,000.[1] In this chapter we address rare mutations. Some are associated with clinical disease; others are interesting solely for the biological principles they illustrate. A current listing of variant human hemoglobins is maintained in the HbVar database at http://globin.cse.psu.edu/, and the journal *Hemoglobin* (Taylor & Francis, Philadelphia) is a rich source for reports of new variants. Both are invaluable resources for clinicians and investigators with interests in unusual hemoglobin disorders.

Globin gene mutations, which include nearly every class of mutation so far described, except trinucleotide repeats and other nucleotide expansions associated with neuromuscular disorders, provided an early catalog of the mutations that can cause genetic disease. Clinically important but rare mutants affect hemoglobin stability causing premature red cell destruction; interfere with normal oxygen binding kinetics producing erythrocytosis; and permit heme iron oxidation, causing cyanosis. Most rare variants have no phenotype and are of biological and diagnostic interest only.

Comparatively few globin residues are critical for maintaining the structural integrity and functional performance of the molecule (Chapter 6). Hemoglobin gene mutations are, as a rule, not associated with hematological or clinical abnormalities and escape detection, especially when they are chromatographically silent.

Large-scale population screening programs have defined the worldwide prevalence of medically important hemoglobinopathies and thalassemias. Most of the hemoglobin variants known today were discovered as a byproduct of this extensive effort. Unlike some thalassemia mutations and HbS, HbE, and HbC, almost none of these variant hemoglobins are polymorphic because they are genetically neutral and their carriage does not provide a selective advantage. Sometimes, in population isolates, there is a founder effect leading to a higher than expected prevalence of a particular mutation. The geographical distribution of hemoglobin variants in the Americas, Europe, Africa, the former USSR, the Middle East, India, southeast Asia, China, Japan, the Antipodes, and Oceania have been cataloged.[2] It is unlikely that new globin mutations that reach polymorphic frequencies will be found. In unexamined population isolates, some new variants present at high frequency might yet be uncovered and sporadic examples of new and already described variants will continue to be unearthed.

Mutation Distribution

More than 90% of hemoglobinopathies result from point mutations. Some globin gene codons are associated with as many as seven different mutations; others have one or no described mutations, suggesting both mutational "hot spots" and sites resistant to mutation.

Mutations have been described in approximately 75% and 95% of α- and β-globin gene codons. Multiple different mutations are described in amino acid residues that are functionally important so that a clinical phenotype brings the substitution to clinical attention. For example, seven mutations have been described at β99, all associated with high oxygen affinity variants and erythrocytosis. Four of the six variants of α141 for which information is available have increased oxygen affinity. Six mutations at β92 are all associated with unstable hemoglobins and hemolytic anemia. In contrast, the five mutations described at the β22 codon are all stable and functionally normal. It is not known if these sites are particularly prone to mutational events or if we are witnessing a bias of ascertainment in which some these mutations are identified because of their obvious phenotype.

Only 20% of the possible globin gene mutations have been described. Clinically silent variants are still likely to escape notice, and many variants that cause a change in the charge of the molecule, simplifying their detection, have been already delineated. Neutral substitutions in which the charge of the molecule is unchanged and a phenotype is not present are rarely detected.

Among hemoglobin mutants, β-globin gene variants are most frequently described whereas α-, γ-, and δ-globin gene variants are reported 65%, 20%, and 10% as often, respectively. This preponderance of β-globin gene variants might reflect the fact that with only two β-globin genes, the intracellular concentration of β-globin variants exceeds that of α-globin variants so they are more likely to be clinically apparent (Chapter 13). For example, a high oxygen affinity variant present at 40%–50% total hemoglobin, the level of most β-globin gene mutants, is more likely to cause clinically apparent erythrocytosis than a similar α-globin

Table 24.1. Sites of globin mutation that are associated with increased oxygen affinity. In addition to single amino acid substitutions, these mutations can include small deletions and insertions of amino acids, reading frameshifts, fusion globins, and elongated globin chains

$\alpha1\beta2$ interface contacts (sliding contact) connecting $\alpha1\beta1$ and $\alpha2\beta2$ dimers
$\alpha1\beta1$, $\alpha2\beta2$ interface
Mutations that reduce 2,3-BPG binding
Heme pocket mutations
Miscellaneous

gene variant present at the usual level of 20%–25%. Some α-globin variants might go unnoticed because of their low levels in the blood. Certain α-globin mutations are more likely to be lethal because α chains are also essential for the functional hemoglobins of the embryo and fetus (Chapter 7). α-Globin chains must also bind three types of non-α-globin chains, β-, γ-, and δ-globin chains to form tetramers, increasing their chance of being functionally incompetent if mutated.

Very low concentrations of HbA_2 and HbF in adults often preclude the detection of an abnormal variant of the δ and γ-globin genes (Chapter 7). Only rarely do γ-globin chain abnormalities have a clinical phenotype in neonates and this usually is due to methemoglobinemia and cyanosis. Structural variants of the embryonic ε- and ζ-globin chains have not been described.

HEMOGLOBINS WITH ALTERED OXYGEN AFFINITY

High Oxygen Affinity Hemoglobins

Globin gene mutations can increase the affinity of the hemoglobin molecule for oxygen and cause erythrocytosis transmitted as a dominant trait. Approximately 100 high oxygen affinity variants have been reported.[3] Although familial erythrocytosis is a valuable clue to the presence of a high oxygen affinity hemoglobin variant, new mutations cause isolated cases. These α- or β-globin chain mutations are expressed clinically in the heterozygote; they might be lethal in homozygotes if they affect the α-globin chain as this will affect embryonic and fetal hemoglobins. Several homozygotes for β-globin high oxygen affinity variants have been described and these individuals might have more severe disease.[4–7] High oxygen affinity hemoglobins have also been described with β^0 thalassemia, and as HbA is not present, they mimic homozygosity for the variant.

Pathophysiology. Stabilization of the relaxed (R) state of the hemoglobin tetramer (high oxygen affinity) or destabilization of the tense (T) state (low oxygen affinity) is caused by mutations in critical areas of the globin chain affecting the R-T transition (Table 24.1) (see Chapter 6).

The increased avidity for oxygen (low P_{50}) of these variants reduces oxygen delivery to tissues stimulating erythropoietin production and increasing red cell mass. Patients with high oxygen affinity hemoglobins and the erythrocytosis that results from relative tissue hypoxia had normal urine erythropoietin levels but showed increases in erythropoietin when phlebotomized to a normal red cell mass. They might be reasonably compensated for the low P_{50} by the increased red cell mass and probable increases in tissue blood flow, along with changes in perfusion patterns in selected regions of the body that negate any adverse effect of increased blood viscosity. Oxygen consumption and arterial pO_2 are normal but occasionally there is reduced mixed venous pO_2 and decreased resting cardiac output.

Diagnosis. The diagnosis of high oxygen affinity hemoglobins is suggested by the following: isolated erythrocytosis without accompanying leukocytosis, thrombocytosis and splenomegaly that is typical in polycythemia vera; a family history of erythrocytosis; reduced P_{50} (partial pressure of oxygen where hemoglobin is half-saturated Fig. 24.1). DNA sequencing defines the mutation. Not unexpectedly, the *JAK2* V617F mutation found in most individuals with polycythemia vera is absent in patients with high oxygen affinity hemoglobin variants.[8]

Determination of the red cell oxygen equilibrium curve (Fig. 24.1) is the benchmark for the diagnosis of erythrocytosis due to high oxygen affinity hemoglobins. The oxygen-binding characteristics of hybrid tetramers ($\alpha_2\beta^A\beta^{var}$) are likely to be intermediate between purified HbA and purified variant and the shape of the hemoglobin oxygen dissociation curve can at times be biphasic. Measurement of blood P_{50} confirms the shift in the hemoglobin–oxygen dissociation curve. Rarely, the whole blood P_{50} is normal, requiring study of dialyzed purified hemoglobin. An accurate P_{50}

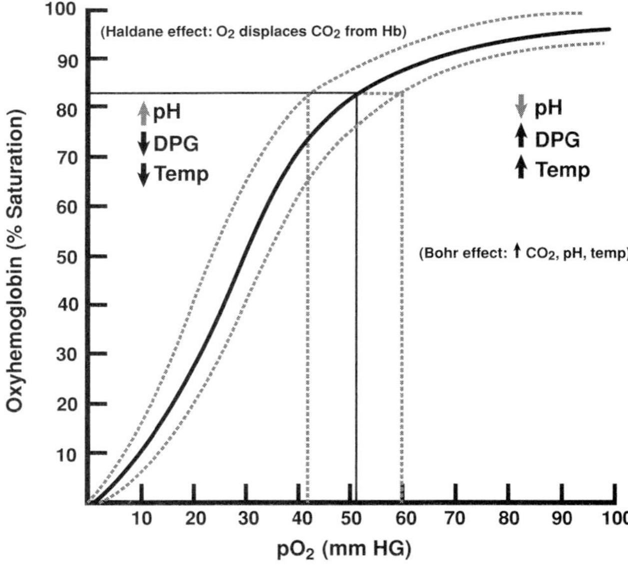

Figure 24.1. Hemoglobin–oxygen dissociation curve. As the P_{50} drops (the curve is left-shifted) the affinity of hemoglobin for oxygen increases. An increased P_{50} decreases hemoglobin–oxygen affinity.

value cannot be "calculated" from pO_2 data and directly measuring the saturation of hemoglobin and pO_2 is necessary. P_{50} measurements are not widely available but can be done with several instruments.

Both erythrocytes and purified dialyzed hemoglobin will have high oxygen affinity and 2,3-BPG concentrations should be normal, suggesting that altered oxygen affinity is not caused by reduced levels of this heterotopic modulator of hemoglobin function (Chapter 6). When 2,3-BPG mutase deficiency is present, red cell levels of 2,3-BPG will be low and whereas erythrocytes or whole blood will have high oxygen affinity red cells, the oxygen affinity of the purified hemolysate stripped of this intermediate will be normal.

In addition to high oxygen affinity hemoglobins, disorders expressed in the erythrocyte that cause isolated erythrocytosis include, 2,3-BPG mutase mutations that reduce the synthesis of this modulator of hemoglobin–oxygen affinity, some instances of methemoglobinemia and chronic carbon monoxide poisoning (Chapter 25).

The search for the mutation is initiated by high-performance liquid chromatography (HPLC) analysis of hemoglobin but normal studies do not exclude the diagnosis of a high-affinity hemoglobin that can migrate with HbA. As with all evaluations for abnormal hemoglobins, determining the DNA sequence of the globin genes provides the definitive information.

Some examples of high oxygen affinity hemoglobins, illustrating the varying mechanisms and heterogeneous clinical findings seen with these variants, are discussed later. A detailed understanding of the structure of hemoglobin and the importance of each residue in determining function allows a molecular explanation of most of the clinical abnormalities observed.

α-Globin Chain Variants. Because of a gene dosage effect, most stable α-globin variants form approximately 25% of the total hemoglobin. As a result, the clinical effects of α-globin variants are less striking than those of similar β-globin variants that usually comprise 50% of total hemoglobin, although coincident thalassemia can modulate the concentration of variant hemoglobins.

The first report of a high oxygen affinity hemoglobin was that of a patient aged 81 years with erythrocytosis, an abnormal hemoglobin detected by hemoglobin electrophoresis, and erythrocytes with increased oxygen affinity (Hb Chesapeake; *HBA* arg92leu). Fifteen members of the proband's family were similarly affected.[9] Hb Chesapeake represented approximately 20% of the total hemoglobin. With a P_{50} of 19 mm Hg (normal ~26 mm Hg), Hb Chesapeake produced moderate erythrocytosis. The mutation affected an invariant residue that stabilized the R-state at the $\alpha_1\beta2$ area of contact, making the T conformer less favored.

Hb Nunobiki (*HBA1* arg141cys) is one of four mutations of this invariant residue, all of which exhibit high oxygen affinity and moderate to mild erythrocytosis. This group of mutations represents an interesting cluster of variants that illustrate the effects of different mutations at the same amino acid residue. As a mutant of the 3′ *HBA1* gene that is expressed to a lesser extent than 5′ *HBA2* gene, Hb Nunobiki makes up approximately 13% of the hemolysate and is accompanied by only mild erythrocytosis. High oxygen affinity is due to the breaking of the C terminal–C terminal salt bridge indispensable for the stabilization of the T-state, favoring the R-state.

β-Globin Chain Variants. All possible single base mutations of the β99 site disturbing the α1β2 area of contact have been described and include Hb Kempsey (*HBB* asp99asn), Hb Yakima (asp99his), Hb Radcliffe (asp99ala), Hb Ypsilanti (asp99tyr), Hb Hotel-Dieu (asp99gly), Hb Chemilly (asp99val), and Hb Coimbra (asp99glu). As expected for stable β-globin chain variants, all are present at 40%–50% of the hemolysate, exhibit moderately high oxygen affinity, and are characterized clinically by erythrocytosis. Other properties of this group of mutants include: moderately decreased response to 2,3-BPG with Hbs Kempsey and Radcliffe and slightly decreased response to 2,3-BPG in Hb Hotel Dieu. Hbs Ypsilanti and Radcliffe form stable hybrid tetramers in the hemolysates in which the abnormal β chains coexist with normal β chains.

Six of the possible seven mutations of the C-terminal CAC (tyr) codon have also been described. One of them, Hb Cochin-Port Royal (tyr146arg), has nearly normal oxygen affinity but decreased 2,3 BPG interaction and Bohr effect.

Three mutations of β82 lys have been described: Hb Rahere (lys82thr), Hb Helsinki (lys82met), and Hb Providence (lys82asn). All have moderately high oxygen affinity and moderate erythrocytosis. These mutants have drastically reduced 2,3-BPG binding due to the elimination of one of the normal binding sites for this allosteric effector.

Hb Porto Alegre (*HBB* ser9cys) has high oxygen affinity and a tendency to aggregate (see later) but erythrocytosis is not present. Oligomerization of this mutant diminishes heme–heme interaction and increases the oxygen affinity.

Hb Tak (*HBB* 147[+AC], modified C-terminal sequence 147thr-lys-leu-ala-phe-leu-leu-ser-asn-phe-157tyr-COOH) is elongated by 11 amino acid residues. It forms 40% of the hemolysate and has a very high oxygen affinity with no cooperativity and no allosteric interaction with pH or 2,3-BPG. The C-terminal of the β-globin chain is actively involved in the conformational changes of the hemoglobin molecule by stabilizing the T-state. By having these stabilizing interactions disrupted, Hb Tak is totally frozen in the R-state. It is also slightly unstable. Despite these severe functional abnormalities, the heterozygous patient did not have erythrocytosis. The extreme biphasic nature of the hemoglobin–oxygen affinity curve observed in mixtures of Hb Tak and HbA suggested that hybrid tetramer ($\alpha_2\beta^A\beta^{Tak}$) formation is absent. The top portion of the oxygen equilibrium curve is normal and begins to be abnormal only below 40% saturation. Because physiological oxygen exchange occurs most commonly above that level of saturation, the tissues might not be hypoxic, removing the stimulus for increased erythropoiesis.

Clinical Aspects. Patients with high-affinity hemoglobins and erythrocytosis have a benign clinical course and rarely have complications, apart from a ruddy complexion. Splenomegaly is typically absent. Hemoglobin concentration and packed cell volume are increased variably, and usually only moderately, suggesting that modulation by variations in other genes might affect the physiological response to hypoxia. Some patients with Hb Malmo (*HBB* his97gln) have been reported to be symptomatic and to benefit from phlebotomy and the transfusion of normal blood, but this is an exception.

Many cases of high oxygen affinity hemoglobins are diagnosed during a routine hematological examination or when the family of a proband known to have erythrocytosis is examined. In very limited studies, exercise capacity in the laboratory and the indices of working capacity and cardiac tolerance were similar in patients with high oxygen affinity hemoglobins and controls. It has been suspected that carriers' of these variants could have enhanced athletic performance under some circumstances and this has lead to the unfortunate and sometimes fatal use of erythropoietin or transfusion to enhance performance in competitive athletics.

If high-affinity hemoglobins are diagnosed early, unnecessary invasive diagnostic procedures and inappropriate therapeutic interventions such as cardiac catheterization can be avoided. Patients have received phosphorus-32 treatment based on a mistaken diagnosis of polycythemia vera.

Increased morbidity or mortality in mothers or their offspring with high oxygen affinity hemoglobins has not been observed, suggesting that the affinity of the mother's hemoglobin is irrelevant with respect to oxygen delivery to the fetus. Low ambient pO_2, as in unpressurized airplanes and ascent to altitude, does not represent a risk because high-affinity hemoglobins are avid for oxygen. Hypothetically, carriers would be less prone to "the bends" during deep sea diving because of slower oxygen release during ascension.

Treatment. Patients with high oxygen affinity hemoglobins have reasonable compensation for their abnormality with adequate tissue oxygen delivery despite increases in blood viscosity. Intervention is therefore rarely required. Exercise studies before and after phlebotomy in patients with Hb Osler (*HBB* tyr145asn), a variant with a P_{50} of 10–11 mm Hg and a hemoglobin concentration of approximately 22 g/dL, did not show impairment after phlebotomy.[10] Limited studies have suggested that phlebotomy does not improve exercise performance.

Although individuals seldom benefit from phlebotomy, unknown factors might interfere with their normal compensation for high hemoglobin oxygen affinity, and increased blood viscosity might become a burden. Prudence dictates that before embarking on a regimen of chronic phlebotomy, one should be conservative and review the hematological and physiological findings at 6-month intervals during the first few years after diagnosis. In older patients special attention should be directed to the adequacy of blood flow to the heart and central nervous system.

Variants with Low Oxygen Affinity

Hemoglobin variants with reduced affinity for oxygen are in many respects the clinical obverse of high oxygen affinity variants. Expressed in the heterozygotes, with homozygosity likely to be embryonic lethal, these variants, which are far less common than variants with high oxygen affinity, are associated with anemia and at times are accompanied by cyanosis.

Pathophysiology. Alterations of critical molecular regions directly involved in the R-T transition result in the stabilization of the T-state or destabilization of the R-state. Low oxygen affinity hemoglobins deliver more oxygen to the tissues per gram of hemoglobin, and this is reflected by an oxygen–hemoglobin dissociation curve shifted toward the right of normal, and an increase in P_{50} (Fig. 24.1). When hemoglobin has a right-shifted or low affinity curve, the difference between oxygen binding in the lungs at pO_2 levels of 100 mm Hg and unloading in the tissues at 40 mm Hg can be twice as great as the differences in a hemoglobin with a normal oxygen equilibrium curve. Patients with moderately right-shifted oxygen equilibrium curve (P_{50} between 35 and 55 mm Hg) could be anemic. With a further right shift (P_{50} ~80) anemia is not present.

A right-shifted oxygen equilibrium curve leads to an increase in the synthesis of 2,3-BPG and decrease in its destruction.

Diagnosis. Approximately half as many low oxygen affinity variants have been described compared with high oxygen affinity variants. The first report of such a hemoglobin was Hb Kansas (*HBB* asn102thr) in a patient who presented with asymptomatic cyanosis without anemia or hemolysis. Detection of a low oxygen affinity hemoglobin is part of the differential diagnosis of patients with cyanosis. Before undertaking extensive diagnostic procedures in cases of cyanosis that are not clearly due to cardiovascular or pulmonary disease, obtaining hemoglobin HPLC and measuring blood P_{50} is advisable. A search for low affinity hemoglobins as an explanation for anemia without cyanosis is less compelling but if other investigations prove fruitless, unexplained normocytic anemia without reticulocytosis might be evaluated by measuring P_{50}.

A simple bedside test to distinguish cyanosis due to low oxygen affinity hemoglobins and cardiopulmonary cyanosis from that of methemoglobinemia, M hemoglobins, and sulfhemoglobinemia (Chapter 25) is to expose blood to pure oxygen. Blood from carriers of low oxygen affinity hemoglobins or patients with cardiopulmonary disease will turn from purple-greenish to the bright red. Blood of patients with methemoglobinemia, sulfhemoglobinemia, and M hemoglobins will remain abnormally colored.

Clinically apparent cyanosis is only observed in carriers of low oxygen affinity variants with greatly right-shifted curves and in whom the variant comprises a substantial portion of the hemolysate. Cyanosis is present from birth in some low oxygen affinity hemoglobins due to α-globin chain mutants. In carriers of β-globin chain mutants, cyanosis can appear from the middle to the end of the first year of life as γ-globin gene expression and HbF synthesis wanes and is replaced by β-globin gene expression and HbA. Globin gene sequencing is the sole means of definitive diagnosis

Clinical Features. Three low oxygen affinity variants have been described at β102. Hb Kansas, the best-studied variant, has a whole blood P_{50} of approximately 70 mm Hg, decreased cooperativity, and a normal Bohr effect. The β102 asn residue is invariant among β-globin chains and participates in the only hydrogen bond between asn102 and asp 94 across the α1β2 interface in oxyhemoglobin. This bond is broken when the molecule assumes the T-state. The new thr residue is incapable of forming this bond and low oxygen affinity results from destabilization of the R conformer. The changes induced by this substitution at the α1β2 interface allow Hb Kansas to dissociate into αβ dimers, the near opposite of the high oxygen affinity Hb Chesapeake.

Hb Beth Israel (*HBB* asn102ser) was found in a patient with cyanosis of the fingers, lips, and nail beds. The P_{50} was 88 mm Hg and arterial blood was only 63% saturated despite a normal pO_2. The hemolysate also had a low oxygen affinity and a normal Bohr effect. Erythrocyte 2,3-BPG was mildly elevated. The molecular mechanism of reduced oxygen affinity is the same as for Hb Kansas, although the defect might be more disruptive locally as the serine side chain is shorter than that of threonine.

Hb Bologna (*HBB* lys61met) was informative as it was present as a compound heterozygote with β^0 thalassemia and comprised 90% of the hemolysate. During development, the effects of this mutation were unlikely to be manifest because of high HbF concentrations and adults were neither cyanotic nor anemic despite Hb Bologna forming nearly 50% of the hemolysate and having a P_{50} of 37.6 mm Hg.

Hb Bruxelles (phe42del) is a deletion of the most conserved amino acid residue of hemoglobin. Phenylalanine residues at β41 and β42 are conserved in all normal mammalian non-α-globin chains and are indispensable for the structural integrity and oxygen-binding functions of the molecule. From age 4 years, the index case of Hb Bruxelles had severe hemolytic anemia and cyanosis, requiring blood transfusion once. Later in life, her hemoglobin concentration stabilized at 10 g/dL. Reasons for this "switch" of phenotype are unknown. Other mutations of β41 and β42, which are predominately unstable hemoglobins, are discussed later.

In individuals with low oxygen affinity variants, the oxygen saturation measured using pulse oximetry can be spuriously reduced.[6,11] Attention should be paid to measurement of blood oxygen saturation when any hemoglobin variant is present. Blood oxygen saturation can be measured using an arterial blood gas analyzer, by pulse oximetry, and by using a CO oximeter. The first method measures blood partial pressure of dissolved oxygen and provides the paO_2 and saO_2. The convenient pulse oximeter provides a transcutaneous measure of absorbance at two wavelengths (660 and 940 nm) but is inaccurate when dyshemoglobins, such as methemoglobin (hemoglobin with oxidized [Fe^{+3}] heme iron), carboxyhemoglobin, and sulfhemoglobin are present. CO oximetry, the most accurate of all the methods, can be inaccurate in cases of M hemoglobins.[12]

Oxygen saturation calculated from pH and pO_2 should be interpreted with caution as the algorithms used assume normal hemoglobin oxygen affinity, normal 2,3-BPG concentrations, and no dyshemoglobin such as methemoglobin or hemoglobinopathies. CO oximeter reports should include the dyshemoglobin fractions besides the oxyhemoglobin fraction. In cases of an increased methemoglobin fraction, pulse oximeter values trend toward 85%, underestimating the actual oxygen saturation. Hemoglobin M variants can have normal methemoglobin levels and increased carboxyhemoglobin or sulfhemoglobin fractions measured by CO oximetry.

Treatment. Treatment for these variants is not needed. The importance of the early diagnosis is to avoid unnecessary work-up and to alleviate concern for the patient and family.

UNSTABLE HEMOGLOBINS

Globin chain mutations can cause hemoglobin tetramer instability and intracellular precipitation of its globin subunits. These mutants, sometimes called collectively, congenital Heinz body hemolytic anemia, cause intraerythrocytic precipitates that are detectable by supravital staining, and that appear as globular aggregates called Heinz bodies (Fig. 24.2). The inclusions reduce variably the life of the erythrocyte by binding to the membrane, decreasing cell deformability, and increasing membrane permeability. Erythrocyte enzyme deficiencies can also cause Heinz bodies and hemolysis. More than 135 unstable variants of both the β- and α-globin chains with widely varying clinical severity have been reported (Fig. 24.3), usually as heterozygotes, although some homozygous cases have been reported. Anemia, reticulocytosis, pigmenturia, and splenomegaly are the major clinical features.[13]

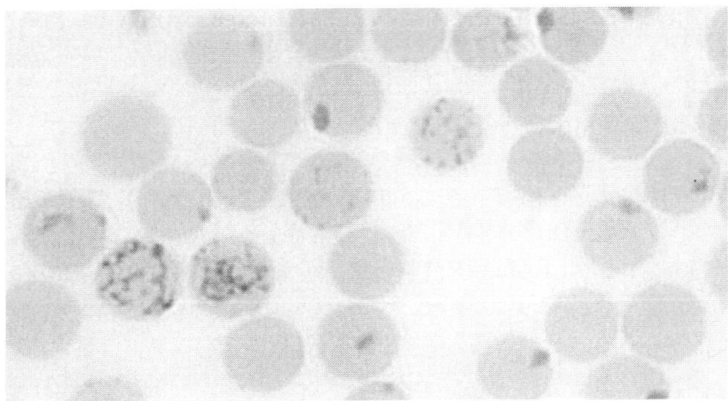

Figure 24.2. Heinz bodies. Heinz bodies are the large, single basophilic inclusions inside erythrocytes. Other red cell inclusions represent reticulocytes. (See color plate 24.2.)

Pathophysiology

Mutations that change the primary structure of globin, depending on the substitution and its location, can alter the secondary (α-helical), tertiary (folding of the globin chain) or quaternary (interactions within the hemoglobin tetramer) structure of hemoglobin by mechanisms shown in Table 24.2.

Heme–globin interactions are vital for oxygen delivery but also contribute to molecular stability. For example, introduction of a charged amino acid residue into the heme pocket, a site normally formed by residues with nonpolar side chains, deletions involving residues that directly interact with the heme, mutations other than to a tyrosine residue of the (F8) proximal histidine or (E7) distal histidine, all cause molecular instability.

Disruption of the secondary structure reduces subunit solubility and is often a result of the introduction of proline residue that cannot be accommodated into α-helix except in its first two positions. α-Helices comprise approximately 70% of the globin subunit and must be folded into a globin motif. Introduction of water into the molecule destroys its stability and this can be caused by substitution of a charged residue, for example, leucine, for a nonpolar residue, like arginine.

Table 24.2. Sites of globin mutation that are associated with unstable hemoglobins. In addition to single amino acid substitutions, these mutations can include small deletions and insertions of amino acids, reading frameshifts, fusion globins, and elongated globin chains

Weakening or modification heme–globin interactions
Interference with the secondary structure of a globin subunit
Interference with the tertiary structure of the subunit
Altered subunit interactions interfering with the quaternary structure

Loss of intersubunit contact hydrogen bonds or salt bridges in the α1β1 contact area will also reduce stability. Dissociation of α1β1 dimers into monomers is normally minimal as it generates methemoglobin and consequent instability. Dissociation of chains along the α1β1 contact generates α- and β-globin chains that uncoil, loosening their heme–globin interaction and favoring methemoglobin formation. Mutations affecting the α1β1 interface tend to be more unstable than those affecting the α1β2 contact.

Heme loss is inhibited by maintaining heme iron in the reduced ferrous (Fe^{2+}) state by the action of methemoglobin reductases and detoxification of oxygen radicals. Therefore, dimerization and the dispersion and precipitation of free heme is minimalized. Hemoglobin dimers autoxidize and lose heme more readily than tetramers. Generation of methemoglobin increases the thermoinstability of hemoglobin, suggesting that the pathways and events accompanying the conversion of ferrous to ferric heme are important for hemoglobin stability.

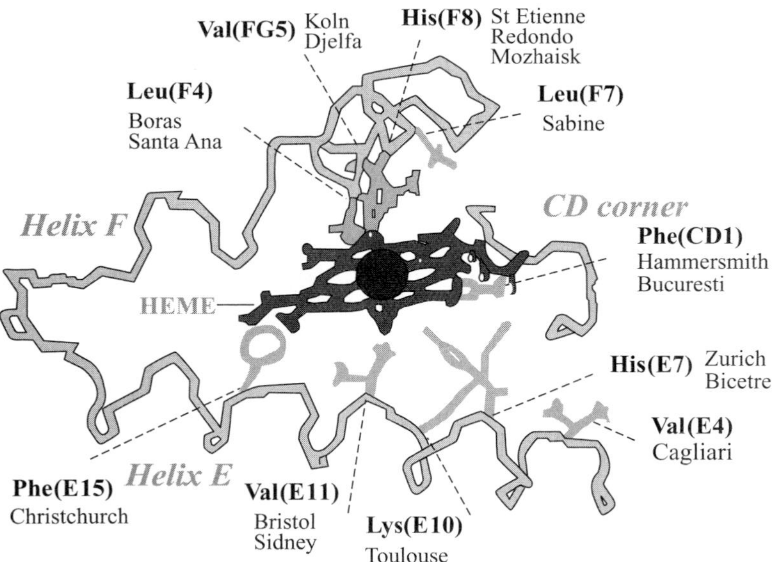

Figure 24.3. Mutation sites of some unstable hemoglobins. Mutations shown are near the heme moiety.

Heinz bodies are the product of hemoglobin denaturation. First suggested to be heme-depleted globin chains, these inclusions were subsequently identified as hemichromes, derivatives of ferric hemoglobin that have the sixth coordination position occupied by a ligand provided by the globin. Hemichromes are generated when the heme is dissociated from the heme pocket and rebinds elsewhere in the globin after the α or the β chains have denatured. Irreversible hemichromes are a stage in the formation of Heinz bodies. Membranes prepared from the red cells of patients with Hb Köln (*HBB* val98met) who have had a splenectomy contain aggregates composed of disulfide-linked spectrin, band 3 (Chapter 9), globin and

Table 24.3. Some hemoglobin variants with elongated globin chains

Variant	Mutation	Mechanism	Phenotype
NH_2-Terminal Extension			
South Florida[51]	*HBB* val1met	Initiator met retained, chain extended by 1 residue	Acetylated at the NH_2 terminus and appears as HbA_1C
Doha[52]	*HBB* val1glu	Initiator met retained, chain extended by 1 residue	21% in heterozygote, acetylated
Long Island	*HBB* his2pro	Initiator met retained, chain extended by 1 residue	No clinical phenotype but appears as HbA_1C
Thionville[53]	*HBA1* val1glu	Initiator met retained, chain extended by 1 residue	50% in heterozygote, acetylated
Insertions			
Catonsville[54]	Insertion between α37 and α38	glu inserted	Increased O_2 affinity, unstable
Zaïre	Insertion between α116 and 117	5 residues inserted	Normal
Grady	Insertion between α118 and 119	3 residues inserted	Normal
Koriyama[55]	Insertion between β95 and 96	5 residues inserted by possible out of frame base pairing. In Hb Gun Hill the same 15-bp segment is deleted	Severe instability and anemia. Resembles a thalassemic hemoglobinopathy
COOH-Terminal Extensions			
α-Globin gene termination mutants	See Chapter 13	Termination codon mutations	α Thalassemia
Tak	β147 (+AC)	2-bp insertion and frameshift	~Normal
Wayne	α139 (−A)	1-bp deletion and frameshift	See Table 24.5

high-molecular-weight complexes composed in part of denatured spectrin.

Hemichrome can bind band 3 of the erythrocyte membrane. Decreased deformability of the erythrocyte leads to preferential trapping in the spleen where Heinz bodies are removed. The coincident loss of small amounts of membrane gradually converts discoid cells into spherocytes that are eventually removed from the circulation. Membrane damage might also result from lipid peroxidation and protein cross-linking due to free radical formation that is a result of Fenton chemistry.

When the mutation is such that heme dissociates from the abnormal globin chain, as in the example of Hb Köln, the partially heme-deficient molecule is susceptible to reversible and irreversible hemichrome formation with subsequent denaturation. Precipitates tend to be pale, and the pattern found during hemoglobin electrophoresis was characterized by multiple bands unless stabilized by the addition of hemin. Dipyrroluria was present, suggesting that free heme was converted to dipyrroles rather than bilirubin.

By different mechanisms, hemoglobin chains might be extended beyond their expected length. Small insertions and deletions are caused by slipped mispairing at the replication fork of DNA at the site of direct repeats or inverted repeats. Nonsense to missense mutations at the termination codon, reading frameshifts, failure to cleave the initiator methionine residue from the amino terminus of globin, amino acid insertions, and combined deletions and insertions have been reported. Although many resulting variants are not associated with hematological abnormalities, some are accompanied by hemolytic anemia that can be severe. Not unexpectedly, distortion of tertiary structure because of chain elongation can provoke different degrees of globin instability. Table 24.3 highlights other variants with extended globin chains.

Almost without exception, the deletion of one or more amino acid residues results in an unstable globin. When one or two residues are missing, the clinical phenotype is usually mild with slight anemia. When more than one or two amino acids are deleted the phenotype is apt to be more severe. Hb Bruxelles (*HBB* phe41 or 42del) is accompanied by severe Heinz body hemolytic anemia.

Alpha hemoglobin-stabilizing protein (AHSP) binds free α-globin chains protecting them from precipitation (Chapter 4). In vitro studies suggest that the impaired interaction of AHSP with α-globin variants where the mutation lies in the molecular sites where ASHP binds α globin might affect the stability of the variant.[14,15] In these studies, recombinant Hb Groen Hart (*HBA* pro119ser), Hb Diamant (*HBA* pro119leu), and α-globin termination mutants had impaired interactions with AHSP. These observations suggest an additional mechanism for unstable α-globin variants.

Hyperunstable hemoglobins are an uncommon class of variants where the mutation, usually in the third exon of the globin gene, leads often to a truncated globin that is barely detectable or undetectable. These hemoglobins, creating the phenotype of dominant inherited thalassemia, are discussed in Chapter 16.

Chronic hemolysis has been associated with dysregulated nitric oxide (NO) biochemistry and reduced NO bioavailability. This subject is discussed in Chapter 11.

Diagnosis

Multiple tests are used to diagnose unstable hemoglobins. Patients with unstable hemoglobins might have characteristically dark urine or pigmenturia. This is due to the presence of dipyrroles that are also present in Heinz bodies. The absence of pigmenturia does not exclude the diagnosis of unstable hemoglobin and the severity of the hemolysis is unrelated to pigmenturia. For example, carriers of Hb Köln and Hb Zürich (*HBB* his63arg) can have pigmenturia but hemolysis can be severe with Hb Köln and is usually very mild with Hb Zürich. The P_{50} of unstable hemoglobins is quite variable and can be normal, low, or high. This is a result of different mutations variously affecting heme–globin interaction, and the tertiary and quaternary structures of the molecule.

Blood Smear and Heinz Body Preparation. Abnormalities of the blood smear are often present but are nonspecific. They might include anisocytosis, basophilic stippling, Howell–Jolly bodies, nucleated red blood cells and microspherocytes. Fragmented cells can appear to have had "a bite" taken from them and are thought to result from the phagocytosis of Heinz bodies during passage of the cell through the spleen. The mean corpuscular hemoglobin concentration can be as low as 25 g/dL because of heme loss or Heinz body formation. Some reported values for reticulocytes might be factitiously high as inclusion bodies are mistaken for reticulocytes.

Heinz bodies in circulating red cells are usually found only after splenectomy or during an acute hemolytic episode (Fig. 24.2). Under such circumstances, more than 50% of the cells typically contain one large, spherical inclusion. Heinz body detection requires the incubation of erythrocytes with a supravital stain such as new methylene blue or crystal violet. They appear as single or multiple inclusions of 2 μ in diameter or less and often appear membrane attached. Heinz bodies can be found in fresh blood, but usually, incubation for 24 hours without glucose is required for their formation. A normal control should always be run simultaneously.

Hemoglobin Stability Tests. The isopropanol test, a good screening test for unstable hemoglobins, can give false positive results when the sample contains more than 5% HbF.

In the heat denaturation test, a hemolysate is incubated for 1 or 2 hours at 50°C. Hemoglobin instability is suggested by a visible precipitate. Although simple, the results of this test vary because of different concentrations of the abnormal variant and different temperatures need for their denaturation. A control with a normal, stable hemolysate is vital for correct interpretation.

Detection of the Variant Hemoglobin and Mutation Analysis. If clinical and hematological studies suggest an unstable variant, the determination of the molecular defect becomes the final step in diagnosis. Approximately a quarter of unstable hemoglobins are not detectable by commonly used methods of hemoglobin separation, and an unstable variant might be reflected only by a diffuse peak. DNA analysis is the best approach to defining the globin mutation. New mutations are common, thus a family history need not be present.

Clinical Aspects

The presence of an unstable hemoglobin should always be prime consideration when hemolytic anemia is present and its cause is not clearly defined. Chronic hemolysis due to unstable hemoglobins can be associated with all of the known complications of hemolysis such as aplastic crisis, jaundice with cholelithiasis, leg ulcers, pulmonary hypertension, splenomegaly, and hypersplenism, along with special features of unstable hemoglobins such as pigmenturia and drug-induced and fever-associated increases in anemia.[16,17] Dusky cyanosis has been described in some patients with unstable hemoglobins predisposed to methemoglobin formation. In one case where the γ-globin chain of HbF was affected (HbF-Poole; *HBG2* trp130gly), hemolytic anemia was present in the newborn but disappeared as the γ- to β-globin switch was completed. Sometimes, the disease is seen in early childhood; it can be found in adults incidentally or when fever or drug treatment induces hemolysis.

Many unstable hemoglobin variants produce mild hemolytic disease with minimal or no anemia in the steady state and a reticulocyte count between 4% and 10%. Splenomegaly might or might not be present. Most patients with mild disease are first seen during a hemolytic crisis induced by drugs or infection. More than one-half of the unstable variants are associated with no hematological abnormality and were detected through screening programs.

Although most differences in clinical phenotypes are explained by nature of the amino acid substitution, as in many single gene disorders, other genetic and some environmental factors might modulate the severity of disease. For example, investigation of the basis for intrafamilial variation in drug-related hemolysis with Hb Zürich disease suggested that tobacco smoking ameliorated hemolysis, probably because the high affinity of Hb Zürich for CO stabilized the hemoglobin tetramer.

B19 parvovirus infection can temporarily shut down erythropoiesis, rapidly worsening the anemia and causing aplastic crisis. Anemia might also increase during infection and after treatment with oxidant drugs such as sulfonamides. The intensity of hemolysis is variable and is dependent on the mutation and fraction of abnormal hemoglobin present.

Hb Köln, described in multiple kindreds, is the most common unstable hemoglobin and is characterized by anemia, reticulocytosis, splenomegaly, and 10%–25% Hb Köln. It is not associated with oxidant drug-induced hemolysis. The independent occurrence of this variant in so many apparently unrelated individuals suggests that the Hb Köln mutation, located at a methylated CpG dinucleotide sequence of the β-globin gene, can act as a "hotspot" for mutation through the deamination of the methylcytosine nucleotide to form thymine.

Hb Zürich has also been reported often. This variant, forming approximately 25% of the hemolysate, is accompanied by mild anemia exacerbated by oxidant drugs, pigmenturia, and increased affinity for CO. The latter protects the β-globin heme group from oxidation and increased instability. Carriers have a special susceptibility to sulfonamide-induced hemolytic crisis. Hb Hasharon (*HBA2* asp47his) is another more common variant affecting the α-globin chain, found in Ashkenazi Jews, and causing hemolysis in newborns but not in most adults. This variant comprises 15%–20% of the hemolysate and inclusion bodies were not found.

Some unstable hemoglobins are linked to α- or β-thalassemia genes: the α-chain mutants Hb Suan-Dok (*HBA2* leu109arg) and Hb Petah Tikva (*HBA* ala110asp) coexist in *cis* with α thalassemia and some β-chain mutants like Hb Leiden (*HBB* glu6 or 7del), Hb Duarte (*HBB* ala62pro), and HbG-Ferrara (*HBB* asn57lys) coexist with a β^0-thalassemia mutation in trans.

Miscellaneous. A 10-year-old girl with hemolytic anemia due to Hb Bristol-Alesha (*HBB* val68met) had moyamoya and transient ischemic attacks. The authors suggested that chronic hypoxemia might be the cause of occlusive moyamoya in unstable hemoglobinopathies or in hemoglobins with altered oxygen affinity.[18]

Hyperunstable Hemoglobins

Some uncommon globin mutations are hyperunstable. Although these mutants are synthesized in normal amounts, they are unable to form stable tetramers or even dimers and are rapidly catabolized. These variants therefore have features of both an unstable hemoglobins and thalassemias and have been called thalassemic hemoglobinopathies.[19] The dominant phenotype is that of severe, dominantly inherited β thalassemia because the effected globin chain fails to accumulate and participate in tetramer formation. These mutations are discussed in Chapters 13 and 16.

Treatment. Unstable hemoglobinopathies are generally mild disorders and do not require therapy except for supportive and preventive measures. Administration of folic acid to prevent megaloblastic arrest of erythropoiesis might be warranted, although access to a nutritious diet is probably satisfactory. The possibility of fever-associated hemolysis should be recognized and oxidant drugs should be avoided, including acetaminophen and sulfonamides, especially when history suggests they can provoke hemolysis, and there are other management considerations. Chronic hemolysis is associated with a high incidence of cholelithiasis although this alone is not an indication for surgery.

Severe hemolysis raises the question of splenectomy. Undoubtedly, the spleen plays an important pathophysiological role in the destruction of Heinz body containing red cells. This must be balanced with the role of the spleen as a defense against pneumococcal infections early in life and the need for antipneumococcal vaccines and prophylactic penicillin in cases in which splenectomy is performed in childhood. On balance, splenectomy might be beneficial for some severe unstable hemoglobinopathies, and partial correction of the anemia is sometimes achieved. Nevertheless, predicting the response to splenectomy is difficult. Hydroxyurea has been used to stimulate HbF production and help repair anemia in two cases of unstable hemoglobin disease.[20]

M HEMOGLOBINS

Cyanosis is the major clinical feature of amino acid substitutions causing methemoglobinemia. These rare disorders are not noted for their clinical severity; misdiagnosis, and unneeded treatment are their major hazards. Other causes of methemoglobinemia are discussed in Chapter 25.

Pathophysiology

In the M (met) hemoglobins, the mutant globin chain creates an abnormal microenvironment for the heme iron, displacing the equilibrium toward the oxidized or ferric (Fe^{3+}) state (Fig. 24.4). A combination of Fe^{3+} and its abnormal coordination with the substituted amino acid generates a visible spectrum that resembles but is clearly different from methemoglobin not due to a globin gene mutation, where the heme iron is oxidized but an associated amino acid substitution is absent (Chapter 25).

In the Iwate prefecture of Japan, "black children" had been observed for more than 160 years and this was associated with a brownish colored hemoglobin in the hemolysate of a patient that was eventually characterized as HbM Iwate (*HBA* his87tyr).[21] Four β-, two α-, and two γ-globin HbM variants have been reported. In five of the eight described HbM variants, the mutation involves the substitution of the distal (E7) or proximal (F8) histidine interacting with the heme iron via tyrosine. With HbM Milwaukee (*HBB* val67glu), the longer side chain of the glutamic acid residue can reach and perturb the heme iron.

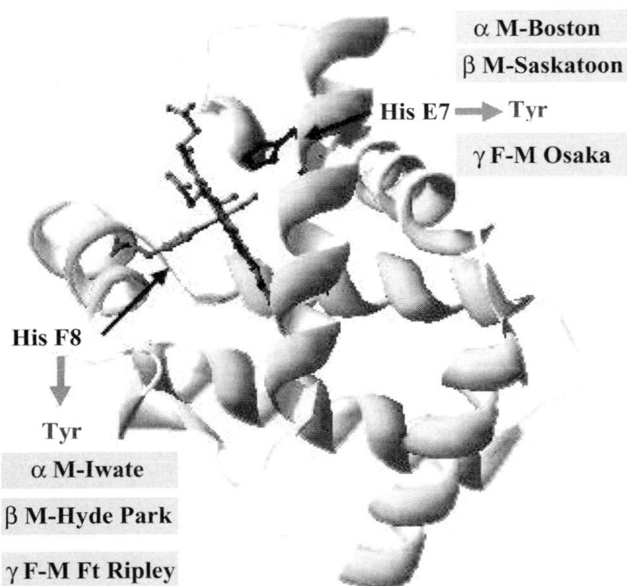

Figure 24.4. Mutation sites of some hemoglobin M variants.

Some properties of M hemoglobins are shown in Table 24.4. The strength of attachment of ferric heme to globins differs among M hemoglobins. The γ-globin gene HbM variants, HbF-M Osaka (*HBG2* his63tyr), and HbF-M Fort Ripley (*HBG* his92tyr) have been associated with neonatal "cyanosis" that disappears with maturation.

HbM Milwaukee is the sole example of an M hemoglobin not caused by mutation of the proximal or distal histidine residues but by the nearby β67 (E11) val. When this residue is replaced by a residue with an appropriate side chain, as happens with the glutaminyl residue, it perturbs the heme iron and generates an M hemoglobin. Other mutations of that site, such as Hb Bristol (val67asp) or Hb Sidney (val67ala), are unstable or have low affinity but do not lead to heme iron oxidation. X-ray crystallography showed that the carboxylic group of the new glutaminyl residue in Hb Milwaukee occupies the sixth coordination position of the iron, and that the proximal histidine maintains its role as the tenant of the fifth coordinating position, stabilizing the abnormal ferric state of HbM Milwaukee.

Oxygen-binding Properties and the R→ T Transition of M Hemoglobins. HbM Milwaukee, Hyde Park (*HBB* his92tyr), and Hb Boston (*HBA* his58tyr) all adopt deoxy or deoxy-like conformation upon the deoxygenation of the two normal chains although the abnormal chains cannot off load oxygen. This, and crystallographic, electron paramagnetic resonance, and nuclear magnetic resonance spectroscopy, and 2,3-BPG binding studies affirm that after two heme groups become deoxygenated, the entire molecule adopts the deoxy T conformation.

A normal Bohr effect and P_{50} strongly suggest that in HbM Milwaukee, HbM Saskatoon (*HBB* his63tyr), and HbM Hyde Park the molecule adopts the R-state when the two normal chains are oxygenated, a finding supported by nuclear magnetic resonance studies of HbM Milwaukee. In contrast, HbM Iwate is in the crystallographic T configuration when its normal heme groups are in the ferric state, explaining its decreased oxygen affinity; the molecule does not shift to the R-state when the normal heme groups are liganded and remains in the low affinity T-state. A similar situation probably exists in HbM Boston, as the habit of the deoxy crystal remains intact after oxygenation, suggesting that no conformational change has occurred that would require a different crystal structure.

HbM Saskatoon and HbM Boston have different properties despite the common substitution of the distal histidine because the former variant does not change its conformation when oxygenated, whereas the latter variant does. Why properties of the β-globin chains differ from that of the α-globin chain when their distal histidine is substituted is unresolved.

Iron Oxidation and Spectral Characteristics. In all M hemoglobins, the affected heme groups are stabilized in the ferric state and have an abnormal microenvironment. They exhibit an abnormal visible absorption spectrum that can be easily distinguished from methemoglobin. This characteristic separates these variants from some unstable hemoglobin mutants that also have a tendency to form methemoglobin.

Heme iron in the abnormal subunits of the M hemoglobin exhibit abnormally low redox potential. They are oxidized more rapidly by molecular oxygen and are resistant, to a variable degree, to reduction by dithionite. Differences exist in the rate of reduction of the five M hemoglobins with various reductases, including the enzyme active in the normal erythrocyte, NADH-cytochrome

Table 24.4. Hematological features of HbM variants of the α- and β-globin chains

Variant	Percent	Hb (g/dL)	Reticulocytes (%)	P_{50}	Bohr effect
HbM Hyde Park (Milwaukee-2)(β)	23–32	10–13	4–6	Normal	Present
HbM Iwate (α)	19	17	–	Decreased	Decreased
HbM Boston (α)	20–30	–	–	Decreased	Decreased
HbM Milwaukee (β)	50	14–15	1–2	Decreased	Present
HbM Saskatoon (β)	35	13–16	0.8–3.2	Normal	Present
HbM Chile (β)	17	13.2	1.2	–	–

b_5 reductase (*CYB5R3*). HbM Iwate, HbM Hyde Park, and HbM Boston are not reduced at all; HbM Milwaukee is reduced slowly and HbM Saskatoon is reduced normally by this reductase. These last two variants might be less oxidized in vivo than expected. Full ferric conversion might occur only in vitro, due to the high autoxidation rate of these abnormal hemoglobins. Older red cells might, nevertheless, have fully oxidized abnormal chains consistent with the presence of clinically apparent cyanosis.

Clinical Aspects and Diagnosis

Clinically, the skin and mucous membranes of HbM carriers have an appearance similar to but not identical with cyanosis, sometimes called pseudocyanosis. Skin and mucosal surfaces are brownish/slate colored, more like methemoglobinemia, but not as slate blue-purple as true cyanosis. This distinction is subtle and might not be apparent without simultaneously comparing the two conditions. Skin reflects hemoglobin molecules with an abnormal ferric heme and abnormal spectrum, because cyanosis is caused by the presence of more than 5 g/dL of deoxyhemoglobin. Pseudocyanosis is present from birth in α-globin chain abnormalities and from the middle of the first year of life in the β-chain mutants. A mixture of the abnormal pigment and true cyanosis, due to hemoglobin desaturation of the normal chains, is observed in the low oxygen affinity HbM Boston and HbM Iwate. Pseudocyanosis, is not associated with dyspnea or clubbing and carriers have a normal life expectancy. A mild hemolytic anemia and reticulocytosis has been observed in HbM Hyde Park and can be explained by the instability of the hemoglobin induced by partial heme loss.

HbM should be considered in all patients with abnormal homogeneous coloration of the skin and mucosa, particularly if pulmonary and cardiac function is normal. The diagnosis can be suspected by observing an abnormal brown coloration of the blood in a tube. To distinguish this coloration from methemoglobin, the addition of KCN to the hemolysate is useful. KCN will turn blood containing methemoglobin red, but has little if any effect on HbM-containing hemolysates. Lack of color conversion with KCN is diagnostic of HbM.

A spectrophotometrical recording of the visible spectrum of the hemolysate is critical for the diagnosis. M hemoglobins do not have an absorbance peak at 630–635 nm, which is typical of methemoglobin A (Fig. 24.5). In the presence of HbM, accurate measurement of oxygen saturation and CO hemoglobin is difficult with most instruments. Absorption maxima at different wavelengths of all hemoglobin M variants have been reported.

Treatment. Treatment is neither possible nor necessary. A correct diagnosis is most important because this will forestall therapeutic and diagnostic misadventures.

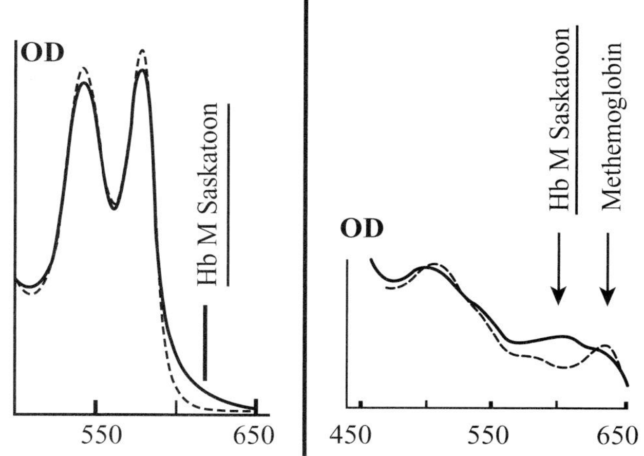

Figure 24.5. Absorption spectra of HbM Saskatoon. The left panel shows a fresh hemolysate and the right panel, a hemolysate totally oxidized.

RARE MUTATIONS WITHOUT A PHENOTYPE OR WITH MINOR HEMATOLOGICAL CHANGES

Posttranslational Modifications

Posttranslational modifications of globin are broadly illustrative of the secondary changes possible in all proteins and form an interesting group of hemoglobinopathies.

Deamidation. Under certain conditions, mutant asparaginyl residues can be deamidated to aspartate and result in two species of globin caused by a single mutation (Table 24.5).[22] Aspartic acid to asparagine mutants could be deamidated, reducing levels of the asparagine-containing globin. Usually, deamidation occurs when a histidine residue is adjacent to the asparagine substitution or when changes in the tertiary structure of a variant globin can bring a histidine into the proximity of an asparagine residue. Other factors favoring asparagine deamidation are glycine, serine, or alanine residues with nonbulky side chains on either side of the asparagine or brought near the asparagine, a basic or acidic residue on one side and a serine or cysteine on the other side of asparagine and peptide chain flexibility. Not all aspartic acid to asparagine mutants are subject to posttranslational deamidation. Two abnormal hemoglobins can be present when variants susceptible to deamidation are analyzed: a native form containing the encoded asparagine and a deamidated form containing aspartic acid. When a variant of this type is present in a compound heterozygote with another variant hemoglobin, a confusing HPLC profile with three hemoglobin bands representing two globins resulting from the asparagine substitution and another from the other β-globin gene variant can exist.

Oxidation. A young girl with hemolytic anemia was found to have two unstable hemoglobins: Hb Sidney (*HBB* val67asp) and a new variant called Hb Coventry (*HBB* leu141del) that formed less than 10% of the hemolysate.

Table 24.5. Hemoglobin variants with deamidated asparaginyl residues

Variant	DNA mutation	Phenotype
La Roche-sur-Yon (*HBB* leu81his)	CTC→CAC (?)	Unstable, decreased P_{50}, mild hemolysis. leu81his facilitates β80 asn deamidation
Providence (*HBB* lys82asn)	AAG→AAC/T (?)	Increased O_2 affinity but normal packed cell volume
Redondo (*HBB* his92asn)	CAC→AAC (?)	Heme loss, unstable, hemolysis, migrates like HbS and HbA_2
Osler (*HBB* tyr145asn)	TAT→AAT	Increased O_2 affinity, migrates like HbJ and HbA
J Sardegna (*HBA* his50asn)	CAC→AAC	Functionally normal. Present in 0.09% of Sardinians
J-Singapore (*HBA2* ala79gly)	GCG→GGG	Normal, ~22%. The *HBA2* ala79gly mutation allows deamidation of α78 asn[56]
Wayne (*HBA* 139 -A)	-A in either *HBA2 or HBA1* with 5 codon elongation	Normal hematology, either ~14% or ~6% present

As the patient also had HbA, three β-globin genes were postulated, one being a βδ gene.[23] Another patient with unstable hemoglobin hemolytic anemia was also found with three putative β-globin chains: Hb Atlanta (*HBB* leu75pro), Hb Coventry, and β^A. These observations, and a third instance of Hb Coventry in a similar clinical setting, suggested that this variant was widespread and only became apparent when present with another unstable hemoglobin. It was proposed that the two mutations were in a single β-globin gene (*HBB* leu75pro; leu141del), that was the product of a βδ anti-Lepore gene, the leucine 141 being deleted in the crossover event.[24] Two genetic events must have occurred to explain these findings; a de novo β75 leu→pro mutation and a sister chromatid exchange in a somatic cell. When DNA techniques were applied to study the structure of the β-globin gene cluster and the nucleotide sequence of the β-globin genes, only two normal β-globin genes were found. The expected leu75pro mutation was found but the codon for β141 was intact in genomic DNA and in mRNA. Mass spectroscopy demonstrated the peptide containing β141 leucine to contain a novel amino acid of 129 D instead of the 113 D of the leucine peptide and was postulated to be hydroxyleucine. Hydroxyleucine cannot be detected by amino acid analysis so its presence remains conjectural. It was proposed that perturbation of the heme pocket by the leu75pro mutation in the E helix, perhaps via the generation of activated oxygen species, lead to oxidation of some β141 leucine residues. This notion provides a parsimonious explanation for the existence of the Hb Coventry anomaly in the same globin chain as Hb Atlanta and other unstable variants.[25]

Acetylation. Hb Raleigh (*HBB* val1ala) is acetylated and migrates with HbA_1C.[26] Proteins with an NH_2-terminal alanine are often acetylated. Acetylation of a retained N-terminal methionyl occurs when normal cleavage of this residue malfunctions (see later). Acetylated hemoglobins can be mistaken for Hb A_1C.

N-Terminal Elongated Globins

Several mutations of the NH_2-terminal valine of both the α- and β-globin chain and a *HBB* his2pro mutation result in a globin elongated by one residue because of the failure to cleave the initiator methionyl (Table 24.3). A hematological phenotype is not present but the NH_2-terminal methionine is acetylated and appears as HbA_1C by some methods of hemoglobin separation.

Interesting β-Globin Gene Variants with Point Mutations

Hemoglobin G Coushatta (HBB glu22ala). This β-globin chain variant has no clinical or hematological manifestations and has been found in geographically separated racial and ethnic groups.[27] It is common in China and North American Coushatta Indians and has also been described in Japan, Korea, and Turkey. It is the most common variant hemoglobin described along the Chinese Silk Road. Its presence in Asia, the Old World, and in American Indians raised the question of whether this variant had a unicentric origin and spread to the New World over the ancient Bering land bridge or originated multicentrically in Asia and in Amerindians. When the haplotype of the β-globin gene cluster was examined in Louisiana Coushatta Indians and native Chinese who carried Hb G Coushatta, these groups had different haplotypes and β-globin gene framework associated with the identical HbG Coushatta mutation. Both the HbG Coushatta mutation (GAA→GCA) and the codon 2 CAC→CAT polymorphism are normal δ-globin gene sequences, suggesting the possibility of gene conversion. HbG Coushatta had at least two independent origins

Table 24.6. Mutations encoded on HBA_2 and HBA_1

Variant	*HBA2*	Genotype	%	*HBA1*	Genotype	%
J-Paris (ala12asp)	GCC→GAC	$\alpha^X\alpha/\alpha\alpha$	24	GCC→GAC	$\alpha\alpha^X/\alpha\alpha$	20.7
Hekinan (glu27asp)	GAG→GAC	$\alpha^X\alpha/\text{-}\alpha$	27.9	GAG→GAT	$\alpha\alpha^X/\alpha\alpha$	13.9
G-Philadelphia (asn68lys)*	AAC→AAA	$\alpha^X\alpha/\alpha\alpha$	25.1	AAC→AAG	$\alpha\alpha/\text{-}\alpha^{X*}$	33.4
J-Broussais (lys90asn)	AAG→AAT	$\alpha^X\alpha/\alpha\alpha$	25	AAG→AAC	$\alpha\alpha^X/\alpha\alpha\alpha$	18
Manitoba ser102arg)	AGC→CGC	$\alpha^X\alpha/\alpha\alpha$	18.7	AGC→AGA	$\alpha\alpha^X/\alpha\alpha^X$	23.9
J-Meerut (ala120glu)	GCG→GAG	$\alpha^X\alpha/\alpha\alpha$	23	GCG→GAG	$\alpha\alpha^X/\alpha\alpha$	18.4

* This variant is usually present on the -$\alpha^{3.7}$ rightward deletion chromosome.

that could be due to two separate mutations at codon β22, a mutation at this codon and a β→δ gene conversion or two β→δ gene conversion events.[28] The β-globin gene haplotype predominant in Thailand and in Koreans suggesting yet other possible origins for this ostensibly genetically "neutral" variant.[29,30,31]

Hemoglobin Vicksburg (HBB leu75del). It was proposed that Hb Vicksburg arose as a stem cell mutation on a β^+-thalassemia chromosome.[32] When first studied, only Hb Vicksburg was present, then both HbA and Hb Vicksburg were found, and finally, only HbA was present. This suggested that over time there were at least two clones of erythroid progenitors contributing to erythropoiesis.[33] A leucine deleted in Hb Vicksburg recalls the origin of Hb Coventry so it remains possible that a technical artifact was responsible for the failure to find a β75 leucine residue when Hb Vicksburg was present.

Support for the notion of a somatic mutation leading to traces of abnormal hemoglobin comes from studies of the stable variant, Hb Costa Rica (*HBB* his77arg). Six percent to 8% Hb Costa Rica was found in a young woman but not in any of her relatives. A mutation corresponding to the CAC→CGC transversion expected to code for this variant could not be detected in her genomic DNA. Yet, small amounts of Hb Costa Rica mRNA were present in reticulocytes. Globin gene structure was normal. A somatic mutation causing genetic mosaicism was hypothesized. In follow-up studies in which burst-forming unit erythrocytes were grown from the blood of this patient, only 12%–15% of these erythroid colonies contained both HbA and Hb Costa Rica mRNA, whereas the remainder had mRNA only for HbA.

HBB mutations in *cis* to a β^+-thalassemia mutation was the explanation for unusually low levels of HbS and the rare variant, Hb Dhofar (*HBB* pro58arg).[34]

Interesting α-Globin Gene Variants with Point Mutations

Mutations can occur in either or both the 5′ *HBA2* or the 3′ *HBA1* genes. Where information is available, mutations are equally divided between both α-globin genes.[35] Depending on whether they are encoded on the *HBA2* or the *HBA1* gene, there is a small difference in the levels of stable α-globin gene mutants. *HBA2* mutants usually form approximately 24% and *HBA1* mutants approximately 20% of the hemolysate, a difference explained by the transcription rate of each α-globin gene, translational efficiency of the mRNA from each gene, the assembly of αβ dimers, the presence of deleted or triplicated α-globin loci, and the presence of nondeletion types of α thalassemia (Chapter 13). Some identical amino acid substitutions encoded on both the α_1- and α_2-globin genes, often by different mutations, are shown in Table 24.6.

Hemoglobin G-Philadelphia (HBA asn68ys). HbG Philadelphia is the most common α-globin gene variant in blacks and is found in approximately one in 5,000 African Americans. A clinical phenotype is not present, but because it is usually found with α thalassemia and can be present on many different α-globin gene arrangements, its level in the hemolysate varies widely and it has a bimodal or trimodal distribution.[36,37] Interactions of HbG-Philadelphia with sickle cell anemia are discussed in Chapter 23. Most often, in the black population, HbG-Philadelphia is present on the -$\alpha^{3.7}$ chromosome as an AAC→AAG transversion. It is also found in Italians on the *HBA2* gene in a normal α-globin gene locus ($\alpha^G\alpha/\alpha\alpha$) where the mutation is AAC→AAA.[38,39] Different proportions of HbG-Philadelphia found with different α-globin gene haplotypes are shown in Table 24.7. In addition to the α-globin genotypes shown, it is likely that HbG-Philadelphia will be found in trans to chromosomes with both α-globin genes deleted and associated

Table 24.7. Levels of HbG-Philadelphia in different α-globin genotypes

α-Globin genotype	% HbG-Philadelphia
$\alpha^G\alpha/\alpha\alpha$	25
$-\alpha^G/\alpha\alpha$	33
$-\alpha/\alpha^G\alpha$	33
$-\alpha/-\alpha^G$	50
$-\alpha^G/-\alpha^G$	100
$-\alpha^T/-\alpha^{G*}$	100
$-/-\alpha^{G\dagger}$	HbG+HbH

* α^T denotes a dysfunctional α-globin gene that is not expressed because of a frameshift and new in-phase termination codon.

† In HbG/HbH disease, both HbH and HbG are present.

with triplicated and quadruplicated α-globin loci. In the latter case, the percent of HbG should be lower than usual.

Other α-globin gene variants present at levels near 50% are probably also present on an α thalassemia-2 chromosome. HbJ-Tongariki (*HBA* ala115asp) is commonly found in Melanesians and always on a $-\alpha^{3.7}$ chromosome. Heterozygotes have approximately 50% and homozygotes, nearly 100% of this variant. This mutation was likely to have occurred on a $-\alpha^{3.7}$ thalassemia chromosome that is prevalent in Vanuatuans.

Hb Setif (HBA2 asp22tyr) Pseudosickling and Hemoglobin Oligomerization. Only hemoglobin variants with the *HBB* glu6val mutation polymerize when deoxygenated and cause vasoocclusive disease. Hb Setif, a variant found in North Africa and the Middle East, forms pseudosickled cells in vitro but not in vivo, when it is oxygenated. This is due to the aggregation of Hb Setif.[40–44] Pseudosickled Hb Setif cells can be distinguished from sickled HbS-containing cells by many physical characteristics although they have several features in common. The C_{sat} of a 40%/60% hemolysate of Hb Setif/HbA at 290 mOsm was 24 g/dL at 24°C. During incubation in NaCl buffer at 450 mOsm, polymer in pseudosickled cells required more than 30 minutes to begin formation; after 24 hours, nearly all cells contained aggregated Hb Setif. In contrast, HbS polymer forms in fractions of a second to seconds. Deoxygenation promotes HbS polymerization but inhibits pseudosickling of Hb Setif cells. Pseudosickled Hb Setif cells have been described as twisted cigars with a monotonous morphology in contrast to the eclectic conformation of sickle cells (Fig. 24.6). In common with HbS erythrocytes, cell deformability decreased with increasing Hb Setif concentrations and increasing osmolality of the suspending buffer, whereas the amount of Hb Setif polymer increased under these conditions.

Pseudosickling of Hb Setif is strictly an in vitro phenomenon. Whether Hb Setif was present at levels of less than 20%, attributable to mild instability, or found at concentrations near 40%, because of a coexistent α thalassemia deletion, there was no evidence of hemolysis and vasoocclusive disease. Urine-concentrating ability in carriers of Hb Setif seemed unimpaired, whereas this is abnormal in sickle cell trait and sickle cell anemia.

Hemoglobin Porto Alegre (*HBB* ser9cys) contains an extra thiol group oriented toward the molecule's exterior and spontaneously oligomerizes during storage by forming intermolecular disulfide bridges. Although other substitutions introducing a cysteine residue have been described, only Hb Mississippi (*HBB* ser44cys), Hb Harrow (*HBB* phe118cys), and Hb Ta-Li (*HBB* gly83cys) are also known to form low concentrations of oligomers.[45] None of these variants are associated with cell sickling.

HbI (HBA2 lys16glu). HbI has been encoded on both *HBA2* and *HBA1* of a single individual and considered an example of concerted evolution (the parallel development of related closely linked genes). In a hematologically normal black woman, 65% of the hemolysate was HbI. Her α-globin gene haplotype revealed a normal α-globin gene locus and an α-globin gene locus with the common $-\alpha^{3.7}$ deletion. Genetic studies showed she transmitted to a daughter who had only HbA, the $\alpha^{-3.7}$ deletion, suggesting that HbI was encoded on the normal α-globin gene locus. When mRNAs from the *HBA1* and *HBA2* were selectively isolated and translated in vitro, both encoded a glutaminyl residue at position 16, whereas the *HBA1* mRNA also encoded normal mRNA, the product of the chromosome with the $\alpha^{3.7}$ deletion. These observations suggested a gene conversion event between the highly homologous α-globin genes. Two of the

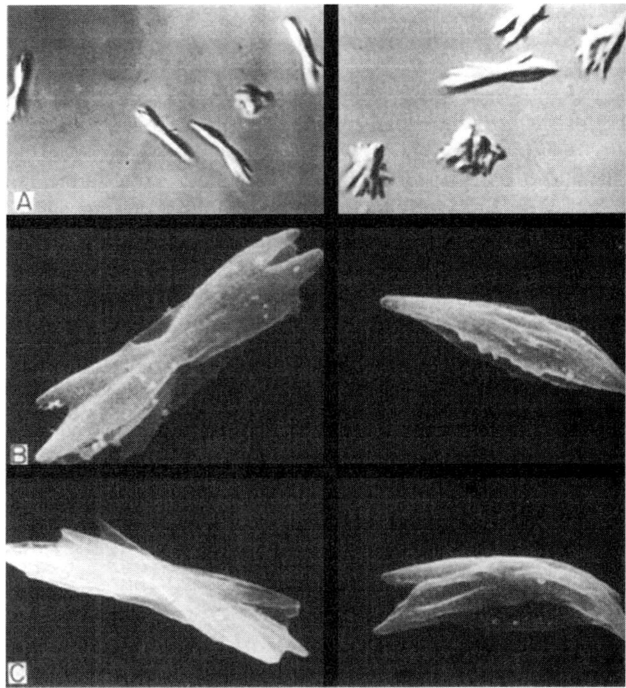

Figure 24.6. Pseudosickling of HbSetif erythrocytes by **(A)** light microscopy and Nomarski optics **(B** and **C)** and scanning electron microscopy. (From ref. 43 with permission.)

Table 24.8. β-Globin gene variants with two amino acid substitutions*

Variant	Substitutions	Hemoglobins involved	Hematology
Arlington Park	glu6lys; lys95glu	HbC; HbN Baltimore	Normal
HbC-Rothschild	glu6lys; trp37arg	HbC; Hb Rothschild	Normal
HbC-New Cross	glu6lys; gly83asp	HbC; ?	Mild instability?
HbC-Ndjamena	glu6lys; trp37gly	HbC; ?	Compound heterozygote with HbS causing sickle cell disease
HbD-Agri	ser9tyr; glu121gln	Hb Brem-sur-Mer; HbD Punjab	?
HbO-Tibesti	val11ile; glu121lys	Hb Hamilton; HbO Arab	Compound heterozygote with HbS causing sickle cell disease
T-Cambodia	glu26lys; glu121gln	HbE; Hb D-Los Angeles	?
Corbeil	glu26lys; arg104thr	HbE; Hb Sherwood Forest	Normal
Grenoble	pro51ser; glu52lys	?; Hb Osu Christiansborg	?
Poissy	gly56arg; ala86pro	Hamadan; ?	erythrocytosis, hemolysis
Hb Casablanca	lys65met: phe122leu	Anakya; Bushey	Normal
Villeparisis	his77tyr; asn80ser	Fukuyama; ?-	Normal
Duino	his92pro; arg104ser	Newcastle; Camperdown	Hemolysis
Medicine Lake	val98met; leu32gln	Köln; ?	Severe β thalassemia
Fannin-Lubbock	val111leu; gly119asp	?	Normal
Masuda	leu114met; gly119asp	Zengcheng; ?	Normal
Cleveland	glu121gln; cys93arg	D-Los Angeles; Okazaki	Normal

* Variants with the sickle cell mutation and another amino acid substitution are discussed in Chapter 23. Details and references at http://globin.cse.psu.edu.

three α-globin genes present in the proband produced HbI, accounting for the very high concentration of the variant.

A report of HbI associated with "sickled" cells contains many unknowns, including the structure of the abnormal globin and whether there is some sort of hemoglobin polymer in the cell. Some features of HbI appear to resemble those of Hb Setif.

Five stable α-globin variants formed by mutations of codon 6, Hb Sarawa (asp6ala), Hb Dunn (asp6asn), Hb Ferndown (asp6val), Hb Woodville (asp6tyr), and Hb Swan River (asp6gly) are all present at a concentration of 10%. Four stable to mildly unstable α-globin variants at codon 27 mutations, Hb Fort Worth (glu27gly), Hb Spanish Town (glu27val), Hb Shuanfeng (glu27lys), and Hb Hekinan (glu27asp) are present at concentrations of 4%–14%. In no case has it been established whether the mutant is on *HBA2* or *HBA1* or whether the α-globin gene loci are duplicated. Other than Hb Dunn, whose asparaginyl residue might be deamidated, it is not clear why these variants with uncommonly low blood levels are clustered at these sites.

Two Point Mutations in a Globin Chain

Examples of two point mutations in a single β-globin chain, where one mutation codes for HbS, are discussed in Chapter 23. β-Globin gene variants with two amino acid substitutions in *cis* are shown in Table 24.8. There are two putative origins for these double-substitution variants: recombination between homologous chromosomes each containing a different mutation and a new mutation in a gene already containing one mutation. When both mutations are common in a population, like HbC and HbN-Baltimore that in *cis* characterize Hb Arlington Park, or HbE and HbD-Los Angeles that are found in HbT-Cambodia, then the doubly substituted variant most likely arose by recombination. De novo mutation could explain instances where a rare variant is present along with a polymorphic one, such as HbC or HbE. Occasionally, both mutations are rare.

Hb Medicine Lake (β98 val→met; β32 leu→gln) has the phenotype of severe β thalassemia because the β-globin chain, containing both the Hb Köln and the β32 mutation, is likely to be highly unstable and rapidly catabolized (Chapter 13). Lacking a detectable protein, it was not possible to explore directly the properties of the abnormal hemoglobin containing the β32 CTG→CAG mutation. It was predicted that because the leu→gln mutation does not alter the charge of the β subunit, the electrophoretic mobility of Hb Medicine Lake might not differ from Hb Köln. A hydrophilic glutamine residue contains an uncharged polar side chain that could distort the B helix. Also, perturbation of the adjacent β31 leucine that contacts the heme group could result in instability. A definitive assessment of the inheritance of Hb Medicine Lake was not possible, but the most plausible cause of this abnormal hemoglobin was a new mutation in the germ cell of the father or in the proband.

Seven variants of *HBG1* contain the ile75thr polymorphism (HbF-Sardinia, Chapter 6) and an additional mutation. Curiously, no α-globin chain or *HBG2* variants with two point mutations have been described.

Table 24.9. $\beta\delta$ and $\gamma\beta$ fusion chains

Variant	Crossover	Features
Miyada	β through 12 δ from 12	17% in heterozygotes; normal hematology
P-Congo	β through 22 δ from 116	Normal hematology
P-Nilotic*	β through 22 δ from 50	Normal hematology
P-India	β through 87 δ from 116	23% in heterozygotes
Kenya	$^{A}\gamma$ through 81 β from 86	6% in heterozygotes; 5% HbF (100%$^{G}\gamma$); normal hematology
Hong Kong	within 54 bp of CAP site and exon 1	Protein is identical to δ globin. β-globin like in 5′ untranslated portion. HbA^2 16–20%[56]
Parchman	δ through 12 β from 22–50 δ from 86	1.6%; stable; found in a patient with α thalassemia

* Hb Lincoln Park is identical to HbP-Nilotic but is associated with reticulocytosis. It contains a deletion of δ137 valine and was hypothesized to result from multiple crossing over events.

References to variant described before 2000 can be found in http://globin.cse.psu.edu.

Nonthalassemic Fusion Globins

Anti-Lepore $\beta\delta$ fusion globins and Hb Kenya, a $\gamma\beta$ fusion globin, are not usually associated with hematological abnormalities because a normal β-globin gene is present on the chromosome along with the hybrid gene. These variants are shown in Table 24.9.

NOVEL COMPOUND HETEROZYGOUS CONDITIONS

With the widespread use of hemoglobin screening and increasingly sensitive methods of hemoglobin separation, many interesting but rare compound heterozygous conditions have been described. Although most of these have no hematological abnormalities they could, if not correctly diagnosed, lead to misinformed genetic counseling. As expected, most of these compound heterozygotes include HbS, HbC, and HbE but other interesting combinations have been reported.

RECOMBINANT HEMOGLOBINS

Recombinant hemoglobins can be produced in bacterial and yeast expression systems and in transgenic animals. Hundreds of variants have been engineered and used to study hemoglobin structure, function,[46] HbS polymerization, and its inhibition[47] and for potential therapeutic purposes.[32] As hemoglobin-based blood substitutes, recombinant hemoglobins could provide a shelf-storable oxygen carrying solution for use in surgery, trauma, and other emergencies without the need for blood typing and cross matching. Free hemoglobins have been difficult to develop as blood substitutes. They must not scavenge NO and form methemoglobin (Chapters 10 and 11), they should overcome the very high oxygen affinity of free hemoglobin, they should not readily dissociate into dimers, and they should be retained in the vasculature.[48] None of these conditions have been sufficiently realized to the point of producing a product for late phase clinical trials.

A recombinant human β-globin variant with gly16asp, glu22ala, and thr87gln was designed as an antisickling protein. The gly16asp substitution increased affinity for α-globin, whereas the other mutations inhibited deoxyHbS polymerization. This variant binds oxygen cooperatively and has an oxygen affinity that is comparable with HbF. Delay time experiments showed that it is a potent inhibitor of HbS polymerization. When knockout transgenic mice that expressed only this variant were bred with knockout transgenic sickle mice, hematological abnormalities and organ pathology were abolished, suggesting the value of a variant like this in diminishing the pathology of sickle cell disease.[49]

REFERENCES

1. Huisman THJ, Carver MFH, Efremov GD. A Syllabus of Human Hemoglobin Variants. 2nd ed. Augusta: Sickle Cell Anemia Foundation; 1998.
2. *Hemoglobin Variants in Human Populations.* Boca Raton: CRC Press; 1986.
3. Wajcman H, Galacteros F. Hemoglobins with high oxygen affinity leading to erythrocytosis. New variants and new concepts. *Hemoglobin.* 2005;29(2):91–106.
4. Williamson D, Beresford CH, Langdown JV, Anderson CC, Green AR. Polycythaemia associated with homozygosity for the abnormal haemoglobin Sherwood Forest (beta 104 (G6)Arg-->Thr). *Br J Haematol.* 1994;86(4):890–892.
5. Tanphaichitr VS, Viprakasit V, Veerakul G, Sanpakit K, Tientadakul P. Homozygous hemoglobin Tak causes symptomatic secondary polycythemia in a Thai boy. *J Pediatr Hematol Oncol.* 2003;25(3):261–265.
6. Bruns CM, Thet LA, Woodson RD, Schultz J, Hla KM. Hemoglobinopathy case finding by pulse oximetry. *Am J Hematol.* 2003;74(2):142–143.
7. Papassotiriou I, Traeger-Synodinos J, Marden MC, et al. The homozygous state for Hb Crete [beta129 (H7) Ala-->Pro] is associated with a complex phenotype including erythrocytosis and functional anemia. *Blood Cells Mol Dis.* 2005; 34(3):229–234.
8. McClure RF, Hoyer JD, Mai M. The JAK2 V617F mutation is absent in patients with erythrocytosis due to high oxygen affinity hemoglobin variants. *Hemoglobin.* 2006;30(4):487–489.
9. Charache S, Weatherall DJ, Clegg JB. Polycythemia associated with a hemoglobinopathy. *J Clin Invest.* 1966;45(6):813–822.
10. Charache S, Achuff S, Winslow R, Adamson J, Chervenick P. Variability of the homeostatic response to altered p50. *Blood.* 1978;52(6):1156–1162.

11. Deyell R, Jackson S, Spier S, Le D, Poon MC. Low oxygen saturation by pulse oximetry may be associated with a low oxygen affinity hemoglobin variant, hemoglobin Titusville. *J Pediatr Hematol Oncol.* 2006;28(2):100–102.
12. Haymond S, Cariappa R, Eby CS, Scott MG. Laboratory assessment of oxygenation in methemoglobinemia. *Clin Chem.* 2005;51(2):434–444.
13. Williamson D. The unstable haemoglobins. *Blood Rev.* 1993;7:146–163.
14. Vasseur-Godbillon C, Marden MC, Giordano P, Wajcman H, Baudin-Creuza V. Impaired binding of AHSP to alpha chain variants: Hb Groene Hart illustrates a mechanism leading to unstable hemoglobins with alpha thalassemic like syndrome. *Blood Cells Mol Dis.* 2006;37(3):173–179.
15. Turbpaiboon C, Limjindaporn T, Wongwiwat W, et al. Impaired interaction of alpha-haemoglobin-stabilising protein with alpha-globin termination mutant in a yeast two-hybrid system. *Br J Haematol.* 2006;132(3):370–373.
16. Rother RP, Bell L, Hillmen P, Gladwin MT. The clinical sequelae of intravascular hemolysis and extracellular plasma hemoglobin: a novel mechanism of human disease. *JAMA.* 2005;293(13):1653–1662.
17. Gladwin MT. Unraveling the hemolytic subphenotype of sickle cell disease. *Blood.* 2005;106:2925–2926.
18. Brockmann K, Stolpe S, Fels C, Khan N, Kulozik AE, Pekrun A. Moyamoya syndrome associated with hemolytic anemia due to Hb Alesha. *J Pediatr Hematol Oncol.* 2005;27(8):436–440.
19. Thein SL. Structural variants with a β-thalassemia phenotype. In: Steinberg MH, Forget BG, Higgs DR, Nagel RL, eds. *Disorders of Hemoglobin: Genetics, Pathophysiology, and Clinical Management.* 1st ed. Cambridge: Cambridge University Press; 2001:342–355.
20. Rose C, Bauters F. Hydroxyurea therapy in highly unstable hemoglobin carriers. *Blood.* 1996;88:2807–2808.
21. Percy MJ, McFerran NV, Lappin TR. Disorders of oxidised haemoglobin. *Blood Rev.* 2005;19(2):61–68.
22. Wright HT. Sequence and structure determinants of nonenzymatic deamidation of asparagine and glutamine residues in proteins. *Protein Eng.* 1991;4:283–294.
23. Casey R, Kynoch AM, Lang A, Lehmann H, Nozari G, Shinton NK. Double heterozygosity for two unstable hemoglobins: Hb Sydney (β67[E11] Val->Ala) and Hb Coventry (β141[H9] Leu deleted. *Br J Haematol.* 1978;38:195–209.
24. Moo-Penn W, Bechtel K, Jue D, et al. The presence of hemoglobin S and C Harlem in an individual in the United States. *Blood.* 1975;46:363–367.
25. Brennan SO, Shaw JG, George PM, Huisman THJ. Post-translational modification of β141 Leu associated with the b75(E19)Leu–>Pro mutation in Hb Atlanta. *Hemoglobin.* 1993;17:1–7.
26. Moo-Penn W, Bechtel K, Schmidt RM, et al. Hemoglobin Raleigh (β1 valine->acetylalanine). structural and functional characterization. *Biochemistry.* 1977;16:4872–4879.
27. Schneider RG, Haggard ME, McNutt CW, Johnson CW, Bowman JE, Barnett DR. Hemoglobin GCoushatta: a new variant in an American Indian family. *Science.* 1964;143: 197.
28. Li J, Wilson D, Plonczynski M, et al. Genetic studies suggest a multicentric origin of Hb G Coushatta [β22(B4)Glu~Ala]. *Hemoglobin.* 1999;23: 57–67.
29. Itchayanan D, Svasti J, Srisomsap C, Winichagoon P, Fucharoen S. Hb G-Coushatta [beta22(B4)Glu-->Ala] in Thailand. *Hemoglobin.* 1999;23(1):69–72.
30. Chinchang W, Viprakasit V. Further identification of Hb G-Coushatta [beta22(B4)Glu-->Ala (GAA-->GCA)] in Thailand by the polymerase chain reaction-single-strand conformation polymorphism technique and by amplification refractory mutation system-polymerase chain reaction. *Hemoglobin.* 2007;31(1):93–99.
31. Lee ST, Kim MS, Choi DY, Kim SK, Ki CS. Incidence of variant hemoglobin (Hb) and increased fetal Hb concentrations and their effect on Hb A1c measurement in a Korean population. *Clin Chem.* 2006;52(7):1445–1446.
32. Steinberg MH, Nagel RL. Native and recombinant hemoglobins of biological interest. In: Steinberg MH, Forget BG, Higgs DR, Nagel RL, eds. *Disorders of Hemoglobin: Genetics, Pathophysiology, and Clinical Management.* 1st ed. Cambridge: Cambridge University Press; 2001:1195–1211.
33. Abkowitz JL, Linenberger ML, Newton MA, Shelton GH, Ott R, Guttorp P. Evidence for the maintenance of hematopoiesis in a large animal by sequential activation of stem-cells. *Proc Natl Acad Sci USA.* 1990;87(9062):9066.
34. Williamson D, Brown KP, Langdown JV, Baglin TP. Haemoglobin Dhofar is linked to the codon 29 C --> T (IVS- 1 nt- 3) splice mutation which causes β^+ thalassaemia. *Br J Haematol.* 1995;90:229–231.
35. Molchanova TP, Pobedimskaya DD, Huisman THJ. The differences in quantities of α2- and α1-globin gene variants in heterozygotes. *Br J Haematol.* 1994;88:300–306.
36. Milner PF, Huisman THJ. Studies on the proportion and synthesis of haemoglobin G Philadelphia in red cells of heterozygotes a homozygote and a heterozygote for both haemoglobin G and α thalassaemia. *Br J Haematol.* 1976;34:207–220.
37. Baine RM, Rucknagel DL, Dublin PA, Adams JG III. Trimodality in the proportion of hemoglobin G Philadelphia in heterozygotes: evidence for heterogeneity in the number of human alpha chain loci. *Proc Natl Acad Sci USA.* 1976;73:3633–3636.
38. Brudzinski CJ, Sisco KL, Ferrucc SJ, Rucknagel DL. The occurrence of the αG Philadelphia-globin allele on a double-locus chromosome. *Am J Hum Genet.* 1984;36:101–109.
39. Molchanova TP, Pobedimskaya DD, Ye Z, Huisman THJ. Two different mutations in codon 68 are observed in Hb G- Philadelphia heterozygotes. *Am J Hematol.* 1994;45:345–346.
40. Wajcman H, Belkhodja O, Labie D. Hb Setif: G1(94)asp->tyr. A new alpha chain hemoglobin variant with substitution of the residue involved in a hydrogen bond between unlike subunits. *FEBS Let.* 1972;27:298.
41. Drupt F, Poillot M-H, Leclerc M, Lavollay B, Allard C, Bach C. Hemoglobine instable (mutant alpha) se singularisant par la formation de pseudo-drapanocytes in vitro. *Nouv Presse Med.* 1976;5:1066.
42. Raik E, Powell E, Fleming P, Gordon S. Hemoglobin Setif and in vitro pseudosickling noted in a family with co-existent alpha and beta thalassemia. *Pathology.* 1983;15:453.
43. Charache S, Raik E, Holtzclaw D, Hathaway PJ, Powell E, Fleming P. Pseudosickling of hemoglobin Setif. *Blood.* 1987;70:237–242.
44. Noguchi CT, Mohandas N, Blanchette-Mackie J, Mackie S, Raik E, Charache S. Hemoglobin aggregation and

pseudosickling in vitro of hemoglobin Setif-containing erythrocytes. *Am J Hematol.* 1991;36:131–139.

45. Baudin-Creuza V, Fablet C, Zal F, et al. Hemoglobin Porto Alegre forms a tetramer of tetramers superstructure. *Protein Sci.* 2002;11(1):129–136.

46. Cheng Y, Shen TJ, Simplaceanu V, Ho C. Ligand binding properties and structural studies of recombinant and chemically modified hemoglobins altered at beta 93 cysteine. *Biochemistry.* 2002;41(39):11901–11913.

47. Li X, Briehl RW, Bookchin RM, et al. Sickle hemoglobin polymer stability probed by triple and quadruple mutant hybrids. *J Biol Chem.* 2002;277(16):13479–13487.

48. Olson JS, Foley EW, Rogge C, Tsai AL, Doyle MP, Lemon DD. NO scavenging and the hypertensive effect of hemoglobin-based blood substitutes. *Free Radic Biol Med.* 2004;36(6):685–697.

49. Levasseur DN, Ryan TM, Reilly MP, McCune SL, Asakura T, Townes TM. A recombinant human hemoglobin with anti-sickling properties greater than fetal hemoglobin. *J Biol Chem.* 2004;279(26):27518–27524.

50. Hutt PJ, Donaldson MH, Khatri J, et al. Hemoglobin S hemoglobin Osler: A case with 3 β globin chains. DNA sequence (AAT) proves that Hb Osler is β 145 Tyr-->Asn. *Am J Hematol.* 1996;52:305–309.

51. Boissel J-P, Kasper TJ, Shah SC, Malone JI, Bunn HF. Amino-terminal processing of proteins: Hb South Florida a variant with retention of initiator methionine and N^a-acetylation. *Proc Natl Acad Sci USA.* 1985;82:8448–8452.

52. Kamel K, el-Najjar A, Chen SS, Wilson JB, Kutlar A, Huisman THJ. Hb Doha or alpha 2 beta 2[X-N-Met-1(NA1)val->glu] a new beta-chain abnormal hemoglobin observed in a Qatari female. *Biochim Biophys Acta.* 1985;831:257–260.

53. Vasseur C, Blouquit Y, Kister J et al. Hemoglobin thionville. An α-chain variant with a substitution of a glutamate for valine at NA-1 and having an acetylated methionine NH2 terminus. *J Biol Chem.* 1992;267:12682–12691.

54. Kavanaugh JS, Moo-Penn WF, Arnone A. Accommodation of insertions in helices: The mutation in hemoglobin Catonsville (Pro 37 alpha-Glu-Thr 38 alphaα) generates a 3(10) --> alpha bulge. *Biochemistry.* 1993;32:2509–2513.

55. Kawata R, Ohba Y, Yamamoto K, et al. Hyperunstable hemoglobin Korriyama anti-Hb Gun Hill insertion of five residues in the β chain. *Hemoglobin.* 1988;12:311–321.

56. So CC, Chan AY, Tsang ST, et al. A novel beta–delta globin gene fusion, anti-Lepore Hong Kong, leads to overexpression of delta globin chain and a mild thalassaemia intermedia phenotype when co-inherited with beta(0)-thalassaemia. *Br J Haematol.* 2007;136(1):158–162.

25

Dyshemoglobinemias

Neeraj Agarwal, Ronald L. Nagel, and
Josef T. Prchal

Hemoglobin can bind gases other than oxygen (O_2). These include carbon monoxide (CO) and nitric oxide (NO). Carboxyhemoglobin (COHb) precludes normal O_2 transport and is toxic. Nitrosohemoglobin has critical physiological functions discussed in Chapter 10. Normal hemoglobin can be oxidized to methemoglobin and sulfhemoglobin by exogenous agents and these hemoglobin forms can also be found as a result of germline mutations. In aggregate, these modified hemoglobins, referred as dyshemoglobinemias, are the basis of a group of acquired and genetic disorders that are rare but can have serious clinical implications.

METHEMOGLOBINEMIA

Methemoglobin is formed when the iron of the heme group is oxidized or converted from the ferrous (Fe^{2+}) to the ferric (Fe^{3+}) state. The ferric hemes of methemoglobin are unable to reversibly bind O_2. In addition, the presence of ferric heme increases the O_2 affinity of the accompanying ferrous hemes in the hemoglobin tetramer.[1] This leads to a left shift in the hemoglobin–O_2 dissociation curve, which impairs tissue delivery of O_2. Normally, methemoglobin is generated and then reduced physiologically to maintain a very low steady-state blood methemoglobin level of 1% or less of the total hemoglobin. The half-life of methemoglobin is approximately 1 hour if the reductase mechanism is normal.[2] Methemoglobinemia occurs when there is imbalance between methemoglobin production and methemoglobin reduction. Methemoglobinemia can have both inherited and acquired causes; hemoglobin oxidation has been recently reviewed.[3]

Pathophysiology of Methemoglobinemia

Production of Methemoglobin. O_2 binds the ferrous form of iron present in hemoglobin to form oxyhemoglobin. During this process, one electron is partially transferred from iron to the bound O_2, forming a ferric–superoxide (Fe^{+3}-O_2) anion complex.[4] At the time of tissue delivery of O_2, some leaves as a superoxide (O_2^-) radical. The partially transferred electron is not returned to the iron moiety, thus leaving the iron in the ferric state and forming methemoglobin (Fig. 25.1). This physiological autooxidation of hemoglobin occurs spontaneously at a slow rate, creating 0.5%–3% methemoglobin per day.[5] Oxidation of heme iron can occur by other nonphysiological means. These include 1) reactions with free radicals and endogenous compounds, including hydrogen peroxide (H_2O_2), NO, O_2- and hydroxyl radical (OH•);[6,7] and 2) oxidation by exogenous compounds or their metabolic derivatives.

Antioxidant protein 2, the product of the *PRDX6* gene, is present in high concentrations in red cells and prevents methemoglobin formation. This member of the peroxiredoxin protein family binds to hemoglobin and prevents spontaneous and oxidant-induced methemoglobin formation. Mutations of this gene or its acquired deficiency are potential candidates responsible for congenital and acquired methemoglobinemia; however, to our knowledge, this has not been yet described.[8]

Reduction of Methemoglobin. The ferric form of methemoglobin can be reduced to the ferrous form via the following metabolic pathways.

1) Cytochrome b5 reductase (*CYB5R3*) pathway: Cytochrome b5 reductase (previously termed diaphorase and NADH methemoglobin reductase) is the only physiologically meaningful way of reduction of methemoglobin. Cytochrome b5 reductase, a housekeeping enzyme and a member of the flavoenzyme family of dehydrogenases–electron transferases, is involved in the transfer of electrons from reduced nicotine adenine dinucleotide (NADH) generated by glyceraldehyde-3-phosphate reduction in the glycolytic pathway to cytochrome b5.[9,10] In red cells, NAD is reduced to NADH during glycolysis. Flavine adenine dinucleotide (FAD) is a noncovalently bound prosthetic group in the cytochrome b5 reductase, which acts as an acceptor and donor of electrons. NADH donates an electron and reduces FAD to FADH.[11–13] In turn, FADH reduces the heme protein of the cytochrome b5, which donates an electron to reduce methemoglobin to ferrous hemoglobin (Fig. 25.2).

Besides reducing methemoglobin to hemoglobin by donating an electron, cytochrome b5 also serves as an electron donor in cells with mitochondria. In these cells, a reaction catalyzed by stearyl–coenzyme A (CoA) desaturase transfers electrons from cytochrome b5 to stearyl-CoA in the outer mitochondrial membrane and endoplasmic reticulum.[14] These reactions play an important role in fatty acid desaturation and drug metabolism.

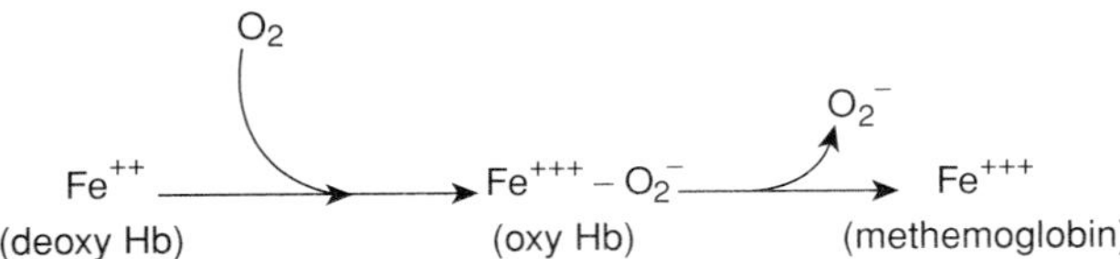

Figure 25.1. Generation of methemoglobin from hemoglobin: O_2 binds easily to the ferrous form of iron present in hemoglobin (Hb Fe^{2+}) to form oxyhemoglobin. During this process, one electron is partially transferred from iron to the bound O_2, forming a ferric–superoxide (Fe^{3+}–O_2) anion complex. At the time of tissue delivery of O_2, some of the O_2 leaves as a superoxide (O_2^-) radical. The partially transferred electron is not returned to the iron moiety, thus leaving the iron in the ferric state and forming methemoglobin (Hb Fe^{3+}).

2) NADPH-methemoglobin reductase pathway: Normally NADPH, an essential coenzyme for this reductase (an electron donor), is generated by glucose-6-phosphate dehydrogenase (G6PD) in the hexose monophosphate (pentose phosphate) shunt. There is no electron carrier in red blood cells to accept an electron directly from NADPH-methemoglobin reductase. This is possible, however, in the presence of the pharmacologically provided electron acceptors such as methylene blue or riboflavin that can link electron transfer from NADPH coenzyme of this reductase to methemoglobin.[15–18] Because these electron acceptors are not physiological, NADPH-methemoglobin reductase does not play a role in vivo in the reduction of methemoglobin. Nonetheless, this is a very important pathway during treatment of toxic methemoglobinemia when the physiological pathway is overwhelmed (Fig. 25.3).

Hereditary Methemoglobinemia

In 1845, Francois[19] reported the first case of congenital methemoglobinemia in a patient with chronic congenital cyanosis without obvious cardiac or pulmonary disease. A familial incidence of "autotoxic cyanosis" and methemoglobinemia was later described by Hitzenberger[20] and accounts of the early work on this disorder have been published.[21–23]

There are three types of hereditary methemoglobinemia. Two, cytochrome b5 reductase deficiency and cytochrome b5 deficiency, are inherited as autosomal recessive traits. The third type, inherited as an autosomal dominant disorder, is caused by globin gene mutations (HbsM), is discussed in Chapter 24. Due to the rarity of hereditary methemoglobinemia, it is not clear which of these forms is most common. Nevertheless, even discounting endemic Navajo, Athabascan, and Yakutsk congenital methemoglobinemia due to cytochrome b5 reductase deficiency, the published reports of congenital methemoglobinemia due to cytochrome b5 reductase deficiency far exceed cases of HbM. Furthermore, in our experience in a referral laboratory, more than 20 subjects with unrelated hereditary methemoglobinemia were due to cytochrome b5 reductase deficiency compared with only one case of HbM. Only a single, well documented family with methemoglobinemia (and other systemic defects) due to cytochrome b5 deficiency has been reported.

Cytochrome b5 Reductase Deficiency. The gene for cytochrome b5 reductase (*CYB5R3*) is on chromosome 22 and is 31 kb in length, containing nine exons and eight introns.[24,25] There are more than 40[3,26–28] mutations described that result in either type I or type II cytochrome b5 reductase deficiency. Although most of the mutants have been found in Caucasians, five unique mutations were found in Chinese,[29] at least three in Thai,[30,31] two in African Americans,[32] and one in an Asian Indian.[33] The cytochrome b5 reductase mutations that cause endemic methemoglobinemia in Yakutsk, Navajo, and Athabascans have not been defined, due in part to the reluctance of tribal authorities to consent to studies. An additional mutation of cytochrome b5 reductase (T116S) is not a disease-causing mutation but a high-frequency African-specific polymorphism that does not cause any appreciable disruption of the cytochrome b5 reductase secondary structure.[34]

The cytochrome b5 reductase gene has several potential transcripts generating multiple isoforms. Differences at the 5′ end of rat liver and reticulocyte cDNAs indicate the use of alternative promoters for the production of all forms of cytochrome b5 reductase.[35] Two putative promoters with different characteristics have been well described. A constitutive promoter region has similarities with housekeeping genes as it does not contain a TATA box or CAAT box but instead contains five GC box sequences (GGGCGG and CCGCCC), representing potential binding sites for the transcription factor Sp1.[25] The erythroid-specific promoter region contains several possible regulatory elements found in erythroid promoter regions, including a TATA box, CAAT-like sequences, two binding sites for the erythroid-specific transcription factor GATA-1, and a GT box.[36] Two additional promoter regions have been identified but not yet fully characterized.[37]

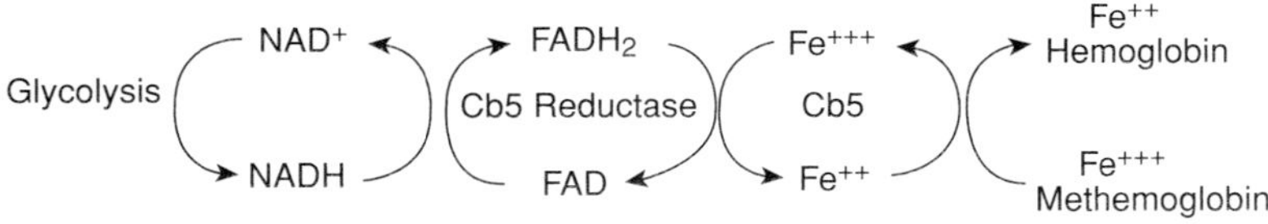

Figure 25.2. Physiological reduction of methemoglobin to hemoglobin: NADH is generated from glycolysis and reduces FAD to $FADH_2$. $FADH_2$ reduces ferric (Fe^{3+} to ferrous (Fe^{2+}) form in the cytochrome b5, which in turn reduces methemoglobin (Fe^{3+}) to hemoglobin (Fe^{2+}).

Multiple isoforms of cytochrome b5 reductase are generated from a single gene by a combination of alternative promoters and alternative initiation of translation.[36–38] One isoform, found in nonerythroid cells and reticulocytes but not in mature erythrocytes, is a membrane-associated isoform located on the endoplasmic reticulum membrane and the outer mitochondrial membrane.[39,40] This

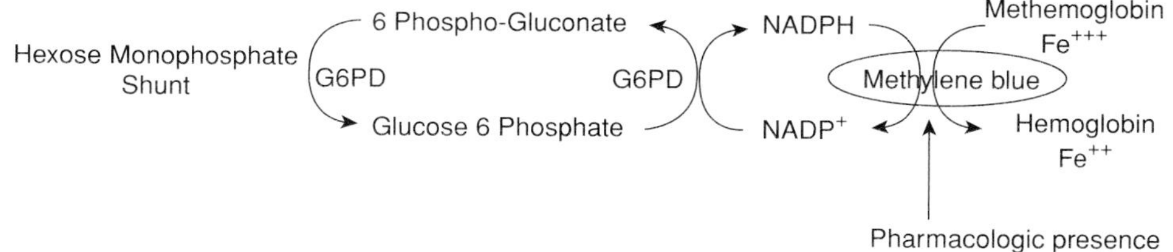

Figure 25.3. Reduction of methemoglobin by methylene blue: NADPH is generated by glucose-6-phosphate dehydrogenase (G6PD) in the hexose monophosphate shunt (pentose phosphate pathway). NADPH, in the presence of pharmacologically supplied electron acceptor such as methylene blue, reduces methemoglobin (Fe^{3+}) to hemoglobin (Fe^{2+}).

membrane-bound isoform consists of a 275–amino acid hydrophilic moiety that contains the active site and a hydrophobic domain at the N-terminal end that anchors the protein to the membrane.[41–43] Two other isoforms are found only in erythroid cells.

The isoform involved in methemoglobin reduction in erythroid cells is soluble and consists of the same 275 hydrophilic amino acids found in the ubiquitously expressed membrane-associated isoform.[18,44] The other erythroid-specific isoform is membrane-associated with an N-terminal hydrophobic sequence that differs from the sequence found in the ubiquitously expressed isoform.[36] Although it contributes only 20%–25% of erythrocyte cytochrome b5 reductase activity in adult humans, it represents a greater proportion in infants.[45]

In type I cytochrome b5 reductase deficiency (see later) only erythrocytes have decreased enzyme activity. This enzyme is heat labile and presumably is unstable and easily degraded. Thus, although cytochrome b5 reductase is abnormal in all cells in type I deficiency, only mature red cells, which cannot synthesize proteins and replace the enzyme, are significantly affected. Because cytochrome b5 reductase is coded by a single gene, it is hypothesized that type I cytochrome b5 reductase deficiency results from mutations producing an unstable enzyme, whereas mutations in type II deficiency (see later) either affect the catalytic function or cause underproduction of the enzyme, resulting in a generalized decrease in functional cytochrome b5 reductase activity.[46]

Type I Cytochrome b5 Reductase Deficiency. Most cases of enzymopenic congenital methemoglobinemia are type I, in which the functional deficiency of cytochrome b5 reductase is limited to erythrocytes. Homozygotes or compound heterozygotes[47,48] have methemoglobin concentrations of 10%–35% and appear cyanotic. Homozygotes, because of the chronic nature of their methemoglobinemia, are usually physiologically adapted to their disease state and are asymptomatic even with methemoglobin levels up to 40%.[49] Headache and easy fatigability are occasionally reported symptoms. Life expectancy is normal and pregnancy is unaffected. Significant compensatory erythrocytosis (polycythemia) is rarely observed. The cyanosis is of cosmetic significance only and can be treated with methylene blue or ascorbic acid, both of which facilitate the reduction of methemoglobin through alternate pathways.[50]

In contrast to the asymptomatic, chronically methemoglobinemic homozygotes (or compound heterozygotes) for type I cytochrome b5 reductase deficiency, heterozygous individuals are at risk for developing acute, symptomatic methemoglobinemia after exposure to exogenous methemoglobin-generating agents. Cohen and colleagues[51] report of acute toxic methemoglobinemia in US military personnel receiving malarial prophylaxis in Vietnam is a classic description of this phenomenon.

This form of cytochrome b5 reductase deficiency is distributed worldwide but is endemic in the Athabascan Alaskans,[52,53] Navajo Indians,[54] and Yakutsk natives of Siberia.[55,56] The Navajo Indians and the Athabascan Indians of Alaska are known to share a common ancestor; thus, the high frequency of cytochrome b5R deficiency suggests a common origin for all three of these populations. It remains to be determined if the molecular defect resulting in cytochrome b5R deficiency is identical in these populations. In other ethnic and racial groups the defect occurs sporadically. Although cyanosis is difficult to detect due to skin pigmentation, type I deficiency has been reported in two unrelated African American families.[57]

Point mutations in patients with type I cytochrome b5R deficiency all have been missense mutations, resulting in an amino acid substitution. Most of these mutations are found in the 5′ end of the cytochrome b5 reductase gene.[58,59] A one mutation, a G to A transition in exon 8 (E212K) in an African American family, occurs in the 3′ end.[32] As discussed, the T116S polymorphism in exon 5 in African Americans with type I cytochrome b5 reductase deficiency[34] is unlikely to be the disease-causing mutation as the amino acid substitution causes no readily appreciable disruption of the enzyme secondary structure and is not associated with methemoglobinemia. Rather, it is one of the most common African-specific polymorphisms known.

Type II Cytochrome b5 Reductase Deficiency. Unlike type I mutations that are confined to the red cell, type II mutations are associated with cytochrome b5 reductase deficiency of all cells. Type II cytochrome b5 reductase deficiency represents 10%–15% of cases of enzymopenic congenital methemoglobinemia and has a sporadic distribution. In addition to methemoglobinemia and cyanosis, the affected infants have mental retardation and developmental delay with failure to thrive and typically die during the first year of life.[60] Other associated neurological features include microcephaly, opisthotonus, athetoid movements, strabismus, seizures, and spastic quadriparesis. The mechanism resulting in the neurological problems is currently unknown but might be due to abnormal lipid elongation and desaturation in the central nervous system[61] or perhaps due to impairment of ferric-iron reduction of other cellular globins.[57] Type II mutations have been reported in both the 5′ and 3′ ends of the cytochrome b5 reductase gene[62–68] and are heterogeneous, including deletions, point mutations, splicing site mutations, and premature stop codons.

Cytochrome b5 Deficiency. Deficiency of cytochrome b5 is an extremely rare disorder that causes congenital methemoglobinemia. Only one well-documented case of cytochrome b5 deficiency has been described, compared with more than 500 reported cases of cytochrome b5 reductase deficiency,[69] and the large number of uncounted subjects affected in the endemic areas. This patient, a product of an Israeli consanguineous marriage, was also a male pseudohermaphrodite. Further analysis revealed that he was homozygous for a splicing mutation in the cytochrome b5 gene, resulting in a premature stop codon and a truncated protein molecule.[70] Another family with probable cytochrome b5 deficiency was described prior to the recognition of this entity;[71] however, the inheritance pattern in this family was autosomal dominant.

Acquired Methemoglobinemia

Most cases of methemoglobinemia are acquired, resulting from increased methemoglobin formation due to exposure to exogenous agents (Table 25.1).[72–75] Medication overdose or chemical ingestion causes methemoglobinemia by increasing the production of methemoglobin. Perhaps even more often, standard doses of medication cause methemoglobinemia in either normal individuals or those with partial deficiencies of cytochrome b5 reductase.[51,76] Use of multiple drugs together has also been implicated in the development of methemoglobinemia.[77] In one study of 138 cases of acquired methemoglobinemia, use of dapsone accounted for 42% of all affected patients, with a mean level of methemoglobin of 7.6% (range 2%–34%).[78] Xylocaine and related compounds appear to be the most common cause of drug-induced acquired methemoglobinemia; the most severe cases were seen after the use of 20% benzocaine spray for topical anesthesia (mean peak methemoglobin level 44%, range 19%–60%). Benzocaine is used during commonly performed endoscopic procedures such as bronchoscopy and endoscopy.[79] The estimated incidence in a population undergoing transesophageal echocardiography was 0.115%.[80] The molecular mechanism underlying this association has not been elucidated, as previous or subsequent exposure might not be associated with methemoglobinemia. The true incidence of drug-induced methemoglobinemia due to less frequently used agents is not known. Furthermore, it is unknown whether the development of methemoglobinemia is dose related or idiosyncratic. During surgery, methemoglobinemia should be suspected in the presence of clinical "cyanosis," a normal paO_2 and/or the presence of "chocolate brown blood."

Table 25.1. Drugs and agents that might cause methemoglobinemia

Anesthetics (local): benzocaine, lidocaine, procaine, prilocaine
Antimalarials: chloroquine, primaquine, quinacrine
Aniline dyes
Chlorates
Dapsone
Diarylsulfonylureas
Doxorubicin
Metoclopramide
Nitric and nitrous oxide
Nitrates and nitrites (amynitrate, isobutyl nitrite, nitroglycerine, sodium and silver nitrate)
Nitrobenzenes (shoe and floor polish and in paint solvents)
Nitroethane (nail polish remover, propellent, fuel additive)
Nitrofurantoin (furadantin)
Pyridium (phenazopyridine)
Phenacetin (acetaminophen)
Phenylhydrazine
Rasburicase
Sulfonamides (sulfacetamide, sulfamethoxazole, sulfanilamide, sulfapyridine)

Infants, especially those born premature, are particularly susceptible to development of methemoglobinemia because their erythrocytes contain only 50%–60% of adult cytochrome b5 reductase activity.[81–83] Although cytochrome b5 reductase levels rise to those of an adult within months of birth, young infants are unusually vulnerable to developing toxic methemoglobinemia following exposure to a number of otherwise relatively harmless medications, local ointments, and dyes used on diapers. This problem can be especially severe upon ingestion of nitrates. Nitrates do not oxidize hemoglobin directly; intestinal bacteria convert the nitrates to nitrites, which then oxidize hemoglobin to methemoglobin. In the United States, formula and food prepared from well water contaminated with nitrates have been implicated in development of methemoglobinemia in infants and children.[84–86] The nitrate nitrogen concentration of water should be less than 10 ppm to avoid methemoglobinemia. Methemoglobinemia does not occur in breast-fed infants of mothers who ingest nitrate-contaminated water because nitrates do not concentrate in breast milk. Methemoglobinemia has also been associated with diarrheal illnesses in infants without known exposure to toxins.[87,88] The exact mechanism leading to methemoglobinemia is unknown but could be due to metabolic acidosis induced by diarrhea, increased endogenous nitrite production, milk intolerance, or unique bacterial pathogens producing nitrites.[89] Other predisposing factors associated with development of methemoglobinemia in infants with diarrhea are low admission weight percentiles, failure to thrive, and diarrhea lasting for more than 7 days.[90,91] Administration of over-the-counter local anesthetic for teething has also been reported to cause methemoglobinemia in infants.[92]

Systemic infection can predispose to methemoglobinemia. NO is a free radical that is synthesized from L-arginine by NO synthases (Chapter 10). During bacteremia and sepsis, proinflammatory cytokines and bacterial lipopolysaccharide stimulate the production of inducible nitric oxide synthase (*NOS2*) from a variety of cell types including endothelial cells.[93–95] Increase in circulating NO leads to increased production of methemoglobin.[96,97] Symptomatic methemoglobinemia can also occur as a result of concomitant use of drugs predisposing to methemoglobinemia during infection and inflammation. Methemoglobinemia has been described in a burn patient with necrotizing fasciitis after prolonged application of topical 0.5% silver nitrate solution.[98] Methemoglobin production is enhanced by reactions with free radicals and endogenous compounds including H_2O_2. Reduced glutathione (GSH) in red cells helps in decreasing the level of methemoglobin by eliminating free radicals and H_2O_2. Intercellular parasites such as *Plasmodium* sp. are associated with reduced levels of erythrocyte GSH. A progressive decrease in GSH level has been shown to occur with increasing parasitemia.[99] Oxidative stress caused by medications used to treat malaria such as primaquine can also contribute to development of methemoglobinemia. Prophylaxis with primaquine alone, in absence of malarial infection, has been shown to cause mild asymptomatic methemoglobinemia.[100]

Clinical Features of Methemoglobinemia

Most individuals with congenital, chronically elevated methemoglobin concentrations are generally asymptomatic even with methemoglobin levels up to 40% of total hemoglobin.[49] Headache and easy fatigability are occasionally reported. The main clinical feature is "cyanosis" or a slate-blue color of the skin and mucous membranes, a finding that is due to the different absorbance spectrum of methemoglobin compared with oxyhemoglobin and is of only cosmetic importance. Significant polycythemia (erythrocytosis) is rarely observed.[51] Life expectancy is not shortened and pregnancies occur normally. Although cyanosis associated with cytochrome b5 reductase deficiency is readily corrected with methylene blue, this therapy is not effective for methemoglobinemia due to HbM disease.

In comparison to the general lack of symptoms in patients with chronic methemoglobinemia, patients with acute acquired methemoglobinemia are symptomatic due to acutely impaired O_2 delivery to tissues that does not allow sufficient time for physiological compensation to occur. Early symptoms include headache, fatigue, dyspnea, and lethargy. At higher levels, respiratory depression, altered consciousness, shock, seizures, and death can occur.[73] Most individuals presenting with acute acquired methemoglobinemia are not heterozygous for cytochrome b5 reductase deficiency.[101]

Cyanosis is clinically detected when the absolute concentration of methemoglobin exceeds 1.5 g/dL, which is equivalent to 8%–12% methemoglobin at normal hemoglobin concentrations.[49] In contrast, the more common cause of cyanosis, due to decreased hemoglobin O_2 saturation, is observed when the absolute level of deoxygenated hemoglobin exceeds 4–5 g/dL, as in severe respiratory failure or cardiac abnormalities due to right-to-left shunts. This form of cyanosis cannot be clinically differentiated from that due to methemoglobinemia, and laboratory analysis is required for its distinction from methemoglobinemia and sulfhemoglobinemia (see later).

The general lack of symptoms other than cyanosis, and the normal life expectancy in patients with cytochrome b5 reductase deficiency applies only to the more common type I disease in which the enzymatic deficiency is limited to the red cells. All cells are affected in patients with type II disease who exhibit neurological and developmental abnormalities.[60]

Diagnosis of Methemoglobinemia

Methemoglobinemia can be clinically suspected by the presence of clinical "cyanosis" in the face of normal paO_2. Unlike deoxyhemoglobin, the dark color of the blood in methemoglobinemia does not change with the addition of O_2. Historically pulse oximetry has been considered inaccurate in monitoring O_2 saturation in the presence of methemoglobinemia; however, the presence of methemoglobin can be suspected when the O_2 saturation as measured by pulse oximetry is significantly less than the O_2 saturation calculated from arterial blood gas analysis ("saturation gap").[78,102]

The laboratory diagnosis of methemoglobinemia is based on analysis of its absorption spectra, which have peak absorbance at 631 nm. A fresh specimen should always be obtained, as methemoglobin levels tends to increase with storage. The standard method of assaying methemoglobin utilizes a microprocessor-controlled, fixed-wavelength cooximeter. This instrument interprets all readings in the 630-nm range as methemoglobin so that false positives can occur in the presence of other pigments including sulfhemoglobin and methylene blue.[103,104] Hence, methemoglobin detected by the cooximeter should be confirmed by the specific Evelyn–Malloy method.[105] This assay involves the addition of cyanide, which binds to the positively charged methemoglobin, eliminating the peak at 630–635 nm in direct proportion to the methemoglobin concentration. Subsequent addition of ferricyanide converts the entire specimen to cyanomethemoglobin for measurement of the total hemoglobin concentration. Methemoglobin is then expressed as a percentage of the total concentration of hemoglobin.

Recently, a new eight-wavelength pulse oximeter, Masimo Rad-57 (the Rainbow-SET Rad-57 Pulse CO-Oximeter, Masimo Inc, Irvine, CA), has been reported to be accurate in measuring carboxyhemoglobin and methemoglobin. The Rad-57 uses eight wavelengths of light instead of the usual two and is thereby able to measure more than two species of human hemoglobin.[106] It is approved by the US Food and Drug Administration for the measurement of both carboxyhemoglobin and methemoglobin. In addition to the usual SpO_2 value, the Rad-57 displays SpCO and SpMet, which are the pulse oximeter's estimates of carboxyhemoglobin and methemoglobin percentage levels, respectively. In a study on healthy human volunteers in whom controlled levels of methemoglobin and carboxyhemoglobin were induced, the Rad-57 measured carboxyhemoglobin with an uncertainty of $\pm$ 2% within the range of 0%–15% and measured methemoglobin with an uncertainty of 0.5% within the range of 0%–12%.[106]

Distinguishing the hereditary forms of congenital methemoglobinemia requires interpretation of family pedigrees followed by biochemical analyses. Cyanosis in successive generations suggests the presence of HbM disease, whereas normal parents but possibly affected siblings imply the presence of the autosomal recessive cytochrome b5 reductase deficiency or, rarely, cytochrome b5 deficiency.

Incubation of blood with methylene blue distinguishes cytochrome b5 reductase deficiency from HbM disease as this results in the rapid reduction of methemoglobin through the NADPH–flavin reductase pathway in cytochrome b5 reductase deficiency.[107–109]

Measurement of the level of cytochrome b5 reductase activity, or cytochrome b5 if cytochrome b5 reductase activity is normal, is required to distinguish cytochrome b5 reductase deficiency from cytochrome b5 deficiency; however, the assay for cytochrome b5 is not commercially available.

Assays of Enzyme Activity. Types I and II cytochrome b5 reductase deficiency are distinguished by clinical phenotype and analysis of enzymatic activity in erythroid and nonerythroid cells. Reports of decreased cytochrome b5 reductase activity are difficult to compare because several different assays of cytochrome b5 reductase activity, varying in their substrate and in their normal values, have been used.[6,47,57,65,66,110,111] These assays also vary in their technical difficulty. The first widely accepted cytochrome b5 reductase activity assay used a difficult to produce and standardize methemoglobin–ferrocyanide complex and its reduction by an enzyme containing tissue homogenate.[110] The most rigorous cytochrome b5 reductase enzyme activity is based on partial purification of the enzyme by ultracentrifugation and uses the physiological enzyme substrate (cytochrome b5 prepared by a recombinant DNA technology)[42]; this assay is not readily available and is too complex for nonspecialized research laboratories. The most convenient assay uses readily available ferricyanide[111] and easily differentiates type I and type II cytochrome b5 reductase deficiency because patients with type I deficiency have normal enzyme activity in platelets, fibroblasts, Epstein–Barr virus–transformed lymphocytes, and granulocytes whereas, in type II deficiency, the activity in nonerythroid tissues is markedly to moderately decreased.[32,57,64,111] Because the enzyme defect is also found in fibroblasts and amniotic cells, analysis of cytochrome b5 reductase activity in cultured amniotic cells for the purpose of prenatal diagnosis of type II disease is possible.[112,113]

Two families with "type III" deficiency have been described in whom cytochrome b5 reductase activity was allegedly decreased not only in erythrocytes but in also in platelets and leukocytes.[114,115] The existence of this entity is difficult to accept because these individuals did not exhibit the neurological abnormalities characteristic of type II deficiency. Reevaluation of one of the patients with a rigorous assay using recombinant cytochrome b5 confirmed sufficient b5 reductase activity in the platelets, leukocytes, and fibroblasts and this analysis was consistent with the presence of type I deficiency.[116]

Treatment of Methemoglobinemia

Treatment of methemoglobinemia depends on the clinical setting. Is the onset acute and due to drugs or other toxic agents or is there congenital life-long methemoglobinemia? All patients with hereditary methemoglobinemia should avoid exposure to aniline derivatives, nitrates, and other agents that could, even in normal individuals, induce methemoglobinemia (Table 25.1). Known heterozygotes for cytochrome b5 reductase deficiency should be similarly counseled.[117] Treatment of HbM disease is neither possible nor necessary.

Hereditary methemoglobinemia. In most cases, congenital methemoglobinemia results in chronic cyanosis, except when acute methemoglobinemia occurs in heterozygotes for cytochrome b5 reductase deficiency, in which case it should be treated like acquired methemoglobinemia. Treatment of the cyanosis in these individuals is indicated for cosmetic reasons only. Options include methylene blue (100–300 mg/day orally) or ascorbic acid (300–1,000 mg/day orally in divided doses). Concerns about kidney stone formation with ascorbic acid therapy remain unproven but high-dose therapy can be associated with the theoretical nephrolithiasis risk. Riboflavin (20–30 mg/day) has also been used with some success,[118] although clinical experience with its use is very limited. Although effective for the cyanosis, neither methylene blue nor ascorbic acid has any effect on the neurological abnormalities in type II disease. Theoretically, a bone marrow or liver transplant would alleviate these neurological problems if they were due to a problem with circulating fatty acids; however, these approaches have not yet been tested.

Acquired Methemoglobinemia. Offending agents in acquired methemoglobinemia should be discontinued (Table 25.1). This condition can be life-threatening when methemoglobin comprises more than 30% of total hemoglobin. Blood transfusion or exchange transfusion might be helpful in patients who are in shock. In lesser degrees of methemoglobinemia, no therapy other than discontinuation of the offending agent(s) might be required. If the patient is symptomatic, which is often the case in deliberate or accidental overdoses or toxin ingestion, specific therapy is indicated.

Methylene blue is given intravenously in a dose of 1–2 mg/kg over 5 minutes. Methylene blue, as mentioned previously, provides an artificial electron acceptor for the reduction of methemoglobin via the NADPH-dependent reductase pathway (Fig. 25.4). The response is usually rapid; the dose can be repeated in hourly, but this is frequently not necessary. Maximum cumulative dose should not exceed 7 mg/kg as overdose can cause dyspnea and chest pain, as well as hemolysis in some susceptible subjects.[119,120] Because cooximetry detects methylene blue as methemoglobin, this technique cannot be used to follow the response of methemoglobin levels to treatment with methylene blue. If needed, the more specific Evelyn–Malloy method should be used to discriminate between methemoglobin and methylene blue and to follow response to therapy with methylene blue.

Methylene blue should not be administered to patients with G6PD deficiency because the reduction of methemoglobin by methylene blue is dependent on NADPH generated by G6PD (Fig. 25.3). As a result, methylene blue can be ineffective and is potentially dangerous because it has oxidant potential that could further produce hemolysis.[121] To avoid these problems, pretreatment screening of populations with a high incidence of G6PD deficiency (e.g., African Americans, patients of Mediterranean descent, and southeast Asians) is reasonable, although not usually practical. If methylene blue is contraindicated, only moderate doses of ascorbic acid, 300–1,000 mg/day orally in divided doses, should be given, as this drug can also cause oxidant hemolysis in G6PD-deficient patients when given in very high doses. Hyperbaric O_2 and exchange transfusion have been used with success in severe cases.[122]

Marked methemoglobinemia can occur after treatment of dermatitis herpetiformis or *Pneumocystis carinii* infection with dapsone. Cimetidine, used as a selective inhibitor of N-hydroxylation, might be effective in this setting when taken on a regular basis and lowers the methemoglobin level by more than 25%.[117,123] Because it works slowly, cimetidine is not helpful for the management of acute symptomatic methemoglobinemia arising from the use of dapsone.

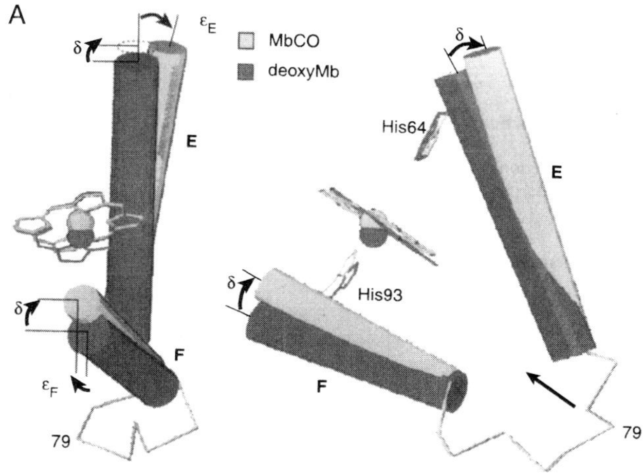

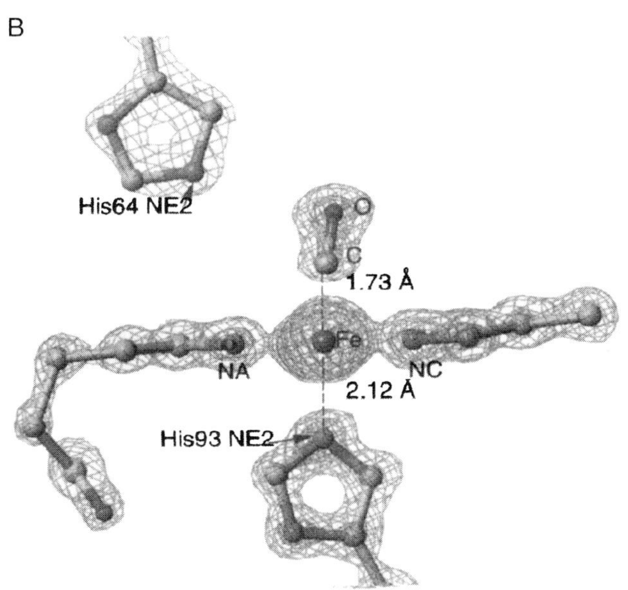

Figure 25.4. CO binding to myoglobin. **(A)** Binding of CO at the heme group. **(B)** CO binding to heme is possible because the E helix (and His 64) moves away, making space for the CO molecule without the need for bending.

CARBON MONOXIDE POISONING: CARBOXYHEMOGLOBINEMIA

CO, a toxic gas, is unusually dangerous because it is odorless, colorless, and tasteless, increasing the probability of serious and life-threatening accidents when high concentrations are unknowingly present in the environment.[124]

Epidemiology

CO intoxication is one of the most common causes of morbidity due to poisoning in the United States. Although deaths from CO poisoning had decreased in the United States, the total burden (fatal and nonfatal) might not have significantly changed in the past two decades.[125] In the United States, CO poisoning results in approximately 40,000 emergency department visits per year.[126,127] Approximately 500 accidental deaths due to CO poisoning are reported to occur annually in the United States and the number of intentional CO-related deaths is 5–10 times higher.[128,129] To examine unintentional, nonfire-related CO exposures, the Centers for Disease Control and Prevention analyzed 2001–2003 data on emergency department visits from the National Electronic Injury Surveillance System All Injury Program and 2001–2002 death certificate data from the National Vital Statistics System.[130] This analysis determined that each year, approximately 15,000 U.S. residents' visit emergency departments for unintentional, non-fire-related CO exposure and approximately 500 die from this exposure. Primary sources of CO were home appliances, and the majority of exposures occurred during the fall and winter months, when persons are more likely to use gas furnaces and heaters. During warmer months, boating activities were another source of exposure. Males were more likely to die from CO poisoning than females, which was consistent with previous findings.[131] Death rate was highest among persons aged older than 65 years. The increased death rate in elderly can be attributed to delayed diagnosis because symptoms often resemble those of associated comorbidities.[132]

The exhaust produced by the typical home-use 5.5-kW generator contains as much CO as that of six idling automobiles.[133] A survey of generator use after the 2004 Florida hurricane season reported that 4.6% of persons using generators had used them inside their home or garage. During this 2004 Florida hurricane season (13 August–25 September 2004), there were 167 persons requiring treatment for CO poisoning in 10 hospitals and six deaths were attributed to CO poisoning.[134]

Although most of the aforementioned causes more often result in acute CO intoxication, cigarette smoking is a common cause of chronic CO intoxication and can increase the COHb level by as much as 15%. By increasing hemoglobin–O_2 affinity, COHb can cause erythrocytosis (polycythemia) in smokers. Houses with defective heating exhaust systems and vehicles that leak CO into the passenger compartment, either because of mechanical failure or driving with the rear hatch-door open, are the second most common cause of chronic CO exposure. Occupations that involve a high risk for CO intoxication include garage work with improper ventilation, toll booth attendants, tunnel workers, firefighters, and workers exposed to paint remover, aerosol propellant, or organic solvents containing dichloromethane.[135]

Pathophysiology of CO Poisoning

CO has low solubility in water and is relatively inert because of its extremely high bond enthalpy. Still, it combines with high affinity with the heme of hemoglobin – and with lesser affinities to myoglobin and cytochromes – at the iron core, a site that it shares with O_2.[136] Its affinity to cytoglobin and neuroglobin has not yet been studied. Binding of CO to hemoglobin is the basis of its toxicity. An excellent summary of CO chemistry is provided by Bunn and Forget.[137]

At equilibrium in physiological conditions, CO affinity for hemoglobin is approximately 240 times greater than that of O_2. This very high equilibrium constant is the result of reaction kinetics. Contrary to popular belief, CO reacts more slowly than O_2 with the heme of hemoglobin. At 20°C and pH 7.0, the "on" rate for CO is 20 mol/L/sec compared with 470 mol/L/sec for O_2. The steric constraints present in the heme pocket make it more difficult for CO to reach the heme group. Indeed, x-ray crystallography and neutron crystal structure showed that the Fe-C-O geometry was not "linear," but "bent," an unfavorable position for CO binding.[138] Once CO is bound to heme, its "off" rate is only 0.015 mol/L/sec in contrast to 35 mol/L/sec for O_2.[136] This extraordinarily slow-release process produces a very high affinity constant of CO for heme and a life-threatening danger for individuals exposed to high levels of CO. An alternative picture has been proposed of the steric mechanisms involved in the inhibition of CO binding to heme proteins.[139] These investigators compared unliganded myoglobin and CO myoglobin at a resolution of 1.15 Å, and found perfect linearity of the Fe-C-O complex, not a "bent" configuration. This geometry was possible because a concerted motion of heme, iron, and helices E and F relieved the steric constraints (Fig. 25.4). Once two molecules of CO are bound to hemoglobin, the molecule switches to the relaxed (R) state, further endangering those exposed to CO, and the two globin chains that remain capable of binding O_2 will be in their high-affinity conformation. This high ligand affinity will make more difficult the delivery of O_2 to the tissues by the remaining O_2 binding sites. As a consequence of this phenomenon, called the Darling–Roughton effect,[1] the hemoglobin O_2 affinity increases in parallel with increasing CO levels.

In the absence of environmental CO, the blood of adults contains approximately 1%–2% COHb. This represents approximately 80% of the total body CO, the remainder probably sequestered in myoglobin and other heme binding proteins. This CO is endogenously produced,[140] originating from the degradation of heme by the rate-limiting heme oxygenase–cytochrome P-450 complex, which produces CO and biliverdin. CO levels in expired air have been used as an index of hemolysis, although the difficulty of standardization and the availability of simpler means of assessing red cell destruction have hampered the widespread use of this technique.[141,142] Further degradation of biliverdin to bilirubin by biliverdin reductase renders a stoichiometry in which one molecule of hemoglobin, by oxidation of the α-methane bridge of the tetrapyrrole ring, generates one molecule of CO and one molecule of biliverdin.

Endogenous CO levels differ among individuals. Caloric restriction, dehydration, infancy, and the genetic variations reported in Japanese and Native Americans generate higher endogenous levels of CO. Hemolytic anemia, hematomas, and infection tend to increase CO production up to threefold. Fetuses and newborns have double the normal adult levels of COHb, and levels can be much higher with hemolytic disease of the newborn. Not all endogenous CO is the product of normal metabolism. Drugs such as diphenylhydantoin and phenobarbital, by inducing the cytochrome P-450 complex, increase CO production, as does any drug that causes hemolysis. Endogenous CO production might have important physiological consequences.[143] Like its analog, NO, CO can bind to the heme of soluble guanylate cyclase and to the iron/sulfur centers of macrophage enzymes. Guanylate cyclase regulates cyclic guanosine-3′,5′-monophosphate, a second messenger involved in many cellular functions. The exact physiological significance of CO in these reactions remains to be determined.

Exogenous sources of CO include atmospheric CO, which is a product of incomplete combustion and oxidation of hydrocarbons, and natural sources.[144] High-altitude polycythemia (erythrocytosis) and hypoxemia prolong CO excretion that increases COHb levels and further compounds our imperfect adaptation to high altitude associated with decreased tissue O_2 delivery.[145]

Although the normal adult level of COHb is less than 1% or 2%, this low concentration is rarely found in urban centers because of air pollution. Hemolysis can produce COHb levels of more than 2%. Levels more than 3% must have an exogenous origin, except for rare conditions as occur in carriers of abnormal hemoglobins such as Hb Zurich. The affinity of Hb Zurich for CO is approximately 65 times that of normal hemoglobin.[146] The U.S. Environmental Protection Agency considers an acceptable exposure time to be 1 hour to 25 ppm CO or an 8 hours exposure to 9 ppm. This exposure would raise the COHb by 1.5%. Pregnant women and fetuses are particularly at risk,[147] because they already have higher levels of COHb. CO readily crosses the placenta and half life of CO in the fetus is as much as five times longer than it is in the mother. This results in approximately 15% higher fetal COHb level than the maternal COHb level.[148] The O_2 affinity of HbF is shifted to the left[149,150] owing to its lack of 2,3-BPG binding, making the Darling–Roughton effect particularly pernicious, yet another reason why cigarette smoking during pregnancy is hazardous to the fetus.

Clinical Features of CO Poisoning

Acute intoxication with CO rapidly affects the central and peripheral nervous systems and cardiopulmonary functions. Cerebral edema is common, as are alterations of sensory and peripheral nerve function. CO induces increased permeability in the lung resulting in acute pulmonary edema. Cardiac arrhythmias, generalized hypoxemia, and respiratory failure are the common causes of CO-related death; COHb levels more than 40% are found in these cases. In survivors, considerable neurological deficits might remain. Patients with less severe acute cases have the same type of clinical features as patients with chronic intoxication. Myocardial ischemia, lactic acidosis, convulsions, and coma can sometimes occur. An interesting complication observed several days after the exposure to CO are patches of necrotic skin induced by localized hypoxia. Levels of COHb that can elicit any of these symptoms vary widely among patients. Acute CO intoxication in children[151] is responsible for approximately 400 deaths a year, is more severe, and sometimes has unique symptomatology resembling gastroenteritis. Surviving children are more likely to have severe sequelae such as leukoencephalopathy (white cerebral matter destruction), and severe myocardial ischemia.[152]

Chronic intoxication in adults might result in irritability, nausea, lethargy, headaches, and sometimes a flu-like condition. Higher COHb levels produce somnolence, palpitations, cardiomegaly, and hypertension and could contribute to atherosclerosis. Chronic CO poisoning can produce erythrocytosis, the magnitude of which varies with the level of COHb. By increasing red cell production, chronic CO poisoning can mask the mild anemia of acquired or congenital hemolytic disorders.

Diagnosis and Treatment of CO Poisoning

CO poisoning is a clinical diagnosis that is confirmed by laboratory testing. Signs and symptoms consistent with CO poisoning in certain circumstances should raise the suspicion of its presence. A higher index of suspicion should attend the simultaneous presentation of multiple patients from the same family or housing complex. The eight-wavelength pulse oximeter (Masimo Rad-57) has been reported to be accurate in measuring CO.[106] Because CO has a relatively short half-life in vivo, the levels obtained in the emergency setting often do not correlate directly with symptoms.

The most important step in the treatment for CO poisoning is prompt removal of patients from the source of CO followed by administering 100% supplemental O_2 via a tight-fitting mask. The CO molecule reversibly binds to hemoglobin and is eliminated through the lungs. The serum elimination half-life of CO is 5 hours when breathing room air and 30 minutes with O_2 therapy (100% O_2 at 3 atm).[148]

For mild to moderate cases of CO poisoning, which more often happens with chronic intoxication, removing the patient from the source of environmental CO is usually curative. If the COHb level is high, breathing 100% O_2 will increase the rate of CO removal.

In severe cases of CO poisoning, which more often occur with acute intoxication, after identification and removal of the source of CO, 100% O_2 should be administered with cardiac monitoring. Endotracheal intubation should be done in any patient with impaired mental status and other interventions should be dictated by the symptomatology.

Hyperbaric O_2, which has complications of its own such as bronchial irritation and pulmonary edema, should be reserved for exceptional cases of CO intoxication. Most often, by the time the patient is brought into a hyperbaric chamber, the simple breathing of 100% O_2 has reduced COHb sufficiently to make it unnecessary. Because of conflicting evidence, there is no absolute indication for the use of hyperbaric O_2 treatment for patients with CO poisoning. Hyperbaric O_2 might be indicated in patients who have obvious neurological abnormalities, have a history of loss of consciousness with their exposure, have cardiac dysfunction, have persistent symptoms despite normobaric O_2, or have metabolic acidosis.[153] Locations of hyperbaric chambers throughout the world and in the United States can be found at the Undersea and Hyperbaric Medical Society web site, www.uhms.org under "chamber directory."

Pregnant women exposed to CO are at particularly high risk. CO poisoning is especially dangerous to the fetus because CO readily crosses the placenta and half-life of CO in the fetus is as much as five times longer than it is in the mother. For these reasons treatment with hyperbaric O_2 should be carried during pregnancy when the COHb levels exceed 15%. In limited number of studies done on pregnant patients, hyperbaric O_2 does not seem to adversely affect the fetus.[154,155]

SULFHEMOGLOBINEMIA

Definition and Pathogenesis

Sulfhemoglobin is a modification of the hemoglobin molecule that produces a bright green color because a sulfur atom is incorporated into the porphyrin ring. It has been associated with the use of certain "oxidant" medications, with drug abuse,[156–161] with occupational exposure to sulfur compounds,[162] and with exposure to polluted air.[163] Heme modification by the addition of sulfur is associated with a drastic right shift in the hemoglobin–O_2 dissociation curve in the physiologically relevant PO_2 range, rendering the molecule totally ineffective for O_2 transport.[164] Fully sulfurated tetramers seem to have no cooperativity. In most cases, only a fraction of the hemes are modified and full saturation of the unaltered hemes in the lungs and enhanced O_2 unloading in tissues would be expected. Because this right shift would ameliorate any decrease in functional hemoglobin mass, sulfuration of hemes might have little physiological significance as long as sufficient proportion of hemoglobin with some unmodified hemoglobin subunits remains.

An understanding of the molecular basis of the right-shifted oxygenation curve emerges from isoelectric focusing data. In a clinical sample that contained only 12% modified heme[165] the distribution of these hemes among partially sulfurated tetramers resulted in a larger percentage of the tetramers being abnormal. Between 24% and 48% of the hemoglobin tetramers in a clinical sample were abnormal and contributed to the shift of the hemoglobin–O_2 dissociation curve.[166] The actual effect that these partially modified molecules have on this curve depends on their conformation. Because the half-sulfurated, half-liganded tetramers have an isoelectric point between deoxyhemoglobin and oxyhemoglobin and bind 2,3-BPG under conditions when oxyhemoglobin does not, their conformation must be closer to the T-state (deoxy state) than that of oxyhemoglobin. Whereas in methemoglobinemia some tetramers have subunits fixed in an oxidized R-like state (Darling–Roughton effect),[1] in sulfhemoglobinemia some tetramers have subunits fixed in a deoxidized T-like state because they remain unliganded at physiological pO_2. In the former case, a left-shifted oxygenation curve and impaired O_2 delivery results, whereas in the latter case, a right-shifted curve and enhanced O_2 delivery occur. The slightly higher 2,3-BPG in the blood of patients with sulfhemoglobinemia probably reflects increased binding to the T-like sulfurated tetramers rather than an actual increase in free 2,3-BPG.[166,167]

Clinical Presentation, Diagnosis, and Treatment

Sulfhemoglobin in concentrations greater than 0.5 g/dL also causes "cyanosis" with a normal paO_2 and might be erroneously measured as methemoglobin. Sulfhemoglobin can be distinguished from methemoglobin by its peak absorption at 620 nm, which unlike methemoglobin is not abolished by the addition of cyanide. Sulfhemoglobin and methemoglobin have been reported to coexist in a number of cases of drug-induced acute toxic methemoglobinemia.[156–161] The lists of chemicals and drugs reported to produce these syndromes overlap. Acetanilid, usually in the form of Bromo Seltzer, and phenacetin were the main offenders in 62 cases of sulfhemoglobinemia seen at the Mayo Clinic in 1951.[157] The aryl hydroxylamine metabolites of these drugs can serve as reducing agents in a cyclic process capable of generating both sulfhemoglobin[165] and methemoglobin.[168] The origin of the sulfur atom in the former case remains unclear, but both H_2S generated by intestinal flora[169] and glutathione[170,171] have been suggested. Laboratory assays used for detection of methemoglobinemia are often inadequate to detect sulfhemoglobin, so it is likely that sulfhemoglobinemia is underdiagnosed.[172] Although acetanilid was removed from Bromo Seltzer a number of years ago and the Food and Drug Administration removed phenacetin from the United States market, sulfhemoglobinemia is not likely to vanish. Sulfonamides, dapsone, and sulfur-containing ointments are reported offenders[162,173,174] and are still widely used. Some drugs reported to produce methemoglobin, including acetaminophen, might be found to also produce sulfhemoglobin when more careful analysis is done. Sulfhemoglobinemia, which has been associated with constipation, possibly because sulfides produced by an expanded intestinal flora when stasis exists, converts methemoglobin to sulfhemoglobin. Treatment of this cause of sulfhemoglobinemia is to treat constipation.

Accidents involving occupational exposure to hydrogen sulphide (H_2S) are expected to increase.[175] Because exposure of red blood cells to H_2S produces sulfhemoglobin within minutes, it is likely that occupational exposure to H_2S poisoning in industrial societies, particularly emerging ones, will increase. A fatal case of a shrimp fisherman exposed to high levels of ambient H_2S emanating from the dithionite-treated catch has been reported.[165] In Alberta, Canada, there were 221 cases of exposure to H_2S over 4 years, with an overall mortality of 6%. Hospital admission was required for 65% of the victims.[175] Acute problems were coma, ataxia, and respiratory insufficiency with pulmonary edema. Sulfhemoglobin is seldom suspected in this setting and thus likely underdiagnosed. Increased interest in occupational and environmental pollutants and screening of populations at risk could reveal many more subclinical cases. Although CO_2 was thought to be the cause of death in the Lake Nyos African disaster that claimed nearly 2,000 lives as a cloud of toxic gases erupted from the bottom of this tropical lake, H_2S was among the liberated gases that could have modified hemoglobin and contributed to this calamity.[176] Significant exposure to H_2S can occur in workers at sulphurous thermal baths. Blood sulfhemoglobin levels has been shown to be a reliable measure of individual exposure to H_2S.[177] One case report described the false diagnosis of "methemoglobinemia," which on further analysis, because of refractoriness to methylene blue, was found to be sulfhemoglobinemia.[72] The patient had applied 4 oz of dimethyl sulfoxide to her abdomen to treat interstitial cystitis. Within 24 hours she developed fatigue, cyanosis, and dyspnea with mild exertion.

Although sulfhemoglobinemia is probably a relatively nontoxic syndrome in individuals with HbA, it might prove to be a surprisingly toxic syndrome in individuals with HbS, especially compared with methemoglobinemia, which would be expected to ameliorate sickling because of left-shifted hemoglobin dissociation curve associated with methemoglobinemia. The presence of sulfurated subunits will shift the conformation of HbS tetramers toward the unliganded, polymerizing T form, even in the presence of high pO_2, thus leading to polymerization of HbS. Microvascular occlusion could be exacerbated by these tetramers remaining in the polymerizing conformation in both the arterial and venous circulation. This hypothetical scenario has yet to be reported.

Congenital sulfhemoglobinemia has been reported but is rare and a fraction of sulfhemoglobin has been described with an unstable hemoglobin.[137]

Diagnosis of sulfhemoglobinemia is suspected when a patient who is cyanotic with normal to near-normal O_2 tension and the clinical and laboratory diagnosis of methemoglobinemia does not respond to therapy with methylene blue. With the eight-wavelength pulse oximeter capable of measuring methemoglobin more accurately, diagnosis of sulfhemoglobinemia will likely be made earlier without requiring waiting for therapy with methylene blue treatment to fail. With equivalent amounts of abnormal pigment, the patient with sulfhemoglobinemia appears more cyanotic than the patient with methemoglobinemia as a result of spectral differences between the pigments, but is less symptomatic as a result of the differences in P_{50}. This is fortunate, as there is no known treatment analogous to methemoglobin reduction for reconverting sulfhemoglobin to functional hemoglobin; exchange transfusion is the sole therapeutic option, if therapy is needed.

In summary, sulfhemoglobin is a green-pigmented protein that can be accurately identified by spectrophotometry and isoelectric focusing. At low concentrations, sulfurated tetramers are shifted toward the deoxy or T form, producing a right shift of the O_2 equilibrium curve. For this reason, dyspnea is absent unless the levels of sulfhemoglobin are extraordinarily high. Mild cases that are typically undiagnosed might be revealed in screening studies looking for toxic effects of drugs and environmental pollutants. Awareness of this entity and modern, widely used, simple equipment could allow us to determine the true prevalence of sulfhemoglobinemia.

CONCLUSIONS

COHb, methemoglobin, and sulfhemoglobin are present in normal red cells in very low concentrations. Mutations or environmental conditions can increase the concentrations of these liganded or oxidized hemoglobins, producing a dyshemoglobinemia. Although rare, increased levels of dyshemoglobins can be life threatening so that their presence should be identified in a timely fashion to permit effective treatment. The distinction between environmental and genetic dyshemoglobinemia is often blurred because many acquired dyshemoglobins are, in effect, the consequence of both an environmental challenge and a genetic predisposition.

REFERENCES

1. Darling R, Roughton F. The effect of methemoglobin on the equilibrium between oxygen and hemoglobin. *Am J Physiol.* 1942;137:56.
2. Olsen M, McEvoy GK. Methemoglobinemia induced by topical anesthetics. *Am J Hosp Pharm.* 1981;38:89–93.
3. Percy MJ, McFerran NV, Lappin TR. Disorders of oxidised haemoglobin. *Blood Rev.* 2005;19:61–8.
4. Misra H, Fridorich I. The generation of superoxide radical during the autoxidation of hemoglobin. *J Biol Chem.* 1972;247:6960.
5. Jaffe E, Neumann, G. A comparison of the effect of mendione, methylene blue, and ascorbic acid on the reduction of methemoglobin in vivo. *Nature.* 1964;202:607.
6. Jaffe E, Hultquist D. Cytochrome b5 reductase deficiency and enzymopenic hereditary methemoglobinemia. In: Scriver C, Beaudet A, Sly W, Valle D, eds. *The Metabolic and*

Molecular Bases of Inherited Disease. 7th ed., New York: McGraw Hill; 1995;2:3399.

7. Feelisch M, Kubitzek, D, Werringloer, J. The oxyhemoglobin assay. In: Feelisch M, Stamler J, eds. *Methods in Nitric Oxide Research*; New York: John Wiley and Sons;1996:453.
8. Stuhlmeier K, Kao, JJ, Wallbrandt P, et al. Antioxidant protein 2 prevents methemoglobin formation in erythrocyte hemolysates. *Eur J Biochem.* 2003;270:334–41.
9. Strittmatter P. The reaction sequence in electron transfer in the reduced nicotinamide adenine dinucleotide-cytochrome b5 reductase system. *J Biol Chem.* 1965;240:4481.
10. Iyanagi T, Watanabe, S, Anan, KF. One-electron oxidation-reduction properties of hepatic NADH-cytochrome b5 reductase. *Biochemistry.* 1984;23:1418–25.
11. Scott EM, Mc GJ. Purification and properties of diphosphopyridine nucleotide diaphorase of human erythrocytes. *J Biol Chem.* 1962;237:249–52.
12. Kuma F, Ishizawa S, Hirayama K, et al. Studies on methemoglobin reductase. I. Comparative studies of diaphorases from normal and methemoglobinemic erythrocytes. *J Biol Chem.* 1972;247:550.
13. Passon P, Hultquist D. Soluble cytochrome b5 reductase from human erythrocytes. *Biochim Biophys Acta.* 1972;275:62.
14. Hackett C, Strittmatter P. Covalent cross-linking of the active sites of vesicle-bound cytochrome b5 and NADH-cytochrome b5 reductase. *J Biol Chem.* 1984;259:3275.
15. Warburg O, Kubowitz F, Christian W. Uber die katalytische wirkung von methlenblau in lebenden zellen. *Biochem Z.* 1930;227:245.
16. Kiese M. *Die reduktion des hamiglobins.* 1944;316:264.
17. Yubisui T, Takeshita M, Yoneyama Y. Reduction of methemoglobin through flavin at the physiological concentration by NADPH-flavin reductase of human erythrocytes. *J Biochem (Tokyo).* 1980;87:1715.
18. Yubisui T, Miyata T, Iwanaga S, et al. Complete amino acid sequence of NADH-cytochrome b5 reductase purified from human erythrocytes. *J Biochem.* 1986;99:407.
19. Francois. A case of congenital cyanosis without an apparent cause. *Bull Acad Roy Med Belg.* 1845;4:698.
20. Hitzenberger K. Autotoxic cyanosis due to intraglobular methemoglobinemia. *Wien Arch Med.* 1932;23:85.
21. Gibson Q. Historical note: methemoglobinemia-long ago and far away. *Am J Hematol.* 1993;42:3–6.
22. Gibson Q. Introduction: congenital methemoglobinemia revisited. *Blood.* 2002;100:3445.
23. Percy M, Gillespie M, Savage G, et al. Familial idiopathic mutations in NADH-cytochrome b5 reductase. *Blood.* 2002;100:3447.
24. Bull P, Shephard E, Povey S, et al. Cloning and chromosomal mapping of human cytochrome b5 reductase (DIA1). *Ann Hum Genet.* 1988;52:263.
25. Tomatsu S, Kobayashi Y, Fukumaki Y, et al. The organization and the complete nucleotide sequence of the human NADH-cytochrome b5 reductase gene. *Gene.* 1989;80:353–361.
26. Percy MJ, Oren H, Savage G, Irken G. Congenital methaemoglobinaemia Type I in a Turkish infant due to a novel mutation, Pro144Ser, in NADH-cytochrome b5 reductase. *Hematol J.* 2004;5(4):367–370.
27. Percy MJ, Crowley LJ, Davis CA, et al. Recessive congenital methaemoglobinaemia: functional characterization of the novel D239G mutation in the NADH-binding lobe of cytochrome b5 reductase. *Br J Haematol.* 2005;129(6):847–853.
28. Percy MJ, Crowley LJ, Boudreaux J, et al. Expression of a novel P275L variant of NADH:cytochrome b5 reductase gives functional insight into the conserved motif important for pyridine nucleotide binding. *Arch Biochem Biophys.* 2006;447(1):59–67.
29. Wang Y, Wu Y, Zheng P, et al. A novel mutation in the NADH-cytochrome b5 reductase gene of a Chinese patient with recessive congenital methemoglobinemia. *Blood.* 2000; 95:3250.
30. Higasa K, Manabe J, Yubisui T, et al. Molecular basis of hereditary methaemoglobinaemia, types I and II: two novel mutations in the NADH-cytochrome b5 reductase gene. *Br J Haematol.* 1998;103:922.
31. Shotelersuk V, Tosukhowong P, Chotivitayatarakorn P, et al. A Thai boy with hereditary enzymopenic methemoglobinemia type II. *J Med Assoc Thai.* 2000;83:1380.
32. Jenkins M, Prchal J. A novel mutation found in the 3′ domain of NADH-cytochrome b5 reductase in an African-American family with type I congenital methemoglobinemia. *Blood.* 1996;87:2993–2999.
33. Nussenzveig R, Lingam HB, Gaikwad A, et al. A novel mutation of the cytochrome-b5 reductase gene in an Indian patient: the molecular basis of type I methemoglobinemia. *Haematologica.* 2006;91:1542–1545.
34. Jenkins M, Prchal J. A high frequency polymorphism of NADH-cytochrome b5 reductase in African-Americans. *Hum Genet.* 1997;99:248–250.
35. Pietrini G, Carrera P, Borgese N. Two transcripts encode rat cytochrome b5 reductase. *Proc Natl Acad Sci USA.* 1988;85:7246–7250.
36. Pietrini G, Aggujaro D, Carrera P, et al. A single mRNA, transcribed from an alternative erythroid-specific promoter, codes for two non-myristylated forms of NADH-cytochrome b5 reductase. *J Cell Biol.* 1992;117:975.
37. Mota Vieira L, Kaplan J-C, Kahn A, et al. Heterogeneity of the rat NADH-cytochrome-b5-reductase transcripts resulting from multiple alternative first exons. *FEBS.* 1994;220:729.
38. Bulbarelli A, Valentini A, DeSilvestris M, et al. An erythroid-specific transcript generates the soluble form of NADH-cytochrome b5 reductase in humans. *Blood.* 1998;92:310–319.
39. Borgese N, Pietrini G. Distribution of the integral membrane protein NADH-cytochrome b5 reductase in rat liver cells, studied with a quantitative radioimmunoblotting assay. *Biochem J.* 1986;239:393–403.
40. Tamura M, Yubisui T, Takeshita M, et al. Structural comparison of bovine erythrocyte, brain, and liver NADH-cytochrome b5 reductase by HPLC mapping. *J Biochem (Tokyo).* 1987;101:1147–1159.
41. Ozols J, Korza G, Heinemann, FS, et al. Complete amino acid sequence of steer liver microsomal NADH-cytochrome b5 reductase. *J Biol Chem.* 1985;260:11953–11961.
42. Yubisui T, Naitoh Y, Zenno S, et al. Molecular cloning of cDNAs of human liver and placenta NADH-cytochrome b5 reductase. *Proc Natl Acad Sci USA.* 1987;84:3609–3613.
43. Zenno S, Hattori M, Misumi Y, et al. Molecular cloning of a cDNA encoding rat NADH-cytochrome b5 reductase and the corresponding gene. *J Biochem (Tokyo).* 1990;107:810–816.

44. Hultquist D, Passon P. Catalysis of methemoglobin reduction by erythrocyte cytochrome b5 and cytochrome b5 reductase. *Nature.* 1971;229:252.
45. Kitajima S, Yasukochi Y, Minakami S. Purification and properties of human erythrocyte membrane NADH-cytochrome b5 reductase. *Arch Biochem Biophys.* 1981;210:330.
46. Dekker J, Eppink M, van Zwieten R, et al. Seven new nucleotides in the nicotinamide adenine dinucleotide reduced-cytochrome b(5) reductase gene leading to methemoglobinemia type I. *Blood.* 2001;97:1106–1114.
47. Gonzalez R, Estrada M, Wade M, et al. Heterogeneity of hereditary methaemoglobinaemia: a study of 4 Cuban families with NADH-Methaemoglobin reductase deficiency including a new variant (Santiago de Cuba variant). *Scand J Haematol.* 1978;20(5):385–393.
48. Board P, Petcock M. Methaemoglobinaemia resulting from heterozygosity for two NADH-methaemoglobin reductase variants: characterization as NADH-ferricyanide reductase. *Br J Haematol.* 1981;47:361–370.
49. Jaffe E. Hereditary methemoglobinemias associated with abnormalities in the metabolism of erythrocytes. *Ann J Med.* 1962;32:512.
50. Waller H. Inherited methemoglobinemia (enzyme deficiencies). *Humangenetik.* 1970;9:217.
51. Cohen R, Sachs J, Wicker D, et al. Methemoglobinemia provoked by malarial chemoprophylaxis in Vietnam. *New Engl J Med.* 1968;279:1127.
52. Scott E, Hoskins D. Hereditary methemoglobinemia in Alaskan Eskimos and Indians. *Blood.* 1958;13:795.
53. Scott E. The relation of diaphorase of human erythrocytes to inheritance of methemoglobinemia. *J Clin Invest.* 1960;39:1176.
54. Balsamo P, Hardy W, Scott E. Hereditary methemoglobinemia due to diaphorase deficiency in Navajo Indians. *J Pediatr.* 1964;65:928.
55. Ilinskaia I, Derviz G, Lavrova O, et al. Enzymatic methemoglobinemia. In: Papers of the Symposium: Biological Problems of the North State University, Yakutsk, and 1974: 226.
56. Andreeva A, Dmitrieva M, Levina A, et al. Molecular basis for disorders in the functional properties of hemoglobin in patients with enzymopenic methemoglobinemia. Papers of the 49th Scientific Session of the Central Scientific Research Institute of Hematology and Blood Transfusion. 1979;SSSR:73.
57. Prchal J, Borgese N, Moore M, et al. Congenital methemoglobinemia due to methemoglobin reductase deficiency in two unrelated American black families. *Am J Med.* 1990;89:516.
58. Katsube T, Sakamoto N, Kobayashi Y, et al. Exonic point mutations in NADH-cytochrome B5 reductase genes of homozygotes for hereditary methemoglobinemia, types I and III: putative mechanisms of tissue-dependent enzyme deficiency. *Am J Hum Genet.* 1991;48(4):799–808.
59. Shirabe K, Yubisui T, Borgese N, et al. Enzymatic instability of NADH-cytochrome b5 reductase as a cause of hereditary methemoglobinemia type I (red cell type). *J Biol Chem.* 1992;267:20416–20421.
60. Leroux A, Junien C, Kaplan J-C, et al. Generalised deficiency of cytochrome b5 reductase in congenital methaemoglobinaemia with mental retardation. *Nature.* 1975;258:619.
61. Takeshita M, Tamura M, Kugi M, et al. Decrease of palmitoyl-CoA elongation in platelets and leukocytes in the patient of hereditary methemoglobinemia associated with mental retardation. *Biochem Biophys Res Commun.* 1987;148:384–391.
62. Kobayashi Y, Fukumaki Y, Yubisui T, et al. Serine-proline replacement at residue 127 of NADH-cytochrome b5 reductase causes hereditary methemoglobinemia, generalized type. *Blood.* 1990;75:1408–1413.
63. Shirabe K, Fujimoto Y, Yubisui T, et al. An in-frame deletion of codon 298 of the NADH-cytochrome b5 reductase gene results in hereditary methemoglobinemia type II (generalized type). A functional implication for the role of the COOH-terminal region of the enzyme. *J Biol Chem.* 1994;269:5952–5957.
64. Jenkins M, Prchal J. A novel mutation found in the NADH-cytochrome b5 reductase gene in African-American family with type I congenital methemoglobinemia. *Blood.* 1995;86:649.
65. Shirabe K, Landi M, Takeshita M, et al. A novel point mutation in a 3′ splice site of the NADH-cytochrome b5 reductase gene results in immunologically undetectable enzyme and impaired NADH-dependent ascorbate regeneration in cultured fibroblasts of a patient with type II hereditary methemoglobinemia. *Am J Hum Genet.* 1995;57:302–310.
66. Vieira L, Kaplan JC, Kahn A, et al. Four new mutations in the NADH-cytochrome b5 reductase gene from patients with recessive congenital methemoglobinemia type II. *Blood.* 1995;85:2254–2262.
67. Manabe J, Arya R, Sumimoto H, et al. Two novel mutations in the reduced nicotinamide adenine dinucleotide (NADH)-cytochrome b5 reductase gene of a patient with generalized type, hereditary methemoglobinemia. *Blood.* 1996;88:3208–3215.
68. Owen E, Berens J, Marinaki AM, et al. Recessive congenital methaemoglobinaemia type II a new mutation which causes incorrect splicing in the NADH-cytochrome b5 reductase gene. *J Inherit Metab Dis.* 1997;20:610.
69. Hegesh E, Hegesh J, Kaftory A. Congenital methemoglobinemia with a deficiency of cytochrome b5. *N Engl J Med.* 1986;314:757.
70. Giordano S, Kaftory A, Steggles A. A splicing mutation in the cytochrome b5 gene from a patient with congenital methemoglobinemia and pseudohermaphrodism. *Hum Genet.* 1994;93:568.
71. Townes P, Morrison M. Investigation of the defect in a variant of hereditary methemoglobinemia. *Blood.* 1962;19:60.
72. Mansouri A, Lurie AA. Concise review: methemoglobinemia. *Am J Hematol.* 1993;42:7–12.
73. Coleman M, Coleman NA. Drug-induced methaemoglobinaemia. Treatment issues. *Drug Saf.* 1996;14:394–405.
74. Hadjiliadis D, Govert J. Methemoglobinemia after infusion of ifosfamide chemotherapy: first report of a potentially serious adverse reaction related to ifosfamide. *Chest.* 2000;118:1208.
75. Kizer N, Martinez E, Powell M. Report of two cases of rasburicase-induced methemoglobinemia. *Leuk Lymphoma.* 2006;47:2648–2650.
76. Daly J, Hultquist D, Rucknagel D. Phenazopyridine induced methaemoglobinaemia associated with decreased activity of erythrocyte cytochrome-b5 reductase. *J Med Genet.* 1983;20:307.

77. Linden C, Burns MJ. Poisoning and drug overdosage. In: Braunwald E FA, Kasper D, Hauser S, Longo D, Jameson J, et al., eds. *Harrison's Principles of Internal Medicine* 15th ed: New York: McGraw-Hill; 2001:2612.
78. Ash-Bernal R, Wise R, Wright SM. Acquired methemoglobinemia: a retrospective series of 138 cases at 2 teaching hospitals. *Medicine (Baltimore)*. 2004;83:265.
79. Moore T, Walsh CS, Cohen MR. Reported adverse event cases of methemoglobinemia associated with benzocaine products. *Arch Intern Med*. 2004;164:1192–1196.
80. Novaro G, Aronow H, Militello M, et al. Benzocaine-induced methemoglobinemia: experience from a high-volume transesophageal echocardiography laboratory. *J Am Soc Echocardiogr*. 2003;16:170.
81. Ross J. Deficient activity of DPNH-dependent methemoglobin diaphorase in cord blood erythrocytes. *Blood*. 1963; 21:51.
82. Bartos H, Desforges J. Erythrocyte DPNH-dependent diaphorase levels in infants. *Pediatrics*. 1966;37:991.
83. Eng L, Loo M, Fah FK. Diaphroase activity and variants in normal adults and newborns. *Br J Haematol*. 1972;23:419.
84. Comly H. Cyanosis in infants caused by nitrates in well water. *JAMA*. 1945;129:112.
85. Kross B, Ayebo A, Fuortes L. Methemoglobinemia: nitrate toxicity in rural America. *Am Fam Physician*. 1992;46:183.
86. Greer F, Shannon M. Infant methemoglobinemia: the role of dietary nitrate in food and water. *Pediatrics*. 2005;116:784–786.
87. Heyman I. Methemoglobinemia in infants. *Harefuah*. 1954; 46:144.
88. Yano S, Danish E, Hsia Y. Transient methemoglobinemia with acidosis in infants. *J Pediatr*. 1982;100:415.
89. Hegesh E, Shiloah, J. Blood nitrates and infantile methemoglobinemia. *Clin Chim Acta*. 1982;125:107.
90. Pollack E, Pollack CJ. Incidence of subclinical methemoglobinemia in infants with diarrhea. *Ann Emerg Med*. 1994;24:652.
91. Hanakoglu A, Danon P. Endogenous methemoglobinemia associated with diarrheal disease in infancy. *J Pediatr Gastroenterol and Nutr*. 1996;23:1.
92. Carlson G, Negri E, McGrew A, et al. Two cases of methemoglobinemia from the use of topical anesthetics. *J Emerg Nurs*. 2003;29:106–108.
93. Kilbourn R, Belloni P. Endothelial cell production of nitrogen oxides in response to interferon gamma in combination with tumor necrosis factor, interleukin-1, or endotoxin. *J Natl Cancer Inst*. 1990;82:772–776.
94. Moncada S, Palmer, RMJ, Higgs EA. Nitric oxide: Physiology, pathophysiology, and pharmacology. *Pharmacol Rev*. 1991;43:109–142.
95. Szabo C, Thiemermann C. Role of nitric oxide in haemorrhagic, traumatic and anaphylactic shock and in thermal injury. *Shock*. 1994;2:145–155.
96. Sharma V, Isaacson RA, John ME, et al. Reaction of nitric oxide with heme proteins: Studies on metmyoglobin, opossum methemoglobin and microperoxidase. *Biochemistry*. 1983;22:3897–3902.
97. Wennmalm A, Benthin G, Patersson AS. Dependence of the metabolism of nitric oxide in healthy human whole blood on the oxygenation of its red cell hemoglobin. *Br J Pharmacol*. 1992;106:507–508.
98. Chou T, Gibran NS, Urdahl K, et al. Methemoglobinemia secondary to topical silver nitrate therapy-a case report. *Burns*. 1999;25:549–552.
99. Bhattacharya J, Swarup-Mitra, S. Role of Plasmodium vivax in oxidation of haemoglobin in red cells of the host. *Indian J Med Res*. 1986;83:111–113.
100. Baird J, Lacy MD, Basri H, et al. Randomized, parallel placebo-controlled trial of primaquine for malaria prophylaxis in Papua, Indonesia. *Clin Infect Dis*. 2001;33:1990–1997.
101. Maran J, Guan Y, Ou CN, et al. Heterogeneity of the molecular biology of methemoglobinemia: a study of eight consecutive patients. *Haematologica*. 2005;90:687.
102. Barker S, Tremper K, Hyatt J. Effects of methemoglobinemia on pulse oximetry and mixed venous oximetry. *Anesthesiology*. 1989;70:112.
103. Kelner M, Bailey D. Mismeasurement of methemoglobin ("methemoglobin revisited"). *Clin Chem*. 1985;31:168.
104. Molthrop D, Wheeler, R, Hall K, et al. Evaluation of the methemoglobinemia associated with sulofenur. *Invest New Drugs*. 1994;12:99.
105. Evelyn K, Malloy H. Microdetermination of oxyhemoglobin, methemoglobin, and sulfhemoglobin in a single sample of blood. *J Biol Chem*. 1938;126:655.
106. Barker S, Curry J, Redford D, et al. Measurement of carboxyhemoglobin and methemoglobin by pulse oximetry: a human volunteer study. *Anesthesiology*. 2006;105:892–897.
107. Beutler E, Baluda M. Methemoglobin reduction: Studies of the interaction between cell populations and of the role of methylene blue. *Blood*. 1963;22:323.
108. Jaffe E. Hereditary methemoglobinemias associated with abnormalities in the metabolism of erythrocytes. *Am J Med*. 1966;41:786.
109. Jaffe E, Hsieh H. DPNH-methemoglobin reductase deficiency and hereditary methemoglobinemia. *Semin Hemat*. 1971;8:417.
110. Hegesh E, Calmanovici N, Avron M. New method for determining ferrihemoglobin reductase (NADH-methemoglobin reductase) in erythrocytes. *J Lab Clin Med*. 1968;72:339.
111. Board P. NADH-ferricyanide reductase, a convenient approach to the evaluation of NADH-methaemoglobin reductase in human erythrocytes. *Clin Chim Acta*. 1981;109: 233.
112. Kaftory A, Freundlich E, Manaster J, et al. Prenatal diagnosis of congenital methemoglobinemia with mental retardation. *Isr J Med Sci*. 1986;22:837.
113. Leroux A, Leturcq F, Deburgrave N, Szajnert MF. Prenatal diagnosis of recessive congenital methaemoglobinaemia type II: novel mutation in the NADH-cytochrome b5 reductase gene leading to stop codon read-through. *Eur J Haematol*. 2005;74:389–395.
114. Arnold H, Botcher H, Hufnagel D, et al. Hereditary methemoglobinemia due to methemoglobin reductase deficiency in erythrocytes and leukocytes without neurological symptoms (abstract). In: *XVII Congress of the International Society of Hematology*. Paris; 1978:752.
115. Tanishima K, Tanimoto K, Tomoda A, et al. Hereditary methemoglobinemia due to cytochrome b5 reductase deficiency in blood cells without associated neurologic and mental disorders. *Blood*. 1985;66:1288.

116. Nagai T, Shirabe K, Yubisui T, et al. Analysis of mutant NADH-cytochrome b5 reductase: apparent "type III" methemoglobinemia can be explained as type I with an unstable reductase. *Blood.* 1993;81:808.
117. Beutler E. Methemoglobinemia and other causes of cyanosis. In: Beutler E, Lichtman MA, Coller B, Kipps, TJ, eds. *Williams' Hematology.* 5th ed. New York: McGraw-Hill; 1995:654.
118. Kaplan J, Chirouze M. Therapy of recessive congenital methaemoglobinemia by oral riboflavin. *Lancet.* 1978;2:1043.
119. Goluboff N, Wheaton, R. Methylene blue induced cyanosis and acute hemolytic anemia complicating the treatment of methemoglobinemia. *J Pediatr.* 1961;58:86.
120. Harvey J, Keitt A. Studies of the efficacy and potential hazards of methylene blue therapy in aniline-induced methemoglobinemia. *Br J Haematol.* 1983;54:29.
121. Rosen P, Johnson C, McGehee WG, et al. Failure of methylene blue treatment in toxic methemoglobinemia: associations with glucose-6-phosphate dehydrogenase deficiency. *Ann Intern Med.* 1971;75:83.
122. Goldstein G, Doull J. Treatment of nitrite-induce methemoglobinemia with hyperbaric oxygen. *Proc Soc Experimental Biology and Medicine.* 1971;138:134.
123. Coleman M, Rhodes LE, Scott AK, et al. The use of cimetidine to reduce dapsone-dependent methaemoglobinaemia in dermatitis herpetiformis patients. *Br J Clin Pharmacol.* 1992;34:244.
124. Vreman H, Mahoney JJ, Stevenson DK. Carbon monoxide and carboxyhemoglobin. *Adv Pediatr.* 1995;42:303–325.
125. Hampson N. Trends in the incidence of carbon monoxide poisoning in the United States. *Am J Emerg Med.* 2005;23:838–841.
126. Hampson N. Emergency department visits for carbon monoxide poisoning in the Pacific northwest. *J Emerg Med.* 1998;16:695–698.
127. Weaver L. Carbon monoxide poisoning. *Crit Care Clin.* 1999;15:297–317.
128. Ernst A, Zibrak JD. Carbon monoxide poisoning. *N Engl J Med.* 1998;339:1603–1608.
129. Centres for Disease Control and Prevention C. Carbon monoxide poisoning from hurricane-associated use of portable generators – Florida 2004. *MMWR.* 2005;54:697–700.
130. Centers for Disease Control and Prevention C. Unintentional non-fire-related carbon monoxide exposures–United States, 2001–2003. *MMWR.* 2005;54:36–39.
131. Mott J, Wolfe MI, Alverson CJ, et al. National vehicle emissions policies and practices and declining US carbon monoxide-related mortality. *JAMA.* 2002;288:988–995.
132. Harper A, Croft-Baker J. Carbon monoxide poisoning: undetected by both patients and their doctors. *Age Ageing.* 2004;33:105–109.
133. US Environmental Protection Agency Emission facts: Idling vehicle emissions. US Environmental Protection Agency, Washington, DC; 1998 Publication EPA420-F-98-014 1998.
134. Centers for Disease Control and Prevention Carbon monoxide poisoning from hurricane-associated use of portable generators – Florida 2004. *MMWR.* 2005;54:697–700.
135. Stewart R, Fisher TN, Hosko MJ, et al. Carboxyhemoglobin elevation after exposure to dichloromethane. *Science.* 1972;176:295–296.
136. Antonini E, Brunori M. Hemoglobin and myoglobin in their reactions with ligands. In: Neuberger A, Tatum EL, eds. *Frontiers of Biology.* Amsterdam, London: North-Holland Publishing Company; 1971.
137. Bunn H, Forget BG. *Hemoglobin: Molecular, Genetic and Clinical Aspects.* New York: Saunders; 1986.
138. Cheng X, Schoenborn BP. Neutron diffraction study of carbon- monoxymyoglobin. *J Mol Biol.* 1991;220:381–399.
139. Kachalova G, Popov AN, Bartunik HD. A steric mechanism for inhibition of CO binding of heme proteins. *Science.* 1999;284:473–476.
140. Sjostrand T. Endogenous formation of carbon monoxide in man. *Nature.* 1949;164:580–581.
141. Coburn R, Danielson GK, Blakemore WS, et al. Carbon monoxide in blood: Analytical method and sources of error. *J Appl Physiol.* 1964;19:510–515.
142. Coburn R, Williams WJ, Kahn SB. Endogenous carbon dioxide production in patients with hemolytic anemia. *J Clin Invest.* 1966;44:460–468.
143. EPA. 600/8–90/045F: Air Quality Criteria for Carbon Monoxide. Research Triangle Park, NC, Environmental Criteria and Assessment Office, Office of Health and Environmental Assessment, Office of Research and Development, US Environmental Protection Agency, 1991:1–1 to 12–23.
144. Marks G, Brien JF, Nakatsu K, et al. Does carbon monoxide have a biological function? *Trends Pharmacol Sci.* 1991;12:185–188.
145. McGrath J. Effects of altitude on endogenous carboxyhemoglobin levels. *J Toxicol Environ Health.* 1992;35:127–33.
146. Giacometti G, Brunori, M, Antonini E, et al. The reaction of hemoglobin Zurich with oxygen and carbon monoxide. *J Biol Chem.* 1980;255:6160–6165.
147. Balster R, Ekelund LG, Grover RF. Evaluation of subpopulations potentially at risk to carbon monoxide exposure, in EPA 600/8–90/045F: Air quality criteria for carbon monoxide. Research Triangle Park, NC, Environmental Criteria and Assessment Office, Office of Health and Environmental Assessment, Office of Research and Development, US Environmental Protection Agency 1991:12–1 to 12–23.
148. Hampson N, Dunford RG, Kramer CC, et al. Selection criteria utilized for hyperbaric oxygen treatment of carbon monoxide poisoning. *J Emerg Med.* 1995;13:227–231.
149. Benesch R, Maeda N, Benesch R. 2,3-Diphosphoglycerate and the relative affinity of adult and fetal hemoglobin for oxygen and carbon dioxide. *Biochim Biophys Acta.* 1972;257:178–182.
150. Engel R, Rodkey FL, O'Neal JD, et al. Relative affinity of human fetal hemoglobin for CO and O2. *Blood.* 1969;33:37–45.
151. Gemelli F, Cattani R. Carbon monoxide poisoning in childhood. *Br Med J.* 1985;291:1197.
152. Lacey D. Neurologic sequellae of acute carbon monoxide intoxication. *Am J Dis Child.* 1981;135:145–147.
153. Kao L, Nanagas KA. Carbon monoxide poisoning. *Emerg Med Clin North Am.* 2004;22:985–1018.
154. Elkharrat D, Raphael JC, Korach JM, et al. Acute carbon monoxide intoxication and hyperbaric oxygen in pregnancy. *Intensive Care Med.* 1991;17:289–292.
155. Koren G, Sharav T, Pastuszak A, et al. A multicenter, prospective study of fetal outcome following accidental carbon monoxide poisoning in pregnancy. *Reprod Toxicol.* 1991;5:397–403.

156. Evans A, Enzer N, Eder HA, et al. Hemolytic anemia with paroxymal methemoglobnemia and sulfhemoglobinemia. *Arch Intern Med.* 1950;86:22.
157. Bradenburg R, Smith HL. Sulfhemoglobinemia: a study of 62 clinical cases. *Am Heart J.* 1951;42:582.
158. Reynolds T, Ware AG. Sulfhemoglobinemia following habitual use of acetanilid. *JAMA.* 1952;149:538–542.
159. Cumming R, Pollock A. Drug induced sulphaemoglobinemia and Heinz body anemia in pregnancy with involvement of the foetus. *Scott Med J.* 1967;12:320–322.
160. Kneezel LD, Kitchens CS. Phenacetin-induced sulfhemoglobinemia: Report of a case and review of the literature. *Johns Hopkins Med J.* 1967;139:175–180.
161. Lambert M, Sonnet J, Mahien P, et al. Delayed sulfhemoglobinemia after acute dapsone intoxication. *Clin Toxicol.* 1982;19:45–49.
162. Ford R, Shkov J, Akman WV, et al. Deaths from asphyxia among fisherman. *PFR: MMWR.* 1978;27:309.
163. Madeiros M, Bechara EJ, Naoum PC, et al. Oxygen toxicity and hemoglobinemia in subjects from a highly polluted town. *Arch Environ Health.* 1983;38:11–15.
164. Carrico R, Blumberg WE, Peisach J J. The reversible binding of oxygen to sulfhemoglobin. *J Biol Chem.* 1978;253:7212–7215.
165. Park C, Nagel RL. Sulfhemoglobinemia. Clinical and molecular aspects. *N Engl J Med.* 1984;310:1579–1584.
166. Park C, Nagel RL, Blumberg WE. Sulfhemoglobin. Properties of partially sulfurated tetramers. *J Bio Chem.* 1986;261:8805–8810.
167. Berzofsky J, Peisach J, Blumberg WE. Sulfheme proteins. II. The reversible oxygenation of ferrous sulfmyoglobin. *J Biol Chem.* 1971;246:7366–7372.
168. Nichol A, Hendry I, Movell DB, et al. Mechanism of formation of sulfhemoglobin. *Biochim Biophys Acta.* 1968;156:97–103.
169. Kiese M. The biochemical production of ferrihemoglobin-forming derivatives from aromatic amines and mechanisms of ferrihemoglobin formation. *Pharmacol Rev.* 1966;18:1091–1161.
170. McCutcheon A. Sulphaemoglobinaemia and glutathione. *Lancet.* 1960;2:290.
171. Gibson Q, Roughton, FJW. The kinetics and equilibria of the reactions of nitric oxide with sheep haemoglobin. *J Physiol.* 1957;136:507–526.
172. Suzuki T, Hayshi A, Shimizu A, et al. The oxygen equilibrium of hemoglobin M Saskatoon. Biochim. *Biophys Acta.* 1966;127:280–282.
173. Basch F. On hydrogen sulfide poisoning from external application of elementary sulfur as an ointment. *Arch Exp Pathol Pharmacol.* 1926;111:126.
174. Glud T. A case of enterogenic cyanosis? Complete recovery from acquired met- and sulfhemoglobinemia following treatment with neomycin and bacitracin. *Ugeskr Laeg.* 1979;141:1410–1411.
175. Burnett E, King EG, Grace M, et al. Hydrogen sulfide poisoning: review of 5 years' experience. *Can Med Assoc.* 1977;117:1277–1280.
176. Afane Ze E, Roche N, Atchou G, et al. Respiratory symptoms and peak expiratory flow in survivors of the Nyos disaster. *Chest.* 1996;110:1278–1281.
177. Ensabella F, Spirito A, Dupre S, et al. Measurement of sulfhemoglobin (S-Hb) blood levels to determine individual hydrogen sulfide exposure in thermal baths in Italy. Italian. *Ig Sanita Pubbl.* 2004;60:201–217.

SECTION SEVEN

SPECIAL TOPICS IN HEMOGLOBINOPATHIES

Martin H. Steinberg

Three chapters in this section, Population Genetics and Global Health Burden, Genetic Modulation of Sickle Cell Disease and Thalassemia, and Developments in Laboratory Methods to Detect Hemoglobinopathies, cover diverse subjects.

Without endemic malaria, the genes for HbS, HbC, HbE, and the thalassemias would not exist at polymorphic frequencies as the selective pressure from *Plasmodium falciparum* is so strong. Weatherall and Williams discuss the "Malaria hypothesis," and the evidence that carriers of thalassemia and HbS, HbC, and HbE are protected from *P. falciparum* infection, although the mechanisms behind such protection are incompletely understood. The health burden of hemoglobinopathies and thalassemia is great, particularly in developing countries, and it is likely to increase as development proceeds. Many obstacles to providing genetic services are discussed, among them, the prioritization of scant healthcare resources and the problems posed by communicable disease and malnutrition, leaving hemoglobin disorders underserved.

Hemoglobinopathy detection is often a part of the evaluation of anemia and microcytosis. It should first be determined, using hemoglobin high-performance liquid chromatography, whether a variant hemoglobin is present, how abundant the variant is, and whether the variant is relevant to the clinical picture. With background information from the patient's history, studies of informative family members, physical examination, blood counts, and erythrocyte indices, high-performance liquid chromatography can suggest the genotype of sickle cell disease. Thalassemia mutations are multitudinous and only DNA-based studies can pinpoint the genotype of this disease. For purposes of genetic counseling, especially when antenatal diagnosis is being considered, DNA-based diagnostics are required, although these tests are not required for managing disease complications in an individual. An accurate prognosis is often facilitated by knowing the genotype of the disease.

Mutations of the β-globin gene usually change only one hemoglobin component and stable variants usually have a concentration of 40%–50%. In contrast, α-globin gene variants should produce abnormal major and minor hemoglobins because, with rare exceptions, all hemoglobin molecules contain α-globin chains. Mutation of a single α-globin gene usually creates variants forming 20%–25% of the total hemoglobin, and a variant minor hemoglobin fraction, but the actual amounts of different hemoglobin types that accumulate can vary. γ-Globin gene mutants are important only in the fetus and usually "disappear" postnatally, when γ-globin gene expression is nearly extinguished. α-Globin chain abnormalities are expressed at birth and can produce signs of disease neonatally. Characteristically, β-globin chain mutations are clinically apparent only after the first few months of life, although their mutations can be detected beforehand.

Although a prototypical mendelian, single gene disease, the clinical heterogeneity of sickle cell anemia resembles that of a complex multigenic trait. Similarly, genotype–phenotype correlations are often difficult to establish in thalassemia. Modifying genes must affect the pathogenesis of these disorders and modulate their phenotypes. Candidate gene association studies have linked several genes and pathways with some subphenotypes of sickle cell anemia, including stroke, leg ulceration, priapism, pulmonary hypertension, and osteonecrosis. Genome-wide association studies now permit an "unbiased" assessment of all genes that could modulate disease. To be successful, this work requires precise definitions of phenotypes or heritable quantitative traits, samples of sufficient size to provide reasonable power to detect associations, knowledge of linkage disequilibrium patterns in the study populations, the availability of economically feasible high-throughput genotyping platforms, and sophisticated analytical techniques. These conditions have now been largely met, and some results are beginning to be published but this remains a "discovery" process.

Although it is still early in this quest, we can envision a time when disease diagnosis might include the use of tests for polymorphic modifier genes that will allow the treating physician to predict the future level of severity and complications likely to occur in an individual. This knowledge would help rationalize the use of antenatal diagnosis and the selection of patients for risky treatments and procedures. It might also allow a prediction of drug response, preclude exposing some patients to toxic therapies, and identify new pathways to which therapy could be targeted.

26

Population Genetics and Global Health Burden

David J. Weatherall and Thomas N. Williams

It is now widely accepted that the hemoglobinopathies are the most common monogenic diseases in humans. In this chapter we discuss the possible reasons for their very high frequency and uneven distribution among the world's population and describe recent attempts to determine their global health burden and how this might be managed.

FREQUENCY AND DISTRIBUTION

Frequency

A number of attempts have been made to review or determine the global frequency and annual birth rates of homozygotes or compound heterozygotes for the important inherited disorders of hemoglobin.[1–8] Composite data from these reports for the frequency and distribution by World Health Organization (WHO) regions are summarized in Table 26.1 and similar data for the estimated annual birth rate of severe forms of hemoglobinopathy are summarized in Figure 26.1. As we will discuss later in this chapter, such summaries are based on imperfect data and should be viewed with some caution; nevertheless, it is now generally acknowledged that as a group the hemoglobinopathies represent the most common monogenic diseases of humans.

Any explanation for the extremely high gene frequencies of the inherited disorders of hemoglobin must take into account a number of unusual features about their world distribution. The high-frequency regions stretch across the tropical belt of the Old World or areas into which there has been a high rate of migration from this region. None of the hemoglobinopathies have been found in the indigenous populations of the New World despite the fact that some of its populations have existed in tropical conditions over thousands of years. Furthermore, the different hemoglobinopathies are unevenly distributed in the tropical belt of the Old World. For example, HbS reaches its highest frequencies in Africa, parts of the Middle East, and the Indian subcontinent but is not observed further east, whereas HbE occurs at extremely high frequencies in Southeast Asia, Myanmar, Bangladesh, and parts of the eastern borders of the Indian subcontinent, yet does not extend further west (Fig. 26.2), and every population with a high frequency of different forms of thalassemia has its own particular set of mutations. These observations, which suggest that these conditions have arisen de novo with local expansion, are not compatible with older theories about their distribution, which suggested that it reflects massive population movements in an eastward or westward direction.[4]

As well as the heterogeneous distribution of the hemoglobinopathies, there are certain other generalizations that can be made about their frequency, which also have to be taken into account in any explanation for why these conditions are so common. The sickle cell (HbS) and β thalassemia genes (Figs. 26.2 and 26.3), although they occur at varying frequencies in different populations, rarely are found in more than 20% of the population. The α^0 thalassemias occur at similar frequencies to the β thalassemias. On the other hand, the α^+ thalassemias occur at much higher frequencies, achieving up to 70%–80% of the population in some regions (Fig. 26.4) and, similarly, the carrier rates for HbE greatly exceed those of HbS, reaching as high as 70% in some parts of Asia including northern Thailand and Cambodia. Further details of these gene frequencies, together with the appropriate references and data that underline these generalizations are reviewed in more detail elsewhere.[4]

In short, the hemoglobinopathies only occur at very high frequencies in warm or tropical climates, their distribution is extremely heterogeneous, and the maximum population frequencies that are achieved appear to vary considerably between different forms of thalassemia and structural hemoglobin variants.

Why Do the Hemoglobinopathies Occur at Such a High Frequency?

The high-frequency populations for the hemoglobinopathies are mainly those of developing countries or countries that have only recently made the demographic and epidemiological transitions from the effects of extreme poverty. There is considerable evidence that genetic diseases and congenital malformations occur more frequently in countries with a low per capita gross national income for which a number of explanations have been put forward. These include increased rates of consanguinity, increased parental age, population migration, and natural selection.[6]

Although it is difficult to obtain accurate data, it is clear that consanguineous marriage is still practiced in many parts of the world and may be acceptable to a minimum of 20% of the world's population.[9,10] This practice is especially common throughout the eastern Mediterranean, North Africa, and the Indian subcontinent, and to a lesser extent in parts of South America and subsaharan Africa.[9–11] There is clear evidence that the birth prevalence of autosomal

Table 26.1. Percent carrier frequencies for common hemoglobin disorders, by WHO region (1–7)

Region	HbS	HbC	HbE	β Thalassemia	α^0 Thalassemia	α^+ Thalassemia
Americas	1–20	0–10	0–20	0–3	0–5	0–40
Eastern Mediterranean	0–60	0–3	0–2	2–18	0–2	1–80
Europe	0–30	0–5	0–20	0–19	1–2	0–12
Southeast Asia Africa	40	0	0–70	0–11	1–30	3–40
Western Pacific	0	0	0	0–13	0	2–60

Note: Many of these data are derived from small population samples.

recessive diseases is increased by this mechanism in these populations.[6] The percentage of pregnant women aged older than 35 years is also high in middle- and low-income countries, although the major consequence of this appears to be an increase in the number of live births of infants with chromosomal defects or developmental abnormalities.[6] A large population movement from areas of high frequency for single gene effects also has the effect of introducing these disorders into new populations, as evidenced by the spread of the hemoglobin disorders to the Americas, the Caribbean, and Europe by the slave trade and later migrations. Although all of these mechanisms might undoubtedly have been responsible for increasing the frequency of autosomal recessive disorders and others over time, they cannot account for the remarkably high gene frequencies of the hemoglobinopathies in these populations, and the evidence is now overwhelming that the principle factor in maintaining these high gene frequencies is natural selection working through the relative protection of heterozygotes for the common hemoglobinopathies against *Plasmodium falciparum* malaria.

NATURAL SELECTION AND THE HEMOGLOBINOPATHIES; THE MALARIA HYPOTHESIS

Historical Background

The notion that variation in host response to infection might have a genetic basis is not new;[12,13] however, it was not until the late 1940s, and through the remarkable insight of J.B.S. Haldane, that a plausible genetic protective mechanism was first suggested.

During the period just after World War II, independent studies in Italy and in Mediterranean immigrants in the

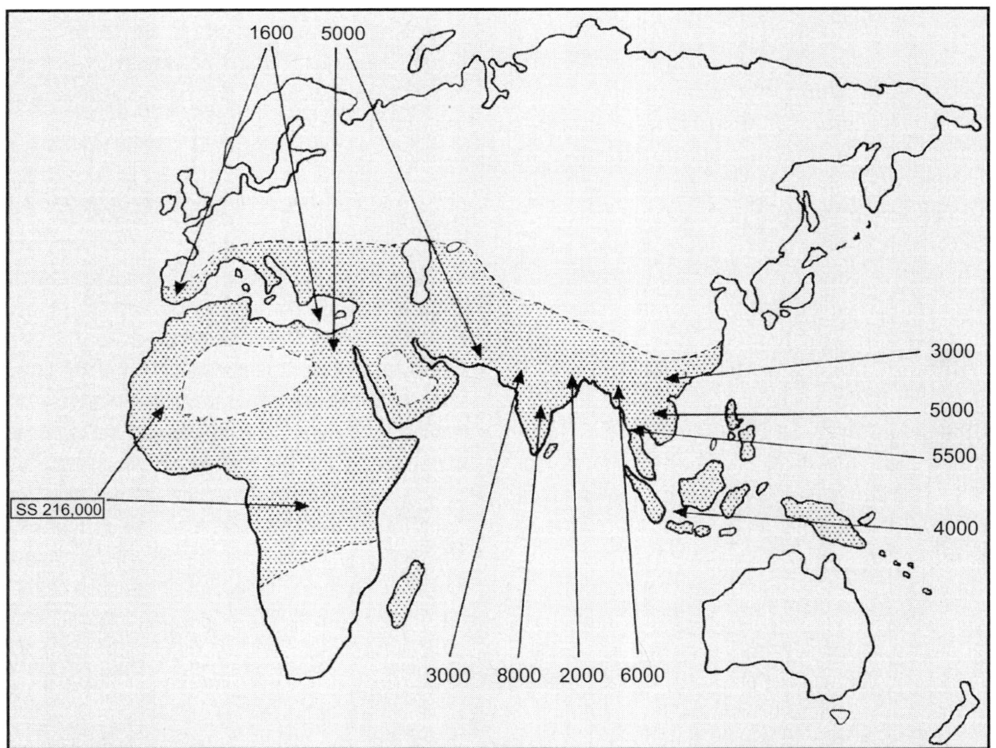

Figure 26.1. Estimated annual births of hemoglobinopathies. Data from references 2–5. The SS box shows sickle cell disease in Africa; other figures are for β thalassemia. These data are currently being revised and extended; in many cases they may underestimate the birth rates. (From ref. 4.)

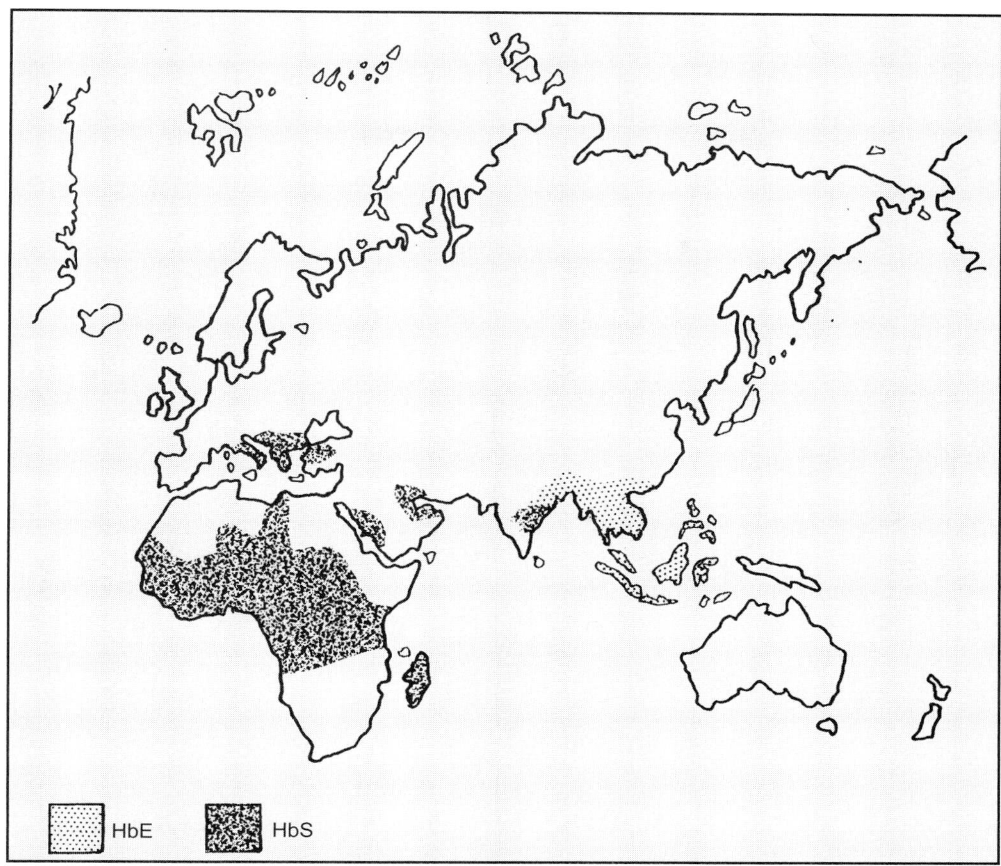

Figure 26.2. The world distribution of hemoglobins S and E. (From ref. 4.)

United States highlighted a remarkably high frequency of thalassemia in these populations.[14,15] Influenced by the intense interest in human mutation rates following studies of the survivors of the atomic bombs in Hiroshima and Nagasaki, workers on both sides of the Atlantic suggested that this might reflect a high rate of mutation and, because they appeared to be restricted to certain populations, that the mutation rate might differ between different ethnic groups.

At the 8th International Congress of Genetics in Stockholm in 1948, Neel and Valentine, to explain the high frequency of thalassemia in immigrant populations in the United States, calculated a mutation rate for thalassemia of 1:2500. Haldane felt that this was unlikely and that these remarkable gene frequencies were more likely to be the result of heterozygote selection. Furthermore, he went on to suggest, "The corpuscles of anemic heterozygotes are smaller than normal, and more resistant to hypertonic solutions. It is at least conceivable that they are also more resistant to attacks by the sporozoa which cause malaria, a disease prevalent in Italy, Sicily and Greece, where the gene is frequent."[16]

In essence, what became known as the "malaria-hypothesis" intimated that diseases like thalassemia can be considered balanced polymorphisms – conditions in which the gene frequency for the advantageous heterozygous state increases until it is balanced by the loss of disadvantaged homozygotes from the population. Haldane's great contribution to this field was to encourage geneticists and hematologists to analyze the high frequency of common genetic diseases of the blood as putative polymorphisms of this kind. Although, over the years, the hypothesis has stood the test of time, as we shall see in subsequent sections it has not always been easy to substantiate Haldane's ideas in human populations.

It is beyond the scope of this chapter to review in detail all the population and experimental work that has followed from Haldane's original idea. In particular, it has not been possible to review the evidence suggesting that polymorphisms other than the hemoglobinopathies have also come under selection by malaria. Readers who wish to explore this aspect of the topic further are referred to several recent reviews.[17–19]

Malaria in Human Populations

Malaria has decimated large populations in the past and is still one of the world's most common causes of mortality. Currently, close to 50% of the world's population are at risk of transmission, more than 3 billion people live in malarious areas and the disease causes between 1 and 3 million deaths per year.[20] Four different species of

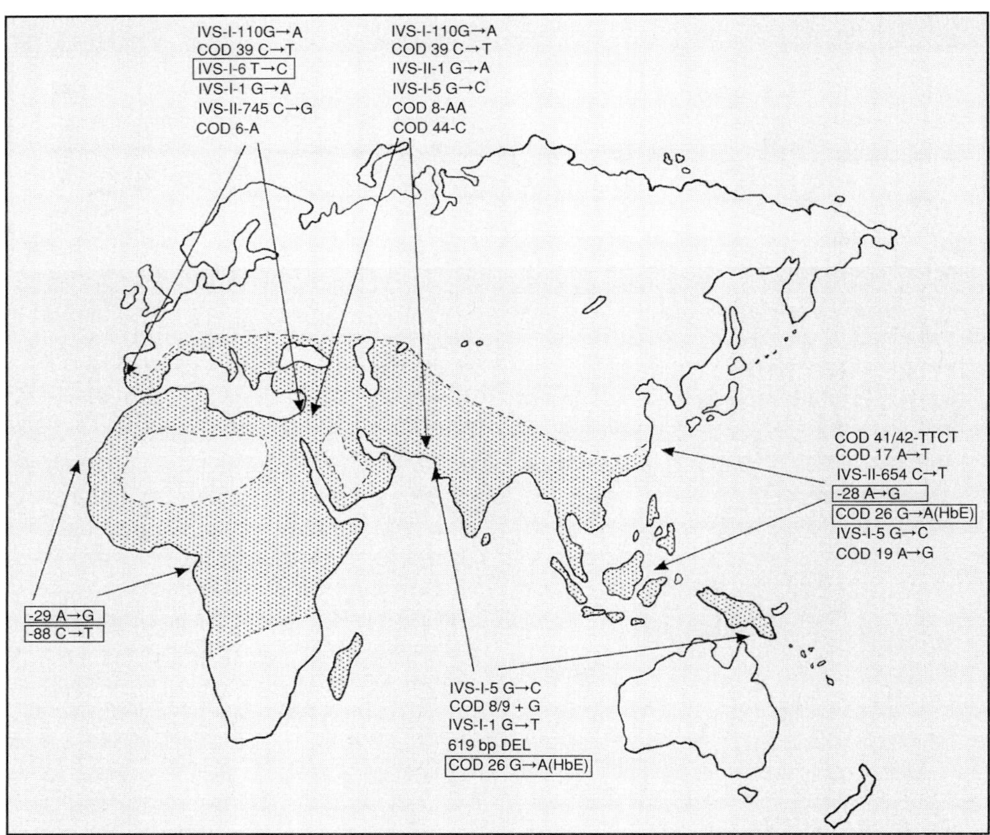

Figure 26.3. The world distribution and different mutations that cause β thalassemia. Those shown in boxes are milder mutations. Hemoglobin E is included in the milder mutation because of its β thalassemic phenotype. (From ref. 4.)

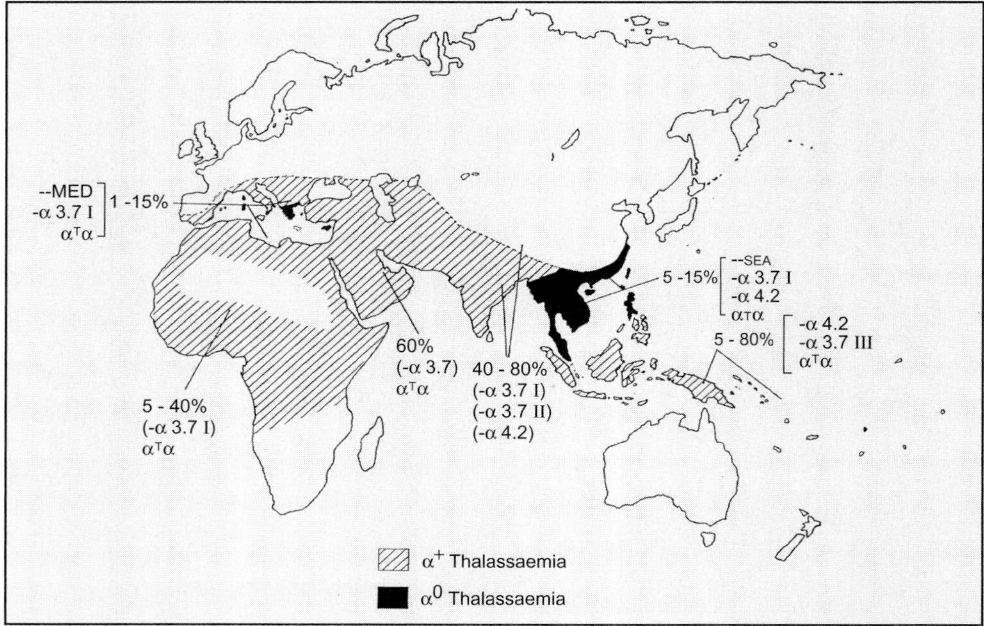

Figure 26.4. The world distribution of the α thalassemias. The α^0 thalassemias are only found at high frequencies in Asia and some Mediterranean countries. The α^+ thalassemias have a much broader distribution. Some of the different subtypes of α^0 and α^+ thalassemia are shown. - -SEA indicates the Southeast Asian deletion form of α^0 thalassemia. $-\alpha^{4.2}$ or $-\alpha^{3.7}$ relate to different forms of α^+ thalassemia with their particular deletion sizes, $-\alpha^{3.7}$ is further subdivided into types I, II, and III, again depending on the different deletion sizes. α^T denotes nondeletion α thalassemia. (From ref. 4.)

Plasmodium cause human infections: *P. falciparum, P. vivax, P. ovale*, and *P. malariae*. Although the majority of deaths are caused by *P. falciparum* malaria, *P. vivax* malaria is a common cause of chronic ill health, particularly in children.

Infection occurs when a female anopheline mosquito inoculates sporozoites into humans where they mature in the liver and are then released into the blood stream as merozoites. The latter invade red cells, causing both their destruction and also adhesion to the walls of blood vessels.

The complex interactions of malarial parasites and red blood cells, that have to be understood for a full appreciation of the complexities of the potential protective effects of the hemoglobin disorders have been reviewed recently.[18,19]

Hemoglobin S

Because, paradoxically, it was the structural hemoglobin variants, notably HbS, for which Haldane's hypothesis was first explored we will consider this condition first and then discuss how far his hypothesis has stood up in the case of the thalassemias (see Chapter 22).

Early studies on the relationship of the high frequency of the HbS gene to *P. falciparum* malaria are summarized elsewhere.[21] In short, analyses of parasite rates and densities in children with the sickle cell trait (HbAS) and non-affected controls, together with observations of the rarity of sickling in patients with severe malaria and the distribution of the sickle cell gene combined to provide convincing evidence that HbAS offers at least some degree of protection against severe malarial infection. More recent studies in east and west Africa suggest that the greatest impact of HbS is against fatal or severe malaria, that is profound anemia or cerebral malaria, having no discernible effect on infection rates per se.[22–24] Indeed, case-control studies suggest that HbS heterozygotes have a level of protection of approximately 60%–80% against the severe complications of malaria.

Some progress has also been made in determining the mechanisms of protection of those with HbAS against *P. falciparum* malaria, although many questions remain unanswered. Early studies demonstrated that in those with HbAS the rate of sickling is significantly greater in parasitized than in unparasitized red cells,[25] findings that were later confirmed and extended under more physiological conditions.[26] These studies suggested that the parasites cause a "suicidal infection;" because parasitized HbAS red cells sickle and are more likely to be removed from the circulation. At approximately the same time it was also demonstrated independently by two groups that parasitized HbAS cells maintained at low oxygen tension do not support the growth of malaria parasites as effectively as normal cells at similar oxygen tensions.[27,28] Later it was suggested that this effect might be due to the increased loss of potassium or water from the HbAS cells.[29]

Recent studies have also been compatible with the early suggestion[21] that there might also be an immune component involved in the protection of individuals with HbAS. In a cohort study of mild clinical malaria in Kenya, the protection attributable to HbAS showed a significant increase with age.[30] Compatible with these findings, it was demonstrated in two studies that those with HbAS had significantly higher titers of immunoglobulin G antibodies to a variety of malarial antigens than normal children.[31,32]

Thus although there are a number of feasible mechanisms at both the cellular and immunological levels for protection of HbAS individuals against *P. falciparum* malaria the precise mechanisms of these complex interactions that result in such a remarkable protective effect remain to be determined.

Hemoglobin C

Although early studies were not convincing, more recent work conducted in West Africa indicates that the relatively high frequencies of HbC in that region have been maintained by resistance to *P. falciparum* malaria (see Chapter 21).[33] In this case there is evidence that protection is greater in homozygotes (90%) than in heterozygotes (30%), suggesting that, unlike the sickle cell mutation, HbC may be an example of a transient polymorphism – one that would move to fixation under continued selective pressure. This hypothesis is based on the assumption that, in itself, homozygosity for HbC has no adverse consequences. If this were the case, however, it is difficult to understand why the frequency of HbC is not higher in African populations. Furthermore, the fitness (in the Darwinian sense) of homozygotes for this variant is not completely established; further work will be required to confirm this interesting suggestion.

Although a number of early studies suggested that the protective mechanism of HbC might be mediated through the inability of parasites to grow and develop in affected red cells, this mechanism is not supported by studies of parasite densities in vivo (summarized in ref. 19). More recently it has been shown that the expression of PfEMPI, an important parasite-encoded red cell adhesion protein, is reduced in HbC-containing red cells, an effect that is most marked in homozygotes.[34,35] It should be remembered, however, that HbC-containing red cells have a number of abnormal properties including rheological abnormalities and increased levels of oxidant stress; clearly, the final story about the definitive protective mechanism remains to be determined.[36]

Hemoglobin E

Because of its extremely high frequency in Asia, HbE has always seemed to be a good candidate for a malaria-protection polymorphism (see Chapter 18). Many of the early population studies that were conducted failed to show a clear relationship between HbE and malaria.[4] It is possible that some of these studies may have been bedeviled by the very high frequency of α thalassemia that occurs in many populations with a high frequency of HbE.

Recent extended linkage-disequilibrium analyses of the HbE gene suggest that it is of relatively recent origin and must have come under intense selection.[37] In keeping with this observation it has been found that the presence of HbE trait is associated with a reduced severity of disease in adults admitted with acute *P. falciparum* malaria.[38] Furthermore, in vitro culture studies using mixtures of normal and variant red cells have shown that those from HbAE individuals, although not those from HbE homozygotes or different forms of α thalassemia, are more resistant to invasion by the parasite.[39]

Although these findings are suggestive, a major gap in our information about HbE and malaria is the absence of adequate data from case-control studies of the kind that have been so successful in demonstrating the magnitude of the protective effects of HbS and HbC. Thus, although it seems almost certain that HbE is in some way protective against malaria, a great deal more work needs to be done before we will have any clear understanding of the magnitude of the effect or its mechanism.

α Thalassemia

The frequency of α^+ thalassemia in the southwest Pacific follows a clinal distribution from north/west to south/east, with the highest frequency in northern Papua New Guinea and the lowest in New Caledonia (see also Chapters 13 and 14). This distribution shows a strong correlation with malarial endemicity; similar relations are not observed with other genetic polymorphisms in this region.[40] The possibility that α thalassemia has been introduced from the mainland populations of Southeast Asia, and that its frequency has been diluted as populations moved south, has been largely excluded by finding that the molecular forms of α thalassemia in Melanesia and Papua New Guinea are different from those of the mainland and are set in different α-globin gene haplotypes.[40] One feature of the distribution of α thalassemia in this region that, on the face of it, does not fit with the malaria hypothesis was that it is also found in Fiji in the west, Tahiti and beyond in the east, and in Micronesian atolls, populations in which malaria has never been recorded. It has been found that a single mutation, which has been previously defined in Vanuatu, accounts for virtually all the cases of α^+ thalassemia that have so far been described in Polynesia, indicating that the presence of α thalassemia in these nonmalarious areas has almost certainly resulted from population migration rather than selection.[41]

These population data were augmented by prospective case-control studies in northern Papua New Guinea, where it was found that compared with normal children, the risk of contracting strictly defined severe malaria was 0.4 for α^+ thalassemia homozygotes and 0.66 for α^+ thalassemia heterozygotes.[42] Similar findings have since been reported from studies conducted in two African populations.[43,44] Although some progress has been made toward an understanding of the mechanisms of malaria protection afforded by α thalassemia, the overall picture is still far from clear. Paradoxically, early studies in Papua New Guinea suggested that very young children with α^+ thalassemia might be slightly more prone to uncomplicated malaria than normal children.[45] Later studies conducted in Vanuatu appear to support this conclusion, showing that the incidence of uncomplicated malaria and the prevalence of splenomegaly, an index of malaria infection, were both significantly higher in children with α thalassemia than in normal children. Moreover, the effect was most marked in the youngest children and in those affected by the nonlethal parasite, *P. vivax*.[46] It was suggested that the early susceptibility to *P. vivax*, which may reflect the more rapidly turning over red cells of α thalassemic infants,[47] could be acting as a natural vaccine by inducing cross-species protection against *P. falciparum*. These intriguing observations require further study in other populations.

There has also been some progress toward determining how protection might be mediated at a cellular level. Overall, there is no evidence for a reduced rate of invasion or growth of *P. falciparum* in red cells of the genotype -α/αα or -α/-α, the mild forms of α thalassemia that have been shown to be protective by case-control studies. It has been found that these cells consistently bind more malaria-immune globulin than normal red cells.[48,49] When infected with parasites, α thalassemic red cells are less able than normal red cells to form rosettes, an in vitro phenomenon whereby uninfected red cells bind to infected cells. It has been demonstrated that complement receptor 1 expression, which is required for rosette formation, is reduced on α thalassemia red cells,[50] offering a convincing potential mechanism for reduced rosetting.[51,52] In addition, infected α thalassemic red cells are less able than normal red cells to adhere to human umbilical vein endothelial cells.[51] Because rosetting and cytoadherence are mechanisms that underlie sequestration of infected red blood cells and are associated with virulence of infection, these observations suggest that malaria protection by α thalassemia might be determined by specific red cell membrane abnormalities that are associated with this condition. In an extensive series of studies to define other membrane components involved, it was suggested that altered red cell membrane band 3 could also be a target for enhanced antibody binding to α thalassemic cells infected with parasites.[49]

Thus, although there are a number of tantalizing clues as to possible mechanisms of protection against malaria by the milder forms of α thalassemia, a coherent picture of how they fit together remains to be produced.

β Thalassemia (Chapters 16 and 17)

In their now classic studies conducted in the 1960s, Siniscalco and colleagues[53] found that the population frequencies of thalassemia carriers in Sardinia, a considerable number of whom must have been β thalassemia carriers, correlated with altitude. Although malaria was no longer endemic in Sardinia at that time, historically, its incidence had been correlated closely with altitude. Similar correlations were found later in Melanesia.[54] In addition, a relatively small case-control study in Northern Liberia suggested that the β thalassemia trait is protective against severe malaria.[55] Thus, although a number of other population studies, mostly analyzing parasite rates or densities, failed to show any correlations between β thalassemia and malaria (see ref. 4), such epidemiological data that are available certainly point to a protective effect of the β thalassemia trait (see also Chapters 16 and 17).

Another finding in favor of the concept that β thalassemia is a protective polymorphism is the observation that in every country in which this disease is common there is a different set of mutations. Studies of β-globin gene haplotypes (Chapter 27) and their relationship to β thalassemia mutations have been particularly interesting in this respect. Unlike the α-globin gene haplotypes there is a "hot-spot" for recombination between the 5′ and 3′ ends of the β gene haplotypes (Chapter 27). Over time there seems to have been admixture between the 5′ and 3′ haplotypes among human populations but this has not occurred in the case of thalassemia; the thalassemia mutations, which occur in the 3′ haplotype, are almost invariably associated with the same 5′ haplotype, indicating that in evolutionary terms they are much more recent and that there has not been time for mixing the 5′ and 3′ ends of haplotypes that carry these mutations (see ref. 4). This suggests a fairly recent selective pressure, possibly approximately 5,000 years, which is in agreement with current estimations of the time that human populations have been exposed to pathogenic forms of *Plasmodium* (see later).

Very little is known about the potential mechanisms of protection against malaria in the case of β thalassemia. In vitro studies have shown that β thalassemic red cells are invaded at the same rate as normal red cells and that the rate of parasite growth is also indistinguishable from normal. One potential explanation is that protection is related to levels of fetal hemoglobin (HbF) that are associated with this condition. There is clear evidence that the rate of decline of HbF levels after birth is delayed in β thalassemia heterozygotes (see ref. 4) and studies conducted in both humans[56] and in transgenic mice[57] have found defective development of *P. falciparum* or *P. yoelii*, respectively, in red cells that contain human HbF. This could provide a mechanism for protection by β thalassemia during the first year of life, but not thereafter (see later section).

A more general hypothesis for why β thalassemia heterozygotes might be protected against malaria has also been proposed.[58] In short, it is known that these cells are under increased oxidative stress due to globin chain imbalance; it is suggested therefore that the further stress imposed by the parasite might render these cells prone to damage and rapid removal from the circulation, a mechanism reminiscent of that outlined earlier for the protective effect of HbAS.

Epistatic Interactions Between Protective Polymorphisms

Because different hemoglobin disorders that offer protection against malaria frequently occur together in the same population it is becoming increasingly important to determine whether they interact with one another and, in particular, the effect that this might have on changing the pattern of susceptibility to malarial infection.

The term epistasis is used to describe nonadditive interactions between two or more different genetic loci. A study in East Africa has provided intriguing information that suggests that there is negative epistasis between the HbS and α thalassemia genes with respect to protection against *P. falciparum* malaria. Although those with HbAS or heterozygous or homozygous for α^+ thalassemia alone have been found to have a highly significant protection against *P. falciparum* malaria (see previous sections) this effect was completely nullified in individuals who had HbAS and were homozygous or heterozygous for α^+ thalassemia.[59] Although the numbers involved in this study were relatively small, results from a recent case-control study conducted in Ghana were compatible with the same conclusion.[60] Considering current uncertainty about the precise mechanism of protection mediated by either of these variants alone, it is difficult to explain this remarkable epistatic interaction. Phenotypically, the major difference between HbAS individuals and those who, in addition to HbS, carry α thalassemia is that the doubly affected persons have significantly lower levels of HbS in their red cells (see ref. 4). It is possible therefore that protection in HbAS persons may require a critical level of HbS. In this context it should be noted that these doubly affected individuals have reduced mean corpuscular hemoglobin (MCH) and mean corpuscular volume (MCV) values associated with the particular α thalassemia genotype (Chapter 22). In uncomplicated sickle cell trait HbS accounts for approximately 40% of total red cell hemoglobin and the MCH is 30 pg, giving an absolute amount of HbS per cell of approximately 12 pg. On the other hand, in those with the HbAS who are also homozygous for α^+ thalassemia, the level of HbS is reduced to approximately 25% and the MCH to only 20 pg, giving an absolute level of HbS of only 5 pg per cell; a more than 50% reduction in the absolute amount of HbS per cell could, therefore, have an important effect on the degree of protection enjoyed by individuals of different genetic combinations.

It seems very likely that other interactions of this type occur. Apart from their intrinsic interest in the population genetics of these conditions their further study may provide valuable information about the protective mechanisms of some of the hemoglobinopathies.

Summary

From the data summarized in the previous sections, it is clear that, at least at the population level, there is reasonably convincing evidence that the five major groups of hemoglobin disorders that occur at very high frequencies in different populations are all associated with protection against *P. falciparum* malaria in the heterozygous, and, in some cases, homozygous states. The clinical and parasitological evidence for protection varies widely; in some cases there appears to be a genuine reduction in parasite densities, whereas in others the effects seem to be mediated almost entirely by protection against the severe complications of malaria.

Perhaps it is not surprising that progress has been much slower in trying to determine the protective mechanisms involved. The studies that have been conducted are asking questions of an enormously complex biological system; transmission rates of malaria vary widely, populations differ in whether one type of parasite predominates or whether there are several. There is a wide difference in antigenic strains of parasite and many of the in vitro techniques that have been used are extremely difficult to standardize between different laboratories. Added to this, the cellular pathophysiology of these different hemoglobinopathies, although there might be some features in common, is undoubtedly different. Against this complex background, however, certain generalizations are beginning to appear. For example, a reduction in rosette formation seems to be common to several different hemoglobinopathies, suggesting that changes in the red cell membrane associated with particular differences in antigen presentation may be at least one common pathophysiological mechanism. No doubt more will be found.

An even more difficult question, and one posed by the increasing evidence for an additional immune basis to protection, is how the primary protective mechanisms at the level of the red cell might be associated with enhanced immune response. Clearly this question requires a great deal more work.

It is beyond the scope of this chapter to discuss the increasing list of protective polymorphisms associated with malaria. They are the subject of several recent reviews.[13,17,18] As in the case of the hemoglobinopathies, in the majority of cases the protective mechanisms have not been fully worked out. There is one notable exception however. Epidemiological studies, first in Africa[61] and later in Papua New Guinea[62] showed a high frequency of the Duffy-negative phenotype in populations in which malaria is common. Further studies suggested that the Duffy blood group antigen might be the receptor for *P. vivax*. Later studies demonstrated that the Duffy antigen chemokine receptor (DARC) is not expressed on red cells when there is a promoter mutation that alters a GATA-1 binding site. In cells carrying this mutation DARC expression is abolished and therefore DARC-mediated entry of *P. vivax* is inhibited. This receptor is expressed predominantly on reticulocytes and young red cells and hence this observation is in keeping with the proposal discussed earlier in this chapter regarding the possible immune basis for protection against α thalassemia, at least in populations where *P. vivax* is common. The finding of increased susceptibility to both *P. vivax* and *P. falciparum* in babies with α thalassemia in Papua New Guinea, possibly because of the relative increase in young red cells in their blood, might allow early immunization against *P. vivax* and, because there is cross immune response between the two species, later protection against *P. falciparum*.[46]

Some other interesting similarities to observations in the hemoglobinopathies are also appearing in relationship to other protective polymorphisms. For example, evidence has been emerging for several years that individuals of blood group O are protected against *P. falciparum* malaria (reviewed in ref. 63). Interestingly, as in the case of some of the hemoglobinopathies, individuals of blood group O show significantly reduced rosette formation compared with nongroup O individuals. It appears therefore that there could be common pathways among the malaria-related protective polymorphisms, and further work of this kind might help to clarify some of the protective mechanisms involved in the hemoglobinopathies.

POPULATION AND EVOLUTIONARY IMPLICATIONS

The picture that is emerging is that the extremely common hemoglobin disorders occur at a high frequency in those parts of the world in which malaria was, or still is, a major cause of mortality. These protective polymorphisms are extremely patchy in their distribution; the HbS mutation occurs across Africa, the Middle East and the eastern side of India, but not further east; the HbE mutation occurs at an extremely high frequency in many of the populations stretching from the eastern part of the Indian subcontinent throughout the rest of Asia. Every high-frequency population for thalassemia has its own mutations and, at least in the case of HbS and HbE, there is evidence that they may have arisen de novo on more than one occasion.

These observations are best explained by the occurrence of local mutations with rapid selection; the lack of homogenization of some of these highly protective polymorphisms suggests that exposure of populations to malaria has been, at least in evolutionary terms, a fairly recent event. Although ancestral forms of the malaria species that infect humans arose many millions of years ago, it is likely that *P. falciparum* arose from its closest ancestor approximately 10 million years ago.[64] After approximately 10 million years of development in Africa, modern humans emigrated out of Africa 40,000–100,000 years ago, probably carrying at least some polymorphisms that evolved from selection against *P. falciparum*.[65] It is likely that death due to malaria increased very rapidly between 5,000 and 10,000 years ago with the development of agriculture and settlements that would have greatly facilitated the transmission of the disease by mosquitoes.[66] These observations are all compatible with a fairly recent appearance of the malaria-resistant polymorphisms such as the hemoglobinopathies. This interpretation is certainly in keeping with recent studies of haplotype diversity and linkage disequilibrium at the human glucose-6-phosphate dehydrogenase locus.[67]

These concepts also go some way toward explaining the absence of common hemoglobinopathies in the indigenous populations of the new world. Presumably the selective factors leading to the high frequency of the thalassemias in Asian populations had not been present before their early migrations into the New World. Currently, it is not clear when malaria reached this region, although it has been suggested that it was as recently as the early Spanish conquests. Hence there might not have been time for selection to generate high frequencies of malaria-resistant polymorphisms in these populations.

Another interesting aspect of the population genetics of the hemoglobin disorders is how different polymorphic genes interact in the same population to produce present day frequencies.[4,21] Mutations like those for HbS and β thalassemia, which are alleles, interact to produce compound heterozygotes, HbS–β thalassemia, which can have clinically severe phenotypes. In this case, selection will not only act against those with sickle cell anemia and homozygous β thalassemia, but also to some extent against compound heterozygotes with HbS–β thalassemia. Early theoretical analyses of this type of situation[21] concluded that a stable equilibrium would be obtained provided that heterozygotes for both genes enjoyed a selective advantage. A consequence of selection acting in this way is that the more advantageous heterozygous state, in this case HbAS, would tend to come under much stronger selection and therefore the HbS and β thalassemia alleles would tend to be mutually exclusive in populations. Although this is not entirely the case, it mirrors broadly the pattern of distribution of these alleles in Africa. In the case of HbE and β thalassemia in many Asian populations, there is an inverse relationship between the frequency of β thalassemia and HbE, although because both are so common there still is a high frequency of compound heterozygotes.

POPULATION DYNAMICS AND IMPLICATIONS FOR THE CONTROL OF THE HEMOGLOBINOPATHIES

Population Dynamics

In the interests of public health planning a number of attempts have been made to predict the future burden of the inherited disorders of hemoglobin at local, regional, and global scales. As we will discuss later, such predictions suggest that we will be unlikely to see a significant decline in their current frequencies for the foreseeable future and the hemoglobinopathies will therefore assume increasing importance in many countries in development as they go through their demographic transition.

The population dynamics of the hemoglobinopathies are related to a number of issues including potential changes in the factors that result in selective advantage, the rates of epidemiological and demographic transitions in the developing countries, population migration, and the potential role of medical intervention. Predicting what might happen to the gene frequencies of the hemoglobinopathies in the face of a reduction in the incidence of malaria is complex and discussed in detail elsewhere.[68] In short, even if malaria were eradicated completely it would take many generations before the frequency of these diseases fell significantly. Furthermore, it is still not clear whether relative protection against malaria is the only factor that has maintained the hemoglobinopathies at their present high level. Studies conducted in Papua New Guinea suggested that the α thalassemias might offer protection against the infectious diseases of childhood,[42] although this effect has not been seen in other populations.

The Epidemiological Transition and the Frequency of Severe Forms of Hemoglobinopathy

During the last decade of the twentieth century, gross domestic product per head in the developing countries grew by 1.6% each year, and the proportion of people living on less than $1 a day fell from 29% to 23%. These statistics are reflected in improvements in the overall health of a number of populations in the developing world and in declines in childhood mortality, most notably in South America and the Caribbean, east Asia and the Pacific, the Mediterranean region, the Middle East and parts of North Africa.[6]

The consequences of such epidemiological transition for the recognition of the importance of genetic disease in developing countries were shown graphically in Cyprus after World War II. Thalassemia was not known to occur on the island until 1944, at which time the clinical findings in 20 patients were reported.[69] This study highlights the difficulty in identifying diseases of this type against the background of chronic malaria and other infections; it was published at the end of an extremely successful program to control mosquito breeding and other improvements in public health. Hence, during this remarkably short period it became clear that there was a high frequency of genetic anemia. By the early 1970s it was estimated that, if no steps were taken to control the disease, in approximately 40 years the blood required to treat all the children with thalassemia would amount to 78,000 U/year, 40% of the population would need to be donors, and the total cost to the health services would equal or exceed the island's health budget.[4] A similar trend is occurring at present throughout many Asian countries and will undoubtedly be repeated in subsaharan Africa as social conditions improve. A more detailed analysis of the effects of both demographic and epidemiological transitions has been summarized recently.[70]

The potential effects of improvements in the medical management of the hemoglobinopathies on the size of their gene pools is also complex and difficult to predict. In the short term, such improvements have been shown to result in treatment-seeking migration of affected individuals from high-frequency regions to countries with stronger medical services, potentially widening the geographic range of these diseases. Although improved treatments for the more serious forms that allow patients to survive to reproductive age might have a modest effect on their overall population frequencies, the most contentious issue is the so-called dysgenic effect of programs for the control of these disorders by prenatal diagnosis and termination of affected pregnancies. This important issue is discussed in detail elsewhere[4,11,68,71] and will only be outlined here. The dysgenic effect of prenatal diagnosis is based on the premise that if most pregnancies that carry severely affected infants were aborted, the gene frequency for the particular disorder will steadily increase in the population. This is because homozygotes are replaced by healthy individuals, two thirds of whom are heterozygous and hence will pass on their genes. This assumes, of course, that couples undergoing prenatal diagnosis will attain the population norm for their final family size. But such evidence as there is suggests that this might not be the case; studies in Cyprus, for example, have shown that approximately 25% of the decrease in thalassemic births is due to limited reproduction.[71] Indeed, as elegantly summarized by Bodmer and Cavalli-Sforza, the changes in the size of the thalassemic gene pool that might follow interventions of this kind are likely to be extremely small: "It would seem therefore that the dysgenic effect of medicine is not a real threat. By the time that it may have a clearly perceptive global effect, 200 or 300 years from now – when the incidence of severe genetic disease may have doubled on average – our descendants almost certainly will have discovered simple methods of therapy."[68]

There have been few efforts to convert the health burden of the hemoglobin disorders into disability-adjusted life years, the only measure that the international public health community will accept as an approach to assessing the comparative health burden of different diseases. Recent and very preliminary analyses of this kind[70] have shown that the thalassemias pose a health burden comparable to some common communicable diseases in Asia; however, they encountered major difficulties because of lack of information about the gene frequency of some of the hemoglobin disorders in particular developing countries. In the future, it will be essential to improve these data and to obtain the help of health economists to assess the true health burden of the hemoglobinopathies.

In short therefore, in planning for the future public health measures required for the control and management of the hemoglobinopathies it can be assumed that as the developing countries continue to pass through the epidemiological transition they will impose an ever increasing burden on health services.

Control and Management Issues

The main approaches to the control and clinical management of the hemoglobinopathies are discussed in other chapters. Here, some of the particular problems relating to the control of the hemoglobinopathies are discussed in the light of their global distribution and peculiarities in their population genetics. The development of approaches to the global control and management of genetic disease in general,[72] and of the hemoglobin disorders in particular[4,73–75] have been discussed in detail recently.

The particular problems relating to the control of the hemoglobinopathies reflect their widespread heterogeneity and extremely uneven distribution even over relatively short geographical distances, their high frequency in rural populations of the developing countries, and inadequacies of education and medical services in these populations. These issues raise problems in bioethics, counseling, education, and the provision of medical care that are not encountered in the developed countries.

Ethical and Counseling Issues. Ethical issues in genetic research, screening, and testing in developing countries are discussed in detail in a report by the WHO[73] and in reports by the Nuffield Council on Bioethics.[76,77] They are also considered in a recent review.[72] There are major ethnic differences in how the nature of disease is interpreted. In many societies in which the level of education is limited it is viewed as being the action of evil spirits or other external forces, a belief that might be encouraged by visits to local healers. In these circumstances, even the simplest explanations of the nature of genetic disease might be extremely difficult to communicate. In many patriarchal societies, genetic disease raises particular problems for women who are carriers or who have affected children. Despite careful explanation of the mechanisms of inheritance, husbands frequently blame their wives for having a child with a genetic disease, often leading to the break up of the family and to a high rate of suicide. Genetic information may be used to discriminate or stigmatize in the context of social practices, particularly in countries in which arranged marriages are still common. In short, a screening program that has demonstrated that a woman is a carrier for a genetic disease can make her unmarriageable. Children with genetic diseases in developing countries can be severely stigmatized and even ostracized by their communities. Informed consent for any procedure is extremely difficult to establish and in many developing countries there are no regulatory or ethical bodies.

All these issues, and many others, need to be taken into account when developing genetic services of any kind in the developing countries. Although the principles of genetic counseling are the same as in the developed countries, their application is quite different and must be developed hand in hand with those who have a full knowledge of the local scene. Indeed, a great deal more research is required about the appreciation of disease in different ethnic groups and how this may be best approached by sensitive counseling.

Genetic Services in Developing Countries. There have been several reviews of the problems of developing services for the control of genetic and congenital disorders in the developing countries.[6,73,74] Establishing programs for the hemoglobinopathies presents particular problems because this field has never come under the auspices of clinical genetics and usually requires special training in centers with experience of the field for appropriate pediatricians, hematologists, and technical staff. Once these personnel are in place, training of appropriate counselors and the development of public education programs can proceed. Next, based on local social and religious beliefs, decisions need to be made about whether community control will be achieved by prenatal diagnosis or community education alone. At a later stage, prenatal screening programs can be developed. Each country requires one or more centers with expertise in both the laboratory diagnosis and clinical management of the hemoglobinopathies, depending on its size.

In the current climate it is extremely difficult to achieve any of these developments in developing countries. Their governments are unwilling or unable to give priority to these conditions because of the many other more pressing problems of communicable disease, often associated with a concomitant increase in their health burdens by a rapidly rising rate of noncommunicable disease. Currently, very few governments in Asia or subsaharan Africa are able to support any form of hemoglobinopathy program and hence without some form of external international help it will be a long time before these diseases come under control in many parts of the world.

In a report published by the WHO[73] and in a follow-up article,[78] suggestions were made about how the international medical and scientific community could help the developing countries in establishing programs for the control of hemoglobinopathies. These concepts were based in part on the success of the hemoglobin field over the past 30 years in evolving programs for the control of the thalassemias in several developing countries by the development of north/south partnerships, that is a partnership between experts in centers in the developed countries and those in whom the skills were lacking in the developing world. The natural evolution of north/south partnerships is the development of south/south partnerships in which those developing countries that have gained skills in the diagnosis and treatment of genetic disorders can form partnerships with countries in which these skills are lacking. Currently, several of the centers in developing countries that were established by north/south partnerships are taking forward the concept of helping neighboring countries.

None of these developments will move forward successfully without some form of external support from international health organizations. Like many of the developing country governments, to date these bodies have prioritized more immediate health problems such as those posed by communicable disease, malnutrition, and dysfunctional healthcare systems and, as a consequence, have shown little interest in the hemoglobinopathies. At the time of writing there does appear to be at least some recognition on their part of the increasing health burden posed by the common inherited disorders of hemoglobin. For example, the next phase of the Global Burden of Disease study will include the hemoglobinopathies in its assessment of the relative roles of different diseases in the overall economic burden of disease.[79]

REFERENCES

1. Livingstone FB. *Frequencies of Hemoglobin Variants.* New York: Oxford University Press; 1985.
2. WHO. *Guidelines for the Control of Haemoglobin Disorders.* Geneva: World Health Organization; 1994.
3. Angastiniotis M, Modell B. Global epidemiology of hemoglobin disorders. *Ann NY Acad Sci.* 1998;850:251–269.
4. Weatherall DJ, Clegg JB. *The Thalassaemia Syndromes.* 4th ed. Oxford: Blackwell Science; 2001.
5. Weatherall DJ, Clegg JB. Inherited haemoglobin disorders: an increasing global health problem. *Bull WHO.* 2001;79:704–712.
6. Christiansen A, Howson CP, Modell B. *March of Dimes Global Report on Birth Defects.* New York: March of Dimes Birth Defects Foundation; 2006.
7. WHO. *Primary Health Care Approaches for Prevention and Control of Congenital and Genetic Disorders.* Geneva: World Health Organization; 2000.
8. Modell B, Boulyjenkov V. Distribution and control of some genetic disorders. *World Health Stat Quart.* 1988;41:209–218.
9. Bittles AH, Mason WM, Greene J, Rao NA. Reproductive behavior and health in consanguineous marriages. *Science.* 1991;252(5007):789–794.
10. Bittles AH. Consanguineous marriage: current global incidence and its relevance to demographic research. Research Report No. 90-186. University of Michigan, Detroit, US: Population Studies Center; 1990.
11. Modell B, Kuliev AM. Impact of public health on human genetics. *Clin Genet.* 1989:36:286–298.
12. Lederberg J, Haldane JBS. On infectious disease and evolution. *Genetics.* 1999;153:1–3.
13. Cooke GS, Hill AVS. Genetics of susceptibility to human infectious disease. *Nat Rev Genet.* 2001;2:967–977.
14. Valentine WN, Neel JV. Hematologic and genetic study of transmission of thalassemia (Cooley's anemia: Mediterranean anemia). *Arch Intern Med.* 1944;74:185–196.
15. Silvestroni E, Bianco I. Sulla frequenza dei porta tori di malatia di morbo di Cooley e primi observazioni sulla frequenza dei portatore di microcitemia nel Ferrarese e inakune region! limitrofe. *Boll Atti Acad Med.* 1947;72:32.
16. Haldane JBS. The rate of mutation of human genes. *Proc VIII Int Cong Genetics Hereditas.* 1949;35:267–273.

17. Weatherall DJ, Clegg JB. Genetic variability in response to infection. Malaria and after. *Genes Immun.* 2002;3:331–337.
18. Kwiatkowski DP. How malaria has affected the human genome and what human genetics can teach us about malaria. *Am J Hum Genet.* 2005;77(2):171–192.
19. Williams TN. Red blood cell defects and malaria. *Mol Biochem Parasitol.* 2006;149(2):121–127.
20. WHO. *Shaping the Future.* Geneva: World Health Organization; 2003.
21. Allison AC. Population genetics of abnormal haemoglobins and glucose-6-phosphate dehydrogenase deficiency. In: Jonxis JHP, ed. *Abnormal Haemoglobins in Africa.* Oxford: Blackwell Scientific Publications; 1965:365.
22. Hill AVS, Allsopp GEM, Kwiatkowski D, et al. Common west African HLA antigens are associated with protection from severe malaria. *Nature.* 1991;352:595–600.
23. Williams TN, Mwangi TW, Wambua S, et al. Sickle cell trait and the risk of Plasmodium falciparum malaria and other childhood diseases. *J Infect Dis.* 2005;192(1):178–186.
24. Aidoo M, Terlouw DJ, Kolczak MS, et al. Protective effects of the sickle cell gene against malaria morbidity and mortality. *Lancet.* 2002;359(9314):1311–1312.
25. Luzzatto L, Nwachiku-Jarrett ES, Reddy S. Increased sickling of parasitised erythrocytes as mechanism of resistance against malaria in the sickle-cell trait. *Lancet.* 1970;i:319.
26. Roth EF, Jr., Friedman M, Ueda Y, Tellez L, Trager W, Nagel RL. Sickling rates of human AS red cells infected in vitro with Plasmodium falciparum malaria. *Science.* 1978;202:650–652.
27. Friedman MJ. Erythrocytic mechanism of sickle cell resistance to malaria. *Proc Natl Acad Sci USA.* 1978;75:1994.
28. Pasvol G, Weatherall DJ, Wilson RJM. A mechanism for the protective effect of haemoglobin S against *P. falciparum.* *Nature.* 1978;274:701–703.
29. Friedman MJ, Roth EF, Nagel RL, Trager W. Plasmodium falciparum: physiological interactions with the human sickle cell. *Exp Parasitol.* 1979;47:73.
30. Williams TN, Mwangi TW, Roberts DJ, et al. An immune basis for malaria protection by the sickle cell trait. *PLoS Med.* 2005;2(5):e128.
31. Cabrera G, Cot M, Migot-Nabias F, Kremsner PG, Deloron P, Luty AJ. The sickle cell trait is associated with enhanced immunoglobulin G antibody responses to Plasmodium falciparum variant surface antigens. *J Infect Dis.* 2005;191(10):1631–1638.
32. Marsh K, Otoo L, Hayes RJ, Carson DC, Greenwood BM. Antibodies to blood stage antigens of Plasmodium falciparum in rural Gambians and their relation to protection against infection. *Trans R Soc Trap Med Hyg.* 1989;83(3):293–303.
33. Modiano D, Luoni G, Sirima BS, et al. Haemoglobin C protects against clinical Plasmodium falciparum malaria. *Nature.* 2001;414:305–308.
34. Fairhurst RM, Fujioka H, Hayton K, Collins KF, Wellems TE. Aberrant development of Plasmodium falciparum in hemoglobin CC red cells: implications for the malaria protective effect of the homozygous state. *Blood.* 2003;101(8):3309–3315.
35. Fairhurst RM, Baruch Dl, Brittain NJ, et al. Abnormal display of PfEMP-1 on erythrocytes carrying haemoglobin C may protect against malaria. *Nature.* 2005;435(7045):1117–1121.
36. Duffy PE, Fried M. Red blood cells that do and red blood cells that don't: how to resist a persistent parasite. *Trends Parasitol.* 2006;22(3):99–101.
37. Ohashi J, Naka I, Patarapotikul J, et al. Extended linkage disequilibrium surrounding the hemoglobin E variant due to malarial selection. *Am J Hum Genet.* 2004;74(6):1198–1208.
38. Hutagalung R, Wilairatana P, Looareesuwan S, Brittenham GM, Aikawa M, Gordeuk VR. Influence of hemoglobin E trait on the severity of Falciparum malaria. *J Infect Dis.* 1999;179(1):283–286.
39. Chotivanich K, Udomsangpetch R, Pattanapanyasat K, et al. Hemoglobin E: a balanced polymorphism protective against high parasitemias and thus severe P. falciparum malaria. *Blood.* 2002;100(4):1172–1176.
40. Flint J, Hill AVS, Bowden DK, et al. High frequencies of alpha-thalassaemia are the result of natural selection by malaria. *Nature.* 1986;321:744–749.
41. O'Shaughnessy DF, Hill AVS, Bowden DK, Weatherall DJ, Clegg JB, with collaborators. Globin genes in Micronesia: origins and affinities of Pacific Island peoples. *Am J Hum Genet.* 1990;46:144–155.
42. Allen SJ, O'Donnell A, Alexander NDE, et al. α^+-thalassemia protects children against disease due to malaria and other infections. *Proc Natl Acad Sci USA.* 1997;94:14736–14741.
43. Mockenhaupt FP, Ehrhardt S, Gellert S, et al. Alpha(+)-thalassemia protects African children from severe malaria. *Blood.* 2004;104(7):2003–2006.
44. Williams TN, Wambua S, Uyoga S, et al. Both heterozygous and homozygous α^+ thalassemias protect against severe and fatal Plasmodium falciparum malaria on the coast of Kenya. *Blood.* 2005;106(1):368–371.
45. Oppenheimer SJ, Hill AV, Gibson FD, Macfarlane SB, Moody JB, Pringle J. The interaction of alpha thalassaemia with malaria. *Trans Roy Soc Trop Med Hyg.* 1987;81:322–326.
46. Williams TN, Maitland K, Bennett S, et al. High incidence of malaria in α-thalassaemic children. *Nature.* 1996;383:522–525.
47. Rees DC, Williams TN, Maitland K, Clegg JB, Weatherall DJ. Alpha thalassemia is associated with increased soluble transferrin receptor levels. *Br J Haematol.* 1998;103:365–370.
48. Luzzi GA, Merry AH, Newbold CL, Marsh K, Pasvol G, Weatherall DJ. Surface antigen expression on Plasmodium falciparum-infected erythrocytes is modified in α- and β-thalassemia. *J Exp Med.* 1991;173:785–791.
49. Williams TN, Weatherall DJ, Newbold CL. The membrane characteristics of Plasmodium falciparum-infected and -uninfected heterozygous alpha(0)thalassaemic erythrocytes. *Br J Haematol.* 2002;118(2):663–670.
50. Cockburn IA, MacKinnon MJ, O'Donnell A, et al. A human complement receptor 1 polymorphism that reduces Plasmodium falciparum resetting confers protection against severe malaria. *Proc Natl Acad Sci USA.* 2004;101(1):272–277.
51. Udomsangpetch R, Sueblinvong T, Pattanapanyasat K, Dharmkrong-at A, Kittilayawong A, Webster HK. Alteration in cytoadherence and rosetting of *Plasmodium falciparum*-infected thalassemic red blood cells. *Blood.* 1993;82:3752–3759.
52. Carlson J, Nash GB, Gabutti V, Al-Yaman F, Wahlgren M. Natural protection against severe *Plasmodium falciparum* malaria

due to impaired rosette formation. *Blood.* 1994;84:3909–3914.

53. Siniscalco M, Bernini L, Latte B, Motulsky AG. Favism and thalassaemia in Sardinia and their relationship to malaria. *Nature.* 1961;190:1179–1180.
54. Hill AVS, Bowden DK, O'Shaughnessy DF, Weatherall DJ, Clegg JB. β-thalassemia in Melanesia: association with malaria and characterization of a common variant (IVSI nt 5 G-C). *Blood.* 1988;72:9.
55. Willcox MC, Bjorkman A, Brohult J, Persson P-O, Rombo L, Bengtsson E. A case-control study in northern Liberia of Plasmodium falciparum malaria in haemoglobin S and β-thalassaemia traits. *Ann Trop Med Parasit.* 1983;77:239–246.
56. Pasvol G, Weatherall DJ, Wilson RJ. Effects of foetal haemoglobin on susceptibility of red cells to Plasmodium falciparum. *Nature.* 1977;270:171–173.
57. Shear HL, Grinberg L, Oilman J, et al. Transgenic mice expressing human fetal globin are protected from malaria by a novel mechanism. *Blood.* 1998;92(7):2520–2526.
58. Nagel RL. Malaria and hemoglobinopathies. In: Steinberg MH, Forget BG, Higgs DR, Nagel RL, eds. *Disorders of Hemoglobin.* Cambridge: Cambridge University Press; 2001:832–860.
59. Williams TN, Mwangi TW, Wambua S, et al. Negative epistasis between the malaria-protective effects of α^+-thalassemia and the sickle cell trait. *Nat Genet.* 2005;37(11):1253–1257.
60. May J, Evans JA, Timmann C, et al. Hemoglobin variants and disease manifestations in severe falciparum malaria. *JAMA.* 2007;297(20):2220–2226.
61. Miller LH, Mason SJ, Clyde DF, McGinniss MH. The resistance factor to *Plasmodium vivax* in Blacks. *N Eng J Med.* 1976;295:302–304.
62. Zimmerman PA, Woolley I, Masinde GL, et al. Emergence of FY*A(null) in a Plasmodium vivax-endemic region of Papua New Guinea. *Proc Natl Acad Sci USA.* 1999;96(24):13973–13977.
63. Cserti CM, Dzik WH. The ABO blood group system and plasmodium falciparum malaria. *Blood.* 2007;110(7):2250–2258.
64. Dronamraju KR, Arese P. Malaria: genetic and evolutionary aspects. In: Rich SM, Ayala FJ, eds. *Evolutionary Origins of Human Malaria Parasites.* Chapter 6. New York: Springer; 2006.
65. Cavalli-Sforza LL, Feldman MW. The application of molecular genetic approaches to the study of human evolution. *Nat Genet.* 2003;33 Suppl:266–275.
66. Carter R, Mendis KN. Evolutionary and historical aspects of the burden of malaria. *Clin Microbiol Rev.* 2002;15(4):564–594.
67. Tishkoff SA, Varkonyi R, Cahinhinan N, et al. Haplotype diversity and linkage disequilibrium at human G6PD: recent origin of alleles that confer malarial resistance. *Science.* 2001;293:455–462.
68. Bodmer WF, Cavalli-Sforza LL. *Genes, Evolution and Man.* San Francisco: W. H. Freeman and Co; 1976.
69. Fawdry AL. Erythroblastic anaemia of childhood (Cooley's anaemia) in Cyprus. *Lancet.* 1944;i:171–176.
70. Weatherall DJ, Akinyanju O, Fucharoen S, Olivieri NF, Musgrove P. Inherited disorders of hemoglobin. In: Jamison D, et al, eds. *Disease Control Priorities in Developing Countries.* New York: Oxford University Press and the World Bank; 2006:663–680.
71. Modell B, Petrou M, Layton M, et al. Audit of prenatal diagnosis for haemoglobin disorders in the United Kingdom: the first 20 years. *Br M S.* 1997;315:779–784.
72. Weatherall DJ. Genetic medicine and global health. In: Vogel F, Motulsky AG, Antonarakis SE, Speicher M, eds. *Human Genetics – Principles and Approaches.* 4th ed. Berlin/Heidelberg: Springer-Verlag; 2009:in press.
73. WHO. *Genomics and World Health.* Geneva: WHO; 2002.
74. Alwan A, Modell B. Community control of genetic and congenital disorders. EMRO Technical Publication Series 24, WHO, Alexandria, 1997.
75. Christiansen AL, Modell B. Medical genetics in developing countries. *Annul Re Gen Hum Genet.* 2004;5:219–265.
76. Nuffield Council on Bioethics. The ethics of patenting DNA. A discussion paper. London: Nuffield Council on Bioethics; 2002.
77. Nuffield Council on Bioethics. The ethics of research related to healthcare in developing countries. London: Nuffield Council on Bioethics; 2002.
78. Weatherall DJ. Genomics and global health: time for a reappraisal. *Science.* 2003:302:597–599.
79. Institute for Health Metrics and Evaluation. *Global Burden of Disease.* Available at: www.globalburden.org. Accessed August 2008.

27

Genetic Modulation of Sickle Cell Disease and Thalassemia

Martin H. Steinberg and Ronald L. Nagel

INTRODUCTION

Sickle cell anemia is a typical mendelian, single gene disease. Nevertheless, because of its characteristic phenotypic heterogeneity it resembles a multigenic trait. That is, the mutation in *HBB* is necessary, but alone insufficient to account for the phenotypic differences among patients, and other genes and the environment are likely to modulate its phenotype. In β thalassemia, and even in HbH disease, genotype–phenotype correlations are also often difficult to establish. Modulation of the phenotypes of these disorders by epistatic and other modifying genes has been a subject of increasing interest. Although studies based on candidate-modulating genes – genes chosen for study on the basis of their possible affects on a phenotype – have started to suggest genes and pathways that might modulate the phenotype of sickle cell anemia, a complete picture of genetic modulators should emerge as genome-wide association studies mature.

It is likely that fetal hemoglobin (HbF) concentration, and its distribution among erythrocytes is the major genetic modulator of both sickle cell disease and the β thalassemias. The coincidence of α thalassemia with sickle cell anemia or β thalassemia is another powerful modulatory influence. Individually, other genetic modulators are likely to have small effects, yet together the interactions of modulatory genes (and environmental factors) might have an important influence on morbidity and mortality.

In this chapter we will first discuss HbF and the genetic elements and genes that might modulate its levels and then the effects of α thalassemia in sickle cell disease and β thalassemia. Finally we will look at genetic association studies that have attempted to link polymorphisms in many genes with the phenotypes of sickle cell disease and thalassemia. As in other chapters, we will try to summarize and consolidate information available in the first edition of this book and concentrate on more recent data.

HbF

HbF ($\alpha_2\gamma_2$) is the best-known modulator of sickle cell anemia and β thalassemia. Its effect in sickle cell disease is mediated principally by its ability to inhibit HbS polymerization. In β thalassemia, HbF compensates for the reduced expression of the β-globin gene, with the resulting deficit of HbA and severe anemia.

HbF concentrations vary considerably among patients with sickle cell disease and β thalassemia, suggesting that there is genetic regulation of γ-globin gene (*HBG1, HBG2*) expression and HbF levels.[1–5]

Initially, only very high levels of HbF were considered capable of influencing the phenotype of sickle cell anemia. Further epidemiological studies suggested that any increment in HbF was clinically and perhaps therapeutically important.[6–8]

Haplotypes of the β-Globin (*HBB*) Genelike Cluster in Sickle Cell Anemia and β Thalassemia

An important event for understanding the genetic heterogeneity of sickle cell anemia was the discovery that the β^S-globin gene (*HBB* glu6val) was in linkage disequilibrium (LD) with a polymorphic site in its 3′ flanking region that was identifiable by a Hpa I restriction endonuclease cleavage site (Fig. 27.1). The complexity of this linkage was suggested by the finding that the Hpa I single nucleotide polymorphism (SNP), a recognition site for cleavage of DNA by this restriction endonuclease, was territorially segregated in Atlantic West Africa, Bantu-speaking central Africa and central west Africa, where this SNP was either negatively or positively linked to the HbS mutation (Fig. 27.1). A β-globin gene cluster haplotype was based on a series of restriction endonuclease–defined SNPs in and surrounding this gene cluster.[9,10]

The β^S-globin gene was present on three different haplotypes, and each haplotype was localized to one of three geographical regions of Africa.[11] This suggested that the β^S gene had at least three origins, with subsequent expansion of the frequency of the abnormal gene in each area of origin (Fig. 27.1). Other independent origins of the HbS mutation occurred in Cameroon (Cameroon haplotype) and in the Indian subcontinent (Arab–Indian haplotype). The origins of the HbS gene in Africa, its expansion within Africa, the role of *Plasmodium falciparum* in the selection of this gene, its spread throughout the world, and the genetic differences among HbS gene haplotypes have been extensively reviewed.[12–18]

A C-T polymorphism 158 bp 5′ to *HBG2* (rs7482144) in carriers of Senegal and Arab–Indian haplotypes is strongly associated with HbF levels. Nevertheless, there is considerable diversity of HbF levels in carriers of this SNP, suggesting that other modulatory elements could have an effect. One study suggested that the β-globin gene cluster

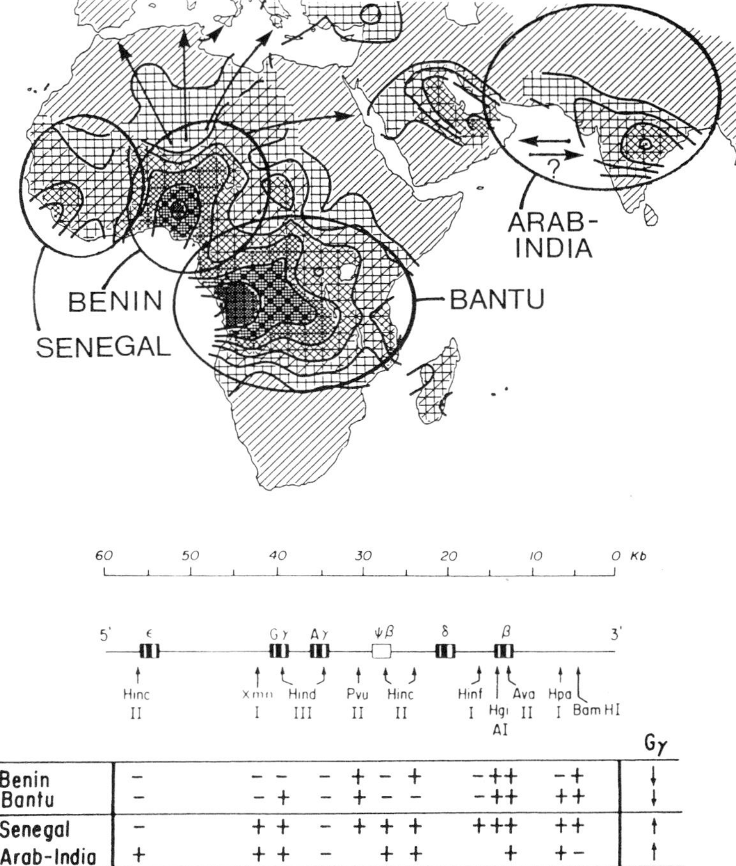

Figure 27.1. Haplotypes of the β-like globin gene cluster. (Above) Africa, the Mideast, and India showing regions of greatest frequency of their cognate haplotypes and the fall in this frequency moving outward from the center. Arrows depict possible routes of gene flow. (Below) This group of genes and their associated regulatory elements corresponds to a 60-kb stretch of DNA that contains the β-globin gene (*HBB*) and other highly homologous globin genes including the $^{G}\gamma$- and $^{A}\gamma$-globin genes (*HBG2*, *HBG1*, the δ-globin gene [*HBD*], the ε-globin gene [*HBE1*], and some pseudogenes). It is generally inherited en bloc but a "hot spot" of recombination has been located around the ψβ-δ region. Depicted by arrows are also the location of the sites that are polymorphic in human populations and cleaved by several restriction endonucleases. Haplotypes correspond to a set of SNPs identified by the presence or absence of selected restriction endonuclease cleavage sites. Although approximately 20 different haplotypes are found in different ethnic groups, only five–seven of them are frequent.

haplotype, independent of HbF level, is a correlate of survival in hydroxyurea-treated sickle cell anemia patients.[19] How this might occur is unclear; other modifying genes or elements might be linked to the β-globin like cluster, although to date, a haplotype-associated effect on HbF concentration is the sole known modulating factor.

Molecular Characteristics of the African and Indo–European β^s-linked Haplotypes. SNPs that define a haplotype are present in a 63-kb stretch of DNA subdivided into a 34-kb 5′, 19-kb 3′, and 9 kb central domain. Many other SNPs are present in these haplotype blocks and some could modulate the expression of the γ-globin genes and the accumulation of HbF; however, a mechanism for modulation of HbF gene expression is still lacking.

Atypical haplotypes in sickle cell anemia usually result from recombination between common and rare haplotypes. In African Americans, because of their genetic diversity, many atypical haplotypes are found.[20] In the central domain, 5′ to the δ-globin gene, is a "hot spot" for recombination.

When a 5′ subhaplotype, including the β-globinlike gene cluster locus control region (LCR, Chapter 5), becomes linked to a β^S-globin gene by recombination, polymorphisms in the LCR or any region 5′ to the site of recombination need not be the same as that linked to the β^S-globin gene in the original haplotype. For example, a 5′ Benin subhaplotype from a β^A chromosome might contain SNPs distinct from those of the 5′ Benin subhaplotype linked to the β^S-globin gene. This is a consequence of the relatively short time the β^S-globin gene has been linked to the 5′ Benin haplotype compared with the β^A-globin gene. This longer period of evolution allows for many more SNPs to be associated with the LCR. In some atypical haplotypes of African Americans, the 5′ subhaplotype is likely to be of Caucasian origin, further uncoupling the β^S-globin gene from the influence of genetic elements that could have co-evolved to maintain high HbF levels.

LD between the β^S-globin gene and the Arab–Indian haplotype was discovered independently in sickle cell anemia patients inhabiting the eastern oasis of Saudi Arabia. This haplotype is also linked to the C-T SNP 5′ to *HBG2*. The Arab–Indian haplotype also has a unique $(AT)_9T_5$ repeat sequence 5′ to the β gene and an unusual sequence in HS-2 of the LCR. The $(AT)_9T_5$ motif lies within a negative regulatory region between nucleotides −610 and −490, and binds the protein BP-1, a putative repressor of gene expression, which was postulated to influence the fractional concentration of HbS in sickle cell trait (HbAS).[21,22] Nevertheless,

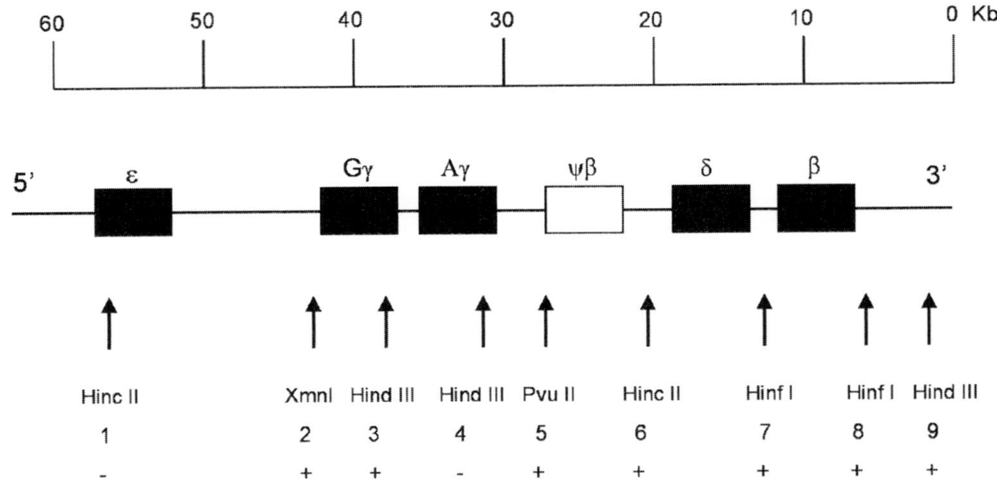

Figure 27.2. The β-like globin gene cluster and the 5′ $^{G}\gamma$-158 C-T SNP. The restriction endonuclease sites defining the β-like globin gene cluster are shown, including the 5′ $^{G}\gamma$-158 C-T SNP (rs7482144) (site number 2) that characterizes the Senegal and Arab–India haplotype. Sickle cell anemia patients who are compound heterozygotes for a Senegal and Benin chromosome typically have between 6% and 10% HbF, whereas homozygotes can have up to 20% HbF. These numbers are modulated by age, sex, hydroxyurea treatment, and likely, other genetic differences among patients.

although Indian subjects with HbAS have a lower percentage of HbS than subjects of African descent, this might be a result of α thalassemia or even iron deficiency (Chapter 23). In 5′ HS-2 of the Arab–Indian haplotype, the AT repeat region has the unique form $(AT)_{10}$ACACATATACGT$(AT)_{12}$. How and if these and other polymorphisms modulate HbF and $^{G}\gamma$-globin chain levels in the Arab–Indian and Senegal haplotypes is unclear.

In β thalassemia, different mutations were associated with each haplotype and more than one haplotype was linked to the same thalassemia mutation.

Effects of β-Globin Gene Cluster Haplotype on HbF

Sickle Cell Anemia. Any effect of the β-globin gene cluster haplotype on the phenotype of sickle cell anemia and β thalassemia appears to be dependent on the HbF level associated with a haplotype. This, in turn, is associated with the presence of the 5′ *HBG2* C-T SNP (rs7482144) and perhaps other *cis*-acting elements (Fig. 27.2). Other studies have suggested that regions 5′ to the γ-globin genes have regulatory importance. Multiple point mutations in the promoters of the γ-globin genes have been found to modulate γ-globin gene expression and cause the nondeletion HPFH phenotype (Chapter 7).

Erythroid colonies derived from precursor cells obtained from carriers of HbAS with the Arab–Indian haplotype and normal HbF concentration synthesize more HbF than colonies derived from controls.[23,24] Erythroid colony growth in vitro might mimic the perturbed erythropoiesis that occurs with hemolysis, suggesting that hematopoietic stress might be needed for the −158 *HBG2* C-T SNP to increase levels of HbF. In normal adults and neonates, the −158 C-T SNP is also associated with small but statistically significant increases in the synthesis of HbF and $^{G}\gamma$-globin chains.[25,26]

The Cameroon haplotype and Mediterranean haplotypes II and VI have in common a high $^{G}\gamma$:$^{A}\gamma$ ratio but lack the −158 C-T SNP. Haplotype II is linked to β thalassemia and to a 4-bp deletion (AGCA) in the region of a GCA repeat at −124 to −127 bp relative to the $^{A}\gamma$ CAP-site.[27] This 4-bp deletion has been reported in the promoters of the $^{A}\gamma$ alleles on both β^{A} and β^{S} chromosomes; no effect on the expression of the $^{A}\gamma$-globin gene was noted however.[28] It was suggested that the 4-bp deletion is a common polymorphism linked to the $^{A}\gamma$ gene (see later). Other polymorphisms that might be associated with HbF level have been called the pre-γ framework.[29]

β Thalassemia. Many different mutations cause β thalassemia, making an understanding of the molecular basis of HbF modulation in β thalassemia more difficult. Most studies suggest that the −158 C-T *HBG2* SNP is a major modulating factor.[28,30,31] One study of polymorphisms related to high HbF suggested that a haplotype of the $^{A}\gamma$-δ-globin intergenic region, the motif $(TA)_9N_{10}(TA)_{10}$ in HS-2, and the pre-$^{G}\gamma$ haplotype were sufficient but not necessary for high HbF expression. The genetic determinant(s) of high HbF without HPFH was linked to a specific $^{A}\gamma$-δ intergenic haplotype.[32]

In HbE–β thalassemia, the Senegal haplotype but not the (AT)(x)T(y) 5′ to the β-globin gene was linked to the high-HbF phenotype.[33]

More detailed studies of HbE–β^{0} thalassemia examined 67 SNPs within the β-globin genelike cluster in two groups of unrelated patients, all of whom had a normal α-globin genotype. Approximately 200 patients had mild disease and 300 had severe disease when severity was graded by a clinical scoring system.[34] The SNPs associated with disease severity and HbF comprised two distinct LD blocks, one containing the β-globin gene and the other extending from the LCR to the δ-globin gene, and they were separated by a recombination hotspot in the region of the β-globin gene promoter. Forty-five SNPs within the interval, including the LCR region and the δ-globin gene, showed strong association with disease severity. The strongest association was observed with the −158 C-T *HBG2* SNP, but this explained only approximately 5% and 8% of the HbF variation in the two groups. Carriers of the T allele were more likely to have a milder disease course and higher level HbF in both the mild and severe patient groups. The T allele was always in *cis* with the HbE allele. Although it seems likely that the association with disease severity is mediated through the effect on HbF level (severe cases, 32.7% ± 11.7%; mild cases, 39.2% ± 11.6%), these differences are small and a mechanistic explanation for the differences in HbF is still lacking.

Genetic Modulation of HbF

HbF expression is regulated by complex interactions among chromosome remodeling activities, transcription factors, genes modulating erythropoiesis, and elements linked to the β-globin gene cluster (Chapters 4 and 5). This complexity provides many sites for modulation of HbF level in sickle cell disease and thalassemia.

LCR and HbF. With rare exceptions, the only *cis*-acting SNP consistently associated with HbF levels in sickle cell anemia has been the aforementioned −158 C-T transversion 5′ to *HBG2*. Most studies of the influence of the LCR on HbF production have focused on 5′ HS-2, which appears to be the only 5′ hypersensitive site that is polymorphic among HbS-associated haplotypes. Because this region probably has some regulatory role in globin gene transcription, it was of interest to see if polymorphisms of this region were associated with phenotypic variation in sickle cell anemia and the results of these studies were previously summarized.[13] To date, SNPs in the LCR associated with HbF in sickle cell anemia have yet to be pinpointed. In a sickle cell anemia patient homozygous for the Benin haplotype with a HbF of 21% and with 65% $^G\gamma$-chains, the sequence of HS-2 was characteristic of the Senegal type but the −158 C-T SNP was absent, suggesting a crossover 5′ to the $^G\gamma$-globin gene. The Senegal HS-2 is distinguished by the presence of Sp1 and GATA-binding sites and a motif similar to that found 5′ to the BP-1–binding site; however, the functional significance of this association is not known. HbF levels in six Benin haplotype homozygotes with a Senegal haplotype HS-2 were between 2.6% and 8.5%, suggesting that this polymorphism alone did not lead to increased levels of HbF of the magnitude often seen in carriers of a Senegal haplotype.

Polymorphisms in a tandem repeat of the sequence $(TA)_xN_{10-12}(TA)_y$ that contains a Hox2-binding site were examined in 100 patients with sickle cell anemia aged 1–18 years.[35] Nearly 8% of chromosomes had a discordance in the HS-2 tandem repeat that was not characteristic of the haplotype.[36,37] A region between −1445 and −1225 5′ to the promoter of the $^G\gamma$-globin gene was found to vary among haplotypes. Senegal–Benin chromosomes associated with modest HbF levels had a likely breakpoint for recombination upstream of −1500 bp 5′ to $^G\gamma$-globin gene promoter. In contrast, when a high HbF was present with the Senegal–Benin chromosome recombination, the breakpoint was 3′ to position −369 to −309 in the $^G\gamma$-globin gene promoter. In HbAS with a Benin haplotype, when the normal chromosome had the HS-2 $(TA)_9$ $N_{12}(TA)_{10}$ structure, HbF (0.9%) and F cells (8.3%) were approximately twice as high as with the presence of other configurations for this region.[38] These data suggest that HbF is influenced by elements 3′ to HS-2 and 5′ to the γ-globin gene promoter.

F-cell numbers in Benin haplotype HbAS carriers were more strongly associated with the $(TA)_9N_{12}(TA)_{10}$ configuration of HS-2 of β^A chromosomes than the −158 C-T SNP.[39] These subjects did not have hemolytic anemia so the results are less likely to reflect differential F cell survival and more likely to estimate HbF production.

Although other *cis*-acting elements, for example, in additional phylogenetically conserved regions of the LCR outside the core sequences of its constituent hypersensitive sites, might partake in the regulation of γ-globin gene transcription; definitive associations have not yet been found.[13]

The activity of constructs containing variant HS-2 enhancers derived from HbS chromosomes was studied to examine the functional effects of these polymorphisms.[40] A relationship of reporter gene activity with HbF and the β-globin gene cluster haplotype was not found. In a multiplex assay permitting simultaneous analysis of three polymorphic *cis*-acting elements spanning 53 kb of the β-globin gene cluster, concordance between polymorphic alleles in γ- and β-globin gene promoters was identified. SNPs in HS-2 of the LCR were found juxtaposed to atypical *cis* alleles in the γ-globin gene promoter. Analysis of many such hybrid haplotype chromosomes suggested that polymorphisms in the γ-globin gene promoter exerted the dominant influence on HbF level in sickle cell disease.[5]

β-Globin Gene Silencer. Located −530 bp 5′ to the β-globin gene is an AT-rich region with the core structure $(AT)_x(T)_y$, which is polymorphic and linked to the β-globin gene cluster haplotype. This element has been proposed as a β-globin gene silencer that might influence the expression of the β-globin gene by variably binding a putative repressor protein, BP-1, depending on the $(AT)_x(T)_y$ composition.[41] BP-1 is a member of the homeobox gene family and the Distal-less subfamily, genes important in early development. BP-1 protein can repress the β-globin gene promoter and in the human erythroid cell line MB-02; its expression decreases upon induction of the β-globin gene.[21] By modulating erythropoiesis, BP-1 might also effect HbF production.[22]

The Arab–Indian motif has a higher affinity for BP-1 than the Bantu haplotype motif. This could be reflected at the protein level by less HbS in Indian carriers of the β^S gene and a normal α-globin genotype, when compared with blacks with HbAS, however, this interpretation, as discussed in Chapter 22, is not clear-cut. $(AT)_9(T)_5$, along with the −158 C-T polymorphism, can be associated with high HbF in some homozygous β thalassemia patients. In these patients, the $(AT)_9(T)_5$ motif was associated with approximately 10 g/dL HbF, whereas $(AT)_7(T)_7$ was accompanied by approximately 5 g/dL of HbF.

Four–base pair Deletion Linked to the $^A\gamma$ Gene. Only the Cameroon haplotype β^S chromosome is associated with an AGCA deletion at nucleotides −222 to −225 5′ to the β-globin gene and is always linked to the $^A\gamma^T$ allele. The effects of this deletion on γ-globin gene expression are controversial and unlikely to affect carriers of other haplotypes. In a study of sickle cell anemia in which a Cameroon haplotype was *trans* to a typical HbS haplotype, HbF levels, packed cell volume (PCV) and mean corpuscular volume was similar whatever the haplotype in *trans*.[20] It was also suggested that the 4-bp deletion was associated with decreased expression of not only the $^A\gamma^T$-globin gene, but also of the $^G\gamma$-globin gene in cis. Studies in β thalassemia in which the 4-bp deletion was present also suggested decreased $^G\gamma$ gene expression in *cis* to the $^A\gamma^T$ allele. Together, these results implicate the region of the 4-bp deletion as a possible *cis*-acting element that augments the expression of both γ-globin genes when combined with a *trans*-acting factor.[42]

$^G\gamma$ Gene 5′ Regulatory Region. Approximately 1.65–1.15 kb 5′ to the $^G\gamma$ gene lies an area of 0.5 kb proposed to be another region that potentially has a regulatory role in γ-globin gene expression.[29] Designated the pre-$^G\gamma$ framework, this region was found to have four polymorphic variants that, like most other *cis*-acting sequences with possible regulatory roles, are linked to the β-gene cluster haplotype. This region contains four GATA-1–binding sites and Sp1 and CRE protein–binding domains. Strongest protein binding was associated with the Senegal pre-$^G\gamma$ framework and the Benin haplotype–linked pre-$^G\gamma$ enhancer activity was sevenfold lower than the Bantu and Senegal type pre-$^G\gamma$ framework. The physiological significance of these findings remains unclear.

A SNP, GA<u>T</u>A→GA<u>G</u>A, in a GATA site that is in a putative silencing element at nucleotide −567 5′ of the $^G\gamma$-globin gene promoter was associated with increased HbF in two otherwise normal individuals. This mutation alters a GATA-1–binding motif to a GAGA sequence. DNA–protein binding assays showed that this GATA motif was capable of binding GATA-1 transcription factor in vitro and in vivo. Truncation analyses of $^G\gamma$-globin gene promoter linked to a luciferase reporter gene revealed a negative regulatory activity present between nucleotides −675 and −526. In addition, the T→G mutation at the GATA motif increased the promoter activity by two- to threefold in transiently transfected erythroid cell lines. The binding motif is uniquely conserved in simian primates with a fetal pattern of γ-globin gene expression. This GATA motif appears to have a functional role in silencing γ-globin gene expression in adults. The T→G mutation in this motif disrupts GATA-1 binding and the associated repressor complex, abolishing its silencing effect and resulting in the up regulation of γ-globin gene expression.[43]

The functional importance of this site was supported by studies in transgenic adult β-YAC mice, where it was shown that during definitive erythropoiesis, γ-globin gene expression is silenced, in part, by binding a protein complex containing GATA-1, FOG-1, and Mi2 at the −566/−567 GATA sites of both γ-globin gene promoters. Chromatin immunoprecipitation assays showed that GATA-1, FOG-1, and Mi2 were recruited to the −566 or the −567 GATA sites of the γ-globin gene promoters when γ-expression was low, but not when these genes were being expressed.[44]

A C-T SNP in 3′ HS1 was associated with increased HbF in 11 β thalassemia intermedia patients lacking other explanations for their mild phenotype.[45] This report is difficult to interpret because the β thalassemia mutations in these cases were diverse and two individuals had HbF levels less than 10%.

Polymorphisms in trans*-acting Regulatory Elements Regulating HbF Expression.* It has been estimated that the −158 SNP 5′ to *HBG2* and other postulated haplotype-associated effects on HbF account for less than 25% the variability of HbF in sickle cell anemia. This suggests that *trans*-acting regulatory elements exert control over HbF levels.

Putative *trans*-acting elements modulating HbF include four quantitative trait loci (QTLs). These are the F cell production locus, a QTL at Xp22 associated with F cell number;[4] a QTL at 6q22.3-23.2 associated with F cell numbers first described in an extended Asian–Indian family;[1,2,46] a QTL at chromosome 8q that appeared to interact with the −158 C → T SNP;[47] and a QTL at 2p16.1, identified in a genome-wide association study of healthy adults that mapped to *BCL11A*, a zinc-finger protein, which accounted for 15% of F cell variance.[48] These elements were first associated with F cells or HbF in individuals with β thalassemia trait or those who did not have a hemoglobinopathy. Further examination of some of these QTLs was undertaken to identify the genes and polymorphisms associated with modulation of HbF in sickle cell anemia and β thalassemia.

A candidate gene screening study in patients with sickle cell anemia showed associations with HbF and SNPs in phosphodiesterase 7 (*PDE7B*), microtubule-associated protein 7 (*MAP7*), mitogen-activated protein kinase kinase kinase 5 (*MAP3K5*), and peroxisomal biogenesis factor 7 (*PEX7*). These genes abut but were not within 6q 23.2.[3] It had been hypothesized that variable expression of a collection of linked genes of functional interdependence might be associated with certain phenotypes,[49] and long-range LD, as seen in this QTL, has been reported for other chromosomal regions.[50]

To refine further the functional importance of the 6q QTL direct sequencing of five protein-coding genes, *ALDH8A1*, *HBS1L*, *MYB*, *AHI1*, and *PDE7B*, within the

1.5-Mb candidate interval of 6q23 was done but failed to detect mutations that could be associated with HbF modulation.[51] The expression profile of these genes in cultured erythroid cells of healthy adults with non-gene deletion hereditary persistence of HbF (HPFH) found that two genes, *MYB* and *HBS1L*, were down regulated. Transfection of K562 cells with cDNA of *MYB* and *HBS1L* showed that overexpression of only *MYB* inhibited γ-globin gene expression. Low levels of *MYB* were associated with low cell expansion and accelerated erythroid differentiation, suggesting that differences in the intrinsic levels of *MYB* might account for some variation in adult HbF levels by its effect on the cell cycle.[52] In northern European families, polymorphisms within and 5′ to *HBS1L* were strongly associated with F cell levels, accounting for 17.6% of the F cell variance. Although mRNA levels of *HBS1L* and *MYB* in erythroid precursors are positively correlated, only *HBS1L* expression correlated with high F cells, suggesting that *HBS1L* variants modulate HbF.[53]

A QTL at chromosome 8q appeared to interact with the −158 C-T SNP to modulate HbF levels in the same Asian–Indian family in which the 6q QTL was first discovered.[2,47] In more than 870 dizygotic twins, effects of the 8q QTL on HbF were also conditional on the genotype of the −158 *HBG2* C-T SNP.[54]

Panels of haplotype tagging SNPs in the β-globin genelike cluster and in QTLs on chromosomes 8q and Xp were genotyped in two independent sickle cell anemia patient groups to study their association with baseline HbF levels. In one group of 327 individuals, three SNPs in *TOX* (thymus high mobility protein; 8q12.1) were associated with HbF. Three additional SNPs in *TOX* showed significant association in a second group of 987 individuals. Joint analysis of all SNPs and covariates confirmed the association with *TOX* and identified SNPs potentially associated with HbF in two genes in the Xp22.2-p22.3 QTL. SNPs in *TOX* and a few other genes were associated with the HbF response to hydroxyurea treatment in sickle cell anemia.[55] *TOX* belongs to a conserved high-mobility group box protein family that binds the minor groove of DNA.

Eight hundred and fifty SNPs in 320 candidate genes in the β-globin genelike cluster, QTL on chromosomes 6q, 8q, and Xp and other candidate genes were studied in a group of 1,518 adults and children with sickle cell anemia and validated in an independent group of 211 adults. HbF concentration was modeled as a continuous variable with values in a finite interval by using a novel Bayesian approach. In individuals aged 24 years or older, five SNPs in *TOX*, two SNPs in the β-globin genelike cluster, two SNPs in the Xp QTL, and one SNP in chromosome 15q22 were associated with HbF. Four SNPs in 15q22 were associated with HbF only in the larger patient sample. When patients younger than 24 years were examined, additional genes, including four with roles in nitric oxide (NO) metabolism, were associated with HbF level. These observations raise the possibility that different genes might modulate the rate of decline of HbF and the final HbF levels in sickle cell anemia.[56]

The results of this analysis confirmed work where more traditional analytical approaches showed associations of SNPs in *TOX*, *GPM6B*, and the β-globin genelike cluster with HbF levels. Included in the 15q22-21 interval are *MAP2K1*, *SMAD3*, and *AQP9*. None of these genes have a known connection to HbF synthesis or erythropoiesis, and this region is not a known QTL associated with HbF.

Genome-wide association studies focused on HbF concentration in normal individuals and patients with β thalassemia trait, β thalassemia intermedia, and sickle cell anemia, have been reported.[57] Six SNPs in *BCL11A* (2p16.1) were first found to be associated with F cells in 179 normal adults[58] with the highest and lowest 5% of F cell numbers. *BCL11A*, is a highly conserved zinc-finger protein, and codes for a transcription factor containing three C2H2-type zinc finger motifs, a proline rich region, and an acidic domain.[48] Similar associations of SNPs in *BCL11A* were found in Sardinian β thalassemia patients and by focused genotyping, in more than 1,200 patients with sickle cell anemia. In the β thalassemia patients the C allele of SNP rs1188686 was associated with higher HbF in the general population and in patients with thalassemia intermedia compared with thalassemia major.

With genome-wide association studies of 113 parents of Thai HbE-β thalassemia patients and 255 unrelated African Americans with sickle cell anemia, and by focused genotyping of 250 parents of β thalassemia major patients from Hong Kong, association of HbF and F cells were found with SNP rs766432, one of the same SNPs of *BCL11A* previously reported. In the patients with sickle cell anemia, homozygotes for the C allele of SNP rs766432 had an average of 7% HbF compared with 3% HbF in patients homozygous for the A allele. These findings in at least four different populations are consistent with an aboriginal *BCL11A* variant in Yorubans that is highly conserved among ancestral populations, even as the haplotype blocks containing this gene have diverged. Together, these observations suggest that possible functional motifs responsible for modulating HbF level or F cells might reside within or immediately adjacent to a 3-kb region bounded by rs1427407 and rs4671393 in intron 2 of *BCL11A*.

A small guanosine triphosphate (GTP)-binding protein, secretion-associated and RAS-related (*SAR1A*) protein is inducible by hydroxyurea and might play a pivotal role in induction of γ-globin gene expression via its role in erythroid maturation. Polymorphisms in the *SAR1A* promoter were associated with differences HbF levels or the HbF response to hydroxyurea in patients with sickle cell anemia. Three SNPs in the upstream 5′ untranslated region (−809 C-T, −502 G-T and −385 C-A) were significantly associated with the HbF response in sickle cell anemia patients treated with hydroxyurea and four SNPs (rs2310991, −809 C-T, −385 C-A and rs4282891) were significantly associated with the change in absolute HbF level after 2 years of treatment.[59,60]

Effects of β-Globin Gene Cluster Haplotype on the Phenotype of Sickle Cell Disease. Generally, a haplotype is associated with characteristic hematological and clinical findings, although there is considerable heterogeneity within any haplotype. For example, carriers of the HbS gene on Senegal or Arab–Indian haplotype usually have the highest HbF level and PCV and the mildest clinical course. Individuals with Bantu haplotypes have the lowest HbF level and PCV and the most severe clinical course. Carriers of the Benin haplotype have intermediate features (reviewed in ref. 13).

Studies of small numbers of African patients with sickle cell anemia and different β-globin gene cluster haplotypes who had distinct hematological characteristics first suggested that haplotype could be a marker for the phenotypic heterogeneity of sickle cell anemia. In most of Africa, the environmental, nutritional, and infectious obstacles make it difficult to distinguish the role of haplotype in modulating the course of disease, but clinical differences have been noted. It appears that Africans with the Senegal haplotype fare better than those with other common haplotypes, but there are too few clinical data to permit dogmatism.[61]

Most of the detailed and larger studies of the clinical and hematological effects of haplotype in sickle cell anemia have been in regions where the HbS gene arrived by gene flow, and after many years of genetic admixture, patients in such regions are usually haplotype heterozygotes, which complicates interpretation of the association of haplotype with phenotype. Reports of the clinical and hematological effects of haplotype in sickle cell anemia should be interpreted carefully because often few patients were studied, the patient's ages differed among series, clinical events might not have been sharply defined, and distinctions between haplotype homozygotes and heterozygotes were often not clearly drawn.

In longitudinal studies from the United States, the Senegal haplotype was associated with fewer hospitalizations and painful episodes.[62,63] An effect of the Senegal haplotype on reducing episodes of acute chest syndrome was of marginal significance. The Bantu haplotype was associated with the highest incidence of organ damage, and renal failure was strongly associated with this haplotype.[64] Both sex and haplotype affect HbF levels in sickle cell anemia. PCV was higher in males with Benin and Bantu haplotypes. Among carriers with a Senegal haplotype, the PCV in males and females was equal and females had the highest HbF. Females with the Senegal haplotype and high HbF can have less hemolysis and therefore higher PCV.[65] Most work suggests that the Arab–Indian haplotype is also associated with milder disease although vasoocclusive events do occur.[66–69]

Lacking a reasonable hypothesis about how the haplotype of the β-globin gene cluster could modify disease severity, other than via an effect on HbF, it seems most reasonable to conclude that the effect of haplotype on the phenotype of disease is mediated through a *cis*-acting effect on HbF.

EFFECTS OF α THALASSEMIA IN SICKLE CELL DISEASE AND β THALASSEMIA

Sickle Cell Disease

Approximately a third of patients with sickle cell anemia have coincidental α thalassemia (Chapter 23). These individuals have less hemolysis, higher PCV, lower mean corpuscular volume, and lower reticulocyte counts (see Table 23.9, Chapter 23). Coincident α thalassemia results in longer erythrocyte lifespan because of the reduction of dense and rigid red cells (Table 23.8, Chapter 23).

α Thalassemia decreased the risk of organ failure in carriers of a Bantu haplotype. In Jamaicans, the absence of α thalassemia coupled with a high HbF presaged benign disease.[70] When phenotypes of sickle cell anemia were clustered into two or three phenotype groups, neither α thalassemia nor the β-globin gene cluster haplotype appeared to influence the clinical events defining the groups.[71]

The benefits and liabilities afforded by the presence or absence of α thalassemia in sickle cell anemia is very likely to be due to its effects on hemolysis. Recent work suggests that concurrent α thalassemia reduces the incidence of stroke, priapism, leg ulceration, and pulmonary hypertension but has little effect or increases the chances of developing osteonecrosis, acute chest syndrome, and painful episodes.[72–75] As discussed in Chapter 11, hemolysis is associated with a proliferative vasculopathy due to decreased bioavailable NO.

β Thalassemia

Concurrent α thalassemia or the presence of α-globin gene duplications modifies the phenotype of β thalassemia. As the pathophysiology of β thalassemia is largely determined by imbalance globin chain synthesis (Chapter 17), concurrent α thalassemia, by reducing the accumulation of α-globin chains, tends to balance the deficit in β-globin chains and causes a milder disease. A sufficient α-globin gene deficit can cause a thalassemia intermedia phenotype in homozygotes or compound heterozygote for severe β-thalassemia mutations where the expected phenotype would be thalassemia major.

Conversely, extra α-globin genes, as seen with chromosomes containing triplicated or quadruplicated α-globin loci, by increasing the imbalance in α:β synthesis, can convert a heterozygote for β thalassemia into a symptomatic thalassemia intermedia.[76,77] One might hypothesize that with an improvement in the α:β globin synthesis ratio and reduced hemolysis, hemolysis-related complications of β thalassemia, which also include pulmonary hypertension, leg ulcers, and perhaps priapism, might also be reduced; however, there are no data on this subject.

Role of α-Hemoglobin Stabilizing Protein. α-Hemoglobin stabilizing protein (*ERAF*, 16p11.2), by binding free α-globin chains, prevents their proteolysis and preserves their ability to form α:β dimers.[78] In β thalassemic mice that

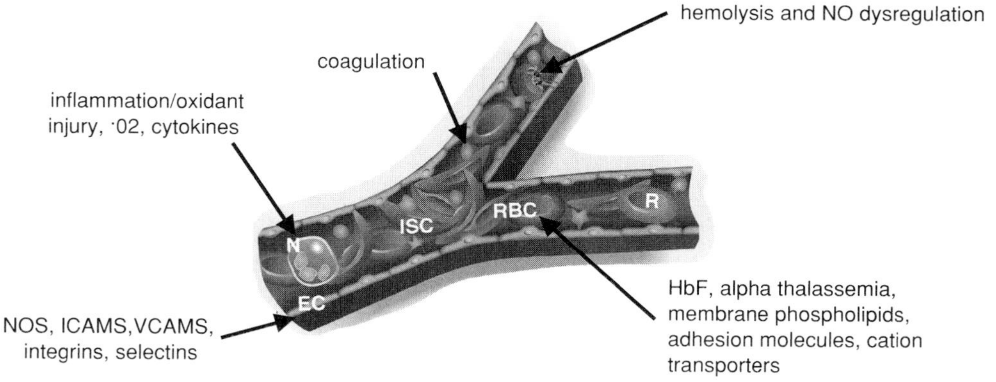

Figure 27.3. Some facets of sickle cell disease pathobiology that might be genetically modulated. (See color plate 27.3.)

are also deficient in α-hemoglobin–stabilizing protein, the phenotype of the β thalassemia was more severe.[79]

The role of α-hemoglobin–stabilizing protein as a modulator of β thalassemia is less conclusive, with no relationship found between haplotypes of α-hemoglobin–stabilizing protein and the severity of HbE–β thalassemia.[80,81] In a study of more than 100 healthy individuals, expression of α-hemoglobin–stabilizing protein was measured. Among six common variants of this protein, four were strongly associated with its expression. In nine anemic patients with heterozygous β thalassemia who also had a triplicated α-globin locus, one variant of α-hemoglobin–stabilizing protein was more common than expected, suggesting that variation in the protein could contribute to some heterogeneity in β thalassemia.[82]

HEMOGLOBIN A_2

HbA_2, a tetramer of α-and δ-globin chains (Chapter 7), impairs the polymerization of HbS to the same extent as the γ-globin chain of HbF. HbA_2 has the advantage of being evenly distributed in all red cells, whereas HbF is sequestered in F cells. The naturally low level of HbA_2 makes it an inconsequential contributor to the total hemoglobin concentration but there are instances when the level of HbA_2 is increased far beyond its usual values. Some exceptionally high HbA_2 levels are the result of deletions that remove the β-globin gene promoters. When HbA_2 and HbF levels are high, their combination might modulate sickle cell disease and cause a milder phenotype, but few patients with these genotypes are available to establish conclusively its phenotype (Chapter 23). With these rare exceptions, it is unlikely that variation in HbA_2 level affects the phenotype of sickle cell anemia.

MODULATION OF THE PHENOTYPE OF SICKLE CELL ANEMIA

Genetic Polymorphisms as Predictors of Disease Severity

The diversity of sickle cell anemia cannot be explained solely by HbF and α-globin gene–linked modulation. Modifying or epistatic genes that potentially affect the pathogenesis of sickle cell anemia and modulate the phenotype of disease include: mediators of hemolysis; vascular remodeling; inflammation; oxidant injury; NO biology; vasoregulation; cell–cell interaction; blood coagulation and hemostasis; growth factors; cytokines and receptors; and transcriptional regulators (Fig. 27.3). These genes have modifying affects independent of effecting HbS polymerization, the mechanism by which both HbF and α thalassemia impact the phenotype of disease (Fig. 27.4). Polymorphisms have been found in candidate genes that might affect the phenotype of sickle cell disease (Table 27.1).[83]

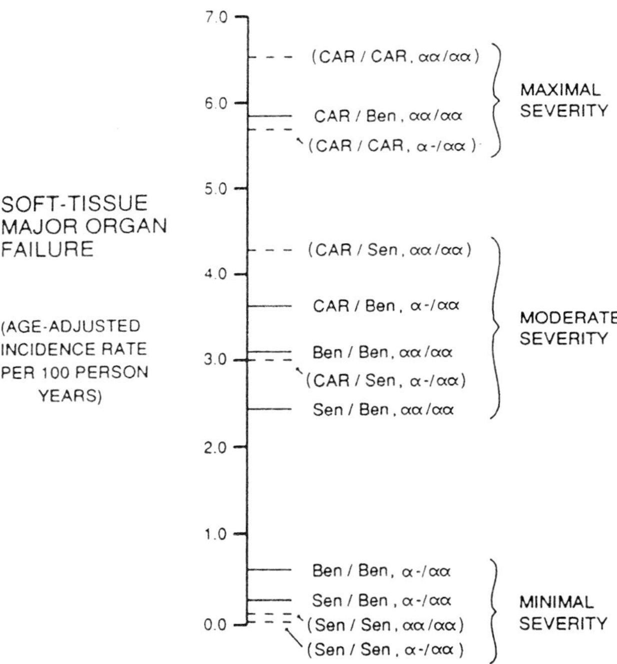

Figure 27.4. The relationships between β-like globin gene cluster haplotypes and clinical features of sickle cell anemia. PCV connotes packed cell volume. The clinical features include events such as osteonecrosis, acute chest syndrome, renal failure, and other common disease complications. These associations of haplotype and phenotype in sickle cell anemia are only generalities, and within each haplotype group there is considerable heterogeneity whose cause is unknown.[168]

Table 27.1. Genetic polymorphisms affecting some phenotypes of sickle cell anemia and β thalassemia

Phenotype	Gene/SNP marker	References
Sickle cell anemia		
Stroke	*VCAM1*/ G1238C	91
	VCAM1/T-1594C	92
	IL4R/S503P	92
	TNFA/G-308S	92
	LDLR/NcoI +/−	92
	ADRB2/Q/27E	92
	AGT/AG repeats	96
	HLA genes	94,95
	Multiple genes	72
Osteonecrosis	*MTHFR*/C677T *BMP6, ANXA2*	104–106, 165, 166
Acute chest syndrome	*NOS3*/T-786C	117
	NOS1/AAT repeats	167
	TGFBR3, SMAD1, KL, NRCAM, SMAD3, SMAD7 PIK3CG	121
Pulmonary hypertension	TGFβ/BMP pathway genes	116
Cholelithiasis	*UGT1A*/promoter repeats	122, 123, 125
Priapism	*KL, TGFBR3, AQP1, ITGAV*	101, 102
Leg ulcers	*KL, TEK,* TGFβ/BMP pathway genes	74
Bacteremia	TGFβ/BMP pathway genes	107
β Thalassemia		
Cholelithiasis	*UGT1A*	see text
Iron overload	*HFE*	151, 152
Bone disease	COl1A1, *VDR*	156–159
Cardiovascular disease	*APOE*	160

Other genetic variants, some mentioned in the text, have been studied and have shown no associations.

A unifying theme emerging from these studies is that polymorphisms in genes of the transforming growth factor–β/bone morphogenetic protein (TGFβ/BMP) pathway appear involved in several subphenotypes of disease and could reflect the hitherto unappreciated role of this very large pathway in the pathobiology of disease.[84]

The first approaches to understanding how genetic polymorphism might modulate the phenotype of sickle cell anemia were based on the selection of candidate genetic modifiers. A candidate gene–based approach is limited by the imagination needed to define likely candidates and alone cannot provide a complete picture of the genetic heterogeneity that must account for the complex pathobiology of any disease. In some studies, picking the "wrong" SNP or choosing insufficient numbers of SNPs in large genes might have lead to false-negative results. Nonsynonymous coding region SNPs are an obvious first choice to examine, but they are the least common. Recent studies suggest that by affecting protein folding, even synonymous SNPs might modulate a genes' function,[85] and genome-wide association studies have yield surprising results in other diseases in which the strongest associations of genotype with phenotype have occurred in gene-poor regions.[86] SNPs that effect gene expression might be even more important, but it is difficult to identify all of these by in silico analysis.

Genome-wide association studies are just beginning and have the promise of unbiased interrogation of the entire genome for an association with a phenotype. Copy number variants can also be assessed with the available technology. Analytical methods for genetic association studies are evolving, and dealing with the problem of false-positive results can be vexing when more than 1 million SNPs can be genotyped across the genome of thousands of cases.[87] Other issues that must be considered in genome-wide association studies include: LD with causative polymorphisms; interpretation of associations with SNPs without an obvious function; gene–gene interaction; gene–environment interaction; and precise phenotype definition.

Painful Episodes. Acute painful episodes are the major clinical event in sickle cell disease. These episodes are one measure of disease severity, and a predictor of early death in adults.[6] The rate of painful episodes varies widely among patients; highest pain rates are found in patients with high PCV and low HbF. In addition to HbF concentration and a possible role of α thalassemia, a genetic basis for the heterogeneous distribution of painful episodes among patients has not been described. Case-control studies are problematic because nearly all patients will have pain, therefore, finding genes that modify the risk of pain will be difficult. SNPs modulating HbF levels in sickle cell anemia were genotyped in the CSSCD patients and a smaller number of patients from Brazil. SNPs in *BCL11A*, *HBS1L-MYB* and the C-T polymorphism 158 bp 5′ to *HBG2* (rs7482144) were strongly associated with HbF and the rate of painful episodes.[88]

Patient response to opioid analgesics varies considerably, and the efficacy of these drugs is known to depend on genetic variability of their catabolic enzymes and receptors.[89] How this might affect the treatment of the sickle cell acute painful episode is unknown.

Stroke. Most genetic association studies in sickle cell anemia have examined the stroke phenotype (Chapter 19). A family predisposition to stroke in sickle cell disease suggested that inherited modulation of this phenotype was possible.[90] Among the genes associated with stroke in sickle cell anemia, two alleles of vascular adhesion molecule–1 (*VCAM1*), G1238C in the coding region of immunoglobulin domain 5, and, T-1594C, an intronic SNP, had an association with stroke. The coding region SNP was protective, whereas the intronic SNP predisposed to small-vessel stroke.[91,92] Preliminary studies also suggested that the *VCAM1* G1238C SNP was protective for developing high transcranial Doppler flow velocity, which is a strong predictor of stroke in children (Chapter 19).[93] VCAM1 is approximately 19,000 bp long and has nine exons and at least 200 SNPs. Clearly, choosing the "right" SNP is not trivial and an association is likely to identify LD.

Six SNPs in the intercellular adhesion molecule–1 and CD 36 genes (*ICAM1; CD36*) were not associated with stroke.[91] When stroke was subdivided into large- and small-vessel disease based on imaging studies, SNPs in the interleukin-4 receptor gene (*IL4R;* nonsynonymous coding region, S503P) predisposed to large vessel stroke, whereas TNFα gene (*TNFA;* noncoding G308A) and β-adrenergic receptor 2 (*ADRB2;* nonsynonymous coding region, Q27E) SNPs were protective. In the small-vessel stroke group, a low-density lipoprotein receptor (*LDLR;* untranslated region) SNP was protective. Homozygosity for the combination of *TNFA* -308 GG and the *IL4R* 503P heterozygosity was associated with a strong predisposition to large-vessel stroke.[92] The endothelium and vascular response to regulators might distinguish small from large blood vessels but a continuum must exist, making the pathophysiological basis of these observations enigmatic.

Human leukocyte antigen (HLA) genes might be risk factors for vascular disease. In sickle cell anemia patients with cerebral infarction, the HLA DRB1*0301 and *0302 alleles increased the risk of stroke and the DRB1*1501 protected from stroke. DQB1*0201, in LD with DRB1*0301, was associated with stroke and DQB1*0602, in LD with DRB1*1501, was protective. HLA genotyping was performed in patients with large-vessel stroke and with small-vessel stroke.[94,95] In the small-vessel stroke group, HLA DPB1*0401 was associated with stroke, whereas DPB1*1701 was protective. In the large-vessel stroke patients, DPB1*0401 was associated with susceptibility, and DPB1*1701 was associated with a trend toward protection. Also, HLA-A*0102 and A*2612 caused susceptibility to stroke and A*3301 was protective.

Other genes have been studied in the stroke phenotype. These include the C1565T mutant of the platelet glycoprotein IIIa (*ITPG3*) gene, angiotensinogen (*AGT*), cystathionine B synthase (*CBS*; 278thr 68-bp insertion), cholesterol ester transfer protein (*CETP*; −628A), apolipoprotein C III (*APOC3*; −641A) the C677T polymorphism in 5,10-methylenetetrahydrofolate reductase (*MTHFR*) the plasminogen activator inhibitor–1 gene (*PAI1*), TGFβ receptor 3 (*TGFBR3*), and adenine cyclase 9 (*ADCY9*).[96–99] These studies were all equivocal or negative; however, the sample size was usually insufficient for a definitive result.

It seems unlikely that a still undiscovered gene polymorphisms in any single gene will have a dominant effect on a phenotype of disease. To examine the interactions among genes and their SNPs and to develop a prognostic model for stroke in sickle cell anemia, a bayesian network was developed to analyze SNPs in candidate genes in 1,398 unrelated patients with sickle cell anemia (Fig. 27.5).[72] SNPs in 11 genes and four clinical variables, including α thalassemia and HbF, interacted in a complex network of dependency to modulate the risk of stroke. This network of interactions included three genes, *BMP6*, *TGFBR2*, and *TGFBR3* with a functional role in the TGFβ/BMP pathway and P-selectin (*SELP*). The model was validated in a different population by predicting the occurrence of stroke in unrelated individuals with 98.2% accuracy, predicting the correct outcome for all stroke patients, and for 98% of the nonstroke patients. This gave a 100% true positive rate, a 98.14% true negative rate, and a predictive accuracy of 98.2%. As traditional analytical methods are often inadequate for the discovery of the genetic basis of complex traits in large association studies, bayesian networks are a promising approach. The predictive accuracy of this stroke model is a step toward the development of prognostic tests that are better able to identify patients at risk for stroke. The association in the general population of genes like *SELP* and genes in the TGFβ pathway with stroke suggest that predisposition to stroke might be shared by both sickle cell anemia patients and stroke victims overall.

Gene expression studies have also contributed to understanding predisposition to stroke.[100] When individuals at risk for stroke, estimated based on the presence of circle of Willis disease or history of stroke, were compared with controls, transcripts in genes of inflammation-related pathways expressed in blood-outgrowth endothelial cells were most strongly associated with stroke or predisposition to stroke.

Priapism. SNPs in 44 candidate genes were examined for their association with priapism in 148 patients with sickle cell anemia with priapism and controls who had not developed priapism. Polymorphisms in Klotho (*KL*) showed an association with priapism by genotypic and haplotype analyses.[101] *KL* has a role in NO biochemistry and directly or indirectly promotes endothelial NO production.

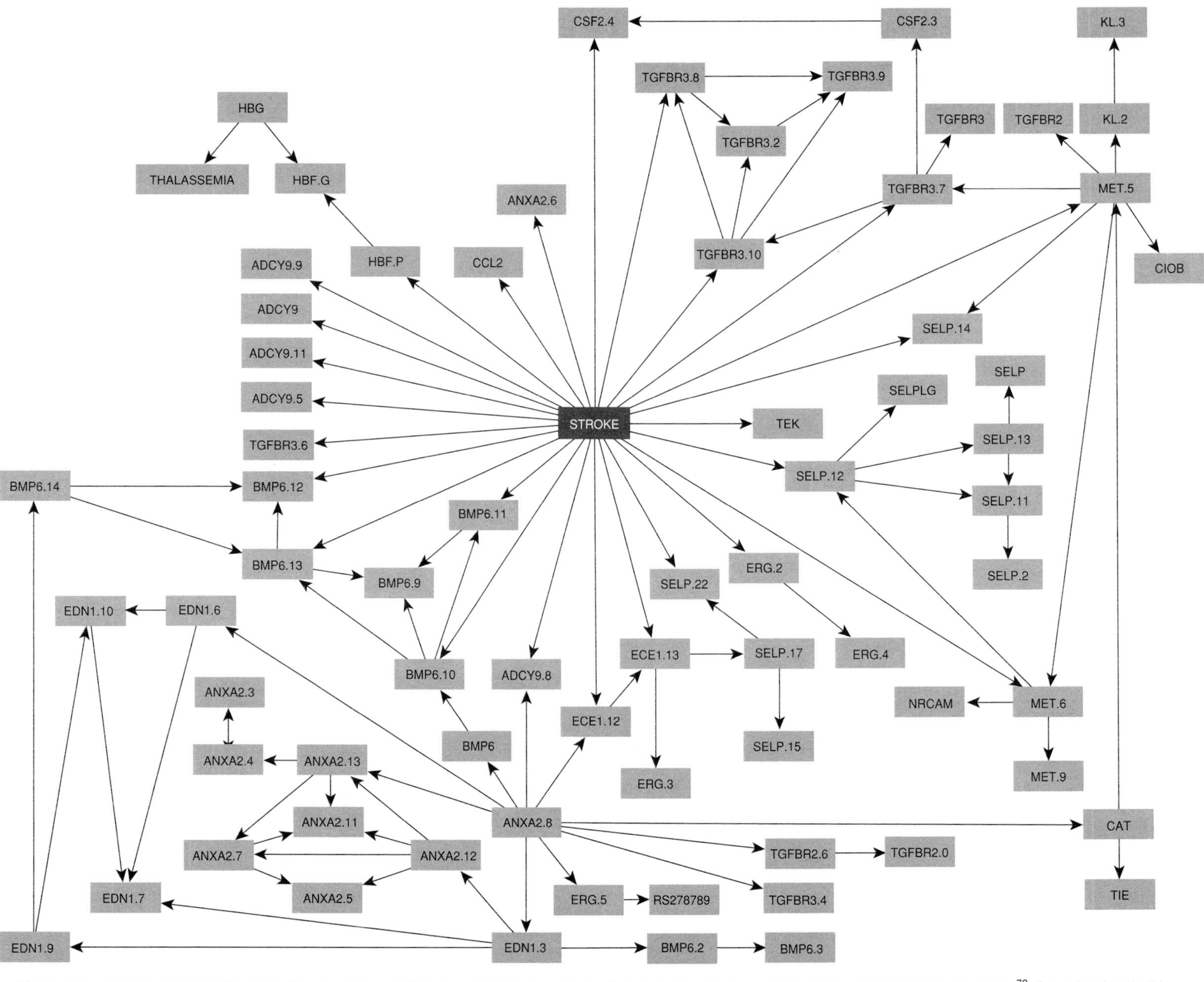

Figure 27.5. A bayesian network describing the associations of SNPs in candidate genes with the likelihood of developing nonhemorrhagic stroke in sickle cell anemia.[72] (See color plate 27.5.)

A strong association was also found between the prevalence of priapism, the severity of hemolysis, and the presence of α thalassemia.[73] Of approximately 200 men older than 18 years, 83 had a history of priapism. A candidate gene study in this population failed to show an association of priapism with SNPs in *KL*, nevertheless, there were associations with SNPs in *TGFBR3*, *AQP1* and the adhesion molecule, *ITGAV*.[102] Further study of this population, which included 186 men with a mean age of 32.4 years, found that a single coding SNP in *F13A1*, the Factor XIII gene was associated with priapism with an odds ratio of 2.43 for individuals with C/C compared with the C/G genotype.[103]

Osteonecrosis. Osteonecrosis is found in nearly half of all adults with sickle cell anemia. It is one of the so-called vasoocclusive/viscosity-associated phenotypes and it appears to be increased by concurrent α thalassemia (Chapter 19). The C677T polymorphism in *MTHFR* was found in 36% of adults with sickle cell disease and osteonecrosis but only 13% of controls.[94] Nevertheless, other reports failed to confirm this association (reviewed in ref. 78). The C1565T SNP in *ITPB3* and a polymorphism in *PAI1* were not associated with sickle osteonecrosis.[105] These studies all examined small numbers of patients and few SNPs.

When sickle cell anemia patients with osteonecrosis were compared with controls, individuals with osteonecrosis had a higher prevalence of coincident α thalassemia, and there were no differences in PCV or HbF levels. Significant associations were observed with SNPS in seven genes (*BMP6*, *TGFBR2*, *TGFBR3*, *EDN1*, *ERG*, *KL*, and *ECE1*). Additional SNPs, equally distributed within the gene, were typed in all seven genes and a significant association with many SNPs in *KL* and *BMP6* was found.[106] Of the 18 SNPs typed in *KL*, 10 were significantly associated with osteonecrosis. Most of these SNPs were located in the 20-kb region, representing the first half of the first *KL* intron and were in LD with each other. SNPs in *BMP6* (5/14) and *ANXA2* (6/13) were also associated with osteonecrosis; however, these SNPS were distributed throughout the intronic and 3′ untranslated regions of the genes, and disease-associated SNPs tended to be in LD. The distribution of haplotypes of all three genes was significantly different among cases and controls.

These genes might play a role in bone metabolism. Among its many functions, *KL* is a glycosyl hydrolase that participates in a negative regulatory network of the vitamin D endocrine system. BMPs, including *BMP6*, are secreted proteins structurally related to TGFβ and activins and are involved in bone formation and development. *ANXA2*, a member of the calcium-dependent phospholipid-binding protein family, is involved in osteoblast mineralization. Lipid rafts containing annexin-2 seem important for alkaline phosphatase activity in bone. The actual mechanisms by which variants of these genes predispose sickle cell patients to vascular complications are unknown.

Leg Ulcers. Sickle cell leg ulcers are related to hemolysis and associated with SNPs in genes that could affect sickle vasoocclusion. Leg ulcer patients had lower PCV and higher levels of lactate dehydrogenase, bilirubin, aspartate aminotransferase, and reticulocytes than controls. Age-adjusted comparisons showed that sickle cell anemia–α thalassemia was more frequent among controls than cases, suggesting that the likelihood of having leg ulcers was related to the intensity of hemolysis, which is modulated by α thalassemia. In candidate gene association studies, associations were found with SNPs in *KL*, *TEK*, and several genes in the TGFβ/BMP signaling pathway. The *TEK* receptor tyrosine kinase is involved in angiogenesis, whereas the TGFβ/BMP signaling pathway modulates wound healing and angiogenesis, among its other functions.[74]

Bacteremia. Infection, bacteremia, and sepsis are common events in sickle cell anemia. SNPs in candidate genes have been associated with an increased risk of sepsis in other diseases. In a case-control study, bacteremia in sickle cell anemia was associated with SNPs and haplotypes of genes of the TGFβ/BMP pathway such as *BMP6*, *TGFBR3*, *BMPR1A*, *SMAD6*, and *SMAD3*. The TGFβ/BMP pathway might play an important role in immune function.[107]

Renal Disease. Patients with sickle cell anemia associated with a Bantu haplotype are more likely to develop renal failure and other vasoocclusive complications, perhaps because these individuals have the lowest levels of HbF.[64,108]

SNPs in selected candidate genes are also associated with glomerular filtration rate. When the estimated glomerular filtration rate was used as a phenotype of sickle nephropathy, and tagging SNPs in approximately 70 genes of the TGFβ/BMP pathway were studied, four SNPs and three haplotypes in *BMPR1B*, a BMP receptor gene, yielded statistically significant associations. The TGFβ/BMP pathway has been associated with the development of diabetic nephropathy, which has some features in common with sickle cell nephropathy.[109]

Pulmonary Disease. Pulmonary hypertension or pulmonary vascular disease has emerged as an important risk factor for premature death in patients with sickle cell anemia, but its genetic basis has only recently started to be studied.[110,111] Pulmonary hypertension is likely to be modulated by the effects of genes that control NO and oxidant radical metabolism, cell–cell interaction, vasculogenesis, and vasoreactivity. For example, mutations in BMP receptor 2 (*BMPR2*) and other genes have been associated with both familial and idiopathic pulmonary hypertension.[112–114] A study of patients with sickle cell pulmonary hypertension compared with controls found that SNPs in *BMPR2* and *ADCY6* were associated with this phenotype, and follow-up studies suggested that SNPs in *TGFBR3* were associated with this phenotype.[115] Further work by this group involved the study of 297 SNPs in 49 candidate genes in 111 patients screened for pulmonary hypertension, and evidence of an association was primarily identified for genes in the TGFβ/BMP superfamily, including *ACVRL1*, *BMPR2*, and *BMP6*.[116] *BMP6* SNP 449853, associated with pulmonary hypertension, was also associated with stroke and bacteremia in studies of totally different patients, supporting these associations.[72,107]

Acute chest syndrome is a common vasoocclusive complication with, significant morbidity and mortality rates.[111] Both an increased and decreased risk of having acute chest syndrome were associated with a T786C SNP in the endothelial NO synthase gene (*NOS3*); one small study did not replicate either of these observations.[117–119] Exhaled NO levels were reduced in patients with acute chest syndrome compared with controls, and this was associated with the number of AAT repeats in intron 20 of *NOS1*.[120] In follow-up studies, the ATT repeat polymorphism in *NOS1* was associated with acute chest syndrome only in patients without asthma (itself, a risk factor for acute chest syndrome).[119] In this study of 134 children, 64% had at least one acute chest syndrome, and 36% had asthma. This study examined a small number of patients. Also, the relationship between the number of *NOS1* ATT repeats and risk of acute chest syndrome was an unusual curvilinear one. The association was modest, at best, and a plausible reason why this polymorphism should be important only in acute chest syndrome patients without asthma is not obvious. A T8002C SNP in the endothelin-1 gene (*EDN1*) was associated with an increased risk of acute chest syndrome in 173 children in whom sickle cell anemia was detected at birth and patients followed longitudinally.[118] All of these studies examined small numbers of cases and controls; most were limited to children, and few SNPs were examined.

To deal with these issues, a candidate gene association study of acute chest syndrome was performed using data from 1,422 individuals with sickle cell anemia. Because the etiology and clinical course of acute chest syndrome in patients younger than 4 years is different from that in older individuals, the population was dichotomized into pediatric (aged $\leq$ 5 years) and older children and adults (aged $>$ 5 years).[121] There were 170 acute chest syndrome cases and 884 controls in the group younger than 5 years and 388 cases and 819 controls in older group. Using time to first event in an age-, sex-, leukocyte-, reticulocyte-, and platelet count–adjusted analysis, and controlling for the false discovery rate, two SNPs were found to be significantly associated with acute chest syndrome in both patient groups. These SNPs were in *TGFBR3* and in an unknown gene in LD with *SMAD7*, which is also in the TGFβ pathway. Additional SNPs significantly associated with acute chest syndrome in younger cases were in *PIK3CG*, a member of the PI3/PI4 kinase family involved in cell–cell adhesion. Six additional SNPs were associated with acute chest syndrome in older patients were found in *SMAD1*, *KL*, *NRCAM*, and *SMAD3*. The *NOS1* ATT repeat polymorphism, *EDN1*, and *NOS3* SNPs discussed previously were not examined in this study.

Hyperbilirubinemia and Gallstones. Promoter polymorphisms in the uridine diphosphate–glucuronosyltransferase 1A (*UGT1A*) gene are associated with unconjugated hyperbilirubinemia and Gilbert syndrome. Children with sickle cell disease had a significantly higher mean bilirubin level if they carried the 7/7 *UGT1A* genotype compared with the wild-type 6/6 or 6/7 genotypes; patients with the 7/7 genotype were more likely to have had a cholecystectomy. This suggested that symptomatic cholelithiasis is more common in carriers of this genotype.[122,123] Steady-state bilirubin levels are also influenced by the presence of α thalassemia and the HbF level.[124,125] The 7/7 and 7/8 genotype were risk factors for symptomatic gallstones only in older patients with sickle cell disease, and although coincident α thalassemia was associated with less hemolysis, it did not compensate for the *UGT1A* promoter polymorphism.[126,127] α Thalassemia, regardless of the *UGT1A* genotype, was associated with reduced serum bilirubin levels.[125]

Erythrocyte Glucose-6-Phosphate Dehydrogenase (G6PD) Deficiency and the Endothelium. G6PD deficiency is common in sickle cell anemia. Studies of the phenotype of combined G6PD deficiency and sickle cell anemia have given disparate results. In a multiinstitutional study, however, G6PD deficiency was not associated with differential survival, reduced hemoglobin levels, increased hemolysis, more pain crises, septic episodes, or a higher incidence of acute anemic episodes.[128] Using DNA-based methods to detect unequivocally the GdA- allele of *G6PD*, it was reported that the frequencies of GdA$^-$ and of the normal GdB and GdA$^+$ genes were identical in patients with sickle cell anemia and controls.[129] Blood counts were similar in patients with and without G6PD deficiency, although the hemoglobin concentration was lower in sickle cell anemia with the GdA$^-$ gene. The prevalence of GdA$^-$ did not change with age.

Although there is clearly little, if any, modulation of the phenotype of sickle cell anemia by coincident G6PD deficiency, perhaps the "right" phenotype has not been studied. Patients with sickle cell anemia have impaired flow-dependent and independent vasodilation.[130] This might be a consequence of intravascular hemolysis, heme scavenging of NO with decreased NO bioavailability, and oxidant stress (Chapter 11). Adequate availability of G6PD is needed to maintain both NO levels and preserve the proper redox milieu. It has been proposed that a G6PD-deficient phenotype could be present in critical vascular tissues in G6PD-deficient individuals and perhaps even in sickle cell disease patients with a normal G6PD genotype.[131] In sickle cell disease, flux through the pentose phosphate pathway is reduced.[132] G6PD activity in sickle cell disease might be inadequate to maintain intracellular GSH levels, producing in effect, a functional G6PD-deficient state.[133] This same relative deficiency might also occur in endothelium and play a role in the endothelium-related pathophysiology of disease. It has been hypothesized that the hyperaldosteronism of sickle cell anemia might impair vascular reactivity by decreasing endothelial G6PD activity.[134]

Sickle erythrocyte adherence to endothelium is likely to be an important component of the pathophysiology of disease (Chapter 8). One determinant of this interaction is red cell adhesion to laminin, which increases in response to adrenaline stimulation of β_2-adrenergic receptors and adenylate cyclase. Polymorphisms of the β_2-adrenergic receptor (*ADRB2*) and adenylate cyclase (*ADCY6*) genes were associated with increased adhesion, suggesting that this and other features of the interaction of sickle erythrocytes with endothelial cells could be genetically modulated.[135]

Compound Phenotypes and Integrated Measure of Disease Severity. Few studies have combined disease complications and laboratory variables to seek associations with polymorphisms in candidate genes. One small study of patients with histories of stroke, acute chest syndrome, osteonecrosis, and priapism showed that patients with complications had a significantly higher frequency of the HPA-5b allele compared with controls.[136] In this small study, an individual needed only a single complication to be included. Most events were osteonecrosis, and only four individuals had more than a single phenotype.

To produce an integrated disease phenotype, a Bayesian network model was developed that described the complex associations of 25 clinical and laboratory variables, deriving a score to define disease severity as the risk of death within 5 years[137] (Chapter 19). The genetic basis of severity was examined using this score as a phenotype and studying the association of 795 SNPs in 320 candidate genes by using a Bayesian test that compared the genotype distribution among cases with mild and severe disease and calculated the probability that the two distributions were different in 741 HbS homozygotes older than 18 years of age.[138] Positive associations were validated in a smaller independent patient sample. Among the SNPs in genes associated with disease severity, some associations, like *TGFBR3*, confirmed previous findings in stroke and pulmonary hypertension in patients with sickle cell anemia, and support the speculation that dysregulation of the TGFβ/BMP signaling pathway might play a major role in the modulation of disease severity. Other genes in which SNPs were associated with severity, such as *ECE1* and *KL*, are expressed in endothelium or modulate endothelial function. Some associated genes play a less obvious role in the pathobiology of disease, such as *HAO2* and *TOX*, but were strongly associated with sickle cell disease severity and with normal aging. It seems likely that increased oxidative stress and the relentless progression of vasculopathy in sickle cell anemia cause accelerated tissue damage, and this might be modulated by a set of genes similar to those involved in the normal aging process.

As the results of unbiased genome-wide association studies are added to capture polymorphisms not included in candidate gene studies, a predictive network with even greater reliability than one using only clinical and laboratory variables might be developed. To begin this process, 684 mild and severe sickle cell anemia patients, based their severity score, were compared with 877 centenarians and 1,850 younger controls and each SNP was tested for association with the traits of severe or less severe sickle cell anemia and exceptional longevity. The analysis identified 140 SNPs in more than 50 genes and some intergenic regions that showed robust and consistent associations, a number more than twice than expected by chance. Among the most "significant" associations were genes with putative roles in blood circulation, coronary artery disease, type 2 diabetes, triglyceride, and glucose metabolism and sudden death. SNPs in *HAO2* and *MAP2K*, associated with both sickle cell disease severity and exceptional longevity in candidate gene studies, were also associated in the genome-wide association studies. These data further suggest that common metabolic pathways are likely to influence the chance of developing complications of mendelian and multigenic diseases and the likelihood of achieving exceptional longevity.[139] This might explain the commonality of genes whose SNPs are associated with the vascular complications of sickle cell anemia, arteriosclerosis and diabetes. A new paradigm suggests that hitherto unexpected genetic differences modulate a limited number of pathways that form a common route toward determining good health and disease.

Duffy red cell glycoproteins (Fy^a and Fy^b) have been implicated in the clearance of inflammatory cytokines. Duffy negative individuals that include approximately 70% of African Americans might clear these cytokines less efficiently. In adults with sickle cell anemia, end-organ damage and overall disease severity, assessed by a composite score reflecting the presence or absence of injury to a group of organs, were compared between Duffy-positive and -negative patients, as assessed by a SNP (rs2814778) in the promoter of the *DARC* gene. Sixty-five percent of Duffy-negative patients had chronic organ damage and 32% had proteinuria, statistically significant differences from Duffy-positive cases.[140]

GENETIC MODULATION OF THE PHENOTYPIC DIVERSITY OF β THALASSEMIA

Genetic Polymorphisms as Predictors of Disease Severity

Very little is known about the modifiers of the phenotype in β thalassemia other than the roles played by HbF level and α thalassemia.[30]

Hyperbilirubinemia and Gallstones. As with sickle cell anemia, bilirubin levels are modified by promoter polymorphisms of *UGT1A*.[141–146]

Iron Loading. Part of the phenotype of β thalassemia is the tendency for iron loading as a result of chronic hemolytic anemia, increased iron absorption, and blood transfusion. Hereditary hemochromatosis – most often a result of a C282Y mutation in *HFE*, a gene regulating iron metabolism – can also be found in rare cases of β thalassemia and might increase iron loading and its consequences.[147] However, in a larger study of patients with β thalassemia, there was no association of the C282Y *HFE*

SNP with iron overload.[148,149] Concurrent β-thalassemia trait can increase iron loading in classic hereditary hemochromatosis.[150]

Homozygosity for the H63D SNP in *HFE* has been associated with increased serum ferritin in Italian carriers of β thalassemia trait. In northern Indian β thalassemia carriers, this SNP was not associated with iron loading.[151–153]

In the Chinese, classic *HFE* mutations are even less common than in Italians; thus it is unlikely that polymorphisms of this gene would influence iron loading in β thalassemia. Mutations in the transferrin receptor gene (*TFR2*) can cause hemochromatosis. Two polymorphisms of *TFR2* were not associated with ferritin level or transferrin saturation in Chinese patients with transfusion-dependent β thalassemia or in nontransfusion-dependent β-thalassemia intermedia.[154]

Bone Disease. Bone disease and osteoporosis are causes of morbidity in severe β thalassemia, and bone mass is regulated by many genes.[155] In severe β thalassemia, a G-T SNP in the collagen type α1 gene (*COL1A1*) was associated with osteoporosis and in patients with β-thalassemia major and intermedia, an intronic SNP in *VDR*, the vitamin D (1,25-dihydroxyvitamin D3) receptor gene, was associated with a reduction in lower spine bone mineral density.[156–159] SNPs in *TGFB1* were not associated with osteoporosis.[158] Both studies examined a small number of cases and controls and very few SNPs, so these results must be replicated in larger patient samples.

Cardiovascular Disease. Heart failure, a result of iron loading, is the common cause of death in severe β thalassemia. Decreased antioxidant activity of the apolipoprotein E (*APOE*) 4 allele was postulated as a genetic risk factor for the development of left ventricular failure in homozygous β thalassemia. Greek patients with β thalassemia were grouped into 1) patients without heart disease, 2) patients with left ventricular failure, and 3) patients with left ventricular dilation and normal systolic function. Patients with normal hearts had an *APOE* 4 allele frequency similar to that of normal controls. Patients with left ventricular failure had a significantly higher frequency of *APOE* 4 than the controls, suggesting that this allele can represent a genetic risk factor for the development of heart failure.[160]

Two SNPs in the estrogen receptor gene (*ESR1*) were examined in pre- and postpubertal, well-treated, homozygous β thalassemia patients. Individuals lacking an Xba I restriction site polymorphism had higher body mass index, triglycerides, and blood pressure. The authors suggested that this SNP might influence nutrition and could be considered an additional risk factors for later cardiac disease.[161]

GENETIC MODULATION OF THE PHENOTYPIC DIVERSITY OF HbH DISEASE

Heterogeneity of α-globin gene mutations leads to phenotypic diversity of HbH disease.[162] If little is known about the modulation of phenotype in β thalassemia, even less is known about the other modulators of phenotype in HbH disease or Hb Bart's hydrops fetalis caused by identical α-globin gene mutations. As might be expected, polymorphism of the *UGT1A* promoter affects the bilirubin concentration and the likelihood of cholelithiasis.[163]

Iron overload is a cause of disability in HbH disease even in the absence of regular blood transfusion. When polymorphisms of *TFR2* and *HFE* were tested for their association with iron overload in HbH disease, iron loading was similar in patients with and without these mutations. It was concluded that excess iron in HbH disease is most likely a result of increased absorption.[164]

REFERENCES

1. Garner C, Mitchell J, Hatzis T, Reittie J, Farrall M, Thein SL. Haplotype mapping of a major quantitative-trait locus for fetal hemoglobin production, on chromosome 6q23. *Am J Hum Genet.* 1998;62(6):1468–1474.
2. Garner CP, Tatu T, Best S, Creary L, Thein SL. Evidence of genetic interaction between the beta-globin complex and chromosome 8q in the expression of fetal hemoglobin. *Am J Hum Genet.* 2002;70(3):793–799.
3. Wyszynski DF, Baldwin CT, Cleves MA, et al. Polymorphisms near a chromosome 6q QTL area are associated with modulation of fetal hemoglobin levels in sickle cell anemia. *Cell Mol Biol.* 2004;50(1):23–33.
4. Chang YPC, Maier-Redelsperger M, Smith KD, et al. The relative importance of the X-linked FCP locus and β-globin haplotypes in determining haemoglobin F levels: A study of SS patients homozygous for βS haplotypes. *Br J Haematol.* 1997;96:806–814.
5. Ofori-Acquah SF, Lalloz MR, Serjeant G, Layton DM. Dominant influence of gamma-globin promoter polymorphisms on fetal haemoglobin expression in sickle cell disease. *Cell Mol Biol.* 2004;50(1):35–42.
6. Platt OS, Thorington BD, Brambilla DJ, et al. Pain in sickle cell disease-rates and risk factors. *N Engl J Med.* 1991;325:11–16.
7. Platt OS, Brambilla DJ, Rosse WF, et al. Mortality in sickle cell disease. Life expectancy and risk factors for early death. *N Engl J Med.* 1994;330(23):1639–1644.
8. Steinberg MH, Barton F, Castro O, et al. Effect of hydroxyurea on mortality and morbidity in adult sickle cell anemia: risks and benefits up to 9 years of treatment. *JAMA.* 2003;289(13):1645–1651.
9. Orkin SH, Antonarakis SE, Kazazian HH Jr. Polymorphism and molecular pathology of the human beta-globin gene. *Prog Hematol.* 1983;13:49–73.
10. Antonarakis SE, Kazazian HH Jr, Orkin SH. DNA polymorphism and molecular pathology of the human globin gene clusters. *Hum Genet.* 1985;69:1–14.
11. Pagnier J, Mears JG, Dunda-Belkhodja O, et al. Evidence for the multicentric origin of the sickle cell hemoglobin gene in Africa. *Proc Natl Acad Sci USA.* 1984;81:1771–1773.
12. Nagel RL. Origins and dispersion of the sickle gene. In: Embury SH, Hebbel RP, Mohandas N, Steinberg MH, eds. *Sickle Cell Disease: Basic Principles and Clinical Practice.* 1st ed. New York: Raven Press; 1994;353–380.

13. Nagel RL, Steinberg MH. Genetics of the β^S gene: origins, epidemiology, and epistasis. In: Steinberg MH, Forget BG, Higgs DR, Nagel RL, eds. *Disorders of Hemoglobin: Genetics, Pathophysiology, and Clinical Management.* 1st ed. Cambridge: Cambridge University Press; 2001;711–755.
14. Nagel RL, Labie D. DNA haplotypes and the beta S globin gene. *Prog Clin Biol Res.* 1989;316B:371–393.
15. Antonarakis SE, Boehm CD, Serjeant GR, Theisen CE, Dover GJ, Kazazian HH Jr. Origin of the β^S-globin gene in blacks: The contribution of recurrent mutation or gene conversion or both. *Proc Natl Acad Sci USA.* 1984;81:853–856.
16. Öner C, Dimovski AJ, Olivieri NF, et al. β^S Haplotypes in various world populations. *Hum Genet.* 1992;89:99–104.
17. Nagel RL. The sickle haplotypes in Guadeloupe and the African gene flow. *Hemoglobin.* 1996;20:V–VII.
18. Adekile AD. Historical and anthropological correlates of β^S haplotypes and α- and β-thalassemia alleles in the Arabian Peninsula. *Hemoglobin.* 1997;21:281–296.
19. Bakanay SM, Dainer E, Clair B, et al. Mortality in sickle cell patients on hydroxyurea therapy. *Blood.* 2004;105:545–547.
20. Steinberg MH, Lu ZH, Nagel RL, et al. Hematological effects of atypical and Cameroon beta-globin gene haplotypes in adult sickle cell anemia. *Am J Hematol.* 1998;59(2):121–126.
21. Chase MB, Fu S, Haga SB, et al. BP1, a homeodomain-containing isoform of DLX4, represses the beta-globin gene. *Mol Cell Biol.* 2002;22(8):2505–2514.
22. Mpollo MS, Beaudoin M, Berg PE, Beauchemin H, D'Agati V, Trudel M. BP1 is a negative modulator of definitive erythropoiesis. *Nucl Acids Res.* 2006;34(18):5232–5237.
23. Miller BA, Salameh M, Ahmed M, et al. Analysis of hemoglobin F production in Saudi Arabian families with sickle cell anemia. *Blood.* 1987;70:716–720.
24. Miller BA, Olivieri N, Salameh M, et al. Molecular analysis of the high-hemoglobin-F phenotype in Saudi Arabian sickle cell anemia. *N Engl J Med.* 1987;316:244–250.
25. Peri KG, Gagnon J, Gagnon C, Bard H. Association of −158(C−>T) (XmnI) DNA polymorphism in $^G\gamma$-globin promoter with delayed switchover from fetal to adult hemoglobin synthesis. *Pediatr Res.* 1997;41:214–217.
26. Sampietro M, Thein SL, Contreras M, Pazmany L. Variation in HbF and F-cell number with the G-γ XmnI (C->T) polymorphisms in normal individuals. *Blood.* 1992;79:832–833.
27. Gilman JG, Johnson ME, Mishima N. Four base-pair DNA deletion in human Aγ globin gene promoter associated with low Aγ expression in adults. *Br J Haematol.* 1988;68:455–458.
28. Labie D, Pagnier J, Lapoumeroulie C, et al. Common haplotype dependency of high Gγ-globin gene expression and high HbF levels in β-thalassemia and sickle cell anemia patients. *Proc Natl Acad Sci USA.* 1985;82:2111–2114.
29. Pissard S, Beuzard Y. A potential regulatory region for the expression of fetal hemoglobin in sickle cell disease. *Blood.* 1994;84:331–338.
30. Thein SL. Genetic modifiers of beta-thalassemia. *Haematologica.* 2005;90(5):649–660.
31. Thein SL, Wainscoat JS, Sampietro M, et al. Association of thalassaemia intermedia with a beta-globin gene haplotype. *Br J Haematol.* 1987;65(3):367–373.
32. Papachatzopoulou A, Kourakli A, Makropoulou P, et al. Genotypic heterogeneity and correlation to intergenic haplotype within high HbF beta-thalassemia intermedia. *Eur J Haematol.* 2006;76(4):322–330.
33. Bandyopadhyay S, Mondal BC, Sarkar P, Chandra S, Das MK, Dasgupta UB. Two beta-globin cluster-linked polymorphic loci in thalassemia patients of variable levels of fetal hemoglobin. *Eur J Haematol.* 2005;75(1):47–53.
34. Ma Q-L, Abel K, Sripichai O, et al. β-globin gene cluster polymorphisms are strongly associated with severity of Hb E/ β^0 thalassemia. *Clin Genet.* 2007;72(6):497–505.
35. Ofori-Acquah SF, Lalloz MRA, Layton DM. Localisation of *cis* regulatory elements at the β-globin locus: analysis of hybrid haplotype chromosomes. *Biochem Biophys Res Commun.* 1999;254(1):181–187.
36. Ofori-Acquah SF, Lalloz MRA, Layton DM, Luzzatto L. Localization of *cis*-active determinants of fetal hemoglobin level in sickle cell anemia. *Blood.* 1996;88:493a.
37. Lu ZH, Steinberg MH. Fetal hemoglobin in sickle cell anemia: Relation to regulatory sequences cis to the β-globin gene. *Blood.* 1996;87:1604–1611.
38. Merghoub T, Maier-Redelsperger M, Labie D, et al. Variation of fetal hemoglobin and F-cell number with the LCR-HS2 polymorphism in nonanemic individuals. *Blood.* 1996;87:2607–2609.
39. Merghoub T, Perichon B, Maier-Redelsperger M, et al. Dissection of the association status of two polymorphisms in the β-globin gene cluster with variations in F-cell number in non-anemic individuals. *Am J Hematol.* 1997;56(4):239–243.
40. Ofori-Acquah SF, Lalloz MR, Layton DM. Nucleotide variation regulates the level of enhancement by hypersensitive site 2 of the beta-globin locus control region. *Blood Cells Mol Dis.* 2001;27(5):803–811.
41. Elion J, Berg PE, Lapouméroulie C, et al. DNA sequence variation in a negative control region 5′ to the β-globin gene correlates with the phenotypic expression of the βS mutation. *Blood.* 1992;79:787–792.
42. Steinberg MH, Forget BG, Higgs DR, Nagel RL, eds. *Disorders of Hemoglobin: Genetics, Pathophysiology, and Clinical Management.* 1st ed. Cambridge: Cambridge University Press; 2001.
43. Chen Z, Hong-Yuan L, Basran RK, et al. A T-G transversion at NT-567 upstream of the Gγ-globin gene in a GATA-1 binding motif Is associated with elevated HbF. *Mol Cell Biol.* 2008;28(13):4386–4393.
44. Harju-Baker S, Costa FC, Fedosyuk H, Neades R, Peterson, KR. Silencing of Aã-globin gene expression during adult definitive erythropoiesis mediated by GATA-1-FOG-1-Mi2 complex binding at the −566 GATA site. *Mol. Cell. Biol.* 2008;28:3101–3113.
45. Papachatzopoulou A, Kaimakis P, Pourfarzad F, et al. Increased gamma-globin gene expression in beta-thalassemia intermedia patients correlates with a mutation in 3′HS1. *Am J Hematol.* 2007;82(11):1005–1009.
46. Thein SL, Sampietro M, Rohde K, et al. Detection of a major gene for heterocellular hereditary persistence of fetal hemoglobin after accounting for genetic modifiers. *Am J Hum Genet.* 1994;54:214–228.
47. Garner C, Silver N, Best S, et al. A quantitative trait locus on chromosome 8q influences the switch from fetal to adult hemoglobin. *Blood.* 2004;104:2184–2186.

48. Menzel S, Garner C, Gut I, et al. A QTL influencing F cell production maps to a gene encoding a zinc-finger protein on chromosome 2p15. *Nat Genet.* 2007;39(10):1197–1199.
49. de Haan G, Bystrykh LV, Weersing E, et al. A genetic and genomic analysis identifies a cluster of genes associated with hematopoietic cell turnover. *Blood.* 2002;100(6):2056–2062.
50. Liu X, Barker DF. Evidence for effective suppression of recombination in the chromosome 17q21 segment spanning RNU2-BRCA1. *Am J Hum Genet.* 1999;64(5):1427–1439.
51. Close J, Game L, Clark B, Bergounioux J, Gerovassili A, Thein SL. Genome annotation of a 1.5 Mb region of human chromosome 6q23 encompassing a quantitative trait locus for fetal hemoglobin expression in adults. *BMC Genomics.* 2004;5(1):33.
52. Jiang J, Best S, Menzel S, et al. cMYB is involved in the regulation of fetal hemoglobin production in adults. *Blood.* 2006;108(3):1077–1083.
53. Thein SL, Menzel S, Peng X, et al. Intergenic variants of HBS1L-MYB are responsible for a major quantitative trait locus on chromosome 6q23 influencing fetal hemoglobin levels in adults. *Proc Natl Acad Sci USA.* 2007;104(27):11346–11351.
54. Garner C, Menzel S, Martin C, et al. Interaction between two quantitative trait loci affects fetal haemoglobin expression. *Ann Hum Genet.* 2005;69(Pt 6):707–714.
55. Ma Q, Wyszynski DF, Farrell JJ, et al. Fetal hemoglobin in sickle cell anemia: genetic determinants of response to hydroxyurea. *Pharmacogenomics J.* 2007;7:386–394.
56. Sebastiani P, Wang L, Nolan VG, et al. Fetal hemoglobin in sickle cell anemia: Bayesian modeling of genetic associations. *Am J Hematol.* 2008;83(3):189–195.
57. Sedgewick A, Timofeev N, Sebastiani P, et al. *BCL11A* (2p16) is a major HbF quantitative trait locus in three different populations. *Blood Cells Mol. Dis.* 2008;41:255–258.
58. Uda M, Galanello R, Sanna S, et al. Genome-wide association study shows BCL11A associated with persistent fetal hemoglobin and amelioration of the phenotype of beta-thalassemia. *Proc. Natl. Acad. Sci. USA.* 2008;105:1620–1625.
59. Kumkhaek C, Taylor JG, Zhu J, et al. Fetal haemoglobin response to hydroxycarbamide treatment and sar1a promoter polymorphisms in sickle cell anaemia. *Br J Haematol.* 2008;141:254–259.
60. Tang DC, Zhu J, Liu W, et al. The hydroxyurea-induced small GTP-binding protein SAR modulates gamma-globin gene expression in human erythroid cells. *Blood.* 2005;106:3256–3263.
61. Ohene-Frempong K, Nkrumah FK. Sickle cell disease in Africa. In: Embury SH, Hebbel RP, Mohandas N, eds. *Sickle Cell Disease: Basic Principles and Clinical Practice.* 1st ed. New York: Raven Press; 1994;423–435.
62. Powars DR. β^S-Gene-cluster haplotypes in sickle cell anemia: Clinical and hematologic features. *Hematol Oncol Clin North Am.* 1991;5:475–493.
63. Powars DR. Sickle cell anemia: β^S-gene-cluster haplotypes as prognostic indicators of vital organ failure. *Semin Hematol.* 1991;28:202–208.
64. Powars DR, Elliott Mills DD, Chan L. Chronic renal failure in sickle cell disease: risk factors, clinical course, and mortality. *Ann Intern Med.* 1991;115:614–620.
65. Steinberg MH, Hsu H, Nagel RL, et al. Gender and haplotype effects upon hematological manifestations of adult sickle cell anemia. *Am J Hematol.* 1995;48(3):175–181.
66. Padmos MA, Roberts GT, Sackey K, et al. Two different forms of homozygous sickle cell disease occur in Saudi Arabia. *Br J Haematol.* 1991;79:93–98.
67. El-Hazmi MAF. Clinical and haematological diversity of sickle cell disease in Saudi children. *J Trop Pediatr.* 1992; 38:106–112.
68. El-Hazmi MAF. Heterogeneity and variation of clinical and haematological expression of haemoglobin S in Saudi Arabs. *Acta Haematol.* 1992;88:67–71.
69. Adekile AD, Haider MZ. Morbidity, β^S haplotype and α-globin gene patterns among sickle cell anemia patients in Kuwait. *Acta Haematol.* 1996;96:150–154.
70. Thomas PW, Higgs DR, Serjeant GR. Benign clinical course in homozygous sickle cell disease: A search for predictors. *J Clin Epidemiol.* 1997;50:121–126.
71. Alexander N, Higgs D, Dover G, Serjeant GR. Are there clinical phenotypes of homozygous sickle cell disease? *Br J Haematol.* 2004;126(4):606–611.
72. Sebastiani P, Ramoni MF, Nolan V, Baldwin CT, Steinberg MH. Genetic dissection and prognostic modeling of overt stroke in sickle cell anemia. *Nat Genet.* 2005;37(4):435–440.
73. Nolan VG, Wyszynski DF, Farrer LA, Steinberg MH. Hemolysis-associated priapism in sickle cell disease. *Blood.* 2005;106(9):3264–3267.
74. Nolan VG, Adewoye A, Baldwin C, et al. Sickle cell leg ulcers: associations with haemolysis and SNPs in Klotho, TEK and genes of the TGF-beta/BMP pathway. *Br J Haematol.* 2006;133(5):570–578.
75. Kato GJ, Gladwin MT, Steinberg MH. Deconstructing sickle cell disease: Reappraisal of the role of hemolysis in the development of clinical subphenotypes. *Blood Rev.* 2007;21:37–47.
76. Camaschella C, Kattamis AC, Petroni D, et al. Different hematological phenotypes caused by the interaction of triplicated α-globin genes and heterozygous β-thalassemia. *Am J Hematol.* 1997;55:83–88.
77. Traeger-Synodinos J, Kanavakis E, Vrettou C, et al. The triplicated α-globin gene locus in β-thalassaemia heterozygotes: Clinical, haematological, biosynthetic and molecular studies. *Br J Haematol.* 1996;95:467–471.
78. Kihm AJ, Kong Y, Hong W, et al. An abundant erythroid protein that stabilizes free alpha-haemoglobin. *Nature.* 2002; 417(6890):758–763.
79. Kong Y, Zhou S, Kihm AJ, et al. Loss of alpha-hemoglobin-stabilizing protein impairs erythropoiesis and exacerbates beta-thalassemia. *J Clin Invest.* 2004;114(10):1457–1466.
80. Viprakasit V, Tanphaichitr VS, Chinchang W, Sangkla P, Weiss MJ, Higgs DR. Evaluation of alpha hemoglobin stabilizing protein (AHSP) as a genetic modifier in patients with beta thalassemia. *Blood.* 2004;103(9):3296–3299.
81. dos Santos CO, Costa FF. AHSP and beta-thalassemia: a possible genetic modifier. *Hematology.* 2005;10(2):157–161.
82. Lai MI, Jiang J, Silver N, et al. Alpha-haemoglobin stabilising protein is a quantitative trait gene that modifies the phenotype of beta-thalassaemia. *Br J Haematol.* 2006;133(6):675–682.
83. Steinberg MH. Predicting clinical severity in sickle cell anaemia. *Br J Haematol.* 2005;129:465–481.

84. Bertolino P, Deckers M, Lebrin F, ten DP. Transforming growth factor-beta signal transduction in angiogenesis and vascular disorders. *Chest.* 2005;128(6 Suppl):585S–590S.
85. Kimchi-Sarfaty C, Oh JM, Kim IW, et al. A "silent" polymorphism in the MDR1 gene changes substrate specificity. *Science.* 2007;315(5811):525–528.
86. Saxena R, Voight BF, Lyssenko V, et al. Genome-wide association analysis identifies loci for type 2 diabetes and triglyceride levels. *Science.* 2007;316(5829):1331–1336.
87. Balding DJ. A tutorial on statistical methods for population association studies. *Nat Rev Genet.* 2006;7(10):781–791.
88. Lettre G, Sankaran VG, Bezerra MA, et al. DNA polymorphisms at the BCL11A, HBS1L-MYB, and beta-globin loci associate with fetal hemoglobin levels and pain crises in sickle cell disease. *Proc. Natl. Acad. Sci. USA.* 2008;105:11869–11874.
89. Lotsch J, Skarke C, Liefhold J, Geisslinger G. Genetic predictors of the clinical response to opioid analgesics: clinical utility and future perspectives. *Clin Pharmacokinet.* 2004;43(14):983–1013.
90. Driscoll MC, Hurlet A, Styles L, et al. Stroke risk in siblings with sickle cell anemia. *Blood.* 2003;101(6):2401–2404.
91. Taylor JG, Tang DC, Savage SA, et al. Variants in the VCAM1 gene and risk for symptomatic stroke in sickle cell disease. *Blood.* 2002;100(13):4303–4309.
92. Hoppe C, Klitz W, Cheng S, et al. Gene interactions and stroke risk in children with sickle cell anemia. *Blood.* 2004;103(6):2391–2396.
93. Kutlar A, Brambilla D, Clair B, et al. Candidate gene polymorphisms and their association with TCD velocities in children with sickle cell disease. *Blood.* 2007;110:133a.
94. Styles LA, Hoppe C, Klitz W, Vichinsky E, Lubin B, Trachtenberg E. Evidence for HLA-related susceptibility for stroke in children with sickle cell disease. *Blood.* 2000;95(11):3562–3567.
95. Hoppe C, Klitz W, Noble J, Vigil L, Vichinsky E, Styles L. Distinct HLA associations by stroke subtype in children with sickle cell anemia. *Blood.* 2002;101:2865–2869.
96. Tang DC, Prauner R, Liu W, et al. Polymorphisms within the angiotensinogen gene (GT-repeat) and the risk of stroke in pediatric patients with sickle cell disease: a case-control study. *Am J Hematol.* 2001;68(3):164–169.
97. Romana M, Diara JP, Doumbo L, et al. Angiotensinogen gene associated polymorphisms and risk of stroke in sickle cell anemia: additional data supporting an association. *Am J Hematol.* 2004;76(3):310–311.
98. Hoppe C, Cheng S, Grow M, et al. A novel multilocus genotyping assay to identify genetic predictors of stroke in sickle cell anaemia. *Br J Haematol.* 2001;114(3):718–720.
99. Romana M, Muralitharan S, Ramasawmy R, Nagel RL, Krishnamoorthy R. Thrombosis-associated gene variants in sickle cell anemia. *Thromb Haemost.* 2002;87(2):356–358.
100. Hebbel RP, Wei P, Jiang A, et al. Genetic influence on the systems biology of sickle cell stroke risk detected by endothelial cell gene expression. *Blood.* 2008;111(7):3872–3879.
101. Nolan VG, Baldwin CT, Ma Q-L, et al. Association of single nucleotide polymorphisms in *KLOTHO* with priapism in sickle cell anemia. *Br J Haematol.* 2004;128:266–272.
102. Elliott L, Ashley-Koch A, Castro L.D., et al. Genetic polymorphisms associated with priapism in sickle cell disease. *Br J Haematol.* 2007;137:262–267.
103. El-khatib A, Ashley-Koch A, Kail M, et al. Further investigation of the role of factor XIII in priapism associated with SCD. *Blood.* 2007;110:998a.
104. Kutlar F, Tural C, Park D, Markowitz RB, Woods KF, Kutlar A. MTHFR (5, 10-methlylenetetrathydrofolate reductase) 677 C->T mutation as a candidate risk factor for avascular necrosis (AVN) in patients with sickle cell disease. *Blood.* 1998;92:695a.
105. Zimmerman SA, Ware RE. Inherited DNA mutations contributing to thrombotic complications in patients with sickle cell disease. *Am J Hematol.* 1998;59(4):267–272.
106. Baldwin C, Nolan VG, Wyszynski DF, et al. Association of klotho, bone morphogenic protein 6, and annexin A2 polymorphisms with sickle cell osteonecrosis. *Blood.* 2005;106(1):372–375.
107. Adewoye AH, Nolan VG, Ma Q, et al. Association of polymorphisms of IGF1R and genes in the transforming growth factor- beta/bone morphogenetic protein pathway with bacteremia in sickle cell anemia. *Clin Infect Dis.* 2006;43(5):593–598.
108. Powars DR, Chan L, Schroeder WA. Beta S-gene-cluster haplotypes in sickle cell anemia: clinical implications. *Am J Pediatr Hematol Oncol.* 1990;12(3):367–374.
109. Nolan VG, Qian Li M, Cohen HT, et al. Estimated glomerular filtration rate in sickle cell anemia is associated with polymorphisms of bone morphogenetic protein receptor 1B (BMPR1B). *Am J Hematol.* 2007;82:179–184.
110. Gladwin MT, Sachdev V, Jison ML, et al. Pulmonary hypertension as a risk factor for death in patients with sickle cell disease. *N Engl J Med.* 2004;350(9):886–895.
111. Vichinsky EP, Neumayr LD, Earles AN, et al. Causes and outcomes of the acute chest syndrome in sickle cell disease. *N Engl J Med.* 2000;342(25):1855–1865.
112. Ameshima S, Golpon H, Cool CD, et al. Peroxisome proliferator-activated receptor gamma (PPAR gamma) expression is decreased in pulmonary hypertension and affects endothelial cell growth. *Circ Res.* 2003;92(10):1162–1169.
113. Nichols WC, Koller DL, Slovis B, et al. Localization of the gene for familial primary pulmonary hypertension to chromosome 2q31-32. *Nat Genet.* 1997;15(3):277–280.
114. Machado RD, Pauciulo MW, Thomson JR, et al. BMPR2 haploinsufficiency as the inherited molecular mechanism for primary pulmonary hypertension. *Am J Hum Genet.* 2001;68(1):92–102.
115. Ashley-Koch A, DeCastro L, Lennon-Graham F, et al. Genetic polymorphisms associated with the risk for pulmonary hypertension and proteinuria in sickle cell disease. *Blood.* 2004;104:464a.
116. Ashley-Koch AE, Elliott L, Kail ME, et al. Identification of genetic polymorphisms associated with risk for pulmonary hypertension in sickle cell disease. *Blood.* 2008;111(12):5721–5726.
117. Sharan K, Surrey S, Ballas S, et al. Association of T-786C eNOS gene polymorphism with increased susceptibility to acute chest syndrome in females with sickle cell disease. *Br J Haematol.* 2004;124(2):240–243.

118. Chaar V, Tarer V, Etienne-Julan M, Diara JP, Elion J, Romana M. ET-1 and ecNOS gene polymorphisms and susceptibility to acute chest syndrome and painful vaso-occlusive crises in children with sickle cell anemia. *Haematologica.* 2006;91(9):1277–1278.
119. Duckworth L, Hsu L, Feng H, et al. Physician-diagnosed asthma and acute chest syndrome: associations with NOS polymorphisms. *Pediatr Pulmonol.* 2007;42(4):332–338.
120. Sullivan KJ, Kissoon N, Duckworth LJ, et al. Low exhaled nitric oxide and a polymorphism in the NOS I gene is associated with acute chest syndrome. *Am J Respir Crit Care Med.* 2001;164(12):2186–2190.
121. Martinez-Castaldi C, Nolan VG, Baldwin CT, Farrer LA, Steinberg MH, Klings ES. Association of genetic polymorphisms in the TGF-β pathway with the acute chest syndrome of sickle cell disease. *Blood.* 2007;118:666a.
122. Fertrin KY, Melo MB, Assis AM, Saad ST, Costa FF. UDP-glucuronosyltransferase 1 gene promoter polymorphism is associated with increased serum bilirubin levels and cholecystectomy in patients with sickle cell anemia. *Clin Genet.* 2003;64(2):160–162.
123. Passon RG, Howard TA, Zimmerman SA, Schultz WH, Ware RE. Influence of bilirubin uridine diphosphate-glucuronosyltransferase 1A promoter polymorphisms on serum bilirubin levels and cholelithiasis in children with sickle cell anemia. *J Pediatr Hematol Oncol.* 2001;23(7):448–451.
124. Adekile A, Kutlar F, McKie K, et al. The influence of uridine diphosphate glucuronosyl transferase 1A promoter polymorphisms, beta-globin gene haplotype, co-inherited alpha-thalassemia trait and Hb F on steady-state serum bilirubin levels in sickle cell anemia. *Eur J Haematol.* 2005;75(2):150–155.
125. Vasavda N, Menzel S, Kondaveeti S, et al. The linear effects of alpha-thalassaemia, the UGT1A1 and HMOX1 polymorphisms on cholelithiasis in sickle cell disease. *Br J Haematol.* 2007;138(2):263–270.
126. Haverfield EV, McKenzie CA, Forrester T, et al. UGT1A1 variation and gallstone formation in sickle cell disease. *Blood.* 2005;105(3):968–972.
127. Chaar V, Keclard L, Etienne-Julan M, et al. UGT1A1 polymorphism outweighs the modest effect of deletional (−3.7 kb) alpha-thalassemia on cholelithogenesis in sickle cell anemia. *Am J Hematol.* 2006;81(5):377–379.
128. Steinberg MH, West MS, Gallagher D, Mentzer W. Effects of glucose-6-phosphate dehydrogenase deficiency upon sickle cell anemia. *Blood.* 1988;71:748–752.
129. Bouanga JC, Mouélé R, Préhu C, Wajcman H, Feingold J, Galactéros F. Glucose-6-phosphate dehydrogenase deficiency and homozygous sickle cell disease in Congo. *Hum Hered.* 1998;48(4):192–197.
130. Belhassen L, Pelle G, Sediame S, et al. Endothelial dysfunction in patients with sickle cell disease is related to selective impairment of shear stress-mediated vasodilation. *Blood.* 2001;97(6):1584–1589.
131. Forgione MA, Loscalzo J, Holbrook M, et al. The A326G (A+) variant of the glocose-6-phosphate dehydrogenase gene is associated with endothelial dysfunction in African Americans. *J Am Coll Cardiol.* 2003;41:249A.
132. Schrader MC, Simplaceanu V, Ho C. Measurement of fluxes through the pentose phosphate pathway in erythrocytes from individuals with sickle cell anemia by carbon-13 nuclear magnetic resonance spectroscopy. *Biochim Biophys Acta.* 1993;1182(2):179–188.
133. Amer J, Ghoti H, Rachmilewitz E, Koren A, Levin C, Fibach E. Red blood cells, platelets and polymorphonuclear neutrophils of patients with sickle cell disease exhibit oxidative stress that can be ameliorated by antioxidants. *Br J Haematol.* 2006;132(1):108–113.
134. Leopold J, Dam A, Maron BA, et al. Aldosterone impairs vascular reactivity by decreasing glucose-6-phosphate dehydrogenase activity. *Nat Med.* 2007;13:189–197.
135. Eyler CE, Jackson T, Elliott LE, et al. Beta(2)-adrenergic receptor and adenylate cyclase gene polymorphisms affect sickle red cell adhesion. *Br J Haematol.* 2008;141:105–108.
136. Castro V, Alberto FL, Costa RN, et al. Polymorphism of the human platelet antigen-5 system is a risk factor for occlusive vascular complications in patients with sickle cell anemia. *Vox Sang.* 2004;87(2):118–123.
137. Sebastiani P, Nolan VG, A, et al. Predicting severity of sickle cell disease. *Blood.* 2007;110:2727–2735.
138. Sebastiani P, Wang L, Perls T, et al. A repertoire of genes modifying the risk of death in sickle cell anemia. *Blood.* 2007;110:52a.
139. Sebastiani P, Timofeev N, Hartley SH, et al. Genome-wide association studies suggest shared polymorphisms are associated with severity of sickle cell anemia and exceptional longevity. *Blood.* 2008;112:1446a.
140. Afenyi-Annan A, Kail M, Combs MR, et al. Lack of Duffy antigen expression is associated with organ damage in patients with sickle cell disease. *Transfusion.* 2008;48:917–924.
141. Galanello R, Melis MA, Podda A, et al. Deletion delta-thalassemia: the 7.2 kb deletion of Corfu δβ-thalassemia in a non-beta-thalassemia chromosome. *Blood.* 1990;75:1747–1749.
142. Galanello R, Perseu L, Melis MA, et al. Hyperbilirubinaemia in heterozygous beta-thalassaemia is related to co-inherited Gilbert's syndrome. *Br J Haematol.* 1997;99(2):433–436.
143. Galanello R, Piras S, Barella S, et al. Cholelithiasis and Gilbert's syndrome in homozygous beta-thalassaemia. *Br J Haematol.* 2001;115(4):926–928.
144. Sampietro M, Lupica L, Perrero L, et al. The expression of uridine diphosphate glucuronosyltransferase gene is a major determinant of bilirubin level in heterozygous beta-thalassaemia and in glucose-6-phosphate dehydrogenase deficiency. *Br J Haematol.* 1997;99(2):437–439.
145. Huang YY, Huang CS, Yang SS, Lin MS, Huang MJ, Huang CS. Effects of variant UDP-glucuronosyltransferase 1A1 gene, glucose-6-phosphate dehydrogenase deficiency and thalassemia on cholelithiasis. *World J Gastroenterol.* 2005;11(36):5710–5713.
146. Au WY, Cheung WC, Chan GC, Ha SY, Khong PL, Ma ES. Risk factors for hyperbilirubinemia and gallstones in Chinese patients with β thalassemia syndrome. *Haematologica.* 2003;88(2):220–222.
147. Rees DC, Luo LY, Thein SL, Singh BM, Wickramasinghe S. Nontransfusional iron overload in thalassemia: Association with hereditary hemochromatosis. *Blood.* 1997;90(8):3234–3236.

148. Cappellini MD, Fargion SR, Sampietro M, Graziadei G, Fiorelli G. Nontransfusional iron overload in thalassemia intermedia: Role of the hemochromatosis allele. *Blood.* 1998;92(11):4479–4480.
149. Borgna-Pignatti C, Solinas A, Bombieri C, et al. The haemochromatosis mutations do not modify the clinical picture of thalassaemia major in patients regularly transfused and chelated. *Br J Haematol.* 1998;103(3):813–816.
150. Piperno A, Mariani R, Arosio C, et al. Haemochromatosis in patients with β-thalassaemia trait. *Br J Haematol.* 2000;111(3):908–914.
151. Melis MA, Cau M, Deidda F, Barella S, Cao A, Galanello R. H63D mutation in the HFE gene increases iron overload in beta-thalassemia carriers. *Haematologica.* 2002;87(3):242–245.
152. Merryweather-Clarke AT, Pointon JJ, Shearman JD, Robson KJ. Global prevalence of putative haemochromatosis mutations. *J Med Genet.* 1997;34(4):275–278.
153. Garewal G, Das R, Ahluwalia J, Marwaha RK. Prevalence of the H63D mutation of the HFE in north India: its presence does not cause iron overload in beta thalassemia trait. *Eur J Haematol.* 2005;74(4):333–336.
154. Ma ES, Lam KK, Chan AY, Ha SY, Au WY, Chan LC. Transferrin receptor-2 polymorphisms and iron overload in transfusion independent β-thalassemia intermedia. *Haematologica.* 2003;88(3):345–346.
155. Uitterlinden AG, van Meurs JB, Rivadeneira F, Pols HA. Identifying genetic risk factors for osteoporosis. *J Musculoskelet Neuronal Interact.* 2006;6(1):16–26.
156. Wonke B, Jensen C, Hanslip JJ, et al. Genetic and acquired predisposing factors and treatment of osteoporosis in thalassaemia major. *J Pediatr Endocrinol Metab.* 1998;11(Suppl 3):795–801.
157. Pollak RD, Rachmilewitz E, Blumenfeld A, Idelson M, Goldfarb AW. Bone mineral metabolism in adults with β-thalassaemia major and intermedia. *Br J Haematol.* 2000; 111(3):902–907.
158. Perrotta S, Cappellini MD, Bertoldo F, et al. Osteoporosis in β-thalassaemia major patients: analysis of the genetic background. *Br J Haematol.* 2000;111(2):461–466.
159. Arisal O, Deviren A, Fenerci EY, et al. Polymorphism analysis in the COLIA1 gene of patients with thalassemia major and intermedia. *Haematologia.* 2002;32(4):475–482.
160. Economou-Petersen E, Aessopos A, Kladi A, et al. Apolipoprotein E epsilon 4 allele as a genetic risk factor for left ventricular failure in homozygous beta-thalassemia. *Blood.* 1998;92(9):3455–3459.
161. Ferrara M, Matarese SM, Borrelli B, et al. Impact of excess weight and estrogen receptor gene polymorphisms on clinical course of homozygous beta thalassemia. *Hematology.* 2005;10(5):407–411.
162. Chen FE, Ooi C, Ha SY, et al. Genetic and clinical features of hemoglobin H disease in Chinese patients. *N Engl J Med.* 2000;343(8):544–550.
163. Au WY, Cheung WC, Hu WH, et al. Hyperbilirubinemia and cholelithiasis in Chinese patients with hemoglobin H disease. *Ann Hematol.* 2005;84(10):671–674.
164. Chan V, Wong MS, Ooi C, et al. Can defects in transferrin receptor 2 and hereditary hemochromatosis genes account for iron overload in HbH disease? *Blood Cells Mol Dis.* 2003;30(1):107–111.
165. DeCastro L, Rinder HM, Howe JG, Smith BR. Thrombophilic genotypes do not adversely affect the course of sickle cell disease (SCD). *Blood.* 1998;92:161a.
166. Zimmerman SA, Howard TA, Whorton MR, Rosse WF, Ware RE. The A312G polymorphism in α-fibrinogen is associated with stroke and avascular necrosis in patients with sickle cell anemia. *Blood.* 1998;92:36b.
167. Sullivan KJ, Kissoon N, Duckworth LJ, et al. Low exhaled nitric oxide and a polymorphism in the NOS I gene is associated with acute chest syndrome. *Am J Respir Crit Care Med.* 2001;164(12):2186–2190.
168. Powars D, Hiti A. Sickle cell anemia: β^S gene cluster haplotypes as genetic markers for severe disease expression. *Am J Dis Child.* 1993;147:1197–1202.

28

Laboratory Methods for Diagnosis and Evaluation of Hemoglobin Disorders

Mary Fabry and John M. Old

INTRODUCTION

Hemoglobinopathy detection is often a part of the evaluation of anemia, hemolysis, microcytosis, cyanosis, or erythrocytosis. For this purpose, protein (hemoglobin)-, cellular-, and DNA-based approaches to the detection of variant hemoglobins and thalassemias are available. Diagnostic details can be found in each disease-specific chapter, whereas in the following pages we focus on the available methods and their strengths and weaknesses.

Characterization of mutant hemoglobins and thalassemias described throughout this book takes place in different contexts: large newborn screening laboratories that need to identify positively the most common mutants; general hematology laboratories that most often encounter common hemoglobinopathies and thalassemias; and reference or research laboratories that can detect rare mutant globin genes. Approaches that are necessary in one setting might not be practical in others.

Normal adult blood contains predominantly HbA ($\alpha_2\beta_2$) and small amounts of HbF ($\alpha_2\gamma_2$) and HbA_2 ($\alpha_2\delta_2$). After synthesis, monomeric globin chains form α/non-α dimers that do not dissociate under physiological conditions. In the presence of oxygen, hemoglobin tetramers rapidly dissociate into very low concentrations of dimers that can then form new tetramers.[1,2] This implies that when more than one α- or non-α-chain is present, the predominant form in the red cell will be the heterotetramer (for example, in red cells of HbSC disease, the dominant species will be $\alpha_2\beta^S\beta^C$, and $\alpha_2\beta^S\gamma$ heterotetramers form when HbS is present with high levels of HbF (Fig. 28.1). Most hemoglobin separation techniques detect only the homotetramer because the migratory properties of the individual dimers are similar to those of the homotetramers (identical $\alpha\beta$ subunits); hence, following dissociation of the heterotetramer into dimers, the two dimers will move apart toward the region where the respective homotetramers are found and recombine. This process will continue until all heterotetramers have dissociated. Heterotetramers can be detected by conventional separation techniques if oxygen is rigorously excluded because exchange is greatly slowed in deoxyhemoglobin.[1]

PROTEIN- AND CELLULAR-BASED METHODS USED TO IDENTIFY AND STUDY HEMOGLOBIN DISORDERS

Sample Preservation, Preparation, and Laboratory Safety

Analytical techniques depend on the starting materials, which include hemoglobin in dried filter paper blots. Anticoagulated whole blood should be refrigerated and processed within 48 hours. Hemoglobin is best stored as red cells in plasma because the red cell contains methemoglobin reductase, which will convert methemoglobin to deoxyhemoglobin. Plasma glucose and albumin stabilize the red cell and its membrane and ensure that enzyme activity will be maintained. With prolonged storage, methemoglobin will be generated and less stable mutant hemoglobins might be selectively lost.

Hemoglobin for analysis is usually prepared by hypotonic lysis with shaking. Care must be taken that all cells undergo lysis. In sickle cell disease, red cells are heterogeneous in their properties with different hemoglobin compositions (Chapter 7) and can be particularly resistant to lysis. Long-term storage of hemoglobin samples requires first washing the cells in isotonic saline to remove plasma proteins and then immersing them in liquid nitrogen or a freezer at −135°C or below. Hemoglobin stored at higher temperatures gradually loses heme, becomes insoluble, and can form degradation products that complicate analysis.

Safety of personnel working in hematology laboratories is a major consideration with the primary risks of hepatitis and human immunodeficiency virus. All human samples should be regarded as a potential source of infection. The first line of defense is care in sample handling: avoiding aerosol formation; wearing gloves; and observing precautions to avoid transferring material from gloves to other surfaces that may be touched by exposed skin. For more detailed discussion of laboratory safety, see the Occupational Safety and Health Agency web site (www.osha.gov).

Electrophoresis

Electrophoresis was once the most widely used method for initial detection of variant hemoglobins but has been supplanted by high-performance liquid chromatography (HPLC) as the most useful screening approach.

Proteins are composed of amino acids that bear side chains that can ionize. The pH at which a side chain is half ionized is its pK. Proteins are amphoteric; that is, they bear both positively and negatively charged side chains, and the net charge will depend on the pH of the solution and the pKs of its amino acids. Because proteins are charged

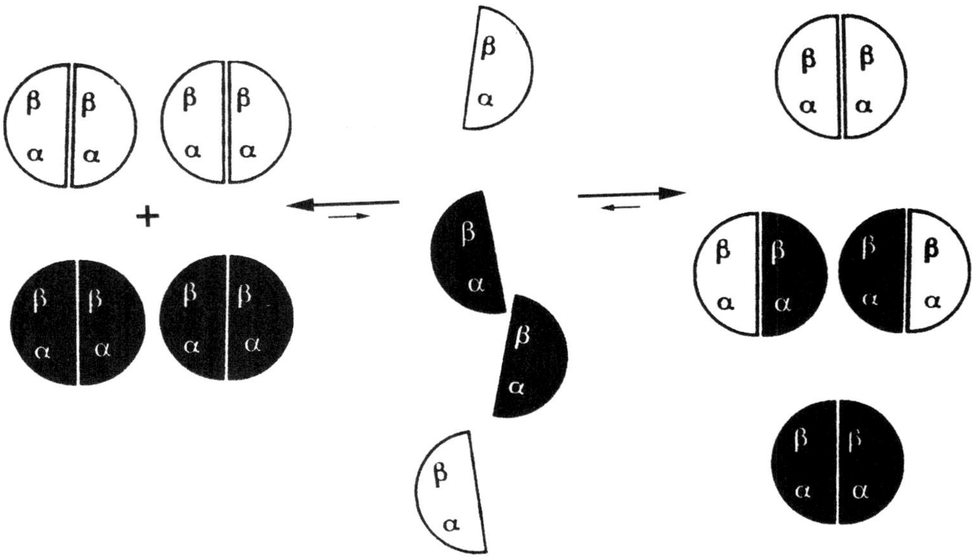

Figure 28.1. Hemoglobin is a tetramer of two αβ dimers that do not dissociate under physiological conditions; however, the tetramers rapidly dissociate and reassociate, generating very low concentrations of dimers under physiological conditions. Mixing two hemoglobins, represented by black and white, rapidly leads to an equilibrium mixture in which the original homotetramers and the heterotetramer exist in a ratio of 1:2:1.

molecules, they will migrate in an electrical field and the relative speed and direction will depend on the sign and magnitude of the net charge.

At pH 8.6, all human hemoglobins will have a net negative charge and will migrate in an electrical field toward the positive pole or anode. Mutations that do not alter the charge may be "silent" and not detectable by electrophoresis; however, interaction with the matrix (such as cellulose acetate or agar) can also affect the rate of migration. Most electrophoretic methods separate hemoglobin tetramers, but only tetramers composed of two identical α-non-α dimers, or homotetramers, are seen at the end of the separation process.

Because many different hemoglobins migrate similarly under a given set of conditions, electrophoresis is usually performed at two different pHs and on two different supporting mediums, but this method is insensitive to many rare variants. The usual choice is cellulose acetate electrophoresis at pH 8.4 and citrate agar electrophoresis at pH 6.0.[3] On citrate agar, in addition to the net charge, there is some selective interaction with the substrate, which further aids in resolution of some hemoglobins. This is based on the interaction of the central cavity of the hemoglobin with agaropectin in agar.[4] In all cases, a set of reference hemoglobins, usually HbA, A_2, F, S, and C should be included with each run. Electrophoresis can also be performed on separated globin chains if denaturing conditions are used.[5–7] Another approach that sometimes allows separation of overlapping hemoglobins, one of which contains cysteine, is treatment of the sample with cystamine.[8]

Most laboratories use commercially prepared kits that contain the hemolyzing agent, buffers, support media, a means for applying multiple samples, and a stain. The sample is lysed and applied to the cathodic or negative side and an electrical field is applied. Gels can be stained with protein- or hemoglobin-specific stains, or the color of the hemoglobin itself can be used for visualization. Quantification of hemoglobin fractions by densitometry is possible but inaccurate when a hemoglobin fraction is present at less than 5%.

Isoelectric Focusing, Capillary Isoelectric Focusing, and Capillary Electrophoresis

Isoelectric focusing (IEF) is capable of much higher resolution than the electrophoretic techniques. If a molecule has two or more ionizable groups, at least one of which has a pK in the acidic range and another in the basic range, then there will be a pH at which the net charge is zero. Proteins and amino acids all have a pH at which the net charge is zero, which is called the isoelectric point (pI) where there is no net movement in the presence of an externally applied electrical field. To separate proteins based on their pIs, a stable pH gradient must be created. This is achieved by applying a set of ampholytes with pIs that cover the range of pIs of the proteins that are to be separated on a support matrix. During the initial period after the current is applied, both the ampholytes and the proteins to be separated move as the pH gradient is formed. If a protein molecule finds itself on the acidic side of its pI it will migrate to the cathode, and if it finds itself on the basic side of its pI, it will migrate toward the anode (hence the term isoelectric focusing). Sharp bands of individual proteins are thus formed. With optimization, methods using free ampholytes can resolve two proteins with a pI difference of approximately 0.01 pH unit (Fig. 28.2).[9] Even higher resolution can

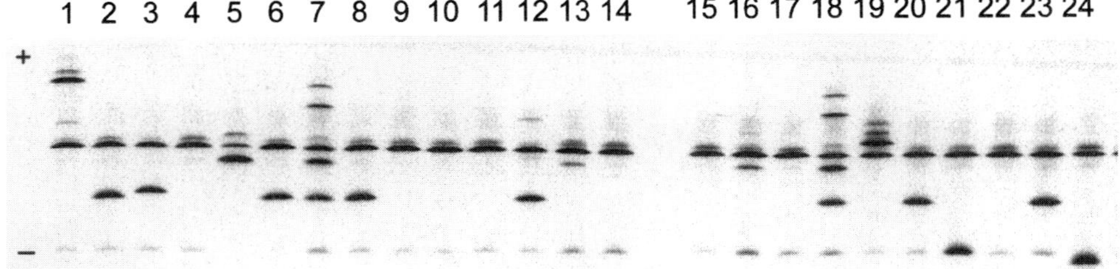

Figure 28.2. Separation of various mutant hemoglobins by IEF. A precast agarose gel (Resolve Systems, Wallac Inc., Akron, OH) was used at 75 mA, 1,200 V, 14°C, for 90 minutes. Present on the gel are: lane 1, HbA–HbN Baltimore; lanes 2, 6, 8, 12, 20, 23, HbAS; lane 3 HbA–HbD Punjab; lane 5 normal newborn; lanes 7, 18 controls (HbA_2, HbS, HbF, HbA, HbJ Baltimore, HbI Texas); lane 16 β thalassemia trait; lane 19 HbA–Hb Hope; lane 21 HbE trait; lane 24 HbC trait. (Gel contributed by H. Wajcman, Director of Research INSERM, Hopital Henri Mondor, Paris, France.)

be attained if the ampholytes are covalently bound to the matrix and the pH gradient is preformed by casting the gel with a two-vessel gradient mixer, thus preforming a stable pH gradient before the protein is applied. This type of gel is capable of resolution of proteins with pIs differing by approximately 0.001 pH units.[10,11] The most commonly used IEF technique is application of multiple samples to a commercially prepared thin-layer gel, which precludes automated technology.

Capillary IEF is performed by using pH gradients in fine capillary tubes. Available commercial systems require small sample size, have good resolving power, are rapid and sensitive, allow automated data analysis, and provide quantitative information. Capillary zone electrophoresis is another alternative in which hemoglobin molecules migrate through a capillary filled with a salt buffer near physiological conditions. There are no matrix interactions to introduce complexities or alter reproducibility, and the system has the potential for automation.[12,13]

Capillary electrophoresis combined with mass spectrometry has been applied to analysis of proteins present in single cells.[14,15] A wide variety of detection systems have been used, including conventional UV/visible detection similar to that used by HPLC instruments,[16] absorption imaging,[17] and mass spectrometry.[18]

High-performance Liquid Chromatography

The techniques described so far depend primarily on the ionization (pKs) of the amino acid side chains of intact hemoglobin molecules and their migration in an electrical field. In HPLC, ionic and hydrophobic interactions of the sample with the supporting matrix are the basis of separation. The sample is applied to the top of the column under conditions wherein it interacts strongly with the matrix. The proteins are then eluted with a developing solution (buffer) of gradually increasing strength, until all of the proteins are eluted. In cation and anion exchange chromatography, the properties of the developing solution that are varied are pH and ionic strength (salt concentration) and in reverse phase chromatography, the hydrophobicity (organic solvent) content is also varied. Hemoglobin may be separated as the intact tetramer or, under denaturing conditions, the individual globin chains can be separated. Human hemoglobins usually have a relatively small number of possible homotetramers and analysis of the intact tetramer generally yields readily interpretable results.

HPLC is currently the standard for the initial evaluation of hemoglobin variants and thalassemia. It is rapid, automated, capable of resolving most of the common and many uncommon variants, and provides reliable measurement of hemoglobin fractions such as HbA_2 and HbF (see later). Dedicated clinical systems based on HPLC separation of tetrameric hemoglobin with very rapid-automated sampling are in widespread use and allow preprogramed detection of hemoglobin variants (see Fig. 23.7, Chapter 23). Hemoglobin from transgenic mice – because of the possible formation of human – mouse chimeric dimers and hence a wide variety of homotetramers – and less common human variants yield a more readily interpretable chromatogram when denaturing conditions are used and the isolated globin chains are detected (Fig. 28.3). In most systems the pumps and the detector are computer controlled and the area under each detectable peak is automatically calculated. Very small internal diameters increase column resolution and decrease the amount of sample required at the cost of increased time per sample.[19]

Under the appropriate conditions HPLC readily separates hemoglobin variants that cannot be resolved by other means. The equipment used for HPLC is expensive, sophisticated, and difficult to maintain compared with that used for electrophoresis or IEF. HPLC screening techniques have been developed in which individual samples can be run in approximately 3 minutes with very high reproducibility.

Mass Spectrometry

Mass spectrometry is rarely used for clinical purposes and DNA-based studies have largely supplanted its use for definitive detection of rare variants. This method can start with a hemolysate and return the molecular weights of individual globin chains to within 1 atomic mass unit (amu). This level of accuracy allows detection of posttranslational

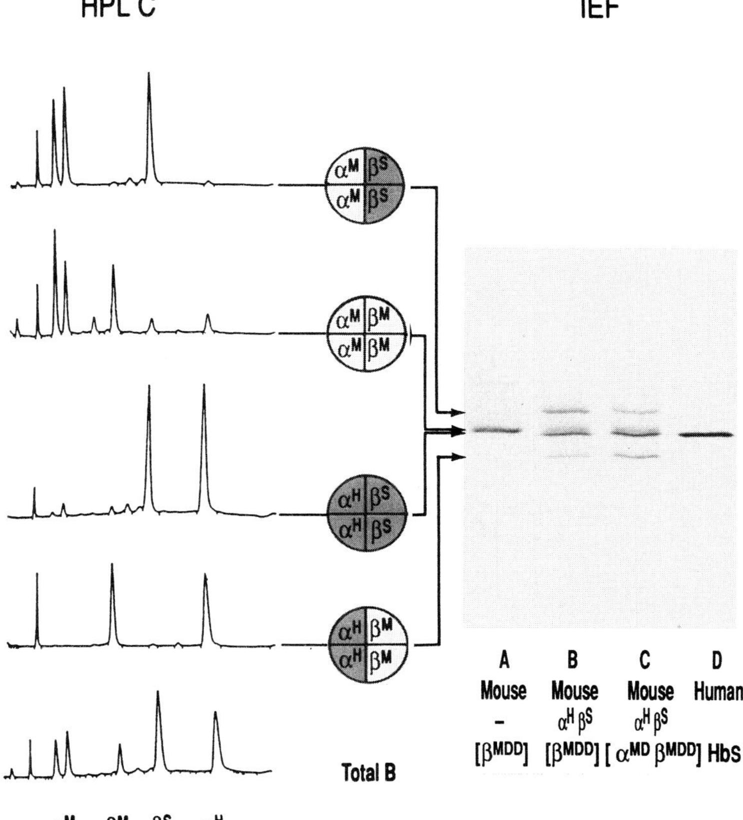

Figure 28.3. IEF and HPLC of hemoglobins from several transgenic mice expressing human HbS and mouse globins. The bands representing homotetramers composed of dimers of mouse α and human β^S chains, mouse α and mouse β chains, human α and human β^S chains, and human α and mouse β chains were separated by IEF, isolated from the gel, and separated by denaturing HPLC to allow identification of the tetramers present in the IEF gel. (From Fabry et al., 1992 Proc Natl Acad Sci, USA 89;1250–1254, with permission.)

modification[20] and verification of mutant and recombinant hemoglobins, and in contrast to electrophoretic techniques, mass spectrometry can separate similarly charged samples. Individual bands or peaks from IEF or HPLC can also serve as the starting sample. Requiring a few picomoles of protein, hemoglobin is an ideal molecule for mass spectrometry because it has a favorable size, an adequate number of protonation sites, distinct mass differences between mutants, and few posttranslational modifications.[21] Mass spectrometry combined with capillary electrophoresis has been applied to analysis of proteins present in single or small numbers of red cells.[15]

This method is based on the principle that charged particles moving through a magnetic field will undergo deflection proportional to the charge/mass ratio. Particles with the smallest charge/mass ratio are the least affected. The sample is first converted to gaseous ions and an accelerating voltage is applied. The particles are focused through a slit into a highly evacuated area, where they are subjected to the magnetic field that causes them to separate. The most important methods of ionization are electrospray ionization (ESI),[22] and matrix-assisted laser desorption (MALDI). ESI is most suitable for intact globin chain analysis and MALDI is the method of choice for peptide identification. ESI allows mass spectrometers to be interfaced with HPLC and capillary IEF devices, which frequently allows immediate positive identification of the separated species and is also useful for identification of small peaks that could represent derivatives or degradation products.[23,24]

Mass spectrometry can be used for complete sequencing of proteins based on identification of fragments that can be produced classically by proteolytic digestion and then exposed to MALDI. The abnormal fragments can be identified, and in many cases, the mutation deduced. With a few exceptions, whole blood hemolysates can be subjected to digestion without further separation. Separation is necessary when the variant is present at a low level, a mass difference of 1 D is suspected, or high levels of HbF are present. In these cases the sample can be purified by IEF or HPLC prior to digestion.[26] Alternatively, the protein can be fragmented in the spectrometer itself without resorting to wet chemistry and the fragments produced in the spectrometer can be used to identify the portion bearing the mutant animo acid.[23–28]

Hemoglobin F

HbF (Chapter 7) in adult blood is normally is less than 1%–2% of total hemoglobin. It is unevenly distributed among red cells. Cells with high levels of HbF are called F cells and, in sickle cell disease, F cells are seldom found among the most dense cells. This implies that when either HbF or F cells are measured, care must be taken to avoid biasing the sample. Careful mixing into the suspension of any cells that have settled at the bottom of the tube is sufficient; however, automated systems for resuspending normal red cells might not be sufficient for blood from patients with any of the sickle hemoglobinopathies.

Several methods may be used for quantitation of HbF, including alkaline denaturation, electrophoresis, or IEF followed by densitometry, disposable minicolumns, and HPLC. HbF is more resistant to denaturation by alkaline conditions than is HbA. In the alkaline denaturation method, potassium hydroxide is added to a known concentration of hemoglobin and, after a predetermined time interval, the reaction is stopped by adding a known volume of ammonium sulfate, which lowers the pH and precipitates the denatured hemoglobin that is removed by filtration. The concentration of hemoglobin remaining in solution is then determined. Two versions of the alkaline denaturation protocol exist: that of Betke et al.,[29] which is reliable for HbF less than 10%–15%, and thereafter systematically underestimates the percentage of HbF, and that of Jonxis and Visser,[30] which is only accurate when HbF is greater than 10%. HPLC allows accurate quantitation of HbF and is currently the most widely used method.[31,32] It is accurate for samples with levels of HbF down to approximately 0.5% and has no upper limit of detection. Some hemoglobin components that are present at low concentrations elute in the position of HbF under some HPLC conditions (Chapter 7). Electrophoresis or IEF followed by densitometry are less reliable than HPLC for HbF quantification. For detection of very low levels of HbF radioimmunoassay,[33,34] and enzyme-linked immunosorbent assay (ELISA)[35] are alternative techniques.

Because HbF is almost always unevenly distributed among erythrocytes – an exception is some types of hereditary persistence of HbF (HPFH) – immunological techniques using flow cytometry that allow the determination of F cells are also useful and can provide a reasonable surrogate for whole blood HbF levels.[36] Measuring F cells is discussed later.

Hemoglobin A_2

HPLC systems that detect many hemoglobin variants are the current standard for measuring HbA_2 levels. Electrophoresis can separate HbA_2 from HbA and HbF, enabling accurate measurement of this minor hemoglobin component but this requires elution from gels or membranes because densitometric scanning is inaccurate.[45,46] Acid agar gel electrophoresis does not resolve HbA_2 from HbA. Refrigeration and freezing may reduce the percentage of HbA_2 in stored hemolysates. The differential elution of HbA_2 in minicolumns is reliable, rapid, and inexpensive.[37]

HbA_2 cannot be separated from hemoglobin variants with similar positive charges, such as HbC and HbE, by electrophoresis or many column-chromatographic methods. In the company of abnormal globins that contain only a single additional positive charge, such as HbS, the HbA_2 level has been reported to be higher than normal but appropriate separation methods can circumvent this overestimation of HbA_2.

Recent improvement allows reasonably accurate measurement of HbA_2 by HPLC even in the presence of HbS as in sickle cell trait (HbAS) or sickle cell anemia, although the level of HbA_2 reported is slightly higher than normal because of the coelution of minor HbS fractions (Chapter 7). HbE, and Hb Lepore have very similar retention time to HbA_2, and these hemoglobins cannot be positively separated. HbC and Hb O-Arab also cannot be definitively distinguished by cation HPLC that affords excellent resolution of HbA_2 from HbS and HbC.

HbA_2 can be measured immunologically[33,38] with high specificity. The levels obtained correlate well with the more traditional methods of measurement.

Capillary IEF has been used to measure HbA_2 in normal subjects and in those with β thalassemia trait, HbAS, and sickle cell anemia.[39,40] Accurate measurements are possible, although in one study HbA_2 levels in HbAS and sickle cell anemia were slightly elevated compared with normal. Nevertheless, they were clearly separated from β thalassemia trait. Glycosylated forms of HbA_2, analogous to the minor components of HbA, are present and can be quantified by HPLC and IEF. Like HbA_{1c}, these glycohemoglobins are elevated in poorly controlled diabetics (Chapter 7).

Functional Properties of Hemoglobin

P_{50} and Other Measurements of Oxygen Saturation

The partial pressure, at which hemoglobin is half saturated with oxygen, or P_{50}, is an important property of hemoglobin in solution and in the red cell. P_{50} is extremely sensitive to the presence of 2,3-bisphosphoglycerate (2,3-BPG), inorganic phosphate or other phosphates, pH (Bohr effect), CO_2, anions, and, in the case of HbS, polymer formation. In dilute solutions, the P_{50} of HbA and HbS are equal. In the red cell and in plasma, HbA has a P_{50} of 25 ± 2 mm Hg when equilibrated with gases containing 5% CO_2. The increase in P_{50} (or decrease in oxygen affinity) is primarily due to the effect of 2,3-BPG on the oxygen affinity of hemoglobin. P_{50} of HbS in the red cell is higher, ranging from 25 to 45 mm Hg. HbS polymerization increases P_{50} in proportion to the amount of polymer formed because polymer has a lower P_{50}.[41] With HbA, the association curve ($Hb \rightarrow HbO_2$) is identical to the dissociation curve ($HbO_2 \rightarrow Hb$); there is no hysteresis. The P_{50} in blood samples with HbS depends on whether equilibrium with polymer has been reached, that is, whether polymer formation or polymer melting is complete before the next level of oxygenation is tested. The delay time for polymer formation is dependent to the 30th power of the deoxyhemoglobin concentration.[42] In the absence of equilibrium there is hysteresis and the P_{50} for the association and dissociation curves will differ. Changing the pO_2 at a slower rate will bring the two curves closer together.

The most common measurements of P_{50} are based on measurement of oxygen association curves. Two parameters are simultaneously measured: pO_2, which is continuously varied, and the percentage of hemoglobin, which is saturated with oxygen. In these measurements, the hemoglobin is first fully deoxygenated and then oxygen is gradually reintroduced, whereas the pO_2 is measured with an oxygen electrode. At the same time, hemoglobin saturation with oxygen is measured optically. The Hemoscan (no longer manufactured) used equilibrated hemoglobin or whole blood samples between layers of gas-permeable membranes and allowed measurement of whole blood P_{50} in plasma. The Hemox-Analyzer (TCS Medical Products) measures percentage of oxyhemoglobin with a dual-wavelength spectrophotometer at 560 nm, which is sensitive to the transition between deoxyhemoglobin and oxyhemoglobin, and at 570 nm, at which the absorption is sensitive to the hemoglobin concentration but insensitive to the oxygenation state. Dual-wavelength systems cannot discriminate between oxyHb and several other forms of hemoglobin such as CO, NO, metHb, or sulfHb, which can lead to systematic errors (Chapter 25).

Blood gas analyzers measure the pH, pO_2, and pCO_2 for samples of whole blood and then calculate hemoglobin saturation with oxygen and a number of other parameters, based on the normal P_{50}. This will systematically overestimate the percentage of oxyhemoglobin present in the blood of sickle cell disease patients and any other hemoglobinopathies that result in elevated P_{50}. Similarly, a low P_{50} such as is found for HbF will result in systematic underestimation of the percentage of oxyhemoglobin. The presence of met- and carbonmonoxy hemoglobin (CO-Hb) are not accounted for in these measurements.

A CO-Oximeter (Instrumentation Laboratories, Lexington, MA) uses multiple wavelengths to measure the hemoglobin concentration, percentage oxyhemoglobin, hemoglobin, percentage metHb, and percentage CO-Hb and can be used in conjunction with blood gas analyzers to give a more accurate, but still incomplete, picture of hemoglobin saturation.

The 2,3-BPG content of the red cell is needed to evaluate the significance of P_{50} measurements because altered P_{50} might be the result of a hemoglobin abnormality or altered 2,3-BPG content.

If a hemoglobin with a P_{50} different from that of HbA is present (such as HbS or HbF), the hemoglobin saturation cannot be obtained from a blood gas analyzer, which uses the P_{50} of HbA to calculate hemoglobin saturation from the measured pO_2.

A useful test for patient monitoring is measurement of the arterial hemoglobin saturation with oxygen that can be measured in vivo by use of a pulse oximeter. The pulse oximeter estimates arterial hemoglobin saturation by measuring the light absorbance of pulsating vascular tissue at two wavelengths. The relationship between measured light absorbance and saturation was developed empirically and is built into the oximeter software. The presence of methemoglobin and CO-Hb will lead to systematic overestimation of oxygen saturation by pulse oximetry (Chapter 25).

Detection and Estimation of Polymer Formation in Red Cells and Solutions Containing HbS

Solubility

The insolubility of deoxyHbS in high-phosphate solutions is the basis of a rapid nonquantitative test that when combined with the results of HPLC provides a positive identification of sickling hemoglobin variants. Solubility tests should never be used for definitive diagnosis. If they are performed correctly, they can identify the presence of a sickling hemoglobin variant (Chapter 23). This could be clinically important when rapidly knowing if HbS is present is imperative, but the need for this knowledge is uncommon.

C_{SAT}

The solubility of a substance is the concentration of that substance in equilibrium with a condensed phase that may be crystalline, polymer, or particulate. In the case of HbS, the solubility is important because it allows estimation of the percentage of the HbS content of the red cell that will be converted to polymer under fully deoxygenated conditions. The concentration of deoxyHbS in equilibrium with the polymer phase (C_{SAT}) is useful for characterizing sickle hemoglobins that contain a second mutation and for characterizing mixtures of HbS with other hemoglobins.

Several methods are used. One method uses quasiphysiological conditions and the other relies on high phosphate to precipitate sickle hemoglobins. Formation of protein crystals and polymers is extremely sensitive to the nature and concentration of the counter ions present. Either the crystal structure itself or the rate of nucleation can be affected. In the low-phosphate method,[43] hemoglobin is concentrated versus 0.1 M potassium phosphate buffer and deoxygenated, first by alternating vacuum and nitrogen, and then by adding enough sodium dithionite solution to give a final concentration equal to three times the heme concentration. The samples are transferred anaerobically to C_{SAT} tubes filled with paraffin oil, incubated overnight in a nitrogen atmosphere, and centrifuged for 2 hours at 35,000 rpm with purified HbS used as a control. The supernatants are removed anaerobically, and concentrations and deoxy pHs are determined; solubility is expressed in grams per deciliter of HbS in equilibrium with the polymer. This is regarded as the reference method.

Another method is based on the turbidity of a microparticulate suspension that is formed when HbS is introduced into a solution at pH 7.0 and 27°C with a high-phosphate concentration that has been deoxygenated with dithionite.[44] A third alternate approach uses 50 mM phosphate in the presence of 70 kD dextran to decrease polymer solubility.[45] Because solubility is determined by the residues in the contact area between the tetramers, this method offers an advantage over the high-phosphate method, in which the insoluble phase does not have a fiber structure. Finally, a method that takes advantage of the observation that polymerization of HbS shifts the P_{50} to the right and that this shift is proportional to the amount of polymer formed is available. Correlation of the C_{SAT} determined by P_{50} with that determined by the centrifugation method has been shown to be good for a wide range of samples[46] and has been applied to suspensions of red cells.[47]

In the high-phosphate method, the pH dependence of solubility is opposite to that found in the minimum gelling concentration method.[48]

Plasma Hemoglobin

The importance of cell free or plasma hemoglobin in sickle cell disease and other hemolytic anemias has recently been emphasized[49,50] (Chapter 11). In plasma, due to the low hemoglobin concentration, all hemoglobin will be dissociated into less stable dimers, and oxidation will result in conversion to methemoglobin with potential loss of heme. The first consideration for measurement of plasma hemoglobin is avoiding artifacts due to technique in blood draws or sample preparation. This is particularly so in sickle cell disease because of the greater fragility of sickle erythrocytes. Small bore needles, rapid flow, and vortexing should be avoided. Red cells and plasma should be separated promptly. In recent studies,[50] blood was collected from artery or vein by using large-bore catheters (18 gauge). The first 3 mL of blood was discarded, and the blood then slowly drawn into heparinized syringes. Blood was spun at 750 G at 4°C for 10 minutes without braking, and the plasma was removed. Plasma was then spun at 14,000 G at 4°C for 10 minutes to eliminate residual erythrocytes and platelets.

Several techniques can be applied to measure cell-free hemoglobin: For relatively high concentrations, plasma can be diluted 1:1 with Drabkin reagent. A more sensitive technique is use of tetramethylbenzidine.[51] Tetramethylbenzidine is noncarcinogenic and more sensitive than benzidine. Samples can be read at 600 nm, at room temperature, and concentrations can be calculated using the slope of the sample and the slope of a calibrator. This method is sensitive to heme in all forms: heme in hemoglobin, bound to albumin, and heme in haptoglobin and hemopexin. An ELISA can also be used.[52]

Both Drabkin reagent and tetramethylbenzidine are inexpensive and do not require complex instrumentation and they are sensitive to heme in all forms. This can lead to overestimation of plasma hemoglobin, but because heme or heme proteins bound to albumin, haptoglobin, or hemopexin are usually present at a relatively low concentration, this might not be a major drawback. The ELISA method is more expensive and is sensitive to all forms of human hemoglobin, including HbF.

Lactate dehydrogenase (LDH) is released from the red cell on hemolysis. There are five isoforms of LDH that come from red cell, heart, kidney, lymphoid cells, platelets, liver, and skeletal muscle. If only LDH isoforms 1 and 2 are measured, the sources are narrowed to red cell, heart, and kidney. A high correlation between serum LDH and plasma heme measured by ELISA exists in sickle cell anemia.[52] Absence of an accepted standard of LDH measurement makes it difficult to compare values between different laboratories, making agreement problematic on a single upper limit of LDH that would identify all cases of high plasma hemoglobin.

CHARACTERIZING THE RED CELL

Complete Blood Count

Blood for a complete blood count (CBC) should be slowly drawn into an anticoagulant, usually EDTA. Prompt but gentle mixing is needed to avoid clotting. This is particularly important for patients with low packed cell volume (PCV) because the amount of anticoagulant may be only marginally sufficient. Red cells from patients with hemoglobinopathies can be fragile, and narrow gauge needles, rapid flow, or violent mixing should be avoided. Whole blood can be stored refrigerated or on wet ice and used within 24 hours and shipped overnight on wet ice. To avoid hemolysis, freezer packs should not be used and should never be placed in direct contact with tubes containing whole blood. Special care may be needed to resuspend whole blood from patients with sickle cell disease because these cells may adhere to each other and resist resuspension.

Manual Methods

Although red cell indices are determined by automated methods in most laboratories, manual methods are still used sometimes. The ratio of hemoglobin to PCV can be used to calculate a mean corpuscular hemoglobin concentration (MCHC) that might be more reliable than that determined by automated measurements. The most accurate way to measure hemoglobin concentration is by the cyanmethemoglobin method, which is insensitive to oxygenation and pH. Hemoglobin is oxidized to methemoglobin by ferricyanide and then interacts with cyanide to form cyanomethemoglobin and its absorbance at 540 nm is read in a spectrophotometer. A dedicated microhematocrit centrifuge that generates a force of 12,000 G and microhematocrit tubes with or without heparin are used to estimate PCV. For samples from patients with high PCV, and those with sickle cell anemia or hereditary spherocytosis, an additional centrifugation might be required. If MCHC is to be calculated from hemoglobin and hematocrit, multiple measurements should be made.

Automated Methods

Current automated CBC methods measure properties of single cells flowing through a detector.[53,54] Two general types of detection are currently used: Coulter-type detectors based on impedance and high-frequency conductivity, and detectors based on optical properties of the cell. Most instruments measure several variables for a large number of cells and present results as an average value; the averaging of samples with red cell heterogeneity, therefore, such as those from sickle cell anemia or hereditary spherocytosis, might yield values that seem normal. All instruments count particles, estimate their size, and hemolyze the cells and measure hemoglobin. The results of the direct measurements (hemoglobin, red blood cell count, white blood cell count, and platelet count) are the most accurate values, but failure to hemolyze all cells can lead to error in hemoglobin concentration in hemoglobinopathies such as sickle cell disease. Failure to resuspend completely all cells in samples of blood that have been stored for several hours can also lead to errors in hemoglobin and PCV. Because identification of erythrocytes and platelets is based on their size, fragmentation might lead to misclassification. Most systems measure hemoglobin by the cyanmethemoglobin method. Coulter detectors are based on the observation that the electrical conductivity of cells is lower than that of saline solutions and measurement of the impedance across a small orifice with cells flowing through allows cell size (mean corpuscular volume [MCV]) to be estimated. Factors that lead to deviations are cellular asymmetry and loss of an intact cell membrane, both of which may be features in samples with abnormal red cells.

Cell volume measurements using light scattering (Mie principle) are based on the observation that the intensity of light scattered at small angles in the forward direction is proportional to cell size. Two major factors lead to deviations: cell shape and variation in refractive index, which is related to hemoglobin concentration. The first problem has been approached by sphering the cells at constant volume, and the second problem has been addressed directly by measuring at two wavelengths, which allows intracellular hemoglobin concentration and refractive index to be estimated. Incomplete sphering is a problem for some samples such as those from sickle cell disease patients. PCV, mean corpuscular hemoglobin (MCH), MCHC, and red cell distribution width (RDW) and other functions that provide information on dense cells are calculated from measured variation in red cell size. For most instruments, the least reliable measurement is the MCHC, which is calculated from the whole blood hemoglobin concentration divided by the mean cell volume times the number of cells. Because the calculation requires three measurements in most instruments, the error from all of them enters into the calculation; the exception to this is the Bayer Advia machine, which measures intracellular hemoglobin concentration directly as cell hemoglobin concentration mean (CHCM).

The major advantages of automated methods are speed, low manpower requirements, and high precision. Comparisons of available instruments have been made.[53–57] Automated systems have high reproducibility; however, the accuracy is sensitive to errors in calibration that systematically affect the results so that absolute values may vary between instruments. All systems generate flags to call attention to unusual values, which may be taken either as indications of pathology or a need to examine the sample more closely. In general all instruments performed all tests satisfactorily with the exception of estimation of MCHC, which was the least reliable. Analyzers using the Mie principle, by measuring density of individual red cells, are able to generate histograms of variation in cell density (cell hemoglobin distribution) of individual red cells in a given blood sample (see later). This is useful for following changes in the distribution of dense red cells in sickle cell anemia.

Reticulocyte Count

Reticulocyte counts, along with PCV, are useful for evaluating hematopoiesis and hemolysis. Reticulocytes contain remnants of mRNA; they continue to synthesize hemoglobin for 1–2 days in the marrow and for another day after release into the circulation. The reticulocyte count may be elevated even in cases where hemoglobin levels are normal, and, in these cases, can serve as a more sensitive indicator of errors in either production or destruction of red cells. The peripheral blood of normal adults has less than 2% reticulocytes, but the count varies with the method. If the individual is under hematopoietic stress, the peripheral blood can contain stress reticulocytes, cells prematurely released from the bone marrow, or even nucleated erythrocytes. All reticulocyte counts are based on the presence of mRNA in the cell. In the manual method, the cells are stained with new methylene blue, which precipitates RNA, rendering it visible. The amount and distribution of the precipitate allow the degree of immaturity of the reticulocyte to be estimated, and stress reticulocytes have a characteristic appearance. After staining, the cells are spread on a microscope slide and reticulocytes are counted as a percentage of all red cells.

Automated reticulocyte counts use fluorescence-stained cells that are read in a flow cytometer, which may be either dedicated to reticulocyte counting or part of a larger automated system. Red cells are usually discriminated from white cells and platelets by size, and a maximum fluorescence gate is usually set that may exclude nucleated red cells. The relative age of reticulocytes can be estimated by the degree of fluorescence. One drawback of these methods is that staining with the most frequently used reagent, thiazole orange, requires approximately 30 minutes incubation and variation in the chosen time of incubation can affect the final reticulocyte count. Based on the intensity of the reaction between the dye Oxazine 750 and reticulocyte mRNA, reticulocytes can be classified as low-, medium-, or high-staining intensity reticulocytes. An increase in the number of high-staining intensity reticulocytes indicates the presence of stress reticulocytes. Reticulocytes can also be stained with a labeled antibody to the transferrin receptor.[58] Bayer Advia counters can also measure reticulocyte volume (MCVr), reticulocyte hemoglobin concentration (CHCMr), and total reticulocyte hemoglobin (retHb), ratio of total hemoglobin to retHb (Hb/retHb), absolute reticulocyte count, mature red cell hemoglobin (rbcHb), rbcHb/retHb ratio, and numbers of erythrocytes with MCHC more than a chosen value. From the absolute reticulocyte count and the CHr, the retHb is calculated, which is expressed in grams per liter, the hemoglobin content of all reticulocytes.[59] The ratio of rbcHb to retHb defines the ratio between the hemoglobin contained in mature red cells and in the reticulocytes. Under steady-state conditions, erythrocyte survival can be estimated indirectly from the ratio of hemoglobin contained in mature red cells and in reticulocytes. A reduction in retHb and a concomitant increase in rbcHb/retHb ratio provide indirect evidence for prolonged red cell survival. Changes in MCVr can provide a much more rapid indication of response of patients to folate or vitamin B12 deficiency.[60]

Measures of Cell Heterogeneity

Most automated counters produce an indication of red cell heterogeneity called the RDW, which is calculated from the measured variation in red cell size by a nonlinear formula that magnifies heterogeneity. Increased reticulocyte count will increase RDW and a correlation between the RDW and percentage of cells in the densest part of density gradient separations has also been shown.[61] Bayer Advia counters also compute a hemoglobin distribution width that is based on the variation of the CHCM, which is directly determined for each cell. Typically hemoglobin distribution width is a much smaller number than RDW.

MCHC has distinct characteristics in many hemoglobinopathies. Small increases in MCHC occur when normal erythrocytes are deoxygenated and this can be visually demonstrated on continuous density gradients.[62,63] Hemoglobin concentration is directly proportional to cell density, but is not necessarily correlated with cell volume unless cells from the same source are compared at different osmolarities. For example, the red cells of patients with HbE are microcytic but have a narrow range of densities identical to that of individuals with HbA.[64] Red cells from normal adults have an MCHC of 33 ± 1.5 g/dL by conventional measurements; however, more sensitive measurements show that there are consistent differences between males and females and between African Americans and Caucasians. Several hemoglobinopathies have altered MCHC with a narrow range of densities. For example, in δβ thalassemia trait the cells are uniformly less dense by approximately 2 g/dL and in homozygous HbC disease, the cells are uniformly denser by approximately 4 g/dL. In other diseases, such as sickle cell disease, hereditary spherocytosis, and some of the thalassemias, there is a broad but characteristic distribution of red cells that include both high- and low-density red cells.

MCHC is the least reliable of all automated measurements and is frequently considered uninformative, so alternative methods are used to analyze and isolate red cells according to density. These can be broken into three broad classes: methods using microhematocrit tubes filled with materials of different densities, methods that rely on discontinuous or layered density of supporting media for separation, and techniques that rely on continuous density gradients. All methods take advantage of the fact that cells will move under the influence of centrifugal force until they find a region of density the same as that of the cell – continuous gradients – or stop when they encounter a region of higher density – at the boundaries in discontinuous gradients.

Discontinuous gradients based on a number of substances have been used in density-based separation. The most successful of these methods are based on substances that are nontoxic to the cell, have a low osmolarity, neutral pH, and low viscosity. Phthalate esters, Percoll®, Hypaque®, Stractan®, (Larex®), and others have all been used for red cell separations. Danon and coworkers[65] devised a simple method of generating density profiles and isolating cells of defined density by using mixtures of phthalate esters that cover the density range of red cells. A disadvantage of this method is that the separated cells are not viable for physiological studies.

Stractan (arabinopolygalactan, now marketed as Larex) is a high-molecular-weight product made from the bark of the larch tree. It is physiologically benign and has a low osmotic contribution, which allows the ionic content of solutions to be adjusted freely.[66] A disadvantage of discontinuous gradients is that they usually have four or fewer densities that can either mask relatively large changes in density of cells at the upper boundary between density levels, or exaggerate small changes in cells at the lower boundary.

Percoll is a commercially available product that spontaneously generates a continuous density gradient when centrifuged. It is composed of silica particles coated with polyvinyl pyrrolidone with range of sizes whose rate of sedimentation by centrifugation force is determined by size. The density at any depth in the tube is determined by the number and size of the particles. For this reason the density profile of Percoll gradients depends on the duration of centrifugation, viscosity (which is temperature dependent), and G force applied. The density range of Percoll is suitable for separation of white cells and needs to be increased before it can be applied to red cells. Renografin® and Percoll can be combined to produce a continuous density gradient capable of separation of red cells by their density.[67] A disadvantage of Renografin is its high osmolarity, which results in a final osmolarity of the mixture of more than

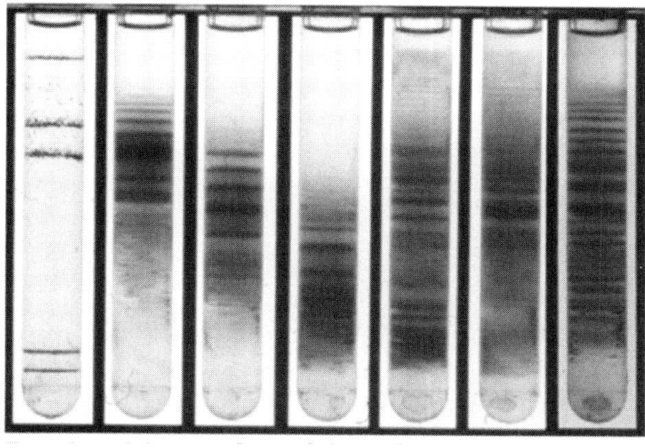

Figure 28.4. Percoll–Larex continuous density gradient. Red cell density is directly proportional to the MCHC. The least dense (lowest MCHC) cells are at the top of the gradient and the highest density cells are at the bottom. This technique provides a method for directly visualizing the distribution of red cell density in a sample of whole blood. The example shows a continuous density gradient with density marker beads and red cells from patients with normal hemoglobin (AA), HbC trait (AC), HbC disease (CC), sickle cell anemia (SS), HbS-O Arab, and hereditary spherocytosis (HS). (See color plate 28.4.)

360 mOsm. Stractan and Percoll can produce continuous density gradients with physiological pH, osmolarity, and ionic composition.[68] These gradients are sensitive to very small changes in red cell density and can be used both preparatively and analytically. Assignment of density is based on position relative to density marker beads and on measured MCHC of cells isolated from defined positions in the gradient. An example of the power of separation of Percoll–Larex gradients is given in Figure 28.4, in which the red cell density distributions of several common hemoglobinopathies are compared.

All separations based on red cell density are sensitive to the pH and osmolarity of the solutions because these variables will change the MCHC of the cells. Sedimentation through the interface may depend on red cell deformability,[69] leading to systematic underestimation of the density of poorly deformable cells. Stractan (Larex) is tedious to prepare, but cells isolated from these gradients are suitable for transport measurements and other protocols requiring physiologically intact cells.

F Cells

With the exception of some forms of HPFH (Chapter 16), HbF is not uniformly distributed among red cell. Erythrocytes with detectable amounts of HbF are called F cells (Chapter 7), and these can be detected by the acid elution method and flow cytometry. The Kleihauer and Betke method relies on resistance of precipitated HbF to acid elution. Cells are spread on a slide, fixed, and then incubated with citric acid–phosphate buffer. HbF remains precipitated while all other hemoglobins are eluted from the cell. When stained with hematoxylin–eosin F cells are stained; in gene deletion HPFH all erythrocytes are uniformly stained.

Development of monoclonal antibodies to HbF in several laboratories allowed a more quantitative detection of HbF. Cells are first lightly fixed and the membrane permeabilized with detergents and/or organic solvents. After fixation and permeabilization, the cells are stained with antibody and may be observed either by microscopy or by flow cytometry[70–72] (Fig. 28.5). Early measurements used immunodiffusion to create a ring of precipitated HbF antibody around the positive cells. Fluorescent labels can be attached directly to the antibodies and cells observed by fluorescence microscopy.[70] Monoclonal antibodies against several hemoglobins including HbF are commercially available. These antibodies can be used for immunofluorescent labeling of F cells in fixed smears on slides, including archival samples.[70]

Globin Chain Synthesis

Incorporation of labeled amino acids into intact cells was first reported more than 50 years ago. Imbalance of synthesis of α- versus non-α-globin chains is the fundamental definition of thalassemia. Globin-chain synthesis can be measured in blood reticulocytes and marrow erythroid precursors, although the results are not always equivalent. The most convenient means of chain separation is

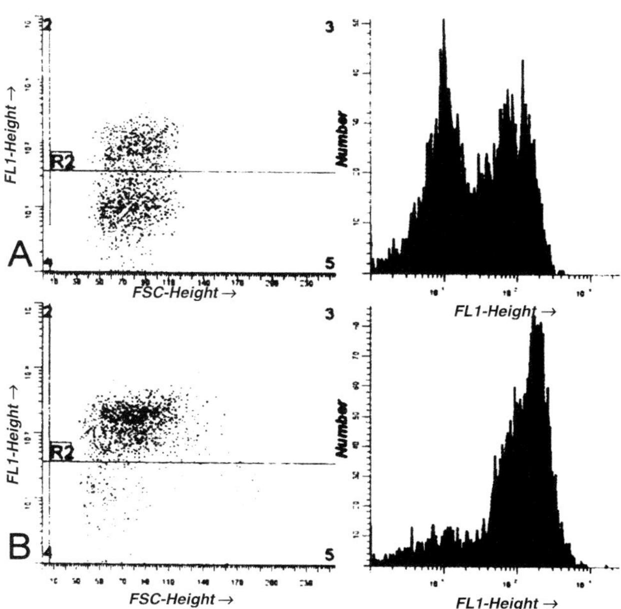

Figure 28.5. Comparison of distribution of γ-globin chains in red cells by fluorescence-activated cell sorting analysis using fluorescein isothiocyanate–labeled antibody specific for human γ-globin chains (supplied by Thomas Campbell of EG&G Wallac). In this case, the examples are two different types of transgenic mice expressing exclusively human hemoglobin and either a low level of γ globin (panel **A**) or a high level of γ globin (panel **B**). Left panels: fluorescence intensity versus cell size; right panels: number of cells versus fluorescence intensity. Note the presence of two populations of red cells that represent non-F cells and F cells (high fluorescence intensity).

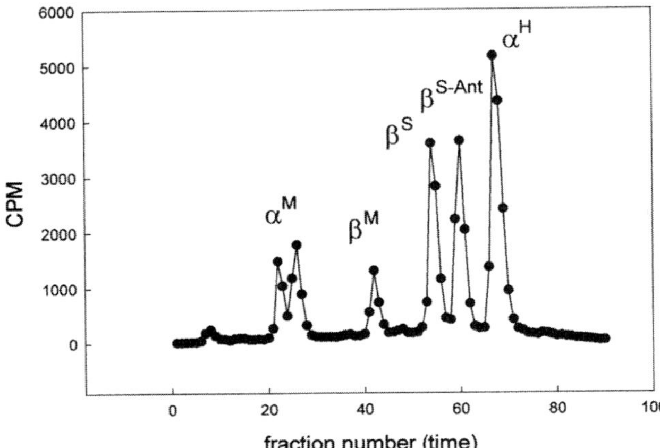

Figure 28.6. Chain synthesis as measured by incorporation of radioactive leucine followed by separation of globin chains by denaturing reverse-phase HPLC. In this case the sample studied was from a transgenic mouse expressing human α, β^S, and $\beta^{S\text{-Antilles}}$ as well as mouse α- and β-globins.

reverse-phase HPLC.[73] Fractions containing globin chains are collected, and the radioactivity incorporated is counted (Fig. 28.6). The efficiency of labeling can be greatly improved if the percentage reticulocytes is enriched by a process such as layering whole blood on a discontinuous Stractan gradient and collecting the lightest fraction that contains the most reticulocytes. Chain synthesis is still the gold standard when trying to elucidate the mechanism(s) by which synthesis of γ-globin is enhanced by butyrate in sickle cell disease.[74,75]

Hemoglobin S Polymerization, Rate of Sickling, and Percentage of HbS Polymer

When the concentration of deoxyHbS exceeds the C_{SAT}, polymer is formed. Polymer formation does not occur immediately because, prior to polymer formation, nucleation must occur, and because the nucleus consists of several hemoglobin molecules, there is a very high concentration dependence (Chapter 6). The time between deoxygenation and the onset of polymer formation is called the delay time[76] that has one of the highest concentration dependencies in biology[77] and may range from values of less than a microsecond at high hemoglobin concentrations to several minutes at low concentrations.

The distortion of the red cell known as sickling is the result of intracellular polymer formation and can be used as an indirect endpoint for polymer formation. Two methods have been used to measure the rate of sickling: manual mixing and continuous flow. In the manual and continuous flow methods, oxygenated red cells are mixed with buffered sodium dithionite, which reacts with the oxygen and, at predetermined intervals, cells are fixed with isotonic formalin; the number of cells that have sickled are counted, and the results plotted as a function of time. The earliest recorded time point for continuous mixing was at 25 msec. Because samples of blood from sickle cell disease patients can contain appreciable numbers of cells with unusual shapes, the number of deformed cells can be counted in a control sample and subtracted from the total of sickled cells. This method is capable of showing that cells from patients with HbSC disease have a stronger response to reduced osmolarity than cells from sickle cell anemia patients and can detect retardation of polymer formation by antisickling agents. Polymer formation can occur much more rapidly than the mixing time in these methods and methods capable of directly studying polymerization in solutions and intact cells have been devised.

These more quantitative methods consist of two parts: 1) rapid generation of high concentrations of nonpolymerized deoxyHbS, and 2) a sensitive, rapid readout. Two methods have been used to generate high concentrations of deoxyhemoglobin: temperature jump and laser photolysis. Readout methods have included optical birefringence, turbidity, light scattering, water proton line width and relaxation time, and differential interference contrast. The temperature jump method makes use of the negative temperature dependence of HbS solubility and is very simple, but requires a minimum of approximately 10 seconds to reach thermal equilibrium and has a resolution of approximately 1 second. In addition, the highest hemoglobin concentration that can be attained at 0°C without polymer is approximately 30 g/dL. The majority of sickle cells have a MCHC exceeding this value.

Because of these limitations a laser photolysis method was developed that allows direct measurement of polymer formation with very high time resolution both in solutions and in red cells. Using laser photolysis of CO-Hb, deoxyHb is produced followed by detection of polymer formation by light scattering. The principle of this measurement is the observation that CO can be completely dissociated from hemoglobin by exposure to a focused laser beam at 514.5 nm, yielding deoxyhemoglobin and that this deoxyhemoglobin can be maintained with continuous photolysis with minimal heating. Polymerization can then be monitored by the method of choice such as light scattering.

New insights into nucleation, fiber growth, and factors affecting red cell shape have been obtained using differential interference contrast and birefringence.[78,79]

Clinical Evaluation of Hemoglobinopathies and Thalassemias using Protein-based and Cellular Diagnostics

When clinical evaluation, family history, or the results of a screening or routine blood count raise the possibility of a hemoglobinopathy or thalassemia, the first approach to diagnosis lies in the further evaluation of the erythrocyte indices, such as MCV or MCH, followed by expert examination of a peripheral blood film. The reticulocyte count, when persistently elevated is highly suggestive of hemolysis. As discussed in individual disease-specific chapters, peripheral blood smear morphology can provide clues to the diagnosis of most of the common hemoglobinopathies and thalassemia.

No single hemoglobin analytical procedure available in most clinical laboratories can distinguish definitively all common and clinically important variant hemoglobins, and rare variants can be especially difficult to resolve. The highest levels of hemoglobin-based diagnostics are limited to reference laboratories. The β thalassemias rely on quantitation of HbA_2 levels to detect heterozygotes, and some α thalassemias are characterized by HbH inclusion bodies. Quantitation of HbF is important for the diagnosis of thalassemia syndromes and HPFH.

If a hemoglobin variant is detected, the major clinical questions to be resolved are, what is the nature and abundance of the variant, and is it relevant to the clinical condition? In general, mutations of the β-globin gene usually cause only a single abnormal hemoglobin fraction, and if stable (Chapter 24), forms half of the total hemoglobin. In contrast, α-globin chain variants cause alterations in all hemoglobins, as all hemoglobins contain an α-globin chain. Usually, mutation of one α-globin gene creates variants forming 20%–25% of the total HbA, and proportionally similar fractions of the total HbA_2 and HbF. γ-Globin variants will alter a single major hemoglobin during fetal and neonatal life, but after the first year of life will alter only the small residual amount of HbF, and as a result, are rarely detected. Mutants of the δ-globin gene will alter only the HbA_2 band. The actual amounts of different hemoglobin types that accumulate in vivo depend on the expression of each globin gene, the stability of the monomer, dimer and tetramer, and on the posttranslational assembly of αβ dimers (Chapter 7).

Not all variant hemoglobins are resolvable using the commonly available protein-based means of detection, and a definitive diagnosis of rare variants is usually not possible with these methods. Therefore, rather than attempt the questionable, when definitive diagnosis is called for, it is best to move to DNA-based diagnostics.

DNA-BASED DIAGNOSIS OF THE HEMOGLOBIN DISORDERS

Hemoglobinopathies were the first genetic diseases to be characterized at the molecular level and consequently have been used as a prototype for the development of new techniques of mutation detection. Many different PCR-based techniques can be used to detect the known globin gene mutations, including dot blot analysis, reverse dot blot analysis, the amplification refractory mutation system (ARMS), denaturing gradient gel electrophoresis (DGGE), mutagenically separated polymerase chain reaction (MS-PCR), gap-PCR, and restriction endonuclease (RE) analysis. Each method has its advantages and disadvantages and the particular one chosen by a laboratory for the diagnosis of point mutations depends not only on the technical expertise available in the diagnostic laboratory but also on the type and variety of the mutations likely to be encountered in the individuals being screened.

The spectrum of α- and β-globin gene mutations is different for each population, and many mutations are regionally specific. Although more than 1,200 different globin gene alleles have been identified, mutation analysis is simplified by the fact that each country has only a few common alleles. Thus, a strategy is required for mutation diagnosis that involves knowledge of the ethnic group of the patient under study, the gene frequencies of the mutations in the ethnic group of the patient, and the appropriate method of mutation detection for those mutations. The following is an overview of the diagnostic methods currently being used worldwide for DNA-based diagnosis, including their use in antenatal diagnosis, and we describe strategies and the methods used in one large national laboratory for the diagnosis of mutations in an ethnically heterogeneous population. The approach used in ethnically homogeneous populations will be different and more focused.

SOURCES OF DNA

Blood

DNA is normally prepared from 5 to 10 mL of peripheral blood that is anticoagulated with heparin or preferably EDTA. The DNA can be isolated by the standard method of phenol–chloroform extraction and ethanol precipitation or by using one of several commercial kits based on salt extraction, protein precipitation etc. Sufficient DNA is obtained for both molecular analysis and subsequent storage in a DNA bank at −20°C.[80] If DNA banking is not required, a much smaller quantity of blood may be used for just PCR techniques. Mutation analysis may be performed by simply adding 1 μL of boiled whole blood to the PCR mixture.[81]

Amniotic Fluid

DNA can be prepared from amniotic fluid cells directly or after culturing. It is prudent to split an amniotic fluid sample into a sample to be sent for culturing and a sample for direct DNA analysis. It takes 2–3 weeks to grow amniocytes to confluence in a 25-mL flask, but culturing has the advantage that a large amount of DNA is obtained (the yield from such a flask has varied from 15 to 45 μg, enough DNA for all types of analyses). This provides a backup for failure with a direct analysis or material for confirmation in case of maternal contamination problems. A diagnosis can be made using DNA from the noncultivated cell sample in most cases. Approximately 2 μg of DNA is obtained from 7 mL of amniotic fluid and this is sufficient for all PCR-based methods of analysis. The method of DNA preparation for both cultured and noncultivated cells is essentially the same as that for chorionic villi.[80]

Chorionic Villi

The two main approaches to chorionic villus sampling, ultrasound-guided transcervical aspiration and ultrasound guided transabdominal sampling, provide good-quality samples of chorionic villi for fetal DNA diagnosis. Sufficient DNA is normally obtained for both PCR and Southern blot analysis of the globin genes. In 200 chorionic villus sampling DNA diagnoses, the average yield of DNA was 46 μg and only in one instance was less than 5 μg obtained.[80]

The main technical problem with this source of fetal DNA is the risk of contamination with maternal DNA, which arises from the maternal decidua that is sometimes obtained along with the chorionic villi. Careful dissection and removal of the maternal decidua with the aid of a phase-contrast microscope, yields pure fetal DNA samples, as shown by a report of 457 first trimester diagnoses for β thalassemia in Italians, without any misdiagnoses.[82] Maternal contamination can be ruled out in most cases by the presence of one maternal and one paternal allele following the amplification of highly polymorphic repeat markers. Originally, variable number tandem repeat (VNTR) polymorphic markers were amplified and analyzed by gel electrophoresis and ethidium bromide staining,[83] but now most laboratories have switched to using short tandem repeat markers or microsatellite polymorphic markers analyzed on a DNA sequencing machine.[84] The risk of misdiagnosis from maternal DNA contamination might be further reduced by the preparation and analysis of DNA from a cleaned single villus frond;[85] however, following a case in which a single frond appeared to give a different sickle cell genotype compared with the remaining chorionic villus sampling material, this techniques was abandoned.

Fetal Cells in Maternal Blood

Fetal cells have long been known to be present in the maternal circulation and they provide an attractive noninvasive approach to prenatal diagnosis, but attempts to isolate the fetal cells as a source of fetal DNA by using immunological methods and cell sorting have had only moderate success in providing a population of cells pure enough for fetal DNA analysis. Until recently, analysis of fetal cells in maternal blood could only be applied for the prenatal diagnosis of β thalassemia in women whose partners carried a different mutation, as reported for the diagnosis of Hb Lepore.[86] The development of the technique of isolation of single nucleated fetal erythrocytes by micromanipulation under microscopic observation[87] has permitted the analysis of both fetal genes in single cells from maternal blood. This approach has now been used successfully for prenatal diagnosis in two pregnancies at risk for sickle cell anemia and β thalassemia.[88] The approach has proved subject to technical difficulties and is costly and time consuming and so is not widely applicable.

Fetal DNA in Maternal Plasma

The analysis of fetal DNA in maternal plasma is a simpler and more robust procedure than the analysis of DNA in fetal nucleated red cells in maternal blood as no enrichment process is involved.[89] Cells are removed from the plasma by simple centrifugation and then the DNA in the plasma can be purified by standard methods.[90] Fetal DNA has been detected in as little as 10 mL of maternal plasma at 11–17 weeks gestation and is cleared very rapidly from the maternal plasma postpartum.[91] The technique is being used for the prenatal diagnosis of sex-linked disease and fetal RhD blood group type. The approach can only be used to detect the paternally inherited mutation and thus for β thalassemia it is limited in that it is only potentially applicable to couples in whom the paternal mutation is different than the maternal mutation. It has been used for the prenatal exclusion of β thalassemia major in eight fetuses at risk, using allele-specific primers for the detection of the CD 41/42 (-CTTT) mutation by real-time PCR[92] and the detection of homozygous α^0 thalassemia.[93] Further development of the method to detect both maternal and paternal linked polymorphisms might allow the technique to exclude maternal β thalassemia mutations.[94]

Preimplantation Diagnosis

Preimplantation genetic diagnosis represents a state-of-the-art procedure that allows at risk couples to have disease-free children without the need to terminate affected pregnancies. PCR-based diagnostic methods can be potentially applied for preimplantation genetic diagnosis using three types of cells: polar bodies from the oocyte/zygote stage, blastomeres from cleavage stage embryos, and trophectoderm cells from blastocysts.[95] Although the technique requires a combined expertise in both reproductive medicine and molecular genetics, a small number of centers around the world can now perform this procedure for hemoglobin disorders, resulting in the birth of more than 50 healthy children. Preimplantation diagnosis has been used successfully for both α[96,97] and β thalassemia.[98,99] The approach is especially useful for couples for whom religious or ethical beliefs will not permit the termination of pregnancy, and for couples who have already had one or more therapeutic abortions.

Nevertheless, preimplantation genetic diagnosis is technically challenging, multistep, and expensive. The PCR protocol must be able to detect accurately the required genotype in single cells, be optimized to minimize PCR failure and avoid the problem of allele drop out, which could lead to misdiagnosis. Protocols designed to monitor the occurrence of allele drop out include multiplex PCR to detect both alleles that contribute to the genotype, such as DGGE, single-strand conformation analysis and real time PCR.[100] The birth of a healthy unaffected baby depends not only on an accurate diagnosis, but also on the success of each of the multiple stages of the assisted reproduction procedure. Overall, the success rate of the procedure is only 20%–30% and thus this approach is not likely to be used routinely for the monitoring of pregnancies at risk for hemoglobin disorders. One specific use of this approach is to allow the birth of a normal child who is HLA identical to an affected sibling, thus permitting a possible cure by stem cell transplantation.[20]

DNA DIAGNOSIS OF α THALASSEMIA

α Thalassemia is almost always a result of mutations affecting either one α-globin gene (α^+ thalassemia) or both α-globin genes on the same chromosome (α^0 thalassemia) (Chapter 13). The majority of the mutations are gene deletions but some point mutations in one of the two α-globin genes resulting in α^+ thalassemia have been described. The deletion breakpoints of the seven most common deletion alleles have been determined, and these deletions can be diagnosed quickly by the technique known as gap-PCR (Table 28.1). The remainder of the deletion alleles used to be diagnosed by Southern blot analysis,[101] but now are diagnosed by the technique called multiplex ligation–dependent probe amplification (MLPA).[102]

Diagnostic Strategy

α^0 Thalassemia is found in mainly patients of Mediterranean or Southeast Asian in origin. Although α^0 thalassemia has been described in patients of Asian Indian or African origin, it is extremely uncommon, and patients with the phenotype of α^0 thalassemia trait usually have the genotype of homozygous α^+ thalassemia. α^+ Thalassemia can reach high gene frequencies in parts of Africa and Asia, with the -$\alpha^{3.7}$ deletion being the predominant mutation in African, Mediterranean, and Asian individuals and the -$\alpha^{4.2}$ being more common in Southeast Asian and the Pacific islands populations. The strategy for screening is based on ethnic origin of the individual, although PCR now makes it easy to screen for all the common deletion mutations in any individual.

In multiethnic countries like the United Kingdom and United States the ethnic origin of carriers of α thalassemia include individuals of African, Indian, Pakistani, Chinese, Southeast Asian, Greek Cypriot, and Turkish Cypriot descent and occasionally members of the indigenous population. In this environment, screening is first done for the -$\alpha^{3.7}$-kb and -$\alpha^{4.2}$-kb α^+ thalassemia deletions by multiplex gap-PCR. If indicated by the MCH, MCV, or suspected HbH disease, screening is next done for α^0 thalassemia deletions by multiplex gap-PCR for either the Mediterranean or Southeast Asian deletions according to an individuals' ethnic origin. If negative results are still obtained, screening for nondeletion mutations by selective DNA sequencing of both α-globin genes for suspected α^+ thalassemia carriers and screening, for other deletions by MLPA analysis in suspected α^0 thalassemia carriers can also be done. All prenatal diagnoses for α^0 thalassemia are carried out by both gap-PCR and MLPA.

Table 28.1. Globin gene disorder deletions diagnosable by gap-PCR

Disorder	Deletion mutation	Distribution
α^0 Thalassemia	--^{SEA}	Southeast Asia
	--^{MED}	Mediterranean
	-(α)$^{20.5}$	Mediterranean
	--^{FIL}	Philippines
	--^{THAI}	Thailand
α^+ Thalassemia	-$\alpha^{3.7}$	Worldwide
	-$\alpha^{4.2}$	Worldwide
β^0 Thalassemia	290-bp deletion	Turkey, Bulgaria
$(\delta\beta)^0$ Thalassemia	532-bp deletion	Africa
	619-bp deletion	India, Pakistan
	1393-bp deletion	Africa
	1605-bp deletion	Croatia
	3.5-kb deletion	Thailand
	10.3-kb deletion	India
	45-kb deletion	Philippines, Malaysia
	Hb Lepore	Mediterranean, Brazil
$(^A\gamma\delta\beta)^0$ Thalassemia	Spanish	Spain
	Sicilian	Mediterranean
	Vietnamese	Vietnam
	Macedonian/Turkish	Macedonia, Turkey
	Indian	India, Bangladesh
	Chinese	Southern China
HPFH	HPFH1	Africa
	HPFH2	Ghana
	HPFH3	India
	Hb Kenya	Africa

Diagnosis of Deletion Mutations by PCR

The two most common α^+ thalassemia gene deletions, the -$\alpha^{3.7}$ and -$\alpha^{4.2}$ alleles, together with 5 α^0 thalassemia deletion genes, the --^{FIL}, --^{THAI}, --^{MED}, -(α)$^{20.5}$, and the --^{SEA} alleles can be diagnosed by gap-PCR[81,103–106] (Table 28.1). Gap-PCR is the simplest of amplification techniques, using two primers complimentary to the sense and antisense strand of the DNA regions that flank the deletion. Amplified product is only obtained from the α thalassemia deletion allele as the primers are located too far apart on the normal DNA sequence for successful amplification. Therefore, the normal allele ($\alpha\alpha$) is detected by amplifying across

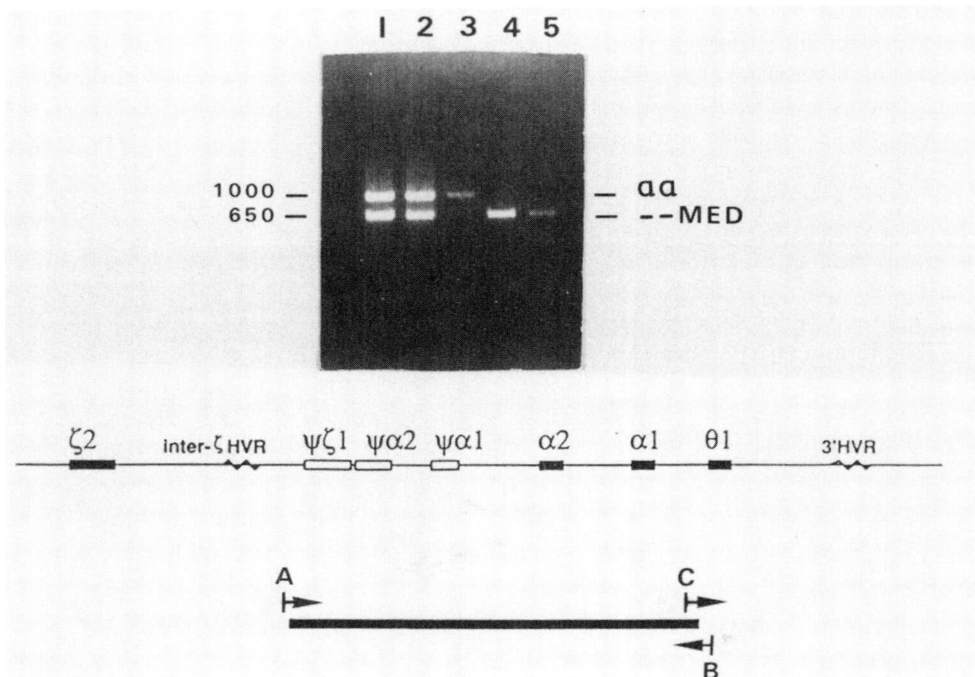

Figure 28.7. Prenatal diagnosis of the --^{MED} α^0 thalassemia allele by using gap-PCR. The amplification products after agarose gel electrophoresis and ethidium bromide staining are shown as follows: track 1, maternal DNA; track 2, paternal DNA; track 3, normal DNA; and tracks 4 and 5, different concentrations of chorionic villi DNA. The diagram below shows the location of the --^{MED} deletion with respect to the α-globin gene cluster. Primers A and B span the deletion and amplify --^{MED} allele to give a 650-bp product; primers B and C span one breakpoint and amplify the normal allele to give a 1000-bp product.

one of the breakpoints, using one primer complimentary to the deleted sequence and one to the normal sequence. An example of the use of gap-PCR for the prenatal diagnosis of the Mediterranean α^0 thalassemia mutation --^{MED} is illustrated in Figure 28.7.

Gap-PCR provides a quick diagnostic test for α^0 thalassemia trait but requires careful application for prenatal diagnosis. Prenatal diagnosis results by gap-PCR should be confirmed by MLPA analysis. Amplification of sequences in the α-globin gene cluster is technically more difficult than that of the β-globin gene cluster, requiring more stringent conditions for success due to the higher GC content of the α-globin gene cluster.[107] For a more reliable diagnosis of the carrier state by gap-PCR, amplification of the GC-rich α-globin locus can be improved by using betaine and dimethyl sulfoxide in the PCR reaction. These agents enhance the reaction by disrupting the base pairing of the GC-rich region and lead to the destabilization of the secondary structure by making the GC and AT base pairs equally stable in the DNA duplex. The application of these agents with redesigned primers has lead to the development of multiplex assays to detect heterozygosity and homozygosity of the seven deletion mutations.[81,108] Experience has shown that great care is still needed in interpreting the results, as some tests still result occasionally in unpredictable reaction failure and allele drop out. Testing several different dilutions of a DNA sample can help resolve this problem, as the inhibition causing allele drop out can be diluted out.

Other approaches have been developed to provide quick, simple, rapid, accurate, and cost effective methods of screening for the deletion mutations. These include the use of real-time quantitative PCR analysis for the Southeast Asian α^0 thalassemia deletion in Taiwan,[109] the use of denaturing HPLC to diagnose the 4.2-kb α^+ thalassemia deletion gene in Chinese individuals,[110] real-time quantitative PCR to detect the Southeast Asian α^0 thalassemia deletion,[93] and the use of an oligonucleotide microarray to detect the Southeast Asian α^0 thalassemia deletion and the -$\alpha^{3.7}$-kb and -$\alpha^{4.2}$ -kb α^+ thalassemia deletions.[111,112] The most useful recent development for the diagnosis of deletion mutations is MLPA.[102] In this method, two sets of 35 probes have been developed to detect all known deletions located in the α-globin gene cluster on chromosome 16p13.3. This method will detect rare and novel forms of deletional α thalassemia that cannot be diagnosed by gap-PCR and provides an excellent back-up screening method for the common deletion mutations. In some cases, MLPA can replace Southern blotting for the routine diagnosis of α^0 thalassemia deletions.

Diagnosis of Point Mutations by PCR

The nondeletion α^+ thalassemia mutations can be identified by PCR techniques following the selective amplification of the α-globin genes.[113] This technique allows the amplified product from each α-globin gene to be analyzed for the expected known mutation according to the ethnic origin of the patient or for the gene to be sequenced to identify new mutations. Selective amplification followed by DNA sequence analysis is a reasonable approach for the diagnosis of all nondeletion α^+ thalassemia mutations.

Several of the nondeletion α^+ thalassemia mutations create or destroy a restriction enzyme site and can be analyzed for by restriction enzyme digestion of the amplified product. For example, Hb Constant Spring mutation can be diagnosed by *Mse* I digestion.[114] In theory, any technique for the direct detection of point mutations such as allele specific oligonucleotide hybridization or allele specific priming can be used for the diagnosis of nondeletion α^+ thalassemia mutations. No simple strategy to diagnose all the known mutations has been developed however. The only published approach to date is a complex strategy involving the combined application of the indirect detection methods of DGGE and single-strand conformation analysis, followed by direct DNA sequencing.[115]

DNA DIAGNOSIS OF β THALASSEMIA

Although more than 200 different β-globin gene mutations have been associated with the phenotype of thalassemia, only approximately 30 mutations are found in at risk groups at a frequency of 1% or greater (as listed in Table 28.2), and thus just a small number account for the majority of the mutations worldwide.[116] All of the mutations are regionally specific and the spectrum of mutations has now been determined for most at risk populations.[117] Each population has been found to have just a few of the common mutations together with a larger and more variable number of rare mutations. This makes it easy to screen for β thalassemia mutations in most cases if the ethnic origin of the patient is known.

Diagnostic Strategy

The strategy for identifying β thalassemia mutations in most diagnostic laboratories is to screen for the common ones first using a PCR-based technique that allows the detection of multiple mutations simultaneously. This approach will identify the mutation in more than 90% of cases. Further screening for the possible rare mutation will identify the defect in most of the remaining cases. Mutations remaining unknown after this second screening are characterized by direct DNA sequence analysis. The β-globin gene can be amplified simultaneously in three sections of approximately 500 bp in length for direct DNA sequence analysis using an automatic DNA sequencer. Alternatively, the site of the mutation can be localized first by the application of a nonspecific detection method such as DGGE and then the mutation identified using just one sequencing reaction. Although a bewildering variety of PCR techniques have been described for the molecular diagnosis of point mutations, most diagnostic laboratories are using one or more of the techniques described herein.

Panels of primers for the detection of the common mutations in each ethnic group can be developed by the primer-specific amplification method known as ARMS. Panels for the common Mediterranean, Asian Indian, Chinese, and African mutations are available along with a panel for the most common silent or normal HbA_2 β thalassemia mutations. Rare or novel mutations are then diagnosed by DNA sequence analysis. Prenatal diagnosis results for β thalassemia are confirmed by a second method, either by restriction enzyme analysis of amplified product (RE-PCR), or more usually, by DNA sequence analysis.

Allele-specific Oligonucleotide PCR

The hybridization of allele-specific oligonucleotide (ASOs) probes to amplified genomic DNA bound to a nylon membrane in the form of dots was the first PCR method to be developed. This method, known as dot blotting, is based on the use of two oligonucleotide probes for each mutation, one complimentary to the mutant DNA sequence and the other complimentary to the normal β-globin gene sequence at the same position. The probes are usually 5′ end-labeled with ^{32}P-labeled deoxynucleoside triphosphates, biotin, or horseradish peroxidase. The genotype of the DNA sample is diagnosed by observing the presence or absence of a hybridization signal from the mutation specific and normal probes. The technique has been applied in many laboratories with great success, especially for populations with just one common and a small number of rare mutations, as in the example of Sardinia.[118] When screening for a large number of different mutations, this method becomes limited by the need for separate hybridization and washing step for the detection of each mutation.

To overcome this problem of screening for multiple mutations, the technique of reverse dot blotting has been developed in which the roles of the oligonucleotide probe and the amplified genomic DNA are reversed.[119] Unlabeled oligonucleotide probes complementary to the mutant and normal DNA sequences are fixed to a nylon membrane strip in the form of dots or slots. Amplified genomic DNA, labeled by either the use of end-labeled primers or the internal incorporation of biotinylated deoxyuridine triphosphate, is then hybridized to the filter. This allows multiple mutations to be tested in one hybridization reaction. It has been applied to the diagnosis of β thalassemia mutations in Mediterranean individuals,[120] African Americans,[121] and Thais,[122] using a two-step procedure with one nylon strip for the common and another for the less common mutations.

Reverse hybridization screening is the only technique for the diagnosis of β thalassemia mutations to have been developed commercially with some success and there are currently there are two competing systems on the market. One uses a strip with oligonucleotide probes for eight common Mediterranean mutations affixed together with probes to detect HbS and HbC mutations in amplified DNA. Another uses nucleotides complementary to mutant and

Table 28.2. The distribution of the common β thalassemia mutations expressed as percentage gene frequencies of the total number of thalassemia chromosomes studied

	Mediterranean			Indian		Chinese		African
Mutation	Italy	Greece	Turkey	Pakistan	India	China	Thailand	African-American
-88 (C$\rightarrow$T)					0.8			21.4
-87 (C$\rightarrow$G)	0.4	1.8	1.2					
-30 (T$\rightarrow$A)			2.5					
-29 (A$\rightarrow$G)						1.9		60.3
-28 (A$\rightarrow$G)						11.6	4.9	
CAP + 1 (A$\rightarrow$C)					1.7			
CD5 (-CT)		1.2	0.8					
CD6 (-A)	0.4	2.9	0.6					
CD8 (-AA)		0.6	7.4					
CD8/9 (+G)				28.9	12.0			
CD15 (G$\rightarrow$A)				3.5	0.8			0.8
CD16 (-C)				1.3	1.7			
CD17 (A$\rightarrow$T)						10.5	24.7	
CD24 (T$\rightarrow$A)								7.9
CD30 (G$\rightarrow$A)				0.9				
CD30 (G$\rightarrow$C)				3.5	0.9			
CD39 (C$\rightarrow$T)	40.1	17.4	3.5					
CD41/42 (-TCTT)				7.9	13.7	38.6	46.4	
CD71/72 (+A)						12.4	2.3	
IVSI-1 (G$\rightarrow$A)	4.3	13.6	2.5					
IVSI-1 (G$\rightarrow$T)				8.2	6.6			
IVSI-5 (G$\rightarrow$C)				26.4	48.5	2.5	4.9	
IVSI-6 (T$\rightarrow$C)	16.3	7.4	17.4					
IVSI-110 (G$\rightarrow$A)	29.8	43.7	41.9					
IVSII-1(G$\rightarrow$A)	1.1	2.1	9.7					
IVSII-654 (C$\rightarrow$T)						15.7	8.9	
IVSII-745 (C$\rightarrow$G)	3.5	7.1	2.7					
619-bp deletion				23.3	13.3			
Others	4.1	2.2	9.7	0.5	0.9	6.8	7.9	10.6

CD = Codon; IVS = intervening sequence.

normal sequences immobilized in the wells of a microplate and thus is more complex, requiring a dedicated microplate incubator, washer, and reader. Two kits, one for eight common Mediterranean mutations and one for the eight most common Southeast Asian β-thalassemia mutations, including HbE, are available.

Oligonucleotide Microarrays

The principle of reverse dot blotting has been brought up to date by the development of microarrays for the simultaneous detection of multiple β thalassemia mutations. Several groups have now published details of a DNA chip platform that has been used to genotype β thalassemia carriers and patients.[112,123] The approach of tagged single-based extension and hybridization to glass or flow-through arrays has been developed for the detection of 17 β-globin gene mutations[124] and a similar approach of arrayed primer extension has been used to detect 23 mutations.[125] It is not clear whether these state-of-the-art methods will be economically viable and replace conventional techniques in the future. This will depend on the market for thalassemia mutation chips, especially for the diagnosis of mutations in populations with just one or two very common mutations that can be easily screened for by rapid low-technology methods and for which the additional screening capacity on the chip would be redundant.

Primer-specific Amplification

Different diagnostic methods have been developed based on the principle of primer-specific amplification, where

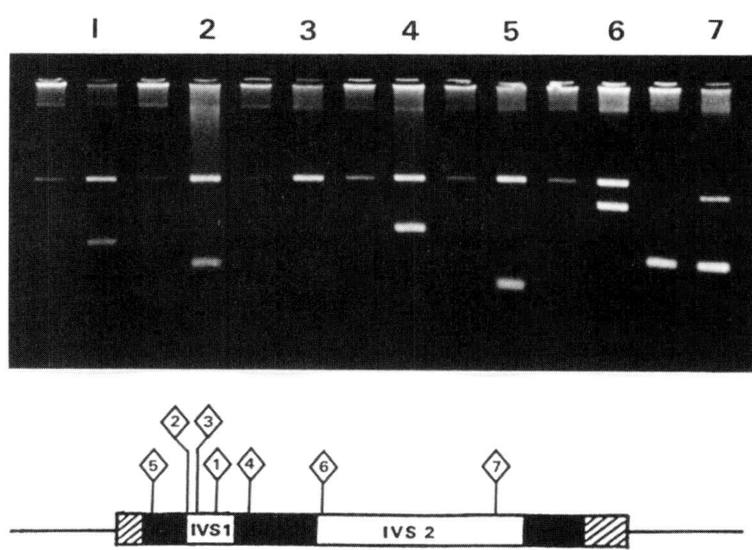

Figure 28.8. ARMS-PCR screening of a DNA sample for seven common Mediterranean mutations. The gel shows alternating tracks containing the amplification products from DNA of a patient with β thalassemia trait and those from control DNA for each of the seven mutations (labeled 1–7). The mutations screened for are: 1, IVSI-110 (G→A); 2, IVSI-1 (G→A); 3, IVSI-6 (T→C); 4, codon 39 (C→T); 5, codon 6 (-A); 6, IVSII-1 (G→A); 7, IVSII-745 (C→G); as shown in the diagram of the β gene. In the first 12 tracks, the control primers D and E (Table 28.4) were used (producing an 861-bp fragment), and in the last 2 tracks, the $^{G}\gamma$-*Hind* III RFLP control primers were used (producing a 323-bp fragment).

a perfectly matched PCR primer is much more efficient in annealing and directing primer extension than a mismatched primer. The most widely used method is ARMS, in which a primer will only permit amplification to take place when it perfectly matches the target DNA sequence at the 3′ terminal nucleotide.[126] The target DNA is amplified using a common primer and either of two allele specific primers, two complimentary to the mutation to be detected (the β thalassemia primer) and the other complimentary to normal DNA sequence at the same position. The method provides a quick screening assay that does not require any form of labelling as the amplified products are visualized by agarose gel electrophoresis and ethidium bromide staining. ARMS primers were first developed for the screening and prenatal diagnosis of β thalassemia mutations in the Asian Indian and Cypriot populations in the United Kingdom.[127] Subsequently, ARMS primers have been designed to screen for the common mutations of all ethnic groups.[128] Figure 28.8 shows the results of a screening a Cypriot individual with β thalassemia trait for seven common mutations by ARMS-PCR. Details of the mutation-specific and normal sequence-specific primers used to diagnose the common β thalassemia mutations are presented in Tables 28.3 and 28.4. ARMS-PCR is currently the main approach for mutation detection and prenatal diagnosis for β thalassemia, HbE–thalassemia, and the sickling disorders in the United Kingdom. The technique has been established in nations such as India because of its rapidity and economy, making realistic for the first time the development of a prenatal diagnostic service in developing countries.[129]

Other variations on the primer-specific amplification theme are multiplex ARMS, competitive oligonucleotide priming (COP)–PCR and mutagenetically separated (MS)-PCR. More than one mutation can be screened for at the same time in a single PCR reaction by multiplexing the ARMS primers provided that they are coupled with the same common primer.[130] Fluorescent labeling of the common primer allows the sizing of the amplification products on an automated DNA fragment analyzer.[131] If the normal and mutant ARMS primers for a specific mutation are coamplified in the same reaction they compete with each other to amplify the target sequence. This technique is called COP and requires the two ARMS primers to be labeled differently. Fluorescent labels permit a diagnosis to be made by means of a color complementation assay.[132] A variation of this method is to use ARMS primers that differ in length instead of the label. The primers compete with each other to produce fragments that can be distinguished simply by agarose gel electrophoresis. Normal, heterozygous and homozygous DNAs are diagnosed by simple analysis of the presence or absence of the two products. This technique, called MS-PCR, has been applied to the prenatal diagnosis of β thalassemia in Taiwan.[133]

Restriction Enzyme PCR

This is a useful but limited technique because very few β thalassemia mutations create or abolish a restriction endonuclease site and generate diagnosable products (Table 28.5). The presence or absence of the enzyme recognition site is determined from the pattern of fragments of digested fragments after agarose or polyacrylamide gel electrophoresis. Mutations that do not naturally create or abolish restriction sites may be diagnosed by the technique of amplification created restriction sites. This method uses primers that are designed to insert new bases into the amplified product to create a restriction enzyme recognition site adjacent to the mutation sequence. This technique

Table 28.3. Primer sequences used for the detection of common mutations for β thalassemia and β-globin chain variants by the allele-specific priming technique

Mutation	Oligonucleotide sequence	Second primer	Product size (bp)
β-Thalassemia			
-88 (C→T)	TCACTTAGACCTCACCCTGTGGAGCCTCAT	A	684
-87 (C→G)	CACTTAGACCTCACCCTGTGGAGCCACCCG	A	683
-30 (T→A)	GCAGGGAGGGCAGGAGCCAGGGCTGGGGAA	A	626
-29 (A→G)	CAGGGAGGGCAGGAGCCAGGGCTGGGTATG	A	625
-28 (A→G)	AGGGAGGGCAGGAGCCAGGGCTGGGCTTAG	A	624
CAP + 1 (A→G)	ATAAGTCAGGGCAGAGCCATCTATTGGTTC	A	597
CD5 (-CT)	TCAAACAGACACCATGGTGCACCTGAGTCG	A	528
CD6 (-A)	CCCACAGGGCAGTAACGGCAGACTTCTGCC	B	207
CD8 (-AA)	ACACCATGGTGCACCTGACTCCTGAGCAGG	A	520
CD8/9 (+G)	CCTTGCCCCACAGGGCAGTAACGGCACACC	B	225
CD15 (G→A)	TGAGGAGAAGTCTGCCGTTACTGCCCAGTA	A	500
CD16 (-C)	TCACCACCAACTTCATCCACGTTCACGTTC	B	238
CD17 (A→T)	CTCACCACCAACTTCAGCCACGTTCAGCTA	B	239
CD24 (T→A)	CTTGATACCAACCTGCCCAGGGCCTCTCCT	B	262
CD30 (G→A)	TAAACGTGTCTTGTAACCTTGATACCTACT	B	280
CD30 (G→C)	TAAACCTGTCTTGTAACCTTGATACCTACG	B	280
CD39 (C→T)	CAGATCCCCAAAGGACTCAAAGAACCTGTA	B	436
CD41/42 (-TCTT)	GAGTGGACAGATCCCCAAAGGACTCAACCT	B	439
CD71-72 (+A)	CATGGCAAGAAAGTGCTCGGTGCCTTTAAG	C	241
IVSI-1 (G→A)	TTAAACCTGTCTTGTAACCTTGATACCGAT	B	281
IVSI-1 (G→T)	TTAAACCTGTCTTGTAACCTTGATACCGAAA	B	281
IVSI-5 (G→C)	CTCCTTAAACCTGTCTTGTAACCTTGTTAG	B	285
IVSI-6 (T→C)	TCTCCTTAAACCTGTCTTGTAACCTTCATG	B	286
IVSI-110 (G→A)	ACCAGCAGCCTAAGGGTGGGAAAATAGAGT	B	419
IVSII-1 (G→A)	AAGAAAACATCAAGGGTCCCATAGACTGAT	B	634
IVSII-654 (C→T)	GAATAACAGTGATAATTTCTGGGTTAACGT*	D	829
IVSII-745 (C→G)	TCATATTGCTAATAGCAGCTACAATCGAGG*	D	738
β-variants			
β^{S}CD6 (A→T)	CCCACAGGGCAGTAACGGCAGACTTCTGCA	B	207
β^{C}CD6 (G→A)	CCACAGGGCAGTAACGGCAGACTTCTCGTT	B	206
β^{E}CD26 (G→A)	TAACCTTGATACCAACCTGCCCAGGGCGTT	B	236
$\beta^{D\text{-}Punjab}$CD121 (G→C)	TCTGTGTGCTGGCCCATCACTTTGGCAAGC	E	250
$\beta^{D\text{-}Iran}$CD22 (G→C)	CAACCTGCCAGGGCCTCACCACCAACATG	B	255

The above primers are coupled as indicated with primers A, B, C, or D.
A: CCCCTTCCTATGACATGAACTTAA
B: ACCTCACCCTGTGGAGCCAC
C: TTCGTCTGTTTCCCATTCTAAACT
D: GAGTCAAGGCTGAGAGATGCAGGA
E: GGCAGAATCCAGATGCTCAAGGCCCTTC
F: CAATGTATCATGCCTCTTTGCACC
The control primers used for all the above mutation-specific ARMS primers except the two marked * are primers D plus F. For IVSII-654(C→T) and IVSII-745(C→G), the $^{G}\gamma$-*Hind* III RFLP primers (listed in Table 28.6) are used as control primers.

Table 28.4. Primer sequences used for the detection of normal DNA sequence by the allele-specific priming technique

Mutation	Oligonucleotide sequence	Second primer	Product size (bp)
-88 (C→T)	TCACTTAGACCTCACCCTGTGGAGCCACTC	A	684
-87 (C→G)	CACTTAGACCTCACCCTGTGGAGCCACCCC	A	683
CD5 (-CT)	CAAACAGACACCATGGTGCACCTGACTCCT	A	528
CD6 (-A)	CACAGGGCAGTAACGGCAGACTTCTCCTCA	B	207
CD8 (-AA)	ACACCATGGTGCACCTGACTCCTGAGCAGA	A	520
CD8/9 (+G)	CCTTGCCCCACAGGGCAGTAACGGCACACT	B	225
CD15 (G→A)	TGAGGAGAAGTCTGCCGTTACTGCCCAGTA	A	500
CD30 (G→C)	TAAACCTGTCTTGTAACCTTGATACCTACC	B	280
CD39 (C→T)	TTAGGCTGCTGGTGGTCTACCCTTGGTCCC	A	299
CD41/42 (-TCTT)	GAGTGGACAGATCCCCAAAGGACTCAAAGA	B	439
IVSI-1 (G→A)	TTAAACCTGTCTTGTAACCTTGATACCCAC	B	281
IVSI-1 (G→T)	GATGAAGTTGGTGGTGAGGCCCTGGGTAGG	A	455
IVSI-5 (G→C)	CTCCTTAAACCTGTCTTGTAACCTTGTTAC	B	285
IVSI-6 (T→C)	AGTTGGTGGTGAGGCCCTGGGCAGGTTGGT	A	449
IVSI-110 (G→A)	ACCAGCAGCCTAAGGGTGGGAAAATACACC	B	419
IVSII-1 (G→A)	AAGAAAACATCAAGGGTCCCATAGACTGAC	B	634
IVSII-654 (C→T)	GAATAACAGTGATAATTTCTGGGTTAACGC	D	829
IVSII-745 (C→G)	TCATATTGCTAATAGCAGCTACAATCGAGC	D	738
β-variants			
^{S}CD6 (A→T)	AACAGACACCATGGTGCACCTGACTCGTGA	A	527
$β^{E}$CD26 (G→A)	TAACCTTGATACCAACCTGCCCAGGGCGTC	B	236

See Table 28.3 legend for details of primers A–D and control primers.

has been applied to the detection of Mediterranean β thalassemia mutations.[134]

Other Methods for Point Mutations

Many other techniques for the diagnosis of known β-globin gene point mutations have been published, including the use of denaturing high-performance liquid chromatography (DHPLC), the DNA ligase reaction, minisequencing, real-time PCR and multiplex primer extension technology. For example, DHPLC has been used for the analysis of polymorphic duplexes created by allele-specific priming,[135] the analysis of five common Southeast Asian mutations by multiplex minisequencing,[136] multiplex primer extension analysis for 10 Taiwanese mutations[137] and the most common Chinese mutations,[138] and the screening for 11 most common Greek mutations.[139] Real-time PCR quantification and melting curve analysis using LightCycler technology have been used to provide rapid genotyping for a panel of the 10 most frequent Greek mutations[100] and six Lebanese mutations.[140] The DNA ligase method has been updated by the development of a novel piezoelectrical method for detection of a single base mutation in codon 17 of the β-globin gene using nano-gold-amplified DNA probes.[141] All provide rapid and accurate genotyping of the common mutations and are worth considering as alternative diagnostic approaches for point mutations.

Gap-PCR and MLPA

Deletions in the β-globin gene cluster are detected by gap-PCR and/or MLPA analysis. Table 28.1 lists the deletions detectable by gap-PCR. Small deletion mutations in the β-globin gene sequence may be detected by PCR using two primers complimentary to the sense and antisense strand in the DNA regions that flank the deletion.[142–149] For large deletions, amplified product using flanking primers is obtained only from the deletion allele because the distance between the two primers is too great to amplify normal DNA. As is the case with the α thalassemia deletions, the normal allele may be detected by amplifying sequences spanning one of the breakpoints, using a primer complimentary to the deleted sequence and one complimentary to flanking DNA.

PCR Methods for Unknown Mutations

A number of techniques have been applied for the characterization of β-thalassemia mutations without prior knowledge of the molecular defect. The most widely used

Table 28.5. β-thalassemia mutations detectable by RE-PCR

Position	Mutation	Ethnic group	Affected site
-88	C→T	African/Asian Indian	+*Fok* I
-87	C→G	Mediterranean	-*Avr* II
-87	C→T	Italian	-*Avr* II
-87	C→A	African/Yugoslavian	-*Avr* II
-86	C→G	Lebanese	-*Avr* II
-86	C→A	Italian	-*Avr* II
-29	A→G	African/Chinese	+*Nla* III
+43 to +40	(-AAAC)	Chinese	+*Dde* I
Initiation CD	T→C	Yugoslavian	-*Nco* I
Initiation CD	T→G	Chinese	-*Nco* I
Initiation CD	A→G	Japanese	-*Nco* I
CD 5	(-CT)	Mediterranean	-*Dde* I
CD 6	(-A)	Mediterranean	-*Dde* I
CD 15	(-T)	Asian Indian	+*Bgl* I
CD 17	A→T	Chinese	+*Mae* I
CD 26	G→T	Thai	-*Mnl* I
CD 26	G→A	Southeast Asian	-*Mnl* I
CD 27	G→T	Mediterranean	-*Sau*96 I
CD 29	C→T	Lebanese	-*Bsp*M I
CD 30	G→C	Tunisian/African	-*Bsp*M I
CD 30	G→A	Bulgarian	-*Bsp*M I
IVSI-1	G→A	Mediterranean	-*Bsp*M I
IVSI-1	G→T	Asian Indian/Chinese	-*Bsp*M I
IVSI-2	T→G	Tunisian	-*Bsp*M I
IVSI-2	T→C	African	-*Bsp*M I
IVSI-2	T→A	Algerian	-*Bsp*M I
IVSI-5	G→A	Mediterranean	+*Eco*R V
IVSI-6	T→C	Mediterranean	+*Sfa*N I
IVSI-116	T→G	Mediterranean	+*Mae* I
IVSI-130	G→C	Turkish	-*Dde* I
IVSI-130	G→A	Egyptian	-*Dde* I
CD 35	C→A	Thai	-*Acc* I
CD 37	G→A	Saudi Arabian	-*Ava* II
CD 38/39	(-C)	Czechoslovakian	-*Ava* II
CD 37/8/9	(-GACCCAG)	Turkish	-*Ava* II
CD 39	C→T	Mediterranean	+*Mae* I
CD 43	G→T	Chinese	-*Hinf* I
CD 47	(+A)	Surinamese	-*Xho* I
CD 61	A→T	African	-*Hph* I
CD 74/75	(-C)	Turkish	-*Hae* III
CD 121	G→T	Polish, French, Japanese	-*Eco*R I
IVSII-1	G→A	Mediterranean	-*Hph* I
IVSII-4,5	(-AG)	Portuguese	-*Hph* I
IVSII-745	C→G	Mediterranean	+*Rsa* I

of these methods is DGGE, which allows the separation of DNA fragments differing by a single base change according to their melting properties.[150] The technique involves the electrophoresis of double-stranded DNA fragments through a linearly increasing denaturing gradient until the lowest melting temperature domain of the fragment denatures, creating a branched molecule that effectively becomes stationary in the gel matrix. DNA fragments differing by 1 bp in the low melting temperature domain have different melting temperatures and can be separated in most but not all cases. The β-globin gene is amplified in segments using five–seven pairs of primers, one of each pair having a GC-rich sequence added to it to create a high melting domain. Heterozygous DNA creates four bands, two heteroduplexes of normal and mutant sequence and two homoduplexes, one of normal sequence and the other of mutant sequence. DGGE has been used for prenatal diagnosis of β thalassemia in India[151] and also for the analysis of point mutations resulting in δ thalassemia and nondeletion HPFH.[152,153]

Another approach by heteroduplex analysis is using nondenaturing gel electrophoresis. Unique heteroduplex patterns can be generated for each mutation by annealing an amplified target DNA fragment with an amplified heteroduplex generator molecule, a synthetic oligonucleotide of approximately 130 bases in length containing deliberate sequence changes or identifiers at known mutation positions.[154] Other methods such as mismatch cleavage, single-strand conformation polymorphism, and protein truncation test have been used to detect unknown mutations but they have not been applied specifically to the diagnosis of hemoglobinopathies or thalassemias. These techniques simply pinpoint the presence of a mutation or DNA polymorphism in the amplified target sequence. Sequencing of the amplified product can then be performed manually or automatically to identify the localized mutation. This can now be done very efficiently with an automated DNA sequencing machine and fluorescence detection technology.

Although it is clear that many novel detection methods have been developed and used, many large laboratories prefer direct DNA sequencing of amplified product as the primary method of identifying rare or unknown β thalassemia mutations. Once a rare or novel mutation has been identified through DNA sequencing, the DNA sample can be used as a control for the development of ARMS primers to provide a more rapid and cheaper screening of further cases.[155]

β-Globin Gene Haplotype Analysis

At least 18 restriction fragment length polymorphisms (RFLPs) have been characterized within the β-globin gene cluster.[156] Conveniently, most of these RFLP sites are nonrandomly associated with each other and they combine to produce just a handful of haplotypes[157] (Chapter 27). In particular, they form a 5′ cluster from the ε-globin gene to the δ-globin gene and a 3′ cluster around the β-globin gene, with a relative hot spot for meiotic recombination in between.[158] Each β thalassemia mutation is strongly associated with just one or two common haplotypes, and haplotype analysis has been used extensively to study the origin of globin gene mutations found in different ethnic groups[159] (Chapter 27).

The β-globin gene cluster haplotype normally consists of five RFLPs located in the 5′ cluster (*Hin*d II/ε-gene; *Hin*d III/$^G\gamma$-gene; *Hin*d III/$^A\gamma$-gene; *Hin*d II/3′ψβ; and *Hin*d II/5′ψβ) and two RFLPs in the 3′ cluster (*Ava* II/β-gene; *Bam*H I/β-gene). All the RFLPs can be easily analyzed by RE-PCR except the *Bam*H I polymorphism, for which a *Hin*f I RFLP located just 3′ to the β-globin gene is used instead, because these two RFLPs have been found to exist in linkage disequilibrium.[160] The primer sequences together with the sizes of the fragments generated are listed in Table 28.6. Primers for three other useful RFLPs are also listed: an *Ava* II RFLP in the ψβ-gene; a *Rsa* I RFLP located just 5′ to the β-globin gene; and the $^G\gamma$-*Xmn* I RFLP C→T polymorphism at position −158 5′ to the $^G\gamma$-globin gene that acts as a nondeletion HPFH allele under conditions of erythropoietic stress, raising the HbF level in patients with β thalassemia or sickle cell anemia (Chapters 27 and 30).

DNA DIAGNOSIS OF δβ THALASSEMIA, Hb LEPORE, AND HPFH

The δβ thalassemia, Hb Lepore, and HPFH deletion mutations were characterized originally by restriction endonuclease mapping and Southern blotting, but gap-PCR is now used for the diagnosis of the common mutations (Table 28.1). This technique is useful for the diagnosis of Hb Lepore,[86] six δβ-thalassemia alleles, and three HPFH deletion mutations[161] and has also been used for the diagnosis of Hb Kenya. It provides a useful and simple screening method for distinguishing HPFH from δβ thalassemia in Asian Indian, African and Mediterranean individuals. Those testing negative and carrying novel or rare δβ thalassemia, εγδβ thalassemia, and HPFH deletion mutations can now be examined by MLPA analysis.[102] Fifty probes have been developed to cover a region of 500 kb of the β-globin gene cluster, including the locus control region. This enables all large deletions to be identified, including the εγδβ thalassemias, that leave the β-globin genes intact and are not easily detected by conventional techniques.

DNA DIAGNOSIS OF ABNORMAL HEMOGLOBINS

More than 1,000 hemoglobin variants have been described to date, although only a few are clinically important and require routine diagnosis by DNA-based methods. These variants are HbS, HbC, HbE, HbD-Punjab, and HbO-Arab. The mutations for these five abnormal hemoglobins can be diagnosed by a variety of methods.

Sickle Hemoglobin

The HbS mutation destroys the recognition site for three restriction enzymes, *Mnl* I, *Dde* I, and *Mst* II. *Mst* II was used for detection of the β^S allele by Southern blot analysis because it cuts infrequently around the β-globin gene producing large DNA fragments. For PCR, the enzyme *Dde* I is the enzyme of choice (Fig. 28.9). The primer sequences are listed in Table 28.7. The β^S mutation can also be detected by a variety of other PCR-based techniques such as ASO/dot blotting or ARMS. Prenatal diagnosis of sickle cell disease should always be done using two methods, ARMS-PCR and *Dde* I PCR, with careful attention being paid to the intensity of the stained bands on electrophoresis. The ratio of intensity between the mutant band and the control or normal bands must be identical to those of all the control samples. Fainter bands indicate possible maternal DNA contamination; stronger bands may indicate PCR product contamination.

Hemoglobin C

The HbC mutation does not abolish the recognition site for *Dde* I or *Mst* II because the mutation occurs at a nonspecific nucleotide in the enzyme recognition sequences. Thus another method such as ASO/dot blotting or the ARMS technique must be used. The primer sequences used for the ARMS method are included in Table 28.3.

Hemoglobin D-Punjab and Hemoglobin O-Arab

The mutations giving rise to the abnormal variants HbD Punjab (*HBB* glu121gln) and HbO-Arab (*HBB* glu121lys) both abolish an *Eco*R I site at codon 121. Mutation detection is conducted very simply by RE-PCR using *Eco*R I. The primer sequences used for this approach are listed in Table 28.7. This assay does not distinguish the two variants, so this test must be combined with hemoglobin HPLC. HbD-Punjab can be detected by ARMS (Table 28.3).

Hemoglobin E

The HbE mutation abolishes a *Mnl* I site and may be diagnosed by amplification of exon 1 and restriction enzyme analysis. The primer sequences used for this approach are listed in Table 28.7. The HbE mutation may also be diagnosed easily using ASO probes or ARMS primers (Tables 28.3 and 28.4).

Other Variants

A definitive identification of the other abnormal variants requires either DNA sequencing or analysis of the amino

Table 28.6. Primers used for the analysis of β-globin gene cluster RFLPs

RFLP and Primer Sequences 5′–3′	Product size (bp)	Coordinates on GenBank sequence U01317	Absence of site (bp)	Presence of site (bp)	Annealing temperature (°C)
*Hin*d II/ε					55°
TCTCTGTTTGATGACAAATTC	760	18652–18672	760	315	
AGTCATTGGTCAAGGCTGACC		19391–19411		445	
Xmn I /Gγ					55°
AACTGTTGCTTTATAGGATTTT	657	33862–33883	657	455	
AGGAGCTTATTGATAACCTCAGAC		34495–34518		202	
*Hin*d III /Gγ					65°
AGTGCTGCAAGAAGAACAACTACC	326	35677–35700	326	235	
CTCTGCATCATGGGCAGTGAGCTC		35981–36004		91	
*Hin*d III /Aγ					65°
ATGCTGCTAATGCTTCATTAC	635	40357–40377	635	327	
TCATGTGTGATCTCTCAGCAG		40971–40991		308	
*Hin*d II /5′ψ β					55°
TCCTATCCATTACTGTTCCTTGAA	795	46686–46709	795	691	
ATTGTCTTATTCTAGAGACGATTT		47457–47480		104	
Ava II /ψ β					55°
Sequence as for Hind 5′ψ β RFLP	795	46686–46709	795	440	
		47457–47480		355	
*Hin*d II /3′ ψ β					55°
GTACTCATACTTTAAGTCCTAACT	913	49559–49582	913	479	
TAAGCAAGATTATTTCTGGTCTCT		50448–50471		434	
Rsa I /β					55°
AGACATAATTTATTAGCATGCATG	1200	61504–61527	411	330 & 81	
CCCCTTCCTATGACATGAACTTAA		62680–62703	plus	plus	
			694 & 95	694 & 95	
Ava II /β					65°
GTGGTCTACCCTTGGACCCAGAGG	328	62416–62439	328	228	
TTCGTCTGTTTCCCATTCTAAACT		62720–62743		100	
*Hin*f I /β					55°
GGAGGTTAAAGTTTTGCTATGCTGTAT	474	63974–64001	320	213 & 107	
GGGCCTATGATAGGGTAAT		64429–64447	plus	plus	
			154	154	

Table 28.7. Oligonucleotide primers for the detection of β^S, β^E, β^D Punjab, and β^0 Arab mutations as RFLPs

Mutation and affected RE site	Primer sequences 5′–3′	Annealing temperature (°C)	Product size, bp	Absence of site, bp	Presence of site, bp
β^SCD6 (A→T)	ACCTCACCCTGTGGAGCCAC	65	443	386/67	201/175/67
(Loses *Dde* I site)	GAGTGGACAGATCCCCAAAGGACTCAAGGA	65			
β^ECD26 (G→A)	ACCTCACCCTGTGGAGCCAC	65	443	231/89/56/35/33	171/89/60/35/33
(Loses *Mnl* I site)	GAGTGGACAGATCCCCAAAGGACTCAAGGA	65			
β^DPunjab CD121 (G→C)	CAATGTATCATGCCTCTTTGCACC	65	861	861	552/309
(Loses *Eco*R I site)	GAGTCAAGGCTGAGAGATGCAGGA	65			
β^0 Arab CD121 (G→A)	CAATGTATCATGCCTCTTTGCACC	65	861	861	552/309
(Loses *Eco*R I site)	GAGTCAAGGCTGAGAGATGCAGGA	65			

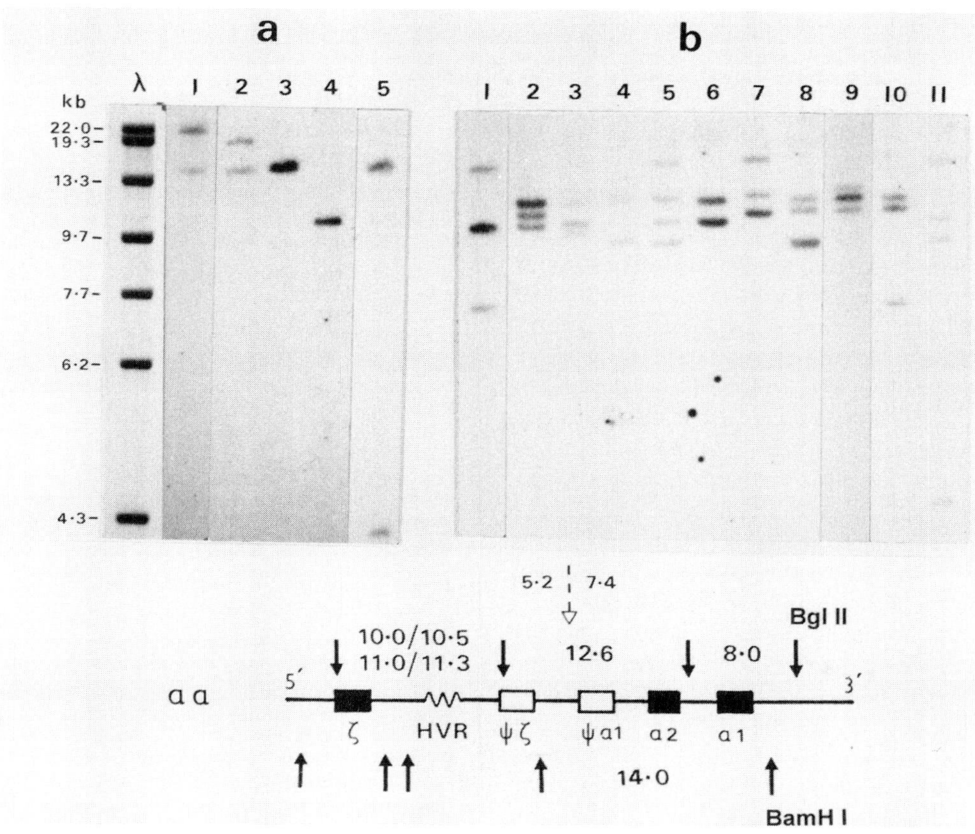

Figure 28.9. The diagnosis of the HbS gene mutation by *Dde* I digestion of amplified DNA. The gel shows *Dde* I–digested fragments of: HbAS individuals (tracks 2, 3, and 5); normal HbA individual (track 6); and sickle cell anemia (track 4). Track 1 contains ϕX174 – *Hae* III DNA markers. The primers used are listed in Table 28.7. The *Dde* I site 5′ to the one at codon 6 (marked by the dotted arrow) is a rare polymorphic site caused by the sequence change G→A at position −83 to the β-globin gene. When present the fragment of 175 bp is cleaved to give 153-bp and 27-bp fragments as shown in track 2.

acid change by mass spectrometry, although a few have had other quick diagnostic tests developed, such as the ARMS technique for the α-chain variant HbQ-India[162] and HbD-Iran (Table 28.3). DNA sequence analysis can be performed in the same manner as that described for the identification of α-chain and α thalassemia point mutations, or more simply through the use of just one sequencing reaction, by sequencing cDNA produced by the reverse transcription of globin mRNA.[84] For the future, the ultimate goal of the identification of all known and unknown hemoglobin variants, by a DNA chip containing every possible codon mutation is within technological reach, but again, this attractive "one stop" method of total variant identification might never find a market as most variants have no clinical significance and identification is often of academic interest only.

ANTENATAL DIAGNOSIS

An antenatal screening program for detection of at risk couples should be able to identify by hematological and DNA testing the majority of carrier states for α thalassemia, β thalassemia, δβ thalassemia, and common variant hemoglobins such as HbS, HbC, HbD-Punjab, HbO-Arab, and Hb Lepore.[163] Strategies for antenatal screening depend on the programs' context. In multiethnic countries such as the United Kingdom or United States, two strategies are applied; one based on universal screening in high prevalence areas for thalassemia or a hemoglobinopathy and one based on ethnic origin of the woman and her partner in low prevalence areas. For example, in the United States, neonatal screening for the HbS gene is universal. The screening algorithms and guidelines for referral of patients for DNA analysis in the United Kingdom can be found on the NHS Sickle Cell and Thalassaemia Screening Programme web site (http://www.kcl-phs.org.uk/haemscreening).

PCR-based techniques provide a quick and relatively simple method for the prenatal diagnosis of homozygous α^0 thalassemia, β thalassemia, and sickle cell disease. The techniques have proven to be reliable and accurate as long as careful attention is given to all potential diagnostic pitfalls and best-practice guidelines are followed.[164,165] These include using two different mutation detection methods whenever possible and excluding maternal DNA contamination by the analysis of VNTR or STR polymorphisms. Kits for profiling 12 or more STR markers simultaneously by using an ABI or Beckman DNA sequencer are now available and recommended for checking maternal contamination of fetal DNA.[84]

WHICH TECHNIQUES TO USE?

The variety of techniques for the DNA-based diagnosis of hemoglobinopathies and thalassemia creates a problem for laboratories wishing to start molecular analysis of globin gene mutations: What is the best method to adopt? It is clear that ASO hybridization and the ARMS currently form the linchpins for the diagnosis of β thalassemia. Both offer a rapid, cheap, and convenient method to test for multiple mutations simultaneously. Whether one chooses the dot blot method or the reverse dot blot approach will depend on a number factors, including the range of mutations to be diagnosed, the ability to use radioactivity, or the need to use a nonisotopic approach (and thus to consider the use of one of the kits on the market). The laboratory also needs to become proficient in a number of other techniques such as gap-PCR and be able to sequence a β-globin gene for the rare cases in which no common mutations can be identified in individuals with clear-cut phenotypic evidence of β thalassemia. In addition, when these techniques are used for prenatal diagnosis a number of precautionary measures have to be implemented, such as the analysis of fetal DNA samples for maternal DNA contamination when necessary and the confirmation of a diagnosis by a different approach. Therefore, the answer to the question is that each laboratory must carry out preliminary studies using a number of these approaches and work out for itself which techniques are best suited to its needs and the mutations found in the population.

REFERENCES

1. Park CM. The dimerization of deoxyhemoglobin and of oxyhemoglobin. Evidence for cleavage along the same plane. *J Biol Chem.* 1970;245:5390–5394.
2. Shaeffer JR, McDonald MJ, Turci SM, Dinda DM, Bunn HF. Dimer-monomer dissociation of human hemoglobin A. *J Biol Chem.* 1984;259(23):14544–14547.
3. Dacie JV, Lewis SM. *Practical Hematology.* 8th ed. Edinburgh: Churchill Livingstone; 1995.
4. Winter WP, Yodh J. Interaction of human hemoglobin and its variants with agar. *Science.* 1983;221(4606):175–178.
5. Ueda S, Schneider RG. Rapid differentiation of polypeptide chains of hemoglobin by cellulose acetate electrophoresis of hemolysates. *Blood.* 1969;34(2):230–235.
6. Schneider RG, Hosty TS, Tomlin G, Atkins R. Identification of hemoglobins and hemoglobinopathies by electrophoresis on cellulose acetate plates impregnated with citrate agar. *Clin Chem.* 1974;20(1):74–77.
7. Schneider RG. Differentiation of electrophoretically similar hemoglobins – such as S, D, G, and P, or A2, C, E, and O – by electrophoresis of the globin chains. *Clin Chem.* 1974;20(9):1111–1115.
8. Whitney JB. Simplified typing of mouse hemoglobin (Hbb) phenotypes using cystamine. *Biochem Genet.* 1978;16:667–672.
9. Righetti PG, Gianazza E, Bjellqvist B. Modern aspects of isoelectric focusing: two-dimensional maps and immobilized pH gradients. [Review]. *J Biochem Biophys Methods.* 1983;8(2):89–108.
10. Righetti PG, Gelfi C, Chiari M. Isoelectric focusing in immobilized pH gradients. *Methods Enzymol.* 1996;270:235–255.
11. Righetti PG, Bossi A. Isoelectric focusing in immobilized pH gradients: recent analytical and preparative developments. *Anal Biochem.* 1997;247(1):1–10.
12. Jenkins MA, Ratnaike S. Capillary isoelectric focusing of haemoglobin variants in the clinical laboratory. *Clin Chim Acta.* 1999;289(1–2):121–132.
13. Gulbis B, Fontaine B, Vertongen F, Cotton F. The place of capillary electrophoresis techniques in screening for haemoglobinopathies. *Ann Clin Biochem.* 2003;40(Pt 6):659–662.
14. Hofstadler SA, Swanek FD, Gale DC, Ewing AG, Smith RD. Capillary electrophoresis-electrospray ionization Fourier transform ion cyclotron resonance mass spectrometry for direct analysis of cellular proteins. *Anal Chem.* 1995;67(8):1477–1480.
15. Cao P, Moini M. Separation and detection of the alpha- and beta-chains of hemoglobin of a single intact red blood cell using capillary electrophoresis/electrospray ionization time-of-flight mass spectrometry. *J Am Soc Mass Spect.* 1999;10(2):184–186.
16. Mario N, Baudin B, Aussel C, Giboudeau J. Capillary isoelectric focusing and high-performance cation-exchange chromatography compared for qualitative and quantitative analysis of hemoglobin variants. *Clin Chem.* 1997;43(11):2137–2142.
17. Wu J, Pawliszyn J. Application of capillary isoelectric focusing with absorption imaging detection to the quantitative determination of human hemoglobin variants. *Electrophoresis.* 1995;16(4):670–673.
18. Banks JF. Recent advances in capillary electrophoresis/electrospray/mass spectrometry. *Electrophoresis.* 1997;18(12–13):2255–2266.
19. Joutovsky A, Hadzi-Nesic J, Nardi MA. HPLC Retention time as a diagnostic tool for hemoglobin variants and hemoglobinopathies: a study of 60000 samples in a clinical diagnostic laboratory. *Clin Chem.* 2004;50(10):1736–1747.
20. Zurbriggen K, Schmugge M, Schmid M, et al. Analysis of minor hemoglobins by matrix-assisted laser desorption/ionization time-of-flight mass spectrometry. *Clin Chem.* 2005;51(6):989–996.
21. Shackleton CH, Witkowska HE. Characterizing abnormal hemoglobin by MS. *Anal Chem.* 1996;68(1):29A–33A.
22. Yamashita M, Fenn JB. Electrospray ion source. Another viriation on the free-jet theme. *J Phys Chem.* 1984;88:4451–4459.
23. Motos GA, Hernandez JA, Hernandez JM, Rovira JM, Fluvia L, Bosch A, et al. Identification and characterization by high-performance liquid chromatography/electrospray ionization mass spectrometry of a new variant hemoglobin, Mataro [beta134(H12) Val > Ala. *J Mass Spectrom.* 2001;36(8):943–949.

24. Motos A, Hernandez JM, Fluvia L, Hernandez JA, Pastor MC. Direct peptide mapping of real samples containing sickle-cell and fetal hemoglobin by electrospray mass spectrometry. *Rapid Commun Mass Spectrom.* 2000;14(23):2328–2329.
25. Rai DK, Alvelius G, Landin B, Griffiths WJ. Electrospray tandem mass spectrometry in the rapid identification of alpha-chain haemoglobin variants. *Rapid Commun Mass Spectrom.* 2000;14(14):1184–1194.
26. Daniel YA, Turner C, Haynes RM, Hunt BJ, Dalton RN. Quantification of hemoglobin A2 by tandem mass spectrometry. *Clin Chem.* 2007;53(8):1448–1454.
27. Caruso D, Crestani M, Mitro N, Da Riva L, Mozzi R, Sarpau S, et al. High pressure liquid chromatography and electrospray ionization mass spectrometry are advantageously integrated into a two-levels approach to detection and identification of haemoglobin variants. *Clin Lab Haematol.* 2005;27(2):111–119.
28. Basilico F, Di Silvestre D, Sedini S, et al. New approach for rapid detection of known hemoglobin variants using LC-MS/MS combined with a peptide database. *J Mass Spectrom.* 2007;42(3):288–292.
29. Betke K, Marti HQ, Schlicht I. Estimation of small percentages of foetal haemoglobin. *Nature.* 1959;184:877.
30. Jonxis JHP, Visser HKA. Determination of low percentages of fetal hemoglobin in blood of normal children. *Am J Dis Child.* 92;588. 1956.
31. Papassotiriou I, Ducrocq R, Prehu C, Bardakdjian-Michau J, Wajcman H. Gamma chain heterogeneity: determination of Hb F composition by perfusion chromatography. *Hemoglobin.* 1998;22(5–6):469–481.
32. Prehu C, Ducrocq R, Godart C, Riou J, Galacteros F. Determination of Hb F levels: the routine methods. *Hemoglobin.* 1998;22(5–6):459–467.
33. Garver FA, Jones CS, Baker MM, et al. Specific radioimmunochemical identification and quantitation of hemoglobins A2 and F. *Am J Hematol.* 1976;1(4):459–469.
34. Rutland PC, Pembrey ME, Davies T. The estimation of fetal haemoglobin in healthy adults by radioimmunoassay. *Br J Haematol.* 1983;53(4):673–682.
35. Epstein N, Epstein M, Boulet A, Fibach E, Rodgers GP. Monoclonal antibody-based methods for quantitation of hemoglobins: application to evaluating patients with sickle cell anemia treated with hydroxyurea. *Eur J Haematol.* 1996;57(1):17–24.
36. Steinberg MH. Determinants of fetal hemoglobin response to hydroxyurea. *Semin Hematol.* 1997;34(3:Suppl 3):Suppl-14.
37. Steinberg MH, Adams JG. Hemoglobin A2: origin, evolution, and aftermath. *Blood.* 1991;78(9):2165–2177.
38. Garver FA, Singh H, Moscoso H, Kestler DP, McGuire BSJ. Identification and quantification of hemoglobins A2 and Barts with an enzyme-labeled immunosorbent assay. *Clin Chem.* 1984;30(7):1205–1208.
39. Jenkins MA, Hendy J, Smith IL. Evaluation of hemoglobin A2 quantitation assay and hemoglobin variant screening by capillary electrophoresis. *J Capillary Electrophoresis.* 1997;4(3): 137–143.
40. Cotton F, Lin C, Fontaine B, Gulbis B, Janssens J, Vertongen F. Evaluation of a capillary electrophoresis method for routine determination of hemoglobins A2 and F. *Clin Chem.* 1999;45(2):237–243.
41. Benesch RE, Edalji R, Kwong S, Benesch R. Oxygen affinity as an index of hemoglobin S polymerization: a new micromethod. *Anal Biochem.* 1978;89(1):162–173.
42. Eaton WA, Hofrichter J. Sickle cell hemoglobin polymerization. *Adv Protein Chem.* 1990;40:63–279.
43. Magdoff-Fairchild B, Poillon WN, Li T, Bertles JF. Thermodynamic studies of polymerization of deoxygenated sickle cell hemoglobin. *Proc Natl Acad Sci USA.* 1976;73(4):990–994.
44. Adachi K, Asakura T. The solubility of sickle and non-sickle hemoglobins in concentrated phosphate buffer. *J Biol Chem.* 1979;254:4079–4084.
45. Bookchin RM, Balazs T, Wang Z, Josephs R, Lew VL. Polymer structure and solubility of deoxyhemoglobin S in the presence of high concentrations of volume-excluding 70-kDa dextran. *J Biol Chem.* 1999;274:6689–6697.
46. Fabry ME, Acharya SA, Suzuka SM, Nagel RL. Solubility measurement of the sickle polymer. *Methods Mol Med.* 2003;82:271–287.
47. Fabry ME, Desrosiers L, Suzuka SM. Direct intracellular measurement of deoxygenated hemoglobin S solubility. *Blood.* 2001;98(3):883–884.
48. Adachi K, Asakura T. Gelation of deoxyhemoglobin A in concentrated phosphate buffer. Exhibition of delay time prior to aggregation and crystallization of deoxyhemoglobin A. *J Biol Chem.* 1979;254:12273–12276.
49. Reiter CD, Wang X, Tanus-Santos JE, et al. Cell-free hemoglobin limits nitric oxide bioavailability in sickle-cell disease. *Nat Med.* 2002;8(12):1383–1389.
50. Rother RP, Bell L, Hillmen P, Gladwin MT. The clinical sequelae of intravascular hemolysis and extracellular plasma hemoglobin: a novel mechanism of human disease. *JAMA.* 2005;293(13):1653–1662.
51. Lijana RC, Williams MC. Tetramethylbenzidine – a substitute for benzidine in hemoglobin analysis. *J Lab Clin Med.* 1979;94(2):266–276.
52. Kato GJ, McGowan VR, Machado RF, et al. Lactate dehydrogenase as a biomarker of hemolysis-associated nitric oxide resistance, priapism, leg ulceration, pulmonary hypertension and death in patients with sickle cell disease. *Blood.* 2006;107: 2279–2285.
53. Bentley SA, Johnson A, Bishop CA. A parallel evaluation of four automated hematology analyzers. *Am J Clin Pathol.* 1993;100(6):626–632.
54. Ward PC. The CBC at the turn of the millennium: an overview. *Clin Chem.* 2000;46(8 Pt 2):1215–1220.
55. Gulati GL, Hyun BH, Ashton JK. Advances of the past decade in automated hematology. *Am J Clin Pathol.* 1992;98(4 Suppl 1):Suppl-6.
56. Jones RG, Faust AM, Matthews RA. Quality team approach in evaluating three automated hematology analyzers with five-part differential capability. *Am J Clin Pathol.* 1995;103(2):159–166.
57. Buttarello M. Quality specification in haematology: the automated blood cell count. *Clin Chim Acta.* 2004;346(1):45–54.
58. Frazier JL, Caskey JH, Yoffe M, Seligman PA. Studies of the transferrin receptor on both human reticulocytes and nucleated human cells in culture: comparison of factors regulating receptor density. *J Clin Invest.* 1982;69:853–865.
59. Brugnara C, Zelmanovic D, Sorette M, Ballas SK, Platt O. Reticulocyte hemoglobin: an integrated parameter for

evaluation of erythropoietic activity. *Am J Clin Pathol.* 1997;108(2):133–142.
60. Brugnara C. Use of reticulocyte cellular indices in the diagnosis and treatment of hematological disorders. *Int J Clin Lab Res.* 1998;28(1):1–11.
61. Lawrence C, Fabry ME, Nagel RL. Red cell distribution width parallels dense red cell disappearance during painful crises in sickle cell anemia. *J Lab Clin Med.* 1985;105(6):706–710.
62. Ponder E. *Hemolysis and Related Phenomena.* New York: Grune & Stratton; 1948.
63. Fabry ME, Nagel RL. The effect of deoxygenation on red cell density: significance for the pathophysiology of sickle cell anemia. *Blood.* 1982;60:1370–1377.
64. Nagel RL, Raventos Suarez C, Fabry ME, Tanowitz H, Sicard D, Labie D. Impairment of the growth of Plasmodium falciparum in HbEE erythrocytes. *J Clin Invest.* 1981;68:303–305.
65. Marikovsky Y, Lotan R, Lis H, Sharon N, Danon D. Agglutination and labeling density of soybean agglutinin on young and old human red blood cells. *Exp Cell Res.* 1976;99(2):453–456.
66. Clark MR, Morrison CE, Shohet SB. Monovalent cation transport in irreversibly sickled cells. *J Clin Invest.* 1978;62:329–337.
67. Vettore L, Zanella A, Molaro GL, De Matteis MC, Pavesi M, Mariani M. A new test for the laboratory diagnosis of spherocytosis. *Acta Haematol.* 1984;72(4):258–263.
68. Fabry ME, Nagel RL. Heterogeneity of red cells in the sickler: a characteristic with practical clinical and pathophysiological implications. *Blood Cells.* 1982;8:9–15.
69. Corry WD, Meiselman HJ. Modification of erythrocyte physiochemical properties by millimolar concentrations of glutaraldehyde. *Blood Cells.* 1978;4:465–480.
70. Thein SL, Reittie JE. F cells by immunofluorescent staining of erythrocyte smears. *Hemoglobin.* 1998;22(5–6):415–417.
71. Amoyal I, Fibach E. Flow cytometric analysis of fetal hemoglobin in erythroid precursors of beta-thalassemia. *Clin Lab Haematol.* 2004;26(3):187–193.
72. Porra V, Bernaud J, Gueret P, et al. Identification and quantification of fetal red blood cells in maternal blood by a dual-color flow cytometric method: evaluation of the Fetal Cell Count kit. *Transfusion.* 2007;47(7):1281–1289.
73. Galanello R, Satta S, Pirroni MG, Travi M, Maccioni L. Globin chain synthesis of high performance liquid chromatography in the screening of thalassemia syndromes. *Hemoglobin.* 1998;22(5&6):501–508.
74. Weinberg RS, Ji X, Sutton M, Perrine S, Galperin Y, Li Q, et al. Butyrate increases the efficiency of translation of gamma-globin mRNA. *Blood.* 2005;105(4):1807–1809.
75. Fathallah H, Weinberg RS, Galperin Y, Sutton M, Atweh GF. Role of epigenetic modifications in normal globin gene regulation and butyrate-mediated induction of fetal hemoglobin. *Blood.* 2007;110(9):3391–3397.
76. Eaton WA, Hofrichter J. Hemoglobin S gelation and sickle cell disease. *Blood.* 1987;70:1245–1266.
77. Cao Z, Ferrone FA. A 50th order reaction predicted and observed for sickle hemoglobin nucleation. *J Mol Biol.* 1996;256(2):219–222.
78. Galkin O, Vekilov PG. Mechanisms of homogeneous nucleation of polymers of sickle cell anemia hemoglobin in deoxy state. *J Mol Biol.* 2004;336(1):43–59.
79. Christoph GW, Hofrichter J, Eaton WA. Understanding the shape of sickled red cells. *Biophys J.* 2005;88(2):1371–1376.
80. Old JM. Fetal DNA analysis. In: Davies KE, ed. *Human Genetic Disease Analysis: A Practical Approach.* 2nd ed. Oxford: IRL Press; 1993;1–19.
81. Liu YT, Old JM, Fisher CA, Weatherall DJ, Clegg JB. Rapid detection of α-thalassaemia deletions and α-globin gene triplication by multiplex PCRs. *Br J Haematol.* 2000;108:295–299.
82. Rosatelli MC, Tuveri T, Scalas MT, et al. Molecular screening and fetal diagnosis of β-thalassaemia in the Italian population. *Hum Genet.* 1992;89:585.
83. Decorte R, Cuppens H, Marynen P, Cassiman JJ. Rapid detection of hypervariable regions by the polymerase chain reaction technique. *DNA Cell Biol.* 1990;9:461–469.
84. Stojikovic-Mikic T, Mann K, Docherty Z, Ogilvie CM. Maternal cell contamination of prenatal samples assessed by QF-PCR genotyping. *Prenatal Diag.* 2005;25:79–83.
85. Cariolou MA, Kokkofitou A, Manoli P, Ioannou P. Prenatal diagnosis for beta-thalassemia by PCR from single chorionic villus. *Biotechniques.* 1993;15:32–34.
86. Camaschella C, Alfarano A, Gottardi E, et al. Prenatal diagnosis of fetal hemoglobin Lepore-Boston disease on maternal peripheral blood. *Blood.* 1990;75:2102–2106.
87. Sekizawa A, Watanabe A, Kimwa T, et al. Prenatal diagnosis of the fetal RhD type using a single fetal nucleated erythrocyte from maternal blood. *Obstet Gynaecol.* 1996;87:501–505.
88. Cheung MsC, Goldberg JD, Kan YW. Prenatal diagnosis of sickle cell anemia and thalassemia by analysis of fetal cells in maternal blood. *Nat Genet.* 1996;14:264–268.
89. Lo YM. Fetal DNA in maternal plasma. *Ann NY Acad Sci.* 2000;906:141–147.
90. Chiu RW, Lui WB, El-Sheikah A, et al. Comparison of protocols for extracting circulating DNA and RNA from maternal plasma. *Clin Chem.* 2005;51:2209–2210.
91. Lo YM, Zhang J, Leung TN, et al. Rapid clearance of fetal DNA from maternal plasma. *Am J Hum Genet.* 1999;64:18–24.
92. Chiu RW, Lau TK, Leung TN Chow KC, Chui DH, Lo YM. Prenatal exclusion of β-thalassaemia major by examination of maternal plasma. *Lancet.* 2002;360:998–1000.
93. Tungwiwat W, Fucharoen S, Fucharoen G, Ratanasiri T, Sanchaisuriya K. Development and application of a real-time quantitative PCR for prenatal detection of fetal alpha(0)-thalassemia from maternal plasma. *Ann NY Acad Sci.* 2006; 1075:103–107.
94. Lo YM. Recent developments in fetal nucleic acids in maternal plasma: implications to noninvasive prenatal fetal blood group genotyping. *Transfusion Clin Biol.* 2006;13:50–52.
95. Kanavakis E, Traeger-Synodinos J. Preimplantation genetic diagnosis in clinical practice. *J Med Genet.* 2002;39:6–11.
96. Chan V, Ng EH, Yam I, Yeung WS, Ho PC, Chan TK. Experience in preimplantation genetic diagnosis for exclusion of homozygous α^0 thalassemia. *Prenatal Diag.* 2006;26:1029–1036.
97. Deng J, Peng WL, Li J, et al. Successful preimplantation genetic diagnosis for alpha- and beta-thalassemia in China. *Prenatal Diag.* 2006;26:1021–1028.
98. Monni G, Cau G, Usai V, et al. Preimplantation genetic diagnosis for beta-thalassaemia: the Sardinian experience. *Prenatal Diag.* 2004;24:949–954.
99. Kuliev A, Rechitsky S, Verlinsky O, et al. Preimplantation diagnosis and HLA typing for haemoglobin disorders. *Reprod Biomed Online.* 2005;11:362–370.

100. Vrettou C, Traegaer-Synodinos J, Tzetis M, Palmer G, Sofocleous C, Kanavakis E. Real-time PCR for single-cell genotyping in sickle cell and thalassemia syndromes as a rapid, accurate, reliable, and widely applicable protocol for preimplantation genetic diagnosis. *Hum Mutat.* 2004;23:513–521.
101. Old J. DNA-based diagnosis of the hemoglobin disorders. In: Steinberg MH, Forget BG, Higgs DR, Nagel RL, eds. *Disorders of Hemoglobin: Genetics, Pathophysiology, and Clinical Management.* Cambridge: Cambridge University Press; 2001:941–957.
102. Harteveld Cl, Voskamp A, Phylipsen M, et al. Nine unknown rearrangements in 16p13.3 and 11p15.4 causing alpha- and beta-thalassaemia characterised by high resolution multiplex ligation-dependent probe amplification. *J Med Genet.* 2005;42:922–931.
103. Bowden DK, Vickers MA, Higgs DR. A PCR-based strategy to detect the common severe determinants of α-thalassaemia. *Br J Haematol.* 1992;81:104–108.
104. Dode C, Krishnamoorthy R, Lamb J, Rochette J. Rapid analysis of –α3.7 thalassaemia and ααα anti 3.7 triplication by enzymatic amplification analysis. *Br J Haematol.* 1992;82:105–111.
105. Baysal E, Huisman THJ. Detection of common deletional α-thalassaemia-2 determinants by PCR. *Am J Hematol.* 1994;46:208–213.
106. Ko TM, Li S-F. Molecular characterization of the –FIL determinant of alpha-thalassaemia (corrigendum for Ko et al 1998). *Am J Hematol.* 1999;60:173.
107. Ko T-M, Tseng L-H, Hsu P-M, et al. Molecular characterization of β-thalassemia in Taiwan and the identification of two new mutations. *Hemoglobin.* 1997;21:131–142.
108. Chong SS, Boehm CD, Higgs DR, Cutting GR. Single-tube multiplex-PCR screen for common deletional determinants of α-thalassemia. *Blood.* 2000;95:360–362.
109. Sun CF, Lee CH, Cheng SW, et al. Real-time quantitative PCR analysis for alpha-thalassemia-1 of Southeast Asian type deletion in Taiwan. *Clin Genet.* 2001;60:305–309.
110. Ou-Yang H, Hua L, Mo HQ, Xu Xm. Rapid, accurate genotyping of the common alpha (4.2) deletion based on the use of denaturing HPLC. *J Clin Pathol.* 2004;57:159–163.
111. Zesong L, Ruijun G, Wen Z. Rapid detection of deletional alpha-thalassemia by an oligonucleotide microarray. *Am J Hematol.* 2005;80:306–308.
112. Bang-Ce Y, Hongqiong L, Zhuanfong Z, Zhensong L, Jiangling G. Simultaneous detection of alpha-thalassemia and beta-thalassemia by oligonucleotide microarray. *Haematologica.* 2004;89:1010–1012.
113. Molchanova TP, Pobedimskaya DD, Postnikov YV. A simplified procedure for sequencing amplified DNA containing the α-2 or α-1 globin gene. *Hemoglobin.* 1994;18:251–255.
114. Ko TM, Tseng LH, Hsieh FJ, Lee TY. Prenatal diagnosis of HbH disease due to compound heterozygosity for south-east Asian deletion and Hb Constant Spring by polymerase chain reaction. *Prenatal Diag.* 1993;13:143–146.
115. Harteveld CL, Heister AJGAM, Giordano PC, Losekoot M, Bernini LF. Rapid detection of point mutations and polymorphisms of the α-globin genes by DGGE and SSCA. *Hum Mutat.* 1996;7:114–122.
116. Huisman THJ. Frequencies of common β-thalassaemia alleles among different populations: variability in clinical severity. *Br J Haematol.* 1990;75:454–457.
117. Distribution and population genetics of the thalassaemias. In: Weatherall DJ, Clegg JB, eds. *The Thalassaemia Syndromes.* 4th ed. Oxford: Blackwell Scientific; 2001:237–286.
118. Ristaldi MS, Pirastu M, Rosatelli C, Cao A. Prenatal diagnosis of β-thalassaemia in Mediterranean populations by dot blot analysis with DNA amplification and allele specific oligonucleotide probes. *Prenatal Diag.* 1989;9:629–638.
119. Saiki RK, Walsh PS, Levenson CH, Erlich HA. Genetic analysis of amplified DNA with immobilized sequence-specific oligonucleotide probes. *Proc Natl Acad Sci USA.* 1989;86:6230–6234.
120. Maggio A, Giambona A, Cai SP, Wall J, Kan YW, Chehab FF. Rapid and simultaneous typing of hemoglobin S, hemoglobin C and seven Mediterranean β-thalassaemia mutations by covalent reverse dot-blot analysis: application to prenatal diagnosis in Sicily. *Blood.* 1993;81:239–242.
121. Sutcharitchan P, Saiki R, Huisman THJ, Kutlar A, McKie V, Embury SH. Reverse dot-blot detection of the African-American β-thalassaemia mutations. *Blood.* 1995;86:1580–1585.
122. Sutcharitchan P, Saiki R, Fucharoen S, Winchagoon P, Erlich H, Embury SH. Reverse dot-blot detection of Thai beta-thalassaemia mutations. *Br J Haematol.* 1995;90:809–816.
123. Gemignani F, Perra C, Landi S, et al. Reliable detection of beta-thalassemia and G6PD mutations by a DNA microarray. *Clin Chem.* 2002;48:2051–2054.
124. Van Moorsel CH, van Wijngaraarden EE, Fokkema IF, et al. β-Globin mutation detection by tagged single-base extension and hybridization to universal glass and flow-through microarrays. *Eur J Hum Genet.* 2004;12:567–573.
125. Lu Y, Kham SK, Tan PL, Quah TC, Heng CK, Yeoh AE. Arrayed primer extension: a robust and reliable genotyping platform for the diagnosis of single gene disorders: beta-thalassemia and thiopurine methyltransferase deficiency. *Genet Test.* 2005;9:212–219.
126. Newton CR, Graham A, Heptinstall LE. Analysis of any point mutation in DNA. The amplification refractory mutation system (ARMS). *Nucl Acids Res.* 1989;17:2503–2516.
127. Old JM, Varawalla NY, Weatherall DJ. The rapid detection and prenatal diagnosis of β thalassaemia in the Asian Indian and Cypriot populations in the UK. *Lancet.* 1990;336:834–837.
128. Old J. Haemoglobinopathies. *Prenatal Diag.* 1996;16:1181–1186.
129. Saxena R, Jain PK, Thomas E, Verma IC. Prenatal diagnosis of β-thalassaemia: experience in a developing country. *Prenatal Diag.* 1998;18:1–7.
130. Tan JA, Tay JS, Lin LI, et al. The amplification refractory mutation system (ARMS): a rapid and direct prenatal diagnostic technique for β-thalassaemia in Singapore. *Prenatal Diag.* 1994;14:1077–1082.
131. Zschocke J, Graham CA. A fluorescent multiplex ARMS method for rapid mutation analysis. *Mol Cell Probes.* 1995;9:447–451.
132. Chehab FF, Kan YW. Detection of specific DNA sequence by fluorescence amplification: a colour complementation assay. *Proc Natl Acad Sci USA.* 1989;86:9178–9178.
133. Chang JG, Lu JM, Huang JM, Chen JT, Liu HJ, Chang CP. Rapid diagnosis of β-thalassaemia by mutagenically separated polymerase chain reaction (MS-PCR) and its application to prenatal diagnosis. *Br J Haematol.* 1995;91:602–607.

134. Linderman R, Hu SP, Volpato F, Trent RJ. (1991) Polymerase chain reaction (PCR) mutagenesis enabling rapid non-radioactive detection of common β thalassaemia mutations in Mediterraneans. *Br J Haematol.* 1991;78:100–104.
135. Webster MT, Wells RS, Clegg JB. Analysis of variation in the human beta-globin gene cluster using a novel DHPLC technique. *Mutat Res.* 2002;501:99–103.
136. Yip SP, Pun SF, Leung KH, Lee SY. Rapid, simultaneous genotyping of five common Southeast Asian beta-thalassemia mutations by multiplex minisequencing and denaturing HPLC. *Clin Chem.* 2003;49:1656–1659.
137. Su YN, Lee CN, Hung CC, et al. Rapid detection of beta-globin gene (HBB) mutations coupling heteroduplex and primer-extension analysis by DHPLC. *Hum Mutat.* 2003;22:326–336.
138. Wu G, Hua L, Zhu J, Mo QH, Xu XM. Rapid, accurate genotyping of beta-thalassaemia mutations using a novel multiplex primer extension/denaturing high-performance liquid chromatography assay. *Br J Haematol.* 2003;122:311–316.
139. Bournazos SN, Tserga A, Patrinos GP, Papadakis MN. A versatile denaturing HPLC approach for human beta-globin gene mutation screening. *Am J Hematol.* 2007;82:168–170.
140. Naja RP, Kaspar H, Shabakio H, Chakar N, Makhoul Nj, Zalloua PA. Accurate and rapid prenatal diagnosis of the most frequent East Mediterranean beta-thalassemia mutations. *Am J Hematol.* 2004;75:220–224.
141. Pang L, Li J, Jiang J, Shen G, Yu R. DNA point mutation detection based on DNA ligase reaction and nano-Au amplification: a piezoelectric approach. *Anal Biochem.* 2006;358: 99–103.
142. Craig JE, Kelly SJ, Barnetson R, Thein SL. Molecular characterisation of a novel 10.3 kb deletion causing β-thalassaemia with unusually high Hb A2. *Br J Haematol.* 1992;82:735–744.
143. Dimovski AJ, Efremove DG, Jankovic L, Plaseska D, Juricic D, Efremov GD. A β^0 thalassaemia due to a 1605 bp deletion of the 5′ β-globin gene region. *Br J Haematol.* 1993;85:143–147.
144. Faa V, Rosatelli MC, Sardu R, Meloni A, Toffoli C, Cao A. A simple electrophoretic procedure for fetal diagnosis of β-thalassaemia due to short deletions. *Prenatal Diag.* 1992;12:903–908.
145. Waye JS, Cai S-P, Eng B, et al. High hemoglobin A2 β^0 thalassaemia due to a 532 bp deletion of the 5′ β-globin gene region. *Blood.* 1991;77:1100–1103.
146. Waye JS, Eng B, Hunt JA, et al. Filipino β-thalassaemia due to a large deletion: identification of the deletion endpoints and polymerase chain reaction (PCR)-based diagnosis. *Hum Genet.* 1994;94:530–532.
147. Old JM, Petrou M, Modell B, Weatherall *Prenatal Diag.* D. J. Feasibility of antenatal diagnosis of β-thalassaemia by DNA polymorphisms in Asian Indians and Cypriot populations. *Br J Haematol.* 1984;57:255–263.
148. Thein SL, Hesketh C, Brown KM, Anstey AV, Weatherall DJ. Molecular characterisation of a high A2 β thalassemia by direct sequencing of single strand enriched amplified genomic DNA. *Blood.* 1989;73:924–930.
149. Lynch JR, Brown JM, Best S, Jennings MW, Weatherall DJ. Characterisation of the breakpoint of a 3.5 kb deletion of the β-globin gene. *Genomics.* 1991;10:509–511.
150. Losekoot M, Fodde R, Harteveld CL, Van Heeren H, Giordano PC, Bernini LF. Denaturing gradient gel electrophoresis and direct sequencing of PCR amplified genomic DNA: a rapid and reliable diagnostic approach to beta thalassaemia. *Br J Haematol.* 1991;76:269–274.
151. Gorakshaker AC, Lulla CP, Nadkarni AH, et al. Prenatal diagnosis of β-thalassemia using denaturing gradient gel electrophoresis among Indians. *Hemoglobin.* 1997;21:421–435.
152. Gottardi E, Losekoot M, Fodde R, Saglio G, Camaschella C, Bernini LF. Rapid identification of denaturing gradient gel electrophoresis of mutations in the γ-globin gene promoters in non-deletion type HPFH. *Br J Haematol.* 1992;80:533–538.
153. Papadakis M, Papapanagiotou E, Loutradi-Anagnostou A. Scanning methods to identify the molecular heterogeneity of δ-globin gene especially in δ-thalassemias: detection of three novel substitutions in the promoter region of the gene. *Hum Mutat.* 1997;9:465–472.
154. Savage DA, Wood NAP, Bidwell JL, Fitches A, Old JM, Hui KM. Detection of β-thalassaemia mutations using DNA heteroduplex generator molecules. *Br J Haematol.* 1995;90:564–571.
155. Old JM, Khan SH, Verma I, et al. A multi-center study in order to further define the molecular basis of beta-thalassemia in Thailand, Pakistan, Sri Lanka, Mauritius, Syria, and India, and to develop a simple molecular diagnostic strategy by amplification refractory mutation system-polymerase chain reaction. *Hemoglobin.* 2001;25:397–407.
156. Kazazian HH Jr, Boehm CD. Molecular basis and prenatal diagnosis of β-thalassemia. *Blood.* 1988;72:1107–1116.
157. Antonarakis SE, Boehm CD, Diardina PJV, Kazazian HH Jr. Non-random association of polymorphic restriction sites in the β-globin gene cluster. *Proc Natl Acad Sci USA.* 1982;79: 137–141.
158. Chakravarti A, Buetow KH, Antonarakis SE, Waber PG, Boehm CD, Kazazian HH. Non-uniform recombination within the human β-globin gene cluster. *Am J Hum Genet.* 1984;36:1239–1258.
159. Varawalla NY, Fitches AC, Old JM. Analysis of beta-globin gene haplotypes in Asian Indians: origin and spread of beta-thalassaemia on the Indian subcontinent. *Hum Genet.* 1992;90:443–449.
160. Semenza GL, Dowling CE, Kazazian HH Jr. Hinf I polymorphisms 3′ to the human β globin gene detected by the polymerase chain reaction (PCR). *Nucl Acids Res.* 1989;17:2376.
161. Craig JE, Barnetson RA, Prior J, Raven JL, Thein SL. Rapid detection of deletions causing δ β thalassemia and hereditary persistence of fetal hemoglobin by enzymatic amplification. *Blood.* 1994;83:1673–1682.
162. Abraham R, Thomas M, Britt R, Fisher C, Old J. Hb Q-India; an uncommon variant diagnosed in three Punjabi patients with diabetes is identified by a novel DNA analysis test. *J Clin Pathol.* 2003;56:296–299.
163. Old JM. Screening and genetic diagnosis of haemoglobinopathies. *Scand J Clin Lab Invest.* 2006;66:1–16.
164. The Globin Gene Disorder Working Party of the BCSH General Haematology Task Force. Guidelines for the fetal diagnosis of globin gene disorders. *J Clin Pathol.* 1994;47:199–204.
165. Old JM. Best practice recommendations. In: *Prevention of Thalassaemias and Other Haemoglobin Disorders.* Vol 2. Nicosia, Cyprus: Thalassaemia International Federation; 2005:1–16.

SECTION EIGHT

NEW APPROACHES TO THE TREATMENT OF HEMOGLOBINOPATHIES AND THALASSEMIA

Martin H. Steinberg

The treatment of hemoglobin disorders is evolving and clinical trials of many new agents are underway. Hydroxyurea is used to increase fetal hemoglobin (HbF) levels, stem cell transplantation has the potential for cure, and a larger repertory of iron chelators might make long-term transfusion more feasible. In this section of five chapters, three cover clinically available treatments, discussing in detail aspects of HbF induction, blood transfusion with iron chelation, and stem cell transplantation. One chapter focuses on innovative treatment approaches that remain, at the time of writing, investigative. Treatments include antioxidants, statins, antiinflammatory agents, transport channel inhibitors, antiadhesive agents, and therapeutic methods of increasing nitric oxide bioavailability. The first patients have been treated in a gene therapy trial in which lentiviral vectors containing therapeutic β-like globin genes are used to counter the results of the sickle or β thalassemia mutation, and a final chapter brings this field up to date.

Transfusions are not innocuous and are complicated by alloimmunization, the transmission of unsuspected viral diseases, and iron overload. Controlled, randomized trials of the utility of transfusions for specific complications are sparse. When transfusion is contemplated, expert opinion, with its pitfalls, is relied on in most instances. Usually, it is unclear if simple transfusion or exchange transfusion yields superior results for sickle cell disease complications such as stroke in children or the acute chest syndrome. Strong personal feelings among clinicians regarding the method of transfusion make the chance of definitive clinical trials dim. Since our last edition, efficacious new oral iron chelators have been approved in many countries. Deferiprone might have special benefit for the iron-overloaded heart, but it is not approved for use in the United States. Deferasirox, an oral agent, has efficacy similar to desferrioxamine, the standard for chelating agents. If long-term experience shows that the toxicities of deferiprone and deferasirox are manageable, they will be major adjuncts in dealing with transfusion-induced iron overload.

Stem cell transplantation has been used successfully in sickle cell anemia and β thalassemia. Pioneers in the development of transplantation for sickle cell disease and β thalassemia discuss criteria for patient selection, conditioning regimens, complications and their management, and the most recent results of transplantation. Transplantation is a dynamic field and its future includes the use of cord blood stem cells, inducing stable mixed chimerism, and new possibilities for immunosuppression. Stem cell transplantation, if successful, provides the sole cure for β thalassemia and sickle cell disease, but with the risk, albeit small, of transplant-related death.

The efficacy of hydroxyurea has been proven in a randomized controlled trial in which its use was associated with a nearly 50% reduction in the incidence of pain crisis, acute chest syndrome, frequency of hospitalization, and the use of blood transfusion. Moreover, during a 10-year follow-up period that was no longer randomized or controlled, mortality appeared to be reduced by 40% and toxicity was minor. This cytotoxic agent could have other therapeutic mechanisms in addition to inducing HbF with effects on erythrocytes and vasculature. Studies of hydroxyurea in very young children, in whom therapeutic benefits should be greatest, are nearing completion and the results awaited eagerly. In children, the HbF response is greater than seen in adults with levels near 20% achieved after 6 months–1 year of treatment and with minimal short-term toxicity. Early interruption of the vasoocclusive and hemolytic processes in young patients might also prevent damage to the central nervous system, lungs, kidneys, and bones that end in neurocognitive damage, pulmonary hypertension, disability, and premature death.

We do not yet know the long-term negative effects of hydroxyurea – is it mutagenic, carcinogenic, or leukemogenic? Whether or not the incidence of neoplasia is increased is not known, but in seriously ill patients, small risks are likely to be dominated by the benefits of treatment. In the very young, in whom this agent is likely to be used for decades one must consider longer-term toxicities. In HbSC disease, hydroxyurea appeared to reduce hemolysis but a clinical a trial of this agent in HbSC has not been done.

Studies of butyrate given by short-term pulses have shown remarkable increases in HbF that could be synergistic with those of hydroxyurea. Butyrate was the first agent whose effects could be mediated by epigenetic mechanisms, and work on orally available agents of this general class of drug is continuing. Finally, decitabine, a less toxic analog of 5-azacytidine, the drug that began the effort to induce HbF synthesis, has shown promising results in sickle cell anemia, and development of an oral form is progressing.

The principles of gene therapy approaches to sickle cell disease and β thalassemia are discussed along with the current problems of this approach, foremost among them, how to achieve safe, stable and robust transgene expression.

Until cures of disease by stem cell transplantation or gene therapy become feasible and widely applicable, drug treatment will remain in the forefront. A single agent that will prevent or reverse the disease pathophysiology seems an unlikely possibility, except for the still unachievable goal of an agent that will increase HbF to sufficient concentrations in each sickle erythrocyte to totally prevent HbS polymerization and its consequences. Any other class of drug used alone is unlikely to be sufficient. Trials of combined treatments should be undertaken and include one or more HbF-inducing agent and drugs that target facets of pathophysiology other than HbS polymerization. One can imagine clinical trials that combine agents that increase nitric oxide bioavailability, reduce intercellular interactions, reduce hemolytic anemia, and are antiinflammatory used along with HbF-inducing drugs.

29

Transfusion and Iron Chelation Therapy in Thalassemia and Sickle Cell Disease

Janet L. Kwiatkowski and John B. Porter

TRANSFUSION

Thalassemia Major (Cooley Anemia)

Eighty years ago, Dr. Thomas Cooley and his colleagues at the Children's Hospital of Michigan administered blood transfusions to children with a newly recognized clinical entity whose features included severe anemia, splenomegaly, and peculiar facies.[1] Five years later, Cooley's name had become indelibly associated with the disease, and transfusions were administered along with ferrous carbonate, ultraviolet rays, and extract of pituitary gland.[2] Not surprisingly, given the state of crossmatching at the time, the response to transfusion was poor. Another 30 years elapsed before improvements in blood banking and recognition of the benefits of a higher hemoglobin level came together to initiate the era of modern transfusion therapy for thalassemia major.

Transfusion Programs

In 1963, the results of an evaluation of 35 children with thalassemia major, aged 12 years or younger, whose pretransfusion hemoglobin levels fell into three categories – 4.0–5.9 g/dL, 6.0–7.9 g/dL, or 8.0–9.9 g/dL – were described.[3] Children in the highest hemoglobin group had better linear growth, less enlargement of the liver and spleen, less facial and skull bony abnormalities, fewer fractures, and less cardiomegaly than children in the two lowest hemoglobin groups. Two patients who received regular red cell transfusions to maintain their hemoglobin level above 10 g/dL at all times were also reported.[4] More than 40 years later, this regimen – hypertransfusion – remains the standard of care for the treatment of thalassemia major. General guidelines for hypertransfusion therapy are presented in Tables 29.1 and 2.

By 1968, several reports confirmed the benefits of hypertransfusion[5–7] and that patients were leading normal, active lives. Their satisfaction with the benefits of hypertransfusion therapy was tempered by a growing appreciation of the problem of transfusional iron overload and the need for iron chelation therapy.

Hemoglobin Level and Physiological Parameters

The target pretransfusion hemoglobin level varies among thalassemia centers, but usually falls between 9.0 and 10.5 g/dL. The goal is to select a hemoglobin level that achieves the important physiological benefits while minimizing the rate of iron accumulation. In regard to the first issue, no significant difference in appearance, cardiac size, occurrence of splenomegaly, or feeling of well-being has been identified with higher or lower hemoglobin levels in a hypertransfusion regimen. Because some of the complications of thalassemia might be related to erythroid hyperplasia in the bone marrow, the level of bone marrow suppression achieved by different target hemoglobin levels could have clinical significance. Both ferrokinetic studies and measurements of soluble serum transferrin receptor levels have demonstrated an inverse relationship between mean pretransfusion hemoglobin level and marrow erythroid activity.[8–10] When anemia is severe – hemoglobin levels 4–7 g/dL – the marrow erythroid activity increases to 10 times normal. One important clinical consequence is impaired bone metabolism with osteoporosis;[11] however, when the selected mean pretransfusion hemoglobin level is 9 g/dL rather than 10.5 g/dL, erythroid activity increases only threefold,[9] and this level of erythroid expansion is associated with little or no impairment of bone metabolism.[11] Thus, no significant physiological difference between target pretransfusion hemoglobin levels of 9 and 10.5 g/dL is known at this time.

Hemoglobin Level and Blood Requirements

The relationship between target hemoglobin level, blood requirements and rate of iron accumulation in patients with thalassemia major is controversial. In 166 splenectomized and nonsplenectomized patients, transfusion requirements remained constant at mean transfusion hemoglobin levels of 10–14 g/dL (equivalent to pretransfusion hemoglobin levels of ~8–12 g/dL).[12] A subsequent expansion of this study to include 392 patients confirmed the earlier findings and concluded that the maintenance of higher hemoglobin levels in transfusion programs for thalassemia major did not necessitate a higher blood requirement.[13] Additional supportive evidence came from a study of "supertransfusion," in which maintenance of pretransfusion hematocrits of 27% and 35% required similar amounts of blood.[14]

Nevertheless, several studies found that maintenance of higher hemoglobin levels requires more blood. Transfusion requirements in 14 patients were directly proportional to the mean hemoglobin levels and nearly doubled

Table 29.1. General guidelines for transfusion. Therapy for thalassemia major

Variable	Range
Pretransfusion Hb level	9–10.5 g/dL
Blood product	Leukoctye-depleted red cells
Amount of blood	1–3 units
Interval between transfusions	2–4 wk

between 9.6 and 13.4 g/dL.[15] Among 3,468 patients, transfusion requirements in 1,985 were proportional to mean hemoglobin level in both splenectomized and nonsplenectomized individuals.[16] Only one large study is reported in which the annual transfusion requirement has been measured repeatedly in the same patients under two different transfusion regimens.[17] From 1982 to 1986, when the mean pretransfusion hemoglobin level of 32 patients was 11.3 g/dL, the mean annual transfusion requirement was 137 mL/kg[17] (Table 29.3). Following modification of the transfusion regimen in 1987–1992, the mean transfusion hemoglobin level fell to 9.4 g/dL, and the mean blood requirement decreased to 104 mL/kg. Of note, the change in target hemoglobin level from 11.3 to 9.4 g/dL was associated with a reduction in serum ferritin levels from a mean level of 2,448 to 1,187 μg/L. The improvement in overall iron status at the lower hemoglobin level might have been a combined effect of decreased transfusional iron loading, enhanced desferrioxamine-induced iron excretion, and maintenance of an acceptable level of gastrointestinal iron absorption.

Beginning Transfusion Therapy

The decision to begin chronic transfusion therapy in an infant or young child with homozygous β thalassemia is based on a combination of laboratory and clinical data. The specific molecular defect may provide general, albeit imperfect, prognostic clues, and the course of an affected sibling might also be helpful. Steady-state hemoglobin levels that remain below 7 g/dL on at least two measurements are one indication for transfusion, particularly in children, but this is not the only consideration. Clinical factors and other laboratory findings in addition to the hemoglobin level will determine whether a chronic hemolytic anemia or

Table 29.2. Estimation of blood requirements according to hematocrit of donor unit

Hematocrit of packed red cell units (%)	Amount of packed red cells to raise Hb by 1 g/dL (mL/kg)
60	3.7
65	3.5
70	3.2
75	3.0

Table 29.3. Effect of target hemoglobin level on transfusion requirements in thalassemia

Years	Mean pretransfusion Hb level (g/dL)	Mean transfusion requirement (mL/kg/y)	Median serum ferritin (μg/L)
1981–1986	11.31 ± 0.5	137 ± 26	2,280
1987–1992	9.4 ± 0.4	104 ± 23	1,004

From ref. 17.

a chronic transfusion program better serves the interests of the patient. For example, the development of Cooley facies, growth retardation, pathological fractures, or persistent fatigue is a strong indication for transfusion, even when the hemoglobin level is 8 g/dL. On the other hand, for a patient with none of these problems despite a lower hemoglobin level, the marginal benefits of transfusions might be outweighed by the associated risks. Clinicians should regularly assess growth, and in conjunction with the family, the overall well-being of the child. In addition, the nucleated red cell count and/or other laboratory indicators of the degree of erythropoiesis such as soluble transferrin receptor levels should be monitored because the consequences of excessive bone marrow expansion could be as important as those of anemia in prompting regular transfusions. Later initiation of transfusion therapy might delay the need for iron chelation therapy until an age at which side effects are less common. Earlier initiation of transfusion therapy might prevent irreversible facial changes and lower the risk of alloimmunization. When the indications for transfusion therapy are equivocal but a decision is made to proceed, the treatment should be reevaluated if the patient later undergoes splenectomy. Sometimes, removal of the spleen makes the difference between transfusion dependency and nondependency.

Choice of Blood Product

Patients with thalassemia should receive leukocyte-reduced red blood cells to decrease or eliminate febrile reactions. The reduction of white cells to less than 5×10^6 per unit of red cells could carry the additional benefit of delaying sensitization to human leukocyte antigens in patients who might later be candidates for bone marrow transplantation. Filtration of the blood product, before storage, or at the time of administration, is the method most commonly used for leukocyte reduction. Prestorage leukocyte reduction is usually more efficient than bedside filtration.[18] Prestorage leukocyte reduction might also decrease cytokine accumulation in the blood during storage, further diminishing the chance of a febrile reaction. One study has suggested that prestorage leukocyte reduction has the additional advantage of reducing the proliferation of *Yersinia enterocolitica* in blood products inoculated with the organism.[19] Because infection with *Y. enterocolitica* can be a serious event in patients with iron overload on chelation therapy, decreasing the likelihood of its transmission from asymptomatic donors might reduce the risk of one of the more serious infectious complications of thalassemia. Whether leukocyte reduction removes prions from potentially infected units remains under investigation.[20]

Even after 42 days of storage, red cell recovery 24 hours after transfusion is 75% or greater.[21] Little information is available, however, regarding the survival of these red cells after this time. Earlier studies showed that the survival of red cells stored in acid-citrate-dextrose for 28 days was reduced in comparison with red cells stored for 14 days.[22] Although this difference is not important for patients with acute or one-time indications for transfusions, it might have a marked effect on the overall blood requirements of patients receiving long-term transfusion. Until more is known about the effect of storage time on posttransfusion red cell survival, it seems prudent to use red cells less than 14–21 days old for patients with thalassemia major.

Frequency and Amount of Transfusion

When using donor units with a hematocrit of 75%, transfusion of 10–15 mL of red cells per kilogram body weight at 3- or 4-week intervals usually maintains a minimum hemoglobin level of 9.0–10.5 g/dL. New additive solutions have reduced the hematocrit of packed red cells from 75%–80% to 55%–65%, and larger volumes of the blood product are therefore necessary to achieve the same target hemoglobin level. This can pose problems for small children or for older patients with heart disease, and in these instances, hemoconcentration of the donor units can be used. Although intervals between transfusions of 3–4 weeks accommodate the school or work schedule of most patients with thalassemia major, shorter intervals would more closely mimic the physiological situation by reducing fluctuations in hemoglobin level. Moreover, mathematical modeling suggests that maintenance of a pretransfusion hemoglobin level of 9 g/dL with transfusions every 2 weeks rather than every 4 weeks would reduce overall blood requirements by 20%.[23] In a large group of splenectomized patients, however, a shorter interval of 2 weeks between transfusions had no measurable effect on transfusion requirements in comparison with an interval of 3 or 4 weeks.[24]

Other conditions might increase the frequency of transfusion or the amount of blood needed to maintain the target hemoglobin level. For example, transfusion requirements rise during pregnancy in women with β thalassemia major.[25,26] Patients undergoing treatment of hepatitis C infection with ribavirin need additional blood due to drug-induced hemolysis; transfusion requirements rise by a median of approximately 40% (range 25%–136%), compared with pretreatment transfusion requirements.[27,28] Transfusion requirements also appear to show seasonal variation. In patients from four thalassemia centers, pretransfusion hemoglobin levels were significantly lower in the summer months in all centers except the one where monthly temperatures varied the least.[29] Possible explanations include hemodilution from expanded plasma volume in the patients and lower hemoglobin levels in donor blood in the summer months.

Young Red Cells

Several groups have evaluated the effect of young red cell (neocyte) transfusions on overall blood requirements, and therefore on the rate of iron loading. The theoretical benefit of this modified blood product lies in the assumption that although all red cells contribute the same amount of iron upon senescence, younger red cells from the donor will circulate longer in the recipient before their iron is released. Thus, enhancement of the blood product for younger donor red cells should reduce the transfusion requirements and the rate of iron loading. Studies in animals have confirmed that age-dependent separation of red cells by density gradient centrifugation has a marked effect on red cell survival.[30] Both simple centrifugation of single donor units and neocyte enhancement during continuous centrifugation apheresis of the donor have yielded red cells with younger estimated mean ages, and in labeled erythrocyte survival studies, longer half-lives than conventional units.[10,31–34] Several factors have impeded the clinical application of young red cell transfusions. In particular, preparation of neocytes by continuous flow centrifugation is costly, and trials using neocytes prepared from single donor units have been disappointing. In three studies, the reduction in the rate of iron loading was only 13%–20%, and both the preparation costs and donor exposures were significantly higher in transfusion regimens in which neocytes were used.[35–38]

Partial Exchange Transfusion

Partial exchange transfusion, whether performed manually or by erythrocytapheresis, decreases the net blood requirement by combining the administration of donor red cells with the removal of red cells from the patient. The rationale for the use of partial exchange transfusion to prevent complications of sickle cell disease is straightforward. Donor HbA-containing cells directly replace endogenous HbS-containing cells, and because the goal of lowering the HbS level is largely independent of the total hemoglobin level, little or no net gain of red cells occurs. The goal of transfusion therapy for thalassemia major differs from that for sickle cell disease. The critical outcome in thalassemia is maintaining a particular hemoglobin level. Although the rationale for the use of partial exchange transfusion for this purpose is less obvious, some studies support this approach in thalassemia major.[39] Seventeen patients

Table 29.4. Comparison of simple transfusion and red cell exchange transfusion in thalassemia

	Mean pretransfusion Hb level (g/dL)	Mean posttransfusion Hb level (g/dL)	Mean transfusion interval (d)	Transfusion requirement level (mL/kg/d)
Simple transfusion	9.7	14.2	35.7	0.41
Red cell exchange transfusion	9.6	14.5	50.8	0.29

From ref. 39.

with thalassemia, and one each with sickle cell disease and Diamond–Blackfan anemia, underwent regular partial exchange transfusion for 6–7 months. Continuous flow centrifugation was used, and returned blood was enriched for younger red cells. In comparison with simple transfusion, the net rate of iron loading fell by 29% (Table 29.4).[39] The mean interval between transfusions increased from 36 to 51 days. Serum ferritin levels decreased by 20% during partial exchange transfusion therapy in contrast with an increase of 12% during a comparable period of conventional transfusion therapy. The authors noted the disadvantages of a 40%–60% increase in exposure to donor units and a 1.5–2.0-fold increase in transfusion-associated costs. Subsequently, the investigators reported the successful extension of this program without neocyte enrichment.[40]

A preliminary report describing a prospective clinical trial that utilized a crossover design to compare simple transfusion to partial exchange transfusion confirmed these findings. In 16 patients with thalassemia major, automated partial exchange transfusion decreased net red cell requirements, and therefore, transfusional iron loading, by a mean of 29% in comparison with simple transfusion, although with considerable interpatient variability in response.[41] Overall, donor blood exposure increased 2.1–3.7-fold. Age-dependent separation of pretransfusion blood samples by density gradient analysis showed an increase in younger red cells during partial exchange transfusion compared with simple transfusion. This suggests that the benefit of partial exchange transfusion in thalassemia might be derived primarily from the replacement of previously administered donor red cells with new donor red cells that have a younger mean age. By reducing the rate of new iron accumulation, this method of transfusion could enhance the overall management of transfusional iron overload in some patients with β thalassemia.

Sickle Cell Disease

Transfusions are used for both the acute management of complications of sickle cell disease and for chronic therapy to prevent the development or progression of complications. One goal of transfusion in sickle cell disease is to raise the hemoglobin level to improve oxygen carrying capacity. A second goal involves lowering the proportion of HbS-containing erythrocytes to reduce complications related to vasoocclusion and hemolysis. In some situations, such as an acute anemic event related to parvovirus B19 infection (Chapter 19), the former goal predominates; in other situations, such as severe acute chest syndrome, the two goals transfusion therapy overlap. Still for other indications, such as preparation for surgery while receiving general anesthetic, the benefits of transfusion therapy cannot be attributed with certainty to one goal or the other.

Choice of Blood Product

The same considerations of used in selecting a blood product in thalassemia also apply to sickle cell disease and leukocyte reduction is important. Selection of blood with a shorter storage time is as important for chronically transfused patients with sickle cell disease as it is for patients with thalassemia.

Extended red cell antigen typing prior to the first transfusion is particularly important in sickle cell disease because, as discussed later, alloimmunization is common. The use of the original antigen profile to determine accurately the specificity of new antibodies and to eliminate the possibility of an autoantibody helps to guide the choice of an appropriate blood product for future transfusions. In chronically transfused patients, in whom the presence of donor red cells can interfere with serological testing, DNA typing of blood groups can aid in accurate determination of the patient's true red cell antigen genotype.[42]

The choice of the best blood product to use for patients with sickle cell disease has been controversial.[43] Generally, most investigators and clinicians agree that at a minimum, in addition to matching ABO and D, partial antigen matching for C, E, and Kell – the antigens most frequently associated with alloimmunization and delayed hemolytic transfusion reactions in sickle cell disease – should be used when selecting red cell units.[43–45] When this transfusion approach was used in a multicenter primary stroke prevention trial, 8% of children receiving chronic transfusions developed a clinically significant alloantibody.[46] The rate of new red cell alloantibodies or autoantibodies was only 0.5% per unit, compared with a rate of approximately 3% per unit in prior studies.[46–49] Several investigators have advocated the use of blood matched for multiple red cell antigens for patients with sickle cell disease.[49,50] This approach can be particularly useful when the racial composition of the donor and recipient pool differ as they do in the United States and elsewhere where certain blood group antigens are common in donors but rare in recipients. A prospective study showed that the initiation of complete matching of donor blood for the Rh, Kell, Kidd, and Duffy systems with less stringent matching for other minor groups resulted in a 10-fold reduction in the rate of new alloantibody formation per unit.[50] Because of the high cost associated with extended antigen matching, other investigators have proposed using this approach only after patients have developed one or two alloantibodies.[51,52]

Units donated by African Americans have an eightfold greater likelihood of antigen identity than units from predominantly Caucasian donor pools.[53] Programs to increase blood donations by African Americans have been introduced to increase the availability of phenotypically matched blood products for chronically transfused patients with sickle cell disease.[54,55] Such a program has been successful in providing racially matched (as well as C, E, and Kell antigen matched) red cell units for the majority of transfusions to children with sickle cell disease in a large urban sickle cell disease program.[54] Another strategy to reduce alloimmunization is to recruit a limited number of dedicated donors to provide the majority of red cell units used for chronically transfused patients with sickle cell disease, thereby limiting donor exposure.[55] The long-term effect of such programs on alloimmunization rates remains to be seen.

Patients with sickle cell disease in chronic transfusion programs generally should not be given blood from donors with sickle cell trait. As discussed later, the target of chronic transfusion programs is a reduction in the percentage of endogenous HbS-containing cells to a particular level, and this is measured in the laboratory by the relative amounts of HbA (from the donor) and HbS (from the recipient). Although not harmful to the patient, the administration of sickle cell trait blood obscures the laboratory assessment of the proportion of the patient's HbS-containing cells that remain in the circulation.

Transfusion Methods

Simple Transfusion

In the acute setting, red cells often are administered as a simple transfusion, although exchange transfusion also is used emergently for complications such as stroke and severe acute chest syndrome. When administering red cells to relieve anemia, the physician must first determine whether there is accompanying hypovolemia. If the blood volume is reduced, as with acute splenic sequestration, sufficient red cells to raise the hemoglobin concentration to the desired level can be given without concern about circulatory overload. In contrast, in a more slowly developing anemia such as an aplastic episode or with advancing renal disease, the patient's blood volume is maintained, and the volume of administered red cells must be calculated to limit the risk of congestive heart failure. One simple approach is to use the hemoglobin level to determine the volume of the transfusion product. For example, if the hemoglobin level is 3 g/dL, the volume of packed red cells is 3 mL/kg of body weight. In most clinical situations, even a small rise in the hemoglobin level is sufficient to address the immediate problem. As noted, however, the use of newer additive solutions has reduced the hematocrit of donor red cell units, complicating the balance between raising the hemoglobin concentration and preventing volume overload; a diuretic might be helpful in this situation. A further consideration when utilizing simple transfusions in the acute setting is that the posttransfusion hemoglobin level should not exceed 10 g/dL because higher levels can lead to hyperviscosity.[56,57]

Simple transfusion also is frequently used in chronic transfusion programs. In general, the administration of 10–15 mL/kg of red cells every 3 or 4 weeks will maintain the pretransfusion HbS level at less than 30%–50%. The target pretransfusion HbS level is variable, but generally a value of less than 30% is used for primary stroke prevention and for secondary stroke prevention at least for the first few years after the event.[58,59] A switch from a target HbS of 30%–50% after 3 or 4 years of more aggressive transfusion for secondary stroke prevention is used in some centers (see later).[60] A target HbS level of 50% often is used for the prevention of severe chronic pain and acute chest syndrome, although studies to determine the optimal HbS level to manage these complications are lacking. The main benefit of targeting a higher HbS level is the reduction in red cell transfusion requirements, which limits iron loading.[60]

Exchange Transfusion

Exchange transfusion can be performed either manually or by an automated process, erythrocytapheresis. A single partial exchange transfusion is useful for the rapid reduction of HbS levels in the patient with sickle cell disease who has an acute complication such as stroke. Partial exchange transfusion can decrease the HbS level below 30% in less than 2 hours without volume overload or hyperviscosity that would accompany repeated simple transfusions for this purpose.[61,62] In comparison with simple transfusion, manual or automated partial exchange transfusion decreases the net amount of blood needed to lower HbS levels by combining the administration of donor red cells with the removal of the patient's red cells.[60,63–65] This has proven to be a valuable tool in the management of iron overload in patients with sickle cell disease in long-term transfusion programs for prevention of stroke or other complications. New iron accumulation is stopped or greatly reduced. Limitations to exchange transfusion include greater donor exposure, higher cost, less widespread availability due to the need for special expertise, and the need for large intravenous access.[63,64]

Table 29.5. Indications for transfusion in sickle cell disease

	Generally Accepted	Controversial
Episodic transfusion	Stroke Aplastic episode Splenic sequestration Acute chest syndrome Acute multiorgan failure Retinal artery occlusion Prior to surgery with general anesthesia – moderate- to high-risk procedure*	Priapism Prior to surgery with general anesthesia – low risk procedure*
Chronic transfusion	Stroke Abnormal transcranial Doppler ultrasound Recurrent acute chest syndrome Recurrent severe vasoocclusive pain Pulmonary hypertension	Recurrent priapism Pregnancy Silent cerebral infarcts* Recurrent splenic sequestration Leg ulcers

* Currently under study.

Clinical Application of Transfusion Therapy in Sickle Cell Disease

Specific complications of sickle cell disease and their treatment are discussed in Chapter 19. The following focuses on the data for and against transfusion therapy for selected disease complications. Particular attention is devoted to randomized, prospective studies of transfusion therapy, but few such studies are available. The specific clinical indications for transfusion therapy are divided into episodic and chronic therapy and evidence-based recommendations are made when possible (Table 29.5).

Indications for Episodic Transfusions

Transient Aplastic Episode

Patients with sickle cell disease can develop profound anemia in association with transient red cell aplasia caused by infection with parvovirus B19. Furthermore, cerebrovascular events, acute chest syndrome, splenic sequestration, and vasoocclusive pain episodes can occur in association with parvovirus B19 infection.[66,67] Transfusion of red cells is indicated to relieve the severe anemia and to prevent or treat organ complications. When the anemia is milder and the need for a transfusion is uncertain, evidence of imminent bone marrow recovery such as nucleated red cells in the peripheral blood or the reappearance of reticulocytes might favor waiting. The *HBB* genotype of the patient might help predict the eventual need for transfusion: Individuals with sickle cell anemia and HbS–β^0 thalassemia generally maintain a lower baseline hemoglobin level and, thus, often develop more severe anemia with an aplastic episode. Nonetheless, patients with HbSC disease or HbS–S β^+ thalassemia also can require transfusion, so knowledge of the genotype cannot substitute for close clinical and laboratory monitoring. For example, in a retrospective study of 84 patients with aplastic episodes, 72% received transfusion therapy, including 85% of those with sickle cell anemia, 57% with HbSC disease, and 14% with other genotypes.[66] If red cells transfusion is necessary, the slow administration of one or two transfusions of small volume, raising the hemoglobin by 2–3 g/dL over 4–8 hours, is usually sufficient to improve the clinical condition until spontaneous recovery occurs.

Acute Splenic Sequestration

Sudden, massive enlargement of the spleen with pooling of large amounts of blood within the organ can cause profound anemia and hypovolemia. Transfusion therapy carries two benefits: restoration of intravascular volume and improvement in oxygen carrying capacity. Acute splenic sequestration is one of the few complications of sickle cell disease in which rapid administration of red cells is not only safe but can also be lifesaving. Occasionally, transfusion with Rh- and ABO-specific, non-crossmatched blood might be necessary to prevent death from shock and severe anemia. Hypovolemia makes consideration of the volume of the transfused red cells less important; however, small amounts of blood are usually sufficient to reverse the process of sequestration, with subsequent release of trapped blood back into the circulation, which further improves the intravascular volume and the hemoglobin level.

Acute Stroke

Red cell transfusion to lessen the anemia, reduce tissue hypoxia, and reduce the percentage of HbS is the mainstay of treatment for acute infarctive stroke, and red cells should be administered as quickly as possible to patients who develop this complication. Manual or automated exchange transfusion, when available, often is used initially. The goal is to reduce the percentage of HbS to less than 30% of the total hemoglobin and to raise the hemoglobin level to approximately 10 g/dL. No prospective studies have been undertaken to compare simple with exchange transfusion. A multicenter, retrospective study found a fivefold higher incidence of stroke recurrence in children who were treated acutely with simple transfusion compared with those treated with exchange transfusion.[68] Nonetheless, a simple transfusion to raise the hemoglobin level to no higher than 10 g/dL should be given if exchange transfusion cannot be performed within a few hours of presentation.

Acute Chest Syndrome

The use of red cell transfusions in the management of acute chest syndrome can cause a rapid improvement in oxygenation.[69] Both simple and exchange transfusion have been used for this indication. In one multicenter study, no significant difference between simple and exchange transfusion in improvement in oxygen levels in patients with acute chest syndrome was seen, although transfusion method was at the treating physician's discretion and, thus, subject to bias.[69] Given the lack of randomized, controlled trials comparing these two transfusion methods, management usually is based on the patient's clinical condition and physician preference. Simple transfusions often are used as first-line treatment with the administration of 1–2 U to raise the hemoglobin level to no greater than 10 g/dL. In more severe cases, such as patients requiring mechanical ventilation or those developing a worsening clinical condition despite simple transfusion, or for patients with a high baseline hemoglobin level that precludes simple transfusion, exchange transfusion should be considered. Case reports and uncontrolled series describe rapid clinical and radiological improvement and higher paO_2 levels after exchange transfusion.[70–73] In the largest series to date, 35 patients with acute chest syndrome and clinical deterioration underwent exchange transfusion.[74] Thirty-two of the 35 patients, including five of seven on assisted ventilation, had a rapid and dramatic improvement in oxygenation and other clinical parameters, leading the investigators to recommend that exchange transfusion be considered for patients with diffuse pulmonary involvement.

Almost half of all acute chest syndromes follow hospitalization, usually for acute painful episodes.[69] Early transfusion might prevent the development of acute chest syndrome in high-risk patients. Such an approach is preferable because it could help prevent lung injury and associated long-term complications. Elevated secretory phospholipase A_2 levels, particularly in association with fever, predict an increased risk of acute chest syndrome in patients admitted with vasoocclusive pain[75]. In a pilot study, patients with sickle cell disease admitted with pain who developed fever and elevated phospholipase A_2 levels (>100 ng/mL) with a negative chest radiograph were randomized to receive a single transfusion of approximately 10 mL/kg or to standard care.[76] Five of eight (63%) patients randomized to standard care developed acute chest syndrome compared with none of seven patients randomized to receive transfusions. A multicenter study currently is under design to study further the benefit of red cell transfusions in preventing acute chest syndrome.

Table 29.6. Effect of goal of perioperative transfusions on outcome

Complications	Group 1 (HbS < 30%, Hb = 10 g/dL)	Group 2 (Hb = 10 g/dL)
Serious or life-threatening postoperative complications	21%	22%
Acute chest syndrome	10%	10%
Fever or infection	7%	5%
Painful crisis	4%	7%
Neurological event	1%	< 1%
Death	1%	0%
Transfusion-related complications	14%	7%
New antibody	10%	5%
Hemolysis	6%	1%

From ref. 93.

Perioperative Management

The use of transfusions to prevent complications of general anesthetics and surgery is particularly controversial. To reduce the high risk of perioperative complications, some have favored simple transfusions to correct the anemia, whereas others have favored exchange transfusion to decrease the HbS level. Uncontrolled studies of these approaches yielded perioperative complication rates of 0%–20%, and a very low death rate.[58,77–88] Other investigators argued that careful attention to hydration and oxygenation rather than administration of red cells produced an equally successful outcome, at least in minor surgical procedures.[82,89–92] Partial resolution of the role of perioperative transfusion therapy came from a large, multiinstitutional, randomized study of two approaches.[93] Patients in group 1 received simple or exchange transfusions to reduce the HbS level below 30% and to raise the total hemoglobin level to 10 g/dL; patients in group 2 received simple transfusions to raise the total hemoglobin level to 10 g/dL, irrespective of the HbS level. The type of transfusion therapy did not affect the rate of minor or major perioperative complications other than those related to transfusion itself (Table 29.6).[93] Acute chest syndrome occurred in 11% of patients in group 1 and 10% of patients in group 2. Both deaths occurred in group 1. The reduction in HbS level in group 1 required twice as much donor blood as the increase in hemoglobin level in group 2. As a result, patients in group 1 had a significantly higher rate of alloimmunization.

Although this study randomly assigned patients only to one of two transfusion arms, the investigators concurrently followed a group of patients who, for different reasons, did not undergo transfusion.[93] In a subanalysis of patients undergoing cholecystectomy, the most common surgical procedure, the rate of sickling-related complications was higher in the patients who did not undergo transfusion than in those receiving either of the two transfusion protocols.[94] Acute chest syndrome occurred in 19% of the 37 nontransfused patients, and two patients died. In other series of patients who did not routinely receive transfusions preoperatively, retrospective analyses have demonstrated complication rates of 13%–26%.[82,85,95] Adverse events generally were more common in patients undergoing major surgery or emergency surgery.

Questions and controversies remain regarding optimal transfusion practices for patients undergoing surgery. Given the lack of randomization to a no-transfusion treatment arm, it remains unclear if transfusion truly is superior or if meticulous supportive care without transfusion could be equally effective, at least for some surgical procedures. For example, success has been reported using a regimen without preoperative transfusion, but with supportive care measures including continuous positive airway pressure postoperatively in patients with sickle cell disease undergoing cholecystectomy.[92] The benefit of routine preoperative transfusion in those undergoing low-risk surgical procedures also is unclear. In one retrospective study of 34 minor surgical procedures, such as myringotomy, strabismus repair, and dental procedures, performed in children without preoperative transfusion, minor complications were seen in 15% of cases and neither acute chest syndrome nor severe complications developed.[89]

The value and goal of preoperative transfusions in patients with HbSC disease is not established. One multicenter study in which transfusions were administered at the physicians' discretion showed a 20% incidence of sickle cell complications with moderate-risk procedures in patients with HbSC disease who did not receive preoperative transfusion compared with none in transfused cases;[96] no difference was seen between the two groups for low-risk procedures. Currently available data also do not address some issues such as the management of a patient with sickle cell disease who maintains a steady-state hemoglobin level of 10 g/dL or a patient receiving hydroxyurea with good hematological response, and transfusion strategies in these instances vary among sickle cell centers.

Given the lack of a robust randomized clinical trial comparing transfusion to no transfusion in the preoperative period, considerable variability in clinical practice exists. In a recent prospective study involving 31 hospitals in Great Britain, among 114 patients with sickle cell disease who underwent surgery, 43% were not treated with preoperative transfusion, whereas 39% received simple transfusion, and 23% underwent exchange transfusion.[97] Although for hip surgery and otorhinolaryngological procedures, exchange transfusion and simple transfusion, respectively, were used in most cases, for other surgical procedures such as cholecystectomy, preoperative transfusion practices varied widely. In multivariate analysis, moderate/high-risk surgery was the only variable associated with postoperative complications and transfusion was not associated with a lower risk of complications. A randomized, multicenter study has been designed to compare surgical complication rates between groups randomized to receive or not to receive preoperative transfusions, which might provide better guidance for optimal management of the patient with sickle cell disease who needs surgery.

Based on current data, preoperative transfusion to raise the hemoglobin level to 10 g/dL generally appears to be equally as effective as a transfusion program to reduce the HbS below 30%. With either approach, acute chest syndrome remains a substantial risk, especially in patients with a history of lung disease who are undergoing a high-risk operation. Transfusions before minor, elective procedures with short anesthesia times might convey no advantage in patients without chronic lung disease or other significant complications.

Vasoocclusive Pain Episode

The value of transfusion therapy in the management of acute painful episode is uncertain. Partial exchange transfusion to reduce the HbS below 50% improved the clinical condition and reduced the duration of hospitalization in eight patients.[98] No subsequent study has confirmed or disproved these old but intriguing findings. In general, the use of red cell transfusion for the management of acute painful episodes is not indicated; however, acute painful episodes occasionally may progress to catastrophic multiorgan failure associated with a falling hemoglobin level. In 17 such episodes, transfusion therapy rapidly and dramatically improved the encephalopathy, urine output, oxygenation. and general clinical condition.[99]

Priapism

Transfusion therapy for the treatment of acute, prolonged episodes of priapism is also controversial. No randomized, controlled studies exploring the use of this therapeutic modality exist and several small, uncontrolled studies of simple and exchange transfusion in the treatment of priapism have yielded inconsistent results.[100–109] In one recent case series, among six patients treated with exchange transfusion the procedure was "very" effective in five and partially effective in one patient,[109] whereas in another report of seven patients treated with red cell exchange, only one patient improved partially.[103] Overall, no difference between the results with simple and exchange transfusion is readily discernible, aside from descriptions of individual patients who had immediate detumescence or relief of pain during erythrocytapheresis. Importantly, neurological events, including headache, seizures, and strokes, have occurred in a small but worrisome number of patients within 1–14 days of simple or exchange transfusion for priapism (ASPEN syndrome).[104,110–112] Whether the risk of such events is greater after transfusion therapy for priapism than other complications of sickle cell disease is uncertain. The limited benefit of transfusion therapy for priapism and the possible risk of neurological sequelae should be carefully considered in managing this acute problem.

Indications for Chronic Transfusion Therapy

Stroke

Although transfusion therapy has not been studied in a randomized controlled clinical trial for prevention of recurrent stroke, data from several case series[113–115] and two multicenter retrospective studies[59,116] support its beneficial effect. Regular red cell transfusions to maintain the HbS level below 30% reduce the risk of recurrent infarctive stroke from approximately 70%[117] to 10%–20%.[59,116] This finding has led to the recommendation to initiate chronic transfusion therapy after a first stroke in children with sickle cell disease.

Although the value of transfusion in preventing recurrent stroke is clear, the optimal duration of therapy is uncertain. Most recurrences in nontransfused patients are in the first 3 years after the initial event,[117] suggesting that lowering the HbS level is particularly important during this period. This view is supported by the recurrence of stroke in seven of 10 patients who stopped transfusion therapy after 1 or 2 years[118] and in four of 10 patients who stopped after 1–4 years.[119] The benefits of longer transfusion therapy are debatable. In one study, stopping transfusions after periods of 5–12 years resulted in a 50% recurrence rate within 1 year,[120] whereas in another study, stopping transfusions in nine patients after a mean duration of 6 years resulted in no recurrences during the next 3–18 years.[121] Six of the nine patients began hydroxyurea therapy at a median of 4 years after discontinuing transfusions, which might have affected stroke risk. At present, most pediatric sickle cell centers continue transfusion therapy indefinitely for the prevention of recurrent stroke. This therapy, however, frequently ends when patients transfer to adult centers. The determination of the optimal duration of transfusion therapy for prevention of recurrent stroke awaits a prospective, randomized trial that avoids the pitfall of selection bias and that accounts for the potential impact of transfusions administered for other purposes.

Given that the major reason for discontinuing transfusions is the concern about iron overload, an alternative to stopping therapy is to modify the transfusion program to reduce the rate of iron accumulation. In a study of nine patients with no recurrence of stroke and no progressive neurological deterioration during at least 4 years of simple transfusion therapy, a subsequent increase in the pretransfusion HbS level from 30% to 50% reduced blood requirements, and thus the rate of iron loading by approximately 30% without raising the risk of recurrent infarctive stroke.[60] A second study supported the safety and benefits of this modified simple transfusion program.[122] Even greater reductions in net blood requirements have been achieved with manual or automated exchange transfusions (Table 29.7).[60,63,64] Novel transfusion programs that prevent recurrent stroke and reduce the risk of iron overload and new oral chelation treatment options could increase the clinician's level of comfort with long-term therapy.

Table 29.7. Effect of transfusion therapy on prevention of first stroke in children with sickle cell disease and abnormal transcranial doppler ultrasonograph

	Patient-months	Cerebral infarctions	Intracerebral hematoma
Transfusion (n = 63)	1,321	1	0
No Transfusion (n = 67)	1,229	10	1

From ref. 123.

Abnormal Transcranial Doppler Ultrasonography

The screening technique of transcranial Doppler ultrasonography (TCD) now allows the identification of children who are at high risk of developing a first stroke, creating the potential for intervention before overt neurological injury occurs (Chapter 19). In the Stroke Prevention Trial in Sickle Cell Anemia (STOP) 63 children with abnormal TCD studies were randomly assigned to receive regular transfusions to maintain the percentage of HbS less than 30%, and 67 to receive standard care without transfusions.[58] Transfusions were associated with a significantly lower risk of stroke (Table 29.7),[123] which led to early termination of the trial. In the years following the publication of the STOP results, the rate of first stroke in children in California with sickle cell disease fell from a baseline of 0.88 per 100 patient-years to 0.17 per 100 patient-years, suggesting a tremendous impact of TCD screening and transfusion therapy on preventing this devastating complication.[124]

A follow-up study, Optimizing Primary Stroke Prevention in Sickle Cell Anemia (STOP II), was designed to assess whether transfusions could be discontinued in children with a history of abnormal TCD whose TCD studies normalized while receiving transfusions, suggesting a reversion to low-risk of stroke.[125] Children considered to have more severe vasculopathy as demonstrated by moderate to severe vessel stenosis detected by brain magnetic resonance angiography were excluded. Among the 41 children who discontinued transfusions, 14 had a reversion to abnormal TCD studies and an additional two children developed stroke; no TCD reversions or strokes occurred in the 38 children who continued transfusions. This highly significant finding led to the current recommendation to continue transfusion therapy indefinitely for primary stroke prevention. Modified transfusion programs that allow the HbS level to rise to 50% or higher have not been studied in this clinical setting and thus the target pretransfusion HbS level is usually kept at less than 30%.

Silent Cerebral Infarcts

Given that silent infarcts occur commonly in sickle cell anemia, often progress over time, and are associated with neurocognitive abnormalities and a higher risk of overt stroke[126–129] effective treatments are needed. Transfusion therapy has been suggested as a treatment option for patients with silent infarcts who demonstrate neurocognitive abnormalities,[46] but the benefit of such therapy is currently unknown. In the STOP study, among the 37% of randomized subjects who had silent infarcts, those receiving transfusions had a significantly lower risk of progression of silent infarcts than those receiving standard care.[130] Whether transfusions will prevent silent infarct progression and neurological complications in children without abnormal TCD remains to be determined. A pilot study showed that transfusion therapy for children with silent infarcts is feasible[131] and a larger, randomized, controlled trial assessing the effect of transfusions on the prevention of neurological complications in children with silent infarcts is currently underway.[132]

Pregnancy

Transfusions are commonly used in the management of acute complications such as toxemia, severe acute chest syndrome, exacerbation of anemia, stroke, acute renal failure, or when emergency surgery is needed in pregnant women with sickle cell disease.[133] Greater controversy surrounds the use of prophylactic transfusion therapy during pregnancy.[134–142] Assessment of the effectiveness of this approach is hindered by differing transfusion protocols and by retrospective analyses. Even if one limits the additional confounding effect of general improvements in obstetrical care by considering only those studies reported in the past three decades, conclusions differ widely. For example, in a retrospective review of 101 women with sickling disorders treated between 1981 and 1990 at a single institution, the investigators concluded that the early (mean 19 weeks) introduction of partial exchange transfusions to maintain the HbS below 50% resulted in fewer episodes of pain, a lower incidence of pneumonia, a reduction in preterm deliveries, a lower perinatal death rate, and fewer low-birth-weight infants.[138] In contrast, two retrospective British studies covering similar periods found no beneficial effect of prophylactic transfusions on either maternal or fetal outcome.[136,143] One study used partial exchange transfusions from the first or second trimester but no consistent target hemoglobin level or HbS percentage,[136] whereas the other used simple transfusion to reduce the HbS level below 25% and raise the hemoglobin to 11 g/dL.[143]

The most informative data regarding the role of prophylactic transfusions during pregnancy in women with sickle cell disease come from a multicenter, prospective, randomized, controlled study.[137] Thirty-six women received prophylactic simple or partial exchange transfusions beginning before 28 weeks of gestation to maintain the hemoglobin level between 10 and 11 g/dL and to reduce the HbS level to less than 35%. An equal number of women received transfusions only for medical or obstetrical emergencies. Although women receiving prophylactic transfusions had fewer painful episodes and a lower cumulative incidence of sickle cell disease–related complications, the two treatment groups did not differ in obstetrical complications or perinatal outcome, which was high at 10%. Even without a clear benefit of transfusions on perinatal outcome, the lower rate of sickle cell complications could be enough to prompt some physicians to treat pregnant patients with transfusions.

Recurrent Acute Chest Syndrome and Pulmonary Hypertension

The role of transfusion therapy for acute chest syndrome might extend to the prevention of recurrences in patients with severe or repeated episodes. This long-term application is predicated on the finding that recurrent acute chest syndrome might be immediately life threatening or contribute to chronic pulmonary failure, pulmonary hypertension, and cor pulmonale.[144,145] In a retrospective study of 17 children receiving chronic transfusion therapy, 13 for stroke and four for recurrent pain, the rate of hospitalizations for acute chest syndrome was reduced significantly from 0.7 per year before treatment to 0.04 per year on transfusion therapy.[146] These findings were confirmed in an analysis of children participating in the STOP trial: The hospitalization rate for acute chest syndrome was significantly lower in the transfusion group compared with the standard care group (4.8 vs. 15.3 per 100 patient-years).[128] A single retrospective study evaluated the effect of chronic transfusions in children treated for the primary indication of recurrent or severe acute chest syndrome.[147] In that study, transfusions were effective in preventing recurrences of acute chest syndrome. The incidence of acute chest syndrome fell significantly from 1.3 per year before transfusions to 0.1 per year during treatment. Chronic transfusions did not reduce the severity of acute chest syndrome in those who developed recurrent episodes.

The effect of transfusion therapy on late pulmonary outcomes remains unknown. Although studies of red cell transfusions for the management of pulmonary hypertension are lacking, this treatment might be beneficial for some patients who develop this complication. Potential benefits of transfusion include improved oxygen carrying capacity and reduction in the amount of HbS. Maintaining a low HbS level should reduce hemolysis, a factor thought to be central to the pathogenesis of pulmonary hypertension in sickle cell disease.[148,149] In addition, transfusions might prevent other complications of sickle cell disease such as acute chest syndrome and pain, which can exacerbate pulmonary hypertension. Further studies are needed to determine the role of transfusions in the management of pulmonary hypertension.

Recurrent Splenic Sequestration

Short-term chronic transfusion therapy might be beneficial in some infants with recurrent acute splenic sequestration to reduce the risk of recurrence and delay the need for splenectomy until the age of 1–2 years. Given, however, that functional asplenia develops in children with sickle cell anemia and HbS–β^0 thalassemia when they are 6–12 months old,[150] it is unclear if deferring surgical asplenia adds much benefit in the protection against invasive infection. One study of 130 Jamaican patients with sickle cell disease who underwent splenectomy showed no increased risk of bacteremia or death compared with nonsplenectomized control subjects.[151] The study group included 46 young children who underwent splenectomy at a median age of 2.3 years for recurrent splenic sequestration. With the routine use of penicillin prophylaxis and the availability of the pneumococcal conjugate 7-valent vaccine, the benefit of postponing splenectomy in young children is even less clear. Furthermore, recurrences of splenic sequestration occur even while receiving regular transfusions to maintain the HbS below 30% and recurrences are frequent when the transfusion program is interrupted or completed.[152] Thus, the role of a short course of prophylactic transfusions for the prevention of recurrent splenic sequestration remains unproven.

Recurrent Painful Episodes

Five percent of patients with sickle cell disease have three–10 episodes of intense pain resulting in hospitalization each year.[153] No study to date has directly addressed the value of transfusion therapy in reducing the physical and social consequences severe pain; however, the experience gained from transfusion therapy for prevention of primary or recurrent stroke demonstrates that reduction of the HbS level to 30% reduces the rate of vasoocclusive pain episodes seven–10-fold, suggesting that such an approach could be beneficial.[146,154] Randomized, controlled clinical trials are needed to address the effect of transfusion therapy on recurrent or unusually severe pain.

Other Proposed Indications

Long-term transfusion therapy might help prevent recurrent episodes of priapism.[104] Case reports and uncontrolled series also have suggested a possible therapeutic role for red cell transfusions in the management of other complications of sickle cell disease such as leg ulcers, avascular necrosis, and persistent hematuria. In some of these descriptions the benefit of transfusion has appeared to be very dramatic, but specific recommendations must await more extensive clinical trials.

Other Approaches

New approaches to the management of sickle cell disease might redefine the role of transfusion therapy. For example, hydroxyurea therapy is an alternative to transfusions for the treatment of recurrent painful episodes and acute chest syndrome. In addition, a strategy of switching from transfusion therapy to hydroxyurea treatment for secondary stroke prevention showed promising results in a pilot study of 35 children,[155] and a larger, multicenter study is currently underway. Bone marrow transplantation is being offered with increasing frequency as an alternative to transfusion therapy for patients with stroke or other severe or recurrent complications. These advances, as well as progress in the general management of pregnancy, general anesthetics, and other medical and surgical conditions, will require regular reevaluation of the effectiveness and safety of transfusions.

Other Hemoglobinopathies

Patients with unstable hemoglobins might need occasional red cell transfusions during exacerbations of anemia. If the unstable hemoglobin has an increased oxygen affinity, the decision to transfuse reaches a higher level of complexity.[156] In this situation, the chronic hemolysis due to the unstable hemoglobin blocks the usual compensatory erythrocytosis in response to the hemoglobin's abnormally increased oxygen affinity. The resultant "normal" hemoglobin level may have only one-half of the normal oxygen delivery capacity. Simple transfusions to achieve normal oxygen delivery at the time of surgery or acute illnesses might raise the hemoglobin to unacceptably high levels. Alternatively, exchange transfusion carries the dual benefits of improving oxygen delivery while maintaining a normal total hemoglobin level, and replacing the unstable hemoglobin variant with HbA.

COMPLICATIONS OF TRANSFUSION THERAPY

Most adverse consequences of transfusion therapy for thalassemia, sickle cell disease, and other hemoglobinopathies are independent of the underlying blood disorder, although they might occur with differing frequency in each of these diseases because of environmental or other reasons. The following sections focus on complications that are particularly problematic for patients with hemoglobinopathies receiving long-term transfusions. A detailed discussion of other complications such as febrile or allergic reactions and acute hemolytic transfusion reactions can be found in textbooks of transfusion medicine. Iron overload, the leading and most complex clinical problem of long-term transfusion therapy, is discussed in full in the second major section of this chapter.

Alloimmunization

Thalassemia

Alloantibodies have been detected in 3%–37% of patients with thalassemia.[24,157–163] Variations among the protocols practiced at different centers are likely due to several factors. Alloimmunization rates are generally higher when there is a greater discordance of red cell antigen frequencies between donors and recipients. For example, the prevalence of alloimmunization was 20.8% among thalassemia patients of Asian descent treated at a northern California center where donors are primarily Caucasian,[158] whereas lower rates of 5%–10% were reported in more homogeneous populations.[157,159] The degree of antigen matching of blood products also affects alloimmunization rates. Antibodies are most commonly directed against antigens of the Rh and Kell systems.[159–161] In the northern Californian thalassemia population, the alloimmunization rate was only 3% among patients receiving Rh- and Kell-matched blood, compared with 33% in those treated with nonphenotypically matched blood.[158] Extension of antigen matching beyond the Rh and Kell systems might not be helpful.[165] Immune factors, related to both the recipient and to the blood product preparation, could also impact alloimmunization rate. For example, splenectomy might increase the risk of alloimmunization, whereas prestorage leukocyte depletion can lower the rate because leukocytes release potentially immunomodulatory cytokines during storage.[158,161]

The age at which transfusion therapy is initiated in thalassemia major has a consistent effect on the rate of alloimmunization. In two studies from Greece, alloimmunization occurred more than twice as often in children beginning transfusion therapy after age 3 years[160] and four times as often in children beginning transfusion therapy after 1 year of age.[164] In 110 alloimmunized patients in Greece and Italy, alloantibodies developed in fewer than 3% of children who began transfusion therapy in the first year of life, but did occur in more than 15% of children who received their first transfusion after age 4 years.[24] Because alloimmunization by itself is rarely a significant clinical problem in thalassemia, these findings of the influence of age might not have a substantial impact on the decision to initiate or delay transfusion therapy. In some children, however, receiving regular transfusions, alloantibodies are accompanied by red cell autoantibodies, presenting additional and often serious clinical problems. This unusual but severe complication is worthy of consideration in deciding at what age to initiate transfusion therapy in the child with a marginal hemoglobin level or clinical status.

Sickle Cell Disease

Red cell alloimmunization occurs in 3%–76% of patients with sickle cell disease who have been transfused.[46,47,49,50,157,165–169] In the Cooperative Study of Sickle Cell Disease, the overall rate of alloimmunization in 1,814 patients transfused before or after study entry was 18.6%.[167] In a subanalysis of 604 patients who had no alloantibodies at study entry and subsequently underwent transfusion, the investigators found a significantly higher incidence of alloimmunization in patients with sickle cell anemia in comparison with patients with other sickling disorders. A relationship between age and risk of alloimmunization exists in sickle cell disease as it does in thalassemia. Patients with sickle cell disease who received their first transfusion at age 10 years or older had a 20.7% rate of alloimmunization compared with 9.6% in individuals first transfused when aged younger than 10 years. Alloimmunization rose continuously with an increasing number of transfusions. Patients first transfused at a young age consistently required more transfusions to become alloimmunized than those first transfused at older ages.

Red cell antigens causing alloimmunization in patients with sickle cell disease most commonly belong to the Rh, Kell, Duffy, and Kidd systems. Antibodies to E, C, K, Jk^b, and Fy^a account for approximately 80% of clinically significant alloantibodies, reflecting the differences in red cell phenotype between blood donors who are predominantly Caucasian and patients with sickle cell disease who are predominantly of African ancestry.[49,167] The red cell alloimmunization rate was 76% among patients with sickle cell disease who underwent transfusion in the United Kingdom compared with a rate of only 2.6% in patients transfused in Jamaica, where donors and recipients are more genetically similar.[166] Similarly, the rate of alloimmunization among previously transfused Caucasians with sickle cell disease in Italy is only 5.4%.[170]

Red cell autoantibodies also can develop in patients with thalassemia or sickle cell disease, often in association with alloantibodies.[171–173] The mechanism underlying the formation of autoantibodies is unclear, but possible causes include antigenic changes in the erythrocyte membrane or more generalized immune dysregulation. Erythrocyte autoantibodies occur in 5%–8% of multiply transfused children with sickle cell disease but cause hemolysis in only approximately 2%.[46,169,171]

Alloimmunization has consequences that range from additional work and expense in the blood bank to severe hemolysis. Delayed hemolytic transfusion reactions pose a particularly important problem for patients with sickle cell disease.[47,52,174–176] In two prospective studies, delayed hemolytic transfusion reactions occurred in 38% and 44% of newly alloimmunized patients with sickle cell disease.[49,93] Delayed hemolytic transfusion reactions arise when an alloantibody is not present in sufficient quantity to be detected by direct or indirect antiglobulin testing or when the antibody is directed against a low-frequency antigen that is not present on the screening cells used for the indirect antiglobulin test.[177] On reexposure to the offending antigen, an anamnestic response occurs, and hemolysis begins in 3–10 days. Fever, and back, leg, or abdominal pain can accompany the delayed hemolysis, mimicking a vasoocclusive episode.[176,178] In addition to destruction of the transfused cells, the patient's HbS-containing cells also can be destroyed, leading to profound anemia.[173,176,179] Reticulocytopenia might occur and the direct antiglobulin test also can be negative, further complicating the diagnosis. Treatment with steroids, intravenous immunoglobulin, and erythropoietin might be helpful; further transfusions, even using apparently compatible blood, should be carefully considered in light of the risk of life-threatening hemolysis.[176,179]

Transfusion-transmitted Infections

Because patients with thalassemia major and regularly transfused patients with sickle cell disease usually receive 12–50 U of red cells each year, they are at higher risk than most blood recipients for transfusion-transmitted infections such as hepatitis and human immunodeficiency virus (HIV). Rates of seropositivity for hepatitis C have varied from 12% in patients with thalassemia who received treatment in the United Kingdom to 91% in those who were treated in Italy.[180,181] Serological testing of donated blood for hepatitis C, which became available in developed countries in the early 1990s, has reduced the risk of acquiring this infection from transfusion. In a 2004 report from the Thalassemia Clinical Research Network, 35% of 334 North American patients with thalassemia had evidence of hepatitis C exposure.[182] Among children aged younger than 5 years, only 5% had evidence of hepatitis C exposure compared with 70% of patients aged 25 years and older. Antibodies to hepatitis C have been detected in 23%–30% of repeatedly transfused patients with sickle cell disease.[183,184] Nucleic acid testing for hepatitis C, implemented in most developed countries by 2000, is expected to reduce greatly the risk of transfusion-transmitted hepatitis C virus. Viral hepatitis might have particularly grave clinical consequences in regularly transfused patients with hemoglobinopathies because iron overload aggravates the liver damage and can diminish the response to antiviral therapy.[185,186] New cases of transfusion-transmitted hepatitis B are rare in the United States as a result of vaccination programs and blood screening. High rates of hepatitis B infection continue to occur in thalassemia patients in some parts of the world,[187,188] mostly attributable to late or no vaccination. A recent study of children with thalassemia in India infected with hepatitis B found a number of mutations in viral DNA regions involved in reactivity to antihepatitis B surface antibody, raising concern that such mutations might contribute to vaccine failures.[189] This intriguing finding deserves further study.

The risk of transfusion-transmitted HIV infection in patients with thalassemia and sickle cell disease has varied with time and geographical location. In 1984, when donor testing was still unavailable, 12% of patients with thalassemia at one center in New York were seropositive for HIV.[190] In contrast, in a 1987 study of 3,633 patients with thalassemia in Europe, only 1.56% were seropositive for HIV.[191] Following the introduction of routine donor screening programs and serological testing for HIV by enzyme-linked immunosorbent assay, new seroconversions became extremely rare in many countries.[192,193] In a more report from the Thalassemia Clinical Research Network, 2% of North American patients with thalassemia major were positive for HIV.[182] The current risk of acquiring HIV from transfusion is less than 1 in 2 million.[194] In countries with a high prevalence of HIV coupled with inadequate blood safety programs, the risk of HIV infection in repeatedly transfused children with sickle cell disease remains high.[195]

Iron overload, as assessed by serum ferritin level, might contribute to the progression of HIV infection in patients with thalassemia.[196] The iron chelator desferrioxamine, on the other hand, might have a dose-dependent inhibitory effect on disease progression.[197] This observation is supported by in vitro studies of the effect of chelators on HIV infectivity. Both desferrioxamine and deferiprone have an inhibitory effect on HIV-1 replication[198] and more recently, the newer oral chelator, deferasirox has been shown to inhibit HIV-1 transcription.[199]

Red cell transfusions infrequently transmit bacterial infections.[200] *Yersinia enterocolitica*, the organism responsible for seven of the eight fatal red cell–transmitted bacterial infections reported to the Food and Drug Administration between 1986 and 1991, deserves special attention. This contaminant represents a particular problem for chronically transfused patients because iron overload and the iron chelator desferrioxamine enhance its pathogenicity. *Y. enterocolitica* enters the blood supply when blood donation coincides with asymptomatic bacteremia, making efforts at prevention difficult. Evaluating febrile transfusion reactions or persistent unexplained fevers in regularly transfused patients with hemoglobinopathies should include careful consideration of systemic or localized *Y. enterocolitica* infection.

Hypersplenism and Increased Transfusion Requirements

A sustained increase in transfusion requirements is an indication for splenectomy in patients with thalassemia major.[201] When the annual blood requirement exceeds 200 mL of packed red cells (hematocrit 75%) per kilogram body weight, a minimum reduction of at least 20% usually follows removal of the spleen. The role of splenectomy in reducing transfusion requirements might be less important in patients in whom chelation therapy is working well, and should be weighed against potential complications such as postsplenectomy sepsis and thrombosis. Moreover, other causes of increased blood requirements, such as alloimmunization or different preparation of donor units, should be sought before removing the spleen for this purpose. Regular red cell transfusions can have the unintended consequence of reversing partial splenic atrophy in children and adults with sickle cell disease. As the newly restored spleen enlarges, transfusion requirements sometimes increase substantially.[202,203] In such cases, removal of the spleen reduces the need for donor blood and therefore the accumulation of iron by 39%–51%. Careful monitoring of spleen size and annual transfusion requirements assists in identifying patients with hypersplenism who might benefit from surgical intervention.

Hypertension and Encephalopathy

Hypertension, accompanied or followed shortly by headache, or changes in mental status and seizures, is an unusual but potentially devastating complication of transfusion therapy in thalassemia, especially when the hemoglobin is raised from very low levels to normal or high levels.[204,205] This constellation of findings also has been reported after transfusion in sickle cell disease.[111,206] The cause is unknown. Autopsy findings in six cases showed brain edema and congestion, gross or microscopic hemorrhage, and microdissecting aneurysms.[207] No underlying vascular disease distinguished these patients from those without encephalopathy. Similar symptoms of hypertension, seizures, and mental status changes accompanied by reversible T2 hyperintensities on brain magnetic resonance imaging (MRI), constitutes a syndrome known as reversible posterior leukoencephalopathy. This has also have been reported in children with sickle cell disease and severe acute chest syndrome treated with erythrocytapheresis.[208] Complaints of headache or weakness after transfusion should prompt careful evaluation for neurological abnormalities including cerebral hemorrhage; hypertension, if present, should be treated aggressively.

IRON OVERLOAD AND CHELATION THERAPY

Pathophysiology of Iron Overload

Rates of Iron Loading

The average iron content of a healthy human is 40–50 mg/kg of body weight, with 30 mg/kg present in hemoglobin. Approximately 4 mg/kg is found in muscle myoglobin and 2 mg/kg in iron-containing enzymes. The remaining body iron is in the storage form of ferritin or hemosiderin, predominantly in liver, spleen and bone marrow. Mean iron stores are 769 mg in men and 323 mg in women.[209,210] A healthy individual absorbs approximately 10% of the dietary iron, or 1–2 mg daily. This intake is matched by insensible losses through exfoliation of skin, urinary tract, and gut mucosal cells together with gastrointestinal and menstrual loss of red blood cells. Humans have a limited capacity to modulate iron absorption and no physiological mechanism for excreting excess iron.

Iron can accumulate as a consequence of increased gastrointestinal absorption or from repeated red cell transfusions. In thalassemia major, iron loading predominantly derives from blood transfusion but excess iron absorption might also contribute. A unit of red cells, processed from 420 mL of donor blood, contains approximately 200 mg of iron (0.47 mg iron/mL of whole donor blood or 1.16 mg iron/mL of pure red cells). Splenectomized patients with thalassemia major received the red cells derived from approximately 300 mL/kg/year of whole blood per (range 200–400 mL whole blood/kg)[211] to maintain a mean hemoglobin level of 12 g/dL. This volume of transfused blood is equivalent to 0.4 mg/kg of transfused iron daily or 28 mg of iron in an adult weighing 70 kg. Iron loading varies greatly both within a given diagnosis and among diagnoses.[212,213] In thalassemia major with a mean loading rate of 0.4 mg/kg/day[212] there is considerably variability with approximately 20% of patients receiving less than 0.3 mg/kg/day, approximately 60% receiving 0.3–0.5 mg/kg/day, and a further 20% more than 0.5 mg/kg/day. The transfusion requirements in nonsplenectomized patients are generally higher than splenectomized patients and might contribute to an increased rate of iron loading. In one study of patients on hypertransfusion regimens who required more than 250 mL/kg/year of packed red cells, splenectomy decreased the annual iron loading by an average of 39%.[214] Average transfusion requirements in nonspelenectomized thalassemia major patients are 0.43 mg/kg/day compared with 0.33 mg/kg/day in splenectomized patients.[212] In general, hypertransfusion decreases the rate of splenic enlargement,[215] and the early introduction of a hypertransfusion regimen might diminish the extent to which the spleen contributes to an increased blood transfusion requirement.[211]

The contribution of increased iron absorption to iron loading in hemoglobin disorders is variable depending on the underlying condition. In thalassemia major, gastrointestinal iron absorption accounted for a further 1–4 mg daily of net iron loading[216] in a splenectomized adult patient who weighed 70 kg. In thalassemia intermedia, blood transfusion is intermittent or absent, and the increased iron loading is mainly a consequence of excess iron absorption. The amount of excess iron absorption depends on the degree of ineffective erythropoiesis, the extent of erythroid expansion, and the severity of the anemia, all of which are highly variable in thalassemia intermedia. In one study, patients with thalassemia intermedia absorbed 26%–73% of food iron.[217] Patients with this form of thalassemia absorbed 60% (range 17%–90%) of a 5-mg dose of ferrous sulfate, whereas healthy controls absorbed 10% (5%–15%).[217] In another study, absorption varied from 20% to 75% in HbE–β thalassemia and correlated

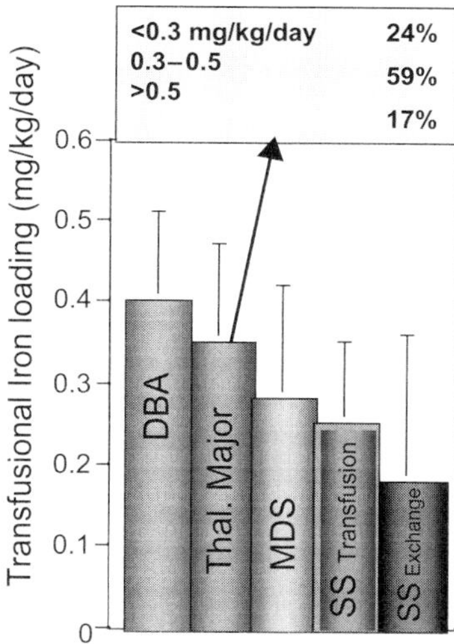

Figure 29.1. Rates of transfusional iron loading by diagnosis. (Original figure derived from data in refs. 212, 225, 246, 453.)

with plasma iron turnover, transferrin saturation, and liver iron concentration.[218] Iron absorption in thalassemia intermedia can thus be as much as five–10 times normal, or 0.1 mg/kg/day.[219]

In sickle cell disease, iron overload does not occur in the absence of blood transfusion.[220] Indeed, a variable proportion of untransfused patients might be iron deficient.[221–223] Repeated simple blood transfusions will inevitably lead to iron overload, but can mitigate iron deficiency.[60,224] The average rate of transfusional iron loading was less in sickle cell disease (0.22 mg/kg/day)[225] than in thalassemia major.[212] Figure 29.1 shows the relative rates of iron accumulation from transfusion measured in clinical trials involving desferrioxamine and deferasirox. Various exchange transfusion rates were highest in Diamond–Blackfan anemia (DBA) and lowest in sickle cell disease. These rates affect the chelation doses that are typically required for each condition.[212,213]

Distribution of Excess Iron

The tissue distribution and clinical manifestations of transfused iron are influenced by the mode and rate of iron loading and by the absolute levels of tissue iron within the body. Increased iron absorption leading to a predominantly parenchymal distribution of iron loading is a feature of genetic hemochromatosis and is also found in many conditions associated with ineffective erythropoiesis.[218,226–228] Postmortem examination of patients with thalassemia major showed a striking variability in iron concentrations among different tissues.[229] In thalassemia major in the pre–chelation era, iron was found at high concentrations in liver, heart, and endocrine glands with very little present in striated muscle[229] and none in the brain and nervous tissue. In the absence of chelation therapy, siderosis in liver macrophages and hepatocytes correlates with the number of units of blood transfused, with age, and with liver iron concentration.[230] With more advanced iron overload or in splenectomized patients, hepatocyte deposition predominates.[230]

Recent evidence in iron-loaded mice suggests that uptake of nontransferrin-bound iron (NTBI) into tissue expressing L-type calcium channels can account for this uneven distribution of iron overload and in particular the uptake into heart and endocrine tissues.[231] Another factor that could influence iron distribution in transfusional iron overload is hepcidin synthesis by the liver. Under relatively normal levels of iron loading, hepcidin is upregulated by increments in iron loading causing decreased iron absorption from the gut and decreased iron release from macrophages by secondary down regulation of ferroportin.[232] This process could occur through increments in transferrin saturation with progressive iron loading.[233] There is evidence, however, that hepcidin synthesis is downregulated by ineffective erythropoiesis as seen in thalassemia[234–236] and at very high levels of iron loading in the liver,[237] possibly through production of reactive oxygen species. This would lead to an increased propensity to distribute iron to the heart and endocrine tissues in conditions associated with high levels of ineffective erythropoiesis and also when liver iron levels reach a point at which increased damage through reactive oxygen species production is seen. Increased alanine aminotransferase values[238] and progression of fibrosis[239] are associated with liver iron concentrations above approximately 15–20 mg/g dry weight. These levels of liver iron loading are also associated with an increased likelihood of myocardial iron deposition in patients who have not undergone intensive chelation treatment.[240,241] In transfusional iron overload, cardiac iron is preferentially distributed to the ventricular compared with atrial myocardium or conducting tissue.[240] In nonthalassemic patients in the pre–chelation era, increased myocardial iron was found at postmortem in approximately 30% of patients after 50–75 U of blood, in 60% of patients who received 65–200 U of blood and in all patients who had received 200–300 U of blood.[240] Ventricular myocardial iron distribution is uneven, being maximal in the subepicardium, intermediate in the subendocardial region and papillary muscles, and least in the middle third of the ventricular myocardium. Focal areas of fibrosis can also be seen in papillary muscles or ventricles.[240] The uneven distribution of iron makes endocardial biopsy an unreliable tool for assessing cardiac iron concentration and iron-mediated cardiac damage.[242,243] The use of cardiac MRI to estimate myocardial iron has added to the understanding of factors affecting myocardial iron uptake and removal with chelation therapy. In adult patients with myelodysplastic syndrome who have not undergone chelation therapy, increased myocardial iron was demonstrated by MRI using signal intensity ratios to skeletal muscle, after 75 U of blood or when the liver iron concentration exceeded 400 μmol/g ($\sim$ 23 mg/g dry wt.).[241] Correlations between liver iron concentration and myocardial iron and between serum ferritin and myocardial iron were seen prior to initiation of chelation in these patients: After 6 months of chelation therapy with desferrioxamine, these correlations were still present but less strong in the case of serum ferritin and myocardial iron. With chronic chelation therapy in thalassemia major, a clear relationship between liver iron and cardiac iron is no longer seen,[244] most likely because the rate of iron removal from the liver by chelation therapy exceeds that from the heart.[245] With modern chelation regimes, as many as 45% of thalassemia major patients still show evidence of myocardial iron loading on MRI.[246] Iron loading in the heart can occur after multiple transfusions in a variety of other conditions such as Diamond–Blackfan anemia and sideroblastic anemia.[246] In sickle cell disease, multiple transfusions are less likely to result in myocardial iron deposition,[246,247] perhaps as a result of lower levels of plasma NTBI compared with thalassemia patients matched for body iron load.[248]

Mechanisms of Iron Overload Toxicity

In the absence of iron overload, iron is unavailable to participate in the generation of harmful free radicals by its binding to physiological ligands such as transferrin. When iron overload develops, these protective mechanisms become saturated, and NTBI[249] and increased quantities of redox-active low-molecular-weight intracellular iron[250] are available to participate in the generation of harmful free radicals. NTBI species are likely to be heterogeneous, consisting of iron citrate monomers, oligomers and polymers and protein-bound forms.[251,252] In experimental models, NTBI is rapidly taken up by hepatocytes[253] and by myocytes.[254] Although the most important effects of NTBI result from its pattern of uptake and subsequent iron accumulation in tissues expressing appropriate receptors,[231] plasma NTBI (or subtractions of it) can generate lipid peroxidation through free radical formation,[255] and depletion of plasma antioxidants is associated with increased NTBI levels.[256] In cultured heart cells, species of NTBI are taken up at 200 times the rate of transferrin iron and generate free radicals, lipid peroxidation, organelle dysfunction, and abnormal rhythmicity.[254,257]

A free radical is defined as any species capable of independent existence that contains one or more unpaired electrons. The products formed sequentially during the reduction of molecular oxygen (O_2) to water are superoxide (O_2-), hydrogen peroxide (H_2O_2) and the hydroxyl radical (·OH), the reduction of the latter resulting in the formation of water. The hydroxyl radical has a great affinity for electrons and will oxidize all substances within its immediate vicinity diffusion radius of 2.3 nm.[258] H_2O_2 is relatively stable and nontoxic by itself. It is, however, an important precursor of ·OH requiring the availability of catalytic trace elements such as iron, copper, or cobalt. Iron is particularly important because it is present at sufficient concentrations in tissues and because of the favorable redox potential of the Fe^{2+}/Fe^{3+} couple (between +0.35 and -0.5 V). The oxidation of Fe^{2+} to Fe^{3+}, with the concomitant generation of the ·OH from water, is referred to as the Fenton reaction.

$$H_2O_2 + Fe^{2+} \rightarrow OH^- + HO' + Fe^{3+} \text{ (Fenton reaction)\#}$$

Within cells are a number of physiological scavengers of toxic oxygen products such as superoxide dismutase, which dismutates O_2- to H_2O_2, and catalase, which scavenges H_2O_2. Tissue damage depends on the relative rates of formation and scavenging of toxic free radicals. ·OH can damage proteins, DNA, and membrane lipids by peroxidation. Particularly important is the initiation of peroxidation of lipid (Lp) by hydrogen abstraction:[259]

$$LpH + HO' \rightarrow Lp' + H2O.$$

Because iron is concentrated in hepatocyte lysosomes in both primary and secondary iron overload, these organelles are particularly susceptible to lipid peroxidation.[260,261] The resulting lysosomal fragility[262] is directly proportional to the degree of iron overload.[263] In cultured heart cells, iron increased lysosomal instability and caused direct damage to mitochondria.[257,264] Lipid peroxidation and damage to organelles and lysosomal fragility might lead to apoptotic cell death[265–267] but might also encourage fibrogenesis. Iron-induced aldehyde lipid peroxidation products such as malondialdehyde[268] and others[269] have been shown to promote collagen gene expression and fibrogenesis in cultured fibroblasts and perisinusoidal stellate (Ito) cells. Fibrogenesis is also associated with autocrine production of transforming growth factor–β (TGFβ) in stellate cells[270] and increased mRNA levels of TGFβ and procollagen al(I) have been observed in a model of iron and alcohol induced fibrogenesis.[271] Increased TGFβ expression and malondialdehyde protein adducts have also been reported in hepatocytes and sinusoidal cells of patients with genetic hemochromatosis,[272] suggesting that iron overload increases both lipid peroxidation and *TGF-β* gene expression, which together might promote hepatic injury and fibrogenesis. In other tissues, similar mechanisms are likely to be involved, although the concentration and distribution of intracellular iron clearly differs among tissues: Tissues that have a high mitochondrial activity could be particularly susceptible to iron toxicity.[273] A scheme for iron-induced cell injury is shown in Figure 29.2.

Clinical Consequences of Transfusional Iron Overload

The consequences of transfusional iron overload and the effects of chelation treatment on these consequences are best described in thalassemia major, in which transfusion typically begins in the first few years of life and transfusional iron loading occurs at a rapid rate. In other forms of transfusional iron overload, the pathological effects of transfusional iron overload are less well documented.

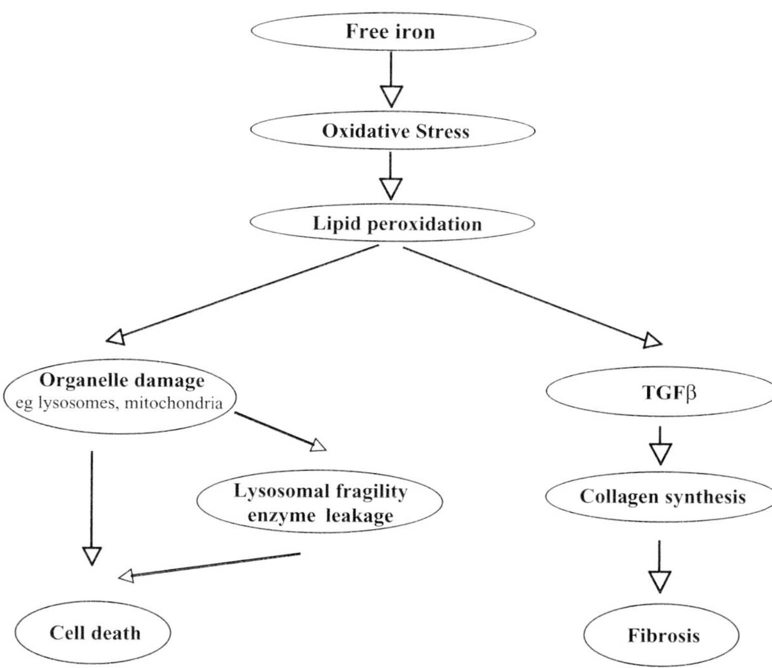

Figure 29.2. Mechanisms of liver damage in iron overload.[277]

Thalassemia Major

In thalassemia major, if chelation treatment is withheld, death from iron-induced cardiac failure is common from the second decade on.[274–276] By contrast, in conditions such as genetic hemochromatosis in which iron loading is slower, cirrhosis is a common presenting feature, usually in the fourth and fifth decades, and commonly leads to death from liver failure or hepatocellular cancer. Cirrhosis is also a common feature in thalassemia major, being present in 50% of patients at postmortem examination, particularly if chronic infective hepatitis (e.g., hepatitis C) is also present. Although cirrhosis was a relatively uncommon cause of death in thalassemia major[275] as patients live longer with improved chelation, cirrhosis and hepatocellular carcinoma[277] are likely to become increasingly common problems. Liver fibrosis can develop early in the course of thalassemia major, even in the absence of infective hepatitis. For example, fibrosis has been observed as early as 3 years after starting transfusion.[278] Fibrosis correlates with age, the number of units of blood transfused, and with liver iron concentration.[230] In these studies there was an exponential increase in hepatic fibrosis with increasing liver iron concentrations. The concentration of liver iron at which fibrosis progresses was examined in ex-thalassemic patients who had received a successful bone marrow transplant.[239] In the absence of active hepatitis C, fibrosis only progressed when liver iron concentrations exceeded 16-mg/g dry weight.

The most common cause of death in thalassemia major remains iron-induced cardiomyopathy but this has been reduced since the introduction of subcutaneous desferrioxamine infusions in the late 1970s[277] (Fig. 29.3). Risk factors for the development of fatal cardiomyopathy include late commencement of chelation therapy,[276,279] failure to maintain serum ferritin below 2,500 μg/L over a period of a decade or more,[277,279–283] failure to control iron concentration below 15 mg/g dry weight,[276,282] poor compliance with chelation therapy,[276,279,281] and a fall in ejection fraction below reference ranges.[279] Development of left ventricular dysfunction is increasingly likely when a myocardial T2* values fall below 20 m sec[244] and especially if T2* values are less than 8 msec.[284]

Hypogonadism commonly occurred in 55% of patients aged more than 12 years[285] and led to disturbances of growth and sexual maturation. The frequency of this complication is falling in progressive birth cohorts treated from an early age with desferrioxamine, so that at age 20 years, 65% of patients born between 1970 and 1974 had evidence of hypogonadism, and this fell to 14% in 1980–1984 birth cohorts[277] (Table 29.8). Hypogonadism is typically secondary to anterior pituitary dysfunction (hypogonadotrophic hypogonadism), and hence in many female thalassemics with secondary amenorrhea,[286] induction of ovulation and successful pregnancy are often achievable.[287] The effects of iron damage to the anterior pituitary with consequent hypogonadotrophic hypogonadism will clearly be more devastating if transfusion begins early in life and damage occurs before growth has ceased and full sexual maturity has been achieved.

Other complications such as diabetes, hypothyroidism,[288] and hypoparathyroidism are seen in a variable proportion of patients, and the frequency of these complications is also falling with improved chelation.

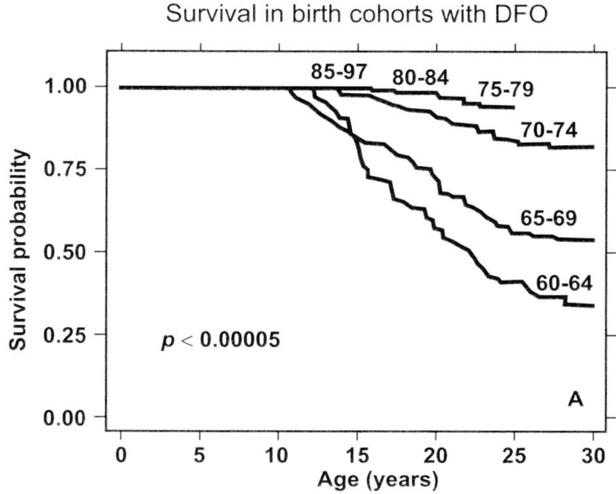

Figure 29.3. Survival by birth cohort in desferrioxamine-treated thalassemia major patients.[277]

Table 29.8. Falling complications since the introduction of DFO chelation therapy patients with thalassemia major born after 1960, n = 977

	Birth 1970–1974*	Birth 1980–1984†
Death at 20 y	5%	1%
Hypogonadism	64.5%	14.3%
Diabetes	15.5%	0.8%
Hypothyroidism	17.7%	4.9%

* DFO intramuscularly, 1975
† DFO subcutaneously, 1980.
In 1995, 121 patients switched to DFP (censored at this time).

The frequency of diabetes at age 20 years has fallen from 16% to 0.8% between birth cohorts from 1970–1974 to 1980–1984[277] (Table 29.8). In optimally treated patients who receive more than 260 infusions of desferrioxamine each year, these complications are absent at 15 years of follow-up.[281] Low levels of adrenal androgen secretion with normal glucocorticoid reserve have also been reported.[289] Other features of iron overload include skin pigmentation, arthropathy, ascorbic acid deficiency and osteoporosis.[219]

Infections are the second most frequent cause of death in thalassemia, occurring particularly commonly in younger age groups.[275] Postsplenectomy sepsis due to encapsulated organisms is an important contributor,[290] but iron overload also appears to play a central role in increasing susceptibility to infection. Reports of infection with *Y. enterocolitica, Vibrio vulnificus, Listeria monocytogenes, Escherichia coli, Candida* sp. and *Klebsiella* can be found.[291–294] The increased infective risk partly results from the saturation of transferrin with iron, depriving the body of an important mechanism to withhold this nutrient from bacteria. Defective neutrophil and macrophage function,[295–297] presumably secondary to the effects of excess iron, might also be important. Some bacteria such as *Yersinia* are able to utilize iron from iron complexes of chelators.[298] This is particularly likely if the chelator is a naturally occurring siderophore such as desferrioxamine.

The relevance of the rate of iron loading to the clinical manifestations of iron overload is further illustrated by the contrasting complications of excessive iron in thalassemia major and thalassemia intermedia. Thalassemia intermedia patients have different transfusion requirements.[218] Because of the slower buildup of iron, damaging levels of iron loading typically develop later than in thalassemia major and might not affect pituitary function until the third or fourth decade or beyond. Therefore, in thalassemia intermedia, growth and sexual development are typically unaffected by iron overload per se, and, when present, are more likely to be the consequences of ineffective erythropoiesis and anemia.

Sickle Cell Disease

In sickle cell disease, in which regular blood transfusions to correct anemia are usually not needed, iron overload only develops in individuals who receive repeated blood transfusions to prevent certain complications. In the minority of patients who receive repeated transfusions sufficient to cause significant iron overload, clinical consequences begin later than in thalassemia major, and thus effects on growth and sexual development are relatively uncommon. The use of the serum ferritin to estimate iron loading is problematic in sickle cell disease. The ferritin level is disproportionately increased in relation to iron loading for several weeks after a painful sickle episode[299] and often correlates poorly with hepatic iron concentration,[300] although under carefully controlled conditions a correlation is seen.[301] Transfusion-induced iron loading in the liver[301] with fibrosis and cirrhosis are seen.[302–304] Portal fibrosis develops quickly: after 21 months of transfusion without chelation, fibrosis was found in the livers of approximately a third of patients; after 4 years of transfusion, with variable chelation, fibrosis was still present in a third of patients with cirrhosis and in one of 29 patients in the absence of hepatitis C infection.[304] The fibrosis score correlates with liver iron concentration[303] but develops at widely varying hepatic iron concentrations of 9–38 mg/g dry weight in the absence of hepatitis C infection.[305]

Postmortem studies have found that cirrhosis was present in nearly half of patients who died with severe liver siderosis.[306] Postmortem studies also show clear evidence of iron deposition in the heart in heavily transfused patients;[240,306] however, MRI evidence suggests that the propensity for myocardial iron deposition[246,247,307] is less than in other forms of transfusional iron overload. A variety of endocrine disturbances have been reported in sickle cell disease,[308,309] including hypothyroidism[310] and increased pancreatic deposition of iron.[311] If sickle cell disease and thalassemia major patients matched for liver iron are compared, the incidence of heart disease, gonadal failure, and endocrine disturbances appears to be less in sickle cell disease patients aged younger than 20 years compared with thalassemia major.[308] Sickle cell disease patients typically begin transfusion later than those with thalassemia, and the rate of transfusion is on average lower, so that without carefully controlled studies the significance of these differences is unclear. At similar levels of iron loading, plasma NTBI values are lower in sickle cell disease than in thalassemia,[248,312] and this could account for decreased iron distribution to organs such as the heart.[247,248,307] Lower plasma NTBI values could result from the existence of a chronic inflammatory state in sickle cell disease[312] that would depress NTBI though increased hepcidin synthesis.

Other Transfusion-dependent Anemias

In multitransfused patients with myelodysplastic disease and a mean transfusional load of 120 U, there was evidence for multiple endocrine disorders including impaired glucose tolerance, decreased gonadotrophins, and impaired ACTH reserve.[313] A functional impact of myocardial iron deposition was suggested by one study in which heart failure was the cause of death in 51% of patients.[314] Among 705 patients followed for 2 years or until death, cardiac comorbidities were seen in 79% of chronically transfused patients, in only 54% of nontransfused patients, and in 42% of a control population.[315] Furthermore overall survival was significantly worse in iron overloaded myelodysplastic disease patients compared with untransfused patients;[316,317] an independent effect of iron loading on survival is uncertain without prospective studies.

Monitoring of Iron Overload

Liver Iron Concentration

Liver iron concentration (LIC) is a key measure of iron overload because its value relates to body iron stores in a well-defined mathematical relationship: body iron stores in mg/kg = 10.6 x the LIC (in mg/g dry weight).[318]

Normal LIC values are up to 1.8-mg/g dry weight and levels up to 7 mg/g dry weight are seen in some nonthalassemic populations without apparent adverse effects.[319] In principle, iron balance with a given chelation regime can be calculated from the change in LIC over time, provided the iron input from transfusion is known. Change in LIC over a given time can also be used to calculate the efficiency of a chelator (i.e. the proportion of administered drug that is excreted in an iron bound form). Thus the change in LIC over a period of time period (6 months–1 year) is useful way to assess the efficiency and effectiveness of an iron chelator regime.

Measurement of LIC also has prognostic and pathophysiological significance. Sustained LIC values more than approximately 15–20 mg/g dry weight over a period of time predict an increased risk of liver fibrosis progression[239] and liver function abnormalities.[238] In patients not receiving chelation therapy, similar LIC values predict an increased risk of myocardial iron deposition[240,241] and iron-induced cardiomyopathy.[276,282] Intensive chelation therapy reduces liver iron faster than cardiac iron so that a simple relationship between LIC and estimated heart iron values is often not seen once long-term or intensive chelation therapy has been used.[245] Patients might develop heart failure after iron has been removed from the liver because excess iron remains in the heart.[320] Although low LIC in previously highly iron overloaded patients does not necessarily guarantee low heart iron concentrations, sustained high levels of LIC has clearly poor prognostic significance.

The use of LIC to follow the progress of transfusional iron overoad is becoming easier because noninvasive approaches to measurement are now more widely available. Liver biopsy to measure iron overload has the obvious disadvantage that it is invasive and carries a small risk of bleeding but in expert hands, using ultrasound guidance, no mortality was seen in more than 1,000 biopsies, with an overall complication rate of 0.5%.[321] Although liver iron is somewhat uneven in distribution,[322] this is not a serious problem provided a sample of 1 mg dry weight (4 mg wet or ~ 2.5 cm in length) is obtained.[318,323] The presence of cirrhosis could increase the unevenness of iron distribution and hence the accuracy of LIC measurement.[323] In expert hands, with established methodology,[324] and with samples of adequate size, and in the absence of cirrhosis the coefficient of variation on duplicate specimens is only 6.6%.[325]

A problem in comparing values between studies is that the measurement of wet and dry weights of samples varies considerably among laboratories. Paraffin-embedded biopsy material can be used to measure LIC[324] but a recent multicenter study has shown that the ratio of wet/dry weight differs using this approach when compared with using fixed nonembedded tissue, being higher in paraffin-embedded tissue (5.9) than vacuum-dried fresh samples (3.8).[326] In many clinics worldwide, the regular measurement of LIC by biopsy is organizationally difficult. Furthermore, many patients who have been monitored successfully for many years by using the serum ferritin level are reluctant to undergo yearly liver biopsies. On the other hand, liver biopsy yields additional information about inflammation and fibrosis that might be particularly important in monitoring the activity of hepatitis C or evaluating experimental chelation regimens. Because of the increased use of LIC to monitor treatment, there is a need to harmonize both the techniques used to measure LIC and the units in which it is expressed. For example, some laboratories weigh the wet samples but use a conversion factor from wet to dry weight and express results in the latter units. A variety of conversion factors from wet to dry weight have been used by different centers. The implementation of an internationally agreed on standard and methodology would be helpful to the interpretation of studies on outcome of chelation treatment.

For these reasons, a noninvasive method to measure LIC that is reliable, standardized, and widely available would be highly desirable. Noninvasive measurement of LIC has been possible for many years by using superconducting quantum interface devices (SQUIDs) but these are expensive and only available in four centers worldwide (west and east coast of the United States, Germany, and Italy) and have been calibrated using different approaches. Excellent correlations with LIC values measured by biopsy were reported in hemochromatosis patients ($r = 0.98$)[327] but less impressive correlations were obtained in thalassemia,[328] possibly because of the diverse methodology for LIC biopsy measurements. Standardization between these devices has been problematic.[329] In recent multicenter trials using SQUID, significant differences in SQUID measurements were obtained from different centers.[213]

The current development of room temperature handheld susceptometric devices would have wider applications. Several MRI techniques for measuring LIC are now available,[330,331] relying on the general principle that tissue iron exerts a paramagnetic effect on surrounding tissues that affects the relaxation time of molecules excited by the application of a magnetic field. There is now a standardized and validated MRI method (FerriScan®) in which there is a linear relationship between the measured value (R2) and LIC by biopsy over a clinically useful range.[330] Further advantages of this method are that it uses standard MRI equipment that is available in most hospitals, can be used with little extra training of local staff, and analysis of data acquired locally is performed at a central facility.

Use and Limitations of Serum Ferritin

Although LIC predicts body iron and this can now be measured noninvasively, the practical advantages of having a blood test for monitoring iron overload that can be repeated with each clinic visit are obvious. Serum ferritin fits many of the requirements as it broadly correlates with iron loading and can be performed frequently and inexpensively. There are limitations to its use and interpretation: Serum ferritin is increased not only by increased body iron stores but also as a result of tissue damage and inflammation; levels are depressed by ascorbate deficiency. Unlike tissue ferritin, serum ferritin is predominantly iron free, being secreted in glycosylated form by macrophages proportional to their iron content, up to values of approximately 3,000 μg/L.[332] Above this value, iron-rich ferritin tends to leak from hepatocytes so that responses to treatment at levels more than 3,000 μg/L might occur at a different rate compared with values below 3,000 μg/L.[333] The relationship between serum ferritin and body iron stores can vary with the chelator being used, and it is important to define such a relationship for each chelation regime so that informed dose adjustments can be made.[334] Serum ferritin is usually measured by immunoassay with reference to an agreed international standard; however, 'kits' for measuring serum ferritin have been optimized for identifying iron deficiency so care must be taken at high ferritin values to ensure that dilutions allow measurements within the linear range of the assay.

In normal subjects[335] and in genetic hemochromatosis[336] a good correlation exists between iron mobilizable stores by quantitative phlebotomy and serum ferritin. With transfusional iron overload in the pre–chelation era, a correlation of serum ferritin with the number of units transfused in thalassemic children was present,[337] but this correlation was reduced in adults.[332] Serum ferritin also correlates with the LIC; in children with thalassemia major, this correlation was present both in those receiving and not receiving chelation therapy ($r = 0.75$).[337] In patients with HbE–β thalassemia and HbH disease, a correlation of $r = 0.82$ was noted between the log of serum ferritin and liver iron measure by SQUID.[218] A very weak correlation between serum ferritin and LIC was seen in a diverse group of patients, many of whom had liver disease ($r = 0.11$). When the serum ferritin was corrected for liver inflammation, by dividing by the aspartate aminotransferase, the correlation was much closer ($r = 0.92$).[338] More recent studies, although confirming the general relationship between serum ferritin and LIC, have emphasized that this is not close enough in multiply transfused thalassemia patients, many of whom have hepatitis C, to give a clinically reliable prediction of LIC.[339,340] In one study, variation in body iron stores accounted for only 57% of the variability in plasma ferritin.[301] The relationship between serum ferritin and iron stores is similar in thalassemia major and sickle cell disease[301] provided serum values are taken several weeks away from a vasoocclusive episode,[224] but in thalassemia intermedia, serum ferritin tends to underestimate the amount of iron overloading.[234]

Depression of serum ferritin occurs in ascorbate deficiency. Subclinical but biochemically demonstrable ascorbate deficiency is common in iron-overloaded patients[256,341] due to the rapid oxidation of ascorbic acid in the presence of redox active iron.[342] In ascorbate-deficient patients, the correlation between serum ferritin and LIC was 0.39, whereas in ascorbate-replete patients it was 0.77[341]. Repletion of ascorbate status increased transferrin saturation and serum ferritin rose in approximately half the treated patients.

In an individual patient with iron overload, long-term control of serum ferritin, at least with desferrioxamine therapy, has prognostic significance. If the ferritin is maintained below 2,500 μg/L on a long-term basis, this is associated with a significantly lower risk of iron-mediated cardiac disease and death.[277,280–282,343] Maintenance of a serum ferritin of 1,000 μg/L might be associated with additional advantages.[277] Serum ferritin has also been used as means of modifying the dose of chelation treatment, based on experience with desferrioxamine therapy in which toxicity due to this agent is more likely in the context of low serum ferritin levels. Dose modification algorithms have been constructed for desferrioxamine under circumstances of falling ferritin values;[340,344] however, the basis for dose modification with other chelation regimens has yet to be established.

Monitoring of the Heart

Iron-mediated cardiomyopathy remains the most common cause of death in thalassemia major;[277] therefore, the identification of patients at the greatest risk is of paramount importance, so that effective intensification of therapy can be introduced.

Long-term quantitative sequential measurement of left ventricular ejection fraction in thalassemia major has shown that a fall below reference values indicated a 35-fold increased risk of cardiac failure and death with a median interval to progression of 3.5 years.[343] Longitudinal monitoring of heart function is best achieved using a method that can be standardized and is not operator dependent. In the hands of an expert, echocardiography is a useful tool for visualizing heart function but it is difficult to quantify left ventricular ejection fraction reproducibly over time. Mulitgated acquisition scanning is well suited to this purpose as it has excellent reproducibility and less operator dependence, but MRI techniques are now widely available and measurement of left ventricular ejection fraction function can now be combined with measurement of heart iron in a single visit.

Little or no role exists for measuring cardiac iron by biopsy because of the uneven distribution of cardiac iron.[240,242,243] MRI can be used to estimate tissue iron because iron overload results in shortening of the T1 and T2 tissue relaxation times on which MRI is based and thus leads to a reduction in signal intensity. The decrease in the intensity of spin echo images with iron overload derives from decrements in the T2 relaxation times.[345,346] This shortening is due mainly to the paramagnetic properties of ferritin iron.[346,347] The problem in measuring heart iron was that levels were considerably lower than in the liver and the heart is rapidly moving. Early approaches lacked sensitivity over a wide enough linear range but several MRI methods have now been developed that are applicable to the heart.[241,244]

Myocardial T2* is a gradient echo method that is now the most widely used to estimate myocardial iron and has been found to be highly reproducible.[348] The T2* gradient echo sequence was first used in imaging of iron deposits in the brain[349] but is particularly applicable to myocardial imaging because a short acquisition time is possible, which is advantageous when measuring a moving tissue. T2 is related to T2* by the formula $1/T2^* = 1/T2 + 1/T'$, where T2 is the tissue relaxation and T' is the magnetic inhomogeneity of the tissue being analyzed. As the T2* becomes shorter implying higher tissue iron concentrations, there is an increased chance of left ventricular function being adversely affected.[244] In one study, the left ventricular ejection fraction was decreased in 10% of patients with T2* less than 20 msec, 18% of patients with T2* values between 8 and 10 msec, 38% of those with T2* of 6 msec, and 70% at 4 msec.[284] Myocardial iron deposition has been found by using this technique in as many as half of adult patients with thalassemia major and in a variety of other forms of transfusional iron overload.[246] Myocardial T2* can be used to identify patients most at risk of myocardial decompensation, which can occur suddenly over a period of a few days, and allow consideration of intensification of chelation therapy in those most at risk prior to decompensation.

Monitoring for the Clinical Effects Iron Overload

The earliest consequence of iron overload in transfused children is hypogonadotrophic hypogonadism, which although not fatal, has severe consequences for growth, sexual development, fertility, and bone health.[286] Close monitoring of growth and sexual development in children is therefore vital so that chelation can be intensified before irreversible effects ensue. In older patients, regular monitoring for the cardiological, endocrinological, and growth and developmental effects of iron overload is an essential part of management of iron overload. For example, monitoring for impaired glucose tolerance might identify patients at most risk of developing diabetes. Monitoring for hypothyroidism and hypoparathyroidism is also advisable, particularly in adults. As there is no clear evidence that damage to these tissues can be reversed, prevention of these complications by adequate control of body iron at all times is the optimal strategy. A scheme for such monitoring is outlined in Table 29.9 showing that monitoring will tend to be predicated by the availability of local resources.

Table 29.9. Monitoring for iron toxicity from transfusion

Observation	Frequency	Expense
Iron intake rate	Each transfusion	(increasing, low to high)
Chelation dose and frequency	3 monthly	
Growth and sexual development	6 monthly children	
Liver function	3 monthly	
Sequential ferritin	3 monthly	
GTT, thyroid, Ca metab.	Yearly in adults	
Liver iron	Yearly	
Heart function	Yearly	
Heart iron (T2*)	Yearly	

Monitoring Tissue Iron in Other Organs

MRI can be used to visualize iron in other organs affected by iron loading such as the anterior pituitary and pancreas. MRI of the pituitary shows a correlation between anterior pituitary size and biochemical markers of anterior pituitary function.[350] More recently T2* MRI has been used to assess iron in the anterior pituitary,[351,352] but prospective studies are required to determine how changes in pituitary T2* relate to biochemical evidence of disturbed gonadotrophin production. Attempts have been made to use MRI to relate changes in pancreatic function to iron deposition and a possible correlation between MRI signal and pancreatic exocrine but not endocrine function was found.[353,354]

Urine Iron Excretion

Measurement of urinary iron has been used with desferrioxamine monotherapy, with deferiprone monotherapy, and with combinations of the two drugs. Because all iron is excreted by the fecal route with deferasirox, urinary iron measurement has not been used with this chelator. A relationship between 24-hour urinary iron excretion following intramuscular desferrioxamine and iron stores was recognized soon after the introduction of the chelator.[355] Later it was suggested that 24-hour urinary iron excretion could be used to titrate an individual's therapy with desferrioxamine by "tailoring the dose"[356] as the dose at which the urinary iron excretion plateaus varies considerably.[356] Several limitations to this approach exist. First, there are practical difficulties for many families in obtaining reliable sequential 24-hour urine collections outside of a hospital setting. Second, there is considerable day-to-day variability in urinary iron excretion when taking desferrioxamine, even under controlled conditions of collection, and this might be compounded by variable daily ascorbate intake.[356] Finally, the proportion of urinary iron excretion relative to fecal iron excretion is not constant. The urinary iron excretion decreases following blood transfusion and suppression of erythropoiesis and is proportionately less at higher doses of desferrioxamine.[357] Whereas fecal iron excretion contributes to at least half of desferrioxamine-induced iron excretion there is little fecal excretion with deferiprone, making urine iron determination a potentially useful tool. When the two drugs are used in combination, however, changes in urinary iron excretion without reference to total iron removal or the fecal excretion are uninterpretable.

Other Markers of Iron Overload

Plasma transferrin saturation increases with increasing iron loading but is also affected by inflammation,[358] hepcidin synthesis,[359] and degree of erythropoiesis,[360] making its use in the management of transfusional iron overload of limited value. NTBI is present when transferrin becomes saturated in iron overload[249] and sometimes before.[361,362] Plasma NTBI negatively correlates with evidence of antioxidant depletion.[256] NTBI is highly labile, being only partially removed with chelation therapy and returning rapidly after elimination of the chelator.[363] NTBI is also affected by factors other than iron overload. For example, fewer iron-loaded thalassemia intermedia patients appear to have higher NTBI levels, which rebound faster after cessation of iron chelation than thalassemia major patients with higher levels of iron loading. This suggests that ineffective erythropoiesis may influence plasma NTBI.[364] Plasma NTBI is heterogeneous, consisting of iron citrate of varying molecular weights and loosely protein bound iron species.[252] Total plasma NTBI can be measured by a number of methods.[365,366] An assay has been developed for a redox active subfraction that has been termed labile plasma iron.[367] Assays for NTBI have variable reference ranges but generally correlate.[365] An assay measuring a labile subfraction, the component capable of accelerating oxidation of a fluorophore, termed labile plasma iron,[367] is convenient for measuring in the presence of chelators. Progressive removal of this subfraction has been seen with deferasirox,[368] consistent with the notion that continuous chelation minimizes exposure to NTBI species.[364] The application of NTBI or labile plasma iron as a way of tailoring chelation therapy on an individual patient basis has yet to be determined. How hepcidin levels can be used to guide chelation management is also unclear.[233,369]

Objectives of Chelation Therapy

Iron Balance

The primary objective of chelation therapy is to balance iron excretion with intake so that tissue iron never reaches damaging levels. If this strategy is successfully applied, iron-mediated tissue damage is prevented. Unfortunately many patients either start treatment too late or fail to maintain effective exposure to iron chelation so that rescue chelation therapy is needed. Rescue therapy has two objectives: to detoxify iron pools promoting acute tissue damage and to remove excess storage iron from affected tissues. The first objective can be achieved rapidly in some circumstances, for example by inducing rapid reversal of heart failure before much storage iron has been removed. The second goal of removing storage iron can take months or years especially in tissue not designed to store iron such as the heart.[245] Because of the difficulty in removing established storage iron overload from heart, pituitary, thyroid, and pancreas, a long-term strategy to prevent primary iron loading is preferable. At lower levels of iron loading, chelation therapy might lead to removal of essential metals required for physiological functions. In this instance, over chelation too early in the iron loading process could lead to unwanted toxicities.[370] Iron chelation requires that iron loading and excretion be balanced and that the intensity of chelation is matched to the level and rate of iron loading.

Maintenance of Safe Tissue Iron Concentrations

How the age iron loading begins, its rate, and how the absolute levels of iron loading contribute to tissue damage or determine the distribution of iron overload are incompletely understood. Thus there is debate about what constitutes "safe" levels of body iron burden. Good evidence supports the notion that control of serum ferritin (mainly iron free), liver iron (iron-rich ferritin and hemosiderin), and myocardial T2* visible iron (iron-rich storage iron) has prognostic significance. This does not mean that these forms of iron are the direct cause of tissue damage however, but rather that these are valuable markers for potential iron-mediated problems. Both biopsy and MRI techniques measure storage iron rather than the small fraction of labile iron that is directly toxic to cells.[264,371,372] The slow accumulation of iron in heterozygotes for hereditary hemochromatosis is typically not associated with liver damage, even though LIC values can approach 7 mg/g dry weight.[319] Conversely, liver fibrosis might develop in transfused and nontransfused,[373] iron-overloaded patients at or around these levels.[303,304] Progressive liver damage and abnormal liver tests in the absence of viral hepatitis are associated with LIC values of more than 16 mg/g dry weight[239] and similar sustained values over a decade or more are associated with an increased risk of cardiomyopathy in thalassemia major.[276] Yet we do not yet understand the relationship between myocardial iron load and LIC, particularly in patients undergoing chelation therapy. In the pre–chelation era, or in patients undergoing only light chelation therapy, there appears to be a relationship between myocardial iron loading and LIC, with myocardial iron appearing after approximately 75 U of blood in

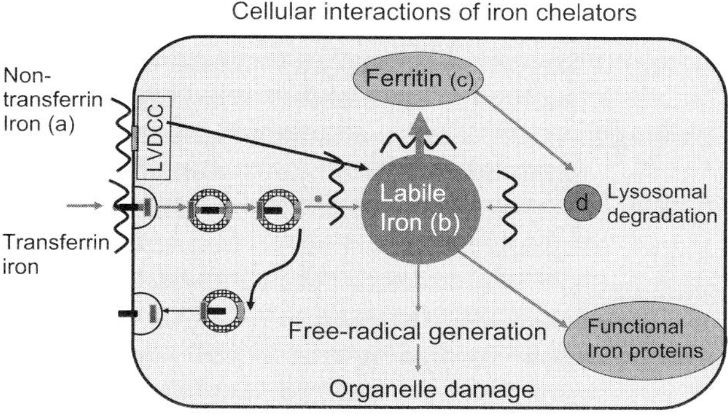

LVDCC = L-type voltage-dependent calcium channel.

Figure 29.4. Mechanism of chelator action at cellular level.[246]

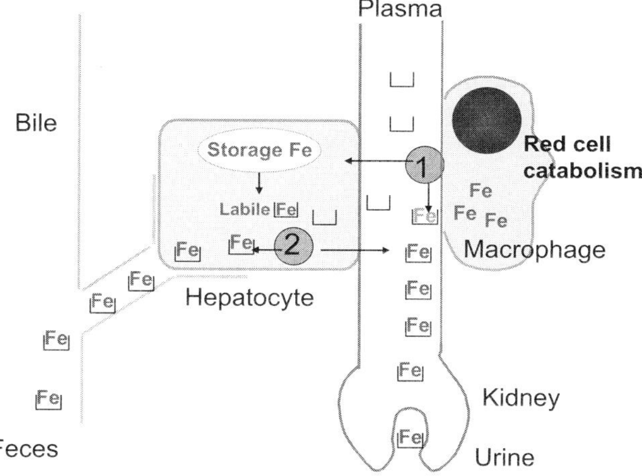

Figure 29.5. Major chelatable iron pools and excretion pathways.[249]

adults (15–20 mg/g dry weight with LIC). Together, the data suggest that it would seem wise to commence chelation therapy before LIC values approach 15 mg/g dry weight, probably at a time when LIC values exceed approximately 7 mg/g dry weight, and to aim to maintain LIC values lower than 7 mg/g dry weight. Whether the maintenance of LIC values lower than 7 mg/g dry weight at all times will prevent myocardial iron loading requires prospective evaluation for which studies are currently ongoing.

Detoxification of Harmful Iron Species

Although it can take months or years to remove all the excess iron from iron-loaded subjects, a well-designed chelator should ideally decrease the iron-mediated damage rapidly and until all the excess storage iron has been removed. To do this, potentially harmful labile iron pools must be removed rapidly and rendered harmless[246] (Fig. 29.4). As iron pools are constantly being turned over, continuous exposure to chelation is theoretically desirable, both in terms of maximizing the efficiency of chelation therapy and minimizing the exposure to harmful free radicals generated by labile iron species. Clinical data supporting the concept of detoxification of iron before storage iron has been changed significantly are seen in studies with intravenous desferrioxamine in which improvement in liver tests is rapid and precedes changes in T2* reflecting storage iron.[246]

Iron Pools Available for Chelation

Labeling of iron pools both in experimental animals[374,375] and in humans[376] suggest that only a small proportion of total body iron is available for chelation at any moment. This is broadly related to two iron turnover pools: red cell catabolism in macrophages (1 in Fig. 29.5): hemosiderin and ferritin catabolism in hepatocytes (2 in Fig. 29.5). This has a fundamental bearing on the strategies adopted for chelation therapy because it follows that escalation of chelation doses will have a finite impact on increasing iron excretion. The reason for this can be appreciated from consideration of both extracellular and intracellular iron turnover.

Extracellular Iron

The major turnover of body iron, amounting to some 20–30 mg/day in healthy individuals, is through the plasma compartment from the breakdown of effete red cells in the reticuloendothelial system. Iron is released onto transferrin for subsequent delivery to erythroid precursors in the bone marrow.[377] This can increase up to sevenfold when hemolysis and ineffective erythropoiesis are pronounced, as in thalassemia intermedia. Considerable evidence both in animal studies[375] and in humans[376] indicates that iron derived from the breakdown of hemoglobin in macrophages is chelated directly by desferrioxamine and other compounds such as DTPA before binding to transferrin[378] (Fig. 29.4). Whether this interception occurs extracellularly or within the macrophages is uncertain, but in vitro studies suggest the former is more likely with desferrioxamine.[379] This will presumably vary depending on rates of access of the chelator in question to intracellular iron pools in macrophages. Studies using selective ^{59}Fe cell–labeling techniques in iron-overloaded rats[374,375,380] and ferrokinetic data in humans[376] suggest that most urinary iron excretion with desferrioxamine is derived from catabolized red cells (1 in Fig. 29.5). Although other chelators used for the treatment of iron overload are excreted though different pathways than desferrioxamine the sources of chelatable iron are essentially the same. Thus with deferasirox, animal studies show that although nearly all iron bound to the chelator is excreted in feces, much of this is derived from red cell breakdown.[381] Deferiprone-bound iron is excreted almost entirely in urine but there is evidence for chelation of iron both from red cell breakdown and from parenchymal stores.[382]

Table 29.10. Characteristics of approved chelating agents

	Deferiprone	Desferrioxamine	Deferasirox
Denticity	Bidentate	Hexadentate	Tridentate
Molecular weight	175	560	373
Iron (III) binding (pM)	19.9	26.6	22.5
Lipid solubility	High	Low	High
Charge free ligand	Neutral	Positive	Negative (1-)
Charge iron complex	Neutral	Positive	Negative (3-)
Absorption route	Oral	Parenteral	Oral
Max. plasma levels	90–450 μM	7 μM (total)	20 μM
Elimination	Rapid	Very rapid	Slow
Route of iron excretion	Urine	Urine + Feces	Feces
Metabolism	Inactive glucuronide	Active metabolites	Active glucuronide

Another potential source of chelatable iron outside cells is transferrin-bound iron (Fig. 29.4). Although this is quantitatively very small (~ 4 mg) at any moment, approximately 20–30 mg pass through this pool every day after iron is released from reticuloendothelial cells. In principle, iron chelators are in competition with transferrin for iron released by reticuloendothelial cells. Because the concentration of transferrin in plasma exceeds that of desferrioxamine, deferasirox, or deferiprone, except at transient peak concentrations, and because the stability constant of transferrin for iron is comparable to that of these chelators, iron binds effectively to transferrin even when chelators are being used. Furthermore, once plasma iron has bound to transferrin it is virtually unavailable for chelation by desferrioxamine.[380] Hydroxypyridinones can remove iron from transferrin but the concentrations required to do so at a significant rate make this an unlikely mode of action in vivo. For example, at 100 μM concentrations of deferiprone, approximately a quarter of the iron is removed from 90% saturated transferrin (50 μM) and only 12% for 30% saturated transferrin after 24 hours.[383] It must also be remembered that iron can be donated to transferrin by bidentate hydroxypyridin-4-ones but not by desferrioxamine at clinically relevant concentrations of transferrin and chelator.[383] This is because the iron complexes of bidentate chelators are inherently less stable than those of hexadentate ligands such as desferrioxamine. Thus, because the plasma concentrations following orally administered chelators such as deferiprone are only transiently above 100 μM[384] (Table 29.10), donation of iron to transferrin might be as likely as iron removal, particularly when transferrin is not saturated in the steady state.

Another important potentially chelatable extracellular iron pool is NTBI (Fig. 29.4). Total NTBI values do not usually exceed approximately 10 μM[364] but the speciation is heterogeneous. These forms are not all equally available for rapid chelation.[252] Iron citrate polymers are more slowly accessed by chelators than monomers and dimers.[252] In plasma of iron-overloaded patients at clinically relevant concentrations, not all NTBI is removed by desferrioxamine.[363] The component of NTBI that is rapidly accessed by desferrioxamine has been termed desferrioxamine-chelatable iron.[385] Only the subfraction of NTBI capable of redox cycling, so-called labile plasma iron, is rapidly available for chelation.[386] The contribution of chelation of NTBI to iron balance has not been determined, but removal of NTBI by chelation therapy is potentially important for iron detoxification. NTBI is only partly removed by chelation with desferrioxamine and rebounds rapidly after cessation of an intravenous infusion[364] or subcutaneous infusion of chelator.[363] Thus, with conventional nightly subcutaneous desferrioxamine infusion, NTBI can enter tissues during the day.[363] Using the labile plasma iron assay, it was found that there is also rapid rebound of labile plasma iron at night with daytime use of deferiprone, but that when deferiprone is given three times a day with desferrioxamine at night, 24-hour coverage can be achieved.[367] A similar degree of 24-hour coverage from labile plasma iron can be achieved with once daily deferasirox because of its longer plasma half-life.[368]

Intracellular Iron

The major source of chelatable intracellular iron derives from the continuous turnover of intracellular ferritin and to a lesser extent hemosiderin (source b in Fig. 29.4 and source 2 in Fig. 29.5). Iron chelators can be considered as interacting potentially with three intracellular iron pools. These are the labile "transit" iron pool or (pool a), which is generally of low molecular weight, finite, and rapidly chelatable; the storage iron pool of hemosiderin and ferritin (pool b), which is relatively slowly chelatable but larger at any moment than pool a; and the functional iron pools (pool c), which are iron-containing molecules essential for normal cellular function (e.g., hemoglobin, myoglobin, enzymes such as lipoxygenase and ribonucleotide reductase). Pool a is in dynamic exchange with the other two pools. The goal of chelation therapy is to chelate pool a without affecting the important functions of iron in pool c (Fig. 29.4). Although some of pool b may be depleted directly, this is relatively slow because chelators cannot remove iron from ferritin cores at a clinically useful rate.

Transit iron can theoretically be chelated at any point during its uptake into cells by receptor-mediated endocytosis of transferrin, liberation from transferrin in the acidic endosome, or egress from the endosome via divalent metal ion transporter 1 (*SLC11A2*).[387] Labile chelatable intracellular iron has been demonstrated in a variety of cells including reticulocytes, marrow cells, intestinal epithelial cells, blood leukocytes, alveolar macrophages, and hepatocytes, although evidence has been largely indirect and the nature of the pool is uncertain.[371,388–391] It is clear that iron entering the cell, either from transferrin or by other mechanisms, becomes transiently chelatable before incorporation into ferritin.[392] Early studies in Chang cells showed approximately 20% of cellular iron was present as a nonheme, nonferritin soluble form after 24-hour incubation[393] and was rapidly chelatable with EDTA, desferrioxamine, or transferrin.[394] Quantification of this pool from tissue homogenate iron extracted by desferrioxamine showed a correlation with an ultrafilterable fraction bound to low-molecular-weight ligand(s).[395] Studies using the fluorescent probe calcein in K562 cells suggested that the labile intracellular iron pool is present at 0.4 μM with an estimated transit time of 24 hours.[390] Similar values have been obtained with rat hepatocytes labeled with $^{59}FeCl_3$ and analyzed for desferrioxamine-chelatable ^{59}Fe[396] and using electron paramagnetic resonance in K562 cells.[397] The magnitude of the labile iron pool is assumed to be sensed by a cytosolic iron-responsive protein so that increments in labile plasma iron increase ferritin mRNA translation and decrease transferrin receptor mRNA stability,[398] thereby having homeostatic effects on labile plasma iron concentrations. When cells become heavily iron loaded or the rate of uptake of NTBI into cells exceeds an as-yet undetermined rate, the sequestrating capacity of cellular ferritin is exceeded,[390] leading to an expanded labile plasma iron that is an obvious target of intracellular iron chelation therapy by drugs that are able to cross the cytoplasmic membrane. The same properties of chelators that favor mobilization of intracellular iron[399] such as lipid solubility, also favor chelation of the labile intracellular pool[400–402]. Thus hydroxpyridinones access labile iron pools more rapidly than desferrioxamine[372,397,400,403] the latter taking approximately 4 hours, whereas hydroxpyridinones may take only a few minutes. Deferasirox appears to access labile intracellular iron rapidly and have access to iron pools within organelles.[372,402]

With respect to pool b, iron can be mobilized from ferritin by desferrioxamine in vitro but the rate is less than 0.5%/hour, even when desferrioxamine is present in 15-fold molar excess.[404] Furthermore, acidic pH values, such as those present in the lysosome, do not appear to enhance this rate.[405] Bidentate hydroxypyridinones can gain access to the ferritin core directly by virtue of their smaller size.[406] At neutral pH values, iron mobilization from rat ferritin is still only 1%/hour even in the presence of 15-fold chelator excess.[405] Thus access by chelators to ferritin iron will occur at useful rates in vivo only when this protein is being degraded by proteolysis with the subsequent release of iron to the labile intracellular transit pool. It has been estimated that ferritin is turned over intracellularly with a half-life of approximately 72 hours[407] and that proteolysis is predominantly lysosomal rather than cytosolic.[408]

With respect to pool c, it is clear that the physicochemical properties of chelators have a major influence on their rate of access to iron. Desferrioxamine, by virtue of its hexadentate structure, relatively high molecular weight (Table 29.10), and its hydrophilicity compared with the clinically studied hydroxypyridinones, accesses intracellular iron and iron within organelles more slowly than hydroxypyridinones.[400,409] Furthermore, interaction with key enzymes in pool c such as lipoxygenase[410] and ribonucleotide reductase[411] is significantly slower for desferrioxamine than hydroxypyridinones. Because of the pivotal role of ribonucleotide reductase in DNA synthesis and cell proliferation, its rapid inhibition by hydroxypyridinones is a putative mechanism for the leukopenia and marrow hypoplasia associated with these agents.[411–413]

Constraints of Chelator Design

To be unavailable to participate in the generation of free radicals, iron must be fully coordinated at each of its six ligand-binding sites. If any of these remain partially coordinated, iron may participate in the Fenton reaction, resulting in lipid peroxidation with organelle and cell damage. The design of a chelator is crucial to preventing these events. In general, hexadentate ligands, which have six coordination sites and hence bind iron in a 1:1 ratio, scavenge iron at low chelator concentrations more efficiently and are more stable in their iron complexed forms than bidentate or tridentate chelators (Fig. 29.6). The latter chelator classes have two or three iron-coordinating sites per ligand, respectively, and therefore require three or two chelating molecules, respectively, to coordinate iron (III) completely. EDTA, which only coordinates one free electron, does not diminish the reactivity of iron salts in the Fenton reaction and indeed might catalyze such reactions.[259] By contrast the hexadentate desferrioxamine and physiological ligands such as lactoferrin and transferrin that surround the iron more completely are powerful inhibitors of lipid peroxidation in several systems.[414] The iron–chelate complexes of bidentate hydroxypyridinones, being less stable than the hexadentate desferrioxamine, can generate free radicals and damage cell membranes with increased lipid peroxidation and loss of cell viability, particularly if the chelators have high lipid solubility.[406] The effect can be "designed out" by synthesizing hydroxypyridinones with high pM (-log of the uncoordinated metal [iron] concentration calculated at pH 7.4, 10-μM ligand concentration and 1-μM iron[III] values).[415] Deferasirox, a tridentate chelator, is inherently less stable than ferrioxamine but is unlikely to participate in redox cycling of iron because Fe deferasirox

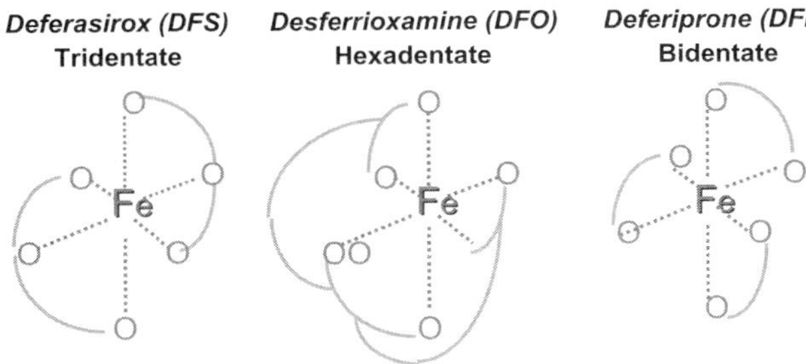

Figure 29.6. Denticity of iron chelation.[213]

is a very weak oxidizing agent, making its reduction under physiological conditions unlikely.[416]

Hexadentate chelators tend to have the advantage over bidentate and tridentate ligands of a greater ability to scavenge iron at low concentrations, a lesser potential to redistribute iron and a slower access to iron in pool c. Conversely, lower molecular weight bidentate and tridentate ligands have a potential to be absorbed from the gut and to access intracellular iron pools more rapidly. It is difficult to design hexadentate molecules with molecular weights less than 400, thus severely limiting their absorption from the gastrointestinal tract.[417] Consequently no hexadentate chelators have yet been identified with sufficient oral bioavailability for clinical use. Many bidentate and tridentate chelators have sufficiently low molecular weights for acceptable oral bioavailability. To minimize the inherent disadvantages of their lower denticity, novel chelators with greater stability of the iron–chelate complex are being sought.

Clinically useful iron chelators should possess a sufficiently high iron binding (stability) constant[409,417] and have specificity of iron binding over other essential metals like zinc and copper. A more clinically relevant expression of iron binding than the stability constant is the pM (Table 29.10). This measure takes into account the tendency of bidentate chelators to dissociate at low concentrations and is a more useful indicator of the ability of a chelator to scavenge iron at low chelator concentrations. Chelators with high pM values are therefore desirable.

The distribution of chelators to different tissues and subcellular compartments will also inevitably affect their toxicity. Ideally a compound should have low penetration of the central nervous system, where adverse effects have been observed with desferrioxamine (see later) and should have a high extraction of iron from liver cells where iron is present in high concentrations.[417,418] The rate at which chelators gain access to intracellular iron pools is determined by their lipid solubility, charge, shape, and molecular weight.[401,409,419] Once within cells, the structure of iron chelators also determines the rate of interaction with key iron-containing enzymes in pool 3. Larger and less lipophilic molecules tend to interact with intracellular metalloenzymes more slowly than small lipid soluble molecules.[403,411,420]

Finally, the pharmacokinetics and metabolism of an iron chelator are critical to its success. The metabolism of chelators has been shown to have a key bearing on their efficacy and toxicity.[421–424] As the majority of body iron is not directly chelatable, increasing the chelator dose might not have a proportionately increased effect on iron excretion while increasing the risk of toxicity disproportionately due to an excess of free chelator. This relative unavailability limits the efficiency of chelation therapy, where chelation efficiency refers to the proportion of the drug that ends up being excreted in the iron-bound form. In iron-overloaded humans, the efficiency of desferrioxamine is approximately 13%, deferiprone is approximately 4%, and deferasirox is approximately 27%.[425,426] The relatively low efficiency of deferiprone is likely to be explained not only by the rapid metabolism to forms that do not bind iron but also by its rapid elimination.[427] Conversely, the long plasma half-life of deferasirox contributes to the higher efficiency of this drug.[428] Thus iron excretion with deferasirox[429] as with desferrioxamine[363,430] is directly proportional to the area under the curve of the drugs. A further advantage of slow chelator elimination is that 24-hour protection from labile iron species in plasma or within cells can be achieved.[364,367]

CHELATION THERAPY WITH DESFERRIOXAMINE

Historical Perspective

Desferrioxamine, a naturally occurring hexadentate siderophore derived from *Streptomyces pilosus*, was discovered by chance in 1960 during work on isolation of the iron-containing antibiotic ferrimycin from *Streptomyces griseoflavus*. Following its isolation, the iron-bound form, ferrioxamine B, was initially investigated as a potential iron donor for iron-deficient subjects, but it was excreted intact in the urine without losing or exchanging its iron. The notion that an iron-free ferrioxamine, desferrioxamine, might be used to chelate excess iron was supported by clinical studies.[431]

Desferrioxamine when first given to thalassemia major patients as single intramuscular injections increased urinary iron excretion in a dose-dependent manner, proportional to iron stores.[432] Once daily intramuscular injections of 500 mg, 6 days a week in thalassemia major children over a period of 7 years, stabilized liver iron at approximately 3% dry weight and also stabilized liver fibrosis compared with untreated comparators.[325] Twenty-four-hour intravenous infusions produced more urinary iron than the same dose given as an intramuscular bolus.[433] The same group and others subsequently showed that 24-hour subcutaneous desferrioxamine infusions resulted in urinary iron excretion nearly equivalent to that achieved with intravenous infusions.[433,434] Urinary iron excretion was similar giving the same dose over 12 rather than 24 hours, and this was generally achieved iron balance.[356,435] Metabolic iron balance studies revealed that between 30% and 50% of total iron excretion with desferrioxamine was in the feces[357] and that the proportion increased with ascending desferrioxamine doses and following suppression of erythropoiesis by blood transfusion.[357] Nightly 8–12-hour subcutaneous infusions of desferrioxamine gradually became standard practice. The use of ascorbate, 2–3 mg/kg daily, on the same day as desferrioxamine administration increased urinary iron excretion,[357] but doses in excess of this were possibly associated with cardiac toxicity.[436] In the 1980s progressively larger doses of desferrioxamine were tried, often by the intravenous route, in attempts to reverse massive iron overload or to reverse cardiac failure.[437–439]

Although some of these objectives were achieved, significant toxicity from desferrioxamine began to be reported, most noticeably retinal[440] and auditory toxicity.[441] Later, effects on bone and growth were reported in children.[442,443] From these and other studies, a "standard" dosing regimen for desferrioxamine has emerged, aimed at balancing the beneficial effects of chelation with unwanted effects of excessive dosing. It must be made clear however that some aspects of "standard therapy" recommendations, such a when to begin and the dose recommended to maximize growth potential, have been arrived at by empirical retrospective analysis rather than prospective randomized trials.

Chemistry and Pharmacology of Desferrioxamine

The hexadentate structure of desferrioxamine necessitates a relatively high-molecular-weight structure of 560 (or when administered clinically as the mesylate, 657) that limits its absorption from the gut, and therefore only parenteral routes of administration are realistic. Its hexadentate structure helps desferrioxamine to scavenge Fe^{3+} particularly at low concentrations of iron, as evidenced by the high pM (Table 29.10). A hexadentate structure and high pM also contribute to stabilization of the iron complex, and iron redistribution or partial iron complexation is insignificant. Other metals are bound with a much lower affinity; only the chelation of aluminum has clinical significance. Desferrioxamine has been successfully used to treat aluminum overload in renal dialysis patients at doses of 5–10 mg/kg/week.[444] Entry of desferrioxamine into most cell types and into subcellular compartments is retarded by two mechanisms, its relatively high molecular weight and its highly hydrophilic nature.[400,411] in hepatocytes, however, there appears to be a facilitated uptake mechanism.[363] The free drug is positively charged, as is the iron complex. This latter property accounts for the slow egress of the iron complex from cells.[411]

Elimination of desferrioxamine from plasma is fast, with an initial half-life of 0.3 hours and a terminal half-life of 3 hours.[445] With an intravenous infusion of 50 mg/kg/day, mean steady-state concentrations of 7.4 μM are achieved[445] (Table 29.10). Desferrioxamine and its major metabolites are cleared by the liver and the kidney in their iron-free forms. Once iron is bound to form ferrioxamine in the plasma, clearance is almost exclusively renal because ferrioxamine is not cleared by the liver. In renal disease, levels of ferrioxamine may therefore accumulate; however, ferrioxamine is highly stable and does not redistribute iron significantly within the body. With 24-hour infusion, the duration of protection from NTBI and labile plasma iron is continuous, but plasma levels still rarely exceed 10 μM at conventional doses.[364] Metabolism of the iron-free drug but not the iron complex occurs within hepatocytes, so that an increase in metabolites indicates a decrease in the availability of chelatable iron.[363,446]

Fecal iron excretion as ferrioxamine is almost entirely due to intrahepatic iron chelation, whereas urinary iron is mainly derived from plasma iron turnover[380] (Fig. 29.5). Uptake of desferrioxamine into hepatocytes results in chelation of cytosolic and possibly lysosomal iron to form ferrioxamine that is then excreted in the bile.[374] At conventional doses approximately a third of the iron is excreted through this route into the feces, and this amount increases with higher desferrioxamine doses,[447] reflecting a greater proportion of intrahepatic chelation.

Evidence of Efficacy of Desferrioxamine

Effects on Iron Balance and Liver Iron

Iron balance can be estimated from metabolic balance studies with measurement of iron excretion in urine and feces and iron input in the diet[357] or by measuring the change in LIC over time and relating this change to the Angelucci formula, which relates LIC to total body iron stores.[318] Early studies suggested that iron balance, based on urine iron alone, could be achieved at a dose of approximately 30 mg/kg/day when given as a 12-hour infusion.[356] In patients not previously receiving chelation therapy, the quantity of urine iron excreted correlated with transferrin saturation,[448] the number of transfusions,[448] and the dose of desferrioxamine[356,432,448] Fecal excretion contributes a further 30%–50% to total desferrioxamine-induced iron output.[357] Formal metabolic iron balance studies suggested that daily 12-hour infusions at 30 mg/kg could achieve iron balance in thalassemia major, particularly if oral ascorbic acid was supplemented at the equivalent of 2–3 mg/kg/day.[357]

Intramuscular desferrioxamine was more effective at stabilizing liver iron at 6 years follow-up in thalassemia major.[325] Using subcutaneous infusions of 40 mg/kg, more maintained liver iron at safe levels.[449–452] Intensification of therapy by combining subcutaneous and intravenous therapy can normalize liver iron levels.[438] Surprisingly, detailed studies of the dose effect of desferrioxamine on LIC and hence on iron balance have only become available recently as a byproduct of prospective 1-year comparisons with deferasirox, in which changes in LIC over a 1-year period were measured in 290 patients receiving sliding scale doses of desferrioxamine between 25 mg/kg/day and 60 mg/kg/day 5 nights a week.[453] These studies have revealed the critical importance of dose and transfusion rate on iron balance.[212] Importantly at doses of desferrioxamine used in many recent studies, and at average transfusional iron loading rates of 0.3–0.5 mg/kg/day, negative iron balance was achieved in only half of patients prescribed 40 mg/kg/day 5 days per week. When doses of 50 mg/kg or higher were given, 86% of patients were in negative iron balance, even at high transfusional rates of 0.5 mg/kg/day or higher.[212] The proportions of patients in iron balance might be even less during routine clinical where compliance is likely to be poorer.

Effects on Serum Ferritin

Dose-dependent reductions of serum ferritin with desferrioxamine have been recognized for several decades, and the value of maintaining serum ferritin at less than 2,500 μg/L has been linked to protection from heart disease and with survival.[280] Formal trials relating changes in serum ferritin to dosage have been scarce. Recent studies comparing desferrioxamine with other chelators have added some important information about its effects on ferritin. In interpreting these findings it is critical to know what treatment patients received prior to the formal study as a change in ferritin is unlikely if patients simply continue the same dosage of drug.

In a prospective study of 290 patients with thalassemia major mainly treated with desferrioxamine prior to the trial and followed for 1 year, those receiving a daily dose of 40 mg/kg five times per week had mean decreased serum ferritin of approximately 360 μg/L, whereas a dose of 50 mg/kg decreased serum ferritin by approximately 1,000 μg/L.[453] These are average effects, and dose should be increased if the transfusional iron intake exceeds the average.

Long-term Effects on Survival

Because no other chelation treatment was available when desferrioxamine was introduced, the pattern of survival in progressive birth cohorts gives a clear indication of its impact on survival as well as its cardioprotective effects. The impact of desferrioxamine on overall survival began to emerge in the 1980s[454] but the full impact was clearly documented only later.[275–277,280,281] Only 70% of patients born before 1970, and hence prior to the modern era of iron chelation, survived to age 20 years compared with 89% of patients born after 1970 who received effective chelation treatment from an early age.[455] In nearly 1,000 Italian patients born between 1970 and 1974, mortality was 5% by age 20 years and this fell to 1% in cohorts born between 1980 and 1984 when desferrioxamine was widely used.[277] The age of starting treatment has been shown to be a key factor in outcome,[276,277,343] although the optimal age has not been assessed in prospective studies. Compliance with nightly infusions is key to long-term survival. Life table analysis shows that patients who comply well with treatment can have a 100% survival rate to age 25 years, whereas survival for patients who comply poorly is only 32%.[276] For patients who administer subcutaneous infusions of desferrioxamine more than 250 times a year, survival to age 30 years is 95%. If the frequency of infusion falls below 250 times a year, or approximately five times a week, survival to age 30 years is only 12%.[281] The environment in which patients are treated has an important effect on compliance and survival. In thalassemic patients treated at a single thalassemia center, 83% of patients survived to age 40 years, and all compliant patients born after 1975 survived to age 25 years.[320] The effect of compliance on survival has not been reported with other chelators. The provision of comprehensive care that delivers the necessary practical and psychological lifelong support to patients on chronic transfusion is therefore vital.

Effects on the Heart

Because iron-induced cardiomyopathy remains the most common cause of death in thalassemia major, the effects of desferrioxamine on heart disease and survival will be considered together. Perhaps the most persuasive evidence for the cardioprotective effects of desferrioxamine is the ability to reverse preexisting cardiomyopathy. Improvement in left ventricular function after 1 year of treatment was first noted in a small group of thalassemia patients with subclinical heart disease in response to intensive subcutaneous desferrioxamine[456] and was sustained with long-term follow-up.[439] This effect was confirmed in other studies.[457] Evidence for reversal of clinically overt heart failure in thalassemia major was first shown in three of five patients treated with intravenous doses of desferrioxamine of up to 200 mg/kg/day.[437] Later work using a discontinuous, high-dose regimen of 6–12 g of desferrioxamine over 12 hours daily[458] showed improvement in symptoms and echocardiographic parameters in one patient with congestive cardiac failure and another with a severe ventricular arrhythmia. Other experience with discontinuous therapy has been variable. No improvement in the cardiac status of two patients was seen at 100 mg/kg over 8–12 hours[459] but improvements were observed in eight thalassemic patients followed-up for 6.5 years while using high-dose administration via an indwelling central venous line for 8–10 hours daily.[460]

Experience with continuous 24-hour therapy has been more consistent, having the theoretical advantages of continuous removal of NTBI[364] and of reestablishing good compliance.[333,461] In one study, four patients were treated with continuous 24-hour therapy with improvement in left ventricular ejection fraction in two and reversal in atrial fibrillation in a third.[457] In nine other patients, not only did continuous 24-hour infusions produce superior urinary iron excretion compared with an equivalent subcutaneous 12-hour regimen, but the intravenous regimen encouraged excellent compliance.[461] Longer-term studies have established that continuous intravenous therapy is a safe, lifesaving therapeutic option in the management of high-risk thalassemia: 25 intravenous devices were inserted into 17 patients over a 16-year period, and desferrioxamine, usually at 50 mg/kg/day, was infused continuously over 24 hours, 6–7 days a week.[333] Resting ejection fraction improved significantly from 36%–49% in seven of nine patients with previously documented deterioration in left ventricular function. This occurred in some cases within a few days of starting treatment and therefore cannot be attributed to normalization of iron stores but to the depletion of a limited toxic labile iron pool. Atrial fibrillation was reversed in all six patients in whom this was present within 12 months; in one patient, cardioversion occurred within 5 days without the need for conventional antiarrhythmic drugs. Drug toxicity was limited to a single early case of reversible retinopathy in a patient with preexisting diabetes mellitus who had been on an initial dose of 80 mg/kg/day. Long-term follow-up showed 62% survival at 13 years in those with demonstrable cardiac disease. Deaths occurred in patients whose compliance was not maintained. Large doses such as those initially used to reverse heart failure and that were associated with severe retinal problems[437,440] might not be necessary and doses of 50–60 mg/kg/day could be sufficient.[333] The risk of overdosing can be minimized by adjusting the dose as the ferritin falls, maintaining the therapeutic index of desferrioxamine to serum ferritin ratio of 0.025 as recommended for conventional subcutaneous desferrioxamine treatment.[333]

Reversal of left ventricular dysfunction similar to that achieved with continuous intravenous therapy has also been shown with 24-hour subcutaneous therapy,[343] although this is demanding and only suitable for some patients. With the increasing use of T2* to estimate myocardial iron, there is now evidence that desferrioxamine, when given at sufficient doses and with sufficient frequency and duration can improve myocardial T2*. Patients with severe myocardial iron overload and a mean T2* less than 6 msec, with advanced myocardial dysfunction, when given continuous desferrioxamine infusions at 50 mg/kg/day or more showed improved T2* values of 3 msec over 1 year.[245] During this same observation period, liver iron levels were nearly normalized and left ventricular function normalized within 3 months of treatment, suggesting that heart function can be improved by continuous desferrioxamine even when heart storage iron remains high. It might take several years, however, to normalize heart iron when T2* values begin less than 10 msec.[320] It might not be necessary to use intravenous treatment to improve myocardial T2* values if myocardial iron loading is only mild: improvement in cardiac T2* even at low, intermittent doses has been confirmed in two prospective randomized studies,[462,463] even in people on a previous similar treatment regime. Using subcutaneous treatment at relatively low doses of 35 mg/kg patients with baseline T2* values between 8 and 20 msec showed improvement in T2* of 1.8 msec over 1 year;[462] doses of 40–50 mg/kg 5 days a week lead to an improvement of 3 msec over 1 year.[464]

Other Long-term Effects on Morbidity

Other effects of desferrioxamine therapy include: improvement in liver fibrosis,[325] decreased severity of hypogonadism,[465] improved glucose tolerance,[466] and decreased incidence of diabetes,[276] and hyperparathyroidism.[277] The onset of glucose intolerance is delayed and glucose intolerance can be improved[466] by the timely use of desferrioxamine. Hypothyroidism might also be reversed.[469] Introduction of subcutaneous infusions of desferrioxamine before age 10 years significantly reduces gonadal dysfunction, with improvement in pubertal status and growth.[465] Concomitant improvement in fertility has also been seen, although secondary amenorrhea is still common.[286]

Unlike heart failure,[467,468] once advanced endocrine dysfunction has developed, reversal has not been documented. Intramuscular desferrioxamine at relatively modest doses stabilizes hepatic fibrosis and there is no progression over an 8-year period in patients receiving subcutaneous infusions of desferrioxamine in the absence of histological evidence of active hepatitis.[451]

Tolerability of Desferrioxamine

General

Most of the toxic effects of desferrioxamine are dose related; effects on growth, skeletal changes, audiometric, and retinopathic effects are more likely at higher doses of the drug. Toxicity from desferrioxamine in thalassemia major is very unlikely at doses up to 40 mg/kg/day. The risk of toxicity at any given dose is greater in patients with low levels of iron loading than in those with high levels of iron loading so that as serum ferritin falls, particularly below 1000 μg/L, it is wise to consider reducing the dose.[344,470] It is clear that some unwanted effects such a those on growth and bone development are mostly applicable to children in whom special care must be taken to avoid doses of greater than 40 mg/kg/day. These patients should be monitored particularly carefully with the consideration of dose lowering as iron levels fall.

Injection Site Reactions

Local mild reactions can occur with skin reddening and soreness at the site of subcutaneous infusions. These are often caused by desferrioxamine being reconstituted above the recommended concentration of 10%. Increasing the volume of water used to dilute the desferrioxamine can substantially decrease reactions. On occasions when local reactions remain a problem, the addition of 5–10 mg hydrocortisone to the desferrioxamine solution can help.

Effects on Growth and Bone

Although desferrioxamine usually improves growth in thalassemia major by decreasing iron overload, excessive amounts might cause growth retardation. The risk factors are, age younger than 3 years at commencement of treatment, higher doses of desferrioxamine,[442] and lower levels of iron overload. It is advisable to monitor height velocity as well as sitting and standing height twice yearly and adjust dosing as necessary. A quick resumption in growth follows reduction in desferrioxamine dosing without the need to stop treatment.[443] Rickets-like bone abnormalities have been described in association with decreased growth[442] and radiographic abnormalities of the distal ulnar, radial, and tibial metaphases appear to be associated features. Vertebral growth retardation or milder changes involving vertebral demineralization and flatness of vertebral bodies have also been noted in patients receiving chelation therapy.[281] It might be advisable to undertake regular surveillance for the toxic effects of desferrioxamine on bone[471] with annual radiological assessment of the thoracolumbar–sacral spine and the forearm and knees and to reduce the dose of the chelator if significant changes are noted.

Renal and Auditory Toxicity

Retinal and optic nerve disturbances, sometimes associated with pigmentary retinal changes, were originally described in patients receiving 125 mg/kg/day[440] and are rare at currently recommended doses. Other abnormalities that have been linked to excessive use of desferrioxamine include blurred vision, loss of central vision, night blindness, and optic neuropathy.[441] The risk might be higher in patients with diabetes or other factors affecting the blood–retinal barrier,[472] so these groups should be monitored more carefully by using electroretinographic techniques. Desferrioxamine therapy should be withdrawn until symptoms partially or fully resolved and then resumed at a reduced dose with close monitoring by electroretinography.

High-frequency sensorineural hearing loss was initially described in approximately 25% of patients on high-dose desferrioxamine regimens.[441] This complication might be reversible if diagnosed early.[344] The risk is greatest in patients with low degrees of iron overload receiving high doses of desferrioxamine. By keeping the therapeutic index[344] below 0.025 and by monitoring audiometry regularly, the risks can be minimized. It is advisable to perform audiometry before starting treatment and approximately once a year during treatment.

Infections

There is an increased risk of *Yersinia* infection in iron overload, and this risk increases further with desferrioxamine treatment as *Yersinia* does not make a natural siderophore and uses iron from ferrioxamine to facilitate its growth.[473,474] Patients who present with diarrhea, abdominal pain, or fever should stop taking desferrioxamine until *Yersinia* infection can reasonably be excluded by appropriate stool samples, blood cultures, and serological testing. If *Yersinia* infection is proven or seriously suspected, desferrioxamine should be withheld until the infection has been eliminated by antibiotic treatment. Prolonged treatment with an antibiotic such a ciprofloxacin is occasionally necessary to prevent recurrence, but it is rarely necessary to withhold desferrioxamine after the initial infection has been treated. Very rarely, other infections such as *Pneumocystis carinii*[475] and *mucormycosis*[476] have been associated with desferrioxamine. In any patient with undiagnosed fever it is wise to consider stopping the desferrioxamine until the cause is identified.

Miscellaneous Effects

Generalized reactions such as fever, muscle aches, and arthralgia occur rarely. True systemic allergic reactions are uncommon but can include anaphylaxis. Some patients can be successfully desensitized using published procedures,[477,478] Renal impairment, characterized by a reduction in the glomerular filtration rate, has been reported in occasional patients given high doses[479] and a clinically significant decrease in glomerular filtration rate occurred in 40% of patients receiving subcutaneous desferrioxamine that was reversible on its discontinuation.[480] A fatal acute respiratory distress syndrome–like syndrome has been described in patients with acute iron poisoning given 15 mg/kg/hour desferrioxamine infusions for periods in excess of 24 hours; lower doses and shorter infusions are recommended for acute iron poisoning.[481] Pulmonary injury with fibrosis has also been reported in patients with chronic iron overload receiving doses of 10–22 mg/kg/hour.[482]

In noniron-overloaded patients, the use of desferrioxamine potentiated the action of prochlorperazine, a phenothiazine derivative, leading to reversible coma in two patients.[483] Lens opacities, observed rarely in patients receiving high doses of desferrioxamine, improved when the chelator was withdrawn.[437] In a recent randomized study comparing desferrioxamine with deferasirox, five of 290 patients randomized to desferrioxamine without lens opacities at baseline appeared to develop them over a 1-year period. In the context of the knowledge that clinically significant lens opacities are uncommon in patients on long-term desferrioxamine, these findings need interpreting with caution. Thrombocytopenia has been observed with desferrioxamine in two patients on renal dialysis.[484] It is important to avoid a sudden bolus infusion of desferrioxamine in patients receiving intravenous treatment through an indwelling catheter or during blood transfusions because this can lead to nausea, vomiting, hypotension with acute collapse,[485] or even transient aphasia.[486]

General Treatment Recommendations for Thalassemia Major

Standard Therapy

Guidelines aim to achieve a balance between the unwanted effects of under or over chelation, and advise what is most practical for the patient. Standard current practice for commencing desferrioxamine in β thalassemia major is to begin at the age of 3 years or when the ferritin reaches 1,000 μg/L, whichever is sooner, and not to exceed 30 mg/kg until response to this regimen can be assessed. Although it is clear that the introduction of desferrioxamine at excessive doses or too early increase the risks of toxicity, the optimal dosing and timing have not been the subjects of prospective, randomized trials, and recommendations are therefore to some extent empirically based. Delay in treatment until after age 3 years has been recommended because of observations of poor growth and metaphyseal dysplasia when started earlier.[442,471,487–489] Conversely, delay in starting treatment increases the risk of iron-mediated toxicity as hepatic fibrosis associated with liver iron loading has been reported in children as young as age 3 years.[278,490] It is possible that very low doses given from an earlier age could prevent accumulation of liver iron without concomitant desferrioxamine toxicity, but there are presently no data that address this directly. Furthermore, failure to start treatment sufficiently early increases the risk of growth retardation due to the well-established effects of iron overload on growth and sexual development.

Downward dose adjustment is advisable with young age and low levels of iron loading. In patients younger than age 5 years, doses in excess of 35 mg/kg/day might be inadvisable. Ferritin can be used as an approximate indicator of falling iron levels, and doses of desferrioxamine should be reduced accordingly keeping the therapeutic index less than 0.025 (mean daily dose in mg/kg, divided by the serum ferritin in μg/L).[344,370] If liver iron quantitation is available, a scheme for dose adjustment has been suggested.[340] Liver iron determinations are unlikely to be available more frequently than yearly, even in centers performing these measurement routinely, therefore, ferritin measurements will still be useful in dose adjustment.

Upward dose adjustment should be considered in patients with rates of transfusional iron intake greater than 0.5 mg/kg/day. Doses of 50–60 mg/kg/day will be necessary for negative iron balance in approximately half of these patients.[212] Even at intermediate transfusion rates between 0.3 and 0.5 mg/kg/day, approximately a quarter of all patients will require doses higher than 50 mg/kg/day to achieve negative iron balance. Doses less than 35 mg/kg/day result in positive iron balance even in patients with a transfusional iron loading rate of less than 0.3 mg/kg/day.[212] Therefore, in adults, doses above 40 mg/kg/day and typically 50–60 mg/kg/day are often necessary. Ascorbate supplementation of 2–3 mg/kg/day is another useful way of increasing iron excretion and it is recommended for patients who are stable and not in heart failure or do not have an arrhythmia on the days that desferrioxamine is given. Patients with mild myocardial iron loading and T2* of 10–20 msec can also benefit from modest increments in desferrioxamine dose or frequency. With T2* less than 10 seconds or with left ventricular dysfunction, a greater degree of intensification is required.

Rescue Therapy

For patients with acute heart failure, continuous desferrioxamine infusion is recommended. This is usually most conveniently achieved by diluting desferrioxamine in 500 mL of saline and infusing through a peripheral vein. For longer-term infusions, once the patient has been stabilized, an indwelling line is usually necessary, although 24-hour infusion has been successfully achieved by the subcutaneous route in selected cases.[343] Doses in excess of 50–60 mg/kg/day have been used successfully but increase the risk of pulmonary[482] and retinal toxicity.[440] Complications associated with the use of central venous access lines include infection and thrombosis.[333] To limit the thrombotic complications of central venous access lines, close monitoring and prophylactic anticoagulant therapy have been suggested. Intensification, as described previously, has also been successfully used in very severe iron overload without myocardial dysfunction or as a way of reestablishing compliance with chelation therapy with good long-term outcome if compliance is maintained.[333] With evidence of moderately increased myocardial loading or T2* of 10–20 msec, improvement in these measures might be achieved by increasing the dose or duration of exposure or compliance with subcutaneous desferrioxamine above that given for standard therapy. With severe myocardial iron loading and T2* less than10 msec, but without heart failure, intensification of therapy is necessary and can include increasing the dose and/or duration of desferrioxamine exposure without[245,343] or with the addition of deferiprone.

Methods of Delivery for Desferrioxamine

The mode of delivery of standard desferrioxamine is critical to compliance and hence the success of therapy. It is usually infused at night via a thin subcutaneous needle inserted into the abdomen, arm, or lateral thigh region, which is connected to a portable pump over 8–12 hours, five–seven times per week at a daily dose of 20–60 mg/kg. The infusion site needs to be rotated nightly and a solution infused should not damage tissues. The most widely delivery system has been the battery-operated syringe driver, delivering between 10 and 30 mL, depending on the manufacturer. These are best suited to subcutaneous infusions for 8–12 hours daily, but some can also be used for intravenous infusions. Lighter or smaller systems have been developed that might be better suited to continuous

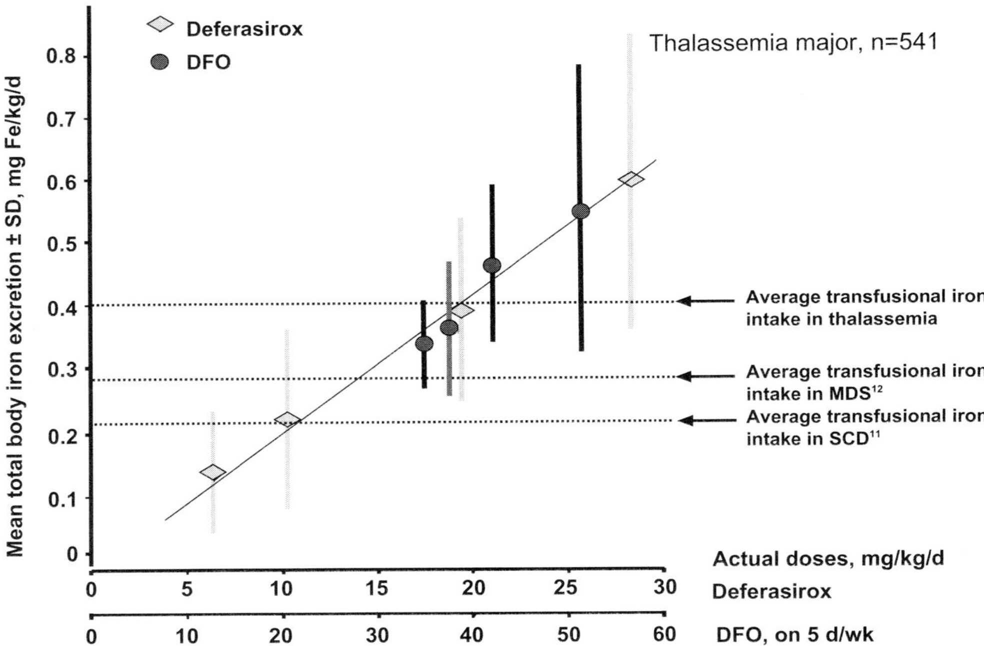

Figure 29.7. Dose–response comparison of DFO and DFX.[212]

infusion. Some battery-operated pumps can take 50–100 mL of desferrioxamine solution, allowing continuous intravenous treatment for up to 1 week. An alternative is to use disposable pumps that expel fluid under the pressure produced by filling an expandable balloon.[491] These devices are light and silent, making them attractive to patients who need continuous infusions, but disposable pumps are expensive. Recently introduced mechanical delivery devices and gas-operated systems are also lighter and more compact than conventional syringe driver models.

Subcutaneous bolus injections have been evaluated as an alternative approach to chelation therapy if pumps are unavailable or impractical. Studies suggest that iron excretion with twice daily subcutaneous injections of desferrioxamine might be comparable to that observed with the same total dose given as an 8-hour subcutaneous infusion.[492,493] In a randomized comparison of twice daily bolus injections and subcutaneous infusion, similar decrements of serum ferritin and approximate liver iron values were seen in both groups of thalassemia patients.[494] This approach might be an alternative when pumps are not available and when patients are prepared to inject twice daily.

Use of Desferrioxamine in Sickle Cell Disease and Thalassemia Intermedia

Sickle Cell Disease

Patients with sickle cell disease who receive long-term transfusion therapy to prevent the complications will eventually require iron chelation therapy unless exchange transfusions are used in preference to simple transfusions. A variety of chronic anemias associated with iron loading, in which regular transfusion is not necessary but erythropoietic reserve might be marginal, such as pyruvate kinase deficiency, sideroblastic anemias, and thalassemia intermedia, may also benefit from chelation therapy if venesection is not feasible.

The optimal dose to achieve iron balance can be referred to the rate of iron loading from transfusion that can easily be calculated from the number of blood units given over a given time period. On the basis of the transfusional loading rate, the optimal dose can be referred to a graph[212] relating dose to iron balance. Thus the dose of desferrioxamine to obtain iron balance will on average be lower in sickle cell disease (20 mg/kg/day) than in thalassemia major (40 mg/kg/day) (see Fig. 29.7).

Although in sickle cell disease, iron distribution to endocrine organs and to the heart is less common than in thalassemia major, chelation therapy is still necessary to maintain iron balance and decrease the risks of iron overload. Iron balance with desferrioxamine and the proportions of fecal and urinary iron excretion appear similar to those seen in thalassemia syndromes.[495] The rate of iron loading varies considerably between patients and depending whether simple transfusion or erythrocytapheresis is used. In a recent multicenter study the average rate of transfusional iron loading was less in sickle cell disease (0.22 mg/kg/day).[225] The use of ferritin for dose adjustment is more problematic in sickle cell disease as discussed previously. LICs above 7 mg/g dry weight are a clear indication for starting treatment because the risk of liver fibrosis increases above this value,[304] which will typically be exceeded after 21 months of simple transfusion.[303,304] Maximal doses should not exceed those given in thalassemia syndromes, and careful monitoring for toxicity is advisable.

Thalassemia Intermedia

In thalassemia intermedia, iron overload might result from increased iron absorption up to five times the normal rate[217,218] or from sporadic transfusions. Serum ferritin tends to underestimate the degree of iron overloading[234] so that liver iron determination is particularly helpful in planning the optimal regime. In general, because of the lack of regular transfusion, negative iron balance can be achieved at relatively modest doses or frequency of chelation. By referring to the dose response for other diseases (Fig. 29.7), a mean daily dose of desferrioxamine at 10 mg/kg/day would maintain iron balance or put patients into negative iron balance. In practice, iron can be decreased steadily and safely by giving standard doses (40 mg/kg) of desferrioxamine twice or three times a week in such patients, thus achieving mean daily doses of 10–20 mg/kg/day.

Because of the discordance of serum ferritin from body iron burden in both thalassemia intermedia and sickle cell disorders, it might be advisable to quantitate liver iron before making a decision to initiate chelation therapy and to repeat liver iron quantitation at regular intervals during treatment.

ORAL CHELATION THERAPY

Although desferrioxamine is highly efficacious, complying with long-term administration has been problematic for an important subset of patients limiting its effectiveness. This has driven the development of orally absorbed chelators. Inconveniently, the very properties that encourage oral absorption also increase the access of chelators to iron or other metal pools that are necessary for normal physiological functions. Many promising compounds have been discarded because preclinical animal toxicology or clinical evaluation has shown too narrow a margin between the therapeutic and the toxic effects. Two orally absorbed iron chelators are now in widespread clinical use: deferiprone and deferasirox.

Deferiprone

Historical Perspective

The hydroxypyridinones were first described in 1982.[496] Initial clinical trials were conducted without the backing of a major pharmaceutical company and showed promising effects on urinary iron excretion in myelodysplasia and patients with transfusional iron overload.[497,498]

Animal toxicology demonstrated a dose-dependent and time-dependent suppression of the bone marrow, both in iron overloaded and nonoverloaded states.[419,499,500] Several cases of agranulocytosis were also reported in humans.[501–503] Other effects in animal models, such as redistribution of iron from the liver to the heart and liver fibrosis, were later reported with the closely related hydroxypyridine, CP94, in an iron-overloaded gerbil model.[504,505] Thymic atrophy and teratogenic effects at doses close to the effective clinical therapeutic range were later identified.[506] Further development led to trials to establish the efficacy of deferiprone and the frequency of complications, but the original efficacy study was discontinued following disagreements between the pharmaceutical company and clinical investigators.[340] The results of a 4-year toxicity trial have been reported.[507] More recently, prospective randomized studies have been undertaken, particularly focusing on the cardioprotective effects of the drug.[462] Deferiprone was licensed as second-line therapy for transfusional iron overload in Europe in 1999 but is not licensed in North America. The drug is licensed in India under the trade name Kelfer.

Chemistry and Pharmacology

Deferiprone (1,2-dimethyl-3-hydroxypyrid-4-one) (L1, CP20, Kelfer, Ferriprox) is a member of the family of 3-hydroxypyrid-4-one bidentate chelators[496] that bind to iron in a 3:1 ratio. It is less hydrophilic than desferrioxamine with approximately one-third of the molecular weight (139). Although the stability constant for iron (III) is approximately six orders of magnitude higher than desferrioxamine, the pM of 20 is lower than that of desferrioxamine at 26.6.[418] As a consequence, iron (III) coordination is most efficient at high concentrations of the chelator but at concentrations of 1 μM iron and 10 μM chelator, desferrioxamine will scavenge iron more efficiently. The lower stability at lower concentrations of drug also increases the potential to redistribute iron within the body[508] and leads to the potential formation of incomplete 1:1 and 1:2 iron–chelate complexes at low chelator concentrations. Such incomplete complexes have the potential to participate in the generation of hydroxyl radicals.[406] Unlike desferrioxamine, which is positively charged both in its iron free and complexed forms, deferiprone and its 3:1 iron complex are both neutrally charged. This neutral charge, and the less hydrophilic nature of the iron chelator and its complex, encourages a rapid diffusion of the free chelator into cells and its iron complex out of cells. Thus, unlike desferrioxamine, which slowly accumulates within cells at concentrations above those in the plasma with ferrioxamine egressing only slowly, the iron complex of deferiprone egresses relatively quickly.[363,400,411]

Following oral administration, absorption is rapid with the drug appearing in plasma within 5–10 minutes of ingestion. High concentrations are achieved at commonly prescribed doses, reaching levels in excess of 300 μM after oral ingestion of a 50 mg/kg dose.[384,427] These levels are 5–10 times higher than infused desferrioxamine[445,509] (Table 29.10). In vitro studies in myocytes show that these high concentrations, together with a more rapid access to intracellular iron, might favor the scavenging of chelatable iron by deferiprone.[402] It has been suggested that at clinically relevant desferrioxamine concentrations of 10 μM, the effects of desferrioxamine on preventing and reversing cardiac pathology might result more from prevention of iron uptake into myocytes than from rapid iron removal.[402] With deferiprone, however, these high levels are short-lived with an elimination $t_{1/2}$ of 1.52 hours,[427] and if given three times daily, are punctuated by low levels between doses and negligible nocturnal levels. The drug is metabolized in hepatocytes to the inactive glucuronide, which is the predominant form recovered in the urine.[384,510] In contrast to desferrioxamine, iron excretion with deferiprone is almost exclusively in the urine.[495,509,511] The rapid inactivation of deferiprone in the liver by glucuronidation[421] might explain the relatively less impressive effect of deferiprone on liver iron removal compared with desferrioxamine,[426] but in other cells such as myocytes this would be less of a limitation and could explain why deferiprone appears to be more effective in the heart than the liver. In contrast, the highly hydrophilic nature and high molecular weight will tend to retard access to intracellular iron pools,[372,400,403] and the positive charge of the iron complex will retard egress from cells.[400,411]

Evidence of Efficacy of Deferiprone

Evidence of efficacy with deferiprone has been based on the effects of the drug on iron excretion, serum ferritin, LIC, and more recently the iron-induced cardiomyopathy.

Effects on Iron Excretion and Balance

Early observations demonstrated that urinary iron excretion in response to deferiprone 75 mg/kg was comparable to that with desferrioxamine infused subcutaneously over 8–12 hours at a dose of 40–50 mg/kg.[509] Urinary iron excretion correlated with the serum ferritin and desferrioxamine-induced urinary iron excretion.[509] Formal iron balance studies showed that total iron excretion at 75 mg/kg was 62% of that achieved with subcutaneous desferrioxamine at 50 mg/kg given over 8 hours.[495] Urinary iron excretion did not change significantly in a group of patients receiving 75 mg/kg/day with a mean follow-up of 39 months.[512] Dose equivalence for desferrioxamine and deferiprone has not been determined in iron balance studies.

Effects on Serum Ferritin

Many early small nonrandomized studies have examined the effects of deferiprone on serum ferritin. Ferritin values fell in the most heavily iron overloaded subjects with serum ferritin of 5,000 μg/L and more,[502] but in patients with levels below 2,500 μg/L levels did not typically fall. In a study in India, serum ferritin fell from initially very high levels by an average of more than 3,500 μg/L over 20 months.[513] In a Canadian study of 21 patients given a dose of 75 mg/kg/day, the serum ferritin declined from 3,975 to 2,546 μg/L after a mean follow-up of 3 years.[339] Changes were most marked in patients starting with high ferritin values, whereas in those patients starting with ferritin values below 2,500 μg/L there was no significant further change. In a study from London, there was no overall change in serum ferritin in 26 patients treated for 3 years at 75 mg/kg (initial value 2,937 μg/L, final value 2,323 μg/L).[512] In 52 patients from Turin with a median pretreatment ferritin value of 1,826 μg/L, there was no significant change in the serum ferritin level after 2 years of therapy with deferiprone at a dose of 75 mg/kg/day.[514] Randomized prospective comparisons of desferrioxamine and deferiprone have been undertaken more recently with a combined total 235 patients.[462,515–518] Due to differences in previous treatments, baseline ferritin values, and dosing regimes, pooled comparisons were not particularly revealing. Nevertheless, statistically significant decrease in serum ferritin in favor of desferrioxamine was seen at 6 months[516,517] with no difference at 12 months.[515]

Effect on Liver Iron

Relatively few prospective studies have examined changes in liver iron. Early studies measured LIC after periods of treatment but not before, making interpretation of results difficult. For example, hepatic iron was above 15 mg/g dry weight in 10 of 17 patients (58%) in a 2–4-year follow-up study and below 7 mg/g dry weight in only two patients.[512] In another study of 52 previously well chelated patients treated for 2 years at 75 mg/kg/day, the hepatic iron concentration increased in 69% of patients by a mean of 43%[514] and mean values had increased by 56% from 5.1 to 8.0 mg/g dry weight after 3 years. In a nonrandomized report with 7–8-year follow-up of seven patients, there was an "unexplained resurgence" of serum ferritin after 4–5 years, associated with a concomitant increase in liver iron in three.[519] In 21 patients given deferiprone, LICs were followed prospectively initially for 3.1 years;[339] in 10 previously suboptimally chelated patients, LICs fell from 23 mg/g dry weight to 11 mg/g dry weight ($P < 0.005$) with values above 15 mg/g dry weight in only two patients. In 11 patients in whom desferrioxamine had been effectively taken prior to use of deferiprone, hepatic iron concentrations remained below 15 mg/g dry weight; at 4.6 years, hepatic iron was above 15 mg/g dry wt in seven of 18 patients (39%).[452]

A combined systematic analysis of several randomized studies in a total of 143 subjects has been reported.[518] The patient selection, dosing, and scheduled period of follow-up varied considerably between studies, as did the findings. In a Canadian study, at 33 months of treatment at 75 mg/kg, a mean increase in liver iron of 5 mg/g dry weight in 18 patients was noted with deferiprone compared with a 1 mg/g dry weight increase with desferrioxamine.[520] In an

Italian study, a comparable decrease in LIC was seen with both deferiprone (21 patients) and with desferrioxamine (15 patients) at 30 months.[515] In a 1-year study of other Italian patients given 100 mg/kg daily, a mean decrease of 0.93 mg/g dry weight was seen with deferiprone (27 patients) compared with a decrease of 1.54 mg/g dry weight with desferrioxamine, at a dose of 43 mg/kg five–seven times a week (30 patients).[462] In a small 6-month randomized study, where baseline LIC values were higher than in the aforementioned studies, a greater decrease in LIC was reported with deferiprone (75 mg/kg) (6.6 mg/g dry weight, n = 6) than with desferrioxamine (30–60 mg/kg 5–7 days/week) (2.9 mg/g dry weight).[517] As with ferritin findings, patients with initially high LICs might respond better than those with lower values. Apparent loss of response with time could also reflect changes in compliance with longer periods of observation. Other factors that might account for the variable response between studies are differences in the rate of drug inactivation by glucuronidation or differences in transfusion rates.

Effects on the Heart

Initial data of the effects on myocardial dysfunction, myocardial iron, and the prevalence of heart disease gave conflicting results, most likely reflecting the retrospective nature of patient allocation and differences in prestudy chelation histories. More recently prospective studies have demonstrated a beneficial effect on both heart function and myocardial T2*, particularly at higher doses.

An early study showed continued cardiac mortality in 51 thalassemia patients who previously were poorly chelated with desferrioxamine. Four died of cardiac causes[512] leading to the authors to conclude that in the face of pre-existing severe iron overload, deferiprone cannot reliably protect patients from cardiomyopathic mortality. In a large retrospective analysis of 532 Italian thalassemia major patients, nine died of heart failure while being treated with deferiprone.[521] On the other hand, a retrospective study of survival in 157 Italian patients treated with deferiprone between 1995 and 2003 for a median of 4.3 years reported significantly better survival in this group than in 369 patients treated with desferrioxamine. As patients were not randomized to desferrioxamine or to deferiprone the possibility of selection bias cannot be excluded. Furthermore the dropout rate of 31% was particularly high in deferiprone-treated patients. Another Italian study compared cardiac complications and survival over 6 years in 54 deferiprone-treated patients with 75 retrospectively allocated desferrioxamine-treated patients.[522] Three deaths occurred in the desferrioxamine group and none in the deferiprone-treated group; however, the three deaths were in patients who started chelation at a late age. Furthermore, five patients in the desferrioxamine group had New York Heart Association class II–IV cardiac disease at baseline compared with only one in the deferiprone group. Another retrospective analysis of 539 thalassemic patients from Cyprus born after 1960 and followed from 1980 to 2004 showed an increased trend in cardiac mortality between 1980 and 2000 with a subsequent decline after 2000, which the authors attributed to increased deferiprone use.[523] A possible beneficial effect of deferiprone on myocardial T* was first suggested[524] in a retrospective nonrandomized study of 15 patients treated with deferiprone compared with 30 desferrioxamine-treated patients. Desferrioxamine patients were retrospectively matched for serum ferritin from a large group of 160 patients.[524] The authors concluded that the lower incidence of reduced T2* in the deferiprone group was likely to be due to deferiprone treatment rather than any unintentional selection bias resulting from retrospective allocation of comparator groups.

To clarify the apparent inconsistencies between the aforementioned studies, prospective studies are needed. Two studies examining the effect of deferiprone monotherapy have been published. In one prospective randomized trial, 71 patients treated with deferiprone at conventional doses of 75 mg/kg/day were compared with 73 patients treated with standard-dose desferrioxamine. After 1 year, both groups showed a similar and significant improvement in cardiac nuclear MRI signal.[515] By contrast, in a prospective randomized study,[462] 61 thalassemic patients with moderate cardiac siderosis and T2* 8–20 msec were randomized to continue on desferrioxamine at an average dose of 43 mg/kg/day or deferiprone at a higher than usual mean dose of 92 mg/kg/day. In the standard-dose desferrioxamine group, the T2* improved 13%, whereas improvement was 27% in the deferiprone group. Although the ejection fraction was in the normal range at baseline in both groups, it improved significantly in the deferiprone- compared with the desferrioxamine-treated patients (3.1% vs. 0.3%). Taken together, these studies suggest that high-dose deferiprone might be more effective at improving myocardial T2* than standard-dose intermittent desferrioxamine 5 days a week, but at standard doses of deferiprone this advantage is more difficult to show. If patients have evidence of shortened T2* values, particularly with T2* values less than 10 msec, standard doses of desferrioxamine or deferiprone are not recommended; either high-dose deferiprone or intensified desferrioxamine by continuous infusion is recommended. An alternative approach, discussed later, would be to combine the two treatments.

Unwanted Effects of Deferiprone

Neutropenia and Agranulocytosis

Agranulocytosis was initially reported in 3%–4% of patients treated with deferiprone, and mild neutropenia occurred in an additional 4%.[502,525] Neutropenia can last from 4–124 days.[501,526,527] In 532 thalassemic patients treated for a total of 1,154 patient-years, the rates of agranulocytosis and neutropenia were 0.43 and 2.08 per 100 patient-years, respectively.[521] In a study designed to establish the frequency of agranulocytosis defined as neutrophils 0.0–0.5 × 10^9/L, only one of 187 patients (0.5%) developed agranulocytosis.[527] Nine patients (4.8%) developed milder neutropenia (absolute neutrophil count 0.5–1.5 × 10^9/L). No additional cases of agranulocytosis occurred, but seven new cases of mild neutropenia developed during the next 3 years of treatment.[507] The lower incidence of agranulocytosis compared with some earlier estimates suggests that this might be decreased by monitoring the white count weekly and stopping therapy in a timely manner. There are very few data on evaluation of deferiprone in children aged younger than 6 years, and a study of 44 patients showed no cases of agranulocytosis occurred, but thrombocytopenia was seen in 45% 3 months–1 year after starting deferiprone and was reversible on cessation of treatment.[528] As this was not a randomized study, the significance of this observation is difficult to gauge and further studies are needed in this age group.

The mechanism of agranulocytosis is unclear. It has been suggested that this occurs though a dose-dependent inhibition of DNA synthesis and ribonucleotide reductase[411] or possibly though a zinc-depletion mechanism.[529] Alternatively the effect in humans might be idiosyncratic; however, several observations do not fit this mechanism. First, bone marrow hypoplasia is dose dependent in animal studies,[413] which is not typical of an idiosyncratic response and dose–response studies have not been conducted in humans. Agranulocytosis might appear as a late event after more than 1 year of therapy and can be preceded by previous episodes of neutropenia,[521] a pattern also not characteristic of idiosyncratic reactions. The involvement of other hematopoietic lineages in both animal studies[413,419] and humans[528,530,531] would also be more consistent with a general effect on hematopoietic progenitors. Milder forms of neutropenia might be related to hypersplenism and intercurrent infections rather than to drug toxicity.[532]

Other Unwanted Effects

The largest prospective clinical study designed to characterize the safety profile of deferiprone included 187 patients.[532] Nausea and vomiting were relatively common in the first year of therapy, occurring in 24% of patients, with abdominal pain in 14%, and arthralgia in 13%. Analysis after 4 years of treatment demonstrated that additional gastrointestinal symptoms were infrequent but the overall dropout rate increased from 15% after 1 year to 55% at 4 years.[507] Arthralgia and arthropathy vary greatly among studies, with an incidence 30%–40%[513,533] in the developing world and less than 5% in Italy.[521] The higher iron load in the patients from the developing world might increase the risk of iron redox cycling by incomplete chelate complexes in the joints. The risk of arthropathy appears to increase with the duration of treatment and increased from 6% at 1 year to 13% at 4 years.[507]

In a pooled analysis, fluctuations in liver tests were reported in 44% of patients.[525] Accelerated liver fibrosis was reported in a randomized study comparing deferiprone- (n = 19) with desferrioxamine-treated patients (n = 20) over 3.5 years,[452] and some progression of liver fibrosis was also found in other reports.[519,534] No progression was seen in 34 of 187 patients with available biopsies who were treated for 3.5 years[535] or in a randomized 1-year study with desferrioxamine.[515] None of these studies were designed to evaluate progression of liver fibrosis, and interpretation of the findings is limited by a number of factors such as unclear hepatitis C mRNA status,[452] variations in the duration of treatment,[534] failure to record baseline liver fibrosis,[512,519] and lack of clarity about changes in LIC.[535] Thus long-term prospective data comparing liver fibrosis with desferrioxamine has not been reported.[518] Small decreases in plasma zinc[532] and cases of zinc deficiency[525] not requiring cessation of therapy have been reported.

Recommended Dosing

Formal safety studies have only been conducted at 75 mg/kg in three divided doses and this is the usual dose given. Published tolerability data at 100 mg/kg, a dose also licensed in the European Union, are confined to a single 1-year prospective study in 32 patients.[462] As no excess toxicity was reported, it might be reasonable to increase the dose in otherwise unresponsive patients. Nevertheless it is not known whether tolerability issues such as neutropenia and agranulocytosis increase at doses above 75 mg/kg/day. Few data are available in young children, and this is reflected in the licensing in the European Union, which is confined to patients older than 6 years.

Combined Chelation Therapy: Deferiprone and Desferrioxamine

Pharmacology

When control of iron load or iron distribution is inadequate with monotherapy, the combined use of two chelators might be useful. In principle, two chelators can be given simultaneously or sequentially and the pharmacological implications differ. The use of more than one chelator, often referred to as mixed-ligand therapy,[536] is well established.[536,537] There is often a marked synergism of metal removal when a small kinetically labile ligand is combined with a larger hexadentate chelator. Typical examples are nitrilotriacetate/desferrioxamine for iron removal, penicillamine/DTPA for copper removal[538] and salicylic acid/EDTA for plutonium removal.[536]

Mixed-ligand therapy with deferiprone and desferrioxamine relies on the principle of the low-molecular-weight bidentate deferiprone rapidly accessing chelatable iron pools unavailable to desferrioxamine and subsequently "shuttling" the chelated iron onto a desferrioxamine "sink."[382,539,540] Although this might increase net iron excretion, it could also increase unwanted effects due to shuttling from key metalloenzymes. If chelators are given sequentially, for example desferrioxamine by night and deferiprone by day, the main effect will be to provide a greater period of chelation exposure, increasing the protection time without significant shuttling of metals and with less risk of interactive toxicities. For example whereas monotherapy with desferrioxamine at night or deferiprone during the day only provides intermittent decrements in labile plasma iron, by alternating desferrioxamine at night with deferiprone by day decreases in labile iron can be obtained. Although deferasirox could also be used together with other chelators, at this time experience is very limited so that the discussion of combined treatment will be limited to desferrioxamine and deferiprone.

Clinical Regimens Assessed in Combined Therapy

Many combinations have been given with various degrees of pharmacological overlap, even within a given study. Combined treatment has often been given as a way of helping patients who comply poorly with desferrioxamine monotherapy or have a poor response with deferiprone monotherapy to achieve more exposure to chelation. For example, a patient with inadequate ferritin or liver iron control on deferiprone given as 75 mg/kg/day in three divided doses would take additionally desferrioxamine two–three times a week. Another group that has been considered for mixed treatment is high-risk cases with particularly low myocardial T2* values or with very high levels of iron overload. The regimens used have tended to have a greater degree of overlap of chelators. For patients with cardiac dysfunction, the additional value of combined therapy over intensive desferrioxamine treatment is presently under investigation in a randomized trial. The effects of combined therapy in controlled trials have recently been included in a systematic review[518] in which the considerable variability in responses between studies has been attributed to the diverse nature of the regimens used and differences in the prestudy treatments.

Effects on Serum Ferritin and Liver Iron

Several prospective randomized studies have now compared the use of various combined treatments with that of desferrioxamine or deferiprone monotherapy. In a small study, no significant difference in serum ferritin was seen between standard desferrioxamine monotherapy 5 nights a week compared with 7 days of deferiprone and 2 nights of desferrioxamine.[541] In another study, effects on ferritin and liver iron were similar with desferrioxamine monotherapy 5 nights a week compared with deferiprone 7 days a week plus 2 nights of desferrioxamine.[542] In a study in which desferrioxamine was given five times a week in the combination arm, the serum ferritin and liver T2* decreased more in the combined group of desferrioxamine five times a week plus deferiprone 7 days a week than with desferrioxamine monotherapy five times a week.[463] Together, these studies suggest that deferiprone given 7 days a week combined with desferrioxamine 2 nights a week will have similar effects on serum ferritin as desferrioxamine monotherapy given 5 nights but a greater effect than with deferiprone monotherapy at 75 mg/kg/day. When patients were randomized to one of three regimens, monotherapy of deferiprone or desferrioxamine or to combined deferiprone 7 days a week with desferrioxamine 2 nights a week, the greatest ferritin decrease was seen with desferrioxamine monotherapy and the least with deferiprone monotherapy.[516] A similar three-armed study is in broad agreement with these findings. Desferrioxamine monotherapy 5 nights a week was compared with deferiprone monotherapy 7 days a week or the same treatment plus desferrioxamine twice a week.[543] This 1-year study measured LIC at baseline and at the end of the study, allowing calculation of iron balance and total iron excretion based on the known transfusion rate. The combination therapy ($n = 8$) produced a significantly larger decrease in LIC and serum ferritin and a higher total iron excretion that deferiprone monotherapy ($n = 12$) and a similar effect to desferrioxamine monotherapy ($n = 12$). Decrease in LIC was only seen in 42% of patients on deferiprone monotherapy but in 88% of patients on combined treatment. These studies suggest that control of iron balance with monotherapy is more likely to be achieved with desferrioxamine than with deferiprone. Combined therapy with daily deferiprone plus desferrioxamine at least 2 nights a week is roughly equivalent to desferrioxamine given five times a week.

Effect on the Heart

Initial observational studies with a variety of combined regimens suggested possible beneficial effects on myocardial T2* or on heart function. In 79 patients treated with deferiprone 7 days a week with a variable desferrioxamine regimen, improvement in left ventricular ejection fraction was found compared with the previous noncompliant desferrioxamine monotherapy.[544] In another observational study, 42 patients given deferiprone 7 days a week plus desferrioxamine 2–6 nights a week over 3–4 years showed improvement in the left ventricular shortening.[545] More recently, a randomized controlled study of 65 patients with moderate heart iron loading and T2* 8–20 msec was undertaken comparing monotherapy with standard desferrioxamine five times a week with the same desferrioxamine treatment plus deferiprone 7 days a week.[463] Despite the relative conservative monotherapy desferrioxamine regimen, T2* improved 3 msec in 1 year but this increased to 6 msec with combined treatment. Although all patients had left ventricular ejection fraction of more than 56%

at baseline, left ventricular ejection fraction increased by approximately 2.5% in the combination arm and 0.5% in the monotherapy arm. In another small randomized study in patients with normal left ventricular ejection fraction at baseline, no difference was found with combination treatment after 1 year or with deferiprone monotherapy, but a small decrease was found with desferrioxamine monotherapy.[543] Interestingly, desferrioxamine was given only twice a week, whereas in the study in which an improvement in left ventricular ejection fraction was seen, desferrioxamine was given five times a week in the combination arm.[463] Prospective studies in patients with abnormal left ventricular ejection fraction are needed but until such data are available, it is recommended that desferrioxamine is given with or without deferiprone for the maximum practicable duration when patients have evidence of decreased left ventricular function.

Safety of Combined Treatment

Formal safety data on combined treatment are limited. In general, alternating regimens are less likely to be an issue for toxicity compared with regimens in which chelation is simultaneous or overlapping. A meta-analysis of the incidence of agranulocytosis with combined regimens compared with deferasirox monotherapy suggested that the risk might be increased several-fold, although the numbers of evaluable patients are small (Macklin, IND submission to FDA, 2004); the increased incidence appeared to occur mostly in those regimens in which the drugs were administered simultaneously. In a recently reported prospective study, one case of agranulocytosis and two of neutropenia were seen at 1 year in the combination arm containing 32 patients.[463] No excess in arthropathy was seen in the combination arm and no new tolerability issues that were not recognized with monotherapy have been reported.

Deferasirox (ICL670, Exjade)

Historical Perspective

Deferasirox is a member of a new class of tridentate (Fig. 29.6) iron-selective synthetic chelators, the bis-hydroxyphenyl-triazoles. Unlike the clinical development of desferrioxamine and deferiprone that were predominantly clinician led, deferasirox has been taken through a development program that complies with modern regulatory processes involving over 1,000 patients in phase I–IV studies. Preregistration phase I-III trials were designed to last 1 year but many have been extended to 3 years or more. The drug is now licensed for the treatment of transfusional iron overload, including children older than 2 years in most countries. The long-term tolerability profile and longer-term effects on complications of iron overload are still being evaluated.

Chemistry and Pharmacology

The tridentate structure with 2:1 chelator:iron binding results in an iron complex coordinated by four oxygen and two nitrogen atoms with the chemical formula: 4-[3,5-bis(2-hydroxyphenyl)-1,2,4-triazol-1-yl]benzoic acid and a molecular weight of 373. The stability of this complex as estimated by the pM values is intermediate between desferrioxamine and deferiprone (Table 29.10). Deferasirox is lipophilic but highly protein bound in plasma, which appears to confer good tissue penetration with faster mobilization of tissue iron than desferrioxamine.[546] In culture systems, mobilization of myocyte iron appears to be efficient.[381,402] This has been confirmed in studies with iron-overloaded gerbils.[547] The drug has low solubility in water and is given once daily as an oral suspension.

Pharmacokinetics were examined in the first phase I study of single oral doses of deferasirox involving 24 patients with thalassemia major. In this randomized, double-blind study, patients received single oral doses of dispersible tablets ranging from 2.5 to 80 mg/kg.[428] Deferasirox was absorbed promptly and was detectable in the blood for 24 hours. A plasma half-life of 11–19 hours was found, supporting once-daily oral administration. The area under the curve (AUC) at 0–24 hours and C_{max} of deferasirox increased nearly proportionally with the dose. At doses between 10 and 40 mg/kg/day the AUC of the iron complex of deferasirox was approximately 20%–30% of that of the iron free drug. A later study showed that with once daily repeated dosing at 20 mg/kg, peak plasma levels reach a mean of 80 μM with trough values of 20 μM (Table 29.10).[548] The urinary excretion of deferasirox and its iron complex was less than 0.1% of the dose. A further study of using single doses of ^{14}C deferasirox showed that metabolism occurred at several sites with glucuronidation in the liver.[549] Elimination of this and other metabolites was predominantly fecal. It was concluded that the final elimination process of deferasirox, the Fe-complex, and metabolites was by hepatobiliary anion transport and that the metabolic drug interaction potential via cytochrome p450 enzymes was low.

Effects on Iron Balance, LIC, and Ferritin

Initial iron balance studies entailed formal metabolic balance studies. Twenty-four patients randomly allocated to one of three doses or to placebo showed that excretion averaged 0.13, 0.34, and 0.56 mg/kg/day at deferasirox doses of 10, 20, and 40 mg/kg/day, respectively, predicting equilibrium or negative iron balance at daily doses of 20 mg and above.[429] The fraction of iron in the urine was less than 6% of total iron elimination with the majority occurring in the feces. These studies also showed that iron excretion in each patient was linearly related to exposure to the drug as measured by the AUC.

Iron balance over 1 year was assessed in a series of studies which used the Angelucci principle,[318] relating LIC to body iron stores, together with the measured transfusion rate to calculate net iron balance in a range of conditions associated with transfusional iron overload. The pivotal phase III study in 586 thalassemia major patients aged 2–53 years compared changes in LIC, serum ferritin, and net iron balance in 290 patients treated with desferrioxamine with 296 patients treated with deferasirox[453] In this and other similar studies in sickle cell disease[225] and other rare anemias[213] the dosing regimen chosen was conservative, with the dose chosen on the basis of baseline LIC obtained by biopsy or by SQUID. Although this was an understandable precaution to avoid overchelation in patients with a low iron load (LIC <7 mg/g dry weight), it meant that patients who received less than 20 mg/kg/day generally had a positive iron balance.[213,453] At 20 mg/kg/day, iron balance was typically achieved, whereas 30 mg/kg/day resulted in significant reductions in LIC averaging 10 mg/g dry weight over 1 year.[453] A 1-year randomized study in sickle cell disease[225] and a 1-year prospective study in myelodysplastic syndrome, Diamond–Blackfan anemia, and in other rare anemias[213] showed that the dose–response effects and trends in serum ferritin were similar to those in thalassemia, although because the transfusional iron loading rates differed between disease categories, the effective doses varied. In sickle cell disease, the effective doses for iron balance or negative iron balance were less on average than in thalassemia (Fig. 29.7). It is important to point out that there was considerable overlap between patient groups.[213] The efficiency of chelation, or the proportion of administered drug excreted in the iron bound form, was 27%–34% and was essentially the same across all diagnoses and doses tested,[213] being significantly higher than for desferrioxamine in the same studies. Changes in LIC were paralleled proportional to changes in serum ferritin across a range of diagnoses,[213] allowing the trend in serum ferritin to be used as a way of following changes in body iron loading.

Analysis of the combined data from studies in thalassemia, sickle cell disease, and rare anemias has revealed that other factors influence iron balance as seen with desferrioxamine. The most important of these is the transfusional iron-loading rate. The proportion of patients in negative iron balance at 20 mg/kg was 75% at low transfusion rates of less than 0.3 mg/kg/day, but fell to 55% and 47%, respectively, at intermediate (0.3–0.5 mg/kg/day) and high (>0.5 mg/kg/day) transfusion rates.[212] At 30 mg/kg, 96% of patients with a low iron-loading rate were in negative iron balance but at intermediate and high transfusional loading rates, the proportion fell to 80% of patients.[212]

Effects on the Heart

Thus far, experience of the effects of deferasirox on the heart are confined to cell culture, animal data, and preliminary clinical studies. Cell culture[402] and animal studies[548,592] suggested that deferasirox would be effective at accessing myocardial iron. Although studies on myocardial iron estimation were not included as part of the phase II and III trials, preliminary data obtained during these studies in 27 patients treated at doses of 10–30 mg/kg/day showed an improved myocardial T2* at 1 year from 18.7 to 23 msec and improvement was significant for both patients with baseline T2* values below and above 20 msec.[464,550] Prospective studies are ongoing to examine the effects of deferasirox on myocardial iron as measured by T2*. Preliminary results in one of these studies have been reported.[551] Eighteen patients receiving 30 mg//kg for 6 months showed a significant mean improvement in myocardial T2* from 9.5 to 11.2 msec, with improvement in 14 of 18 patients. Randomized comparison of the effects with those of desferrioxamine is also in progress. No data on patients with preexisting myocardial dysfunction are yet available.

Unwanted Effects and their Management

In the key registration phase III study, deferasirox was well tolerated[453] with 5.7% discontinuing drug over 1 year. Common adverse events were generally mild, including transient gastrointestinal events in 15% and skin rash in 11%. The drug is now licensed in European Union and the United States for use in children aged 2 years and older with transfusional iron overload. Follow up data in the five core phase II/III studies are now at a median of 3.5 years with no evidence of new or progressive toxicities.[552] Understandably, it is too early yet to allow any statements on the impact of deferasirox on survival. Recommended patient monitoring includes monthly creatinine and liver function and annual auditory and ophthalmic examinations, including slit-lamp examination and funduscopy.

Gastrointestinal Disturbances

Gastrointestinal disturbances such as diarrhea, constipation, nausea, or vomiting were often self-limiting but in persistent cases were managed by dose modification or by changing the timing of the dose from morning to evening.

Skin Rash

Mild to moderate skin rashes were usually managed by temporary dose reductions followed by subsequent return to the therapeutic dose. Severe skin rashes were usually managed by dose interruptions followed by gradual reintroduction at a smaller dose. Occasional cases of angioedema have been seen for which cessation of drug is recommended.

Renal Effects

Dose-dependent increases in serum creatinine of a third or more above baseline were observed in 38% of patients. These generally remained within the normal range and never exceeded two times the upper limit of normal. Increases in creatinine typically occurred within a few weeks of starting or increasing therapy, were not progressive, and reversed or stabilized with dose adjustment when necessary. In older myelodysplastic syndrome patients in whom baseline creatinine values were just below the upper limit of normal, some patients increased values above normal but these were managed by dose modification. No cases of progressive increments above the normal range were seen in these studies. Proteinuria has been described with deferasirox but is also seen in thalassemia major patients who are not receiving chelation therapy[553] and in sickle cell disease, and therefore baseline testing for proteinuria should be performed before starting treatment. Monthly testing for proteinuria is recommended. If positive, quantitation might be helpful and if this exceeds 1 mg/mL creatinine on more than one occasion treatment should be temporarily withheld or adjusted.

Liver Function

In general the alanine aminotransferase values were observed to fall as LIC values fell with treatment. Increased liver enzymes judged to be related to deferasirox were observed in two patients in the core studies.[453] Outside core studies, other cases of transaminitis have been seen that respond to dose reduction or drug cessation. Monthly liver monitoring is therefore recommended.

Effects in Children

In five phase II and III studies, approximately half of the 703 patients were children younger than 16 years and included children as young as age 2 years. With follow-up at approximately 3 years, no adverse effects on growth or skeletal development have been found and no specific tolerability issues for children have been identified. Evaluation of pediatric patients has shown that growth and development proceeded normally while on deferasirox, lending support to its use in very young patients.

Other Effects

Deafness, neurosensory deafness, and hypacusis were reported as adverse events irrespective of drug relationship in thalassemia major patients in the 1-year core trial in eight patients on deferasirox and seven on desferrioxamine.[453] Cataracts or lenticular opacities were reported as adverse events irrespective of drug relationship in two patients on deferasirox and five on desferrioxamine. Overall the tolerability profile compared favorably with desferrioxamine.[453] The results of the 4-year extension will be useful in interpreting the significance of these findings. Importantly, no drug-related agranulocytosis was observed in thalassemia or sickle cell disease patients from the core studies.[225,453]

Recommended Dosing Regimen

Deferasirox is taken as a suspension in 100–200 mL of water, orange, or apple juice stirred with a nonmetallic utensil. The relationship between dose and iron balance has been studied in large studies over a 1-year period. A decision needs to be made at the time of therapy whether iron balance alone is sufficient or whether negative iron balance is desirable. Recommended starting dose for iron balance is 20 mg/kg, but as can be seen from Figure 29.7, the required dose can be adjusted upward or downward depending on the iron-loading rate. In patients with low transfusion rates of less than 0.3 mg/kg/day a daily dose of 20 mg/kg should be sufficient to maintain iron balance, whereas the doses for intermediate (0.3–0.5) and high (>0.5) loading rates are 25 mg and 30 mg/kg, respectively.[212] Response rates in myelodysplastic syndrome, rare anemias,[213] and sickle cell disease[225] are consistent with those in thalassemia with respect to dose dependency of LIC and ferritin response. The effective dose in milligram/kilogram is approximately half that obtained with subcutaneous desferrioxamine five times per week. In the first 4 weeks after starting deferasirox, weekly serum creatinine and liver function tests are advisable and repeated monthly thereafter. If the dose is adjusted upward, it is advisable to monitor these same variables for 4 weeks after dose increments. Studies are ongoing at doses up to 40 mg/kg/day to assess the safety and efficacy of such doses for the small proportion of patients who fail to respond to lower doses. The proportion of patients with ferritin values less than 1,000 μg/L in extension studies up to 3 years is falling, but this has not been associated with increased toxicity.[554] At 42 months of deferasirox treatment, 25% of patients had ferritin levels less than 1,000 μg/L, and some patients achieve levels less than 500 μg/L, below which the drug is not licensed. To avoid a stop-go approach, it is sensible to reduce the dose slightly as values fall below 1,000 μg/L so ferritin can be kept between 500 and 1,000 μg/L without stopping treatment.

Future Perspectives with Chelation Therapy

The immediate future for chelation therapy is likely to be exciting as results of prospective studies become available with monotherapy and combined therapies using the currently available iron chelators. With three chelators now licensed in many countries, there is considerable scope for assessing how best to use these in combination if monotherapy fails. Unless this is done in a systematic way, however, the true risks and benefits are likely to remain unclear. New chelators continue to be synthesized and evaluated[555] but have yet to reach beyond phase II of clinical evaluation. Intravenous depot desferrioxamine is an interesting concept that still requires formal evaluation beyond phase I clinical studies.[556] The prospective evaluation of MRI to characterize iron distribution and its relationship to transfusional iron loading and to the relative effects of different chelation regimens will be valuable in defining how best to use the tools now available for managing transfusional iron overload.

REFERENCES

1. Cooley T, Witwer E, Lee P. Anemia in children with splenomegaly and peculiar changes in the bones. *Am J Dis Child.* 1927;34:347–363.
2. Whipple GH, Bradford WL. Racial or familial anemia of children. *Am J Dis Child.* 1932;44:336–365.
3. Wolman IJ. Transfusion therapy in Cooley's anemia: growth and health as related to long-range hemoglobin levels. A progress report. *Ann NY Acad Sci.* 1964;119:736–747.
4. Schorr JB, Radel E. Transfusion therapy and its complications in patients with Cooley's anemia. *Ann NY Acad Sci.* 1964;119:703–708.
5. Beard MEJ, Necheles TF, Allen DM. Clinical experience with intensive transfusion therapy in Cooley's anemia. *Ann NY Acad Sci.* 1969;165:415–422.
6. Piomelli S, Danoff SJ, Becker MH, Lipera MJ, Travis SF. Prevention of bone malformations and cardiomegaly in Cooley's anemia by early hypertransfusion regimens. *Ann NY Acad Sci.* 1969;165:427–436.
7. Wolman IJ, Ortolani M. Some clinical features of Cooley's anemia patients as related to transfusion schedules. *Ann NY Acad Sci.* 1969;165:407–414.
8. Cavill I, Ricketts C, Jacobs A, Letsky E. Erythropoiesis and the effect of transfusion in homozygous ß-thalassemia. *N Engl J Med.* 1978;298(14):776–778.
9. Cazzola M, De Stefano P, Ponchio L, et al. Relationship between transfusion regimen and suppression of erythropoiesis in beta-thalassaemia major. *Br J Haematol.* 1995;89(3):473–478.
10. Propper RD, Button LN, Nathan DG. New approaches to the transfusion management of thalassemia. *Blood.* 1980;55(1):55–60.
11. Pootrakul P, Hungsprenges S, Fucharoen S, et al. Relation between erythropoiesis and bone metabolism in thalassemia. *N Engl J Med.* 1981;304:1470–1473.
12. Gabutti V, Piga A, Fortina P, Miniero R, Nicola P. Correlation between transfusion requirement, blood volume and haemoglobin level in homozygous beta-thalassaemia. *Acta Haematol.* 1980;64(2):103–108.
13. Gabutti V, Piga A, Nicola P, et al. Haemoglobin levels and blood requirement in thalassaemia. *Arch Dis Child.* 1982;57(2):156–158.
14. Propper RD, Button LN, Nathan DG. New approaches to the transfusion management of thalassemia. *Blood.* 1980;55(1):55–60.
15. Brunengo MA, Girot R [Transfusion requirements and mean annual hemoglobin level in thalassemia major]. *Nouv Rev Fr Hematol* 1986;28(5):309–313.
16. Rebulla P, Modell B. Transfusion requirements and effects in patients with thalassaemia major. *Cooleycare Programme. Lancet.* 1991;337(8736):277–280.
17. Cazzola M, Borgna-Pignatti C, Locatelli F, Ponchio L, Beguin Y, De Stefano P. A moderate transfusion regimen may reduce iron loading in beta-thalassemia major without producing excessive expansion of erythropoiesis. *Transfusion.* 1997;37(2):135–140.
18. Sprogoe-Jakobsen U, Saetre AM, Georgsen J. Preparation of white cell-reduced red cells by filtration: comparison of a beside filter and two blood bank filter systems. *Transfusion.* 1995;35:421–426.
19. Buchholz DH, AuBuchon JP, Snyder EL, et al. Removal of yersinia enterocolitica from AS-1 red cells. *Transfusion.* 1992;32:667–672.
20. Gregori L, McCombie N, Palmer D, et al. Effectiveness of leucoreduction for removal of infectivity of transmissible spongiform encephalopathies from blood. *Lancet.* 2004;364(9433):529–531.
21. Hogman CF. Preparation and preservation of red cells. *Vox Sanguinis.* 1998;74 (Suppl 2):177–187.
22. Mollison PL, Engelfriet CP, Contreras M. *Blood Transfusion in Clinical Medicine*, 10th ed. Oxford: Blackwell Science; 1997.
23. Levin TL, Sheth SS, Hurlet A, et al. MR marrow signs of iron overload in transfusion-dependent patients with sickle cell disease. *Pediatr Radiol.* 1995;25(8):614–619.
24. Rebulla P, Modell B. Transfusion requirements and effects in patients with thalassaemia major. *Lancet.* 1991;337:277–280.
25. Kumar RM, Khuranna A. Pregnancy outcome in women with beta-thalassemia major and HIV infection. *Eur J Obstet Gynecol Reprod Biol.* 1998;77(2):163–169.
26. Skordis N, Christou S, Koliou M, Pavlides N, Angastiniotis M. Fertility in female patients with thalassemia. *J Pediatr Endocrinol Metab.* 1998;11 (Suppl 3):935–943.
27. Butensky E, Pakbaz Z, Foote D, Walters MC, Vichinsky EP, Harmatz P. Treatment of hepatitis C virus infection in thalassemia. *Ann NY Acad Sci.* 2005;1054:290–299.
28. Telfer PT, Garson JA, Whitby K, et al. Combination therapy with interferon alpha and ribavirin for chronic hepatitis C virus infection in thalassemic patients. *Br J Haematol.* 1997;98:850–855.
29. Borgna-Pignatti C, Cappellini MD, De Stefano P, et al. Cardiac morbidity and mortality in deferoxamine- or deferiprone-treated patients with thalassemia major. *Blood.* 2006;107(9):3733–3737.
30. Piomelli S, Seaman C, Reibman J, et al. Separation of younger red cells with improved survival in vivo: an approach to chronic transfusion therapy. *Proc Natl Acad Sci USA.* 1978;75(7):3474–3478.
31. Bracey AW, Klein HG, Chambers S, Corash L. Ex vivo selective isolation of young red blood cells using the IBM-2991 cell washer. *Blood.* 1983;61(6):1068–1071.
32. Corash L, Klein H, Deisseroth A, et al. Selective isolation of young erythrocytes for transfusion support of thalassemia major patients. *Blood.* 1981;57(3):599–606.
33. Graziano JH, Piomelli S, Seaman C, et al. A simple technique for preparation of young red cells for transfusion from ordinary blood units. *Blood.* 1982;59:865–868.
34. Klein HG. Transfusions with young erythrocytes (neocytes) in sickle cell anemia. *Am J Pediatr Hematol Oncol.* 1982;4(2):162–165.
35. Cohen AR, Schmidt JM, Martin MB, Barnsley W, Schwartz E. Clinical trial of young red cell transfusions. *J Pediatr.* 1984;104(6):865–868.
36. Collins AF, Goncalves-Dias C, Haddad S, et al. Comparison of a transfusion preparation of newly formed red cells and

standard washed red cell transfusions in patients with homozygous beta-thalassemia. *Transfusion.* 1994;34(6):517–520.

37. Marcus RE, Wonke B, Bantock HM, et al. A prospective trial of young red cells in 48 patients with transfusion-dependent thalassaemia. *Br J Haematol.* 1985;60:153–159.
38. Spanos T, Ladis V, Palamidou F, et al. The impact of neocyte transfusion in the management of thalassaemia. *Vox Sang.* 1996;70(4):217–233.
39. Berdoukas VA, Kwan YL, Sansotta ML. A study on the value of red cell exchange transfusion in transfusion dependent anaemias. *Clin Lab Haematol.* 1986;8:209–20.
40. Berdoukas VA, Moore R. Automated red cell exchange transfusions in transfusion dependent anemias. In: 5th Annual Meeting of the Cooleycare Group, Athens, Greece; 1990.
41. Friedman DF, Jawad AF, Martin MB, Horiuchi K, Mitchell CF, Cohen AR. Erythrocytapheresis to reduce iron loading in thalassemia. *Blood.* 2003;102(11):121a.
42. Castilho L, Rios M, Bianco C, et al. DNA-based typing of blood groups for the management of multiply-transfused sickle cell disease patients. *Transfusion.* 2002;42(2):232–238.
43. Afenyi-Annan A, Willis MS, Konrad TR, Lottenberg R. Blood bank management of sickle cell patients at comprehensive sickle cell centers. *Transfusion.* 2007;47(11):2089–2097.
44. Osby M, Shulman IA. Phenotype matching of donor red blood cell units for nonalloimmunized sickle cell disease patients: a survey of 1182 North American laboratories. *Arch Pathol Lab Med.* 2005;129(2):190–193.
45. Castro O, Sandler SG, Houston-Yu P, Rana S. Predicting the effect of transfusing only phenotype-matched RBCs to patients with sickle cell disease: theoretical and practical implications. *Transfusion.* 2002;42(6):684–690.
46. Vichinsky EP, Luban NL, Wright E, et al. Prospective RBC phenotype matching in a stroke-prevention trial in sickle cell anemia: a multicenter transfusion trial. *Transfusion.* 2001;41(9):1086–1092.
47. Cox JV, Steane E, Cunningham G, Frenkel EP. Risk of alloimmunization and delayed hemolytic transfusion reactions in patients with sickle cell disease. *Arch Intern Med.* 1988;148(11):2485–2489.
48. Orlina AR, Unger PJ, Koshy M. Post-transfusion alloimmunization in patients with sickle cell disease. *Am J Hematol.* 1978;5:101–106.
49. Vichinsky EP, Earles A, Johnson RA, Hoag MS, Williams A, Lubin B. Alloimmunization in sickle cell anemia and transfusion of racially unmatched blood. *N Engl J Med.* 1990;322(23):1617–1621.
50. Ambruso DR, Githens JH, Alcorn R, et al. Experience with donors matched for minor blood group antigens in patients with sickle cell anemia who are receiving chronic transfusion therapy. *Transfusion.* 1987;27:94–98.
51. Luban NL. Variability in rates of alloimmunization in different groups of children with sickle cell disease: effect of ethnic background. *Am J Pediatr Hematol Oncol.* 1989;11(3):314–319.
52. Orlina AR, Sosler SD, Koshy M. Problems of chronic transfusion in sickle cell disease. *J Clin Apheresis.* 1991;6:234–240.
53. Sosler SD, Jilly BJ, Saporito C, Koshy M. A simple, practical model for reducing alloimmunization in patients with sickle cell disease. *Am J Hematol.* 1993;43:103–106.
54. Sesok-Pizzini DA, Friedman DF, Smith-Whitley K, Nance SJ. Transfusion support of patients with sickle cell disease at the Children's Hospital of Philadelphia. *Immunohematology.* 2006;22(3):121–125.
55. Isaak EJ, LeChien B, Lindsey T, Debaun MR. The Charles Drew program in Missouri: a description of a partnership among a blood center and several hospitals to address the care of patients with sickle cell disease. *Immunohematology.* 2006;22(3):112–116.
56. Jan K, Usami S, Smith JA. Effects of transfusion on rheological properties of blood in sickle cell anemia. *Transfusion.* 1982;22:17–20.
57. Schmalzer EA, Lee JO, Brown AK, Usami S, Chien S. Viscosity of mixtures of sickle and normal red cells at varying hematocrit levels. Implications for transfusion. *Transfusion.* 1987;27:228–233.
58. Adams DM, Ware RE, Schultz WH, Ross AK, Oldham KT, Kinney TR. Successful surgical outcome in children with sickle hemoglobinopathies: the Duke University experience. *J Pediatr Surg.* 1998;33(3):428–432.
59. Pegelow CH, Adams RJ, McKie V, et al. Risk of recurrent stroke in patients with sickle cell disease treated with erythrocyte transfusions. *J Pediatr.* 1995;126:896–899.
60. Cohen AR, Martin MB, Silber JH, Kim HC, Ohene-Frempong K, Schwartz E. A modified transfusion program for prevention of stroke in sickle cell disease. *Blood.* 1992;79(7):1657–1661.
61. Janes SL, Pocock M, Bishop E, Bevan DH. Automated red cell exchange in sickle cell disease. *Br J Haematol.* 1997;97:256–258.
62. Klein HG, Garner RJ, Miller DM, Rosen SL, Statham NJ, Winslow RM. Automated partial exchange transfusion in sickle cell anemia. *Transfusion.* 1980;20:578–584.
63. Adams DM, Schultz WH, Ware RE, Kinney TR. Erythrocytapheresis can reduce iron overload and reduce the need for chelation therapy in chronically transfused pediatric patients. *J Pediatr Hematol Oncol.* 1996;18:46–50.
64. Hilliard LM, Williams BF, Lounsbury AE, Howard TH. Erythrocytapheresis limits iron accumulation in chronically transfused sickle cell patients. *Am J Hematol.* 1998;59:28–35.
65. Kim HC, Dugan NP, Silber JH, et al. Erythrocytapheresis therapy to reduce iron overload in chronically transfused patients with sickle cell disease. *Blood.* 1994;83:1136–1142.
66. Smith-Whitley K, Zhao H, Hodinka RL, et al. Epidemiology of human parvovirus B19 in children with sickle cell disease. *Blood.* 2004;103(2):422–427.
67. Wierenga KJ, Serjeant BE, Serjeant GR. Cerebrovascular complications and parvovirus infection in homozygous sickle cell disease. *J Pediatr.* 2001;139(3):438–442.
68. Hulbert ML, Scothorn DJ, Panepinto JA, et al. Exchange blood transfusion compared with simple transfusion for first overt stroke is associated with a lower risk of subsequent stroke: a retrospective cohort study of 137 children with sickle cell anemia. *J Pediatr.* 2006;149(5):710–712.
69. Vichinsky EP, Neumayr LD, Earles AN, et al. Causes and outcomes of the acute chest syndrome in sickle cell disease. *National Acute Chest Syndrome Study Group. N Engl J Med.* 2000;342(25):1855–1865.
70. Davies SC, Luce PJ, Win AA, Riordan JF, Brozovic M. Acute chest syndrome in sickle-cell disease. *Lancet.* 1984;1(8367):36–38.

71. Emre U, Miller ST, Gutierez M, Steiner P, Rao SP, Rao M. Effect of transfusion in acute chest syndrome of sickle cell disease. *J Pediatr.* 1995;127(6):901–904.
72. Kleinman S, Thompson-Breton R, Breen D, Hurvitz C, Goldfinger D. Exchange red blood cell pheresis in a pediatric patient with severe complications of sickle cell anemia. *Transfusion.* 1981;21(4):443–446.
73. Mallouh AA, Asha A. Beneficial effect of blood transfusion in children with sickle cell chest syndrome. *Am J Dis Child.* 1988;142(2):178–182.
74. Wayne AS, Kevy SV, Nathan DG. Transfusion management of sickle cell disease. *Blood.* 1993;81(5):1109–1123.
75. Styles LA, Aarsman AJ, Vichinsky EP, Kuypers FA. Secretory phospholipase A(2) predicts impending acute chest syndrome in sickle cell disease. *Blood.* 2000;96(9):3276–3278.
76. Styles LA, Abboud M, Larkin S, Lo M, Kuypers FA. Transfusion prevents acute chest syndrome predicted by elevated secretory phospholipase A2. *Br J Haematol.* 2007;136(2):343–344.
77. Bhattacharyya N, Wayne AS, Kevy SV, Shamberger RC. Perioperative management for cholecystectomy in sickle cell disease. *J Pediatr Surg.* 1993;28:72–75.
78. Bischoff RJ, Williamson A, Dalali MJ, Rice JC, Kerstein MD. Assessment of the use of transfusion therapy perioperatively in patients with sickle cell hemoglobinopathies. *Ann Surg.* 1988;207:434–438.
79. Coker NJ, Milner PF. Elective surgery in patients with sickle cell anemia. *Arch Otolaryngol.* 1982;108:574–576.
80. Derkay CS, Bray G, Milmoe GJ, Grundfast KM. Adenotonsillectomy in children with sickle cell disease. *South Med J.* 1991;84:205–208.
81. Fullerton MW, Philippart AI, Lusher JM. Preoperative exchange transfusion in sickle cell disease. *J Pediatr Surg.* 1981;16:297–300.
82. Griffin TC, Buchanan GR. Elective surgery in children with sickle cell disease without preoperative blood transfusion. *J Pediatr Surg.* 1993;28:681–685.
83. Halvorson DJ, McKie V, McKie K, Ashmore PE, Porubsky ES. Sickle cell disease and tonsillectomy. Preoperative management and postoperative complications. *Arch Otolaryngol Head Neck Surg.* 1997;123(7):689–692.
84. Holzmann L, Finn H, Lichtman HC, Harmel MH. Anesthesia in patients with sickle cell disease: A review of 112 cases. *Anesth Analg.* 1969;48:566–572.
85. Homi J. General anaesthesia in sickle-cell disease. *Br Med J.* 1979;2(6192):739.
86. Janik J, Seeler RA. Perioperative management of children with sickle hemoglobinopaty. *J Pediatr Surg.* 1980;15:117–120.
87. Lanzkowsky P, Shende A, Karayalcin G, Kim YJ, Aballi AJ. Partial exchange transfusion in sickle cell anemia. Use in children with serious complications. *Am J Dis Child.* 1978;32(12):1206–1208.
88. Morrison JC, Whybrew WD, Bucovaz ET. Use of partial exchange transfusion perioperatively in patients with sickle hemoglobinopathies. *Am J Obstet Gynecol.* 1978;132:59–63.
89. Fu T, Corrigan NJ, Quinn CT, Rogers ZR, Buchanan GR. Minor elective surgical procedures using general anesthesia in children with sickle cell anemia without pre-operative blood transfusion. *Pediatr Blood Cancer.* 2005;45(1):43–47.
90. Oduro A, Searle JF. Anaesthesia in sickle cell states: a please for simplicity. *Br J Med.* 1972;4:596–598.
91. Serjeant GR. Chronic transfusion programmes in sickle cell disease: problem or panacea? *Br J Haematol.* 1997;97:253–255.
92. Leff DR, Kaura T, Agarwal T, Davies SC, Howard J, Chang AC. A nontransfusional perioperative management regimen for patients with sickle cell disease undergoing laparoscopic cholecystectomy. *Surg Endosc.* 2007;21(7):1117–1121.
93. Vichinsky EP, Haberkern CM, Neumayr L, et al. A comparison of conservative and aggressive transfusion regimens in the perioperative management of sickle cell disease. The Preoperative Transfusion in Sickle Cell Disease Study Group. *N Engl J Med.* 1995;333(4):206–213.
94. Haberkern CM, Neumayr LD, Orringer EP, et al. Cholecystectomy in sickle cell anemia patients: Perioperative outcome of 364 cases from the National Preoperative Transfusion Study. *Blood.* 1997;89(5):1533–1542.
95. Koshy M, Weiner SJ, Miller ST, et al. Surgery and anesthesia in sickle cell disease. Cooperative study of sickle cell diseases. *Blood.* 1995;86(10):3676–3684.
96. Neumayr L, Koshy M, Haberkern C, et al. Surgery in patients with hemoglobin SC disease. Preoperative Transfusion in Sickle Cell Disease Study Group. *Am J Hematol.* 1998;57(2):101–108.
97. Buck J, Casbard A, Llewelyn C, Johnson T, Davies S, Williamson L. Preoperative transfusion in sickle cell disease: a survey of practice in England. *Eur J Haematol.* 2005;75(1):14–21.
98. Brody JI, Goldsmith MH, Park SK, Soltys HD. Symptomatic crises of sickle cell anemia treated by limited exchange transfusion. *Ann Intern Med.* 1970;72:327–330.
99. Hassell KL, Eckman JR, Lane PA. Acute multi-organ failure syndrome: a potentially catastrophic complication of severe sickle cell pain episodes. *Am J Med.* 1994;96:155–162.
100. Baron M, Leiter E. The management of priapism in sickle cell anemia. *J Urol.* 1978;119:610–611.
101. Hamre MR, Harmaon EP, Kirkpatrick DV. Priapism as a complication of sickle cell disease. *J Urol.* 1991;145:1–5.
102. Kinney TR, Harris MB, Russell MO. Priapism in association with sickle hemoglobinopathies in children. *J Pediatr.* 1975;86:241–242.
103. McCarthy LJ, Vattuone J, Weidner J, et al. Do automated red cell exchanges relieve priapism in patients with sickle cell anemia? *Ther Apher* 2000;4(3):256–258.
104. Miller ST, Rao SP, Dunn EK, Glassberg KI. Priapism in children with sickle cell disease. *J Urol.* 1995;154:844–847.
105. Noe HN, Wilimas J, Jerkins GR. Surgical management of priapism in children with sickle cell anemia. *J Urol.* 1981;126:770–771.
106. Rifkind S, Waisman J, Thompson R, Goldfinger D. RBC exchange pheresis for priapism in sickle cell disease. *JAMA.* 1979;242:2317–2318.
107. Seeler RA. Intensive transfusion therapy for priapism in boys with sickle cell anemia. *J Urol.* 1973;110:360–361.
108. Tarry WF, Duckett JW, Snyder HM. Urological complications of sickle cell disease in a pediatric population. *J Urol.* 1987;138:592–594.
109. Adeyoju AB, Olujohungbe AB, Morris J, et al. Priapism in sickle-cell disease; incidence, risk factors and complications – an international multicentre study. *Br J Urol Int.* 2002;90(9):898–902.

110. Rackoff WR, Ohene-Frempong K, Month S. Neurological events after partial exchange transfusion for priapism in sickle cell disease. *J Pediatr.* 1992;120:882–885.

111. Royal JE, Seeler RA. Hypertension, convulsions, and cerebral haemorrhage in sickle-cell anaemia patients after blood transfusions. *Lancet.* 1978;2:1207.

112. Siegel JF, Rich MA, Brock WA. Association of sickle cell disease, priapism, exchange transfusion and neurological events: ASPEN syndrome. *J Urol.* 1993;150:1480–1482.

113. Lusher JM, Haghighat H, Khalifa AS. A prophylactic transfusion program for children with sickle cell anemia complicated by CNS infarction. *Am J Hematol.* 1976;1(2):265–273.

114. Russell MO, Goldberg HI, Reis L, et al. Transfusion therapy for cerebrovascular abnormalities in sickle cell disease. *J Pediatr.* 1976;88(3):382–387.

115. Sarnaik S, Soorya D, Kim J, Ravindranath Y, Lusher J. Periodic transfusions for sickle cell anemia and CNS infarction. *Am J Dis Child.* 1979;133(12):1254–1257.

116. Scothorn DJ, Price C, Schwartz D, et al. Risk of recurrent stroke in children with sickle cell disease receiving blood transfusion therapy for at least five years after initial stroke. *J Pediatr.* 2002;140(3):348–354.

117. Powars D, Wilson B, Imbus C, Pegelow C, Allen J. The natural history of stroke in sickle cell disease. *Am J Med.* 1978;65:461–471.

118. Wilimas J, Goff JR, Anderson HR, Jr., Langston JW, Thompson E. Efficacy of transfusion therapy for one to two years in patients with sickle cell disease and cerebrovascular accidents. *J Pediatr.* 1980;96(2):205–208.

119. de Montalembert M, Beauvais P, Bacir D, Galacgteros F, Girot R. Cerebrovascular accidents in sickle cell disease. Risk factors and blood transfusion influence. *Eur J Pediatr.* 1993;152:201–204.

120. Wang W, Kovnar EH, Tonkin IL, et al. High risk of recurrent stroke after discontinuance of five to twelve years of transfusion therapy in patients with sickle cell disease. *J Pediatr.* 1991;118:377–382.

121. Rana S, Houston PE, Surana N, Shalaby-Rana EI, Castro OL. Discontinuation of long-term transfusion therapy in patients with sickle cell disease and stroke. *J Pediatr.* 1997;131:757–760.

122. Miller ST, Jensen D, Rao SP. Less intensive long-term transfusion therapy for sickle cell anemia and cerebrovascular accident. *J Pediatr.* 1992;120:54–57.

123. Adams RJ, McKie VC, Hsu L, et al. Prevention of a first stroke by transfusions in children with sickle cell anemia and abnormal results on transcranial doppler ultrasonography. *N Engl J Med.* 1998;339:5–11.

124. Fullerton HJ, Adams RJ, Zhao S, Johnston SC. Declining stroke rates in Californian children with sickle cell disease. *Blood.* 2004;104(2):336–339.

125. Adams RJ, Brambilla D. Discontinuing prophylactic transfusions used to prevent stroke in sickle cell disease. *N Engl J Med.* 2005;353(26):2769–2778.

126. Pegelow CH, Macklin EA, Moser FG, et al. Longitudinal changes in brain magnetic resonance imaging findings in children with sickle cell disease. *Blood.* 2002;99:3014–3018.

127. Steen RG, Miles MA, Helton KJ, et al. Cognitive impairment in children with hemoglobin SS sickle cell disease: relationship to MR imaging findings and hematocrit. *AJNR Am J Neuroradiol* 2003;24(3):382–389.

128. Miller ST, Macklin EA, Pegelow CH, et al. Silent infarction as a risk factor for overt stroke in children with sickle cell anemia: a report from the Cooperative Study of Sickle Cell Disease. *J Pediatr.* 2001;139(3):385–390.

129. Berkelhammer LD, Williamson AL, Sanford SD, et al. Neurocognitive sequelae of pediatric sickle cell disease: a review of the literature. *Child Neuropsychol.* 2007;13(2):120–131.

130. Pegelow CH, Wang W, Granger S, et al. Silent infarcts in children with sickle cell anemia and abnormal cerebral artery velocity. *Arch Neurol.* 2001;58(12):2017–2021.

131. King AA, Noetzel M, White DA, McKinstry RC, Debaun MR. Blood transfusion therapy is feasible in a clinical trial setting in children with sickle cell disease and silent cerebral infarcts. *Pediatr Blood Cancer.* 2008;50(3):599–602.

132. Kirkham FJ, Lerner NB, Noetzel M, et al. Trials in sickle cell disease. *Pediatr Neurol.* 2006;34(6):450–458.

133. Koshy M, Burd L. Management of pregnancy in sickle cell syndromes. *Hematol Oncol Clin North Am.* 1991;5:585–596.

134. Charache S, Scott J, Niebyl J, Bonds D. Management of sickle cell disease in pregnant patients. *Obstet Gynecol.* 1980;55:407–410.

135. Cunningham FG, Pritchard JA, Mason R. Pregnancy and sickle cell hemoglobinopathies: results with and without prophylactic transfusions. *Obstet Gynecol.* 1983;62(4):419–424.

136. Howard RJ, Tuck SM, Pearson TC. Pregnancy in sickle cell disease in the UK: Results of a multicentre survey of the effect of prophylactic blood transfusion on maternal and fetal outcome. *Br J Obstet Gynaecol.* 1995;102:947–951.

137. Koshy M, Burd L, Wallace D, Moawad A, Baron J. Prophylactic red-cell transfusions in pregnant patients with sickle cell disease. A randomized cooperative study. *N Engl J Med.* 1988;319:1447–1452.

138. Morrison JC, Morrison FS, Floyd RC. Use of continuous flow erythrocytapheresis in pregnant patients with sickle cell disease. *J Clin Apheres.* 1991;6:224–229.

139. Morrison JC, Schneider JM, Whybrew WD. Prophylactic transfusions in pregnant patients with sickle hemoglobinopathies: Benefit versus risk. *Obstet Gynecol.* 1980;56:274–280.

140. Morrison JC, Wiser WL. The use of prophylactic partial exchange transfusion in pregnancies associated with sickle cell hemoglobinopathies. *Obstet Gynecol.* 1976a;48:516–520.

141. Tuck SM, Studd J. Sickle haemoglobin and pregnancy. *Br Med J (Clin Res Ed).* 1983;287(6399):1143–1144.

142. Gilli SC, De Paula EV, Biscaro FP, Marques JF, Costa FF, Saad ST. Third-trimester erythrocytapheresis in pregnant patients with sickle cell disease. *Int J Gynaecol Obstet.* 2007;96(1):8–11.

143. Tuck SM, James CE, Brewster EM. Prophylactic blood transfusion in maternal sickle cell syndromes. *Br J Obstet Gynaecol.* 1987;94:121–125.

144. Collins FS, Orringer EP. Pulmonary hypertension and cor pulmonale in the sickle hemoglobinopathies. *Am J Med.* 1982;73(6):814–821.

145. Powars D, Weidman JA, Odom-Maryon T, Niland JC, Johnson C. Sickle cell chronic lung disease: prior morbidity and the risk of pulmonary failure. *Medicine.* 1988;67(1):66–76.

146. Styles LA, Vichinsky E. Effects of a long-term transfusion regimen on sickle cell-related illnesses. *J Pediatr.* 1994;125:909–911.

147. Hankins J, Jeng M, Harris S, Li CS, Liu T, Wang W. Chronic transfusion therapy for children with sickle cell disease and

recurrent acute chest syndrome. *J Pediatr Hematol Oncol.* 2005;27(3):158–161.

148. Castro O, Gladwin MT. Pulmonary hypertension in sickle cell disease: mechanisms, diagnosis, and management. *Hematol Oncol Clin North Am* 2005;19(5):881–896, vii.
149. Machado RF, Gladwin MT. Chronic sickle cell lung disease: new insights into the diagnosis, pathogenesis and treatment of pulmonary hypertension. *Br J Haematol.* 2005;129(4):449–464.
150. Pearson HA, Gallagher D, Chilcote R, et al. Developmental pattern of splenic dysfunction in sickle cell disorders. *Pediatrics.* 1985;76(3):392–397.
151. Wright JG, Hambleton IR, Thomas PW, Duncan ND, Venugopal S, Serjeant GR. Postsplenectomy course in homozygous sickle cell disease. *J Pediatr.* 1999;134(3):304–309.
152. Kinney TR, Ware RE, Schultz WH, Filston HC. Long-term management of splenic sequestration in children with sickle cell disease. *J Pediatr.* 1990;117:194–199.
153. Platt OS, Thorington BD, Brambilla DJ, et al. Pain in sickle cell disease. *N Engl J Med.* 1991;325:11–16.
154. Miller ST, Rao SP. Acute chest syndrome, transfusion, and neurologic events in children with sickle cell disease. *Blood.* 2003;102(4):1556.
155. Ware RE, Zimmerman SA, Sylvestre PB, et al. Prevention of secondary stroke and resolution of transfusional iron overload in children with sickle cell anemia using hydroxyurea and phlebotomy. *J Pediatr.* 2004;145(3):346–352.
156. Larson PJ, Freidman DF, Reilly MP, et al. The presurgical management with erythrocytapheresis of a patient with a high-oxygen-affinity, unstable Hb variant (Hb Bryn Mawr). *Transfusion.* 1997;37:703–707.
157. Coles SM, Klein HG, Holland PV. Alloimmunization in two multitransfused patient populations. *Transfusion.* 1981;21(4):462–466.
158. Singer ST, Wu V, Mignacca R, Kuypers FA, Morel P, Vichinsky EP. Alloimmunization and erythrocyte autoimmunization in transfusion-dependent thalassemia patients of predominantly Asian descent. *Blood.* 2000;96(10):3369–3373.
159. Sirchia G, Zanella A, Parravicini A, Morelati F, Rebulla P, Masera G. Red cell alloantibodies in thalassemia major. Results of an Italian cooperative study. *Transfusion.* 1985;25(2):110–112.
160. Spanos T, Karageorga M, Ladis V, Peristeri J, Hatziliami A, Kattamis C. Red cell alloantibodies in patients with thalassemia. *Vox Sang.* 1990;58(1):50–55.
161. Ameen R, Al-Shemmari S, Al-Humood S, Chowdhury RI, Al-Eyaadi O, Al-Bashir A. RBC alloimmunization and autoimmunization among transfusion-dependent Arab thalassemia patients. *Transfusion.* 2003;43(11):1604–1610.
162. Bilwani F, Kakepoto GN, Adil SN, Usman M, Hassan F, Khurshid M. Frequency of irregular red cell alloantibodies in patients with thalassemia major: a bicenter study. *J Pak Med Assoc.* 2005;55(12):563–565.
163. Wang LY, Liang DC, Liu HC, et al. Alloimmunization among patients with transfusion-dependent thalassemia in Taiwan. *Transfusion Med.* 2006;16(3):200–203.
164. Michail-Merianou V, Pamphili-Panousopoulou L, Piperi-Lowes L, Pelegrinis E, Karaklis A. Alloimmunization to red cell antigens in thalassemia: comparative study of usual versus better-match transfusion programmes. *Vox Sang.* 1987;52 (1–2):95–98.
165. Olujohungbe A, Hambleton I, Stephens L, Serjeant B, Serjeant G. Red cell antibodies in patients with homozygous sickle cell disease: a comparison of patients in Jamaica and the United Kingdom. *Br J Haematol.* 2001;113:661–665.
166. Patten E, Patel SN, Soto B, Gayle RA. Prevalence of certain clinically significant alloantibodies in sickle cell disease patients. *Ann NY Acad Sci.* 1989;565:443–445.
167. Rosse WF, Gallagher D, Kinney TR. Transfusion and alloimmunization in sickle cell disease. *Blood.* 1990;76:1431–1437.
168. Sarnaik S, Schornack J, Lusher JM. The incidence of development of irregular red cell antibodies in patients with sickle cell anemia. *Transfusion.* 1986;26:249–252.
169. Aygun B, Padmanabhan S, Paley C, Chandrasekaran V. Clinical significance of RBC alloantibodies and autoantibodies in sickle cell patients who received transfusions. *Transfusion.* 2002;42:37–43.
170. Russo-Mancuso G, Sciotto A, Munda SE, Romano V, Schiliro G. Alloimmunization and autoimmunity in caucasian patients with sickle cell disease. *Intl J Pediatr Hematol Oncol.* 1998;5(6):443–447.
171. Castellino SM, Combs MR, Zimmerman SA, Issitt PD, Ware RE. Erythrocyte autoantibodies in paediatric patients with sickle cell disease receiving transfusion therapy: frequency, characteristics and significance. *Br J Haematol.* 1999;104:189–194.
172. Chaplin H, Jr., Zarkowsky HS. Combined sickle cell disease and autoimmune hemolytic anemia. *Arch Intern Med.* 1981;141(8):1091–1093.
173. King KE, Shirey RS, Lankiewicz MW, Young-Ramsaran J, Ness PM. Delayed hemolytic transfusion reactions in sickle cell disease: simultaneous destruction of recipients' red cells. *Transfusion.* 1997;37:376–381.
174. Petz LD, Calhoun L, Shulman IA, Johnson C, Herron RM. The sickle cell hemolytic transfusion reaction syndrome. *Transfusion.* 1997;37:382–392.
175. Syed SK, Sears DA, Werch JB, Udden MM, Milam JD. Delayed hemolytic transfusion reaction in sickle cell disease. *Am J Med Sci.* 1996;312:175–181.
176. Talano JA, Hillery CA, Gottschall JL, Baylerian DM, Scott JP. Delayed hemolytic transfusion reaction/hyperhemolysis syndrome in children with sickle cell disease. *Pediatrics.* 2003;111(6 Pt 1):e661–665.
177. Larson PJ, Lukas MB, Freidman DF, Manno CS. Delayed hemolytic transfusion reaction due to anti-Go(a), an antibody against the low-prevalence gonzales antigen. *Am J Hematol.* 1996;53(4):248–250.
178. Diamond WJ, Brown FL, Bitterman P, Klein HG, Davey RJ, Winslow PM. Delayed hemolytic reaction presenting as sickle cell crisis. *Ann Intern Med.* 1980;93:231–233.
179. Win N, Doughty H, Telfer P, Wild BJ, Pearson TC. Hyperhemolytic transfusion reaction in sickle cell disease. *Transfusion.* 2001;41(3):323–328.
180. Rebulla P, Mozzi F, Contino G, Locatelli E, Sirchia G. Antibody to hepatitis C virus in 1,305 Italian multiply transfused thalassaemics: a comparison of first and second generation tests. *Transfusion Med.* 1992;2:69–70.
181. Wonke B, Hoffbrand AV, Brown D, Dusheiko G. Antibody to hepatitis C virus in multiply transfused patients with thalassaemia major. *J Clin Pathol.* 1990;43:638–640.

182. Cunningham MJ, Macklin EA, Neufeld EJ, Cohen AR. Complications of beta-thalassemia major in North America. *Blood.* 2004;104(1):34–39.

183. DeVault KR, Friedman LS, Westerberg S. Hepatitis C in sickle cell anemia. *J Clin Gastroenterol.* 1994;18:206–209.

184. Hasan MF, Marsh F, Posner G, et al. Chronic hepatitis C in patients with sickle cell disease. *J Clin Gastroenterol.* 1996;91(6):1204–1206.

185. Clemente MG, Congia M, Lai ME, et al. Effect of iron overload on the response to recombinant interferon-alfa treatment in transfusion-dependent patients with thalassemia major and chronic hepatitis C. *J Pediatr.* 1994;125(1):123–128.

186. Di Marco V, Lo Iacono O, Camma C, et al. A randomized controlled trial of high-dose maintenance interferon therapy in chronic hepatitis C. *J Med Virol.* 1997;51(1):17–24.

187. Irshad M, Peter S. Spectrum of viral hepatitis in thalassemic children receiving multiple blood transfusions. *Indian J Gastroenterol.* 2002;21(5):183–184.

188. Mollah AH, Siddiqui MA, Anwar KS, et al. Seroprevalence of common transfusion-transmitted infections among blood donors in Bangladesh. *Public Health.* 2004;118(4):299–302.

189. Singh NP, Mandal SK, Thakur A, et al. Efficacy of GM-CSF as an adjuvant to hepatitis B vaccination in patients with chronic renal failure–results of a prospective, randomized trial. *Renal Fail.* 2003;25(2):255–266.

190. Robert-Guroff M, Giardina PJ, Robey WG, et al. HTLV-III neutralizing antibody development in transfusion-dependent seropositive patients with beta-thalassemia. *J Immunol.* 1987;138(11):3731–3736.

191. Lefrere JJ, Girot R. HIV infection in polytransfused thalassemic patients. *Lancet.* 1987;2:686. (Letter)

192. Lefrere JJ, Girot R. Risk of HIV infection in polytransfused thalassemic patients. *Lancet.* 1989;2:813. (Letter)

193. Mozzi F, Rebulla P, Lillo F, et al. HIV and HTLV infections in 1305 transfusion-dependent thalassemis in Italy. *AIDS.* 1992;6(5):505–508.

194. Stramer SL. Current risks of transfusion-transmitted agents: a review. *Arch Pathol Lab Med.* 2007;131(5):702–707.

195. Tshilolo LM, Mukendi RK, Wembonyama SO. Blood transfusion rate in Congolese patients with sickle cell anemia. *Indian J Pediatr.* 2007;74(8):735–738.

196. Salhi Y, Costagliola D, Rebulla P, et al. Serum ferritin, desferrioxamine, and evolution of HIV-1 infection in thalassemic patients. *J AIDS Hum Retrovirol.* 1998;18(5):473–478.

197. Costagliola DG, de Montalembert M, Lefrere JJ, et al. Dose of desferrioxamine and evolution of HIV-1 infection in thalassaemic patients. *Br J Haematol.* 1994;87(4):849–852.

198. Georgiou NA, Van Der Bruggen T, Oudshoorn M, Nottet HS, Marx JJ, van Asbeck BS. Inhibition of human immunodeficiency virus type 1 replication in human mononuclear blood cells by the iron chelators deferoxamine, deferiprone, and bleomycin. *J Infect Dis.* 2000;181(2):484–490.

199. Georgiou NA, Van Der Bruggen T, Oudshoorn M, Hider RC, Marx JJ, van Asbeck BS. Human immunodeficiency virus type 1 replication inhibition by the bidentate iron chelators CP502 and CP511 is caused by proliferation inhibition and the onset of apoptosis. *Eur J Clin Invest* 2002;32 (Suppl 1):91–96.

200. Menitove JE. Transfusion-transmitted infections: update. *Semin Hematol.* 1996;33:290–301.

201. Cohen A, Markenson AL, Schwartz E. Transfusion requirements and splenectomy in thalassemia major. *J Pediatr.* 1980;97(1):100–102.

202. Campbell PJ, Olatunji PO, Ryan KE, Davies SC. Splenic regrowth in sickle cell anaemia following hypertransfusion. *Br J Haematol.* 1997;96:77–79.

203. Cohen AR, Buchanan GR, Martin M, Ohene-Frempong K. Increased blood requirements during long-term transfusion therapy for sickle cell disease. *J Pediatr.* 1991;118(3):405–407.

204. Wasi P, Na-Nakorn S, Pootrakul P, Sonakul D, Piankijagum A, Pacharee P. A syndrome of hypertension, convulsion, and cerebral haemorrhage in thalassaemic patients after multiple blood-transfusions. *Lancet.* 1978;2(8090):602–604.

205. Yetgin S, Hicsonmez G. Hypertension, convulsions and purpuric skin lesions after blood-transfusions. *Lancet.* 1979;1:610. (Letter)

206. Warth JA. Hypertension and a seizure following transfusion in an adult with sickle cell anemia. *Arch Intern Med.* 1984;144:607–608.

207. Sonakul D, Fucharoen S. Brain pathology in 6 fatal cases of post-transfusion hypertension, convulsion and cerebral hemorrhage syndrome. *SE Asian J Trop Med Public Health.* 1992;23(Supplement 2):116–119.

208. Henderson JN, Noetzel MJ, McKinstry RC, White DA, Armstrong M, DeBaun MR. Reversible posterior leukoencephalopathy syndrome and silent cerebral infarcts are associated with severe acute chest syndrome in children with sickle cell disease. *Blood.* 2003;101(2):415–419.

209. Jacobs A. The pathology of iron overload. *Iron in Biochemistry and Medicine.* London: Academic Press; 1974.

210. Bothwell T, Charlton RW, Cook JD, Finch CA. *Iron Metabolism in Man.* Oxford: Blackwell; 1979.

211. Modell B. Total management of thalassaemia major. *Arch Dis Childhood.* 1977;52:485–500.

212. Cohen AR, Glimm E, Porter JB. Effect of transfusional iron intake on response to chelation therapy in β-thalassemia major. *Blood.* 2008;111(2):583–587.

213. Porter J, Galanello R, Saglio G, et al. Relative response of patients with myelodysplastic syndromes and other transfusion-dependent anaemias to deferasirox (ICL670): a 1-yr prospective study. *Eur J Haematol.* 2008;80(2):168–176.

214. Graziano JH, Piomelli S, Hilgartner M, et al. Chelation therapy in beta-thalassemia major. III. The role of splenectomy in achieving iron balance. *J Pediatr.* 1981;99(5):695–699.

215. O'Brien RT, Pearson HA, Spencer RP. Transfusion-induced decrease in spleen size in thalassemia major: documentation by radioisotopic scan. *J Pediatr.* 1972;81(1):105–107.

216. Pippard M, Weatherall D. Iron absorption in iron-loading anaemias. *Haematologica.* 1984;17:407–414.

217. Pippard MJ, Callender ST, Warner GT, Weatherall DJ. Iron absorption and loading in beta-thalassaemia intermedia. *Lancet.* 1979;2(8147):819–821.

218. Pootrakul P, Kitcharoen K, Yansukon P, et al. The effect of erythroid hyperplasia on iron balance. *Blood.* 1988;71(4):1124–1129.

219. Gordeuk VR, Bacon BR, Brittenham GM. Iron overload: causes and consequences. *Annu Rev Nutr.* 1987;7:485–508.

220. O'Brien RT. Iron burden in sickle cell anemia. *J Pediatr.* 1978;92(4):579–588.

221. Vichinsky E, Kleman K, Embury S, Lubin B. The diagnosis of iron deficiency anemia in sickle cell disease. *Blood.* 1981;58(5):963–968.

222. Davies S, Hentroth JS, Brozovic M. Effect of blood transfusion on iron status in sickle cell anaemia. *Clin Lab Haematol.* 1984;6:17–22.

223. Rao KRP, Ashok RP, McGinnis P, Patel MK. Iron stores in adults with sickle cell anemia. *J Lab Clin Med.* 1984;103:792–797.
224. Porter JB, Huehns ER. Transfusion and exchange transfusion in sickle cell anaemias, with particular reference to iron metabolism. *Acta Haematol.* 1987;78(2–3):198–205.
225. Vichinsky E, Onyekwere O, Porter J, et al. A randomised comparison of deferasirox versus deferoxamine for the treatment of transfusional iron overload in sickle cell disease. *Br J Haematol.* 2007;136(3):501–508.
226. Cavill I. Internal regulation of iron absorption. *Nature.* 1975;256:328–329.
227. Pippard MJ, Weatherall DJ. Iron absorption in non-transfused iron loading anaemias: prediction of risk for iron loading, and response to iron chelation treatment, in beta thalassaemia intermedia and congenital sideroblastic anaemias. *Haematologia.* 1984;17(1):17–24.
228. Zanella A, Berzuini A, Colombo MB, et al. Iron status in red cell pyruvate kinase deficiency: study of Italian cases. *Br J Haematol.* 1993;83(3):485–490.
229. Modell B, Mathews R. Thalassaemia in Britain and Australia. *Birth Defects Orgin Art Series.* 1976;12:13–29.
230. Risdon RA, Barry M, Flynn DM. Transfusional iron overload: the relationship between tissue iron concentration and hepatic fibrosis in thalassaemia. *J Pathol.* 1975;116(2):83–95.
231. Oudit GY, Sun H, Trivieri MG, et al. L-type Ca2+ channels provide a major pathway for iron entry into cardiomyocytes in iron-overload cardiomyopathy. *Nat Med.* 2003;9(9):1187–1194.
232. Nemeth E, Tuttle MS, Powelson J, et al. Hepcidin regulates cellular iron efflux by binding to ferroportin and inducing its internalization. *Science.* 2004;306(5704):2090–2093.
233. Lin L, Valore EV, Nemeth E, Goodnough JB, Gabayan V, Ganz T. Iron transferrin regulates hepcidin synthesis in primary hepatocyte culture through hemojuvelin and BMP2/4. *Blood.* 2007;110(6):2182–2189.
234. Origa R, Galanello R, Ganz T, et al. Liver iron concentrations and urinary hepcidin in beta-thalassemia. *Haematologica.* 2007;92(5):583–588.
235. Kattamis A, Papassotiriou I, Palaiologou D, et al. The effects of erythropoetic activity and iron burden on hepcidin expression in patients with thalassemia major. *Haematologica.* 2006;91(6):809–812.
236. Tanno T, Bhanu NV, Oneal PA, et al. High levels of GDF15 in thalassemia suppress expression of the iron regulatory protein hepcidin. *Nat Med.* 2007;13(9):1096–1101.
237. Shah FT. The relationship between non transferrin bound iron and iron overload in thalassaemia and sickle syndromes. MD Thesis, University of London, 2008.
238. Jensen PD, Jensen FT, Christensen T, Nielsen JL, Ellegaard J. Relationship between hepatocellular injury and transfusional iron overload prior to and during iron chelation with desferrioxamine: a study in adult patients with acquired anemias. *Blood.* 2003;101(1):91–96.
239. Angelucci E, Muretto P, Nicolucci A, et al. Effects of iron overload and hepatitis C virus positivity in determining progression of liver fibrosis in thalassemia following bone marrow transplantation. *Blood.* 2002;100(1):17–21.
240. Buja LM, Roberts WC. Iron in the heart. Etiology and clinical significance. *Am J Med.* 1971;51(2):209–221.
241. Jensen PD, Jensen FT, Christensen T, Eiskjaer H, Baandrup U, Nielsen JL. Evaluation of myocardial iron by magnetic resonance imaging during iron chelation therapy with deferrioxamine: indication of close relation between myocardial iron content and chelatable iron pool. *Blood.* 2003;101(11):4632–4639.
242. Fitchett DH, Coltart DJ, Littler WA, et al. Cardiac involvement in secondary haemochromatosis: a catheter biopsy study and analysis of myocardium. *Cardiovasc Res.* 1980;14(12):719–724.
243. Barosi G, Arbustini E, Gavazzi A, Grasso M, Pucci A. Myocardial iron grading by endomyocardial biopsy. A clinicopathologic study on iron overloaded patients. *Eur J Haematol.* 1989;42(4):382–388.
244. Anderson LJ, Holden S, Davis B, et al. Cardiovascular T2-star (T2*) magnetic resonance for the early diagnosis of myocardial iron overload. *Eur Heart J.* 2001;22(23):2171–2179.
245. Anderson LJ, Westwood MA, Holden S, et al. Myocardial iron clearance during reversal of siderotic cardiomyopathy with intravenous desferrioxamine: a prospective study using T2* cardiovascular magnetic resonance. *Br J Haematol.* 2004;127(3):348–355.
246. Porter JB. Concepts and goals in the management of transfusional iron overload. *Am J Hematol.* 2007;82(12 Suppl):1136–1139.
247. Wood JC, Tyszka JM, Carson S, Nelson MD, Coates TD. Myocardial iron loading in transfusion-dependent thalassemia and sickle cell disease. *Blood.* 2004;103(5):1934–1936.
248. Shah F, Westwood MA, Evans PJ, Porter JB. Discordance in MRI assessment of iron distribution and plasma NTBI between transfusionally iron loaded adults with sickle cell and thalassaemia syndromes. *Blood.* 2002;100:468a.
249. Hershko C, Graham G, Bates G, Rachmilewitz E. Non-specific serum iron in thalassaemia; an abnormal serum fraction of potential toxicity. *Br J Haematol.* 1978;40:255–263.
250. Breuer W, Epsztejn S, Cabantchik ZI. Iron acquired from transferrin by k562 cells is delivered into a cytoplasmic pool of chelatable iron (II). *J Biol Chem.* 1995;270:24209–24215.
251. Grootveld M, Bell JD, Halliwell B, Aruoma OI, Bomford A, Sadler PJ. Non-transferrin-bound iron in plasma or serum from patients with idiopathic hemochromatosis. Characterization by high performance liquid chromatography and nuclear magnetic resonance spectroscopy. *J Biol Chem.* 1989;264(8):4417–4422.
252. Evans RW, Rafique R, Zarea A, et al. Nature of non-transferrin-bound iron: studies on iron citrate complexes and thalassemic sera. *J Biol Inorg Chem.* 2008;13(1):57–74.
253. Brissot P, Wright TL, Ma WL, Weisiger RA. Efficient clearance of non-transferrin-bound iron by rat liver. Implications for hepatic iron loading in iron overload states. *J Clin Invest.* 1985;76(4):1463–1470.
254. Link G, Pinson A, Kahane I, Hershko C. Iron loading modifies the fatty acid composition of cultured rat myocardial cells and liposomal vesicles: effect of ascorbate and alpha-tocopherol on myocardial lipid peroxidation. *J Lab Clin Med.* 1989;114:243–249.
255. Gutteridge J, Rowley D, Griffiths E, Halliwell B. Low molecular weight iron complexes and oxygen radical reactions in idiopathic haemochromatosis. *Clin Sci.* 1985;68:463–467.
256. De Luca C, Filosa A, Grandinetti M, Maggio F, Lamba M, Passi S. Blood antioxidant status and urinary levels of catecholamine metabolites in beta-thalassemia. *Free Radic Res.* 1999;30(6):453–462.

257. Link G, Pinson A, Hershko C. Iron loading of cultured cardiac myocytes modifies sarcolemmal structure and increases lysosomal fragility. *J Lab Clin Med.* 1993;121(1):127–134.
258. Marx JJM, van Asbeck BS. Use of chelators in preventing hydroxyl radical damage: adult respiratory distress syndrome as an experimental model for the treatment of oxygen-radical-mediated tissue damage. *Acta Haematol.* 1996;95:49–62.
259. Gutteridge J, Halliwell B. Iron toxicity and oxygen radicals. *Bailliere Clin Haematol.* 1989;2:195–256.
260. Kornbrust DJ, Mavis RD. Microsomal lipid peroxidation. 1. Characterisation of the role of iron and NADPH. *Mol Pharmacol.* 1980;17:400–407.
261. Bacon BR, Tavill AS, Brittenham GM, Park CH, Recknagel RO. Hepatic lipid peroxidation in vivo in rats with chronic iron overload. *J Clin Invest.* 1983;71(3):429–439.
262. Myers BM, Prendergast FG, Holman R, Kuntz SM, LaRusso NF. Alterations in the structure, physicochemical properties, and pH of hepatocyte lysosomes in experimental iron overload. *J Clin Invest.* 1991;88(4):1207–1215.
263. Le Sage GD, Kost LJ, Barham SS, LaRusso NF. Biliary excretion of iron from hepatocyte lysosomes in the rat: a major excretory pathway in experimental iron overload. *J Clin Invest.* 1986;77:90–97.
264. Link G, Saada A, Pinson A, Konijn AM, Hershko C. Mitochondrial respiratory enzymes are a major target of iron toxicity in rat heart cells. *J Lab Clin Med.* 1998;131(5):466–474.
265. Zhao M, Laissue JA, Zimmermann A. Hepatocyte apoptosis in hepatic iron overload diseases. *Histol Histopathol.* 1997;12(2):367–374.
266. Jacob AK, Hotchkiss RS, Swanson PE, Tinsley KW, Karl IE, Buchman TG. Injection of iron compounds followed by induction of the stress response causes tissue injury and apoptosis. *Shock.* 2000;14(4):460–464.
267. Antunes F, Cadenas E, Brunk UT. Apoptosis induced by exposure to a low steady-state concentration of H2O2 is a consequence of lysosomal rupture. *Biochem J.* 2001;356(Pt 2):549–555.
268. Houglum K, Filip M, Witztum JL, Chojkier M. Malondialdehyde and 4-hydroxynonenal protein adducts in plasma and liver of rats with iron overload. *J Clin Invest.* 1990; 86(6):1991–1998.
269. Parola M, Pinzani A, Casini E, et al. Stimulation of lipid peroxidation or 4-hydroxynonenal treatment increased procollagen (I) gene expression in human fat storing cells. *J Biol Chem.* 1993;264:16957–16962.
270. Bissell DM, Wang SS, Jarnagin WR, Roll FJ. Cell specific expression of transforming growth factor-ß in the rat liver. *J Clin Invest.* 1995;96:447–455.
271. Tsakamota H, Horne W, Kamimura S, Niemela O, Parkkila S, Yia-Herttuala S. Experimantal liver cirrhosis induced by alcohol and iron. *J Clin Invest.* 1995;96:620–630.
272. Houglum K, Ramm GA, Crawford DH, Witztum JL, Powell LW, Chojkier M. Excess iron induces hepatic oxidative stress and transforming growth factor beta1 in genetic hemochromatosis. *Hepatology.* 1997;26(3):605–610.
273. Eaton JW, Qian M. Molecular bases of cellular iron toxicity. *Free Radic Biol Med* 2002;32(9):833–840.
274. Wolfe L, Olivieri N, Sallan D, et al. Prevention of cardiac disease by subcutaneous deferoxamine in patients with thalassemia major. *N Engl J Med.* 1985;312(25):1600–1603.
275. Zurlo MG, De Stefano P, Borgna-Pignatti C, et al. Survival and causes of death in thalassaemia major. *Lancet.* 1989;2(8653):27–30.
276. Brittenham GM, Griffith PM, Nienhuis AW, et al. Efficacy of deferoxamine in preventing complications of iron overload in patients with thalassemia major [see comments]. *N Engl J Med.* 1994;331(9):567–573.
277. Borgna-Pignatti C, Rugolotto S, De Stefano P, et al. Survival and complications in patients with thalassemia major treated with transfusion and deferoxamine. *Haematologica.* 2004;89(10):1187–1193.
278. Angelucci E, Baronciani D, Lucarelli G, et al. Liver iron overload and liver fibrosis in thalassemia. *Bone Marrow Transplant.* 1993;12(Suppl 1):29–31.
279. Davis B, O'Sullivan C, Porter J. Value of LVEF monitoring in the long-term management of beta-thalassaemia. 8th International Conference on Thalassemia and the Hemoglobinopathies (Athens) 2001.Abstract 056: 147.
280. Olivieri NF, Nathan DG, MacMillan JH, et al. Survival in medically treated patients with homozygous beta-thalassemia. *N Engl J Med.* 1994;331(9):574–578.
281. Gabutti V, Piga A. Results of long-term iron-chelating therapy. *Acta Haematol.* 1996;95(1):26–36.
282. Telfer PT, Prestcott E, Holden S, Walker M, Hoffbrand AV, Wonke B. Hepatic iron concentration combined with long-term monitoring of serum ferritin to predict complications of iron overload in thalassaemia major. *Br J Haematol.* 2000;110(4):971–977.
283. Ladis V, Chouliaras G, Berdousi H, Kanavakis E, Kattamis C. Longitudinal study of survival and causes of death in patients with thalassemia major in Greece. *Ann NY Acad Sci.* 2005;1054:445–450.
284. Westwood MA, Wonke B, Maceira AM, et al. Left ventricular diastolic function compared with T2* cardiovascular magnetic resonance for early detection of myocardial iron overload in thalassemia major. *J Magn Reson Imaging.* 2005;22(2):229–233.
285. Borgna-Pignatti C, Rugolotto S, De Stefano P, et al. Survival and disease complications in thalassemia major. *Ann NY Acad Sci.* 1998;850:227–231.
286. Chatterjee R, Katz M, Cox TF, Porter JB. Prospective study of the hypothalamic-pituitary axis in thalassaemic patients who developed secondary amenorrhoea. *Clin Endocrinol.*1993;39(3):287–296.
287. Chatterjee R, Wonke B, Porter JB, Katz M. Correction of primary and secondary amenorrhoea and induction of ovulation by pulsatile infusion of gonadotrophin releasing hormone (GnRH) in patients with beta thalassaemia major. In: Beuzard Y, Lubin B, Rosa J, eds. *Sickle Cell Disease and Thalassaemia: New Trends in Therapy. Colloq Inserm* 1995;234:451–455.
288. Landau H, Matoth I, Landau-Cordova Z, Golfarb A, Rachmilewitz EA, Glaser B. Cross-sectional and longditudinal study of the pituitary-thyroid axis in patients with thalassaemia major. *Clin Endocrinol.* 1993;38:55–61.
289. Sklar CA, Lew LQ, Yoon DJ, David R. Adrenal function in thalassemia major following long-term treatment with multiple transusions and chelation therapy. Evidence for dissociation of cortisol and adrenal androgen sectretion. *Am J Dis Child.*1987;141:327–330.

290. Pinna AD, Argiolu F, Marongiu L, Pinna DC. Indications and results for splenectomy for beta thalassemia in two hundred and twenty-one pediatric patients. *Surg Gynecol Obstet.* 1988;167(2):109–113.
291. Barry DMJ, Reeve AN. Increased incidence of gram-negative neonatal sepsis with intramuscular iron administration. *Pediatrics.* 1977;60:908–912.
292. Hwang CF, Lee CY, Lee PI, et al. Pyogenic liver abscess in beta-thalassemia major–report of two cases. *Chung Hua Min Kuo Hsiao Erh Ko I Hsueh Hui Tsa Chih.* 1994;35(5):466–467.
293. Wanachiwanawin W. Infections in E-beta thalassemia. *J Pediatr Hematol Oncol.* 2000;22(6):581–587.
294. Li CK, Shing MM, Chik KW, Lee V, Yuen PM. Klebsiella pneumoniae meningitis in thalassemia major patients. *Pediatr Hematol Oncol.* 2001;18(3):229–232.
295. Skoutelis AT, Lianou E, Papavassiliou T, Karamerou A, Politi K, Bassaris HP. Defective phagocytic and bactericidal function of polymorphonuclear leucocytes in patients with beta-thalassaemia major. *J Infect.* 1984;8(2):118–122.
296. Ballart IJ, Estevez ME, Sen L, et al. Progressive dysfunction of monocytes associated with iron overload and age in patients with thalassemia major. *Blood.* 1986;67(1):105–109.
297. Kutukculer N, Kutlu O, Nisli G, Oztop S, Cetingul N, Caglayan S. Assessment of neutrophil chemotaxis and random migration in children with thalassemia major. *Pediatr Hematol Oncol.* 1996;13(3):239–245.
298. Robins-Browne R, Prpic J. Effects of iron and desferrioxamine on infections with Yersinia Enterocolitica. *Infect Immun.* 1985;47:774–779.
299. Brownell A, Lowson S, Brozovic M. Serum ferritin concentration in sickle crisis. *J Clin Pathol.* 1986;39:253–255.
300. Harmatz P, Heyman MB, Cunningham J, et al. Effects of red blood cell transfusion on resting energy expenditure in adolescents with sickle cell anemia. *J Pediatr Gastroenterol Nutr.* 1999;29(2):127–131.
301. Brittenham GM, Cohen AR, McLaren CE, et al. Hepatic iron stores and plasma ferritin concentration in patients with sickle cell anemia and thalassemia major. *Am J Hematol.* 1993;42(1):81–85.
302. Comer GM, Ozick LA, Sachdev RK, et al. Transfusion-related chronic liver disease in sickle cell anemia. *Am J Gastroenterol.* 1991;86(9):1232–1234.
303. Harmatz P, Butensky E, Quirolo K, et al. Severity of iron overload in patients with sickle cell disease receiving chronic red blood cell transfusion therapy. *Blood.* 2000;96(1):76–79.
304. Olivieri NF. Progression of iron overload in sickle cell disease. *Semin Hematol.* 2001;38(1 Suppl 1):57–62.
305. Olivieri NF, Saxon BR, Nisbet-Brown E, et al. Quantitive assessment of tissue iron in patients with sickle cell disease. In: Proceedings of 9th International Conference on Oral Iron Chelation. Hamburg, Germany; 1999:55.
306. Darbari DS, Kple-Faget P, Kwagyan J, Rana S, Gordeuk VR, Castro O. Circumstances of death in adult sickle cell disease patients. *Am J Hematol.* 2006;81(11):858–863.
307. Westwood MA, Shah F, Anderson LJ, et al. Myocardial tissue characterization and the role of chronic anemia in sickle cell cardiomyopathy. *J Magn Reson Imaging.* 2007;26(3):564–568.
308. Vichinsky E, Butensky E, Fung E, et al. Comparison of organ dysfunction in transfused patients with SCD or beta thalassemia. *Am J Hematol.* 2005;80(1):70–74.
309. Fung EB, Harmatz PR, Lee PD, et al. Increased prevalence of iron-overload associated endocrinopathy in thalassaemia versus sickle-cell disease. *Br J Haematol.* 2006;135(4):574–582.
310. Phillips G, Becker B, Keller VA, Hartman J. Hypothyroidism in adults with sickle cell anemia. *Am J Med.* 1992;92(5):567–570.
311. Siegelman ES, Outwater E, Hanau CA, et al. Abdominal iron distribution in sickle cell disease: MR findings in transfusion and nontransfusion dependent patients. *J Comput Assist Tomog.* 1994; 18:63–67.
312. Walter PB, Fung EB, Killilea DW, et al. Oxidative stress and inflammation in iron-overloaded patients with beta-thalassaemia or sickle cell disease. *Br J Haematol.* 2006;135(2):254–263.
313. Schafer AI, Cheron RG, Dluhy R, et al. Clinical consequences of acquired transfusional iron overload in adults. *N Engl J Med.* 1981;304(6):319–324.
314. Malcovati L, Porta MG, Pascutto C, et al. Prognostic factors and life expectancy in myelodysplastic syndromes classified according to WHO criteria: a basis for clinical decision making. *J Clin Oncol.* 2005;23(30):7594–7603.
315. Novel treatment options for transfusional iron overload in patients with myelodysplastic syndromes. *Leuk Res.* 2007; Suppl 3: S16–22.
316. Cazzola M, Malcovati L. Myelodysplastic syndromes–coping with ineffective hematopoiesis. *N Engl J Med.* 2005;352(6):536–538.
317. Malcovati L, Della Porta MG, Cazzola M. Predicting survival and leukemic evolution in patients with myelodysplastic syndrome. *Haematologica.* 2006;91(12):1588–1590.
318. Angelucci E, Brittenham GM, McLaren CE, et al. Hepatic iron concentration and total body iron stores in thalassemia major. *N Engl J Med.* 2000;343(5):327–331.
319. Cartwright GE, Edwards CQ, Kravitz K, et al. Hereditary hemochromatosis. Phenotypic expression of the disease. *N Engl J Med.* 1979;301(4):175–179.
320. Porter JB, Davis BA. Monitoring chelation therapy to achieve optimal outcome in the treatment of thalassaemia. *Best Pract Res Clin Haematol.* 2002;15(2):329–368.
321. Angelucci E, Baronciani D, Lucarelli G, et al. Needle liver biopsy in thalassaemia: analyses of diagnostic accuracy and safety in 1184 consecutive biopsies. *Br J Haematol.* 1995;89(4):757–761.
322. Ambu R, Crisponi G, Sciot R, et al. Uneven hepatic iron and phosphorus distribution in beta-thalassemia. *J Hepatol.* 1995;23(5):544–549.
323. Villeneuve JP, Bilodeau M, Lepage R, Cote J, Lefebvre M. Variability in hepatic iron concentration measurement from needle- biopsy specimens. *J Hepatol.* 1996;25(2):172–177.
324. Barry M, Sherlock S. Measurement of liver-iron concentration in needle biopsy specimens. *Lancet.* 1971;1:100–103.
325. Barry M, Flynn D, Letsky E, Risdon R. Long term chelation therapy in thalassaemia: effect on liver iron concentration, liver histology and clinical progress. *Br Med J.* 1974;2:16–20.
326. Ropert-Bouchet M, Turlin B, Graham G, et al. Drying methods affect the wet dry ratio of liver tissue samples and impact on iron content measurements. *Bioiron* 2005:107: 274 (Abstract).
327. Brittenham GM, Farrell DE, Harris JW, et al. Magnetic-susceptibility measurement of human iron stores. *N Engl J Med.* 1982;307(27):1671–1675.

328. Nielsen P, Fischer R, Engelhardt R, Tondury P, Gabbe EE, Janka GE. Liver iron stores in patients with secondary haemosiderosis under iron chelation therapy with deferoxamine or deferiprone. *Br J Haematol.* 1995;91:827–833.
329. Piga A, R F, T SP, et al. Comparison of LIC obtained from biopsy, BLS and R2-MRI in iron overloaded patients with beta-thalassemia, treated with deferasirox (Exjade®, ICL670). *Blood.* 2005;106(11): 2689a.
330. St Pierre TG, Clark PR, Chua-anusorn W, et al. Noninvasive measurement and imaging of liver iron concentrations using proton magnetic resonance. *Blood.* 2005;105(2):855–861.
331. Gandon Y, Olivie D, Guyader D, et al. Non-invasive assessment of hepatic iron stores by MRI. *Lancet.* 2004;363(9406):357–362.
332. Worwood M, Cragg SJ, Jacobs A, McLaren C, Ricketts C, Economidou J. Binding of serum ferritin to concanavalin A: patients with homozygous beta thalassaemia and transfusional iron overload. *Br J Haematol.* 1980;46(3):409–416.
333. Davis BA, Porter JB. Long-term outcome of continuous 24-hour deferoxamine infusion via indwelling intravenous catheters in high-risk beta-thalassemia. *Blood.* 2000;95(4):1229–1236.
334. Fischer R, Longo F, Nielsen P, Engelhardt R, Hider RC, Piga A. Monitoring long-term efficacy of iron chelation therapy by deferiprone and desferrioxamine in patients with beta-thalassaemia major: application of SQUID biomagnetic liver susceptometry. *Br J Haematol.* 2003;121(6):938–948.
335. Walters GO, Miller R, Worwood M. Serum ferritin concentration and iron stores in normal subjects. *J Clin Pathol.* 1973;26:770–2.
336. Beamish MR, Walker R, Miller F, et al. Transferrin iron, chelatable iron and ferritin in idiopathic haemochromatosis. *Br J Haematol.* 1974;27(2):219–228.
337. Letsky EA, Miller F, Worwood M, Flynn DM. Serum ferritin in children with thalassaemia regularly transfused. *J Clin Pathol.* 1974;27:1213–6.
338. Prieto J, Barry M, Sherlock S. Serum ferritin in patients with iron overload and with acute and chronic liver disease. *Gastroenterology.* 1975;68(3):525–533.
339. Olivieri NF, Brittenham GM, Matsui D, et al. Iron-chelation therapy with oral deferiprone in patients with thalassemia major [see comments]. *N Engl J Med.* 1995;332(14):918–922.
340. Olivieri NF, Brittenham GM. Iron-chelating therapy and the treatment of thalassemia. *Blood.* 1997;89(3):739–761.
341. Chapman RW, Hussain MA, Gorman A, et al. Effect of ascorbic acid deficiency on serum ferritin concentration in patients with beta-thalassaemia major and iron overload. *J Clin Pathol.* 1982;35(5):487–491.
342. Berger TM, Polidori MC, Dabbagh A, et al. Antioxidant activity of vitamin C in iron-overloaded human plasma. *J Biol Chem.* 1997;272(25):15656–15660.
343. Davis BA, O'Sullivan C, Jarritt PH, Porter JB. Value of sequential monitoring of left ventricular ejection fraction in the management of thalassemia major. *Blood.* 2004;104(1):263–269.
344. Porter JB, Jaswon MS, Huehns ER, East CA, Hazell JW. Desferrioxamine ototoxicity: evaluation of risk factors in thalassaemic patients and guidelines for safe dosage. *Br J Haematol.* 1989;73(3):403–409.
345. Leung AW, Steiner RE, Young IR. NMR imaging of the liver in two cases of iron overload. *J Comput Assist Tomogr.* 1984;8(3):446–449.
346. Stark DD. Hepatic iron overload: paramagnetic pathology. *Radiology.* 1991;179(2):333–335.
347. Brown DW, Henkelman RM, Poon PY, Fisher MM. Nuclear magnetic resonance study of iron overload in liver tissue. *Magn Reson Imaging.* 1985;3(3):275–282.
348. Tanner MA, He T, Westwood MA, Firmin DN, Pennell DJ. Multi-center validation of the transferability of the magnetic resonance T2* technique for the quantification of tissue iron. *Haematologica.* 2006;91(10):1388–1391.
349. Helpern JA, Ordidge RJ, Gorell JM, Deniau JC, Welch KM. Preliminary observations of transverse relaxation rates obtained at 3 tesla from the substantia nigra of adult normal human brain. *NMR Biomed.* 1995;8(1):25–27.
350. Chatterjee R, Katz M, Oatridge A, Bydder GM, Porter JB. Selective loss of anterior pituitary volume with severe pituitary – gonadal insufficiency in poorly compliant male thalassemic patients with pubertal arrest. *Ann NY Acad Sci.* 1998;850:479–482.
351. Argyropoulou MI, Kiortsis DN, Efremidis SC. MRI of the liver and the pituitary gland in patients with beta-thalassemia major: does hepatic siderosis predict pituitary iron deposition? *Eur Radiol.* 2003;13(1):12–16.
352. Christoforidis A, Haritandi A, Perifanis V, Tsatra I, Athanassiou-Metaxa M, Dimitriadis AS. MRI for the determination of pituitary iron overload in children and young adults with beta-thalassaemia major. *Eur J Radiol.* 2007;62(1):138–142.
353. Midiri M, Lo Casto A, Sparacia G, et al. MR imaging of pancreatic changes in patients with transfusion-dependent beta-thalassemia major. *AJR Am J Roentgenol.* 1999;173(1):187–192.
354. Au WY, Lam WW, Chu W, et al. A T2* magnetic resonance imaging study of pancreatic iron overload in thalassemia major. *Haematologica.* 2008;93(1):116–119.
355. Balcerzac S, Westerman M, Heihn E, Taylor F. Effect of desferrioxamine and DTPA in iron overload. *Br J Med.* 1968;2:1573–1576.
356. Pippard MJ, Letsky EA, Callender ST, Weatherall DJ. Prevention of iron loading in transfusion-dependent thalassaemia. *Lancet.* 1978;1(8075):1178–1181.
357. Pippard M, Johnson D, Callender S, Finch C. Ferrioxamine excretion in iron loaded man. *Blood.* 1982;60:288–294.
358. Fillet G, Cook JD, Finch CA. Storage iron kinetics. VII. A biologic model for reticuloendothelial iron transport. *J Clin Invest.* 1974;53(6):1527–1533.
359. Frazer DM, Wilkins SJ, Millard KN, McKie AT, Vulpe CD, Anderson GJ. Increased hepcidin expression and hypoferraemia associated with an acute phase response are not affected by inactivation of HFE. *Br J Haematol.* 2004;126(3):434–436.
360. Bradley SJ, Gosriwitana I, Srichairatanakool S, Hider RC, Porter JB. Non-transferrin-bound iron induced by myeloablative chemotherapy [see comments]. *Br J Haematol.* 1997;99(2):337–343.
361. Gosriwatana I, Loreal O, Lu S, Brissot P, Porter J, Hider RC. Quantification of non-transferrin-bound iron in the presence of unsaturated transferrin. *Anal Biochem.* 1999;273(2):212–220.

362. Loreal O, Gosriwatana I, Guyader D, Porter J, Brissot P, Hider RC. Determination of non-transferrin-bound iron in genetic hemochromatosis using a new HPLC-based method [see comments]. *J Hepatol.* 2000;32(5):727–733.

363. Porter JB, Rafique R, Srichairatanakool S, et al. Recent insights into interactions of deferoxamine with cellular and plasma iron pools: implications for clinical use. *Ann NY Acad Sci.* 2005;1054:155–168.

364. Porter JB, Abeysinghe RD, Marshall L, Hider RC, Singh S. Kinetics of removal and reappearance of non-transferrin-bound plasma iron with deferoxamine therapy. *Blood.* 1996;88(2):705–713.

365. Jacobs EM, Hendriks JC, van Tits BL, et al. Results of an international round robin for the quantification of serum non-transferrin-bound iron: Need for defining standardization and a clinically relevant isoform. *Anal Biochem.* 2005;341(2):241–250.

366. Singh S, Hider RC, Porter JB. A direct method for quantification of non-transferrin bound iron (NTBI). *Anal Biochem.* 1990;186:320–323.

367. Cabantchik ZI, Breuer W, Zanninelli G, Cianciulli P. LPI-labile plasma iron in iron overload. *Best Pract Res Clin Haematol.* 2005;18(2):277–287.

368. Daar S, Taher A, Pathare A, et al. Plasma LPI in thalassemia patients before and after treatment with Deferasirox (Exjade®, ICL670). *Blood.* 2005;106(11): 2697a.

369. Nemeth E, Valore EV, Territo M, Schiller G, Lichtenstein A, Ganz T. Hepcidin, a putative mediator of anemia of inflammation, is a type II acute-phase protein. *Blood.* 2003;101(7):2461–2463.

370. Porter JB, Huehns ER. The toxic effects of desferrioxamine. *Baillieres Clin Haematol.* 1989;2:459–474.

371. Jacobs A. Low molecular weight intracellular iron transport compounds. *Blood.* 1977;50:433–439.

372. Glickstein H, El RB, Shvartsman M, Cabantchik ZI. Intracellular labile iron pools as direct targets of iron chelators: a fluorescence study of chelator action in living cells. *Blood.* 2005;106(9):3242–3250.

373. Loreal, GET. Liver fibrosis in genetic hemochromatosis: Respective roles of iron and non iron related factors. *J Hepatol.* 1992;16:122.

374. Hershko C. Determinants of fecal and urinary iron excretion in rats. *Blood.* 1978;51:415–423.

375. Hershko C, Grady R, Cerami A. Mechanism of desferrioxamine-induced iron excterion in the hypertransfused rat: definition of two alternative pathways of iron mobilisation. *J Lab Clin Med.* 1978;92:144–151.

376. Hershko C, Rachmilewitz E. Mechanism of desferrioxamine induced iron excretion in thalassaemia. *Br J Haematol.* 1979;42:125–132.

377. Finch CA, Deubelbeiss K, Cook JD, et al. Ferrokinetics in man. *J Clin Invest.* 1970;49:17–53.

378. Hershko C. A study of the chelating agent diethylenetriaminepentacetic acid using selective radioiron probes of reticuloendothelial and parenchymal iron stires. *J Lab Clin Med.* 1975;85:913–921.

379. Saito K, Nishisato T, Grasso JA, Aisen P. Interaction of transferrin with iron loaded rat peritoneal macrophages. *Br J Haematol.* 1986;62:275–286.

380. Hershko C, Cook J, Finch C. Storage iron kinetics III. Study of desferrioxamine action by selective radioiron labels of RE and parenchymal cells. *J Lab Clin Med.* 1973;81:876–886.

381. Hershko C, Konijn AM, Nick HP, Breuer W, Cabantchik ZI, Link G. ICL670A: a new synthetic oral chelator: evaluation in hypertransfused rats with selective radioiron probes of hepatocellular and reticuloendothelial iron stores and in iron-loaded rat heart cells in culture. *Blood.* 2001;97(4):1115–1122.

382. Link G, Konijn AM, Breuer W, Cabantchik ZI, Hershko C. Exploring the "iron shuttle" hypothesis in chelation therapy: effects of combined deferoxamine and deferiprone treatment in hypertransfused rats with labeled iron stores and in iron-loaded rat heart cells in culture. *J Lab Clin Med.* 2001;138(2):130–138.

383. Stefanini S, Chiancone E, Cavallo S, Saez V, Hall AD, Hider RC. The interaction of hydroxypyridinones with human serum transferrin and ovotransferrin. *J Inorg Biochem.* 1991;44(1):27–37.

384. Kontoghiorghes GJ, Goddard JG, Bartlett AN, Sheppard L. Pharmacokinetic studies in humans with the oral iron chelator 1,2-dimethyl-3-hydroxypyrid-4-one. *Clin Pharmacol.* 1990;48:255–261.

385. Breuer W, Ermers MJ, Pootrakul P, Abramov A, Hershko C, Cabantchik ZI. Desferrioxamine-chelatable iron, a component of serum non-transferrin- bound iron, used for assessing chelation therapy. *Blood.* 2001;97(3):792–798.

386. Esposito BP, Breuer W, Sirankapracha P, Pootrakul P, Hershko C, Cabantchik ZI. Labile plasma iron in iron overload: redox activity and susceptibility to chelation. *Blood.* 2003;102(7):2670–2677.

387. Tabuchi M, Yoshimori T, Yamaguchi K, Yoshida T, Kishi F. Human NRAMP2/DMT1, which mediates iron transport across endosomal membranes, is localized to late endosomes and lysosomes in HEp-2 cells. *J Biol Chem.* 2000;275(29):22220–22228.

388. Weaver J, Pollack S. Low Mr iron isolated from guinea pig reticulocytes as AMP-Fe and ATP-Fe complexes. *Biochem J.* 1989;261:787–792.

389. Pollack S, Weaver J, Zhan H. Intracellular iron. *Blood.* 1990;76:15a.

390. Breuer W, Epsztejn S, Cabantchik ZI. Dynamics of the cytosolic chelatable iron pool of K562 cells. *FEBS Lett.* 1996;382(3):304–308.

391. Epsztejn S, Kakhlon O, Glickstein H, Breuer W, Cabantchik I. Fluorescence analysis of the labile iron pool of mammalian cells. *Anal Biochem.* 1997;248(1):31–40.

392. Pippard M, Johnson D, Finch C. Hepatocyte iron kinetics in the rat explored with an iron chelator. *Br J Haematol.* 1982;52:211–224.

393. Bailey-Wood R, White G, Jacobs A. The use of chang cells in votro for the investigation of cellular iron metabolism. *Br J Exp Pathol.* 1975;56:358–362.

394. White GP, Bailey-Wood R, Jacobs A. The effect of chelating agents on cellular iron metabolism. *Clin Sci Mol Med.* 1976;50:145–152.

395. Mulligan M, Althus B, Linder M. Non-ferritin, non-heme iron pools in rat tissues. *Int J Biochem.* 1986;18:791–798.

396. Rothman RJ, Serroni A, Farber JL. Cellular pool of transient ferric iron, chelatable by deferoxamine and distinct from ferritin that is involved in oxidative cell injury. *Mol Pharmacol.* 1992;42(4):703–710.

397. Cooper CE, Porter JB. Ribonucleotide reductase, lipoxygenase and the intracellular low- molecular-weight iron pool. *Biochem Soc Trans.* 1997;25(1):75–80.
398. Klausner R, Rouault T, Harford J. Regulating the fate of mRNA: the control of cellular iron metabolism. *Cell.* 1993 72:19–28.
399. Porter JB, Huehns ER, Hider RC. The development of iron chelating drugs. *Baillieres Clin Haematol.* 1989;2(2):257–292.
400. Hoyes KP, Porter JB. Subcellular distribution of desferrioxamine and hydroxypyridin-4-one chelators in K562 cells affects chelation of intracellular iron pools. *Br J Haematol.* 1993;85(2):393–400.
401. Zanninelli G, Glickstein H, Breuer W, et al. Chelation and mobilization of cellular iron by different classes of chelators. *Mol Pharmacol.* 1997;51(5):842–852.
402. Glickstein H, El RB, Link G, et al. Action of chelators in iron-loaded cardiac cells: Accessibility to intracellular labile iron and functional consequences. *Blood.* 2006;108(9):3195–3203.
403. Kayyali R, Porter JB, Liu ZD, et al. Structure-function investigation of the interaction of 1- and 2- substituted 3-hydroxypyridin-4-ones with 5-lipoxygenase and ribonucleotide reductase. *J Biol Chem.* 2001;15:15.
404. Crichton R, Roman F, Roland F. Iron mobilisation from ferritin by chelating agents. *J Inorg Biochem.* 1980;13:305–316.
405. Brady MC, Lilley KS, Treffry A, Harrison PM, Hider RC, Taylor PD. Release of iron from ferritin molecules and their iron-cores by 3- hydroxypyridinone chelators in vitro. *J Inorg Biochem.* 1989;35(1):9–22.
406. Dobbin PS, Hider RC, Hall AD, et al. Synthesis, physicochemical properties, and biological evaluation of N- substituted 2-alkyl-3-hydroxy-4(1H)-pyridinones: orally active iron chelators with clinical potential. *J Med Chem.* 1993;36(17):2448–2458.
407. Drysdale J, Munro J. Regulation of synthesis and turnover of ferritin in rat liver. *J Biol Chem.* 1966;241:3630–3637.
408. Cooper PJ, Iancu TC, Ward RJ, Guttridge KM, Peters TJ. Quantitative analysis of immunogold labelling for ferritin in liver from control and iron-overloaded rats. *Histochem J.* 1988;20(9):499–509.
409. Porter J, Gyparaki M, Burke L, et al. Iron mobilization from hepatocyte monolayer cultures by chelators: the importance of membrane permeability and the iron binding constant. *Blood.* 1988;72:1497–1503.
410. Abeysinghe RD, Roberts PJ, Cooper CE, MacLean KH, Hider RC, Porter JB. The environment of the lipoxygenase iron binding site explored with novel hydroxypyridinone iron chelators. *J Biol Chem.* 1996;271(14):7965–7972.
411. Cooper CE, Lynagh GR, Hoyes KP, Hider RC, Cammack R, Porter JB. The relationship of intracellular iron chelation to the inhibition and regeneration of human ribonucleotide reductase. *J Biol Chem.* 1996;271(34):20291–20299.
412. Hoyes KP, Hider RC, Porter JB. Cell cycle synchronization and growth inhibition by 3-hydroxypyridin-4- one iron chelators in leukemia cell lines. *Cancer Res.* 1992;52(17):4591–4599.
413. Hoyes KP, Jones HM, Abeysinghe RD, Hider RC, Porter JB. In vivo and in vitro effects of 3-hydroxypyridin-4-one chelators on murine hemopoiesis. *Exp Hematol.* 1993;21(1):86–92.
414. Gutteridge JMC, Richmond R, Halliwell B. Inhibition of iron catalysed formation of hydroxyl radicals from superoxide and of lipid peroxidation by desferrioxamine. *Biochem J.* 1979;184:469–472.
415. Hider RC, Liu ZD. Emerging understanding of the advantage of small molecules such as hydroxypyridinones in the treatment of iron overload. *Curr Med Chem.* 2003;10(12):1051–1064.
416. Steinhauser S, Heinz U, Bartholomä M, Weyhermüller T, Nick H, Hegetschweile K. Complex Formation of ICL670 and Related Ligands with FeIII and FeII. *Eur Inorg Chem.* 2004;21:4177–4192.
417. Hider RC, Epemolu O, Singh S, Porter JB. Iron chelator design. *Adv Exp Med Biol.* 1994;356:343–349.
418. Hider RC, Choudhury R, Rai BL, Dehkordi LS, Singh S. Design of orally active iron chelators. *Acta Haematol.* 1996;95(1):6–12.
419. Porter JB, Morgan J, Hoyes KP, Burke LC, Huehns ER, Hider RC. Relative oral efficacy and acute toxicity of hydroxypyridin-4-one iron chelators in mice. *Blood.* 1990; 76(11):2389–2396.
420. Liu ZD, Kayyali R, Hider RC, Porter JB, Theobald AE. Design, synthesis, and evaluation of novel 2-substituted 3-hydroxypyridin-4-ones: structure-activity investigation of metalloenzyme inhibition by iron chelators. *J Med Chem.* 2002;45(3):631–639.
421. Porter JB, Abeysinghe RD, Hoyes KP, et al. Contrasting interspecies efficacy and toxicology of 1,2-diethyl-3-hydroxypyridin-4-one, CP94, relates to differing metabolism of the iron chelating site. *Br J Haematol.* 1993;85(1):159–168.
422. Lu SL, Gosriwatana I, Liu DY, Liu ZD, Mallet AI, Hider RC. Biliary and urinary metabolic profiles of 1,2-diethyl-3-hydroxypyridin- 4-one (CP94) in the rat. *Drug Metab Dispos.* 2000;28(8):873–879.
423. Liu DY, Liu ZD, Lu SL, Hider RC. Hydrolytic and metabolic characteristics of the esters of 1-(3′- hydroxypropyl)-2-methyl-3-hydroxypyridin-4-one (CP41), potentially useful iron chelators. *Pharmacol Toxicol.* 2000;86(5):228–233.
424. Porter JB, Singh S, Hoyes KP, Epemolu O, Abeysinghe RD, Hider RC. Lessons from preclinical and clinical studies with 1,2-diethyl-3- hydroxypyridin-4-one, CP94 and related compounds. *Adv Exp Med Biol.* 1994;356:361–370.
425. Porter J, Borgna-Pignatti C, Baccarani M, et al. Iron chelation efficiency of Deferasirox (Exjade, ICL670) in patients with transfusional hemosiderosis. *Blood.* 2005;106:2690a.
426. Hoffbrand AV, Cohen A, Hershko C. Role of deferiprone in chelation therapy for transfusional iron overload. *Blood.* 2003;102(1):17–24.
427. al-Refaie FN, Sheppard LN, Nortey P, Wonke B, Hoffbrand AV. Pharmacokinetics of the oral iron chelator deferiprone (L1) in patients with iron overload. *Br J Haematol.* 1995;89(2):403–408.
428. Galanello R, Piga A, Alberti D, Rouan MC, Bigler H, Sechaud R. Safety, tolerability, and pharmacokinetics of ICL670, a new orally active iron-chelating agent in patients with transfusion-dependent iron overload due to beta-thalassemia. *J Clin Pharmacol.* 2003;43(6):565–572.
429. Nisbet-Brown E, Olivieri NF, Giardina PJ, et al. Effectiveness and safety of ICL670 in iron-loaded patients with thalassaemia: a randomised, double-blind, placebo-controlled, dose-escalation trial. *Lancet.* 2003;361(9369):1597–1602.
430. Porter J, Davis B, Weir T, et al. Preliminary findings with single-dose evaluation of a new depot formulation of

deferoxamine (ICL 749B) for transfusion-dependent beta-thalassemia. Florida: The Saratoga Group, Ponte Verde Beach; 2000.
431. Bannerman R, Callender S, Williams D. Effect of desferrioxamine and DTPA in iron overload. *Br Med J.* 1962;2:1573–1576.
432. Sephton-Smith R. Iron excretion in thalassaemia major after administration of chelating agents. *Br Med J.* 1962;2:1577–1580.
433. Propper RL, Cooper B, Rufo RR, et al. Continuous subcutaneous administration of deferoxamine in patients with iron overload. *N Engl J Med.* 1977;297:418–423.
434. Hussain MA, Green N, Flynn DM, Hussein S, Hoffbrand AV. Subcutaneous infusion and intramuscular injection of desferrioxamine in patients withy transfusional iron overload. *Lancet.* 1976;2(7998):1278–1280.
435. Pippard MJ, Callender ST, Weatherall DJ. Intensive iron-chelation therapy with desferrioxamine in iron-loading anaemias. *Clin Sci Mol Med.* 1978;54(1):99–106.
436. Nienhuis AW, Griffith P, Strawczynski H, et al. Evaluation of cardiac function in patients with thalassemia major. *Ann NY Acad Sci.* 1980;344:384–396.
437. Marcus RE, Davies SC, Bantock HM, Underwood SR, Walton S, Huehns ER. Desferrioxamine to improve cardiac function in iron overloaded patients with thalassaemia major. *Lancet.* 1984; 1:392–393.
438. Cohen AR, Mizanin J, Schwartz E. Rapid removal of excessive iron with daily high dose intravenous chelation therapy. *J Pediatr.* 1987; 115:151–155.
439. Freeman AP, Giles RW, Berdoukas VA, Talley PA, Murray IP. Sustained normalization of cardiac function by chelation therapy in thalassaemia major. *Clin Lab Haematol.* 1989;11(4):299–307.
440. Davies SC, Marcus RE, Hungerford JL, Miller HM, Arden GB, Huehns ER. Ocular toxicity of high-dose intravenous desferrioxamine. *Lancet.* 1983;2:181–184.
441. Olivieri NF, Buncic JR, Chew E, et al. Visual and auditory neurotoxicity in patients receiving subcutaneous deferoxamine infusions. *N Engl J Med.* 1986;314(14):869–873.
442. De Virgillis S, Congia M, Frau F, et al. Desferrioxamine-induced growth retardation in patients with thalassaemia major. *J Pediatr.* 1988; 113:661–669.
443. Piga A, Luzzatto L, Capalbo P, Gambotto S, Tricta F, Gabutti V. High dose desferrioxamine as a cause of growth failure in thalassaemic patients. *Eur J Haematol.* 1988;40: 380–381.
444. Andriani M, Nordio M, Saporiti E. Estimation of statistical moments for desferrioxamine and its iron and aluminum chelates: contribution to optimisation of therapy in uremic patients. *Nephron.* 1996;72:218–224.
445. Lee P, Mohammed N, Abeysinghe RD, Hider RC, Porter JB, Singh S. Intravenous infusion pharmacokinetics of desferrioxamine in thalassaemia patients. *Drug Metab Dispos.* 1993;21(4): 640–644.
446. Porter JB, Faherty A, Stallibrass L, Brookman L, Hassan I, Howes C. A trial to investigate the relationship between DFO pharmacokinetics and metabolism and DFO-related toxicity. *Ann NY Acad Sci.* 1998;850:483–487.
447. Pippard MJ. Desferrioxamine-induced iron excretion in humans. *Baillieres Clin Haematol.* 1989;2.2:323–343.
448. Modell CB, Beck J. Long term desferrioxamine therapy in thalassaemia. *Ann NY Acad Sci.* 1974;232:201–210.
449. Cohen A, Martin M, Schwartz E. Response to long term deferrioxamine therapy in thalassemia. *J Pediatr.* 1981;99:689–694.
450. Cohen A, Martin M, Schwartz E. Depletion of excessive iron stores with desferrioxamine. *Br J Haematol.* 1984;58:369–373.
451. Aldouri MA, Wonke B, Hoffbrand AV, et al. Iron state and hepatic disease in patients with thalassaemia major, treated with long term subcutaneous desferrioxamine. *J Clin Pathol.* 1987;40:1353–1359.
452. Olivieri NF, Brittenham GM, McLaren CE, et al. Long-term safety and effectiveness of iron-chelation therapy with deferiprone for thalassemia major [see comments]. *N Engl J Med.* 1998;339(7):417–423.
453. Cappellini MD, Cohen A, Piga A, et al. A phase 3 study of deferasirox (ICL670), a once-daily oral iron chelator, in patients with beta-thalassemia. *Blood.* 2006;107(9):3455–3462.
454. Modell B, Letsky E, Flynn D, Peto R, Weatherall D. Survival and desferrioxamine in thalassaemia major. *Br Med J.* 1982;284:1081–1084.
455. Gabutti V, Borgna-Pignatti C. Clinical manifestations and therapy of transfusional haemosiderosis. *Bailliere Clin Haematol.* 1994;7:919–940.
456. Freeman AP, Giles RW, Berdoukas VA, Walsh WF, Choy D, Murray PC. Early left ventricular dysfunction and chelation therapy in thalassemia major. *Ann Intern Med.* 1983;99(4):450–454.
457. Aldouri MA, Hoffbrand AV, Flynn DM, Ward SE, Agnew JE, Hilson AJW. High incidence of cardiomyopathy in beta-thalassemia patients receiving transfusion and iron chelation: reversal by intensified chelation. *Acta Haematol.* 1990;84:113–117.
458. Cohen AR, Mizanin J, Schwartz E. Rapid removal of excessive iron with daily, high-dose intravenous chelation therapy. *J Pediatr.* 1989;115(1):151–155.
459. Tamary H, Goshen J, Carmi D, et al. Long-term intravenous deferoxamine treatment for noncompliant transfusion-dependent beta-thalassemia patients. *Isr J Med Sci.* 1994;30:658–664.
460. Miskin H, Yaniv I, Berant M, Hershko C, Tamary H. Reversal of cardiac complications in thalassemia major by long-term intermittent daily intensive iron chelation. *Eur J Haematol.* 2003;70(6):398–403.
461. Olivieri NF, Berriman AM, Tyler BJ, Davis SA, Francombe WH, Liu PP. Reduction in tissue iron stores with a new regimen of continuous ambulatory intravenous deferoxamine. *Am J Hematol.* 1992;41(1):61–63.
462. Pennell DJ, Berdoukas V, Karagiorga M, et al. Randomized controlled trial of deferiprone or deferoxamine in beta-thalassemia major patients with asymptomatic myocardial siderosis. *Blood.* 2006;107(9):3738–3744.
463. Tanner MA, Galanello R, Dessi C, et al. A randomized, placebo-controlled, double-blind trial of the effect of combined therapy with deferoxamine and deferiprone on myocardial iron in thalassemia major using cardiovascular magnetic resonance. *Circulation.* 2007;115(14):1876–1884.
464. Porter JB, A. TM, J. PD, P E. Improved Myocardial T2* in Transfusion Dependent Anemias Receiving ICL670 (Deferasirox). *Blood.* 2005;106(11):3600a.
465. Bronspiegel-Weintrob N, Olivieri NF, Tyler B, Andrews DF, Freedman MH, Holland FJ. Effect of age at the start of iron

chelation therapy on gonadal function in beta-thalassemia major. *N Engl J Med.* 1990;323(11):713–719.

466. Fosburg M, Nathan DG. Treatment of Cooleys anaemia. *Blood.* 1990;76:435–444.
467. Rahko PS, Salerni R, Uretsky BF. Successful reversal by chelation therapy of congestive cardiomyopathy due to iron overload. *J Am Coll Cardiol.* 1986;8:436–440.
468. Freeman AP, Giles RW, Berdoukas VA, Talley PA, Murray IP. Sustained normalisation of cardiac function by chelation therapy in thalassaemia major. *Clin Lab Haematol.* 1989;11(4):299–307.
469. Flynn DM, Hoffbrand AV, Politis D. Subcutaneous desferrioxamine: the effect of three years' treatment on liver, iron, serum ferritin, and comments on echocardiography. *Birth Defects Orig Artic Series.* 1982;18(7):347–353.
470. Olivieri NF, Rees DC, Ginder GD, et al. Treatment of thalassaemia major with phenylbutyrate and hydroxyurea. *Lancet.* 1997;350(9076):491–492.
471. De Sanctis V, Pinamonti A, Di Palma A, et al. Growth and development in thalassaemia major patients with severe bone lesions due to desferrioxamine. *Eur J Pediatr.* 1996;155(5):368–372.
472. Arden GB, Wonke B, Kennedy C, Huehns ER. Ocular changes in patients undergoing long term desferrioxamine treatment. *Br J Ophthalmol.* 1984; 68: 873–877.
473. Robins-Browne R, Prpic J. Desferrioxamine and systemic yersiniosis. *Lancet.* 1983;2:1372.
474. Gallant R, Freedman M, Vellend H, Francome W. Yersinia sepsis in patients with iron overload treated with desferrioxamine. *N Engl J Med.* 1986;314:1643.
475. Kouides PA, Slapak CA, Rosenwasser LJ, Miller KB. Pneumocystis carinii. pneumonia as a complication of desferrioxamine therapy. *Br J Haematol.* 1988;70:382–384.
476. Boelaert JR, Verauwe PL, Vandepitte JM. Mucormycosis infections in dialysis patients. *Ann Intern Med.* 1987;107(5):782–783.
477. Miller KB, Rosenwasser LJ, Bessette JM, Beer DJ, Rocklin RE. Rapid desenstitisation for desferrioxamine anaphylactic reaction. *Lancet.* 1981;1:1059. (Letter)
478. Bosquet J, Navarro M, Robert G, Aye P, Michel FB. Rapid desensitisation for desferrioxamine anaphylactoid reaction. *Lancet.* 1983;2:859–860.
479. Koren G, Bentur Y, Strong D, et al. Acute changes in renal function associated with desferrioxamine therapy. *Am J Dis Child.* 1990;143(9):1077–1080.
480. Koren G, Kochavi Atiya Y, Bentur Y, Olivieri NF. The effects of subcutaneous deferoxamine administration on renal function in thalassemia major. *Intl J Hematol.* 1991;54(5):371–375.
481. Tenenbein M, Kowalski S, Sienko A, Bowden DH, Adamson IYR. Pulmonary toxic effects of continuous desferrioxamine administration in acute iron poisoning. *Lancet.* 1992;339:699–701.
482. Freedman MH, Grisaru D, Olivieri NF, MacLusky I, Thorner PS. Pulmonary syndrome in patients with thalassaemia receiving intravenous desferrioxamine infusions. *Am J Dis Child.* 1990; 144:565–569.
483. Blake DR, Winyard P, Lunec J, et al. Cerebral and ocular toxicity induced by desferrioxamine. *Q J Med.* 1985;56:345–355.
484. Walker JA, Sherman RA, Eisinger RP. Thrombocytopenia associated with intravenous desferrioxamine. *Am J Kidney Dis.* 1985;6:254–256.
485. Modell B. Advances in the use of iron-chelating agents for the treatment of iron overload. *Prog Haematol.* 1979;11:267–312.
486. Dickerhoff R. Acute aphasia and loss of vision with desferrioxamine overdose. *J Pediatr Hematol Oncol.* 1987;9:287–288.
487. Olivieri NF, Koren G, Matsui D, et al. Reduction of tissue iron stores and normalization of serum ferritin during treatment with the oral iron chelator L1 in thalassemia intermedia. *Blood.* 1992;79(10):2741–2748.
488. Rodda CP, Reid ED, Johnson S, Doery J, Matthews R, Bowden DK. Short stature in homozygous beta-thalassaemia is due to disproportionate truncal shortening. *Clin Endocrinol.* 1995;42(6):587–592.
489. Piga A, Facello O, Gaglioti G, Pucci A, Pietribiasi F, Zimmerman A. No progression of liver fibrosis in thalassaemia major during deferiprone or desferrioxamine iron chelation. *Blood.* 1998;92 (Supple 2)(10):21b. (Abstract)
490. Berkovitch M, Collins AF, Papadouris D, et al. Need for early, low-dose chelation therapy in young children with transfused homozygous beta thalassemia. *Blood.* 1993;82:359a.
491. Araujo A, Kosaryan M, MacDowell A, et al. A novel delivery system for continuous desferrioxamine infusion in transfusional iron overload. *Br J Haematol.* 1996;93(4):835–837.
492. Jensen PD, Heickendorff L, Pedersen B, et al. The effect of iron chelation on haemopoiesis in MDS patients with transfusional iron overload. *Br J Haematol.* 1996;94(2):288–299.
493. Borgna-Pignatti C, Cohen A. Evaluation of a new method of administration of the iron chelating agent deferoxamine. *J Pediatr.* 1997;130(1):86–88.
494. Yarali N, Fisgin T, Duru F, et al. Subcutaneous bolus injection of deferoxamine is an alternative method to subcutaneous continuous infusion. *J Pediatr Hematol Oncol.* 2006;28(1):11–16.
495. Collins AF, Fassos FF, Stobie S, et al. Iron-balance and dose-response studies of the oral iron chelator 1,2- dimethyl-3-hydroxypyrid-4-one (L1) in iron-loaded patients with sickle cell disease. *Blood.* 1994;83(8):2329–2933.
496. Hider R, Kontoghiorghes G, Silver J. Pharmaceutical Compositions. UK Patent GB 2118176A, 1982.
497. Kontoghiorghes GJ, Aldouri MA, Hoffbrand AV, et al. Effective chelation of iron in beta thalassaemia with the oral chelator 1,2-dimethyl-3-hydroxypyrid-4-one. *Br Med J.* 1987;295(6612):1509–1512.
498. Kontoghiorghes GJ, Aldouri MA, Sheppard L, Hoffbrand AV. 1,2-dimethyl-3-hydroxypyrid-4-one, an orally active chelator for treatment of iron overload. *Lancet.* 1987b;1:1294–1295.
499. Porter J, Hoyes K, Abeysinghe R, Huehns E, Hider R. Animal Toxicology of iron chelator L1. *Lancet.* 1989;2:156. (Letter)
500. Porter JB, Hoyes KP, Abeysinghe RD, Brooks PN, Huehns ER, Hider RC. Comparison of the subacute toxicity and efficacy of 3-hydroxypyridin-4-one iron chelators in overloaded and nonoverloaded mice. *Blood.* 1991;78(10):2727–2734.
501. Hoffbrand A, Bartlett A, Veys P, O'Connor N, Kontoghiorghes G. Agranulocytosis and thrombocytopenia in patient with Blackfan-Diamond anaemia during oral chelator trial. *Lancet.* 1989;2:457.
502. al-Refaie FN, Wickens DG, Wonke B, Kontoghiorghes GJ, Hoffbrand AV. Serum non-transferrin-bound iron in beta-thalassaemia major patients treated with desferrioxamine and L1. *Br J Haematol.* 1992;82(2):431–436.

503. al-Refaie FN, Veys PA, Wilkes S, Wonke B, Hoffbrand AV. Agranulocytosis in a patient with thalassaemia major during treatment with the oral iron chelator, 1,2-dimethyl-3-hydroxypyrid-4-one. *Acta Haematol.* 1993;89(2):86–90.
504. Carthew P, Dorman BM, Edwards RE, Francis JE, Smith AG. A unique rodent model for both cardiotoxic and heptatotoxic effects of prolonged iron overload. *Lab Invest.* 1993;69:217–222.
505. Carthew P, Smith AG, Hider RC, Dorman B, Edwards RE, Francis JE. Potentiation of iron accumulation in cardiac myocytes during the treatment of iron overload in gerbils with the hydroxypyridinone iron chelator CP94. *Biometals.* 1994;7(4):267–71.
506. Berdoukas V, Bentley P, Frost H, Schnebli HP. Toxicity of oral iron chelator L1. *Lancet.* 1993;341(8852):1088.
507. Cohen AR, Galanello R, Piga A, De Sanctis V, Tricta F. Safety and effectiveness of long-term therapy with the oral iron chelator deferiprone. *Blood.* 2003;102(5):1583–1587.
508. Pippard MJ, Pattanapanyssat K, Tiperkae J, Hider RC. Metabolism of the iron chelates of desferrioxamine and hydroxypyridinones in the rat. In: Proceedings of the European Iron Club. Budapest, Hungary; 1989:55.
509. Olivieri NF, Koren G, Hermann C, et al. Comparison of oral iron chelator L1 and desferrioxamine in iron-loaded patients. *Lancet.* 1990;336(8726):1275–1279.
510. Lange R, Lameijer W, Roozendaal KL, Kersten M. Pharmaceutical analysis and pharmacokinetics of the oral iron chelator 1,2-dimethyl-3-hydroxypyridi-4-one (DMHP). In: Proceedings of 4th International Conference on Oral Chelation. Limasol, Cyprus; 1993.
511. Kontoghiorghes G, Sheppard L, Barr J, et al. Iron Balance studies with the oral chelator 1,2,dimethyl-3-hydroxypyridin-4-one. *Br J Haematol.* 1988;69:129a.
512. Hoffbrand AV, Al-Refaie F, Davis B, et al. Long-term trial of deferiprone in 51 transfusion-dependent iron overloaded patients. *Blood.* 1998;91(1):295–300.
513. Agarwal MB, Gupte SS, Viswanathan C, et al. Long-term assessment of efficacy and safety of L1, an oral iron chelator, in transfusion dependent thalassaemia: Indian trial. *Br J Haematol.* 1992;82(2):460–466.
514. Longo F, Fischer R, Engelbert R, Nielsen P, Sachetti L, Piga A. Iron balance in thalassemia patients treated with deferiprone. *Blood.* 1998;92(Suppl 1):235a.
515. Maggio A, D'Amico G, Morabito A, et al. Deferiprone versus deferoxamine in patients with thalassemia major: a randomized clinical trial. *Blood Cells Mol Dis.* 2002;28(2):196–208.
516. Gomber S, Saxena R, Madan N. Comparative efficacy of desferrioxamine, deferiprone and in combination on iron chelation in thalassemic children. *Indian Pediatr.* 2004;41(1):21–27.
517. Ha SY, Chik KW, Ling SC, et al. A randomized controlled study evaluating the safety and efficacy of deferiprone treatment in thalassemia major patients from Hong Kong. *Hemoglobin.* 2006;30(2):263–274.
518. Roberts D, Brunskill S, Doree C, Williams S, Howard J, Hyde C. Oral deferiprone for iron chelation in people with thalassaemia. *Cochrane Database Syst Rev.* 2007(3):CD004839.
519. Tondury P, Zimmermann A, Nielsen P, Hirt A. Liver iron and fibrosis during long-term treatment with deferiprone in Swiss thalassaemic patients. *Br J Haematol.* 1998;101(3):413–415.
520. Olivieri N, Brittenham G. Final Results of the randomised trial of deferiprone and deferoxamine. *Blood.* 1997;90(Suppl 1):264a.
521. Ceci A, Baiardi P, Felisi M, et al. The safety and effectiveness of deferiprone in a large-scale, 3-year study in Italian patients. *Br J Haematol.* 2002;118(1):330–336.
522. Piga A, Gaglioti C, Fogliacco E, Tricta F. Comparative effects of deferiprone and deferoxamine on survival and cardiac disease in patients with thalassemia major: a retrospective analysis. *Haematologica.* 2003;88(5):489–496.
523. Telfer P, Coen P, Christou Sea. Survival of medically treated thalassemia patients in Cyprus. Trends and risk factors over the period 1980–2004. *Haematologica.* 2006;91:1187–1192.
524. Anderson LJ, Wonke B, Prescott E, Holden S, Walker JM, Pennell DJ. Comparison of effects of oral deferiprone and subcutaneous desferrioxamine on myocardial iron concentrations and ventricular function in beta-thalassaemia. *Lancet.* 2002;360(9332):516–520.
525. al-Refaie FN, Hershko C, Hoffbrand AV, et al. Results of long-term deferiprone (L1) therapy: a report by the International Study Group on Oral Iron Chelators. *Br J Haematol.* 1995;91(1):224–229.
526. Hoffbrand AV. Prospects for oral iron chelation therapy. *J Lab Clin Med.* 1994;123(4):492–494.
527. Cohen A, Galanello R, Piga A, Vullo C, Tricta F. A multi-center safety trial of the oral iron chelator deferiprone. *Ann NY Acad Sci.* 1998;850:223–226.
528. Naithani R, Chandra J, Sharma S. Safety of oral iron chelator deferiprone in young thalassaemics. *Eur J Haematol.* 2005;74(3):217–220.
529. Maclean KH, Cleveland JL, Porter JB. Cellular zinc content is a major determinant of iron chelator-induced apoptosis of thymocytes. *Blood.* 2001;98(13):3831–3839.
530. Bartlett AN, Hoffbrand AV, Kontoghiorghes GJ. Long-term trial with the oral iron chelator 1,2-dimethyl-3-hydroxypyrid-4-one (L1). II. Clinical observations. *Br J Haematol.* 1990;76(2):301–304.
531. Cermak J, Brabec V. [Treatment of iron overload states with oral administration of the chelator agent, L1 (Deferiprone)]. *Vnitr Lek.* 1994;40(9):586–590.
532. Cohen AR, Galanello R, Piga A, Dipalma A, Vullo C, Tricta F. Safety profile of the oral iron chelator deferiprone: a multicentre study. *Br J Haematol.* 2000;108(2):305–312.
533. Choudhry VP, Pati HP, Saxena A, Malaviya AN. Deferiprone, efficacy and safety. *Indian J Pediatr.* 2004;71(3):213–216.
534. Berdoukas V, Bohane T, Eagle C, et al. The Sydney Children's Hospital experience with the oral iron chelator deferiprone (L1). *Transfusion Sci.* 2000;23(3):239–240.
535. Wanless IR, Sweeney G, Dhillon AP, et al. Lack of progressive hepatic fibrosis during long-term therapy with deferiprone in subjects with transfusion-dependent beta-thalassemia. *Blood.* 2002;100(5):1566–1569.
536. Schubert J, Derr SK. Mixed ligand chelate therapy for plutonium and cadmium poisoning. *Nature.* 1978;275(5678):311–313.
537. May PM, Williams DR. Computer simulation of chelation therapy. Plasma mobilizing index as a replacement for effective stability constant. *FEBS Lett.* 1977;78(1):134–138.

538. Jackson GE, May PM, Williams DR. The action of chelating agents in the removal of copper from ceruloplasmin: an in vitro study. *FEBS Lett.* 1978;90(1):173–177.
539. Grady R, Giardina P. Iron Chelation: Rationale for Combination Therapy. Florida: The Saratoga Group; 2000.
540. Giardina PJ, Grady RW. Chelation therapy in beta-thalassemia: an optimistic update. *Semin Hematol.* 2001; 38(4):360–366.
541. Mourad FH, Hoffbrand AV, Sheikh-Taha M, Koussa S, Khoriaty AI, Taher A. Comparison between desferrioxamine and combined therapy with desferrioxamine and deferiprone in iron overloaded thalassaemia patients. *Br J Haematol.* 2003;121(1):187–189.
542. Galanello R, Kattamis A, Piga A, et al. A prospective randomized controlled trial on the safety and efficacy of alternating deferoxamine and deferiprone in the treatment of iron overload in patients with thalassemia. *Haematologica.* 2006;91(9):1241–1243.
543. Aydinok Y, Ulger Z, Nart D, et al. A randomized controlled 1-year study of daily deferiprone plus twice weekly desferrioxamine compared with daily deferiprone monotherapy in patients with thalassemia major. *Haematologica.* 2007;92(12):1599–1606.
544. Origa R, Bina P, Agus A, et al. Combined therapy with deferiprone and desferrioxamine in thalassemia major. *Haematologica.* 2005;90(10):1309–1314.
545. Kattamis A, Ladis V, Berdousi H, et al. Iron chelation treatment with combined therapy with deferiprone and deferioxamine: a 12-month trial. *Blood Cells Mol Dis.* 2006;36(1):21–25.
546. Nick H, Acklin P, Lattmann R, et al. Development of tridentate iron chelators: from desferrithiocin to ICL670. *Curr Med Chem.* 2003;10:1065–1076.
547. Wood JC, Otto-Duessel M, Aguilar M, et al. Cardiac iron determines cardiac T2*, T2, and T1 in the gerbil model of iron cardiomyopathy. *Circulation.* 2005;112:535–543.
548. Piga A, Galanello R, Forni GL, et al. Randomized phase II trial of deferasirox (Exjade, ICL670), a once-daily, orally-administered iron chelator, in comparison to deferoxamine in thalassemia patients with transfusional iron overload. *Haematologica.* 2006;91:873–880.
549. Porter J, Waldmeier F, Bruin G, et al. Pharmacokinetics, metabolism and elimination of the iron chelator drug ICL670 in patients, following single oral doses of 1000 mg [14C]labelled drug at steady state. *Blood.* 2003;102:5b: Abstract 3720.
550. Eleftheriou P, Tanner M, Pennell D, Porter J. Response of myocardial T2* to oral deferasirox monotherapy for 1 year in 29 patients with transfusion-dependent anaemias; a subgroup analysis. *Haematologic.* 2006;91 (suppl):Abstract 999.
551. Wood J, Thompson A, Paley C, et al. Exjade® reduces cardiac iron burden in chronically transfused β-thalassemia patients: an MRI T2* Study. *Blood.* 2007;110:Abstract 2781.
552. Cappellini MD, Vichinsky E, Ford JM, Porter J. Long-term safety of deferasirox (Exjade®, ICL670) in the management of blood transfusion-induced iron overload: results after a median reatment duration of 3.5 years. Submitted 2008.
553. Ong-ajyooth L, Malasit P, Ong-ajyooth S, et al. Renal function in adult beta-thalassemia/HB E disease. *Nephron.* 1998:78:156–161.
554. Cappellini M, Vinchinsky E, Ford J, Rabault B, Porter J. Evaluation of deferasirox (Exjade®, ICL670) therapy in patients with transfusional iron overload who achieve serum ferritin (SF) ≤1000 ng/ml in long-term studies. Session type: *Blood.* 2007;110 16b:Abstract 3795.
555. Donovan JM, Plone M, Dagher R, Bree M, Marquis J. Preclinical and clinical development of deferitrin, a novel, orally available iron chelator. *Ann N Y Acad Sci.* 2005;1054:492–449.
556. Dragsten PR, Hallaway PE, Hanson GJ, Berger AE, Bernard B, Hedlund BE. First human studies with a high-molecular-weight iron chelator. *J Lab Clin Med.* 2000;135:57–65.

30

Induction of Fetal Hemoglobin in the Treatment of Sickle Cell Disease and β Thalassemia

Yogen Saunthararajah and George F. Atweh

INTRODUCTION

The beneficial effects of high levels of fetal hemoglobin (HbF) in sickle cell disease and β thalassemia have been recognized for many years. In 1948, Watson et al.[1] noted that newborns with sickle cell disease do not suffer from the clinical complications of their disease until HbF declines to adult levels after the first 6 months of life. Later, it was shown that the majority of patients with sickle cell disease from some regions of Saudi Arabia[2] and India[3] who co-inherit another genetic determinant associated with high HbF levels, have a very mild sickling disorder. More recently, the Cooperative Study of Sickle Cell Disease, a large multicenter study of the natural history of sickle cell disease (see Chapter 19) demonstrated an inverse correlation between HbF levels and the frequency of painful crises and early death.[4,5] These clinical and epidemiological observations are supported by laboratory studies that demonstrate a sparing effect of HbF on polymerization of deoxyhemoglobin S.[6] Similarly, in β thalassemia, an increase in the synthesis of fetal γ-globin chains may decrease the imbalance between α- and non-α-globin chains and ameliorate the severity of the anemia. This appreciation of the beneficial effects of HbF in sickle cell disease and β thalassemia stimulated a great deal of interest in the development of therapeutic agents to increase HbF production in patients with these disorders. In this chapter, we discuss the preclinical and clinical development of the different classes of pharmacological inducers of HbF production including DNA hypomethylating agents such as 5-azacytidine and decitabine, cytotoxic agents such as hydroxyurea, and inhibitors of histone deacetylase such as butyrate.

DNA HYPOMETHYLATING AGENTS

Gene expression is a process that is regulated to an important degree by the packaging of DNA around histones and by methylation of deoxycytosines that precede deoxyguanines (CpG) in the promoters of genes. The DNA methylation patterns that regulate the expression of cell type–specific genes are established by DNA methyltransferase (DNMT) enzymes that recognize and methylate target deoxycytosines. Generally, methylation in the promoter of a tissue-specific gene is associated with nonexpression of the gene. Approximately 65% of all CpG dinucleotides in vertebrate DNA are methylated at the cytosine residue by the action of DNA DNMT enzymes. As would be expected, γ-globin gene promoter DNA is relatively unmethylated at developmental stages when it is expressed, and methylated in adult bone marrow erythroid cells when the genes are not expressed.[7] This suggests that DNA hypomethylating agents might reactivate the expression of the silenced γ-globin gene.

The related compounds 5-azacytidine and decitabine (Fig. 30.1) are cytosine analogs first synthesized more than 40 years ago. Like other nucleoside analogs, they were originally viewed as cytotoxic chemotherapy agents and drug regimens were based on the maximum tolerated dose. It was only with the emergence of the field of epigenetics that inhibition of DNA methylation, reactivation of gene expression, and induction of cellular differentiation were recognized as actions of decitabine (5-azacytidine exerts its DNA hypomethylating effect by being converted to decitabine by ribonucleotide reductase).[8] Importantly, the DNA hypomethylating effect is seen at low and very well-tolerated doses of the drugs.[9] The specific mechanism by which decitabine depletes DNMT in dividing cells explains why low doses of decitabine can hypomethylate DNA without causing cytotoxicity whereas higher doses are toxic: The mechanism of action of decitabine begins with decitabine phosphorylation by deoxycytosine kinase (DCK) and incorporation into the replicating genome, just like natural deoxycytidine. DNMT is covalently trapped as it tries to methylate the 5-N position of the triazene ring of DNA-incorporated decitabine. This covalent trapping/modification depletes cellular DNMT and decreases DNA methylation. At high decitabine doses, hydrolytic cleavage at DNMT–CpG complexes overwhelms the cellular repair machinery, damaging the replicating genome to an extent that results in cell death (cytotoxicity). Lower doses do not overwhelm the cellular repair machinery, and although temporary growth arrest (cytostatic effect) might occur, cell division ultimately continues but with depleted DNMT, DNA hypomethylation, and consequently altered gene expression. 5-Azacytidine, but not decitabine, incorporates into RNA and inhibits protein synthesis. On a mole for mole basis, decitabine is a more potent inhibitor of DNMT than 5-azacytidine.

The γ-globin gene in baboons is structurally and functionally similar to that of human beings. Prompted by the association of γ-globin gene promoter methylation with its developmental silencing, the ability of 5-azacytidine to induce HbF synthesis in baboons was studied.

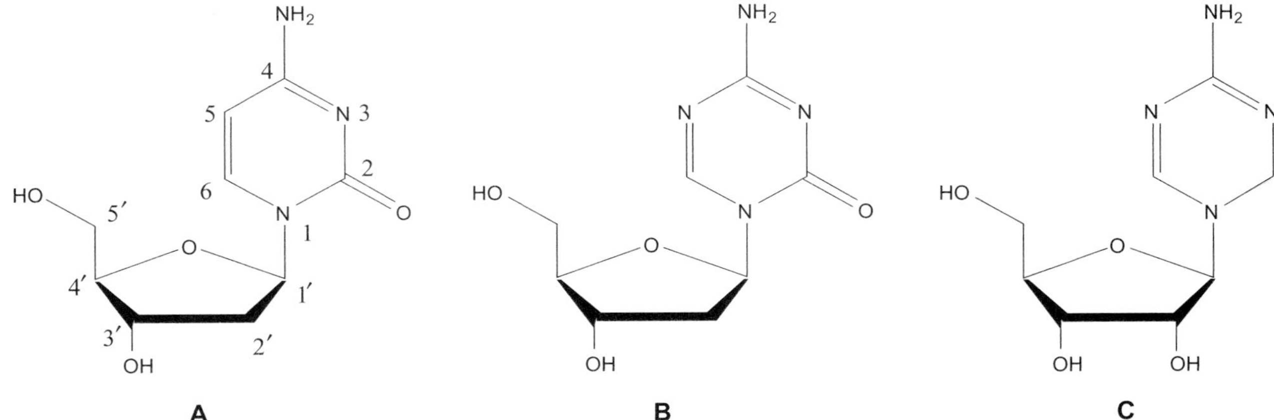

Figure 30.1. Structure of natural deoxycytidine **(A)**, decitabine **(B)**, and 5-azacytidine **(C)**. Decitabine, a deoxynucleotide, is only incorporated into DNA and is a more specific and potent DNA-hypomethylating agent than 5-azacytidine, which is also incorporated into RNA.

5-Azacytidine (injected into anemic baboons at a dose of 2–4 mg/kg/d 5 d/wk for 2 wk) increased HbF levels up to 70% of total hemoglobin (HbF 70%).[11] This effect was achieved at doses of the drug that caused mild neutropenia, but did not seem to change RBC or platelet production. The results in baboons led to a number of clinical studies in patients with sickle cell disease and β thalassemia.[12–14] In two patients with sickle cell disease treated with 5-azacytidine at a dose of 2 mg/kg/day for 5 days, HbF levels increased to 22% without substantial toxicity.[13] The percentage of F cells (Chapter 7) increased up to 80%. There was also improvement in surrogate clinical markers, denoted by decreased irreversibility of sickle cells, dense cells, and indirect bilirubin.[14,15] 5-Azacytidine treatment of three patients with end-stage β thalassemia also produced large increases in total hemoglobin (3–5 g/dL).[16] In these patients with β thalassemia, the total hemoglobin increases consist of HbF. Two of these patients, treated for 30 months (1–2 mg/kg/d, 4 d/wk, 1 time/mo), remained transfusion independent for the duration of treatment.

Despite these very promising early results, further trials with 5-azacytidine were curtailed due to concerns regarding potential carcinogenicity. These concerns were largely based on a study conducted by Carr et al.[17] in the Fisher rat testicular cancer model, which suggested that 5-azacytidine caused tumors in 31 of 70 rats treated with the drug. The study received criticism because the incidence of testicular cancer in the control population of Fisher rats was 0%, which is not in accordance with the usual rate (~20%) of spontaneous testicular cancer development in these rats.[18] Another controversy was whether HbF induction resulted from DNA hypomethylation induced by 5-azacytidine, or cytotoxic effects. If cytotoxicity was the mechanistic basis for HbF induction, then other cytostatic/cytotoxic agents such as the well-tolerated and orally available ribonucleotide reductase inhibitor hydroxyurea might also be effective. This led to studies of hydroxyurea in patients with sickle cell disease and thalassemia, culminating in the Multicenter Study of Hydroxyurea (MSH) in patients with symptomatic sickle cell anemia. The MSH conclusively demonstrated that hydroxyurea reduced the frequency of acute painful episodes, acute chest syndrome, and transfusions.[19]

The historical efficacy of 5-azacytidine in HbF reactivation suggested that DNA-hypomethylating agents could still have a role in the management of sickle cell disease. Decitabine holds two apparent advantages over 5-azacytidine: 1) the majority of preclinical studies suggest chemoprevention of cancer rather than carcinogenicity, and 2) decitabine is exclusively incorporated into DNA (5-azacytidine is also incorporated into RNA) and is a more potent DNA-hypomethylating agent. Therefore, studies are being pursued that focus on the use of decitabine to reactivate HbF synthesis in patients with symptomatic sickle cell disease.

In the first study, eight patients were treated with decitabine at low doses (compared with doses of decitabine used in previous cancer trials) of 0.15 mg/kg–0.30 mg/kg given 5 days per week for 2 weeks.[9] Five of these patients did not have increases in HbF with hydroxyurea treatment (hydroxyurea levels documented compliance), two were low responders to hydroxyurea, and one patient was not in the MSH. The average γ-globin synthesis relative to non–α-globin synthesis prior to therapy was 3.2% and increased to 13.7% after treatment. HbF increased from 3.6% to 13.5%, whereas F cells increased from 21% to 55%. The HbF content per F cell increased from 17% to 24%. Hydroxyurea treatment increased HbF levels in these patients from 2.4% to 2.6%. With decitabine treatment, however, the average HbF increased to 12.7%, and total hemoglobin increased by 1 g/dL in six of eight patients. The only toxicity was transient neutropenia. These studies suggested that the optimal daily dose of decitabine is 0.2 mg/kg, producing greater increases in HbF without much increased risk of neutropenia compared with decitabine 0.15 mg/kg/day.

A follow-up study examined whether increased HbF and total hemoglobin levels could be maintained without toxicity with repeated cycles administered every 6 weeks over a 36-week period.[20] In six sickle cell anemia patients, the average HbF during the last 20 weeks of treatment was 13.9% ± 2.8% (mean ± standard deviation [SD]) compared with a baseline HbF of 3.1% ± 2.8%. Maximum HbF levels were 18.45% ± 4.5% (mean ± SD). Maximum F cell percentages ranged between 58% and 87%. The average hemoglobin value increased from 7.2 g/dL to 8.8 g/dL (mean ± SD). Maximum hemoglobin values were 9.7 ± 0.5 g/dL. The neutrophil nadirs between weeks 16 and 36 were all less than 1,500/μL, occurred at approximately 5–6 weeks of each treatment cycle, and rapidly recovered. Interestingly, a peak in the platelet count mirrored the neutrophil count nadir. With the exception of neutropenia, there were no other toxicities.

In a subsequent study, the objectives were to 1) evaluate whether decitabine is safe and effective if given by a more practical subcutaneous route; 2) assess whether weekly administration could produce cumulative and stable increases in HbF and total hemoglobin levels; 3) measure additional surrogate clinical endpoints (the pathophysiology of vasoocclusive crises in sickle cell disease involves erythrocyte adhesion to endothelium, endothelial damage, and activation of coagulation and inflammatory cascades; therefore, red cell adhesion to thrombospondin and laminin, markers of endothelial damage, coagulation system activation, and inflammatory activity were measured); and 4) confirm that, at the low doses being used, decitabine hypomethylates DNA without typical chemotherapy-associated myelotoxicity. In addition to hematological parameters, bone marrow morphology, and DNA methylation changes were assessed.[21]

Decitabine was administered subcutaneously at 0.2 mg/kg, one–three times/week in two cycles of 6 weeks each, with a 2-week interval between cycles. Eight patients were studied who either did not respond to or did not tolerate hydroxyurea therapy. All patients demonstrated statistically significant increases in HbF (± SD) from 6.5% ± 1.4% to 20.4% ± 2.0%, and F cells from 38.1% ± 7.6% to 71.4% ± 6.5% with treatment. Three hydroxyurea nonresponding patients had lower HbF levels at baseline but demonstrated a rate of increase in HbF similar to that seen in five hydroxyurea responders. The only toxicity noted was neutropenia, which coincided with increases in the platelet count of up to 860 × 10^9/L. Total hemoglobin increased from 7.6 ± 1 g/dL to 9.6 ± 0.9 g/dL. Both the absolute reticulocyte count and total bilirubin decreased during treatment. The reticulocyte count correlated inversely with total hemoglobin, suggesting that the reticulocyte decrease resulted from decreased hemolysis. There were significant improvements in a spectrum of surrogate clinical endpoints that measure the activity of vasoocclusive pathophysiology: 1) RBCs from patients demonstrated decreased adhesion to the matrix molecules thrombospondin and laminin; 2) D-dimer levels, which are a measure of coagulation system activity, decreased; and 3) soluble vascular adhesion molecule–1 and von Willebrand Factor propeptide levels, which are measures of endothelial damage, decreased.

A number of observations suggest that the mechanism by which decitabine produces HbF elevations is DNA hypomethylation. DNA hypomethylation per se is not necessarily cytotoxic,[10] suggesting that low doses of decitabine might hypomethylate DNA without inducing cytotoxicity. The low doses of decitabine used in the clinical trials and in vitro studies were sufficient to produce DNA hypomethylation.[22] Platelet counts increased during therapy, concurrent with a downward trend in neutrophil and monocyte counts. Although there was a decrease in reticulocyte counts during therapy, there was a strong inverse correlation between the decreasing reticulocyte counts and increasing hemoglobin levels, suggesting that the decreased reticulocyte count resulted from decreased hemolysis. Serial bone marrow aspirate specimens obtained during therapy did not demonstrate a decrease in marrow spicule cellularity. Instead, there was an increase in megakaryocyte numbers and a decrease in the myeloid/erythroid ratio (an increase in the proportion of erythroid cells). In vitro studies with decitabine treatment of human CD34+ hematopoietic cells were consistent with the in vivo results, demonstrating an increase in the proportion of mixed colonies (erythroid and myeloid) formed relative to pure granulocyte–macrophage colonies. Thus, decitabine-induced hypomethylation in the γ-globin gene promoter could contribute to the increased HbF with treatment, but hypomethylation at other genes might also be important because the change in pattern of hematopoietic differentiation could be contributing to the increased HbF.

With regard to pharmacological reactivation of HbF, decitabine has a number of advantages when compared with hydroxyurea. All patients treated to date have had clinically significant increases in HbF. The large increases in HbF could translate into more clinical benefits and potentially some protection from organ complications such as pulmonary hypertension and stroke.[23] The noncytotoxic mechanism of action of decitabine might facilitate prolonged administration and durable responses. Decitabine could potentially synergize with other epigenetically active agents, such as histone deacetylase inhibitors.[24] Presently, there are no data regarding the clinical effectiveness of decitabine in sickle cell disease. The trials conducted to date, which have measured surrogate clinical endpoints such as HbF levels, red cell adhesion, coagulation system activation, and endothelial damage, indicate the promise of this drug as a treatment for sickle cell disease.

Extended phase II/III studies evaluating clinical endpoints such as crisis frequency, quality of life, and survival will be required to demonstrate definitively a clinical benefit. As a further incentive to such studies, off-label treatment of patients with severe sickle cell disease on a chronic basis produced notable clinical improvement.[25] Although most preclinical studies show negligible mutagenicity and a chemopreventive rather than carcinogenic effect and no unusual cytogenetic abnormalities have been reported in the many patients with myelodysplastic syndrome treated with decitabine thus far, further studies involving chronic dosing of patients with sickle cell disease or thalassemia should attempt to measure the risks of inducing DNA mutations and chromosome instability, perhaps in comparison to the current standard of care, hydroxyurea, which has a similar risk profile. Decitabine is likely to be teratogenic and could have effects on male fertility; these concerns are significant because many of the target patient population are of reproductive age.

HYDROXYUREA

Interestingly, controversy about the mechanism of activation of fetal γ-globin gene expression by 5-azacytidine led to the identification of hydroxyurea as a second therapeutic agent that can stimulate HbF production. Some investigators hypothesized that 5-azacytidine increases HbF production by accelerating erythroid cell differentiation rather than by hypomethylation of DNA.[26] To support this hypothesis, experiments were performed to show that hydroxyurea, an S-phase–specific chemotherapeutic agent without DNA-demethylating activity, can also increase HbF production in phlebotomized monkeys[27] and in patients with sickle cell disease.[28] These interesting observations, however, did not completely resolve the controversy about the mechanism of action of 5-azacytidine or decitabine because these agents appear to be more potent inducers of HbF production than hydroxyurea. Moreover, decitabine was shown to increase HbF levels in sickle cell patients who were resistant to hydroxyurea, suggesting that the two drugs have different mechanisms of action.[9] Nonetheless, hydroxyurea had some significant advantages, it is an oral agent with a relatively good safety profile and it was already in wide use for the treatment of myeloproliferative disorders. Thus, it quickly replaced 5-azacytidine as the agent of choice for stimulating HbF production in patients with sickle cell disease.

Clinical Use of Hydroxyurea

The clinical use of hydroxyurea was discussed in detail in the first edition of this book and elsewhere more recently.[29–32]

Hydroxyurea was first used in a number of small, nonrandomized clinical trials that confirmed its HbF-inducing activity in sickle cell disease.[33–34] These studies provided the proof of principle and led to the identification of an effective dose schedule for the use of this drug in the treatment of patients with sickle cell disease. These phase I/II studies were followed by a large randomized, placebo-controlled MSH that had well-defined clinical efficacy endpoints.[19] This study was terminated prematurely when interim analysis showed a significant reduction in the frequency of crises and acute chest syndrome in the hydroxyurea-treated group compared with the control group. There was also a reduction in the frequency of blood transfusions in the hydroxyurea-treated group but no changes in the frequency of stroke or death during the 2.5 years of study.[19] The effects of hydroxyurea on quality of life were mixed but most evident in patients with the highest HbF response to treatment.[35] On the basis of the controlled clinical trial, hydroxyurea became the first HbF-inducing drug to be approved by the Food and Drug Administration for the treatment of sickle cell anemia, and as a result, hydroxyurea is now widely used in the United States and Europe.

Hydroxyurea should be used in all adults when indications for this treatment are present (Table 30.1). Unfortunately, for complex and poorly understood reasons, only a fraction of patients who might benefit from treatment receive it. In follow-up studies to the MSH, cumulative mortality was reduced nearly 40% and a favorable result was related to the ability of the drug to increase HbF and reduce painful episodes and acute chest syndrome.[36]

Children have a more robust HbF response to hydroxyurea than do adults.[31,32,37–41] In a study of more than 100 children who received maximal drug doses, HbF increased to almost 20% and the treatment effects were sustained for 7 years without clinically important toxicity.[42] Some have proposed using hydroxyurea for secondary and primary prevention of stroke in children, and recent studies suggest that hydroxyurea, by a mechanism still unknown, can in some individuals reduce transcranial Doppler flow rates into the normal range.[43–47] This issue is now being studied in a controlled clinical trial.

The clinical benefits of hydroxyurea in HbSC disease are unknown, although the drug does have effects on the HbSC disease erythrocyte.[48,49] This topic is also just beginning to be studied in a therapeutic trial.

Although hydroxyurea was associated with reduced mortality in follow-up of the MSH, patients still die of complications of this disease while receiving treatment. In a single-center analysis of the 34 patients who died due to sickle cell disease–related causes, acute chest syndrome was the cause of death in 35%. The deceased and surviving patients did not differ significantly in average hydroxyurea dose or HbF response but were older when hydroxyurea was first started, were more anemic, and had significantly higher serum blood urea nitrogen and serum creatinine levels. They might represent a subgroup of older patients, possibly with more severe disease and organ damage who would benefit from earlier treatment.[50]

Preventing the usual HbF to HbS switch in gene expression early in childhood, before HbF levels decline to subtherapeutic concentrations and sickle vasculopathy results, should "cure" sickle cell anemia. Studies using hydroxyurea beginning in the first year of life are underway and focus on

Table 30.1. A method for treating patients with sickle cell anemia with hydroxyurea. Special caution should be exercised in patients with compromised renal or hepatic function and when patients are habituated to narcotics. Contraception should be practiced by both men and women because hydroxyurea is a teratogen and its effects in pregnancy are unknown. After a stable and nontoxic dose of hydroxyurea is reached, blood counts may be done at 4- to 8-week intervals. Granulocytes should be $\geq$2,000/mm^3, platelets $\geq$80,000/mm^3. A fall in hemoglobin level (in most patients who respond, the hemoglobin level increases slightly) and absolute reticulocyte count to $<$80,000/mm^3 should be carefully evaluated. A hemoglobin $<$5.5 g/dL before treatment is not a contraindication to treatment

Indications for Treatment
Adults, adolescents, and after consultation with parents and expert pediatricians, children with frequent pain episodes, history of acute chest syndrome, other severe vasoocclusive complications. Severe symptomatic anemia
Baseline Evaluation
Blood counts, red cell indices, HbF, serum chemistries, pregnancy test, willingness to adhere to all recommendations for treatment, absence of chronic transfusion program
Initiation of Treatment
Hydroxyurea 10–15 mg/kg/d or 500 mg q A.M. for 6–8 wk, complete blood count q 2 wk, HbF q 6–8 wk
Continuation of Treatment
If counts are acceptable, escalate dose in increments of 500 mg every 6–8 wk
Failure of HbF (or MCV) to Increase
Consider biological inability to respond to treatment or poor compliance with treatment. Increase dose very cautiously to 2,000–2,500 mg/d (maximum dose 30 mg/kg). Absent transfusion support or intercurrent illness suppressing erythropoiesis, a trial period of 6–8 mo is probably adequate
Treatment Endpoints
Less pain, increase in HbF (or MCV), increased hemoglobin level if severely anemic, acceptable toxicity

the prevention of organ damage in the spleen, kidney, and central nervous system.[39]

Hydroxyurea is potentially mutagenic and carcinogenic. Cancer and leukemia have been reported in hydroxyurea-treated sickle cell disease patients but whether the incidence is higher than in the general population is not known.[36] In one study, acquired somatic DNA mutations in peripheral blood mononuclear cells were studied after in vivo exposure to hydroxyurea. Children with sickle cell disease exposed to the drug for 30 months had significantly more immunoglobulin gene VDJ mutations than patients exposed for 7 months or those not taking the drug at all. Overall, the studies suggested that although the mutagenic and carcinogenic potential of hydroxyurea is low, young patients should be monitored serially.[51]

Prediction of Response to Treatment. An ability to predict the therapeutic response to hydroxyurea would be clinically useful. In early studies from the MSH, the best HbF-responding patients had the highest initial neutrophil and reticulocyte counts and the largest treatment-associated decrements in these counts. In children, baseline HbF, leukocyte count and reticulocyte count, and the fall in leukocyte and reticulocyte counts also predicted a higher HbF response.[37]

It is likely that HbF levels at baseline and in response to drug treatment are genetically regulated. Genetic elements linked to the β-globin gene–like cluster and quantitative trait loci (QTL) present on chromosomes 6, 8, and on the X-chromosome as well as other regulatory loci are likely to exist, and epigenetic and cellular factors could also have regulatory importance (see Chapter 27). As the increase of HbF in response to hydroxyurea varies among patients with sickle cell anemia, 29 candidate genes within QTL previously reported to be linked to HbF level (6q22.3–q23.2, 8q11–q12, and Xp22.2–p22.3), involved in metabolism of hydroxyurea, or related to erythroid progenitor proliferation were studied in 137 sickle cell anemia patients treated with hydroxyurea. Three hundred and twenty tagging single nucleotide polymorphisms (SNPs) in candidate genes were selected and the association between SNPs and the change of HbF level after 2 years of drug treatment was analyzed. SNPs in genes within the 6q22.3–23.2 and 8q11–q12 linkage peaks and also the *ARG2, FLT1, HAO2,* and *NOS1* genes were associated with the HbF response to hydroxyurea. These results suggested that polymorphisms in genes regulating HbF expression, erythroid progenitor proliferation, and hydroxyurea metabolism might modulate a patient's response to this agent.[52]

Mechanisms of Action

Although hydroxyurea was shown to have similar HbF-inducing activity to 5-azacytidine in anemic baboons and patients with sickle cell disease, its molecular targets and mechanism(s) of action are still not fully elucidated. It was originally proposed that hydroxyurea might elevate HbF levels by accelerating erythroid differentiation in the bone marrow, leading to the appearance of "fetal-like" cells in the peripheral blood.[26] More recent studies have shown that hydroxyurea generates nitric oxide in vivo, which results in the activation of the nitric oxide–cyclic guanosine monophophate signaling pathway and the up-regulation of γ-globin gene expression in patients with sickle cell disease.[53] Hydroxyurea has other effects that might also benefit patients with sickle cell disease. For example, hydroxyurea was shown to decrease the adhesion of sickle cells to endothelium and to decrease the level of soluble vascular adhesion molecule-1.[54,55] Owing to its myelosuppressive activity, hydroxyurea reduces circulating leukocyte counts, and likely, the number of adherent leukocytes recruited to the wall of small venules.

In one analysis, the reduction of white blood cell counts was correlated with the clinical benefit from hydroxyurea.[56] This report led to widespread speculation in the field that the clinical benefits of hydroxyurea are not related to its effect on HbF production. Since this publication, an additional report was published in which the clinical and laboratory data that were collected as part of the MSH were analyzed in detail. Curiously, the analysis of long-term follow-up failed to show a correlation between the increase in HbF production and the clinical benefit in patients who received hydroxyurea and suggested that study design issues forced the relationship between leukocyte count and the reduction in painful episodes.[36] This study showed a positive correlation between survival and HbF levels in patients who were treated with hydroxyurea, and no correlation between survival and leukocyte counts.[36] We would caution against the premature conclusion that the beneficial effects of hydroxyurea are a result of its effects on blood leukocytes rather than HbF concentration.

INHIBITORS OF HISTONE DEACETYLASES

In 1985, Ginder et al.[57] reported that the administration of butyrate, a well-known inhibitor of histone deacetylases, to chickens pretreated with 5-azacytidine resulted in the induction of embryonic globin gene expression. Shortly thereafter, Perrine et al.[58] and Bard et al.[59] showed that infants born to diabetic mothers had higher HbF levels at birth than their aged-matched controls. Interestingly, the diabetic pregnant mothers had high levels of butyric acid in their plasma. Perrine et al. went on to demonstrate that butyrate infusions in utero in sheep fetuses prevented the switch from HbF to HbA that is normally seen around the time of birth.[60] This was followed by the demonstration that the administration of butyric acid to adult baboons could partially reverse the switch from fetal to adult globin expression.[61] These preclinical observations formed the basis for clinical trials that investigated the therapeutic potential of butyrate as an HbF-inducing agent in patients with sickle cell disease and β thalassemia.

Perrine et al.[62] first evaluated the effects of arginine butyrate on HbF production in six patients with β-globin disorders (three patients with sickle cell disease and three patients with β thalassemia). Treatment with butyrate resulted in an increase in γ-globin chain synthesis in all six patients following a 2-week infusion of the drug. This initial study was followed by another study that was conducted by Sher et al.[63] in which arginine butyrate infusions were given to five patients with sickle cell disease and five patients with β thalassemia. A 10-week dose escalation course of arginine butyrate resulted in a significant increase in HbF levels in two of the five patients with sickle cell disease. This increase in HbF levels, however, was not sustained with continuous high-dose therapy. Moreover, there was no increase in the total hemoglobin levels in any of the five patients with β thalassemia who were enrolled on this regimen.

Sodium phenylbutyrate was also used to induce HbF production in patients with sickle cell disease. All six patients who received the drug orally showed a rapid increase in the number of circulating F reticulocytes.[64] Two of the six patients who received the drug for 5–6 months increased their HbF levels from 10.6% to 18% and 10.4% to 16%, respectively. Because this oral regimen required the intake of 30–40 tablets/day, poor compliance was a major problem that limited the effectiveness of this agent in the outpatient setting.

The potential role of intravenous arginine butyrate in sickle cell disease has recently been revisited.[65] The first six patients who were enrolled in this new study received arginine butyrate infusions 8 hours per day, 5 days per week. The HbF levels increased in half of these patients but the increase in the HbF levels was not sustained with continuous long-term therapy. These observations and those of Sher et al.[63] summarized above suggested that toxicity resulting from long-term exposure to butyrate might be responsible for the loss of the HbF response. Thus, a regimen in which butyrate is given intermittently to allow recovery of the bone marrow from the well-known antiproliferative effects of butyrate was investigated in 11 patients. The HbF levels of the 11 patients enrolled on this regimen increased from a mean of 7.2% at baseline to a mean of 21.0% on intermittent butyrate therapy. This HbF response to butyrate was sustained in all patients, including one patient who received arginine butyrate for more than 6 years [65] Interestingly, all five patients who did not respond to butyrate in both the continuous and intermittent butyrate studies had baseline HbF levels below 2%, whereas all 10 responders had baseline HbF levels of 2% or above.[65]

Because butyrate is an inhibitor of histone deacetylases, it is widely believed, although never proven, that butyrate increases γ-globin gene expression, at least in part, by increasing histone acetylation at its promoter and regulatory elements. Although studies in the murine globin system have shown that butyrate can induce an increase in the acetylation of histone H4 in the globin cluster, those changes were not associated with the reactivation of the silenced genes.[66] The effects of butyrate on the chromatin structure in the γ-globin genes in patients with sickle cell disease and β thalassemia have not yet been investigated.

More recently, it has been recognized that histone deacetylases can exert their effect regionally through their recruitment to DNA in a sequence-specific manner by binding to transcription factor complexes.[67,68] This might explain the specificity of the butyrate effect and also the clinical observation that the HbF-inducing activity of butyrate requires partially active human γ-globin genes whose regulatory elements may already be occupied by transcription complexes. Interestingly, a number of *cis*-acting elements have been identified in the promoter of the γ-globin genes that appear to be necessary for the induction of γ-globin expression by butyrate.[69] Moreover, other studies have demonstrated an important role for the p38 mitogen-activated protein kinase signaling pathway in mediating the transcriptional effects of butyrate.[70] A model was proposed in which butyrate would open the chromatin structure of the γ-globin gene through its effect on histone acetylation and also activate sequence-specific transcription factor binding through its effect on mitogen-activated protein kinase signaling.[71] Recent studies have shown that butyrate can also induce HbF production by increasing the translational efficiency of γ-globin mRNA.[72] More studies are necessary to define clearly the respective roles of these different activities of butyrate on the induction of HbF production in vivo in patients with sickle cell disease and β thalassemia.

CLINICAL EFFICACY OF HbF INDUCTION THERAPY IN SICKLE CELL DISEASE AND β THALASSEMIA AND OTHER HEMOGLOBINOPATHIES

All the pharmacological agents that have been investigated for their HbF-inducing activity in sickle cell disease have also been tested in β thalassemia. This subject has been reviewed in detail elsewhere.[73] Although HbF-inducing activity of these agents has also been demonstrated in patients with β thalassemia, in most, but not all instances, meaningful hematological and/or clinical responses have been much more difficult to demonstrate.[74,75] It is not clear why the increase in HbF levels does not result in the correction of the anemia in a majority of patients with β thalassemia. There are many potential explanations that require more investigation.[76] It is possible that the magnitude of the induction of HbF that can be achieved with the currently available agents might not be sufficient to correct the globin chain imbalance and the resulting anemia. It is also conceivable that the pharmacological agents that are being used might induce the expression of the α-globin genes at the same time that they induce the expression of the γ-globin genes. This will reduce the beneficial effects of the activation of the γ-globin genes on $\alpha/(\beta+\gamma)$ chain imbalance in β thalassemia. Furthermore, the poor responses to pharmacological induction of HbF in β thalassemia could be, at least in part, a result of the suppression of the HbF response by chronic transfusions, which are used much more frequently in β thalassemia than in sickle cell disease. Although sickle cell disease and β thalassemia result from mutations in the same gene, the pathophysiology of the two diseases is quite distinct. Much more research is necessary to understand fully the molecular basis for the different responses to the pharmacological inducers of HbF in patients with sickle cell disease and β thalassemia.

Hydroxyurea has been used to induce HbF expression in patients with HbS–β^+ thalassemia with good success.[77] Although it has also been used to treat rare sickle hemoglobinopathies such as HbSD disease and unstable hemoglobin disorders, too few cases have been reported to allow comment on its clinical efficacy. In HbE–β thalassemia, some patients appear to respond to treatment with an increase in hemoglobin concentration and a reduced or absent transfusion requirement.[78]

COMBINATION THERAPY

Of the five patients in the study previously summarized who were treated with arginine butyrate but did not respond with an increase in HbF levels, three were treated with hydroxyurea. All three increased their HbF levels above 20% in response to hydroxyurea.[65] A majority of patients who do not respond to hydroxyurea increase their HbF levels in response to decitabine.[9] This absence of cross-resistance to the HbF-inducing activities of 5-azacytidine, hydroxyurea, and butyrate confirms the long-held suspicion that these drugs activate γ-globin gene expression by different mechanisms and makes it likely that the use of these agents in combination therapy regimens would induce HbF production in an additive or synergistic manner. This hypothesis has recently been tested in three patients who were enrolled on a combination therapy protocol consisting of hydroxyurea for several months followed by hydroxyurea and butyrate. All three patients had a marked increase in their HbF levels after butyrate was added to hydroxyurea.[23] Thus, the combination of butyrate and hydroxyurea was more effective in these patients than hydroxyurea alone. In one patient who was totally resistant to the effect of butyrate following both weekly and intermittent therapy, addition of butyrate after hydroxyurea therapy resulted in a large-increment increase in the HbF level. This demonstrates that resistance to butyrate is not absolute and can be reversed following pretreatment with hydroxyurea.[23] Similar advantages of combinations of other HbF-inducing agents were previously described in studies of hydroxyurea with erythropoietin[79] and hydroxyurea with sodium phenylbutyrate.[80]

Before conducting large-scale studies of combinations of HbF-inducing agents, it is important to ask if there is a need for the use of combinations of two or more agents in sickle cell disease. The study of the natural history of sickle cell disease had clearly shown that higher HbF levels are associated with a less severe clinical outcome.[5] This, however, does not preclude the possibility that the clinical benefits of increased HbF levels may plateau when the levels exceed 20%. Even though patients from Saudi Arabia whose HbF levels are generally above 20% can have a very mild clinical course, they are not always free of sickling complications.[81] Interestingly, Sutton et al.[82] recently described a patient with sickle cell disease who developed progressive pulmonary hypertension although her HbF level was greater than 20% while receiving hydroxyurea. Addition of butyrate to hydroxyurea in this patient resulted in a peak HbF level of 45% and was associated with in a marked amelioration of the pulmonary hypertension. Although there is no definitive evidence yet that HbF levels of 30%–45% are significantly better than levels of 20%–30%, laboratory data support the hypothesis that such high levels might be necessary to inhibit completely intracellular polymerization of deoxyHbS in red blood cells.[83] Thus, with the current availability of multiple drugs that can activate HbF additively or synergistically, we suggest that the aim of pharmacological therapy should be to achieve the highest possible HbF level rather than to settle for the traditionally accepted level of 20%.

In addition to the drugs that stimulate HbF production, a number of other agents that target different aspects of the pathophysiology of sickle cell disease are under investigation. These include antiadhesive agents, antidehydration agents, and possibly antileukocyte agents (Chapter 31). If these newer agents prove to be effective in clinical trials, it would be of considerable interest to investigate combinations of HbF-inducing agents with these newer agents that target different aspects of the pathophysiology of sickle cell disease. After more than 50 years of intense research on sickle cell disease, we might soon be in a position to select, based on the genotype and/or phenotype of a patient, one or more therapeutic agents that target different aspects of the pathophysiology of sickling. It is gratifying to know that the intense study of the molecular and cellular basis of this disease is finally being translated into novel therapies that could make a significant impact on the lives of patients.

REFERENCES

1. Watson J. The significance of the paucity of sickle cells in newborn negro infants. *Am J Med Sci.* 1948;215:419–423.
2. Perrine RP, Pembrey ME, John P, Perrine S, Shoup F. Natural history of sickle cell anemia in Saudi Arabs. A study of 270 subjects. *Ann Intern Med.* 1978;88(1):1–6.
3. Brittenham G, Lozoff B, Harris JW, Mayson SM, Miller A, Huisman TH. Sickle cell anemia and trait in southern India: further studies. *Am J Hematol.* 1979;6(2):107–123.
4. Platt OS, Thorington BD, Brambilla DJ, et al. Pain in sickle cell disease. Rates and risk factors. *N Engl J Med.* 1991;325(1):11–16.
5. Platt OS, Brambilla DJ, Rosse WF, et al. Mortality in sickle cell disease. Life expectancy and risk factors for early death. *N Engl J Med.* 1994;330(23):1639–1644.
6. Poillon WN, Kim BC, Rodgers GP, Noguchi CT, Schechter AN. Sparing effect of hemoglobin F and hemoglobin A2 on the polymerization of hemoglobin S at physiologic ligand saturations. *Proc Natl Acad Sci USA.* 1993;90(11):5039–5043.
7. Mavilio F, Giampaolo A, Care A, et al. Molecular mechanisms of human hemoglobin switching: selective undermethylation and expression of globin genes in embryonic, fetal, and adult erythroblasts. *Proc Natl Acad Sci USA.* 1983;80(22):6907–6911.
8. Jones PA, Taylor SM. Cellular differentiation, cytidine analogs and DNA methylation. *Cell.* 1980;20(1):85–93.
9. Koshy M, Dorn L, Bressler L, et al. 2-deoxy 5-azacytidine and fetal hemoglobin induction in sickle cell anemia. *Blood.* 2000;96(7):2379–2384.
10. Juttermann R, Li E, Jaenisch R. Toxicity of 5-aza-2′-deoxycytidine to mammalian cells is mediated primarily by covalent trapping of DNA methyltransferase rather than DNA demethylation. *Proc Natl Acad Sci USA.* 1994;91(25):11797–11801.
11. Heller P, DeSimone J. 5-Azacytidine and fetal hemoglobin. *Am J Hematol.* 1984;17(4):439–447.
12. Ley TJ, DeSimone J, Anagnou NP, et al. 5-azacytidine selectively increases gamma-globin synthesis in a patient with beta+ thalassemia. *N Engl J Med.* 1982;307(24):1469–1475.
13. Ley TJ, DeSimone J, Noguchi CT, et al. 5-Azacytidine increases gamma-globin synthesis and reduces the proportion of dense cells in patients with sickle cell anemia. *Blood.* 1983;62(2):370–380.
14. Charache S, Dover G, Smith K, Talbot CC Jr, Moyer M, Boyer S. Treatment of sickle cell anemia with 5-azacytidine results in increased fetal hemoglobin production and is associated with nonrandom hypomethylation of DNA around the gamma-delta-beta-globin gene complex. *Proc Natl Acad Sci USA.* 1983;80(15):4842–4846.
15. Humphries RK, Dover G, Young NS, et al. 5-Azacytidine acts directly on both erythroid precursors and progenitors to increase production of fetal hemoglobin. *J Clin Invest.* 1985; 75(2):547–557.
16. Lowrey CH, Nienhuis AW. Brief report: treatment with azacitidine of patients with end-stage beta-thalassemia. *N Engl J Med.* 1993;329(12):845–848.
17. Carr BI, Reilly JG, Smith SS, Winberg C, Riggs A. The tumorigenicity of 5-azacytidine in the male Fischer rat. *Carcinogenesis.* 1984;5(12):1583–1590.
18. Carr BI, Rahbar S, Asmeron Y, Riggs A, Winberg CD. Carcinogenicity and haemoglobin synthesis induction by cytidine analogues. *Br J Cancer.* 1988;57(4):395–402.
19. Charache S, Terrin ML, Moore RD, et al. Effect of hydroxyurea on the frequency of painful crises in sickle cell anemia. Investigators of the Multicenter Study of Hydroxyurea in Sickle Cell Anemia. *N Engl J Med.* 1995;332(20):1317–1322.
20. DeSimone J, Koshy M, Dorn L, et al. Maintenance of elevated fetal hemoglobin levels by decitabine during dose interval treatment of sickle cell anemia. *Blood.* 2002;99(11):3905–3908.
21. Saunthararajah Y, Hillery CA, Lavelle D, et al. Effects of 5-aza-2′-deoxycytidine on fetal hemoglobin levels, red cell adhesion, and hematopoietic differentiation in patients with sickle cell disease. *Blood.* 2003;102(12):3865–38670.
22. Milhem M, Mahmud N, Lavelle D, et al. Modification of hematopoietic stem cell fate by 5aza 2′deoxycytidine and trichostatin A. *Blood.* 2004;103(11):4102–4110.

23. Atweh GF, DeSimone J, Saunthararajah Y, et al. Hemoglobinopathies. *Am Soc Hematol Educ Program.* 2003:14–39.
24. Rodgers GP, Saunthararajah Y. Advances in experimental treatment of beta-thalassaemia. *Expert Opin Investig Drugs.* 2001;10(5):925–934.
25. Saunthararajah Y, Molokie R, Saraf S, et al. Clinical effectiveness of decitabine in severe sickle cell disease. *Br J Haematol.* 2008;141(1):126–129.
26. Stamatoyannopoulos G. Control of globin gene expression during development and erythroid differentiation. *Exp Hematol.* 2005;33(3):259–271.
27. Letvin NL, Linch DC, Beardsley GP, McIntyre KW, Nathan DG. Augmentation of fetal-hemoglobin production in anemic monkeys by hydroxyurea. *N Engl J Med.* 1984;310(14): 869–873.
28. Platt OS, Orkin SH, Dover G, Beardsley GP, Miller B, Nathan DG. Hydroxyurea enhances fetal hemoglobin production in sickle cell anemia. *J Clin Invest.* 1984;74(2):652–656.
29. Rodgers GP, Steinberg MH. Pharmacologic treatment of sickle cell disease and thalassemia: the augmentation of fetal hemoglobin. In: Steinberg MH, Forget BG, Higgs DR, Nagel RL, eds. *Disorders of Hemoglobin: Genetics, Pathophysiology, and Clinical Management.* 1st ed. Cambridge: Cambridge University Press; 2001:1028–1051.
30. Steinberg MH, Rodgers GP. Pharmacologic modulation of fetal hemoglobin. *Medicine (Baltimore).* 2001;80(5):328–344.
31. Hankins JS, Ware RE, Rogers ZR, et al. Long-term hydroxyurea therapy for infants with sickle cell anemia – the Husoft extension study. *Blood.* 2005;106:2269–2275.
32. Ferster A, Tahriri P, Vermylen C, et al. Five years of experience with hydroxyurea in children and young adults with sickle cell disease. *Blood.* 2001;97(11):3628–3632.
33. Charache S, Dover GJ, Moyer MA, Moore JW. Hydroxyurea-induced augmentation of fetal hemoglobin production in patients with sickle cell anemia. *Blood.* 1987;69(1):109–116.
34. Rodgers GP, Dover GJ, Noguchi CT, Schechter AN, Nienhuis AW. Hematologic responses of patients with sickle cell disease to treatment with hydroxyurea. *N Engl J Med.* 1990;322(15): 1037–1045.
35. Ballas SK, Barton FB, Waclawiw MA, et al. Hydroxyurea and sickle cell anemia: effect on quality of life. *Health Qual Life Outcomes.* 2006;4:59–66.
36. Steinberg MH, Barton F, Castro O, et al. Effect of hydroxyurea on mortality and morbidity in adult sickle cell anemia: risks and benefits up to 9 years of treatment. *JAMA.* 2003;289(13):1645–1651.
37. Ware RE, Eggleston B, Redding-Lallinger R, et al. Predictors of fetal hemoglobin response in children with sickle cell anemia receiving hydroxyurea therapy. *Blood.* 2002;99(1):10–14.
38. Gulbis B, Haberman D, Dufour D, et al. Hydroxyurea for sickle cell disease in children and for prevention of cerebrovascular events: the Belgian experience. *Blood.* 2005;105(7):2685–2690.
39. Wang WC, Wynn LW, Rogers ZR, Scott JP, Lane PA, Ware RE. A two-year pilot trial of hydroxyurea in very young children with sickle-cell anemia. *J Pediatr.* 2001;139(6):790–796.
40. Wang WC, Helms RW, Lynn HS, et al. Effect of hydroxyurea on growth in children with sickle cell anemia: results of the HUG-KIDS Study. *J Pediatr.* 2002;140(2):225–229.
41. de Montelembert M, Brousse V, Elie C, Bernaudin F, Shi J, Landais P. Long-term hydroxyurea treatment in children with sickle cell disease: tolerance and clinical outcomes. *Haematologica.* 2006;91(1):125–128.
42. Zimmerman SA, Schultz WH, Davis JS, et al. Sustained long-term hematologic efficacy of hydroxyurea at maximum tolerated dose in children with sickle cell disease. *Blood.* 2004; 103(6):2039–2045.
43. Ware RE, Zimmerman SA, Schultz WH. Hydroxyurea as an alternative to blood transfusions for the prevention of recurrent stroke in children with sickle cell disease. *Blood.* 1999; 94(9):3022–3026.
44. Zimmerman SA, Schultz WH, Burgett S, Mortier NA, Ware RE. Hydroxyurea therapy lowers transcranial Doppler flow velocities in children with sickle cell anemia. *Blood.* 2007; 110(3):1043–1047.
45. Kratovil T, Bulas D, Driscoll MC, Speller-Brown B, McCarter R, Minniti CP. Hydroxyurea therapy lowers TCD velocities in children with sickle cell disease. *Pediatr Blood Cancer.* 2006; 47(7):894–900.
46. Wang WC. The pathophysiology, prevention, and treatment of stroke in sickle cell disease. *Curr Opin Hematol.* 2007;14(3): 191–197.
47. Ware RE, Zimmerman SA, Sylvestre PB, et al. Prevention of secondary stroke and resolution of transfusional iron overload in children with sickle cell anemia using hydroxyurea and phlebotomy. *J Pediatr.* 2004;145(3):346–352.
48. Miller MK, Zimmerman SA, Schultz WH, Ware RE. Hydroxyurea therapy for pediatric patients with hemoglobin SC disease. *J Pediatr Hematol Oncol.* 2001;23(5):306–308.
49. Steinberg MH, Nagel RL, Brugnara C. Cellular effects of hydroxyurea in Hb SC disease. *Br J Haematol.* 1997;98(4):838–844.
50. Bakanay SM, Dainer E, Clair B, et al. Mortality in sickle cell patients on hydroxyurea therapy. *Blood.* 2004;105:545–547.
51. Hanft VN, Fruchtman SR, Pickens CV, Rosse WF, Howard TA, Ware RE. Acquired DNA mutations associated with in vivo hydroxyurea exposure. *Blood.* 2000; 95(11):3589–3593.
52. Ma Q, Wyszynski DF, Farrell JJ, et al. Fetal hemoglobin in sickle cell anemia: genetic determinants of response to hydroxyurea. *Pharmacogenomics J.* 2007;7:386–394.
53. Cokic VP, Smith RD, Beleslin-Cokic BB, et al. Hydroxyurea induces fetal hemoglobin by the nitric oxide-dependent activation of soluble guanylyl cyclase. *J Clin Invest.* 2003;111(2): 231–239.
54. Saleh AW, Hillen HF, Duits AJ. Levels of endothelial, neutrophil and platelet-specific factors in sickle cell anemia patients during hydroxyurea therapy. *Acta Haematol.* 1999; 102(1):31–37.
55. Bridges KR, Barabino GD, Brugnara C, et al. A multiparameter analysis of sickle erythrocytes in patients undergoing hydroxyurea therapy. *Blood.* 1996;88(12):4701–4710.
56. Charache S, Barton FB, Moore RD, et al. Hydroxyurea and sickle cell anemia. Clinical utility of a myelosuppressive "switching" agent. The Multicenter Study of Hydroxyurea in Sickle Cell Anemia. *Medicine (Baltimore).* 1996;75(6):300–326.
57. Ginder GD, Whitters MJ, Pohlman JK. Activation of a chicken embryonic globin gene in adult erythroid cells by 5-azacytidine and sodium butyrate. *Proc Natl Acad Sci USA.* 1984;81(13):3954–3958.
58. Perrine SP, Greene MF, Faller DV. Delay in the fetal globin switch in infants of diabetic mothers. *N Engl J Med.* 1985; 312(6):334–338.

59. Bard H, Prosmanne J. Relative rates of fetal hemoglobin and adult hemoglobin synthesis in cord blood of infants of insulin-dependent diabetic mothers. *Pediatrics.* 1985;75(6): 1143–1147.
60. Perrine SP, Rudolph A, Faller DV, et al. Butyrate infusions in the ovine fetus delay the biologic clock for globin gene switching. *Proc Natl Acad Sci USA.* 1988;85(22):8540–8542.
61. Constantoulakis P, Papayannopoulou T, Stamatoyannopoulos G. Alpha-amino-N-butyric acid stimulates fetal hemoglobin in the adult. *Blood.* 1988;72(6):1961–1967.
62. Perrine SP, Ginder GD, Faller DV, et al. A short-term trial of butyrate to stimulate fetal-globin-gene expression in the beta-globin disorders. *N Engl J Med.* 1993;328(2):81–86.
63. Sher GD, Ginder GD, Little J, Yang S, Dover GJ, Olivieri NF. Extended therapy with intravenous arginine butyrate in patients with beta-hemoglobinopathies. *N Engl J Med.* 1995;332(24):1606–1610.
64. Dover GJ, Brusilow S, Charache S. Induction of fetal hemoglobin production in subjects with sickle cell anemia by oral sodium phenylbutyrate. *Blood.* 1994;84(1):339–343.
65. Atweh GF, Sutton M, Nassif I, et al. Sustained induction of fetal hemoglobin by pulse butyrate therapy in sickle cell disease. *Blood.* 1999;93(6):1790–1797.
66. Forsberg EC, Downs KM, Christensen HM, Im H, Nuzzi PA, Bresnick EH. Developmentally dynamic histone acetylation pattern of a tissue-specific chromatin domain. *Proc Natl Acad Sci USA.* 2000;97(26):14494–14499.
67. Heinzel T, Lavinsky RM, Mullen TM, et al. A complex containing N-CoR, mSin3 and histone deacetylase mediates transcriptional repression. *Nature.* 1997;387(6628):43–48.
68. Laherty CD, Yang WM, Sun JM, Davie JR, Seto E, Eisenman RN. Histone deacetylases associated with the mSin3 corepressor mediate mad transcriptional repression. *Cell.* 1997;89(3):349–356.
69. Pace BS, Chen YR, Thompson A, Goodman SR. Butyrate-inducible elements in the human gamma-globin promoter. *Exp Hematol.* 2000;28(3):283–293.
70. Pace BS, Qian XH, Sangerman J, et al. p38 MAP kinase activation mediates gamma-globin gene induction in erythroid progenitors. *Exp Hematol.* 2003;31(11):1089–1096.
71. Pace BS, Zein S. Understanding mechanisms of gamma-globin gene regulation to develop strategies for pharmacological fetal hemoglobin induction. *Dev Dyn.* 2006;235(7): 1727–1737.
72. Weinberg RS, Ji X, Sutton M, et al. Butyrate increases the efficiency of translation of gamma-globin mRNA. *Blood.* 2005;105(4):1807–1809.
73. Atweh GF, Loukopoulos D. Pharmacological induction of fetal hemoglobin in sickle cell disease and beta-thalassemia. *Semin Hematol.* 2001;38(4):367–373.
74. Karimi M, Darzi H, Yavarian M. Hematologic and clinical responses of thalassemia intermedia patients to hydroxyurea during 6 years of therapy in Iran. *J Pediatr Hematol Oncol.* 2005;27(7):380–385.
75. Bradai M, Abad MT, Pissard S, Lamraoui F, Skopinski L, De Montalembert M. Hydroxyurea can eliminate transfusion requirements in children with severe beta-thalassemia. *Blood.* 2003;102(4):1529–1530.
76. Fathallah H, Sutton M, Atweh GF. Pharmacological induction of fetal hemoglobin: Why haven't we been more successful in thalassemia? *Ann NY Acad Sci.* 2005;1054:228–237.
77. Loukopoulos D, Voskaridou E, Kalotychou V, Schina M, Loutradi A, Theodoropoulos I. Reduction of the clinical severity of sickle cell/b-thalassemia with hydroxyurea: The experience of a single center in Greece. *Blood Cells Mol Dis.* 2000;26(5):453–466.
78. Singer ST, Kuypers FA, Olivieri NF, et al. Fetal haemoglobin augmentation in E/beta(0) thalassaemia: clinical and haematological outcome. *Br J Haematol.* 2005;131(3):378–388.
79. Rodgers GP, Dover GJ, Uyesaka N, Noguchi CT, Schechter AN, Nienhuis AW. Augmentation by erythropoietin of the fetal-hemoglobin response to hydroxyurea in sickle cell disease. *N Engl J Med.* 1993;328(2):73–80.
80. Olivieri NF, Rees DC, Ginder GD, et al. Treatment of thalassaemia major with phenylbutyrate and hydroxyurea. *Lancet.* 1997;350(9076):491–492.
81. Al-Jam'a AH, Al-Dabbous IA. Hydroxyurea in sickle cell disease patients from Eastern Saudi Arabia. *Saudi Med J.* 2002;23(3):277–281.
82. Atweh GF, Schechter AN. Pharmacologic induction of fetal hemoglobin: raising the therapeutic bar in sickle cell disease. *Curr Opin Hematol.* 2001;8(2):123–130.
83. Noguchi CT, Rodgers GP, Serjeant G, Schechter AN. Levels of fetal hemoglobin necessary for treatment of sickle cell disease. *N Engl J Med.* 1988;318(2):96–99.

31

Novel Approaches to Treatment

Kirkwood A. Pritchard Jr, Alicia Rivera, Cheryl Hillery, and Carlo Brugnara

INTRODUCTION

Sickle cell disease and β thalassemia should be ideal genetic disorders for which to design specific therapies at the cellular, protein, or gene levels. First, normal and abnormal differentiated cells, bone marrow precursors, progenitors, and hematopoietic stem cells are easily obtained for ex vivo studies. Second, specific mutations of the β hemoglobin gene have been characterized; the abnormal structure of sickled hemoglobin (HbS) detailed at atomic resolution is available, the secondary cellular defects and, beyond the erythrocyte itself, the interactions of the defective erythrocytes with other blood or vascular components are better understood. Third, mouse models are available for in vivo evaluation of new therapies. Despite a detailed understanding of the genetics, molecular biology, and biochemistry of HbS and β thalassemia and their effects on the host erythrocyte, the pathogenesis of the organ and vascular dysfunctions observed in both sickle cell disease and β thalassemia remain incompletely understood and likely involve many complex and heterogeneous steps.

The complex pathophysiology of sickle cell disease, as detailed in earlier chapters, involves erythrocyte dehydration and interactions of sickle erythrocytes, leukocytes and platelets with the endothelium, and hemolysis, among many other factors.[1] Severity of disease differs significantly among patients, whereas the HbS mutation is common to all patients (Chapter 27). Therefore, the original idea that a single pathophysiological mechanism, whose basis is polymerization of deoxygenated HbS that leads to sickling, is inadequate to explain the myriad of clinical variations. This has prompted studies of factors that can potentially modulate sickle vasoocclusion and disease severity.[2–4] It is believed that vasoocclusion begins with a delay in the flow of the sickle erythrocyte through the vasculature, thereby allowing HbS sufficient time to polymerize. In this scenario, the integrity of microvascular endothelial cell monolayer and postcapillary venule play important roles in maintaining steady flow and preventing entrapment of dehydrated sickle erythrocytes. Consequently, inflammatory factors that mediate or alter cell adherence to the endothelium and/or modulate erythrocyte hydration status will likely affect vasoocclusion. Some of these factors include cytokines, adhesive receptors, and oxidized proinflammatory lipids that have been found to be elevated in sickle cell disease and often correlate with disease severity. Thus, besides anticellular dehydration therapy, additional therapies targeting adhesion, inflammation as well as oxidation might be required for optimal protecting against sickle vasoocclusion, painful episodes, and chronic organ injury.

As described in other chapters of this book, cellular therapies – transfusions and hematopoietic stem cell transplantation – have important drawbacks and limitations. New agents activating fetal hemoglobin (HbF) expression are very useful; however, these agents are not without risk and up to now have offered minor benefits for patients with β thalassemia. Finally, hemoglobin gene therapy remains a treatment goal for the future. Consequently, therapies aimed at alleviating the cellular and vascular defects of hemoglobinopathies remain an area of intense research.

Hemoglobin Modifiers

Sickle Cell Disease

Initial attempts at developing specific therapies for sickle cell disease were aimed at decreasing HbS polymerization.[5] Nitrite-generating methemoglobin[6] and carbon monoxide (CO)[7] were tested in an attempt to decrease the proportion of HbS molecules in the deoxy conformation, which promotes polymerization. The incidence of painful sickle cell episodes, used as a criterion for efficacy, was not decreased in these clinical trials. After observing that urea inhibited HbS gelation and sickling of erythrocytes[8] clinical trials with urea were undertaken. The results from these studies were disappointing.[9] Cyanate, which is derived from urea in solution, was also shown to inhibit sickling and HbS polymerization[10] and on the basis of these in vitro findings was tested as a potential treatment for sickle cell disease.[11] The initial attempt was encouraging, decreasing hemolysis and anemia. Cyanate-dependent carbamoylation of the N-terminal amino group of both α- and β-globin chains increased directly the oxygen affinity and the solubility of HbS. Nonetheless one of the major goals of the study, reduction in painful sickle cell episodes, was not achieved. Side effects, such as cataracts and peripheral neuropathy also occurred, thereby prompting the end of clinical trials with oral potassium cyanate.

The design of antisickling agents targeting the hemoglobin molecule has improved with the precise knowledge

Table 31.1. Hemoglobin modifiers as antisickling agents

Agents	Drawbacks
Noncovalent reagents	
Nonspecific reagents	
Urea, organic solvent	High concentration required
Aromatic alcohols or acids	Small and nonspecific effects
Stereospecific inhibitors	
Aromatic acid derivatives	Small effects
Peptides	High concentration required
Organic compounds	
Covalent reagents	
Targeting terminal residues (cyanate, pyridoxal, tucaresol)	Toxicity Immunostimulant
Targeting side chains (glyceraldehyde, nitrogen mustard)	Toxicity
Targeting 2,3-BPG binding site (Diaspirin)	Toxicity
Nitric oxide	Under evaluation

of hemoglobin tertiary structure and allosteric conformations at the atomic level.[12–16] Several potential antisickling agents have been investigated. Table 31.1 summarizes the major potential antisickling agents that have been investigated. Various types of chemically reactive compounds were able to inhibit intermolecular contact or increase the oxygen affinity of HbS. Nitrogen mustards and other alkylating agents,[17] pyridoxal and other aldehydes forming Schiff base adducts,[18–21] esterifying agents,[22] Sulfhydryl reagents targeting cysteine β93,[23] and bifunctional agents,[24] which form intra- or intermolecular crosslinks, were found to be efficient antisickling compounds. Bis(3,5-dibromosalicyl)fumarate crosslinked β 82 lysine residues in the central cavity prevent the binding of 2,3 bisphosphoglycerate and stabilize the deoxy conformation of HbS.[25] Unfortunately, the poor specificity and the toxicity of many of these antisickling agents precluded clinical trials.

At one time, the cyclic aldehyde compounds offered more promising treatment strategies. The initial reagent 12C79 (BW12C) was very efficient in increasing the oxygen affinity of sickle erythrocytes in vitro,[26] or when infused in normal adults in a phase I clinical trial.[27] BW12C specifically bound to the N terminus of α-globin chains[28] and prevented hypoxia-induced death in the SAD transgenic model of sickle cell disease (Chapter 12).[29] The orally active derivative 589C80 (Tucaresol) increased the oxygen affinity and reduced hemolysis in six patients with sickle cell anemia.[30] The oxygen affinity of HbS was increased between 10% and 20% in all patients, depending on the dose. Increases in the hemoglobin level (mean + 2.2 g/dL), 50% decreases in irreversibly sickled cells and decreased hemolysis as measured by a drop in lactate dehydrogenase (16%–52%) were obtained within a few days from initiating therapy and lasted for 1–2 weeks. Three patients developed fever and tender lymphadenopathy between days 7 and 11 from the start of the drug. Schiff base formation on specific amines of the T-cell surface provided a costimulatory signal that activated Na^+ and K^+ transport, enhancing T-cell receptor dependent interleukin (IL)-2 production.[31–33] Therefore, there are no ongoing or planned trials of Tucaresol in sickle cell disease. Other cyclic aldehyde compounds have lower T-cell potentiation and maintain very efficient hemoglobin binding and a left shift of the red cell oxygen dissociation curve.[34,35] Agents that increase the oxygen affinity of HbS could also increase the red cell mass and blood viscosity. Thus, their use might be limited to short-term therapy of severe sickle cell crises in hospitalized patients.

Fifty years after the discovery of sickle hemoglobin and despite the many experimental advantages this single gene mutation affords for studying sickle cell disease, none of the hundreds of antisickling agents that were shown to inhibit HbS polymerization in vitro are in clinical use today. One reason these agents might not have worked is that hemoglobin is at very high concentrations within the erythrocyte, approximately 5 mmol, representing nearly a third of the erythrocyte's mass. As abnormal red cells have fast turnovers, large quantities of therapeutic drugs are required for binding to red cell hemoglobin on an ongoing basis. In addition to preventing HbS polymerization, the effective therapeutic agent should not affect the physiological functions of hemoglobin. The agent has to be not only specific for hemoglobin but also nontoxic at its effective dose. Today, tremendous progress in molecular drug design and the recently refined structure of HbS polymer at 2.05 Å resolution[36] make it possible for screening of new hemoglobin modifiers with specific antisickling properties. The specific inhibition of intermolecular contacts within the HbS molecule by agents that do not affect the oxygen affinity of HbS remains a major goal.

β Thalassemia

Hemoglobin modifiers targeting α-globin chains could be useful therapies in β thalassemia major, the severity of which is related to the excess of unpaired α hemoglobin chains, which are cytotoxic. These unstable α chains oxidize, precipitate, and form Heinz bodies in erythroid cells.

Reduction in α chain instability, heme oxidation and release, could transform thalassemia major into a thalassemia intermedia syndrome, as shown by the clinical benefit of increasing the expression of γ-globin chains of HbF or by coinheritance of α thalassemia determinants, both of which decrease the relative excess of α-globin chains.

α Hemoglobin stabilizing protein (AHSP) (Chapter 4) is a recently described abundant erythroid protein that specifically binds to and stabilizes free α-globin, thereby limiting its prooxidant activities.[37] When β-globin subunits are present, AHSP is displaced, permitting the formation of HbA ($\alpha_2\beta_2$). AHSP-deficient mice have hemolytic anemia with hemoglobin precipitates and reticulocytosis, reflecting an essential role for AHSP in erythropoiesis.[37] AHSP appears to function as both a chaperone to optimize the correct folding of newly synthesized α-globin[38] as well as a stabilizer of free α hemoglobin (α-globin with heme), whereby the heme iron becomes detoxified by binding to two histidines within the α-globin polypeptide.[39] In agreement with this protective role, AHSP deficiency exacerbates the β thalassemia phenotype in mice.[40] It is possible that variations in AHSP function or expression could affect the phenotype of human β thalassemia by restraining the toxicity of free α-globin (Chapter 27).[41]

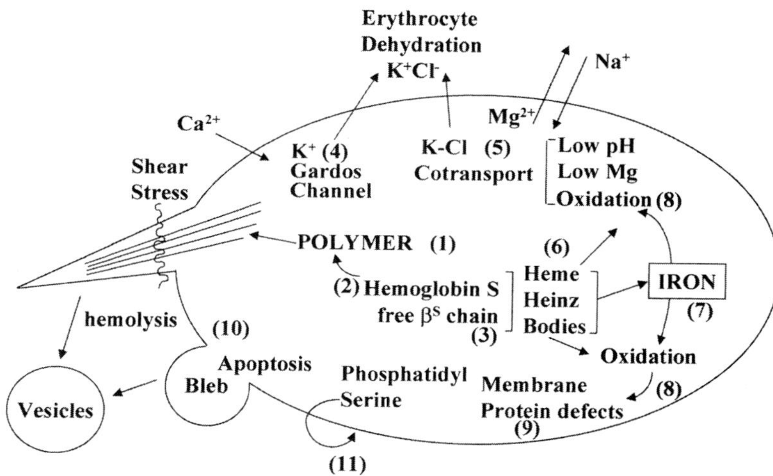

Figure 31.1. Sites of red cell physiology that are targets of experimental therapies. Sickle hemoglobin polymer and free β^S-globin chains, primary defects in sickle cell anemia, are shown in red; secondary defects are shown in green, and tertiary defects in black. (See color plate 31.1.).

In HbH disease, despite a similar degree of hemoglobin chain imbalance, the self-association of β-globin chains into nonfunctional β_4 tetramers, or HbH, induces a less severe anemia, which is mostly hemolytic in contrast to the ineffective erythropoiesis prevalent in β thalassemia major.

Inhibitors of Erythrocyte Dehydration

Sickle Cell Disease

Intracellular concentration of HbS is a major factor for HbS polymerization as the delay time of polymer formation is dependent on the 15th–30th power of hemoglobin concentration.[42] In most physiological conditions hemoglobin polymers are not present in erythrocytes of sickle cell trait carriers who are asymptomatic because the HbS concentration is 13–14 g/dL in cells, which is below the threshold value for polymerization (Chapter 22).

In sickle cell anemia, polymerization of HbS with subsequent cellular dehydration likely plays a major role in the expression of the disease. A substantial number of abnormally dense erythrocytes result from polymerization-induced membrane damage, leading to cell dehydration.[43,44] Because the polymerization process is highly dependent on HbS concentration, these dense erythrocytes are likely to rapidly accumulate HbS polymers at decreased pO2, become distorted and rigid, and contribute to vasoocclusive and hemolytic defects.

Important contributors to sickle cell dehydration are potassium–chloride cotransport (KCl efflux) and the Ca^{2+}-activated K^+ channel, the so-called Gardos channel[45] (Chapter 9). Deoxygenation-induced HbS polymer formation leads to increased membrane permeability to cations, including Ca^{2+} and Mg^{2+}. The transient increase in cellular ionized Ca^{2+} is sufficient to trigger activity of the K^+ channel resulting in water loss. In sickle cell disease, K:Cl cotransport is activated by low pH,[46] low Mg^{2+} content of erythrocytes, oxidative damage, positively charged hemoglobins like HbS, HbC, and HbE, and cell swelling (Fig. 31.1).

Water retention using antidiuretic therapy (desmopressin) and a low-sodium diet was an initial attempt to decrease cellular HbS concentration by inducing hypotonic cell swelling.[47,48] The practical difficulty was in maintaining a significant hyponatremia, and a second trial[49] failed to confirm the initial beneficial results. This nonselective approach to erythrocyte hydration was associated with neurotoxicity. Cetiedil, a membrane active agent that has a low affinity for the Gardos channel and that increases Na^+ permeability, was shown to have some beneficial effects in reducing sickle cell painful events;[50,51] however, no further clinical study of this agent has been conducted. Ca^{2+} channel blockers (Verapamil, Diltiazem, Bepridil, Nifedipine, and Nitrendipine) inhibit sickling and erythrocyte dehydration in vitro [52] but had few effects in vivo. Other membrane modifiers that have an erythrocyte swelling effect, such as Monensin, Tellurite, Nystatin, and Chlorpromazine, have been studied only in vitro.

Blockade of Ca^{2+}-activated K^+ Channel (Gardos Channel)

Clotrimazole and other imidazole antimycotics have been shown to be potent blockers of the Gardos channel in vitro.[53,54] Among imidazoles, clotrimazole is the most potent inhibitor, whereas econazole and miconazole are the most potent inhibitors of plasma membrane Ca^{2+} channels.[53] In vitro studies with human sickle cells indicate that clotrimazole can specifically prevent red cell dehydration and K^+ loss through Gardos channel inhibition.[55]

The efficacy of clotrimazole as a specific inhibitor of the Gardos channel was evaluated in vivo in the SAD mouse (Chapter 12).[56] These mice show clinical and biological features similar to those observed in HbSC disease. The effect of oral administration of clotrimazole was studied during a 4-week period. Oral administration of clotrimazole (160 mg/kg/d) induced a significant inhibition of the Ca^{2+}-activated Rb^+ transport measured in whole blood and restored the red cell volume after 48 hours of administration. These effects persisted during the 28 days of treatment.[56] The inhibition of the Gardos channel was associated with increased erythrocyte K^+ content, decreased mean corpuscular hemoglobin concentration (MCHC), and decreased red cell density. All of these changes were reversible within 2 days after clotrimazole was withdrawn at day 7 or 28 of treatment. No toxicity and side effects were observed.

Studies with normal volunteers taking clotrimazole orally identified a dosage range of 10–20 mg/kg of body weight per day that caused marked inhibition of the Gardos channel.[57] This dosage is substantially lower than that used in the treatment of systemic mycosis (100–160 mg/kg/d).[58,59] Clotrimazole metabolites lacking the imidazole ring were detectable in plasma. These metabolites have no antimycotic effects but they maintain a substantial inhibitory activity on the Gardos channel.

A short-term study was performed in sickle cell anemia patients who were treated with clotrimazole at a dosage of 10–30 mg/kg/day. This treatment induced an inhibition of the Gardos channel, a decrease in red cell dehydration and an increase in red cell K^+ content.[60] The effects of clotrimazole on red cells were more evident in patients with a significant number of dense cells at baseline. Adverse side effects were limited to mild/moderate dysuria in all subjects, likely due to urinary excretion of clotrimazole metabolites, and a reversible increase in plasma alanine transaminase and aspartic transaminase levels in two subjects treated with clotrimazole at the dosage of 30 mg/kg/day.

A novel inhibitor of the Gardos channel (ICA-17043) was developed based on the structure of clotrimazole metabolites. This compound showed increased potency in vitro compared with clotrimazole[61] and favorable pharmacokinetic properties with no serious toxicities.[62] Phase II studies showed that administration of ICA-17043 at the dose of 10 mg/kg/day resulted in significant improvement of anemia and reduction in hemolysis and reticulocytosis in patients with sickle cell disease.[63]

This study was followed by a phase III study (ClinicalTrials.gov identifier: NCT00102791) modeled after the trial that led to the approval of hydroxyurea in early 1990s, with painful events as the primary endpoint. ICA-17403 reduced hemolysis without toxicity, but the trial was terminated prematurely because of the low probability of achieving its primary endpoint, which was a reduction in vasoocclusive events. ICA-17403 is able to reduce the hemolytic rate, probably because it reduces on sickle erythrocyte density. More than 20 years ago, it was noted that coincident α thalassemia, which is associated with reduced cell density and reduced hemolysis in sickle cell anemia, was not associated with a reduction in the number of vasoocclusive events and might have been associated with an increased number of complications that dependent on blood viscosity (Chapters 11 and 19). This suggested that a drug that reduces hemolysis without effecting the intracellular hemoglobin composition might benefit some but not all disease complications. Although some patients enrolled in the phase III trial of ICA-17403 received hydroxyurea, no attempt was made to ensure that HbF levels were maximized. In future trials, it might be wise to craft endpoints that take into account the hemolytic complications of disease, which include premature death, but at this time, no further studies are planned for ICA-17043 in sickle cell disease.

Inhibition of KCl Transport by Mg^{2+}

K:Cl cotransport promotes loss of K^+ and Cl^- with subsequent erythrocyte dehydration and is activated when erythrocytes are exposed to different conditions such as pH lower than 7.40, swelling in hypotonic media, low intracellular Mg^{2+} content and positively charged hemoglobin variants such as HbS or HbC.[64,65] Pharmacological inhibitors of this pathway that could be used to prevent cell dehydration in vivo do not exist. [(Dihydroindenyl)oxy]alkanoic acid can inhibit the K:Cl cotransport system but it is not active at a low enough concentration to be used in vivo.[66]

K:Cl cotransport is exquisitely sensitive to cell Mg^{2+} concentration, and a slight increase in cell Mg^{2+} induces marked inhibition of K:Cl cotransport.[67] When cell Mg^{2+} is increased, Cl^- moves into the cell to compensate for the positively charged ions, with an obligatory osmotic water influx and consequent cell swelling.[68] There have been reports of abnormally low cell Mg^{2+} content in sickle erythrocytes, especially in the dense fractions containing irreversibly sickled cells.[69,70]

The effects of oral Mg^{2+} supplementation have been studied in the SAD mouse.[71] In this mouse strain, oral Mg^{2+} supplementation (1,000 $\pm$ 20 mg/kg of body weight/day) restored red cell Mg^{2+} and K^+ content, and reduced K:Cl cotransport activity, MCHC, and cell density. A Mg^{2+}-deficient diet led to worsening anemia, reticulocytosis, and dehydration of SAD mouse red cells, associated with increased K:Cl cotransport activity. Oral Mg^{2+} supplementation prevented additional erythrocyte dehydration and K^+ loss caused by hypoxemia.

Studies in diabetic patients have shown that dietary Mg^{2+} supplementation with magnesium pidolate can increase red cell Mg^{2+} content.[72,73] Based on the SAD mouse experiments, the effects of oral Mg^{2+} supplementation were evaluated on red cell dehydration in sickle cell anemia.[74] Magnesium pidolate at a dose of 0.6 mEq/kg/day was used as oral supplementation in 10 sickle cell anemia patients. Four weeks of treatment induced an increase in red cell Mg^{2+} and K^+, and a decrease in the activity of K:Cl cotransport. There were no laboratory or clinical signs of hypermagnesemia, and mild, transient diarrhea was the only reported side effect. A pilot study, using magesium pidolate for 6 months, confirmed the beneficial effects on red cell dehydration and demonstrated a 58% reduction in the number of painful days.[75]

Mg^{2+} supplementation remains a promising therapeutic approach for preventing red cell dehydration in sickle cell disease, especially in HbSC disease in which K:Cl transport is most active. Its use in combination with other agents seems most attractive. A maximum tolerated dose for magnesium pidolate of 0.9 mEq/kg/day has been established when combined with hydroxyurea in children with sickle cell anemia.[76] A phase I trial of magnesium pidolate plus hydroxyurea has been completed in children with sickle cell anemia (NCT00143572). As of this writing a randomized, placebo-controlled phase II trial to evaluate the effects of long-term Mg^{2+} supplementation in patients with HbSC disease, as a single agent and in combination with hydroxyurea (NCT00532883) is ongoing.

β Thalassemia

Mg^{2+} supplementation ameliorated the anemia in a mouse model of β thalassemia[77] and decreased red cell dehydration in human β thalassemia intermedia.[78] Because there was no improvement of anemia in human β thalassemia, the relative dehydration of thalassemic cells does not seem to be critical in the pathogenesis of anemia. Thus, Mg^{2+} supplementation is not likely to be a viable therapeutic strategy for the treatment of anemia in thalassemia.

Antiadhesion Therapy

Sickle Cell Disease

The increased adhesion of sickle erythrocytes to vascular endothelium (Chapter 8) in vitro has been described when using both static adhesion assays[79,80] and endothelialized flow chambers.[81] These observations have been confirmed using live animal models by either infusing human sickle erythrocytes into rats[82–84] or by studying transgenic sickle cell mice.[85,86] In addition, leukocyte interactions with sickle erythrocyte and vascular endothelium likely contribute to the vascular pathologies observed in sickle cell disease.[87] The enhanced interactions among sickle erythrocytes, leukocytes, and the vessel wall likely play important roles in the pathogenesis of vascular occlusion in sickle cell disease.

Observations that sickle erythrocytes adhere to the endothelium to a variable degree and that the level of adhesion correlated with the severity of the disease[88] prompted investigation of the specific receptors involved in this interaction and the possible signaling pathways by which this occurs. Reticulocytes from both normal controls and sickle disease patients express the adhesion molecules integrin α4β1[89,90] and CD36 (GP IV).[89,91,92] Various studies have demonstrated that immature reticulocytes have greater levels of adhesion to endothelial cells compared with mature erythrocytes, pointing to a potential role for reticulocyte adhesion under selected experimental conditions.[80,89,92–94] Potential adhesion molecules that remain present on mature sickle erythrocytes include basal cell adhesion molecule–1/Lutheran (BCAM/Lu), intercellular adhesion molecule (ICAM)-4/Landsteiner-Weiner,[95] integrin-associated protein (CD47), phosphatidylserine (PS),[96] and sulfated glycolipids.[97,98] The sickle erythrocyte likely utilizes multiple adhesive pathways, potentially first binding to the endothelium and inducing localized pathological changes, followed by a second adhesive event with the sickle erythrocyte binding to the newly exposed endothelial or subendothelial adhesive ligands.

A disturbed endothelium also contributes to sickle cell adhesion in vivo. Endothelial adhesive molecules that bind sickle erythrocytes include vascular cell adhesion molecule–1 (VCAM-1),[90,99,100] integrin αVβ3,[93,100,101] E-selectin,[100] and P-selectin.[102] Optimal surface expression of these endothelial adhesion molecules requires induction by cytokines, shear stress or other perturbations of the endothelium, and exposure of endothelium to inflammatory agonists is associated with increased erythrocyte adhesion.[103,104] Increased levels of circulating endothelial cells are found in patients with sickle cell disease, with higher levels at the time of vasoocclusive crises;[105] the circulating endothelial cells have an activated phenotype, including increased expression of tissue factor[106] and adhesion molecules.[105] Increased levels of soluble VCAM-1 are found in patients with sickle cell disease at steady state, with a further marked increase during vasoocclusive crises, consistent with participation of endothelial injury in vasoocclusive disease.[107]

Adhesive plasma and extracellular matrix proteins can also contribute to sickle erythrocyte adhesion. Thrombospondin (TSP) is a 450-kD, homotrimeric glycoprotein present in the subendothelial matrix, plasma, and platelet α storage granules; it can be released in high local concentrations by activated platelets.[108] Both soluble and matrix TSP might play a role in sickle erythrocyte adhesion. In its soluble form, TSP might serve as a linker molecule between sickle erythrocytes and endothelial cells.[93,109] TSP also interacts with sickle erythrocyte CD47,[110] sulfated glycolipids,[111] and a normally cryptic domain of the dominant membrane protein, band 3, which is subject to rearrangement in hematological disorders,[112,113] Laminin, a major constituent of the extracellular matrix, is composed of a family of large heterotrimeric glycoproteins that support cell adhesion and migration and modulate gene expression.[114] Sickle erythrocytes avidly bind both immobilized and soluble laminin.[97,115] Vitronectin, fibrinogen, and von Willebrand have also been shown to support sickle cell adherence.[104]

Integrin-associated protein (CD47) functions as both a binding site for TSP and as an agonist receptor in response to soluble TSP in hematopoietic cells.[110,116,117] CD47 is expressed in normal and sickle erythrocytes[110] and protects normal erythrocytes from immune clearance.[118] CD47 on sickle erythrocytes binds immobilized TSP as a result of shear stress–dependent and G protein–mediated signal transduction pathways.[110]

Integrin $\alpha4\beta1$ is a receptor for both fibronectin and VCAM-1.[119] Sickle red cells bind to VCAM-1 on cultured cytokine-stimulated endothelial cells[90] or transfected COS cells[99] and to immobilized fibronectin[120] via $\alpha4\beta1$. The activation state of $\alpha4\beta1$ is regulated by several factors, including divalent cation concentration and agonist-induced cell signaling.[121] The $\alpha4$ cytoplasmic domain is directly phosphorylated in vitro by cyclic adenosine monophosphate–dependent protein kinase A,[122] suggesting a role for protein kinase A on activation of $\alpha4\beta1$. Ligation of CD47 on sickle reticulocytes activates $\alpha4\beta1$ via a protein kinase A–dependent phosphorylation of the $\alpha4$ cytoplasmic tail.[123] In vitro, $\alpha4\beta1$ interaction with endothelial VCAM-1 likely contributed to the adherence of sickle reticulocytes to cytokine-stimulated retinal microvascular endothelial cells.[124] In these studies, sickle erythrocyte binding to cytokine-stimulated retinal endothelium was inhibited by the $\alpha4\beta1$ cyclic peptide antagonist TBC772[125] and monoclonal antibody 9H8 that blocks $\alpha4\beta1$ adhesion.[89,90,99] Thus, integrin-blocking cyclic peptides such as TBC772 could eventually have potential therapeutic application in sickle cell disease.

The Lutheran blood group proteins, BCAM/Lu, are derived by alternative splicing from the same gene and differ only in the length of their cytoplasmic tails. Sickle erythrocytes overexpress BCAM/Lu, which specifically binds to the $\alpha5$ subunit of the extracellular matrix protein laminin.[115,126] Erythrocyte ICAM-4, otherwise known as blood group Landsteiner-Weiner, binds $\beta3$ integrins, including $\alpha v\beta3$ expressed on vascular endothelial cells.[127] In a rat ex vivo microvascular flow model, ICAM-4-specific peptides inhibited human sickle erythrocyte adhesion to the activated ex vivo microvascular endothelium.[128] Interestingly, both BCAM/Lu and ICAM-1 can be activated by epinephrine in a subset of sickle erythrocyte via a cyclic adenosine monophosphate–dependent pathway that likely involves protein kinase A.[95,129]

CD36 is a nonintegrin adhesive receptor that binds TSP and collagen and is present on the surface of endothelial cells, platelets, and a reticulocyte-rich subpopulation of normal and sickle red cells.[89,92] Sickle red cells bind to endothelial cells in the presence of soluble TSP and this adhesion is blocked by anti-CD36 monoclonal antibodies in both static adhesion assays[92] and under flow conditions.[93]

Sulfated glycolipids avidly bind TSP, von Willebrand factor, and laminin and might play a role in sickle red cell adhesion.[97,98,111] Abnormally exposed or altered lipids in the damaged sickle erythrocyte membrane could mediate sickle erythrocyte adhesion to immobilized TSP; this interaction is inhibited by the anionic polysaccharides high-molecular-weight dextran sulfate and glycosaminoglycan chondroitin sulfate A, but not other anionic polysaccharides of similar charge or structure.[97,98] TSP-induced erythrocyte adhesion to cultured human umbilical vein endothelial cells and sickle erythrocyte adhesion within an ex vivo mesocecum of the rat were both reduced by the same two anionic polysaccharides.[111] Thus, anionic polysaccharides could provide a potential therapeutic avenue to reduce pathological sickle erythrocyte interactions with the injured vessel wall.

Phosphatidylserine (PS) is abnormally exposed on the outer surface of sickle erythrocytes (Chapter 9) and also contributes to sickle erythrocyte adhesion to endothelial cells.[96,130,131] When PS translocates to the cell surface, it serves as an anchor for factors in the hemostatic system, promoting the activation of the coagulation cascade.[132] A strong correlation between the level of sickle erythrocyte PS exposure and the activity of the coagulation cascade in human and murine sickle cell disease is present, suggesting that the loss of sickle cell membrane asymmetry might also contribute to the observed prothrombotic state.[133,134] Furthermore, PS exposure on sickle erythrocytes might contribute to shortened erythrocyte survival in both sickle cell disease and thalassemia.[135,136]

With regard to the vessel wall, integrin $\alpha V\beta3$ likely contributes to sickle erythrocyte adhesion to the endothelial cells.[93,100,101] For example, monoclonal antibodies directed against $\alpha V\beta3$ inhibited human sickle erythrocyte adhesion to platelet-activating factor–treated rat mesocecum vasculature ex vivo. The $\alpha V\beta3$ antagonists, EMD 66203 and EMD 270179, also reduced sickle erythrocyte adhesion to human endothelial cell monolayers under venular shear flow conditions.[137] In the same rat ex vivo mesocecum model, these antagonists not only inhibited adhesion, but also abolished related vasoocclusion and maintained flow transit. These results suggest that the use of receptor antagonists could provide a beneficial therapeutic approach to reducing sickle cell adhesion and subsequent vasoocclusion.

P-selectin is an adhesion molecule that is rapidly expressed by activated platelets and endothelial cells.[138,139] Because P-selectin–mediated adhesive events are theorized to occur early in the evolution of sickle cell adhesion and vascular stasis, this pathway could serve as a model for the development of preventive antiadhesive therapy. Thus, P-selectin–blocking agents will likely best be used for preventing painful vasoocclusion rather than treating acute painful events in which numerous selectin-independent processes might already be active. This is accomplished best by using orally absorbable agents because chronic administration of injectable drugs is usually associated with poor compliance. Presently, nearly all of the P-selectin–blocking agents under development must be administered parenterally.[140] Specificity of P-selectin blockage also is critical to these considerations, and experience with selectin knockout mice has shown that chronic deficiency of P-selectin alone is not associated with risks of immune deficiency or hemorrhage,[141] but knockout of two or all three selectins is associated with serious clinical consequences.[142,143] Thus, blockage of P-selectin on a long-term basis must not also block E- or L-selectin.

Heparin also inhibits sickle cell adhesion to endothelial cells, potentially via either inhibition of sickle erythrocyte adhesion to endothelial P-selectin,[144,145] or by blocking the N-terminal heparin binding domain of TSP that can link sickle erythrocytes to endothelial cells.[109] In this regard, unfractionated heparin in sub-anticoagulating concentrations could have the advantage of blocking P-selectin in a concentration-specific manner,[146] but has the disadvantage of being poorly[147] and inconsistently[148] absorbed when administered orally. A preliminary trial of long-term low-dose subcutaneous heparin prophylaxis in four patients with sickle cell disease was reported. Patients experienced a reduction in painful crises while on therapy, with minimal toxicity.[149] To date attempts at developing orally absorbable heparin are still in their infancy.[150,151] The potential of developing oral heparins and other inhibitory compounds for chronic P-selectin inhibition, improved microvascular blood flow, and reduced frequency of painful vasoocclusion hinges on whether formulations with greater and more consistent oral absorption can be created.

RheothRx (poloxamer 188) is a nonionic surfactant copolymer with hemorheological properties that improve microvascular blood flow by lowering viscosity and frictional forces. RheothRx has been shown to block hydrophobic adhesive interactions (cell–cell, cell–protein, and protein–protein) in blood, resulting in the reduction of erythrocyte aggregation, adherence of erythrocytes to vascular endothelium, and an improvement in microvascular flow.[152] In a randomized, double-blind, placebo-controlled, pilot phase II study, RheothRx was well tolerated when 50 patients received 48-hour infusions of either RheothRx or placebo for moderate or severe pain lasting at least 4 hours, but less than 18 hours after presentation to the hospital.[153] A 48-hour infusion at doses of 30 mg/kg/hour of RheothRx significantly reduced total analgesic use, pain intensity, and showed trends to shorter duration of painful episodes and total days of hospitalization. This first formulation of poloxamer 188 was, however, associated with reversible nephrotoxicity in patients with heart failure. This toxicity was shown to be due to impurities in the formulation. Studies of a new highly purified version of poloxamer 188, Flocor™, were tested and found to be safe, but not efficacious for the general treatment of sickle cell disease vasoocclusive episodes, although children younger than 15 years and patients already taking hydroxyurea appeared to have a benefit from treatment (NCT00004408).[154]

Although the use of antiadhesive therapy is still in its infancy for many diseases, antiintegrin agents are already well-established therapies for the treatment of myocardial ischemia syndromes.[155] The ability to design rational approaches to inhibit the pathological adhesive properties of the sickle erythrocyte is dependent on a more complete understanding of the predominant pathological adhesive interactions in this disease. Furthermore, these findings suggest the possibility of selectively modulating adhesive interactions so that unwanted interactions associated with pathology can be ameliorated without compromising other functions.

Antithrombotic Therapy

Sickle Cell Disease and β Thalassemia

Individuals with either sickle cell disease or thalassemia have increased risk for thromboembolic complications and laboratory evidence for increased activity of platelets and the coagulation pathway.[156–158] There is increased thrombin generation in steady-state sickle cell disease with elevated levels of thrombin–antithrombin complexes, fibrinopeptide A, prothrombin fragment 1+2, and fibrin D-dimer levels that tend to increase further during acute vasoocclusive episodes.[158,159] Increased tissue factor activity with decreased factor VII levels consistent with higher factor VII turnover is also found.[159] Activated endothelial cells and monocytes with increased levels of tissue factor expression might contribute to this observation. Increased expression of tissue factor was found in circulating endothelial cells recovered from individuals with sickle cell disease.[106] Furthermore, increased levels of tissue factor–positive microparticles, derived from both monocytes and endothelial cells, were present in the plasma;[160] the levels of tissue factor–positive microparticles increased further during acute vasoocclusive events.[160] In different murine models of sickle cell disease, increased levels of endothelial tissue factor expression on pulmonary veins were found in the more severe models.[161] Exposure to hypoxia followed by oxygenation increased the expression of tissue factor of the milder sickle cell disease mice to levels similar to the more severe Berkeley mice.[161]

Increased exposure of PS on sickle and thalassemic erythrocytes promotes surface-dependent coagulation reactions and correlates with increased activity of coagulation parameters in sickle cell disease.[133,156,162,163] Furthermore, the levels of the natural anticoagulants, protein C and protein S, are decreased in patients with sickle cell disease and thalassemia.[164]

Platelet numbers and activity are increased in individuals with either sickle cell disease[158,165–167] or thalassemia.[156] As noted, the release of TSP by activated platelets might contribute to sickle erythrocyte adhesion. Alternatively, sickle erythrocyte adhesion to endothelial cells could damage the endothelium,[100] increase tissue factor expression,[168] and initiate the procoagulant activity.

Few clinical trials of anticoagulation in sickle cell disease have been reported. In one study, high-dose warfarin therapy minimally reduced painful vasoocclusive episodes but was associated with major bleeding complications.[169] In another, low-dose warfarin therapy successfully reduced the prothrombin fragment 1+2 level by 50% in seven patients;[170] however, clinical efficacy was not addressed. More recently, a pilot study of low-dose acenocoumarol in 22 patients with sickle cell disease demonstrated significant decreases in prothrombin fragment 1+2 levels, thrombin–antithrombin complexes, and D-dimer fragments but found no effect on the incidence of vasoocclusive episodes.[171] In 19 of these 22 patients on low-dose acenocoumarol, there was no difference in their measured levels of soluble VCAM-1, soluble cellular fibronectin, and von Willebrand factor antigen.[172]

Despite the evidence for platelet activation and consumption during vasoocclusive events, there has been no clear clinical benefit in small, nonrandomized clinical studies of aspirin,[173,174] ticlopidine,[175] or aspirin plus dipyrimadole.[176] Antiplatelet therapies have not been specifically tested for the primary or secondary prevention of arterial disease, such as sickle cell stroke or pulmonary hypertension. These limited observations are insufficient to establish the efficacy of anticoagulation therapy in preventing sickle vasoocclusion.

Given the overwhelming biochemical evidence for increased activity of the coagulation pathways linked with the higher incidence of thromboembolic complications in both sickle cell disease and thalassemia,[156–158] it makes sense to initiate large well-designed clinical trials to study the safety and efficacy of anticoagulation therapies.

Antiinflammatory Therapy

Sickle cell disease is a proinflammatory condition. The leukocyte count is elevated and correlates with a more severe clinical course, including increased risk of stroke and early death.[177–180] Moreover, patients have chronically elevated acute phase proteins, which increase further during acute events.[181] The plasma levels of the proinflammatory cytokines IL-1β, IL-6, interferon-γ, and tumor necrosis factor–α have been also reported elevated in at steady state with further increases during acute vasoocclusive events.[182,183] Endothelin-1 (ET-1),[184,185] transforming growth factor–β,[186] stem cell factor,[186] serum transferrin receptor,[186] IL-8,[187] and platelet activating factor[188,189] have been reported to be increased. These cytokines and chemokines might induce activation of the vascular endothelium, circulating erythrocytes, leukocytes, and platelets and contribute to the pathogenesis of painful vasoocclusive episodes.[183,190]

Sulfasalazine and Nuclear Factor–κB

Murine models of sickle cell disease have proven useful in the study of the inflammatory components of this disease. The more severe sickle cell disease mice exhibit an inflammatory response profile that is similar to that in humans and is characterized by increased expression of endothelial adhesion molecules[191] and activation of nuclear factor–κB (NF-κB).[192,193] Intravital examination studies showed activation of vascular endothelium and increased leukocyte–endothelium interactions that should cause abnormal blood flow and vasoocclusive episodes. These findings parallel observations in humans with sickle cell disease that showed that vasoocclusive crisis is often preceded by infection.[194–196] Inflammation elicits increased generation of oxidants that activate NF-κB, which in turn increases expression of endothelial adhesion molecules involved in leukocyte–endothelium interactions.[197,198] These experimental studies suggest that the use of targeted antiinflammatory therapy could be an effective means of decreasing inflammation and sickle vasoocclusion.

A small pilot study was conducted to evaluate the potential effect of the antiinflammatory molecule, sulfasalazine, on endothelial activation.[191] Sulfasalazine is an antiinflammatory agent that has been used to treat inflammatory bowel disease in humans. Its antiinflammatory effects are attributed to its ability to inhibit NF-κB activation.[199,200] Sulfasalazine decreased the expression of VCAM, ICAM, and E-selectin in human circulating endothelial cells.[191] The effects of sulfasalazine on endothelial cell activation were studied in transgenic sickle mice.[201] Although sulfasalazine can decrease expression of endothelial adhesion molecules in humans and transgenic sickle cell disease mice, it does not appear to decrease tissue factor expression.[191] In transgenic mice, sulfasalazine attenuated leukocyte adhesion and improved microvascular flow. Treatment of sickle cell mice with the antioxidant polynitroxyl albumin, which inhibits NF-κB activity, decreased the expression of VCAM-1, ICAM-1 in the liver and lung, and limited leukocyte rolling and vascular stasis in dorsal skin microvessels following hypoxia reoxygenation.[202] The level of inhibition of NF-κB activation correlated with the level of reduction in cell adhesion molecule expression and improved vascular flow.[202] These results support the concept that inflammation plays an important role in the pathogenesis of sickle vasoocclusion and they warrant further investigation.[105,106,192]

Targeting Endothelin-1

Sickle erythrocytes can interact with vascular endothelial cells, stimulate the release of ET-1, and modulate the expression of ET-1 in cultured endothelial cells.[203] ET-1 can also activate the Gardos channel through a protein kinase C–dependent mechanism in mouse erythrocytes.[204] These data suggest that activation of the Gardos channel might be coupled to receptors such as C-X-C (PAF), C-C (RANTES), and ET receptor subtype B-1, which implies an important role for inflammatory cytokines in the activation of the endothelium and erythrocyte dehydration.[204–206] In vivo treatment of sickle mice with the ET-1 receptor antagonist BQ-788 decreased MCHC and the percentage of dense cells while increasing mean cellular volume and decreasing Gardos channel activity.[207] These results provide strong evidence that ET-1 receptor antagonists represent a compelling target for the development of novel therapies to inhibit red cell sickling and endothelial cell activation.

Further support for the idea of using ET-1 receptor antagonists to treat complications associated with sickle cell disease comes from the fact that ET-1 receptor antagonists are already being used to treat pulmonary hypertension and asthma. As in sickle cell disease, these conditions are associated with increased plasma levels of ET-1.[208–210] In a mouse model of pulmonary hypertension, ET-1 receptor antagonists prevented pulmonary vascular remodeling and even reversed hypoxia-induced pulmonary remodeling. Furthermore, treatment with bosentan, a nonselective blocker of ET-1 receptors, was reported to reduce the levels of proinflammatory molecules that are associated with the development of asthma.[209] A phase III clinical trial testing the safety and efficacy of the ET-1 receptor blocker, bosentan, in sickle cell disease patients diagnosed with pulmonary hypertension has been started (ASSET-2; NCT00313196).

Antioxidant Therapy Targeting the Vasculature

HbS appears to undergo autooxidation at faster rates than HbA.[211,213] It is argued that because of the higher rates of autooxidation sickle erythrocytes experience significantly greater levels of oxidative stress as indicated by their increased susceptibility to lipid peroxidation.[213] Sickle erythrocytes also have increased ability to generate reactive oxygen species.[214] This is important because reactive oxygen species are well recognized for depleting cells of their natural antioxidants. Chronic increases in oxidative stress and inflammation as a result of increased HbS autooxidation and xanthine oxidase and nicotinamide adenine dinucleotide phosphate (NADPH) oxidase activity are believed to play a key role in the mechanisms eroding antioxidant defenses of the vessel wall. Indeed, increased reactive oxygen species production has been shown to oxidize a variety of proteins, lipids, and DNA. Taken together the ability of hemoglobin to undergo autooxidation coupled with chronic shifts in the balance of nitric oxide (NO) and superoxide should have adverse effects on the vessel wall.

Nitric Oxide

NO biology is discussed in detail in Chapter 10. NO is a chain-breaking antioxidant, which explains its ability to inhibit low-density lipoprotein oxidation and subsequently, inflammation.[215,216] The major source of NO in the vessel wall is endothelial nitric oxide synthase (eNOS). NO plays important protective roles in maintaining normal blood flow and vascular function. Therapies aimed at improving endothelial cell function and eNOS-dependent NO generation might have a major impact on vascular function in sickle cell disease and thalassemia.

Loss of NO bioactivity is one the earliest changes in vascular physiology associated with vascular injury. eNOS requires tetrahydrobiopterin (BH4), Ca^{2+}/calmodulin, L-arginine, hsp90–dependent chaperone activity and post-translational phosphorylation for optimal activity.[217–220] Interestingly, disruption of signaling mechanisms, loss of essential cofactors (BH4 and L-arginine) or chaperone-dependent activity leads to the uncoupling of eNOS activity from L-arginine oxidation and therefore increases production of superoxide anion ($O_2^{\bullet}$) rather than NO. Such observations and the fact that sickle cell disease patients have lower L-arginine levels due to increased release of red cell arginase[221] provided some of the earliest rationale for treating sickle cell disease with L-arginine. L-Arginine supplementation in murine models of sickle cell disease increased total NO production, decreased lipid peroxidation and increased glutathione (GSH) levels, superoxide dismutase, catalase, and GSH peroxidase activity.[222] The importance of restoring eNOS-coupled activity is underscored by yet another study showing that BH4 supplementation with sepiapterin improved eNOS function and decreased vascular endothelial cell activation.[223] Such observations support the notion that preserving coupled eNOS activity plays an important role in increasing NO bioactivity that inhibits lipid peroxidation and decreases oxidative stress. Several clinical studies are examining the efficacy of BH4 or L-arginine supplementation in the treatment of sickle cell disease patients. In a phase II trial of arginine supplementation in children and adults with sickle cell disease (NCT00513617) in which the primary endpoints were NO levels, Gardos channel activity, and erythrocyte density, no effect was seen. Arginine has also been studied for its effect on chronic leg ulceration (NCT00004412).

Chronic release of hemoglobin in sickle cell disease inhibits vascular NO activity by scavenging NO and converts it to nitrate, which is ineffective for promoting vasodilation.[224] Second, free hemoglobin increases production of lipid peroxides that further increase vascular instability.[225]

The importance of NO to the sickle red cell was suggested by studies showing that low concentrations of NO specifically increase the oxygen affinity of sickle erythrocytes.[226] The left shift of the oxygen dissociation curve was obtained within 45 minutes after exposure of deoxygenated sickle cells to NO and was dose dependent in the range 20–80 ppm of NO. Breathing NO (80 ppm for 45 minutes) restored normal oxygen dissociation curves to sickle cells in eight of nine patients with sickle cell anemia.

In contrast, NO did not affect the oxygen affinity of normal erythrocytes in vitro or in vivo and the formation of methemoglobin was negligible. Unfortunately, these studies have not been confirmed and the effects of inhaled NO on the sickle erythrocyte and hemoglobin remain controversial.

Nevertheless, a randomized, placebo-controlled trial of 20 patients demonstrated that inhaled NO reduced the duration of acute painful events in young patients and decreased the amounts of opioids used; further phase II trials of inhaled NO for acute painful events in adults and children are ongoing (NCT00094887 and NCT00142051).[227] Inhaled NO prevented some of the changes induced by hypoxia and reoxygenation in transgenic sickle mice.[228] Transgenic sickle cell mice treated with the NO-donor S-nitroso albumin showed decreased hypoxia-induced pulmonary injury based on lung histology and gene expression profiling.[229]

Therapies aimed at preserving eNOS-dependent NO production might have beneficial effects at several levels: 1) at the erythrocyte level, by possibly decreasing polymer formation, 2) at the leukocyte level by decreasing adherence, 3) at the platelet level by decreasing aggregation, 4) at the vascular level by increasing vasodilation and decreasing endothelial cell activation, and 5) at the inflammation level by inhibiting lipid peroxidation and oxidative stress. Because this line of research continues to yield insight into the mechanisms by which endothelial cells maintain eNOS function, new therapies targeting eNOS function could improve vascular function in both sickle cell disease and β thalassemia.

Apolipoprotein A-I Mimetics

As chronic increases in oxidative stress seem to be one of the primary mechanisms by which sickle cells impair vascular function, an alternative approach might be to protect vascular function by improving high-density lipoprotein (HDL) function. Recent reports indicate that small peptides, mimicking defined structures of apolipoprotein (Apo) A-I, improve vascular function[230] and decrease lesion formation in murine models of hypercholesterolemia.[231,232] When sickle mice were treated with L-4F, marked increases in endothelial- and eNOS-dependent vasodilation were observed.[230] Binding studies reveal that the 4F peptide has a 10,000 higher affinity for oxidized phospholipids than unaltered phospholipids.[233] This property is not shared by apo A-I. Such findings begin to explain why 4F, when added to plasma, partitions the HDL particle into two particles with the oxidized lipids accompanying 4F and the unaltered lipid remaining with the native HDL particle.[234] These studies indicate that the 4F acts as a molecular sponge preferentially binding oxidized phospholipids over native lipids. The importance of this unique property is that where an antioxidant might scavenge a lipid peroxide, the antioxidant has no mechanism to remove the modified lipid from the site of inflammation. In contrast, the 4F peptide not only binds oxidized lipids but also decreases their accumulation in vascular tissues and HDL.[235] Failure to remove the oxidized lipid species means that it is still able to induce inflammation in the vessel wall. For these reasons treatment of sickle mice and potentially patients with 4F represents a novel and effective means of decreasing the accumulation of oxidized lipids in the vessel wall and, therefore, improving endothelial- and eNOS-dependent NO production. Changes in the vessel wall might help attenuate vasoocclusive crises. Presently, L-4F is in phase II clinical trials for healthy volunteers and patients with coronary heart disease (NCT00568594).

Other apo A-I mimetics might also act by similar mechanisms. For example 37pA, a dimer of 18A, has been found to promote cholesterol efflux by an *ABCA1*-dependent and -independent mechanisms.[236] On the basis of these observations, this small peptide might also protect the vessel wall in animal models of vascular disease. Small, thiol-bearing peptides patterned after apo $A\text{-}I_{Milano}$ have been shown to retain the antioxidant activity of the apo $A\text{-}I_{Milano}$.[237] No studies have been reported addressing the ability of these peptides to inhibit vascular disease in animal models.[237,238] Finally, synthetic HDL has been successfully used to decrease lesion size not only in animals but also humans;[239] however, the expense associated with producing sufficient quantities of recombinant HDL for chronic treatments precludes its use on a large scale.[240]

Statins

Pretreatment with lovastatin reduced significantly the expression of tissue factor expression after hypoxia–reoxygenation to induce ischemia–reperfusion injury in sickle transgenic mice.[161] It has been proposed that statins might be beneficial in sickle cell disease not only for their antiinflammatory properties but also for their ability to increase eNOS and eNOS-dependent production of NO.[241] These studies suggest a provocative new idea for using statins to treat sickle vasculopathy, based on the ability of statins to attenuate reperfusion injury and the effects of vasoocclusive-inducible factors.

Xanthine Oxidase Inhibitors

Vascular injury due to increased oxidative stress can occur through a number of different mechanisms. Based on histological studies showing depletion of xanthine oxidase in sickle cell disease mouse hepatocytes accompanied by increased xanthine oxidase staining of sickle cell disease mouse vascular endothelium, it was proposed that chronic and repeated bouts of vasoocclusive injury to the liver resulted in the release of hepatic xanthine oxidase stores and accumulation of endothelial-associated xanthine oxidase at distant sites.[242] As xanthine oxidase accumulates on the vessel wall, it creates a new region of increased superoxide anion production that subsequently increases consumption of vascular NO and impairs vasodilation.[242] Likewise, release of myeloperoxidase from neutrophils increases the nitration of vascular surface tyrosine residues to increase vascular inflammation.[243] Although there are higher circulating levels of xanthine oxidase in both human and murine sickle cell disease with associated vascular injury[242] and evidence for oxidative injury in both sickle cell disease and thalassemia,[244] there have been no reported clinical trials testing the safety and efficacy of xanthine oxidase inhibitors as a therapeutic strategy for the treatment of individuals affected with either sickle cell disease or thalassemia.

Hypoxia–reoxygenation induces greater endothelial oxidant generation in sickle mice compared with controls, which was significantly reduced by antioxidant therapy.[201] Allopurinol, an inhibitor of xanthine oxidase activity, reduced the inflammatory effect of hypoxia–reoxygenation in sickle transgenic mice. Furthermore, pretreatment of these mice with superoxide dismutase and catalase inhibited the increased oxidant production and subsequent leukocyte accumulation following hypoxia–reoxygenation.[201] Although allopurinol might target xanthine oxidase and therefore superoxide, this study found that treating with superoxide dismutase and catalase at the onset of reoxygenation was more effective than allopurinol alone in restoring the microvascular flow and endothelial-dependent vascular function to control values.[201] The fact that superoxide dismutase and catalase effectively scavenge both superoxide anion and H_2O_2, the substrate for myeloperoxidase, during hypoxia suggests that the mechanisms by which sickle cell disease impairs vascular function are more complex than just an increase in xanthine oxidase and that broader approaches are needed to inhibit vascular oxidative stress effectively in sickle cell disease.

Antioxidant Therapy Targeting the Erythrocyte

Deferiprone (L1)

Increased lipid peroxidation and protein thiol oxidation due to generation of reactive oxygen species could also arise from an increase in intracellular iron levels and unstable heme moieties in both sickle and thalassemic erythrocytes.[211,245] Thus, the membrane abnormalities observed in these erythrocytes might be in part due to iron-mediated oxidative damage.[246] Accordingly, agents that target free iron and protect the erythrocyte from oxidative damage should be of therapeutic benefit in both sickle cell disease and thalassemia. Deferiprone (L1) is an oral iron-chelating agent with an enhanced ability to permeate cell membranes (Chapter 29). Therefore, L1 should limit iron-mediated oxidative damage to the erythrocyte membrane. Preincubation of erythrocytes with L1 effectively reduced H_2O_2-mediated damage to both sickle and thalassemic erythrocyte membranes.[247] Furthermore, treatment of six patients with β thalassemia with L1 reduced membrane free iron and reduced lipid peroxidation and malonyldialdehyde production in their erythrocytes.[247] These data demonstrate that binding free iron removes what appears to be a significant portion of redox-active iron from erythrocyte membranes and in so doing significantly attenuates free iron–mediated oxidant damage.

Oral Glutamine

Sickle erythrocytes cells have decreased levels of reduced nicotinamide adenine dinucleotide (NADH) and increased total NAD+.[248] Sickle cell disease patients with pulmonary hypertension had decreased levels of GSH and glutamine. It was hypothesized that defects in GSH and glutamate metabolism were involved in red cell hemolysis and NO consumption.[249] Supplementation with a precursor of NADH, L-glutamine, might increase NADH in sickle erythrocytes.[250] Oral L-glutamine therapy increased NADH levels in sickle erythrocytes and was associated with a subjective improvement in chronic pain and energy level of patients.[251,252] These data suggested that glutamine could play a role in increasing sickle erythrocytes defenses against oxidative damage with attendant positive clinical effects. Although the mechanism for this improvement is unclear, it was postulated that glutamine might act an antioxidant through the GSH pathway.[252] L-glutamine therapy also reduces sickle erythrocyte adhesion to cultured endothelial cells, providing additional potential therapeutic benefit.[251] Although the exact mechanisms by which glutamine supplementation improves erythrocyte function are not known, glutamine-induced increases in NADPH might help restore erythrocyte GSH levels.[249]

Oral N-Acetyl-Cysteine Therapy

Reduced GSH is key factor for the antioxidant activity of erythrocytes. Its depletion might contribute to the increase in oxidative damage in both sickle cell disease and thalassemia. N-acetyl-cysteine is an effective precursor of cysteine for cellular GSH synthesis.[253] Several other antioxidants such as vitamin C and vitamin E have also been shown to decrease oxidative damage in sickle cell disease, suggesting that antioxidant treatment of patients with sickle cell disease could reduce oxidative damage to blood cells and the vasculature, thus potentially reducing sickle cell–induced pathologies.[254,255] In sickle cell disease, in vitro studies have found that N-acetyl-cysteine blocked dense cell and irreversible sickle cell formation in vitro.[256,257] A phase II double-blind, randomized clinical trial found that N-acetyl-cysteine therapy reduced sickle dense cell, but not irreversible sickle cell formation, and enhanced erythrocyte GSH levels.[258] N-acetyl-cysteine was also associated with a reduction in the frequency of vasoocclusive episodes.[258] Because N-acetyl-cysteine has minimal toxicity and is inexpensive, it is a good candidate for future phase III clinical studies in human sickle cell disease.

Based on the aforementioned preliminary studies, targeting oxidant generation might constitute another promising therapeutic approach for the treatment of both erythrocyte and vascular dysfunction in sickle cell disease.

CONCLUSION

Therapeutic approaches to reduce the incidence and severity of vascular obstruction and hemolysis in sickle cell disease are derived from the current knowledge of the disease pathophysiology and will continue to evolve. Murine models of hemoglobin disorders have been essential to accelerate answers to specific questions and confirm proof of principle in vivo, before performing clinical trials. Now it is possible to change a single genetic or treatment factor in transgenic mice to modulate the expression of the disease and to define or confirm therapeutic targets. The major studies to date have been designed to reduce the primary event of HbS polymerization, including antisickling agents, induction of HbF synthesis, and rehydration of the sickle erythrocyte. Therapies designed to ameliorate the more complex secondary pathological effects of HbS, including the enhanced adhesive properties of the sickle erythrocyte, the severe vascular pathologies and the increased activity of the coagulation and inflammatory pathways are in promising initial stages of investigation. Because the vascular dysfunction and organ pathologies observed in sickle cell disease and thalassemia are the culmination of a complex multifactorial process, short of a genetic cure, an array of therapies, targeting both the abnormal erythroid cell and the myriad secondary vascular and systemic pathologies, should be beneficial for improving the survival and function of diseased erythrocytes, organ function and life expectancy and the quality of life in the many individuals who suffer from severe hemoglobin disorders.

REFERENCES

1. Elion JE, Brun M, Odievre MH, Lapoumeroulie CL, Krishnamoorthy R. Vaso-occlusion in sickle cell anemia: role of interactions between blood cells and endothelium. *Hematol J.* 2004;Suppl 3:S195–S198.
2. Lee K, Gane P, Roudot-Thoraval F, et al. The nonexpression of CD36 on reticulocytes and mature red blood cells does not modify the clinical course of patients with sickle cell anemia. *Blood.* 2001;98:966–971.
3. Steinberg MH, Brugnara C. Developing treatment for sickle cell disease. *Expert Opin Invest Drugs.* 2002;11:645–659.
4. Vichinsky E. New therapies in sickle cell disease. *Lancet.* 2002;360:629–631.
5. Dean J, Schechter AN. Sickle-cell anemia:molecular and cellular bases of therapeutic approaches. *N Engl J Med.* 1978;299:752–763.
6. Beutler E, Mikus BJ. The effect of sodium nitrite and para-aminopropriophenone administration on blood methemoglobin levels and red blood cell survival. *Blood.* 1961;18: 455–467.
7. Sirs JA. The use of carbon monoxide to prevent sickle-cell formation. *Lancet.* 1963;1:971–972.
8. Murayama M. Molecular mechanism of red cell "sickling." *Science.* 1966;153:145–149.
9. Cooperative Urea Trials Group. Treatment of sickle cell crisis with urea in invert sugar. A controlled trial. Cooperative urea trials group. *JAMA.* 1974;228:1125–1128.
10. Cerami A, Manning JM. Potassium cyanate as an inhibitor of the sickling of erythrocytes in vitro. *Proc Natl Acad Sci USA.* 1971;68:1180–1183.
11. Castro O, Brambilla DJ, Thorington B, et al. The acute chest syndrome in sickle cell disease:incidence and risk factors. The Cooperative Study of Sickle Cell Disease. *Blood.* 1994;84:643–649.
12. Benesch RE, Kwong S, Benesch R. The effects of alpha chain mutations cis and trans to the β6 mutation on the polymerization of sickle cell haemoglobin. *Nature.* 1982;299:231–234.
13. Dykes G, Crepeau RH, Edelstein SJ. Three-dimensional reconstruction of the fibres of sickle cell haemoglobin. *Nature.* 1978;272:506–510.
14. Nagel RL, Johnson J, Bookchin RM, et al. Beta-chain contact sites in the haemoglobin S polymer. *Nature.* 1980;283:832–834.
15. Perutz RR, Liquori AM, Eirich F. X-ray and solubility studies of the haemoglobin of sickle-cell anaemia patients. *Nature.* 1951;167:929–931.
16. Wishner BC, Ward KB, Lattman EE, Love WE. Crystal structure of sickle-cell deoxyhemoglobin at 5 A resolution. *J Mol Biol.* 1975;98:179–194.
17. Fung LW, Ho C, Roth EF Jr, Nagel RL. The alkylation of hemoglobin S by nitrogen mustard. High resolution proton nuclear magnetic resonance studies. *J Biol Chem.* 1975; 250:4786–4789.
18. Abraham EC, Stallings M, Abraham A, Garbutt GJ. Modification of sickle hemoglobin by acetaldehyde and its effect on oxygenation, gelation and sickling. *Biochim Biophys Acta.* 1982;705:76–81.
19. Acharya AS, Manning JM. Reactivity of the amino groups of carbonmonoxyhemoglobin S with glyceraldehyde. *J Biol Chem.* 1980;255:1406–1412.
20. Benesch R, Benesch RE, Edalji R, Suzuki T. 5′-deoxypyridoxal as a potential anti-sickling agent. *Proc Natl Acad Sci USA.* 1977;74:1721–1723.
21. Zaugg RH, Walder JA, Klotz IM. Schiff base adducts of hemoglobin. Modifications that inhibit erythrocyte sickling. *J Biol Chem.* 1977;252:8542–8548.
22. Seetharam R, Manning JM, Acharya AS. Specific modification of the carboxyl groups of hemoglobin S. *J Biol Chem.* 1983;258:14810–14815.
23. Garel MC, Domenget C, Caburi-Martin J, Prehu C, Galacteros F, Beuzard Y. Covalent binding of glutathione to hemoglobin. *I.* Inhibition of hemoglobin S polymerization. *J Biol Chem.* 1986;261:14704–14709.
24. Chao TL, Berenfeld MR, Gabuzda TG. Inhibition of sickling by methyl acetimidate. *FEBS Lett.* 1976;62:57–59.
25. Chatterjee R, Walder RY, Arnone A, Walder JA. Mechanism for the increase in solubility of deoxyhemoglobin S due to cross-linking the beta chains between lysine-82 beta 1 and lysine-82 beta 2. *Biochemistry.* 1982;21:5901–5909.

26. Keidan AJ, Franklin IM, White RD, Joy M, Huehns ER, Stuart J. Effect of BW12C on oxygen affinity of haemoglobin in sickle-cell disease. *Lancet.* 1986;1:831–834.
27. Philip PA, Thompson CH, Carmichael J, et al. A phase I study of the left-shifting agent BW12C79 plus mitomycin C and the effect on the skeletal muscle metabolism using 31P magnetic resonance spectroscopy. *Cancer Res.* 1993;53:5649–5653.
28. Wireko FC, Abraham DJ. X-ray diffraction study of the binding of the antisickling agent 12C79 to human hemoglobin. *Proc Natl Acad Sci USA.* 1991;88:2209–2211.
29. Trudel M, De Paepe ME, Chretien N, et al. Sickle cell disease of transgenic SAD mice. *Blood.* 1994;84:3189–3197.
30. Arya R, Rolan PE, Wootton R, Posner J, Bellingham AJ. Tucaresol increases oxygen affinity and reduces haemolysis in subjects with sickle cell anaemia. *Br J Haematol.* 1996;93: 817–821.
31. Chen H, Hall S, Heffernan B, Thompson NT, Rogers MV, Rhodes J. Convergence of Schiff base costimulatory signaling and TCR signaling at the level of mitogen-activated protein kinase ERK2. *J Immunol.* 1997;159:2274–2281.
32. Rhodes J. Covalent chemical events in immune induction:fundamental and therapeutic aspects. *Immunol Today.* 1996;17:436–441.
33. Rhodes J, Chen H, Hall SR, et al. Therapeutic potentiation of the immune system by costimulatory Schiff-base-forming drugs. *Nature.* 1995;377:71–75.
34. Abraham DJ, Mehanna AS, Wireko FC, Whitney J, Thomas RP, Orringer EP. Vanillin, a potential agent for the treatment of sickle cell anemia. *Blood.* 1991;77:1334–1341.
35. Abraham DJ, Safo MK, Boyiri T, Danso-Danquah RE, Kister J, Poyart C. How allosteric effectors can bind to the same protein residue and produce opposite shifts in the allosteric equilibrium. *Biochemistry.* 1995;34:15006–15020.
36. Harrington DJ, Adachi K, Royer WE Jr. The high resolution crystal structure of deoxyhemoglobin S. *J Mol Biol.* 1997;272: 398–407.
37. Kihm AJ, Kong Y, Hong W, et al. An abundant erythroid protein that stabilizes free alpha-haemoglobin. *Nature.* 2002; 417:758–763.
38. Yu X, Kong Y, Dore LC, et al. An erythroid chaperone that facilitates folding of alpha-globin subunits for hemoglobin synthesis. *J Clin Invest.* 2007;117:1856–1865.
39. Feng L, Zhou S, Gu L, et al. Structure of oxidized alpha-haemoglobin bound to AHSP reveals a protective mechanism for haem. *Nature.* 2005;435:697–701.
40. Kong Y, Zhou S, Kihm AJ, et al. Loss of alpha-hemoglobin-stabilizing protein impairs erythropoiesis and exacerbates beta-thalassemia. *J Clin Invest.* 2004;114:1457–1466.
41. Lai MI, Jiang J, Silver N, Best S, Menzel S, Mijovic A, Colella S, Ragoussis J, Garner C, Weiss MJ, Thein SL. Alpha-haemoglobin stabilising protein is a quantitative trait gene that modifies the phenotype of β-thalassaemia. *Br J Haematol.* 2006;133:675–682.
42. Eaton WA, Hofrichter J. Hemoglobin S gelation and sickle cell disease. *Blood.* 1987;70:1245–1266.
43. Glader BE, Nathan DG. Cation permeability alterations during sickling:relationship to cation composition and cellular hydration of irreversibly sickled cells. *Blood.* 1978;51:983–989.
44. Joiner CH. Cation transport and volume regulation in sickle red blood cells. *Am J Physiol.* 1993;264:C251–C270.
45. Lew VL, Freeman CJ, Ortiz OE, Bookchin RM. A mathematical model of the volume, pH, and ion content regulation in reticulocytes. Application to the pathophysiology of sickle cell dehydration. *J Clin Invest.* 1991;87:100–112.
46. Brugnara C, Bunn HF, Tosteson DC. Regulation of erythrocyte cation and water content in sickle cell anemia. *Science.* 1986;232:388–390.
47. Rosa RM, Bierer B, Thomas R, et al. Prevention and treatment of sickle cell crisis by induced hyponatremia. *Trans Assoc Am Physicians.* 1980;93:164–174.
48. Rosa RM, Bierer BE, Thomas R, et al. A study of induced hyponatremia in the prevention and treatment of sickle-cell crisis. *N Engl J Med.* 1980;303:1138–1143.
49. Charache S, Walker WG. Failure of desmopressin to lower serum sodium or prevent crisis in patients with sickle cell anemia. *Blood.* 198158:892–896.
50. Benjamin LJ, Berkowitz LR, Orringer E, et al. A collaborative, double-blind randomized study of cetiedil citrate in sickle cell crisis. *Blood.* 1986;67:1442–1447.
51. Berkowitz LR, Orringer EP. Effects of cetiedil on monovalent cation permeability in the erythrocyte:an explanation for the efficacy of cetiedil in the treatment of sickle cell anemia. *Blood Cells.* 1982;8:283–288.
52. Benjamin LJ. Membrane modifiers in sickle cell disease. *Ann NY Acad Sci.* 1989;565:247–261.
53. Alvarez J, Montero M, Garcia-Sancho J. Cytochrome P-450 may link intracellular Ca2+ stores with plasma membrane Ca2+ influx. *Biochem J.* 1991;274(Pt 1):193–197.
54. Brugnara C. Erythrocyte dehydration in pathophysiology and treatment of sickle cell disease. *Curr Opin Hematol.* 1995;2:132–138.
55. Brugnara C, de FL, Alper SL. Inhibition of Ca(2+)-dependent K+ transport and cell dehydration in sickle erythrocytes by clotrimazole and other imidazole derivatives. *J Clin Invest.* 1993;92:520–526.
56. De Franceschi L, Saadane N, Trudel M, Alper SL, Brugnara C, Beuzard Y. Treatment with oral clotrimazole blocks Ca(2+)-activated K+ transport and reverses erythrocyte dehydration in transgenic SAD mice. A model for therapy of sickle cell disease. *J Clin Invest.* 1994;93:1670–1676.
57. Brugnara C, Armsby CC, Sakamoto M, Rifai N, Alper SL, Platt O. Oral administration of clotrimazole and blockade of human erythrocyte Ca(++)-activated K+ channel:the imidazole ring is not required for inhibitory activity. *J Pharmacol Exp Ther.* 1995;273:266–272.
58. Sawyer PR, Brogden RN, Pinder RM, Speight TM, Avery GS. Clotrimazole: a review of its antifungal activity and therapeutic efficacy. *Drugs* 1975;9:424–447.
59. Seo M, iida H, Miura Y. Basic experiments with clotrimazole administered orally. *Curr Med Res Opin.* 1977;5:169–178.
60. Brugnara C, Gee B, Armsby CC, et al. Therapy with oral clotrimazole induces inhibition of the Gardos channel and reduction of erythrocyte dehydration in patients with sickle cell disease. *J Clin Invest.* 1996;97:1227–1234.
61. Stocker JW, De Franceschi L, McNaughton-Smith GA, Corrocher R, Beuzard Y, Brugnara C. ICA-17043, a novel Gardos channel blocker, prevents sickled red blood cell dehydration in vitro and in vivo in SAD mice. *Blood.* 2003; 101:2412–2418.

62. Ataga KI, Orringer EP, Styles L, Vichinsky EP, Swerdlow P, Davis GA, Desimone PA and Stocker JW. Dose-escalation study of ICA-17043 in patients with sickle cell disease. *Pharmacotherapy* 2006;26:1557–1564.
63. Ataga KI, Smith WR, De Castro LM, et al. Efficacy and safety of the Gardos channel blocker, senicapoc (ICA-17043), in patients with sickle cell anemia. *Blood.* 2008;111:3991–3997.
64. Brugnara C, Armsby CC, De Franceschi L, Crest M, Euclaire MF and Alper SL. Ca(2+)-activated K+ channels of human and rabbit erythrocytes display distinctive patterns of inhibition by venom peptide toxins. *J Membr Biol* 1995;147:71–82.
65. Canessa M, Spalvins A, Nagel RL. Volume-dependent and NEM-stimulated K+,Cl- transport is elevated in oxygenated SS, SC and CC human red cells. *FEBS Lett.* 1986;200:197–202.
66. Vitoux D, Olivieri O, Garay RP, Cragoe EJ Jr, Galacteros F, Beuzard Y. Inhibition of K+ efflux and dehydration of sickle cells by [(dihydroindenyl)oxy]alkanoic acid:an inhibitor of the K+ Cl- cotransport system. *Proc Natl Acad Sci USA.* 1989;86:4273–4276.
67. Brugnara C, Tosteson DC. Inhibition of K transport by divalent cations in sickle erythrocytes. *Blood.* 1987;70:1810–1815.
68. Bookchin RM, Balazs T, Lew VL. Measurement of the hemoglobin concentration in deoxyhemoglobin S polymers and characterization of the polymer water compartment. *J Mol Biol.* 1994;244:100–109.
69. Olukoga AO, Adewoye HO, Erasmus RT, Adedoyin MA. Erythrocyte and plasma magnesium in sickle-cell anaemia. *E Afr Med J.* 1990;67:348–354.
70. Ortiz OE, Lew VL, Bookchin RM. Deoxygenation permeabilizes sickle cell anaemia red cells to magnesium and reverses its gradient in the dense cells. *J Physiol.* 1990;427:211–226.
71. De Franceschi L, Beuzard Y, Jouault H, Brugnara C. Modulation of erythrocyte potassium chloride cotransport, potassium content, and density by dietary magnesium intake in transgenic SAD mouse. *Blood.* 1996;88:2738–2744.
72. Borella P, Ambrosini G, Concari M, Bargellini A. Is magnesium content in erythrocytes suitable for evaluating cation retention after oral physiological supplementation in marginally magnesium-deficient subjects? *Magnes Res.* 1993;6: 149–153.
73. Paolisso G, Scheen A, Cozzolino D, et al. Changes in glucose turnover parameters and improvement of glucose oxidation after 4-week magnesium administration in elderly noninsulin-dependent (type II) diabetic patients. *J Clin Endocrinol Metab.* 1994;78:1510–1514.
74. De Franceschi L, Bachir D, Galacteros F, et al. Oral magnesium supplements reduce erythrocyte dehydration in patients with sickle cell disease. *J Clin Invest.* 1997;100:1847–1852.
75. De Franceschi L, Bachir D, Galacteros F, et al. Oral magnesium pidolate:effects of long-term administration in patients with sickle cell disease. *Br J Haematol.* 2000;108:284–289.
76. Hankins JS, Wynn LW, Brugnara C, Hillery CA, Li CS, Wang WC. Phase I study of magnesium pidolate in combination with hydroxycarbamide for children with sickle cell anaemia. *Br J Haematol.* 2008;140:80–85.
77. De Franceschi L, Brugnara C, Beuzard Y. Dietary magnesium supplementation ameliorates anemia in a mouse model of beta-thalassemia. *Blood.* 1997;90:1283–1290.
78. De Franceschi L, Cappellini MD, Graziadei G, et al. The effect of dietary magnesium supplementation on the cellular abnormalities of erythrocytes in patients with beta thalassemia intermedia. *Haematologica.* 1998;83:118–125.
79. Hebbel RP, Yamada O, Moldow CF, Jacob HS, White JG, Eaton JW. Abnormal adherence of sickle erythrocytes to cultured vascular endothelium:possible mechanism for microvascular occlusion in sickle cell disease. *J Clin Invest.* 1980;65:154–160.
80. Mohandas N, Evans E. Adherence of sickle erythrocytes to vascular endothelial cells:requirement for both cell membrane changes and plasma factors. *Blood.* 1984;64:282–287.
81. Barabino GA, McIntire LV, Eskin SG, Sears DA, Udden M. Rheological studies of erythrocyte-endothelial cell interactions in sickle cell disease. *Prog Clin Biol Res.* 1987;240:113–127.
82. Fabry ME, Rajanayagam V, Fine E, Holland S, Gore JC, Nagel RL, Kaul DK. Modeling sickle cell vasoocclusion in the rat leg: quantification of trapped sickle cells and correlation with 31P metabolic and 1H magnetic resonance imaging changes. *Proc Natl Acad Sci USA.* 1989;86:3808–3812.
83. French JA, Kenny D, Scott JP, et al. Mechanisms of stroke in sickle cell disease:sickle erythrocytes decrease cerebral blood flow in rats after nitric oxide synthase inhibition. *Blood.* 1997;89:4591–4599.
84. Kaul DK, Fabry ME, Nagel RL. Microvascular sites and characteristics of sickle cell adhesion to vascular endothelium in shear flow conditions: pathophysiological implications. *Proc Natl Acad Sci USA.* 1989;86:3356–3360.
85. Kaul DK, Fabry ME, Costantini F, Rubin EM, Nagel RL. In vivo demonstration of red cell-endothelial interaction, sickling and altered microvascular response to oxygen in the sickle transgenic mouse. *J Clin Invest.* 1995;96:2845–2853.
86. Wood KC, Hebbel RP, Granger DN. Endothelial cell P-selectin mediates a proinflammatory and prothrombogenic phenotype in cerebral venules of sickle cell transgenic mice. *Am J Physiol Heart Circ Physiol.* 2004;286:H1608–H1614.
87. Turhan A, Weiss LA, Mohandas N, Coller BS, Frenette PS. Primary role for adherent leukocytes in sickle cell vascular occlusion: a new paradigm. *Proc Natl Acad Sci USA.* 2002;99:3047–3051.
88. Hebbel RP, Boogaerts MA, Eaton JW, Steinberg MH. Erythrocyte adherence to endothelium in sickle-cell anemia. A possible determinant of disease severity. *N Engl J Med.* 1980;302:992–995.
89. Joneckis CC, Ackley RL, Orringer EP, Wayner EA, Parise LV. Integrin alpha 4 beta 1 and glycoprotein IV (CD36) are expressed on circulating reticulocytes in sickle cell anemia. *Blood.* 1993;82:3548–3555.
90. Swerlick RA, Eckman JR, Kumar A, Jeitler M, Wick TM. Alpha 4 beta 1-integrin expression on sickle reticulocytes: vascular cell adhesion molecule-1-dependent binding to endothelium. *Blood.* 1993;82:1891–1899.
91. Browne PV, Hebbel RP. CD36-positive stress reticulocytosis in sickle cell anemia. *J Lab Clin Med.* 1996;127:340–347.
92. Sugihara K, Sugihara T, Mohandas N, Hebbel RP. Thrombospondin mediates adherence of CD36+ sickle reticulocytes to endothelial cells. *Blood.* 1992;80:2634–2642.
93. Brittain HA, Eckman JR, Swerlick RA, Howard RJ, Wick TM. Thrombospondin from activated platelets promotes sickle erythrocyte adherence to human microvascular endothelium under physiologic flow: a potential role for platelet activation in sickle cell vaso-occlusion. *Blood.* 1993;81:2137–2143.

94. Fabry ME, Fine E, Rajanayagam V, et al. Demonstration of endothelial adhesion of sickle cells in vivo: a distinct role for deformable sickle cell discocytes. *Blood.* 1992;79:1602–1611.
95. Zennadi R, Hines PC, De Castro LM, Cartron JP, Parise LV, Telen MJ. Epinephrine acts through erythroid signaling pathways to activate sickle cell adhesion to endothelium via LW-alphavbeta3 interactions. *Blood.* 2004;104:3774–3781.
96. Setty BN, Kulkarni S, Stuart MJ. Role of erythrocyte phosphatidylserine in sickle red cell-endothelial adhesion. *Blood.* 2002;99:1564–1571.
97. Hillery CA, Du MC, Montgomery RR, Scott JP. Increased adhesion of erythrocytes to components of the extracellular matrix:isolation and characterization of a red blood cell lipid that binds thrombospondin and laminin. *Blood.* 1996;87:4879–4886.
98. Joneckis CC, Shock DD, Cunningham ML, Orringer EP, Parise LV. Glycoprotein IV-independent adhesion of sickle red blood cells to immobilized thrombospondin under flow conditions. *Blood.* 1996;87:4862–4870.
99. Gee BE, Platt OS. Sickle reticulocytes adhere to VCAM-1. *Blood.* 1995;85:268–274.
100. Natarajan M, Udden MM, McIntire LV. Adhesion of sickle red blood cells and damage to interleukin-1 beta stimulated endothelial cells under flow in vitro. *Blood.* 1996;87:4845–4852.
101. Kaul DK, Tsai HM, Liu XD, Nakada MT, Nagel RL, Coller BS. Monoclonal antibodies to alphaVbeta3 (7E3 and LM609) inhibit sickle red blood cell-endothelium interactions induced by platelet-activating factor. *Blood.* 2000;95:368–374.
102. Matsui NM, Borsig L, Rosen SD, Yaghmai M, Varki A, Embury SH. P-selectin mediates the adhesion of sickle erythrocytes to the endothelium. *Blood.* 2001;98:1955–1962.
103. Manodori AB. Sickle erythrocytes adhere to fibronectin-thrombospondin-integrin complexes exposed by thrombin-induced endothelial cell contraction. *Microvasc Res.* 2001;61:263–274.
104. Wick TM, Eckman JR. Molecular basis of sickle cell-endothelial cell interactions. *Curr Opin Hematol.* 1996;3:118–124.
105. Solovey A, Lin Y, Browne P, Choong S, Wayner E, Hebbel RP. Circulating activated endothelial cells in sickle cell anemia. *N Engl J Med.* 1997;337:1584–1590.
106. Solovey A, Gui L, Key NS, Hebbel RP. Tissue factor expression by endothelial cells in sickle cell anemia. *J Clin Invest.* 1998;101:1899–1904.
107. Stuart MJ, Setty BN. Sickle cell acute chest syndrome: pathogenesis and rationale for treatment. *Blood.* 1999;94:1555–1560.
108. Santoro SA, Frazier WA. Isolation and characterization of thrombospondin. *Methods Enzymol.* 1987;144:438–446.
109. Gupta K, Gupta P, Solovey A, Hebbel RP. Mechanism of interaction of thrombospondin with human endothelium and inhibition of sickle erythrocyte adhesion to human endothelial cells by heparin. *Biochim Biophys Acta.* 1999;1453:63–73.
110. Brittain JE, Mlinar KJ, Anderson CS, Orringer EP, Parise LV. Integrin-associated protein is an adhesion receptor on sickle red blood cells for immobilized thrombospondin. *Blood.* 2001;97:2159–2164.
111. Barabino GA, Liu XD, Ewenstein BM, Kaul DK. Anionic polysaccharides inhibit adhesion of sickle erythrocytes to the vascular endothelium and result in improved hemodynamic behavior. *Blood.* 1999;93:1422–1429.
112. Sherman IW, Crandall I, Smith H. Membrane proteins involved in the adherence of Plasmodium falciparum-infected erythrocytes to the endothelium. *Biol Cell.* 1992;74:161–178.
113. Thevenin BJ, Crandall I, Ballas SK, Sherman IW, Shohet SB. Band 3 peptides block the adherence of sickle cells to endothelial cells in vitro. *Blood.* 1997;90:4172–4179.
114. Tryggvason K. The laminin family. *Cell Biol.* 1993;5:877–882.
115. Udani M, Zen Q, Cottman M, et al. Basal cell adhesion molecule/lutheran protein. The receptor critical for sickle cell adhesion to laminin. *J Clin Invest.* 1998;101:2550–2558.
116. Brittain JE, Mlinar KJ, Anderson CS, Orringer EP, Parise LV. Activation of sickle red blood cell adhesion via integrin-associated protein(CD47-induced signal transduction. *J Clin Invest.* 2001;107:1555–1562.
117. Gao AG, Lindberg FP, Finn MB, Blystone SD, Brown EJ, Frazier WA. Integrin-associated protein is a receptor for the C-terminal domain of thrombospondin. *J Biol Chem.* 1996;271:21–24.
118. Oldenborg PA, Zheleznyak A, Fang YF, Lagenaur CF, Gresham HD, Lindberg FP. Role of CD47 as a marker of self on red blood cells. *Science.* 2000;288:2051–2054.
119. Humphries MJ, Sheridan J, Mould AP, Newham P. Mechanisms of VCAM-1 and fibronectin binding to integrin alpha 4 beta 1: implications for integrin function and rational drug design. *Ciba Found Symp.* 1995;189:177–191.
120. Kasschau MR, Barabino GA, Bridges KR, Golan DE. Adhesion of sickle neutrophils and erythrocytes to fibronectin. *Blood.* 1996;87:771–780.
121. Han J, Rose DM, Woodside DG, Goldfinger LE, Ginsberg MH. Integrin alpha 4 beta 1-dependent T cell migration requires both phosphorylation and dephosphorylation of the alpha 4 cytoplasmic domain to regulate the reversible binding of paxillin. *J Biol Chem.* 2003;278:34845–34853.
122. Goldfinger LE, Han J, Kiosses WB, Howe AK, Ginsberg MH. Spatial restriction of alpha4 integrin phosphorylation regulates lamellipodial stability and alpha4beta1-dependent cell migration. *J Cell Biol.* 2003;162:731–741.
123. Brittain JE, Han J, Ataga KI, Orringer EP, Parise LV. Mechanism of CD47-induced alpha4beta1 integrin activation and adhesion in sickle reticulocytes. *J Biol Chem.* 2004;279:42393–42402.
124. Setty BN, Stuart MJ. Vascular cell adhesion molecule-1 is involved in mediating hypoxia-induced sickle red blood cell adherence to endothelium:potential role in sickle cell disease. *Blood.* 1996;88:2311–2320.
125. Vanderslice P, Ren K, Revelle JK, et al. A cyclic hexapeptide is a potent antagonist of alpha 4 integrins. *J Immunol.* 1997;158:1710–1718.
126. Parsons SF, Lee G, Spring FA, et al. Lutheran blood group glycoprotein and its newly characterized mouse homologue specifically bind alpha5 chain-containing human laminin with high affinity. *Blood.* 2001;97:312–320.
127. Parsons SF, Spring FA, Chasis JA, Anstee DJ. Erythroid cell adhesion molecules Lutheran and LW in health and disease. *Baillieres Best Pract Res Clin Haematol.* 1999;12:729–745.

128. Kaul DK, Liu XD, Zhang X, et al. Peptides based on alphaV-binding domains of erythrocyte ICAM-4 inhibit sickle red cell-endothelial interactions and vaso-occlusion in the microcirculation. *Am J Physiol Cell Physiol.* 2006;291:C922–C930.
129. Hines PC, Zen Q, Burney SN, et al. Novel epinephrine and cyclic AMP-mediated activation of BCAM(Lu-dependent sickle (SS) RBC adhesion. *Blood.* 2003;101:3281–3287.
130. Manodori AB, Barabino GA, Lubin BH, Kuypers FA. Adherence of phosphatidylserine-exposing erythrocytes to endothelial matrix thrombospondin. *Blood.* 2000;95:1293–1300.
131. Schlegel RA, Prendergast TW, Williamson P. Membrane phospholipid asymmetry as a factor in erythrocyte-endothelial cell interactions. *J Cell Physiol.* 1985;123:215–218.
132. Zwaal RF, Schroit AJ. Pathophysiologic implications of membrane phospholipid asymmetry in blood cells. *Blood.* 1997;89:1121–1132.
133. Setty BN, Kulkarni S, Rao AK, Stuart MJ. Fetal hemoglobin in sickle cell disease:relationship to erythrocyte phosphatidylserine exposure and coagulation activation. *Blood.* 2000;96:1119–1124.
134. Setty BN, Rao AK, Stuart MJ. Thrombophilia in sickle cell disease: the red cell connection. *Blood.* 2001;98:3228–3233.
135. de Jong K, Emerson RK, Butler J, Bastacky J, Mohandas N, Kuypers FA. Short survival of phosphatidylserine-exposing red blood cells in murine sickle cell anemia. *Blood.* 2001;98:1577–1584.
136. Kuypers FA, Yuan J, Lewis RA, et al. Membrane phospholipid asymmetry in human thalassemia. *Blood.* 1998;91:3044–3051.
137. Finnegan EM, Barabino GA, Liu XD, Chang HY, Jonczyk A, Kaul DK. Small-molecule cyclic alpha V beta 3 antagonists inhibit sickle red cell adhesion to vascular endothelium and vasoocclusion. *Am J Physiol Heart Circ Physiol.* 2007;293:H1038–H1045.
138. Hattori R, Hamilton KK, Fugate RD, McEver RP, Sims PJ. Stimulated secretion of endothelial von Willebrand factor is accompanied by rapid redistribution to the cell surface of the intracellular granule membrane protein GMP-140. *J Biol Chem.* 1989;264:7768–7771.
139. Stenberg PE, McEver RP, Shuman MA, Jacques YV, Bainton DF. A platelet alpha-granule membrane protein (GMP-140) is expressed on the plasma membrane after activation. *J Cell Biol.* 1985;101:880–886.
140. Lowe JB, Ward PA. Therapeutic inhibition of carbohydrate-protein interactions in vivo. *J Clin Invest.* 1997;99:822–826.
141. Mayadas TN, Johnson RC, Rayburn H, Hynes RO, Wagner DD. Leukocyte rolling and extravasation are severely compromised in P selectin-deficient mice. *Cell.* 1993;74:541–554.
142. Bullard DC, Kunkel EJ, Kubo H, et al. Infectious susceptibility and severe deficiency of leukocyte rolling and recruitment in E-selectin and P-selectin double mutant mice. *J Exp Med.* 1996;183:2329–2336.
143. Frenette PS, Mayadas TN, Rayburn H, Hynes RO, Wagner DD. Susceptibility to infection and altered hematopoiesis in mice deficient in both P- and E-selectins. *Cell.* 1996;84:563–574.
144. Embury SH, Matsui NM, Ramanujam S, et al. The contribution of endothelial cell P-selectin to the microvascular flow of mouse sickle erythrocytes in vivo. *Blood.* 2004;104:3378–3385.
145. Matsui NM, Varki A, Embury SH. Heparin inhibits the flow adhesion of sickle red blood cells to P-selectin. *Blood.* 2002;100:3790–3796.
146. Koenig A, Norgard-Sumnicht K, Linhardt R, Varki A. Differential interactions of heparin and heparan sulfate glycosaminoglycans with the selectins. Implications for the use of unfractionated and low molecular weight heparins as therapeutic agents. *J Clin Invest.* 1998;101:877–889.
147. Hirsh J, Raschke R, Warkentin TE, Dalen JE, Deykin D, Poller L. Heparin:mechanism of action, pharmacokinetics, dosing considerations, monitoring, efficacy, and safety. *Chest.* 1995;108:258S–275S.
148. Hiebert LM, Wice SM, Ping T. Increased plasma anti-Xa activity and recovery of heparin from urine suggest absorption of orally administered unfractionated heparin in human subjects. *J Lab Clin Med.* 2005;145:151–155.
149. Chaplin HJ, Monroe MC, Malecek AC, Morgan LK, Michael J, Murphy WA. Preliminary trial of minidose heparin prophylaxis for painful sickle cell crises. *E African Med J.* 1989;66:574–584.
150. Hiebert LM. Oral heparins. *Clin Lab.* 2002;48:111–116.
151. Mousa SA, Zhang F, Aljada A, et al. Pharmacokinetics and pharmacodynamics of oral heparin solid dosage form in healthy human subjects. *J Clin Pharmacol.* 2007;47:1508–1520.
152. Smith CM, Hebbel RP, Tukey DP, Clawson CC, White JG, Vercellotti GM. Pluronic F-68 reduces the endothelial adherence and improves the rheology of liganded sickle erythrocytes. *Blood.* 1987;69:1631–1636.
153. Adams-Graves P, Kedar A, Koshy M, et al. RheothRx (poloxamer 188) injection for the acute painful episode of sickle cell disease: a pilot study. *Blood.* 1997;90:2041–2046.
154. Gibbs WJ, Hagemann TM. Purified poloxamer 188 for sickle cell vaso-occlusive crisis. *Ann Pharmacother.* 2004;38:320–324.
155. Tricoci P, Newby LK, Kandzari DE, Harrington RA. Present and evolving role of eptifibatide in the treatment of acute coronary syndromes. *Expert Rev Cardiovasc Ther.* 2007;5:401–412.
156. Ataga KI, Cappellini MD, Rachmilewitz EA. Beta-thalassaemia and sickle cell anaemia as paradigms of hypercoagulability. *Br J Haematol.* 2007;139:3–13.
157. Eldor A, Rachmilewitz EA. The hypercoagulable state in thalassemia. *Blood.* 2002;99:36–43.
158. Francis RB Jr. Platelets, coagulation, and fibrinolysis in sickle cell disease: their possible role in vascular occlusion. *Blood Coagulat Fibrinolysis.* 1991;2:341–353.
159. Kurantsin-Mills J, Ofosu FA, Safa TK, Siegel RS, Lessin LS. Plasma factor VII and thrombin-antithrombin III levels indicate increased tissue factor activity in sickle cell patients. *Br J Haematol.* 1992;81:539–544.
160. Shet AS, Aras O, Gupta K, et al. Sickle blood contains tissue factor-positive microparticles derived from endothelial cells and monocytes. *Blood.* 2003;102:2678–2683.
161. Solovey A, Kollander R, Shet A, et al. Endothelial cell expression of tissue factor in sickle mice is augmented by hypoxia/reoxygenation and inhibited by lovastatin. *Blood.* 2004;104:840–846.
162. Franck PFH, Bevers EM, Lubin BH, et al. Uncoupling of the membrane skeleton from the lipid bilayer:the cause of accelerated phospholipid flip-flop leading to an enhanced

procoagulant activity of sickle cells. *J Clin Invest.* 1985;75: 183–190.

163. Kuypers FA, Lewis RA, Hua M, et al. Detection of altered membrane phospholipid asymmetry in subpopulations of human red blood cells using fluorescently labeled Annexin V. *Blood.* 1996;87:1179–1187.
164. Peters M, Plaat BE, ten Cate H, Wolters HJ, Weening RS, Brandjes DP. Enhanced thrombin generation in children with sickle cell disease. *Thromb Haemost.* 1994;71:169–172.
165. Kurantsin-Mills J, Ibe BO, Natta CL, Raj JU, Siegel RS, Lessin LS. Elevated urinary levels of thromboxane and prostacyclin metabolities in sickle cell disease reflects activated platelets in the circulation. *Br J Haematol.* 1994;87:580–585.
166. Setty BN, Chen D, Stuart MJ. Sickle cell vaso-occlusive crisis is associated with abnormalities in the ratio of vasoconstrictor to vasodilator prostanoids. *Pediatr Res.* 1995;38:95–102.
167. Wun T, Paglieroni T, Tablin F, Welborn J, Nelson K, Cheung A. Platelet activation and platelet-erythrocyte aggregates in patients with sickle cell anemia. *J Lab Clin Med.* 1997;129:507–516.
168. Solovey A, Gui L, Ramakrishnan S, Steinberg MH, Hebbel RP. Sickle cell anemia as a possible state of enhanced anti-apoptotic tone:survival effect of vascular endothelial growth factor on circulating and unanchored endothelial cells. *Blood.* 1999;93:3824–3830.
169. Salvaggio JE, Arnold CA, Banov CH. Long-term anticoagulation in sickle cell disease. *N Engl J Med.* 1963;269:182–186.
170. Wolters HJ, ten Cate H, Thomas LL, et al. Low-intensity oral anticoagulation in sickle-cell disease reverses the prethrombotic state:promises for treatment? *Br J Haematol.* 1995;90:715–717.
171. Schnog JB, Kater AP, Mac Gillavry MR, et al. Low adjusted-dose acenocoumarol therapy in sickle cell disease: a pilot study. *Am J Hematol.* 2001;68:179–183.
172. Schnog JB, Mac Gillavry MR, Rojer RA, et al. No effect of acenocoumarol therapy on levels of endothelial activation markers in sickle cell disease. *Am J Hematol.* 2002;71:53–55.
173. Greenberg J, Ohene-Frempong K, Halus J, Way C, Schwartz E. Trial of low doses of aspirin as prophylaxis in sickle cell disease. *J Pediatr.* 1983;102:781–784.
174. Zago MA, Costa FF, Ismael SJ, Tone LG, Bottura C. Treatment of sickle cell diseases with aspirin. *Acta Haematol.* 1984;72:61–64.
175. Semple MJ, Al-Hasani SF, Kioy P, Savidge GF. A double-blind trial of ticlopidine in sickle cell disease. *Thromb Haemost.* 1984;51:303–306.
176. Chaplin HJ, Alkjaersig N, Fletcher AP, Michael JM, Joist JH. Aspirin-dipyridamole prophylaxis of sickle cell disease pain crises. *Thromb Haemost.* 1980;43:218–221.
177. Balkaran B, Char G, Morris JS, Thomas PW, Serjeant BE, Serjeant GR. Stroke in a cohort of patients with homozygous sickle cell disease. *J Pediatr.* 1992;120:360–366.
178. Kinney TR, Sleeper LA, Wang WC, et al. Silent cerebral infarcts in sickle cell anemia:a risk factor analysis. The Cooperative Study of Sickle Cell Disease. *Pediatrics.* 1999;103:640–645.
179. Miller ST, Sleeper LA, Pegelow CH, et al. Prediction of adverse outcomes in children with sickle cell disease. *N Engl J Med.* 2000;342:83–89.
180. Platt OS, Brambilla DJ, Rosse WF, et al. Mortality in sickle cell disease. Life expectancy and risk factors for early death. *N Engl J Med.* 1994;330:1639–1644.
181. Stuart J, Stone PC, Akinola NO, Gallimore JR, Pepys MB. Monitoring the acute phase response to vaso-occlusive crisis in sickle cell disease. *J Clin Pathol.* 1994;47:166–169.
182. Pathare A, Al Kindi S, Alnaqdy AA, Daar S, Knox-Macaulay H, Dennison D. Cytokine profile of sickle cell disease in Oman. *Am J Hematol.* 2004;77:323–328.
183. Pathare A, Kindi SA, Daar S, Dennison D. Cytokines in sickle cell disease. *Hematology.* 2003;8:329–337.
184. Graido-Gonzalez E, Doherty JC, Bergreen EW, Organ G, Telfer M, McMillen MA. Plasma endothelin-1, cytokine, and prostaglandin E2 levels in sickle cell disease and acute vaso-occlusive sickle crisis. *Blood.* 1998;92:2551–2555.
185. Rybicki AC, Benjamin LJ. Increased levels of endothelin-1 in plasma of sickle cell anemia patients. *Blood.* 1998;92:2594–2596.
186. Croizat H, Nagel RL. Circulating cytokines response and the level of erythropoiesis in sickle cell anemia. *Am J Hematol.* 1999;60:105–115.
187. Duits AJ, Schnog JB, Lard LR, Saleh AW, Rojer RA. Elevated IL-8 levels during sickle cell crisis. *Eur J Haematol.* 1998;61:302–305.
188. Bourantas KL, Dalekos GN, Makis A, Chaidos A, Tsiara S, Mavridis A. Acute phase proteins and interleukins in steady state sickle cell disease. *Eur J Haematol.* 1998;61:49–54.
189. Oh SO, Ibe BO, Johnson C, Kurantsin-Mills J, Raj JU. Platelet-activating factor in plasma of patients with sickle cell disease in steady state. *J Lab Clin Med.* 1997;130:191–196.
190. Khodorova A, Navarro B, Jouaville LS, et al. Endothelin-B receptor activation triggers an endogenous analgesic cascade at sites of peripheral injury. *Nat Med.* 2003;9:1055–1061.
191. Solovey AA, Solovey AN, Harkness J, Hebbel RP. Modulation of endothelial cell activation in sickle cell disease: a pilot study. *Blood.* 2001;97:1937–1941.
192. Belcher JD, Bryant CJ, Nguyen J, et al. Transgenic sickle mice have vascular inflammation. *Blood.* 2003;101:3953–3959.
193. Osarogiagbon UR, Choong S, Belcher JD, Vercellotti GM, Paller MS, Hebbel RP. Reperfusion injury pathophysiology in sickle transgenic mice. *Blood.* 2000;96:314–320.
194. Barrett-Connor E. Bacterial infection and sickle cell anemia. An analysis of 250 infections in 166 patients and a review of the literature. *Medicine (Baltimore).* 1971;50:97–112.
195. Lachant NA, Sun NC, Leong LA, Oseas RS, Prince HE. Multicentric angiofollicular lymph node hyperplasia (Castleman's disease) followed by Kaposi's sarcoma in two homosexual males with the acquired immunodeficiency syndrome (AIDS). *Am J Clin Pathol.* 1985;83:27–33.
196. Platt OS. Sickle cell anemia as an inflammatory disease. *J Clin Invest.* 2000;106:337–338.
197. Collins T, Read MA, Neish AS, Whitley MZ, Thanos D, Maniatis T. Transcriptional regulation of endothelial cell adhesion molecules:NF-kappa B and cytokine-inducible enhancers. *FASEB J.* 1995;9:899–909.
198. Grisham MB, Granger DN, Lefer DJ. Modulation of leukocyte-endothelial interactions by reactive metabolites of oxygen and nitrogen:relevance to ischemic heart disease. *Free Radic Biol Med.* 1998;25:404–433.
199. Wahl C, Liptay S, Adler G, Schmid RM. Sulfasalazine:a potent and specific inhibitor of nuclear factor kappa B. *J Clin Invest.* 1998;101:1163–1174.

200. Weber CK, Liptay S, Wirth T, Adler G, Schmid RM. Suppression of NF-kappaB activity by sulfasalazine is mediated by direct inhibition of IkappaB kinases alpha and beta. *Gastroenterology.* 2000;119:1209–1218.
201. Kaul DK, Liu XD, Choong S, Belcher JD, Vercellotti GM, Hebbel RP. Anti-inflammatory therapy ameliorates leukocyte adhesion and microvascular flow abnormalities in transgenic sickle mice. *Am J Physiol Heart Circ Physiol.* 2004;287:H293–H301.
202. Mahaseth H, Vercellotti GM, Welch TE, Bowlin PR, Sonbol KM, Hsia CJ, Li M, Bischof JC, Hebbel RP, Belcher JD. Polynitroxyl albumin inhibits inflammation and vasoocclusion in transgenic sickle mice. *J Lab Clin Med.* 2005;145:204–211.
203. Hammerman SI, Kourembanas S, Conca TJ, Tucci M, Brauer M, Farber HW. Endothelin-1 production during the acute chest syndrome in sickle cell disease. *Am J Respir Crit Care Med.* 1997;156:280–285.
204. Rivera A, Rotter MA, Brugnara C. Endothelins activate Ca(2+)-gated K(+) channels via endothelin B receptors in CD-1 mouse erythrocytes. *Am J Physiol.* 1999;277:C746–C754.
205. de Winter RJ, Manten A, de Jong YP, Adams R, van Deventer SJ, Lie KI. Interleukin 8 released after acute myocardial infarction is mainly bound to erythrocytes. *Heart.* 1997;78:598–602.
206. Neote K, Mak JY, Kolakowski LF Jr, Schall TJ. Functional and biochemical analysis of the cloned Duffy antigen: identity with the red blood cell chemokine receptor. *Blood.* 1994;84:44–52.
207. Rivera A. Reduced sickle erythrocyte dehydration in vivo by endothelin-1 receptor antagonists. *Am J Physiol Cell Physiol.* 2007;293:C960–C966.
208. Eddahibi S, Raffestin B, Clozel M, Levame M, Adnot S. Protection from pulmonary hypertension with an orally active endothelin receptor antagonist in hypoxic rats. *Am J Physiol.* 1995;268:H828–H835.
209. Finsnes F, Lyberg T, Christensen G, Skjonsberg OH. Effect of endothelin antagonism on the production of cytokines in eosinophilic airway inflammation. *Am J Physiol Lung Cell Mol Physiol.* 2001;280:L659–L665.
210. Pearl JM, Wellmann SA, McNamara JL, Lombardi JP, Wagner CJ, Raake JL, Nelson DP. Bosentan prevents hypoxia-reoxygenation-induced pulmonary hypertension and improves pulmonary function. *Ann Thorac Surg.* 1999;68:1714–1721.
211. Hebbel RP, Morgan WT, Eaton JW, Hedlund BE. Accelerated autoxidation and heme loss due to instability of sickle hemoglobin. *Proc Natl Acad Sci USA.* 1988;85:237–241.
212. Sheng K, Shariff M, Hebbel RP. Comparative oxidation of hemoglobins A and S. *Blood.* 1998;91:3467–3470.
213. Chiu D, Lubin B, Shohet SB. Erythrocyte membrane lipid reorganization during the sickling process. *Br J Haematol.* 1979;41:223–234.
214. Hebbel RP, Eaton JW, Balasingam M, Steinberg MH. Spontaneous oxygen radical generation by sickle erythrocytes. *J Clin Invest.* 1982;70:1253–1259.
215. Hogg N, Kalyanaraman B, Joseph J, Struck A, Parthasarathy S. Inhibition of low-density lipoprotein oxidation by nitric oxide. Potential role in atherogenesis. *FEBS Lett.* 1993;334:170–174.
216. Hogg N, Struck A, Goss SP, et al. Inhibition of macrophage-dependent low density lipoprotein oxidation by nitric-oxide donors. *J Lipid Res.* 1995;36:1756–1762.
217. Garcia-Cardena G, Fan R, Shah V, et al. Dynamic activation of endothelial nitric oxide synthase by Hsp90. *Nature.* 1998;392:821–824.
218. Lin MI, Fulton D, Babbitt R, et al. Phosphorylation of threonine 497 in endothelial nitric-oxide synthase coordinates the coupling of L-arginine metabolism to efficient nitric oxide production. *J Biol Chem.* 2003;278:44719–44726.
219. Vasquez-Vivar J, Kalyanaraman B, Martasek P, et al. Superoxide generation by endothelial nitric oxide synthase:the influence of cofactors. *Proc Natl Acad Sci USA.* 1998;95:9220–9225.
220. Xu H, Shi Y, Wang J, et al. A heat shock protein 90 binding domain in endothelial nitric-oxide synthase influences enzyme function. *J Biol Chem.* 2007;282:37567–37574.
221. Morris CR, Morris SM Jr, Hagar W, et al. Arginine therapy: a new treatment for pulmonary hypertension in sickle cell disease? *Am J Respir Crit Care Med.* 2003;168:63–69.
222. Dasgupta T, Hebbel RP, Kaul DK. Protective effect of arginine on oxidative stress in transgenic sickle mouse models. *Free Radic Biol Med.* 2006;41:1771–1780.
223. Wood KC, Hebbel RP, Lefer DJ, Granger DN. Critical role of endothelial cell-derived nitric oxide synthase in sickle cell disease-induced microvascular dysfunction. *Free Radic Biol Med.* 2006;40:1443–1453.
224. Reiter CD, Wang X, Tanus-Santos JE, et al. Cell-free hemoglobin limits nitric oxide bioavailability in sickle-cell disease. *Nat Med.* 2002;8:1383–1389.
225. Nath KA, Shah V, Haggard JJ, et al. Mechanisms of vascular instability in a transgenic mouse model of sickle cell disease. *Am J Physiol Regul Integr Comp Physiol.* 2000;279:R1949–R1955.
226. Head CA, Brugnara C, Martinez-Ruiz R, et al. Low concentrations of nitric oxide increase oxygen affinity of sickle erythrocytes in vitro and in vivo. *J Clin Invest.* 1997;100:1193–1198.
227. Weiner DL, Hibberd PL, Betit P, Cooper AB, Botelho CA, Brugnara C. Preliminary assessment of inhaled nitric oxide for acute vaso-occlusive crisis in pediatric patients with sickle cell disease. *JAMA.* 2003;289:1136–1142.
228. De Franceschi L, Baron A, Scarpa A, et al. Inhaled nitric oxide protects transgenic SAD mice from sickle cell disease-specific lung injury induced by hypoxia/reoxygenation. *Blood.* 2003;102:1087–1096.
229. De Franceschi L, Malpeli G, Scarpa A, et al. Protective effects of S-nitrosoalbumin on lung injury induced by hypoxia-reoxygenation in mouse model of sickle cell disease. *Am J Physiol Lung Cell Mol Physiol.* 2006;291:L457–L465.
230. Ou J, Ou Z, Jones DW, et al. L-4F, an apolipoprotein A-1 mimetic, dramatically improves vasodilation in hypercholesterolemia and sickle cell disease. *Circulation.* 2003;107:2337–2341.
231. Navab M, Anantharamaiah GM, Hama S, et al. Oral administration of an Apo A-I mimetic Peptide synthesized from D-amino acids dramatically reduces atherosclerosis in mice independent of plasma cholesterol. *Circulation.* 2002;105:290–292.
232. Navab M, Anantharamaiah GM, Reddy ST, et al. Human apolipoprotein AI mimetic peptides for the treatment of atherosclerosis. *Curr Opin Invest Drugs.* 2003;4:1100–1104.

233. Van Lenten BJ, Wagner AC, Jung CL, Lehrer RI, Navab M, Fogelman AM. The ability of apolipoprotein A-I mimetic peptides to improve HDL anti-inflammatory properties is due to their remarkable binding affinities for oxidized lipids. *Circulation.* 2007;116:581.
234. Navab M, Anantharamaiah GM, Reddy ST, et al. Oral D-4F causes formation of pre-beta high-density lipoprotein and improves high-density lipoprotein-mediated cholesterol efflux and reverse cholesterol transport from macrophages in apolipoprotein E-null mice. *Circulation.* 2004;109:3215–3220.
235. Weihrauch D, Xu H, Shi Y, et al. Effects of D-4F on vasodilation, oxidative stress, angiostatin, myocardial inflammation, and angiogenic potential in tight-skin mice. *Am J Physiol Heart Circ Physiol.* 2007;293:H1432–H1441.
236. Remaley AT, Thomas F, Stonik JA, et al. Synthetic amphipathic helical peptides promote lipid efflux from cells by an ABCA1-dependent and an ABCA1-independent pathway. *J Lipid Res.* 2003;44:828–836.
237. Jia Z, Natarajan P, Forte TM, Bielicki JK. Thiol-bearing synthetic peptides retain the antioxidant activity of apolipoproteinA-I(Milano). *Biochem Biophys Res Commun.* 2002;297:206–213.
238. Bielicki JK, Oda MN. Apolipoprotein A-I(Milano) and apolipoprotein A-I(Paris) exhibit an antioxidant activity distinct from that of wild-type apolipoprotein A-I. *Biochemistry.* 2002;41:2089–2096.
239. Shah PK, Yano J, Reyes O, et al. High-dose recombinant apolipoprotein A-I(milano) mobilizes tissue cholesterol and rapidly reduces plaque lipid and macrophage content in apolipoprotein e-deficient mice. Potential implications for acute plaque stabilization. *Circulation.* 2001;103:3047–3050.
240. Shah PK. High-density lipoprotein mimetics: focus on synthetic high-density lipoprotein. *Am J Cardiol.* 2007;100:S62–S67.
241. Brouet A, Sonveaux P, Dessy C, Moniotte S, Balligand JL, Feron O. Hsp90 and caveolin are key targets for the proangiogenic nitric oxide-mediated effects of statins. *Circ Res.* 2001; 89:866–873.
242. Aslan M, Ryan TM, Adler B, et al. Oxygen radical inhibition of nitric oxide-dependent vascular function in sickle cell disease. *Proc Natl Acad Sci USA.* 2001;98:15215–15220.
243. Baldus S, Eiserich JP, Brennan ML, Jackson RM, Alexander CB, Freeman BA. Spatial mapping of pulmonary and vascular nitrotyrosine reveals the pivotal role of myeloperoxidase as a catalyst for tyrosine nitration in inflammatory diseases. *Free Radic Biol Med.* 2002;33:1010.
244. Schrier SL, Centis F, Verneris M, Ma L, Angelucci E. The role of oxidant injury in the pathophysiology of human thalassemias. *Redox Rep.* 2003;8:241–245.
245. Shinar E, Rachmilewitz EA. Haemoglobinopathies and red cell membrane function. *Baillieres Clin Haematol.* 1993; 6:357–369.
246. Repka T, Hebbel RP. Hydroxyl radical formation by sickle erythrocyte membranes: role of pathologic iron deposits and cytoplasmic reducing agents. *Blood.* 1991;78:2753–2758.
247. Shalev O, Repka T, Goldfarb A, et al. Deferiprone (L1) chelates pathologic iron deposits from membranes of intact thalassemic and sickle red blood cells both in vitro and in vivo. *Blood.* 1995;86:2008–2013.
248. Zerez CR, Lachant NA, Lee SJ, Tanaka KR. Decreased erythrocyte nicotinamide adenine dinucleotide redox potential and abnormal pyridine nucleotide content in sickle cell disease. *Blood.* 1988;71:512–515.
249. Morris CR, Suh JH, Hagar W, et al. Erythrocyte glutamine depletion, altered redox environment, and pulmonary hypertension in sickle cell disease. *Blood.* 2008;111:402–410.
250. Niihara Y, Zerez CR, Akiyama DS, Tanaka KR. Increased red cell glutamine availability in sickle cell anemia: demonstration of increased active transport, affinity, and increased glutamate level in intact red cells. *J Lab Clin Med.* 1997;130:83–90.
251. Niihara Y, Matsui NM, Shen YM, et al. L-glutamine therapy reduces endothelial adhesion of sickle red blood cells to human umbilical vein endothelial cells. *BMC Blood Disord.* 2005;5:4.
252. Niihara Y, Zerez CR, Akiyama DS, Tanaka KR. Oral L-glutamine therapy for sickle cell anemia: I. Subjective clinical improvement and favorable change in red cell NAD redox potential. *Am J Hematol.* 1998;58:117–121.
253. Wu G, Fang YZ, Yang S, Lupton JR, Turner ND. Glutathione metabolism and its implications for health. *J Nutr.* 2004;134:489–492.
254. Amer J, Ghoti H, Rachmilewitz E, Koren A, Levin C, Fibach E. Red blood cells, platelets and polymorphonuclear neutrophils of patients with sickle cell disease exhibit oxidative stress that can be ameliorated by antioxidants. *Br J Haematol.* 2006;132:108–113.
255. Udupi V, Rice-Evans C. Thiol compounds as protective agents in erythrocytes under oxidative stress. *Free Radic Res Commun.* 1992;16:315–323.
256. Gibson XA, Shartava A, McIntyre J, et al. The efficacy of reducing agents or antioxidants in blocking the formation of dense cells and irreversibly sickled cells in vitro. *Blood.* 1998;91:4373–4378.
257. Goodman SR. The irreversibly sickled cell: a perspective. *Cell Mol Biol.* 2004;50:53–58.
258. Pace BS, Shartava A, Pack-Mabien A, Mulekar M, Ardia A, Goodman SR. Effects of N-acetylcysteine on dense cell formation in sickle cell disease. *Am J Hematol.* 2003;73:26–32.

32

Stem Cell Transplantation

Emanuele Angelucci and Mark Walters

INTRODUCTION

Homozygous β thalassemia is characterized by absent or defective β-globin chain synthesis. This defect causes imbalance in chain production and accumulation of unstable α-globin tetramers in red blood cells or their precursors, leading to intramedullary destruction, apoptosis and hemolytic anemia (chapter 17). Regular transfusions and iron chelation has, in developed countries, transformed this disease from one fatal in infancy to a chronic disease with prolonged survival.[1–3] Medical treatment is expensive and requires a complex multidisciplinary approach. In underdeveloped countries, where most patients reside, thalassemia remains fatal early in life because of poor access to modern medical treatment. Curing β thalassemia by hematopoietic cell transplantation, with the cost efficiencies inherent in this approach, is therefore an attractive option.

As in β thalassemia major, the objective of hematopoietic cell transplantation for sickle cell disease is to replace recipient erythropoiesis, or to reduce its clinical impact, by the expression of donor β-globin chains. The clinical benefit of this cellular replacement is the elimination, or significant amelioration, of the clinical complications caused by polymerized sickle hemoglobin. More than a decade ago, the initial clinical trials of hematopoietic cell transplantation for sickle cell disease indicated that the replacement of donor for sickle erythropoiesis might eliminate not only the hematological manifestations of the underlying disorder, but also stabilize and even reduce the organ damage caused by recurrent vasoocclusion occlusion and hemolysis.[4–7] As in malignant disorders, there is utility in assigning a risk-based approach to applying transplantation for sickle cell disease. Unfortunately, defining risk characteristics is difficult in the absence of randomized, prospective trials that compare therapeutic interventions among high-risk patients. Nonetheless, the appropriate broader application of hematopoietic cell transplantation hinges on three important objectives. The first is to identify those patients who have the greatest risk of developing sickle-related complications and who are most likely to benefit from hematopoietic cell transplantation. The second is to reduce transplant-related complications by minimizing the short- and long-term toxicities of hematopoietic cell transplantation, but in such a way that does not diminish the likelihood of a successful transplantation outcome. The third, which is common to sickle cell disease and β thalassemia, is to increase the availability of hematopoietic cell transplantation to potential recipients by expanding the pool of suitable donors, either by using alternate sources of hematopoietic stem cells or by overcoming human leukocyte antigen (HLA) disparity and its formidable barrier to donor–host immunological tolerance.

HEMATOPOIETIC STEM CELL TRANSPLANTATION FOR β THALASSEMIA

In simple terms, the purpose of treating β thalassemia by allogeneic hematopoietic stem cell transplantation is to affect a "cure," that is, to replace ineffective erythropoiesis with effective erythropoiesis capable of producing sufficient number of circulating red cells that contain an adequate amount of hemoglobin. This simple statement, however, implies several major problems, which are biological, clinical, and ethical.[8]

The First Cases

In December 1981, a 14-month-old child with β thalassemia, who had undergone transfusion with a total of 250 mL of packed red blood cells, received a bone marrow transplant in Seattle, Washington from his HLA identical sister.[9] The transplant was successful and the patient is now more than 25 years old and in excellent health without any manifestations of β thalassemia. Two weeks later, a 14-year-old patient with advanced thalassemia who had received more than 150 red blood cell transfusions underwent transplantation in Pesaro, but had recurrence of β thalassemia after rejection of the graft.[10]

The Pesaro Experience

In the early 1980s, the initial Pesaro studies were concentrated on patients with advanced β thalassemia. Of the first six patients who were aged 16 years or older and who underwent transplantation after receiving high doses of cyclophosphamide and total body irradiation, four died of causes related to graft-versus-host disease (GVHD) within the first 100 days; one died of infection 235 days after hematopoietic cell transplantation; and one had recurrence of thalassemia 48 days after hematopoietic cell transplantation, dying of thalassemia-related cardiac disease more than 6 years later.[10]

In view of this experience, subsequent studies concentrated on enrolling patients who were younger than 17 years. Results in young patients were encouraging[10–12] and in 1990 the Pesaro group reported experience through August 1988 in treating 222 consecutive patients younger than 16 years.[13] All of these patients received HLA-identical marrow allografts: in 10 cases from parents and in the other cases from siblings. All patients were prepared for transplantation after conditioning with regimens that contained busulfan (14 mg/kg) and cyclophosphamide (200 mg/kg). In this series, the probabilities of survival and thalassemia-free survival plateaued after 1 year at 82% and 75%, respectively.[13] Analysis of the influence of pretransplant characteristics on the outcome of transplantation was conducted in 116 patients who were all treated similarly. This analysis demonstrated that hepatomegaly and portal fibrosis were associated with a significantly reduced probability of survival. In a multivariate analysis, history of poor compliance with iron chelation therapy could not be distinguished from hepatomegaly as a predictor of survival and thalassemia-free survival. The influence of pretransplant characteristics on the outcome of transplantation was reexamined in late 1989[14] by which time 161 patients younger than 17 years had been treated with the same regimen. The quality of chelation therapy was characterized as regular when deferoxamine therapy was initiated not later than 18 months after the first transfusion and administered subcutaneously for 8–10 hours continuously for at least 5 days each week. Chelation therapy was defined as irregular for any deviation from this requirement. The degree of hepatomegaly (> or <2 cm), the presence or absence of portal fibrosis in the pretransplant liver biopsy,[15] and the quality of chelation (regular or irregular) given through the years before transplantation were identified as variables permitting the categorization of patients younger than 17 years into three risk classes: class 1 patients had none of these adverse risk factors; class 3 patients had all three; and class 2 patients had one or two adverse risk factors.

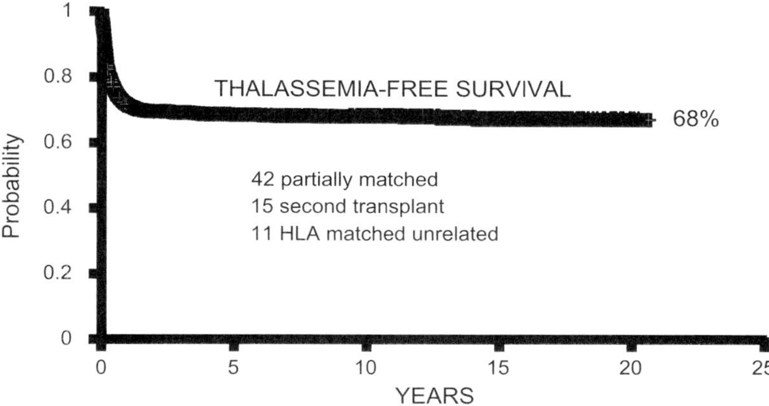

Figure 32.1. A total of 1,003 consecutive thalassemia patients between the ages of 1 and 35 years underwent transplantation in Pesaro from 1981 to January 2003. This survival curve includes 950 patients who underwent transplantation from an HLA-identical donor, 42 patients from a partially matched-related donor, and 11 from a matched-unrelated donor.

Between 17 December 1981 and 31 January 2003, a total of 1,003 consecutive patients, aged from 1 to 35 years, underwent transplantation in Pesaro (950 from an HLA-identical related donor, 42 from partially matched related donor, and 11 from a matched unrelated donor). Overall, the greater than 20-year Kaplan–Meier probability of thalassemia-free survival was 68% (Fig. 32.1).[16]

With regard to predictors of transplant outcome, patients younger than 17 years were stratified on the basis of the risk factors of hepatomegaly, a history of irregular chelation, and hepatic fibrosis. Class 1 (low risk) and 2 (intermediate risk) patients underwent transplantation after conditioning with the combination of busulphan (14 mg/kg) and cyclophosphamide (200 mg/kg). This conditioning regimen has remained unmodified since 1985. Class 3 patients (advanced disease) underwent transplantation based on protocols that included lower dosages of cyclophosphamide (120–160 mg/kg). These results are shown in Table 32.1. Transplantation in class 3 children, with treatment of a reduced dose of cyclophosphamide, was characterized by a 30% risk of thalassemia recurrence.[17] In contrast, in adults with the same dose of cyclophosphamide, thalassemia recurrence was only 4%, but there was a 35% transplant-related mortality.[18]

Because class 3 children had the problem of thalassemia recurrence whereas adults had the problem of transplant-related mortality, a new preparative regimen was introduced for class 3 patients with the aim of increasing the rate of sustained engraftment while decreasing transplant-related mortality. This regimen was characterized by a 30-day preconditioning period designed to produce erythroid cytoreduction and immunosuppression before a conditioning regimen using a reduced dose of cyclophosphamide. In a pilot study of 33 consecutive class 3 thalassemia children, the 5-year Kaplan–Meier probability of survival and disease-free survival was 93% and 85%, respectively.[19]

Table 32.1. Transplant outcome. Pesaro results in children and adults

Class of risk	Regimen	% Survival	% Thalassemia-free survival
1	Bu 14-Cy 200	93	90
2	Bu 14-Cy 200	87	84
3	Bu 14-Cy 120–160	79	58
Adults	Bu 14-Cy 120–160	66	62

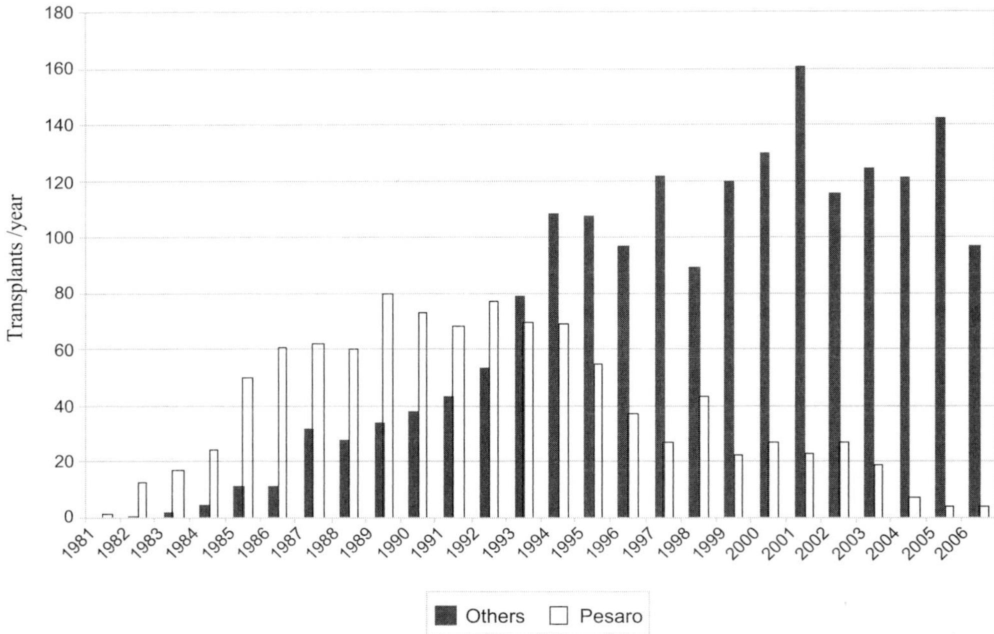

Figure 32.2. Hematopoietic stem cell transplants for hemoglobinopathies performed between 1981 and 2006 in centers reporting data to the European Group for Blood and Bone Marrow Transplantation. Transplants performed in Pesaro versus all other centers (2006 data incomplete).

ALTERNATIVE SOURCE OF HEMATOPOIETIC STEM CELLS

The results reported in the previous section were obtained using bone marrow derived, unmanipulated hematopoietic stem cells, and today, most centers continue to use bone marrow hematopoietic stem cells in lieu of mobilized peripheral blood progenitor cells. From a survey conducted by the European Group for Blood and Bone Marrow Transplantation (unpublished data), approximately 10% of the transplants performed for hemoglobinopathies involved the use of mobilized peripheral blood progenitor cells. Even in the absence of a randomized clinical trial to compare these two sources of hematopoietic cells in thalassemia, it is reasonable to predict that a reduced incidence of chronic GVHD is a very good reason to choose bone marrow hematopoietic stem cells for this nonmalignant disorder for which GVHD offers no benefit.

Recently confirmatory results have been reported when using cord blood as a source of HLA genotypically identical hematopoietic stem cells for class 1 and 2 children[20] with a 2-year survival and disease-free survival of 100% and 79%, respectively.

Reduced-intensity Transplants

Because of the excellent results of conventional transplantation for β thalassemia, no systematic study of reduced-intensity or nonmyeloablative transplantation has been reported. The relatively high incidence of thalassemic recurrence in children after conventional myeloablative hematopoietic stem cell transplantation[16] makes it is reasonable to suppose that a nonmyeloablative regimen will have to contend with very high frequencies of thalassemic recurrence. If an investigation is to be proposed, additional tools to ensure sustained engraftment such as donor lymphocyte infusions will probably be necessary.

Experience of Other Transplant Centers

Following the Pesaro experience, hematopoietic cell transplant programs for thalassemia have been established in several parts of the world where the disease is prevalent. Overall, approximately 80% of patients survive long term and of these, nearly 90% are "cured."[21]

The recently developed hemoglobinopathy registry of the European Group for Blood and Bone Marrow Transplantation provides demonstration of the diffusion of the procedure worldwide (Fig. 32.2). Preliminary outcome data analyses confirm reproducibility of Pesaro Class of risk in a multicentric setting and demonstrate a 90% 5-year survival rate for patients who underwent transplantation in the 1990s.

Alternative Donors

Approximately 60%–70% children with β thalassemia do not have HLA-identical family members[22] and therefore are not candidates for transplantation. Expanding the number of available donors would have a major impact on the management of this disease.

HLA-nonidentical Related Donor Transplant. The use of HLA-nonidentical family member donors in the treatment of β thalassemia has not been comprehensively studied in recent years because the results in leukemia were not sufficiently promising to justify a large trial. The results reported are anecdotal and therefore it is difficult to extrapolate useful information.

As of December 1998 in Pesaro, 29 thalassemia patients were transplanted from a family member donor who was not an HLA-identical sibling. The number of mismatched HLA antigens was one in 15 cases, two in five cases, and three in three cases. Results have been unrewarding, with only six successes, 10 transplant-related deaths, and 13 patients who had recurrence of thalassemia.[23]

Between 1969 and 1996, 60 cases were reported by 22 different teams to the International Bone Marrow Transplant Registry but only 11 (17%) underwent transplantation after 1993. Forty-seven of the 60 patients survived and 16 of the survivors had recurrence of thalassemia. In this group of 60 patients, 24 received a transplant from an HLA phenotypically matched parental donor, 11 had related donors with one HLA mismatch, and four had donors with two HLA mismatches.[24] Although most of these patients would not have benefited from improved supportive care techniques and DNA typing technologies that were established after 1993, it is clear that HLA-mismatched related donor transplantation is not a favored option at present in the early management of patients who can access and tolerate medical therapy. A pilot study involving the use of the mother as an HLA haploidentical donor is ongoing but results have not yet been published.

Transplant From Matched Unrelated Donors. Unrelated donor transplantation has significant potential in thalassemia because of the possibility for many patients to remain healthy for a long time under medical treatment until an "optimal" hematopoietic stem cell donor is identified. In recent years, improvements in HLA typing technology, improved control of GVHD and infectious diseases, and expanded pools of unrelated volunteer donors together have generated significant improvements in the outcome after unrelated marrow transplantation in patients affected by malignancies and by inborn errors of metabolism. In leukemia, unrelated transplant results are now very similar to those achieved using an related HLA-identical donor. On the basis of this finding, an investigation of HLA-matched unrelated donor transplantation for β thalassemia that included six Italian transplant centers was established in 1996. Patients with pretransplant evidence of cirrhosis or cardiac disease were excluded, and a high degree of histocompatibility between patient and the potential donor was required. The clinical trial also required extended HLA–haplotype identity, which means that matching donor/recipient HLA alleles extending from locus HLA-A to locus HLA-Dq on the same chromosome is required.

Thus far, 68 patients (median age 15, range 2–37 years) have been transplanted in the unrelated donor trial. With a median follow-up of 30 months, nine patients (13%) had recurrence of thalassemia, 14 (20%) died, and 45 (67%) had successful transplants.[25] The incidence of acute GVHD grades II–IV was 40% and that of chronic GVHD 18%. After a median follow-up of 40 months, overall and disease-free survival rates were 79% and 65%, respectively. In the 30 patients who were classified as class 1–2, overall survival and disease-free survival rates were both 97%. These data confirm the relevance of the patients' condition to transplant outcome in the setting of matched-unrelated and matched-related donor transplant, and once again, emphasize the adverse clinical characteristics of advanced thalassemia major. Nevertheless, hematopoietic cell transplantation from HLA-matched unrelated donors is still an approach that should be limited to experienced transplant centers. As a public health issue, the probability of finding a closely matched unrelated marrow donor would be higher than in the general population if representative marrow donor registries were established in areas with the highest incidence of thalassemia.

The Thalassemia Patient Undergoing Bone Marrow Transplantation

Patient Selection and Classes of Risk. All patients who require chronic red cell transfusions are potential candidates for hematopoietic cell transplantation. Patients with advanced liver [Child–Pugh grades B–C] and cardiac disease are ineligible for transplantation. Thalassemia intermedia patients can be considered for marrow transplantation in selected situations.[26]

The development of a regimen of regular transfusions combined with regular iron chelation therapy has transformed the prognosis for thalassemia children in industrialized countries from a disease fatal in infancy to a chronic disease permitting prolonged survival.[27–29] The critical factor for survival of thalassemic patients undergoing transfusion and chelation therapy is control of the iron overload (Chapter 29). If good compliance is achieved with chelation therapy, iron overload can be controlled but not abolished.[1,3,30] Nevertheless, hematopoietic cell transplantation remains the only definitive curative approach and any clinical decision must be approached with this assumption.

Classification of patients in pretransplant classes of risk permits an assessment of an individual's probability of "cure" by hematopoietic cell transplantation independent of the patient's response to treatment, and therefore adequate information can be obtained from survival curves. The clinical significance of the Pesaro classification has sometimes been misinterpreted. This classification was developed for transplant purposes only and reflects progression of disease severity. Although it is based primarily on the liver status, it does not predict a liver-related cause of death. Liver status must be considered as a "window" on the patient's global health situation. A major criticism of the Pesaro classification is that two of the variables, chelation and hepatomegaly, are qualitative and subject to intra- and interobserver variability.[31] This is a valid criticism and quantitatively defined risk factors based on a defined unit of measure would obviously increase the precision and accuracy of the classification. It is hoped that such criteria could be introduced in the future, but so far all attempts to identify such criteria have failed. Variables such as serum ferritin or hepatic iron concentration did not achieve significance in the statistical analyses as predictors of transplant outcome. This reflects the complexity in assessing the global clinical condition of a thalassemic patient. Any quantitative laboratory value reflecting iron overload, for example, serum ferritin or hepatic iron concentration, reflects the situation at a certain moment in life and does not necessarily reflect the impact on tissue damage of years of exposure to a toxic element like iron.

The inclusion of a patient in class 2 and particularly, in class 3, represents failure of conventional therapy and this reflects the clinically progressive nature of the disease whose optimal treatment is based on a delicate balance among the degree of anemia, body iron content, and iron chelation.

Recurrence of Thalassemia. In a variable percentage of cases, the patient can reject the graft. Rejection can be followed by persistent marrow aplasia or by return of thalassemia. The first situation is relatively rare and can be reversed only with a second transplant. By analogy to the behavior of malignant tissue, it might be supposed that a largely expanded hematopoietic tissue mass would be difficult to eradicate and likely to recur after transplantation. Leukemic relapse is, however, characterized by the reappearance of leukemia in the presence of a persistent immune system of donor origin. In contrast, the return of thalassemia usually occurs in the context of a return of host-type immune reconstitution. This event has aspects of both rejection and relapse.

Mixed Chimeric State. An important finding that became evident during the Pesaro transplant experience was the demonstration that in a significant group of patients, the clinical control of the disease was achieved with a partial engraftment. This defines mixed chimerism – the simultaneous presence in the bone marrow of cells of both donor and host origin. Although early chimerism is a risk factor for thalassemia recurrence, late chimerism, detected at least 2 years after transplantation, is a stable condition called persistent chimerism.[32] All 31 patients with persistent chimerism studied yearly for up to 11 years of follow-up had stable engraftment. Despite limited allogeneic engraftment – some patients had only 20% donor cells – these patients had normal hemoglobin values, were transfusion free, and had no signs of ineffective erythropoiesis.[32]

Effect of Bone Marrow Transplantation on Thalassemia

Transplantation in thalassemia provides what appears to be a permanent cure of the marrow defect in nearly all patients. Thalassemia patients who have acquired normal bone marrow as a result of transplantation cannot be accurately described as "cured" per se. They have homozygosity for the mutant gene in every cell of the body except in the hematopoietic cells and carry all the clinical complications there were acquired during years of transfusion and chelation therapy before transplantation. The treatment of patients with thalassemia is not always completed after a successful hematopoietic cell transplant has been achieved. Good health and a normal life expectancy can only be achieved after the organ damage acquired during years with thalassemia and its treatment is reversed. These features are mainly iron overload and hepatitis C virus infection. Thus, the care of patients after transplantation should be divided into transplant-related complications and thalassemia-related complications.

Transplant-related Complications. Transplant-related complications include chronic GVHD and secondary malignancy. The most serious long-term marrow transplant complication is GVHD, which is associated with significant morbidity and mortality. A retrospective study was performed in Pesaro that included 734 consecutive thalassemic patients, 614 of whom were evaluable for chronic GVHD.[33] The overall incidence of chronic GVHD was 27.3% (168 of 614 evaluable patients). The probabilities of mild, moderate, and severe chronic GVHD were 20%, 8%, and 2%, respectively. In 67% of the affected patients, chronic GVHD was limited and in 33% it was extensive. No difference in incidence was observed among the three classes of risk. Of the 168 patients who developed chronic GVHD, 85.1% recovered from the complication, 8.9% died, and 6% were still being treated at the end of the study.

As of August 2005, four cases of early malignancies, defined as occurring within the first year after transplantation, were recorded in patients from Pesaro. These included three cases of B-cell lymphoproliferative disease and one case of cardiac myxoma. Two of the patients with lymphoproliferative disease died of progressive disease and one is alive and well more than 15 years after radiotherapy. The patient with cardiac myxoma died 6 years later in a car accident while in continuous remission after surgical removal of the tumor.[34] Five cases of late, solid tumors have been recorded. One patient developed Kaposi sarcoma while receiving treatment for mild chronic GVHD that spontaneously reversed after discontinuation of immunosuppressive therapy.[35] A second patient with chronic GVHD developed lip spinocellular cancer and died of progressive cancer 13 years after hematopoietic cell transplantation. Another patient with resolved mucosal chronic GVHD developed lip carcinoma 17 years after transplantation. Two other cases were registered in patients without chronic GVHD (one osteochondroma and one colon cancer 7 and

20 years after transplantation, respectively). These last three patients are alive and well after combined surgical and medical treatment. Overall, the incidence of secondary solid tumors in thalassemia after transplantation is less than 10/100,000 patient-years, a rate that does not appear higher than that reported in patients undergoing medical treatment for β thalassemia.[36–38] These findings are consistent with data reported by the International Bone Marrow Transplant Registry; patients undergoing hematopoietic cell transplantation for nonmalignant diseases had an incidence of secondary malignancies that was not significantly increased when compared with the expected value in the normal population.[39] Thus, a concern about late malignancy is not a reason to deny transplantation.

Thalassemia-related Complications. Thalassemia-related complications are those acquired during years of thalassemia and its treatment.

Iron Overload

Hematopoietic cell transplantation will not eliminate excess iron acquired during treatment.

Iron overload causes significant morbidity and mortality and progression of liver disease to cirrhosis after transplantation has been documented.[40,41] A prospective analysis of annual liver biopsies in patients not treated by iron chelation and in whom thalassemia was cured by hematopoietic cell transplantation demonstrated that iron overload and hepatitis C virus infection were independent and mutually reinforcing risk factors for progressive liver fibrosis. Patients who were hepatitis C virus positive and also had very high levels of hepatic iron had an 80% risk of developing progressive hepatic fibrosis 10–12 years after successful transplantation. Conversely, patients with a liver iron level less than 16 mg iron/g liver dry weight and who were also free of evidence of active hepatitis C virus infection,showed no signs of progressive hepatic fibrosis.

Due to the presence of normal erythropoiesis, phlebotomy in the posttransplant thalassemia recipient appeared to be the appropriate method for rapidly removing excess iron.[42] Phlebotomy is safe, inexpensive, and highly efficient, and therefore it is the treatment of choice in this situation even in patients who received a transplant from a donor with thalassemia minor. With this approach, excess iron can be completely mobilized from the body without any relevant side effect (Figs. 32.3 and 32.4). Following completion of the phlebotomy program, significant improvement in liver function was observed, particularly in patients infected with hepatitis C virus.[42] Several cases of reversion of pretransplant severe hepatic fibrosis and even early cirrhosis have been reported.[43] Patients with early cardiac involvement characterized by left ventricular diastolic dysfunction and impaired left ventricular contractility demonstrated regression of subclinical cardiac disease after iron depletion.[43] In posttransplantation thalassemic patients with high iron levels who cannot be treated by phlebotomy because of young age or difficult peripheral venous access, daily subcutaneous administration of desferrioxamine has proved to be useful in reducing iron stores.[44] Because of the development of deferasirox, an effective oral chelator with no reported marrow toxicity (Chapter 29) there is no reason to use desferrioxamine as a second-line therapy for patients who cannot have repeated phlebotomies.

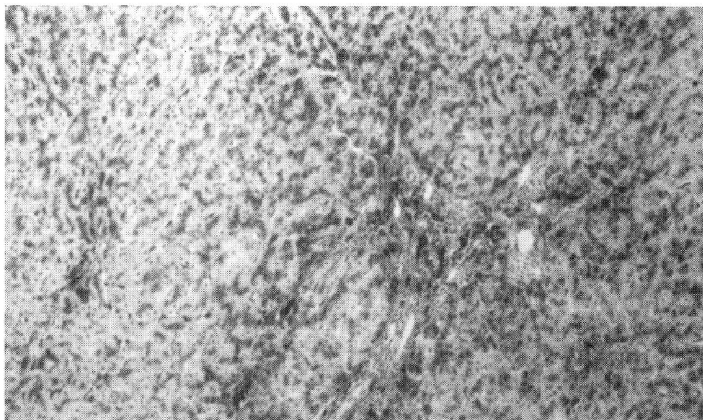

Figure 32.3. Pretransplant liver biopsy of a thalassemia patient. The biopsy was prepared using Perls technique. Hepatic iron concentration was 23 mg/g dry weight. (See color plate 32.3.)

Hepatitis

After hematopoietic cell transplantation, patients with thalassemia have a life expectancy that approaches normal, and mild chronic liver disease has to be considered with this perspective. Viral liver disease is probably the only significant factor that might limit survival in ex-thalassemics, thus avoiding progression of liver damage and cirrhosis in follow-up over 20–30 years is fundamental. In approximately half of hepatitis C–seropositive patients, transaminase levels normalized and the histological activity index significantly improved after iron depletion,[45] resulting in the dilemma of whether to recommend interferon therapy

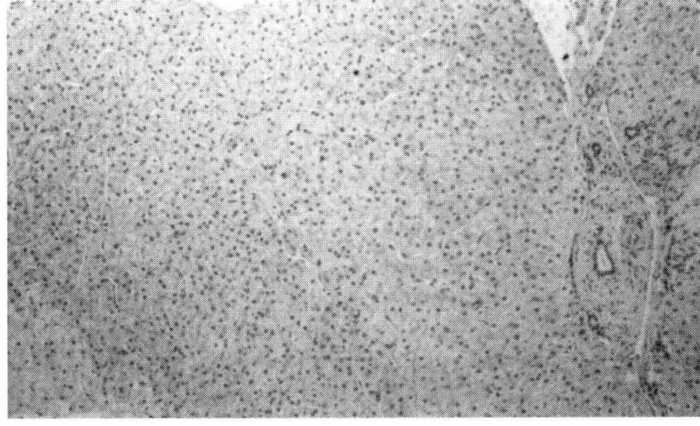

Figure 32.4. Liver biopsy (Perls technique) of the same patient as in Fig. 32.3 years after BMT. Hepatic iron concentration was 1.41 mg/g dry weight, normal value <1.6 mg/g (Weinfeld, 1964). The patient had been treated by a course of sequential phlebotomies starting during the third year after transplant. (See color plate 32.4.)

routinely. Also, in patients presenting with active hepatitis after iron removal, interferon treatment has proven to be a rational approach several years after transplant, with a success rate not different from that obtained in the normal population.[46] The absence of thalassemia and of iron overload makes it easier to treat other complications such as viral hepatitis, somewhat contradicting the assessment that the "cure" of thalassemia by transplantation does not modify the other complications acquired before hematopoietic cell transplantation.[31]

Endocrine Dysfunction

Hypogonadism is the most common endocrine disorder in medically treated patients with thalassemia major, affecting approximately half the patients.[47,48] In a study involving 68 children after hematopoietic cell transplantation, 32% reached an advanced or complete puberty spontaneously (34% of girls and 63% of boys),[49] despite clinical and hormonal evidence of gonadal impairment in most cases. In this group, iron overload and the conditioning regimen were the major factors influencing endocrine function. Preliminary observations in young children who undergo transplantation in the early phase of thalassemia indicate a good prognosis for growth and fertility. In a case report, a woman who was treated at age 10 years became pregnant naturally and delivered a healthy child.[50] Subsequently, five young men and four young women had normal and spontaneous paternity/maternity 3–12 years following allogeneic hematopoietic cell transplantation.

Impaired glucose tolerance and diabetes mellitus are common complications of iron overload. The administration of busulfan, cyclophosphamide, and cyclosporine after transplantation did not appear to have an adverse affect on pancreatic β cell function. In a prospective, unpublished study of 93 patients, only three with impaired oral glucose tolerance test and cirrhosis before transplant demonstrated worsening of glucose intolerance, whereas more than half of those with impaired glucose tolerance before transplant demonstrated improved pancreatic β cell function after transplantation.

HEMATOPOIETIC CELL TRANSPLANTATION FOR SICKLE CELL DISEASE

Unlike β thalassemia major, where the genotype directs a reasonably reliable phenotype in the vast majority of cases, the clinical expression of sickle cell anemia is quite variable and difficult to predict based upon the hemoglobin genotype alone (Chapter 27). Thus, in standard practice, hematopoietic cell transplantation for sickle cell disease currently is reserved almost exclusively for patients with clinical features that portend a poor outcome or significant sickle-related morbidity, in part due to the toxicity of this intensive therapy.[51] These clinical indications, which were adapted from the multicenter investigation of bone marrow transplantation for sickle cell disease, are listed in Table 32.2. These criteria have been applied almost exclusively to children, for whom the risk–benefit ratio is most advantageous in terms of years-of-life gained among those who survive with sustained engraftment of donor cells. Less certain is how to apply inclusion criteria to adults with sickle cell anemia, in whom the experience of transplantation is limited, but for whom the risk of significant transplantation-related toxicity remains substantial. For all patients, clinicians must carefully weigh therapeutic alternatives to hematopoietic cell transplantation, with particular attention to safety, efficacy, availability, and the cost of intervention.[52–55]

Table 32.2. Indications of hematopoietic cell transplantation for sickle cell disease

Patients with sickle cell anemia or HbS–β^0 thalassemia, aged <16 y
One or more of the following complications:
Stroke or central nervous system event lasting >24 h
Impaired neuropsychological function with abnormal cerebral MRI and angiography
Recurrent acute chest syndrome
Stage I or II sickle lung disease
Recurrent vasoocclusive painful episodes or recurrent priapism
Sickle nephropathy (glomerular filtration rate 30%–50% of predicted normal)
Other indications to consider:
Abnormal transcranial Doppler
Pulmonary hypertension
Silent cerebral infarction

Current Results of Hematopoietic Cell Transplantation for Sickle Cell Disease

The worldwide experience of conventional myeloablative hematopoietic cell transplantation for sickle cell disease is summarized in Table 32.3.[5–7,57,59,60,63] In the collective experiences of these studies, the transition of hematopoietic cell transplantation from an experimental intervention reserved for severely affected patients, to one in which younger children with early signs of sickle-related morbidity are targeted, has been observed. Several series in Europe and North America have reported very similar results after HLA-identical sibling transplantation.[4,5,7] The principal aim of these multicenter clinical studies was to define more completely the risks and benefits of this therapy, and to characterize the natural history of those surviving free of sickle cell disease. The results of transplantation were best when performed in children with sickle cell disease who had HLA-identical sibling donors. Even though many children who received allografts had significant sickle-related complications such as stroke and recurrent episodes of acute chest syndrome, the disease-free

Table 32.3. Hematopoietic cell transplantation for sickle cell disease with myeloablative preparation[5–7,57,59,60,63]

	US collaborative	French	Belgian	CIBMTR
No. of patients	59	87	50	67
Median patient age (range in y)	9.9 (3.3–15.9)	9.5 (2–22)	7.5 (0.9–23)	10 (2–27)
Conditioning regimen (dose) [no. of patients]	BU/CY/ATG [55]; BU/CY/Campath [4]	BU/CY [12]; BU/CY/ATG [65]	BU/CY [30]; BU/CY/TLI [6]; BU/CY/ATG [14]	BU + CY ± other [63]; other [4]
Source of stem cells (no. of patients)	Marrow	Marrow (74); CBSC (10); CBSC + marrow (2); PBHC (1)	Marrow (48); CBSC (2)	Marrow (54); PBHC (9); CBSC (4)
Induction of mixed chimerism	Yes	Yes	Yes	Yes
No. with graft rejection/ disease recurrence	5 (8.5%)	7 (8%)	5 (10%)	9 (13%)
No. with GVHD	Acute 25%, chronic 12%	Acute 20%, chronic 12.6%	Acute 40%, chronic 20%	Acute 10%, chronic 22%
No. of deaths	4 (7%)	6 (7%)	2 (4%)	3 (4.5%)
No. with event-free survival	50 (85%)	74 (85%)	43 (86%)	55 (82%)

ATG = antithymocyte globulin; CY = cyclophosphamide; TLI = total lymphoid irradiation; CBSC = umbilical cord blood.

survival rate was 80%–85% in several series; however, 5%–10% of patients died of complications related to transplantation, with GVHD and its treatment the leading cause of death.

In the multicenter investigation of hematopoietic cell transplantation for sickle cell disease, 59 children aged between 3.3 and 15.9 years (median 9.9 years) received HLA-identical sibling allografts between September 1991 and April 2000.[7] Patients received a myeloablative combination of busulfan, cyclophosphamide, and equine antithymocyte globulin, and most received a combination of methotrexate and cyclosporine after hematopoietic cell transplantation to prevent GVHD. Fifty of 59 children survive disease-free after hematopoietic cell transplantation. The Kaplan–Meier probabilities of survival and disease-free survival are 93% and 84%, respectively (Fig. 32.5). A recent publication from the Center for International Blood and Marrow Transplantation Research reported very similar results.[59] Outcomes after HLA-matched sibling hematopoietic cell transplantation in 67 patients with sickle cell disease between 1989 and 2002 were described, in which the leading indications for transplantation were stroke and recurrent vasoocclusive crisis occurring in 38% and 37% of patients, respectively. The median age at transplantation was 10 years. Ninety-two percent received busulfan and cyclophosphamide in the conditioning regimen and bone marrow was the predominant source of hematopoietic cells. Most patients achieved hematopoietic recovery and there were no deaths during the early post transplantation period. Rates of acute and chronic GVHD were 10% and 22%, respectively. Sixty-four of 67 patients are alive; 5-year probabilities of disease-free and overall survival rates are 85% and 97%, respectively.

Results among 101 patients who received conventional myeloablative HLA-identical sibling hematopoietic cell transplantation in Europe were remarkably similar, with an overall survival probability of 88% and disease-free survival rate of 80%.[5] A recent update included 87 consecutive patients treated between November 1988 and December 2004 at 14 centers in France.[60] The median age was 9.5 years and the leading indication for hematopoietic cell transplantation was stroke or transient ischemic attack (n = 36) and the development of abnormal cerebral arterial flow velocity as detected by transcranial Doppler flow studies (n = 8). Five of the 18 patients who did not receive antithymocyte globulin had graft rejection. One patient with 50% mixed chimerism developed aplastic anemia 15 months posttransplantation and received a second successful allograft, whereas the other four patients had autologous reconstitution and recurrent sickle cell disease. The rate of

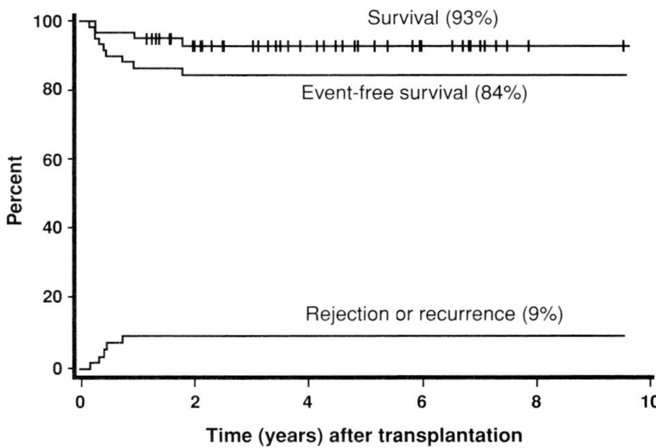

Figure 32.5. Kaplan–Meier estimates of survival and event-free survival after hematopoietic cell transplantation for sickle cell anemia. Events were defined as death, sickle cell disease recurrence, and graft rejection. A cumulative incidence curve for graft rejection and return of sickle cell disease is also shown.

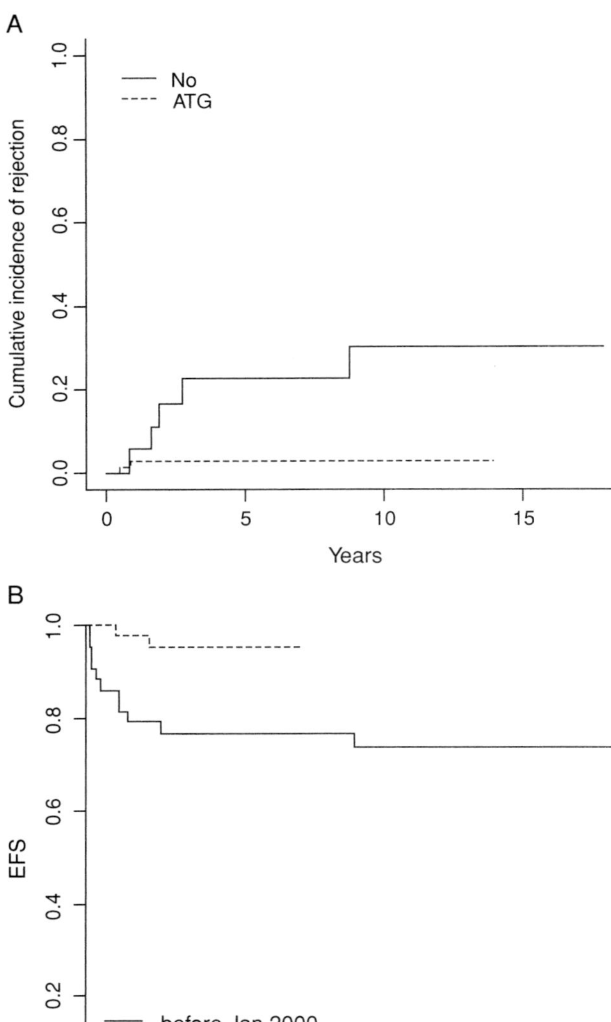

Figure 32.6. **(A)** Comparison of the cumulative incidence of rejection in patients conditioned with and without antithymocyte globulin (ATG). **(B)** Comparison of event-free survival (EFS) in patients who underwent transplantation before (43 patients) and after January 2000 (44 patients).

graft rejection declined from 22.6% to 2.9% after the addition of antithymocyte globulin to the conditioning regimen (Fig. 32.6A). The Kaplan–Meier estimate of event-free survival at 5 years was 86.1%. Multivariate analysis showed that the date of transplantation was the only significant risk factor. The 5-year event-free survival rate was 95.3% in patients treated after January 2000 compared with 76.7% in patients treated earlier (Fig. 32.6B).

A retrospective review of 24 Belgian patients with sickle cell disease analyzed the impact of pretransplant antithymocyte globulin and hydroxyurea on outcome. When hydroxyurea was received before hematopoietic cell transplantation, there was a significantly lower rate of graft rejection compared with patients who did not receive hydroxyurea, but the administration of antithymocyte globulin before transplantation did not affect the rate of engraftment. Overall, 20 of 24 patients had stable engraftment of donor cells after hematopoietic cell transplantation, but none of those who received hydroxyurea before transplantation with antithymocyte globulin in the conditioning regimen had graft rejection or a late recurrence of sickle cell disease. This suggests that the augmentation of pretransplantation immunosuppression might be necessary to overcome the immunological barrier of tolerance to donor histocompatibility antigens. The propensity for graft rejection even after HLA-identical sibling hematopoietic cell transplantation supports the hypothesis that multiple transfusion exposures before hematopoietic cell transplantation induce sensitization to minor histocompatibility antigens expressed on the surface of transfused cells. It appears possible that leukocytes present in blood products are not alone in this ability to cause sensitization because erythrocytes might also present histocompatibility antigens via the HLA Class I pathway to elicit expansion and activation of host CD8+ T cells.[61]

Stable Donor–Host Chimerism After Myeloablative Hematopoietic Cell Transplantation for Sickle Cell Disease. As in thalassemia major, the observation of donor–host hematopoietic chimerism after conventional myeloablative hematopoietic cell transplantation has lent substantial support to the notion that persistence of even a fraction of normal erythropoiesis might elicit a curative clinical effect.[62] The basis of this effect appears to be twofold: improved survival of healthy donor erythrocytes in the blood compared with sickle erythrocytes, and ineffective erythropoiesis in the sickle cell disease marrow that lends a competitive advantage to normal donor erythroid progenitors. Approximately 25% of children with sickle cell disease developed stable mixed chimerism after HLA-identical sibling hematopoietic cell transplantation.[63] In the multicenter investigation of bone marrow transplant for sickle cell anemia, five patients had a proportion of donor cells that ranged from 11% to 74%. Their hemoglobin levels varied between 11.2 and 14.2 g/dL (median 11.3; mean 12.0). None experienced painful events or other clinical complications related to sickle cell disease after transplantation. One patient who had a stroke before transplantation had no further strokes after transplantation and magnetic resonance imaging (MRI) demonstrated stable brain abnormalities, despite having only 10% donor cells detectable in peripheral blood. In the French series, low levels of residual host hematopoiesis were observed significantly more frequently in patients who did not receive antithymocyte globulin before hematopoietic cell transplantation ($P = 0.04$ at 12 months and $P = 0.002$ at 24 months posttransplant).[60] A higher fraction of residual host cells was observed in patients who received antithymocyte

Table 32.4. Hematopoietic cell transplantation for sickle cell disease with nonmyeloablative preparation[61,64,66–68,71]

	Minimal-toxicity conditioning regimen	Reduced-intensity conditioning regimen
No. of patients	11†	18‡
Median patient age (range in y)	10 (3–28)	12.4 (1.8–56)
Conditioning regimen (dose) {no. of patients}	Flu(90–150)/TBI (200) {5}; Flu(125–150)/ATG/TBI (200){6}	Flu(175)/BU(8)/ATG/TLI (500) {5}; Flu (120)/Mel(140)/ATG {2}; Flu(120)/CY(120) {1}; Flu(120)/Mel(140/70)/Campath {2}; Flu(120)/BU(3.2) {2}; Campath/FLU(150)/Mel(140) {2}; Flu (180)/BU(6.4)/ATG {4}*
Source of stem cells (no. of patients)	Marrow (9); PBHC (2)	Marrow (8);* CBSC (1); PBHC (10)
Induction of mixed chimerism	Yes (transient in 10)	Yes
No. with graft rejection/disease recurrence	10 (91%)	5 (28%)
No. with GVHD	Acute 1 (grade I), chronic, none	Acute 5 (grade II–IV), chronic, 4 (3 fatal)
No. of deaths	1 (after a 2nd hematopoietic cell transplantation)	4 (22%)
No. with event-free survival	1 (9%)	9 (50%)

* HLA-matched unrelated donor PBHCs were used for hematopoietic cell transplantation.
† Includes two patients with thalassemia major.
‡ Includes three patients with thalassemia major.
ATG = antithymocyte globulin; CY = cyclophosphamide; Flu = fludarabine; Mel = melphalan; PBHC = peripheral blood stem cells; TBI = total body irradiation; TLI = total lymphoid irradiation; CBSC = umbilical cord blood.

globulin ($P = 0.03$ at 12 months and $P = 0.001$ at 24 months posttransplant), and this level of donor–host chimerism remained stable in the long term. These observations are consistent with the idea that chimerism, even with a minority of donor cells, can have a significant ameliorative effect so that full engraftment of donor cells is not a requirement for successful hematopoietic cell transplantation and that the donor chimerism fraction remains stable 12 months and longer after hematopoietic cell transplantation.

Nonmyeloablative Hematopoietic Cell Transplantation for Sickle Cell Disease. Due in part to the observations discussed in the previous section, it was reasoned that pretransplantation therapy might be adjusted to promote stable engraftment of a threshold fraction of donor cells that would be sufficient to prevent sickle vasoocclusion and that this regimen could be administered more safely than conventional myeloablative conditioning. Toward this end, several groups have attempted to apply nonmyeloablative stem cell transplantation to sickle cell disease, utilizing conditioning regimens of varying intensity.[61,64–68] Although these investigations are continuing, it has been difficult to identify a regimen that is sufficiently immunosuppressive to ensure stable engraftment of donor cells from HLA-identical siblings, yet also meets the objective of "reduced toxicity" with a risk that is distinguishable from conventional allografting. A minimally toxic regimen was first developed in a large-animal model and translated successfully into human trials for older adult patients with hematological malignancies. When applied to sickle cell disease, this approach was safe, generated little or no acute GVHD, and in most cases was associated with an initial period of donor engraftment. Unfortunately, in nearly all cases, withdrawal of postgrafting immunosuppression was followed by graft rejection with disease recurrence (Table 32.4). In another series of nonmyeloablative hematopoietic cell transplantation, there was a twofold higher expression of donor β-globin RNA compared with total genomic DNA in the blood after nonmyeloablative hematopoietic cell transplantation. Direct bone marrow analysis revealed ineffective erythropoiesis of recipient erythroblasts, with a progressive increase in representation of donor erythrocytes during erythrocyte maturation.[69,70] These findings were associated with clinical benefit after transplantation, and with improvements in hemolysis, endothelial function, and nitric oxide bioavailability; however, they did not persist after graft rejection.

An increasing number of patients have received regimens that are less intense than a myeloablative regimen, but retain a moderate degree of the myelosuppressive effect to suppress the host-versus-graft reaction and promote engraftment. These regimens require hospitalization, and their risk of regimen-related toxicity is related to the profound immunosuppression of the regimens and an accompanying risk of opportunistic infection. A group of older sickle cell patients who received such "reduced-intensity" conditioning regimens also received augmented pregrafting immunosuppression to facilitate donor cell engraftment. Nevertheless, three of 12 recipients experienced graft rejection (Table 32.3). Acute and chronic GVHD were also more frequent (4 of 12 patients) in this group, and GVHD was fatal in two cases. Thus, in older recipients the problem of transplant-related mortality was not eliminated by the reduced-intensity conditioning regimen. In contrast, donor chimerism was successfully established in children who received a reduced-intensity regimen consisting of busulfan, fludarabine, antithymocyte globulin, and total lymphoid irradiation (500 cGy).[66] Five patients who were aged between 6 and 18 years received HLA-identical sibling bone marrow transplantation with cyclosporine and mycophenolate mofetil for postgrafting immunosuppression. Treatment-related toxicity was minimal, and all the patients had evidence of stable donor engraftment. Another study that included 16 children with nonmalignant disorders included one patient with sickle cell anemia.[71] The patients received melphalan, fludarabine, and an anti–T cell antibody, Campath-1, before transplantation and included seven patients who received unrelated or HLA-mismatched related donor allografts. Twelve of the 16 (75%) patients survive disease-free after transplantation and none of the surviving patients had graft rejection. These encouraging results in younger patients suggest that future application of reduced-intensity conditioning regimens should focus on children who already have or are at risk for symptomatic disease.

Effect of Donor Hematopoiesis on Sickle Vasoocclusion

After successful hematopoietic cell transplantation for sickle cell disease, patients with stable engraftment of donor cells have not experienced clinical complications or required transfusions after transplantation, even when there was stable mixed donor–host hematopoietic chimerism.[4,5,63] In addition, investigators have reported improvements in splenic function and osteonecrosis.[72,73] Patients treated by hematopoietic cell transplantation also had stabilization of the underlying cerebrovascular disease. Forty-six of 55 patients who were enrolled in the multicenter study underwent cerebral MRI performed a median of 25.4 months after transplantation. These studies were compared with pretransplantation baseline examinations in all but four of the patients. Among those 29 who had a history of stroke before transplantation, one patient with graft rejection had a second stroke and 28 survive stroke free. Of the 28 patients with stroke studied after transplantation, all but the patient with a second stroke had a stable or improved appearance on cerebral MRI. Ten patients had evidence of silent cerebral infarction before transplantation, and of these, all eight with posthematopoietic cell transplantation studies had stable or improved appearance. There were no strokes after hematopoietic cell transplantation in this group. Sixteen patients had no documented central nervous system disease before transplantation. MRI appearance was normal in all 10 patients in this group after hematopoietic cell transplantation and none had stroke. Together, these observations suggest that there is stabilization of cerebral vasculopathy after hematopoietic cell transplantation. These data also suggest that in those with silent cerebral infarction who are at risk of developing stroke, there is protection from disease progression and a first stroke.

A similar experience was reported by the French group.[60] Among the 36 patients with a history of stroke before hematopoietic cell transplantation, two had a recurrent stroke. One patient experienced a transient ischemic attack 10 days after hematopoietic cell transplantation whereas the other, who had severe cerebrovascular injury with Moyamoya disease, had a fatal intracranial hemorrhage 32 days after hematopoietic cell transplantation. With a median follow-up of 6 years, the risk of recurrent stroke was 5.6%, which mirrors the rate of second stroke observed in sickle cell disease patients treated by regular transfusion therapy after a first stroke. Vascular occlusions tended to persist after hematopoietic cell transplantation and the long-term outcome varied somewhat: In five, the arterial stenosis resolved, in 16 there was no change, and in two cases, there was progression. None of the patients had a clinical stroke or silent ischemic lesion among those with durable donor engraftment, including the two patients who had progressive cerebrovascular narrowing. Cortical atrophy worsened in two cases. In addition, the cerebral artery blood flow velocity was significantly decreased ($P < 0.001$) 1 year after hematopoietic cell transplantation in the 49 patients in whom a pre-hematopoietic cell transplantation transcranial Doppler examination was performed. The transcranial Doppler velocity declined from 138 $\pm$ 50 cm/s before hematopoietic cell transplantation to 100 $\pm$ 34 cm/s as measured in the right middle cerebral artery, and 138 $\pm$ 46 to 103 $\pm$ 40 cm/s in the left middle cerebral artery. The transcranial Doppler velocity also normalized by 3 months after hematopoietic cell transplantation in two patients who had abnormal measurements before hematopoietic cell transplantation, even though both had been treated by regular transfusions before transplantation.

In other series, patients with stroke before hematopoietic cell transplantation have experienced transient ischemic attacks and intracranial hemorrhages in the era before measures to prevent these adverse events were instituted.[74–76] After the institution of preventive measures, neurological complications still occurred after transplantation, but these tended to be self-limited events such as seizures, with no long-term sequelae. More recently, one group observed radiographic changes in some patients with sickle cell anemia who underwent hematopoietic cell transplantation for stroke.[77] Five of nine patients had either new or slightly increased size of cerebral lacunae or leukoencephaly that stabilized 2–7.5 years after hematopoietic cell transplantation. Thus, it is possible that these observations reflect the evolution of cerebrovascular disease that existed before transplantation. Of interest, these cerebral MRI changes were not associated with progressive neurocognitive deficits.

Table 32.5. *P* values from each comparison of the hematopoietic cell transplantation cohort to CSSCD and HUG-KIDS groups

	Height				Weight			
	Baseline		Velocity		Baseline		Velocity	
Comparison group	Male	Female	Male	Female	Male	Female	Male	Female
CS sickle cell disease	0.37	0.22	0.01*	0.12	0.30	0.02†	0.0004‡	0.08
HUG–KIDS (Pre)	0.06‖*	0.72	0.15	0.72	0.89	0.66	0.73	0.53
HUG–KIDS (HU)	0.15	0.87	0.68	0.25	0.01§	0.51	0.30	0.92

* Between the baseline ages of 3.3 years and 11.6 years, the linear height velocity was greater for the hematopoietic cell transplantation group than the predicted velocity for the CSSCD group.

† Three females older than 11 years in the hematopoietic cell transplantation group had low baseline weight, creating an illogical decreasing trend in the baseline weight curve.

‡ Until the baseline age of 12.1 years, the linear weight velocity during follow-up in the hematopoietic cell transplantation group was greater than the predicted linear velocity during follow-up for the CSSCD disease group.

‖ The males in the HUG-KIDS (Pre) group tended to be approximately 4.0 cm taller than the males in the hematopoietic cell transplantation group, regardless of age.

§ The males in the HUG-KIDS (HU) group tended to be 2.7 kg heavier than the males in the hematopoietic cell transplantation group, regardless of age.

Growth and Development after Hematopoietic Cell Transplantation for Sickle Cell Disease

There remains concern about possible growth impairment after hematopoietic cell transplantation for sickle cell anemia. The potential for growth impairment stems, in part, from the gonadal toxicity associated with myeloablative doses of busulfan, particularly in females. Although it is difficult to predict the impact of busulfan on linear growth in patients with sickle cell anemia, there is also the possibility that by removing the energy requirements associated with the hemolytic anemia of sickle cell anemia,[78] growth might improve after transplantation.[79] A recent report compared four groups of children with sickle cell anemia in an analysis of growth after hematopoietic cell transplantation. Children who were enrolled in the Cooperative Study of Sickle Cell Disease (CSSCD) comprised one supportive therapy comparison group. Children who were enrolled in the HUG-KIDS trial, a study of hydroxyurea in children with sickle cell anemia made up the remaining two comparison groups.[80] These two groups included children who had pretreatment growth measurements (HUG-KIDS Pre) and the same children who again had measurements for at least 1 year after achieving the maximum tolerated dose of hydroxyurea (HUG-KIDS HU).

There were no statistically significant differences in the estimated height (weight) velocity curves between the hematopoietic cell transplantation and the three comparison groups among females; however, there were significant differences between males in the hematopoietic cell transplantation and CSSCD groups (Table 32.5, Fig. 32.7). An age-dependent growth effect in the secondary analysis of the CSSCD/hematopoietic cell transplantation height and weight comparisons in boys appeared to exist. The predicted height velocity during follow-up in the hematopoietic cell transplantation group was greater than the velocity in the CSSCD disease group aged between 3.3 years and 11.6 years. After this period of 8.4 years, there was no apparent growth benefit associated with hematopoietic cell transplantation. As a result, the predicted height velocity in hematopoietic cell transplantation males who were more than 12 years of age at transplantation was less than the velocity in CSSCD males. Similarly, until the baseline age of 12.1 years, the linear weight velocity in the hematopoietic cell transplantation group was greater than in the CSSCD group. In the HUG-KIDS Pre and hematopoietic cell transplantation male height comparison, secondary analysis showed a statistically significant group effect on linear height velocity during follow-up after adjusting for estimated baseline height ($P = 0.04$). In summary, growth after transplantation for sickle cell anemia was not impaired, except in older boys. These data suggest that conventional myeloablative hematopoietic cell transplantation generally had no adverse effect on height or weight gain in young children.

Gonadotropin and sex hormone levels of surviving patients have also been monitored, and these confirm the toxic effect of busulfan on gonadal function. Among seven surviving females in the multicenter study who were aged more than 13 years after hematopoietic cell transplantation, an interim analysis showed that five had primary amenorrhea and five had corresponding elevated luteinizing hormone (LH) and follicle stimulating hormone (FSH) levels that were associated with decreased serum estradiol levels in four. One individual receiving hormonal replacement therapy had elevated LH and FSH levels and a normal serum estradiol. One postpubertal female had normal serum FSH and estradiol levels. Of seven males who were more than 13 years old, none of four tested had elevated serum LH/FSH levels. Two males who were aged

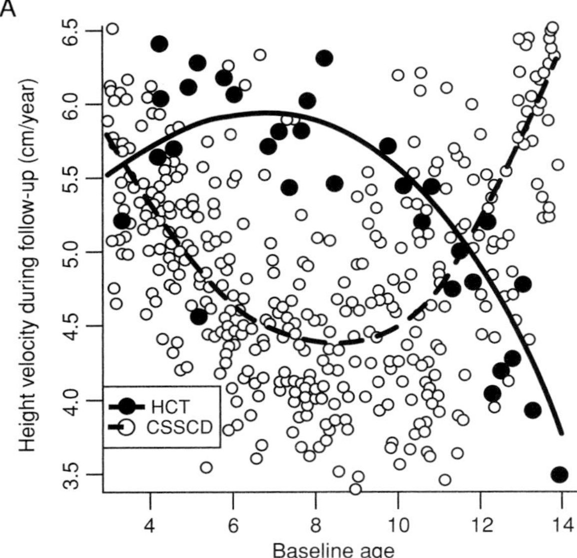

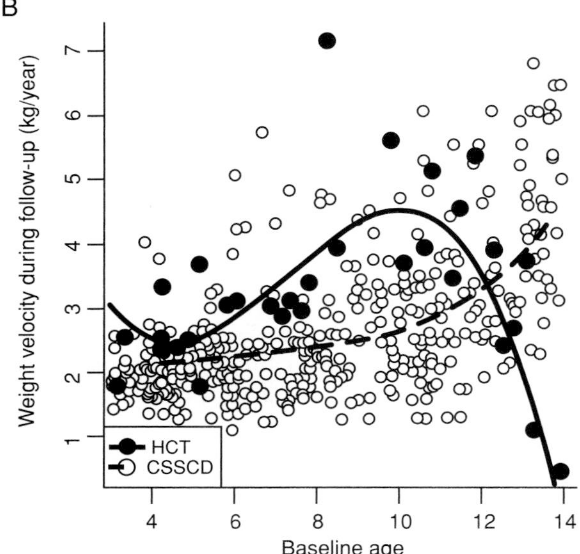

Figure 32.7. (A) Height velocity during follow-up in sickle cell disease. The height velocity in centimeter/year is depicted as a function of the baseline age during the follow-up period. The open circles represent height velocities as determined by an HLM for the male CSSCD comparison group and the accompanying dashed line shows the predicted velocity curve. The solid circles represent height velocities as determined by an HLM for the male hematopoietic cell transplantation group and the accompanying solid line represents the predicted velocity curve. **(B)** Weight velocity during follow-up in sickle cell disease. The weight velocity in kilogram/year is depicted as a function of the baseline age during the follow-up period. The open circles represent weight velocities as determined by an HLM for the male CSSCD comparison group and the accompanying dashed line shows the predicted velocity curve. The solid circles represent weight velocities as determined by an HLM for the male hematopoietic cell transplantation group and the accompanying solid line represents the predicted velocity curve.

14 and 16 years had low testosterone levels that were correlated with gonadotropin levels in the prepubertal range. Among six evaluable prepubertal girls in the Belgian cohort, five had primary amenorrhea with elevated serum LH and FSH.[5] Two postpubertal females developed secondary amenorrhea. Testicular function was also adversely affected in four of six evaluable boys who demonstrated decreased testosterone and elevated FSH levels. In the French series, seven postpubertal females, aged 13–22 years, developed amenorrhea after hematopoietic cell transplantation with decreased serum estradiol and elevated LH and FSH levels and received hormone replacement therapy.[60] In addition, most girls who were prepubertal before hematopoietic cell transplantation received hormone replacement therapy to promote the development of secondary sexual characteristics after they reached a bone age of 13 years. Two younger girls (aged 6.4 and 8.3 years) experienced spontaneous pubertal development, raising the possibility that hematopoietic cell transplantation performed in very young patients might not be associated with delayed puberty. It is anticipated that many, if not most of the females, will require hormonal replacement therapy after hematopoietic cell transplantation.

Alternative Sources of Donor Hematopoietic Cells

The use of umbilical cord blood in lieu of bone marrow in transplantation for sickle cell disease is of interest, primarily because of a lowered risk of GVHD. This benefit is balanced by a higher rate of graft rejection and a longer duration of hematological recovery that accompanies umbilical cord blood transplantation.[81,82] Thus, to overcome these risks, investigators have modulated pre- and postgrafting immunosuppression and intensified supportive care to optimize outcomes. In a report of 44 patients that included 11 with sickle cell disease who received HLA-identical or 1-antigen HLA-mismatched sibling umbilical cord blood allografts, the overall 2-year sickle cell disease-free survival rate was 91% with one patient experiencing recurrent disease.[20] Among patients who received thiotepa or fludarabine in addition to the busulfan/cyclophosphamide backbone, and who did not receive methotrexate with postgrafting immunosuppression, the outcome after umbilical cord blood transplantation was superior, particularly among recipients with β thalassemia major. In addition, only four of 44 patients experienced acute, and two, chronic GVHD after umbilical cord blood transplantation, and there were no deaths related to GVHD. In another series of related donor umbilical cord blood transplantation for hemoglobinopathies, 18 of 22 patients survive event free after transplantation.[83] Thus, it is possible that umbilical cord blood might be utilized as an effective source of hematopoietic stem cells in hemoglobinopathies. The current experience with unrelated donor umbilical cord blood transplantation for sickle cell disease is quite limited, but it illustrates the potential for success and the challenges yet to be investigated. In one series, seven patients were conditioned with myeloablative (n = 4) or reduced-intensity preparative regimens.[84] The indication for cord blood transplantation was stroke, and all received cord blood grafts that were mismatched at two HLA antigens. Five of seven patients (71%) experienced significant adverse events of graft rejection or death. Currently, 43% survive disease free after umbilical cord blood transplantation due to a successful second cord blood transplantation in one patient, and one of seven (14%) subjects died of transplant-related causes. These preliminary findings suggest the possibility of success after unrelated donor cord blood transplantation in high-risk patients. It is the introduction of transplantation in patients like these at risk of progressive neurovascular injury, and who are also very likely to need long-term transfusion support with its attendant risk of life-threatening transfusional iron overload, where risk–benefit considerations might achieve a suitable balance. To tip the balance in favor of transplantation, the problems of graft rejection and GVHD after unrelated donor cord blood transplantation will require better control.

That the broader application of hematopoietic cell transplantation for sickle cell disease is limited can be illustrated by the observation that only 14% of sickle cell anemia recipients are likely to have an HLA-identical sibling donor.[85] Not surprisingly, lacking a suitable donor is the major barrier to hematopoietic cell transplantation for sickle cell anemia.[86] An expanded availability of HLA-compatible unrelated donor sources is necessary to pursue hematopoietic cell transplantation as a therapeutic option in most patients with sickle cell disease. Donors who are matched at six (HLA-A, B and DRB1 loci) to 10 HLA-antigens (including HLA-C and DQB1 loci) can be identified via the National Marrow Donor Program in approximately 80% of Caucasian recipients; however, the likelihood of identifying a similarly HLA-matched unrelated donor is less likely in other ethnic groups due to underrepresentation of these groups in the volunteer donor pool. The reduced likelihood of identifying a suitable donor is a difficult problem in hematopoietic cell transplantation for sickle cell disease and can limit the application of hematopoietic cell transplantation among those who might benefit most.[87,88] The feasibility of identifying suitable donors was suggested by surveys in which 60% of sickle cell disease patients had at least one potential suitable unrelated donor and 26% had three or more potential donors. The challenge of identifying a donor might also be mitigated by the possibility of umbilical cord blood transplantation. An unrelated donor search for 40 sickle cell disease patients showed that 100% and 50% had HLA 4/6 and 5/6 antigen-matched unrelated donor cord blood units, respectively.[89]

Thus, it appears feasible to pursue alternate donors suitably matched at HLA alleles in the treatment of individuals with severe sickle cell disease. It is quite possible and even likely that the successful translation of unrelated donor hematopoietic cell transplantation for sickle cell disease will hinge on our ability to establish bidirectional donor–host immunological tolerance and that this will involve the administration of more intensive immunosuppression than we are accustomed to using in this clinical setting. This represents a shift from the notion that marrow ablation and elimination of sickle cell progenitor cell populations are the principle objectives in performing a successful hematopoietic cell transplantation. There are many reasons for this, not the least of which is that the immunological milieu of sickle cell disease is one of inflammation, in which innate stimulation of graft-versus-host and host-versus-graft reactions is very likely to occur. In the course of inhibiting these reactions by pharmacological means, controlling the emergence of opportunistic viral and other infections will take on greater importance than has been appreciated previously after transplantation for hemoglobin disorders. These concerns have been taken into consideration in the design and implementation of the United States trial to study unrelated donor hematopoietic cell transplantation in children with severe sickle cell disease.

SUMMARY

In general, the experience of hematopoietic cell transplantation from HLA-identical sibling donors to treat clinically significant hemoglobin disorders has been outstanding. Most individuals with sickle cell disease and β thalassemia survive after hematopoietic cell transplantation without anemia or the need for blood transfusion support. In survivors with sickle cell disease, new vasoocclusive episodes do not occur. It is also possible to treat preexisting complications such as transfusional iron overload after hematopoietic cell transplantation and thereby eliminate the risk of disease-related morbidity. The experience of hematopoietic cell transplantation for thalassemia is more extensive than in sickle cell disease, which reflects the greater reliability of the genoptype–phenotype relationship in β thalassemia. Thus, indications of hematopoietic cell transplantation for sickle cell disease continue to evolve as the genotype–phenotype relationship is more completely defined. With the possibility of alternate donor hematopoietic cell transplantation, the availability of hematopoietic cell transplantation is likely to expand, thereby opening the possibility of hematopoietic cell transplantation where none existed previously. The application of hematopoietic cell transplantation in adults with β thalassemia and sickle cell disease has been less successful, due in part to the higher risk of transplant-related mortality that occurs in high-risk recipients. Decisions about treatment options in the future are very likely to be influenced by perceptions about the nature of these chronic illnesses, and whether the short-term risk of mortality inherent to hematopoietic cell transplantation is balanced by the possibility of survival without symptoms or treatment. Ideally, future clinical trials about interventions for both disorders would focus on addressing these decision-making considerations.

REFERENCES

1. Olivieri NF, Brittenham GM. Iron-chelating therapy and the treatment of thalassemia. *Blood.* 1997;89(3):739–761.
2. Giardini C. Treatment of beta-thalassemia. *Curr Opin Hematol.* 1997;4(2):79–87.
3. Cappellini MD, Cohen A, Piga A, et al. A phase 3 study of deferasirox (ICL670), a once-daily oral iron chelator, in patients with beta-thalassemia. *Blood.* 2006;107(9):3455–3462.
4. Bernaudin F, Souillet G, Vannier JP, et al. Report of the French experience concerning 26 children transplanted for severe sickle cell disease. *Bone Marrow Transplant.* 1997;19(Suppl 2):112–115.
5. Vermylen C, Cornu G, Ferster A, et al. Haematopoietic stem cell transplantation for sickle cell anaemia: the first 50 patients transplanted in Belgium. *Bone Marrow Transplant.* 1998; 22(1):1–6.
6. Walters MC, Patience M, Leisenring W, Eckman JR, Scott JP, Mentzer WC, et al. Bone marrow transplantation for sickle cell disease. *N Engl J Med.* 1996;335(6):369–376.
7. Walters MC, Storb R, Patience M, et al. Impact of bone marrow transplantation for symptomatic sickle cell disease: an interim report. *Blood.* 2000;95(6):1918–1924.
8. Giardini C. Ethical issue of bone marrow transplantation for thalassemia. *Bone Marrow Transplant.* 1995;15(5): 657–8.
9. Thomas ED, Buckner CD, Sanders JE, Papayannopoulou T, Borgna-Pignatti C, De Stefano P, et al. Marrow transplantation for thalassaemia. *Lancet.* 1982 Jul 31;2(8292): 227–9.
10. Lucarelli G, Polchi P, Izzi T, Manna M, Agostinelli F, Delfini C, et al. Allogeneic marrow transplantation for thalassemia. *Exp Hematol.* 1984 Sep;12(8):676–81.
11. Lucarelli G, Polchi P, Galimberti M, et al. Marrow transplantation for thalassaemia following busulphan and cyclophosphamide. *Lancet.* 1985;1(8442):1355–1357.
12. Lucarelli G, Galimberti M, Polchi P, et al. Marrow transplantation in patients with advanced thalassemia. *N Engl J Med.* 1987;316(17):1050–1055.
13. Lucarelli G, Galimberti M, Polchi P, et al. Bone marrow transplantation in patients with thalassemia. *N Engl J Med.* 1990;322(7):417–421.
14. Lucarelli G, Galimberti M, Polchi P, et al. Bone marrow transplantation in thalassemia. *Hematol Oncol Clin North Am.* 1991;5(3):549–556.
15. Angelucci E, Baronciani D, Lucarelli G, et al. Needle liver biopsy in thalassaemia: analyses of diagnostic accuracy and safety in 1184 consecutive biopsies. *Br J Haematol.* 1995;89(4): 757–761.
16. Schrier SL, Angelucci E. New strategies in the treatment of the thalassemias. *Annu Rev Med.* 2005;56:157–171.
17. Lucarelli G, Clift RA, Galimberti M, et al. Marrow transplantation for patients with thalassemia: results in class 3 patients. *Blood.* 1996;87(5):2082–2088.
18. Lucarelli G, Clift RA, Galimberti M, et al. Bone marrow transplantation in adult thalassemic patients. *Blood.* 1999;93(4): 1164–1167.
19. Sodani P, Gaziev D, Polchi P, et al. New approach for bone marrow transplantation in patients with class 3 thalassemia aged younger than 17 years. *Blood.* 2004;104(4):1201–1203.
20. Locatelli F, Rocha V, Reed W, et al. Related umbilical cord blood transplantation in patients with thalassemia and sickle cell disease. *Blood.* 2003;101(6):2137–2143.
21. Lawson SE, Roberts IA, Amrolia P, Dokal I, Szydlo R, Darbyshire PJ. Bone marrow transplantation for beta-thalassaemia major: the UK experience in two paediatric centres. *Br J Haematol.* 2003;120(2):289–295.
22. Delfini C, Donati M, Marchionni D, et al. HLA compatibility for patients with thalassemia: implications for bone marrow transplantation. *Int J Cell Cloning.* 1986;4(4):274–278.
23. Gaziev D, Galimberti M, Lucarelli G, et al. Bone marrow transplantation from alternative donors for thalassemia: HLA-phenotypically identical relative and HLA-nonidentical sibling or parent transplants. *Bone Marrow Transplant.* 2000;25(8):815–821.
24. Sullivan KM, Anasetti C, Horowitz M, et al. Unrelated and HLA-nonidentical related donor marrow transplantation for thalassemia and leukemia. A combined report from the Seattle Marrow Transplant Team and the International Bone Marrow Transplant Registry. *Ann NY Acad Sci.* 1998;850:312–324.
25. La Nasa G, Argiolu F, Giardini C, et al. Unrelated bone marrow transplantation for beta-thalassemia patients: The experience of the Italian Bone Marrow Transplant Group. *Ann NY Acad Sci.* 2005;1054:186–195.
26. Baronciani D, Angelucci E, Agostinelli F, et al. Bone marrow transplantation in a thalassemia patient with congenital heart disease. *Bone Marrow Transplant.* 1996;17(1):119–120.
27. Zurlo MG, De Stefano P, Borgna-Pignatti C, et al. Survival and causes of death in thalassaemia major. *Lancet.* 1989; 2(8653):27–30.
28. Modell B, Khan M, Darlison M. Survival in beta-thalassaemia major in the UK: data from the UK Thalassaemia Register. *Lancet.* 2000;355(9220):2051–2052.
29. Borgna-Pignatti C, Rugolotto S, De Stefano P, et al. Survival and complications in patients with thalassemia major treated with transfusion and deferoxamine. *Haematologica.* 2004;89(10):1187–1193.
30. Borgna-Pignatti C, Cappellini MD, De Stefano P, et al. Cardiac morbidity and mortality in deferoxamine- or deferiprone-treated patients with thalassemia major. *Blood.* 2006;107(9): 3733–3737.
31. Splendiani GTC, Mazzarella V, Casciani CU, et al. Deferoxamine in thalassemia major. *N Engl J Med.* 1995;332:270–273.
32. Andreani M, Nesci S, Lucarelli G, et al. Long-term survival of ex-thalassemic patients with persistent mixed chimerism after bone marrow transplantation. *Bone Marrow Transplant.* 2000;25(4):401–404.
33. Gaziev D, Polchi P, Galimberti M, et al. Graft-versus-host disease after bone marrow transplantation for thalassemia: an analysis of incidence and risk factors. *Transplantation.* 1997;63(6):854–860.
34. Baronciani D, Angelucci E, Polchi P, et al. An unusual marrow transplant complication: cardiac myxoma. *Bone Marrow Transplant.* 1998;21(8):825–827.
35. Erer B, Angelucci E, Muretto P, et al. Kaposi's sarcoma after allogeneic bone marrow transplantation. *Bone Marrow Transplant.* 1997;19(6):629–631.
36. Borgna-Pignatti C, Rugolotto S, De Stefano P, et al. Survival and disease complications in thalassemia major. *Ann NY Acad Sci.* 1998;850:227–231.

37. Das Gupta A, Nair L, Shah A, Barbhaya SA. Association of hematologic malignancies with hemoglobinopathies. *Am J Hematol.* 1988;28(2):130–131.
38. Miniero R, Pastore G, Saracco P, Terracini B. Homozygous beta thalassemia and cancer. *Haematologica.* 1985;70(1):78–79.
39. Curtis RE, Rowlings PA, Deeg HJ, et al. Solid cancers after bone marrow transplantation. *N Engl J Med.* 1997;336(13): 897–904.
40. Niederau C, Fischer R, Sonnenberg A, Stremmel W, Trampisch HJ, Strohmeyer G. Survival and causes of death in cirrhotic and in noncirrhotic patients with primary hemochromatosis. *N Engl J Med.* 1985;313(20):1256–1262.
41. Angelucci E, Muretto P, Nicolucci A, et al. Effects of iron overload and hepatitis C virus positivity in determining progression of liver fibrosis in thalassemia following bone marrow transplantation. *Blood.* 2002;100(1):17–21.
42. Angelucci E, Muretto P, Lucarelli G, et al. Phlebotomy to reduce iron overload in patients cured of thalassemia by bone marrow transplantation. Italian Cooperative Group for Phlebotomy Treatment of Transplanted Thalassemia Patients. *Blood.* 1997;90(3):994–998.
43. Muretto P, Angelucci E, Lucarelli G. Reversibility of cirrhosis in patients cured of thalassemia by bone marrow transplantation. *Ann Intern Med.* 2002;136(9):667–672.
44. Giardini C, Galimberti M, Lucarelli G, et al. Desferrioxamine therapy accelerates clearance of iron deposits after bone marrow transplantation for thalassaemia. *Br J Haematol.* 1995;89(4):868–873.
45. Angelucci E, Muretto P, Lucarelli G, et al. Treatment of iron overload in the "ex-thalassemic". Report from the phlebotomy program. *Ann NY Acad Sci.* 1998;850:288–293.
46. Giardini C, Galimberti M, Lucarelli G, et al. Alpha-interferon treatment of chronic hepatitis C after bone marrow transplantation for homozygous beta-thalassemia. *Bone Marrow Transplant.* 1997;20(9):767–772.
47. De Sanctis V, Eleftheriou A, Malaventura C. Prevalence of endocrine complications and short stature in patients with thalassaemia major: a multicenter study by the Thalassaemia International Federation (TIF). *Pediatr Endocrinol Rev.* 2004;2(Suppl 2):249–255.
48. Raiola G, Galati MC, De Sanctis V, et al. Growth and puberty in thalassemia major. *J Pediatr Endocrinol Metab.* 2003;16(Suppl 2):259–266.
49. De Sanctis V. Growth and puberty and its management in thalassaemia. *Horm Res.* 2002;58(Suppl 1):72–79.
50. Borgna-Pignatti C, Marradi P, Rugolotto S, Marcolongo A. Successful pregnancy after bone marrow transplantation for thalassaemia. *Bone Marrow Transplant.* 1996;18(1):235–236.
51. Hoppe CC, Walters MC. Bone marrow transplantation in sickle cell anemia. *Curr Opin Oncol.* 2001;13(2):85–90.
52. Nietert PJ, Abboud MR, Silverstein MD, Jackson SM. Bone marrow transplantation versus periodic prophylactic blood transfusion in sickle cell patients at high risk of ischemic stroke: a decision analysis. *Blood.* 2000;95(10):3057–3064.
53. Nietert PJ, Silverstein MD, Abboud MR. Sickle cell anaemia: epidemiology and cost of illness. *Pharmacoeconomics.* 2002; 20(6):357–366.
54. Wayne AS, Schoenike SE, Pegelow CH. Financial analysis of chronic transfusion for stroke prevention in sickle cell disease. *Blood.* 2000;96(7):2369–2372.
55. Woods K, Karrison T, Koshy M, Patel A, Friedmann P, Cassel C. Hospital utilization patterns and costs for adult sickle cell patients in Illinois. *Public Health Rep.* 1997;112(1):44–51.
56. Atkins RC, Walters MC. Haematopoietic cell transplantation in the treatment of sickle cell disease. *Expert Opin Biol Ther.* 2003;3(8):1215–1224.
57. Cornu G, Vermylen C, Ferster A, et al. Hematopoietic stem cell transplantation in sickle cell anemia. *Arch Pediatr.* 1999;6(Suppl 2):345s–347s.
58. Mentzer WC. Bone marrow transplantation for hemoglobinopathies. *Curr Opin Hematol.* 2000;7(2):95–100.
59. Panepinto JA, Walters MC, Carreras J, et al. Matched-related donor transplantation for sickle cell disease: report from the Center for International Blood and Transplant Research. *Br J Haematol.* 2007;137(5):479–485.
60. Bernaudin F, Socie G, Kuentz M, et al. Long-term results of related, myeloablative stem cell transplantation to cure sickle cell disease. *Blood.* 2007;110(7):2749–2756.
61. Horan JT, Liesveld JL, Fenton P, Blumberg N, Walters MC. Hematopoietic stem cell transplantation for multiply transfused patients with sickle cell disease and thalassemia after low-dose total body irradiation, fludarabine, and rabbit anti-thymocyte globulin. *Bone Marrow Transplant.* 2005; 35(2):171–177.
62. Andreani M, Nesci S, Lucarelli G, et al. Long-term survival of ex-thalassemic patients with persistent mixed chimerism after bone marrow transplantation. *Bone Marrow Transplant.* 2000;25(4):401–404.
63. Walters MC, Patience M, Leisenring W, et al. Stable mixed hematopoietic chimerism after bone marrow transplantation for sickle cell anemia. *Biol Blood Marrow Transplant.* 2001;7(12):665–673.
64. Iannone R, Casella JF, Fuchs EJ, et al. Results of minimally toxic nonmyeloablative transplantation in patients with sickle cell anemia and beta-thalassemia. *Biol Blood Marrow Transplant.* 2003;9(8):519–528.
65. Krishnamurti L, Venkataramanan R, Wu C. A pilot study of hematopoietic transplantation for sickle cell disease following a nonmyeloablative conditioning regimen. *Proceedings of the 27th Meeting of the National Sickle Cell Disease Program.* 2004:172.
66. Krishnamurti L, Wu C, Baker S, Goyal R, Yeager AM, Wagner JE. Hematopoietic stem cell transplantation from a matched sibling donor for high risk patients with sickle cell disease using a reduced intensity conditioning regimen is well tolerated and can lead to long term stable engraftment. *Proceedings of the 28th Meeting of the National Sickle Cell Disease Program.* 2005:21.
67. van Besien K, Bartholomew A, Stock W, et al. Fludarabine-based conditioning for allogeneic transplantation in adults with sickle cell disease. *Bone Marrow Transplant.* 2000;26(4): 445–449.
68. Schleuning M, Stoetzer O, Waterhouse C, Schlemmer M, Ledderose G, Kolb HJ. Hematopoietic stem cell transplantation after reduced-intensity conditioning as treatment of sickle cell disease. *Exp Hematol.* 2002;30(1):7–10.
69. Walters M, Woolfrey A, Torok-Storb B, et al. Enrichment of donor erythroid cells after non-myeloablative bone marrow transplantation (BMT) for sickle cell anemia (sickle cell anemia). *Blood.* 2001;98(11):490a.

70. Wu CJ, Gladwin MT, Krishnamurti L, et al. Mixed chimerism following nonmyeloablative stem cell transplantation for sickle cell disease prevents intravascular hemolysis and restores endothelial function. *Blood.* 2004;104(11):467a.
71. Shenoy S, Grossman WJ, DiPersio J, et al. A novel reduced-intensity stem cell transplant regimen for nonmalignant disorders. *Bone Marrow Transplant.* 2005;35(4):345–352.
72. Hernigou P, Bernaudin F, Reinert P, Kuentz M, Vernant JP. Bone-marrow transplantation in sickle-cell disease. Effect on osteonecrosis: a case report with a four-year follow-up. *J Bone Joint Surg Am.* 1997;79(11):1726–1730.
73. Ferster A, Bujan W, Corazza F, et al. Bone marrow transplantation corrects the splenic reticuloendothelial dysfunction in sickle cell anemia. *Blood.* 1993;81(4):1102–1105.
74. Walters MC, Sullivan KM, Bernaudin F, et al. Neurologic complications after allogeneic marrow transplantation for sickle cell anemia. *Blood.* 1995;85(4):879–884.
75. Ferster A, Christophe C, Dan B, Devalck C, Sariban E. Neurologic complications after bone marrow transplantation for sickle cell anemia. *Blood.* 1995;86(1):408–409.
76. Abboud MR, Jackson SM, Barredo J, Holden KR, Cure J, Laver J. Neurologic complications following bone marrow transplantation for sickle cell disease. *Bone Marrow Transplant.* 1996;17(3):405–407.
77. Woodard P, Helton KJ, Khan RB, et al. Brain parenchymal damage after haematopoietic stem cell transplantation for severe sickle cell disease. *Br J Haematol.* 2005;129(4):550–552.
78. Singhal A, Davies P, Sahota A, Thomas PW, Serjeant GR. Resting metabolic rate in homozygous sickle cell disease. *Am J Clin Nutr.* 1993;57(1):32–34.
79. Wang WC, Morales KH, Scher CD, et al. Effect of long-term transfusion on growth in children with sickle cell anemia: results of the STOP trial. *J Pediatr.* 2005;147(2):244–247.
80. Eggleston B, Patience M, Edwards S, et al. Effect of myeloablative bone marrow transplantation on growth in children with sickle cell anemia: results of the multicenter study of Hematopoietic Cell Transplantation for Sickle Cell Anemia. *Br J Haematol.* 2007;136(4):673–676.
81. Wagner JE, Kernan NA, Steinbuch M, Broxmeyer HE, Gluckman E. Allogeneic sibling umbilical-cord-blood transplantation in children with malignant and non-malignant disease. *Lancet.* 1995;346:214–219.
82. Rocha V, Wagner JE Jr, Sobocinski KA, Klein JP, Zhang MJ, Horowitz MM, et al. Graft-versus-host disease in children who have received a cord-blood or bone marrow transplant from an HLA-identical sibling. Eurocord and International Bone Marrow Transplant Registry Working Committee on Alternative Donor and Stem Cell Sources. *N Engl J Med.* 2000;342(25):1846–1854.
83. Walters MC, Quirolo L, Trachtenberg ET, et al. Sibling donor cord blood transplantation for thalassemia major: experience of the sibling donor cord blood program. *Ann NY Acad Sci.* 2005;1054:206–213.
84. Adamkiewicz TV, Mehta PS, Boyer MW, et al. Transplantation of unrelated placental blood cells in children with high-risk sickle cell disease. *Bone Marrow Transplant.* 2004;34(5):405–411.
85. Mentzer WC, Heller S, Pearle PR, Hackney E, Vichinsky E. Availability of related donors for bone marrow transplantation in sickle cell anemia. *Am J Pediatr Hematol Oncol.* 1994;16(1):27–29.
86. Walters MC, Patience M, Leisenring W, et al. Barriers to bone marrow transplantation for sickle cell anemia. *Biol Blood Marrow Transplant.* 1996;2(2):100–104.
87. Krishnamurti L, Abel S, Maiers M, Flesch S. Availability of unrelated donors for hematopoietic stem cell transplantation for hemoglobinopathies. *Bone Marrow Transplant.* 2003;31(7):547–550.
88. Maiers M, Flesch S. Unrelated donor hematopoietic stem cell transplantation for hemoglobinopathies facilitated by NMDP. National Marrow Donor Program: Minneapolis. 2002.
89. Adamkiewicz TV, Boyer MW, Bray R, Haight A, Yeager AM. Identification of unrelated cord blood units for hematopoietic stem cell transplantation in children with sickle cell disease. *J Pediatr Hematol Oncol.* 2006;28(1):29–32.

33

Prospects for Gene Therapy of Sickle Cell Disease and Thalassemia

Derek A. Persons, Brian P. Sorrentino, and Arthur W. Nienhuis

INTRODUCTION

It has been four decades since the concept of gene therapy for human disease began to be considered and discussed in earnest. With the advent of recombinant DNA technology in the 1970s and the concurrent discovery that viruses could carry novel genetic information into target cells, gene therapy was seen as having significant future potential. A major step in the development of gene therapy for hematopoietic disorders occurred in 1985 when the laboratories of Bernstein and Anderson simultaneously showed that the genome of mouse hematopoietic stem cells (HSCs) could be permanently modified using a genetically engineered retrovirus capable of integrating into host cell DNA.[1,2] These results suggested that a patient's own HSCs could be harvested, genetically modified ex vivo, and then returned, perhaps following administration of radiation or chemotherapy to eradicate the diseased HSCs. From that time, it took almost a decade before functional correction of human disease model was demonstrated using retroviral-mediated, HSC-targeted gene transfer. The first such description was that of Heard and colleagues[3] when they demonstrated the successful treatment of a murine model of the lysosomal disorder, mucopolysaccharidosis type VII. Subsequently, murine models of two immunodeficiencies – chronic granulomatous disease[4] and a form of severe combined immunodeficiency due to *JAK3* deficiency[5] – were also successfully treated using gene therapy. These successes seemed to fulfill the stated goals of the Orkin and Motulsky NIH panel,[6] which called for more basic science research into gene therapy and the use of murine disease models to demonstrate efficacy prior to clinical trials.

After improvements in conditions for transducing primitive hematopoietic cells, these results were translated into successful clinical trials for severe combined immunodeficiencies (SCID). As recently reviewed[7] and discussed in more detail later in this chapter, more than 30 patients with SCID secondary to deficiency of the common γ chain of interleukin-2 or secondary to adenosine deaminase deficiency (ADA) have been successfully treated by ex vivo transduction and reinfusion of autologous primitive hematopoietic cells. Vector-mediated insertional activation of nearby protooncogenes initiated the development of leukemia in five patients, highlighting the importance of vector design to enhance the safety of gene therapy.[7] These otherwise successful trials do establish the potential efficacy of stem cell–targeted gene therapy for hemoglobin disorders. Globin gene vectors with the required regulatory elements have proved challenging to design and produce.[8–12] In this chapter we will review the viral vector systems relevant to HSC-targeted gene therapy, the issues relevant to obtaining efficient gene transfer into human HSCs, the factors unique to globin vector design, the recent remarkable progress in human clinical trials, and the prospects for eventual successful treatment of hemoglobin disorders such as sickle cell disease and β thalassemia.

THE SCIENCE OF VIRAL VECTORS

Successful gene therapy for hemoglobin disorders will require permanent genetic modification of pluripotent HSCs with long-term repopulating ability (Fig. 33.1). Among the various viral vector systems that have been considered, only efficiently integrating retroviruses that become a permanent part of the genome of the target cell and its progeny are potentially useful. As recently reviewed,[13] retroviruses share several features that are of interest for gene delivery. The characteristic that defines retroviruses is their ability to convert their single-stranded RNA genome into double-stranded DNA prior to integration of their genome into a host-cell chromosome. The initial vectors used in clinical gene therapy trials were γ-retroviruses derived from murine leukemia viruses (MLV). In the context of their clinical use, such vectors had the most advanced packaging systems for generating vector particles. Complex lentiviruses such as the human immunodeficiency virus (HIV) have many potential advantages including the ability to transduce nonmitotic cells. Furthermore, the mechanisms that have evolved to facilitate transport of unspliced HIV RNA species to the cytoplasm allow the assembly of vectors having complex genomes. The third class of retroviruses that have been considered for gene therapy applications are the spumaviruses including the human foamy virus (HFV). This virus is also able to transduce quiescent cells with relative efficiency.

Other vector systems without well-developed integration mechanisms nonetheless have important potential clinical applications. Recombinant adeno-associated viral (rAAV) vectors have been shown to transfer and express human γ-globin genes upon transduction of human erythroleukemia cells[14] or human erythroid progenitors,[15] and

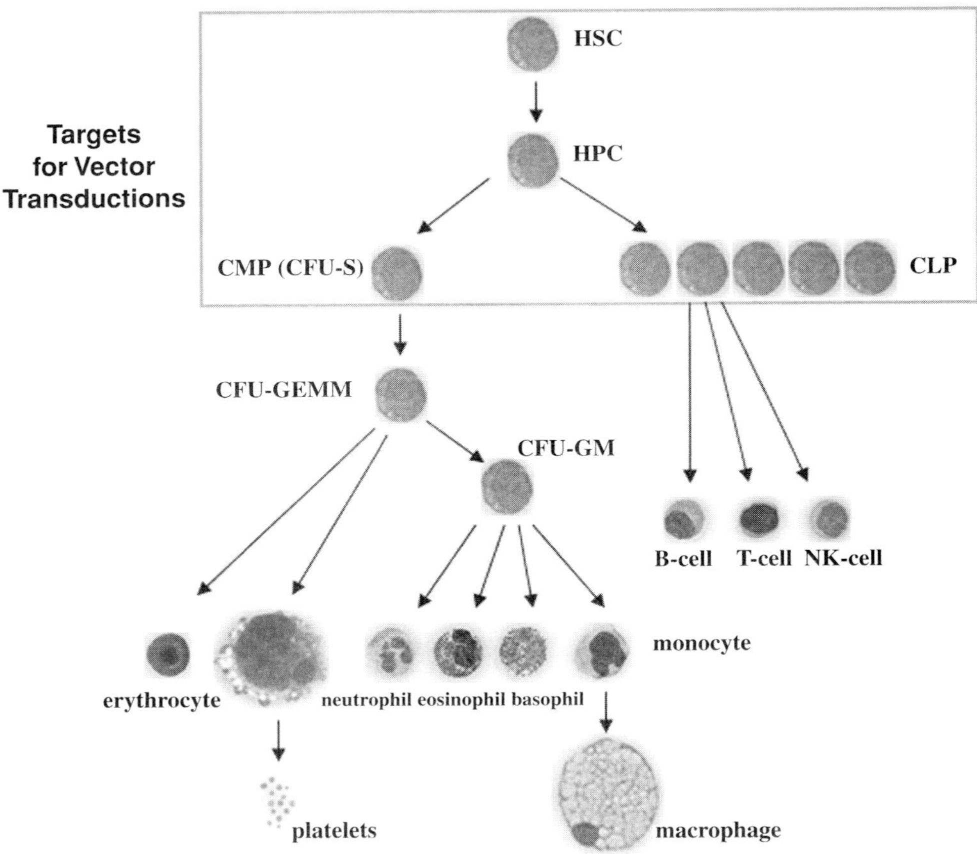

Figure 33.1. Hematopoietic cell targets for gene therapy. This figure shows the general hierarchical structure of hematopoiesis. Hematopoietic stem cells (HSCs) give rise to primitive progenitor cells (HPC), which in turn generate common myeloid progenitors (CMP) and common lymphoid progenitors (CLP). These progenitor cells then give rise to all formed elements of the blood through a number of intermediates including the granulocyte/erythrocyte/monocyte/macrophage colony forming unit (CFU-GEMM) and the granulocyte/monocyte colony forming unit (CFU-GM). The cells contained within the green outline are the desired targets for retroviral vectors because they all give rise to multiple mature cell types and because, to greater or lesser degrees, they can self-renew and lead to the persistence of genetically modified cells over time. The target cell population can differ for various diseases. For instance, for SCID, targeting of the CLP with an appropriate vector will result in long-term reconstitution of all lymphocyte subsets. In contrast, treatment of hemoglobin disorders required targeting of the most primitive HSC to have long-term persistence of stably modified erythrocytes after transplantation. The biology and frequency of the various target cell populations differs and are variable in determining the gene transfer efficiency. (See color plate 33.1.)

transient gene expression can be achieved in more primitive hematopoietic cells.[16] Some have argued that stable transduction of stem cells can be achieved with rAAV vectors[17] but the weight of evidence suggests that stable integration occurs infrequently in dividing cell populations. The ability of rAAV vectors to transduce nondividing cells in vivo with resulting long-term gene expression make them potentially useful for treating a wide variety of diseases as summarized in the recent review.[19] Other viral vector systems such as adenoviral vectors[20] Herpes simplex viral vectors,[21,22] and SV40 viral vectors[23] all have important potential clinical applications and interested readers are directed to recent reviews about each. A hybrid adenoviral/AAV vector containing a large fragment from the human β-globin gene locus has the interesting property of preferential integration into the cellular β-globin locus,[24] although the overall efficiency of integration appears to be relatively low.

Murine Retroviral Vectors

During the two decades following the discovery of reverse transcriptase,[25,26] much was learned about the biology of the retroviral life cycle as summarized in a review published in 1988.[27] Attention focused on the γ-retroviruses of mice that have the capacity to induce tumors and therefore were of great interest in efforts to understand cancer pathogenesis. Such viruses initiate cell entry by interaction with one or more specific proteins that act as a receptor (Fig. 33.2). Entry of the core of the viral vector into the cell

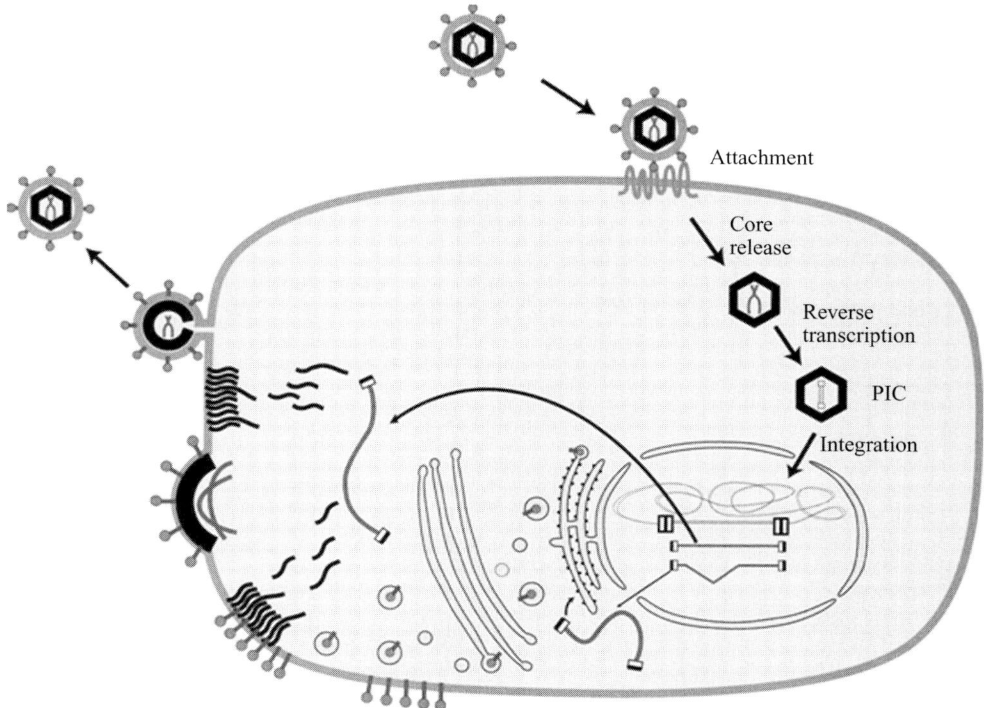

Figure 33.2. Retroviral life cycle. Entry of a retrovirus into a cell is initiated by interaction of its envelope proteins with one or more cellular membrane proteins that act as a receptor followed by internalization through membrane fusion or phagocytosis. The vector core is released and the RNA serves as a template for formation of the reverse transcription complex (RTC). The RTC includes additional viral proteins and is moved by the microtubule system from the cell periphery to the nucleus as it matures to become the preintegration complex (PIC). The PIC gains access to chromatin during mitosis, or in the case of lentiviruses, by ingress through the nuclear membrane. Following integration into host-cell DNA, the retroviral genome is expressed in RNA molecules that are transported to the cytoplasm to serve as a template for synthesis of new viral proteins and, in the case of unspliced RNA species, as a substrate for formation of new viral particles. (See color plate 33.2.)

then is accomplished either by endocytosis or fusion with the cell membrane depending on the envelope protein with which the particle was formed. Retroviruses have a unique capacity to convert their single-stranded RNA genome into a double-stranded DNA molecule, which is then integrated through the action of host cell and viral proteins, particularly viral integrase, into a cellular chromosome. Upon integration, the viral genome may be expressed into spliced and unspliced transcripts. Spliced and unspliced transcripts serve as templates for protein synthesis and unspliced transcripts may also be packaged into new viral particles. Ultimately the viral particles are assembled on the cell surface and new viral particles are released.

Increasing knowledge about the organization of the genome of murine γ-retroviruses suggested strategies for deriving vector particles free of replication-competent retroviruses[28,29] that were potentially useful for gene therapy applications. The fundamental principle underlying the use of potentially pathogenic viruses as therapeutic vectors reflects the ability to express viral proteins from independent genetic elements and deleting most or all of the coding information from the vector genome and replacing it with a therapeutic transgene. Coexpression of the vector genome and viral proteins in cultured cells leads to the production of vector particles encoding the therapeutic transgene without replication-competent retroviral particles (Fig. 33.3).

Only the long terminal repeats (LTRs) and sequences at the 5′ end of the viral genome are required for efficient packaging of RNA molecules into γ-retroviral vector particles. The GAG, POL, and envelope (ENV) gene products are cleaved by cellular and viral proteases to yield multiple proteins. GAG products make up the viral capsid and the POL-derived products include a protease, the integrase, and reverse transcriptase.[13] The coding sequences for these viral proteins can largely be eliminated from the vector genome. Conversely, expression cassettes for the viral proteins have been constructed that allow their expression in packaging cells as RNA molecules that lack both the LTRs and packaging sequences.[28,30] Separating the GAG and POL genes from the ENV gene on two separate transcriptional units (so-called split packaging lines) substantially reduced the possibility for regeneration of replication-competent retrovirus.[31,32] Second- and third-generation vector genomes contain a larger packaging signal that extends into the GAG coding region, thereby

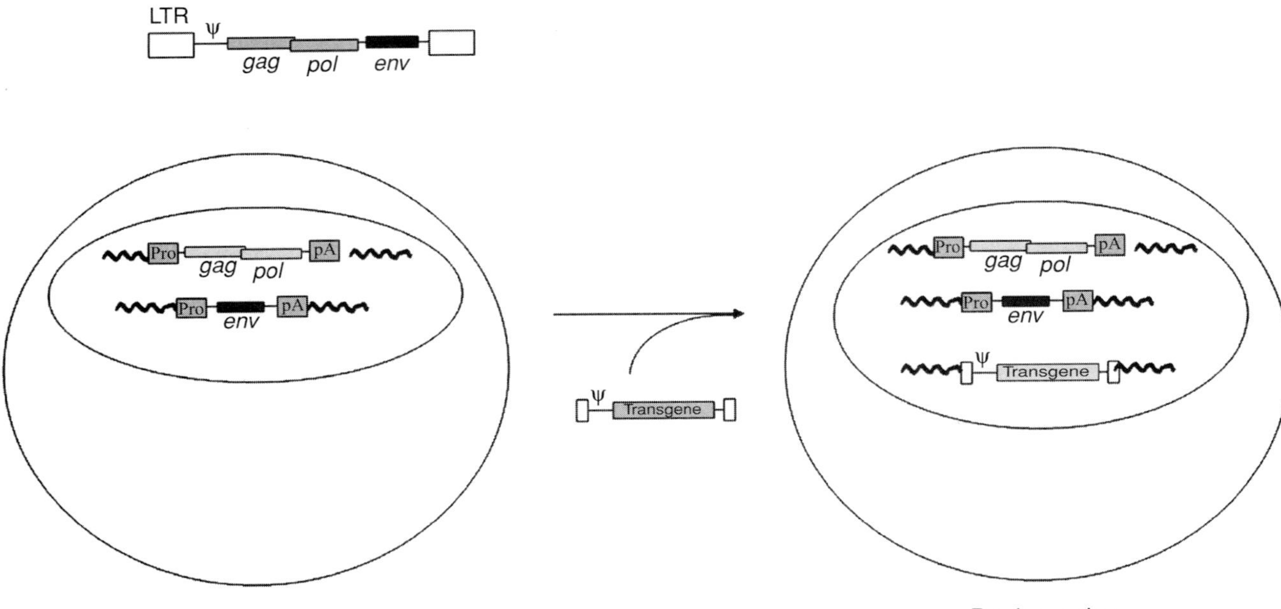

Figure 33.3. Production of retroviral vector particles. This figure illustrates the concept of the strategy used to derive retroviral vector preparations free of replication-competent virus. The diagram at the top shows the organization of a retroviral genome. Murine oncoretroviruses have coding sequences for matrix proteins (gag), reverse transcriptase, integrase and protease (pol), and envelope proteins (env). The LTR contains the viral promoter and enhancer. Immediately downstream is a sequence essential for packaging the genomic RNA (ψ). To reduce the risk of recombination and generation of replication-competent particles, these coding sequences are separated on two or more expression cassettes before transfer into a tissue culture cell line. The coding sequences for viral proteins are replaced by the coding sequences for the intended therapeutic protein in the vector. Various strategies are used for introducing the vector genome into the packaging cell that initiates production of replication-defective retroviral vector particles that can be used to introduce the therapeutic transgene into target cells. In the packaging and producer cells, the viral protein constructs are driven by exogenous promoters (Pro). (See color plate 33.3.)

improving vector production.[33] Despite this extended overlap with the transcriptional unit encoding GAG, the risk of emergence of replication-competent retrovirus by homologous recombination has been controlled by introduction of mutations into the GAG sequences of the vector genome[34] and by using split-function packaging lines. Most packaging lines and producer clones have been based on murine 3T3 fibroblast cell lines, but packaging lines based on human cells have also been generated using this general strategy.[35,36] The vector particles produced by such cell lines are more resistant to destruction by human complement and thus may prove more useful for various gene therapy applications.

Different classes of viruses use different proteins for receptors. For example, ecotropic viruses that infect murine and other rodent cells rely on a cationic amino acid transporter to initiate cellular entry,[37,38] whereas amphotropic viruses, whose broader host range includes human cells, use a sodium-dependent phosphate transporter.[39,40] Over the years, γ-retroviral particles have been assembled or pseudotyped with a number of different envelope proteins including that from gibbon ape leukemia (GAL) retrovirus,[41] the feline endogenous retrovirus (RD114),[42] and the feline leukemia virus type C retrovirus (FLVC).[43] GAL pseudotyped particles have been used in one of the successful clinical trial for X-SCID. The FLVC receptor is expressed at higher levels on primitive hematopoietic cells than are the receptors for other envelope proteins,[43] focusing attention on the evaluation of this particular envelope for pseudotyping vector particles for HSC-targeted gene transfer. A useful review summarizing strategies to target γ-retroviral and lentiviral vectors should be consulted for further information.[44]

The viral core is released into the cell cytoplasm following fusion of the virion membrane with either the cytoplasmic membrane or internal endosome membrane.[45] In the case of MLV, the capsid proteins remain associated with the viral genome in a reverse transcription complex (RTC) that associates with the cytoskeleton.[46] The RTC is actively moved by cytoskeletal components through the viscous cytoplasm, ultimately reaching the nucleus where the capsid proteins disassociate from the final preintegration complex. Movement of the viral genome with associated matrix proteins and enzymatic activities into the nucleus requires dissolution of the nuclear membrane during mitosis.[47] Thus, retroviral vectors that are based on the Moloney virus and other murine γ-retroviruses require cell division for genome integration. Furthermore, the preintegration nucleoprotein complex of oncoretroviruses is highly unstable;[48] therefore successful transduction requires genome integration within hours of exposure of target cells to the retroviral vector particles. Various cells possess innate mechanisms that restrict retroviral infection,[49–51] which undoubtedly complicate and restrict gene transfer with retroviral vectors. These mechanisms include the apolipoprotein B mRNA–editing catalytic polypeptide-like 3 (APOBEC3) factor that has cytosine demethylating activity and the TRIM5α protein, which interacts with the viral capsid proteins.

After integration, expression of the genes encoded by the proviral genome requires continued activity of promoter and enhancer sequences within the LTR. Unfortunately, silencing is all too common and may be mediated both by methylation[52] of proviral sequences and at the level of chromatin structure.[53] MLV LTRs seem particularly prone to silencing in embryonic stem cells and in primitive hematopoietic cells. Later vectors have been designed to resist such silencing. Such vectors include one based on the murine stem cell virus (MSCV)[54] and another based on the myeloproliferative sarcoma virus.[55] The latter vector has also been modified to eliminate a negative control region from the LTR and has a substituted primer-binding site that also enhances expression. A recent version of the MSCV has a self-inactivating (SIN) design in which the enhancer/promoter is eliminated from the 3′ LTR. During reverse transcription and vector genome integration, the 3′ LTR is duplicated to create the 5′ LTR of the integrated provirus. Thus, the SIN vectors lack an enhancer/promoter in both LTRs and depend on an internal promoter to express the transgene. The modified SIN MSCV vector achieved stable γ-retroviral expression during embryonic stem cell–derived in vitro hematopoietic development, a very stringent test of vector silencing.[56] Production of SIN γ-retroviral vectors has been problematic in stable producer clones but substitution of a stronger or an inducible promoter for the viral transcript improves titer.[57] Recently a SIN γ-retroviral vector having an internal cellular promoter has been derived for treatment of X-SCID due to common γ-chain deficiency.[58]

Expression of more than one gene product from a proviral genome is often desirable. Several designs have been tested for creating multigene vectors. One that has been tested extensively is the insertion of a second promoter downstream from the first open reading frame followed by the second open reading frame. Unfortunately, promoter interference often results in poor expression from the internal promoter.[59] Another technique that has been much more successful involves the inclusion of an internal ribosomal entry site between the two open reading frames, creating a vector genome that encodes a polycistronic transcript.[60] Using this design, several genes have been expressed in tandem with the coding sequences for green fluorescent protein, a readily assayable and selectable marker.[61,62] Self-cleaving peptides such as the 2A peptide from Picornavirus have also been used to obtain expression of multiple protein products from a single vector transcript.[63]

Another approach is to place a complete transcriptional unit in reverse orientation within the 3′ LTR of the proviral genome.[64] After replication of such a genome and insertion into a target cell, the transcriptional unit within the 3′ LTR is duplicated, becoming part of the integrated 5′ LTR. Such double-copy vectors often result in a much higher level of expression than can be achieved with an internal promoter configuration, particularly when a deletion mutation is introduced in the 3′ LTR to create a "self-inactivating vector" that lacks LTR promoter activity in target cells.[64]

As discussed in detail later, low levels of globin mRNA are generated by γ-retroviral vectors that contain globin cDNA sequences. Vectors that incorporate an intact genomic globin gene in reverse transcriptional orientation with associated regulatory elements[65–68] have been tested extensively in an effort to achieve therapeutically useful levels of globin in target hematopoietic cells, but these efforts have not met with ultimate success.

Lentiviral Vectors

A major breakthrough in efforts to develop gene therapy for hemoglobin disorders was made by the laboratory of Michel Sadelain in 2000 when they demonstrated that lentiviral vectors could be used to transfer and express a globin gene in the erythroid cells of thalassemic mice.[69] In contrast to simple γ-retroviral vectors, complex vectors such as HIV encode multiple protein products in addition to the products of the GAG, POL, and ENV coding sequences. The tat protein is involved in enhancing transcription, the rev protein interacts with the rev responsive element to facilitate nuclear to cytoplasmic transport of unspliced mRNA species and the vif, vpr, vpu, and nef proteins are virulence factors. Also, in contrast to γ-retroviruses, lentiviruses can transduce nondividing cells.[48] Multiple nuclear localization signals within the matrix, vpr, and integrase proteins and in the central polypurine tract of the viral transcript were thought to mediate transport into the nucleus via nuclear pores.[70–73] Recent evidence, however, has cast doubt on the relevance of these nuclear localization signals.[74] Addition of a nuclear localization signal to the matrix of spleen necrosis virus does not allow efficient gene transfer into quiescent cells with a vector based on this virus.[75] In addition, elimination of all of the known nuclear localization signals from the HIV genome and proteins showed that no combination of the virally encoded nuclear localization signals is essential for the ability of HIV to infect nondividing cells.[76] Evidence has recently been presented for direct involvement of the capsid protein, CA, in HIV infection of nondividing cells. Its role in conferring this property to HIV may occur following nuclear entry of the preintegration complex.[77,78] The preintegration complex of lentiviral vectors is relatively

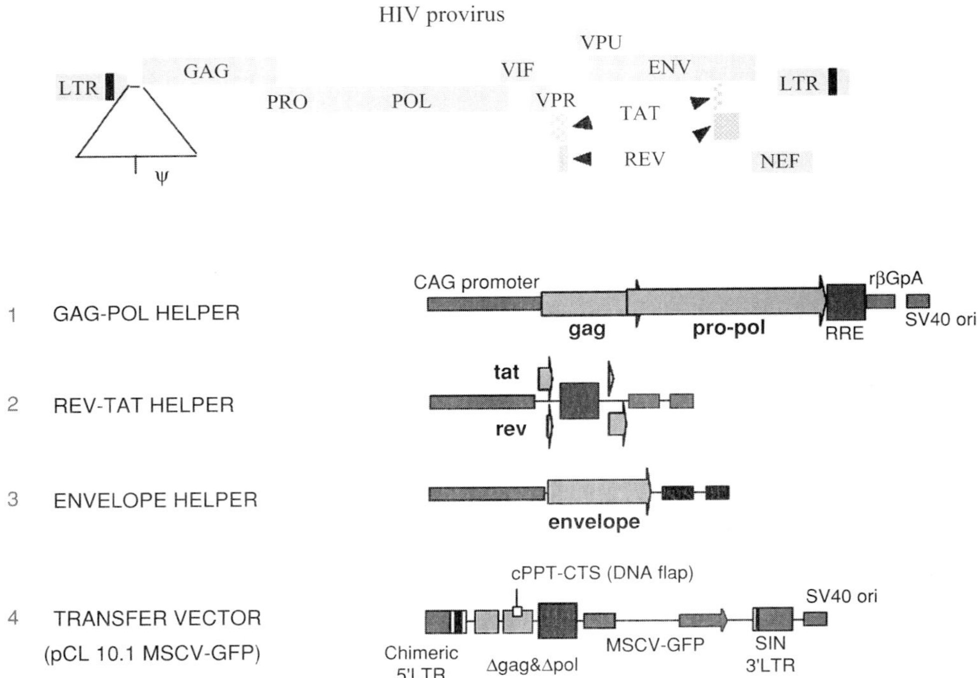

Figure 33.4. Organization of the HIV provirus and development of a packaging system for generation of vector particles free of replication-competent retrovirus. The HIV-1 genome encodes 15 proteins as shown in the top row of this figure. The GAG polyprotein is processed to yield viral core proteins including MA (matrix), CA (capsid), NC (nucleocapsid), and p6. The ENV protein product is processed to yield two proteins, SU (surface) and TM (transmembrane) components of the mature envelope proteins. The POL region encodes the enzymes PR (protease), RT (reverse transcriptase), and IN (integrase). TAT and REV are regulatory proteins that facilitate transcription or nuclear to cytoplasmic transport of unspliced RNA species, respectively. The accessory proteins NEF, VIF, VPR, and VPU are viral virulence factors, which are not required for vector particle formation. Shown below in rows 1–4 are components of a system developed to generate vector particles. Each of the transcriptional units encoding viral proteins includes the powerful chimeric CMV enhance/β-actin promoter, the β-globin large intron (CAG promoter), the rabbit β-globin polyadenylation sequence (rβGpA), and the rev responsive element (RRE), which facilitate nuclear to cytoplasmic transport. The SV40 origin of replication (ORI) is included in each expression plasmid to allow its amplification in cells expressing SV40T antigen. Three separate helper plasmids are used as shown in 1–3. The transfer vector includes a portion of the gag region required for packaging and a portion of the pol region, which includes the central polypurine tract (cPPT) and the central termination sequence (CTS). These elements together constitute the DNA flap that was described as a crucial determinate for lentiviral vector nuclear import and gene transduction of primitive human hematopoietic cells. The U3 region of the 5′ LTR in the vector has been replaced with the CMV enhancer and a deletion in the U3 region of the 3′ LTR renders the vector SIN. Not shown is the fact that a portion of the U5 region of the 3′ LTR has been removed and replaced with rabbit β-globin polyadenylation site to enhance safety and improve the efficiency of vector production. Vector production occurs when a mixture of the four plasmid DNAs are transfected into human embryonic kidney (293T) cells and conditioned media is harvested over the next 3–4 days. Depending on the envelope used, the vector preparation may be concentrated by ultracentrifugation or ultrafiltration. (See color plate 33.4.)

stable. For example, a partial reverse transcriptase product formed in quiescent T lymphocytes can be rescued by cell activation for at least 7–8 days postinfection. In contrast, the nucleoprotein complex of oncoretroviruses disappears within 24 hours of infection of nondividing cells.[48]

HIV-based vector development uses a general strategy similar to that used successfully with murine retroviral vectors (Fig. 33.4). The vector genome includes *cis* active sequences necessary for generation of the RNA form of the viral genome and the sequences required for efficient packaging, reverse transcription, and integration. Needed for these purposes are portions of the LTRs, the 5′ end of the genome, which includes the 5′ splice donor site, a portion of the GAG gene required for efficient packaging, and ENV sequences that contain the rev responsive element needed for nuclear to cytoplasmic transport of the unspliced RNA species.[79–81] Advanced versions of lentiviral vectors[82] now include the central polypurine track[72,73] and the central termination sequence.[83] Fortunately, the coding sequences for the virulence genes can all be deleted from the vector genome.[84] The packaging genome contains the sequences for GAG and POL under the control of a heterologous promoter (e.g., the cytomegalovirus [CMV] promoter and heterologous RNA processing signals). Codon optimization of the GAG and POL genes whereby the codons found in highly expressed mRNAs are used to assemble the coding sequences enhances production of the viral proteins and eliminates homology between the packaging and vector plasmids, thereby improving the safety of the packaging system.[85] The rev coding sequences have also been codon optimized in a separate expression plasmid to enhance expression and to eliminate overlap of the tat and rev coding sequences. Because native HIV viral particles have a limited host range that is dependent on cell surface expression of CD4, alternative envelope proteins are used to generate vector particles. Pseudotyping of vector particles with the ENV protein of amphotropic γ-retrovirus or vesicular stomatitis virus creates vector particles with a broader host range. To date, most vector preparations have been derived by cotransfection of three[82] or more[86] helper plasmids encoding viral proteins along with a vector plasmid into human kidney (293T) cells.[87] Typically titers are approximately 10^7 infectious units (IU)/mL.

Several of the HIV proteins are toxic, limiting the ability to derive packaging lines in which the helper components are stably integrated. This limitation has been overcome by placing both the GAG-POL and envelope genomes under the control of tetracycline-modulatable promoters.[88] As noted previously, it is possible to eliminate coding sequences for the accessory proteins, vif, vpr, vpu, and nef, and still generate vector particles capable of transducing quiescent cells.[84,89] Elimination of these genes increases the safety of HIV-based lentiviral particles because each has a role in the pathogenicity of HIV. Another innovation in the development of stable packaging lines and producer clones has been the introduction of the coding sequences for the viral proteins in the form of γ-retroviral vector genomes.[90,91] This modification eliminates plasmid sequences that have the potential to attract silencing mechanisms.[92] A recent report describes inducible packaging cells for large-scale production of lentiviral vectors in serum-free suspension culture.[93] Our colleague at St. Jude Children's Research Hospital, Dr. John Gray, has also recently succeeded in deriving a fully inducible producer clone for a SIN vector encoding the marker GFP that yields titers in excess of 10^7 IU/mL (Gray J, unpublished observations). He has also derived globin vector producer clones that yield titers of 10^6 IU/mL. Such producer clones should be highly useful for mass cultures to generate sufficient vector particles for downstream processing and purification of vector particles.

Safety will be a paramount concern as HIV-based vectors gain clinical application. As noted, elimination of the accessory and ENV genes greatly reduces the potential pathogenicity of any replication-competent retroviruses that might arise during packaging. As constructed, the vector and packaging genomes with codon optimization have limited homology, greatly reducing the probability of generating replication-competent retroviruses by homologous recombination. HIV is dependent on the expression of the *trans*-acting proteins, tat and rev, that are absent from the target cell population. The HIV LTR, because of its dependence on tat, is naturally at least partially "self-inactivating." Nonetheless, most modern vectors have a SIN design in that they are constructed by removing the enhancer/promoter sequences from the 3′ LTR so that both LTRs of the integrated proviral genome lack transcriptionally active sequences. Further improvement in safety may be sought by improving the transcriptional termination of HIV vectors.[94]

Another safety modification involves the addition of a chromatin insulator to the 3′ LTR in the vector plasmid. By placing an insulator in the 3′ LTR, it is copied over into the 5′ LTR so that the integrated proviral genome has insulator elements flanking an internal gene. Insulator elements have both enhancer blocking and chromatin barrier functions[95] and therefore have the potential to enhance the safety of retroviral vectors by shielding nearby cellular genes from the actions of transcriptional elements within the vector genome and also may improve vector function by preventing silencing.[96] Recent evidence supports the enhanced safety of such a vector design in that a SIN-insulated vector with an internal γ-retroviral LTR exhibited diminished clonal dominance, presumed secondary to gene activation by integrated vector genomes, compared with the control vector without the insulator in short-term cultures of transduced lymphoid cells.[97] Furthermore, the insulator element was shown to block promoter activation by an integrated γ-retroviral LTR in lymphoid cells in which the integration event in the first intron of the LMO2 gene in one of the X-SCID patients with leukemia had been recreated.[18]

Lentiviral vectors are proving highly useful for deriving transcriptional units that rely on expression from cellular promoters. For example, a retroviral vector has been constructed using the native proximal promoter for the Wiskott-Aldrich Syndrome (WAS) protein to achieve hematopoietic-specific expression of the WAS protein coding sequences, which is intended for use in a planned gene therapy trial for WAS.[98] A recent study suggests that adding the distal promoter in tandem enhances WAS protein expression in myeloid cells.[99] Lentiviral vectors have been found to transduce efficiently quiescent cell populations in vivo, including myocytes and hepatocytes,[100] neurons,[81,101,102] and retinal cells.[103] Lentiviral vectors can transduce quiescent human primitive hematopoietic cells that are capable of establishing human hematopoiesis in immunodeficient mice.[80,82,99,104]

A recently reported screen that was based on small interfering RNAs resulted in the identification of more than 250 host HIV dependency factors (HDFs).[105] Two hundred and thirty-seven of these HDFs had not been implicated in the HIV life cycle previously whereas 36 host factors were known to be important to HIV pathogenicity. Individual HDFs were involved in the nuclear pore complex, retrograde vesicular transport, nuclear transport, and HIV transcription. Although the primary screen was performed in HeLa cells, 33% of the HDFs were enriched for genes with high expression in immune cells.[105] Thus the interaction of lentiviral vectors with the intended target population is likely to be highly complex with relatively high expression of host factors that are required favoring transduction and the relatively high level of expression of factors that confer resistance to transduction such as the APOBEC3 factor and the TRIM5α protein[50,51,106] diminishing transduction. One example of the complexity of these interactions is the identification of a mutation in the HIV capsid protein which significantly diminishes infection of nondividing HeLa cells but has little effect in reducing infection of nondividing monocytes suggesting a role for a cell-type specific factor.[78] Another example is the fact that cells from the monkey species, *Macaca nemestrina,* lack a functional TRIM5α and are highly susceptible to HIV infection whereas cells from rhesus macaques express a variant of TRIM5α that renders them highly resistant to HIV infection.[107] Undoubtedly, many such potential target cell specific vector interactions that may influence transducability of specific target cells remain to be discovered.

Foamy Virus Vectors

Human foamy virus (HFV), a retrovirus that is a member of the Spumavirus family, is also being explored for potential gene therapy applications.[108] Its advantages and disadvantages, relative to γ-retroviral and lentiviral vectors have recently been reviewed.[109] Although HFV was isolated from a human nasopharyngeal carcinoma, its origin is now thought to be from a chimpanzee as a result of an early trans-species transmission.[110] Foamy virus infections have frequently been reported in persons occupationally exposed to nonhuman primates,[110] but person-to-person transmission of foamy viruses has not been reported.[109] Foamy viruses are nonpathogenic both in nonhuman primates and in humans.

The originally isolated foamy virus known as HFV has been the focus of most work on this family of viral vectors, although a suggestion has been made because it originated from a non-human primate, that it be redesignated prototype FV (PFV).[109] Foamy viral (FV) vectors are of interest to those focused on developing gene therapy for hemoglobin disorders because of their broad host range which includes human clonogenic progenitors[111] as well as long-term mobilized peripheral blood–derived cells capable of establishing human hematopoiesis in immunodeficient mice.[112] Indeed a direct comparison of the three retroviral vector systems for transduction of these primitive human hematopoietic cells suggests superiority with respect to efficiency for the FV vector tested compared with γ-retroviral and lentiviral vectors.[113] These results have been obtained despite an early report suggesting that there was low-level expression of functional foamy virus receptor on hematopoietic progenitor cells.[114] Indeed a recent report describes FV-mediated gene transfer into canine repopulating cells[115] and canine leukocyte adhesion deficiency has been successfully treated with an FV vector.[116]

The organization of the FV genome is described in a recent review.[109] Like all retroviruses, it includes GAG, POL, and ENV coding sequences. In addition, it encodes several bel proteins, one of which (also called tas) is a DNA-binding protein that activates both an internal promoter and the LTR, whereas a different bel protein (called bet) may sequester APOBEC from being incorporated into vector particles. *Cis*-acting RNA signals have been identified in both GAG and POL coding sequences and both are absolutely required for packaging of a vector genome. FV vector particles cannot be pseudotyped with any other envelope protein. In keeping with this observation, the organization of the FV envelope protein is significantly different than that of other retroviral viruses of interest to gene therapists.[109] Packaging systems in which the GAG, POL, and ENV coding sequences are present on individual plasmids and the vector genome has a Tas independent promoter have been described.[117–119] The FV proteins are toxic to cells and no stable packaging cells or producer clones have been derived. Reverse transcription of FV genome begins in the packaging cell and indeed vector genomes can be integrated in such cells.[109] Full-length vector genomes can also be found in vector particles and the DNA/RNA ratio is higher in FV vector particles than in either γ-retroviral or lentiviral vector particles. Indeed the ability of FV to transduce quiescent cells that divide rarely is thought to reflect the stability of the DNA genome in target cells where it may persist for several days before cell division occurs.[120] FV vectors accommodate more than 9 kb of foreign DNA and therefore it should be possible to construct vectors encoding globin along with the required erythroid-specific regulatory elements although none have yet been reported.

RETROVIRAL-MEDIATED GENE TRANSFER INTO HEMATOPOIETIC STEM CELLS

Gene Therapy for Hemoglobinopathies Will Require High-Level Gene Transfer into Hematopoietic Stem Cells

Arguably, the most important current obstacle to effective gene therapy for hemoglobinopathies is the need for relatively efficient, stable gene transfer into HSCs. Although current gene therapy methodologies are sufficient to correct several of the severe immunodeficiency disorders,[121,122] the strong selective advantage for corrected cells in these disorders negates the requirement for highly efficient HSC transduction. Data from X-SCID patients that have undergone natural reversions of their original mutation suggests that even a single normal HSC is sufficient to correct the immunodeficiency disorder. In these patients, all lymphocytes contain the reverted, normal allele although the proportion of this clone in myeloid cells, which display no advantage for the revertant clone, is extremely low.[123] This appears to also be true in X-SCID gene therapy patients, where the proportion of transduced myeloid cells is less than 1% whereas virtually all the T cells contain the vector.[124]

In contrast, the degree of selective advantage for normal stem cell clones in hemoglobinopathy patients is significantly less. Based on preclinical mouse models[125] and clinical data from sickle cell patients that have partial chimerism after allogeneic transplant,[126] it is estimated that between 15% and 20% of all engrafted stem cells would be required to be transduced with a therapeutic globin-expressing vector to achieve clinical benefit.

There has been steady progress in increasing HSC transduction efficiency in human and nonhuman primate HSCs. In a rhesus macaque gene therapy model, recent results when using SIV-based lentiviral vectors show gene-marking levels in peripheral blood granulocytes ranging between 5% and 15%.[127] Considering that this result was achieved with a simple GFP vector rather than a complicated, lower-titer globin vector it seems likely that further advances in HSC transduction efficiency will be required to cure humans with sickle cell anemia or severe β thalassemia. Fortunately, new information is rapidly emerging regarding HSC biology, vector development, and in vivo selection of transduced cells that may allow for such an advance in the foreseeable future.

Biological Obstacles for Transducing Human Hematopoietic Stem Cells

Early enthusiasm for a gene therapy approach to hemoglobinopathies was in part based on successful retroviral-mediated gene transfer into murine HSCs. Using γ-retroviral vectors based on MLV, it is possible to achieve routinely gene transfer and expression in 80%–90% of blood cells in transplanted mice. What has become clear is that transduction of human and nonhuman primate HSCs is fundamentally more difficult and less efficient. Although all the critical differences are not well understood, several biological differences between mouse and primate cells have been identified as being important. The first step in HSC transduction involves binding of the vector particle to specific receptors on the cell surface. In the mouse model, investigators have utilized vectors that express the ecotropic envelope protein, which binds to the ecotropic receptor, a relatively abundant amino acid transporter on murine HSCs. The ortholog for this transporter in human cells does not function as a receptor for ecotropic retroviruses so that alternate envelope proteins are necessary for transduction of human cells. Commonly used viral envelopes for human cell transduction are the amphotropic envelope protein and the GAL virus protein. Although the receptors for these proteins are expressed in human HSCs, the overall level of expression is low compared with the ecotropic receptor.[128] To circumvent this limitation, alternative envelope proteins have been explored for human HSC transduction. One envelope is the RD114 protein, which has yielded relatively efficient transduction of human and rhesus reconstituting cells when used with γ-retroviral vectors. Another promising choice is the envelope from FLVC, which has been shown to yield an increased transduction efficiency of human HSCs in a xenogeneic sheep model.[43] Another choice more suitable for use in lentiviral vectors is the envelope protein from the vesicular stomatitis virus-G (VSV-G). This envelope protein has been widely used and has the advantage that it utilizes a ubiquitously available membrane phospholipid for cell entry. This property also confers concentration-dependent toxicity due to its ability to induce cell fusion and syncytias, particularly in concentrated vector preparations. Another potential issue is that the membrane fusion entry mechanism used by VSV-G is different from the endocytic internalization process associated with the other viral envelope receptors. At this point, it is not clear what the optimum viral envelope protein is to achieve cell entry. This is particularly important in the context of lentiviral vectors in which alternate envelopes may lead to a decrease in infectious titers.[82]

Another important difference between mouse and primate HSCs is that fewer primate HSCs are in cycle at any point in time and that nonhuman primate HSCs cycle much more slowly.[129,130] This is most relevant to transduction with γ-retroviral vectors that require breakdown of the nuclear membrane during mitosis to gain access to chromosomes. It is also relevant to lentiviral vectors, which despite a relatively enhanced ability to transduce nondividing cells, still display some degree of cell cycle sensitivity.[131] One approach to increase transduction efficiency is to enhance cycling of HSCs in culture while exposing them to vector particles, however the challenge is to induce specific self-renewal divisions rather than induce the production of differentiated progeny. Hematopoietic cytokines have been used to induce self-renewal during culture and result in a modest degree of HSC expansion that is nevertheless self-limited over time.[132]

New Approaches for Transduction of Human Hematopoietic Stem Cells

Recently, a number of novel factors have been identified that can be used to expand HSCs in culture.[133] Investigators are now testing these factors to determine if they can be used to improve HSC transduction efficiency. Some of the more promising examples include a membrane traversing form of the HOXB4 transcription factor,[134] mediators of canonical Wnt signaling pathway,[135] and angiopoietin-like ligands and insulin growth factor binding protein 2.[136,137] These factors have been shown to lead to expansion of murine and human HSCs during in vitro culture, and many are now being tested in the context of HSC transduction protocols. Even when the correct signaling moieties are identified for HSC expansion, other modalities may be necessary to prevent loss of HSCs during the culture phase. It has recently been recognized that HSCs are sensitive to oxidative stress, which limits their lifespan.[138] This oxidative stress activates DNA damage repair pathways that can cause loss of HSCs.[139,140] This may be a particular problem during the hyperoxic conditions associated with cell culture and may require the use reducing compounds such as N-acetylcysteine to reduce accumulation of reactive oxygen species in cultured HSCs.

Another obstacle to be considered is the potential to induce engraftment defects in cultured HSCs. Induction of cycling in HSCs causes an engraftment defect during the S/M/G_2 phase of the cell cycle.[141] This has led to approaches that induce a "resting phase" after transduction that allows transduced HSCs to return to the G_0/G_1 phase of the cell cycle. Data from monkeys that have undergone transplantation indicates that culturing transduced HSCs in stem cell factor alone induced quiescence and led to an increase in engraftment of transduced cells.[142] Another consideration regarding engraftment is the induction of CD26, a peptidase on the surface of HSCs that can disrupt SDF1-mediated migration and adhesion of stem cells.[143] Treatment of human cells with CD26 inhibitors leads to enhanced engraftment in immunodeficient mice.[144] This approach may be useful as an adjuvant for engraftment of genetically modified cells.

Vector Titer and Multiplicity of Infection: Critical Variables for Hematopoietic Stem Cell Transduction

The titer of the vector is an important consideration for HSC transduction efficiency. When titers are adequately high, cells can be cultured at a high multiplicity of infection, which leads to efficient transduction of the target cells. This issue is of particular importance to globin gene transfer protocols because the titers of globin vectors are often relatively low. For example, simple lentiviral vectors that contain a viral promoter and a GFP reporter gene can typically be produced at titers of $1–2 \times 10^7$ transducing particles per milliliter. In contrast, lentiviral vectors containing all the globin regulatory elements usually have much lower titers that require high degrees of concentration when using techniques such as ultracentrifugation or membrane dialysis.[145] Although higher concentrations of vector particles can be achieved, the degree to which these procedures can be used in large-scale production protocols has yet to be established. Another concern is that these procedures may also concentrate interfering activities or toxic components of the supernatant that will interfere with efficient transduction. Further advances in the technical aspects of globin vector production, such as the derivation of stable producer clones, are likely to be necessary to achieve efficient stem cell production.

In Vivo Selection Strategies to Enrich for Transduced Hematopoietic Stem Cells

Another method to compensate for inefficient transduction of HSCs is the use of in vivo selection strategies to amplify and enrich a minor component of transduced HSCs. By including an appropriate selective marker into the vector and then treating the transplant recipient with the selective agent, it is possible to increase the proportion of transduced HSCs in a variety of preclinical models.[146] One approach has been to use drug resistance genes that have been identified in studies on tumor cell drug resistance. Studies using dihydrofolate reductase variants together with antifolate drugs have been shown to be useful for in vivo selection of HSCs in transplanted mice;[147] however, analogous studies in nonhuman primates have not led to stable selection of HSCs using dihydrofolate reductase vectors.[148] This is probably due to differences in the biological properties of mouse versus primate HSCs such as the lower percentage of cycling cells in primates and the lower baseline marking obtained in primate versus mouse systems.

To date, the most promising selection system is based on the methylguanine methyltransferase (MGMT) drug resistance gene which confers resistance to several potent hematopoietic toxins such as BCNU and temozolomide. Point mutations in MGMT have been identified that confer resistance to MGMT depletion due to 6-benzylguanine (6-BG), allowing for drug combinations that can kill cells expressing wild-type MGMT but not the vector-encoded, mutant forms.[149] Cells expressing MGMT have the ability to repair the DNA lesions caused by these drugs prior to the induction of apoptosis. Normal HSCs express relatively low levels of endogenous MGMT and are therefore generally sensitive to these drugs; which is one of the reasons for the efficacy of MGMT systems for in vivo selection of HSCs. Murine transplant studies from several laboratories have confirmed the ability to select transduced HSCs to a high degree of efficiency by using either BCNU plus 6-BG[150] or temozolomide plus 6-BG.[151]

This approach has been used to achieve therapeutic numbers of transduced HSCs in a mouse model of β thalassemia.[152] When bone marrow cells from normal mice were transduced with a MGMT vector and transplanted into β thalassemic recipient mice, low levels of engraftment were obtained and there was no evidence of a therapeutic effect. When some of these mice were then treated with temozolomide and 6-BG to select for normal HSCs, there was a significant increase in peripheral erythrocytes that expressed the normal β-globin genes. Most important, drug treatment resulted in a significant increase in hemoglobin concentration that corresponded with correction of red blood cell abnormalities in the peripheral blood smear. This study provides proof of principle that in vivo selection may be useful in hemoglobin gene therapy applications.

Selection of HSCs using the MGMT system has been validated in several large-animal models. Work done using a dog transplant model has shown that allogeneic HSCs can be enriched by treating with BCNU and 6-BG to select for cells expressing a oncoretroviral vector containing the P140K MGMT cDNA.[153] In a subsequent study from the same group, selection of autologous HSCs in dogs was demonstrated using temozolomide and 6-BG, providing a proof of principal for the anticipated use of selection for treating genetic diseases with gene therapy.[154] High levels of stable polyclonal selection were obtained in this study. Currently, studies are in progress to determine whether MGMT-mediated selection can be successfully implemented in nonhuman primate models. Issues that remain to be resolved is which of the available drugs are most useful in primate models, what degree of selection can be obtained, whether there is a minimal marking frequency necessary for in vivo selection, and what toxicities will be apparent from the drug selection protocol.

PRECLINICAL DEVELOPMENT OF GLOBIN LENTIVIRAL VECTORS

Initial Efforts to Develop Integrating Globin Retroviral Vectors

The hemoglobin disorders of β-thalassemia and sickle cell disease were prime contenders for the development of gene therapy as retroviral vectors were developed in the 1980s, given that the molecular defects of the β-globin gene in both were well-defined at the time and the β-globin gene cluster had been cloned.[155–165] For β-thalassemia, in which little or no β-globin is produced in developing erythroid cells, transfer of an exogenous β- or γ-globin gene into HSCs with subsequent high-level expression in erythroid progeny could be therapeutic. Similarly in the context of sickle cell disease, transfer and high-level expression of γ-globin chains, when coupled with endogenous α-globin chains, could augment fetal hemoglobin (HbF), a potent antisickling molecule, to therapeutic levels. Several attempts using γ-retroviral vectors in the late 1980's were made to transfer and express a human β-globin gene under the transcriptional control of a minimal β-globin promoter in mouse transplant models.[8,166] Unfortunately, poor gene transfer was obtained and the vectors produced very low levels of β-globin mRNA, at most only a few percent of that of the endogenous β-globin gene.

Discovery of Globin Gene Locus Regulatory Elements Essential for High-level Expression

Contemporaneously, investigators were in the process of identifying powerful DNA enhancer elements from the β-globin locus control region (LCR),[10,11,167,168] located on human chromosome 11, that were necessary for the nearby globin genes to be expressed at the very high levels required in erythroid cells. Tuan showed that these elements, termed "hypersensitive sites," were requisite for active transcription of the downstream globin genes.[167] These "hypersensitive sites" consisted of regions of chromatin, located upstream from the globin genes, that were exceedingly sensitive to the enzyme micrococcal nuclease. This suggested that the chromatin was likely in an "open" configuration, such as that which occurs when protein complexes are bound to the DNA. Grosveld[11] showed in transgenic mice that these sequences could be used to direct high-level, copy number–dependent β-globin gene expression, in some instances near endogenous levels. Forrester[168] demonstrated that deletion of this region led to silencing of the transcription of the globin genes. Thus, it became clear that the β-globin LCR was essential to high-level globin gene expression. The LCR, now defined as an approximate 15-kb region approximately 50–60 kb upstream of the β-globin gene, encompasses four or five separate 200–400 core sequences that constitute the hypersensitive sites. These findings led investigators to incorporate these elements, or portions thereof, into the globin γ-retroviral vector design. Including these sequences led to genetic instability of the viral vector and poor vector production.[12] Ultimately, after much molecular optimization, vectors were derived that were capable of transmitting the genome containing the globin gene in an unrearranged fashion.[66,67] Both vector titers and expression levels still remained subtherapeutic in mouse transplant models.

The Development of Mouse Models of β Thalassemia and Sickle Cell Disease

Critical to the preclinical evaluation of globin vectors was the prior development of murine models of both β thalassemia and sickle cell disease. The first mouse model for β thalassemia was described in 1983 as a naturally occurring mutant mouse strain.[169] Mice have two β-globin genes – β-major and β-minor or β^s and β^t – depending on the strain, which reside in tandem on each chromosome 7. This strain had an approximate 3.3-kb deletion of the regulatory and coding sequences for the β-major globin gene. Mice homozygous for this deletion demonstrated a hypochromic, microcytic anemia with anisocytosis and poikilocytosis. Although these mice had moderate anemia, subsequent generation of additional mouse strains bearing different genetically engineered alterations led to a more severe β thalassemia phenotype. In 1995, two groups generated mice having a large deletion of both the murine β-major and β-minor globin genes on chromosome 7. Mice homozygous for this deletion did not survive due to the lack of adult hemoglobin production in late gestation. Heterozygous mice, however, demonstrated a severe anemia akin to that of classical β thalassemia intermedia.[170] All three of these models were subsequently used to test globin lentiviral vectors.[69,152,172,173]

The first attempts at developing a murine model of sickle cell disease led to the generation of mice with high levels of human α- and β^S-globin chains.[174,175] These mice and several others subsequently, although showing some sickle cell disease pathology, retained the mouse hemoglobins that inhibited full expression of the sickle phenotype.[176] Subsequently, Fabry and colleagues[177] developed the first mouse in which a deletion of mouse β-major was present, thereby increasing the levels of the human globins. Although this mouse showed enhanced pathological attributes, the presence of the murine α-chain, which partially inhibits polymerization of HbS,[178] did not allow the full phenotype to become manifest. In 1995, two groups generated mice with a deletion of the adult α-globin genes.[179,180] These mice, like the described β thalassemia strains, were critical to the eventual development of a sickle cell mouse lacking both murine α- and β-globin chains. Such a sickle transgenic/mouse globin gene knockout strain was subsequently described by two groups in 1997.[181,182] These strains were derived by microinjection of DNAs consisting of a β-globin LCR fragment linked to human γ-β globin fragment and also, in a separate fragment, to an α-globin DNA fragment. These mice expressed adequate amounts of human γ-globin during late gestational development to allow significant numbers of affected animals to survive. These mice have extensive pathology and a severe hemolytic anemia. One of the strains, termed the BERK strain, has a modest α- to β-globin chain imbalance, resulting in a phenotype more representative clinically of sickle–β thalassemia. In contrast, several lines in the second strain appear to have more balanced α- and β-globin chain production. All of the mice demonstrate vasoocclusion and thrombosis in several organs, glomerulosclerosis and renal dysfunction, cardiomegaly, and vascular ectasia representative of that in human in sickle cell disease. The BERK strain can be bred in numbers that are experimentally useful and has been used by a variety of investigators in the field.[182–187]

In 1998, another transgenic knockout strain was developed in which a yeast artificial chromosome was used to deliver a 240-kb β-globin locus containing the γ-globin and β^S-globin genes in their natural context.[188] The result was inadequate γ-globin expression during late gestation, leading to significant prenatal and perinatal death of affected animals. Although the few surviving mice had severe disease, the inability to obtain sufficient numbers of mice has limited the utility of this strain.

In 2001, Fabry et al.[189] reported the derivation of the NYC1-knockout model, which also lacked all mouse globins. These mice, having balanced chain synthesis, were developed to also express some human γ-globin to allow survival. In fact, three derivative strains expressing γ-globin at varying levels, resulted in dose-dependent amelioration of sickle cell pathology.[183,190] Thus far, no gene therapy studies have been reported in which this unique model was used.

β-Globin Lentiviral Vectors: Correction of Murine Models of β Thalassemia and Sickle Cell Disease

A major advance in the globin gene therapy field was the derivation of an HIV-based, globin lentiviral vector for correction of mouse β thalassemia (Fig. 33.5).[69,191] It is believed that the HIV rev responsive element contained within the vector backbone, in the context of the rev protein in the vector producer cells, suppressed potential vector genome splicing and rearrangement from occurring. This allowed significant production of unrearranged vector mRNA, which in turn allowed production of vector particles capable of faithful genome transmission. In these studies, long-term hematological and pathological correction of the severe β thalassemia mouse model was demonstrated.[191,69] β-globin transgene mRNA levels of 16% that the level of one copy of an endogenous allele were obtained, which resulted in chimeric hemoglobin molecules (murine α_2, human β_2) comprising approximately 21% of the total hemoglobin in red cells. This level was obtained in the context of virtually every transplanted HSC being genetically modified with the globin vector.

In a subsequent study by Humphries and colleagues,[173] using a β-globin vector containing 2.7 kb of LCR sequences, disease correction was also achieved, but this time improvement depended on a relatively high vector copy number of three in the transplanted HSCs. In fact, animals having only one vector copy per HSC had little or no improvement and expressed the human β-globin gene at low levels in only 30% of the erythroid progeny. In another later study, using the most severe model of murine β thalassemia, which relies on transplanting fetal liver HSCs lacking both endogenous β-globin alleles, Rivella et al.[192] remarkably achieved nearly complete correction of the phenotype in one animal; however, all other animals in the study remained severely anemic with Hb levels of 4.2–7.5 g/dL despite all HSCs likely having at least one vector copy. Together these studies highlighted the significant accomplishment of phenotypic correction of severe β-thalassemia using globin lentiviral vectors containing LCR elements. Importantly, one or more vector copies on average were needed in each HSC, suggesting inconsistent, variable expression from individual globin vector integration sites. This phenomenon, know as position effect variegation, was first demonstrated in mice in the setting of transgenic animals in which different lines containing transgenes at differing chromosomal sites displayed varying expression of the integrated transgene. Using a γ-globin vector, Persons et al.[152] demonstrated that globin vector site of integration heavily influences subsequent expression in erythroid progeny. The development of vectors containing elements designed to diminish this effect has subsequently been the focus of an intensive effort by several laboratories.

Subsequent to the initial finding that lentiviral vectors could mediate therapeutic gene therapy in murine β thalassemia, Leboulch and colleagues[183] used a lentiviral vector containing an antisickling human β-globin gene to ameliorate the disease phenotype in mouse models of sickle cell disease. The β-globin gene that was used contained a mutation at amino acid 87 that corresponds to the residue in γ-globin that is thought to mediate its antisickling activity. A 2.7-kb configuration of LCR sequences was used to drive expression of the variant β-globin gene. High levels of expression of the antisickling β-globin chain were achieved in the context of three vector copies per HSC, which led to

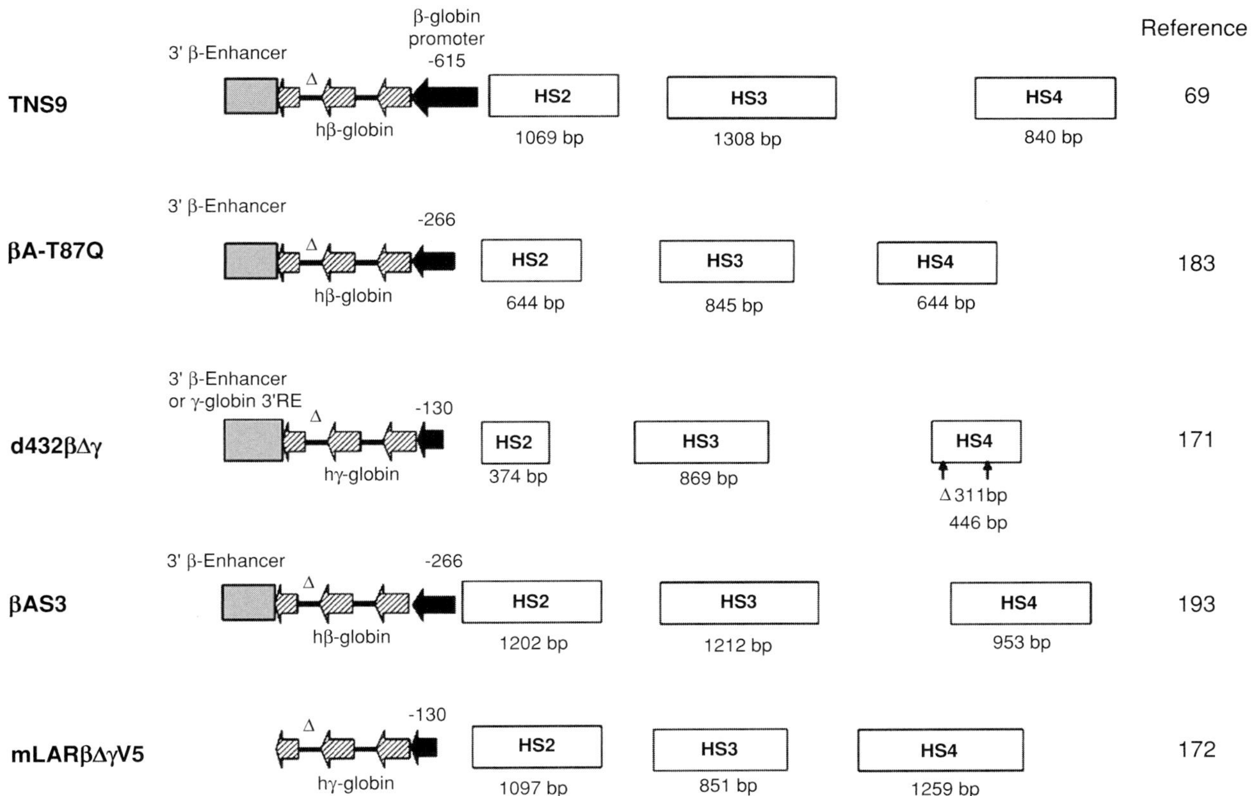

Figure 33.5. Schematic representation of various lentiviral globin vectors used to correct murine models of β thalassemia and sickle cell disease. DNA fragments containing the hypersensitive sites and flanking sequences are shown as open horizontal rectangles, the solid horizontal arrow indicates the β-globin promoter, and the hatched horizontal arrows indicate the genomic β- or γ-globin sequences contained in the mature mRNA. The solid lines connecting the three arrows represent intronic sequences; all of the vectors utilized a deletion in intron 2 to improve vector performance. The solid gray rectangle indicates the 3′ β-globin enhancer sequence or the 3′ γ-globin regulatory element (RE). The fragment sizes of the DNA elements derived from the β-globin LCR that contain the indicated hypersensitive sites (HS) and form the "enhancer" activity are shown below each horizontal rectangle, and the GenBank coordinates (accession number U01317) of the sequences are shown above each rectangle. Self-inactivating lentiviral vectors (SIN) include the d432βΔγ, β^{AS3}, and mLARβΔγV5 vectors. All vectors except TNS9 contain the DNA flap/central polypurine tract element from HIV-1, which can confer improved titer. (Reproduced with permission, from ref. 231.)

levels of the mutant β-globin chain in some mice equaling that of the endogenous β^s allele. Resolution of anemia and diminishment in end-organ damage was observed. Evaluation of vector expression in clonal populations of erythroid cells however demonstrated that there was significant variability of expression with copies number per cell ranging from two to five, again consistent with position effect variegation. Using a different model of sickle cell disease characterized by more severe anemia, Townes and colleagues[193] evaluated a vector encoding 3.4 kb of LCR sequences and an anti-sickling β-globin gene containing the above change at amino acid residue at position 87, and, additionally, two other mutations designed to enhance effectiveness (Fig. 33.5). With an average vector copy number of 2.2 in every HSC, they were able to achieve expression of the globin protein at approximately 20%–25% that of endogenous β^s allele, resulting in an improvement of the Hb level from 2.7 g/dL to 7.3 g/dL. Although still anemic, organ damage was ameliorated in treated mice.

γ-Globin Lentiviral Vectors

Because increased levels of HbF can significantly ameliorate β thalassemia as well as sickle cell disease, both γ-globin γ-retroviral vectors and γ-globin lentiviral vectors have been the focus of study by several groups of investigators. Bodine and colleagues[194] were able to use a γ-retroviral vector that, instead of LCR sequences, utilized ankyrin enhancer/promoter regulatory sequences to drive expression of human γ-globin. Message RNA levels of 3%–8% that of endogenous globin were obtained in wild type mice. Emery and colleagues[195] also obtained similar levels of γ-globin mRNA using a γ-retroviral vector utilizing an α-globin enhancer element coupled to a minimal β-globin promoter. No data are yet available regarding the performance of these vectors in the disease models. Using a lentiviral vector containing a 1.7-kb LCR configuration and a minimal β-globin promoter (Fig. 33.5), Persons et al.[171] were able to obtain significant disease correction in a severe model of β thalassemia intermedia. Animals with vector copy numbers of 2.4 in HSC displayed an average level of 21% HbF protein, which resulted in a 2.5 g/dL increase in the Hb level. This study also provided direct evidence of chromosomal position effects on vector expression by utilizing an analysis of clonal populations of transduced erythroid clones. Many vector integrations did not result in significant expression. Subsequently, this group showed that by including extended sequences surrounding the core enhancers of the LCR HS sites (Fig. 33.5), much more consistent expression could be obtained, and with it improved therapeutic efficacy.[172] In fact, the majority of animals could be essentially cured with one vector copy per HSC.

Recently, this same laboratory has shown that an optimized γ-globin lentiviral vector effectively cured the BERK model of murine SCD through HSC-targeted gene transfer and transplantation.[196] Mice receiving transplants of lineage depleted, steady-state sickle cell bone marrow cells transduced with the globin vector showed hematological correction, compared to animals receiving transplants of cells transduced with a control vector. Importantly, secondary organ damage was prevented by gene therapy, including renal, pulmonary, hepatic and splenic disease. Renal function was found to preserved as determined by the ability to concentrate urine following exposure to limited access to water. These results reinforce the concept that permanent high level expression of HbF is therapeutic for SCD.

Correction of Human β Thalassemia Erythroid Cells

Globin lentiviral vectors have also recently been evaluated in cells from patients with β-thalassemia major. Malik and colleagues[145] demonstrated that the β thalassemia phenotype could be corrected in cultures of erythroid cells derived from patients' $CD34^+$ cells after transduction with a β-globin vector concentrated 10,000-fold. On average, this correction required 2.2 vector copies per cell. This study utilized a β-globin vector containing 3.1 kb of LCR sequences and a 250-bp β-globin promoter. A unique feature of this vector was that it also included a 1.2-kb element from the chicken β-globin LCR HS4 region. This element had previously been described as a genetic insulator element which acts to block interactions between neighboring chromosomal DNA regions.[95,197] Subsequent work by this group confirmed the function of this insulator in diminishing the negative effect on expression of position effect variegation.[198]

The Conundrum of Position Effects Dampening Globin Vector Expression

A major finding from all these studies is that significant phenotypic correction required multiple vector genomes in virtually all of the primitive cells from which the erythroid cells were derived. This fact, and direct experimental data, highlight that consistent expression of globin vectors is problematic and could impact negatively on the potential for clinical success. Although improved expression, as described previously, can be obtained with insulators, this change in vector design caused a significant diminishment in titer of the globin vector as well as other vectors. Encouragingly, recent efforts indicate that a small portion of the 1.2-kb insulator used above may have nearly equivalent functional activity and may not cause as significant a diminishment in vector titer.[199] Further testing of a globin vector with the smaller insulator element in animal models is needed to verify this potential solution.

PROGRESS AND PROBLEMS IN HUMAN STEM CELL GENE THERAPY

Successful Treatment of Patients with Immunodeficiencies

Immunodeficiency disorders were among the first diseases to be identified as candidates for gene therapy because of the low numbers of corrected cells estimated to be necessary and because appropriate expression of the transgene was relatively easy to achieve.[200] Several trials were performed throughout the 1990s in patients with ADA deficiency; however, these pioneering studies did not yield convincing evidence of efficacy.[201,202] In these studies, low levels of marking were observed and clinically significant immune reconstitution was not seen. It was recognized that at least part of the problem was that concomitant enzyme replacement therapy blunted the selective advantage for corrected cells.[203] Another problem was that the engraftment level of transduced HSCs was very low in the absence of myeloablative conditioning. There appeared to be no significant toxicity due to the gene therapy vectors or the transduction procedure.

A groundbreaking study in France that was reported in 2000 showed the first convincing proof that gene therapy could be used successfully to treat patients with SCID.[204,124] This study focused on X-linked SCID, which is caused by mutations in the common γ_c gene that is necessary for multiple cytokine signaling receptors required for normal development of T, B, and natural killer lymphocytes. Studies of rare patients that showed spontaneous recovery of immune function revealed that reversion of mutations that presumably occurred in single stem cells was sufficient for phenotypic correction, illustrating the strong selective advantage for low numbers of corrected cells.[123] This natural selection for corrected cells bypasses the requirement for transducing larger proportions of repopulating cells and can be demonstrated directly in animal models.[205]

In the French study, CD34+ bone marrow cells were collected from patients, usually within the first year of life, and were transduced with a simple MLV vector that expressed the γ_c cDNA under control of the viral promoter in the LTR. Transduced cells were then infused back into the patients without any myeloablative conditioning. In the majority of cases, there was significant recovery of T- and B-cell function and clear clinical improvement with resistance to opportunistic infections. Immune reconstitution was stable in patients with more than 5 years of follow-up.[124] A parallel trial was performed in the United Kingdom that showed similar results with unequivocal immune reconstitution in most patients.[206] Another important advance was the successful treatment of infants with ADA-deficient SCID by gene therapy. In a trial done in Italy, bone marrow CD34+ cells were transduced with a MLV vector expressing an ADA cDNA, but unlike earlier trials, patients were preconditioned with a subablative dose of busulfan to increase engraftment of transduced HSCs. Patients were then followed without enzyme replacement therapy and in all cases were shown to have increased T- and B-cell function as well as partial reconstitution of ADA enzyme levels in blood cells.[207] These patients have remained stably corrected for up to 4 years.[208]

The Unexpected Occurrence of Insertional Mutagenesis in Immunodeficiency Gene Therapy Trials

The stunning success of stem cell–targeted gene therapy for treating SCID disorders has provided strong proof of principle that this approach may be extrapolated to other genetic blood disorders. These pioneering clinical studies have also revealed an important and unanticipated toxicity, the occurrence of insertional mutagenesis leading to leukemia. In 2002, two of the patients in the French X-SCID trial developed a progressive accumulation of phenotypically mature, monoclonal T cells in the peripheral blood.[209] This disorder behaved like an acute T-cell leukemia and was successfully treated using standard cytotoxic chemotherapy. With time, two more patients in the French trial have developed T-cell leukemia and it has recently been reported that a fifth patient in the UK trial has developed leukemia. Although all the molecular data have not been published, it is clear that most cases involve activation of the LMO2 oncogene due to local vector insertion sites.[209,210,215] In the first two patients, the vector was inserted either in a sense orientation immediately upstream of the first exon or in an antisense orientation within the first intron. LMO2 has been identified as a oncogene in translocations seen in T-cell leukemia and functions as part of a transcription factor complex.[211] Constitutive activation of Lmo2 in transgenic mice results in a differentiation block in the thymus, followed by a delayed development of leukemia.[212] It seemed likely that at least some of these cases of oncogene activation are the direct result of interactions of the strong enhancer within the γ-retroviral LTR with the LMO2 promoters. This has now been directly demonstrated by inserting the MLV LTR in a reverse orientation into the first intron of LMO2 in a human T cell line, in the same site noted in one of the patients who developed leukemia.[18] This study directly demonstrated the ability of the enhancer within the LTR to activate cellular LMO2 promoters. Interestingly, no transformation has yet been seen in the small number of ADA patients who have been successfully treated with γ-retroviral vectors, although some of these patients have been shown to harbor vector insertions within the LMO2 gene of circulating blood cells.[208]

There are several reasons why the field did not expect this complication. First, it was widely assumed that integration of γ-retroviral vectors would occur randomly throughout the genome and that the probability of insertions within an oncogene was too low to be significant. Subsequent studies have shown that γ-retroviral vectors preferentially integrate at the transcription start site of actively transcribed genes.[213] Furthermore, in human CD34+ cells, 21% of all γ-retroviral integrations occur in recurrent insertion sites that are enriched for protooncogenes.[214] In contrast, lentiviral vectors have a distinct pattern of integration that is less likely to localize to a potentially dangerous region of the genome,[215] a characteristic that may reduce the risk associated with lentiviral globin vectors.

T-cell leukemias were not seen in studies of gene therapy in X-SCID mouse models probably because of the relatively low frequency of transformation and the small numbers of mice used in these studies.[217] A recent mouse model has been described that is highly sensitive to vector-induced transformation and recapitulates many of the aspects of this leukemic syndrome.[218] Mice that have homozygous ablation of the γ_c gene and homozygous deletion of the Arf tumor suppressor gene have been used as bone marrow cell donors. Deletion of the Arf tumor suppressor gene was based on the fact that it is universally mutated in human T-cell leukemia.[219] When these cells are transduced with γ-retroviral vectors expressing the γ_c gene and transplanted into recipients, approximately 85% of the animals develop T-cell lymphomas/leukemia after 1 year. In most cases, these leukemias were associated with retroviral integrations into known murine oncogenes, although interestingly, Lmo2 integrations were not detected.

One important finding using this model was that the X-SCID background itself is a significant risk factor for transformation. When cells were used from $\gamma_c^{+/+}$, $Arf^{-/-}$ mice, the incidence of leukemia was significantly lower than that seen using $\gamma_c^{-/-}$, $Arf^{-/-}$ cells. This observation suggests that X-SCID gene therapy may carry a uniquely elevated risk of transformation and that gene therapy for other disorders, such as hemoglobinopathies, may carry less risk. This conclusion is consistent with a review of large animals that have been transplanted with MLV-derived vectors.[220] This study examined the consequences of transduction with MLV vectors in 42 rhesus macaques, 23 baboons, and 17 dogs with significant levels of gene transfer. These animals were transplanted in various centers and followed for a median of 3.5 years. In this report, no cases of abnormal hematopoiesis or leukemia were noted. Two years following this report, one case of a vector-induced tumor was observed in a rhesus macaque that had undergone transplantation.[221] In contrast to the T-cell leukemias that have been noted in X-SCID patients and animal models, this case presented as a myeloid tumor with an insertion into BCL2-A1, an antiapoptotic gene.

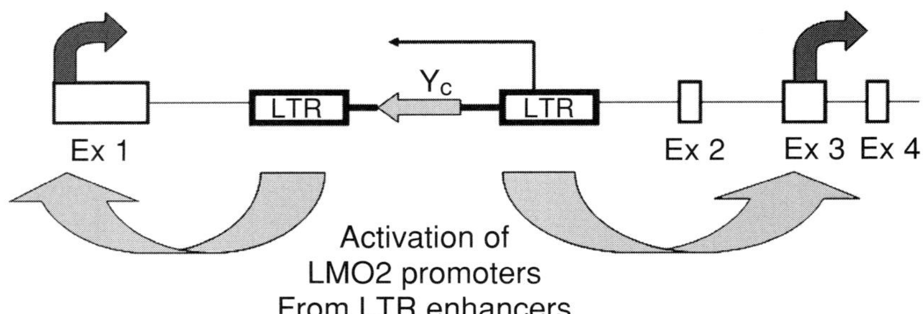

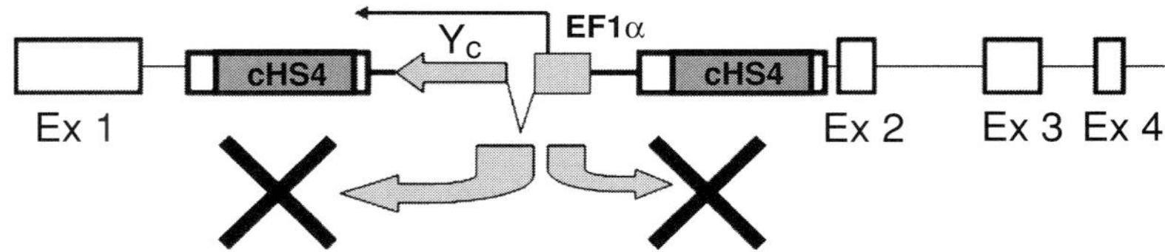

Figure 33.6. Safety design considerations for lentiviral vectors. **(A)** The upper diagram shows the safety problems associated with using γ-retroviral vectors with intact LTRs in the French X-SCID trial.[209] In this case, the vector has integrated into the first intron of the LMO2 gene in a reverse orientation. The strong viral enhancers present in the LTRs activate both cellular LMO2 promoters as shown by the blue and red arrows. This results in oncogene expression in cells that normally would not express LMO2.[18] **(B)** This is a safety modified lentiviral vector that has inactivating mutations in the viral LTRs creating a so-called self-inactivating or SIN design. A copy of the cHS4 chromatin insulator is present in each LTR so that any internal enhancer activity will be blocked from interacting with adjacent cellular promoters (large X). The γ_c transgene is expressed from a single cellular promoter, in the case from the EF1α gene. This promoter itself has much little enhancer activity on its own. This design has been shown to result in no significant LMO2 activation when inserted into the LMO2 locus in a human T cell line.[18] (See color plate 33.6.)

The genetics of insertional transformation for X-SCID versus myeloid disorders are likely to be specific and fundamentally different. In a German gene therapy trial for chronic granulomatous disease, two patients exhibited clonal expansion based on insertions into the MDS1/EVI, PRDM16, and SETBP1 genes.[222] In particular, the MDS1/EVI locus has been identified as a hot spot for MLV insertions in mice[223] and in transplanted rhesus monkeys.[224] Perhaps this is not surprising given that this locus was initially identified as a MLV insertion site. Therefore, just as in the case of other human leukemias, the genetics for lymphoid and myeloid leukemia due to insertional mutagenesis appear to be distinct, with a favoring for LMO2 in lymphoid tumors from X-SCID patients and for MDS/EVI1 in myeloid disorders.

Moving Forward: Can Insertional Mutagenesis be Avoided?

Much work in the field is now focused on generating safer vector systems that are less prone to causing insertional mutagenesis. It is clear from the clinical cases that have been studied to date that the most common mechanism for inducing transformation is activation of oncogene promoters by the strong viral enhancer in the MLV LTRs. This can be avoided by deleting these sequences from the retroviral vector to create SIN vectors. This design requires the use of an appropriate internal promoter to drive expression of the therapeutic transgene (Fig. 33.6). In the case of globin vectors, this is typically the β-globin promoter; however, other erythroid promoters may be useful.[194] A second approach that can be used together with SIN vectors is the use of chromatin insulators to block potential interactions of vector-encoded enhancers with adjacent cellular promoters. A widely used insulator, cHS4, is derived from the chicken β-globin locus and has been shown to be useful both for blocking vector-induced alterations in adjacent cellular genes and in improving expression of the vector-encoded globin gene by shielding the transgene from chromatin effects leading to position site variegation.[195] A 1.2-kb version of cHS4 has been shown to reduce substantially LMO2 activation due to insertion of a MLV-based LTR into the first intron,[18] suggesting that this strategy may also be useful in designing newer vectors for X-SCID. Another question is whether lentiviral vectors may be less prone to inducing insertional mutagenesis due to their intrinsically different pattern of insertion site preferences.[214,225] In this regard, it is notable that no evidence of lentiviral insertions have been reported into either the LMO2 or the MDS1/Evi locus to date. Further evidence for increased safety with lentiviral vectors has recently been generated in a tumor-prone mouse model.[226]

Much effort has been dedicated to developing appropriate assays for insertional mutagenesis to test whether modified vectors are in fact safer than their original MLV counterparts. Previously existing assays that have been used to identify oncogenes commonly utilize replication competent MLV as the mutagen.[227] This system results in continuous virus production in vivo and relatively high viral copy numbers in transduced cells. In contrast, much lower copy numbers are obtained using replication-incompetent vectors so that a challenge has been to develop systems of adequate sensitivity. One approach has been to use tumor-prone mice to assay for an increase in the basal transformation rate. This approach has been successful using mice deleted for Ink4a[226] and Arf [218] and investigators are currently developing appropriately sensitive models for erythroid transformation.

Recent work in our laboratory has directly addressed the issue of the potential genotoxicity of lentiviral vectors containing globin regulatory elements.[228] The question was addressed in primary, clonal murine β thalassemic erythroid cells present in spleen colonies derived from primitive, transduced hematopoietic progenitors. Eleven percent of all genes analyzed within a 600-kb region surrounding vector-insertion sites demonstrated altered expression; however, there was no indication that perturbation of expression interfered with hematopoiesis or was associated with clonal dominance. These results are in keeping with other studies in which it was shown that globin regulatory elements enhanced promoter activation and expression of a trapping cassette in an erythroleukemia cell line but not in nonerythroid (HeLa) cells.[229] Promoter activation in erythroleukemia cells by vectors containing globin regulatory elements was significantly reduced by addition of flanking insulator elements. Studies have also been performed in a mutant mouse strain (Spi1) that suggest that a lentiviral vector with globin regulatory elements and an insulator in the LTRs does not enhance the rate or frequency of leukemia in vivo in this mouse model. Overall, the data suggest that globin vectors will be relatively safe, although additional safety studies are planned.

Recently published work from Jaenisch and Townes demonstrated the ability to generate embryonic stem cell-like cells, termed induced pluripotent stem cells (iPS) from primary fibroblasts derived from SCD mice.[230] These iPS cells could be successfully targeted by homologous recombination to correct the sickle mutation. Subsequent derivation and transplantation of HSCs from these corrected iPS was shown to correct the SCD mouse model. This study highlights the potential for correcting the mutation while minimizing or significantly reducing the issue of vector insertional mutagenesis. However, this technique did rely on the use of a HOXB4 retroviral vector to facilitate production of HSCs from the genetically corrected iPS clone. Future research will determine whether factors can be identified that can substitute for the use of HOXB4 gene transfer to generate HSCs. Additional studies are also needed to determine the quality of HSCs so generated.

FUTURE PROSPECTS

Success in the treatment of immunodeficiencies by gene transfer provides encouragement that the hemoglobin disorders will also ultimately be amenable to gene therapy intervention. If this can be achieved, it would significantly increase the number of patients who would be eligible for a curative, transplantation-based treatment. Indeed, a phase I/II clinical trial has begun to enroll patients with thalassemia or sickle cell disease in France and undoubtedly this trial will yield important information as to whether the current methodologies for vector production and stem cell transduction are amenable to a positive therapeutic outcome. Our own perspective is that a transition to the use of stable producer clones with the ability to generate large volumes of conditioned media for downstream processing and purification of vector particles, advances which seem within our grasp, will make success in a clinical trial more probable. The need to transduce approximately 20% of the stem cells remains a challenge. Amplification of a minority population of gene corrected red cells is likely to enhance efficacy in thalassemia but perhaps less so in patients with sickle cell disease. Since the introduction of lentiviral vectors for globin gene transfer approximately a decade ago, progress has been steady in that hematological correction in the murine models of thalassemia and sickle cell anemia has been achieved as has the correction of the ineffective erythropoiesis in human thalassemic red cells in vitro. These advances and growing knowledge of stem cell biology and the interactions of vectors with cells make us confident that success in the use of gene therapy for the treatment of hemoglobin disorders will come in the future.

REFERENCES

1. Dick JE, Magli MC, Huszar D, Phillips RA, Bernstein A. Introduction of a selectable gene into primitive stem cells capable of long-term reconstitution of the hemopoietic system of W/Wv mice. *Cell.* 1985;42:71–79.
2. Eglitis MA, Kantoff P, Gilboa E, Anderson WF. Gene expression in mice after high efficiency retroviral-mediated gene transfer. *Science.* 1985;230:1395–1398.
3. Marechal V, Naffakh N, Danos O, Heard JM. Disappearance of lysosomal storage in spleen and liver of mucopolysaccharidosis VII mice after transplantation of genetically modified bone marrow cells. *Blood.* 1993;82:1358–1365.

4. Mardiney M III, Jackson SH, Spratt SK, Li F, Holland SM, Malech HL. Enhanced host defense after gene transfer in the murine p47phox-deficient model of chronic granulomatous disease. *Blood.* 1997;89:2268–2275.
5. Bunting KD, Sangster MY, Ihle JN, Sorrentino BP. Restoration of lymphocyte function in Janus kinase 3-deficient mice by retroviral-mediated gene transfer. *Nat Med.* 1998;4:58–64.
6. Orkin SH, Motulsky AG. Report and recommendations of the panel to assess the NIH investment in research on gene therapy. 1995.
7. Nienhuis AW. Development of gene therapy for blood disorders. *Blood.* 2008;111:4431–4444.
8. Karlsson S, Bodine DM, Perry L, Papayannopoulou T, Nienhuis AW. Expression of the human beta-globin gene following retroviral-mediated transfer into multipotential hematopoietic progenitors of mice. *Proc Natl Acad Sci USA.* 1988;85:6062–6066.
9. Dzierzak EA, Papayannopoulou T, Mulligan RC. Lineage-specific expression of a human beta-globin gene in murine bone marrow transplant recipients reconstituted with retrovirus-transduced stem cells. *Nature.* 1988;331:35–41.
10. Tuan D, Solomon W, Li Q, London IM. The "beta-like-globin" gene domain in human erythroid cells. *Proc Natl Acad Sci USA.* 1985;82:6384–6388.
11. Grosveld F, van Assendelft GB, Greaves DR, Kollias G. Position-independent, high-level expression of the human beta-globin gene in transgenic mice. *Cell.* 1987;51:975–985.
12. Novak U, Harris EA, Forrester W, Groudine M, Gelinas R. High-level beta-globin expression after retroviral transfer of locus activation region-containing human beta-globin gene derivatives into murine erythroleukemia cells. *Proc Natl Acad Sci USA.* 1990;87:3386–3390.
13. Baum C, Schambach A, Bohne J, Galla M. Retrovirus vectors: toward the plentivirus? *Mol Ther.* 2006;13:1050–1063.
14. Hargrove PW, Vanin EF, Kurtzman GJ, Nienhuis AW. High-level globin gene expression mediated by a recombinant adeno-associated virus genome that contains the 3′ γ-globin gene regulatory element and integrates as tandem copies in erythroid cells. *Blood.* 1997;89:2167–2175.
15. Miller JL, Donahue RE, Sellers SE, Samulski RJ, Young NS, Nienhuis AW. Recombinant adeno-associated virus (rAAV)-mediated expression of a human γ-globin gene in human progenitor-derived erythroid cells. *Proc Natl Acad Sci USA.* 1995;91:10183–10187.
16. Nathwani AC, Hanawa H, Vandergriff J, et al. Efficient gene transfer into human cord blood CD34+ cells and the CD34+CD38– subset using highly purified recombinant adeno-associated viral vector preparations that are free of helper virus and wild-type AAV. *Gene Ther.* 2000;7:183–195.
17. Zhong L, Zhao W, Wu J, et al. Adeno-associated virus-mediated gene transfer in hematopoietic stem/progenitor cells as a therapeutic tool. *Curr Gene Ther.* 2006;6:683–698.
18. Ryu BY, Evans-Galea MV, Gray JT, et al. An experimental system for the evaluation of retroviral vector design to diminish the risk for proto-oncogene activation. *Blood.* 2008;111:1866–1875.
19. Wu Z, Asokan A, Samulski RJ. Adeno-associated virus serotypes:vector toolkit for human gene therapy. *Mol Ther.* 2006;14:316–327.
20. Douglas JT. Adenoviral vectors for gene therapy. *Mol Biotechnol.* 2007;36:71–80.
21. Wang Y. HSV-1 amplicon vectors are an efficient gene transfer system for skeletal muscle cells. *Curr Gene Ther.* 2006;6:371–381.
22. Berges BK, Wolfe JH, Fraser NW. Transduction of brain by herpes simplex virus vectors. *Mol Ther.* 2007;15:20–29.
23. Kimchi-Sarfaty C, Gottesman MM. SV40 pseudovirions as highly efficient vectors for gene transfer and their potential application in cancer therapy. *Curr Pharm Biotechnol.* 2004;5:451–458.
24. Sova P, Wang H, Bomsztyk K, Stamatoyannopoulos G, Lieber A. Role of chromatin structure in integration of helper-dependent adenoviral vectors containing the beta-globin locus control region. *Hum Gene Ther.* 2008;19:153–166.
25. Baltimore D. RNA-dependent DNA polymerase in virions of RNA tumour viruses. *Nature.* 1970;226:1209–1211.
26. Temin HM, Mizutani S. RNA-dependent DNA polymerase in virions of Rous sarcoma virus. *Nature.* 1970;226:1211–1213.
27. Varmus H. Retroviruses. *Science.* 1988;240:1427–1435.
28. Mann R, Mulligan RC, Baltimore D. Construction of a retrovirus packaging mutant and its use to produce helper-free defective retrovirus. *Cell.* 1983;33:153–159.
29. Watanabe S, Temin HM. Construction of a helper cell line for avian reticuloendotheliosis virus cloning vectors. *Mol Cell Biol.* 1983;3:2241–2249.
30. Cone RD, Mulligan RC. High-efficiency gene transfer into mammalian cells: generation of helper-free recombinant retrovirus with broad mammalian host range. *Proc Natl Acad Sci USA.* 1984;81:6349–6635.
31. Markowitz D, Goff S, Bank A. A safe packaging line for gene transfer: Separating viral genes on two different plasmids. *J Virol.* 1988;62:1120–1124.
32. Markowitz D, Goff S, Bank A. Construction and use of a safe and efficient amphotropic packaging cell line. *Virology.* 1988;167:400–406.
33. Bender MA, Palmer TD, Gelinas RE, Miller AD. Evidence that the packaging signal of Moloney murine leukemia virus extends into the gag region. *J Virol.* 1987;61:1639–1646.
34. Miller AD, Rosman GJ. Improved retroviral vectors for gene transfer and expression. *Biotechniques.* 1989;7:980–990.
35. Ory DS, Neugeboren BA, Mulligan RC. A stable human-derived packaging cell line for production of high titer retrovirus/vesicular stomatitis virus G pseudotypes. *Proc Natl Acad Sci USA.* 1996;93:11400–11406.
36. Davis BM, Reese JS, Koc ON, et al. Selection for G156A O6-methylguanine DNA methyltransferase gene-transduced hematopoietic progenitors and protection from lethality in mice treated with O6-benzylguanine and 1,3-Bis(2-chloroethyl)-1-nitrosourea. *Cancer Res.* 1997;57:5093–5099.
37. Kim JW, Closs EI, Albritton LM, Cunningham JM. Transport of cationic amino acids by the mouse ecotropic retrovirus receptor. *Nature.* 1991;352:725–728.
38. Wang H, Kavanaugh MP, North RA, Kabat D. Cell-surface receptor for ecotropic murine retroviruses is a basic amino-acid transporter. *Nature.* 1991;352:729–731.
39. Kavanaugh MP, Miller DG, Zhang W, et al. Cell-surface receptors for gibbon ape leukemia virus and amphotropic murine retrovirus are inducible sodium-dependent phosphate symporters. *Proc Natl Acad Sci USA.* 1994;91:7071–7075.
40. Miller DG, Edwards RH, Miller AD. Cloning of the cellular receptor for amphotropic murine retroviruses reveals

homology to that for gibbon ape leukemia virus. *Proc Natl Acad Sci USA.* 1994;91:78–82.

41. Miller AD, Garcia JV, von Subh N, et al. Construction and properties of retrovirus packaging cells based on gibbon ape leukemia virus. *J Virol.* 1991;65:2220–2224.
42. Kelly PF, Vandergriff J, Nathwani A, Nienhuis AW, Vanin EF. Highly efficient gene transfer into cord blood nonobese diabetic/severe combined immunodeficiency repopulating cells by oncoretroviral vector particles pseudotyped with the feline endogenous retrovirus (RD114) envelope protein. *Blood.* 2000;96:1206–1214.
43. Lucas ML, Seidel NE, Porada CD, et al. Improved transduction of human sheep repopulating cells by retrovirus vectors pseudotyped with feline leukemia virus type C or RD114 envelopes. *Blood.* 2005;106:51–58.
44. Sandrin V, Russell SJ, Cosset FL. Targeting retroviral and lentiviral vectors. *Curr Top Microbiol Immunol.* 2003;281: 137–178.
45. Anderson JL, Hope TJ. Intracellular trafficking of retroviral vectors: obstacles and advances. *Gene Ther.* 2005;12:1667–1678.
46. Naghavi MH, Goff SP. Retroviral proteins that interact with the host cell cytoskeleton. *Curr Opin Immunol.* 2007;19:402–407.
47. Miller DG, Adam MA, Miller AD. Gene transfer by retrovirus vectors occurs only in cells that are actively replicating at the time of infection [published erratum appears in *Mol Cell Biol.* 1992;12:433]. *Mol Cell Biol.* 1990;10:4239–4242.
48. Lewis PF, Emerman M. Passage through mitosis is required for oncoretroviruses but not for the human immunodeficiency virus. *J Virol.* 1994;68:510–516.
49. Goff SP. Retrovirus restriction factors. *Mol Cell.* 2004;16:849–859.
50. Bieniasz PD. Intrinsic immunity: a front-line defense against viral attack. *Nat Immunol.* 2004;5:1109–1115.
51. Harris RS, Liddament MT. Retroviral restriction by APOBEC proteins. *Nat Rev Immunol.* 2004;4:868–877.
52. Challita PM, Kohn DB. Lack of expression from a retroviral vector after transduction of murine hematopoietic stem cells is associated with methylation in vivo. *Proc Natl Acad Sci USA.* 1994;91:2567–2571.
53. Chen WY, Bailey EC, McCune SL, et al. Reactivation of silenced, virally transduced genes by inhibitors of histone deacetylase. *Proc Natl Acad Sci USA.* 1997;94:5798–5803.
54. Cheng L, Du C, Lavau C, et al. Sustained gene expression in retrovirally transduced, engrafting human hematopoietic stem cells and their lympho-myeloid progeny. *Blood.* 1998;92:83–92.
55. Halene S, Wang L, Cooper RM, et al. Improved expression in hematopoietic and lymphoid cells in mice after transplantation of bone marrow transduced with a modified retroviral vector. *Blood.* 1999;94:3349–3357.
56. Ramezani A, Hawley TS, Hawley RG. Stable gamma retroviral vector expression during embryonic stem cell-derived in vitro hematopoietic development. *Mol Ther.* 2006;14:245–254.
57. Schambach A, Mueller D, Galla M, et al. Overcoming promoter competition in packaging cells improves production of self-inactivating retroviral vectors. *Gene Ther.* 2006;13:1524–1533.
58. Thornhill SI, Schambach A, Howe SJ, et al. Self-inactivating gammaretroviral vectors for gene therapy of X-linked severe combined immunodeficiency. *Mol Ther.* 2008;16:590–598.
59. Emerman M, Temin HM. Genes with promoters in retrovirus vectors can be independently suppressed by an epigenetic mechanism. *Cell.* 1984;39:459–467.
60. Morgan RA, Couture L, Elroy-Stein O, et al. Retroviral vectors containing putative internal ribosome entry sites: development of a polycistronic gene transfer system and applications to human gene therapy. *Nucl Acids Res.* 1992;20:1293–1299.
61. Persons DA, Allay JA, Allay ER, et al. Retroviral-mediated transfer of the green fluorescent protein gene into murine hematopoietic cells facilitates scoring and selection of transduced progenitors in vitro and identification of genetically modified cells in vivo. *Blood.* 1997;90:1777–1786.
62. Persons DA, Allay JA, Riberdy JM, et al. Utilization of the green flourescent protein gene as a marker to identify and track genetically-modified hematopoietic cells. *Nat Med.* 1998;4:1201–1205.
63. Szymczak AL, Workman CJ, Wang Y, et al. Correction of multi-gene deficiency in vivo using a single 'self-cleaving' 2A peptide-based retroviral vector. *Nat Biotechnol.* 2004;22:589–594.
64. Hantzopoulos PA, Sullenger BA, Ungers G, Gilboa E. Improved gene expression upon transfer of the adenosine deaminase minigene outside the transcriptional unit of a retroviral vector. *Proc Natl Acad Sci USA.* 1989;86:3519–3523.
65. Plavec I, Papayannopoulou T, Maury C, Meyer F. A human beta-globin gene fused to the human beta-globin locus control region is expressed at high levels in erythroid cells of mice engrafted with retrovirus-transduced hematopoietic stem cells. *Blood.* 1993;81:1384–1392.
66. Leboulch P, Huang GM, Humphries RK, et al. Mutagenesis of retroviral vectors transducing human beta-globin gene and beta-globin locus control region derivatives results in stable transmission of an active transcriptional structure. *EMBO J.* 1994;13:3065–3076.
67. Sadelain M, Wang CH, Antoniou M, et al. Generation of a high-titer retroviral vector capable of expressing high levels of the human beta-globin gene. *Proc Natl Acad Sci USA.* 1995;92:6728–6732.
68. Ren S, Wong BY, Li J, et al. Production of genetically stable high-titer retroviral vectors that carry a human γ-globin gene under the control of the alpha-globin locus control region. *Blood.* 1996;87:2518–2524.
69. May C, Rivella S, Callegari J, et al. Therapeutic haemoglobin synthesis in beta-thalassaemic mice expressing lentivirus-encoded human beta-globin. *Nature.* 2000;406:82–86.
70. Bukrinsky MI, Haggerty S, Dempsey MP, et al. A nuclear localization signal within HIV-1 matrix protein that governs infection of non-dividing cells. *Nature.* 1993;365:666–669.
71. Heinzinger NK, Bukinsky MI, Haggerty SA, et al. The Vpr protein of human immunodeficiency virus type 1 influences nuclear localization of viral nucleic acids in nondividing host cells. *Proc Natl Acad Sci USA.* 1994;91:7311–7315.
72. Zennou V, Petit C, Guetard D, et al. HIV-1 genome nuclear import is mediated by a central DNA flap. *Cell.* 2000;101:173–185.
73. Sirven A, Pflumino F, Zennou V, et al. The human immunodeficiency virus type-1 central DNA flap is a crucial determinant for lentiviral vector nuclear import and gene

transduction of human hematopoietic stem cells. *Blood.* 2000;96:4103–4110.

74. Yamashita M, Emerman M. Retroviral infection of non-dividing cells: old and new perspectives. *Virology.* 2006; 334:88–93.
75. Caron MC, Caruso M. A nuclear localization signal in the matrix of spleen necrosis virus (SNV) does not allow efficient gene transfer into quiescent cells with SNV-derived vectors. *Virology.* 2005;338:292–296.
76. Yamashita M, Emerman M. The cell cycle independence of HIV infections is not determined by known karyophilic viral elements. *PLoS. Pathog.* 2005;1:e18.
77. Yamashita M, Emerman M. Capsid is a dominant determinant of retrovirus infectivity in nondividing cells. *J Virol.* 2004;78:5670–5678.
78. Yamashita M, Perez O, Hope TJ, Emerman M. Evidence for direct involvement of capsid protein in Hiv infection of non-dividing cells. *PLoS Pathog.* 2007;3:1502–1510.
79. Parolin C, Taddeo B, Palu G, Sodroski J. Use of cis- and trans-acting viral regulatory sequences to improve expression of human immunodeficiency virus vectors in human lymphocytes. *Virology.* 1996;222:415–422.
80. Akkina RK, Walton RM, Chen ML, et al. High-efficiency gene transfer into CD34+ cells with a human immunodeficiency virus type 1-based retroviral vector pseudotyped with vesicular stomatitis virus envelope glycoprotein G. *J Virol.* 1996;70:2581–2585.
81. Naldini L, Blomer U, Gally P, et al. In vivo gene delivery and stable transduction of nondividing cells by a lentiviral vector. *Science.* 1996;272:263–267.
82. Hanawa H, Kelly PF, Nathwani AC, et al: Comparison of various envelope proteins for their ability to pseudotype lentiviral vectors and transduce primitive hematopoietic cells from human blood. *Mol.Ther.* 2002;5:242–251.
83. Charneau P, Marambeau G, Roux P, et al. Hiv-1 reverse transcription. A termination step at the center of the genome. *J Mol Biol.* 1994;241:651–662.
84. Zufferey R, Nagy D, Mandel RJ, et al. Multiply attenuated lentiviral vector achieves efficient gene delivery in vivo. *Nat. Biotechnol.* 1997;15:871–875.
85. Fuller M, Anson DS. Helper plasmids for production of HIV-1-derived vectors. *Hum Gene Ther.* 2001;12:2081–2093.
86. Westerman KA, Ao Z, Cohen EA, Leboulch P. Design of a trans protease lentiviral packaging system that produces high titer virus. *Retrovirology.* 2007;4:96–110.
87. Cockrell AS, Kafri T. Gene delivery by lentivirus vectors. *Mol Biotechnol.* 2007;36:184–204.
88. Kafri T, van Praag H, Ouyang L et al. A packaging cell line for lentivirus vectors. *J Virol.* 1999;73:576–584.
89. Kim VN, Mitrophanous K, Kingsman SM, Kingsman AJ. Minimal requirement for a lentivirus vector based on human immunodeficiency virus type 1. *J Virol.* 1998;72:811–816.
90. Ikeda Y, Takeuchi Y, Martin F, et al. Continuous high-titer HIV-1 vector production. *Nat Biotechnol.* 2003;21:569–572.
91. Strang BL, Ikeda Y, Cosset FL, Collins MK, Takeuchi U. Characterization of HIV-1 vectors with gammaretrovirus envelope glycoproteins produced from stable packaging cells. *Gene Ther.* 2004;11:591–598.
92. Hwang LH, Gilboa E. Expression of genes introduced into cells by retroviral infection is more efficient than that of genes introduced into cells by DNA transfection. *J Virol.* 1984;50:417–424.
93. Broussau S, Jabbour N, Lachapelle G, et al. Inducible packaging cells for large-scale production of lentiviral vectors in serum-free suspension culture. *Mol Ther.* 2008;16:500–507.
94. Schambach A, Galla M, Maetzig T, Loew R, Baum C. Improving transcriptional termination of self-inactivating gamma-retroviral and lentiviral vectors. *Mol Ther.* 2007;15:1167–1173.
95. Gaszner M, Felsenfeld G. Insulators: exploiting transcriptional and epigenetic mechanisms. *Nat Rev Genet.* 2006;7: 703–713.
96. Ramezani A, Hawley TS, Hawley RG. Performance-and safety-enhanced lentiviral vectors containing the human interferon-beta scaffold attachment region and the chicken beta-globin insulator. *Blood.* 2003;101:4717–4724.
97. Evans-Galea, MV, Wielgosz, MM, Hanawa, H, et al. Suppression of clonal dominance in cultured human lymphoid cells by addition of the cHS4 insulator to a lentiviral vector. *Mol Ther.* 2007;15:801–809.
98. Charrier S, Dupre L, Scaramuzza S, et al. Lentiviral vectors targeting WASp expression to hematopoietic cells, efficiently transduce and correct cells from WAS patients. *Gen Ther.* 2007;14:415–428.
99. Frecha C, Toscano MG, Costa C, et al. Improved lentiviral vectors for Wiskott-Aldrich syndrome gene therapy mimic endogenous expression profiles throughout haematopoiesis. *Gene Ther.* 2008;Mar 6;[Epub ahead of print].
100. Kafri T, Blomer U, Peterson DA, et al. Sustained expression of genes delivered directly into liver and muscle by lentiviral vectors. *Nat Genet.* 1997;17:314–317.
101. Naldini, L, Blomer, U, Gage, FH et al. Efficient transfer, integration, and sustained long-term expression of the transgene in adult rat brains injected with a lentiviral vector. *Proc Natl Acad Sci USA.* 1996; 93:11382–11388.
102. Blomer U, Naldini L, Kafri T, et al. Highly efficient and sustained gene transfer in adult neurons with a lentivirus vector. *J Virol.* 1997;71:6641–6649.
103. Miyoshi H, Takahashi M, Gage FH, Verma IM. Stable and efficient gene transfer into the retina using an HIV-based lentiviral vector. *Proc Natl Acad Sci USA.* 1997;94:10319–10323.
104. Miyoshi H, Smith KA, Mosier DE, et al. Efficient transduction of human CD34+ cells that mediate long-term engraftment of NOD/SCID mice by HIV vectors. *Science.* 1999;283:682–686.
105. Brass AL, Dykxhoorn DM, Benita Y, et al. Identification of host proteins required for HIV infection through a functional genomic screen. *Science.* 2008;319:921–926.
106. Goff SP. Host factors exploited by retroviruses. *Nat Rev Microbiol.* 2007;5:253–263.
107. Brennan G, Kozyrev Y, Kodama T, Hu SL. Novel TRIM5 isoforms expressed by Macaca nemestrina. *J Virol.* 2007;81: 12210–12217.
108. Russell DW, Miller AD. Foamy virus vectors. *J Virol.* 1996;70: 217–222.
109. Rethwilm A. Foamy virus vectors: an awaited alternative to gammaretro- and lentiviral vectors. *Curr Gene Ther.* 2007;7:261–271.
110. Switzer WM, Bhullar V, Shanmugam V, et al. Frequent simian foamy virus infection in persons occupationally exposed to nonhuman primates. *J Virol.* 2004;78:2780–2789.

111. Hirata RK, Miller AD, Andrews RG, Russell DW. Transduction of hematopoietic cells by foamy virus vectors. *Blood.* 1996;88:3654–3661.
112. Josephson NC, Trobridge G, Russel DW. Transduction of long-term and mobilized peripheral blood-derived NOD/SCID repopulating cells by foamy virus vectors. *Hum Gene Ther.* 2004;15:87–92.
113. Leurs C, Jansen M, Pollok KE, et al. Comparison of three retroviral vector systems for transduction of nonobese diabetic/severe combined immunodeficiency mice repopulating human CD34+ cord blood cells. *Hum Gene Ther.* 2003;14:509–519.
114. von Laer D, Lindemann D, Roscher S, et al. Low-level expression of functionally foamy virus receptor on hematopoietic progenitor cells. *Virology.* 2001;288:139–144.
115. Kiem HP, Allen J, Trobridge G, et al. Foamy-virus-mediated gene transfer to canine repopulating cells. *Blood.* 2007;109:65–70.
116. Bauer TR Jr, Allen JM, Hai M, et al. Successful treatment of canine leukocyte adhesion deficiency by foamy virus vectors. *Nat Med.* 2008;14:93–97.
117. Trobridge G, Josephson N, Vassilopoulos G, Mac J, Russell DW. Improved foamy virus vectors with minimal viral sequences. *Mol Ther.* 2002;6:321–328.
118. Heinkelein M, Dressler M, Jarmy G, et al. Improved primate foamy virus vectors and packaging constructs. *J Virol.* 2002;76:3774–3783.
119. Bastone P, Romen F, Liu W, et al. Construction and characterization of efficient, stable and safe replication-deficient foamy virus vectors. *Gene Ther.* 2007;14:613–620.
120. Trobridge G, Russell DW. Cell cycle requirements for transduction by foamy virus vectors compared to those of oncovirus and lentivirus vectors. *J Virol.* 2004;78:2327–2335.
121. Gaspar HB, Thrasher AJ. Gene therapy for severe combined immunodeficienies. *Expert Opin Biol Ther.* 2005;5:1175–1182.
122. Fischer A, Nacein-Bey-Albina S, Cavazzana-Calvo M. Gene therapy for immunodeficiency diseases. *Semin Hematol.* 2004;41:272–278.
123. Stephan V, Wahn V, Le Deist F, et al. Atypical Xlinked severe combined immunodeficiency due to possible spontaneous reversion of the genetic defect in T cells. *N Engl J Med.* 1996;335:1563–1567.
124. Hacein-Bey-Abina S, Le Deist F, Carlier F, et al. Sustained correction of X-linked severe combined immunodeficiency by ex vivo gene therapy. *N Engl J Med.* 2002;346:1185–1193.
125. Persons DA, Allay ER, Sabatino DE, Kelly P, Bodine DM, Nienhuis AW: Functional requirements for phenotypic correction of murine beta-thalassemia: implications for human gene therapy. *Blood.* 2001;97:3275–3282.
126. Walters MC, Storb R, Patience M, et al. Impact of bone marrow transplantation for symptomatic sickle cell disease: an interim report. Multicenter investigation of bone marrow transplantation for sickle cell disease. *Blood.* 2000;95:1918–1924.
127. Hanawa H, Hematti P, Keyvanfar K, et al. Efficient gene transfer into rhesus repopulating hematopoietic stem cells using a simian immunodeficiency virus-based lentiviral vector system. *Blood.* 2004;103:4062–4069.
128. Orlic D, Girard LJ, Jordan CT, Anderson SM, Cline AP, Bodine DM. The level of mRNA encoding the amphotropic retrovirus receptor in mouse and human hematopoietic stem cells is low and correlates with the efficiency of retrovirus transduction. *Proc Natl Acad Sci USA.* 1996;93:11097–11102.
129. Cheshier SH, Morrison SJ, Liao X, Weissman IL. In vivo proliferation and cell cycle kinetics of long-term self-renewing hematopoietic stem cells. *Proc Natl Acad Sci USA.* 1999;96:3120–3125.
130. Mahmud N, Devine SM, Weller KP, et al. The relative quiescence of hematopoietic stem cells in nonhuman primates. *Blood.* 2001;97:3061–3068.
131. Zhang S, Joseph G, Pollok K, et al. G2 cell cycle arrest and cyclophilin A in lentiviral gene transfer. *Mol Ther.* 2006;14:546–454.
132. Conneally E, Cashman J, Petzer A, Eaves C. Expansion in vitro of transplantable human cord blood stem cells demonstrated using a quantitative assay of their lympho-myeloid repopulating activity in nonobese diabetic-scid/scid mice. *Proc Natl Acad Sci USA.* 1997;94:9836–9841.
133. Sorrentino BP. Clinical strategies for expansion of haematopoietic stem cells. *Nat Rev Immunol.* 2004;4:878–888.
134. Amsellem S, Pflumio F, Bardinet D, et al. Ex vivo expansion of human hematopoietic stem cells by direct delivery of the HOXB4 homeoprotein. *Nat Med.* 2003;9:1423–1427.
135. Willert K, Brown JD, Daneberg E, et al. Wnt proteins are lipid-modified and can act as stem cell growth factors. *Nature.* 2003;423:448–452.
136. Zhang CC, Kaba M, Ge G, et al. Angiopoietin-like proteins stimulate ex vivo expansion of hematopoietic stem cells. *Nat Med.* 2006;12:240–245.
137. Zhang CC, Kaba M, Iizuka S, Huynh H, Lodish HF. Angiopoietin-like 5 and IGFBP2 stimulate ex vivo expansion of human cord blood hematopoietic stem cells as assayed by NOD/SCID transplantation. *Blood.* 2008 Jan 17 [Epub ahead of print]
138. Ito K, Hirao A, Arai F, et al. Reactive oxygen species act through p38 MAPK to limit the lifespan of hematopoietic stem cells. *Nat Med.* 2006;12:446–451.
139. Ito K, Hirao A, Arai F, et al. Regulation of oxidative stress by ATM is required for self-renewal of haematopoietic stem cells. *Nature.* 2004;431:997–1002.
140. Tothova Z, Kollipara R, Huntly BJ, et al. FoxOs are critical mediators of hematopoietic stem cell resistance to physiologic oxidative stress. *Cell.* 2007;128:325–333.
141. Lambert JF, Liu M, Colvin GA, et al. Marrow stem cells shift gene expression and engraftment phenotype with cell cycle transit. *J Exp Med.* 2003;197:1563–1572.
142. Takatoku M, Sellers S, Agricola BA, et al. Avoidance of stimulation improves engraftment of cultured and retrovirally transduced hematopoietic cells in primates. *J Clin Invest.* 2001;108:447–455.
143. Christopherson KW 2nd, Hangoc G, Mantel CR, Broxmeyer HE. Modulation of hematopoietic stem cell homing and engraftment by CD26. *Science.* 2004;305(5686):1000–1003
144. Christopherson KW 2nd, Paanessi LA, Napier S, Porecha NK. CD26 inhibition on CD34+ or lineage-human umbilical cord blood donor hematopoietic stem cells/hematopoietic progenitor cells improves long-term engraftment into NOD/SCID/beta2-null immunodeficient mice. *Stem Cells Dev.* 2007;16:355–360.

145. Puthenveetil G, Scholes J, Carbonell D, et al. Successful correction of the human beta-thalassemia major phenotype using a lentiviral vector. *Blood.* 2004;104:3445–3453.
146. Neff T, Beard BC, Kiem HP. Survival of the fittest: in vivo selection and stem cell gene therapy. *Blood.* 2006;107:1751–1760.
147. Allay JA, Persons DA, Galipeau J, et al. In vivo selection of retrovirally transduced hematopoietic stem cells. *Nat Med.* 1998;4:1136–1143.
148. Persons DA, Allay JA, Bonifacino A, et al. Transient in vivo selection of transduced peripheral blood cells using antifolate drug selection in rhesus macaques that received transplants with hematopoietic stem cells expressing dihydrofolate reductase vectors. *Blood.* 2004;103:796–803.
149. Liu L, Gerson SL. Targeted modulation of MGMT: clinical implications. *Clin Cancer Res.* 2006;12:328–331.
150. Ragg S, Xu-Welliver M, Bailey J, et al. Direct reversal of DNA damage by mutant methyltransferase protein protects mice against dose-intensified chemotherapy and leads to in vivo selection of hematopoietic stem cells. *Cancer Res.* 2000;60:5187–5195.
151. Sawai N, Zhou S, Vanin EF, Houghton P, Brent TP, Sorrentino BP. Protection and in vivo selection of hematopoietic stem cells using temozolomide, O6-benzylguanine, and an alkyltransferase-expressing retroviral vector. *Mol Ther.* 2001;3:78–87.
152. Persons DA, Allay ER, Sawai N, et al. Successful treatment of murine beta-thalassemia using in vivo selection of genetically modified, drug-resistant hematopoietic stem cells. *Blood.* 2003;101:506–513.
153. Neff T, Horn PA, Peterson LJ, et al. Methylguanine methyltransferase-mediated in vivo selection and chemoprotection of allogeneic stem cells in a large-animal model. *J Clin Invest.* 2003;112:1581–1588.
154. Neff T, Beard BC, Peterson LJ, Anandakumar P, Thompson J, Kiem HP. Polyclonal chemoprotection against temozolomide in a large-animal model of drug resistance gene therapy. *Blood.* 2005;105:997–1002.
155. Williams DA, Lemischka IR, Nathan DG, Mulligan RC. Introduction of new genetic material into pluripotent haematopoietic stem cells of the mouse. *Nature.* 1984;310:476–480.
156. Ingram VM. Abnormal human haemoglobins. III. The chemical difference between normal and sickle cell haemoglobins. *Biochim Biophys Acta.* 1959;36:402–411.
157. Maniatis T, Kee SG, Efstratiadis A, Kafatos FC. Amplification and characterization of a beta-globin gene synthesized in vitro. *Cell.* 1976;8:163–182.
158. Lawn RM, Fritsch EF, Parker RC, Blake G, Maniatis T. The isolation and characterization of linked delta- and beta-globin genes from a cloned library of human DNA. *Cell.* 1978;15:1157–1174.
159. Blattner FR, Blechl AE, Denniston-Thompson K, et al. Cloning human fetal gamma globin and mouse alpha-type globin DNA: preparation and screening of shotgun collections. *Science.* 1978;202:1279–1284.
160. Smithies O, Blechl AE, Denniston-Thompson K, et al. Cloning human fetal gamma globin and mouse alpha-type globin DNA: characterization and partial sequencing. *Science.* 1978;202:1284–1289.
161. Efstratiadis A, Posakony JW, Maniatis T, et al. The structure and evolution of the human beta-globin gene family. *Cell.* 1980;21:653–668.
162. Tiemeier DC, Tilghman SM, Polsky FI, et al. A comparison of two cloned mouse beta-globin genes and their surrounding and intervening sequences. *Cell.* 1978;14:237–245.
163. Ramirez F, Natta C, O'Donnell JV, et al. Relative numbers of human globin genes assayed with purified alpha and beta complementary human DNA. *Proc Natl Acad Sci USA.* 1975;72:1550–1554.
164. Ottolenghi S, Lanyon WG, Williamson R, Weatherall DJ, Clegg JB, Pitcher CS. Human globin gene analysis for a patient with beta-o/delta beta-thalassemia. *Proc Natl Acad Sci USA.* 1975;72:2294–2299.
165. Fritsch EF, Lawn RM, Maniatis T. Molecular cloning and characterization of the human beta-like globin gene cluster. *Cell.* 1980;19:959–972.
166. Bender MA, Gelinas RE, Miller AD. A majority of mice show long-term expression of a human beta-globin gene after retrovirus transfer into hematopoietic stem cells. *Mol Cell Biol.* 1989;9:1426–1434.
167. Tuan D, London IM. Mapping of DNase I-hypersensitive sites in the upstream DNA of human embryonic epsilon-globin gene in K562 leukemia cells. *Proc Natl Acad Sci USA.* 1984;81:2718–2722.
168. Forrester WC, Novak U, Gelinas R, Groudine M. Molecular analysis of the human beta-globin locus activation region. *Proc Natl Acad Sci USA.* 1989;86:5439–5443.
169. Skow LC, Burkhart BA, Johnson FM, et al. A mouse model for beta-thalassemia. *Cell.* 1983;34:1043–1052.
170. Yang B, Kirby S, Lewis J, Detloff PJ, Maeda N, Smithies O. A mouse model for beta 0-thalassemia. *Proc Natl Acad Sci USA.* 1995;92:11608–11612.
171. Persons DA, Hargrove PW, Allay ER, Hanawa H, Nienhuis AW. The degree of phenotypic correction of murine beta-thalassemia intermedia following lentiviral-mediated transfer of a human gamma-globin gene is influenced by chromosomal position effects and vector copy number. *Blood.* 2003;101:2175–2183.
172. Hanawa H, Hargrove PW, Kepes S, Srivastava DK, Nienhuis AW, Persons DA. Extended beta-globin locus control region elements promote consistent therapeutic expression of a gamma-globin lentiviral vector in murine beta-thalassemia. *Blood.* 2004;104:2281–2290.
173. Imren S, Payen E, Westerman KA, et al. Permanent and pan-erythroid correction of murine beta thalassemia by multiple lentiviral integration in hematopoietic stem cells. *Proc Natl Acad Sci USA.* 2002;99:14380–14385.
174. Greaves DR, Fraser P, Vidal MA, et al. A transgenic mouse model of sickle cell disorder. *Nature.* 1990;343:183–185.
175. Ryan TM, Townes TM, Reilly MP, et al. Human sickle hemoglobin in transgenic mice. *Science.* 1990;247:566–568.
176. Trudel M, Saadane N, Garel MC, et al. Towards a transgenic mouse model of sickle cell disease: hemoglobin SAD. *EMBO J.* 1991;10:3157–3165.
177. Fabry ME, Costantini F, Pachnis A, et al. High expression of human beta S- and alpha-globins in transgenic mice: erythrocyte abnormalities, organ damage, and the effect of hypoxia. *Proc Natl Acad Sci USA.* 1992;89:12155–12159.

178. Roy RP, Nagel RL, Acharya AS. Molecular basis of the inhibition of beta s-chain-dependent polymerization by mouse alpha-chain. Semisynthesis of chimeras of human and mouse alpha-chains. *J Biol Chem.* 1993;268:16406–16412.
179. Paszty C, Mohandas N, Stevens ME, et al. Lethal alpha-thalassaemia created by gene targeting in mice and its genetic rescue. *Nat Genet.* 1995;11:33–39.
180. Chang J, Lu RH, Xu SM, et al. Inactivation of mouse alpha-globin gene by homologous recombination: mouse model of hemoglobin H disease. *Blood.* 1996;88:1846–1851.
181. Ryan TM, Ciavatta DJ, Townes TM. Knockout-transgenic mouse model of sickle cell disease. *Science.* 1997;278:873–876.
182. Paszty C, Brion CM, Manci E, et al. Transgenic knockout mice with exclusively human sickle hemoglobin and sickle cell disease. *Science.* 1997;278:876–878.
183. Pawliuk R, Westerman KA, Fabry ME, et al. Correction of sickle cell disease in transgenic mouse models by gene therapy. *Science.* 2001;294:2368–2371.
184. Kaul DK, Hebbel RP. Hypoxia/reoxygenation causes inflammatory response in transgenic sickle mice but not in normal mice. *J Clin Invest.* 2000;106:411–420.
185. Dasgupta T, Hebbel RP, Kaul DK. Protective effect of arginine on oxidative stress in transgenic sickle mouse models. *Free Radic Biol Med.* 2006;41:1771–1780.
186. Belcher JD, Mahaseth H, Welch TE, Otterbein LE, Hebbel RP, Vercellotti GM. Heme oxygenase-1 is a modulator of inflammation and vaso-occlusion in transgenic sickle mice. *J Clin Invest.* 2006;116:808–816.
187. Turhan A, Weiss LA, Mohandas N, Coller BS, Frenette PS. Primary role for adherent leukocytes in sickle cell vascular occlusion: a new paradigm. *Proc Natl Acad Sci USA.* 2002;99:3047–3051.
188. Chang JC, Lu R, Lin C, et al. Transgenic knockout mice exclusively expressing human hemoglobin S after transfer of a 240-kb betas-globin yeast artificial chromosome: A mouse model of sickle cell anemia. *Proc Natl Acad Sci USA.* 1998;95:14886–14890.
189. Fabry ME, Suzuka SM, Weinberg RS, et al. Second generation knockout sickle mice: the effect of HbF. *Blood.* 2001;97:410–418.
190. Kaul DK, Liu XD, Chang HY, Nagel RL, Fabry ME. Effect of fetal hemoglobin on microvascular regulation in sickle transgenic-knockout mice. *J Clin Invest.* 2004;114:1136–1145.
191. May C, Rivella S, Chadburn A, Sadelain M. Successful treatment of murine beta-thalassemia intermedia by transfer of the human beta-globin gene. *Blood.* 2002;99:1902–1908.
192. Rivella S, May C, Chadburn A, Riviere I, Sadelain M. A novel murine model of Cooley anemia and its rescue by lentiviral-mediated human beta -globin gene transfer. *Blood.* 2003;101:2932–2939.
193. Levasseur DN, Ryan TM, Pawlik KM, Townes TM. Correction of a mouse model of sickle cell disease: lentiviral/antisickling beta-globin gene transduction of unmobilized, purified hematopoietic stem cells. *Blood.* 2003;102:4312–4329.
194. Sabatino DE, Seidel NE, Aviles-Mendoza GJ, et al. Long-term expression of gamma-globin mRNA in mouse erythrocytes from retrovirus vectors containing the human gamma-globin gene fused to the ankyrin-1 promoter. *Proc Natl Acad Sci USA.* 2000;97:13294–13299.
195. Emery DW, Yannaki E, Tubb J, Nishino T, Li Q, Stamatoyannopoulos G. Development of virus vectors for gene therapy of beta chain hemoglobinopathies: flanking with a chromatin insulator reduces gamma-globin gene silencing in vivo. *Blood.* 2002;100:2012–2019.
196. Pestina TI, Hargrove PW, Jay D, Gray JT, Boyd KM, and Persons DA. Correction of murine sickle cell disease using a novel γ-globin lentiviral vector to mediate high level expression of fetal hemoglobin. Accepted for publication. Molecular Therapy, 2008.
197. Chung JH, Bell AC, Felsenfeld G. Characterization of the chicken beta-globin insulator. *Proc Natl Acad Sci USA.* 1997;94:575–580.
198. Arumugam PI, Scholes J, Perelman N, Xia P, Yee JK, Malik P. Improved human beta-globin expression from self-inactivating lentiviral vectors carrying the chicken hypersensitive site-4 (cHS4) insulator element. *Mol Ther.* 2007;15:1863–1871.
199. Aker M, Tubb J, Groth AC, et al. Extended core sequences from the cHS4 insulator are necessary for protecting retroviral vectors from silencing position effects. *Hum Gene Ther.* 2007;18:333–343.
200. Weinberg KI, Kohn DB. Gene therapy for congenital lymphoid immunodeficiency diseases. *Semin Hematol.* 1998;35:354–366.
201. Blaese RM, Culver KW, Miller AD, et al. T lymphocyte-directed gene therapy for ADA- SCID: initial trial results after 4 years. *Science.* 1995;270:475–480.
202. Kohn DB, Weinberg KI, Nolta JA, et al. Engraftment of gene-modified umbilical cord blood cells in neonates with adenosine deaminase deficiency. *Nat Med.* 1995;1:1017–1023.
203. Kohn DB, Hershfield MS, Carbonaro D, et al. T lymphocytes with a normal ADA gene accumulate after transplantation of transduced autologous umbilical cord blood CD34+ cells in ADA-deficient SCID neonates. *Nat Med.* 1998;4:775–780.
204. Cavazzana-Calvo M, Hacein-Bey S, de Saint Basile G, et al. Gene therapy of human severe combined immunodeficiency (SCID)-X1 disease. *Science.* 2000;288:669–672.
205. Otsu M, Sugamura K, Candotti F. In vivo competitive studies between normal and common gamma chain-defective bone marrow cells: implications for gene therapy. *Hum Gene Ther.* 2000;11:2051–2056.
206. Gaspar HB, Parsley KL, Howe S, et al. Gene therapy of X-linked severe combined immunodeficiency by use of a pseudotyped gamma retroviral vector. *Lancet.* 2004;364:2181–2187.
207. Aiuti A, Slavin S, Aker M, et al. Correction of ADA-SCID by stem cell gene therapy combined with nonmyeloablative conditioning. *Science.* 2002;296:2410–2413.
208. Aiuti A, Cassani B, Andolfi G, et al. Multilineage hematopoietic reconstitution without clonal selection in ADA-SCID patients treated with stem cell gene therapy. *J Clin Invest.* 2007;117:2233–2240.
209. Hacein-Bey-Abina S, Von Kalle C, Schmidt M, et al. LMO2-associated clonal T cell proliferation in two patients after gene therapy for SCID-XI. *Science.* 2003;301:2526–2527.
210. Fischer A, Abina SH, Thrasher A, von Kalle C, Cavazzana-Calvo M. LMO2 and gene therapy for severe combined immunodeficiency. *N Engl J Med.* 2004;350(24):2526–2527.

211. McCormack MP, Rabbitts TH. Activation of the T-cell oncogene LMO2 after gene therapy for X-linked severe combined immunodeficiency. *N Engl J Med.* 2004;350:913–922.
212. Larson RC, Fisch P, Larson TA, et al. T cell tumours of disparate phenotype in mice transgenic for Rbtn-2. *Oncogene.* 1994;9:3675–3681.
213. Wu X, Li Y, Crise B, Burgess SM. Transcription start regions in the human genome are favored targets for MLV integration. *Science.* 2003;300:1749–1751.
214. Cattoglio C, Facchini G, Sartori D, et al. Hot spots of retroviral integration in human CD34+ hematopoietic cells. *Blood.* 2007;110:1770–1778.
215. Mitchell RS, Beitzel BF, Schroder AR, et al. Retroviral DNA integration: ASLV, HIV, and MLV show distinct target site preferences. *PLoS Biol.* 2004 Aug;2:E234.
216. Lo M, Bloom ML, Imada K, et al. Activation of the T-cell oncogene LMO2 after gene therapy for X-linked severe combined immunodeficiency. *N Engl J Med.* 2004;350:913–922.
217. Soudais C, Shiho T, Sharara LI, et al. Stable and functional lymphoid reconstitution of common cytokine receptor gamma chain deficient mice by retroviral-mediated gene transfer. *Blood.* 2000;95:3071–3077.
218. Shou Y, Ma Z, Lu T, Sorrentino BP. Unique risk factors for insertional mutagenesis in a mouse model of XSCID gene therapy. *Proc Natl Acad Sci USA.* 2006;10:11730–11735.
219. Gardie B, Cayuela JM, Martini S, Sigaux F. Genomic alterations of the p19ARF encoding exons in T-cell acute lymphoblastic leukemia. *Blood.* 1998;91:1016–1020.
220. Kiem HP, Sellers S, Thomasson B, et al. Long-term clinical and molecular follow-up of large animals receiving retrovirally transduced stem and progenitor cells: no progression to clonal hematopoiesis or leukemia. *Mol Ther.* 2004;9:389–395.
221. Seggewiss R, Pittaluga S, Adler RL, et al. Acute myeloid leukemia is associated with retroviral gene transfer to hematopoietic progenitor cells in a rhesus macaque. *Blood.* 2006;107:3865–3867.
222. Ott MG, Schmidt M, Schwarzwaelder K, et al. Correction of X-linked chronic granulomatous disease by gene therapy, augmented by insertional activation of MDS1-EVI1, PRDM16 or SETBP1. *Nat Med.* 2006;12:401–409.
223. Kustikova O, Fehse B, Modlich U, et al. Clonal dominance of hematopoietic stem cells triggered by retroviral gene marking. *Science.* 2005;308:1171–1174.
224. Calmels B, Ferguson C, Laukkanen MO, et al. Recurrent retroviral vector integration at the Mds1/Evi1 locus in nonhuman primate hematopoietic cells. *Blood.* 2005;106:2530–2533.
225. Hematti P, Hong BK, Ferguson C, et al. Distinct genomic integration of MLV and SIV vectors in primate hematopoietic stem and progenitor cells. *PLoS Biol.* 2004;2:e423.
226. Montini E, Cesana D, Schmidt M, et al. Hematopoietic stem cell gene transfer in a tumor-prone mouse model uncovers low genotoxicity of lentiviral vector integration. *Nat Biotechnol.* 2006;24:687–696.
227. Akagi K, Suzuki T, Stephens RM, Jenkins NA, Copeland NG. RTCGD: retroviral tagged cancer gene database. *Nucl Acids Res.* 2004;32(Database issue):D523–527.
228. Hargrove PW, Kepes S, Hanawa H, Obenauer JC, et al. Globin lentiviral vector insertions can perturb the expression of endogenous genes in beta-thalassemic hematopoietic cells. *Mol Ther.* 2008;16:525–533.
229. Evans-Galea MV, Wielgosz MM, Hanawa H, Srivastava DK, Nienhuis AW. Suppression of clonal dominance in cultured human lymphoid cells by addition of the cHS4 insulator to a lentiviral vector. *Mol Ther.* 2007;15:801–809.
230. Hanna J, Wernig M, Markoulaki S, Sun CW, et al. Treatment of sickle cell anemia mouse model with iPS cells generated from autologous skin. *Science.* 2007;318:1920–3.
231. Persons DA, Tisdale JF. Gene therapy for hemoglobin disorders. *Semin Hematol.* 2004;41:279–286.

Index